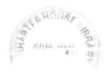

ANDREWS'

DISEASES *of the* SKIN

CLINICAL DERMATOLOGY

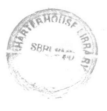

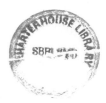

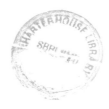

ANDREWS'

DISEASES *of the* SKIN

CLINICAL DERMATOLOGY

RICHARD B. ODOM, M.D.

Professor of Clinical Dermatology
Associate Dean of Continuing Medical Education
University of California, San Francisco
San Francisco, California

WILLIAM D. JAMES, M.D.

Albert M. Kligman Professor of Dermatology
University of Pennsylvania
Philadelphia, Pennsylvania

TIMOTHY G. BERGER, M.D.

Professor of Clinical Dermatology
University of California, San Francisco
San Francisco, California

NINTH EDITION

with 1271 *illustrations*

W.B. SAUNDERS COMPANY

A Harcourt Health Sciences Company

Philadelphia   London   New York   St. Louis   Sydney   Toronto

W.B. SAUNDERS COMPANY
A Harcourt Health Sciences Company

The Curtis Center
Independence Square West
Philadelphia, Pennsylvania 19106

Acquisitions Editor: Elizabeth M. Fathman
Developmental Editor: Ellen Baker Geisel
Project Manager: Patricia Tannian
Senior Production Editor: Anne Salmo
Book Design Manager: Gail Morey Hudson
Cover Designer: Teresa Breckwoldt

Library of Congress Cataloging-in-Publication Data

Odom, Richard B., 1937-
Andrews' diseases of the skin : clinical dermatology.—9th ed./Richard B. Odom,
William D. James, Timothy G. Berger.

p. cm.
Includes bibliographical references and index.

ISBN 0-7216-5832-6

1. Skin—Diseases.   2. Dermatology.   I. Title: Diseases of the skin.
II. James, William D. (William Daniel), 1950- .   III. Berger, Timothy G.   IV. Title.

RL71 .A76 2000

616.5—dc21   99-058324

ANDREWS' DISEASES OF THE SKIN, 9TH EDITION   ISBN 0-7216-5832-6

Last digit is the print number: 9   8   7   6   5   4   3   2   1

Contributors

ROY C. GREKIN, M.D.
Clinical Professor
Co-Director, Dermatologic Surgery and Laser Center
University of California, San Francisco
San Francisco, California

CURT P. SAMLASKA, M.D., F.A.C.P.
Clinical Professor of Dermatology
University of Nevada School of Medicine
Las Vegas, Nevada

KIRSTEN VIN-CHRISTIAN, M.D.
Clinical Instructor
Dermatologic Surgery and Laser Center
University of California, San Francisco
San Francisco, California

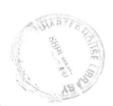

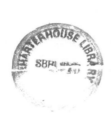

Preface

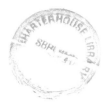

Andrews' remains as it was from the beginning: an authored text that consists of one volume jam-packed with clinical signs, symptoms, diagnostic tests, and therapeutic pearls. The authors have remained general clinical dermatologists in an era of subspecialists in academia. They are committed to keeping *Andrews'* as a reference for anyone who needs help to diagnose a patient with a clinical conundrum or to treat a patient with a therapeutically challenging disease. The advantages of limited authorship are consistent, concise discussions without redundancy and an ability to bring to the text a unified philosophy in caring for patients with skin disease.

As with all previous editions of *Andrews'* our primary goal was to maintain it as a single volume so that it may be used in the clinical setting on the desktop, not as an after-the-fact, library resource. Its intended primary audience is the practicing dermatologist. Residents have always found it to be readily digestible for a yearly curriculum of study, and we are hopeful that another decade of trainees will learn clinical dermatology from the clinical descriptions, disease classifications, and treatment insights that define *Andrews'*. We believe that students, interns, residents, internists and other medical specialists, family practitioners, and other healthcare professionals who desire a comprehensive dermatology textbook will find that ours meets their needs in understanding and managing their patients.

Many major changes have been made in this edition. Harry Arnold died soon after the eighth edition was published. Tim Berger agreed to co-author this revision and has worked diligently to update and improve the organization of the text. Curt Samlaska also participated in revising several of the chapters, and his contributions have been invaluable. Finally, Kirsten Vin-Christian and Roy Grekin have combined the radiotherapy and dermatologic surgery chapters and added the vast array of new surgical techniques to their chapter.

Since our last edition was published a decade ago, medical science has advanced with meteoric speed. Molecular investigative techniques have been a major impetus in gaining insight into skin disease. Inherited conditions are understood at the subcellular level and give us a broader view of the mechanisms leading to tumor formation, immunologic responsiveness, and cell adhesion. Immunodiagnostics continue to sort tumor biology into new classification schemes, especially visible in lymphoma and bullous disease research. Technologic breakthroughs have given us lasers, narrowband ultraviolet therapy, and epiluminescence microscopy. New medications have found their place in the formulary: a multitude of retinoids, calcipitriol, mycophenolate mofetil, topical metronidazole, topical tacrolimus, the rebirth of thalidomide as an immunomodulator, finasteride, and improved systemic antifungals, antivirals (and retrovirals), antibiotics, and antihistamines are some examples.

Extensive revision of the text was necessary to include the wealth of new information. Just as advances in understanding led to additions, older concepts needed to be selectively discarded. These offsetting alterations allow us to maintain the total volume of information constant. Old, oftentimes, classic references are not cited in favor of new ones. When available, references that can readily be found on the practicing dermatologist's shelf, such as recent volumes of the *Journal of the American Academy of Dermatology* and the *Archives of Dermatology,* are cited. The seminal but older references are to be found in these sources.

More than 75 new entities, numerous new diagnostic tests, several new infections, and many new associations appear for the first time in the ninth edition. This sea of new knowledge is presented to be navigated easily and enjoyed.

Many thank yous are in order on completion of a task of this magnitude. Judy Fletcher and Melissa (Dudlick) Messersmith at W.B. Saunders and Liz Fathman, Ellen Baker Geisel, and Anne Salmo at Mosby helped keep us on task and brought our ideas into print. Curt Samlaska's placing his second novel on hold to assist us with this ninth edition leaves us in his debt.

We hope you enjoy this edition of *Andrews'* as we begin to collect new knowledge from the year 2000 literature to present to you in the upcoming tenth edition!

Richard B. Odom, M.D.
William D. James, M.D.
Timothy G. Berger, M.D.

I would just like to dedicate my professional efforts to my family members and thank the many patients who extended the privilege of allowing me to participate in their care.

RBO

My wife, Ann, and my children, Dan and Becca, have supported this effort and my career with their love and patience; the faculty, residents, and patients at Walter Reed and the University of Pennsylvania continued to teach me every day over the years. Dick Odom and Tim Berger continue to provide me with examples to emulate.

WDJ

My efforts in this text are dedicated to Dr. Richard B. Odom, my mentor, colleague, and friend in dermatology for a quarter century. And to Jessica, the love of my life.

TGB

Contents

ANDREWS'

DISEASES *of the* SKIN

CLINICAL DERMATOLOGY

CHAPTER 1

The Skin: Basic Structure and Function

The skin is composed of three layers: epidermis, dermis, and subcutaneous tissue (fat). The epidermis, the outermost layer, is directly contiguous with the environment. It is formed by an ordered arrangement of cells called *keratinocytes,* whose basic function is to synthesize keratin, a filamentous protein that serves a protective function. The dermis is the middle layer. Its principal constituent is the fibrillar structural protein collagen. The dermis lies on the panniculus of subcutaneous tissue, which is composed principally of lobules of lipocytes (Fig. 1-1).

All skin sites are composed of these three anatomically distinct layers, although there is considerable regional variation in their relative thickness. The epidermis is thickest on the palms and soles, measuring approximately 1.5 mm. It is very thin on the eyelid, where it measures less than 0.1 mm. The dermis is thickest on the back, where it is 30 to 40 times as thick as the overlying epidermis. The amount of subcutaneous fat is generous on the abdomen and buttocks compared with the nose and sternum, where it is meager.

EPIDERMIS

During the first weeks of fetal life, the epidermis consists of a single sheet of contiguous, undifferentiated cells that subsequently assume the characteristics of keratinocytes. Adnexal structures, particularly follicles and eccrine sweat units, originate during the third month of fetal life as downgrowths from the developing epidermis. Later, apocrine sweat units develop from the upper portion of the follicular epithelium and sebaceous glands and ducts from the midregion of the follicle. The development of adnexal structures at specific skin sites, such as the regional variation in thickness of the three skin layers, is genetically modulated.

The adult epidermis is composed of three basic cell types: keratinocytes, melanocytes, and Langerhans' cells (Fig. 1-2). An additional cell, the Merkel cell, can be found in the basal layer of the palms and soles, the oral and genital mucosa, the nail bed, and the follicular infundibula. The Merkel cells, located directly above the basement membrane, contain intracytoplasmic neurosecretory-like granules, and, through their association with neurites, act as slow adapting touch receptors. They have direct connections with adjacent keratinocytes by desmosomes and contain intermediate filaments composed of low–molecular-weight keratin. Whether these cells originate from the neural crest or from within the epidermis is still unknown.

Keratinocyte

The keratinocyte, or squamous cell, is the principal cell of the epidermis. It is a cell of ectodermal origin that has the specialized function of producing keratin, a complex filamentous protein that not only forms the surface coat (stratum corneum) of the epidermis but also is the structural protein of hair and nails. Multiple distinct keratin genes have been identified and consist of two subfamilies, acidic and basic. The product of one basic and one acidic keratin gene combines to form the multiple keratins that occur in many tissues. The mixture of these keratins vary with cell type and degree of differentiation.

The epidermis may be divided into the following zones, beginning with the innermost layer: basal layer, malpighian or prickle layer, granular layer, and horny layer, or stratum corneum (Fig. 1-3). These names reflect the changing appearance of the keratinocyte as it differentiates into a cornified cell.

A proportion of the basal cells proliferate, differentiate, and move in a stepwise fashion through the full thickness of the epidermis. As the cell moves upward through the epidermis, it changes morphologically. It flattens out, and eventually the nucleus disappears.

Just as there is regional variation in the thickness of the anatomic layers of the skin, so also is there variation in the thickness of the different zones of the epidermis according to skin site. The horny layer and granular layer are thickest on the palms and soles, and virtually absent on the more delicate skin of the flexor aspect of the forearms and the abdomen. The basal layer, however, is generally one cell thick, regardless of the skin site examined.

During keratinization, the keratinocyte first passes through a synthetic and then a degradative phase on its way to becoming a horn cell. In the synthetic phase, the

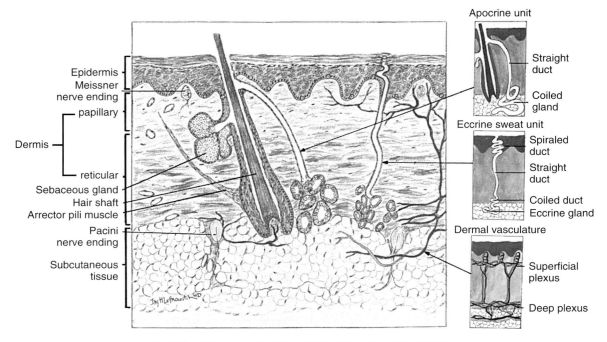

Fig. 1-1 Diagrammatic cross section of the skin and panniculus.

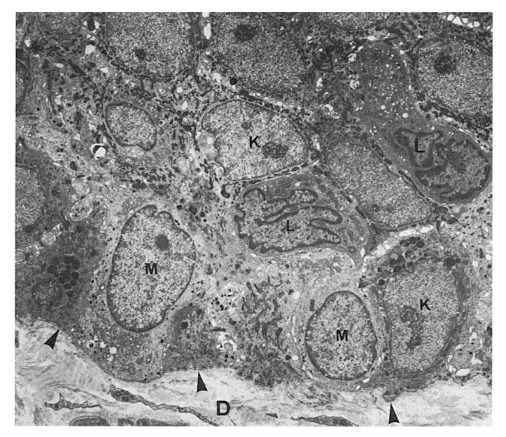

Fig. 1-2 Electron micrograph illustrating the three basic cell types in the epidermis and their relationships. Most of the cells are keratinocytes (prickle cells and basal cells), some labeled *(K)*. Langerhans' cells *(L)* with their characteristic cribriform nuclei are distributed among the keratinocytes in the malpighian layer. Melanocytes *(M)* are located in the basal layer of the epidermis, which is separated from (and attached to) the dermis *(D)* by the basement membrane zone *(arrows)*.

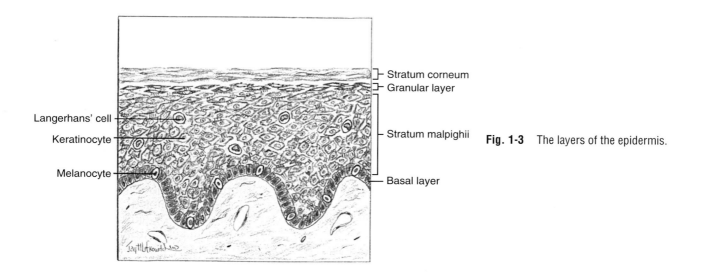

Langerhans' cell

Keratinocyte

Melanocyte

Stratum corneum
Granular layer
Stratum malpighii
Basal layer

Fig. 1-3 The layers of the epidermis.

keratinocyte accumulates within its cytoplasm intermediate filaments composed of a fibrous protein, keratin, arranged in an alpha-helical coiled-coil pattern. These tonofilaments are fashioned into bundles, which converge on and terminate at the plasma membrane, where they end in specialized attachment plates called *desmosomes* (Fig. 1-4). The degradative phase of keratinization is characterized by the disappearance of cell organelles and the consolidation of all contents into a mixture of filaments and amorphous cell envelopes (Fig. 1-5).

The plasma membranes of adjacent cells are separated by an intercellular space. Electron microscopic histochemical studies have shown that this interspace contains glycoproteins and lipids. Lamellar granules function in this space, primarily at the interface between the granular and cornified cell layers.

Keratinocytes of the granular zone contain, in addition to the keratin filament system, keratohyaline granules, composed of amorphous particulate material of high sulphur-protein content. This material, called profilaggrin, is a precursor to filaggrin, so named because it is thought to be responsible for keratin filament aggregation. Conversion to filaggrin takes place in the granular layer, and this forms the electron-dense interfilamentous protein matrix of mature epidermal keratin.

Lamellated organelles called *Odland bodies,* also referred to as membrane-coating granules or keratinosomes, are found intracellularly in upper-level keratinocytes. Their contents are discharged into the extracellular space at the junction of the granular and horny layers. This establishes a barrier to water loss and, with filaggrin, mediate stratum corneum cell cohesion.

Keratinocytes play a role in the immune function of the skin, and they participate in communication, interaction, and regulation of cell systems collaborating in the induction of the immune response. Keratinocytes secrete a wide array of cytokines and inflammatory mediators. They also can express molecules on their surface such as ICAM-1 and MHC Class II molecules, which demonstrates that keratinocytes actively respond to immune effector signals.

Melanocyte

The melanocyte is the pigment-producing cell of the epidermis. It is derived from the neural crest, and by the eighth week of development can be found within the fetal epidermis. In normal adult epidermis, melanocytes reside in the basal layer at a frequency of approximately 1 for every 10 basal keratinocytes. The number of melanocytes in the epidermis is the same, regardless of the person's race or color; it is the number and size of the melanosomes or pigment granules, continuously synthesized by these melanocytes, that determine differences in skin color (Fig. 1-6).

In histologic sections of skin routinely stained by hematoxylin and eosin, the melanocyte appears as a clear cell in the basal layer of the epidermis. The apparent halo is an artefact caused by separation of the melanocyte from adjacent keratinocytes during fixation of the specimen. This occurs because the melanocyte, lacking tonofilaments, cannot form desmosomal attachments with keratinocytes.

The melanocyte is actually a dendritic cell, a feature rarely appreciated at the light-microscope level. Its dendrites extend for long distances within the epidermis, and any one melanocyte is therefore in contact with a great number of keratinocytes; together they form the so-called epidermal melanin unit.

Melanosomes are synthesized in the Golgi zone of the cell and pass through a series of stages in which the enzyme tyrosinase acts on melanin precursors to produce the densely pigmented granules. While this is occurring, the melanosome migrates to the tip of a dendrite, where it is transferred to an adjacent keratinocyte. Keratinocytes are the reservoir for melanin in the skin.

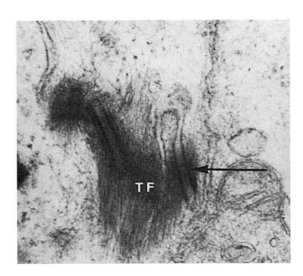

Fig. 1-4 Ultrastructural appearance of the desmosome *(arrow),* the specialized attachment plate between adjacent keratinocytes. Tonofilaments *(TF)* within the cytoplasm of adjacent keratinocytes converge on the plasma membrane of each cell, where they condense to form an electron-dense zone.

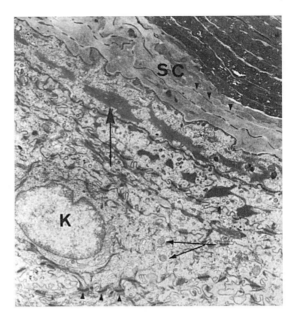

Fig. 1-5 The upper portion of the epidermis. Keratinocytes *(K)* are flatter than those of the lower portion (see Fig. 1-2), and contain keratinosomes *(thin arrows).* Desmosomes *(short arrows)* become more obvious as the ratio of nucleus to cytoplasm increases. Keratinocytes of the granular layer have developed keratohyalin granules *(broad, long arrow).* The stratum corneum *(SC)* is composed of horny plates that retain only filaments and amorphous material enveloped in a thickened cell membrane. Horny cells, like other keratinocytes, are joined by desmosomes *(short arrowheads).*

Fig. 1-6 The epidermal melanin unit in dark *(left)* and light *(right)* skin.

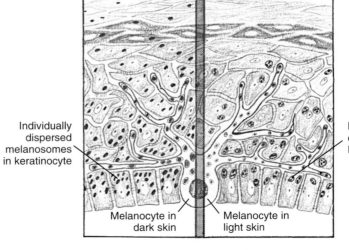

Individually dispersed melanosomes in keratinocyte

Melanosome complex in keratinocyte

Melanocyte in dark skin

Melanocyte in light skin

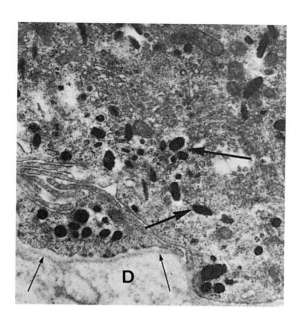

Fig. 1-7 Portion of a melanocyte from dark skin, illustrating melanosomes *(broad arrows)* at various stages of development. Basement membrane zone *(thin arrow)* and dermis *(D)* are also seen.

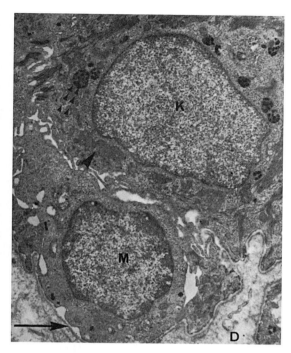

Fig. 1-8 The relationship between melanocytes *(M)* and basal keratinocytes *(K)* in light skin. Melanocytes synthesize pigment granules (melanosomes), which are transferred to keratinocytes, where they are contained within membrane-bound melanosome complexes *(small arrowheads)*. Bundles of tonofilaments *(broad arrowhead)* identify the cell as a keratinocyte. The basement membrane zone *(arrow)* separates epidermis from dermis *(D)*.

Melanocytes of dark skin synthesize melanosomes larger than those produced in light skin. The size of the melanosome is the principal factor in determining how the melanosomes will be distributed within the keratinocytes. The larger melanosomes of dark skin are individually dispersed within the cytoplasm of keratinocytes; smaller melanosomes of light skin are packaged in membrane-bound complexes within the keratinocyte (Figs. 1-7 and 1-8). Chronic sun exposure can stimulate the melanocyte to produce larger melanosomes, thereby making the distribution of melanosomes within keratinocytes resemble the pattern seen in dark-skinned individuals.

Areas of leukoderma or whitening of skin can be caused by very different phenomena. In vitiligo, the affected skin becomes white because of destruction of melanocytes. In albinism, the number of melanocytes is normal; however, they are unable to synthesize fully pigmented melanosomes because of defects in the enzymatic formation of melanin. Local areas of increased pigmentation can result from a variety of causes. The typical freckle results from a localized increase in production of pigment by a normal number of melanocytes. Nevi are benign proliferations of melanocytes. Melanomas are their malignant counterpart. Frequently, though, skin lesions are not pigmented because of hyperplasia or hyperactivity of melanocytes. Rather, they

are colored by pigment within the keratinocyte. Seborrheic keratosis is a common example of such a benign pigmented epithelial neoplasm.

The Langerhans' Cell

Langerhans' cells are normally found scattered among keratinocytes of the stratum spinosum, or prickle cell layer of the epidermis. They constitute 3% to 5% of the cells in this layer. Like the melanocyte, they are not connected to adjacent keratinocytes by the desmosomes. At the light-microscopic level, Langerhans' cells are difficult to detect in routinely stained sections; however, they appear as dendritic cells in sections impregnated with gold chloride, a stain specific for Langerhans' cells. They can also be stained with peroxidase-labeled monoclonal antibody CD1a or S100. Ultrastructurally they are characterized by a folded nucleus and distinct intracytoplasmic organelles called *Langerhans'* or *Birbeck granules* (Fig. 1-9). In their fully developed form, the organelles are rod shaped with a vacuole at one end and resemble a tennis racquet.

Functionally, Langerhans' cells are of the monocyte-macrophage lineage and originate in bone marrow. They play a role in induction of graft rejection, primary contact sensitization, and immunosurveillance. If skin is depleted of them by exposure to ultraviolet radiation, it loses the ability

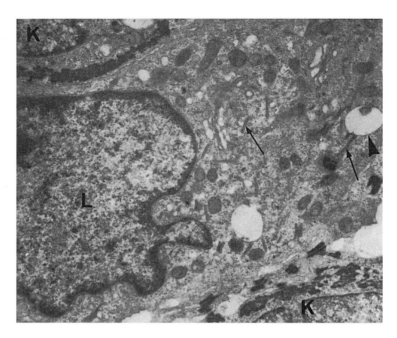

Fig. 1-9 Ultrastructural appearance of the Langerhans' cell *(L)*. The characteristic intracytoplasmic Langerhans' (Birbeck) granules have a rod-shaped handle *(thin arrow)* and a wide head *(broad arrowhead)*. The Langerhans' cell is not connected to adjacent keratinocytes *(K)* by desmosomes.

to be sensitized until its population of Langerhans' cells is replenished. Langerhans' cells function primarily in the afferent limb of the immune response by providing for the recognition, uptake, processing, and presentation of antigens to sensitized T lymphocytes.

Boissy RE, et al: Molecular basis of congenital hypopigmentary disorders in humans. *Pigment Cell Res* 1997, 10:12.

Choi KL: The role of Langerhans cell and keratinocyte in epidermal immunity. *J Leukocyte Biol* 1986, 39:343.

Chu A, et al: Immunoelectron microscopic identification of Langerhans cells using a new antigenic marker. *J Invest Dermatol* 1980, 78:177.

Hanau D: Langerhans cell in allergic contact dermatitis. *Dermatologica* 1986, 172:2.

Katz SI: The skin as an immunologic organ. *J Am Acad Dermatol* 1985, 12:530.

Moll J, et al: Formation of epidermal and dermal Merkel cells during human fetal skin development. *J Invest Dermatol* 1986, 87:779.

Moll J, et al: Intraepidermal formation of Merkel cells in xenografts of human fetal skin. *J Invest Dermatol* 1990, 94:359.

Niedecken H, et al: Differential expression of major histocompatibility complex class II antigens on human keratinocytes. *J Am Acad Dermatol* 1988, 19:1030.

Osborn M: Components of the cellular cytoskeleton. *J Invest Dermatol* 1984, 82:443.

Prota G: Regularity mechanisms of melanogenesis. *J Invest Dermatol* 1993, 100:1565.

Scott GA, et al: Homeobox genes and skin development. *J Invest Dermatol* 1993, 191:3.

Skov L, et al: Susceptibility to effects of UVB irradiation on induction of contact sensitivity, relevance of number and function of Langerhans cells and epidermal macrophages. *Photochem Photobiol* 1998, 67:714.

Smack D, et al: Keratins and keratinization. *J Am Acad Dermatol* 1994, 30:85.

Steinman RM: The dendritic cell system and its role in immunogenicity. *Annu Rev Immunol* 1991, 9:271.

Toews GB, et al: Epidermal Langerhans cell density determines whether contact hypersensitivity or unresponsiveness follows skin painting with DNFB. *J Immunol* 1980, 124:445.

Wakefield PE, et al: Colony stimulating factors. *J Am Acad Dermatol* 1990, 23:903.

Wakefield PE, et al: Tumor necrosis factor. *J Am Acad Dermatol* 1991, 24:675. ▲

THE EPIDERMAL-DERMAL JUNCTION

The junction of epidermis and dermis is formed by the basement membrane zone (see Fig. 1-2). Ultrastructurally, this zone is composed of four components: the plasma membranes of the basal cells with the specialized attachment plates (hemidesmosomes); an electron-lucent zone called the lamina lucida; the basal lamina; and the fibrous components associated with the basal lamina, including anchoring fibrils, dermal microfibrils, and collagen fibers (Fig. 1-10). At the light-microscopic level, the so-called PAS-positive basement membrane is composed of the fibrous components. The basal lamina is synthesized by the basal cells of the epidermis. Uitto et al and Fine have reviewed in detail the many component layers of the basement membrane zone, the ultrastructural localization of the various immunoreactants in the chronic bullous dermatoses, and the abnormalities of the molecular structural proteins in both acquired and inherited blistering diseases.

The basement membrane zone is considered to be a porous semipermeable filter, which permits exchange of cells and fluid between the epidermis and dermis. It further serves as a structural support for the epidermis and holds the epidermis and dermis together. The basement membrane zone serves the same functions for the skin appendages.

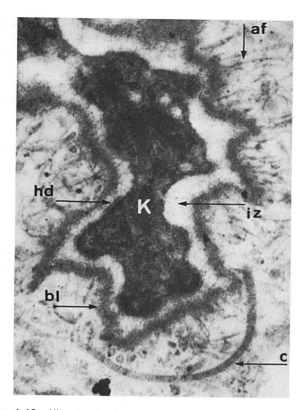

Fig. 1-10 Ultrastructural appearance of the basement membrane zone at the junction of epidermis and dermis. The zone comprises four layers: the plasma membrane of basal keratinocytes *(K)* with their specialized attachment plates, the hemidesmosomes *(hd);* the clear lamina lucida or intermembranous space *(iz);* the basal lamina (bl); and the dermal fibrous components, including anchoring fibrils *(af)* and collagen fibers *(c).*

Fine JD: Structure and antigenicity of the skin basement membrane zone. *J Cutan Pathol* 1991, 18:401.

Katz SI: The epidermal basement membrane zone-structure, ontogeny, and role in disease. *J Am Acad Dermatol* 1984, 11:1025.

Uitto J, et al: Molecular complexity of the cutaneous basement membrane zone. *Mol Biol Rep* 1996, 23:35.

Uitto J, et al: Molecular genetics of the basement membrane zone. *J Clin Invest* 1992, 90:687. _____ ▲

EPIDERMAL APPENDAGES: THE ADNEXA

Eccrine and apocrine glands and ducts and pilosebaceous units constitute the skin adnexa. Embryologically, they originate as downgrowths from the epidermis and are therefore ectodermal in origin. Melanocytes and other cells that are seen in the adult epidermis can be found within the adnexa. While the various adnexal structures serve specific functions, they all can function as reserve epidermis in that reepithelialization after injury to the surface epidermis occurs principally by virtue of the migration of keratinocytes from the adnexal epithelium along the skin surface. It is not surprising, therefore, that skin sites such as the face or scalp, which contain pilosebaceous units in abundance, reepithelialize more rapidly than do skin sites such as the back, where adnexa of all types are comparatively scarce. Since those sites that contain numerous adnexa are also abundantly endowed with a rich network of nerves and blood vessels within the surrounding dermis, wound healing in general is more rapid there.

The Eccrine Sweat Unit

The eccrine sweat unit is composed of three sections that are modified from the basic tubular structure that formed during embryogenesis as a downgrowth of surface epidermis (see Fig. 1-1). The intraepidermal component of the unit, the acrosyringium, which opens directly onto the skin surface, is called the spiral duct. It is derived from dermal duct cells through mitosis and upward migration. The duct consists of a single layer of inner or luminal cells and two or three outer rows of cells. Cornification takes place within the duct, and the horn cells become part of the stratum corneum of the epidermis. The straight dermal portion of the duct is composed of a double layer of cuboidal epithelial cells and is lined by an eosinophilic cuticle on its luminal side.

The secretory acinar portion of the unit, or coil gland, is found within the panniculus near the junction of dermis and subcutaneous fat. An inner layer of epithelial cells, the secretory portion of the gland, is surrounded by a layer of flattened myoepithelial cells. The secretory cells are of two types: glycogen-rich, large pale cells and smaller, darker-staining cells. The pale glycogen-rich cells are thought to initiate the formation of sweat. The darker cells may function in a manner similar to that of cells of the dermal duct, which actively reabsorb sodium, thereby modifying sweat from a basically isotonic solution to a hypotonic one by the time it reaches the skin surface. Sweat is similar in composition to plasma, containing the same electrolytes, though in a more dilute concentration.

Eccrine sweat units are found at virtually all skin sites. They are most abundant on the palms, soles, forehead, and axillae. Some eccrine glands in the axillae, especially in patients with hyperhidrosis, may have widely dilated secretary coils that contain apocrine-appearing cells. Secretion of sweat occurs as a result of many factors and is mediated by cholinergic innervation. Heat is a prime stimulus to increased sweating, but other physiologic stimuli, including emotional stress, are important as well. Increased sweat production in response to heat is part of the thermoregulatory system of the body; together with in-creased cutaneous blood flow, it can effectively dissipate excessive body heat. At friction surfaces, such as the palms and soles, eccrine secretion is thought to assist tactile sensibility and improve adhesion.

The Apocrine Unit

Adult apocrine units develop as outgrowths, not of the surface epidermis, but of the infundibular or upper portion of the hair follicle (see Fig. 1-1). They are therefore intimately related, at least anatomically, to pilar units. Although immature apocrine units are found covering the entire skin surface of the human fetus, these regress and are absent by the time the fetus reaches term. The straight excretory portion of the duct, which opens into the infundibular portion of the hair follicle, is composed of a double layer of cuboidal epithelial cells. The coiled secretory gland is located at the junction of the dermis and subcutaneous fat. It is lined by a single layer of cells, which vary in appearance from columnar to cuboidal. This layer of cells is surrounded by a layer of myoepithelial cells.

The apexes of the columnar cells project into the lumen of the gland and in histologic cross section appear as if they are being extruded (decapitation secretion). Controversy exists about the mode of secretion in apocrine secretory cells, whether merocrine, apocrine, holocrine, or all three. The composition of the product of secretion is only partially understood. Protein, carbohydrate, ammonia, lipid, and iron are all found in apocrine secretion. It appears milky and is odorless until it reaches the skin surface, where it is altered by bacteria, which makes it odoriferous. Apocrine secretion is mediated by adrenergic innervation and by circulating catecholamines of adrenomedullary origin. Excretion, or the propulsion of the secretion through the duct, is episodic, although the actual secretion of the gland is continuous. Apocrine gland secretion in humans serves no known function. In other species it has a protective as well as a sexual function, and in some species, it is important in thermoregulation as well.

Although occasionally found in an ectopic location, apocrine units of the human body are generally confined to the following sites: axillae, areolae, the anogenital region, the external auditory canal (ceruminous glands), and the eyelids (glands of Moll). The glands do not begin to function until puberty.

The Hair Follicle

During embryogenesis, mesenchymal cells in the fetal dermis collect immediately below the basal layer of the epidermis. Epidermal buds grow down into the dermis at these sites. The developing follicle forms at an angle to the skin surface and continues its downward growth. At this base, the column of cells widens and surrounds the small collections of mesenchymal cells forming the bulb. The hair is formed from cells just above the bulb, which also give rise to concentric zones of differentiated epithelial cells destined to form the inner and outer root sheaths. Along one side of the follicle, two buds are formed: an upper, which develops into the sebaceous gland, and a lower, which becomes the attachment for the arrector pili muscle. At skin sites destined to have apocrine units, a third epithelial bud develops from the opposite side of the follicle above the level of the sebaceous gland anlage. The uppermost portion of the follicle, which extends from its surface opening to the entrance of the sebaceous duct, is called the infundibular segment. The portion of the follicle between the sebaceous duct and the insertion of the arrector pili muscle is the isthmus. The matrix, or inferior portion, includes the lowermost part of the follicle and the hair bulb.

Hair follicles develop sequentially in rows of three. Primary follicles are surrounded by the appearance of two secondary follicles; other secondary follicles subsequently develop around the principal units. The density of pilosebaceous units decreases throughout life, mainly because of the poor development of the secondary follicles.

The actual hair shaft, as well as an inner and outer root sheath, develops from the mitotically active undifferentiated cells of the matrix portion of the hair bulb (Fig. 1-11). The sheaths and contained hair are derived from different regions of the bulb, and they form concentric cylindrical layers. The hair shaft and inner root sheath move together as the hair grows toward the surface: the outer root sheath remains fixed in position. The epidermis of the upper part of the follicular canal is contiguous with the outer root sheath and includes the infundibular and isthmus zones of the follicle. This portion of the follicle is permanent; the portion of the follicle between the bulb and the upper limit of the inner root sheath is completely replaced at each new cycle of hair growth.

The rate of hair growth depends on mitotic activity of the cells of the bulb matrix. The cross-sectional shape of the hair depends on the arrangement of cells in the bulb. The scalp hair of whites is round; pubic hair, beard hair, and eyelashes are oval. The scalp hair of blacks is also oval, and it is this, plus a curvature of the follicle just above the bulb, that causes black hair to be curly.

Basic hair color depends on the distribution of melanosomes within hair bulb cells, which become the cells of the hair shaft. Melanocytes of the hair bulb synthesize melanosomes and transfer them to the cells of the bulb matrix in a fashion similar to the transfer of melanosomes from melanocytes to keratinocytes in the surface epidermis. Larger melanosomes are found in the hair of blacks; smaller melanosomes, which are aggregated within membrane-bound complexes, are found in the hair of whites. Red hair is characterized by spherical melanosomes. The intensity of color is most likely a reflection of the number of fully melanized melanosomes produced by the melanocytes. Graying of hair is a result of a decreased number of melanocytes, which produce fewer melanosomes. Lerner has likened the pathogenesis of graying of the hair to that of vitiligo. Both conditions show a decreased number of melanocytes in affected sites.

Human hair growth is cyclical, but each follicle functions as an independent unit. Therefore, humans do not shed hair synchronously, as most animals do. Each hair follicle undergoes intermittent stages of activity and quiescence (Fig. 1-12).

During the growing phase or anagen, the cells of the hair

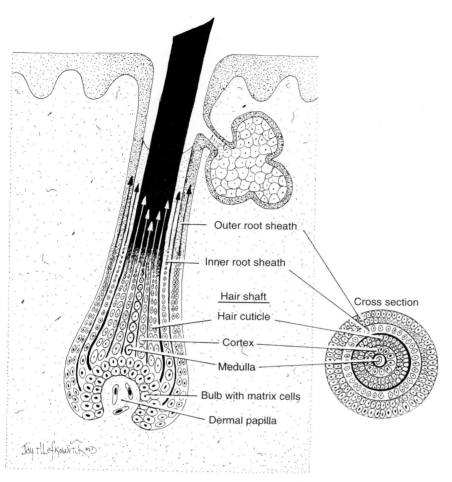

Outer root sheath

Inner root sheath

Hair shaft

Hair cuticle

Cortex

Medulla

Bulb with matrix cells

Dermal papilla

Cross section

Fig. 1-11 Diagrammatic anatomy of the hair follicle.

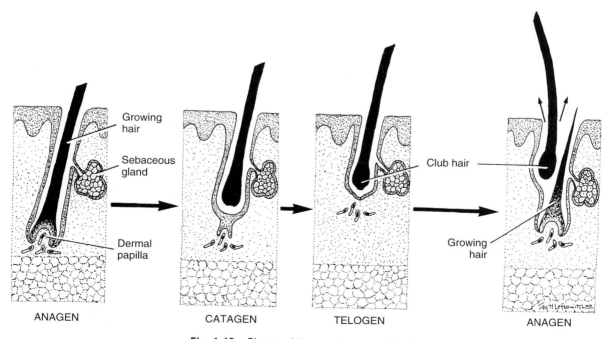

Growing hair

Sebaceous gland

Dermal papilla

Club hair

Growing hair

ANAGEN

CATAGEN

TELOGEN

ANAGEN

Fig. 1-12 Phases of the growth cycle of a hair.

bulb actively divide and produce the growing hair. As this phase ceases, the follicle goes into the catagen, or transitional phase of activity, the matrix cells stop dividing and the hair develops a brushlike zone (club hair) owing to incomplete keratinization of the cells. During catagen, the lower portion of the follicle disappears, leaving behind a thin strand of epithelial cells surrounded by a thick basement membrane zone. During the telogen or resting phase of the hair cycle, the epithelial strand subsequently shortens to the level of the arrector pili muscle and leaves in its wake a small aggregate of epithelial cells exposed to surrounding dermis. The club hair remains within the foreshortened follicle until a new anagen follicle develops in a fashion recapitulating its formation during embryogenesis, and the newly formed hair shaft dislodges the club hair.

The temporal profile of the hair cycle is variable for hairs in different regions of the body. In humans, the average period of growth of a scalp hair is 3 to 4 years, and the involutional and resting phases last for approximately 3 months. Normally, approximately 85% to 90% of all scalp hairs are in the anagen phase, a figure that decreases with age and decreases faster in individuals with male pattern baldness.

Various exogenous and endogenous physiologic factors can modulate the hair cycle. An example is pregnancy, which is often accompanied by retention of an increased number of scalp hairs in the anagen phase. Three or 4 months after pregnancy ends, the normal complement of resting hairs plus those which had been temporarily retained in the anagen phase are lost, producing a transient effluvium. Patients on chemotherapy often have hair loss because the drugs interfere with the mitotic activity of the hair matrix, leading to the formation of a thin shaft, which breaks within the follicle.

The Sebaceous Gland

The sebaceous gland is formed embryologically as an outgrowth from the upper portion of the hair follicle. It is composed of lobules of pale-staining cells with abundant lipid in their cytoplasm. At the periphery of the lobules are several layers of cells that resemble basal cells of the epidermis and are called germinative cells. These germinative cells give rise to the lipid-filled pale cells, which are continuously being extruded through the short sebaceous duct into the infundibular portion of the hair follicle (see Fig. 1-1).

Sebaceous glands are found in greatest abundance on the face and scalp, though they are distributed throughout all skin sites except the palms and soles. They are always associated with hair follicles except at the following sites: the eyelids (meibomian glands), the buccal mucosa and vermilion border of the lip (Fordyce's spots), the prepuce (Tyson's glands), and the female areolas (Montgomery's tubercles).

Although sebaceous glands are independent miniorgans

in their own right, they are anatomically and functionally related to the hair follicle. Cutaneous disorders attributed to sebaceous glands, such as acne vulgaris, are really disorders of the entire pilosebaceous unit. The clinical manifestations of acne, namely the comedo, papule, pustule, and cyst, would not form, regardless of increased sebaceous gland activity, as long as the sebaceous duct and infundibular portion of the hair follicle remained patent and lipid and cell debris (sebum) were able to reach the skin surface.

Bell M: The ultrastructure of human axillary apocrine glands after epinephrine injection. *J Invest Dermatol* 1974, 63:147.

Knutson DD: Ultrastructural observations in acne vulgaris: the normal sebaceous follicle and acne lesions. *J Invest Dermatol* 1974, 62:228.

Montagna W: An introduction to sebaceous glands. *J Invest Dermatol* 1974, 62:120.

Paus R, et al: The biology of hair follicles. *N Engl J Med* 1999, 341:491.

Robertshaw D: Neural and humoral control of apocrine glands. *J Invest Dermatol* 1974, 63:160.

Sato K, et al: Biology of sweat glands and their disorders. *J Am Acad Dermatol* 1989, 20:537.

Sperling LC: Hair anatomy for the clinician. *J Am Acad Dermatol* 1991, 25:1.

Stenn KS, et al: Hair follicle biology, the sebaceous gland, and scarring alopecias. *Arch Dermatol* 1999, 135:973.

Strauss JS, et al: The sebaceous glands: twenty-five years of progress. *J Invest Dermatol* 1976, 67:90. _____ ▲

THE NAILS

Nails act to assist in grasping small objects and in protecting the fingertip from trauma. The matrix keratinization leads to the formation of the nail plate. The keratin types found in the nail are a mixture of epidermal and hair types, with the hair types predominating. Fingernails grow an average of 0.1 mm per day, requiring about 4 to 5 months to replace a complete nail plate. The growth rate is much slower for toenails, with 12 to 18 months required to replace the great toenail. Abnormalities of the nail may serve as important clues to cutaneous and systemic disease and may provide the astute clinician information about disease or toxic exposures that occurred several months in the past.

Achten G, et al: The normal and pathologic nail. *Intern J Dermatol* 1983, 22:556.

Albert SF: Disorders of the nail unit. *Clin Podiatr Med Surg* 1996, 13:1.

Cohen PR: The lunula. *J Am Acad Dermatol* 1996, 34:943.

Ditre CM, et al: Surgical anatomy of the nail unit. *J Dermatol Surg Oncol* 1992, 18:665.

Norton LA: Nail disorders. *J Am Acad Dermatol* 1980, 2:451. _____ ▲

THE DERMIS

The constituents of the dermis are mesodermal in origin except for nerves, which, like melanocytes, derive from the neural crest. Until the sixth week of fetal life, the dermis is merely a pool of acid-mucopolysaccharide–containing, scattered dendritic-shaped cells, which are the precursors of fibroblasts. By the twelfth week, fibroblasts are actively synthesizing reticulum fibers, elastic fibers, and collagen. A vascular network develops, and by the twenty-fourth week, fat cells have appeared beneath the dermis.

The principal component of the dermis is collagen, a family of fibrous proteins comprising at least 15 genetically distinct types in human skin. Collagen serves as the major structural protein for the entire body; it is found in tendons, ligaments, and the lining of bones as well as in the dermis. It represents 70% of the dry weight of skin.

The fibroblast synthesizes the procollagen molecule, a helical arrangement of specific polypeptide chains that are subsequently secreted by the cell and assembled into collagen fibrils. Collagen is rich in the amino acids hydroxyproline, hydroxylysine, and glycine. The fibrillar collagens are the major group found in the skin. The structure of type I collagen is uniform in width, and each fiber displays characteristic cross striations with a periodicity of 68 nm. Collagen fibers are loosely arranged in the upper (papillary) portion of the dermis. They are tightly bundled in a fascicle-like pattern within the lower, or reticular, portion of the dermis. Type IV collagen is found in the basement membrane zone. Type VII collagen is the major structural component of anchoring fibrils and is produced predominately by keratinocytes. Abnormalities in type VII collagen are seen in dominant and recessive dystrophic epidermolysis bullosa and autoantibodies to this collagen type characterize acquired epidermolysis bullosa. Collagen fibers are continuously being degraded by proteolytic enzymes called collagenases, and replaced by newly synthesized fibers. Additional information on collagen types and diseases produced by abnormalities of them may be found in Chapter 25.

The fibroblast also synthesizes elastic fibers, as well as the ground substance of the dermis, which is composed of glycosaminoglycans or acid mucopolysaccharides. Elastic fibers differ both structurally and chemically from collagen. They consist of aggregates of two components: protein filaments and elastin, an amorphous protein. The amino acids desmosine and isodesmosine are unique to elastic fibers. Elastic fibers in the papillary dermis are fine, whereas those in the reticular dermis are coarse. The extracellular matrix or ground substance of the dermis is composed of acid mucupolysaccharide, principally hyaluronic acid, chondroitin sulfate and dermatan sulfate, neutral mucopolysaccharides, and electrolytes.

Collagen is the major stress-resistant material of the skin. Elastic fibers contribute very little to resisting deformation and tearing of skin, but have a role in maintaining elasticity. Although *connective tissue disease* is a term generally used to refer to a clinically heterogeneous group of autoimmune diseases, including lupus erythematosus, scleroderma, and dermatomyositis, only scleroderma involves a detectable abnormality in the metabolism of collagen. Like scleroderma, keloid and hypertrophic scar formation reflect abnormalities in the rates of collagen synthesis and degradation.

Defects in collagen synthesis have been described in a number of inheritable diseases, including Ehlers-Danlos syndrome, X-linked cutis laxa, and osteogenesis imperfecta. Defects in elastic tissue are seen in another group of hereditary diseases such as Marfan syndrome and pseudoxanthoma elasticum.

Vasculature

The dermal vasculature consists principally of two important intercommunicating plexuses: the subpapillary plexus, or upper horizontal network, courses within the papillary portion of the dermis parallel to the epidermis and furnishes a rich supply of capillaries, end arterioles, and venules to the dermal papillae. The deeper, lower horizontal plexus is found at the dermal-subcutaneous interface and is composed of larger blood vessels than those of the superficial plexus (see Fig. 1-1). The vasculature of the dermis is particularly well developed at sites of adnexal structures. Associated with the vascular plexus are the dermal lymphatics.

Muscles

Smooth muscle occurs in the skin as arrectores pilorum (erectors of the hairs), as the tunica dartos (or dartos) of the scrotum, and in the areolas around the nipples. The arrectores pilorum are attached to the hair follicles below the sebaceous glands and, in contracting, pull the hair follicle upward, producing gooseflesh.

Striated (voluntary) muscle occurs in the skin of the neck as the platysma muscle and in the skin of the face as the muscles of expression.

Specialized aggregates of smooth muscle cells found between arterioles and venules are called glomus bodies. These serve to shunt blood from the arterial to the venous side of the vascular system, thereby avoiding the capillaries, where exchange of oxygen and heat takes place. Arteriovenous anastomoses are best developed in the digits.

Nerves

The dermis is rich in nerves. Touch and pressure are mediated by Meissner corpuscles and in the dermal papillae, particularly on the palms and soles, and by Vater-Pacini corpuscles located in the deeper portion of the dermis of weight-bearing surfaces. Mucocutaneous end-organs are found in the papillary dermis of modified hairless skin at the mucocutaneous junctions, namely, the glans, the prepuce, the clitoris, the labia minora, the perianal region, and the vermilion border of the lips. Temperature, pain, and itch sensation are transmitted by unmyelinated nerve fibers which terminate in the papillary dermis and around hair follicles. Impulses pass to the central nervous system by way of the dorsal root ganglia.

Postganglionic adrenergic fibers of the autonomic nervous system regulate vasoconstriction, apocrine gland secretions, and contraction of arrector pili muscles of hair follicles. Cholinergic fibers mediate eccrine sweat secretion.

Mast Cells

An important cellular constituent of the dermis is the mast cell. Six to 12 microns in diameter, it is distinguished by containing up to 1000 granules, each measuring 0.6 to 0.7 microns in diameter. On the cell's surface are 100,000 to 500,000 glycoprotein receptor sites for immunoglobulin E (IgE). There is heterogeneity to mast cells with type I or connective tissue mast cells found in the dermis and submucosa and type II or mucosal mast cells found in the bowel and respiratory tract mucosa.

Mast cell granules stain metachromatically because of their high content of heparin. They also contain histamine, neutrophil chemotactic factor, eosinophil chemotactic factor of anaphylaxis, tryptase, kininogenase, and beta-glucosaminidase. Slow reacting substance of anaphylaxis (leukotrienes C4 and D4), leukotriene B4, platelet activating factor, and prostaglandin D2 are formed only after IgE-mediated release of granules.

Dermal Dendrocyte

This highly dendritic cell of the dermis possesses phenotypic characteristics of macrophages, including strong HLA-DR expression. They are found in a perivascular network and may serve as the antigen presenting cell which initiates immune responses to antigens delivered through the circulation.

Ansel JC, et al: Skin-nervous system interactions. *J Invest Dermatol* 1996, 106:198.
Braverman IM: Ultrastructure and organization of the cutaneous microvasculature in normal and pathologic states. *J Invest Dermatol* 1989, 93:2S.
Clark RAF: Cutaneous tissue repair. *J Am Acad Dermatol* 1985, 13:701.
Headington JT, et al: Dendritic cells and the dermis. *Am J Dermatopathol* 1990, 12:217.
Mecham R: Elastin synthesis and fiber assembly. *Ann NY Acad Sci* 1990, 58:137.
Melman SA: Mast cells and their mediators. *Int J Dermatol* 1987, 26:335.
Miyachi Y, et al: Mast cells in clinical dermatology. *Australas J Dermatol* 1998, 39:14.
Prockop DJ, et Al: Collagens. *Annu Rev Biochem* 1995, 64:403.
Ryan TJ: Structure and function of lymphatics. *J Invest Dermatol* 1989, 93:185.
Serafin WE, et al: Mediators of immediate hypersensitivity. *N Engl J Med* 1987, 317:30.
Sontheimer RD: Perivascular dendritic macrophages as immunological constituents of the human dermal micro-vascular unit. *J Invest Dermatol* 1989, 93:96S.
Uitto J, et al: Molecular biology and pathology of human elastin. *Trans Biochem Soc* 1991, 19:824. ▲

SUBCUTANEOUS TISSUE (FAT)

Beneath the dermis lies the panniculus, lobules of fat calls or lipocytes separated by fibrous septa composed of collagen and large blood vessels. The collagen in the septa is continuous with the collagen in the dermis. Just as the epidermis and the dermis vary in thickness according to skin site, so does the subcutaneous tissue. Certain inflammatory dermatoses, known as the panniculitides, principally affect this level of the skin, producing subcutaneous nodules. The pattern of the inflammation, specifically whether it primarily affects the septa or the fat lobules themselves, serves to distinguish various conditions which clinically may resemble one another.

Ryan TJ, et al: Hypertrophy and atrophy of fat. *Clin Dermatol* 1989, 7:93.
Ryan TJ, et al: Panniculitis. *Dermatol Clin* 1989, 7:120.
Ryan TJ, et al: The structure of fat. *Clin Dermatol* 1989, 7:37. ▲

CHAPTER 2

Cutaneous Symptoms, Signs, and Diagnosis

The various diseases that affect the human skin may present similar symptoms and signs, such as pruritus and erythema. In many instances, the appearance of skin lesions may be so distinctive that the diagnosis is clear at a glance. In other cases, subjective symptoms and clinical signs in themselves are inadequate, and a complete history and laboratory examinations, including a biopsy, are essential to arrive at a diagnosis.

The same disease may show variations under different conditions and in different individuals. The appearance of the lesions may have been modified by previous treatment or obscured by extraneous influences, such as scratching or secondary infection. Subjective symptoms may be the only evidence of a disease, as in pruritus, and the skin appearance may be generally unremarkable. Although history is important, in dermatology, the diagnosis is most frequently made based on the objective physical characteristics and location or distribution of one or more lesions that can be seen or felt. Therefore, careful physical examination of the skin is paramount in dermatologic diagnosis.

CUTANEOUS SYMPTOMS

Subjective symptoms consist of pruritus (itching), sensations of heat (burning), cold (tingling), prickling, biting, formication, pain, and numbness.

Pruritus

Pruritus is defined by *Dorland's Medical Dictionary* as "an unpleasant cutaneous sensation which provokes the desire to scratch or rub the skin." Pruritus is by far the most common cutaneous symptom. The sensation of pruritus is carried from the skin by unmyelinated C fibers. Endogenous opioids may be pathogenically important in pruritus associated with some systemic diseases.

Pruritus may be described by the patient as a mere prickling, tingling, or formication, or its severity may be so intense as to be intolerable. The quality of the pruritus may be useful in determining the diagnosis. For example, the itch of notalgia paresthetica is described as deep, below where one can scratch; whereas patients with delusions, depres-

sion, and sometimes those with a metabolic basis of pruritus describe their pruritus as being "like a worm crawling under the skin."

There are regional and individual differences in the perception of and reaction to pruritus. This may be in part related to the psychologic state at the time (i.e., anxiety and depression appear to lower the pruritus threshold). The anogenital area is especially prone to pruritus, hence the frequency of pruritus ani, vulvae, and scroti. Pruritus is encountered more or less in all inflammatory dermatoses but is especially common in patients with eczematous dermatitis, urticaria, contact dermatitis, dermatitis herpetiformis, scabies, lichen planus, mycosis fungoides, pediculosis, and xerosis. Winter pruritus and pruritus in persons over age 60 is often caused by dryness of the skin (xerosis). Pruritus is common in patients with HIV disease, especially those with AIDS. HIV-associated pruritus is usually caused by an associated inflammatory condition, most commonly a pruritic folliculitis.

Pruritus may result from or be associated with systemic diseases. Among these are hepatobiliary diseases, especially biliary obstructive disease, severe renal insufficiency, iron-deficiency anemia, endocrine disorders, and internal malignancy (especially lymphoma).

Endocrine disorders, especially thyroid dysfunction, and, less commonly, parathyroid disease may cause pruritus. Although diabetes mellitus is frequently listed as a cause of pruritus, most individuals with diabetes do not itch. In a patient with diabetes who has pruritus, other causes should be excluded before the pruritus is attributed to the diabetes. Pruritus of the anogenital area, especially in women with diabetes, may be associated with *Candida* infection.

In Hodgkin's disease, non-Hodgkin's lymphoma, and leukemia, pruritus may be severe, although the skin remains totally normal in appearance. There are no primary lesions. Erythroderma may be a manifestation of the specific lymphoma, usually cutaneous T-cell lymphoma, causing the severe pruritus.

Pruritus associated with severe renal failure (so-called uremic pruritus) is generalized and often associated with the appearance of hyperkeratotic prurigo nodulelike lesions (Kyrle's disease or the perforating disorder of renal failure or dialysis). It occurs whether or not the patient is receiving dialysis treatments and may not improve if a patient with renal failure goes on dialysis. Renal transplantation resolves uremic pruritus. Gilchrist demonstrated the efficacy of UVB phototherapy in uremic pruritus, and this is currently the most common management approach used when simple measures have failed. Intravenous lidocaine (200 mg in 100 ml of physiologic saline), naltrexone, erythropoietin therapy, and correction of abnormalities of calcium and phosphorus with phosphate-binding antacids may also be beneficial.

Pruritus of liver disease, although classically described and more common in patients with a high bilirubin level, is not restricted to this group. Associated hepatitis C virus infection should always be sought in patients with pruritus. The pathogenesis of the pruritus associated with obstructive hepatobiliary disease seems to relate to abnormal endogenous opiate metabolism in the central nervous system. Opiate antagonists may improve this form of pruritus.

Such pharmacologic agents as antidepressants, belladonna alkaloids, opiates, and oral contraceptives may induce pruritus, even without producing a dermatitis. In addition to standard pharmacologic agents, recreational drugs, especially amphetamines and cocaine, are associated with pruritus-like symptoms (cocaine bug). These are often described as a crawling sensation.

Psychologic disease, most frequently anxiety/depression or obsessive compulsive disorder, may be associated with pruritus. This form of itching is typically associated with aggressive scratching leading to scarring. Treatment of the underlying psychologic disorder will lead to improvement or resolution. In addition, anxiety/depression reduces the itch threshold, so that pruritic disorders may be more severe in situations or persons with such a psychologic profile.

Bergasa NV, et al: Effects of naloxone infusions in patients with the pruritus of cholestasis. *Ann Intern Med* 1995, 123:161.
Goicoechea M, et al: Uremic pruritus. *Nephron* 1999, 82:73.
Greaves MW, et al: Pathophysiology of itching. *Lancet* 1996, 348:938.
Peer G, et al: Randomized crossover trial of naltrexone in uraemic pruritus. *Lancet* 1996, 348:1552.
Savin JA: How should we define itching? *J Am Acad Dermatol* 1998, 39:268. _____ ▲

Other Symptoms

Pain may be deep-boring and burning, lancinating or shooting, or throbbing as in furuncles, carbuncles, and cellulitis. Allodynia (the production of pain by normally trivial stimuli such as the clothes touching the skin) is seen frequently in postherpetic neuralgia. Abnormal sensation, either hypesthesia or hyperesthesia, may be seen. Loss of specific sensations (temperature as opposed to pain) may be typical of certain diseases, especially Hansen's disease but is also a feature, though an inconstant one, of follicular mucinosis. Reversal of the perception of heat and cold is characteristic of Ciguatera fish poisoning.

CUTANEOUS SIGNS

Typically, most skin diseases produce or present with lesions with more or less distinct characteristics. They may be uniform or diverse in size, shape, and color, and may be in different stages of evolution or of involution. The original lesions are known as the *primary lesions,* and identification of such lesions is the most important aspect of the dermatologic physical examination. They may continue to full development or be modified by regression, trauma, or other extraneous factors, producing *secondary lesions.*

PRIMARY LESIONS

Primary lesions are of the following forms—macules (or patches), papules (or plaques), nodules, tumors, wheals, vesicles, bullae, and pustules.

Macules (Maculae, Spots)

Macules are variously sized, circumscribed changes in skin color, without elevation or depression (nonpalpable). They may be circular, oval or irregular, and may be distinct in outline or fade into the surrounding skin.

Macules may constitute the whole or part of the eruption, or may be merely an early phase. If the lesions become slightly raised, they are then designated papules, or sometimes, as morbilliform eruptions.

Patches

A patch is a large macule, 1 cm or greater in diameter, as may be seen in nevus flammeus or vitiligo.

Papules (Papulae)

Papules are circumscribed, solid elevations with no visible fluid, varying in size from a pinhead to 1 cm. They may be acuminate, rounded, conical, flat-topped, or umbilicated, and may appear white (as in milium), red (as in eczema), yellowish (as in xanthoma), reddish brown (as in lupus vulgaris), or black (as in melanoma).

Papules may be centered in the dermis, around sebaceous glands, at the orifices of the sweat ducts, or at the hair follicles. They may be of soft or firm consistency. The surface may be smooth or rough. If capped by scales, they are known as *squamous papules,* and the eruption is called *papulosquamous.*

Some papules are discrete and irregularly distributed, as in papular urticaria, whereas others are grouped, as in lichen nitidus. Some persist as papules, whereas those of the inflammatory type may progress to vesicles and even to pustules, or may erode or ulcerate before regression takes place.

The term *maculopapular* should not be used. There is no such thing as a maculopapule, but there may be both macules and papules in an eruption. Most typically these eruptions are morbilliform.

Plaques

A plaque is a broad papule (or confluence of papules), 1 cm or more in diameter. It is generally flat, but may be centrally depressed. The center of a plaque may be normal skin.

Nodules

Nodules are morphologically similar to papules, but they are more than 1 cm in diameter. They most frequently are centered in dermis or the subcutaneous fat.

Tumors

Tumors are soft or firm and freely movable or fixed masses of various sizes and shapes (but in general greater than 2 cm in diameter). General usage dictates that the word "tumor" means a neoplasm. They may be elevated or deep seated, and in some instances are pedunculated (fibromas). Tumors have a tendency to be rounded. Their consistency depends on the constituents of the lesion. Some tumors remain stationary indefinitely, whereas others increase in size, or break down.

Wheals (Hives)

Wheals are evanescent, edematous, plateaulike elevations of various sizes. They are usually oval or of arcuate contours, pink to red, and surrounded by a pink areola. They may be discrete or may coalesce. These lesions often develop quickly. Because the wheal is the prototypic lesion of urticaria, diseases in which wheals are prominent are frequently described as "urticarial" (e.g., urticarial vasculitis). Dermographism, or pressure-induced whealing, may be evident.

Vesicles (Blisters)

Vesicles are circumscribed, fluid-containing, epidermal elevations 1 to 10 mm in size. They may be pale or yellow from serous exudate, or red from serum mixed with blood. The apex may be rounded, acuminate, or umbilicated as in eczema herpeticum. Vesicles may be discrete, irregularly scattered, grouped as in herpes zoster, or linear as in poison ivy dermatitis. They may arise directly or from a macule or papule, and generally lose their identity in a short time, breaking spontaneously or developing into bullae through coalescence or enlargement, or developing into pustules. When the contents are of a seropurulent character, the lesions are known as *vesicopustules*. Vesicles consist of either a single cavity (unilocular) or of several compartments (multilocular), containing fluid.

Bullae

Bullae are rounded or irregularly shaped blisters containing serous or seropurulent fluid. They differ from vesicles only in size, being larger than 1 cm. They are usually unilocular but may be multilocular. Bullae may be located superficially in the epidermis, so that their walls are flaccid and thin and subject to rupture spontaneously or from slight injury. After rupture, remnants of the thin walls may persist and, together with the exudate, may dry to form a thin crust; or the broken bleb may leave a raw and moist base, which may be covered with seropurulent or purulent exudate. More rarely, irregular vegetations may appear on the base (as in pemphigus vegetans). When the bullae are subepidermal, they are tense, and ulceration and scarring may result.

Nikolsky's sign refers to the diagnostic maneuver of putting lateral pressure on unblistered skin in a bullous eruption and having the epithelium shear off. Asboe-Hansen's sign refers to the extension of a blister to adjacent unblistered skin when pressure is put on the top of the blister. Both of these signs demonstrate the principle that in some diseases, the extent of microscopic vesiculation is more than is evident by simple inspection. These findings are useful in evaluating the severity of pemphigus vulgaris and severe bullous drug reactions. Hemorrhagic bullae are common in pemphigus, herpes zoster, severe bullous drug reactions, and lichen sclerosus et atrophicus. The cellular contents of bullae may be useful in confirming the diagnosis of pemphigus, herpes zoster, and herpes simplex.

Pustules

Pustules are small elevations of the skin containing purulent material (usually necrotic inflammatory cells). They are similar to vesicles in shape and usually have an inflammatory areola. They are usually white or yellow centrally, but may be red if they also contain blood. They may originate as pustules or may develop from papules or vesicles, passing through transitory early stages, during which they are known as *papulopustules* or *vesicopustules*.

SECONDARY LESIONS

Secondary lesions are of many kinds; the most important are scales, crusts, erosions, ulcers, fissures, and scars.

Scales (Exfoliation)

Scales are dry or greasy laminated masses of keratin. The body ordinarily is constantly shedding imperceptible tiny, thin fragments of stratum corneum. When the formation of epidermal cells is rapid or the process of normal keratinization is interfered with, pathologic exfoliation results, producing scales. These vary in size, some being fine, delicate, and branny, as in tinea versicolor, others being coarser, as in eczema and ichthyosis, while still others are stratified, as in psoriasis. Large sheets of desquamated epidermis are seen in toxic epidermal necrolysis, staphylococcal scalded skin syndrome, and infection-associated (toxin-medicated) desquamations, such as scarlet fever. Scales vary in color from white-gray to yellow or brown from the admixture of dirt or melanin. Occasionally, they have a silvery sheen from trapping of air between their layers: these are micaceous scales, characteristic of psoriasis. When scaling occurs, it usually implies that there is some pathologic process in the epidermis, and parakeratosis is often associated histologically.

Crusts (Scabs)

Crusts are dried serum, pus, or blood, usually mixed with epithelial and sometimes bacterial debris. They vary greatly in size, thickness, shape, and color, according to their origin, composition, and volume. They may be dry, golden yellow, soft, friable, and superficial, as in impetigo; yellowish, as in favus; thick, hard, and tough as in third-degree burns; or lamellated, elevated, brown, black, or green masses, as in late syphilis. The latter have been described as oyster-shell (ostraceous) crusts and are known as *rupia*. When crusts become detached, the base may be dry or red and moist.

Excoriations and Abrasions (Scratch Marks)

An excoriation is a punctate or linear abrasion produced by mechanical means, usually involving only the epidermis but not uncommonly reaching the papillary layer of the dermis. Excoriations are caused by scratching with the fingernails in an effort to relieve itching in a variety of diseases (eczema, scabies). If the skin damage is the result of mechanical trauma or constant friction, the term *abrasion* may be used. Frequently there is an inflammatory areola around the excoriation or a covering of yellowish dried serum or red dried blood over it. Excoriations may provide access for pyogenic microorganisms and the formation of crusts, pustules, or cellulitis occasionally associated with enlargement of the neighboring lymphatic glands. In general, the longer and deeper excoriations are, the more severe was the pruritus that provoked them. Lichen planus is an exception, however, in which pruritus is severe, but excoriations are rare.

Fissures (Cracks, Clefts)

A fissure is a linear cleft through the epidermis, or into the dermis. These lesions may be single or multiple and vary from microscopic to clefts several centimeters in length with sharply defined margins. They may be dry or moist, red, straight, curved, irregular, or branching. They occur most commonly when the skin is thickened and inelastic from inflammation and dryness, especially in regions subjected to frequent movement. Such areas are the tips and flexural creases of the thumbs, fingers, and palms; the edges of the heels; the clefts between the fingers and toes; at the angles of the mouth; the lips; and about the nares, auricles, and anus. When the skin is dry, exposure to cold, wind, water, and cleaning products (soap, detergents) may produce a stinging, burning sensation indicating microscopic fissuring is present. This may be referred to as *chapping,* as in "chapped lips." When fissuring is present, pain is often produced by movement of the parts, which opens or deepens the fissures or forms new ones.

Erosions

Loss of all or portions of the epidermis alone, as in impetigo or herpes zoster or simplex after vesicles rupture, produces an erosion. It may or may not become crusted, but it heals without a scar.

Ulcers

Ulcers are rounded or irregularly shaped excavations that result from complete loss of the epidermis plus some portion of the dermis. They vary in diameter from a few millimeters to several centimeters. They may be shallow, involving little beyond the epidermis, as in dystrophic epidermolysis bullosa, the base being formed by the papillary layer, or they may extend deep into the dermis or even reach into the subcutaneous structures, as in basal cell cancer or decubitus. They heal with scarring.

Scars

Scars are composed of new connective tissue that replaced lost substance in the dermis or deeper parts as a result of injury or disease, as part of the normal reparative process. Their size and shape are determined by the form of the previous destruction. Scarring is characteristic of certain inflammatory processes and is therefore of diagnostic value. The pattern of scarring may be characteristic of a particular disease. Lichen planus and discoid lupus erythematosus, for example, have inflammation that is in relatively the same area anatomically, yet discoid lupus characteristically causes scarring as it resolves, whereas lichen planus rarely results in scarring of the skin. Both processes, however, cause scarring of the hair follicles when they occur on the scalp. Scars may be thin and atrophic, or the fibrous elements may develop into neoplastic overgrowths, as in keloids. Some individuals and some areas of the body, such as the anterior chest, are especially prone to scarring. Cicatrices may be smooth or rough, pliable or firm, and tend at first to be pink or violaceous, later becoming white, glistening, and rarely, pigmented.

Scars are persistent but tend to become less noticeable in the course of time. On the other hand, sometimes they grow thick, tough, and corded, forming a hypertrophic scar or keloid, and may cause severe pruritus.

GENERAL DIAGNOSIS

Interpretation of the clinical picture may be difficult, because identical manifestations may result from widely different causes. Moreover, the same etiologic factors may give rise to a great diversity of eruptions. There is one great advantage in dermatology, namely, that of dealing with an organ that can be seen and felt. Smears and cultures may be readily made for bacteria and fungi. Biopsy and histologic examination of skin lesions are usually very minor procedures, making histopathology an important component of the evaluation in many clinical situations.

History

Knowledge of the patient's age, health, occupation, hobbies, living conditions, and the onset, duration, and course of the disease and its response to previous treatment are important. The family history of similar disorders and other related diseases may be useful.

A complete drug history is one of the most important aspects of a thorough history. Drug reactions are frequently seen and may simulate many different diseases. Sedatives such as the barbiturates; laxatives such as phenolphthalein; antiinflammatory agents, steroidal or nonsteroidal; and antibacterial agents such as the sulfas and penicillin may all produce distressing cutaneous changes. All these may simulate entities not usually attributed to drugs. It is equally important to inquire about topical agents that have been applied to the skin and mucous membranes for medicinal or cosmetic purposes, for these agents may cause cutaneous or systemic reactions.

Other illnesses, travel abroad, the patient's environment at home and at work, seasonal occurrences and recurrences of the disease, the temperature, humidity, and weather exposure of the patient are all important items in a dermatologic history. Habitation in certain parts of the world predisposes one to distinctive diseases for that particular geographic locale. San Joaquin Valley fever (coccidioidomycosis), leprosy, leishmaniasis, and histoplasmosis are examples. Sexual orientation and practices may be relevant, as in genital ulcer diseases, HIV infection, and infestations (e.g., scabies, pubic lice).

Examination

Examination should be conducted in a well-lit room. Natural sunlight is the ideal illumination. Fluorescent bulbs that produce wavelengths of light closer to natural sunlight than standard fluorescent bulbs are commercially available. Abnormalities of melanin pigmentation, for example vitiligo and melasma, are more clearly visible under ultraviolet light. A Wood's light (365 nm) is most commonly used and is also valuable for the diagnosis of some types of tinea capitis, tinea versicolor, and erythrasma.

A magnifying lens is of inestimable value in examining small lesions. It may be necessary to palpate the lesion for firmness and fluctuation; rubbing will elucidate the nature of scales; scraping will reveal the nature of the lesion's base. Pigmented lesions, especially in infants, should be rubbed in an attempt to elicit Darier's sign (whealing) as seen in urticaria pigmentosa.

The entire eruption must be seen to evaluate distribution and configuration. This is optimally done by having the patient completely undressed and viewing the patient from a distance to take in the whole eruption at once. "Peek-a-boo" examination, by having the patient expose one anatomic area after another while remaining clothed, is not optimal, because the examination of the skin will be incomplete, and the overall distribution is hard to determine.

After the patient is viewed at a distance, individual lesions are examined to identify primary lesions and determine the evolution of the eruption and the presence of secondary lesions.

Diagnostic Details of Lesions

Distribution. Lesions may be few or numerous, and in arrangement they may be discrete or may coalesce to form patches of peculiar configuration. They may appear over the entire body, or follow the lines of cleavage (pityriasis rosea), dermatomes (herpes zoster), or along Blaschko's lines (epidermal nevi). Lesions may form groups, rings, crescents, or unusual linear patterns. A remarkable degree of bilateral symmetry is characteristic of certain diseases such as dermatitis herpetiformis, vitiligo, and psoriasis.

Evolution. Some lesions appear fully evolved. Others develop from smaller lesions, then may remain the same during their entire existence (e.g., warts). When lesions succeed one another in a series of crops, as they do in varicella and dermatitis herpetiformis, a polymorphous eruption results, with lesions in various stages of development or involution all present at the same time.

Involution. Certain lesions disappear completely, whereas others leave characteristic residual pigmentation or scarring. Residual dyspigmentation, although a significant cosmetic issue, is not considered a scar. The pattern in which lesions involute may be useful in diagnosis, the typical keratotic papule of pityriasis lichenoides varioliformis acuta for example.

Grouping. Grouping is a characteristic of dermatitis herpetiformis, herpes simplex, herpes zoster, and late syphilitic eruptions. Small lesions arranged around a large one are said to be in a *corymbose* arrangement. Concentric annular lesions are typical of borderline leprosy and erythema multiforme. These are sometimes said to be in a *cockade* pattern, like the tricolor cockade hats worn by French revolutionists. Flea and other arthropod bites are usually grouped and linear (breakfast-lunch-and-dinner sign). Grouped lesions of various sizes may be termed agminated.

Configuration. Certain terms are used to describe the configuration that an eruption assumes either primarily or by enlargement or coalescence. Lesions in a line are called *linear,* and they may be confluent or discrete. Lesions may form a complete circle *(annular),* a portion of a circle *(arcuate),* or may be composed of several intersecting portions of circles *(polycyclic).* If the eruption is not straight but does not form parts of circles, it may be *serpiginous.* Round lesions may be small, like drops, called *guttate;* or larger, like a coin, called *nummular.* Unusual configurations that do not correspond to these patterns or to normal anatomic or embryonic patterns should raise the possibility of an exogenous dermatosis or factitia.

Color. The color of the skin is determined by melanin, oxyhemoglobin, reduced hemoglobin, and carotene. Not only do the proportions of these components affect the color, but also their depth within the skin and the thickness of the epidermis and hydration also play a role. The Tyndall effect modifies the color of skin and the color of lesions by the selective scattering of light waves of different wavelengths. The blue nevus and mongolian spots are examples of this light dispersion effect.

It is not advisable to place too much reliance on the color of lesions as a diagnostic factor, because it is difficult to describe colors, and they appear differently to different individuals; but they may at least serve as a corroborative aid. Interface reactions such as lichen planus or lupus erythematosus are described as *violaceous*. Lipid containing lesions are yellow, as in xanthomas or steatocystoma multiplex. The orange-red color of pityriasis rubra pilaris is characteristic.

Patches lighter in color than the normal skin may be completely depigmented or have lost only part of their pigment (hypopigmented). This is an important distinction, since certain conditions are or may be hypopigmented such as tinea versicolor, nevus anemicus, leprosy, hypomelanotic macules of tuberous sclerosis, hypomelanosis of Ito, seborrheic dermatitis, and idiopathic guttate hypomelanosis. True depigmentation should be distinguished from this; it suggests vitiligo, nevus depigmentosus, halo nevus, scleroderma, morphea, or lichen sclerosus et atrophicus.

Hyperpigmentation may be result from epidermal or dermal causes. It may be related either to increased melanin or deposition of other substances. Epidermal hyperpigmentation occurs in nevi, melanoma, café au lait spots, melasma, and lentigines. These lesions are accentuated when examined with a Wood's light. Dermal pigmentation occurs subsequent to many inflammatory conditions (postinflammatory hyperpigmentation) or from deposition of metals, medications, medication-melanin complexes, or degenerated dermal material (ochronosis). These conditions are not enhanced when examined by a Wood's light. The hyperpigmentation following inflammation is most commonly the result of dermal melanin deposition, but in some conditions, such as lichen aureus, is caused by iron. Dermal iron deposition appears more yellow-brown or golden than dermal melanin.

Consistency. Palpation is an essential part of the physical examination of lesions. Does the lesion blanch on pressure? If not, it may be purpuric. Is it fluctuant? If so, it may have free fluid in it. Is it cold or hot? If there is a nodule or tumor, does it sink through a ring into the panniculus, like a neurofibroma? Is it hard enough to make one suspect calcification, or merely very firm, like a keloid or

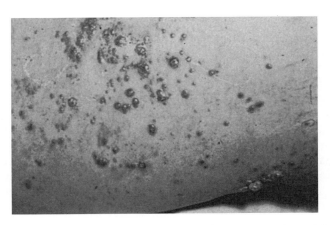

Fig. 2-1 Metastasis to the skin of the upper thigh from endometrial carcinoma, removed 4 years earlier.

dermatofibroma? Or brawny, like scleredema? Or doughy, like the proximal muscles in dermatomyositis?

CUTANEOUS FINDINGS IN SYSTEMIC DISEASE

The human skin may mirror the presence of benign or malignant systemic disease in many different ways. At times an unusual skin eruption may be a clue to some internal disorder that may not be obvious.

Nodules

Subcutaneous or dermal metastatic nodules are common and easily detected manifestations of metastatic carcinoma (Fig. 2-1). Although these nodules may arise anywhere on the skin, the most favored site is the trunk or scalp. They may be present for long periods without evidence of other metastatic disease. These nodules most frequently are metastases from carcinoma of the breast, gastrointestinal tract, lung, melanoma, ovary, or uterus. Sister Mary Joseph's nodule is a deep subcutaneous nodule that occurs in the umbilicus. It usually indicates the presence of an intraperitoneal cancer, frequently gastric adenocarcinoma.

The skin lesions of multicentric reticulohistiocytosis are multiple, symmetrical, firm, red, brown, or yellow nodules 2 to 10 mm in diameter, occurring most frequently on the fingers and hands and, less often, over joints and bony prominences. Internal malignancy may be present in up to 25% of cases.

Gardner's syndrome, a hereditary syndrome of intestinal polyposis and colon cancer, has many cutaneous manifestations, including fibromas, epidermoid cysts (appearing before puberty, and not in acne-prone areas), osteomas, and desmoid tumors.

Vascular Lesions

Petechiae, ecchymoses, "pinch purpura," and caput medusae are some of the vascular lesions associated with malignancies. "Pinch purpura," hemorrhage-induced by mild, often subclinical trauma, is a characteristic presentation of primary systemic amyloidosis of the skin. Similar periorbital hemorrhage following proctoscopy or pulmonary function testing, "postproctoscopic purpura" also typifies the vascular fragility induced by systemic amyloidosis. This is to be distinguished from actinic purpura, easy bruising on chronically sun-exposed skin of the forearms, a frequent finding in the elderly. Systemic steroid treatment may result in similar easy bruisibility. Purpura is a common sign of acute leukemia. Splinter hemorrhages may be present under the nails.

Flushing

Episodic flushing, especially of the face, lasting some 10 to 30 minutes, is a consistent sign of carcinoid syndrome. Bronchial carcinoid tumors may be manifested by severe and prolonged flushing episodes, facial and periorbital edema, excessive lacrimation, salivation, tachycardia, and hypotension.

Pruritus

Generalized pruritus may be seen in many myeloproliferative diseases, but it is most characteristic of lymphoma (especially Hodgkin's disease) or polycythemia vera. The pruritus may be the sole cutaneous reaction and may persist for years before the underlying cause can be identified. Liver disease, renal failure, iron deficiency, and thyroid or parathyroid disease are other systemic diseases in which pruritus may be prominent.

Eczema

A unilateral eczematous eruption on one nipple, though most commonly a dermatitis, may be Paget's disease of the breast with underlying intraductal carcinoma. Paget's disease in the groin may present similarly. The early manifestation of cutaneous T-cell lymphoma (mycosis fungoides) may resemble an eczema with intense pruritus. Years may pass before the diagnosis of cutaneous T-cell lymphoma can be confirmed, despite multiple biopsies. An eczematous eruption involving the hands, feet, nose, and ears is characteristic of Bazex's syndrome, a sign of an underlying malignant neoplasm of the aerodigestive tract.

Vesicles and Bullae

Dermatitis herpetiformis (Duhring's disease) presents with intense pruritus and a vesicular eruption. It is associated with a usually asymptomatic gluten-sensitive enteropathy. Patients not on gluten-free diets not only have increased activity of their skin disease, but are also at increased risk for the development of gastrointestinal lymphoma.

Grouped vesicles on an erythematous base occurring unilaterally are indicative of herpes zoster. It is a common early or initial manifestation of HIV infection. It is only very rarely a sign of an undiagnosed internal malignancy, however.

Erythroderma (Exfoliative Dermatitis)

Universal erythroderma, generally accompanied by scaling, may be associated with malignancy, usually lymphoma. This is characteristic of Sézary syndrome. A severe drug reaction may also be the cause.

Erythema and Edema

Erythema, edema, and a purple (heliotrope) discoloration of the eyelids are indicative of dermatomyositis. Red or violaceous patches and plaques may be present on other areas of the skin. Characteristic papules are present over the knuckles (Gottron's papules). While proximal muscle weakness is usually present, the skin lesions can precede the myositis by weeks to years. Dermatomyositis in the adult is associated with an increased risk of cancer.

Tender, erythematous, edematous plaques that may centrally vesiculate on the upper part of the body associated with fever and leukocytosis characterize Sweet's syndrome. This may be the presenting sign of myelogenous leukemia.

Erythematous Nodules

Erythema nodosum may rarely be associated with Hodgkin's disease and metastatic carcinoma. It may also be seen in tuberculosis, sarcoidosis, histoplasmosis, coccidioidomycosis, blastomycosis, ulcerative colitis, and with use of some medications. The most common cause is preceding streptococcal pharyngitis.

Hyperkeratosis

Sézary's erythroderma, Hodgkin's disease, and lymphocytic leukemia may be accompanied by hyperkeratosis of the palms and soles, as may Bazex's syndrome. Howel-Evans' syndrome is a hereditary esophageal carcinoma syndrome. Hyperkeratosis of the palms and soles identifies those members of the kindreds in whom the carcinoma may develop. Keratosis punctata palmaris et plantaris has been linked to adenocarcinoma of the colon in one family by Bennion et al.

Hyperpigmentation

In metastatic melanoma a generalized darkening of the skin (diffuse melanosis cutis) may occur. Usually melanuria is also present. Pituitary tumors may also cause generalized hyperpigmentation as a result of increased secretion of melanocyte-stimulating hormone (MSH). Addison's disease is associated with a similar pattern of hyperpigmentation. Bronze hyperpigmentation is seen in hemochromatosis and arsenic intoxication.

Acanthosis nigricans presents with gray-brown hyperpigmentation and velvety texture of the skin of the axilla, neck, and over the knuckles. The vast majority of cases are benign and occur around puberty in obese adolescents (pseudoacanthosis nigricans). Hereditary or syndromal acanthosis nigricans is often associated with endocrine diseases and insulin resistance. Malignant acanthosis nigricans occurs in adults and is associated with internal malignancy, most frequently in the gastrointestinal tract. It is usually more extensive and may have mucosal involvement. In malignant acanthosis nigricans, patients may also develop numerous seborrheic keratosis or skin tag–like lesions, demonstrating a partial overlap with Leser-Trélat syndrome.

Alopecia

When follicular mucinosis occurs in lesions of mycosis fungoides, affected areas on the scalp or beard may present with sharply circumscribed plaques of alopecia. Alopecia may also occur in syphilis, thyroid disease, and iron deficiency.

Hirsutism and Hypertrichosis

Adrenal or ovarian carcinomas may be the cause of excessive hair growth. Malignant down is an excessive growth of lanugo-like hair, which is associated with malignant disease of the lung, colon, gallbladder, and uterus.

Urticaria

In most cases of chronic urticaria, an underlying trigger is not found. Hodgkin's disease may be accompanied by urticaria. Cold urticaria with cryoglobulinemia is seen in multiple myeloma.

Sulfur-Yellow Plaques on the Shins

Necrobiosis lipoidica (with or without diabetes) presents as bilateral, well-defined plaques with a smooth, glistening surface and a yellow color.

Bennion SD, et al: Keratosis punctata palmaris et plantaris and adenocarcinoma of the colon. *J Am Acad Dermatol* 1984, 10:587.

Dubrevil A, et al: Umbilical metastasis on Sister Mary Joseph's nodule. *Int J Dermatol* 1998, 37:7.

Esperanza LE, et al: Hyperandrogenism, insulin resistance, and acanthosis nigricans (HAIR-AN) syndrome: spontaneous remission in a 15-year-old girl. *J Am Acad Dermatol* 1996, 34:892.

Eyster ME, et al: Human immunodeficiency virus–related conditions in children and adults with hemophilia: rates, relationship to CD4 counts, and predictive value. *Blood* 1993, 81:828.

Fanning J, et al: Paget's disease of the vulva. *Am J Obstet Gynecol* 1999, 180:24.

Jemec GBE: Hypertrichosis lanuginosa acquisita. *Arch Dermatol* 1986, 122:805.

Kurzrock R, et al: Cutaneous paraneoplastic syndromes in solid tumors. *Am J Med* 1995, 99:662.

Langlois JC, et al: Erythema gyratum repens unassociated with internal malignancy. *J Am Acad Dermatol* 1985, 12:911.

Lewis HM, et al: Protective effect of gluten-free diet against development of lymphoma in dermatitis herpetiformis. *Br J Dermatol* 1996, 135:363.

Loucas EL, et al: Genetic and acquired cutaneous disorders associated with internal malignancy. *Int J Dermatol* 1995, 34:749.

Murata Y, et al: Under pants-pattern erythema. *J Am Acad Dermatol* 1999, 40:949.

Pecora AL, et al: Acrokeratosis paraneoplastica (Bazex's syndrome). *Arch Dermatol* 1983, 119:820.

Robson KJ, et al: Cutaneous manifestations of systemic diseases. *Med Clin North Am* 1998, 82:1359.

Schwartz RA: Sign of Leser-Trélat. *J Am Acad Dermatol* 1996, 35:88.

Wilkin JK: The red face: flushing disorders. *Clin Dermatol* 1993, 11:211.

CHAPTER 3

Dermatoses Resulting from Physical Factors

The body requires a certain amount of heat, but beyond definite limits, insufficient or excessive amounts are injurious. The local action of excessive heat causes burns or scalds; on the other hand, undue cold causes chilblains, frostbite, and congelation. Thresholds of tolerance exist in all body structures sensitive to electromagnetic wave radiation of varying frequencies, such as x-rays and ultraviolet rays. The eye, which is sensitive to visible light, is an example of a special sense organ that has similar limits. The skin, which is exposed to so many external physical forces, is more subject to injuries caused by them than is any other organ.

Page EH, et al: Temperature-dependent skin disorders. *J Am Acad Dermatol* 1988, 18:1003. ▲

HEAT INJURIES
Thermal Burns

Dermatitis of varying intensity may be caused by the action of excessive heat on the skin. If this heat is extreme, the skin and underlying tissue may be destroyed. The changes in the skin resulting from dry heat or scalding are classified in four degrees.

A first-degree burn of the skin results merely in an active congestion of the superficial blood vessels, causing an erythema that may be followed by epidermal desquamation (peeling). Ordinary sunburn is the most common example of a first-degree burn. The pain and increased surface heat may be severe, and it is not rare to have some constitutional reaction if the involved area is large.

Second-degree burns are subdivided into superficial and deep forms. In the superficial type there is a transudation of serum from the capillaries, which causes edema of the superficial tissues. Vesicles and blebs are formed by the serum gathering beneath the outer layers of the epidermis. Complete recovery without scar formation or other blemish is usual in burns of this kind. The deep second-degree burn is pale and anesthetic. Injury to the reticular dermis compromises blood flow and destroys appendages, so that healing takes over 1 month to occur and results in scarring.

In third-degree burns loss of tissue of the full thickness of the skin and often some of the subcutaneous tissues occurs. Since the skin appendages are destroyed, there is no epithelium available for regeneration of the skin. An ulcerating wound is produced, which in healing leaves a scar.

Fourth-degree burn is the destruction of the entire skin and subcutaneous fat with any underlying tendons. Both third- and fourth-degree burns require grafting for closure. All third- and fourth-degree burns are followed by constitutional symptoms of varied gravity, their severity depending on the size of the involved surface, the depth of the burn, and particularly the location of the burned surface. It appears that the more vascular the involved area, the more severe the symptoms.

Symptoms of shock may appear within 24 hours after a burn injury, followed by symptoms of toxemia from absorption of destroyed tissue on the surface of the wound. Then symptoms from wound infection may develop as a result of contamination with pyogenic organisms. The symptoms of these three conditions may merge so that differentiation is difficult.

The prognosis is poor for any patient in whom a large area of skin surface is involved. It is particularly serious if more than two thirds of the body surface has been burned. In addition to the infection of the wound and surrounding tissue (cellulitis), sepsis, with seeding of internal organs, such as the meninges, lungs, or kidneys, may occur. Irregularities in electrolytes and fluid balance and loss of serum proteins can further complicate the patient's condition.

Excessive scarring, with either keloidlike scars or flat scars with contractures, may produce deformities and dysfunctions of the joints as well as chronic ulcerations because local circulation is impaired. Chetty et al and Compton reviewed the frequent problem of delayed postburn blistering. It occurs in partial-thickness wounds and skin graft donor sites, is most common on the lower extremities, and is self-limited. Burn scars may be the site of development of carcinoma or sarcoma. With modern reconstructive surgery these unfortunate end results can be minimized.

TREATMENT. Immediate first aid for minor thermal burns consists of prompt cold applications (ice water, or cold tap water if no ice is at hand) continued until pain does not return on stopping them.

The vesicles or blebs of second-degree burns should not be opened but should be protected from injury, since they form a natural barrier against contamination by microorganisms. If they become tense and unduly painful, the fluid may be evacuated under strictly aseptic conditions by puncturing the wall with a sterile needle, allowing the blister to collapse onto the underlying wound, and then applying a topical antibiotic agent. In severe deep burns, silver sulfadiazine (Silvadene) ointment has been found effective in the control of burn wound infections. Recently developed skin substitutes that employ collagen-synthetic bilaminate membranes are enjoying increasing use in coverage of these wounds. In many centers, cultured epidermal grafts, both autologous and allogeneic, are being used, with promising results.

Morbidity and mortality following severe burns are often caused by bacterial and fungal infection; therefore, treatment should be directed against this complication. Definitive therapy consists of antishock measures, debridement of loose skin and dirt, and the application of silver sulfadiazine ointment. Antibiotics and fluid and electrolyte support are given, and good nutrition is maintained with supplemental vitamins.

Expedient primary excision of deep dermal and full-thickness burn wounds with subsequent grafting is the standard of care. Green et al describe a method to guide surgeons in estimating more accurately the depth of burn using indocyanine green fluorescence. Severe second- and third-degree burns require specialized teams of physicians working together to provide the most effective treatment.

Electrical Burns.
Electrical burns are of two varieties, contact and flash. A contact burn is small but deep, causing some necrosis of the underlying tissues (Fig. 3-1). Flash burns usually cover a large area and, being similar to any surface burn, are treated as such. Volinsky et al recently reviewed lightning injuries. Lightning may cause burns after a direct strike, where an entrance and exit wound are visible. This is the most lethal type of strike, and cardiac arrest or other internal injuries may occur. Other types of strikes are indirect and result in burns that are either linear in areas at which sweat was present; are in a feathery or arborescent pattern, which is believed to be pathognomonic (Fig. 3-2); are punctate with multiple, deep, circular lesions; or are thermal burns from ignited clothing or heated metal.

Hot Tar Burns.
Demling has reported that the polyoxyethylene sorbitan in Neosporin ointment is an excellent dispersing agent that facilitates the removal of hot tar from burns.

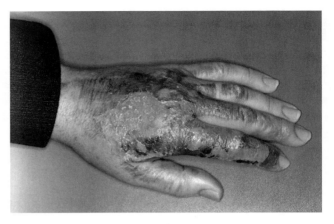

Fig. 3-1 Electrical burn.

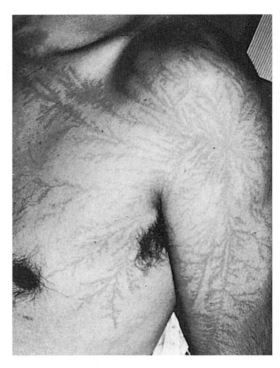

Fig. 3-2 "Christmas tree" pattern in the skin, a characteristic marker of being struck by lightning. (Courtesy Dr. C.W. Bartholome.)

Chetty BV, et al: Blisters in patients with burns. *Arch Dermatol* 1992, 128:181.

Compton CC: The delayed postburn blister. *Arch Dermatol* 1992, 128:249.

Demling R, et al: Management of hot tar burns. *J Trauma* 1980, 20:242.

Edwards MJ, et al: Squamous cell carcinoma arising in previously burned or irradiated skin. *Arch Surg* 1989, 124:115.

Falanga VL: Occlusive wound dressings. *Arch Dermatol* 1988, 124:872.

Green HA, et al: Burn depth estimation using indocyanine green fluorescence. *Arch Dermatol* 1992, 128:43.

Limova M, et al: Synthetic membranes and cultured keratinocyte. *J Am Acad Dermatol* 1990, 23:713.

Phillips TJ, et al: Burn scar carcinoma. *Dermatol Surg* 1998, 24:561.

Ryan TJ: Wound dressing. *Dermatol Clin* 1993, 11:207.

Tamir G, et al: Synchronous appearance of keratoacanthomas in burn scar and skin graft donor site shortly after injury. *J Am Acad Dermatol* 1999, 40:870.

Volinsky JB, et al: Picture of the mouth. *Arch Pediatr Adolesc Med* 1994, 148:529.

Ward CG: Burns. *J Am Coll Surg* 1998, 186:123. ———————————— ▲

Miliaria

Miliaria, the retention of sweat as a result of occlusion of eccrine sweat ducts and pores, produces an eruption that is common in hot, humid climates such as the tropics and during the hot summer months in temperate climates. Mowad et al showed that *Staphylococcus epidermidis*, which produces an extracellular polysaccharide substance, could induce miliaria in an experimental setting. They hypothesized that it is this polysaccharide substance that obstructs the delivery of sweat to the skin surface in miliaria. The occlusion prevents normal secretion from the sweat glands, and eventually the backed-up pressure causes rupture of the sweat gland or duct at different levels. The escape of sweat into the adjacent tissue produces miliaria. Depending on the level of the injury to the sweat gland or duct, several different forms of miliaria are recognized.

Miliaria Crystalline (Sudamina). Miliaria crystalline is characterized by small, clear, and very superficial vesicles with no inflammatory reaction. It appears in bedridden patients in whom fever produces increased perspiration or in situations in which clothing prevents dissipation of heat and moisture, as in bundled children (Fig. 3-3). The lesions are asymptomatic and their duration is short lived because they tend to rupture at the slightest trauma. The lesions are self-limited; no treatment is required.

Miliaria Rubra (Prickly Heat, Heat Rash). The lesions of miliaria rubra appear as discrete, extremely pruritic, erythematous papulovesicles accompanied by a sensation of prickling, burning, or tingling. They later may become confluent on a bed of erythema. The sites most frequently affected are the antecubital and popliteal fossae, the trunk, the inframammary areas (especially under pendulous breasts), the abdomen (especially at the waistline), and the inguinal regions; these sites frequently become macerated because evaporation of moisture has been impeded. The site of injury and sweat escape is in the prickle cell layer, where spongiosis is produced.

Miliaria Pustulosa. Miliaria pustulosa is always preceded by some other dermatitis that has produced injury, destruction, or blocking of the sweat duct. The pustules are distinct, superficial, and independent of the hair follicle (Fig. 3-4). The pruritic pustules occur most frequently on the intertriginous areas, on the flexure surfaces of the extremities, on the scrotum, and on the back of bedridden patients. Contact dermatitis, lichen simplex chronicus, and intertrigo are some of the associated diseases, although pustular miliaria may occur several weeks after the disease has subsided.

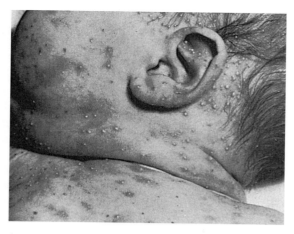

Fig. 3-3 Miliaria crystallina: uniform, minute crystal-clear vesicles. (Courtesy Dr. Axel W. Hoke.)

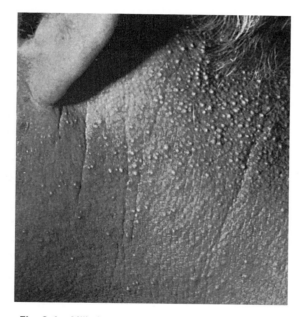

Fig. 3-4 Miliaria pustulosa: red papules and pustules.

Usually the contents of the pustules are sterile, but they may contain nonpathogenic cocci.

Miliaria Profunda. Nonpruritic, flesh-colored, deep-seated, whitish papules characterize this form of miliaria. It is asymptomatic, usually lasts only 1 hour after overheating has ended, and is concentrated on the trunk and extremities. Except for the face, axillae, hands, and feet, where there may be compensatory hyperhidrosis, all the sweat glands are nonfunctional. The occlusion is in the upper dermis. This form is observed only in the tropics and usually follows a severe bout of miliaria rubra.

Postmiliarial Hypohidrosis. Postmiliarial hypohidrosis results from occlusion of sweat ducts and pores and may be severe enough to impair one's ability to perform sustained work in a hot environment. Affected persons may show decreasing efficiency, irritability, anorexia, drowsiness, vertigo, and headache; they may wander in a daze.

It has been shown that hypohidrosis invariably follows miliaria, and that the duration and severity of the hypohidrosis are related to the severity of the miliaria. Further, sweating may be depressed to half the normal amount for as much as 3 weeks following miliaria.

Tropical Anhidrotic Asthenia. This is a rare form of miliaria with long-lasting poral occlusion, which produces anhidrosis and heat retention.

Occlusion Miliaria. Miliaria may be produced with accompanying anhidrosis and increased heat stress susceptibility after the application of extensive polyethylene film occlusion for 48 or more hours.

TREATMENT. The most effective treatment for miliaria is to place the patient in a cool environment. Even a single night in an air-conditioned room helps to alleviate the discomfort. Next best is the use of circulating air fans to cool the skin.

Anhydrous lanolin resolves the occlusion of pores and may help to restore normal sweat secretions. Hydrophilic ointment also helps to dissolve keratinous plugs and facilitates the normal flow of sweat.

Soothing, cooling baths containing Aveeno colloidal oatmeal or cornstarch are beneficial if used in moderation. Mild cases may respond to dusting powders, such as cornstarch or baby talcum powder. A lotion containing 1% menthol and glycerin and 4% salicylic acid in 95% alcohol is also effective. This should be dabbed on the affected areas several times daily until desquamation sets in. An oily "shake" lotion such as calamine lotion, with 1% or 2% phenol, may be effective.

Kirk JF, et al: Miliaria profunda. *J Am Acad Dermatol* 1996, 35:854.

Mowad CM, et al: The role of extracellular polysaccharide substance produced by *Staphylococcus epidermidis* in miliaria. *J Am Acad Dermatol* 1995, 33:729.

Sato K, et al: Biology of sweat glands and their disorders. *J Am Acad Dermatol* 1989, 20:713.

Sulzberger MB, et al: Miliaria and anhidrosis. *Arch Dermatol* 1972, 105:845.

Wenzel FG, et al: Nonneoplastic disorders of the eccrine glands. *J Am Acad Dermatol* 1998, 38:1. ▲

Erythema (Pigmentatio) Ab Igne

Erythema ab igne, or "toasted skin" syndrome, is a persistent erythema—or the coarsely reticulated residual pigmentation resulting from it—that is usually produced by long-continued exposure to excessive heat without the production of a burn. It begins as a mottling caused by local hemostasis and becomes a reticulated erythema, leaving pigmentation. All the various phases usually are simultaneously present in a patch, the color varying from pale pink to old rose or dark purplish brown. After the cause is

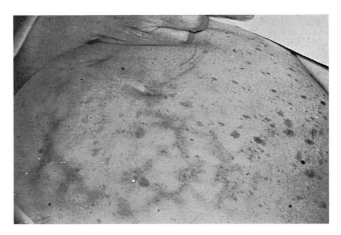

Fig. 3-5 Erythema (pigmentatio) ab igne from years of application of a hot water bottle to the abdomen.

removed, the affection tends to disappear gradually, but sometimes the pigmentation is permanent.

Histologically, an increased amount of elastic tissue in the dermis is noted. The changes in erythema ab igne are similar to those of actinic elastosis, and it has been suggested these changes be called *thermal elastosis*.

Erythema ab igne is most common on the legs of women as a result of habitually warming them in front of open fireplaces, radiators, or heaters. Similar changes may be produced with a hot water bag or electric heating pad (Fig. 3-5). The condition occurs also in cooks, stokers, invalids, and others exposed over long periods to the direct action of moderate heat. Epithelial atypia, including one instance of Bowen's disease, has rarely been reported to occur overlying erythema ab igne. Sahl et al reported 5-fluorouracil cream treatment to be effective in reversing this epidermal alteration.

The use of bland emollients is helpful. There is no effective treatment, although Kligman's combination of 5% hydroquinone in hydrophilic ointment containing 0.1% retinoic acid and 0.1% dexamethasone may help reduce unsightly pigmentation.

Arrington JH, et al: Thermal keratosis and squamous cell carcinoma in situ associated with erythema ab igne. *Arch Dermatol* 1979, 115:1226.

Dvoretsky I, et al: Reticular erythema of the lower back. *Arch Dermatol* 1991, 127:405.

Galvin SA, et al: Rectangular reticulate patches on the pretibial areas. *Arch Dermatol* 1990, 126:385.

Meffert JJ, et al: Furniture-induced erythema ab igne. *J Am Acad Dermatol* 1996, 34:516.

Sahl WJ, et al: Erythema ab igne. *J Am Acad Dermatol* 1992, 27:109. ▲

COLD INJURIES

Local cold injuries are divided into chilblain, frostbite, and immersion foot. Whereas chilblain and frostbite occur sporadically in civil life, immersion foot is encountered almost entirely in the armed forces. However, Wrenn has documented its occurrence in homeless persons.

Intense vasoconstriction resulting from the local action of cold and reflex vasoconstrictor stimulation is reinforced by the passage of cold blood through the vasomotor center. Vasoconstriction provokes tissue anoxia. Decreased muscular activity further diminishes the blood supply. Ice crystal formation in the blood vessels does not usually occur, but when it does, necrosis ensues.

Chilblains (Pernio)

Chilblains is a recurrent, localized erythema and swelling caused by exposure to cold. Blistering and ulcerations may develop in severe cases. In people predisposed by poor peripheral circulation, even moderate exposure to cold may produce chilblains. Acute chilblains is the mildest form of cold injury. This occurs chiefly on the hands, feet, ears, and face, especially in children; onset is enhanced by dampness. Patients are usually unaware of the injury at first, but later burning, itching, and redness call it to their attention. The areas are bluish red, the color partially or totally disappearing on pressure, and are decidedly cool to the touch (Fig. 3-6). Sometimes the extremities are clammy because of excessive sweating.

Chronic chilblains occurs repeatedly during cold weather and disappears during warm weather. The affected extremities are cold, cyanotic, and often hyperhidrotic. Cryoglobulinemia may be present and chilblainlike lesions may occur in discoid and systemic lupus erythematosus.

A condition was described by Toback et al in which painful plaques and vesicles developed on the hands of a group of campers who lived on a boat where there was exposure to cold and moisture. They called this *pulling boat* (the name of their open rowing/sailing craft) hands.

TREATMENT. Nifedipine, 20 mg three times daily, has been shown to be effective. Vasodilators such as nicotinamide, 100 mg three times a day, or dipyridamole, 25 mg three times a day, are used to improve circulation. Systemic corticoid therapy is useful in chilblain lupus erythematosus. Pentoxifylline may be effective.

The parts should be cleansed with water and massaged gently with warm oil each day and should be protected against further injury and exposure to cold or dampness. If the feet are affected, woolen socks should be worn at night during the cold months. Judicious use of electric pads may be used to warm the parts. Smoking is strongly discouraged.

Crowson AN, et al: Idiopathic perniosis and its mimics. *Hum Pathol* 1997, 28:478.

Fisher DA, et al: Violaceous rash of dorsal fingers in a woman. Diagnosis: chilblain lupus erythematosus (perniosis). *Arch Dermatol* 1996, 132:459.

Goette DK: Chilblains. *J Am Acad Dermatol* 1990, 23:257.

Herman EW, et al: A distinctive variant of pernio. *Arch Dermatol* 1981, 117:26.

Toback AC, et al: Pulling boat hands. *J Am Acad Dermatol* 1985, 12:649.

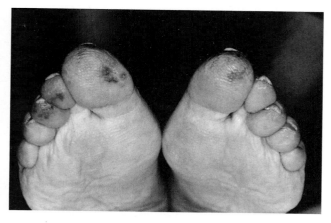

Fig. 3-6 Chilblains (pernio).

Frostbite (Congelation)

When soft tissue is frozen and locally deprived of blood supply, the damage is called *frostbite*. The ears, nose, cheeks, fingers, and toes are most often affected. The frozen part painlessly becomes pale and waxy. Various degrees of tissue destruction similar to those caused by burns are encountered. These are erythema and edema, vesicles and bullae, superficial gangrene, deep gangrene, and injury to muscles, tendons, periosteum, and nerves (Fig. 3-7). The Arolla index is a recently developed formula that links duration of exposure, defined by both temperature and wind chill index, with frostbite.

TREATMENT. Early treatment of frostbite before swelling develops should consist of covering the part with clothing or with a warm hand or other body surface to maintain a slightly warm temperature so that adequate blood circulation can be maintained. Rapid rewarming in a water bath between 100° and 110° F is the treatment of choice for all forms of frostbite. Slow thawing results in more extensive tissue damage. Analgesics, unless contraindicated, should be administered because of the considerable pain experienced with rapid thawing. When the skin flushes and is pliable, thawing is complete. Supportive measures such as bed rest, a high-protein/high-calorie diet, wound care, and avoidance of trauma are imperative. Any rubbing of the affected part should be avoided, but gentle massage of proximal portions of the extremity that are not numb may be helpful.

After swelling and hyperemia have developed, the patient should be kept in bed with the affected limb slightly flexed, elevated, and at rest. Exposing the affected limb to air at room temperature relieves pain and helps prevent tissue damage. Protection by a heat cradle may be desirable.

The use of anticoagulants to prevent thrombosis and gangrene has been advocated. Papaverine or nicotinic acid may be administered to reduce vasospasm. Antibiotics should be given as a prophylactic measure against infection, and tetanus immunization should be updated. Recovery may

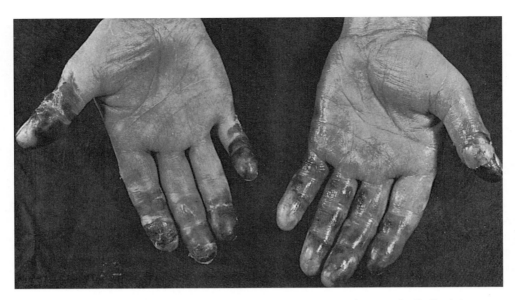

Fig. 3-7 Frostbite. Note highlights, caused by hyperhidrosis. (Courtesy Dr. H. Shatin.)

take many months. Prognostic factors have been reviewed by Urschel.

Corbett DW: Cold injuries. In James WD, ed: Military dermatology, Washington, DC, 1994, Office of the Surgeon General.
Rigo AM: The Arolla index. *J Chir* (Paris) 1988, 125:239.
Urshel JD: Frostbite. *J Trauma* 1990, 30:340, 1990. _____ ▲

Immersion Foot Syndromes

Trench Foot. Trench foot results from prolonged exposure to cold, wet conditions without immersion or actual freezing. The term is derived from trench warfare in World War I, when soldiers stood, sometimes for hours, in trenches with a few inches of cold water in them. The lack of circulation produces edema, paresthesias, and damage to the blood vessels. Gangrene may occur in severe cases. Treatment consists of removal from the causal environment, bed rest, and restoration of the circulation. Other measures, such as those used in the treatment of frostbite, should be employed.

Warm Water Immersion Foot. Exposure of the feet to warm, wet conditions for 48 hours or more may produce a syndrome characterized by maceration, blanching, and wrinkling of the soles and sides of the feet. Itching and burning with swelling may persist a few days after removal of the cause, but disability is temporary. It was commonly seen in military service members in Vietnam but has also been seen in persons wearing insulated boots, the so-called moon-boot syndrome.

This condition should be differentiated from tropical immersion foot, seen after continuous immersion of the feet in water or mud of temperatures above 71.6° F (22° C) for 2 to 10 days. This was known as "paddy foot" in Vietnam. This involves erythema, edema, and pain of the dorsal feet, as well as fever and adenopathy. Resolution occurs 3 to 7 days after the feet have been dried.

Warm-water immersion foot can be prevented by allowing the feet to dry for a few hours out of every 24 or by greasing the soles with a silicone grease once a day. Recovery from it is usually rapid if the feet are thoroughly dried for a few hours.

Adnot J, et al: Immersion foot syndromes. In James WD, editor: Military dermatology, Washington, DC, 1994, Office of the Surgeon General.
Wrenn K: Immersion foot. *Arch Intern Med* 1991, 151:785. _____ ▲

Dermatoses with Cold Hypersensitivity

Exposure to cold may produce abnormal reactions in several disease states. The reactions are mediated most frequently through abnormal globulins such as cryoglobulin and cryofibrinogen. In addition, histamine, serotonin, leukotrienes, prostaglandins, kinins, and cold hemolysins may be involved.

Erythrocyanosis Crurum. Various names have been given to this and similar diseases in which the chief characteristics are a slight swelling and a bluish pink tint of the skin of the legs and thighs of young girls and women. The disease may be unilateral. Atypical varieties are common, some presenting cinnabar red spots, bullae, indurations, and lichenoid papules. There may be a history of cramps in the legs at night. Small tender nodules may be found on palpation. These nodules may break down and form small, often multiple ulcers, as in erythema induratum. As a rule, the affected limbs are cold to the touch. The disease is seen mostly in northern countries and is considered to be an abnormal reaction of the blood vessels to prolonged exposure to cold.

Acrocyanosis. Acrocyanosis is a persistent cyanosis with coldness and hyperhidrosis of the fingers and hands. It may also be present on the toes and feet. It occurs chiefly in young women, but it is not rare in young men. At times, on exposure to cold, a digit becomes stark white and insensitive (acroasphyxia). Cyanosis increases as the temperature decreases and changes to erythema with elevation of the dependent part. The cause is unknown. Smoking, coffee, and tea should be avoided.

Burlina et al described four neurologically impaired male infants who had acrocyanosis and swelling of the extremities only when held upright (orthostatic acrocyanosis). They found relapsing petechiae, chronic diarrhea, and ethylmalonic aciduria to be present. Hoegl et al described an HIV-infected patient with livid macules with underlying swelling of the nose, ears, and dorsal hands. Inhalation of butyl nitrite was the cause of acrocyanosis in this case.

Remitting necrotizing acrocyanosis is a term applied to functional vascular spasm or organic occlusion that produces pain in the hands and feet, with areas of coldness, cyanosis, and necrosis of the tops of the fingers and toes. This has been reported to occur without prodromal or constitutional symptoms.

Bigby M, et al: Reddish-blue hands and feet. *Arch Dermatol* 1988, 124:263.

Burlina AB, et al: A new syndrome with ethylmalonic aciduria and normal fatty acid oxidation in fibroblasts. *J Pediatr* 1994, 124:79.

Hoegl L, et al: Butyl nitrite-induced acrocyanosis in an HIV-infected patient. *Arch Dermatol* 1999, 135:90.

Olson JC, et al: Painful digital vesicles and acrocyanosis in a toddler. *Pediatr Dermatol* 1992, 9:77. _____ ▲

Cold Panniculitis. After exposure to severe cold, well-demarcated erythematous warm plaques may develop, particularly on the cheeks of young children. The lesions usually develop within a few days after exposure, and the induration resolves spontaneously in about 2 weeks.

The lesions are readily reproducible by placing an ice cube on the volar aspect of the forearm for 2 minutes. This type of panniculitis is seen mostly in young children whose fat contains more high saturated fatty acids, which have a higher melting point and lower solidification point than an adult's less saturated fat. Patients outgrow this susceptibility. No treatment is indicated.

Popsicle dermatitis is a temporary redness and induration of the cheek in children resulting from sucking Popsicles. Beacham et al described a variant of cold panniculitis presenting as indurated, red, tender plaques on the upper, outer thighs of young women who went horseback riding in winter.

Beacham BE, et al: Equestrian cold panniculitis in women. *Arch Dermatol* 1980, 116:1025.

Ter Poorten JC, et al: Cold panniculitis in a neonate. *J Am Acad Dermatol* 1995, 33:383. _____ ▲

ACTINIC INJURY
Sunburn and Solar Erythema

The solar spectrum has been divided into different parts by wavelength. The parts of the solar spectrum important in photomedicine include ultraviolet radiation (below 400 nm), visible light (400 to 760 nm), and infrared radiation (beyond 760 nm). Visible light has little biologic activity, except for stimulating the retina. Infrared radiation is experienced as radiant heat. Below 400 nm is the ultraviolet spectrum, divided into three bands: UVA, 320 to 400 nm; UVB, 290 to 320 nm; and UVC, 200 to 290 nm. UVA is divided into two subcategories: UVA I (340 to 400 nm) and UVA II (320 to 340 nm). Virtually no UVC reaches the earth's surface, because it is absorbed by the ozone layer above the earth.

The minimal amount of a particular wavelength of light capable of inducing erythema on an individual's skin is called the *minimal erythema dose* (MED). Although UVA radiation is 100 times greater than UVB radiation during midday hours, since UVB is 1000 times more erythemogenic than UVA, most solar erythema is caused by UVB. Sunlight early and late in the day contains relatively more UVA. UVA is reflected from sand, snow, or ice to a greater degree than UVB is. Therefore, sun exposure, under certain circumstances, may produce erythema with a greater contribution by UVA. Since most sunscreen products are more efficient in the UVB range, exposure under these conditions may lead to erythema, even with the use of a sunscreen.

The amount of ultraviolet exposure increases at higher altitudes, is substantially greater in temperate climates in the summer months, and is greater in tropical regions. A large portion of UVA and UVB may be reflected from sand, snow, ice, and water. Cloud cover, although blocking substantial amounts of visible light, is a poor UV absorber. All these factors must be taken into account when evaluating apparent solar injury.

The usual ultraviolet light source, the mercury-vapor lamp or sunlamp bulb, produces mostly UVB, which is the strongest inducer of erythema (sunburn). *Photochemotherapy* (PUVA) uses bulbs that produce only UVA (mostly UVA I), so that burning may be avoided at therapeutic doses.

CLINICAL SIGNS AND SYMPTOMS. Sunburn is the normal cutaneous reaction to sunlight in excess of an erythema dose (i.e., the amount that will induce reddening). UVB erythema peaks at 12 to 24 hours after exposure, but the onset is sooner and the severity greater with increased exposure. The erythema is followed by tenderness, and in severe cases,

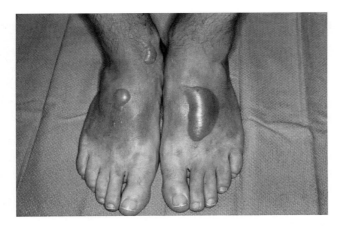

Fig. 3-8 Second-degree sunburn.

TABLE	3-1

Skin Types (Phototypes)

Skin Type	Baseline Skin Color	Sunburn and Tanning History
I	White	Always burns, never tans
II	White	Always burns, tans minimally
III	White	Burns moderately, tans gradually
IV	Olive	Minimal burning, tans well
V	Brown	Rarely burns, tans darkly
VI	Dark brown	Never burns, tans darkly black

blistering, which may become confluent (Fig. 3-8). Discomfort may be severe; edema commonly occurs in the extremities and face; chills, fever, nausea, tachycardia, and hypotension may be present. In severe cases such symptoms may last for as long as a week. Desquamation is common about a week after sunburn, even in areas that did not blister.

After ultraviolet exposure, skin pigment undergoes two changes: immediate pigment darkening (IPD, Meirowsky phenomenon) and delayed melanogenesis. IPD is maximal immediately after sun exposure and results from changes in the melanin already in the skin. It occurs after exposure to long-wave UVB, UVA, and visible light. With large doses of UVA, the initial darkening is prolonged and may blend into the delayed melanogenesis. Delayed tanning is induced by the same wavelengths of UVB (and UVC) that induce erythema, begins 2 to 3 days after exposure, and lasts 10 to 14 days. Although delayed tanning does provide some protection from further solar injury, it is at the expense of damage to the epidermis and dermis. Tanning is not recommended for sun protection. An individual's inherent ability to tan and the ease with which they burn are described as their "skin type." Skin type (Table 3-1) is used to determine starting doses of phototherapy, sunscreen recommendations, and reflects the risk of development of skin cancer.

Exposure to UVB and UVA causes an increase in the thickness of the epidermis. This increased epidermal thickness, especially of the stratum corneum, leads to increased tolerance to further solar radiation. Patients with vitiligo may increase their sun exposure without burning by this mechanism.

TREATMENT. Because prostaglandins are important mediators of sunburn, in addition to cool compresses, 10 grains of aspirin every 2 hours or an equivalent dose of indomethacin may have benefit. In general, a sunburn victim experiences at least 1 or 2 days of discomfort and even pain before much relief occurs. A topical remedy for treatment of severe sunburn is the following:

Indomethacin 100 mg
Absolute ethanol 57 ml
Propylene glycol 57 ml
Sig.: Spread widely over burned area with palms and let dry.

PROPHYLAXIS. Sunburn is best prevented by avoiding sun exposure during the periods of highest UVB intensity; i.e., between 10 AM and 2 PM. Barrier protection with hats and clothing is effective and strongly recommended. Avoidance plus physical barriers, when used with currently available sunscreens, can virtually always prevent sunburn. Use of the UV index, published daily by the National Weather Service for many U.S. cities and found in many newspapers, facilitates taking adequate precautions to prevent solar injury.

A sunscreen's efficacy in blocking the UVB (sunburn-inducing) radiation is expressed as a *sun protection factor* (SPF). This is a ratio of the number of MEDs of radiation required to induce erythema through a thin film of sunscreen, compared with unprotected skin. Sunscreening agents include UV-absorbing chemicals (chemical sunscreens) and UV-scattering or -blocking agents (physical sunscreens). Currently available sunscreens may contain chemical sunscreens (such as para-aminobenzoic acid [PABA], PABA esters, cinnamates, salicylates, anthranilates, benzophenones), physical agents (such as titanium dioxide), or combinations. They are available in sprays, gels, emollient creams, and wax sticks. Sunscreens may be water resistant (maintaining their SPF after 40 minutes of water immersion) or waterproof (maintaining their SPF after 80 minutes of water immersion).

For skin types I to III (see Table 3-1), daily application of a sunscreen with an SPF of 6 to 15 in a facial moisturizer, foundation, or aftershave is recommended. For outdoor exposure, a sunscreen of SPF 15 or higher is recommended for regular use. In persons with severe photosensitivity and at times of high sun exposure, high-intensity sunscreens of SPF 30+ or physical blocking agents (titanium dioxide) may be required. Application of the sunscreen at least 20 minutes before sun exposure is recommended.

If UVA protection is needed, sunscreens containing benzophenones or dibenzoylmethanes may be effective. A combination of physical agents and UVA chemical sunscreens may also be used in such instances.

Gallagher RP, et al: Sunlight exposure, pigmentary factors, and risk of nonmelanocytic skin cancer. *Arch Dermatol* 1995, 131:157.

Gschnait F, et al: Topical indomethacin protects from UVB and UVA radiation. *Arch Derm Res* 1984, 276:131.

Jevtic AP: The sun protective effect of clothing, including beachwear. *Australas J Dermatol* 1990, 31:5.

Koh HK, et al: Prevention and early detection strategies for melanoma and skin cancer. *Arch Dermatol* 1996, 132:436.

Lowe NJ: Photoprotection. *Semin Derm* 1990, 9:78.

Marks R, et al: The effect of regular sunscreen use on vitamin D levels in an Australian population. *Arch Dermatol* 1995, 131:415.

Naylor MF, et al: High sun protection factor sunscreens in the suppression of actinic neoplasia. *Arch Dermatol* 1995, 131:170.

Pathak MA: Advances in photomedicine: photoprotection and sunscreens. *Photochem Photobiol* 1991, 53(S):66.

Pathak MA: Sunscreens, topical and systemic. *J Am Acad Dermatol* 1982, 7:285.

Schaefer H, et al: Recent advances in sun protection. *Semin Cutan Med Surg* 1998, 17:266. _____ ▲

Ephelis (Freckle)

Freckles are small (<0.5 cm) brown macules that occur in profusion on the sun-exposed skin of the face, neck, shoulders, and backs of the hands. They become prominent during the summer when exposed to sunlight and subside, sometimes completely, during the winter when there is no exposure. Blondes and redheads, with blue eyes, of Celtic origin (skin types I or II) are especially susceptible. *Ephelides* may be genetically determined and may recur in successive generations in similar locations and patterns. They usually appear around age 5.

Ephelis must be differentiated from *lentigo simplex.* The lentigo is a benign discrete hyperpigmented macule appearing at any age and on any part of the body, including the mucosa. The intensity of the color is not dependent on sun exposure. The solar lentigo (frequently misnamed "liver spot") appears at a later age, mostly in persons with long-term sun exposure. The backs of the hands and the face (especially the forehead) are favored sites.

Histologically, the ephelis shows increased production of melanin pigment by a normal number of melanocytes. Otherwise the epidermis is normal, whereas the lentigo has elongated rete ridges that appear to be club shaped.

Azizi E, et al: Skin type, hair color, and freckles are predictors of decreased minimal erythema ultraviolet radiation dose. *J Am Acad Dermatol* 1988, 19:32.

Wilson PD, et al: Experimental induction of freckles by ultraviolet B. *Br J Dermatol* 1982, 106:401. _____ ▲

Photoaging (Dermatoheliosis)

The characteristic changes induced by chronic sun exposure are called *photoaging* or *dermatoheliosis.* An individual's risk for developing these changes correlates with his/her baseline pigmentation (constitutive pigmentation) and ability to resist burning and tan following sun exposure (facultative pigmentation). Individuals can be divided into six skin types (or phototypes); these are listed in Table 3-1.

Risk for melanoma and nonmelanoma skin cancer are also related to skin type. The most susceptible to the deleterious effects of sunlight are those of skin type I—blue-eyed, fair-complexioned persons who do not tan. They are frequently of Irish or other Celtic or Anglo-Saxon descent. Individuals who have developed photoaging have the genetic susceptibility and have had sufficient actinic damage to develop skin cancer and therefore require more frequent and careful cutaneous examinations.

Many of the changes now known to be caused by chronic sun exposure were formerly ascribed to chronologic aging. The areas primarily involved are those regularly exposed to the sun: the V area of the neck and chest, back and sides of the neck, the face, and the backs of the hands and extensor arms. The skin becomes atrophic, scaly, wrinkled, inelastic, or leathery with a yellow hue (Milian's citrine skin). In some persons of Celtic ancestry, dermatoheliosis produces profound epidermal atrophy without wrinkling, resulting in an almost translucent appearance of the skin through which hyperplastic sebaceous glands and prominent telangiectasias are seen. These persons appear to be at high risk for nonmelanoma skin cancer. Pigmentation is uneven, with a mixture of poorly demarcated hyperpigmented and white atrophic macules observed. The photodamaged skin appears generally darker because of these irregularities of pigmentation, plus dermal hemosiderosis from actinic purpura (see below). Solar *lentigines,* sharply marginated brown macules, occur on the face and dorsa of the hands.

Many of the textural and tinctorial changes in sun-damaged skin are caused by alterations in the upper dermal elastic tissue and collagen. This process is called *solar (actinic) elastosis,* which imparts a yellow color to the skin. Many variants of solar elastosis have been described, and an affected individual may simultaneously have many of these changes. Small yellowish papules and plaques may develop along the sides of the neck. They have been variably named *striated beaded lines* (the result of sebaceous hyperplasia) or *fibroelastolytic papulosis* of the neck (pseudoxanthoma elasticum–like papillary dermal elastolysis), which is caused by solar elastosis. At times, usually on the face or chest, this elastosis may form a macroscopic, translucent papule with a pearly color that may closely resemble a basal cell carcinoma (Dubreuilh's elastoma, actinic elastotic plaque). Similar plaques may occur on the helix or antihelix of the ear (elastotic nodules of the ear). *Poikiloderma of Civatte* refers to reticulate hyperpigmentation with telangi-

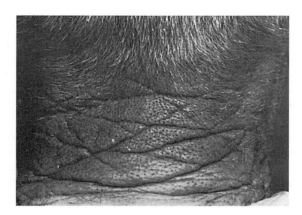

Fig. 3-9 Cutis rhomboidalis nuchae, seen in men after years of exposure to sunlight. (Courtesy Dr. A. Kaminsky.)

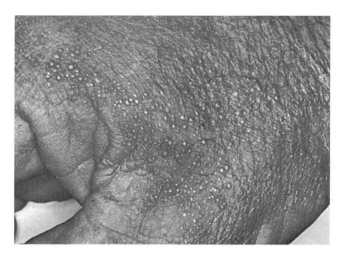

Fig. 3-11 Colloid milium on dorsum of hand, a frequent site, in an oil well worker from Texas. (Courtesy Dr. P. C. Holzberger.)

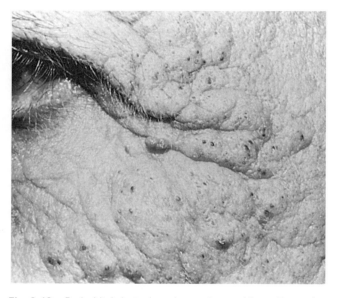

Fig. 3-10 Periorbital elastosis and comedones of Favre-Racouchot syndrome. (Courtesy Dr. Axel W. Hoke.)

ectasia, and slight atrophy of the sides of the neck, lower anterior neck, and V of the chest. The submental area, shaded by the chin, is spared. Poikiloderma of Civatte frequently presents in fair-skinned men and women in their middle to late thirties or early forties. *Cutis rhomboidalis nuchae* (sailor's neck or farmer's neck) is characteristic of long-term, chronic sun exposure. The skin on the back of the neck becomes thickened, tough, and leathery and the normal skin markings are exaggerated (Fig. 3-9). Nodular elastoidosis with cysts and comedones occurs on the inferior periorbital and malar skin *(Favre-Racouchot syndrome)* (Fig. 3-10) or on the forearms (actinic comedonal plaque).

In both situations, the lesions consist of thickened yellow plaques studded with comedones and keratinous cysts. Treatment is the removal of the large comedones and cystic lesions. Retinoic acid cream 0.05% applied nightly is effective in clearing the comedones, especially when combined with mechanical removal (acne surgery). Surgical removal of cysts and redundant skin may lead to substantial cosmetic improvement.

Telangiectasias over the cheeks, ears, and sides of the neck may develop. Because of the damage to the connective tissue of the dermis, skin fragility is prominent, and patients note skin tearing from trivial injuries. Most commonly patients complain that even minimal trauma to their extensor arms leads to an ecchymosis, a phenomenon called *actinic purpura.* As the ecchymoses resolve, dusky brown macules remain for months, increasing the mottled appearance of the skin. White *stellate pseudoscars* on the forearms are a frequent complication of this enhanced skin fragility. In some patients soft, flesh-colored to yellow papules and nodules coalesce on the forearms to form cordlike band extending from the dorsal to the flexural surfaces *(solar elastotic bands).*

Histologically, chronically sun-exposed skin demonstrates homogenization and a faint blue color of the connective tissue of the upper reticular dermis, so-called *solar elastosis.* This "elastotic" material is derived largely from elastic fibers. Characteristically, there is a zone of normal connective tissue immediately below the epidermis.

Adult-Onset Colloid Milium. Translucent, flesh-colored, or slightly yellow 1- to 2-mm papules appear in the sun-exposed areas of the hands, face, neck, and ears in middle-aged adults (Fig. 3-11). Chronic sun exposure of the affected areas is provocative. Refinery workers and persons using high-concentration hydroquinone creams may also develop colloid degeneration. Histologically, homogenous, fissured masses occupy the upper dermis, resembling amyloid. The source of this material is unknown.

PREVENTION OF PHOTOAGING. Although it appears that most photoaging occurs from UVB exposure, UVA may also contribute to chronic sun damage, especially the dermal changes, since UVA penetrates deeper. Because sun damage, like other forms of radiation damage, appears to be cumulative, reducing the total lifetime UV exposure is the goal. The guidelines outlined in the discussion of sunburn prophylaxis on p. 28 should be followed. Patients should avoid sun exposure during the midday, use barrier clothing, and apply a sunscreen daily. Sun protection is important for both adults and children.

Even after photoaging has occurred, the preventive strategies outlined above are still important. Regular use of sunscreen will reduce the number of precancerous and nonmelanoma skin cancers, even in those with prior skin cancers. The regular use of emollients or moisturizing creams to the areas of sun damage will reduce scaling and may improve fragility by making the skin more pliable.

Weiss and other researchers at the University of Michigan have shown that the use of topical tretinoin cream can reverse the changes of photoaging. Changes are slow, and irritation may occur from the high concentrations of tretinoin recommended. Removal of the damaged skin is also effective treatment, and may be accomplished with dermabrasion, chemical peeling, or ultrapulse laser ablation. These procedures can only be done on the face and scalp.

Balus L, et al: Fibroelastolytic papulosis of the neck: a report of 20 cases. *Br J Dermatol* 1997, 137:461.

Benedetto AV, et al: Dermabrasion: therapy and prophylaxis of the photoaged face. *J Am Acad Dermatol* 1992, 27:439.

Calderone DC, Fenske NA: The clinical spectrum of actinic elastosis. *J Am Acad Dermatol* 1995, 32:1016.

Cotton J, et al: Histologic evaluation of preauricular and postauricular human skin after high-energy, short-pulse carbon dioxide laser. *Arch Dermatol* 1996, 132:425.

Council Report: Harmful effects of ultraviolet radiation. *JAMA* 1989, 262:380.

Fisher GJ, et al: Pathophysiology of premature skin aging induced by ultraviolet light. *N Engl J Med* 1997, 337:1419.

Kang S, et al: Photoaging therapy with topical tretinoin. *J Am Acad Dermatol* 1998, 39:S55.

Manuskiatti W, et al: Long term effectiveness and side effects of carbon dioxide laser resurfacing for photoaged facial skin. *J Am Acad Dermatol* 1999, 40:401.

Sharkey MJ, et al: Favre-Racouchot syndrome: a combined therapeutic approach. *Arch Dermatol* 1992, 128:615.

Touart DM, et al: Cutaneous deposition diseases. Part I. *J Am Acad Dermatol* 1998, 39:149.

Weiss JS, et al: Topical tretinoin improves photoaged skin. *JAMA* 1988, 259:527. ▲

PHOTOSENSITIVITY

Photosensitivity includes cutaneous reactions that are chemically induced (from an exogenous source), metabolic (inborn errors such as the porphyrias, resulting in the production of endogenous photosensitizers), idiopathic, and light-exacerbated disorders (genetic and acquired).

Chemically Induced Photosensitivity

A number of substances known as *photosensitizers* may induce an abnormal reaction in skin exposed to sunlight or its equivalent. These substances may be delivered to the skin externally (by contact) or internally by enteral or parenteral administration. The result may be a markedly increased sunburn response without prior allergic sensitization called *phototoxicity*. Phototoxicity may occur from both externally applied (phytophotodermatitis and berloque dermatitis) or internally administered chemicals (phototoxic drug reaction). In contrast, *photoallergic* reactions are true allergic sensitizations triggered by sunlight, produced by either internal administration (photoallergic drug reaction) or by external contact (photoallergic contact dermatitis). Chemicals capable of inducing phototoxic reactions may also produce photoallergic reactions.

In the case of external contactants, the distinction between phototoxicity and photoallergy is usually straightforward: the former occurs on initial exposure, has an onset of less than 48 hours, occurs in the vast majority of persons exposed to the phototoxic substance and sunlight, and shows a histologic pattern similar to sunburn. By contrast, photoallergy occurs only in sensitized persons, may have a delayed onset (up to 14 days—a period of sensitization), and shows histologic features of contact dermatitis.

ACTION SPECTRUM. Chemicals known to cause photosensitivity (photosensitizers) are usually resonating compounds with a molecular weight of less than 500. Absorption of radiant energy (sunlight) by the photosensitizer produces an excited state, which in returning to a lower energy state gives off energy through fluorescence, phosphorescence, charge transfer, heat, or formation of free radicals. Each photosensitizing substance absorbs only specific wavelengths of light called its *absorption spectrum*. The specific wavelengths of light that evoke a photosensitive reaction are called the *action spectrum*. The action spectrum is included in the absorption spectrum of the photosensitizing chemical. The action spectrum for photoallergy is mostly in the long ultraviolet (UVA) region and may extend into the visible light region (320 to 425 nm).

Photosensitivity reactions occur only when there is sufficient concentration of the photosensitizer in the skin, and the skin is exposed to a sufficient intensity and duration of light in the action spectrum of that photosensitizer. The intensity of the photosensitivity reaction is, in general, dose dependent and is worse with a greater dose of photosensitizer and greater light exposure.

Phototoxic Reactions. A phototoxic reaction is a nonimmunologic reaction that develops after exposure to a specific wavelength and intensity of light in the presence of a photosensitizing substance. It is a sunburn-type reaction, with erythema, tenderness, and even blistering occurring only on the sun-exposed parts. This type of reaction can be elicited in many persons who have no previous history of exposure or sensitivity to that particular substance, but individual susceptibility varies widely. In general, to elicit a phototoxic reaction, a considerably greater amount of the photosensitizing substance is necessary than to induce a photoallergic reaction. The erythema begins (like any sunburn) within 2 to 6 hours but worsens for 48 to 96 hours before beginning to subside. Exposure of the nail bed may lead to onycholysis, called *photo-onycholysis*. Phototoxic reactions, especially from topically applied photosensitizers, may cause marked hyperpigmentation, even without significant preceding erythema. The action spectrum for most phototoxic reactions is in the UVA range.

PHOTOTOXIC TAR DERMATITIS. Coal tar, creosote, crude coal tar, or pitch, in conjunction with sunlight exposure, may induce a sunburn reaction associated with a severe burning sensation (tar "smarts" or "flashes"). Direct contact may not be required, since these volatile hydrocarbons may be airborne. The burning and erythema may continue for 1 to 3 days. While up to 70% of whites exposed to such a combination develop this reaction, persons with type V and VI skin are protected by their constitutive skin pigmentation. Following the acute reaction, hyperpigmentation occurs, which may persist for years. Coal tar or its derivatives may be found in cosmetics, drugs, dyes, insecticides, and disinfectants. In the Goeckerman therapy of psoriasis, the phototoxic effect is utilized to advantage.

PHYTOPHOTODERMATITIS. The furocoumarins in many plants may cause a phototoxic reaction when these plants come in contact with moist skin that is then exposed to UVA light. This is called *phytophotodermatitis*. Several hours after exposure, a burning erythema occurs, followed by edema and the development of vesicles or bullae. An intense residual hyperpigmentation results that may persist for weeks or months. The intensity of the initial phototoxic reaction may be mild and may not be recalled by the patient despite significant hyperpigmentation.

Most phototoxic plants are in the families *Umbelliferae, Rutaceae* (rue), *Compositae,* and *Moraceae*. Incriminated plants include agrimony, angelica, atrillal, bavachi, blin weed, buttercup, common rice, cowslip, dill, fennel, fig, garden and wild carrot, garden and wild parsnip, gas plant, goose foot, lime and Persian lime, lime bergamot, masterwort, mustard, parsley, St. John's wort, and yarrow (Fig. 3-12). In Hawaii the anise-scented mokihana berry *(Pelea anisata)* was known to natives for its phototoxic properties (the mokihana burn). Like the lime, it is a member of the rue family.

Occupational disability from exposure to the pink rot

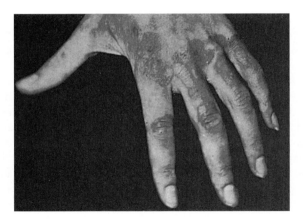

Fig. 3-12 Phytophotodermatits from squeezing limes.

fungus *(Sclerotinia sclerotiorum)* present on celery roots, occurred in celery farmers in upper Michigan and Florida. In addition, disease-resistant celery contains furanocoumarins and was the probable source of phytophotodermatitis in grocery workers.

Dermatitis bullosa striata pratensis (grass or meadow dermatitis) is a phytophotodermatitis caused by contact not with grass, but with yellow-flowered meadow parsnip or a wild, yellow-flowered herb of the rose family. The eruption consists of streaks and bizarre configurations with vesicles and bullae that heal with residual hyperpigmentation. The usual cause is sunbathing in fields containing the phototoxic plants.

Blistering phytophotodermatitis must be differentiated from *rhus dermatitis.* The vesicles and bullae of rhus are not necessarily limited to the sun-exposed areas, and itching is the most prominent symptom. Lesions continue to occur in rhus dermatitis for a week or more. In phytophotodermatitis the reaction is limited to sun-exposed sites, a burning pain appears within 48 hours, and marked hyperpigmentation results.

Treatment of a severe, acute reaction is similar to the management of a sunburn, with cool compresses, mild analgesics if required, and topical emollients. The hyperpigmentation is best managed by "tincture of time."

BERLOQUE (BERLOCKE, PERFUME) DERMATITIS. In 1916 Freund described a peculiar hyperpigmentation that appeared with the use of eau de cologne during sunbathing. Clinically, this pigmentary disturbance is characterized by *lavaliere* (hanging drop) -shaped pigmented patches. The word for pendant in French is *berloque,* and in German it is *berlocke.* This condition is seen most frequently on the sides of the neck and in the retroauricular areas in women (Fig. 3-13). In addition, the shoulders, breasts, face, and other areas may be involved. In men it is usually in the beard area and is caused by aftershave lotion. While this hyperpigmentation is caused by a phototoxic reaction, the initial inflammation is often mild or subclinical, so most patients present at the stage of hyperpigmentation.

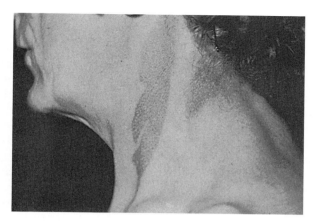

Fig. 3-13 Berloque dermatitis on the side of the neck from perfume.

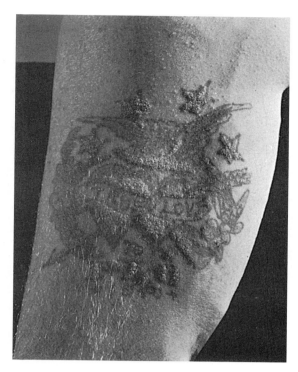

Fig. 3-14 Cadmium sulfide photosensitivity in red portions of tattoo done with red mercuric sulfide "brightened" with cadmium sulfide. Note rough inflammatory crusts from the eczematous reaction. (Courtesy Dr. H. Shatin.)

The chief cause, oil of bergamot, contains a furocoumarin (bergapten), a potent photosensitizer. However, since such compounds have been removed from most perfumes and lotions, berloque dermatitis is now rarely seen. The diagnosis is based largely on the unusual pattern of the pigmentation, leading to a search for a product the patient has applied that contains bergamot.

PHOTOSENSITIVITY IN TATTOOS. Yellow cadmium sulfide may be used as a yellow dye or may be incorporated into red mercuric sulfide pigment to produce a brighter red color for tattooing. When exposed to 380, 400, and 450 nm wavelengths of light, these areas in tattoos may swell, develop erythema, and become verrucose (Fig. 3-14). If this occurs, either the tattooed person must avoid sunlight exposure or the yellow or red parts of the tattoo must be removed.

PHOTOTOXIC DRUG REACTIONS. Most phototoxic drug reactions occur from the following classes of medications: tetracyclines, nonsteroidal antiinflammatory drugs (NSAIDs), amiodarone, and phenothiazines. The action spectrum for all is in the UVA range. In the tetracycline group, demethylchlortetracycline and doxycycline have the greatest phototoxic potential. Among the NSAIDs, piroxicam is the most potent photosensitizer, but ibuprofen and naproxen, the most widely used in the class, also cause phototoxic reactions (Fig. 3-15). In the case of amiodarone and chlorpromazine, while typical phototoxic reactions (resembling sunburn) may occur, hyperpigmentation is a well-recognized pattern of phototoxicity. It causes a slate blue (amiodarone) or slate gray (chlorpromazine) coloration, resulting from deposition of the drug in the tissue. In the case of chlorpromazine, it is complexed with melanin.

Photoallergy. Photoallergic dermatitis is caused by a photosensitizing substance plus sunlight exposure in a sensitized person. If the photosensitizer is delivered internally, it is called a *photoallergic drug reaction;* if it comes

to the skin externally, a *photoallergic contact dermatitis.* Clinically, the patient develops a pruritic eruption, initially in sun-exposed areas. With persistence, lichenification is common, leading to thick plaques. The face and dorsa of the hands, neck, and forearms are most frequently involved (Fig. 3-16). With time the dermatitis may spread to sun-protected areas, so it is critical in taking the history to elicit where the eruption originally began. Removal of the offending photosensitizer may not lead to resolution of the photoallergic reaction, a condition referred to as *persistent light reaction.* This may occur with both topical and systemic photosensitizers. Persistent light reaction is a part of the chronic actinic dermatitis spectrum.

The clinical and histopathologic findings in photoallergy are classically similar to those of an allergic contact dermatitis. It differs only in that sunlight must be present to induce the reaction. The nature of the allergenic substances is similar in that both types are low–molecular-weight compounds. However, in photoallergic dermatitis light photochemically alters the hapten. This newly created hapten then reacts with a cutaneous protein (carrier protein) to form a complete antigen. The remainder of the reaction is similar to other types of delayed type hypersensitivity. The exact mechanism of the development of photoallergic reactions is unknown. The frequent occurrence of these reactions in patients with AIDS suggests that classic

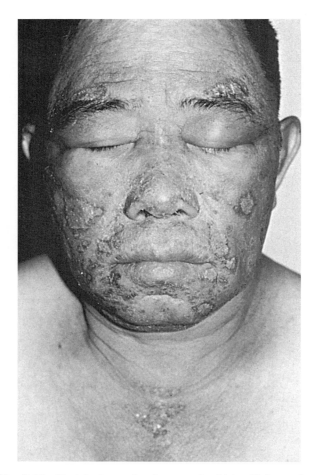

Fig. 3-15 Phototoxic reaction to a nonsteroidal antiinflammatory drug.

sensitization through helper T cells may not be the only possible mechanism.

PHOTOSENSITIZING SUBSTANCES

Phenothiazine and related compounds. Phenothiazines may produce both phototoxic and photoallergic reactions. Photoallergic contact dermatitis may occur when phenothiazines are used as insecticides, or chlorpromazine (Thorazine) and promethazine (Phenergan) for injection are handled by medical personnel. Systemic ingestion of these medications may also result in photoallergic drug reactions.

Sulfonamides. Sulfanilamide and sulfamethoxazole may produce both phototoxic and photoallergic drug reactions. Much less frequently, sulfadiazine and sulfathiazole produce photosensitivity reactions. The thiazide diuretics and the sulfonylurea oral hypoglycemic agents are substituted sulfonamides and are common causes of photoallergic drug reactions. The development of these reactions may be additive, because patients may be receiving one or even two medications from this class without developing photosensitivity, but may develop a photoallergic response with the addition of another sulfonamide. While in most patients the histology is that of acute or chronic dermatitis, lichen planus–like histologic features are a common finding with thiazide diuretics.

Nonsteroidal antiinflammatory drugs. Following the ingestion of medications in this class, especially piroxicam, naproxen, and the now-withdrawn benoxaprofen, phototoxic reactions are common. In some patients, the pattern of reaction closely resembles a photoallergic drug reaction, with marked pruritus, lichenification, and a histologic structure resembling that of acute or chronic allergic contact dermatitis. In some patients the histology is identical to lichen planus—a lichenoid photodermatitis.

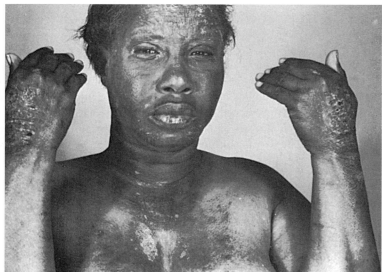

Fig. 3-16 Photoallergic dermatitis on sun-exposed areas. (Courtesy Dr. C. Ames.)

Quinidine. Quinidine may produce photoallergic dermatitis with histologic features of either dermatitis or lichen planus. In addition quinidine may rarely produce an unusual photosensitive livedo reticularis (racemosa) –like eruption, usually on the legs of women.

External photoallergic agents (photosensitizers). The halogenated salicylanilides produced an epidemic of photoallergic dermatitis until they were withdrawn from the market. Other topical antimicrobials capable of producing photoallergy include hexachlorophene, dichlorophen, bithionol, and fenticlor. The most common agents now causing photoallergic contact dermatitis are sunscreens and fragrances. Para-aminobenzoic acid (PABA), PABA esters, the benzophenones, digalloyl trioleate, dibenzoylmethanes, and the cinnamates are all causes of photocontact dermatitis. In fragrances, musk ambrette and 6-methylcoumarin are the most common photosensitizers. Reactions to the former may be particularly persistent. Photosensitization to oil of sandalwood, a common ingredient in aftershave lotions, may also occur.

TESTING FOR PHOTOALLERGY. Although there are numerous techniques suitable for photopatch testing, the most practical office procedure is that each of the suspected photosensitizers is applied in duplicate to two symmetrical sites on the back that have not been exposed to sunlight. The usual concentration used for the patch test is 1% in petrolatum. After 48 hours, one set is removed and examined for reactions as a contactant without exposure to light. Then the site is exposed to 5 to 15 J/cm^2 (usually 10 J/cm^2) of UVA and covered with opaque material. After another 48 hours, the irradiated site is compared with the other patch test site, which has not been exposed to light.

When both sites are equally positive, there is contact sensitivity. When both sides are negative, there is no contact sensitivity or photoallergy. When the irradiated site alone is positive, there is only photoallergy. When the irradiated site is more positive than the unirradiated site, there is both allergic contact and photocontact dermatitis.

TREATMENT. Both acute and chronic photosensitivity are treated similarly to any other inflammatory dermatitis, with topical corticosteroids. In addition, potential photosensitizers should be identified by history and phototesting if necessary. Potential photosensitizing medications should be stopped and potential photoallergen use halted. Sun exposure must be avoided as much as possible; protective clothing is essential. Sunscreens with the broadest UVA coverage are recommended. The treatment of persistent light reaction is discussed under chronic actinic dermatitis.

Addo HA, et al: Thiazide-induced photosensitivity: study of 33 subjects. *Br J Dermatol* 1987, 116:749.

Berkeley SF, et al: Dermatitis in grocery workers associated with high natural concentrations of furocoumarins in celery. *Ann Intern Med* 1986, 105:351.

Bruce S, et al: Quinidine-induced photosensitive livedo reticularis–like eruption. *J Am Acad Dermatol* 1985, 12:332.

Epstein JH: Phototoxicity and photoallergy in man. *J Am Acad Dermatol* 1983, 8:141.

Gonzalez E, et al: Drug photosensitivity, idiopathic photodermatoses, and sunscreens. *J Am Acad Dermatol* 1996, 35:871.

Gould JW, et al: Cutaneous photosensitivity diseases induced by exogenous agents. *J Am Acad Dermatol* 1995, 33:551.

Schauder S, et al: Contact and photocontact sensitivity to suncreens. *Contact Dermatitis* 1997, 37:221.

Vassileva SG, et al: Antimicrobial photosensitive reactions. *Arch Intern Med* 1998, 158:871. ▲

Idiopathic Photosensitivity Disorders

This group includes the photosensitivity diseases for which no cause is known. They are not associated with external photosensitizers (except for some cases of chronic actinic dermatitis) or inborn errors of metabolism to date.

Polymorphous Light Eruption. Polymorphous light eruption (PLE, PMLE) is the most common form of photosensitivity. In various studies among Northern European whites, a history of PLE can be elicited in between 5% and 20% of the adult population. All races and skin types can be affected. The onset is typically in the first three decades of life, and females outnumber males by 2 or 3 to 1. The pathogenesis is unknown, but a family history may be elicited in between 10% and 50% of patients.

Clinically, the eruption may have several different morphologies, although in the individual patient the morphology is usually constant. The papular (or erythematopapular) variant is the most common, but papulovesicular, eczematous, erythematous and plaquelike lesions also occur. Plaquelike lesions are more common in elderly patients and may closely simulate lupus erythematosus, with indurated, erythematous, fixed, scaling lesions. Scarring and atrophy do not occur; however, in darkly pigmented races, marked postinflammatory hyperpigmentation may occur. In some patients, pruritus only without an eruption may be reported (polymorphous light eruption sine eruption). Some of these patients will develop typical PLE later in life.

The lesions of PLE appear most typically 1 to 4 days after exposure to sunlight. Patients may report itching and erythema during sun exposure, and development of lesions within the first 24 hours. A change in the amount of sun exposure appears to be more critical than the absolute amount of radiation. Patients living in tropical climates may be free of eruption, only to develop disease when they move to temperate zones, in which there is more marked seasonal variation in UV intensity. Areas of involvement include the face, the V area of the chest, the neck, and the arms. In general, for each individual certain areas are predisposed. However, typically areas protected during the winter, such as the extensor forearms, are particularly affected, whereas areas exposed all year (face and dorsa of hands) may be relatively spared. The eruption appears most commonly in the springtime. Often the eruption improves with continued sun exposure (hardening) so that patients may be clear of the condition in the summer or autumn.

PLE is induced by ultraviolet light, but the wavelengths responsible are variable. In some patients the action spectrum is in the UVB range, while UVA is the inducing spectrum in the majority of patients. Visible light does not induce PLE. Standard phototesting usually does not demonstrate an abnormal MED response in patients with PLE. If an abnormal response occurs it is in general only erythema, and MED testing does not generally reproduce the eruption. Provocation testing with repeated exposures may be required. Most patients react more in affected sites, and in some, lesions can only be induced in affected areas. In some patients provocation tests may be negative.

Two unusual variants of PLE are *juvenile spring eruption of the ears* and *solar purpura*. Juvenile spring eruption occurs most commonly in boys ages 5 to 12 years. It presents in the spring with grouped small papules or papulovesicles on the helices. It is self-limited and does not scar. UVA is the inducing spectrum, and some of the patients also have lesions of PLE elsewhere. The histologic picture is identical to that of PLE. Solar purpura is a rare variant of PLE, presenting as macular or palpable purpura on the legs. It is also UVA induced, but its distribution suggests that other factors, such as high hydrostatic pressure, are required.

In establishing the differential diagnosis, the following should be considered: lupus erythematosus, lymphocytic infiltration of Jessner, mycosis fungoides, prurigo nodularis, contact dermatitis, and photosensitive contact dermatitis. Histopathologic examination, antinuclear antibody testing, and direct immunofluorescence are helpful in distinguishing the above diseases. The differentiation from lupus erythematosus (LE) of the subacute type may be difficult, and SSA/Ro testing should be ordered to help exclude this form of LE.

Therapeutically, most patients with mild disease can be managed by avoiding the sun and using barrier protection and high SPF broad-spectrum sunscreens. These measures are critical for all patients, since they are free of toxicity and reduce the amount and duration of other therapies required. Patient education is very important in the management of this disease, and phototesting may be required to convince the patient that he or she is UV sensitive. It will also determine the action spectrum. The use of topical steroids, frequently of super or high potency, in several day to weekly pulses is successful in controlling the pruritus and clearing the eruption. Antihistamines (hydroxyzine, diphenhydramine, or doxepin [Sinequan]) may be used for pruritus. Systemic corticosteroids may be necessary, especially in the springtime. In patients whose condition is not controlled by the measures just mentioned, hydroxychloroquine sulfate (Plaquenil), 200 to 400 mg daily, may be used. It has a

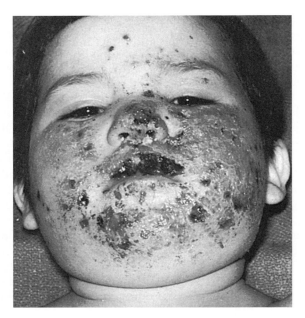

Fig. 3-17 Actinic prurigo in Native American boy. (Courtesy Dr. A.R. Birt.)

delayed onset and is best instituted in the late winter to prevent springtime outbreaks. Chloroquine or quinacrine may be effective if hydroxychloroquine is not, but in general the antimalarials are inferior to phototherapy. PUVA, long wave UVA (340 to 400 nm), and UVB therapy are extremely beneficial, PUVA being superior. Frequently there is an exacerbation of the eruption during phototherapy, and concomitant systemic steroid therapy may be required. Thalidomide is an alternative in patients failing the above regimens. For patients with the most severe disease, azathioprine is often effective.

Actinic Prurigo. Actinic prurigo probably represents a variant of PLE; it is most commonly seen in Native Americans of North and Central America and Columbia. The incidence in Mexico has been reported to be between 1.5% and 3.5%. It has been reported in Europe and Japan as well. The female-to-male ratio is 2 or 3 to 1. Actinic prurigo in Native Americans begins before age 10 in 45% of cases and before age 20 in 72%. Up to 75% of cases have a positive family history (hereditary PLE of Native Americans). In Europe, 80% of cases occur before age 10.

In childhood, lesions begin as small papules or papulovesicles that crust and become impetiginized (Figs. 3-17 and 3-18). They are intensely pruritic and frequently excoriated. In children the cheeks, distal nose, ears, and lower lip are typically involved. Cheilitis may be the initial and only feature for years. Conjunctivitis is seen in 10% to 20% of patients. Lesions of the arms and legs are also common but usually exhibit a prurigo nodule configuration. The eruption may extend to involve sun-protected areas,

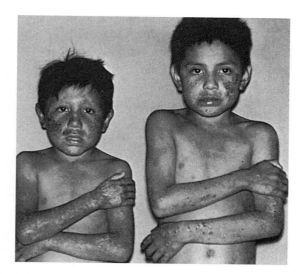

Fig. 3-18 Actinic prurigo in Native American brothers. (Courtesy Dr. A.R. Birt.)

especially the buttocks, but the lesions in these areas are always less severe. In adults, chronic, dry papules and plaques are most typical, and cheilitis and crusting occur much less frequently. Skin lesions tend to persist throughout the year in the tropics, although they are clearly worse during periods of increased sun exposure. In temperate and high-latitude regions, lesions occur from March through the summer and substantially remit in the winter. Hardening as seen with PLE does not occur. In up to 60% of patients with actinic prurigo that presents before the age of 20, the condition improves or resolves within 5 years, whereas adults usually continue to have the disease throughout life.

Phototesting gives normal results in one third, a reduced MED to UVA and UVB in one third, and a reduced MED to UVA alone in one third. Predominantly UVB sensitivity has been reported by some, but patients often report eruptions following sun exposure through window glass, suggesting UVA alone may be sufficient to induce the eruption in some cases. IgE levels may be elevated. Patients with actinic prurigo are more commonly positive for HLA-A24 and Cw4 and negative for A3 than are control subjects. Actinic prurigo is treated identically to PLE. Thalidomide has been used extensively in this setting, with excellent results.

Addo HA, et al: UVB photochemotherapy and phototherapy in the treatment of PMLE and solar urticaria. *Br J Dermatol* 1987, 116:539.

Fotiades J, et al: Results of evaluation of 203 patients for photosensitivity in a 7.3-year period. *J Am Acad Dermatol* 1995, 33:51.

Fusaro, et al: Hereditary polymorphic light eruption of American Indians: occurrence in non-Indians with polymorphic light eruption. *J Am Acad Dermatol* 1996, 34:612.

Hasan T, et al: Disease associations in PMLE. *Arch Dermatol* 1998, 134:1081.

Holzle E, et al: Hydroxychloroquine in PMLE. *Br J Dermatol* 1987, 116:379.

Holzle E, et al: Polymorphous light eruption. *J Am Acad Dermatol* 1982, 7:1110.

Murphy GM, et al: Prophylactic PUVA and UVB in PMLE. *Br J Dermatol* 1987, 116:531.

Ross JS, et al: Sesquiterpene lactone contact sensitivity: clinical patterns of Compositae dermatitis and relationship to chronic actinic dermatitis. *Contact Dermatitis* 1993, 29:84.

Sheridan DP, et al: HLA typing in actinic prurigo. *J Am Acad Dermatol* 1990, 22:1019. _____ ▲

Brachioradial Pruritus. Patients develop lichenified, intermittently itchy disorder of the skin of the lateral elbow-bends. Walcyk and Elpern reported 42 cases seen in Hawaii over a 2-year period. In some patients nerve damage from cervical spine disease had been proposed as the cause. However, 60% of Walcyk and Elpern's patients under age 50 had no cervical abnormality by x-ray, and the lesions are limited to a much smaller area than that served by any nerve. In most patients, brachioradial pruritus result from chronic sunlight exposure. Treatment with topical corticosteroids, capsaicin and photoprotection leads to improvement.

Goodless DR, Eaglstein WH: Brachioradial pruritus: treatment with topical capsaicin. *J Am Acad Dermatol* 1993, 29:783.

Walcyk PJ, Elpern DJ: Brachioradial summer pruritus: a tropical dermopathy. *Br J Dermatol* 1986, 115:177. _____ ▲

Solar Urticaria. Solar urticaria (SU) is most common in females aged 20 to 40. Within seconds to minutes after light exposure, typical urticarial lesions appear and resolve in 1 to 2 hours. Delayed reactions rarely occur. Chronically exposed sites may have some reduced sensitivity. In severe attacks syncope, bronchospasm, and anaphylaxis may occur.

Patients with SU are sensitive to wavelengths of light from UVB through visible light. The wavelengths of sensitivity and the minimal urticarial doses may vary with anatomic site and over time within the same patient. Classification was originally by wavelength of sensitivity, but Leenutaphong et al divided SU into two types. A circulating photoallergen formed by absorption of light energy by a precursor has been demonstrated in SU patients. In type I solar urticaria, this photoallergen precursor is an abnormal endogenous substance; in type II it is a normal skin component. Type I SU has an action spectrum in the visible range; in type II the action spectrum is variable.

Histologically, early lesions contain eosinophils and neutrophils. Mast cell degranulation occurs, and elevated levels of histamine are present in vessels draining lesions. Large amounts of eosinophil major basic protein are deposited in affected sites.

Diagnosis of solar urticaria is usually straightforward. Lupus erythematosus and erythropoietic protoporphyria should be excluded with appropriate tests. Phototesting is useful in SU to determine the wavelengths of sensitivity.

Various light sources, including lasers and natural sunlight, may be used to elicit positive reactions.

Because many patients have sensitivity in the UVA or even visible range, standard sunscreens are of limited benefit. Antihistamines, especially the nonsedating H_1 agents loratadine, cetirizine HCl, and fexofenadine may increase the minimal urticarial dose tenfold or more. These plus sun avoidance are the first-line therapy. Doxepin may be added if the above agents are insufficient. Antimalarials can help some patients. PUVA or increasing UVA exposures are effective in more difficult cases, the former having greater efficacy. For the most difficult cases, plasmapheresis may be used to remove the circulating photoallergen, allowing PUVA to be given leading to remission.

Alora MB, et al: Solar urticaria. *J Am Acad Dermatol* 1998, 38:341.

Leenutaphong V, et al: Pathogenesis and classification of solar urticaria: a new concept. *J Am Acad Dermatol* 1989, 21:237.

Ryckaert S, et al: Solar urticaria. *Arch Dermatol* 1998, 134:71.

▲

Hydroa Vacciniforme. Hydroa vacciniforme (HV) is a rare, chronic photodermatosis with onset in childhood that favors females in a ratio of 2 or 3 to 1. Lesions tend to appear in crops with disease free intervals. Attacks may be preceded by fever and malaise. The ears, nose, cheeks, and extensor arms and hands are affected. Within 6 hours of exposure stinging may occur. At 24 hours or sooner erythema and edema appear, followed by the characteristic 2- to 4-mm vesicles. Over the next few days these lesions rupture, become centrally necrotic, and heal with a smallpoxlike scar (Fig. 3-19). Lesions may become confluent, forming bullae, and recurrent disease may lead to contractures of the digits. Conjunctivitis with photophobia may occur and corneal ulcers and opacities may result. The natural history is for improvement by the end of the second decade, often with complete resolution.

Histologically, early lesions show intraepidermal vesiculation and dermal edema that evolves into a subepidermal blister. Necrotic lesions show reticular degeneration of keratinocytes, with epidermal necrosis flanked by spongiosis with a dense perivascular infiltrate of neutrophils and lymphocytes. Dermal vessels may be thrombosed, simulating vasculitis. Sonnex et al and many others have shown that lesions may be reproduced by repetitive UVA, with the action spectrum in the 330 to 360 nm range.

The differential diagnosis includes PLE, actinic prurigo, and erythropoietic protoporphyria (EPP). Porphyrin levels are normal in hydroa vacciniforme. In EPP the burning typically begins within minutes of sun exposure, and healing is with diffuse, thickened, waxlike scarring, rather than the smallpoxlike scars of hydroa vacciniforme. Histologic evaluation is useful in distinguishing these two conditions. Treatment is principally to avoid sunlight exposure and to use broad-spectrum or barrier sunscreens that block

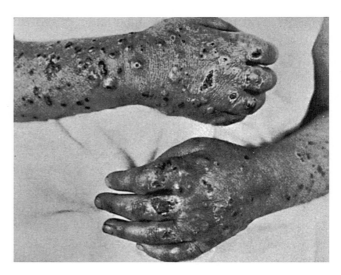

Fig. 3-19   Hydroa vacciniforme. The face was also involved. (Courtesy Dr. B.M. Kesten.)

in the UVA range. Hydroxychloroquine and prophylactic PUVA may be partially effective.

Halasz CLG, et al: Hydroa vacciniforme: induction of lesions with ultraviolet A. *J Am Acad Dermatol* 1983, 8:171.

Sonnex T, et al: Hydroa vacciniforme. *Br J Dermatol* 1988, 118:101.

▲

Chronic Actinic Dermatitis. Chronic actinic dermatitis (CAD) is a disease concept in evolution. It has replaced the terms *persistent light reactivity*, *actinic reticuloid*, *photosensitive eczema*, and *chronic photosensitivity dermatitis*. The basic components of this disease are (1) a persistent, chronic, eczematous eruption in the absence of exposure to known photosensitizers; (2) decreased MED to UVA, and/or UVB (required by some authors), and/or visible light; and (3) histology consistent with a chronic dermatitis with or without features of lymphoma.

Clinically, the disease affects middle-aged or elderly men predominantly. In the United States, patients with skin types V and VI may be disproportionately affected. Skin lesions consist of edematous, scaling, thickened patches and plaques that tend to be confluent. Lesions occur primarily or most severely on the exposed skin and may spare the upper eyelids, behind the ears, and the bottoms of wrinkles. Involvement of unexposed sites often occurs, progressing to erythroderma in the most severe cases. Marked depigmentation resembling vitiligo may result. Patients may not realize their condition is exacerbated by exposure to light, since it may persist in all seasons.

The pathogenesis of this syndrome is unknown. In some patients a preceding topical or oral photosensitizer may be implicated, but the condition fails to improve with discontinuation of the inciting agent. In about one third of patients, photopatch testing yields a positive response to previously applied agents, especially musk ambrette, sunscreen ingredients, and hexachlorophene. Patch testing to standard agents may have a positive result in about 30% of patients, but no particular relevance is found. However, in up to 85% of cases, *sesquiterpene lactone* contact sensitivity from *Compositae* has been identified in Europe. In addition, more than 75% of men over age 60 with sesquiterpene lactone sensitivity have abnormal phototesting results. CD8 (suppressor/cytotoxic) T cells are disproportionately represented in the cutaneous infiltrates in the majority of cases, and less commonly, in the peripheral blood. IgE levels may be elevated.

The diagnosis of chronic actinic dermatitis is established by histologic evaluation and phototesting. Phototesting often reproduces the lesions. PLE, photoallergic contact dermatitis, photoallergic drug reaction, airborne contact dermatitis, and mycosis fungoides or Sézary syndrome must be excluded. PLE is excluded by the reduced MED and reproduction of the lesions by phototesting in CAD, although some patients may begin with a PLE-like disease that later meets the criteria for chronic actinic dermatitis. Contact dermatitis is excluded by patch and photopatch testing. Mycosis fungoides may be difficult to differentiate from CAD in cases with atypical histology. Phototesting is critical in these cases. Mycosis fungoides should have a T-cell receptor rearrangement in lesional skin or peripheral blood and usually shows a CD4 (helper) T cell predominance in the lesions, and in peripheral blood in the case of Sézary syndrome.

Therapy for chronic actinic dermatitis is difficult. Possible topical photosensitizers should be identified by photopatch testing. Maximum sun avoidance and broad-spectrum sunscreens are essential. Topical and systemic steroids are effective in some cases, but chronic toxicity of systemic steroids limits chronic usage. Azathioprine, 50 to 200 mg daily, is the most reproducibly effective treatment and may be required annually during periods of increased sun intensity. The use of danazol, 600 mg daily, was dramatic in one patient. Hydroxychloroquine may be added to systemic steroids or azathioprine for additional benefit. Low-dose PUVA is beneficial but may not be tolerated, even when used with topical and systemic steroids. Cyclosporine is the treatment of last resort but is effective even in the most severe cases. Unfortunately, it is associated with acute and chronic toxicity and relapse occurs rapidly after discontinuation.

Humbert P, et al: Chronic actinic dermatitis responding to danazol. *Br J Dermatol* 1991, 124:195.

Lim HW, et al: Chronic actinic dermatitis. *Arch Dermatol* 1998, 38:108.

Murphy GM, et al: Azathioprine treatment in chronic actinic dermatitis. *Br J Dermatol* 1989, 121:639.

Ross JS, et al: Sesquiterpene lactone contact sensitivity. *Contact Dermatitis* 1993, 29:84.

Von Den Driesch P, et al: Chronic actinic dermatitis with vitiligo-like depigmentation. *Clin Exp Dermatol* 1992, 17:38. _____ ▲

Photosensitivity and HIV Infection.

Photosensitivity resembling PLE, actinic prurigo, or chronic actinic dermatitis may be seen in HIV-infected persons. In general, photosensitivity is seen when the CD4 count is below 200, except in persons with a genetic predisposition (Native Americans) in whom actinic prurigo–like lesions may be the initial manifestation of HIV disease. Photosensitivity may be associated with ingestion of a photosensitizing medication, especially NSAIDs or trimethoprim/sulfamethoxazole. The eruption may not improve even when the medication is discontinued. Histologically, the lesions may show subacute or chronic dermatitis often with an dense infiltrate with many eosinophils. Histology identical to PLE, lichen planus, or lichen nitidus may also occur. When the CD4 count is below 50, especially in black patients, chronic actinic dermatitis with features of actinic prurigo is typical. Therapy is difficult, but thalidomide may be beneficial.

Berger TG, et al: Lichenoid photoeruptions in human immunodeficiency virus infection. *Arch Derm* 1994, 130:609.

Pappert A, et al: Photosensitivity as the presenting illness in four patients with human immunodeficiency viral infection. *Arch Derm* 1994, 130:618. _____ ▲

Dermatoses with Photoexacerbation or Photosensitivity

Photosensitivity may be seen as a component of many skin diseases. The mechanisms by which these conditions are worsened by sun exposure are diverse. Some are heritable disorders of increased sensitivity to ultraviolet cellular or DNA damage such as xeroderma pigmentosum, Bloom syndrome, and Cockayne's disease. In others ultraviolet light seems to act by a Koebner's phenomenon, as in Darier's, and perhaps pemphigus foliaceus. Patients with lupus erythematosus and dermatomyositis, among the connective tissue diseases, often exhibit photosensitivity. The mechanism may involve UV alteration of cellular cytoplasmic or nuclear antigen expression, allowing these antigens to interact with circulating autoantibodies. Patients with diseases characterized by a deficiency of protective pigmentation, such as albinism, piebaldism, and vitiligo, are photosensitive. Disorders of metabolism that are inherited (such as the porphyrias and Hartnup disease), toxin induced (such as porphyria after insecticide ingestion), or related to absence of required nutrients (such as pellagra from niacin deficiency), may all exhibit photoexacerbation. Basal cell nevus syndrome and familial melanoma, atypical mole syndrome (dysplastic nevus syndrome) represent cancer syndromes in which ultraviolet irradiation is an important cofactor in the development of the cancers. In others disorders, such as actinic granuloma and some cases of atopic dermatitis, the mechanism of photoexacerbation is unknown.

Hensley DR, et al: Pediatric photosensitivity disorders. *Dermatol Clin* 1998, 16:571. _____ ▲

RADIODERMATITIS

The major target within the cell by which radiation damage occurs is the DNA. The effects of ionizing radiation on the cells depend on the amount of radiation, its intensity (exposure rate), and the characteristics of the individual cell. Rapidly reproducing cells and anaplastic cells in general have increased radiosensitivity when compared with normal tissue. When radiation therapy is delivered, it is frequently fractionated—divided into small doses called fractions. This allows the normal cells to recover between doses.

In small amounts, the effect is insidious and cumulative. When the dose is large, cell death results. When it is sublethal, many changes occur. Mitosis is arrested temporarily, with consequent retardation of growth. The exposure rate affects the number of chromosome breaks. The more rapid the delivery of a certain amount of radiation, the greater the number of chromosome breaks. The number of breaks is increased also by the presence of oxygen.

Acute Radiodermatitis. When an "erythema dose" of ionizing radiation is given to the skin, there is a latent period of up to 24 hours before visible erythema appears. This initial erythema lasts 2 to 3 days but may be followed by a second phase beginning up to 1 week after the exposure and lasting up to 1 month. When the skin is exposed to a large amount of ionizing radiation, an acute reaction develops, the extent of which will depend on the amount, quality, and duration of exposure. Such radiation reaction occurs in the treatment of malignancy and in accidental overexposure. The reaction is manifested by initial erythema, followed by a second phase of erythema at 3 to 6 days. Vesiculation, edema, and erosion or ulceration may occur, accompanied by pain. The skin develops a dark color that may be mistaken for hyperpigmentation, but that desquamates. This type of radiation injury may subside in several weeks to several months, again depending on the amount of radiation exposure. Skin which receives a large amount of radiation will never return to normal. It will lack adnexal structures, be dry, atrophic, and smooth, and be hypopigmented or depigmented.

Eosinophilic, Polymorphic, and Pruritic Eruption Associated with Radiotherapy. Rueda et al reported that 17% of women receiving cobalt radiotherapy for internal cancer developed a pruritic eruption that favored the extremities. Acral excoriations, erythematous papules, vesicles, and bullae occurred. Histologically, a superficial and deep

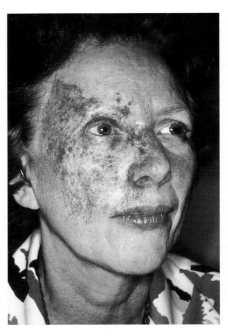

Fig. 3-20 Chronic radiodermatitis in a woman 45 years after ionizing radiation therapy for a nevus flammeus.

perivascular lymphohistiocytic infiltrate with eosinophils was present.

Chronic Radiodermatitis. Chronic exposure to "suberythema" doses of ionizing radiation over a prolonged period will produce varying degrees of damage to the skin and its underlying parts after a variable latent period of from several months to several decades. In the past this type of radiation reaction occurred most frequently in roentgenologists and radiation technicians who were constantly exposed to ionizing radiation. It may also occur through overtreatment of various dermatoses with ionizing radiation and through excessive use of fluoroscopy and roentgenography for diagnostic purposes.

Telangiectasia, atrophy, and hypopigmentation with residual focal increased pigment (freckling) may appear (Fig. 3-20). The skin becomes dry, thin, smooth, and shiny. Subcutaneous fibrosis, thickening and binding of the surface layers to deep tissues may present as tender, erythematous plaques 6 to 12 months after radiation therapy. It may resemble erysipelas or inflammatory metastases. The nails may become striated, brittle, and fragmented. The capacity to repair injury is substantially reduced, resulting in ulceration from minor trauma. The hair becomes brittle and sparse. In the more severe cases these chronic changes may be followed by radiation keratoses and carcinoma.

Radiation Cancer. After a latent period averaging 20 to 40 years, various malignancies may develop. Most frequent are basal cell carcinomas, followed by squamous cell carci-

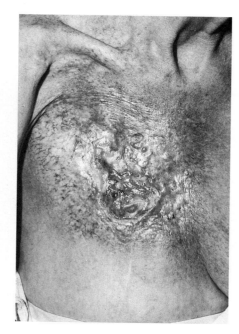

Fig. 3-21 Squamous cell carcinoma developing in a chronic radiation ulcer on the chest.

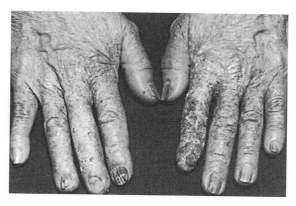

Fig. 3-22 Chronic radiodermatitis with actinic keratoses and basal and squamous cell carcinomas.

noma (SCC) (Figs. 3-21 and 3-22). These may appear in sites of prior radiation, even if there is no evidence of chronic radiation damage. Sun damage may be additive to radiation therapy, increasing the appearance of nonmelanoma skin cancers. SCCs arising in sites of radiation therapy metastasize more frequently than purely sun-induced SCCs. In some patients either type of tumor may predominate. Location plays some role; SCCs are more common on the arms and hands, whereas basal cell carcinomas are seen on the head and neck and lumbosacral area. Other cancers induced by radiation include angiosarcoma, malignant fibrous histiocytoma, sarcomas, and thyroid carcinoma. The incidence of malignant neoplasms increases with the passage of time.

TREATMENT. Radiodermatitis without carcinoma requires little or no attention except protection from sunlight and the extremes of heat and cold. Careful cleansing with mild soap and water, the use of emollients, and, on occasion, corticosteroid ointments, especially hydrocortisone, are the only requirements for good care.

The early removal of precancerous keratoses and ulcerations is helpful in preventing the development of cancers. For radiation keratoses treatment with cryosurgery may be sufficient. If the keratosis feels infiltrated, a biopsy is indicated. Radiation ulcerations should be studied by excisional or incisional biopsy if they have been present for three or more months. Complete removal by excision is frequently required to obtain healing and exclude focal carcinoma in the ulceration. Radiation-induced nonmelanoma skin cancers are managed by standard methods. The

higher risk of metastasis from radiation-induced SCCs mandates careful follow up and regular regional lymph node evaluation.

Davis MM, et al: Skin cancer in patients with chronic radiation dermatitis. *J Am Acad Dermatol* 1989, 20:608.

Goette DK, et al: Post-irradiation malignant fibrous histiocytoma. *Arch Dermatol* 1985, 121:535.

Goldschmidt H, et al: Reactions to ionizing radiation. *J Am Acad Dermatol* 1980, 3:551.

James WD, et al: Late subcutaneous fibrosis following megavoltage radiotherapy. *J Am Acad Dermatol* 1980, 3:616.

Lichenstein DA, et al: Chronic radiodermatitis following cardiac catheterization. *Arch Dermatol* 1996, 132:663.

Rueda RA, et al: Eosinophilic, polymorphic, and pruritic eruption associated with radiotherapy. *Arch Dermatol* 1999, 135:804.

Stone MS, et al: Subacute radiation dermatitis from fluoroscopy during coronary artery stenting. *J Am Acad Dermatol* 1998, 38:333.

Stone NM, et al: Postirradiation angiosarcoma. *Clin Exp Dermatol* 1997, 22:46. ▲

MECHANICAL INJURIES TO THE SKIN

Mechanical factors may induce distinctive skin changes. Pressure, friction, and the introduction of foreign substances (such as by injection) are some of the means by which skin injuries may occur.

Callus

Callus is a nonpenetrating, circumscribed hyperkeratosis produced by pressure. It occurs on parts subject to intermittent pressure, particularly on the palms and soles, and especially over the bony prominences of the joints. Verbov et al report ankle callosity overlying the talus to be common and asymptomatic. Those engaged in various sports and certain occupations develop callosities of distinctive size and location as stigmata of their occupation. Rimmer et al describe such lesions in musicians.

The callus differs from the clavus in that it has no penetrating central core and is a more diffuse thickening. It

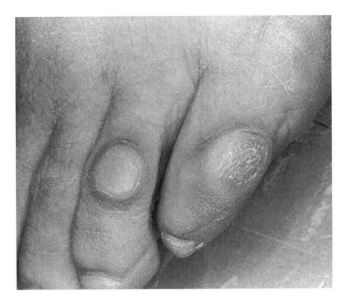

Fig. 3-23 Hard corns.

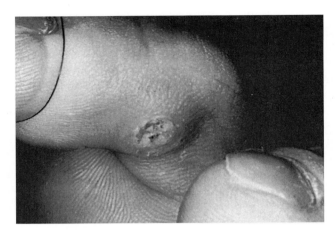

Fig. 3-24 Soft corn on side of toe. (Courtesy Dr. Axel W. Hoke.)

tends to disappear spontaneously when the pressure is removed. Most problems are encountered with calluses on the soles. Ill-fitting shoes and orthopedic problems of the foot caused by aging are some of the etiologic factors to be considered in painful callosities of the feet.

Padding to relieve the pressure, paring of the thickened callus, and the use of keratolytics such as 40% salicylic acid plasters are some of the effective means of relieving painful callosities. Twelve percent ammonium lactate lotion (Lac-Hydrin) is often helpful. Calluses may also be softened by moistening them nightly with 2 parts propylene glycol to 1 part water under snug plastic occlusion (a plastic baggie and a sock will do). This is especially effective with fissured calluses of the heels.

Clavus (Corns)

Corns are circumscribed, horny, conical thickenings with the base on the surface and the apex pointing inward and pressing on subjacent structures. There are two varieties: the hard corns, which occur on the dorsa of the toes or on the soles (Fig. 3-23), and the soft corns, which occur between the toes and are softened by the macerating action of sweat (Fig. 3-24). In a hard corn, the surface is shiny and polished and, when the upper layers are shaved off, a core is noted in the densest part of the lesion (Fig. 3-25). It is this core that causes the dull/boring or sharp/lancinating pain by pressing on the underlying sensory nerves. Corns arise at sites of friction or pressure, and when these causative factors are removed, they may spontaneously disappear. Frequently a bony spur or exostosis is present beneath both hard and soft corns of long duration, and unless this exostosis is removed cure is unlikely. The soft interdigital corn usually occurs in the fourth interdigital space of the foot. Frequently there is

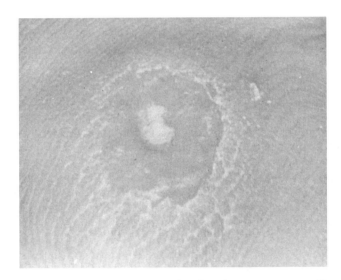

Fig. 3-25 White keratinous core deep in a plantar corn, exposed by shaving. (Courtesy Dr. Axel W. Hoke.)

an exostosis at the metatarsal-phalangeal joint that causes pressure on the adjacent toe. These are soft, soggy, and macerated so that they appear white. Treatment by simple excision may be effective.

Plantar corns must be differentiated from plantar warts, and in most cases this can be done with confidence only by paring off the surface keratin until either the pathognomonic elongated dermal papillae of the wart with its blood vessels, or the clear horny core of the corn, can be clearly seen. Additionally, porokeratosis plantaris discreta is a sharply marginated, cone-shaped, rubbery lesion that commonly occurs beneath the metatarsal heads. Multiple lesions may occur. It has a 3-to-1 female predominance, is painful, and is frequently confused with a plantar wart or corn. Keratosis punctata of the palmar creases may be seen in the creases of the digits of the feet where it may be mistaken for a corn.

TREATMENT. The relief of pressure or friction by corrective footwear is of primary importance; however, this step alone frequently does not cure the corns. Salicylic acid and dichloroacetic acid have been favorite methods of treatment, and are successful when carefully and diligently used. After careful paring of the corn with emphasis on removing the center core, 40% salicylic acid plaster is applied. After 48 hours the plaster is removed, the white macerated skin is rubbed off, and a new plaster is reapplied. This is continued until the corn is gone.

Sometimes it is more feasible to use a salicylic acid—lactic acid in collodion rather than the plaster. The collodion medication is carefully painted on the pared site of the corn and allowed to dry each day until cure. Soaking the foot for half an hour before reapplying the medication enhances the effect. This treatment is especially effective for interdigital soft corns.

Soaking the feet in hot water and paring the surface by means of a scalpel blade or pumice stone leads to symptomatic improvement. The application of a ring of soft felt wadding around the region of the corn will often bring a good result. It should be stressed that removal of any underlying bony abnormality, if present, is often necessary to effect a cure.

Surfer's Nodules

Nodules 1 to 3 cm (rarely as much as 5 or 6 cm) in diameter, sometimes eroded or even ulcerated, may develop on the tops of the feet or over the tibial tubercles of surfboard riders who paddle their boards in a kneeling position, as is customary in the cold water off the California coast (Fig. 3-26). In warmer waters, as in Hawaii, the prone position is customary, and such nodules seldom occur. These nodules slowly involute over the months when there is no surfing. They respond readily to intralesional corticosteroid injections.

Pseudoverrucous Papules and Nodules

Goldberg et al reported striking 2- to 8-mm, shiny, smooth, red, moist, flat-topped, round lesions in the perianal area of five children. They felt it to be a result of encopresis or urinary incontinence. They pointed out the similarity to similar lesions reported by Borglund et al in one fifth of their 57 urostomy patients. Protection of the skin will help eliminate them.

Coral Cuts

A severe type of skin injury may occur from the cuts of coral skeletons. The abrasions and cuts are painful, and local therapy may sometimes provide little or no relief. Healing may take months. As a rule, if secondary infection

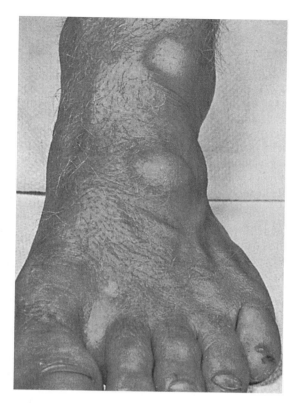

Fig. 3-26 Surfer's nodules on instep and ankle, over bony prominences. (Courtesy Dr. E.A. Taylor.)

is guarded against, such cuts heal as well as any others. The possibility of *Mycobacterium marinum* infection must be considered in persistent lesions.

Pressure Ulcers (Decubitus)

The bedsore, or decubitus, is a pressure ulcer produced anywhere on the body by prolonged pressure. The pressure sore is caused by ischemia of the underlying structures of the skin, fat, and muscles as a result of sustained and constant pressure. Usually it occurs in chronically debilitated persons who are unable to change position in bed. The bony prominences of the body are the most frequently affected sites. Ninety-five percent of all pressure ulcers develop on the lower body, with 65% in the pelvic area and 30% on the legs. The ulcer usually begins with erythema at the pressure point; in a short time a "punched-out" ulcer develops. Necrosis with a grayish pseudomembrane is seen, especially in the untreated ulcer. Potential complications of pressure ulcers include sepsis, local infection, osteomyelitis, fistulas, and squamous cell carcinoma.

Yarkony et al proposed a classification system with good reliability that may be used to teach prevention activities. The U.S. Department of Health and Human Services has released a clinical practice guideline for the treatment of pressure ulcers. They used a four-stage classification system that was developed at a consensus conference. These guidelines are available from HHS, Rockville, Maryland. Ask for Clinical Practice Guideline number 15 (AHCPR No. 95-0652).

Treatment consists of relief of the pressure on the affected parts by frequent change of position, meticulous nursing care, and the use of air-filled products, liquid-filled flotation devices or foam products. Other measures include ulcer care, managing bacterial colonization and infection, operative repair if necessary, continual education, ensuring adequate nutrition, managing pain, and providing psycho-social support.

Ulcer care is critical. Debridement may be accomplished by sharp, mechanical, enzymatic, and/or autolytic measures. In some cases operative care will be required. Stable heel ulcers are an exception; they do not need debridement if only a dry eschar is present. Wounds should be cleaned initially and at each dressing change by a nontraumatic technique. Normal saline rather than peroxide or povidone-iodine is best. Selection of a dressing should ensure that the ulcer tissue remains moist and the surrounding skin dry.

Occlusive dressings such as film and hydrocolloid dressings are often utilized. Surgical debridement with reconstructive procedures may be necessary. Adjuvant therapies such as ultrasound, laser, ultraviolet, hyperbaric oxygen, the application of growth factors, cultured kerati-nocyte grafts, skin substitutes, and miscellaneous topical and oral agents are being investigated to determine their place in the treatment of these ulcers. Electrical stimulation of refractory stage III and IV ulcers may be beneficial.

At times anaerobic organisms colonize these ulcers and cause a putrid odor. Witkowski et al have shown that topical metronidazole applications eliminated this odor within 36 hours, and that by 5 days, the anaerobic cultures were negative.

Friction Blisters

The formation of vesicles or bullae may occur at sites of combined pressure and friction and may be enhanced by heat and moisture. The feet of military recruits in training, the palms of oarsmen who have not yet developed protective calluses, and beginning drummers ("drummer's digits") are examples of those at risk. The size of the bulla depends on the site of the trauma. If the skin is tense and uncomfortable, the blister should be drained, but the roof should not be completely removed as it may act as its own dressing. In studies on long distance runners and soldiers an acrylic fiber sock (Thor-lo) was found to prevent blisters effectively. The drying action and differential sock thickness of this brand were felt to be important in its success.

Fracture Blisters

These blisters occur overlying sites of closed fractures, especially the ankle. They appear a few days to 3 weeks after the injury, are felt to be caused by vascular compromise and may create complications such as infec-

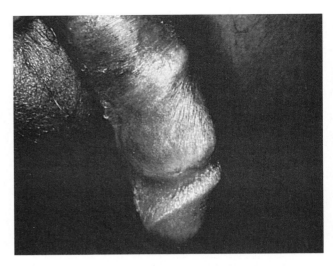

Fig. 3-27 Firm linear cord of sclerosing lymphangitis in coronal sulcus of penis. (Courtesy Dr. Axel W. Hoke.)

tion. They generally heal spontaneously in 5 to 14 days but may result in delay of surgical reduction of the fracture.

Sclerosing Lymphangiitis

This lesion is a cordlike structure encircling the coronal sulcus of the penis, or running the length of the shaft (Fig. 3-27), that has been attributed to trauma during vigorous sexual play. It is produced by a sclerosing lymphangiitis. Treatment is not necessary; it follows a benign, self-limiting course.

Black Heel

Synonyms for black heel include *talon noir, calcaneal petechiae,* and *chromidrose plantaire.* A sudden shower of minute, black, punctate macules occurs most often on the posterior edge of the plantar surface of one or both heels but sometimes distally on one or more toes. Black heel is often seen in basketball, volleyball, tennis, or lacrosse players. Seeming confluence may lead to mimicry of melanoma. The bleeding is caused by shearing stress of sports activities. Paring with a No. 15 blade and perform-ing a guaiac test will confirm the diagnosis. Treatment is unnecessary.

Subcutaneous Emphysema

Free air occurring in the subcutaneous tissues is detected by the presence of cutaneous crepitations. This raises the fear of infection with gas-producing organisms, especially clos-tridial gas gangrene, or leakage of free air from the lungs or gastrointestinal tract. Samlaska et al reviewed the wide variety of causes of subcutaneous emphysema including penetrating and nonpenetrating injuries, iatrogenic causes occurring during various procedures in hospitalized patients, spontaneous pneumomediastinum such as may occur with a violent cough, childbirth, asthma, Boerhaave's

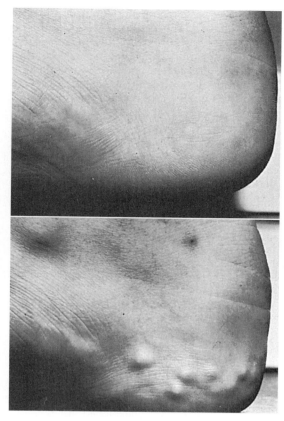

Fig. 3-28 Fat herniation. Papules appear as pressure is put on heel ("piezogenic"). (From Shelley WB, et al: Painful feet due to herniation and fat. *JAMA* 1968, 205:308.)

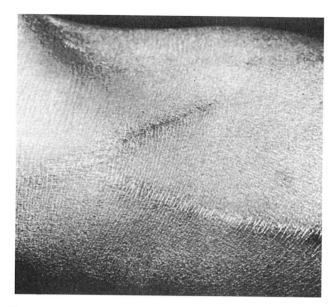

Fig. 3-29 Narcotic dermopathy "tracks"—from phlebitis following intravenous injections of heroin. (Courtesy Dr. Axel W. Hoke.)

syndrome (esophageal rupture after vomiting), or the Heimlich maneuver, intraabdominal causes, such as inflammatory bowel disease, cancer, perirectal abscess, pancreatitis, or cystitis, and factitial disease.

Traumatic Asphyxia

Lowe et al reviewed the skin findings associated with prolonged crushing injuries of the thorax or upper abdomen that reverses blood flow in the superior vena cava or its tributaries. It is characterized by cervicofacial cyanosis and edema, multiple petechiae of the face, neck, and upper chest, and bilateral subconjunctival hemorrhage.

Painful Fat Herniation

Also called *painful piezogenic pedal papules,* this rare cause of painful feet represents fat herniations through thin fascial layers of the weight-bearing parts of the heel. These dermatoceles become apparent when weight is placed on the heel and disappear as soon as the pressure is removed (Fig. 3-28). The extrusion of the fat tissue together with its blood vessels and nerves initiates pain on prolonged standing. Avoidance of prolonged standing is the only means of obtaining relief from this pain. These fat herniations are

present in many people but no symptoms are experienced by the majority. Laing et al found 76% of 29 subjects had pedal papules, and interestingly, by placing pressure on the wrists found 86% to have piezogenic wrist papules.

Narcotic Dermopathy

Heroin (diacetylmorphine) is a narcotic prepared for injection by dissolving the heroin powder in boiling water and then injecting it. The favored route of administration is intravenous. This results in thrombosed, cordlike, thickened veins at the sites of injection (Fig. 3-29). Subcutaneous injection ("skin popping") can result in multiple, scattered ulcerations, which heal with discrete atrophic scars (Fig. 3-30). In addition, amphetamines, cocaine, and other drugs may be injected. Subcutaneous injection may result in infections, complications of bacterial abscess and cellulitis or sterile nodules, apparently acute foreign body reactions to the injected drug, or the adulterants mixed with it. These lesions may ulcerate (Fig. 3-31). Chronic persistent, firm nodules, a combination of scar and foreign body reaction, may result. If cocaine is being injected it may cause ulcers because of its direct vasospastic effect. Addicts will continue to inject heroin and cocaine into the chronic ulcer bed.

The cutaneous manifestations of injection of heroin and other drugs also include camptodactylia, edema of the eyelids, persistent nonpitting edema of the hands, urticaria, abscesses, atrophic scars, and hyperpigmentation. Intramuscular pentazocine abuse leads to a typical clinical picture of tense, woody fibrosis, irregular punched-out ulcerations, and a rim of hyperpigmentation at the sites of injections.

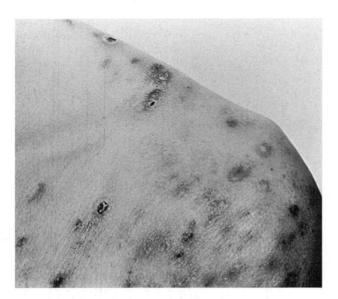

Fig. 3-30 Narcotic dermopathy: scars from "skin popping"—injecting deliberately darkened heroin intracutaneously. (Courtesy Dr. Axel W. Hoke.)

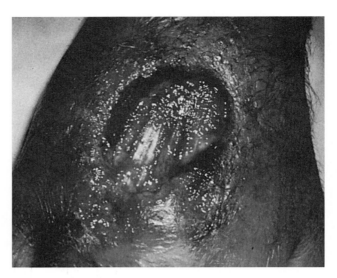

Fig. 3-31 Narcotic dermopathy: ulcer from extravascular injection of "speed" (amphetamine). (Courtesy Dr. Axel W. Hoke.)

Extensive calcification may occur within the thickened sites.

FOREIGN BODY REACTIONS
Tattoo

Tattooing is the introduction of insoluble pigments into the skin to produce permanent inscriptions and figures. Pigment is applied to the skin and then needles pierce the skin to force the material into the dermis. The pigments inserted may be carmine, indigo, vermilion, India ink, chrome green, manganese, Venetian Red, aluminum, titanium or zinc oxide, lead carbonate, logwood, cobalt blue, cinnabar (mercuric sulfide), and cadmium sulfide. The latter, used for yellow color or to brighten the cinnabar red, causes photosensitive reactions.

In addition to the photosensitivity that may develop from tattoos, numerous other reactions can occur. Unsanitary tattooing methods have resulted in inoculation of syphilis, infectious hepatitis, tuberculosis, HIV, and leprosy. Occasionally the tattoo marks may become keloidal. Accidental tattoo marks may be induced by narcotic addicts who sterilize the needles for injection by flaming the needle with a lighted match. The carbon formed on the needle is then tattooed into the skin as the needle is inserted. Discoid lupus erythematosus has been reported to occur in the red-pigmented portion of tattoos. Also, sarcoid nodules and granuloma annulare–like lesions have also been seen. Dermatitis in areas of red (mercury), green (chromium), or blue (cobalt) have been described in patients patch-test positive to these metals. McFadden et al reported a patient who developed aluminum-induced granulomas in an area of purple pigment. Patients have developed this type reaction to aluminum at vaccination sites.

Treatment by excision is satisfactory when the lesions are small enough and situated so that ellipsoid excisions are feasible. Traditional treatment modalities such as dermabrasion, salabrasion, cryosurgery, tangential planing, and older lasers such as the continuous wave carbon dioxide and argon lasers cause tissue destruction and result in scarring. Laser treatment of tattoos has been successful with the Q-switched lasers, which allows for removal of tattoos without scarring. Anderson et al reported five patients' white, flesh-colored and pink-red cosmetic tattoos darkened after treatment. Apparently, ferrous oxide is formed and patients should be forewarned of this potential adverse result.

Paraffinoma (Sclerosing Lipogranuloma)

At one time the injection of paraffin into the skin for cosmetic purposes, such as the smoothing of wrinkles and the augmentation of breasts, was popular. Injection of oils such as paraffin, camphorated oil, cottonseed or sesame oil, and beeswax may produce plaquelike indurations with ulcerations after a time lapse (Fig. 3-32). Another reaction may be inflammatory, with mild erysipeloid attacks and marked tenderness. Human adjuvant disease, which usually presents with scleroderma-like findings, may also occur. Present treatment methods are unsatisfactory. When these tumors are treated surgically it is necessary to remove them widely and completely.

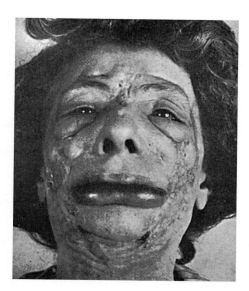

Fig. 3-32   Paraffinoma. The masses fluoresce under a Wood's light.

Granulomas

Silicone Granuloma. Liquid silicones, composed of long chains of dimethyl siloxy groups, are biologically inert. They have been used for the correction of wrinkles, for the reduction of scars, and for building up of atrophic depressed areas of the skin. For breast augmentation, it was also used as silastic implants. If trauma causes rupture of the bag, subcutaneous fibrotic nodules develop. Human adjuvant disease and sclerodermatous reactions after such events have been reported; however, large reviews have failed to establish an etiologic link to silicone and connective tissue disease. These implants are no longer available in the United States.

Bioplastique consists of polymerized silicone particles dispersed in a gel carrier. When used for lip augmentation, nodules may develop. Histologically, these are foreign body granulomas.

Mercury Granuloma. Lupton et al reviewed these lesions, which occur as foreign-body giant cell granulomas. Systemic toxicity may develop from cutaneous injury and may result in death.

Beryllium Granuloma. This is seen as a chronic, persistent, granulomatous inflammation of the skin with ulceration which may follow accidental laceration by an old-fashioned broken fluorescent lightbulb coated with zinc beryllium silicate. Modern bulbs do not contain beryllium.

Zirconium Granuloma. This papular eruption involving the axillae is sometimes seen as an allergic reaction in those shaving their armpits and using a deodorant containing zirconium lactate. Although zirconium was eliminated from aerosol-type deodorants in 1978, Skelton et al and Mon-

temarano et al reported the occurrence of a hypersensitive granuloma to aluminum-zirconium complex in antiperspirants. It may also be seen following the application of various poison ivy lotions containing zirconium compounds. The lesions are brownish red, dome-shaped, shiny papules suggestive of sarcoidosis. This is an acquired, delayed-type, allergic reaction resulting in a granuloma of the sarcoidal type. After many months the lesions involute spontaneously.

Silica Granuloma. Automobile and other types of accidents may produce tattooing of dirt (silicon dioxide) into the skin, which induces silica granulomas. These are usually black or blue papules or macules arranged in a linear fashion and are extremely unsightly, especially on the face. At times the granulomatous reaction to silica may be delayed for many years, until sensitization develops, and the ensuing dermatitis may be both chronic and disfiguring. They may be caused by amorphous or crystalline silicon dioxide (quartz), by magnesium silicate (talcum) or by complex polysilicates (asbestos). Talcum granulomas of the skin and peritoneum may develop after surgical operations from the talcum powder used on surgical gloves. Kasper et al present evidence of talc granulomas surrounding silicone gel–containing breast implants.

The removal of these granulomas is fraught with difficulties. The best method of care is immediate and complete removal to prevent these reactions. Excision and systemic steroids have been used but recurrences are common. Borenmyer et al report that some reactions may subside spontaneously after 1 to 12 months. Dermabrasion is a satisfactory method for the removal of dirt accidentally embedded into the skin of the face or scalp.

Carbon Stain

Discoloration of the skin from embedded carbon usually occurs in children from the careless use of firearms or firecrackers or from a puncture wound by a pencil, which may leave a permanent black mark of embedded graphite, easily mistaken for a metastatic melanoma. The carbon is deposited at various depths to produce a connective tissue reaction and even keloids.

Carbon particles may be removed immediately after their deposition by the use of a toothbrush and forceps. This expeditious and meticulous early care results in the best possible cosmetic result. If the particles are left in place long enough, they are best removed by the use of the Q-switched neodymium-YAG laser. Suzuki reported success in 50 of 51 treated tattoos with an average of 1.7 treatments. Alternatively, dermabrasion may be used.

Injectable Collagen Reactions

Barr et al reviewed the granulomatous reactions one may encounter with injectable enzyme-digested purified bovine collagen solution. The major histologic differential diagnosis is granuloma annulare. Hanke et al reported abscess formation and local necrosis of the glabellar region after Zyderm or Zyplast collagen injections. This may be on a vascular basis. These were both rare—on the order of 4 to 9 per 10,000 patients. Artecoll consists of polymethylmethacrylate microspheres suspended in bovine collagen. Palpable thickening and nodules may occur when it is used for lip augmentation. Histologically, they are granulomas.

Abidin MA, et al: Injection of illicit drugs into the granulation tissue of chronic ulcers. *Ann Plast Surg* 1990, 24:268.

Alper JC, et al: Use of vapor-permeable membrane for cutaneous ulcers: details of application and side effects. *J Am Acad Dermatol* 1984, 11:858.

Alster T: Cosmetic laser surgery. *Adv Dermatol* 1996, 11:51.

Anderson RR, et al: Cosmetic tattoo ink darkening. *Arch Dermatol* 1993, 129:1010.

Ballo F, et al: Fracture blisters. *J Am Acad Dermatol* 1994, 30:1033.

Barr RJ, et al: Delayed skin test reaction to injectable collagen implant (Zyderm). *J Am Acad Dermatol* 1984, 10:652.

Barr RJ, et al: Necrobiotic granulomas in bovine collagen test injection sites. *J Am Acad Dermatol* 1982, 6:867.

Bergstrom N, et al: Pressure ulcer treatment: clinical practice guideline No 15, Rockville, MD, USDHHS, PHS, Agency for Health Care Policy and Research. AHCPR Pub No 95-0563, December 1994.

Bito L, et al: Unusual complications of mercurial (cinnabar) tattoo. *Arch Dermatol* 1967, 96:165.

Bohlerk et al: Treatment of traumatic tattoos with various brushes. *J Am Acad Dermatol* 1992, 26:749.

Borenmyer DA, et al: Spontaneous resolution of silica granuloma. *J Am Acad Dermatol* 1990, 23:322.

Borglund E, et al: Classification of peristomial skin changes in patients with urostomy. *J Am Acad Dermatol* 1988, 19:623.

Brod M, et al: A randomized comparison of poly-HEMA and hydrocolloid dressings for treatment of pressure sores. *Arch Dermatol* 1990, 126:969.

Erickson JG, et al: Surfer's nodules and other complications of surfboarding. *JAMA* 1967, 201:134.

Furner BB: Parenteral pentazocine. *J Am Acad Dermatol* 1990, 22:694.

Gibbs RC, et al: Abnormal biomechanics of the feet and the cause of hyperkeratoses. *J Am Acad Dermatol* 1982, 6:1061.

Goldberg NS, et al: Perianal pseudoverrucous papules and nodules on children. *Arch Dermatol* 1992, 128:240.

Hanke CW, et al: Abscess formation and local necrosis after treatment with Zyderm or Zyplast collagen implant. *J Am Acad Dermatol* 1991, 25:319.

Heng MCY, et al: Erythematous cutaneous nodules caused by adulterated cocaine. *J Am Acad Dermatol* 1989, 21:520.

Herring KM, et al: Friction blisters and sock fiber composition. *J Am Podiatr Med Assoc* 1990, 80:63.

Hoffman C, et al: Adverse reactions after cosmetic lip augmentation with permanent biologically inert implant materials. *J Am Acad Dermatol* 1999, 40:106.

James WD, et al: Treatment of wounds received during live fire exercises. *J Assoc Milit Dermatol* 1984, 10:32.

Kanj LF, et al: Pressure ulcers. *J Am Acad Dermatol* 1998, 38:517.

Kasper CS, et al: Talc deposition in skin and tissues surrounding silicone-gel containing prosthetic devices. *Arch Dermatol* 1994, 130:48.

Kilmer L, et al: The Q-Switched ND:YAG laser effectively treats tattoos. *Arch Dermatol* 1993, 129:971.

Kirsch N: Malignant melanoma developing in a tattoo. *Arch Dermatol* 1967, 99:596.

Laing VB, et al: Piezogenic wrist papules. *J Am Acad Dermatol* 1991, 24:415.

Lazarus GS, et al: Definitions and guidelines for assessment of wounds and evaluation of healing. *Arch Dermatol* 1994, 130:489.

Lerchin E, et al: Discoid lupus erythematosus occurring in red pigment of tattoos. *J Assoc Milit Dermatol* 1976, 1:19.

Leventhal LC, et al: An asymptomatic penile lesion (circular indurated lymphangitis). *Arch Dermatol* 1993, 129:365.

Levine JJ, et al: Sclerodermalike esophageal disease in children breast-fed by mothers with silicone breast implants. *J Am Acad Dermatol* 1994, 271:213.

Lowe L, et al: Traumatic asphyxia. *J Am Acad Dermatol* 1990, 23:972.

Lupton GP, et al: Cutaneous mercury granuloma. *J Am Acad Dermatol* 1985, 12:296.

Magee KL, et al: Extensive calcinosis as a late complication of pentazoane injections. *Arch Dermatol* 1991, 127:159l.

McFadden N, et al: Aluminum induced granuloma in a tattoo. *J Am Acad Dermatol* 1989, 20:903.

Minkin W, et al: Dermatologic complications of heroin addiction. *N Engl J Med* 1967, 277:473.

Modojana RM, et al: Porokeratosis plantaris discreta. *J Am Acad Dermatol* 1984, 10:679.

Monry RG, et al: Cutaneous silica granuloma. *Arch Dermatol* 1991, 127:692.

Montemarano AD, et al: Cutaneous granulomas caused by an aluminum-zirconium complex. *J Am Acad Dermatol* 1997, 37:496.

Padilla RS, et al: Cutaneous and venous complications of pentazocine abuse. *Arch Dermatol* 1979, 115:975.

Posner DI, et al: Cutaneous foreign body granulomas associated with intravenous drug abuse. *J Am Acad Dermatol* 1985, 13:869.

Rimmer S, et al: Dermatologic problems of musicians. *J Am Acad Dermatol* 1990, 22:657.

Sahn EE, et al: Scleroderma following augmentation mammoplasty. *Arch Dermatol* 1990, 120:1198.

Samlaska CP, et al: Subcutaneous emphysema. *Adv Dermatol* 1996, 11:117.

Sau P, et al: Cutaneous reaction from a broken thermometer. *J Am Acad Dermatol* 1991, 25:915.

Signore RJ: Dermatologic problems of musicians. *J Am Acad Dermatol* 1991, 24:321.

Skelton HG, et al: Zirconium granuloma resulting from an aluminum zirconium complex. *J Am Acad Dermatol* 1993, 28:874.

Suzuki H: Treatment of traumatic tattoos with the Q-switched neodymium: YAG laser. *Arch Dermatol* 1996, 132:1226.

Varga J, et al: Augmentation mammoplasty and scleroderma. *Arch Dermatol* 1990, 126:1221.

Verbov JL, et al: Talar callosity. *Clin Exp Dermatol* 1991, 16:118.

Witkowski JA, et al: Topical metronidazole gel. *Int J Dermatol* 1991, 126:1221.

Wood SM, et al: A multicenter study of the use of pulsed low-intensity direct current for healing chronic stage II and III decubitus ulcers. *Arch Dermatol* 1993, 129:999.

Yarkony GM, et al: Classification of pressure ulcers. *Arch Dermatol* 1990, 126:1218. ▲

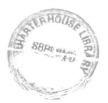

CHAPTER 4

Pruritus and Neurocutaneous Dermatoses

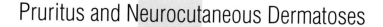

PRURITUS

Pruritus, commonly known as itching, is a sensation exclusive to the skin. It may be defined as the sensation that produces the desire to scratch. It has been determined that there are no specific anatomic fibers for each of the cutaneous sensations, but rather that itch, touch, temperature (hot and cold), and pain sensations are all mediated by the same receptors. These sensations arise in fine unmyelinated C nerve fiber endings in the subepidermal area and are then transmitted via the lateral spinothalamic tract to the thalamus and sensory cortex. Central itch mechanisms may be as important as peripheral cutaneous mediators, as suggested by the increased effectiveness of sedating over nonsedating antihistamines in the treatment of atopic dermatitis and the reported success of parenteral administration of naloxone in patients with severe cholestasis.

Itching may be elicited by many normally occurring stimuli, such as light touch, temperature change, and emotional stress. Chemical, mechanical, thermal, and electrical stimuli may also elicit itching. Pruritus is mediated by the release of chemical substances such as histamine, kinins, and proteases. Prostaglandin E lowers the threshold for histamine-induced pruritus, while enkephalins, pentapeptides which bind to opiate receptors in the brain, modulate pain and itching centrally. Substance P is an 11 amino acid peptide that has been implicated in causing itching in some disorders. There are no specific antagonists of substance P; however, capsaicin depletes cutaneous nociceptor nerve endings of substance P after repeated topical application. The use of 5-hydroxytryptamine (5-HT), which may regulate specific 5-HT receptors and blocking by antagonists, such as ondansetron, has been therapeutic in treating cholestatic itching disorders. Interleukins have also been implicated, particularly in atopic dermatitis.

Patterns of Itching

There are great variations from person to person; indeed, in the same person there may be a variation in reactions to the same stimulus. Psychologic trauma, stress, absence of distractions, anxiety, and fear may all enhance itching. It is apt to be most severe at the time of undressing for bed. Variations also occur by regions of the skin. The ear canals, eyelids, nostrils, and perianal and genital areas are especially susceptible to pruritus.

Bernhard JD, editor: Itch: mechanisms and management of pruritus. New York, 1994, McGraw-Hill.

Greaves MW: New pathophysiological and clinical insights into pruritus. *J Dermatol* 1993, 20:735.

Greaves MW, et al: Pathophysiology of itching. *Lancet* 1996, 348:938.

▲

Treatment

There are many oral agents available to treat pruritus. The tricyclic antidepressants are potent H_1 antagonists, and as such may be effective in certain forms of pruritus. Doxepin, in both oral and topical forms, and amitriptyline can be used for control of pruritus when topical therapy and standard antihistamines are insufficient. Antihistamines, especially promethazine, trimeprazine, diphenhydramine, hydroxyzine, methdilazine, and azatadine maleate are first-line therapies. Second-generation, nonsedating H_1 antagonists such as loratadine, fexofenadine, acrivastine, azelastine, and cetirizine may also be effective; however, the value of nonsedating antihistamines in the treatment of pruritus other than urticaria is not well studied.

Relief of pruritus with topical remedies may be accomplished with the use of numerous medications. Application of an ice bag or the opposite, a hot water bottle, to the affected area is a primitive but sometimes effective remedy—especially when nothing else is available. The "caine" preparations, such as benzocaine, procaine, and lidocaine (Xylocaine) 5% ointments, are excellent antipruritics, but prolonged use may produce contact sensitization. Topical doxepin cream or pramoxine may be effective for mild pruritus when used alone. Their best use appears to be in combination with topical steroids whose antipruritic effects they potentiate. Lotions containing phenol (Sarna), menthol, or camphor are effective topical antipruritics when used with or without topical steroids.

In the severest forms of recalcitrant pruritus, such as that found in HIV disease, chronic renal failure, and liver disease, intravenous lidocaine may be effective. The practical use of lidocaine, however, is limited by its short duration of action, often only a few hours, and because it may cause hypotension. Naloxone and ondansetron have been used successfully in treating the pruritus of cholestasis. The value of these agents in the treatment of other chronic pruritic dermatoses has been suggested but are yet to be defined. Downs et al reported a successful response of recalcitrant palmoplantar pruritus to 8 mg/day of ondansetron hydrochloride.

Downs AMR, et al: Successful treatment of intractable palmoplantar pruritus with ondansetron. *Arch Dermatol* 1998, 134:925.

Drake LA, et al: The antipruritic effect of 5% doxepin cream in patients with eczematous dermatitis. *Arch Dermatol* 1996, 132:1130.

Fishman SM, et al: Intravenous lidocaine for treatment-resistant pruritus. *Am J Med* 1997, 102:584.

Meltzer EO: Comparative safety of H₁ antihistamines. *Ann Allergy* 1991, 67:625. _____ ▲

Paroxysmal Pruritus

Severe, persistent, or recurrent pruritus, with or without prior skin lesions, is often paroxysmal in character: sudden in onset, irresistibly severe, frequently awakening the patient, and stopping instantly and completely as soon as pain is induced by scratching. The pleasure of scratching is so intense that the patient—despite the realization that he or she is damaging the skin—is often unable to stop short of inflicting such damage.

Itching of this distinctive type is characteristic of only a few dermatoses: lichen simplex chronicus, atopic dermatitis, nummular eczema, dermatitis herpetiformis, neurotic excoriations, eosinophilic folliculitis, uremic pruritus, subacute prurigo, and prurigo nodularis. In general, only these disorders produce such intense pruritus and scratching as to induce bleeding. In individual cases, other diseases may manifest such severe symptoms. Koeppel et al reported a case of paroxysmal pruritus in a patient with multiple sclerosis. Magnetic resonance imaging of the cervical spinal cord showed a lesion at a level corresponding to the dermatomal location of the pruritus.

Arnold HL, Jr: Paroxysmal pruritus. *J Am Acad Dermatol* 1984, 11:322.

Koeppel MC, et al: Paroxysmal pruritus and multiple sclerosis. *Br J Dermatol* 1993, 129:597. _____ ▲

Internal Causes of Pruritus

Itching may be present as a symptom in a number of internal disorders. The intensity and duration of itching vary from one disease to another. Among the most important internal causes of itching are liver disease (especially obstructive), hepatitis C (with or without evidence of jaundice or liver failure), renal failure (uremic pruritus), hypothyroidism and hyperthyroidism, iron-deficiency anemia, intestinal parasites, polycythemia vera, malignant lymphoma (especially Hodgkin's disease), leukemia, myeloma, internal malignancies, carcinoid, multiple sclerosis, and neuropsychiatric diseases (anorexia nervosa). Diabetes mellitus is frequently listed as an internal cause of pruritus. Most persons with diabetes do not itch. If a diabetic patient has pruritus with no primary skin lesions, other causes of pruritus should be investigated.

The pruritus of Hodgkin's disease is usually continuous and at times is accompanied by severe burning. The incidence of pruritus is between 10% and 25% and is the first symptom of this disease in 7% of patients. Its cause is unknown. The pruritus of leukemia, except for chronic lymphocytic leukemia, has a tendency to be generalized and less severe than in Hodgkin's disease.

It has been reported that internal cancer may be found in 3% to 47% of patients with generalized pruritus that is unexplained by skin lesions. However, Paul et al confirmed the finding of Kantor et al that no significant overall increase of malignant neoplasms can be found in patients with idiopathic pruritus, and no general efforts at cancer screening are warranted. A suggested workup for chronic, generalized pruritus includes taking a complete history and performing a thorough physical examination; tests include a CBC and differential, thyroid, liver, and renal panels, hepatitis C serology, and chest x-ray evaluation.

Fisher DA, et al: Pruritus as a symptom of hepatitis C. *J Am Acad Dermatol* 1995, 32:629.

Kantor GR, et al: Generalized pruritus and systemic disease. *J Am Acad Dermatol* 1983, 9:375.

Lober CW: Pruritus and malignancy. *Clin Dermatol* 1993, 11:125.

Paul R, et al: Itch and malignancy prognosis in generalized pruritus: a 6-year follow-up of 125 patients. *J Am Acad Dermatol* 1987, 16:1179.

Peterson AO, et al: Pruritus and nonspecific nodules preceding myelomonocytic leukemia. *J Am Acad Dermatol* 1980, 2:496.

Taniguchi S, et al: Generalized pruritus in anorexia nervosa. *Br J Dermatol* 1996, 134:510.

Valsecchi R, et al: Generalized pruritus: a manifestation of iron deficiency. *Arch Dermatol* 1983, 119:630. _____ ▲

Polycythemia Vera

More than one third of patients with polycythemia vera report pruritus; it is usually induced by temperature changes. There is no correlation with circulating basophils or whole-blood histamine levels. The cause is unknown.

Aspirin has been shown to provide immediate relief from itching; however, there is a risk of hemorrhagic complications, and low doses are recommended. Jeanmougin et al have reported good responses to PUVA. Interferon alfa-2b has been shown to be effective for treating the underlying disease and associated pruritus. Myelosuppressive therapy is useful for long-term control of symptoms. Conventional therapy, such as antihistamines and H$_2$ blockers, are usually ineffective.

Jackson N, et al: Skin mast cells in polycythemia vera: relationship to the pathogenesis and treatment of pruritus. *Br J Dermatol* 1987, 116:21.

Jeanmougin M, et al: Efficacy of photochemotherapy on severe pruritus in polycythemia vera. *Ann Hematol* 1996, 73:91.

Muller EW, et al: Long-term treatment with interferon-alpha 2b for severe pruritus in patients with polycythaemia vera. *Br J Haematol* 1995, 89:313. ▲

Biliary Pruritus

Chronic liver disease with obstructive jaundice may cause severe generalized pruritus; 20% to 50% of patients with jaundice have pruritus. This itching is probably caused by central mechanisms. This is suggested by elevated CNS opioid peptide levels, down-regulation of opioid peptide CNS receptors, and the therapeutic effectiveness of naloxone. The serum-conjugated bile acid levels do not correlate with the severity of pruritus.

Primary Biliary Cirrhosis. Primary biliary cirrhosis occurs almost exclusively in women older than 30 years of age. Itching may begin insidiously; with time, extreme pruritus develops. This almost intolerable itching is accompanied by jaundice and a striking melanotic hyperpigmentation of the entire skin; the patient may turn almost black, except for a hypopigmented "butterfly" area in the upper back (Fig. 4-1). Xanthomatosis in the form of plane xanthomas of the palms, xanthelasmas, and tuberous xanthomas over the joints may be seen.

Dark urine, steatorrhea, and osteoporosis occur frequently. The serum bilirubin, alkaline phosphatase, serum ceruloplasmin, serum hyaluronate, and cholesterol values are increased. The antimitochondrial antibody test is positive.

The disease is usually relentlessly progressive with the development of hepatic failure and esophageal varices. The latter may produce hemorrhage and even death. Several cases have been accompanied by scleroderma.

To treat the pruritus, randomized placebo-controlled studies have shown cholestyramine, rifampin, naloxone, S-adenosylmethionine, prednisolone, colchicine, ursodeoxycholic acid, and propofol to be effective in treating primary biliary cirrhosis as well as other forms of hepatobiliary pruritus. Vuoristo et al reported significant improvement in pruritus in patients treated with ursodeoxycholic acid over colchicine. In an open trial, Bergasa et al showed responses in pruritus and fatigue symptoms in patients treated with low-dose methotrexate, but only in patients with early disease.

Liver transplantation is becoming more common for patients with primary biliary cirrhosis. In a series by Navasa evaluating 29 patients, jaundice (96%) and pruritus (92%) were the most frequent symptoms before transplantation.

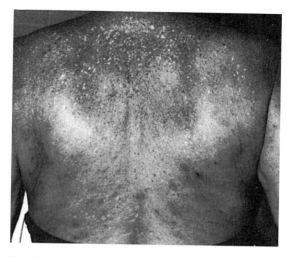

Fig. 4-1 Melanotic pigmentation and depigmentation, and excoriations, caused by intractable generalized pruritus from primary biliary cirrhosis, in a 50-year-old woman.

Twenty-six of the 29 patients survived 2 years after surgery and 76% noted improved well-being, decreased pruritus, and increased ability to perform usual daily activities. Currently liver transplantation is the only definitive treatment available for end-stage disease.

Bergasa NV, et al: Pilot study of low dose oral methotrexate treatment for primary biliary cirrhosis. *Am J Gastroenterol* 1996, 91:295.

Coyle S, et al: Hepatobiliary pruritus: what are effective treatments? *J Am Acad Dermatol* 1995, 33:801.

Goldman RD, et al: The "butterfly" sign. *Arch Dermatol* 1983, 119:183.

Heathcote J: Treatment of primary biliary cirrhosis. *J Gastroenterol Hepatol* 1996, 11:605.

Jones EA, et al: The pathogenesis and treatment of pruritus and fatigue in patients with PBC. *Eur J Gastroenterol Hepatol* 1999, 11:623.

Jones EA, et al: The pruritus of cholestasis and the opioid system. *JAMA* 1992, 268:3359.

Navasa M, et al: Quality of life, major medical complications and hospital service utilization in patients with primary biliary cirrhosis after liver transplantation. *J Hepatol* 1996, 25:129.

Vuoristo M, et al: A placebo-controlled trial of primary biliary cirrhosis treatment with colchicine and ursodeoxycholic acid. *Gastroenterology* 1995, 108:1470. ▲

Chronic Renal Failure and Uremic Pruritus

Chronic renal failure is the most common internal systemic cause of pruritus; 15% to 49% of patients with chronic renal failure have pruritic symptoms. Fifty percent to 90% of patients undergoing dialysis will develop pruritus within 6 months after initiation of therapy, and 65% will experience persistent itching. Uremic pruritus is often generalized, intractable, and severe. Dialysis-associated pruritus may be episodic, mild, or localized to the dialysis catheter site, face, or legs, and effective dialysis does not always improve the itching.

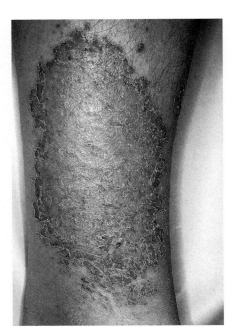

Fig. 4-2 Asteatotic eczema.

The mechanism of pruritus associated with chronic renal failure and uremia may be multifactorial. Xerosis, atrophy of the sweat glands, secondary hyperparathyroidism, increased serum histamine levels, hypervitaminosis A, iron-deficiency anemia, and neuropathy have been implicated. Substance P may be an important neurotransmitter in uremic pruritus. Complications such as Kyrle's disease, lichen simplex chronicus, and prurigo nodularis may develop and contribute to the degree and severity of pruritus.

A systematic approach is recommended by Robertson et al. Renal dialysis should be optimized, and patients with a sensitivity to ethylene oxide should be identified. Dietary restrictions and phosphate-binding therapy should be encouraged. Anemia is best treated with erythropoietin. If xerosis is detected, use of emollients should be emphasized. The use of topical capsaicin cream may be beneficial. Antihistamines or ketotifen (2 mg orally twice daily) can be useful. If pruritus persists, UVB therapy may be attempted (with caution in patients receiving photosensitizing drugs). In recalcitrant disease, the next options include cholestyramine, activated charcoal, and finally, combination therapy consisting of UVB and cholestyramine or activated charcoal. Thalidomide and intravenous lidocaine have also been used.

Breneman DL, et al: Topical capsaicin for treatment of hemodialysis-related pruritus. *J Am Acad Dermatol* 1992, 26:91.

Liu HN, et al: Uremic pruritus: roles of parathyroid hormone and substance P. *J Am Acad Dermatol* 1997, 36:538.

Peer G, et al: Randomized crossover trial of naltrexone in uraemic pruritus. *Lancet* 1996, 348:1552.

Robertson KE, et al: Uremic pruritus. *Am J Health Syst Pharm* 1996, 53:2159.

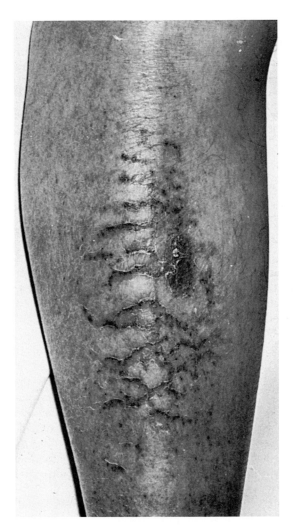

Fig. 4-3 Eczema craquelé, weeping and crusted.

Tan JK, et al: Identifying effective treatments for uremic pruritus. *J Am Acad Dermatol* 1991, 25:811. _____ ▲

PRURITIC DERMATOSES
Winter Itch

Asteatotic eczema, eczema craquelé, pruritus hiemalis, and xerotic eczema are other names given to this pruritic condition. It is characterized by generalized body pruritus that is usually most severe on the arms and shins (Fig. 4-2). The skin is dry, and fine flakes are often generalized, but the condition tends to spare the face, scalp, groin, and axilla. The pretibial regions are particularly susceptible and may develop eczema craquelé, exhibiting fine cracks in the eczematous area that resemble the cracks in old porcelain dishes (Fig. 4-3).

Frequent and lengthy bathing with plenty of soap during the wintertime is the most frequent cause. This is especially prevalent in elderly persons, whose skin has a decreased rate of repair of the epidermal water barrier. Low humidity in overheated rooms during cold weather contributes to this condition. In a study of 584 elderly individuals, the prevalence of asteatosis (28.9%) was second to seborrheic dermatitis as the most common finding.

Treatment consists of educating the patient regarding the factors listed, using soap only in the axilla and inguinal area, and lubrication of the skin immediately after bathing with bath oils. Lactic acid preparations such as 12% ammonium lactate lotion (Lac-Hydrin) are helpful after-bath applications for some patients. However, lactic acid preparations may cause irritation and worsening of itching in patients with erythema and eczema.

Rogers RS III, et al: Comparative efficacy of 12% ammonium lactate lotion and 5% lactic acid lotion in the treatment of moderate to severe xerosis. *J Am Acad Dermatol* 1990, 23:769.

Weismann K, el al: Prevalence of skin diseases in old age. *Acta Derm Venereol* 1980, 60:352. ▲

Pruritus Ani

Pruritus is often centered in the anal or genital area (less commonly, in both), with little or no pruritus elsewhere. Anal neurodermatitis is characterized by paroxysms of violent itching, at which time the patient may tear at the affected area until bleeding is induced. Manifestations are identical with those of lichen simplex chronicus elsewhere on the body. One should always search thoroughly for other etiologic factors.

Allergic contact dermatitis from local anesthetics used in suppositories for hemorrhoids or irritational contact dermatitis from gastrointestinal contents, such as hot spices or cathartics; or failure to adequately cleanse the area after bowel movements may be causes. Anatomic factors may lead to leakage of rectal mucus onto perianal skin and thus promote irritation. Physical changes such as hemorrhoids, anal tags, fissures, and fistulas may aggravate or produce pruritus. Anal warts and condyloma latum (syphilis) may be causative agents, although these rarely itch. Anal gonorrhea, especially in men, is frequently overlooked when pruritus is the only symptom.

Mycotic pruritus ani is characterized by fissures and white, sodden epidermis. Scrapings from the anal area are examined directly with potassium hydroxide mounts for fungi. Cultures for fungi are also taken. *Candida albicans, Epidermophyton floccosum,* and *Trichophyton rubrum* are frequent causative fungi in this area. Other sites of fungal infection, such as the groin, toes, and nails, should also be investigated. Erythrasma in the groin and perianal regions may also occasionally produce pruritus. The diagnosis is established by coral red fluorescence under the Wood's light. Beta-hemolytic streptococcal infections have also been implicated. The use of tetracyclines may cause pruritus ani, most often in women, by inducing candidiasis. Diabetic patients are susceptible to perianal candidiasis.

Seborrheic dermatitis of the anal area may cause pruritus ani. It also involves other areas, such as the inguinal regions, scalp, chest, and face. Similarly, lichen planus may involve the perianal region. Anal psoriasis may cause itching. The perianal lesions are usually sharply marginated, and psoriatic lesions may be present on other parts of the body. Other frequent sites for psoriasis should be examined, such as the fingernails.

Pinworm infestations may cause pruritus ani, especially in children, and sometimes in their parents. Nocturnal pruritus is most prevalent. Other intestinal parasites such as *Taenia solium, T. saginata,* amebiasis, and *Strongyloides stercoralis* may produce pruritus. Pediculosis pubis may cause anal itching; however, attention is focused by the patient on the pubic area, where itching is most severe. A thorough examination for malignancies should be carried out; extramammary Paget's disease is easily overlooked.

Treatment

Meticulous toilet care should be followed no matter what the cause of the itching. After defecation, the anal area should be cleansed with soft cellulose tissue paper and, whenever possible, washed with mild soap and water. Cleansing with wet toilet tissue is advisable in all cases. Medicated cleansing pads such as Tucks should be used regularly. An emollient lotion, Balneol, is helpful for cleansing without producing irritation.

Except in psychogenic pruritus ani, once the etiologic agent has been found, a rational and effective treatment regimen may be started, such as antifungals and anthelminthics for fungal and helminthic disease, respectively. Topical corticosteroids are most effective for the nonfungal types of pruritus ani. Pramoxine hydrochloride, a nonsteroidal topical anesthetic, is effective, especially a lotion form combined with hydrocortisone (Pramosone).

Redondo P, et al: Pruritus ani in an elderly man. Extramammary Paget's disease. *Arch Dermatol* 1995, 131:952.

Weismann K, et al: Pruritus ani caused by beta-haemolytic streptococci. *Acta Derm Venereol* (Norway) 1996, 76:415. ▲

Pruritus Scroti

The scrotum of an adult is relatively immune to dermatophyte infection, but it is a favorite site for circumscribed neurodermatitis (lichen simplex chronicus). Psychogenic pruritus is probably the most frequent type of itching seen. Why it preferentially affects this area (and also affects the female analog, the vulva) is unclear. Lichenification may result, be extreme, and persist for many years despite intensive therapy.

Infectious conditions may complicate or cause pruritus on the scrotum but are less common than idiopathic scrotal pruritus. Fungal infections, except candidiasis, usually spare

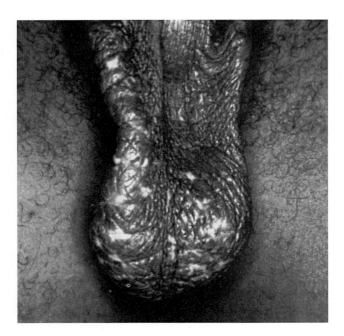

Fig. 4-4 Pruritus scroti, analogous to pruritus vulvae in a woman.

the scrotum. When candidal infection affects the scrotum, burning rather than pruritus is frequently the primary symptom. The scrotum is eroded, weepy, or crusted (Fig. 4-4). The scrotum may be secondarily and to a lesser degree affected in cases of pruritus ani, but this pruritus usually affects the midline, extending from the anus along the midline to the base of the scrotum, rather than the dependent surfaces of the scrotum, where pruritus scroti usually occurs. Scrotal pruritus may be associated with allergic contact dermatitis from gold and topical medications, including topical steroidal agents.

Topical corticosteroids are the mainstay of treatment, but caution should be exercised. "Red balls," or "addicted scrotum syndrome," is caused by the use of high-potency topical steroidal agents. Although this is usually seen after chronic use, even short-term high-potency steroid medications may produce this syndrome. As with facial skin, high-potency steroids used on the scrotum can result in addictive skin: every time the patient attempts to taper off the steroid, severe burning and redness occurs. The scrotum is frequently in contact with inner thigh skin, producing areas of occlusion, which increases the penetration and effectiveness of topical steroidal agents. For these reasons, lower potency topical steroids should be used in treating the scrotum. Topical pramoxine (Pramosone) or doxepin (Zonalon) are useful adjuncts.

Pruritus Vulvae

The vulva is also a common site for pruritus of different causes. Pruritus vulvae is the counterpart of pruritus scroti, and the same mechanisms may be responsible. In a prospec-

tive series of 141 women with chronic vulvar symptoms, the most common causes were unspecified dermatitis (54%), lichen sclerosus (13%), chronic vulvovaginal candidiasis (10%), dysesthetic vulvodynia (9%), and psoriasis (5%).

Vaginal candidiasis is a frequent cause of pruritus vulvae. This is true especially during pregnancy and when oral antibiotics are taken. The inguinal, perineal, and perianal areas may be affected. Microscopic examination for *Candida albicans* and cultures for fungus should be performed. *Trichomonas vaginitis* may cause vulvar pruritus. For the detection of *Trichomonas vaginalis,* examination of vaginal secretions is often diagnostic. The organism is recognized by its motility, its size (somewhat larger than a leukocyte), and its piriform shape.

Contact dermatitis from sanitary pads, contraceptives, douche solutions, fragrance, colophony, corticosteroids, and a partner's condoms are some of the causes of vulvar pruritus. Urinary incontinence and diabetes mellitus should also be considered. Lichen sclerosus is another frequent cause of pruritus in the genital area in middle-aged and elderly women. Lichen planus may involve the vulva, resulting in pruritus and mucosal changes, including resorption of the labia minora and atrophy.

Treatment

Candidiasis is treated with topical anticandidal agents. Fluconazole 150 mg daily for 5 days followed by 150 mg weekly for several months is effective in treating chronic vaginal candidiasis. *Trichomonas* infection is best treated with metronidazole (Flagyl) in an oral form or by vaginal inserts. Lichen sclerosus responds best to high-potency topical steroids (see Chapter 12). Topical steroidal agents may be used to treat psychogenic pruritus or irritant or allergic reactions. High-potency topical steroids are effective in treating lichen planus, but other options are also available (see Chapter 12). Topical lidocaine, pramoxine, or an oral tricyclic antidepressant may be helpful in select cases. Any chronic skin disease that does not appear to be responding to therapy should prompt a biopsy. Referral to a physician specializing in vulvar diseases should be considered for patients whose condition is unresponsive to therapy. In chronic idiopathic forms hypnosis therapy may be useful.

Eisen D, et al: The vulvovaginal-gingival syndrome of lichen planus. *Arch Dermatol* 1994, 130:1379.

Lewis FM, et al: Contact sensitivity in pruritus vulvae: a common and manageable problem. *Contact Dermatitis* (Denmark) 1994, 31:264.

Lewis FM, et al: Vulval involvement in lichen planus. *Br J Dermatol* 1996, 135:89.

Rucklidge JJ, et al: Hypnosis in a case of long-standing idiopathic itch. *Psychosom Med* 1999, 61:355. ▲

Puncta Pruritica (Itchy Points)

"Itchy points" consists of one or two intensely itching spots in clinically normal skin, sometimes followed by the appearance of seborrheic keratoses at exactly the same site. Others believe puncta pruritica is a variant of Astwarzarutow's otalgia or notalgia paresthetica. Curettage, cryosurgery, or punch biopsy of the itching point may cure the condition.

Boyd AS, et al: Puncta pruritica. *Int J Dermatol* 1992, 31:370.
Crissey JT: Puncta pruritica. *Int J Dermatol* 1991, 30:722.
Crissey JT: Puncta pruritica. *Int J Dermatol* 1992, 31:166. ━━━━━ ▲

Aquagenic Pruritus and Aquadynia

Aquagenic pruritus is itching evoked by contact with water of any temperature. Increased degranulation of mast cells and increased concentration of histamine and acetylcholine in the skin after contact with water are found. In most cases there is severe, prickling discomfort within minutes of exposure to water or on cessation of exposure to water, and there is often a family history of similar symptoms.

Aquagenic pruritus must be distinguished from xerosis or asteatosis. The condition may be associated with polycythemia vera, hypereosinophilic syndrome, juvenile xanthogranuloma, and myelodysplastic syndrome. Treatment options include the use of antihistamines, systemic steroids, sodium bicarbonate dissolved in bath water, topical capsaicin cream, transdermal nitroglycerin, propranolol, ethanol ingestion, and ultraviolet phototherapy.

Shelley et al reported two patients with widespread burning pain that lasted 15 to 45 minutes after water exposure. The authors called this reaction *aquadynia* and consider the disorder a variant of aquagenic pruritus. Clonidine and propranolol seemed to provide some relief.

du Peloux Menage H, et al: Aquagenic pruritus. *Semin Dermatol* 1995, 14:313.
Lotti T, et al: Treatment of aquagenic pruritus with topical capsaicin cream. *J Am Acad Dermatol* 1994, 30:232.
Martinez-Escribano JA, et al: Treatment of aquagenic urticaria with PUVA and astemizole. *J Am Acad Dermatol* 1997, 36:118.
Norris JF: Treatment of aquagenic pruritus with alcohol. *Br J Dermatol* 1998, 138:927.
Shelley WB, et al: Aquadynia. *J Am Acad Dermatol* 1998, 38:357.
Wolf R, et al: Variations in aquagenic pruritus and treatment alternatives. *J Am Acad Dermatol* 1988, 18:1081. ━━━━━ ▲

Scalp Pruritus

Pruritus of the scalp, especially in elderly persons, is rather common. When excoriations, scaling, or erythema is not found, seborrheic dermatitis, psoriasis, or lichen simplex chronicus cannot be diagnosed. The cause of this is unknown in most cases, but some represent chronic folliculitis. Treatment is difficult. Topical tar shampoos, salicylic acid shampoos, corticosteroid topical gels and liquids, and in severe cases, an intralesional injection of corticosteroid

suspension can sometimes provide relief. Antihistamines internally may occasionally be helpful.

Drug-Induced Pruritus

Medications should be considered a possible cause of protracted pruritus with or without a skin eruption. Osifo reported a series of 109 patients treated for malaria in which 60% developed chloroquine-induced pruritus without associated cutaneous findings. The pruritic reaction was generalized, with a peak intensity 25 hours after dosing. Antihistamines were ineffective. The pruritus at times can be severe enough to necessitate withdrawal of the medication. Others have reported chloroquine- and amodiaquine-induced pruritus in 8% to 15% of patients in the acute, febrile stages of malaria.

Hydroxyethyl starch (HES) is used as a volume expander, a substitute for human plasma. It has recently been recognized that one third of all patients so treated will develop severe pruritus with long latency of onset (3 to 15 weeks) and persistence. Up to 30% of patients have localized symptoms. Antihistamines are ineffective. HES deposits are found in the skin of all patients tested, distributed in dermal macrophages, endothelial cells of blood and lymph vessels, perineural cells, endoneural macrophages of larger nerve fascicles, keratinocytes, and Langerhans cells. Substance P release from macrophages is not increased, and basophil degranulation test results are negative, suggesting that the actions of HES-induced pruritus result from direct stimulation of cutaneous nerves.

Gall H, et al: Clinical and pathophysiological aspects of hydroxyethyl starch-induced pruritus evaluation of 96 cases. *Dermatology* (Switzerland) 1996, 192:222.
Jurecka W, et al: Hydroxyethyl starch deposits in human skin: a model for pruritus? *Arch Dermatol Res* 1993, 285:13.
Osifo NG: Chloroquine-induced pruritus among patients with malaria. *Arch Dermatol* 1984, 120:80. ━━━━━ ▲

Chronic Pruritic Dermatoses of Unknown Cause

Chronic prurigo is variously called *prurigo simplex (papular dermatitis, subacute prurigo, "itchy red bump" disease,* and *Rosen's papular eruption* in black men) (Fig. 4-5). The term *prurigo* continues to lack nosologic precision. Descriptions such as melanotic prurigo of Pierini and Borda, prurigo of Hebra, pruriginous dermatoses, prurigo mitis, and prurigo agria have been abandoned. Regional descriptions, such as reports from Europe and Japan, further add to the confusion of classification and definition.

Prurigo is characterized by the lesion known as the *prurigo papule,* which is dome-shaped and topped with a small vesicle. The vesicle is usually present only transiently because of its immediate removal by scratching, so that a crusted papule is more frequently seen. The prurigo papules are present in various stages of development and are seen mostly in middle-aged or elderly persons of both sexes. The

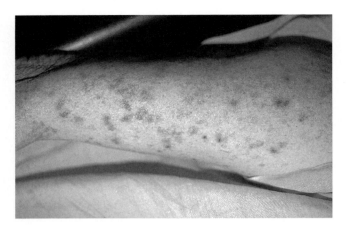

Fig. 4-5 Papular dermatitis, also called *itchy red bump disease.*

trunk and extensor surfaces of the extremities are favorite sites, symmetrically distributed. Other areas include the face, neck, lower trunk, and buttocks, and the lesions usually appear in crops, so that papulovesicles and the late stages of scarring may be seen at the same time. Papular dermatitis, subacute prurigo, "itchy red bump" disease, and Rosen's papular eruption in black men most likely represent variations of prurigo simplex. The cause is unknown.

The histopathology of prurigo simplex is nonspecific. Spongiosis accompanied by a perivascular mononuclear infiltrate with some eosinophils is often found.

Many conditions may cause pruritic erythematous papules. Scabies, atopic dermatitis, insect bite reactions, papular urticaria, dermatitis herpetiformis, contact dermatitis, pityriasis lichenoides et varioliformis acuta (PLEVA), transient acantholytic dermatosis (TAD), papuloerythroderma of Ofuji, dermatographism, and physical urticarias should be considered. Biopsy may be helpful in differentiating dermatitis herpetiformis, PLEVA, TAD, and, on occasion, scabies (a scabies preparation is less invasive).

Treatment

The medications used for initial treatment of prurigo simplex and its variants should be topical corticosteroids and oral antihistamines. Early in the disease process, moderate strength steroids should be used; if the condition is found to be unresponsive, a change to high-potency forms is indicated. Intralesional injection of triamcinolone will eradicate individual lesions. Rebound may occur. For more recalcitrant disease, UVB or PUVA therapy may be beneficial.

Clark AR, et al: Papular dermatitis (subacute prurigo, "itchy red bump" disease). *J Am Acad Dermatol* 1998, 38:929.
Streit V, et al: Foil bath PUVA in the treatment of prurigo simplex subacuta. *Acta Derm Venereol* (Norway) 1996, 76:319. _____ ▲

Prurigo Pigmentosa. Prurigo pigmentosa is a rare dermatosis of unknown cause characterized by the sudden onset of erythematous papules that leave reticulated hyperpigmentation when they heal. The condition mainly affects Japanese women and occurs in the spring and summer. Only a few cases have been reported in whites. Recurrence or exacerbations are common; the areas most frequently involved are the upper back, nape, clavicular region, and chest. Mucous membranes are spared. Histology reveals a lichenoid dermatitis with variable psoriasiform hyperplasia. Direct immunofluorescence yields negative findings. The cause is unknown. Minocycline 100 to 200 mg daily is the treatment of choice and may prevent recurrences. Dapsone is also effective.

Liu MT, et al: Prurigo pigmentosa. *Dermatology* 1994, 188:219.
Roehr P, et al: A pruritic eruption with reticular pigmentation. Prurigo pigmentosa. *Arch Dermatol* 1993, 129:370.
Schepis C, et al: Prurigo pigmentosa: a misdiagnosed dermatitis in Sicily. *Cutis* 1999, 63:99.
Yanguas I, et al: Prurigo pigmentosa in a white woman. *J Am Acad Dermatol* 1996, 35:473. _____ ▲

Papuloerythroderma of Ofuji. A rare disorder most commonly found in Japan, papuloerythroderma of Ofuji is characterized by pruritic papules that spare the skinfolds, producing bands of uninvolved cutis, the so-called deck-chair sign. Frequently there is associated blood eosinophilia. This condition is considered a form of erythroderma in the elderly by some and a paraneoplastic syndrome by others. Skin biopsies reveal a dense lymphohistiocytic infiltrate, eosinophils in the papillary dermis, and increased Langerhans cells (S-100 positive). Reported malignancies include T-cell lymphomas, B-cell lymphomas, Sézary syndrome, and visceral carcinomas. Not enough cases have been reported to determine a true association with malignancies.

The differential diagnosis is the same as for prurigo simplex. Systemic steroids are the treatment of choice, and may result in long-term remissions. Topical steroids, tar derivatives, emollients, systemic retinoids, and PUVA may also be therapeutic.

Depaire F, et al: Ofuji's papuloerythroderma: report of a new case responding to PUVA. *Acta Derm Venereol* (Norway) 1996, 76:93.
Nazzari G, et al: Papuloerythroderma (Ofuji). *J Am Acad Dermatol* 1992, 26:499.
Schepers C, et al: Papuloerythroderma of Ofuji. *Dermatology* 1996, 193:131.
Tay YK, et al: Papuloerythroderma of Ofuji and cutaneous T-cell lymphoma. *Br J Dermatol* 1997, 137:160. _____ ▲

Lichen Simplex Chronicus. As a result of long-continued rubbing and scratching, more vigorously than a normal pain threshold would permit, the skin becomes thickened and leathery. The normal markings of the skin become exaggerated, so that the striae form a criss-cross pattern, and between them a mosaic is produced composed of flat-topped, shiny, smooth, quadrilateral facets (Fig. 4-6). This change, known as *lichenification,* may originate on seemingly normal skin or may develop on skin that is the site of another disease, such as eczema or ringworm. Paroxysmal pruritus is the main symptom. This is known as *lichen simplex chronicus* (neurodermatitis circumscripta).

Lichen simplex chronicus, also known as neurodermatitis circumscripta, is characterized by circumscribed, lichenified, pruritic patches that may develop on any part of the body. However, the disease has a predilection for the back and sides of the neck, and the extremities—especially the wrists and ankles. At times, the eruption is decidedly papular, resembling lichen planus; in other instances, the patches are excoriated, slightly scaly or moist, and, rarely, nodular.

Several distinctive types are recognized. Lichen simplex nuchae occurs on the back of the neck (Fig. 4-7). It is not unusual to find this area excoriated and bleeding. Nodular neurodermatitis of the scalp of Ayres consists of multiple pruritic and excoriated papules and may be called prurigo of the scalp. The nodules or papules may ooze and form crusts and scales. The vulva, scrotum, and anal area can be sites of severe neurodermatitis. Seldom, however, are genital and anal areas involved at the same time. An upper eyelid, the orifice of one or both ears, or a palm or sole may also be involved; the ankle flexure is also a favorite site. Persistent rubbing of the shins or upper back may result in dermal deposits of amyloid and the subsequent development of macular and lichen amyloidosis, respectively.

To what extent mechanical trauma plays a role in producing the original irritation is not known. The onset of this dermatosis is usually gradual and insidious. Chronic scratching of a localized area is a response to unknown factors; however, stress and anxiety have long been thought important.

TREATMENT. Essentially, cessation of pruritus is the goal. It is important to stress the need for the patient to avoid scratching the areas involved. Only in this way will the habitual itch-scratch cycle be broken. Recurrences are frequent, even after the most thorough treatment, and there are instances in which the clearance of one lesion will see the onset of another elsewhere. High-potency agents such as clobetasol propionate (Temovate), diflorasone diacetate (Psorcon), or betamethasone dipropionate (Diprolene) cream or ointment should be used initially but not indefinitely because of the potential for steroid-induced atrophy. Occlusion of medium-potency steroids may be beneficial. Use of a tape containing a steroidal agent (Cordran) to provide both occlusion and antiinflammatory effects may have benefit. Topical doxepin cream (Zonalon) provides significant antipruritic effects and is good adjunctive therapy. Topical capsaicin cream has also been shown to be effective. Treatment can be shifted to the use of

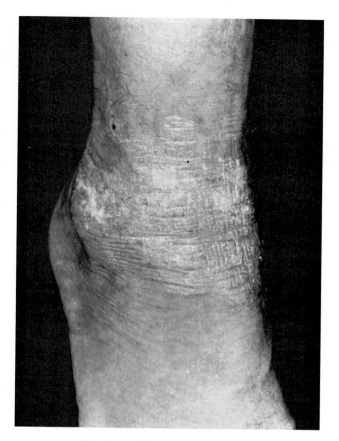

Fig. 4-6 Lichen simplex chronicus.

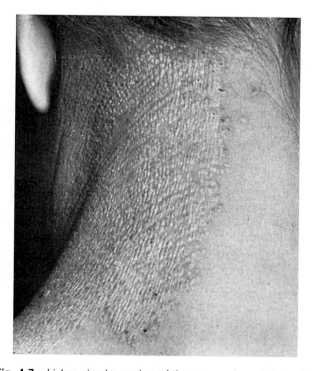

Fig. 4-7 Lichen simplex nuchae of the nape, a characteristic site.

medium- to lower-strength topical steroids as the lesions resolve.

Intralesional injections of triamcinolone suspension, using a concentration of 5 or (with caution) 10 mg per milliliter may be required. Too superficial injection invites the twin risks of epidermal and dermal atrophy and depigmentation, which may last for many months. The suspension should not be injected into infected lesions, for fear of causing abscesses. In the most severe cases, complete occlusion with an Unna boot may break the cycle.

Drake LA, et al: The antipruritic effect of 5% doxepin cream in patients with eczematous dermatitis. *Arch Dermatol* 1995, 131:1403.

Jacob CI, et al: Strongyloides stercoralis infection presenting as generalized prurigo nodularis and lichen simplex chronicus. *J Am Acad Dermatol* 1999, 41:357.

Jones RO: Lichen simplex chronicus. *Clin Podiatr Med Surg* 1996, 13:47.

Kantor GR, et al: Treatment of lichen simplex chronicus with topical capsaicin cream. *Acta Derm Venereol* 1992, 76:161.

Woodruff PW, et al: Psychiatric illness in patients referred to a dermatology-psychiatry clinic. *Gen Hosp Psychiatry* 1997, 19:29. ▲

Prurigo Nodularis. Prurigo nodularis is a disease with multiple itching nodules situated chiefly on the extremities, especially on the anterior surfaces of the thighs and legs (Fig. 4-8). A linear arrangement is common. The individual lesions are pea-sized or larger, firm, and erythematous or brownish. When fully developed they become verrucous, or fissured. The course of the disease is chronic, and the lesions evolve slowly. Itching is severe but usually confined to the lesions themselves. Bouts of extreme pruritus occur when these patients are under stress. Prurigo nodularis is one of the disorders in which the pruritus is characteristically paroxysmal: intermittent, unbearably severe, and relieved only by scratching to the point of damaging the skin, usually inducing bleeding and often scarring.

The cause of prurigo nodularis is unknown. Emotional stress, atopic dermatitis, anemia, hepatic diseases (including hepatitis C), HIV disease, pregnancy, renal failure, photodermatitis, gluten enteropathy, and insect bites have been considered as contributing or causal factors. Pemphigoid nodularis may be confused with prurigo nodularis clinically.

The histologic findings are those of markedly lichenified chronic dermatitis with compact hyperkeratosis, irregular acanthosis, and a perivascular mononuclear cell infiltrate in the dermis. Dermal collagen may be increased, especially in the dermal papillae, and subepidermal fibrin may be seen, both evidence of excoriation. In cases associated with renal failure transepidermal elimination of degenerated collagen may be found.

TREATMENT. Treatment is difficult and challenging. Local measures include antipruritic lotions and emollients. Administration of antihistamines, cyproheptadine, or tranquilizers is of moderate benefit in allaying symptoms. The initial treatment of choice is intralesional or topical admin-

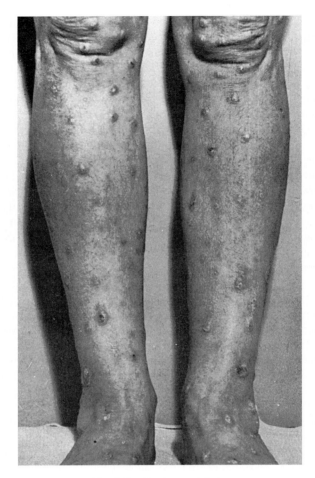

Fig. 4-8 Prurigo nodularis.

istration of steroids. Usually, superpotent topical products are required, but at times lower strength preparations used with occlusion may be beneficial. The use of steroids in tape (Cordran) and prolonged occlusion with semipermeable dressings, such as used for treating nonhealing wounds, can be useful in limited areas. Intralesional steroids will usually eradicate individual lesions, but unfortunately many patients have too extensive disease for these local measures. PUVA has also been shown effective in some cases. Vitamin D₃ ointment applied topically twice daily may be therapeutic and steroid sparing. Accutane, 1 mg/kg/day for 2 to 5 months, may benefit some patients.

Good results have been obtained with thalidomide and cyclosporine. With thalidomide the onset may be rapid or slow, and sedation may occur. The initial dose is 100 mg daily, titered to the lowest dose required. Patients treated with thalidomide are at risk of developing a dose-dependent neuropathy at cumulative doses of 40 to 50 g. Combination therapy with sequential UVB and thalidomide has been reported. Cyclosporine at doses of 3 to 4.5 mg/kg/day has also been shown to be safe and effective in treating recalcitrant disease. Cryotherapy has been used adjunctively.

Berger TG, et al: Prurigo nodularis and photosensitivity in AIDS: treatment with thalidomide. *J Am Acad Dermatol* 1995, 33:837.

Berth-Jones J, et al: Nodular prurigo responds to cyclosporin. *Br J Dermatol* 1995, 132:795.

Ferrandiz C, et al: Sequential combined therapy with thalidomide and narrow-band (TL01) UVB in the treatment of prurigo nodularis. *Dermatology* 1997, 195:359.

Katayama I, et al: Topical vitamin D$_3$ (talcalcitol) for steroid-resistant prurigo. *Br J Dermatol* 1996, 135:237.

Neri S, et al: Hyde's prurigo nodularis and chronic HCV hepatitis. *J Hepatol* 1998, 28:161.

Setoyama M, et al: Prurigo as a clinical prodrome to adult T-cell leukaemia/lymphoma. *Br J Dermatol* 1998, 138:137.

Stephanie T, et al: Rediscovering thalidomide: a review of its mechanism of action, side effects, and potential uses. *J Am Acad Dermatol* 1996, 35:969.

Waldinger TP, et al: Cryotherapy improves prurigo nodularis. *Arch Dermatol* 1984, 120:1598. _____ ▲

Distinctive Exudative Discoid and Lichenoid Dermatitis (DEDLE)

In 1937, Sulzberger and Garbe reported a psychosomatic disease encountered mostly in middle-aged or older patients of Jewish heritage, commonly called "oid-oid" disease. Since then it has been seen frequently by some observers and not at all by others, and its existence has been questioned.

Frank SB: EDLCD: does it exist or should it be discarded? *Int J Dermatol* 1989, 28:59 (letter).

Rebetti A: Sulzberger-Garbe disease in Europe. *Int J Dermatol* 1989, 28:22.

Rongioletti F: EDLCD: a fictional disease? *Int J Dermatol* 1989, 28:40.

Trueb RM: Exudative discoid and lichenoid chronic Sulzberger-Garbe dermatosis ("Oid-Oid disease"): reality or fiction? *Hautarzt* 1993, 44:488. _____ ▲

PSYCHODERMATOLOGY

There are purely cutaneous disorders that are psychiatric in nature, their cause being directly related to psychopathologic causes in the absence of primary dermatologic or other organic causes. Delusions of parasitosis, neurotic excoriations, factitial dermatitis, and trichotillomania compose the major categories of psychodermatology. The differential diagnosis for these four disorders is twofold, requiring the exclusion of (1) organic causes and (2) definition of a potential underlying psychologic disorder. Other delusional disorders include bromidrosiphobia and body dysmorphic disorder.

Psychosis is characterized by the presence of delusional ideation, which is defined as a fixed misbelief that is not shared by the patient's subculture. Monosymptomatic hypochondriacal disorder is a form of psychosis characterized by delusions regarding a particular hypochondriacal concern. In contrast to schizophrenia, there are no other mental deficits, such as auditory hallucination, loss of interpersonal skills, or presence of other inappropriate actions. Patients with monosymptomatic hypochondriacal psychosis often function appropriately in social settings, except for a single fixated belief that there is a serious problem in their skin or other parts of their bodies.

SKIN SIGNS OF PSYCHIATRIC ILLNESS. The skin is a frequent target for the release of emotional tension. Self-injury by the same prolonged compulsive repetitious acts may produce various mutilations, depending on the act and the site of injury.

Self-biting may be manifested by biting the nails (onychophagia), by skin-biting (most frequently the forearms, hands, and fingers) and by lip-biting. Dermatophagia, also known as "wolf biter," is a habit or compulsion, which may be conscious or subconscious, to bite one's own skin. Bumping of the head produces lacerations and contusions, which may be so severe as to produce cranial defects and life-threatening complications. Compulsive repetitive handwashing may produce an irritant dermatitis of the hands.

Bulimia, with its self-induced vomiting, results in crusted papules on the dorsa of the dominant hand from cuts by the teeth. Clenching of the hand produces swelling and ecchymosis of the fingertips and subungual hemorrhage. Self-inflicted lacerations may be of suicidal intent. They are sometimes seen in adolescents who are trying to demonstrate their bravery. Lip-licking produces increased salivation and thickening of the lips. Eventually the perioral area becomes red and produces a distinctive picture resembling the exaggerated mouth makeup of a clown. Pressure produced by binding the waistline tightly with a cord will eventually lead to atrophy of the subcutaneous tissue.

Evidence is mounting in support of a neurobiologic basis for the causes of compulsive obsessive disorders. Psychopharmacologic agents such as clomipramine, fluoxetine, fluvoxamine, sertraline, paroxetine, and venlafaxine and behavioral therapy alone or in combination with these agents are the treatments of choice.

Delusions of Parasitosis

Delusions of parasitosis (acarophobia, dermatophobia, parasitophobia, entomophobia) are firm fixations in a person's mind that he or she suffers from a parasitic infestation of the skin. The belief is so fixed that the patient may pick small pieces of epithelial debris from the skin and bring them to be examined, always insisting that the offending parasite is contained in such material. Samples of alleged parasites enclosed in assorted containers, paper tissue, or sandwiched between adhesive tape are so characteristic that it is referred to as the "matchbox sign." Probably the only symptom will be pruritus. Cutaneous findings may range from none at all to excoriations, prurigo nodularis, and frank ulcerations.

Frequently these patients have paranoid tendencies, seen usually in middle-aged or elderly women. Women are affected 2:1 over men. Classification is controversial, ranging from DSM-III-R to monosymptomatic hypochondriacal psychosis. It has also been reported to be associated with schizophrenia, bipolar disorders, depression, anxiety disorders, and obsessional states. A variety of organic causes have been suggested to include cocaine and amphetamine abuse, dementia, malignancies, cerebrovascular disease, multiple sclerosis, and vitamin B_{12} deficiency. Some of these may produce cutaneous symptoms, particularly pruritus, which may contribute to the delusion.

The differential diagnosis is influenced by the cutaneous findings and history. Initial steps should be directed at excluding a true infestation, such as scabies, or an organic cause. A thorough history, particularly in reference to therapeutic and recreational drug use (amphetamines and cocaine), review of systems, and physical examination, should be performed. A skin biopsy is frequently performed often more to reassure the patient than to uncover occult skin disease. Screening laboratory tests to exclude systemic disorders should be obtained; these include a complete blood cell count (CBC), urinalysis (UA), liver function tests (LFTs), thyroid function tests (TFT), iron studies, and serum B_{12}, folate, and electrolyte levels. Multiple sclerosis may present with dysesthesia, which may at times be mistaken for infestation. Once organic causes have been eliminated, the patient should be evaluated to determine the cause of the delusions. Schizophrenia, monosymptomatic hypochondriacal psychosis, psychotic depression, dementia, and depression with somatization are considerations in the differential diagnosis. Referral to a psychiatrist is recommended.

Management of this difficult problem varies. Most frequently the patient will reject suggestions to seek psychiatric help. Various prescriptions are accepted, but there is little or no improvement of symptoms when the medication is used. The dermatologist is cautioned against confronting the patient with the psychogenic nature of the disease too early, and care must be exercised to develop trust, which will usually require several visits. Review of 100 years of data indicates that the rate of remissions from psychiatric intervention has increased from 33.9% to 51.9% in the psychopharmacologic era. Pimozide (Orap) in doses ranging from 1 to 12 mg/day has been shown to be effective. Many patients show a response at a dosage of 4 mg/day or less, and to minimize adverse effects, the dosage should be maintained at 10 mg/day or less. Pimozide is an antipsychotic medication approved for the treatment of Tourette's syndrome. The main side effects are stiffness, restlessness, and extrapyramidal signs, which can be controlled with diphenhydramine (Benadryl) or benztropine mesylate (Cogentin). Insufficient evidence exists to state that pimozide is superior to other antipsychotic agents, but its use in treating delusions of parasitosis is believed by many to be superior.

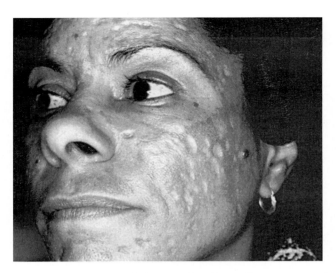

Fig. 4-9 Neurotic excoriations produced to relieve suppressed hostility toward an alcoholic husband. (Courtesy Dr. Axel W. Hoke.)

Neurotic Excoriations

Many persons have unconscious compulsive habits of picking at themselves, and at times the tendency is so persistent and pronounced that excoriations of the skin are produced. The lesions are caused by picking, digging, or scraping, and they usually occur on parts readily accessible to the hands. As a rule the action is unconscious. However, it may be done deliberately, in the belief that it corrects some abnormality of the skin.

The excavations are superficial or deep and are often linear. The bases of the ulcers are clean or covered with a scab (Fig. 4-9). Right-handed persons tend to produce lesions on their left side and left-handed persons on their right side. Many people will persistently pluck at an area until they can "pull a thread" from it. There is evidence of past healed lesions, usually with linear scars, or rounded hyperpigmented or hypopigmented lesions, in the area of the active excoriations. The face is the favorite site for these excoriations. Sometimes this aggravates acne, producing *acne excorie.* The upper arms are also commonly involved.

Most of these patients are otherwise healthy adults. They usually lead normal lives. The organic differential diagnosis is vast and includes any condition that may manifest with excoriations. The most common psychopathologies associated with neurotic excoriations are depression, obsessive-compulsive disorder, and anxiety.

The treatment of choice is doxepin (Sinequan or Adapin) because of its antidepressant and antipruritic effects. Alternatives to doxepin include desipramine (Norpramin, Pertofrane), buspirone (BuSpar), and quick-acting benzodiazepines. Treatment is difficult, often requiring a combination of psychiatric and pharmacologic intervention. It is important to establish a constructive patient-therapist

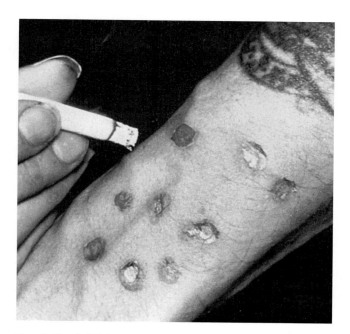

Fig. 4-10 Self-inflicted cigarette burns, done as a means of self-discipline. (Courtesy Dr. Axel W. Hoke.)

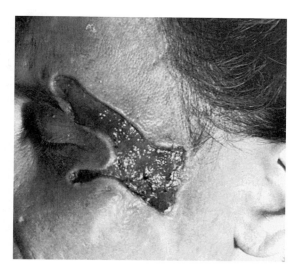

Fig. 4-11 Dermatitis artefacta, produced by acid, self-applied.

alliance. Training in diversion strategies during "scratching episodes" may be helpful. Childhood and adolescent circumstances should be defined and separated from more long-term causes, such as personality disorders. An attempt should be made to identify specific conflicts or stressors preceding onset. The therapist should concentrate on systematic training directed at the behavioral reaction pattern, especially involving aggression management and self-manifestation. Finally, there should be support and advice given with regard to the patient's social situation and social relations.

Factitious Dermatitis (Dermatitis Artefacta)

Factitious dermatitis is the term applied to self-inflicted skin lesions made consciously and often with the intent to elicit sympathy, escape responsibilities, or collect disability insurance. The skin lesions are provoked by mechanical means or by the application of chemical irritants and caustics. The lesions may simulate other dermatoses but usually have a distinctive, clear-cut, bizarre appearance (Fig. 4-10). Frequently the shape and arrangement of lesions are such as are not encountered in any other affection. The lesions are generally distributed on parts easily reached by the hands and have a tendency to be linear and arranged regularly and symmetrically. They are rarely seen on the right hand or right wrist or arm unless the patient is left-handed.

When chemicals are used, one may often see red streaks or guttate marks beneath the principal patch, where drops of the chemical have accidentally run or fallen on the skin. According to the manner of production, the lesions may be erythematous, vesicular, bullous, ulcerative, or gangrenous (Fig. 4-11). The more common agents of destruction used are the fingernails, pointed instruments, hot metal; chemicals such as carbolic, muriatic, nitric, or acetic acid; caustic potash or soda, turpentine, table salt, urine, and feces. The lesions are likely to appear in crops. At times the disorder is manifested only by the indefinitely delayed healing of an operative wound, which is purposely kept open by the patient. Tight cords or clothing tied around an arm or leg may produce factitious lymphedema, which may be mistaken for postphlebitic syndrome, nerve injury, as well as other forms of chronic lymphedema.

Subcutaneous emphysema, manifesting as cutaneous crepitations, may be factitial in origin. Recurrent migratory subcutaneous emphysema involving the extremities, neck, chest, or face can be induced through injections of air into tissue with a needle and syringe. Circular pockets and bilateral involvement without physical findings that suggest a contiguous spread from a single source suggest a factitial origin. Puncturing the buccal mucosa through to facial skin with a needle and puffing out the cheeks can produce alarming results. Neck and shoulder crepitation is also a complication in manic patients that results from hyperventilation and breath-holding.

The organic differential diagnosis depends on the cutaneous signs manifested (e.g., gas gangrene for patients with factitious subcutaneous emphysema, and the various forms of lymphedema for factitious lymphedema). Considerations for psychopathology include malingering, borderline personality disorders, and psychosis.

Proof of diagnosis is sometimes difficult. Occlusive dressings may be necessary to protect the lesions from ready access by the patient. It is usually best not to reveal any suspicion of the cause to the patient and to establish the diagnosis definitely without the patient's knowledge. If the patient is hospitalized a resourceful, cooperative nurse may be useful in helping to establish the diagnosis. When injection of foreign material is suspected, examination of biopsy material by spectroscopy may reveal talc.

Treatment should ideally involve psychotherapy, but most frequently the patient promptly rejects the suggestion and goes to another physician to seek a new round of treatment. It is best for the dermatologist to maintain a close relationship with the patient and provide symptomatic therapy and nonjudgmental support. Pimozide (Orap) has been used with some success. Antidepressants such as fluoxetine (Prozac) may also be beneficial. Consultation with an experienced psychiatrist is prudent.

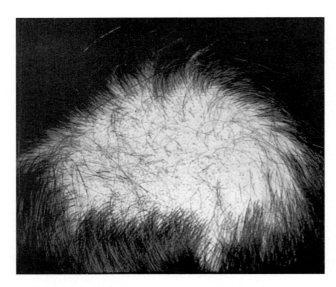

Fig. 4-12 Trichotillomania. (Courtesy Dr. Axel W. Hoke.)

Driscoll MS, et al: Delusional parasitosis. *J Am Acad Dermatol* 1993, 29:1023.

Fruensgaard K: Psychotherapy and neurotic excoriations. *Int J Dermatol* 1991, 30:262.

Koblenzer CS: Neurotic excoriations and dermatitis artefacta. *Dermatol Clin* 1996, 14:447.

Koo J, et al: Delusions of parasitosis and other forms of monosymptomatic hypochondriacal psychosis. *Dermatol Clin* 1996, 14:429.

Samlaska CP, et al: Subcutaneous emphysema. *Adv Dermatol* 1996, 11:117.

Scott MJ, et al: Dermatophagia: "wolf-biter." *Cutis* 1997, 59:19.

Stoberl C, et al: Artificial edema of the extremity. *Hautarzt* 1994, 45:149.

Trabert W: 100 years of delusional parasitosis. *Psychopathology* 1995, 28:238.

Wang CK, et al: Monosymptomatic hypochondriacal psychosis complicated by self-inflicted skin ulceration, skull defect and brain abscess. *Br J Dermatol* 1997, 137:299.

Warnock JK, et al: Obsessive-compulsive disorder. *Dermatol Clin* 1996, 14:456. ▲

Trichotillomania

Trichotillomania is a neurosis characterized by an abnormal urge to pull out the hair. The sites involved are generally the frontal region of the scalp, eyebrows, eyelashes, and the beard. There are irregular areas of hair loss, which may be linear or bizarrely shaped. The classic presentation is the "Friar Tuck" form of vertex and crown alopecia (Fig. 4-12). Hairs are broken and show differences in length. The nails may show evidence of onychophagy (nail biting), but no pits are present. The disease is seven times more common in children than in adults, and girls are affected 2.5 times more often than boys are.

This disease often develops in the setting of psychosocial stress in the family, which may revolve around school problems, sibling rivalry, moving to a new house, hospital-ization of the mother, or a disturbed mother-daughter relationship.

Differentiation from alopecia areata is possible because of the varying lengths of broken hairs present, the absence of nail pitting, the microscopic appearance of the twisted or broken hairs as opposed to the tapered club hairs of alopecia areata, and, if necessary, a biopsy can be performed. Other organic disorders to consider are androgenic alopecia, tinea capitis, monilethrix, pili torti, pseudopelade of Brocq, traction alopecia, syphilis, nutritional deficiencies, and systemic disorders such as lupus and lymphoma. Biopsy can be helpful, the histology showing traumatized hair follicles with perifollicular hemorrhage, fragmented hair in the dermis, empty follicles, and deformed hair shafts (trichomalacia) that may have a ruffled appearance. An alternative technique to biopsy, particularly for children, is to shave a part of the involved area and observe for regrowth of normal hairs. The differential for underlying psychopathology is obsessive-compulsive disorder (most common), depression, and anxiety.

In adults with the problem, psychiatric impairment may be severe. In children one should address the diagnosis openly, and referral to a child psychiatrist for behavioral therapy or psychotherapy should be encouraged. Pharmacotherapy with clomipramine (Anafranil), fluoxetine (Prozac), or venlafaxine may also be helpful for obsessive-compulsive disorder. Other medications may be more appropriate to treat depression or anxiety.

Clark J Jr, et al: Chronic alopecia: Trichotillomania. *Arch Dermatol* 1995, 131:720.

Jefferys D: Trichotillomania: an overview. *Exp Dermatol* 1999, 8:298.

Keuthen NJ, et al: Retrospective review of treatment outcome for 63 patients with trichotillomania. *Am J Psychiatry* 1998, 155:560.

Ninan PT, et al: A controlled trial of venlafaxine in trichotillomania. *Psychopharmacol Bull* 1998, 34:221. ▲

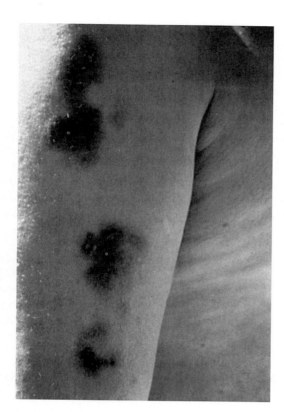

Fig. 4-13 Burises resulting from dermatothlasia. The patient produced one of these lesions as a defense against ulcer pain. (Courtesy Dr. Axel W. Hoke.)

Dermatothlasia

Dermatothlasia (Fig. 4-13) is a cutaneous neurosis characterized by an uncontrollable desire to rub or pinch oneself to form bruised areas on the skin, sometimes as a defense against pain elsewhere.

Bromidrosiphobia

Bromidrosiphobia is a neurosis in which there is the conviction that one's sweat has a repugnant odor that keeps other people away. The patient is unable to accept any evidence to the contrary. Three fourths of patients with bromidrosiphobia are males, with an average age of 25. Pimozide may be beneficial. It may be an early symptom of schizophrenia.

Body Dysmorphic Disorder (Dysmorphic Syndrome, Dysmorphophobia)

Body dysmorphic disorder is the delusion of having an ugly body part. Patients often manifest obsessional features and depression that may present a risk of suicide. The condition may affect up to 1% of the population in the United States. Therapy with selective antidepressants, particularly the serotonergic preparations, have been helpful.

Albertini RS, et al: Thirty-three cases of body dysmorphic disorder in children and adolescents. *J Am Acad Child Adolesc Psychiatry* 1999, 38:453.

Cotterill JA: Body dysmorphic disorder. *Dermatol Clin* 1996, 14:457.

Hanes KR: Body dysmorphic disorder: an underestimated entity? *Australas J Dermatol* 1995, 36:227.

Hollander E, et al: Comorbid social anxiety and body dysmorphic disorder: managing the complicated patient. *J Clin Psychiatry* 1999, 60:27. ▲

NEUROCUTANEOUS DERMATOSES
Burning Mouth Syndrome (Glossodynia, Burning Tongue)

Postmenopausal women are particularly prone to a feeling of burning of the tongue, mouth, and lips, with no objective findings. Symptoms vary in severity but are more or less constant. Patients with burning mouth syndrome often complain that multiple oral sites are involved. It has been blamed on deficiency of B_{12}, iron, or folate; on hypoestrogenism, diabetes, local trauma, and psychologic disturbance. It may be a complication of Sjögren's syndrome. In 130 patients reviewed by Gorsky et al, the most common site was the tongue, and 39% complained of dry mouth. The most effective management in this series was use of mood-altering drugs.

Burning lips syndrome may be a separate entity; it appears to affect both men and women equally and occurs in individuals between the ages of 50 and 70 years. The labial mucosa may be smooth and pale, and the minor salivary glands of the lips are frequently dysfunctional. Treatment with topical steroids has been generally favorable.

Scalp Dysesthesia

Cutaneous dysesthesia syndromes are disorders characterized by chronic cutaneous symptoms without objective findings. It is often difficult to distinguish between pain or burning sensations, since both are carried on the same unmyelinated (slow), afferent, group C nerve fibers. Many patients report coexisting pruritus, or transient pruritus associated with the dysesthesia. A psychiatric cause or overlay is frequently associated with scalp dysesthesia and treatment with antidepressants may be beneficial.

Vulvodynia (Vulvar Vestibulitis Syndrome, Burning Vulva Syndrome)

Vulvodynia is an important syndrome, which in affected patients can lead to severe psychologic sequelae because of its chronic symptoms and disruption of interpersonal relationships. In true vulvar vestibulitis syndrome the discomfort is not usually constant or spontaneous. The definition is a constellation of findings, including (1) severe pain on vestibular touch or attempted vaginal entry, (2) tenderness to pressure localized to the vulvar vestibule, and (3) physical findings of only vulvar erythema of various degrees. This definition should be closely followed. The vulvar symptoms are exacerbated in some patients by stress, depression, or anxiety, perhaps as a result of increased neuropeptide-mediated inflammation associated with these conditions. The exact cause of the syndrome is unknown. Chronic candidiasis (or an abnormal immune response to vaginal candidiasis), subclinical human papilloma virus infection, chronic contact dermatitis (to the numerous topical agents used to treat the symptoms), tissue injury or inflammation produced by the caustics and tissue-destructive agents used to treat HPV, altered vaginal pH (too alkaline, usually), and the presence of urine oxalate crystals have all been proposed as possible causes of this syndrome. In many affected patients, none of these causes can be found—that is, most cases remain idiopathic. Treatment for the above conditions is often of limited benefit.

The vast majority of affected patients are white (92%) and nulliparous (62%), with a mean age of 32 years. Up to 15% of women seen in some gynecologic practices may be affected. The condition is usually chronic, lasting years. The severity of the syndrome can be graded by the degree of dyspareunia it produces (level 3 dyspareunia completely prevents all sexual intercourse). The diagnosis of this syndrome includes initially eliminating other causes of acute or chronic vulvitis, such as candidiasis oratrichomonal infection and contact dermatitis. These conditions are usually more amenable to treatment, and the symptoms often extend beyond the vestibule to the labia minora and majora and other surrounding tissues. There is constant discomfort in the vulva, exacerbated by any contact with the vestibule.

Treatment should be initially supportive and symptomatic, since some proportion of the patients spontaneously improve. Initially, aggressive treatments should be avoided, and topical anesthetics and lubricants such as petrolatum before intercourse should be used. A low-oxalate diet and a daily dose of calcium citrate (200 mg calcium and 950 mg citrate) have been recommended.

Constant searching for possible exacerbating conditions as described above is warranted. These patients require a lot of physician support. Vulvar vestibulitis syndrome may be associated with or lead to depression, which should be treated. Some experts advocate the use of injections of 1 million units of alpha-interferon into the vestibule 3 times weekly for 4 weeks. The response rate is about 50% and may represent spontaneous remission, since it is not specific to patients with evidence of HPV infection. It is cost effective when compared with going directly to surgery for patients with level 3 dyspareunia. Patients with dyspareunia that is preventing all sexual intercourse, who have accurately diagnosed chronic vulvar vestibulitis syndrome, and who wish to have sexual intercourse may respond to surgical removal of the vestibule. Success rates from 60% to above 90% have been reported in carefully selected patients. Consultation with a dermatologist or gynecologist with expertise in this disorder is suggested before recommending surgery.

Notalgia Paresthetica

Notalgia paresthetica is a unilateral sensory neuropathy characterized by infrascapular pruritus, burning pain, hyperalgesia, and tenderness, often in the distribution of the second to sixth thoracic spinal nerves. A pigmented patch localized to the area of pruritus is often found. It has been reported under a variety of titles, such as puzzling posterior pigmented pruritic patches and hereditary localized pruritus. Itchy points (puncta pruritica) may also be a variant of this disorder. Localized, macular amyloidosis may be found on biopsy. The cause is unknown, but nerve trauma and entrapment have long been suspect.

Topical capsaicin has been shown effective; however, relapse occurs in most patients within 4 weeks of discontinuing its use. Local anesthetics and corticosteroids may be helpful and are believed to work by stabilizing neural membranes and suppressing ectopic neural pacemaker activity. Paravertebral blocks provide long remission rates in the severest forms.

Meralgia Paresthetica (Roth-Bernhardt Disease)

This affection is a variety of paresthesia, with persistent numbness and periodic transient episodes of burning or lancinating pain on the anterolateral surface of the thigh. This area is innervated by the lateral femoral cutaneous nerve. The disease occurs most frequently in middle-aged obese men. Aranoff et al report alopecia localized to the area innervated by the lateral femoral nerve to be a sign of this disease. Arthritis of the lumbar vertebrae, a herniated disk, pregnancy, iliac crest bone graft harvesting, seat belt injury associated with motor vehicle accident, diabetes, and rarely, a retroperitoneal tumor are purported causes. The diagnostic test of choice is somatosensory evoked potentials of the lateral femoral cutaneous nerve. Surgical decompression of the lateral femoral cutaneous nerve produces good to excellent outcomes.

Complex Regional Pain Syndrome

Encompassing the descriptors reflex sympathetic dystrophy, causalgia, neuropathic pain, algoneurodystrophy, clenched fist syndrome, Sudek's syndrome, and maintained pain, complex regional pain syndrome (CRPS) is characterized by burning pain, hyperesthesia, and trophic disturbances resulting from injury to a peripheral nerve. It usually occurs in one of the upper extremities. The commonest symptom is burning pain aggravated by movement or friction. The skin of the involved extremity becomes shiny, cold, profusely perspiring, and frequently cracked, and there is usually hyperesthesia and radiographic evidence of osteoporosis. Additional cutaneous manifestations include atrophy, folliculitis, cellulitis, petechiae, erosions, edema, telangiectasias, hyperpigmentation, bullae, and ulcerations.

The intensity of the pain varies from trivial burning to a state of torture accompanied by extreme hyperesthesia and frequently, hyperhidrosis. The part is not only subject to an intense burning sensation, but also a touch or a tap of the finger causes exquisite pain. Exposure to the air is avoided with a care that seems absurd, and the patient walks carefully, carrying the limb tenderly with the sound hand. The patients are tremulous and apprehensive and keep the hand constantly wet, finding relief in the moisture rather than in the temperature of the application. A condition resembling permanent chilblains or even trophic ulcers may be present.

There are three stages to CRPS. The first stage (which lasts about 1 to 3 months) begins with severe, localized, burning pain, focal edema, muscle spasm, rapid growth of hair and nails, stiffness or restricted mobility, hyperesthesia, and vasospasm affecting skin color and temperature. The second stage (3 to 6 months) is associated with a crescendo and diffusion of the pain and edema, diminished hair growth, brittle nails, osteoporosis, joint thickening, and onset of muscle atrophy. The final stage is irreversible trophic changes, intractable pain involving the entire limb, flexor contractures, marked atrophy of the muscles, severe limitation in joint and limb mobility, and severe osteoporosis.

The term *type II CRPS* is used synonymously with reflex sympathetic dystrophy or causalgia and is the most severe form of the illness. There may be a precipitating event, such as a nail biopsy, crush injury, laceration, fracture, sprain, burn, or surgery that produces some degree of soft tissue or nerve complex injury. The most frequent causes include peripheral revascularization of the extremities (5% of cases), hypothermic insult, such as trench foot (5%), myocardial infarction (5%), peripheral nerve injury (2% to 5%), and fractures (1% to 2%). Associations with Munchausen's syndrome and factitial ulcerations have also been reported.

Not all patients will have all of the features of CRPS, and an early diagnosis is essential if the patient is to have any chance of a cure. The five major components are pain, edema, dysregulation of autonomic function, alterations in motor function, and dystrophic changes. A three-phase technetium bone scan is helpful in confirming the diagnosis of CRPS in patients who fail to meet all five of these criteria.

Treatment should be started before central nervous system changes occur and narcotic addiction develops. Consultation with a neurologist or an anesthesiologist specializing in pain is advisable. Osteoporosis is a frequent complication, and studies using biphosphonate (Pamidronate), a powerful inhibitor of bone absorption, have been shown to significantly improve symptoms of pain, tenderness, and swelling. Tricyclic antidepressants and antipsychotic agents are often helpful. Transcutaneous electrical nerve stimulation (TENS) is also useful in the treatment of early disease. Paravertebral block or sympathectomy is most effective, but not without potential complications. In upper extremity disease, axillary blocks with lidocaine and hyaluronidase, rather than stellate ganglionic block, should be considered to eliminate the risk of pneumothorax.

Trigeminal Trophic Lesions

After rhizotomy (or more commonly, alcohol injection) for tic douloureux, a slowly enlarging, uninflamed ulcer may appear on the cheek beside the ala nasi. It may infrequently occur elsewhere on the face, or after other surgery. Onset of ulceration varies from weeks to several years after trigeminal nerve injury. Self-inflicted trauma to the anesthetic skin is believed to be the cause, and the appropriate treatment is to prevent this by persuasion or coercion. It is usually successful, but scarring may be severe.

In addition, the following complications may occur after operation for trigeminal neuralgia: herpes simplex, neuropathic keratitis, corneal ulcer, iritis, conjunctivitis, paresthesias, facial paralysis, and dryness of the nasal mucous membrane.

Postencephalitic Trophic Ulcer. Ulceration of the nose similar to the trigeminal trophic ulcer has been reported following epidemic encephalitis.

Malum Perforans Pedis

Also known as *perforating ulcer of the foot* and *neurotrophic ulcer,* malum perforans is a chronic, trophic, ulcerative disease seen on the sole in the denervating diseases, particularly tabes dorsalis, leprosy, arteriosclerosis, or diabetes, resulting from loss of pain sensation at a site of constant trauma (Fig. 4-14).

The primary cause of the trouble is either in the posterolateral tracts of the cord (in tabes and arteriosclerosis), the lateral tracts (in syringomyelia), or in the peripheral nerves (in diabetes or leprosy). In most cases, malum perforans begins as a circumscribed hyperkeratosis, usually on the ball of the foot. This lesion becomes soft, moist, and malodorous, and later exudes a thin, purulent discharge (Fig. 4-15). A slough slowly develops, and an indolent, necrotic, usually painless but sometimes painful ulcer is left that lasts indefinitely (Fig. 4-16). Deeper perforation and secondary infection often lead to osteomyelitis of the metatarsal or tarsal bones. The process must be differentiated from ulcers caused by suppurating corns and from the ordinary type of diabetic gangrene.

Treatment should consist of relief of pressure on the ulcer by padding and by keeping the patient off his or her feet as much as possible. Administration of local and systemic antibiotics is sometimes helpful. Debridement is recommended.

Sciatic Nerve Injury

Serious sciatic nerve injury can result from improperly performed injections into the buttocks. A paralytic foot drop

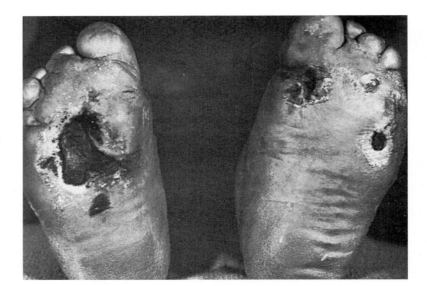

Fig. 4-14 Malum perforans of the feet in a 65-year-old woman with lepromatous leprosy.

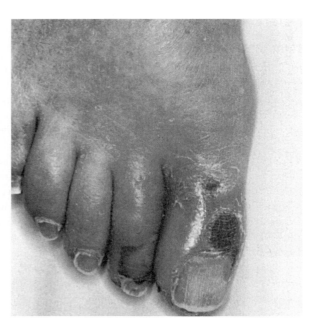

Fig. 4-15 Early diabetic gangrene.

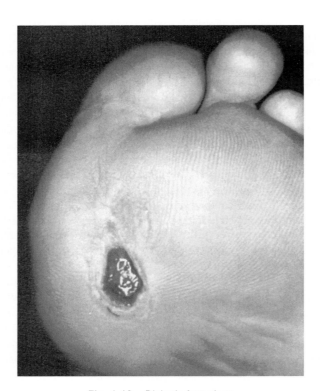

Fig. 4-16 Diabetic foot ulcer.

simulating poliomyelitis is the most common finding. There is sensory loss and absence of sweating over the distribution of the sciatic nerve branches. The skin of the affected extremity becomes thin, shiny, and often edematous. For many years the midanterior or midlateral thigh has been recommended as the preferable site for intramuscular injections in infants and young children because of the risk of sciatic nerve injury. Current guidelines further encourage using the buttock site when large volumes must be given

(e.g., immune globulin). Avoiding the buttocks for vaccinations in pediatric patients is being questioned.

In a retrospective study of 380 patients with sciatic nerve deficiencies, 230 (60%) had causal injuries at the buttock level, with more than half of these (136) attributable to injections. Only 10 patients in this series were in the pediatric age group. Older patients were more susceptible to injection-induced sciatic nerve injury because of their decreased muscle mass and/or debilitating diseases. The most common scenario for nerve damage was improper needle placement, being more medial and/or inferior than the recommended site on the upper, outer quadrant of the buttock. Thigh-level sciatic injury was most often secondary to gunshot wounds, femur fractures, lacerations, or contusions. Surgical exploration, guided by nerve action potentials, with repair of the sciatic nerve is worthwhile in selected cases.

Familial Dysautonomia (Riley-Day Syndrome)

Familial dysautonomia, first recognized by Riley in 1949, has features of defective lacrimation, excessive sweating, drooling, and transient erythema, predominantly on the trunk. In addition, there may be acrocyanosis, especially of the hands. Other major features include decreased pain sensation, impaired temperature and blood pressure regulation, and absent tendon reflexes. There are two interesting features: one is the absence of fungiform and circumvallate papillae of the tongue, and the other is the sensation of tickling of the scalp experienced when the head is stroked lightly. There are measurable deficiencies in taste from water, sweet, bitter, and salty stimuli. Dental features may be prominent and include hypersalivation and orododental trauma progressing to self-mutilation.

The cause is believed to be related to complex interactions between catecholamines. Plasma norepinephrine levels are normal or elevated in a supine position and do not increase with erect posture. Patients with familial dysautonomia have blood pressure readings that correlate with plasma norepinephrine levels when supine and with plasma dopamine levels when upright. DOPA:dihydroxyphenylglycol ratios are above those found in normal subjects. It is not clear how these characteristic neurochemical patterns relate to the well-documented decrease in unmyelinated and small myelinated neuronal populations. The disease is probably inherited as an autosomal recessive trait, most often in Jewish families. The Schirmer test for lacrimal dysfunction is positive. The intradermal histamine test shows a diminished flare, and immersion of the hands in 40° C (104° F) water causes erythematous mottling of the skin. Treatment is supportive.

Syringomyelia

Also known as *Morvan's disease,* syringomyelia results from progressive expansion of the central canal of the spinal cord, compressing the lateral tracts especially and producing sensory and trophic changes on the upper extremities, particularly in the fingers. The disease begins insidiously and gradually causes muscular weakness, hyperhidrosis, and sensory disturbances, especially in the thumb and index and middle fingers. The skin changes are characterized by dissociated anesthesia with loss of pain and temperature sense but with retention of tactile sense. Burns are the most frequent lesions noted. Bullae, warts, and trophic ulcerations occur on the fingers and hands, and

ultimately there are contractures and gangrene. Other unusual features may be hypertrophy of the limbs, hands, or feet and asymmetric scalp hair growth with a sharp midline demarcation. The disease must be differentiated chiefly from leprosy. Unlike leprosy, syringomyelia does not interfere with sweating or block the flare around a histamine wheal.

Congenital Sensory Neuropathy

Also described as congenital sensory neuropathy with anhidrosis and congenital insensitivity to pain with anhidrosis, recurrent acral ulcers, from the time of birth on, characterize this sensory neuropathy that occurs on the hands and feet. Repeated injuries to the hands produce ulcers because of trophic disturbances, progressing to self-mutilation. There may be decreased acral pain perception; however, the sense of touch is present. Complete anhidrosis is a frequent finding.

Treatment of this disorder is symptomatic. Care should be taken to avoid burning, scratching, and the various other traumatic events that can happen in ordinary living.

Adami S, et al: Bisphosphonate therapy of reflex sympathetic dystrophy syndrome. *Ann Rheum Dis* 1997, 56:201.

Allen G, et al: Epidemiology of complex regional pain syndrome: a retrospective chart review of 134 patients. *Pain* 1999, 80:539.

Aranoff SM, et al: Alopecia in meralgia paresthetica. *J Am Acad Dermatol* 1985, 12:176.

Axelrod FB: Familial dysautonomia: a 47-year perspective how technology confirms clinical acumen. *J Pediatr* 1998, 132:S2.

Brown RS, et al: Five cases of burning lips syndrome. *Compend Contin Educ Dent* 1996, 17:927.

Dicken CH: Trigeminal trophic syndrome. *Mayo Clin Proc* 1997, 72:543.

Domingues JC, et al: Congenital neuropathy with anhidrosis. *Pediatr Dermatol* 1994, 11:231.

Edwards-Lee TA, et al: Congenital insensitivity to pain and anhidrosis with mitochondrial and axonal abnormalities. *Pediatr Neurol* 1997, 17:356.

Eisenberg E, et al: Notalgia paresthetica associated with nerve root impingement. *J Am Acad Dermatol* 1997, 37:998.

Esteban A: Lateral femoral cutaneous neuropathy: paresthetic meralgia. *Rev Neurol* 1998, 26:414.

Gadoth N, et al: Taste and smell in familial dysautonomia. *Dev Med Child Neurol* 1997, 39:393.

Goel A: Meralgia paresthetica secondary to limb length discrepancy: case report. *Arch Phys Med Rehabil* 1999, 80:348.

Gorsky M, et al: Clinical characteristics and management outcome in the burning mouth syndrome. *Oral Surg Oral Med Oral Pathol* 1991, 72:192.

Goulden V, et al: Successful treatment of notalgia paresthetica with a paravertebral local anesthetic block. *J Am Acad Dermatol* 1998, 38:114.

Hilz MJ, et al: Cold face test demonstrates parasympathetic cardiac dysfunction in familial dysautonomia. *Am J Physiol* 1999, 276:R1833.

Hoss D, et al: Scalp dysesthesia. *Arch Dermatol* 1998, 134:327.

Koblenzer CS, et al: Chronic cutaneous dysesthesia syndrome: a psychotic phenomenon or a depressive symptom? *J Am Acad Dermatol* 1994, 30:370.

Kline DG, et al: Management and results of sciatic nerve injuries: a 24-year experience. *J Neurosurg* 1998, 89:13.

Lamey PJ, et al: Lip component of burning mouth syndrome. *Oral Surg Oral Med Oral Pathol* 1994, 78:590.

Lipp KE, et al: Reflex sympathetic dystrophy with mutilating ulcerations suspicious of a factitial origin. *J Am Acad Dermatol* 1996, 35:843.

MacDonald N: Does immunization in the buttocks cause sciatic nerve injury? *Pediatrics* 1994, 93:351.

Marbach JJ: Medically unexplained chronic orofacial pain: temporomandibular pain and dysfunction syndrome, orofacial phantom pain, burning mouth syndrome, and trigeminal neuralgia. *Med Clin North Am* 1999, 83:691.

Marinoff SC, et al: Vulvar vestibulitis syndrome. *Dermatol Clin* 1992;10:435.

Mass E, et al: Oro-dental self-mutilation in familial dysautonomia. *J Oral Pathol Med* 1994, 23:273.

Mass E, et al: Dental and oral findings in patients with familial dysautonomia. *Oral Surg Oral Med Oral Pathol* 1992, 74:305.

Myzyka BC, et al: A review of burning mouth syndrome. *Cutis* 1999, 64:29.

Nahabedian MY, et al: Meralgia paresthetica: etiology, diagnosis, and outcome of surgical decompression. *Ann Plast Surg* 1995, 35:590.

Ozbarlas N, et al: Congenital insensitivity to pain with anhidrosis. *Cutis* 1993, 51:373.

Provost TT, et al: Cutaneous manifestations of Sjögren's syndrome. *Rheum Dis Clin North Am* 1991, 18:609.

Raison-Peyron N, et al: Notalgia paresthetica: clinical, physiopathological and therapeutic aspects. *J Eur Acad Dermatol Venereol* 1999, 12:215.

Shea CR, et al: Herpetic trigeminal trophic syndrome. *Arch Dermatol* 1996, 132:613.

Soria E, et al: Asymmetrical growth of scalp hair in syringomyelia. *Cutis* 1989, 43:33.

Sudo K, et al: Syringomyelia as a cause of body hypertrophy. *Lancet* 1996, 347:1593.

Yell JA, et al: Essential vulvodynia. *Br J Dermatol* (Suppl) 1995, 133:45.

Wallengren J: Successful treatment of notalgia paresthetica with topical capsaicin: vehicle-blind, crossover study. *J Am Acad Dermatol* 1995, 32:287. ▲

CHAPTER 5

Atopic Dermatitis, Eczema, and Noninfectious Immunodeficiency Disorders

ATOPIC DERMATITIS

Atopic dermatitis is also known as *atopic eczema, infantile eczema, flexural eczema, disseminated neurodermatitis,* and *prurigo diathsique* (Besnier). In 1925, Coca introduced the term *atopy,* meaning "out of place" or "strange," to signify the hereditary tendency to develop allergies to food and inhalant substances, as manifested by eczema, asthma, and hay fever. In 1933, Wise and Sulzberger detailed the diagnosis of and named atopic dermatitis.

The prevalence of atopic disease appears to be rising, having increased between twofold and tenfold in the last three decades. Atopic dermatitis now affects approximately 10% to 20% of the population. The tendency to develop atopic dermatitis is inherited. In epidemiologic studies, the child is at increased risk to develop atopy, if either parent is affected. More than one fourth of offspring of atopic mothers develop atopic dermatitis in the first 3 months of life. If one parent is atopic, more than half the children develop allergic symptoms by age 2. This rate rises to 79% if both parents are atopic. Some studies have found the risk for inheritance of atopic dermatitis is higher if the mother rather than the father has the disease. However, if the affected parent has moderate to severe atopic dermatitis persisting into adulthood, their risk of transmitting atopic dermatitis to their offspring is equal and about 50%.

Much effort has been put into the study of allergens that may cause or exacerbate atopic dermatitis. Identification of these allergens, their elimination, and hyposensitization to them have been used to study and manage atopy, especially in relation to respiratory disease. Atopic dermatitis patients frequently have high levels of IgE antibodies to house dust mites, and this IgE is bound to Langerhans cells in atopic skin. House dust mites are ubiquitous, and elimination of the mites from the environment leads to improvement of patients with atopic dermatitis. There is no correlation between improvement with house dust mite eradication and prick tests to house dust mite antigen, however. The allergen patch test, or application of the putative allergen to the skin attempting to reproduce the dermatitis, remains controversial as a method to screen for environmental allergens that provoke or perpetuate atopic dermatitis.

Foods clearly exacerbate symptoms in some atopic individuals, and the work of Sampson has convincingly shown that double-blind food challenges can identify inciting foods, especially in children with atopic dermatitis. Unfortunately, such testing is difficult. Prick testing and RAST testing are useful to exclude food allergies, since virtually no atopic individuals who have negative prick test or RAST test results have positive challenge results. Unfortunately, positive results to a food by prick test and RAST test correlates poorly with food challenges because of the large number of false-positive prick and RAST tests. Intracutaneous testing is associated with a risk of anaphylaxis. Eggs, peanuts (other nuts in children older than 3 years of age), and cow's milk represent about 75% of positive test results, but many foods have been incriminated. Elimination diets are useful if targeted, but strict elimination diets must be undertaken with caution in young children because of the risk of malnutrition.

Atopic dermatitis undergoes a clinical and histologic evolution from an acute eczematous eruption in early life to a characteristic lichenified dermatitis seen in older patients. Atopic dermatitis can be divided into three stages: infantile atopic dermatitis, occurring from 2 months to 2 years of age; childhood atopic dermatitis, from 2 to 10 years; and the adolescent and adult stage of atopic dermatitis. In all stages, pruritus is the hallmark of atopic dermatitis. Itching often precedes the appearance of lesions, hence the concept that atopic dermatitis is "the itch that rashes."

The diagnostic criteria of Hanifin and Rajka are useful in classifying cases. These criteria have been simplified as the UK Working Party's Diagnostic Criteria for Atopic Dermatitis.

MAJOR CRITERIA: Must have three of the following:
1. Pruritus
2. Typical morphology and distribution
   a. Flexural lichenification in adults
   b. Facial and extensor involvement in infancy
3. Chronic or chronically relapsing dermatitis
4. Personal or family history of atopic disease (asthma, allergic rhinitis, atopic dermatitis)

MINOR CRITERIA: Must also have three of the following:

Xerosis

Ichthyosis/hyperlinear palms/keratosis pilaris

IgE reactivity (Immediate skin test reactivity, RAST test positive)

Elevated serum IgE

Early age of onset

Tendency for cutaneous infections (especially *S. aureus* and herpes simplex virus)

Tendency to nonspecific hand/foot dermatitis

Nipple eczema

Cheilitis

Recurrent conjunctivitis

Dennie-Morgan infraorbital fold

Keratoconus

Anterior subcapsular cataracts

Orbital darkening

Facial pallor/facial erythema

Pityriasis alba

Itch when sweating

Intolerance to wool and lipid solvents

Perifollicular accentuation

Food hypersensitivity

Course influenced by environmental and/or emotional factors

White dermographism or delayed blanch to cholinergic agents

The diagnostic criteria have been modified for young infants:

Three major features:

Family history of atopic disease

Typical facial or extensor dermatitis

Evidence of pruritus

Three minor features:

Xerosis/ichthyosis/hyperlinear palms

Perifollicular accentuation

Postauricular fissures

Chronic scalp scaling

Infantile Atopic Dermatitis

Sixty percent of cases of atopic dermatitis present in the first year of life, usually after 2 months of age. Eczema in infancy usually begins as an itchy erythema of the cheeks. In the erythematous patches minute intraepidermal vesicles develop, rupture, and produce moist, crusted areas (Fig. 5-1). The eruption may rapidly extend to other parts of the body, chiefly the scalp, neck, forehead, wrists, and extensor extremities. The areas involved correlate with the capacity of the child to scratch or rub the site, and the activities of the infant, such as crawling. The buttocks and diaper area are frequently spared. The eruption may become generalized (often quite suddenly), with erythroderma and considerable desquamation.

Moist lesions are the most common type in infants. The

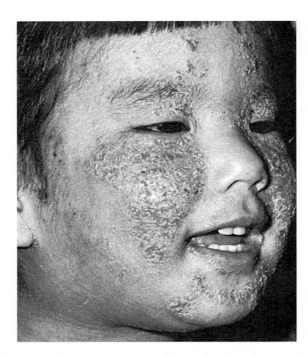

Fig. 5-1 Infantile atopic dermatitis of the face. Note perioral sparing, a frequent feature.

lesions show polymorphism. There may be a significant amount of exudate, and there are many secondary effects from scratching, rubbing, and infection: crusts, pustules, and infiltrated areas. The infiltrated patches eventually take on a characteristic lichenified appearance.

In most infants who suffer from this disease, the skin symptoms disappear toward the end of the second year or sometimes before. The patients are able to eat, without exacerbation, foods that previously seemed to cause flares of dermatitis; they appear to outgrow their sensitivity. Worsening of atopic dermatitis is often observed after immunizations and viral infections. Partial or even complete remission of the dermatitis in summer and relapse in winter are the rule. This may relate to the therapeutic effects of UVB in many atopic patients, and the aggravation by wool and the low humidity of forced air in the winter.

The role of food allergy in infantile and childhood atopic dermatitis has been clarified. In severe atopic dermatitis, Sampson showed that 60% of patients had at least one positive food challenge, and 85% of positive challenges were associated with cutaneous symptoms. The vast majority of positive tests were to egg, peanut, milk, wheat, fish, soy, and chicken. In children over age 3 other nuts were also allergens. The positive challenges correlated with a rise in plasma histamine. If the implicated food was withheld, the patients did better clinically, had a decrease in serum IgE, and 45% lost their reactivity to the food over a 1- to 2-year period. A negative skin prick test was a reliable indicator of absence of food sensitivity. Food allergy, then, may play a significant role in a selected population of young atopic patients. Behavioral symptoms are not associated with positive food challenges, except for irritation from abdominal pain or flare of dermatitis.

Withholding cow's milk foods from infants has been studied with conflicting results, some studies showing dramatic decreases in atopy, others showing no difference in the cumulative prevalence over time. Reports have suggested that mothers eating possible allergens during the second half of pregnancy or during breast feeding may sensitize their children. However, large, randomized trials have failed to show that withholding cow's milk and eggs from mothers reduced the prevalence of atopy in their infants. These restrictive measures may be considered in unique situations in which the risk for atopy in the child is high, or where infantile atopic dermatitis is severe. Particular attention must be paid to the mother's nutritional status if her diet is restricted. Premature discontinuation of breast-feeding should not be advised unless there is clear-cut evidence that breast-feeding is causing or significantly exacerbating the atopic dermatitis.

Childhood Atopic Dermatitis

Throughout childhood, less acute lesions may recur. Such lesions are apt to be less exudative, drier, and more papular. The classic locations are the antecubital and popliteal fossae, the flexor wrists, eyelids, and face, and around the neck (Fig. 5-2). Lesions are quite often lichenified, slightly scaly, or infiltrated plaques. These are intermingled with isolated, excoriated 2- to 4-mm papules that are scattered more widely over the uncovered parts.

Pruritus is a constant feature, and many of the cutaneous changes are secondary to it. Scratching induces lichenification and may lead to secondary infection. A vicious cycle may be established (itch-scratch cycle), as pruritus leads to scratching, the scratching causes thickening of the skin and secondary changes that in themselves cause itching. The scratching impulse is usually beyond the conscious control of the patient. The itching is of exactly the same compelling, paroxysmal type, with inability to feel pain during the paroxysms, that occurs in circumscribed neurodermatitis (lichen simplex chronicus). Indeed, Brocq called atopic dermatitis *neurodermite dissemine.*

Wool irritation appears as pruritus and eczema on the neck, face, hands, wrists, and legs. It is worse every winter and almost disappears during the summer. Feather sensitivity also has its onset in childhood during the second year but is more common in adults. All feather-containing objects, feather comforters, or feather pillows in the house must be discarded or kept out of rooms the child frequents. Sensitivity to cat and dog dander may exacerbate eczema in children.

Severe atopic dermatitis involving more than 50% of the body surface area is associated with growth retardation. This association was not linked to restriction diets or steroid

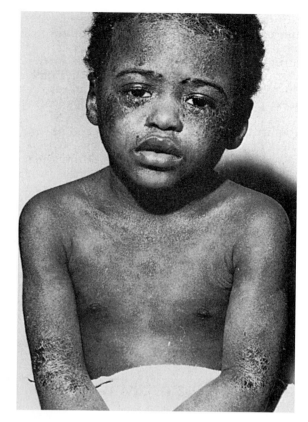

Fig. 5-2 Childhood atopic dermatitis. Lichenification and some scarring have occurred.

usage. Aggressive management of such children with PUVA or phototherapy may allow delayed growth to occur. These children may also have substantial psychologic disturbances, similar to those seen in children with leukemia or epilepsy.

Atopic Dermatitis in Adolescents and Adults

The disease in older patients may occur as localized erythematous, scaly, papular, or vesicular plaques, or in the form of pruritic, lichenified plaques. In adolescents the eruption involves the classic antecubital and popliteal fossae, the front and sides of the neck, the forehead, and the area about the eyes (Fig. 5-3). In older adults the distribution is less characteristic. At times the eruption is generalized, being most severe in the flexures (Fig. 5-4). It is universally lichenified. The typical lesions are dry, slightly elevated, flat-topped papules that tend to coalesce to form lichenified, slightly scaly plaques, which are nearly always excoriated (Fig. 5-5). The plaques are often somewhat erythematous and hyperpigmented. As a result of trauma from scratching, the plaques may become exudative and crusted or infected. The skin, in general, is usually dry and has a tendency to become thickened, and in the widespread type of involvement (disseminated neurodermatitis), there is a leathery quality with exaggerated markings.

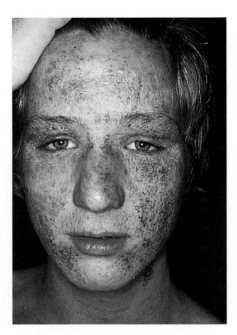

Fig. 5-3 Facial atopic dermatitis in an adolescent.

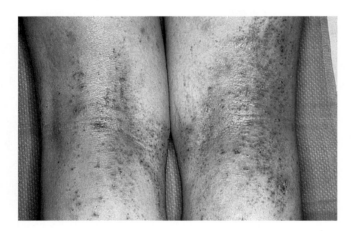

Fig. 5-4 Atopic dermatitis of the popliteal fossae in an adult.

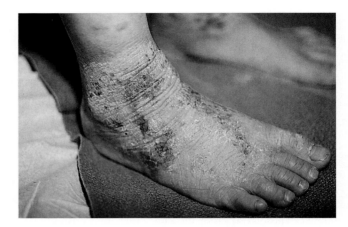

Fig. 5-5 Chronic lichenified acral atopic dermatitis

Itching usually occurs in crises or paroxysms, often in the evening when trying to relax or during the night. Adults frequently complain that flares of atopic dermatitis are triggered by acute emotional upsets. Stress, anxiety, and depression reduce the threshold at which itch is perceived and thus may be a possible mechanism for this finding. Atopic persons may have difficulty delivering sweat to the surface, exacerbating their pruritus when they attempt to exercise. Even in patients with atopic dermatitis in adolescence or early adulthood, improvement usually occurs and atopic dermatitis is uncommon after middle life. In general, throughout life these "resolved atopics" retain mild stigmata of the disease, such as dry skin, easy skin irritation, and itching when they sweat. Unfortunately, they are always

susceptible to a flare of their disease later in life when exposed to the specific allergen or environmental situation. HIV infection is one such trigger, and new onset atopic dermatitis in an at-risk adult should lead to counseling and testing for HIV if warranted.

The hands, including the wrists, are frequently involved in adults. Atopic individuals are at greater risk of developing hand dermatitis than are the rest of the population, about 70% developing it sometime in their life. Atopic individuals represent between 20% and 80% of all patients with hand dermatitis, and patients with severe hand dermatitis tend to be atopic. Hand dermatitis may be the most common problem for adults with a history of prior atopic dermatitis. Atopic hand dermatitis can affect both the dorsal and palmar surfaces. The pattern of hand eczema in atopics, unfortunately, may not be clinically distinguishable from other forms of hand dermatitis, such as contact dermatitis. It is extremely common for atopic hand dermatitis to appear in young women after the birth of their first child, when increased exposure to soaps and water trigger their disease. Hyperlinearity of the palm, long thought to be a marker for atopy, has been recognized both by Lobitz and by Uehara et al to be a manifestation of ichthyosis vulgaris, which accompanies atopic dermatitis in 30% to 40% of cases. Fifty percent of patients with ichthyosis vulgaris have a personal or family history of atopic dermatitis. Keratosis punctata of the creases, a disorder seen almost exclusively in blacks, is more common in atopics.

Associated Features and Complications of Atopic Dermatitis

Cutaneous Stigmata. A linear transverse fold just below the edge of the lower eyelids known as the *Dennie-Morgan fold* is widely believed to be indicative of the "atopic diathesis"—a tendency to or a family history of atopic dermatitis, asthma, or hay fever (Fig. 5-6). A study by Uehara et al of 300 patients with atopic dermatitis and 11 with contact dermatitis showed the fold in 25% of the

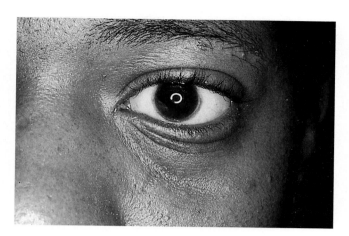

Fig. 5-6   Dennie-Morgan folds.

former and 70% of the latter. He regarded it as a nonspecific consequence of any dermatitis of the lower lids. In atopic patients with eyelid dermatitis, increased folds and darkening under the eyes is common.

The apparently normal skin of atopic dermatitis patients is frequently dry and may be scaly. Transepidermal water loss is increased, although the stratum corneum is thicker. The water barrier is diminished, and the threshold to irritancy is decreased. These suggest that even apparently normal skin is frequently inflamed subclinically. The dry, scaling skin of atopic dermatitis represents low-grade dermatitis.

Pityriasis alba is a form of subclinical dermatitis, frequently atopic in origin. It presents as poorly marginated, slightly scaly patches on the cheeks, upper arms, and trunk, typically in young children. Postinflammatory hypopigmentation is the primary manifestation, and the condition usually responds to mild topical steroids, preferably in an ointment base. Keratosis pilaris, horny follicular lesions of the outer aspects of the upper arms and legs, is commonly associated with the dry skin of atopic dermatitis. It is very refractory to treatment. Moisturizers alone are only partially beneficial, and the keratolytics (salicylic acid and alpha-hydroxy acids) and topical tretinoin easily irritate the skin of atopics. Keratosis pilaris must be distinguished from the permanent "goose bump" appearance of some atopic's skin. There are fine papules identical to cutis anserina that are relatively fixed. Atopic dermatitis and other eczemas are commonly folliculocentric, especially in black patients.

Thinning of the lateral eyebrows, Hertoghe's sign, is sometimes present. Keratosis punctata palmaris et plantaris is a condition seen chiefly in black atopic patients. In a prospective study of 573 patients, Anderson et al found that of 11 affected patients, 9 (82%) had atopy or a family history of atopy. Clover et al described "dirty neck" or reticulated pigmentation of the neck as an adjunctive sign.

Vascular Stigmata. Atopic individuals often exhibit perinasal and periorbital pallor ("headlight sign"); there may be generalized pallor. White dermographism is blanching of the skin at the site of stroking with a blunt instrument. It is best elicited on the brow of an adult with atopic dermatitis. This reaction differs from the triple response of Lewis in that the third response (flaring) is replaced by a blanching to produce a white line. Blanching is caused by the local accumulation of edema, which obscures the color of underlying vessels. When 0.1 ml of a 1:100,000 solution of histamine is injected intradermally, the flare phase of the triple response is absent or diminished.

In atopic dermatitis, 0.1 ml of 1:10,000 acetylcholine injected intradermally will produce in 70% of subjects a delayed blanch phenomenon lasting for some 20 minutes after the injection; moreover, there is increased whealing in response to acetylcholine in atopic dermatitis as well as in those with hay fever or asthma without dermatitis.

Atopics are at increased risk to develop various forms of urticaria, including contact urticaria. Repeated exacerbations of contact urticaria may be followed by typical eczematous lesions.

Ophthalmologic Abnormalities. Up to 10% of patients with atopic dermatitis develop cataracts, either anterior or posterior subcapsular ones. Posterior subcapsular cataracts in atopic individuals are indistinguishable from corticosteroid-induced cataracts. Development of cataracts is more common in patients with severe dermatitis. Keratoconus is an uncommon entity, occurring in approximately 1% of atopic patients. Contact lenses may be of benefit in treating this condition.

Susceptibility to Infection. In lesions of atopic dermatitis, *Staphylococcus aureus* is present abundantly and dominates the skin flora. More than 90% of chronic eczematous lesions contain *S. aureus*, often in large numbers. In addition, the apparently normal nonlesional skin of atopic patients also contains increased numbers of *S. aureus*. A finding of increasing numbers of pathogenic staphylococci is frequently associated with weeping, crusting, folliculitis, and adenopathy. In any flaring atopic the possibility of secondary infection must be considered. Treatment of lesions of atopic dermatitis with topical steroids is associated with reduced numbers of pathogenic bacteria on the surface, even if antibiotics are not used. IgE antibodies directed against staphylococcus and its toxins have been documented in some atopic individuals, a possible mechanism for staphylococcal flares of disease. Staphylococcal production of superantigens is another possible mechanism.

There is increased susceptibility to generalized herpes simplex infection called *eczema herpeticum*. This is seen most frequently in young children and is usually HSV 1 transmitted from a parent or sibling with a cold sore or fever blister. Once infected the atopic may have recurrences of

HSV, and repeat episodes of eczema herpeticum. Eczema herpeticum presents as the sudden appearance of vesicular, pustular, crusted or punched out erosive lesions concentrated in the areas of dermatitis. Secondary staphylococcal infection is frequent and local edema and regional adenopathy commonly occur. If lesions of eczema herpeticum occur on or around the eyelids, ophthalmologic evaluation is recommended. The severity of eczema herpeticum is quite variable, but in all cases systemic acyclovir and an antistaphylococcal antibiotic are recommended.

Vaccination against smallpox is contraindicated in persons with atopic dermatitis, even when the condition is in remission; widespread and even fatal vaccinia can occur.

With or without steroid treatment certain sites of atopic dermatitis, especially the antecubital and popliteal fossae may develop extensive superimposed infections with flat warts and molluscum contagiosum. Because the skin is very easily irritated, chemical treatments such as salicylic acid and cantharidin are poorly tolerated. Destruction with curettage (for molluscum), cryosurgery, or electrosurgery in refractory cases are recommended.

Immunology of Atopic Dermatitis

The immunologic abnormalities identified in atopics result in large part from the T helper cell type 2 (Th2) dominance in tissues affected by atopic disease, including the skin. Th2 cells produce interleukins 4, 5, and 10. IL-4 and IL-5 produce elevated IgE levels and eosinophilia in tissue and peripheral blood. IL-10 inhibits delayed type hypersensitivity. IL-4 downregulates gamma-interferon production. A surprisingly large percentage of these Th2 cells in atopic dermatitis skin may be specific to allergens, such as house dust mites or grass pollen.

Monocytes in the peripheral blood of atopic dermatitis patients produce elevated amounts of prostaglandin E2 (PGE2). PGE2 reduces gamma-interferon production but not IL-4 from helper T cells, enhancing the Th2 dominance. PGE2 also directly enhances IgE production from B cells.

Langerhans cells in the skin of atopic dermatitis are abnormal. They directly stimulate helper T cells without the presence of antigen, selectively activating helper T cells into a Th2 phenotype. Many Langerhans cells in atopic dermatitis have IgE bound onto their surface receptor for IgE, and this IgE is specific to allergens associated with atopic disease, for example, house dust mites.

A mutation in the high affinity IgE receptor has been reported in unrelated cohorts with atopic disease. Inheritance of this mutation from the mother, but not the father, results in an atopic offspring. Atopy mapped to this region of chromosome 11q in 60% of atopic families, and 17% of atopic families had the same specific point mutation in the beta subunit of the high affinity IgE receptor gene. The high affinity IgE receptor exists on mast cells, monocytes, and Langerhans cells and plays a central role in mediating IgE dependent allergic inflammation. Stimulation of this recep-

tor on mast cells results in the production of Th2 cytokines including IL-4, and such stimulated mast cells may directly regulate local B cell IgE synthesis. Mutations in this receptor could result in abnormal stimulation of allergic inflammation.

The Th2-dominant state in atopic skin correlates with the clinical immune defects seen. Reduced Th1 activity (gamma-interferon production) could explain why atopics have decreased sensitivity to topically applied antigens, including DNCB. Toxicodendron sensitivity occurs in only 15% of individuals with atopic dermatitis compared with 61% of nonatopic controls. Atopics may, however, develop allergic contact dermatitis to components of their medicaments, probably because of chronic, long-term exposure. Atopic skin has a reduced capacity to resist dermatophyte and certain viral infections, controlled by Th1 helper T cells.

Abnormalities of cutaneous nerves and the products they secrete (neuropeptides) have been recently identified in atopic dermatitis. These may explain the abnormal vascular responses, reduced itch threshold, and perhaps some of the immunologic imbalances seen in atopic skin.

Differential Diagnosis

Typical atopic dermatitis is not difficult to diagnose because of its predilection for symmetric involvement of face, neck, and antecubital and popliteal fossae. Dermatoses resembling atopic dermatitis may be seborrheic dermatitis (especially in the infant), irritant or allergic contact dermatitis, nummular dermatitis, scabies, and psoriasis (especially palmoplantar). In infants, certain immunodeficiency syndromes discussed later in this chapter may exhibit a dermatitis remarkably similar or identical to atopic dermatitis.

Histopathology

The histology of atopic dermatitis ranges from acute spongiotic dermatitis to lichen simplex chronicus, depending on the morphology of the skin lesion biopsied. Although eosinophils may not be seen in the dermal infiltrate, staining for eosinophil major basic protein, a component unique to the eosinophil granule, demonstrates abundant staining in most cases. These features are nonspecific and do not exclude other forms of dermatitis, so biopsies are only performed when lesions are atypical.

General Management in Infancy and Childhood

Any external irritation may precipitate an attack of eczema—excessive bathing, vigorous rubbing, or chafing; unduly heavy, tight, or soiled clothing; insufficient cleanliness especially in the diaper region, local infections, irritating secretions, or even medicated baby oils. One of the first considerations is the protection of the affected parts from scratching.

Because soap and water may aggravate the disease, olive oil, Cetaphil, Aquanil, or similar products on absorbent cotton may be used for cleansing without water. Particular attention should be given to the genitals and buttocks, and diapers should be changed whenever they are wet or soiled, after the parts have been cleansed.

Antihistaminic drugs are somewhat beneficial, especially if given at night, when the accompanying sedative effects may be helpful. The dosage must be adequate and regular. The nonsedating antihistamines provide little or no benefit in reducing pruritus.

In cases where specific food allergies are implicated, dietary restrictions are in order. Eliminating the foods on a trial basis for several weeks is an alternative to food challenge, but not nearly as accurate. Because food challenges may induce anaphylaxis they must be done under controlled conditions. A general restriction diet for infantile eczema that avoids most of the commonly implicated foods is as follows: for infants under 3 months, milk substitute alone (casein hydrolysates—Nutramigen or Pregestimil); for babies 3 to 6 months, milk substitute and rice cereal; for children 6 months to 2 years, milk substitute with vitamin supplement, rice cereal, applesauce, pears, carrots, squash, and lamb; for older children or adults, add lamb and rice. To confirm food allergy by such elimination diets, the symptoms should improve substantially during the restriction and worsen with reintroduction of incriminated foods. Several cycles may be required to confirm food hypersensitivity.

General Management in Adults

Atopics should avoid extremes of cold and heat. The dry skin of atopics tends to be worse in the winter and should be hydrated daily with moisturizers. Overbathing must be avoided, and soap used only in the axillae, groin, and scalp. The least irritating soaps are Alpha-Keri, Dove, Basis, Neutrogena, and Emulave. Showers should be warm to cool, not hot. Tub soaking is good, if followed by adequate lubrication. Humidifiers in rooms are helpful. The patient should not wear wool, because its fibers are irritating. It is important the patient be aware that emotional stress can be an important factor in causing exacerbations. In adults with atopic disease biofeedback and other psychologic techniques may be adjunctively useful.

Specific Treatment Modalities

Topical Therapy. Corticosteroid therapy is the dominant method of treatment of atopic dermatitis. In infants, low-potency steroid ointments such as hydrocortisone 1% or 2.5% are preferred. Emphasis must be placed on regular application and rubbing the medication in well. In older children and adults, a medium-potency steroid such as triamcinolone are the mainstay, except on the face, where milder steroids are used. For thick plaques and lichen simplex chronicus–like lesions very potent steroids may be necessary. Although the potential for local and even systemic toxicity is real, the steroid must be strong enough

to control the pruritus and remove the inflammation. Even in small children, strong topical steroids may be necessary in pulses to control severe flares. Monitoring of growth parameters should be done in infants and young children with high surface-to-volume ratios. If an atopic patient worsens or fails to improve after the use of topical steroids and moisturizers, the possibility of allergic contact dermatitis to a preservative or even the corticosteroids themselves must be entertained.

For the acute weeping eczematous dermatitis, wet compresses of Burow's solution are the treatment of choice. Burow's solution is available in powder form: Domeboro packets and Aluwets. Alibour's solution and potassium permanganate (1:5000) solution are also effective when applied for 20 to 30 minutes several times daily. Topical steroids or moisturizers are applied immediately after compressing.

For the hydration of xerotic skin of atopic dermatitis, 10% urea in a hydrophilic cream, Eucerin cream, petrolatum, or 1% hydrocortisone in 10% urea cream is effective. Lactic acid–containing moisturizers in concentrations higher than 5% are generally poorly tolerated by atopic patients with active dermatitis.

Crude coal tar 1% to 5% in white petrolatum or hydrophilic ointment USP, or liquor carbonis detergens (LCD) 5% to 10% in hydrophilic ointment USP is helpful. Tar preparations are especially beneficial when used for intensive treatment in an inpatient or day care setting.

Topical FK 506 (tacrolimus) is dramatically beneficial in severe atopic dermatitis when applied as a 0.03% to 0.3% ointment. Alaiti and Rusicka reported that 95% of patients showed at least a good improvement. Burning at the application site and vasodilation were the most common side effects. Systemic accumulation of drug was not detected in most patients. Ascomycin and its derivatives also seem to have similar efficacy with limited toxicity.

Systemic Therapy. Antihistaminics may be used to aid in the relief of the severe pruritus. Hydroxyzine (Atarax or Vistaril), or in more difficult cases, doxepin (Sinequan) in doses of about 25 to 75 mg as a single evening dose is frequently recommended in adults.

S. aureus has long been known to be a frequent resident of both normal and involved skin in atopic dermatitis. Many patients benefit from more or less prolonged courses of antistaphylococcal antibiotics, even when clinical evidence of infection is lacking. Semisynthetic penicillins, first generation cephalosporins, erythromycin (if isolates are sensitive), quinolones, and minocycline are options. Nasal carriage can be treated with topical mupirocin or oral rifampin 600 mg daily for 5 days.

Systemic steroids are effective in the treatment of atopic dermatitis, but their efficacy is frequently complicated by side effects. In general, systemic steroids should be used only to control acute exacerbations, the cause of which can be eliminated, such as a flare resulting from a contact allergen. In patients requiring systemic steroid therapy, the minimum dose, given on alternate days if possible is advised. If doses in excess of 15 to 20 mg on alternate days are required, or if side effects result, consideration should be given to alternative therapies for their steroid sparing effect. Long-term complications of steroids, such as osteoporosis in women, must be considered when choosing chronic oral steroid therapy as a therapeutic option. Preventive strategies such as calcium supplements, vitamin D supplementation, regular exercise, and stopping smoking should be strongly encouraged.

Phototherapy. Photochemotherapy (PUVA) as given for psoriasis, is often helpful in severe atopic dermatitis. UVB therapy, or a Goeckerman with UVB and tar may also be effective. The combination of UVA with UVB is superior to UVB alone, producing complete clearing in half the patients with a 40% lower dose than UVB alone. UVA alone is also effective.

Nonsteroidal Internal Therapy. Cyclosporine is effective in the treatment of severe atopic dermatitis. Its potential side effects and high cost preclude its use in all but the most severe patients. As in other diseases, the condition flares when cyclosporine is discontinued. The immune modulators, interferon gamma and thymopentin, have demonstrated efficacy in atopic dermatitis. Their use is still considered experimental, but experience to date points to more targeted immune therapies for atopic disease. Papaverine has failed to demonstrate efficacy in placebo controlled trials. Traditional Chinese herb mixtures have shown efficacy in children, but the active ingredients and their mechanism of action remain unknown. They are usually delivered as a brewed tea to be drunk daily, but are extremely unpalatable making use difficult. Hepatitis and cardiomyopathy have occurred during herbal treatments.

Management of an Acute Flare of Atopic Dermatitis. Initially, the precipitating cause of the flare should be sought. Secondary infection with *S. aureus* and, less commonly, herpes simplex are identified and treated. Pityriasis rosea and cutaneous coxsackie virus infections may also flare atopic dermatitis. The development of contact sensitivity to an applied medication must be considered. Recent stressful events may be associated with flares.

In the setting of an acute flare, treating triggers identified above may lead to improvement. A short course of systemic steroids may benefit if not contraindicated. "Home hospitalization" may be useful: the patient goes home to bed; large doses of antihistaminics are given to sedate the patient; the patient soaks twice daily in the tub and applies potent steroids two to four times daily. Most important is that the patient gets out of bed only to apply medications or bathe. Meals are prepared for the patient, and the patient is isolated from work and other stressors. Often, 3 to 4 days of

such intensive home "hospitalization" will break a severe flare. Phototherapy and especially day care treatment, as used for psoriasis, will also break flares and result in a more stable disease state following treatment.

Absolon CM, et al: Psychological disturbances in atopic eczema. *Br J Dermatol* 1997, 137:241.

Alaiti S, et al: Tacrolimus FK506 ointment for atopic dermatitis. *J Am Acad Dermatol* 1998, 38:69.

Boiko S, et al: Osteomyelitis of distal phalanges in 3 children with severe atopic dermatitis. *Arch Dermatol* 1988, 124:418.

Businco L, et al: Double-blind crossover trial with oral sodium cromoglycate in children with atopic dermatitis due to food allergy. *Ann Allergy* 1986, 57:433.

Coleman R, et al: Genetic studies of atopy and atopic dermatitis. *Br J Dermatol* 1997, 136:1.

Dahl RE, et al: Sleep disturbances in children with atopic dermatitis. *Arch Pediatr Adolesc Med* 1995, 149:856.

Ferguson JE, et al: Reversible dilated cardiomyopathy following treatment of atopic eczema with Chinese herbal medicine. *Br J Dermatol* 1997, 136:592.

Fitzharris P, et al: House dust mites in atopic dermatitis. *Int J Dermatol* 1999, 38:173.

Friedmann PS: The role of dust mite antigen sensitization and atopic dermatitis. *Clin Exp Allergy* 1999, 29:869.

Gelmetti C: Extracutaneous manifestations of atopic dermatitis. *Pediatr Dermatol* 1992, 9:380.

Goldman AS: Association of atopic diseases with breast feeding. *J Pediatr* 1999, 134:5.

Grewe M, et al: A role for Th1 and Th2 cells in the immunopathogenesis of atopic dermatitis. *Immunol Today* 1998 19:359.

Halbert AR, et al: Atopic dermatitis. *J Am Acad Dermatol* 1995, 33:1008.

Hanifin JM, et al: Biochemical and immunologic mechanisms in atopic dermatitis. *J Am Acad Dermatol* 1999, 41:72.

Larsen FS, et al: The occurrence of atopic dermatitis in North Europe. *J Am Acad Dermatol* 1996, 34:760.

Norris PG, et al: Screening for cataracts in patients with atopic eczema. *Clin Exp Dermatol* 1987, 12:21.

Ogawa H, et al: Atopic dermatitis. *Pediatr Dermatol* 1992, 9:383.

Rothe MJ, et al: Atopic dermatitis: an update. *J Am Acad Dermatol* 1996, 35:1.

Rustin MHA, et al: Chinese herbal therapy in atopic dermatitis. *Dermatologic Therapy* 1996, 1:83.

Ruzicka T, et al: A short-term trial of tacrolimus ointment for atopic dermatitis. *N Engl J Med* 1997, 337:816.

Ruzicka T, et al: Tacrolimus: the drug for the turn of the millennium? *Arch Dermatol* 1999, 135:574.

Sampson HA: Food hypersensitivity and dietary management in atopic dermatitis. *Pediatr Dermatol* 1992, 9: 376.

Sheehan MP, et al: One-year follow up of children treated with Chinese medicinal herbs for atopic dermatitis. *Br J Dermatol* 1994, 130:488.

Strange P, et al: Staphylococcal enterotoxin B applied to intact normal and intact atopic skin induces dermatitis. *Arch Dermatol* 1996, 132:27.

Tan BB, et al: Double-blind controlled trial of effect of housedust-mite allergen avoidance on atopic dermatitis. *Lancet* 1996, 347:15.

Williams HC: Diagnostic criteria for atopic dermatitis. *Arch Dermatol* 1999, 135:583. _____ ▲

ECZEMA

The word *eczema* seems to have originated in AD 543 and is derived from the Greek word *ekzein,* meaning to "boil out" or to "effervesce." Baer described eczema as a "pruritic papulovesicular process which in its acute phase is associated with erythema and edema and which in its more chronic phases, while retaining some of its papulovesicular features, is dominated by thickening, lichenification, and scaling." Ackerman pointed out that the word refers to a group of diseases with no common denominator and calls for its elimination from the dermatologist's vocabulary. If it is recognized that "eczema" is a descriptive term and not a specific diagnosis, the concept has extreme value: it unifies a group of disorders into a morphologic category that is clinically characteristic.

Histologically, the hallmark of all eczematous eruptions is a serous exudate between cells of the epidermis (spongiosis), with an inflammatory infiltrate in the dermis. Spongiosis is very prominent in acute dermatitis of the atopic, infectious eczematoid, dyshidrotic, and contact types and often manifests macroscopic as well as microscopic vesiculation. A scale or crust composed of serous exudate, acute inflammatory cells, and keratin corresponds to the honey-colored crust noted clinically. The dermal infiltrate is usually lymphocytic in nature.

Spongiosis and a mixed-cell inflammatory infiltrate are likewise prominent in nummular eczema, which also shows psoriasiform epidermal hyperplasia. Xerotic eczema is characterized by minimal spongiosis, a scant lymphocytic inflammatory infiltrate, and a change in the appearance of the keratin layer from the normal "basketweave" pattern to a compact one.

Eczema, regardless of cause, will manifest similar histologic changes if allowed to persist chronically. These features, which correspond clinically to lichen simplex chronicus, include hyperkeratosis, irregular acanthosis (hyperplasia) of the epidermis, and thickening of the collagen bundles in the papillary portion of the dermis. The development of lichen simplex chronicus is directly related to persistent rubbing and scratching of the skin.

In these reactions severe pruritus is a common and often the most prominent symptom. The degree of irritation at which itching begins (the itch threshold) is lowered by stress.

Regional Eczemas

Ear Eczema.
Eczema of the ears or otitis externa may involve the helix, postauricular fold, and the external auditory canal. By far the most frequently affected site is the external canal, where many mechanisms join to protect the delicate structures of the internal ear from contamination. Secretions of the ear canal derive from the apocrine and sebaceous glands, which form cerumen. Traumatization of the ear canal by rubbing, wiping, scratching, and picking induces edema and infection with inflammation. Ear eczema is most frequently caused by seborrheic or atopic dermatitis. Infection is usually caused by staphylococci or streptococci. *Pseudomonas aeruginosa* itself will become a pathogen in the wet, damaged skin of the external auditory canal. Contact dermatitis from neomycin, benzocaine, and preservatives may result from topical remedies used to treat these

conditions. Earlobe dermatitis is virtually pathognomonic of nickel allergy and occurs most frequently in women who have pierced ears.

Treatment should be directed to removal of causative agents, such as those already mentioned. Scales and cerumen should be removed by lavage with an ear syringe. Frequent instillation of antibiotic-corticoid preparations, such as Cortisporin, Terra-Cortril, or topical steroid creams or solutions with or without 5% liquor carbonis detergens, are effective treatments. For very weepy lesions, Burow's solution in otic form may be drying and beneficial.

Eyelid Dermatitis.
Eyelid dermatitis of one eye only is most frequently caused by nail polish, and usually affects the upper eyelid. Atopic dermatitis frequently causes eyelid dermatitis of one or both eyes, and both the upper and lower eyelids may be involved. When the lids of both eyes are involved, other allergens such as mascara, eye shadow, eyelash cement, eyeliner, or the rubber-tipped instruments used to apply the cosmetics must be considered. Hair dye, rinse, tint, lacquer, and hair spray contact dermatitis may involve the eyelids, but usually other sites are also involved. Many cases of eyelid contact dermatitis are caused by substances transferred by the hands to the eyelids. Any sensitizer or irritant on the palms or fingers may cause dermatitis of the eyelids long before it affects any other parts of the face.

Volatile gases such as insect sprays, lemon peel oil, benzalkonium chloride, and preservatives in the rinsing solution used in connection with contact lenses, or plastics in spectacle frames containing ethylene glycol monomethyl ether acetate (EGMEA) may all cause eyelid dermatitis.

Breast Eczema (Nipple Eczema).
Eczema of the breasts may affect the nipples, areolae, skin, or the folds beneath. Usually, eczema of the nipples is of the moist type with oozing and crusting (Fig. 5-7). Painful fissuring is frequently seen, especially in nursing mothers.

Circumscribed neurodermatitis, atopic dermatitis, and contact dermatitis must be considered in the differential diagnosis. Nipple eczema if often an isolated manifestation of atopic dermatitis. In those patients in whom the eczema of the nipple or areola has persisted for more than 3 months, especially if it is unilateral, a biopsy is mandatory to rule out the possibility of Paget's disease of the breast. Topical or intralesional corticosteroids are effective in the treatment of non-Paget's eczema of the breast.

Hand Eczema.
The hands may be involved by various dermatoses. Although on other sites, different dermatoses are usually morphologically quite distinct, when the palmar and plantar surfaces are involved, these distinct dermatoses may be difficult or impossible to differentiate. A complete history, careful examination of the rest of the body surface, and often patch testing are required to establish a diagnosis in a patient with hand eczema. Frequently, patients with

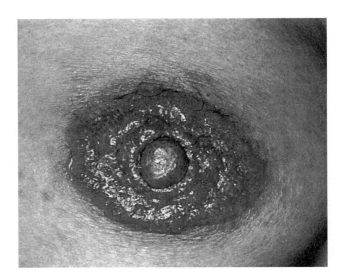

Fig. 5-7 Nipple eczema.

hand eczema have two or more causes for their dermatitis, such as an atopic diathesis plus contact dermatitis resulting from exposure to an environmental allergen. Even so, many cases cannot be definitively diagnosed and are simply labeled "hand eczema."

Hand eczema represents a major occupational problem. Patients with hand eczema frequently miss work and may need to change occupations. It is a major cause of emotional and sometimes financial stress. In health care workers with hand dermatitis who may be exposed to infectious fluids such as blood, the impaired barrier may represent an increased (though very low) risk for infection by blood-borne pathogens.

In most forms of hand dermatitis, atopic patients are disproportionately represented. Hand dermatitis is frequently the initial or only adult manifestation of an atopic diathesis. The likelihood of developing hand eczema is greatest in patients with atopic dermatitis, more common if the atopic dermatitis was severe, but still increased in incidence in patients with only respiratory atopy. Atopic patients should receive career counseling in adolescence to avoid occupations, such as automotive repair, metal, or custodial work, that are likely to induce hand dermatitis.

IRRITANT HAND DERMATITIS. Irritant hand dermatitis is a common disease frequently seen in homemakers, resulting from or at least aggravated by excessive and prolonged exposure to soaps or detergents and water. The eruption usually begins with dryness and redness of the fingers. Dry scales with peeling are evident at the tips of the fingers, "chapping" is seen on the backs of the hands, and erythematous hardening of the palms with fissures develops. Frequently, dermatitis appears around and under rings, especially wedding bands that are not removed when using soap and water.

The defatting action and maceration produced by pro-

longed immersion or frequent washing of the hands may be seen in other occupations, such as bartenders, food service workers, and health care workers, who wash their hands frequently. Irritant hand dermatitis is also frequently seen in occupations in which there is exposure to chemicals, solvents, acids, or alkalis, such as custodians and metal workers. Friction and cold or dry air are other factors that irritate the skin of the hands.

The impaired barrier induced by irritant hand eczema may enhance the development of allergic reactions, which may complicate the hand dermatitis. Such contactants should always be sought by history and patch testing if necessary. In homemakers, there may be allergic sensitization to foods such as garlic, onion, carrot, tomato, spinach, grapefruit, orange, radish, fig, parsnip, or cheese. Some foods may produce contact urticaria, which may manifest as an eczematous reaction 24 to 48 hours after exposure. These include potatoes, flour, fish, shellfish, and cheese. There may be sensitization to rubber gloves, plastic articles, or plants such as the philodendron or *Compositae;* to metals such as nickel; to dyes such as paraphenylenediamine; to colophony resin in newspapers; to formaldehyde in cleaning products; and numerous other allergenic contactants. A careful occupational history is essential to identify possible contactants. Secondary bacterial infection, usually with *S. aureus,* may occur in the fissured areas.

The diagnosis of irritant hand eczema is made by excluding other disorders with which it may be confused, notably patchy pompholyx, allergic contact dermatitis, tinea manum, and psoriasis. Pitting of the nails is characteristic of psoriasis. Palmar tinea is usually unilateral and keratolysis exfoliativa is symmetrical and superficial.

Atopic dermatitis as a primary disorder of the hands or a genetic predisposition to it, is frequently present in many patients with irritant hand dermatitis. It is important when considering psoriasis and atopic dermatitis to take a family history and a personal history of previous related problems and to examine the entire cutaneous surface. The feet should always be examined in evaluating any hand dermatitis.

VESICULOBULLOUS HAND ECZEMA (POMPHOLYX, DYSHIDROSIS). Hand dermatitis commonly presents with a vesicular pattern clinically or spongiosis histologically. Within this group of palm and sole eruptions are acute eruptions (referred to here as *pompholyx*), relapsing or chronic vesiculobullous eruptions, and chronic hand eczemas that are morphologically hyperkeratotic but histologically spongiotic. These classifications are indistinct, but patients can usually be classified into one of these three groups.

Epidemiologically, there appear to be different prevalences of underlying causes in the different groups. *Dyshidrosis* and *dyshidrosiform* are still used as morphologic descriptive terms, but the association with a sweating disorder is no longer held as valid. Palmoplantar hyperhidrosis is common in the acute and subacute forms of vesiculobullous palmoplantar dermatoses.

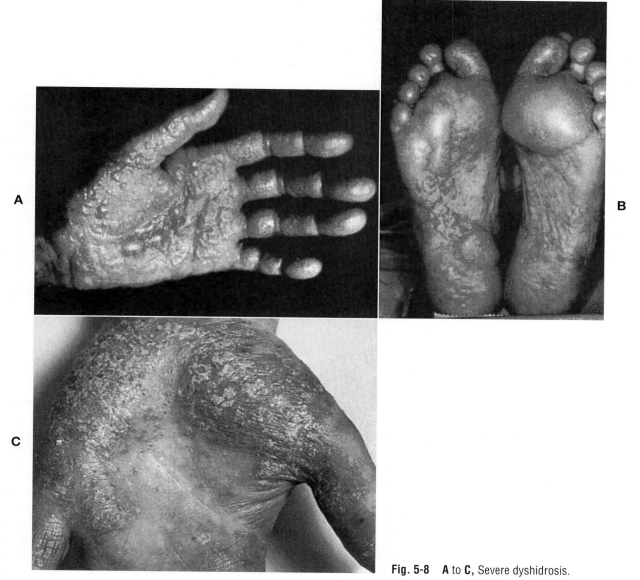

Fig. 5-8 **A** to **C**, Severe dyshidrosis.

Pompholyx. True acute pompholyx, also known as *cheiropompholyx* if it affects the hands, is an uncommon disorder. Patients have severe, sudden outbreaks with often long disease-free periods. Primary lesions are macroscopic, deep-seated vesicles resembling tapioca on the sides of the fingers, palms, and soles (Fig. 5-8). The eruption is symmetrical and pruritic, with pruritus often preceding the eruption. Coalescence of smaller lesions may lead to bulla formation extensive enough to prevent ambulation. Individual outbreaks resolve spontaneously over several weeks. Bullous tinea or an id from a dermatophyte should be excluded, and patch testing should be considered to rule out allergic contact dermatitis.

Chronic vesiculobullous hand eczema. Subacute or chronic vesiculobullous palmoplantar eruptions are com-

mon and difficult to manage. Females outnumber males three to one. All patients present with a vesicular eruption of the palms and soles characterized by eczematous, weeping patches containing intraepidermal vesicles, and often by burning or itching. There is a tendency for the pruritic 1- to 2-mm vesicles to be most pronounced at the sides of the fingers. In long-standing cases the nails may become damaged. The distribution of the lesions is, as a rule, bilateral and roughly symmetrical. Sometimes they are arranged in groups. By coalescence of several contiguous vesicles, bullae may be formed. The contents are clear and colorless but may later become straw-colored or purulent. The disorder may be cyclic, with exacerbations that last a few weeks. Because of the tendency for relapses to occur, the condition may persist for long periods. In chronic cases the lesions may be hyperkeratotic, scaling, and fissured, and the "dyshidrosiform" pattern may be recognized only during exacerbations.

Evaluation of this type of patient requires patience and skill. Atopic dermatitis is found in about 15% of cases but may represent only a cofactor or "fertile soil" for the development of vesicular hand dermatitis. An extremely detailed history for possible contactants and patch testing are usually required if simple therapy does not lead to improvement. Although contact allergens may be found, their relevance is frequently questioned. This is especially true in the case of ingested allergens, such as nickel. Nonetheless, every effort should be made to identify any relevant contactants, because this represents a "curable" cause of the disorder. Tinea pedis must be excluded. Smoking, as in palmoplantar pustulosis, may be a cofactor.

HYPERKERATOTIC DERMATITIS OF THE PALMS. Hersle and Mobacken have described adults with chronic hyperkeratotic eruptions of the palms. Males outnumber females by a ratio of 2:1, and the patients are usually older adults (average age at onset, 45). The eruption presents as hyperkeratotic, fissure-prone, infiltrated lesions of the middle or proximal palm. The volar surfaces of the fingers may also be involved. Plantar lesions occur in about 10% of patients. Histologically, the lesions show chronic spongiotic dermatitis. In this group, atopic dermatitis and allergic contactants are not frequently found. Occasionally, a patient will eventually develop psoriasis. While the evaluation is the same as with other forms of hand eczema, the yield is considerably lower.

Vesicular eruptions of the palms and soles closely resemble each other, so that the clinical features are often inadequate to establish a diagnosis. In addition, patients may have a combination of factors, such as atopic disease plus a contactant, so finding a single cause may not be a sufficient evaluation. Dermatophytid, atopic dermatitis, allergic contact dermatitis, and the palmoplantar pustuloses (pustular psoriasis, acrodermatitis continua, and pustular bacterid) must all be considered. Even the autoimmune bullous disorders may present as vesicular hand dermatitis.

TREATMENT OF HAND ECZEMAS. At times, alleviation of hand dermatitis will tax the ingenuity of the patient and the physician to the limit. In most cases it is impossible for the patient, especially a young mother, to discontinue soap and water exposure. Vinyl gloves should be worn, especially when detergents are used. This avoids the possibility of the development of sensitivity to the rubber in rubber gloves. Although vinyl gloves are protective from chemicals, they do not prevent exposure to heat through the glove or the macerating effect of sweat, which accumulates under the gloves. Wearing white cotton gloves under the vinyl gloves is beneficial. For rough work, such as gardening, wearing protective cloth or leather gloves is essential.

Moisturizing is a critical component of the management of hand dermatitis. Application of a moisturizing protective cream or ointment after each hand washing or water exposure is recommended. At night, even during periods of remission, a heavy moisturizing ointment should be applied to the hands. If palmar dryness is present, occlusion of the moisturizer with vinyl gloves is recommended.

In acute vesicular disease, soaking the hands and feet in a potassium permanganate solution (1:5000) or the use of Burow's solution compresses may have benefit. Superpotent and potent topical steroid agents are the initial therapy; their benefit is variable. Their efficacy may be enhanced by occlusion.

The use of systemic corticosteroids usually results in dramatic improvement. Unfortunately, relapse frequently occurs, so they are recommended in only the most severe cases or to control exacerbations. In most patients, unfortunately, the doses of systemic corticosteroids required to control hand dermatitis are too high to be considered safe in the long term.

Phototherapy in the form of UVA alone or PUVA either topically or systemically has some success and low risk. Topical PUVA is inferior to superficial radiotherapy. Radiotherapy is less time consuming and leads to more rapid improvement. Unfortunately, the doses of radiotherapy published as efficacious can be given only a limited number of times without concern for long-term sequelae. This is one of the benign dermatoses in which superficial radiotherapy may still play a role.

Diaper (Napkin) Dermatitis.
Dermatitis of the diaper area in infants is common cutaneous disorder, with 7% to 35% of infants in diapers affected at any time. The highest prevalence occurs between 6 and 12 months of age. Diaper dermatitis is also seen in elderly incontinent patients and children and adults with urinary or fecal incontinence from Hirschsprung's disease or genitourinary tract anomalies.

In its simplest form, diaper dermatitis is an erythematous and papulovesicular dermatitis distributed over the lower abdomen, genitals, thighs, and the convex surfaces of the buttocks. The folds remain unaffected, since they are not in direct contact with the diaper. Erythematous patches sometimes spread to the legs from contact with the wet diaper. In severe cases there may be superficial erosion. The tip of the penis may become irritated and crusted, with the result that the baby urinates frequently and spots of blood appear on the diaper.

Complications of diaper dermatitis include punched-out ulcers or erosions with elevated borders (Jacquet's erosive diaper dermatitis [Fig. 5-9]); pseudoverrucous papules and nodules; and 0.5 to 4.0 cm violaceous plaques and nodules (granuloma gluteale infantum).

The studies of Leyden et al do not support ammonia as a primary factor in common diaper dermatitis. However, the constant maceration of the skin is critical. The absence of

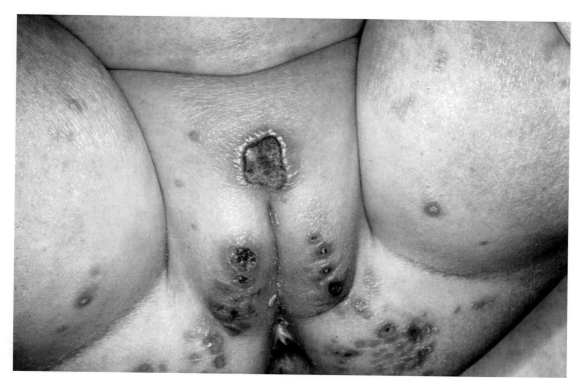

Fig. 5-9 Jacquet's erosive diaper dermatitis.

diaper dermatitis in societies in which children do not wear diapers clearly implicates the diaper environment as the cause of the eruption. Moist skin is more easily abraded by friction of the diaper as the child moves. Wet skin is more permeable to irritants, such as ammonia. Skin wetness also allows the growth of bacteria. Bacteria increase the local pH, increasing the activity of fecal lipases and proteases, which are the major irritants in feces. *Candida albicans* is frequently a secondary invader and when present produces typical satellite pustules at the periphery as the dermatitis spreads.

Napkin psoriasis, seborrheic dermatitis, atopic dermatitis, Langerhans cell histiocytosis, tinea cruris, allergic contact dermatitis, acrodermatitis enteropathica, biotin deficiency, and congenital syphilis should be included in the differential diagnosis.

Prevention is the best treatment. The new diapers that contain superabsorbent gel have been proved effective in preventing diaper dermatitis in both neonates and infants. They work by absorbing the wetness away from the skin and by buffering the pH back toward normal. Cloth diapers and regular disposable diapers are equal to each other in their propensity to cause diaper dermatitis and are inferior to the superabsorbent gel diapers. The frequent changing of diapers is also critical.

Protecting the skin of the diaper area is of great benefit in all forms of diaper dermatitis. Zinc oxide paste or other ointments such as 1-2-3 ointment are excellent:

Burow's solution	1 part
Anhydrous lanolin	2 parts
Lassar's paste without salicylic acid	3 parts
Dispense	120 g

Sig: Apply when changing diapers.

The application of a mixture of equal parts Nystatin ointment and 1% hydrocortisone ointment at each diaper change offers both anticandidal activity and an occlusive protective barrier from urine and stool.

Circumileostomy Eczema. Eczematization or autosensitization of the surrounding skin frequently occurs after an ileostomy (Fig. 5-10). It is estimated that some 75% of ileostomy patients have some postoperative sensitivity as a result of the leakage of intestinal fluid onto unprotected skin. As the consistency of the intestinal secretion becomes viscous, the sensitization subsides. Proprietary medications containing karaya powder have been found to be helpful. Twenty percent cholestyramine (an ion exchange resin) in Aquaphor or topical sucralfate as a powder or emollient at 4 g% concentration have both been effective treatments.

Autosensitization Dermatitis. *Autoeczematization* refers to the development of widespread or distant dermatitis from a

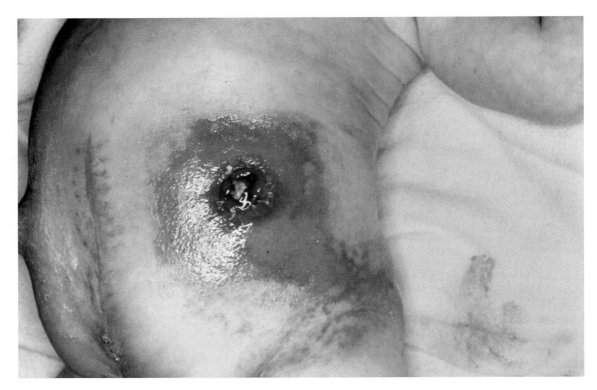

Fig. 5-10 Circumilectomy eczema.

local inflammatory focus. The agent causing the local inflammatory focus is not the direct cause of the dermatitis at the distant sites. Autoeczematization most commonly presents as a generalized acute vesicular eruptions associated with chronic eczema of the legs with or without ulceration. Generalized exfoliative dermatitis subsequent to local dermatitis is also within this context. The "angry back" or "excited skin" syndromes observed with strongly positive patch tests and the local dermatitis seen around infectious foci (infectious eczematoid dermatitis) may represent a limited form of this reaction.

Clinically, autoeczematization occurs after 1 week to several weeks of a localized dermatitis, usually lower leg dermatitis. Often somewhat suddenly widespread, symmetrical, pruritic, erythematous, 1- to 2-mm papulovesicular lesions appear. The palms may be affected in a pattern resembling that of pompholyx. The eruption may spread to confluence, and some areas may become weepy and crusted. The eruption usually persists until the triggering focus is improved. Histologically, the lesions show a spongiotic dermatitis.

Cunningham et al studied a patient with autoeczematization and found an elevated ratio of T helper cells to T suppressor cells, as well as increased circulating activated T cells. This may represent the effect of cytokines produced at the site of local inflammation on the circulating lymphocytes.

Autoeczematization is treated by identifying the original inciting dermatitis and eliminating it. Systemic corticosteroid therapy will clear the eruption, but unless the triggering dermatitis is appropriately managed, the widespread dermatitis is likely to recur. Systemic corticosteroids are often required, but in mild cases topical steroids, soaks, and antipruritics may be adequate. Coexistent infection either secondary or in the original triggering focus (e.g., an infected leg ulcer) should be aggressively treated with oral antibiotics.

Infectious Eczematoid Dermatitis. The eruption may be vesicular, pustular, or crusted, dry, and scaly. It is invariably pruritic. Linear lesions are often present. In mild cases and in the subsiding stages of the more severe cases, the patches may be dry, scaly, and fissured. In the severe types of the disease, there is marked edema, especially of the face and extremities, accompanied by large vesicles and pustulation. The exudation may be extreme, and the skin is easily irritated by mild remedies.

Infectious eczematoid dermatitis is regarded as an example of autosensitization. The disease spreads from a local site by peripheral extension. Often it develops about a discharging abscess, sinus, or ulcer (Fig. 5-11). It may develop from chronic otitis media, a bedsore, a fistula, or from discharges from the eyes, nose, or vagina (Fig. 5-12). Eczematous eruptions during the acute stages of radiodermatitis and about chronic x-ray and radium ulcers belong in this category.

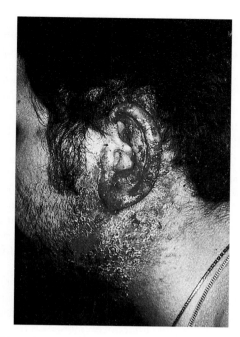

Fig. 5-11 Infectious eczematoid dermatitis. (Courtesy Dr. F. Daniels, Jr.)

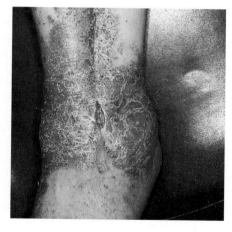

Fig. 5-12 Infectious eczematoid dermatitis, which started in an ulcer on the ankle.

Important considerations in the therapy of this recalcitrant dermatitis are the removal of the focus and antibiotic treatment. A culture with sensitivity testing should be performed. Potassium permanganate or Burow's solution baths are helpful. Acute extensive weeping eczematous eruptions also respond to Aveeno oatmeal baths. Appropriate antibiotic agents may also be given orally or parenterally. Topical antibiotic/corticosteroid creams or ointments or systemic corticosteroid medications are usually beneficial.

Juvenile Plantar Dermatosis. Juvenile plantar dermatosis is an eczematous disorder of children, first described by Enta and Moller in 1972, and named by Mackie in 1976. It

probably is the same disease as symmetrical lividity of the soles described by Pernet in 1925. It usually begins as a patchy, symmetrical, smooth, red, glazed macule on the base or medial surface of the great toes, sometimes with fissuring and desquamation, in children aged 3 to puberty. Lesions evolve into red scaling patches involving the weight-bearing and frictional areas of the feet, usually symmetrically. The forefoot is usually much more involved than the heel. Toe webs and arches are spared. The eruption is disproportionately more common in atopic children.

The disease is caused by the repeated maceration of the feet by occlusive shoes, especially athletic shoes. The affected children's soles remain wet in the rubber bottoms of the shoes. Thin, nonabsorbent, synthetic socks contribute to the problem. The name "toxic sock syndrome" is appropriate and reminds one of the pathogenesis. Sweat gland occlusion as a contributing factor has been proposed.

Histologically there is psoriasiform acanthosis and a sparse, largely lymphocytic infiltrate in the upper dermis, most dense around sweat ducts at their point of entry into the epidermis. Spongiosis is commonly present.

The diagnosis is apparent on inspection, especially if there is a family or personal history of atopy and the toe webs are spared. Shoe dermatitis and dermatophytosis should be considered in the differential diagnosis. Allergic contact dermatitis usually involves the dorsum of the feet, and dermatophytosis will be positive on potassium hydroxide examination.

Treatment consists of getting the children out of the offending shoes. Foot powders, thick absorbent socks, absorbent insoles, and having alternate pairs of shoes to wear to allow the shoes to totally dry out between wearings are all beneficial. Topical steroid medications are of limited value; often they are no more effective than occlusive barrier protection, such as petrolatum, or emollients, such as urea preparations. Most cases clear within 4 years of diagnosis, virtually always resolving at puberty.

Xerotic Eczema

Xerotic eczema is also known as *winter itch, eczema craquelé,* and *asteatotic eczema.* These vividly descriptive terms are all applied to dehydrated skin showing redness, dry scaling, and fine crackling that may resemble crackled porcelain or the fissures in the soil in the bed of a dried lake or pond (Fig. 5-13). The primary lesion is a round, small patch covered with a skin-colored to red adherent scale. As the lesion enlarges, the fine cracks in the epidermis occur concentrically and radially. Tiny foci with eczematous changes may supervene, and a "nummular pattern" may evolve. Xerotic "nummular" eczema is less weepy than classic nummular dermatitis, to which skin dryness also contributes. Favored sites are the normally driest skin areas: the anterior shins, extensor arms, and flank. Elderly persons are particularly predisposed, and xerosis appears to be the most common cause of pruritus in the aged, with no

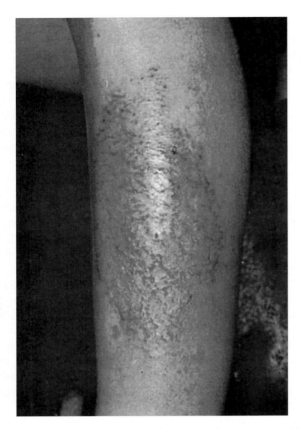

Fig. 5-13 Winter eczema—another cause of eczema craquelé.

underlying etiologic factors identified. Xerotic eczema is seen most frequently during the wintertime, when there is low relative humidity. Excessive bathing with harsh deodorant soaps and hot water contribute. Transepidermal water loss is increased and the epidermal water barrier is impaired, resulting in decreased stratum corneum water content. Xerosis may also be seen in Sjögren's syndrome, reflex sympathetic dystrophy, and myxedema.

Bathing dries the skin. However, with limitation of the use of soap to only the apocrine-bearing areas (axilla and groin), all patients but those with the most severe cases may continue to bathe. The relief and prevention of dryness of the skin is centered on maintenance of proper hydration of the stratum corneum. The rate of water loss from this layer is impeded by using moisturizers. The residual film of oil on the skin prevents or at least impedes evaporation from the surface of the skin and soothes the skin surface to prevent fissuring. The use of bath oils in the bath water or applied to the skin immediately after bathing is recommended. In extremely diffusely dry patients with consequent eczema and itching, soaking in a tub of plain water of comfortable temperature for 20 minutes followed by petrolatum or aquaphor to the wet skin before bedtime will often give immediate relief.

Extremely effective are the modern emollients containing 10% urea and lotions containing 5% lactic acid.

Lac-Hydrin (12% ammonium lactate) is a highly effective lotion in the management of xerosis but may sting when applied to fissured areas. Once erythema and weeping are present, the lactic acid moisturizers may increase irritation. Topical steroids in ointment vehicles are useful for inflamed areas.

Nummular Eczema (Nummular Neurodermatitis)

Nummular eczema usually begins on the lower legs, dorsa of the hands, or extensor surfaces of the arms. Middle-aged men in their sixth and seventh decades are most frequently affected. The primary lesions are discrete, coin shaped, erythematous, edematous, vesicular, and crusted patches from 5 to 50 mm or more in diameter (Figs. 5-14 and 5-15). Most lesions are 20 to 40 mm wide. Lesions may form after trauma (Koebner's phenomenon).

The disease evolves in a characteristic manner. After a single or a few lesions have been present on an extremity for several months, scattered new lesions begin to appear on all extremities, then on the trunk, over a few days to weeks. As new lesions appear, the old lesions expand by tiny papulovesicular satellite lesions appearing at the periphery and fusing with the main plaque. In severe cases the condition may spread into palm-sized or larger patches in which papules or papulovesicles and exudation occur. The plaques sometimes ooze and become thickened and scaly. Although the plaques are usually coin sized, an extensive area may become covered by a single plaque.

Pruritus is usually severe and of the same paroxysmal, compulsive quality and nocturnal timing seen in circumscribed neurodermatitis. Emotional stress may be present in patients with nummular eczema. Some of the worst cases are seen in alcoholics. Atopic dermatitis frequently has nummular morphology in adolescents, but in atopy the lesions tend to be more chronic and lichenified. Histologically, nummular eczema is a subacute dermatitis.

Initial treatment consists of twice-daily applications of a potent or superpotent topical steroid cream or ointment. If secondary staphylococcal infection is present, an antibiotic with appropriate coverage is recommended. Antihistaminics such as hydroxyzine HCl 25 mg three times daily, with a larger dose at bedtime, are useful. If topical steroids are ineffective, management consists of intralesional or systemic corticosteroid therapy. In cases too extensive for intralesional injections, oral prednisone in a tapering dose, beginning at 40 to 60 mg daily, is given. Triamcinolone acetonide administered intramuscularly is also effective in this condition, usually at a dose of 40 mg. Moisturizers and gentle skin care are required, because the whole skin is hyperreactive, resembling autoeczematization. After initial control, the condition tends to relapse or recur. Some of the previously healed or almost healed lesions reactivate. Each recurrence tends to be somewhat milder than the previous one, requiring less-potent therapy for a shorter period. The

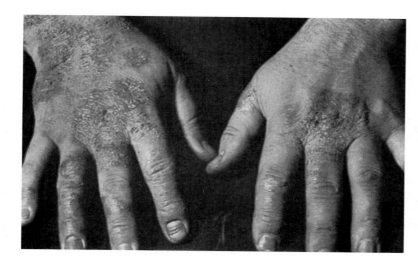

Fig. 5-14 Nummular eczema of the backs of the hands.

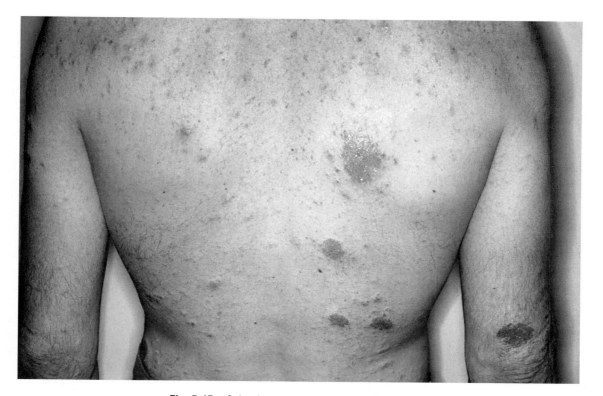

Fig. 5-15 Coin-shaped lesions of nummular eczema.

condition tends to resolve in about 1 to 2 years, but recurrences in the winter and with external irritants are not unusual.

Nutritional Deficiency Eczema

A pattern of eczema with localized, thickened, scaling patches that have some characteristics of nummular eczema, seborrheic dermatitis, and neurodermatitis may be seen in alcoholics. This probably does not represent a discrete entity, but exacerbation of these various dermatoses by poor

hygiene and secondary infection. In addition, in some patients there may be skin findings of pellagra, zinc, and vitamin C deficiencies. Head dermatitis may complicate head lice infestation; body itching and dermatitis may occur because of body lice, and genital involvement may resemble candidal diaper dermatitis associated with urinating and defecating in the clothing. In general, these patients improve rapidly once hospitalized, away from alcohol intake, and are provided access to a well-balanced diet. Persistent areas of dermatitis are treated with topical steroid medications, and in the groin, anticandidal agents. Persistent perlèche, atrophic glossitis, and groin erosions suggest zinc deficiency.

HORMONE-INDUCED DERMATOSES

Autoimmune progesterone dermatitis has been reported to appear as urticaria, urticarial papules, papulovesicular lesions, an eczematous eruption, or erythema multiforme. When urticaria is the predominant skin lesion, there is a generalized distribution, and it may be accompanied by laryngospasm. Pruritus is common. Oral erosions may be present. The eruption typically appears 5 to 10 days before menses and spontaneously clears following menstruation, only to return in the next menstrual period. Many of the reported patients had received artificial progestational agents before the onset of the eruption. In some it appeared after a normal pregnancy. This has been reported as a cause of an eruption early in pregnancy, associated with spontaneous abortion. The eruption may worsen or clear during pregnancy. The pathogenesis is unclear but is felt to be an autoimmunity directed toward one's own progesterone.

In most cases, the diagnosis has been confirmed by intradermal testing with 0.01 ml of aqueous progesterone suspension (50 mg/ml). A positive test may be immediate (30 minutes) or delayed (24 to 96 hours). Flares may be induced by intramuscular or oral progesterone. The most commonly used treatment is oral contraceptives, which suppress ovulation, thereby reducing progesterone levels. Oophorectomy has resulted in resolution. Danazol and tamoxifen may also be effective. In some cases the condition spontaneously resolves.

Autoimmune estrogen dermatitis is a cyclic skin disorder with variable morphologies. Eczematous, papular, urticarial, generalized or localized presentations may occur. Pruritus is typically present. Skin eruptions may be chronic but are exacerbated premenstrually or occur only immediately before the menses. Characteristically, the dermatosis clears during pregnancy and at menopause. Intracutaneous skin testing with estrone produces a papule lasting longer than 24 hours or an immediate urticarial wheal (in cases with urticaria). Injections of progesterone yield negative results, ruling out autoimmune progesterone dermatitis. Treatment with tamoxifen (10 mg one to three times daily for 10 to 14 days before the menses) is reportedly effective in controlling the eruption but may be associated with an increased risk of endometrial carcinoma.

Ackerman AB, et al: A plea to expunge "eczema" from the lexicon of dermatology. *Am J Dermatopathol* 1982, 4:315.

Ashton RE, et al: Juvenile plantar dermatosis: a clinicopathologic study. *Arch Dermatol* 1985, 121:225.

Borglund E, et al: Classification of peristomal skin changes in patients with urostomy. *J Am Acad Dermatol* 1988, 19:623.

Cunningham MJ, et al: Circulating activated T lymphocytes in a patient with autoeczematization. *J Am Acad Dermatol* 1986, 14:1039.

Epstein E: Hand dermatitis: Practical management and current concepts. *J Am Acad Dermatol* 1984, 10:395.

Goldberg NS, Esterly NB, Rothman KF: Perianal pseudoverrucous papules and nodules in children. *Arch Dermatol* 1992, 128:240

Herzberg AJ, Strohmeyer CR, Cirillo-Hyland VA: Autoimmune progesterone dermatitis. *J Am Acad Dermatol* 1995, 32:335.

Jones SK, et al: Juvenile plantar dermatosis. *Clin Exp Dermatol* 1987, 12:5.

Karlberg AT, et al: Colophony (rosin) in newspapers may contribute to hand eczema. *J Dermatol* 1992, 126:161.

Leyden JJ, et al: Role of microorganisms in diaper dermatitis. *Arch Dermatol* 1978, 114:56.

Moller P, et al: Cholestyramine ointment for perianal irritation after ileal anastomosis. *Dis Colon Rectum* 1987, 30:106.

Nilsson E, et al: Density of microflora in hand eczema before and after use of a topical corticosteroid. *J Am Acad Dermatol* 1986, 15:192.

Rietschel RL, et al: Nonatopic eczemas. *J Am Acad Dermatol* 1988, 18:569.

Rosen K, et al: Chronic eczematous dermatitis of the hands. *Acta Derm Venereol* (Stockh) 1987, 67:48.

Rothstein MS: Dermatologic considerations of stomal care. *J Am Acad Dermatol* 1986, 15:411.

Shelley WB, et al: Estrogen dermatitis. *J Am Acad Dermatol* 1995;32:25.

Shelley WB, et al: Symmetrical lividity of the soles. *Cutis* 1999, 64:175.

Sinha SM, et al: Vegetables responsible for contact dermatitis of the hands. *Arch Dermatol* 1977, 113:776.

Srisupalak S, et al: Diaper dermatitis. *Pediatr Rev* 1995, 16:142. ▲

IMMUNODEFICIENCY SYNDROMES

Many of the congenital immunodeficiency syndromes have cutaneous manifestations. The most common of these skin diseases are bacterial or fungal infections (especially mucocutaneous candidiasis), lupus erythematosus–like syndromes, and atopic-like dermatitis. The primary immunodeficiencies may be classified as those with impaired antibody production (B-cell immunodeficiencies), impaired cell-mediated immunity (T-cell immunodeficiencies), and combined B- and T-cell deficiencies.

Some of the many immunodeficiencies with cutaneous involvement are presented in this section. Others such as the acquired immunodeficiency syndrome and chronic mucocutaneous candidiasis will be discussed in later chapters according to the specific infectious agent involved.

Arbiser JL: Genetic immunodeficiencies. *J Am Acad Dermatol* 1995, 33:82.

Hammarstrom L, et al: Molecular basis for human immunodeficiencies. *Curr Opin Immunol* 1993; 5:579

Hong R: Update on immunodeficiency diseases. *Am J Dis Child* 1990, 144:983.

Mallory SB, et al: Congenital immunodeficiency syndrome with cutaneous manifestations. I. *J Am Acad Dermatol* 1990, 23:1153.

Mallory SB, et al: Congenital immunodeficiency syndrome with cutaneous manifestations. II. *J Am Acad Dermatol* 1991; 24:107.

Paller AS: Immunodeficiency syndromes. *Dermatol Clin* 1995, 13:65. ▲

X-Linked Agammaglobulinemia

Also known as *Bruton's syndrome* and *sex-linked agammaglobulinemia,* this rare hereditary immunologic disorder usually becomes apparent after the first 3 to 6 months of life, with increased susceptibility to gram-positive pyogenic infections such as pneumococcal and streptococcal infections. Resistance to viral infections is intact, except for an unusual susceptibility to infections with enteroviruses that may result in vaccine-related paralytic poliomyelitis or a dermatomyositis-meningoencephalitis syndrome. There is an increased tendency in affected boys to develop atopic dermatitis, diffuse vasculitis, and urticaria. Growth failure, chronic diarrhea, and an absence of palpable lymph nodes is characteristic. Fleming et al reported a patient with cutaneous caseating granulomas of unknown cause, similar to cases seen in other immunodeficiency syndromes.

IgA, IgM, IgD, and IgE are virtually absent from the serum, although IgG may be present in small amounts. The spleen and lymph nodes lack germinal centers, and plasma cells are absent from the lymph nodes, spleen, bone marrow, and connective tissues.

Cell-mediated immunity is intact. The T lymphocytes are normal in number, function, and proportion, but B cells are usually completely lacking. Evidence indicates that the defect lies in a maturation block in pre-B-cell to B-cell differentiation. Several groups have mapped the gene locus; it encodes for a novel cytoplasmic protein tyrosine kinase (PTK). The gene is a member of the src family of protooncogenes. Deletions and point mutations have been detected in many unrelated patients, and these result in detrimental effects on the catalytic function of the kinase.

Treatment with gamma globulin is helpful, but it does not completely control the disease. Progressive fatal encephalitis resulting from an enterovirus may develop. Respiratory disease with pulmonary fibrosis is also frequently seen, because there is no means of restoring secretory IgA to mucous membrane surfaces. Lymphoreticular malignancy, especially leukemia, may develop.

Fleming MG, et al: Caseating cutaneous granulomas in a patient with X-linked infantile hypogammaglobulinemias. *J Am Acad Dermatol* 1991, 24:629.

Ochs HD, et al: X-linked agammaglobulinemia. *Medicine* 1996, 75:287.

Vetrie D, et al: The gene involved in X-linked agammaglobulinemia is a member of the src family of protein-tyrosine kinases. *Nature* 1993, 361:226. ————————————————————— ▲

Isolated IgA Deficiency

An absence or marked reduction of serum IgA occurs in approximately 1 in 600 people in the white population; most are entirely well. Of the symptomatic group, half have repeated infections, and one quarter have autoimmune or collagen vascular disease. Allergies such as anaphylactic transfusion reactions, asthma, and atopic dermatitis are common in the symptomatic group. There is an increased association of celiac disease, ulcerative colitis, and regional enteritis. Systemic lupus erythematosus, dermatomyositis, scleroderma, thyroiditis, rheumatoid arthritis, and Sjögren's syndrome have all been reported to occur in these patients. Malignancy is increased in adults with IgA deficiency. Symptomatic IgA deficiency represents 10% to 15% of clinically serious inherited immunodeficiency patients.

It is believed that these patients have a maturation defect of the B lymphocyte as it develops into an IgA-producing plasma cell. The defect can be transmitted as an autosomal dominant or recessive trait. It may also be an acquired deficiency, induced by certain drugs, such as phenytoin.

There have been reports of associated IgG subclass deficiency, as well as decreased levels of IgE, in these patients. The abnormality may be more generalized in symptomatic cases. Patients with associated IgG abnormalities may benefit from immunoglobulin replacement, but more than 40% of these patients have antibodies to IgA, and administration of gamma globulin may cause allergic reactions.

Plebani A, et al: Selective IgA deficiency. *Curr Probl Dermatol* 1989, 18:66. ————————————————————————— ▲

Common Variable Immunodeficiency

Common variable immunodeficiency, also known as *acquired hypogammaglobulinemia,* is a heterogeneous disorder that is the most common immunodeficiency syndrome after IgA deficiency. Children or young adults with higher than expected expression of HLA markers B8 and DR3 are affected, and 11% of family members may have a demonstrable immunoglobulin deficiency. These patients have low levels of most immunoglobulin classes, do not form antibodies to bacterial antigens, and have recurrent sinopulmonary infections. They have a predisposition to autoimmune disorders, such as vitiligo and alopecia areata, to gastrointestinal abnormalities, and to lymphoreticular malignancies. Cutaneous as well as visceral granulomas have been reported in several patients. B cells are present in most patients but do not terminally differentiate. Half of these patients will also have evidence of T cell dysfunction.

Cunningham-Randles C: Clinical and immunologic analysis of 103 patients with CVI. *J Clin Immunol* 1989, 9:22.

Pierson JC, et al: Cutaneous and visceral granulomas in CVI. *Cutis* 1993, 52:221.

Siegfried EC, et al: Cutaneous granulomas in children with combined immunodeficiency. *J Am Acad Dermatol* 1991, 25:761.

Spickett G, et al: Alopecia totalis and vitiligo in CVI. *Postgrad Med J* 1991, 67:291.

Yocum MW, et al: CVI. *Mayo Clin Proc* 1991, 66:83. ——————— ▲

Isolated Primary IgM Deficiency

Eczematous dermatitis is present in about one fifth of the cases with this abnormality. The other immunoglobulin classes are usually present in normal amounts. Isohemagglutinins are absent. Affected persons are predisposed to severe infections, especially those caused by meningococci, pneumococci, and *Haemophilus influenzae*. Verruca vulgaris may occur in great numbers. Thyroiditis, splenomegaly, and hemolytic anemia may occur. Patients with mycosis fungoides, and gluten-sensitive enteropathy may have a secondary IgM deficiency. This disease is probably caused by a defect in the maturation of IgM-producing plasma cells.

Immunodeficiency with Hyper-IgM

This rare disorder is characterized by recurrent infections, low or absent IgG, IgE, and IgA levels, and normal or elevated levels of IgM and IgD. The disorder may be inherited as an autosomal dominant, recessive, or X-linked trait. Respiratory infections, diarrhea, otitis, large painful oral ulcers, widespread therapy-resistant warts, autoimmunity, and recurrent neutropenia are common. Treatment is with intravenous gamma globulin. Allogeneic bone marrow transplantation has been successful.

The X-linked form has been found to be caused by point mutations or deletions in the Xq26.3-27.1 region, which encodes for a ligand of CD40, gp39. Abnormalities of this protein on T cells interferes with the T-cell–B-cell interaction (gp39-CD40 interaction) that signals for immunoglobulin isotype switching.

Aruffo A, et al: The CD40 ligand, gp39, is defective in activated T cells from patients with X-linked hyper-IgM syndrome. *Cell* 1993, 72:291.

Chang MW, et al: Mucocutaneous manifestations of the hyper-IgM immunodeficiency syndrome. *J Am Acad Dermatol* 1998, 38:191.

DeSanto JP, et al: CD40 ligand mutations in X-linked immunodeficiency with hyper-IgM. *Nature* 1993, 361:541.

Thomas C, et al: Correction of X-linked hyper-IgM syndrome by allogeneic bone marrow transplantation. *N Engl J Med* 1995, 333:426. ▲

Thymic Hypoplasia

Congenital thymic hypoplasia, also known as *DiGeorge anomaly* and as *III and IV pharyngeal pouch syndrome,* may be inherited as an autosomal dominant or autosomal recessive trait, or may be a sporadic disorder. It is characterized by a distinctive facies: notched, low-set ears, micrognathia, shortened philtrum, and hypertelorism.

The syndrome includes congenital absence of the parathyroids and thymus, and an abnormal aorta. Neonatal tetany from hypocalcemia is usually the first sign of the disease. Aortic and cardiac defects are the most common cause of death. T-cell defects are present, and cell-mediated immunity is absent or depressed. Fungal and viral infections commonly occur despite usually normal immunoglobulin levels.

DiGeorge anomaly is one of several syndromes associated with deletions within the proximal long arm of chromosome 22. Aubry et al have reported that a gene mapping of the DiGeorge critical region, chromosome 22 qll.2, which encodes for a zinc finger DNA-binding motif, (ZNF74), was hemizygously deleted in 23 of 24 DiGeorge patients.

Aubry M, et al: Isolation of zinc finger gene consistently deleted in DiGeorge syndrome. *Hum Mol Genet* 1993, 2:1583. ▲

Thymic Dysplasia with Normal Immunoglobulins (Nezelof Syndrome)

In Nezelof syndrome there is faulty development of the thymus gland. Onset is in early infancy, with severe, recurrent candidiasis, severe varicella, recurrent bacterial infections of the skin and lungs, or diarrhea.

It is an autosomal recessive disorder. Serum immunoglobulins are normal or increased, but cell-mediated immunity is lacking. The syndrome differs from DiGeorge syndrome in that the thymus is present but underdeveloped, and there are no cardiac abnormalities. One patient was reconstituted to normal immune function by bone marrow transplantation.

Purine Nucleoside Phosphorylase Deficiency

This enzyme defect leads to greatly reduced T-cell counts and depressed cell-mediated immunity, but B cells and antibody formation are intact. Mutations on chromosome 14q13 are responsible. Patients usually present between 3 and 18 months of age with nonbacterial infections involving the lungs, upper airways, skin, and urinary tract. They usually die from overwhelming viral infections.

Edwards NL: Immunodeficiencies associated with errors in purine metabolism. *Med Clin North Am* 1985, 69:505. ▲

Miscellaneous T-Cell Deficiencies

There are many other small subgroups of immunodeficiency disorders being described that affect T cells. Because T- and B-cell interaction is an important facet of the immune response, hypogammaglobulinemia may also characterize some of these disorders. An excellent example of this discussed earlier was immunodeficiency with hyper-IgM.

The bare lymphocyte syndrome is characterized by profound defects in HLA class II expression. Some patients also lack class I expression. The molecular basis for the class II defect is a lack of RF-X, the specific DNA-binding protein that normally binds to the HLA class II promoters.

A deficiency of the T-cell receptor CD3 complex may result from mutations affecting either the gamma or epsilon chains. Many of these patients have relatively benign clinical courses.

Activation of T cells may be deficient. Surface molecules may be deficient, as in the bare lymphocyte syndrome or CD3 deficiency, but also intracytoplasmic signaling molecules are needed to transmit information inside the cell to the nucleus. Zap 70 deficiency is now recognized as a defect in a nuclear factor necessary for activation of T cells.

Cartilage-hair hypoplasia syndrome is an autosomal recessive disorder in which patients with short-limbed dwarfism and fine, sparse, hypopigmented hair have defective cell-mediated immunity.

Omenn's syndrome is an autosomal recessive disorder that closely mimics graft-versus-host disease. Clinical features are exfoliative erythroderma beginning at a few weeks of life, eosinophilia, diarrhea, hepatosplenomegaly, lymphadenopathy, hypogammaglobulinemia with elevated IgE, recurrent infections, and early death (usually by 6 months of age). Both antibody production and cell-mediated immune function are impaired. T-cell receptor rearrangements are severely restricted in patients with Omenn's syndrome, and inefficient and/or abnormal generation of T-cell receptors is a consistent feature of this disease.

Brook EG, et al: T cell receptor analysis in Omenn's syndrome. *Blood* 1999, 93:242.

Klein C, et al: MHC II deficiency. *J Pediatr* 1993, 123:921.

Polmar SH, et al: Cartilage-hair hypoplasia. *Clin Immunol Immunopathol* 1986, 40:87.

Pupo RA, et al: Omenn's syndrome and related combined immunodeficiency syndromes. *J Am Acad Dermatol* 1991, 25:442.

Rybojad M, et al: Omenn's reticulosis associated with nephrotic syndromes. *Br J Dermatol* 1996, 135:124. ⎯⎯⎯⎯⎯⎯ ▲

Severe Combined Immunodeficiency Disease (SCID)

This heterogeneous group of genetic disorders is characterized by severely impaired humoral and cellular immunity. Patients may manifest various cutaneous manifestations, including a simple morbilliform eruption and seborrheic dermatitis. In addition, severe recurrent infections may occur, caused by *Pseudomonas, Staphylococcus, Enterobacteriaceae,* or *Candida.* Moniliasis of the oropharynx and skin, intractable diarrhea, and pneumonia are the triad of findings that commonly lead to the diagnosis of SCID. Overwhelming viral infections are the usual cause of death. Engraftment of maternally transmitted or transfusion-derived lymphocytes can lead to graft-versus-host disease.

SCID is characterized by deficiency or total absence of circulating lymphocytes. Mature T cells are almost invariably absent, but B-cell numbers may be greatly reduced or increased. Immunoglobulin levels are consistently very low. The thymus is very small; its malformed architecture at autopsy is pathognomonic.

The inheritance may be autosomal recessive or X-linked; the most common type of SCID is X-linked. A deficiency of a common gamma chain that is an essential component of the IL-2 receptor is responsible for the profound lymphoid dysfunction in X-linked SCID. This abnormality also has effects on both the IL-4 and IL-7 receptors. The mutation has been mapped to Xq13.1. About half the autosomal recessive cases have a deficiency of adenosine deaminase, the gene for which is located on chromosome 20q13.

Lymphogenic agammaglobulinemia, also known as *Swiss-type* or *hereditary thymic dysplasia,* is inherited as an autosomal recessive trait. The presumed level of the basic cellular defect is in the lymphopoietic stem cell, which fails to differentiate into lymphoid cells. Lymphoid tissue in the body is usually absent.

Prenatal diagnosis and carrier detection are possible for X-linked SCID, and adenosine deaminase deficiency. Short-term replacement therapy is available. The definitive treatment is bone marrow transplantation. Affected patients rarely live longer than age 2 without transplantation. Patients with these diseases are prime candidates for gene therapy.

Flake AW, et al: Treatment of X-linked severe combined immunodeficiency by in utero transplantation of paternal bone marrow. *N Engl J Med* 1996, 335:1806.

Noguchi M, et al: IL-2 receptor gamma chain mutation results in X-linked SCID in humans. *Cell* 1993, 73:147.

Russell SM, et al: IL-2 receptor gamma chain. *Science* 1993, 262:1880.

Santisteban I, et al: Novel splicing, missense, and deletion mutations in several ADA-deficient patients with late/delayed onset SCID. *J Clin Invest* 1993, 92:2291.

Stiehm ER, et al: Bone marrow transplantation in severe combined immunodeficiency from a sibling who had received a paternal bone marrow transplant. *N Engl J Med* 1996, 335:1811. ⎯⎯⎯⎯⎯ ▲

Thymoma with Immunodeficiency

Thymoma with immunodeficiency, also known as *Good's syndrome,* occurs in adults in whom hypogammaglobulinemia, deficient cell-mediated immunity, and benign thymoma may develop almost simultaneously. Recurrent abscesses and pyoderma develop. There is a striking deficiency of B and pre-B cells. Lymphopenia, eosinopenia, thrombocytopenia, anemia, or pancytopenia may occur. Thymectomy does not affect the immunodeficiency.

Verne GN, et al: Chronic diarrhea associated with thymoma and hypogammaglobulinemia (Good's syndrome). *South Med J* 1997, 90:444. ⎯⎯⎯⎯⎯⎯⎯⎯ ▲

Ataxia-Telangiectasia (Louis-Bar's Syndrome)

Distinctive telangiectasia in the bulbar conjunctiva and the flexural surfaces of the arms develops during the fifth year of age (Fig. 5-16). Later, telangiectases appear on the butterfly area of the face, the palate, the ears, and exposed surfaces of skin. Café au lait patches, graying hair, and progeria may also be present. Cohen et al also listed vitiligo, impetigo, recurrent herpetic gingivostomatitis, hirsutism,

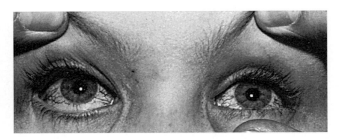

Fig. 5-16 Telangiectasia of the sclerae in ataxia-telangiectasia.

and lipoatrophy among cutaneous problems associated with this disease. Paller et al reported eight patients with cutaneous granulomas of unknown cause. Although necrobiosis was frequently present, histologically the lesions differed from granuloma annulare in that they were persistent erythematous atrophic lesions that frequently became encrusted or ulcerative.

Cerebellar ataxia is the first sign of this syndrome. It begins in the second year of life, usually after the child starts walking. An awkward swaying gait develops and becomes progressively worse. Choreic and athetoid movements are usually present.

The syndrome is transmitted as an autosomal recessive trait. The ataxia-telangiectasia disease gene is located at chromosome 11q22-23, is called the *ATM gene,* and codes for a protein kinase. The majority of mutations are truncating, that is, the absence of a full-length ATM protein is the most common cause of ataxia-telangiectasia.

The ovaries and testicles do not develop normally. There is deficient thymus development, with absence of Hassall's corpuscles, and a lack of T helper cells. Suppressor T cells are normal. In 80% of cases, IgA is absent or deficient, in 75% absent or deficient IgE is seen, and in 50% IgG is very low. Persistently elevated levels of alpha-fetoprotein and carcinoembryonic antigen occur. These may be useful in early diagnosis.

In culture, ataxia-telangiectasia fibroblasts are three times more sensitive to killing by ionizing radiation, but not ultraviolet light. Heterozygous carriers share the defective repair of radiation-induced damage, and there is a threefold to fivefold higher risk for development of neoplasms, especially breast cancer, in heterozygotes under age 45.

Severe pulmonary infections and progressive bronchiectasis complicate the clinical course in most patients. Thirty percent to 40% of affected patients develop cancer; 80% of cases are lymphoid. These are the commonest causes of death.

Cleaver JE, et al: Clinical syndromes associated with DNA repair deficiencies and enhanced sun sensitivity. *Arch Dermatol* 1993, 129:348.

Cohen LE, et al: Common and uncommon cutaneous findings in patients with AT. *J Am Acad Dermatol* 1984, 10:431.

Gatti RA: Ataxia-telangiectasia. *Dermatol Clin* 1995, 13:1.

Murakawa GJ, et al: Chronic plaques in a patient with AT. *Arch Dermatol* 1998, 134:1145.

Paller AS, et al: Cutaneous granulomatous lesions in patients with AT. *J Pediatr* 1991, 119:917.

Peterson RD, et al: Cancer susceptibility in AT. *Leukemia* 1992, 6(Suppl):8.

Sandoval N, et al: Characterization of ATM gene mutations in 66 ataxia telangiectasia families. *Hum Mol Genet* 1999, 8:69.

Swift M, et al: Incidence of cancer in 161 families affected by AT. *N Engl J Med* 1991, 325:1831. ▲

Wiskott-Aldrich Syndrome

The rare Wiskott-Aldrich syndrome, seen exclusively in young boys, consists of a triad: chronic eczematous dermatitis resembling atopic dermatitis; increased susceptibility to recurrent infections, such as pyoderma or suppurative otitis media; and thrombocytopenic purpura, with hepatosplenomegaly. Death occurs usually by age 6, from either infection, or, less often, bleeding. Only a few patients survive to adulthood. They are highly prone to developing lymphoreticular malignancies.

Synthesis of IgA, IgM, and IgE is accelerated; however, accelerated catabolism usually results in low levels of IgM and low or normal levels of IgG. Elevated levels of IgA and IgE are present. There seems to be an intrinsic platelet abnormality. T cells progressively decline in numbers and activity.

Treatment is with platelet transfusions, antibiotics, immunoglobulin, and splenectomy. Bone marrow transplantation from an HLA-identical sibling as early as possible in the disease course provides complete reversal of the platelet and immune dysfunction as well as improvement or clearing of their eczematous dermatitis.

The gene locus for Wiskott-Aldrich syndrome has been mapped to the proximal portion of the short arm of the X chromosome (Xp11). The gene codes for a protein called *WASP,* currently thought to be involved in the reorganization of the actin cytoskeleton in hematopoetic cells in response to external stimuli. The hematopoetic cells of affected patients cannot polarize or migrate in response to physiologic stimuli, accounting for the protean clinical features of the syndrome.

Omerod AD: The Wiskott-Aldrich syndrome (review). *Int J Dermatol* 1985, 24:77.

O'Sullivan E, et al: Wiskott-Aldrich syndrome protein: WASP. *Int J Biochem Cell Biol* 1999, 31:383.

Peacocke M, et al: Wiscott-Aldrich syndrome. *J Am Acad Dermatol* 1992, 27:507. ▲

X-Linked Lymphoproliferative Syndrome

This disorder, also known as *Duncan's disease,* is characterized by an inability of affected individuals to effectively control an Epstein-Barr virus infection. The patients are normal until they develop severe, acute infectious mononucleosis. Necrotic hepatitis and an exanthem are common. Aplastic anemia, chronic infectious mononucleosis, a spectrum of B-cell lymphoproliferative diseases, and acquired hypogammaglobulinemia develop. The locus has been mapped to the Xq26 region.

Schuster V, et al: Epstein-Barr virus-associated lymphoproliferative syndrome. *Cancer Detect Prev* 1991, 15:65. _____ ▲

Chronic Granulomatous Disease

Clinically, chronic granulomatous disease (CGD) is characterized by recurring purulent and granulomatous infections involving long bones, lymphatic tissue, liver, skin, and lungs. It occurs most frequently in boys (because X-linked inheritance is the most frequent type) who have eczema of the scalp, backs of the ears, and face. Ulcerative stomatitis, furunculosis, subcutaneous abscesses, and suppurative lymphadenopathy may occur.

There is decreased ability to destroy catalase-positive bacteria. This is caused by a deficiency in one of the components of the NADPH-oxidase complex, which catalyzes the conversion of molecular oxygen to superoxide. These organisms destroy any hydrogen peroxide they generate, thus leaving the CGD phagocytes, which have a defective ability to generate hydrogen peroxide, without full antimicrobial killing ability. *S. aureus* infection is most frequently seen; infections by streptococci and pneumococci are uncommon. In addition, IgG, IgM, and IgA hyperglobulinemia, neutrophil leukocytosis, and an abnormally low reduction of NBT to blue formazan occur.

The X-linked form, which accounts for 65% of cases, is caused by a lack of the high–molecular-weight subunit of cytochrome b 558(gp 91-phox). In autosomal recessive forms, mutations in the genes encoding for the remaining three oxidase components have been described; p22-phox (chromosome 16), p47-phox (chromosome 7) and p67-phox (chromosome 1) may have deletions, insertions, and point mutations leading to premature stop codons, amino acid substitutions, and splice site defects.

Female carriers of the X-linked form have a mixed population of normal and abnormal cells and therefore show intermediate NBT reduction. There is an increase in infections, discoid lupus–like skin lesions, and often aphthous stomatitis. Kragballe et al reported that two of 10 unselected women with discoid lupus erythematosus were shown to be carriers. Several patients with autosomal recessive disease have developed discoid lupus lesions.

Treatment of infections should be early, aggressive, and prolonged; trimethoprim-sulfamethoxazole prophylaxis significantly prolongs disease-free intervals. Injections of gamma-interferon decrease the frequency of serious infections. Bone marrow transplantation has been successful.

Bolinger AM, et al: Recombinant interferon gamma for treatment of CGD and other disorders. *Clin Pharm* 1992, 11:834.

Curnutte JT: CGD: the solving of a clinical riddle at the molecular level. *Clin Immunol Immunopathol* 1993, 67:S2.

Ezekowitz RAB, et al: Partial correction of CGD by interferon gamma. *N Engl J Med* 1988, 319:146.

Kragballe K, et al: Relation of monocyte and neutrophile oxidative metabolism to skin and oral lesions in carriers of CGD. *Clin Exp Immunol* 1981, 43:390.

Lehrer RI, et al: Neutrophils in human disease. *Ann Intern Med* 1988, 109:127.

Malech HC, et al: Neutrophils in human disease. *N Engl J Med* 1987, 317:687.

Quie PG: CGD of childhood. *Pediatr Infect Dis J* 1993, 12:395.

Sahn EE, et al: Crusted scalp nodule in an infant. *Arch Dermatol* 1994, 130:105.

Smitt JHS, et al: DLE-like skin changes in patients with autosomal recessive CGD. *Arch Dermatol* 1990, 126:1656. _____ ▲

Myeloperoxidase Deficiency

This condition is a relatively common autosomal recessive disorder characterized by an absent or enzymatically inactive myeloperoxidase protein. Myeloperoxidase is normally abundant in neutrophils and monocytes. Cells with this deficiency are unable to terminate their respiratory burst, and patients may be susceptible to systemic and cutaneous candidiasis and bacterial skin infections. Sweet's syndrome and acne may occur despite this deficiency. However, many affected patients are asymptomatic, and usually the life span is unaffected.

Disdier P, et al: Neutrophilic dermatosis despite myeloperoxidase deficiency. *J Am Acad Dermatol* 1991, 24:654.

Nguyen C et al: Myeloperoxidase deficiency manifesting as pustular candidal dermatitis. *Clin Infect Dis* 1997, 24:258. _____ ▲

Leukocyte Adhesion Molecule Deficiency

This rare autosomal recessive disorder is characterized by recurrent bacterial and fungal infections and impaired pus formations as a result of a block of leukocyte migration. Periodontitis or gingivitis and poor wound healing may also occur. The severity of the clinical presentation is variable. There is faulty complexing of the CD11 and CD18 integrins as a result of a defect in the CD18 gene. This leads to absent or severely reduced cell surface expression of the beta-2 leukocyte integrins, resulting in abnormal chemotaxis and opsonization. Death usually occurs in the first 4 years of life unless bone marrow transplantation is undertaken; however, less severe defects may be present, in which case the patient survives into adulthood.

Paller AS, et al: Leukocyte adhesion deficiency. *J Am Acad Dermatol* 1994, 31:316.

Schmalstieg FL: Leukocyte adhesence defect. *Pediatr Infect Dis* 1988, 7:867.

van de Kerkhof PC, et al: Skin manifestations in congenital deficiency of leukocyte-adherence glycoproteins. *Br J Dermatol* 1990, 123:395. ▲

Chédiak-Higashi Syndrome

Chédiak-Higashi syndrome is a progressively degenerative, fatal, familial disease of young children, characterized by partial oculocutaneous albinism, cutaneous and intestinal infections early in childhood, and leukocytes with very large azurophilic granules. The hair of these patients is blond and sparse. The ocular albinism is accompanied by nystagmus and photophobia.

The inheritance is autosomal recessive. Prenatal diagnosis is possible by examining the hairshaft and neutrophils microscopically for large granules. The Chédiak-Higashi gene product has been identified and mapped on chromosome 1q 42-1843.

The defect is in the gene LYST, resulting in defective vesicular transport to and from the lysosome and late endosome and dysregulated homotypic fusion. This causes the giant perinuclear vesicles that characterize this disorder. Patients have increased susceptibility to infections, especially those of enteric bacterial origin. There is a neutropenia and the abnormal neutrophils do not phagocytose normally. Chemotaxis is usually decreased. The immunoglobulins are present in normal amounts. Early death usually occurs, most frequently as a result of malignant lymphoma or other forms of cancer. Bone marrow transplantation may be curative.

Another form of partial albinism and recurrent infections with immunodeficiency is Griscelli's syndrome. Silvery-gray hair, neurologic abnormalities, skin and systemic pyogenic infection, neutropenia, thrombocytopenia, hypogammaglobulinemia, impaired natural killer cell activity, and defective cell-mediated immunity are present. Microscopic analysis of the hair reveals large, unevenly distributed melanin aggregates in the medulla. Skin biopsies show numerous mature melanosomes in melanocytes and few melanosomes in keratinocytes without giant melanosomes. The latter two findings may help in the prenatal diagnosis of Griscelli's syndrome. The genetic locus co-localizes on chromosome 15q21 with the myosin-Va gene which may play a role in membrane transport and organelle trafficking. The age at onset varies from 6 weeks to 4 years, but most patients die by age 5 without bone marrow transplantation. Elejalde syndrome shows similar findings in the hair and frequent fatal central nervous system alterations, but immunodeficiency is not a feature.

Barbosa MD, et al: Identification of the homologous beige and Chédiak-Higashi syndrome genes. *Nature* 1996, 382:262.

Duran-McKinster C, et al: Elejalde syndrome. *Arch Dermatol* 1999, 135:182

Durandy A, et al: Prenatal diagnosis of syndromes associating albinism and immunodeficiency. *Prenat Diagn* 1993, 13:13.

Mancini AJ, et al: Partial albinism with immunodeficiency: Griscelli syndrome. *J Am Acad Dermatol* 1998, 38:295.

Nagle DL, et al: Identification and mutation analysis of the complete gene for Chédiak-Higashi syndrome. *Nat Genet* 1996, 14:307. ▲

Hyperimmunoglobulinemia E Syndrome

This immunodeficiency consists of atopic-like eczematous dermatitis, recurrent pyogenic infection (frequently in the lungs and skin), high levels of serum IgE, elevated IgD levels, IgE antistaphylococcal antibodies, and eosinophilia. The eczematous eruption, seen in more than 80% of patients, is typically found in the sites of predilection for atopic dermatitis. The face is consistently involved. It is chronic and begins early in life (2 months to 2 years of age). Many of the lesions resemble papular prurigo, and there may be keratoderma of the palms and soles. Ichthyosis, urticaria, asthma, and chronic mucocutaneous candidiasis may also occur. The hands and feet may have lesions suggestive of contact dermatitis. Furuncles, carbuncles, and abscesses of variable severity, as well as chronic nasal discharge and recurrent otitis media, are common.

The serum shows an extremely high concentration of IgE (more than 10,000 IU/ml), and eosinophilia is present, with diminished local resistance to staphylococcal infections. Chemotaxis of neutrophils and monocytes is impaired.

Job's syndrome is a subset of hypergammaglobulinemia E syndrome, which occurs mainly in girls with red hair, freckles, blue eyes, and hyperextensible joints. Cold abscesses occur.

Bulengo Ransby SM, et al: Staphylococcal botryomycosis and hyperimmunoglobulin E (Job's) syndrome in an infant. *J Am Acad Dermatol* 1993, 28:109.

Leung DY, et al: Clinical and immunologic aspects of the hyperimmunoglobulin E syndrome. *Hematol Oncol Clin North Am* 1988, 2:81.

Ring L, et al: Hyper-IgE syndrome. *Curr Prob Dermatol* 1989, 18:79. ▲

Complement Deficiency

The complement system is an effector pathway of more than 25 serum proteins that, when activated in a highly regulated and progressive manner, results in three basic types of biologic activity: membrane damage, membrane alteration, and mediator functions such as anaphylatoxin or chemotactic activity. Four major functions result from complement activation: cell lysis, opsonization/phagocytosis, inflammation via vascular responses and neutrophil activation, and immune complex removal.

In the "classic" complement pathway, complement is activated by an antigen-antibody reaction involving IgG or IgM. Some complement components are directly activated by binding to the surface of infectious organisms; this is called the "alternate" pathway. The central component common to both pathways is C3. In the classic pathway, antigen-antibody complexes sequentially bind and activate three complement proteins, Cl, C4, and C2, leading to the formation of C3 convertase, an activator of C3. The alternate pathway starts with direct activation of C3. From activated C3, C5 to C9 are sequentially activated. Cytolysis is induced mainly via the "membrane attack complex," which is made up of the terminal components; opsonization is mainly mediated by a subunit of C3b and inflammation via recruitment of leukocytes is primarily stimulated by the a subunits of C3, C4, and C5. Several regulatory and inhibitory proteins help modulate the system.

In general, deficiencies of the early components of the classic pathway result in connective tissue disease states; deficiency of C3 results in recurrent infections with encapsulated bacteria such as *Pneumococcus, H. influenzae,* and *Streptococcus pyogenes;* and deficiencies of the late components of complement lead to recurrent neisserial sepsis or meningitis. Overlap exists, however, such that patients with late component deficiencies may exhibit connective tissue disease and vice versa. Properdin (a component of the alternate pathway) dysfunction, inherited as an X-linked trait, predisposes to fulminant meningococcemia. Patients deficient in C9 have been identified, but they do not have any of these problems. Regulatory protein defects may also predispose to lupus erythematosus.

Among the complement deficiencies, C2 deficiency is most frequently seen. Most of these patients are healthy. Diseases that occur with increased frequency in persons deficient in C2 are systemic lupus erythematosus (SLE), SLE-like syndrome, frequent infections, anaphylactoid purpura, lethal dermatomyositis, vasculitis, disseminated cutaneous lupus erythematosus, and cold urticaria. C2- and C4-deficient patients with lupus erythematosus commonly have subacute annular morphology, Sjögren's syndrome, and Ro antibodies. They less commonly have ant-dsDNA antibodies and anticardiolipin antibodies.

Inherited deficiencies of complement are usually autosomal recessively transmitted. Deficiencies of all 11 components of the classic pathway, as well as inhibitors of this pathway, have been described. Genetic deficiency of the C1 inhibitor results in hereditary angioedema which is discussed in more detail in Chapter 7. C3 inactivator deficiency, like C3 deficiency, results in recurrent pyogenic infections.

Most of the inherited complement deficiencies are being well characterized on a genetic level. It is being found that individual families have specific mutations, deletions, or insertions in the gene loci controlling the synthesis of the deficient complement component. Many different alterations may give rise to phenotypically identical disease. Additionally, most of these deficiencies may be acquired as an autoimmune phenomenon or a paraneoplastic finding. Examples include acquired angioedema, as when C1-inhibitor is the target, or lipodystrophy and nephritis, when C3 convertase is the target.

When complement deficiency is suspected, a useful screening test is a CH50 (total hemolytic complement level in serum) determination, because deficiency of complement components will usually result in CH50 levels that are markedly reduced or zero. The important exceptions are C9 deficiency, and C1-inhibitor deficiency. The screening laboratory test of choice when the latter is suspected is a serum C4 level assay.

Buckley D, et al: Childhood subacute cutaneous lupus erythematosus associated with homozygous complement 2 deficiency. *Pediatr Dermatol* 1995, 12:327.

Colten HR: Hereditary angioneurotic edema. *N Engl J Med* 1987, 317:43.

Frank MM: Complement in the pathophysiology of human disease. *N Engl J Med* 1987, 316:1525.

Guenther LC: Inherited disorders of complement. *J Am Acad Dermatol* 1983, 9:815.

Heymann WR: Acquired angioedema. *J Am Acad Dermatol* 1997, 36:611.

Jordan RE: The complement system and the skin. *Arch Dermatol* 1982, 118:359.

Ratnoff WD: Inherited deficiencies of complement in rheumatic disease. *Rhem Clin North Am* 1996, 22:75.

Ross SC, et al: Complement deficiency states and infection. *Medicine* 1984, 63:243.

Sjholm AG, et al: Dysfunctional properdin in a family with meningococcal disease. *N Engl J Med* 1988, 319:33.

Wayte J, et al: The clinical significance of partial lipoatrophy and C3 hypocomplementaemia. *Clin Exp Dermatol* 1996, 21:131.

▲

Graft-Versus-Host Disease

Graft-versus-host disease (GVHD) occurs when immunocompetent cells are introduced as a graft or blood transfusion into an antigenically foreign host who is unable to reject these grafted cells. In some instances, however, marrow from the patient (autologous) or from a monozygotic twin (syngeneic) may lead to a limited form of GVHD. Although GVHD occurs most frequently after bone marrow transplantation, it may occur after transfusion of whole blood to immunocompromised patients, in immunocompromised neonates after in utero transfusions, and in pancreas-spleen, small bowel, lung-heart, lung, heart, and liver transplantation. There are two forms: an acute form with cutaneous, hepatic, and gastrointestinal manifestations, and a chronic form with cutaneous manifestations similar to a collagen vascular disorder.

In the acute form the cutaneous eruption begins between the fifth and forty-seventh day, most often between the fourth and fifth weeks after transplantation. It is characterized by an erythematous maculopapular eruption of the face and upper trunk, which may become confluent and result in exfoliative erythroderma. It may begin in a perifollicular distribution. Rarely, a hyperacute form occurs in the first week and is characterized by severe generalized inflammation, fever, hepatitis, fluid retention, and capillary leak, and shock. In patients with liver transplants who develop GVHD, the clinical manifestations differ from that observed after bone marrow transplantation in that liver involvement does not occur and there is early and severe pancytopenia which is the major cause of mortality.

Syngeneic/autologous GVHD usually involves only the skin and is self-limited. This, like chronic GVHD, may result from incomplete elimination of autoreactive T cells directed at epitopes on MHC class II molecules.

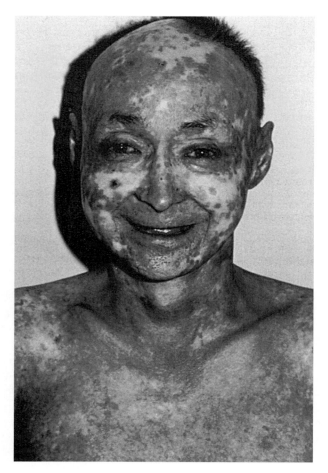

Fig. 5-17 Graft-versus-host disease after bone marrow transplantation for aplastic anemia, showing alopecia, dyspigmentation, and scleroderma. (Courtesy Dr. Axel W. Hoke.)

Although 40% to 50% of HLA-matched allogeneic bone marrow transplantations and 5% to 30% of syngeneic transplants may be followed by acute GVHD, 30% to 50% of long-term survivors develop chronic GVHD. In 80% of the patients who develop chronic GVHD a lichen planus–like eruption occurs 3 to 5 months after grafting, usually beginning on the hands and feet. Sclerosis develops less frequently. It may remain localized, but generalized sclerosis with dyspigmentation, alopecia, atrophy, chronic ulcers, and joint contractures may also be seen (Fig. 5-17). "Parrot-beak" deformity of the nose, sicca syndrome, polymyositis, acquired ichthyosis, eryth-

roderma, and total leukoderma may also be manifestations of chronic GVHD.

Because GVHD occurs so frequently after bone marrow transplantation, efforts to prevent it by giving methotrexate, cyclosporine, or other immunosuppressive or immuno-modulating drugs and by manipulating the donor marrow are being studied. Prevention of posttransfusion GVHD is most safely achieved by irradiating the blood before transfusion.

Glucocorticoids and cyclosporine are used to treat both acute and chronic GVHD. Several reports have anecdotally reported success in treating chronic GVHD with PUVA alone or in combination with methotrexate. Monoclonal antibodies directed against cytokines, gamma globulin infusions, extracorporeal photopheresis, immunotoxins, and receptor antagonists are all being evaluated for therapeutic use in the future.

Aractingi S, et al: Cutaneous graft-versus-host disease. *Arch Dermatol* 1998, 134:602.

Andrews ML, et al: Cutaneous manifestations of chronic graft-versus-host disease. *Australas J Dermatol* 1997, 38:53.

Berger RS, et al: Fulminant transfusion-associated GVHD in a premature infant. *J Am Acad Dermatol* 1989, 20:945.

Capon SM, et al: Transfusion-associated GVHD in an immunocompetent patient. *Ann Intern Med* 1991; 114:1025.

Chosidow O, et al: Sclerodermatous chronic GVHD. *J Am Acad Dermatol* 1992; 26:49.

Connors J, et al: Morbilliform eruption in a liver transplantation patient. *Arch Dermatol* 1996, 132:1161.

Darmstadt GL, et al: Clinical, laboratory, and histopathologic indicators of the development of progressive acute GVHD. *J Invest Dermatol* 1992, 99:397.

Ferrera JLM, et al: GVHD. *N Engl J Med* 1991, 324:667.

Friedman KJ, et al: Acute follicular GVHD. *Arch Dermatol* 1988, 124:688.

Horn TD: Acute cutaneous eruptions after marrow ablation. *J Cutan Pathol* 1994, 21:385.

Jampel RM, et al: PUVA therapy for chronic cutaneous GVHD. *Arch Dermatol* 1991, 127:1673.

Johnson ML, et al: GVH reactions in dermatology. *J Am Acad Dermatol* 1998, 38:369.

Langley RG, et al: Apoptosis is the mode of keratinocyte death in cutaneous graft-versus-host disease. *J Am Acad Dermatol* 1996, 35:187.

Nagler A, et al: Total leucoderma. *Br J Dermatol* 1996, 134:780.

Parker P, et al: Polymyositis as a manifestation of chronic graft-versus-host disease. *Medicine* 1996, 75:279.

Ray TL: Blood transfusions and GVHD. *Arch Dermatol* 1991, 126:1347.

Richter HI, et al: Extracorporeal photopheresis in the treatment of acute graft-versus-host disease. *J Am Acad Dermatol* 1997, 36:787.

Rodu B, et al: Oral manifestations of the graft-versus-host reaction. *JAMA* 1983, 249:504.

Volc-Platzer B, et al: Photochemotherapy improves chronic cutaneous GVHD. *J Am Acad Dermatol* 1990, 23:220. _____ ▲

CHAPTER 6

Contact Dermatitis and Drug Eruptions

CONTACT DERMATITIS

There are two types of dermatitis caused by substances coming in contact with the skin: irritant dermatitis and allergic contact dermatitis. Irritant dermatitis is an inflammatory reaction in the skin resulting from exposure to a substance that causes an eruption in most people who come in contact with it. Allergic contact dermatitis is an acquired sensitivity to various substances that produce inflammatory reactions in those, and only those, who have been previously exposed to the allergen.

Irritant Contact Dermatitis

There are many substances acting as irritants that will produce a nonallergic inflammatory reaction of the skin. This type of dermatitis may be induced in any person if a sufficiently high concentration is used. No previous exposure is necessary, and the effect is evident within minutes, or a few hours at most. The only variation in the severity of the dermatitis from person to person, or from time to time in the same person, is related to the condition of the skin at the time of exposure to a given concentration of the irritant. The skin may be more vulnerable by reason of maceration from excessive humidity, or exposure to water, heat, cold, pressure, or friction. Dry skin is less likely to react to contactants. Thick skin is less reactive than thin. Repeated exposure to some of the milder irritants may, in time, produce a hardening effect. This process makes the skin more resistant to the irritant effects of a given substance.

Alkalis. Irritant dermatitis is often produced by such alkalis as soaps, detergents, bleaches, ammonia preparations, lye, drain pipe cleaners, toilet bowl cleansers, and oven cleansers. Alkalis penetrate and destroy deeply, because these compounds dissolve keratin. Strong solutions are corrosive, and immediate application of a weak acid such as vinegar, lemon juice, or 0.5% hydrochloric acid solution will lessen their effects.

The principal compounds are sodium, potassium, ammonium, and calcium hydroxides. Occupational exposure is frequent among workers in soap manufacturing. Alkalis in the form of soaps, bleaching agents, detergents, and most household cleansing agents figure prominently in the causes of hand eczema. Sodium silicate (water glass) is a caustic used in soap manufacture and paper sizing and for the preservation of eggs. Alkaline sulfides are used as depilatories. Calcium oxide (quicklime) forms slaked lime when water is added. Severe burns may be caused in plasterers.

Acids. The powerful acids are corrosive, whereas the weaker ones are astringent. Hydrochloric acid produces burns that are less deep and more liable to form blisters than injuries from sulfuric and nitric acids. Hydrochloric acid burns are encountered in those who handle or transport the product, and in plumbers and those who work in galvanizing or tin-plate factories. Hydrofluoric acid is used widely in rust remover, in the semiconductor industry, and in germicides, dyes, plastics, and glass etching. Nitric acid is a powerful oxidizing substance that causes deep burns; the tissue is stained yellow. Such injuries are observed in those who manufacture or handle the acid or use it in the making of explosives in laboratories. Sulfuric acid produces a brownish charring of the skin, beneath which is an ulceration that heals slowly. Sulfuric acid is used more widely than any other acid in industry; it is handled principally by brass and iron workers and by those who work with copper or bronze. It is the weapon of so-called vitriol throwers.

Oxalic acid may produce paresthesia of the finger tips, with cyanosis and gangrene. The nails become discolored yellow. Oxalic acid is best neutralized with lime water or milk of magnesia to produce precipitation. Hydrofluoric acid may act insidiously at first, starting with erythema and ending with vesiculation, ulceration, and, finally, necrosis of the tissue. It is one of the strongest inorganic acids, capable of dissolving glass.

Phenol (carbolic acid) is a protoplasmic poison that produces a white eschar on the surface of the skin. It can penetrate deep into the tissue. If a large surface of the skin is treated with phenol for cosmetic peeling effects, the absorbed phenol may produce glomerulonephritis and arrhythmias. Locally, temporary anesthesia may also occur. Phenol is readily neutralized with 65% ethyl or isopropyl alcohol.

Other strong acids that are irritants include acetic, arsenious, chlorosulfonic, chromic, fluoroboric, hydriodic, hydrobromic, iodic, perchloric, phosphoric, salicylic, silicofluoric, sulfonic, sulfurous, tannic, and tungstic acid.

Treatment of burns from these acids consists of immediate rinsing with copious amounts of water and alkalization with sodium bicarbonate, calcium hydroxide (lime water), or soap solutions. Some chemicals require unusual treatment measures. Fluorine is best neutralized with magnesium oxide. Periungual burns should be treated intralesionally with 10% calcium gluconate solution, which deactivates the fluoride ion and averts more tissue damage. Phosphorus burns should be rinsed off with water followed by application of copper sulfate to produce a precipitate.

Titanium hydrochloride is used in the manufacture of pigments. Application of water to the exposed part will produce severe burns. Therefore treatment consists only of wiping away the noxious substance.

Other Irritants. Some metal salts that act as irritants are the cyanides of calcium, copper, mercury, nickel, silver, and zinc, and the chlorides of calcium and zinc. Bromine, chlorine, fluorine, and iodine are also irritants. Herzemans-Boer et al reported on six patients who were occupationally exposed to methyl bromide; these patients developed erythema and vesicles in the axillary and inguinal areas.

Chloracne. Workers in the manufacture of chlorinated compounds may develop chloracne, with small black follicular plugs and papules, chiefly on the malar crescent and retroauricular areas. Another characteristic site is the scrotum. Machinists' use of chlorinated compounds in cutting oils predisposes them to the development of chloracne on their thighs.

The synthetic waxes chloronaphthalene and chlorodiphenyl, used in the manufacture of electric insulators and in paints, varnishes, and lacquers, similarly predispose workers engaged in the manufacture of these synthetic waxes to chloracne. Exposure to 2,6-dichlorobenzonitrile during the manufacture of a herbicide, and to 3,4,3′,4′,tetrachloroazooxybenzene, which occurs as an unwanted intermediate byproduct in the manufacture of a pesticide, may also produce chloracne. Tindall reviewed chloracne and the effects of exposure to the dioxin compounds during the Vietnam War.

Flea-Collar Dermatitis. Dog collars containing an insecticide, 2,2-dichlorovinyl dimethyl phosphate (Vapona), an irritant, have caused dermatitis resembling toxicodendron dermatitis in some individuals who handled dogs wearing such collars. This insecticide is also used in roach powder and hang-up fly repellents and killers. Various other insecticides may act as irritants.

Hunan Hand. The irritation produced by capsaicin in hot peppers used in Korean and North Chinese cuisine may be severe and prolonged. Cold water is not much help: capsaicin is insoluble in water. Acetic acid 5% (white vinegar) may completely relieve the burning even if applied an hour or more after the contact. Soaking should be continued until the area can be dried without return of the discomfort.

Fiberglass Dermatitis. Fiberglass dermatitis is seen after occupational or inadvertent exposure. The small spicules of glass penetrate the skin and cause severe irritation with tiny erythematous papules, scratch marks, and intense pruritus. Usually there is no delayed hypersensitivity reaction. Wearing clothes that have been washed together with fiberglass curtains, handling air conditioner filters, or working in the manufacture of fiberglass material may produce severe folliculitis, pruritus, and eruptions that may simulate scabies or insect or mite bites. Fiberglass is also used in thermal and acoustical installations, padding, vibration isolation, curtains, draperies, insulation for automobile bodies, furniture, gasoline tanks, and spacecraft. A thorough washing of the skin after handling fiberglass is helpful. Talcum powder thoroughly dusted on the flexure surfaces of the arms makes the fibers slide off the skin.

Dermatitis Resulting from Dusts and Gases. Some dusts and gases may irritate the skin in the presence of heat and moisture, such as perspiration. The dusts of lime, zinc, and arsenic may produce folliculitis. Dusts from various woods, such as teak, may incite itching and dermatitis. Dusts from cinchona bark, quinine, and pyrethrum produce widespread dermatitis. Tobacco dust in cigar factories, powdered orris root, lycopodium, and dusts of various nutshells may cause swelling of the eyelids and dermatitis of the face, neck, and upper extremities. Dusts formed during the manufacture of high explosives may cause erythematous, vesicular, and eczematous dermatitis that may lead to generalized exfoliative dermatitis.

TEAR GAS DERMATITIS. Lacrimators such as chloroacetophenone in concentrated form may cause dermatitis, with a delayed appearance some 24 to 72 hours after exposure. Irritation or sensitization, with erythema and severe vesiculation, may result. Treatment consists of lavage of the affected skin with sodium bicarbonate solution and instillation of boric acid solution into the eyes. Contaminated clothing should be removed.

SULFUR MUSTARD GAS. Sulfur mustard gas, also known as *yperite,* is used in chemical warfare. Pierard et al reviewed its skin toxicity after caring for combatants in the Iraq-Iran war. Erythema, vesicles, and bullae, followed by healing with hyperpigmentation over a 1-week period, result from

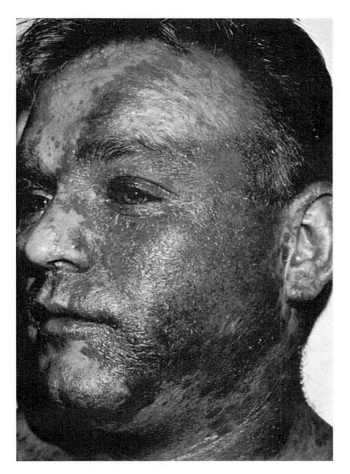

Fig. 6-1 Dermatitis caused by mace.

mild to moderate exposure. Toxic epidermal necrolysis-like appearance may follow more concentrated contact. The earliest and most frequently affected sites are areas covered by clothing and humidified by sweat, such as the groin, axilla, and genitalia.

MACE. Mace is a mixture of tear gas (chloroacetophenone) in trichloroethane and various hydrocarbons resembling kerosene. It is available in a variety of self-defense sprays. It is a potent irritant and may cause allergic sensitization (Fig. 6-1). Treatment consists of changing clothes, washing with oil or a cleansing milk, followed by washing with copious amounts of water.

Dermatitis Resulting from Various Hydrocarbons.
Many hydrocarbons produce skin eruptions. Crude petroleum causes generalized itching, folliculitis, or acneiform eruptions. Irritant properties of petroleum derivatives are directly proportional to fat-solvent properties and inversely proportional to viscosity. Oils of the naphthalene series are more irritating than those of the paraffin series. Refined fractions from petroleum are less irritating than the unrefined products, although benzene, naphtha, and carbon disulfide may cause a mild dermatitis.

Lubricating oils and cutting oils are causes of similar cutaneous lesions. They represent a frequent cause of occupational dermatoses in machine tool operators, machinists, layout men, instrument makers, and set-up men. Water-soluble cutting oils rarely cause dermatitis, whereas chlorinated cutting oils (not water soluble) are very irritating. They were major causes of occupational chloracne, but these types have now been eliminated; other insoluble cutting oils are still responsible for a follicular acneiform eruption on the dorsa of the hands, the forearms, face, thighs, and back of the neck. Scrotal cancer has been found to occur in those exposed to cutting oils. Mule spinners' cancer of the scrotum, formerly an important problem in the cotton industry in England, was caused by certain lubricating oils that are no longer used. Castiglione reported such a case.

Knox described eight cases of an acquired perforating disease in oil field workers. The patients developed tender, umbilicated papules of the forearms that microscopically showed transepidermal elimination of calcium. The drilling fluid was found to contain calcium chloride.

Coal briquette makers develop dermatitis as a result of a tarry residue from petroleum used in their trade. Workers in paraffin show an irritation of the skin that leads to pustules, keratoses, and ulcerations. Shale oil workers develop an erythematous, follicular eruption that eventually leads to keratoses, which may become the sites of carcinoma. It is estimated that 50% of shale oil workers have skin problems.

Impure and low-grade paraffins and mineral oils cause similar skin eruptions. Initially the skin changes are similar to those in chloracne. In due time, a diffuse erythema with dappled pigmentation develops. Gradually, keratoses appear, and after many years some of these are the sites of carcinoma. Melanoderma may occur from exposure to mineral oils and lower-grade petroleum, from creosote, asphalt, and other tar products. Photosensitization may play a role. Creosote is a contact irritant, a sensitizer, and a photosensitizer. Allergy is demonstrated by patch testing with 10% creosote in oil.

Petrolatum dermatitis may appear as a verrucous thickening of the skin caused by prolonged contact with impure petroleum jelly or, occasionally, lubricating oil. A follicular type occurs in which erythematous horny nodules are present, usually on the anterior and inner aspects of the thighs. There are no comedones, and the lesions are separated by apparently normal skin.

Acne corne consists of follicular keratosis and pigmentation resulting from crude petroleum, tar oils, and paraffin. The dorsal aspects of the fingers and hands, the arms, legs, face, and thorax are the areas usually involved. The lesions are follicular, horny papules, often black, and are associated at first with a follicular erythema and later with a dirty brownish or purplish spotty pigmentation, which in severe cases becomes widespread and is especially marked around the genitals. This syndrome may simulate pityriasis rubra pilaris or lichen spinulosus.

Coal tar and pitch and many of their derivatives produce photosensitization and an acneiform folliculitis of the forearms, legs, face, and scrotum. Follicular keratoses (pitch warts) may develop and later turn into carcinoma. Soot, lamp black, and the ash from peat fires produce dermatitis of a dry, scaly character, which in the course of time forms warty outgrowths and cancer. Chimney sweep's cancer was first described in England by Pott in 1790. The cancer occurs under a soot wart and is usually located on the scrotum, where soot, sebum, and dirt collect in the folds of the skin. This form of cancer has virtually disappeared. Asbestos workers develop asbestos warts, but the known carcinogenicity of asbestos has not been described in the skin.

Dermatitis Resulting from Solvents. Solvent sniffers may develop an eczematous eruption about the mouth and nose. There is erythema and edema. It is a direct irritant dermatitis caused by the inhaling of the solvent placed on a handkerchief. Allergic contact dermatitis caused by alcohol is rarely encountered with lower aliphatic alcohols. A severe case of bullous and hemorrhagic dermatitis on the fingertips and on the deltoid region was caused by isopropyl alcohol. Though rare, ethyl alcohol dermatitis may also be encountered. Cetyl and stearyl alcohols provoke an urticaria-like dermatitis.

Baadsgaard O, et al: Mustard gas and the dermatologist. *Int J Dermatol* 1991, 30:684.

Castiglione FM, et al: Mule spinner's disease. *Arch Dermatol* 1985, 121:370.

Finkelstein E, et al: Oil acne. *J Am Acad Dermatol* 1994, 30:491.

Foulds IS, et al: Dermatitis from metal working fluids. *Clin Exp Dermatol* 1990, 25:157.

Garcia-Patos V, et al: Fiberglass dermatitis. *Arch Dermatol* 1994, 130:787.

Herzemans-Boer M, et al: Skin lesions due to methyl bromide. *Arch Dermatol* 1988, 124:917.

Kershenovich J, et al: Dowlins-Degos' disease mimicking chloracne. *J Am Acad Dermatol* 1992, 27:345.

Knox JM, et al: Acquired perforating disease in oil field workers. *J Am Acad Dermatol* 1986, 14:605.

Momeni AZ, et al: Skin manifestations of mustard gas. *Arch Dermatol* 1992, 128:775.

Moshell AN: Workshop on irritant contact dermatitis. *Am J Contact Dermat* 1997, 8:79.

Nickoloff BJ: Immunologic reactions triggered during irritant contact dermatitis. *Am J Contact Dermat* 1998, 9:107.

Pierard GE, et al: Chemical warfare casualties and yperite-induced xerodermoid. *Am J Dermatopathol* 1990, 12:565.

Reguena L et al: Chemical warfare. *J Am Acad Dermatol* 1988, 19:529.

Rietschel RL: Mechanisms in irritant contact dermatitis. *Clin Dermatol* 1997, 15:557.

Rosas-Vasquez E, et al: Chloracne in the 1990s. *Int J Dermatol* 1996, 35:643.

Schmutz JL, et al: Cutaneous accidents due to self-defense sprays. *Ann Dermatol Venereol* 1987, 114:1211.

Smith KJ, et al: Sulfur mustard. *J Am Acad Dermatol* 1995, 32:765.

Tindall JP: Chloracne and chloracnegens. *J Am Acad Dermatol* 1985, 13:539.

Williams SR, et al: Contact dermatitis associated with capsaicin: Hunan hand syndrome. *Ann Emerg Med* 1995, 25:713. _____ ▲

Allergic Contact Dermatitis

Allergic contact dermatitis is also called *dermatitis venenata.* Allergic contact dermatitis results when an allergen comes into contact with previously sensitized skin. Allergic contact dermatitis results from a specific acquired hypersensitivity of the delayed type, also known as *cell-mediated hypersensitivity* or *immunity.* Occasionally, dermatitis may be induced on a sensitized area of skin when the allergen is taken internally; this occurs, for example, with substances such as the antihistaminics or sulfonamides, and is called an *anamnestic* reaction. Persons may be exposed to allergens for years before finally developing hypersensitivity. Once sensitized, however, subsequent outbreaks may result from extremely slight exposure.

The allergens are extremely varied and may be nonprotein in nature. Many substances, such as dyes and their intermediates, oils, resins, coal tar derivatives, chemicals used for fabrics, rubbers, cosmetics, insecticides, the oils and resins of woods and plants, as well as the products or the substances of bacteria, fungi, and parasites, are proven allergens. These sensitizers do not cause demonstrable skin changes on first contact but may produce specific changes in the skin when the patient is reexposed to the allergen at a subsequent time.

Prunieras suggested that the Langerhans' cells might play a major role in the pathogenesis of contact allergy, but how they might act was not known until Silberberg, Baer, and Rosenthal showed in 1976 that in both guinea pigs and humans, during challenge with contact allergens, there is direct apposition of mononuclear cells to the dendrites of the Langerhans' cells, followed by damage to the latter. Langerhans' cells in the dermis are more numerous after such challenges, and they are also found in lymph nodes. Funk and Maibach have reviewed cellular events and immunologic mechanisms leading to the clinical changes of allergic contact dermatitis. They use this framework to discuss current and future therapy.

One must distinguish the eczematous delayed-type hypersensitivity reaction, as exemplified by allergic contact dermatitis and the patch test, from the urticarial immediate type of IgE-mediated reaction (contact urticaria), which is present with urticaria, asthma, and hay fever, and in scratch, intracutaneous, and passive transfer tests. It should be kept in mind, however, that persons who exhibit the latter type of reaction, which is chiefly vascular, may concomitantly have a type IV delayed-type sensitization and eczema from the same allergen.

Although these eruptions involute spontaneously when the cause is identified and removed, some cases prove difficult because the identity of the allergen is not easily ascertained. Typical cases of dermatitis of external origin with erythema, vesiculation, and linear lesions within scratch marks that occur on exposed parts occasionally defy the skill of the dermatologist and require prolonged observation before the causative factor is isolated. In other instances, as among painters, plasterers, and dentists, the cause of the dermatitis may be obvious because of known exposure to specific sensitizing substances.

In some instances impetigo, pustular folliculitis, and irritations or allergic reactions from applied medications are superimposed on the original dermatitis. The cutaneous reaction also may provoke a hypersusceptibility to various other previously innocuous substances, which continues the inflammation indefinitely as eczema.

The most common causes of contact dermatitis in the United States are the following: toxicodendrons (poison ivy, oak, or sumac), nickel, fragrance, thimerosal, quarternium-15, neomycin, formaldehyde and the formaldehyde-releasing preservatives, bacitracin, and rubber compounds. Frequent positive reactions to thimerosal do not often correlate with clinical exposure histories. These reactions are probably related to its use as a preservative in commonly administered vaccines and skin-testing material. It also serves as a marker for piroxicam photosensitivity.

Allergic contact sensitivity to corticosteroids may be acquired. Recent studies document increasing prevalence of allergy to these medicaments. The usual clinical situation in which an allergic reaction to topical corticosteroids should be suspected is one in which a chronic eczema fails to heal. Many cross reactions occur among the various preparations. Patch testing has many pitfalls, but tixicortol pivalate is the best screen. In its absence, testing to 0.5% triamcinolone acetonide ointment or 0.05% fluocinolone ointment has been suggested as a pragmatic screen.

Testing for Sensitivity

PATCH TEST. The patch test is used to detect hypersensitivity to a substance that is in contact with the skin so that the allergen may be determined and corrective measures taken. There are so many allergens causing allergic contact dermatitis that it is impossible to test a person for all of them. In addition, a good history and observation of the pattern of the dermatitis, its localization on the body, and its state of activity are all helpful in determining the cause. The patch test is confirmatory and diagnostic but only within the framework of the history and physical findings; it is rarely helpful if it must stand alone.

The patch test consists of application to the intact uninflamed skin, in nonirritating concentration, of substances suspected to be causes of the contact dermatitis. Patch testing may be administered by the thin-layer rapid-use epicutaneous (TRUE) test or by individually prepared aluminum (Finn) chambers mounted on Scanpor tape. The TRUE test has resulted in more screening for allergic contact dermatitis than in the past; however, if this test does not reveal the allergen for a highly suspect dermatitis, Soni and Sherertz have shown that retesting with an expanded series by the Finn chamber technique may yield relevant allergens in more than half of these patients.

Test substances on the test strips are applied usually to the upper back, although if only one or two are applied, the upper outer arm may be used. Each patch should be numbered to avoid confusion. The patches are removed after 48 hours (or less if itching or burning occur at the site) and read. The patch sites need to be evaluated again at day 4 or 5, because positive reactions may not appear earlier, and some allergens may take up to day 7 to show a reaction. Standard allergens are available that also come with a scale to document the intensity of the reaction. Erythematous papules and vesicles with edema are indicative of allergy. Occasionally, patch tests for potassium iodide, nickel, or mercury will produce pustules at the site of the test application. Usually no erythema is produced; therefore the reaction has no clinical significance.

Strong patch test reactions may induce a state of hyperirritability ("angry back") in which negative tests appear as weakly positive. Because the phenomenon is not limited to the back, Bruynzeel et al have suggested that it be called the excited skin syndrome. They concluded that weakly positive test results in the presence of strong ones do not prove sensitivity. There is wide variation in the ability of the skin and mucous membranes to react to antigens. The oral mucosa is more resistant to primary irritants and is less liable to be involved in allergic reactions. This may be because the keratin layer of the skin more readily combines with haptens to form allergens. Also the oral mucosa is bathed in saliva, which cleanses and buffers the area and dilutes irritants. However, investigations such as those of Shah et al demonstrate the utility of patch testing for various types of oral signs and symptoms, such as swelling, tingling and burning, perioral dermatitis, and the appearance of oral lichen planus.

The ability of the skin to react to allergens also depends on the presence of functional antigen-presenting cells, the Langerhans' cells. Potent topical steroids, ultraviolet light, and acquired immunodeficiency syndrome (AIDS) all have been reported to interfere with the number and function of these key cells. Vitiliginous skin is less reactive than normally pigmented adjacent skin.

PROVOCATIVE USE TEST. The provocative use test will confirm a positive closed patch test reaction to ingredients of a substance, such as a cosmetic; it is used to test the commercial skin product primarily. The material is rubbed onto normal skin of the inner aspect of the forearm several times daily for 7 days.

PHOTOPATCH TEST. The photopatch test is used to evaluate for contact photoallergy to such substances as sulfonamides, phenothiazines, paraaminobenzoic acid, oxybenzone, 6-methyl coumarin, musk ambrette, or tetrachlorsalicylanilide. A standard patch test is applied for 24 hours; this is then exposed to 5 to 15 J/m^2 of UVA and read after another 48 hours. To test for 6-methyl coumarin sensitivity, the patch is applied in the same manner but for only 30 minutes before light exposure, rather than for 24 hours. A duplicate set of nonirradiated patches is used in testing for the presence of routine delayed hypersensitivity reactions.

Also, a site of normal skin is given an identical dose of UVA to test for increased sensitivity to light without prior exposure to chemicals. De Leo et al have reviewed their experience and document the steady increase in incidence of sunscreening agent sensitivity and falling incidence of fragrance photoallergy.

Regional Predilection. Familiarity with certain contactants and the typical dermatitis they elicit on specific parts of the body will assist in diagnosis of the etiologic agent.

HEAD AND NECK. The scalp is relatively resistant to the development of contact allergies; however, involvement may be caused by hair dye, hair spray, shampoo, or permanent-wave solutions. The surrounding glabrous skin including the ear rims and backs of the ears may be much more inflamed and suggestive of the cause. Persistent otitis of the ear canal may be caused by sensitivity to the neomycin that is an ingredient of most aural medications. The forehead of a man may be the site of a hatband dermatitis. The eyelids are the most frequent site for nail polish dermatitis. Volatile gases, false-eyelash cement, fragrances, preservatives, mascara, and eyeshadow cosmetics are also frequently implicated. Rubber allergy to the sponges used to apply eyelid cosmetics commonly cause eyelid dermatitis in our clinics. Perioral dermatitis may be caused by dentifrices, bubble gum, or ordinary chewing gum. Beacham et al warn of the special problem of tartar control dentifrices. Perfume dermatitis may cause redness just under the ears. Nickel sensitivity may be noted at the clasp site of necklaces or earrings. Photocontact dermatitis may involve the entire face and may be sharply cut off at the collar line or extend down onto the sternum in a V shape. There is a typical clear area under the chin where there is little or no exposure to sunlight. In men, in whom shaving lotion fragrances are often responsible, the left cheek and left side of the neck (from sun exposure while driving a left-hand-drive car) may be the first areas involved. Berloque dermatitis is frequently seen on the preauricular areas and sides of the neck.

TRUNK. The trunk is an infrequent site; however, the dye or finish of clothing may cause dermatitis. Fowler et al documented that formaldehyde textile resin allergy should be suspected in truncal eruptions. The axilla may be the site of deodorant and clothing-dye dermatitis. Involvement of the axillary vault suggests the former; of the axillary folds, the latter. In women, brassieres frequently cause dermatitis either from the material itself or from elastic or metal snaps, which seem invariably to be nickel-plated.

ARMS. The wrists may be involved because of jewelry or the backs of watches and clasps, all of which may contain nickel. Wrist bands made of leather are a source of chrome dermatitis.

HANDS. Innumerable substances may cause contact dermatitis of the hands, which typically occurs on the backs of the hands and spares the palms. Poison ivy and other plant dermatitides frequently occur on the hands and arms. Rubber glove sensitivity must be kept constantly in mind.

ABDOMEN. The abdomen, especially the waistline, may be the site of rubber dermatitis from the elastic in pants. The metallic rivets in blue jeans may lead to periumbilical dermatitis in nickel-sensitive patients.

GROIN. The groin is usually spared, but the buttocks and upper thighs may be sites of dermatitis caused by dyes. The penis is frequently involved in poison ivy dermatitis. Condom dermatitis may also occur. The perianal region may be involved from the "caine" medications in suppositories. Lewis et al reported that nearly half of 121 women with pruritus vulvae had one or more relevant allergens. This included many with the itching of lichen sclerosis et atrophicus.

LOWER EXTREMITIES. The shins may be the site of rubber dermatitis from elastic stockings. Feet are sites for shoe dermatitis, most often attributable to rubber sensitivity, chrome-tanned leather, or adhesives. Application of topical antibiotics to stasis ulcers commonly leads to sensitivity and allergic contact dermatitis.

Beacham BE, et al: Circumoral dermatitis and cheilitis caused by tartar control dentifrices. *J Am Acad Dermatol* 1990, 22:1029.

Belsito DV: The rise and fall of allergic contact dermatitis. *Am J Contact Dermat* 1997, 8:193.

Bruynzeel DP, et al: Excited skin syndrome (angry back). *Arch Dermatol* 1986, 122:323.

DeLeo VA, et al: Allergic contact dermatitis. *Arch Dermatol* 1992, 128:1513.

Drake L, et al: Guidelines of care for contact dermatitis. *J Am Acad Dermatol* 1995, 32:109.

Fisher AA: The persulfates: a triple threat. *Cutis* 1985, 27:25.

Fowler JF Jr, et al: Allergic contact dermatitis from formaldehyde resins on permanent press clothing. *J Am Acad Dermatol* 1992, 27:962.

Funk JO, et al: Horizons in pharmacologic intervention in allergic contact dermatitis. *J Am Acad Dermatol* 1994, 31:999.

Kondo S, et al: Epidermal cytokines in allergic contact dermatitis. *J Am Acad Dermatol* 1995, 33:786.

Lauerma AI, et al: Contact allergy to corticosteroids. *J Am Acad Dermatol* 1993, 28:618.

Lewis FM, et al: Contact sensitivity in pruritus vulvae. *Am J Contact Dermat* 1997, 8:137.

Lutz ME, et al: Contact hypersensitivity to tixocortol pivalate. *J Am Acad Dermatol* 1998, 38:691.

Marks JG Jr, DeLeo VA: Contact and occupational dermatology, ed 2, St Louis, 1997, Mosby.

Marks JG, et al: North American Contact Dermatitis Group patch test results for the detection of delayed type hypersensitivity to topical allergens. *J Am Acad Dermatol* 1998, 38:911.

Nethercott JR, et al: A review of 79 cases of eyelid dermatitis. *J Am Acad Dermatol* 1989 21:223.

Rietschel RL: Human and economic impact of allergic contact dermatitis and the role of patch testing. *J Am Acad Dermatol* 1995, 33:812.

Rietschel RL, Fowler JF Jr: Fisher's contact dermatitis, ed 4, Baltimore, 1995, Williams & Wilkins.

Shah MS, et al: Contact allergy in patients with oral symptoms. *Am J Contact Dermat* 1996, 7:146.

Soni BP, et al: Evaluation of previously patch-tested patient referred to a contact dermatitis clinic. *Am J Contact Dermat* 1997, 8:10. ▲

Dermatitis Resulting from Plants.

A large number of plants, including trees, grasses, flowers, vegetables, fruits, and weeds, are potential causes of dermatitis, formerly called *dermatitis venenata*. Eruptions from them vary considerably in appearance but are usually vesicular and accompanied by marked edema. After previous exposure and sensitization to the active substance in the plants, the typical dermatitis results from reexposure. The onset is sudden, a few hours or days after contact. The characteristic linearly grouped lesions are probably produced by brushing the skin with a leaf-edge or a broken twig or by carriage of the allergen under the nails. Contrary to general belief, the contents of vesicles are not capable of producing new lesions.

TOXICODENDRON (POISON IVY) DERMATITIS. Toxicodendron (Rhus) dermatitis includes dermatitis from members of the *Anacrdiaceae* family of plants: poison ivy, poison oak, and poison sumac, the Japanese lacquer tree, the cashew nut tree (the allergen is in the nutshell), mango (the allergen is in the rind, leaves, or sap), Rengas tree, and Indian marking nut tree. The ginkgo (the allergen is in the fruit pulp), the spider flower or silver oak, the *Gluta* species of trees and shrubs in Southeast Asia, the Brazilian pepper tree, also known as Florida holly, and the poisonwood tree contain antigens that are nearly identical.

Toxicodendron dermatitis appears within 48 hours after exposure of a previously sensitized person to the plant. It usually begins on the backs of the fingers, interdigital spaces, wrists, and eyelids, although it may begin on the ankles or other parts that have been exposed (Fig. 6-2). Marked pruritus is the first symptom; then inflammation, vesicles, and bullae may appear. The vesicles are usually grouped and often linear. Large bullae may be present, especially on the forearms and hands. The eyelids are puffy;

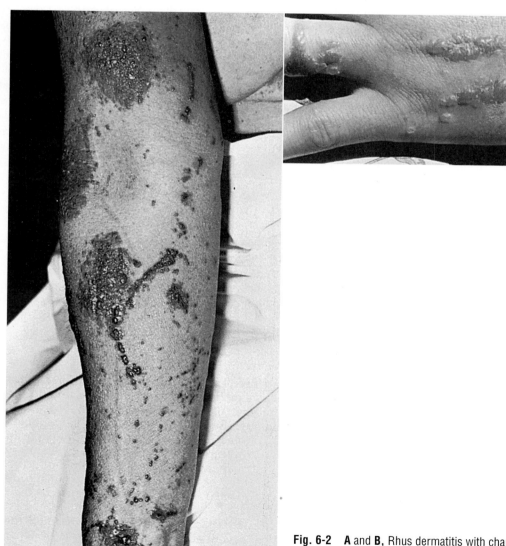

A

B

Fig. 6-2 A and **B,** Rhus dermatitis with characteristic linear groups of vesicles. (**B,** Courtesy Dr. Axel W. Hoke.)

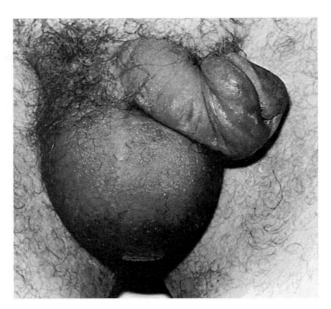

Fig. 6-3 Rhus dermatitis in a common site. (Courtesy Dr. Axel W. Hoke.)

they will be worse in the morning and improve as the day progresses. Pruritus ani and involvement of the genital areas occur frequently (Fig. 6-3). A black lacquer deposit may occur in which the sap of the plant has been oxidized after being bound to the stratum corneum.

The allergen is transferred by the fingers to other parts, especially the forearms and the male prepuce, which become greatly swollen. However, once the causative oil has been washed off, there is no spreading of the allergen and no further spread of the dermatitis. Some persons are so susceptible that direct contact is not necessary, the allergen apparently being carried by the fur of their pets or by the wind. It can also be acquired from golf clubs or fishing rods, or even from furniture that a dog or cat might have occupied after exposure to the catechol. Occasionally, eating the allergen, as occurred in a patient who ingested raw cashew nuts in an imported pesto sauce, may result in the *baboon syndrome* (a deep red-violet eruption on the buttocks, genital area, inner thighs, and sometimes axilla), or a systematized allergic contact dermatitis with the morphology of a generalized erythematous papular eruption.

Repeated attacks do not confer immunity, although a single severe attack may achieve this by what has been called *massive-dose desensitization*. The attacks usually last 2 to 3 weeks, during which time the patches become crusted and dry.

Toxicodendron dermatitis is caused by an oleoresin known as *urushiol*, of which the active agent is a mixture of catechols. This and related resorcinol allergens are present in many plants and are also present in philodendron species, wood from *Persoonia elliptica*, wheat bran, and marine brown algae.

The most striking diagnostic feature is the linearity of the lesions. It is rare to see vesicles arranged in a linear fashion except in plant-induced dermatitis. A history of exposure in the country or in the park to plants that have shiny leaves in groups of three, followed by the appearance of vesicular lesions within two days, usually establishes the diagnosis. Persons with known susceptibility not only should avoid touching plants having the grouped "leaves-of-three" but should also exercise care in handling articles of clothing, tools, toys, and pets that have come in contact with such plants.

Eradication of plants growing in frequented places is one easy preventive measure, as is recognition of the plants in preventing contact. An excellent resource is a pamphlet available from the American Academy of Dermatology. If the individual is exposed, washing with soap and water within 5 minutes may prevent an eruption. Protective barrier creams are available that are somewhat beneficial. Quaternium-18 bentonite has been shown to prevent or diminish experimentally produced poison ivy dermatitis.

Innumerable attempts have been made to immunize against poison ivy dermatitis by ingestion of the leaves, by oral administration of the tincture, or by subcutaneous injections of oily extracts. To date, no accepted method of immunization has evolved. Reginella et al report that 10 of 13 urushiol-sensitive patients lost their patch test positivity after working in a cashew nut shell oil processing plant for several months. Sheard reported the case of a woman who had suffered annual attacks of poison ivy dermatitis for many years but had none after she began chewing six raw cashew nuts daily from February to November.

When the diagnosis is clear and the eruption severe or extensive, systemic steroidal agents are effective, beginning with 40 to 60 mg of prednisone in a single oral dose daily, tapered off over a 3-week period. Improvement should be so rapid that there is seldom a need for wet dressings. When the eruption is limited in extent and severity, local application of topical corticosteroid creams, lotions, or aerosol sprays is superior to any other local application. The time-honored calamine lotion without phenol is helpful and does no harm. Antihistaminic ointments should be avoided because of their sensitization potential. This also applies to the local application of the "caine" topical anesthetics.

OTHER TOXICODENDRON-RELATED DERMATITIS. Lacquer dermatitis is caused by a furniture lacquer made from the Japanese lacquer tree, used on furniture, jewelry, or bric-a-brac. Antique lacquer is harmless, but lacquer less than 1 or 2 years old is highly antigenic. Cashew nutshell oil is extracted from the nutshells of the cashew tree (*Anacardium occidentale*). This vesicant oil contains cardol, a phenol similar to urushiol in poison ivy (Fig. 6-4). The liquid has many commercial applications, such as the manufacture of brake linings, varnish, synthetic glue, paint, and sealer for concrete.

Mango dermatitis is uncommon in natives of mango-

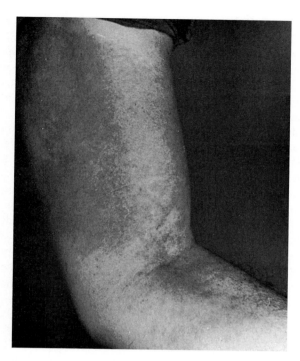

Fig. 6-4 Cashew nutshell oil dermatitis resembling poison ivy dermatitis.

growing countries (the Philippines, Guam, Hawaii, Cuba) who have never been exposed to contact with toxicodendron species. Many persons who have been so exposed, however, whether they had dermatitis from it or not, are sensitized by one or a few episodes of contact with the peel of the mango fruit. Because the palms of the hands are contaminated from the first, the eyelids and the male prepuce are often early sites of involvement. Sponging all contaminated or itchy areas meticulously and systematically with equal parts of ether and acetone at the outset will often remove the oleoresin and ameliorate any worsening of the dermatitis, which can be treated as outlined on p. 102.

Ginkgo tree dermatitis simulates toxicodendron dermatitis with its severe vesiculation, erythematous papules, and edema. The causative substances are ginkgolic acids from the fruit pulp of the ginkgo tree. Ingestion of the gingko fruit may result in perianal dermatitis. Ginkgo biloba given orally for cerebral disturbances is made from a leaf extract so it will not elicit a systemic contact allergy when ingested.

DERMATITIS RESULTING FROM FLOWERS AND HOUSEPLANTS. Among the more common houseplants, the velvety-leafed philodendron, *Philodendron crystallinum* (and its several variants), known in India as the money plant, is a frequent cause of contact dermatitis. The eruption is often seen on the face, especially the eyelids, carried there by hands that have watered or cared for the plant. English ivy follows philodendron in frequency of cases of occult contact

dermatitis. Primrose dermatitis affects the fingers, eyelids, and neck with a punctate or diffuse erythema and edema. It was formerly most frequently encountered in Europe; however, it is now a common houseplant in the United States. Primin, a quinone, is the causative oleoresin abounding in the glandular hairs of the plant *Primula obconica.*

Among the many flowers, the chrysanthemum causes dermatitis most frequently. The eyelids are frequently involved. Florists are most commonly affected. The alpha-methylene portion of the sesquiterpene lactone molecule is the antigenic site, as it is in the other genera of the *Compositae* family. A severe inflammatory reaction with bulla formation may be caused by the prairie crocus (*Anemone patens L.*), the floral emblem of the province of Manitoba. Several species of ornamental "bottle brush" from Queensland, *Grevillea banksii, G. Robyn Gordon,* and *G. robusta,* may cause allergic contact dermatitis. It is being exported to the United States and other Western countries. Menz et al have shown the allergen to be long-chain alkyl resorcinols. A cross sensitivity to toxicodendron has been demonstrated to occur.

Parthenium hysterophorus, a photosensitizing weed, was accidentally introduced into India in 1956 and has spread over most of the country; it is also spreading in Australia, China, and Argentina. The well-deserved reputation of dieffenbachia, a common, glossy-leafed house plant, has for harmfulness rests on the high content of calcium oxalate crystals in its sap, which burn the mouth and throat severely if any part of the plant is chewed or swallowed. Severe edema of the oral tissues may result in complete loss of voice; hence its common nickname, "dumb cane." It does not appear to sensitize.

Florists handling the popular Peruvian lily were reported by Marks to have become sensitized to tuliposide A, the allergen in this plant. It penetrated through vinyl gloves but not through nitrile gloves. In a study of occupational dermatitis among floral shop workers, Thiboutot et al documented that sensitization to this allergen is common. They found that 15 of 57 surveyed workers reported hand dermatitis within the previous 12 months among those who had handled this plant. The castor bean, the seed of *Ricinus communis,* contains ricin, a poisonous substance (phytotoxin). Its sap contains an antigen that may cause anaphylactic hypersensitivity and also dermatitis.

Contact dermatitis may be caused by handling many other flowers, such as the geranium, scorpion flower (*Phacelia crenulata* or *campanularia*), creosote bush (*Larvia tridentata*), Heracula, daffodil, foxglove, lilac, lady slipper, magnolia, and tulip and narcissus bulbs. Fisher noted that poinsettia and oleander almost never cause dermatitis, despite their reputation for it. although they are toxic if ingested. Treatment of all these plant dermatitides is the same as that recommended for toxicodendron dermatitis.

DERMATITIS RESULTING FROM VEGETABLES. Many vegetables may cause contact dermatitis, including asparagus, carrot, celery, cow-parsnip, cucumber, garlic, Indian bean, mushroom, onion, parsley, tomato, and turnip. Onion and celery, among other vegetables, have been incriminated in the production of contact urticaria and even anaphylaxis. Several plants, including celery, fig, lime, and parsley, can cause a phototoxic dermatitis because of the presence of psoralens.

DERMATITIS RESULTING FROM TREES. Some of the trees whose timber and sawdust may produce contact dermatitis are ash, birch, cedar, cocobolo, elm, Kentucky coffee tree, koa, mahogany, mango, maple, mesquite, milo, myrtle, pine, and teak. The latex of the fig and rubber trees may also cause dermatitis, usually of phototoxic type. Melaleuca oil (tea tree oil), which may be applied to the skin to treat a variety of maladies, can cause allergic contact dermatitis, primarily through the allergen d-limonene.

DERMATITIS RESULTING FROM TREE-ASSOCIATED PLANTS. Foresters and lumber workers can be exposed to allergenic plants other than trees. Lichens are a group of plants composed of symbiotic algae and fungi. Foresters and wood choppers exposed to these lichens growing on trees may develop severe allergic contact dermatitis. Exposure to the lichens may also occur from firewood, funeral wreaths, and also as masculine fragrances added to aftershave lotions (oak moss and tree moss). Hypersensitization is produced by the d-usnic acid and other lichen acids contained in lichens. The leafy liverwort (*Frulliana nisquallansis*), a forest epiphyte growing on tree trunks, has produced allergic dermatitis in forest workers. The eruption is commonly called *cedar poisoning*. It resembles toxicodendron dermatitis; its attacks are more severe during wet weather. The allergen is sesquiterpene lactone.

DERMATITIS RESULTING FROM POLLENS AND SEEDS. The pollens in ragweed are composed of two antigens. The protein fraction causes the respiratory symptoms of asthma and hay fever and the oil-soluble portion causes contact dermatitis. Ragweed oil dermatitis is a seasonal disturbance seen mainly during the ragweed growing season from spring to fall. Contact with the plant or with wind-blown fragments of dried plants produces the typical dermatitis. The oil causes swelling and redness of the lids and entire face and a red blotchy eruption on the forearms that, after several attacks, may become generalized, with lichenification; it closely resembles chronic atopic dermatitis, with lichenification of the face, neck, and major flexures, and severe pruritus. The distribution mimics that of photodermatitis, the differentiating point being that in ragweed dermatitis there is involvement of the upper eyelids and the retroauricular and submental areas. Chronic cases may continue into the winter; however, signs and symptoms are most severe at the height of the season. Sesquiterpene lactones are the cause. Coexistent sensitization to pyrethrum may account for prolongation of ragweed dermatitis. Men outnumber

women in hypersensitivity reactions; farmers outnumber patients of all other occupations.

Hypersensitivity reactions to sesame seeds have been noted. Generalized erythema, oral pruritus, wheezing, and shock may be induced. Sesame oil, containing the allergens sesamine and sesamolin, may cause contact urticaria when used on stasis dermatitis.

DERMATITIS RESULTING FROM MARINE PLANTS. Numerous aquatic plants are toxic or produce contact dermatitis. Algae seem to be the worse offenders. Fresh-water plants are rarely of concern. Seaweed dermatitis is a type of swimmer's eruption produced by contact with a marine blue-green alga, which has been identified as *Lyngbya majuscula Gomont*. The onset is within a few minutes after leaving the ocean, with severe itching and burning, followed by dermatitis, blisters, and deep and painful desquamation that affects the areas covered by the bathing suit (in men, especially the scrotum, perineum, and perianal areas; occasionally, in women, the breasts). Patch tests with the alga are neither necessary nor helpful, since it is a potent irritant. The dermatitis may be prevented by bathing in fresh water within 10 or 15 minutes after leaving the ocean. The Bermuda fire sponge may produce contact erythema multiforme. Trawler fishermen in the Dogger Bank area of the North Sea develop allergic dermatitis after contact with *Alcyonidium hirsutism*. This is a seaweedlike animal colony that becomes caught in the fishermen's net and produces erythema, edema, and lichenification on the hands and the wrists.

PLANT-ASSOCIATED DERMATITIS. The role of sunlight-producing photosensitivity contact dermatitis has been discussed. The furocoumarins (psoralens) in certain plants will produce a phototoxic reaction in individuals who have the plant substance on their skin who are exposed to sunlight. The UVA spectrum of light is responsible for producing the phototoxic eruption. This is known as *phytophotodermatitis*. Some of the furocoumarin-containing plants that can produce phytophotodermatitis are celery, dill, fig, lime (Fig. 6-5), lime bergamot, parsley, parsnip, meadow grass, mokihana (*Pelea anisata*) berries, mustard, and St. John's wort. Plants of the *Umbelliferae* family are the most frequent cause of this eruption. Meadow grass (*Agrimonia eupatoria*) produces dermatitis bullosa striata pratensis. It occurs on the hands and legs as irregularly shaped bullae, which heal with pigmented streaks.

The residua of various insecticides on plants may also produce dermatitis. This is especially true of arsenic- and malathion-containing sprays. Randox (2-chloro-N,N-diallyl-acetamide) has been reported as the cause of hemorrhagic bullae on the feet of farmers. Lawn care companies spray herbicides and fungicides throughout the spring, summer, and fall. Dryene, thiuram, carbamates, and chlorothalonil are the potential sensitizers in theses workers, whose clothing frequently becomes wetted while spraying.

Barbs, bristles, spines, thorns, spicules, and cactus

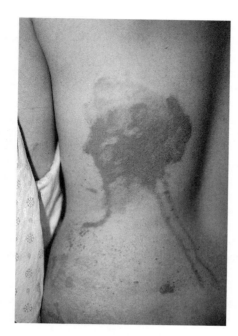

Fig. 6-5 Phytophotodermatitis resulting from lime juice applied to insect bites.

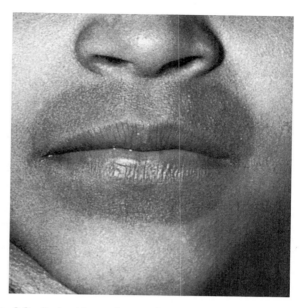

Fig. 6-6 Perioral hyperpigmentation following dermatitis caused by cinnamon in bubble gum.

needles are some of the mechanical accessories of plants that may produce dermatitis. Sabra dermatitis is an occupational dermatitis resembling scabies. It is seen among pickers of the prickly pear cactus plant. It also occurs in persons handling Indian figs in Israel, where the condition is seen from July to November. It is caused by the penetration of minute, invisible thorns into the skin.

DERMATITIS RESULTING FROM PLANT DERIVATIVES. The sensitizing substances derived from plants are found in the oleoresin fractions that contain camphors, essential oils, phenols, resins, and terpenes. The chief sensitizers are the essential oils. They may be localized in certain parts of the plant, such as in the peel of citrus fruits, the leaves of the eucalyptus tree, and the bark of the cinnamon tree. Aromatherapy, an increasingly popular treatment for relief of stress, involves either inhaling or massaging essential oils; this may cause allergic contact dermatitis in therapists or clients.

Cinnamon oil (cassia oil) is a common flavoring agent, especially in pastries. Hand dermatitis in pastry bakers is often caused by cinnamon. It is also used as a flavor for lipstick, bitters, alcoholic and nonalcoholic beverages, toothpaste, and chewing gum. Perioral dermatitis may be caused from cinnamon in chewing gum (Fig. 6-6). A 5% cinnamon solution in olive oil is used for patch testing. Eugenol, clove oil, and eucalyptus oil are used by dentists, who may acquire contact dermatitis from them. Anise, peppermint, and spearmint oils may cause sensitization.

van den Akker et al screened l03 patients for spice allergy and found 10 with allergy, most often to nutmeg, paprika, and cloves. Fragrance-mix was a useful indicator allergen. Lemon oil from lemon peel or lemon wood may cause sensitization in the various handlers of these substances. Citric acid may cause dermatitis in bakers. Lime oil in lime-scented shaving cream or lotion may cause photoallergy. Balsam of Peru contains numerous substances, among which are essential oils similar to the oil of the lemon peel. Balsam of Peru is known to cross-react with vanilla and cinnamon, among many others. Vanillin is derived from the vanilla plant and frequently produces contact dermatitis, vanillism, in those connected with its production and use.

Turpentine frequently acts as an irritant and as an allergic sensitizer (carene). It is contained in paints, paint thinners, varnishes, and waxes.

TESTING FOR PLANT ALLERGIES. The method of testing for plant hypersensitivity is the application of the crushed plant leaf, stem, and petal as a covered patch test. A test should also be performed on several controls to make sure that the leaf is not an irritant. It must be remembered that some of the plants are photosensitizers. Test sites for these must be done in duplicate, with one set kept covered and the other exposed to artificial light or sunlight for the detection of photosensitivity.

Dooms-Goosens A, et al: Airborne contact dermatitis. *Contact Dermatitis* 1991, 25:211.

Fisher AA: Erythema multiforme-like eruptions due to exotic woods and ordinary plants. *Cutis* 1986, 37:101, 158, 262.

Gette MT, et al: Tulip fingers. *Arch Dermatol* 1990, 126:203.

Guin J: Recognizing the toxicodendrons. *J Am Acad Dermatol* 1981, 4:95.

Guin J et al: Compositiae dermatitis in childhood. *Arch Dermatol* 1987, 123:50.

Hamilton TK, et al: Systemic contact dermatitis to raw cashew nuts in a pesto sauce. *Am J Contact Dermat* 1998, 9:51.

Hausen BM: The sensitizing capacity of gingkolic acids in guinea pigs. *Am J Contact Dermat* 1998, 9:146.

Knight TE, et al: Melaleuca oil (tea tree oil) dermatitis. *J Am Acad Dermatol* 1994, 30:423.

Lovell CR: Current topics in plant dermatitis. *Semin Dermatol* 1996, 15:113.

Mallory SB, et al: Toxicodendron radicans dermatitis with black lacquer deposit on the skin. *J Am Acad Dermatol* 1983, 6:363.

Marks JG Jr: Allergic contact dermatitis to *Alstroemeria*. *Arch Dermatol* 1988, 124:914.

Marks JG Jr, et al: Dermatitis from cashew nuts. *J Am Acad Dermatol* 1984, 10:627.

Marks JG Jr, et al: Prevention of poison ivy and poison ask allergic contact dermatitis by quaternium-18 bentonite. *J Am Acad Dermatol* 1995, 33:212.

Mathias CGT: Allergic contact dermatitis from a lawn care fungicide containing Dryene. *Am J Contact Derm* 1997, 8:47.

Menz J, et al: Contact dermatitis from *Greviella Robyn Gordon*. *Contact Dermatitis* 1986, 15:126.

McGovern TW: Alstroemeria L. (Peruvian lily). *Am J Contact Dermat* 1999, 10:172.

Pauli G, et al: Celery allergy. *Ann Allergy* 1988, 60:243.

Reginella AF, et al: Hyposensitization to poison ivy after working in a cashew nutshell oil processing factory. *Contact Dermatitis* 1989, 20:274.

Sheard C: Poison oak/ivy desensitization by chewing raw cashew nuts. *Schoch Letter* May 1987, Item 5.

Stoner JG: Plant dermatitis. *J Am Acad Dermatol* 1983, 9:1.

Thiboutot DM, et al: Dermatoses among flower shop workers. *J Am Acad Dermatol* 1990, 22:54.

van den Akker TW, et al: Contact allergy to spices. *Contact Dermatitis* 1990, 22:267.

Weiss RR, et al: Allergic contact dermatitis from aromatherapy. *Am J Contact Dermat* 1997, 8:250.

Williams JV, et al: Individual variations in allergic contact dermatitis from urushiol. *Arch Dermatol* 1999, 135:1002. _____ ▲

Dermatitis Resulting from Clothing.

A predisposition to contact dermatitis from clothing occurs in persons who perspire freely or who are obese and wear clothing that tends to be tight. Depending on the offending substance, various regions of the body will be affected. Regional location is helpful in identifying the sensitizing substance. The axillary folds are commonly involved; the vaults of the axillae are usually spared. Sites of increased perspiration and sites where evaporation is impeded, such as the intertriginous areas, will tend to leach dyes from fabrics to produce dermatitis. Secondary changes of lichenification and infection occur frequently because of the chronicity of exposure.

Cotton, wool, linen, and silk fabrics were used exclusively before the advent of synthetic fabrics. Most materials are now blended in definite proportions with synthetics to produce superior lasting and aesthetic properties. Dermatitis from cotton is virtually nonexistent. Only the sizing used in cotton to stiffen or glaze the material may sensitize the skin to produce dermatitis. In most instances there is no true sensitization to wool. Wool acts as an irritant because of the barbs on its fibers. These barbs may produce severe pruritus at points of contact with the skin, especially in the intertriginous areas. In sensitive-skinned persons such as those with atopic dermatitis, the use of wool is not advisable because of its mechanical irritative properties. When a positive result is elicited to a wool patch test, it is usually caused by dye or other chemicals rather than the wool itself. Silk is a sensitizer, but rarely; the nature of the allergen is not known.

Numerous types of synthetic fibers are available for clothing and accessory manufacture, all of which again are remarkably free of sensitizing properties. Only the dyes and finishes of these fabrics cause dermatitis. Some of the synthetic fibers are acetates, such as rayon; acrylics such as Orlon and Acrilan; modacrylics such as Dynel, nylon; metallic yarns, olefin, and polyesters such as Dacron, Fortrel, Kodel, Mylar, and Vycron.

Polyvinyl resins are the plastics used in such wearing apparel as raincoats, rainhoods, wristbands, suspenders, plastic mittens, and gloves. These again are only infrequently found to be causes of contact dermatitis. Workers who clean the vats used in producing polyvinyl chloride from vinyl chloride may develop acrosteolysis (bone destruction of the hands and forearms), preceded by Raynaud's phenomenon and thickening and tightening of the hands.

Spandex is a nonrubber (but elastic) polyurethane fiber. It is widely used for garments such as girdles, brassieres, and socks. Dermatitis from Spandex has been reported with brassieres. It was found that Spandex containing mercaptobenzothiazole produced the contact dermatitis. Spandex manufactured in the United States does not contain this and therefore does not produce allergic contact dermatitis.

Aniline and azo dyes are used in textile dyeing. When properly manufactured and used for this purpose, they produce little contact dermatitis; however, cross-sensitization may occur in persons sensitive to paraphenylenediamine or other members of the "para" group, such as paraaminobenzoic acid, benzocaine, procaine, and sulfonamides. Paraphenylenediamine is used in wearing apparel only in fur pieces. However, it is tolerated by patients who are allergic to this chemical, because it is in the fully oxidized form.

Clothing dye dermatitis usually occurs when the patient is subject to hyperhidrosis, which "bleeds" dye from fabrics. However, this bleeding process is extremely rare in today's fabrics because of the superior methods of fixing the dyes. It is usually the various other chemicals used in conjunction with the dyes that cause sensitization. In patch testing for dye sensitivity the test fabric is soaked in 1 ml of water with a drop or two of vinegar for 24 hours; the solute is then applied as a patch test for 48 hours. In testing for axillary dermatitis, the suspected fabric is soaked in 250 ml of water to which a drop of 20% sodium hydroxide has been added and then this is applied to the skin for 48 hours.

Fabric finishes are used to improve the durability, appearance, and feel of a material. Antiwrinkling and crease-holding chemicals are mostly resins, which are incorporated into the fibers as they are being manufactured or applied to the completed (finished) fabric. These resins are cured or polymerized.

Not only are free formaldehyde and formaldehyde resins used extensively in the preparation of fabrics, but they are used in the manufacture of toilet paper, facial tissues, and various other papers to increase their tensile strength. Fabrics are treated with the formaldehydes to make them less vulnerable to the effects of perspiration and of ironing. Clothing may be treated with these substances to make them wrinkle-free and to make them dry rapidly after washing. They are used to make clothing fabrics shrink-resistant and water-repellent as well as stain-repellent. When all these uses are taken into consideration, the low incidence of dermatitis from these formaldehyde-treated materials is remarkable. Improved finishing agents are available that release very little formaldehyde.

The mere presence of free formaldehyde in clothing does not establish the diagnosis of contact dermatitis caused by formaldehyde. A 1% formaldehyde patch test and a positive patch test with the suspected material must also be demonstrated. Also, wearing of the fabric must induce contact dermatitis.

The formaldehyde resins melamine formaldehyde and urea formaldehyde are the most commonly used fabric finishes. Patients suspected of formaldehyde resin hypersensitivity should be tested with 1% formaldehyde in water, 10% urea formaldehyde in petrolatum, 7% melamine formaldehyde in petrolatum, 10% ethylene urea melamine formaldehyde resin in petrolatum, and the material itself. Fowler et al reported 17 patients with formaldehyde resin dermatitis. Several patients had generalized dermatitis with a chronic recalcitrant course. Early in the course of disease the morphology may be erythematous papules. They found ethylene urea melamine formaldehyde resin to be the best screening agent. Many also reacted to the formaldehyde releasing preservatives such as quaternium-15.

Crease-resistant, drip-dry trousers may produce this type of dermatitis. The inner thighs and popliteal spaces are especially involved. Patch testing is done with 1% formaldehyde solution (formalin is a 10% solution). Higher concentrations may cause irritant reactions. Medical personnel may be so sensitive to formaldehyde that even a 0.1% formaldehyde solution patch test will produce a positive reaction.

Treatment is the same as for other types of contact dermatitis—the avoidance of exposure of the skin to formaldehyde resin and free formaldehyde. This is, however, most difficult. New clothes should be thoroughly washed before wearing the first time. Jeans, Spandex, silk, 100% linen, 100% nylon, and 100% cotton that is not wrinkle resistant or colorfast are best tolerated. Tee shirts, sweat shirts, sweat pants, white underclothes suitable for bleaching, and any type of mixed synthetic fibers with cotton fibers that are added to make them drip-dry are most likely to cause problems in these patients.

Arisu K, et al: Tinuvin P in a spandex tape as a cause of clothing dermatitis. *Contact Dermatitis* 1992, 26:311.

Fowler JF Jr, et al: Allergic contact dermatitis from formaldehyde resins in permanent press clothing. *J Am Acad Dermatol* 1992, 27:962.

Guin JD, et al: Clothing dye dermatitis masquerading as mimosa allergy. *Contact Dermatitis* 1999, 40:45.

Hatch K, et al: Textile dye dermatitis. *J Am Acad Dermatol* 1995, 32:631.

Shoe Dermatitis. Footwear dermatitis may begin on the dorsal surfaces of the toes and may remain localized to that area indefinitely. There are erythema and lichenification and, in severe cases, weeping and crusting. Secondary infection is frequent. In severe cases an id reaction may be produced on the hands similar to the reaction from fungus infection of the feet. A diagnostic point is the normal appearance of the skin between the toes, which has no contact with the offending substance. In fungus infections the toe webs are usually involved. Another pattern seen commonly today is involvement of the sole with sparing of the instep and flexural creases of the toes.

Shoe dermatitis is most frequently caused by the rubber accelerators mercaptobenzothiazole and tetramethylthiuram disulfide; by the adhesives used; and by the dichromates in leather. Other causative agents are felt, cork liners, formaldehyde, dyes, asphalt, and tar. Patch testing to determine the offending substance may be helpful so that an individual can purchase footwear that has been made without the sensitizing substances.

Chromate sensitivity is caused by the chrome tanning process most frequently used for tanning leather to make it more resistant to the stresses to which leather is subject (Fig. 6-7). The prevalence of chrome allergy is decreasing in North America, probably as a result of better fixation of chrome to leather. Chromate sensitivity is commonly seen in those with hyperhidrosis of the feet. Tannin is derived from various trees around the world. Vegetable-tanned leather is an acceptable substitute for chromate-sensitive individuals; however, it is not often used in this country because of the time-consuming nature of the process. Aldehydes are used for tanning of white leather. Sensitivity to white shoe leather may be caused by formaldehyde.

Patients with shoe dye sensitivity should avoid redyed shoes because of the usually inadequate binding of the dye with the leather. Artificial leather, synthetic leather, and Corfam materials are excellent substitutes; however, the linings of such shoes may be chrome-tanned and may contain dyes and formaldehyde, which can continue to cause hypersensitivity.

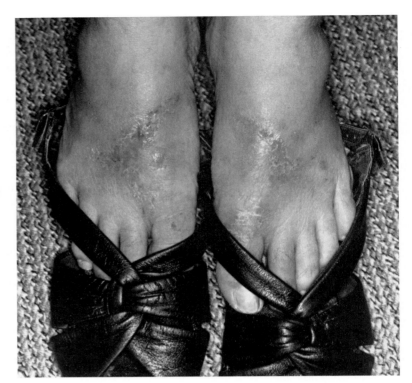

Fig. 6-7 Sandal dermatitis produced by chrome tanning process of leather.

Freeman S: Shoe dermatitis. *Contact Dermatitis* 1997, 36:247.

Gledof B, et al: Clinical aspects of para-tertiary butylphinol-formaldehyde resin allergy. *Contact Dermatitis* 1989, 21:312.

Srinivas C, et al: Footwear dermatitis due to Bisphenol-A. *Contact Dermatitis* 1989, 20:1989.

Trevisan G, et al: Allergic contact dermatitis due to shoes in children. *Contact Dermatitis* 1992, 26:45. _____ ▲

Dermatitis Resulting from Metals and Metal Salts. Metal dermatitis is most frequently caused by nickel, chromates, and mercury. Usually, with the exception of nickel, the pure metals do not cause hypersensitivity; it is only when they are incorporated into salts that they cause reactions. Patch test reactivity to an aqueous solution of the metallic salt does not usually indicate sensitivity to the pure metal. Most objects containing metal or metal salts are combinations of several metals, some of which may have been used to plate the surface, thereby enhancing its attractiveness, durability, or tensile strength. For this reason suspicion of a metal-caused dermatitis should be investigated by doing patch tests on several of the metal salts.

Patients have been reported who developed a wide variety of dermatoses, most often eczematous in type, after placement of an orthopedic implant. Positive diagnosis requires at a minimum the appearance of a chronic dermatitis after placement of the implant, no other cause, corrosion of the implant, healing after removal, and a positive patch test result for the metal.

BLACK DERMATOGRAPHISM. Black or greenish staining under rings, metal wristbands, bracelets, and clasps is caused by the abrasive effect of cosmetics or other powders containing zinc or titanium oxide on the gold jewelry. This skin discoloration is always black because of the deposit of metal particles on skin that has been powdered and that has metal, such as gold, silver, or platinum, rubbing on it. Abrasion of the metal results from the fact that some powders are hard (zinc oxide) and are capable of abrading the metal.

NICKEL DERMATITIS. Because we are all constantly exposed to nickel, nickel dermatitis is a frequent occurrence, especially among women. Nickel produces more cases of allergic contact dermatitis than all other metals combined. Erythematous and eczematous eruptions, sometimes with lichenification, appear beneath earrings, bracelets, hairpins, rings, wristwatches, clasps, eyelash curlers, metallic spectacle frames, brassiere cups, and blue-jeans buttons (Fig. 6-8). Dermatitis stemming from coins containing nickel has always been rare (Fig. 6-9); more common is dermatitis from handles of doors, handbags, and faucets. Nickel dermatitis is seen most frequently on women's earlobes (Fig. 6-10). Piercing the ears with nickel-plated instruments or wearing nickel-plated jewelry readily induces nickel sensitivity. Ears should be pierced only with stainless steel instruments, and only stainless steel earrings should be worn until the ears have healed. Exposure to the metal may not be readily apparent most of the time. Even in gold jewelry the clasps and the solder may contain nickel. The nickel object may be plated with chrome and yet cause nickel dermatitis through the leaching out of some of the nickel through the small pores of the chromium plating.

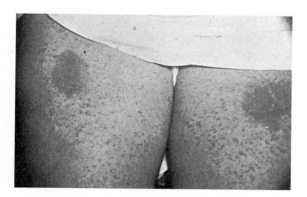

Fig. 6-8 Allergic contact dermatitis from nickel in garters.

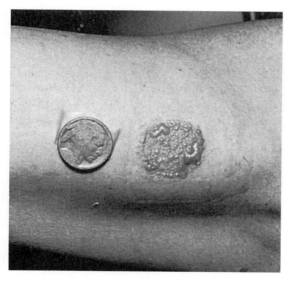

Fig. 6-9 "Money dermatitis." Nickel dermatitis: 3-plus reaction to the application of an Indian head nickel.

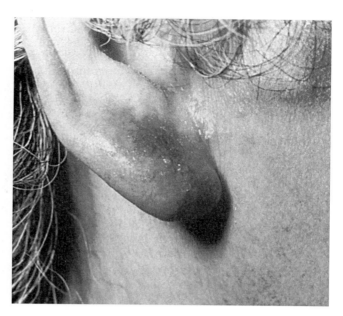

Fig. 6-10 Dermatitis of earlobe caused by nickel-containing earrings. (Courtesy Dr. John R.T. Reeves.)

Nickel oxides occurring in green paints may also produce nickel dermatitis. Sweat containing sodium chloride may combine with nickel to form nickel chloride. This affects the degree of nickel dermatitis, it being more severe in persons who perspire profusely. Prevention of sweating may help to prevent the areas exposed to nickel from developing dermatitis or may at least attenuate the condition.

The diagnosis is established by a positive reaction to a 2.5% nickel sulfate solution patch test. Nickel may be detected by applying a freshly prepared 1% alcohol solution of dimethylglyoxime and a 10% aqueous solution of ammonia separately in equal amounts to the test object. In the presence of nickel, the object will turn orange-pink. A positive test result always means that nickel is present, but a negative test result does not rule out its presence. Sweat, blood, or saline may leach nickel from stainless steel.

Prophylactic measures should include the reduction of perspiration in those sensitive to nickel. Topical corticosteroids applied before exposure to nickel, such as before putting on a brassiere or wristband, has been suggested. Clasps and other objects are available in plastic material so that some of the exposure to nickel may be decreased. Polyurethane varathane 91 (Flecto) applied in three coats will give protection for several months. Treatment of nickel dermatitis consists of the application of topical corticosteroid creams, sprays, or lotions.

Hand eczema in nickel-sensitive patients that has been aggravated by orally ingested nickel in the diet is controversial; however, reports continue to surface, such as the report by Veien et al. He gives a specific low-nickel diet that may be tried in treatment-resistant cases of hand dermatitis.

CHROMIUM DERMATITIS. The chromates are strongly corrosive and irritating to the skin; they may act as primary irritants or as sensitizers to produce allergic contact dermatitis. Aside from occurrence among employees in chromate works, chrome dermatitis is encountered among tanners, painters, dyers, photographers, polishers, welders, aircraft workers, diesel engine workers, and those concerned with the bleaching of crude oils, tallows, and fats. Traces of dichromates in shoe leather and gloves may cause eczema of the feet and hands. Many zippers are chromium-plated, and the nickel underneath the plate may be the causative agent. Chromium metal and stainless steel do not produce contact dermatitis.

Zinc chromate paint is a common source of dermatitis. Matches, hide glues, chrome alloys, cigarette lighters, leather hatbands, and leather sandals or camera cases may cause chrome dermatitis. Anticorrosion solutions used for refrigeration and other recirculation systems often contain chromates that produce dermatitis. Most of those in the cement industry suffering from cement eczema show patch tests positive to dichromates. Cement eczema is often a primary irritant dermatitis complicated by allergic contact dermatitis to the hexavalent chromates. Nickel, arsenic, and cobalt are also in cement.

The skin changes are multiform, ranging from a mild follicular dermatitis to widespread nodular and crusted eruptions, all being worse on exposed parts. Often they are slow to clear up, lasting from a few weeks to 6 months after contact has ceased. Heavy exposure of industrial workers to chromates may produce chrome ulcers (chrome holes) on the backs of the hands and forearms, usually beginning around a hair follicle or in the creases of the knuckles, or in the finger webs. The hole begins as a small abrasion that deepens and widens as its edges grow thick, eventually forming a conical indolent ulceration. Chrome ulcers may also arise on—and perforate—the nasal septum.

Diagnosis of chrome sensitivity is made by a positive patch test to 0.25% potassium dichromate in petrolatum. The hexavalent chrome compounds are the most frequent cause of chrome dermatitis since they penetrate the skin more easily than the trivalent form. Both forms are sensitizers. The chromate-sensitive person should avoid zinc chromate paints, chrome-tanned leather, glue, cement and other chromate-containing objects. Even with avoidance, chromate-induced dermatitis often is persistent.

MERCURY DERMATITIS. The mercurials may not only act as irritants but also as sensitizers. Dermatitis may be caused by the local application of calomel (mercurous chloride) or other mercurial remedies (mercurochrome and ammoniated mercury), or by their internal use. Mercuric chloride, even in weak solutions (1:1000), is irritating, causing dermatitis chiefly among surgeons, nurses, taxidermists, and those using insecticides; 1:2000 is not irritating. Phenylmercuric salts are used as weed killers and as agricultural fungicides and insecticides. Phenylmercuric salts have wide usage in industrial materials (gelatin waving solutions, glue, sizing, starch pastes, bentonite gels, mildew-proofing). Sensitization dermatitis may appear at the site of exposure to the phenylmercuric salts, on the legs after exposure to weed killers, and also on the hands.

Nitrate of mercury produces irritation. The eruptions are encountered among felt-hat workers and those who do etching, embossing, or art metalwork. The manufacturing of thermometers and barometers, the handling of furs, the use of amalgams by dentists, fire gilding, and solder used for dry batteries are all common sources of contamination with mercury, causing various eczematous eruptions. Among the organic mercurial compounds, Merthiolate may be implicated in sensitization reactions. Skin previously sensitized to mercury may react severely when the sensitized person receives a mercurial compound systemically.

COBALT DERMATITIS. Cobalt is frequently combined with nickel as a contaminant. They have similar properties but do not produce cross reactions. Cobalt dermatitis may occur in those involved in the manufacture of polyester resins and paints, in the manufacture of hard metal used for cutting and drilling tools, and in the manufacture and use of cement. Cobalt dermatitis may also occur in producers of pottery, ceramics, metal alloys, glass, carbides, and pigments. One may be exposed to cobalt in hair dye, flypaper, and vitamin B_{12}. Blue tattoo pigment contains cobalt oxide. Rarely, cobalt chloride may cause nonimmunologic local release of vasoreactive materials, with a local urticarial response.

ARSENICAL DERMATITIS. Arsenic is one of the most common chemical causes of dermatitis in those who mine copper and arsenical ores, and in those coming into contact with the artificial dyes used in wallpaper, flowers, and chalk. Arsenical compounds are used in dyeing fabrics and domestic articles, for the preservation of animal skins and hides, and for embalming. Arsenic is an ingredient of some disinfectants and weed exterminators. It is encountered in the manufacture of insecticides, in chemical factories for the manufacture of sulfuric and other acids, in printing establishments where gilt or bronze powder is used, and in farming and gardening. Among those who may incur this disease in the course of their occupation are glucose and candy factory workers, those who use sizing and dextrin, bookbinders, fruit handlers, furriers who handle raw furs, machinists, and metal workers who handle brass, copper, and zinc.

The dermatitis caused by the arsenicals is frequently a folliculitis with secondary pyoderma. Furunculosis is also common. Ulcerations on the extremities and nasal perforation similar to chrome ulcers may occur.

DERMATITIS RESULTING FROM OTHER METALS. Most of the other commonly used metals are not important in causing contact dermatitis. Gold dermatitis may rarely occur from the wearing of gold jewelry. A predisposing factor in such patients is the presence of dental gold. It is the gold salts that are allergenic. It is not infrequent to see positive reactions to gold when patch testing patients with facial or widespread dermatitis of unknown cause. Although it is difficult to make a direct clinical correlation with any one offending piece of jewelry, some patients will clear if they stop wearing all gold jewelry.

A number of cases of dermatitis resulting from gold jewelry, especially gold rings, contaminated with radon and its decay products, have been reported. This may eventuate in radiation dermatitis and squamous cell carcinoma of the finger. Evidently the source of the contaminated gold for the rings had been reclaimed decayed radon gold seeds.

Platinum dermatitis may occur from exposure to platinum salts and sprays in industry. Platinum rings, earrings, white gold spectacles, clasps, and other jewelry cause eruptions resembling those caused by nickel. Zinc, aluminum, copper sulfate, titanium, and antimony dermatitis rarely occur; they may, however, act as irritants.

Bohm I, et al: Comparison of personal history with patch test results in metal allergy. *J Dermatol* 1997, 24:510.

Bruze M, et al: Clinical relevance of contact allergy to gold sodium thiosulfate. *J Am Acad Dermatol* 1994, 31:579.

Burrows D: The dichromatic problem. *Intern J Dermatol* 1984, 23:215.

Christiansen OB: Nickel dermatitis. *Dermatol Clin* 1990, 8:37.

Emmett EA, et al: Allergic contact dermatitis to nickel. *J Am Acad Dermatol* 1988, 19:314.

Fowler JF: Allergic contact dermatitis to metals. *Am J Contact Dermat* 1990, 1:212.

Ho VC, et al: Nickel dermatitis in infants. *Contact Dermatitis* 1986, 15:270.

Kumer P, et al: Metal hypersensitivity in total joint replacement. *Orthopedics* 1983, 6:1455.

Marks JG, et al: North American Contact Dermatitis Group patch test results for the detection of delayed-type hypersensitivity to topical allergens. *J Am Acad Dermatol* 1998, 36:911.

Nethercott JR, et al: Cutaneous nickel sensitivity in Toronto, Canada. *J Am Acad Dermatol* 1990, 22:756.

Nielsen GD, et al: Nickel-sensitive patients with vesicular hand eczema. *Br J Dermatol* 1990, 122:299.

Olsavsky R, et al: Contact sensitivity to chromate. *Contact Dermatitis* 1998, 38:329.

Rostoker G, et al: Dermatitis due to orthopaedic implants. *J Bone Joint Surg* (Am) 1987, 69:1408.

Santosh V, et al: Results of patch testing with dental materials. *Contact Dermatitis* 1999, 40:50.

Shah M, et al: Nickel as an occupational allergen. *Arch Dermatol* 1998, 134:1231.

Stutzman CD, et al: Squamous cell carcinoma from wearing radioactive gold rings. *J Am Acad Dermatol* 1984, 10:1075.

Veien NK, et al: Aluminum allergy. *Contact Dermatitis* 1986, 15:295.

Veien NK, et al: Low nickel diet. *J Am Acad Dermatol* 1993, 29:1002.

Williams SP: Nickel dermatitis from coins. *Contact Dermatitis* 1999, 40:60. ————————————————————————— ▲

Contact Stomatitis.

Contact stomatitis may be seen in cases of sensitivity to metals used in dental fillings and prostheses and to topical therapeutic drugs. Some of these metals known to produce stomatitis include mercury, bismuth, chromium, nickel, gold, copper, and zinc. Mountcastle et al reported a patient who developed allergy to dental impression material. Chewing gums and dentifrices may also produce contact stomatitis. Ingredients thought to be responsible for this are hexylresorcinol, thymol, dichlorophen, oil of cinnamon, and mint.

Dutree-Meulenberg et al investigated the role of contact hypersensitivity in the burning mouth syndrome and found six who were patch-test positive to dental metals and six positive to components used in the production of acrylate-based dentures. Helton et al and Shah et al, however, did not find contact allergy to be a cause for burning symptoms. Shah et al's study was part of a larger investigation of the role of contact allergy in oral symptomatology. They found 30% of their population to have relevant allergens; these were most commonly metals, food additives (flavorings and antioxidants), and dental products.

Clinical signs may be bright erythema of the tongue and buccal mucosa with scattered erosions. Angular cheilitis may also develop. Oral lichenoid lesions may be caused by sensitization to mercury in amalgam fillings. Usually these lesions are adjacent to the dental restoration, and patients are patch-test positive to mercury.

Dutree-Meulenberg ROGM, et al: Burning mouth syndrome. *J Am Acad Dermatol* 1992, 26:935.

Helton J, et al: The burning mouth syndrome. *J Am Acad Dermatol* 1994, 31:201.

Koch P, et al: Oral lesions and symptoms related to metals used in dental restorations. *J Am Acad Dermatol* 1999, 41:422.

Mountcastle EA, et al: Mucosal allergy to dental impression material. *J Am Acad Dermatol* 1986, 15:1055.

Shah M, et al: Contact allergy in patients with oral symptoms. *Am J Contact Dermat* 1996, 7:146.

Tosti A, et al: Contact and irritant stomatitis. *Semin Cutan Med Surg* 1997, 16:314. ————————————————————————— ▲

Rubber Dermatitis.

Rubber dermatitis generally occurs on the hands from wearing rubber gloves (surgeons, nurses, homemakers). The eruption is usually sharply limited to the gloved area but may spread up the forearms. Rubber dermatitis also develops in the axilla from the use of rubber dress shields. Rubber girdles and panties cause pruritus and dermatitis of the areas covered by the girdle, especially the groins and sides of the hips. Antiwrinkle bands may cause dermatitis of the submental region or forehead. Worn cloth coverings, allowing the rubber within to protrude and touch the skin, may explain rubber dermatitis caused by a garment worn for years without trouble. Shoe dermatitis may be caused by rubber allergy to insoles or to sneakers. Wearers of goggles, gas masks, respirators, and other rubber goods sometimes develop rubber dermatitis (Fig. 6-11). Prepatellar dermatitis may be caused by rubber kneeling pads. Rubber sheeting used as bed underpads may cause bizarre eruptions on the trunk. Dermatitis of the glans penis from rubber condoms and vaginitis from pessaries or diaphragms may occur.

Natural and synthetic rubbers are used separately or in combination to make the final rubber product. It is the chemicals added in the rubber manufacturing process, most importantly the accelerators and antioxidants, that are the common causes of allergic contact dermatitis. A similar list of additives is present in neoprene, a synthetic rubber. Elastic in underwear is chemically transformed by laundry bleach, such as Clorox, into a potent sensitizing substance (Fig. 6-12). The allergen is permanent and cannot be removed by washing. The offending garments must be thrown out and the use of bleaches interdicted.

ACCELERATORS. During the manufacturing process, chemicals are used to hasten the vulcanization of rubber. Among

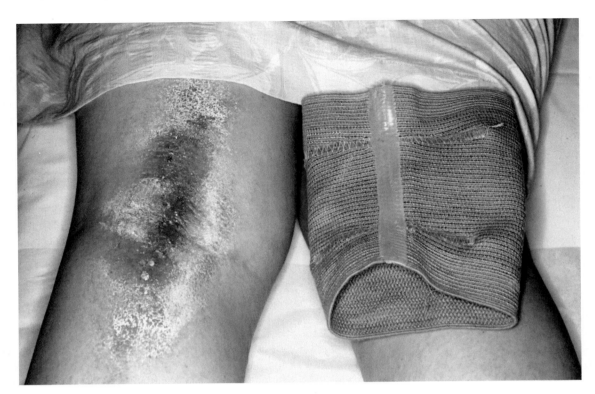

Fig. 6-11 Contact dermatitis resulting from rubber elastic knee supporter.

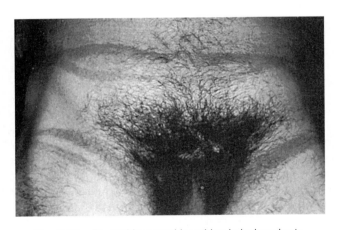

Fig. 6-12 Dermatitis caused by rubber in jockey shorts.

the numerous chemicals available tetramethylthiuram disulfide, mercaptobenzothiazole, and diphenylguanidine are frequently used. Tetramethylthiuram disulfide and its analogs, known as disulfiram and thiuram, may produce contact dermatitis when moist skin is exposed to the finished rubber product. In their 10-year study of 636 cases of allergy to rubber additives, Conde-Salazar et al found thiuram mix to be by far the most common sensitizer. Meriaptobenzathiazole is most often the cause in shoe allergy and thiuram in glove allergy.

ANTIOXIDANTS. To preserve rubber, antioxidants are used. Among the antioxidants the amine type such as phenyl-alpha-naphthylamine is most effective. Hydroquinone antioxidants may cause depigmentation of the skin as well as allergic contact dermatitis. A frequent antioxidant sensitizer, propyl paraphenylenediamine, is used in tires, heavy-duty rubber goods, girdles, boots, and elastic underwear. Rich et al reported two patients who developed allergy to Lowinox 44536, an antioxidant. They generated a useful list of alternative gloves for the patient with type IV hypersensitivity to rubber additives.

Conde-Salazar L, et al: Type IV allergy to rubber additives. *J Am Acad Dermatol* 1993, 29:176.
Fisher AA: Condom dermatitis in either partner. *Cutis* 1987, 39:281.
Johnson RC, et al: Wrist dermatitis. *Am J Contact Dermat* 1997, 8:172.
Rich P, et al: Allergic contact hypersensitivity to two antioxidants in latex gloves. *J Am Acad Dermatol* 1991, 24:37.
Wilkinson SM, et al: Latex: a cause of allergic contact eczema in users of natural rubber gloves. *J Am Acad Dermatol* 1998, 39:36. ▲

Adhesive Dermatitis. Adhesive dermatitis may be caused by cements, glues, and gums (Fig. 6-13). Most of these adhesives are now made of synthetic material, but some may still contain rubber with its accompanying allergenic substances. Formaldehyde resin adhesives contain free formaldehyde, naphtha, glue, and disinfectants. Synthetic

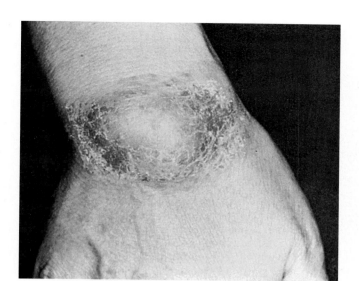

Fig. 6-13 Adhesive dermatitis caused by adhesive bandage.

resin adhesives contain plasticizers; hide glues may contain chromates from the tanned leather while other glues incorporate preservatives such as formaldehyde.

Vegetable gums such as gum tragacanth, gum arabic, and karaya may be used in denture adhesives, hair wave lotions, topical medications, toothpastes, and depilatories, and many cause contact dermatitis. Resins are used in adhesive tapes and in various adhesives such as tincture of benzoin. Compound tincture of benzoin may be a potent sensitizer when applied under occlusion (Fig. 6-14). Turpentine is frequently found in rosin; abietic acid in the rosin is the causative sensitizer.

An ethyl cyanoacrylate adhesive (Krazy Glue) used on the fingernails produced an extensive eruption of scaling plaques that was misdiagnosed as parapsoriasis en plaques; there were vesicular patch test reactions to both Krazy Glue and 5-Second Nail Glue, as reported by Dorinda Shelley.

Many adhesive tape reactions are caused by irritative effects on the skin. Allergic reactions to adhesive tape itself are caused by the rubber components, to accelerators, to antioxidants, and to various resins or turpentine. Some adhesive tapes contain acrylate polymers rather than rubber adhesives; Dermicel, Micropore Surgical Tape, and Steri-Strip are among these. These acrylates may cause allergic contact dermatitis. Pressure-sensitive adhesives are in widespread use in the tape and label industries. Allergens present in these adhesives include rosin, rubber accelerators, antioxidants, acrylates, hydroquinones, lanolin, thiourea compounds, and N-dodecylmaleamic compounds.

Fitzgerald DA, et al: Contact sensitivity to cyanoacrylate nail-adhesive with dermatitis at remote sites. *Contact Dermatitis* 1995, 32:175.

James WD: Allergic contact dermatitis to colophony. *Contact Dermatitis* 1984, 10:6.

Shelley ED, et al: Chronic dermatitis simulating small-plaque parapsoriasis due to cyanoacrylate adhesive. *JAMA* 1984, 252:2455. _____ ▲

Synthetic Resin Dermatitis. The many varieties of synthetic resins preclude adequate discussion of each. The reactions incurred during the manufacture of these substances are more frequent than those encountered in their finished state.

EPOXY RESINS. The epoxy resins in their liquid (noncured, monomene) form may produce severe dermatitis, especially during the manufacturing process. The fully polymerized or cured product is nonsensitizing. Nonindustrial exposure is usually to the epoxy resin glues, to nail lacquers, and to artificial nails. Epoxy resins are used in the home as glues and paints (bathtub and refrigerator). Artists and sculptors frequently use epoxy resins.

Epoxy resins consist of two or more components, the resin and the curing agent. Approximately 90% of allergic reactions are to the resin and 10% to the hardener. There are numerous curing agents such as the amines, phenolic compounds, peroxides, and polyamides. These may be irritants or allergens or both. The resin, based on an acetone and phenol compound known as bisphenol A, in its raw state may cause allergic contact dermatitis. BIS-GMA, a combination of bisphenol A and glycidyl methacrylate, is the allergen in dental bonding agents. One percent epoxy resin in acetone is used for patch testing. Epoxy resins are used also as stabilizers and plasticizers. Their use in the manufacture of polyvinyl chloride (plastic) film has caused dermatitis from plastic handbags, beads, gloves, and panties.

POLYESTER RESINS. Ordinarily, completely cured or polymerized resins are not sensitizers. The unsaturated polyester resins are dissolved and later copolymerized with vinyl monomers. Such polyester resins are used for polyester plasticizers, polyester fibers (Dacron), and polyester film (Mylar). The unsaturated polyester resins, on the other hand, will produce primary irritation in their fabrication. The dermatitis occurs typically as an eczematous eruption on the back of the hands, wrists, and forearms. Polyester resins are commonly incorporated into other plastic material as laminates to give them strength; applications include boat hulls, automobile body putty, safety helmets, fuel tanks, lampshades, and skylights.

ACRYLIC MONOMERS. Multifunctional acrylic monomers may produce allergic or irritant contact dermatitis. Pentaerythritol triacrylate, trimethylolpropane triacrylate, and hexanediol diacrylate are widely used acrylic monomers.

Nethercott et al reported contact dermatitis in 18 cases of printers who handled multifunctional acrylic monomers in printing inks and acrylic printing plates. The clinical manifestations were an erythematous, pruritic eruption, mainly of the hands and arms, swelling of the face, and involvement of the eyelids.

Orthopedic surgeons experience contact dermatitis from the use of acrylic bone cement (methyl methacrylate

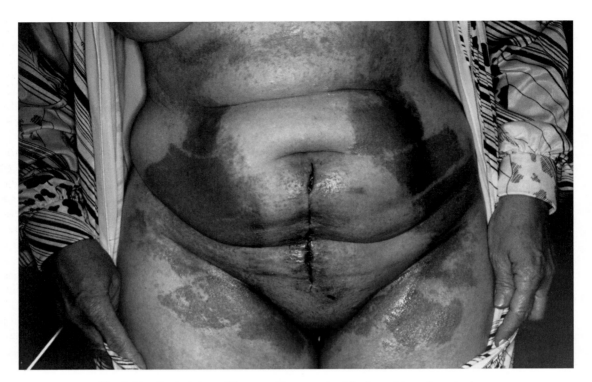

Fig. 6-14 Contact dermatitis caused by compound tincture of benzoin under tape.

monomer) used in mending hip joints. Dentists and dental technicians are exposed when applying this to the teeth. The sensitizer passes through rubber and polyvinyl gloves. In patients who are allergic to their acrylate dental prosthesis, coating them with UV light-cured acrylate lacquer may allow it to be worn without adverse effects.

Benzoyl peroxide is a popular acne remedy. It is also used for bleaching flour and edible oils and for curing plastics, such as acrylic dentures. Infrequently, an allergic contact dermatitis may be caused. Patch testing is done with 1% in petrolatum.

Fisher AA: Adverse nail reactions and paresthesias from photobonded acrylate sculptured nails. *Cutis* 1990, 45:243.

Guill MA, et al: Hearing aid dermatitis. *Arch Dermatol* 1978, 114:1050.

Hemmer W, et al: Allergic contact dermatitis to artificial fingernails prepared from UV light-cured acrylates. *J Am Acad Dermatol* 1996, 35:377.

Kanerva L, et al: Successful coating of an allergenic acrylate-based dental prosthesis. *Am J Contact Dermat* 1995, 6:24.

Nethercott JR, et al: Contact dermatitis in printing tradesman. *Contact Dermatitis* 1986, 14:280. _____ ▲

Cosmetic Dermatitis. Cutaneous reactions to cosmetics may be divided into irritant, allergic hypersensitivity, and photosensitivity reactions. The leading cause of allergic contact dermatitis associated with cosmetics is from fragrance. A close second is preservatives, such as Bronopol (2-bromo-2-nitropropane-1-3-diol), Kathon CG, quater-

nium-15, Euxyl K 400, and imidazolidinyl urea. Third is paraphenylenediamine in hair dye.

AXILLARY ANTIPERSPIRANTS. The aluminum salts, such as aluminum chloride and chlorhydroxide, and the zinc salts, such as zinc chloride, act as primary irritants and may rarely produce a folliculitis (Fig. 6-15). Aluminum chlorhydrate is considered to be the least irritating antiperspirant. Zirconium salt preparations, now removed from all antiperspirants, produced a granulomatous reaction. Zirconium-aluminum complexes have been felt to be nonsensitizing, so they are commonly used as the active ingredient in topical antiperspirants. A patient with cutaneous granulomas from this complex was however reported by Montemarano et al. Quaternary ammonium compounds in some roll-on deodorants may produce allergic contact dermatitis.

AXILLARY DEODORANTS. The chlorinated phenols such as hexachlorophene rarely produce allergic sensitization; the latter may cause photosensitization. This is also true of bithionol.

HAIR DYES. Permanent types of hair dyes incorporate paraphenylenediamine (PPDA), a popular but potent sensitizer that may cross-react with many chemicals. In rinses and tints the azo dyes, acid violet 6B, water-soluble nigrosine, and ammonium carbonate may sensitize and cross-react with PPDA. Exposure to PPDA is the third most common cause of contact dermatitis in cosmetics, after fragrances and preservatives. Those engaged in the manufacture of PPDA, furriers, hairdressers, and those in the photographic and rubber vulcanization industries develop

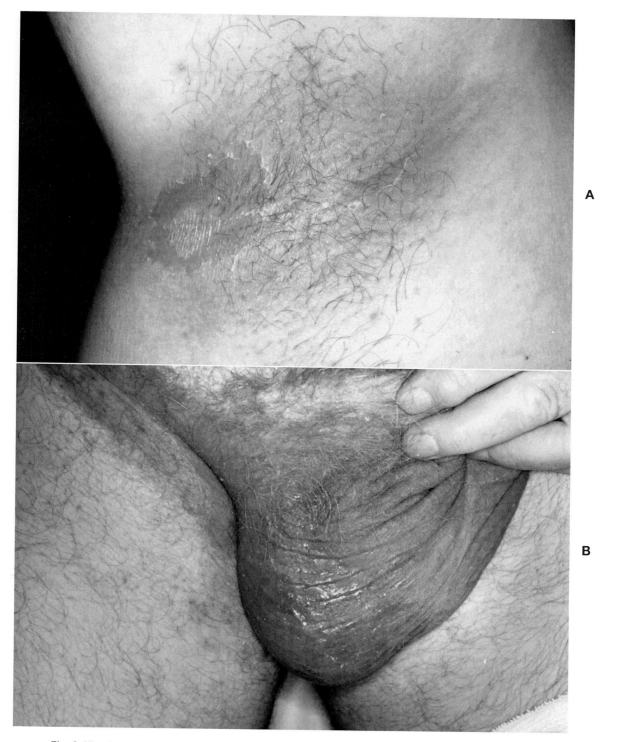

Fig. 6-15 **A** and **B,** Axillary and scrotal irritant dermatitis caused by applications of antiperspirants and deodorants.

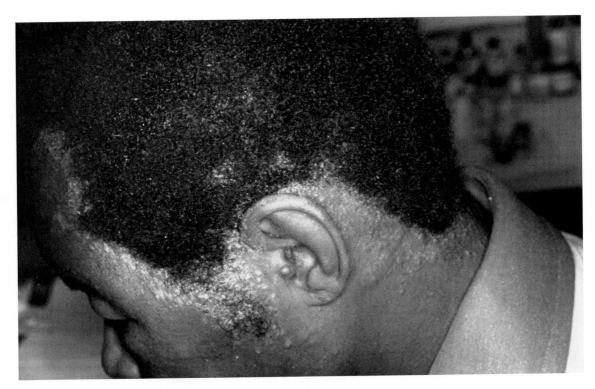

Fig. 6-16   Hair dye dermatitis resulting from paraphenylenediamine.

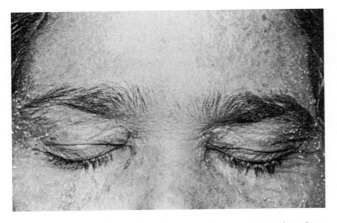

Fig. 6-17   Dermatitis resulting from use of hair dye (paraphenylene-diamine). Eyelid involvement is characteristic. (Courtesy Dr. Axel W. Hoke.)

eruptions at first on the backs of the hands, wrists, forearms, eyelids, and nose, consisting of an eczematous, erythematous, oozing dermatitis. In those whose hair has been dyed, sensitivity is manifested by itching, redness, and puffiness of the upper eyelids, tops of the ears, temples, and back of the neck (Figs. 6-16 and 6-17). Lichenification and scaling are seen in the chronic type.

Patch testing is done with 1% PPDA in petrolatum. The testing material should be stored in dark containers and made fresh at least yearly; if it blackens, new material should be prepared. For the person sensitive to this type of hair dye, use of semipermanent or temporary dyes might be the solution. In the case of sensitivity to the latter, vegetable dyes such as henna may be tried. Metallic dyes are usually not favored by women but are frequently used by men as "hair color restorers." The metallic hair dyes may contain nickel, cobalt, chromium, or lead.

HAIR BLEACHES. Hair bleach products incorporate peroxides, persulfates and ammonia, which may act as primary irritants. Hair bleaches that contain ammonium persulfate, a primary irritant, may produce a local urticarial and a generalized histamine reaction.

PERMANENT WAVE PREPARATIONS. The alkaline permanent wave preparations, which use ammonium thioglycolate, are rarely, if ever, sensitizes and usually cause only hair breakage and irritant reactions. The hot type, or acid perm, first used in the United States in 1973, is far more sensitizing. Storrs reported 12 patients in whom a glyceryl monothioglycolate allergy developed. Cosmetologists are at risk for development of hand dermatitis. The glyceryl thioglycolate persists in the hair for at least 3 months after application and may cause a long-lasting dermatitis. It readily penetrates rubber and vinyl gloves.

HAIR STRAIGHTENERS. The greases and gums are not sensitizers; however, the perfume incorporated in these preparations can be. Thioglycolates are also used, and hair breakage may occur with these products.

HAIR SPRAYS. Shellac, gum arabic, and the synthetic resins are sensitizers, and allergic reactions occur infrequently. Lanolin is frequently incorporated into the aerosol sprays.

DEPILATORIES. Calcium thioglycolate and the sulfides and sulfhydrates may cause primary irritant dermatitis. Mechanical hair removers are the mercaptans, waxes, and resins. The latter may produce allergic dermatitis.

HAIR TONICS AND LOTIONS. Tincture of cinchona produces allergic sensitization; tincture of cantharidin and salicylic acid, primary irritation. Resorcin, quinine sulfate, and perfumes such as bay rum are also sensitizers.

NAIL LACQUERS. These contain sulfonamide-formaldehyde resins (toluene sulfonamide) and are frequent causes of eyelid and neck dermatitis. Polishes free of this resin are now available.

NAIL POLISH REMOVERS. These are solvents such as acetone, which can cause nail brittleness.

ARTIFICIAL NAILS. The acrylic monomers, as well as the ethyl cyanoacrylate glue required to attach the prosthetic nail, may produce allergic sensitivity.

NAIL HARDENERS. Formaldehyde and formaldehyde-releasing agents are the most common of nail hardeners and may produce allergic sensitization. Paronychia, onycholysis, onychomadesis, and subungual hemorrhage may result from use of these hardeners.

LIPSTICKS. Dibromofluorescein and tetrabromofluorescein in the indelible dyes and the perfumes of the lipsticks may cause sensitization reactions (Fig. 6-18). This reaction may be enhanced if allantoin compounds are also included in the lipstick formula.

EYE MAKEUP. In mascara, eye shadow, and eyeliners, the preservative, base wax, and perfumes are the components that may produce sensitization, but this occurs rarely. False-positive reactions to some mascaras occur when a closed patch test is used. This is caused by the irritative qualities of the solvents. An open or nonocclusive patch test is recommended. A provocative use test in the antecubital fossae may ultimately be necessary. The rubber sponges used to apply eye makeup also cause eyelid dermatitis.

SUNSCREENS. Paraaminobenzoic acid (PABA) and its derivatives such as padimate O, padimate A, and glycerol PABA; dibenzoylmethanes, salicylates, cinnamates and benzophenones are photosensitizers as well as sensitizers. If allergy to PABA exists avoidance of its derivatives as well as an awareness that thiazides, sulfonylurea antidiabetic medication, azo dyes, paraaminosalicylic acid, benzocaine, and paraphenylenediamine all may cause dermatitis from cross-reactions should be appreciated.

BLEACHING CREAMS. Ammoniated mercury is a sensitizing agent formerly used in bleaching creams. Hydroquinones are also occasional sensitizers.

LANOLIN. A fatty alcohol, lanolin is rarely a sensitizer on normal skin but may present in atopic patients more frequently. Patch testing must be done with 30% wool wax alcohols in petrolatum.

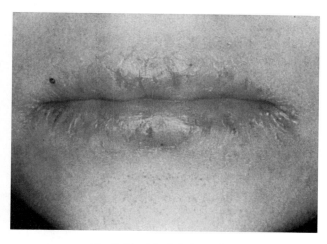

Fig. 6-18 Lipstick dermatitis.

DENTIFRICES AND MOUTHWASHES. Dentifrices and mouthwashes contain sensitizers, such as the essential oils used as flavoring agents and antiseptics (Fig. 6-19). Beacham et al reported 20 women who developed circumoral dermatitis and cheilitis from tartar-control types of dentifrices.

PERFUMES. Almost all cosmetic preparations contain perfumes; even those labeled nonscented often contain a "masking" fragrance that may be a sensitizer. Even "fragrance-free" products have been documented to contain the raw fragrance ingredients, such as the soap that contained "all-natural" products, including rose oil, as Scheinman reported. Fragrances are the most common cosmetic ingredient causing allergic contact dermatitis. Photodermatitis, irritation, contact urticaria, and dyspigmentation are other types of reactions they may produce. The most common individual allergens identified are cinnamic alcohol, hydroxy citronellal, musk ambrette, isoeugenol, geraniol, cinnamic aldehyde, coumarin, and eugenol. Frequently, unspecified allergens are the cause as they are not listed on labels and fragrances are combinations of many different ingredients. Balsam of Peru will identify approximately half of these often unsuspected cases of allergic dermatitis, and fragrance mix will identify nearly 86%. Use testing of new products is often necessary to test tolerance.

COSMETIC INTOLERANCE SYNDROME. Occasionally a patient will complain of intense burning or stinging after applying any cosmetic. Usually there are only subjective symptoms, but objective inflammation may also be present. The underlying cause may be difficult to document, even though thorough patch testing, photo patch testing and contact urticaria testing are completed. Endogenous disease such as seborrheic dermatitis, acne rosacea, or atopic dermatitis may complicate the assessment. Avoidance of all cosmetics with only glycerin being allowed for 6 to 12 months is often necessary to calm the reactive state. Adding back cosmetics one at a time, no more frequently than one per week, may then be tolerated.

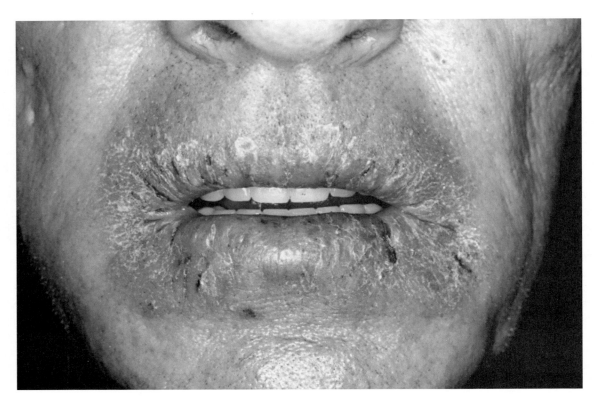

Fig. 6-19 Perioral dermatitis caused by a mouthwash.

Adams RM, et al: A 5-year study of cosmetic reactions. *J Am Acad Dermatol* 1985, 13:1062.

Beacham BE, et al: Circumoral dermatitis and cheilitis caused by tartar control dentifrices. *J Am Acad Dermatol* 1990, 22:1029.

Broeckx W, et al: Cosmetic intolerance. *Contact Dermatitis* 1987, 16:189.

deGroot AC, et al: Contact allergens: what's new? Cosmetic dermatitis. *Clin Dermatol* 1997, 15:485.

deGroot AC, et al: The allergens in cosmetics. *Arch Dermatol* 1988, 124:1525.

deWit FS, et al: An outbreak of contact dermatitis from toluene sulfonamide formaldehyde resin in nail hardener. *Contact Dermatitis* 1988, 18:280.

Dromgoole SH, et al: Sunscreen agent intolerance. *J Am Acad Dermatol* 1990, 22:1068.

Held JL, et al: Consort contact dermatitis due to oak moss. *Arch Dermatol* 1988, 124:261.

Knobler E, et al: Photoallergy to benzophenone. *Arch Dermatol* 1989, 125:801.

Larsen WG: Perfume dermatitis. *J Am Acad Dermatol* 1985, 12:1.

Larsen W, et al: Fragrance contact dermatitis. *Am J Contact Dermat* 1996, 7:77.

Matsunaga K, et al: Occupational allergic contact dermatitis in beauticians. *Contact Dermatitis* 1988, 18:94.

Montemarano AD, et al: Cutaneous granulomas caused by an aluminum-zirconium complex. *J Am Acad Dermatol* 1997, 37:496.

Morrison CH, et al: Persistence of an allergen in hair after GMTG-containing permanent wave solutions. *J Am Acad Dermatol* 1988, 19:52.

Scheinman PL: Allergic contact dermatitis to fragrance. *Am J Contact Dermat* 1996, 7:65.

Scheinman PL: Is it really fragrance-free? *Am J Contact Dermat* 1997, 8:239.

Storrs FJ, et al: Paraphenylenediamine dihydrochloride. *Contact Dermatitis* 1979, 5:126.

Storrs FJ: Permanent wave dermatitis: contact allergy to glyceryl monothioglycolate. *J Am Acad Dermatol* 1984, 11:74. _____ ▲

Preservatives. Preservatives are added to any preparation that contains water to kill microorganisms and prevent spoilage. They are the second leading cause of contact dermatitis in cosmetics. The most important class is formaldehyde and the formaldehyde-releasing compounds; this includes quaternium-15 (the leading preservative sensitizer in the United States), imidazolidinyl urea, diazolidinyl urea, DMDM hydantoin, and 2-bromo-2 nitropropane-l,3, diol. Kathon CG or methyl chloroisothiazolinone/methyl isothiazolinone (MCI/MI) is a biocide that is causing increasing numbers of reports of allergic contact dermatitis. Euxyl K 400 is another preservative that is becoming increasingly important. It causes a typical cosmetic dermatitis. It consists of two active ingredients; dibromodicyanobutane is the component that produces the allergic response. Thimerosal and parabens are other preservatives that may cause allergy.

FORMALDEHYDE AND FORMALDEHYDE-RELEASING AGENTS. Formaldehyde is used in cosmetics, primarily in shampoos. Because it is quickly diluted and washed away, sensitization through this exposure is rare. Formaldehyde releasers are polymers of formaldehyde that may release small amounts of formaldehyde under certain conditions. Allergy may be caused by the formaldehyde-releasing preservatives (which act as antibacterial and antifungal agents in their own right), to the released formaldehyde, or both.

PARABENS. Allergic contact dermatitis may develop from parabens, which are also used in some cosmetics, foods, drugs, dentifrices, and suppositories. The paraben esters (methyl, ethyl, propyl, and butyl parahydroxybenzoates) are used in concentrations below 0.3% as preservatives. Parahydroxybenzoic acid (another paraben) has also been found to cause reactions. Perpetuation of a dermatitis, despite effective topical medication, suggests the possibility of paraben sensitivity or corticosteroid sensitivity, or that another sensitizer may be present. The concentration of paraben (below 0.3%) is too low in the various topical applications to produce a positive patch test to the medication. Therefore testing is done with a 12% paraben mix (methyl, ethyl, propyl, and butyl, 3% each) in petrolatum. Parabens, which are frequently used as bacteriostatic agents, are capable of producing immunologically mediated immediate systemic hypersensitivity reactions.

PARA-CHLORO-META-XYLENOL (PCMX). This chlorinated phenol antiseptic is used in many over-the-counter products with the disinfectant properties of *p*-chloro-meta-cresol. Sensitization occurs primarily through exposure to betamethasone-containing cream. There is cross-reactivity to PCMX.

SORBIC ACID. A rare sensitizer, sorbic acid is tested as 2% in petrolatum. It is a cause of facial flushing and stinging through its action as an inducer of nonimunologic contact urticaria.

deGroot AC, et al: Kathon CG. *J Am Acad Dermatol* 1988, 18:350.

deGroot AC, et al: Methyldibromoglutaronitrile (Euxyl K 400). *J Am Acad Dermatol* 1996, 35:743.

Dooms-Goossens A, et al: Imidazolindinyl urea dermatitis. *Contact Dermatitis* 1986, 14:322.

Fransway AF: The problem of preservation in the 1990s. *Am J Contact Dermat* 1991, 2:6.

Frosch PJ: Contact allergy to Bronopol. *Contact Dermatitis* 1990, 22:24.

Jackson JM, et al: Methyldibromoglutaronitrile. *J Am Acad Dermatol* 1998, 38:934.

Madden SD, et al: Occupationally induced allergic contact dermatitis to MCI/MI among machinists. *J Am Acad Dermatol* 1994, 30:272.

Primka EJ III, et al: Three cases of contact allergy after chemical burns from MCI/MI. *Am J Contact Dermat* 1997, 8:43.

Rietschel RL, et al: MCI/MI reactions in patients screened for vehicle and preservative hypersensitivity. *J Am Acad Dermatol* 1990, 22:739.

Skinner SL, et al: Allergic contact dermatitis to preservatives in topical medicaments. *Am J Contact Dermat* 1998, 9:199.

Storrs FJ, et al: Allergic contact dermatitis to 2-bromo-2-nitropropane l,3-diol in hydrophilic ointment. *J Am Acad Dermatol* 1983, 8:157.

Tosti A, et al: Occupational contact dermatitis due to quaternium-15. *Contact Dermatitis* 1990, 23:41. _____ ▲

Vehicles. Formulation of topically applied products is complex as more additives are blended to make a pleasing base for carriage of the active ingredient to the skin. Various emulsifiers, humectants, stabilizers, surfactants, and surface active agents are used to make aesthetically pleasing preparations. These may cause irritation, erythema and allergy.

PROPYLENE GLYCOL. Propylene glycol is widely used as a vehicle for topical medications, cosmetics, and various emollient lotions. It is used in the manufacture of automobile brake fluid and alky resins, as a lubricant for food machinery, and as an additive for food colors and flavoring agents. It is commonly used in antiperspirants. Propylene glycol must be considered as a sensitizer able to produce contact dermatitis, and it can cause a flare of the contact dermatitis when ingested. It is tested as a 4% aqueous solution, but irritant reactions or false negatives are common. A use test of the implicated propylene glycol–containing products may be required.

ETHYLENEDIAMINE. Ethylenediamine is used as a stabilizer in medicated creams. It may cause contact dermatitis and cross-react with internally taken aminophylline, which consists of theophylline and ethylenediamine. Ash et al reported a patient with a generalized itchy, red eruption that recurred each time hydroxyzine was taken orally. Hydroxyzine is a piperazine derivative that is structurally based on a dimer of ethylenediamine, to which this patient was sensitive.

Ash S, et al: Systemic contact dermatitis to hydroxyzine. *Am J Contact Dermat* 1997, 8:2.

Cantanzaro JM, et al: Propylene glycol dermatitis. *J Am Acad Dermatol* 1991; 24:90

Tosti A, et al: Prevalence and sources of sensitization to emulsifiers. *Contact Dermatitis* 1990, 23:68. _____ ▲

Topical Drug Contact Dermatitis. Drugs, in addition to their pharmacologic and possible toxic action, also possess sensitizing properties. This may not only occur from topical application but also from ingestion. Some, such as the antihistamines, sensitize much more frequently when applied topically than when taken orally. With the advent of transdermal patches for delivery of medications such as nitroglycerin, hormones, clonidine, and scopolamine reports of sensitization are increasing.

Some drugs may produce sensitization of the skin when applied topically; if the medication is later taken internally an acute flare at the site of the contact dermatitis may result. This so-called anamnestic (recalled) eruption or systemic contact dermatitis can occur with antihistaminics, sulfonamides, and penicillin. The same is true of the local anesthetic ointments containing "caine" medications.

Although it is impossible to mention all topical medications that cause irritation or allergic contact dermatitis, some are important enough to be dealt with individually.

HYPERSENSITIVITY TO LOCAL ANESTHETICS. Physicians and dentists may develop allergic contact dermatitis from local anesthetics. In addition, the continued use of these local anesthetics as antipruritic ointments and lotions cause sensitization of the skin. Benzocaine is a frequently used topical antipruritic and is the most common topical sensitizer of this group. Allergy to local anesthetics may induce edema and erythema (especially of the face), severe pruritus, urticaria, and even anaphylactic reaction a few minutes after injection.

Local anesthetics may be divided into two groups: the first includes the para-aminobenzoic acid esters, such as benzocaine, butethemine (Monocaine), chloroprocaine, procaine (Novocain), and tetracaine (Pantocaine); the second, which sensitizes much less frequently, includes the amides, such as dibucaine (Nupercainal), lidocaine (Lido-Mantle, Xylocaine) (least likely to sensitize), mepivacaine (Carbocaine), and prilocaine (Citanest). In addition, the preservative methylparaben, frequently found in these prepared solutions, may cause hypersensitivity reactions that can easily be misattributed to the local anesthetics. Benzocaine sensitivity is determined by a patch test of 5% benzocaine in petrolatum. It should be kept in mind that numerous cross-reactions are seen in benzocaine-sensitive individuals. These are discussed on p. 117 in the section on sunscreens.

ANTIMICROBIAL CONTACT DERMATITIS. Physicians, dentists, nurses, and other medical personnel, as well as patients, may develop contact dermatitis from various antibiotics. Neomycin is a common sensitizer. As a topical antibiotic, neomycin sulfate has been incorporated into innumerable ointments, creams, and lotions. It is present in such preparations as underarm deodorants, otic and ophthalmologic preparations, and antibiotic creams and ointments available without prescriptions. The signs of neomycin sensitivity may be those of a typical contact dermatitis but are often those of a recalcitrant skin eruption that has become lichenified and even hyperkeratotic. This may be because many of the topical agents contain several types of antibiotics but also often have corticosteroids present. This picture may be seen in persistent external otitis, lichen simplex chronicus of the nuchal area, or dermatophytosis between the toes. Patch testing is done with 20% concentration of neomycin in petrolatum. The patch should be observed at day 4, as well as at day 7, for possible delayed reactions.

There has been a dramatic rise in allergy to bacitracin. Its use after minor surgical procedures may account for this. Smack et al showed that white petrolatum was as effective in aiding wound healing after surgical procedures and of course did not carry the allergenic potential. There is a high rate of co-reacting (not cross-reacting) to neomycin because of simultaneous exposures. Contact urticaria and anaphylaxis are reported more often with bacitracin than with other antibiotics.

Allergic dermatitis of the fingertips caused by streptomycin may be encountered in nurses who prepare this infrequently used drug for injection. The dermatitis may become chronic, with eczematization and fissuring. Cross-reactivity to neomycin, gentamicin, and kanamycin may occur. Hypersensitivity develops in many people exposed to contact with streptomycin, as in the handling of the material for injection.

ANTIFUNGAL AGENTS. Allergic contact dermatitis to imidazole antifungal agents may occur. There is a high cross-reactivity rate between miconazole, isoconazole, clotrimazole and oxiconazole because of their common chemical structure. Hydroxyquinolones, nitrofurazone (Furacin), mercury compounds such as ammoniated mercury, thimerosal, and phenylmercuric acetate are sensitizers, as are the sulfonamides, resorcinol, and formaldehyde.

PHENOTHIAZINE DRUGS. Handling injectable solutions and tablets may produce dermatitis in those sensitized to chlorpromazine and other phenothiazine derivatives. The reactions may be photoallergic or nonphotoallergic.

CORTICOSTEROIDS. Numerous reports of large series of patients who have developed allergy to these commonly used preparations emphasize the need for a high index of suspicion when treating patients with chronic dermatitis who fail to improve, or who worsen, when topical steroidal agents are used. Once sensitized to one type of corticosteroid cross-sensitization may occur. The corticosteroids have been separated into four structural classes: class A is the hydrocortisone, tixicortol pivalate group, class B is the triamcinolone acetonide group, class C is the betamethasone group, and class D is the hydrocortisone-17-butyrate group. There are frequent cross-reactions between classes A and C. Tixicortol pivalate and budesonide have been found to be the best screen for such reactions. In the absence of having these agents patch testing to the implicated product with a reading at day 4 may be useful.

Baes H: Contact sensitivity to miconazole with ortho-chloro cross-sensitivity to other midazoles. *Contact Dermatitis* 1991, 24:89.

Coopman S, et al: Identification of cross-reaction patterns in allergic contact dermatitis from topical corticosteroids. *Br J Dermatol* 1989, 121:27.

Cox NH: Contact allergy to clobetasol propionate. *Arch Dermatol* 1988, 124:9ll.

Farley M, et al: Bacitracin anaphylaxis. *Am J Contact Dermat* 1995, 6:28.

Gallenkemper G, et al: Contact sensitization in chronic venous insufficiency. *Contact Dermatitis* 1998, 38:274.

Gette MT, et al: Frequency of post operative allergic contact dermatitis to topical antibiotics. *Arch Dermatol* 1992, 128:365.

Ghadially R, et al: Gentamicin. *J Am Acad Dermatol* 1988, 19:428.

Goh CL, et al: Contact sensitivity to topical medications. *Int J Dermatol* 1989, 28:25.

Grandinetti PJ, et al: Simultaneous contact allergy to neomycin, bacitracin, and polymyxin. *J Am Acad Dermatol* 1990, 23:646.

Grekin RC, et al: Local anesthesia in dermatology surgery. *J Am Acad Dermatol* 1988, 19:599.

Lauerma AJ, et al: Contact allergy to corticosteroids. *J Am Acad Dermatol* 1993, 28:618.

Lepoitterin JP, et al: Studies in patients with corticosteroid contact allergy. *Arch Dermatol* 1995, 131:31.

Lutz ME, et al: Contact hypersensitivity to tixicortal pivalate. *J Am Acad Dermatol* 1998, 38:691.

Marks JG Jr, et al: North American Dermatitis Group standard tray patch test results (1992 to 1994). *Am J Contact Dermat* 1995, 6:160.

McBurney EI, et al: Contact dermatitis to transdermal estradiol system. *J Am Acad Dermatol* 1989, 20:508.

Rietschel RL: Patch testing for corticosteroid allergy in the U.S. *Arch Dermatol* 1995, 131:91.

Sasaki E: Corticosteroid sensitivity and cross-sensitivity. *Contact Dermatitis* 1990, 23:306.

Schillinger BM, et al: Boric acid poisoning. *J Am Acad Dermatol* 1982, 7:667.

Smack DP, et al: Infection and allergy incidence in ambulatory surgery patients using white petrolatum vs. bacitracin ointment. *JAMA* 1996, 276:972.

Trozak DJ: Delayed hypersensitivity to scopolamine delivered by a transdermal device. *J Am Acad Dermatol* 1985, 13:247.

▲

Occupational Contact Dermatitis

Workers in various occupations are prone to contact dermatitis from primary irritants and allergic contactants. In certain occupations it is a common occurrence. Irritant contact dermatitis is more frequent in the workplace, but it tends to be less severe and less chronic than allergic contact dermatitis. Some causative agents are listed below according to occupations:

Agriculture: Cement, cobalt in animal feed, pesticides, plants, rubber, wood preservatives, diesel oil, gasoline, disinfectants

Airplane workers: Glues, chromium, casein, phenol formaldehyde, urea formaldehyde, epoxy and polyester resins, dichromates

Artists: Synthetics such as acrylic and vinyl acrylic resins, epoxy and polyester resins, solvents such as carbon tetrachloride, benzene, toluene, acetone, turpentine, azo dyes, nickel and chromium pigments, clay, plaster

Bakers: Flour, cottonseed oil, potash (used in making pretzels), cardamom, cinnamon, benzoyl peroxide, persulfones

Barbers: Quinine, resorcin, mercury, nickel, paraphenylenediamine, capsicum, arsenic, sulfur

Carpenters and cabinetmakers: Teak, mahogany, rosewood, glues, nickel, plastics, polishes, rubber, turpentine

Compositors: Benzine, dichromates

Cooks: Soap, detergents, vegetables (such as onions, garlic, artichokes, carrots, and potatoes), nickel, insecticides, ammonia

Dentists: Soaps and detergents, acrylic monomers, local anesthetics such as procaine (most frequently) and tetracaine of the paraaminobenzoic acid derivatives, topical anesthetics such as benzocaine and tetracaine (diclonine hydrochloride is recommended instead of these two "caines"), self-curing acrylic resins, essential oils such as eucalyptol, menthol, thymol, eugenol, and methylsalicylate, formaldehyde for disinfection

of instruments, quaternary ammonium compounds such as benzalkonium chloride and benzethonium chloride

Diesel engine workers: Dichromates, lubricating oils, nickel

Dyers: Sodium silicate

Electroplaters: Cyanide, various acids

Exterminators: DDT, arsenic, formalin, sodium fluoride, formaldehyde, pyrethrum

Foresters: Poisonous shrubs, sprays containing arsenic and lead, lichens, moss, wood, oleoresins

Furriers: Arsenic, dyestuffs such as paraphenylenediamine

Gardeners: Plants, arsenic, insecticides, lime dust, fertilizers, formaldehyde, primula, chrysanthemum, tulip, narcissus, manure

Hairdressers: Paraphenylenediamine, soaps, peroxide, ammonium persulfate, glyceryl monothioglycolate, rubber, nickel, perfumes, acrylic plastics

Jewelers: Cyanide, nickel, metal polish

Masons: Chromates and cobalt in cement, leather goods, epoxy resin

Metal polishers: Oxalic acid, turpentine, dichromates

Milliners: Dyes, arsenic

Newspaper production workers: Tertiary butyl catechol in phototypesetting paper (Fardal)

Nurses and other health care workers: Penicillin, streptomycin, codeine, morphine, bichloride formalin, medicated alcohol, lye, hexachlorophene, formaldehyde, chlorpromazine

Painters: Turpentine, varnish remover, arsenic, linseed oil, aniline dyes, paints, benzene, paint thinners, deter-gents, chromates (green, yellow), cobalt (dyes, driers), epoxy resin, formaldehyde, polyester resins

Photographers: Pyrogallol, metal, dichromates, sodium hydroxide, azo compounds, selenium, formaldehyde, chemicals used in color film processing

Physicians: Rubber gloves, soaps

Printers: Arsenic, dichromates, nickel, hydrocarbons in ink, acrylic monomers

Sculptors: Woods such as satin wood, South American box wood, cocobolo, birch, pine, and beech; binders in synthetic materials such as urea, formaldehyde, alkyds, hexamethylenetetramine

Soap makers: Strong alkalis, perfumes

Surgeons: Antiseptics, iodine, mercurials, hexachlorophene, latex (rubber gloves), procaine, formaldehyde, acrylic polymers

Tanners: Dichromate, hydrochloric acid, vegetable tanning agents, glutaraldehyde, antimildew chemicals

Management. Occupational contact dermatitis is managed by eliminating contact of the skin with irritating and sensitizing substances. The work environment should be carefully controlled, with use of all available protective devices to prevent accidental and even planned exposures. Personal protective measures such as frequent clothing changes, cleansing showers, protective clothing, and protective barrier creams should be used as appropriate. Hand cleansing procedures should be thoroughly surveyed, with particular attention paid to the soaps available and also what solvents may be used.

Treatment of the dermatitis follows closely that recommended for toxicodendron dermatitis on p. 102. Topical corticosteroid preparations are especially helpful in the acute phase. When rubber and polyvinyl gloves are not feasible to use against irritant and allergenic substances, skin protective creams may offer a solution, although they are often impractical. A wide variety are available. Two main types of protective creams are used. One is for "wet work": protective against acids, alkalis, water-base paints, coolants, and cutting oils with water. The other type is for "dry work," to protect against oils, greases, cutting oils, adhesive, resins, glues, and wood preservatives.

Unfortunately, despite the best efforts at treatment and prevention the prognosis for occupational skin disease is guarded. One third to one quarter heal, another one third to one half improve, with the remainder the same or worse. Atopics, chromate allergy patients, and those in the construction industry fare the worst.

Adams RM: Occupational skin disease, ed 3, Philadelphia, 1999, WB Saunders.

Fisher AA: Allergic baker's dermatitis due to benzoyl peroxide. *Cutis* 1989, 43:128.

Hogan DJ, et al: The prognosis of contact dermatitis. *J Am Acad Dermatol* 1990, 23:300.

Marks JG Jr, DeLeo VA: Contact and occupational dermatology, ed 2, St Louis, 1997, Mosby.

Mathias GGT: Occupational dermatitis. *J Am Acad Dermatol* 1988, 19:1107.

Nethercott JR, et al: Disease outcome in workers with occupational skin disease. *J Am Acad Dermatol* 1994, 30:569.

Nethercott JR, et al: Follow-up study of workers with occupational contact dermatitis. *Contact Dermatitis* 1990, 23:241.

Nurse DS: Industrial dermatitis. *Int J Dermatol* 1987, 26:434.

Rietschel RL, Fowler JF Jr: Fisher's contact dermatitis, ed 4, Baltimore, 1995, Williams & Wilkins.

Rosen RH, et al: Prognosis of occupational contact dermatitis in New South Wales, Australia. *Contact Dermatitis* 1993, 29:88.

Taylor JS, editor: Occupational dermatoses. *Dermatol Clin* 1988, 6(1):1. ▲

Contact Urticaria Syndrome (Syndrome of Immediate Reactions)

Contact urticaria may be defined as a wheal and flare reaction occurring when a substance is applied to the intact skin. Urticaria is only one of a broad spectrum of immediate reactions, including pruritus, dermatitis, local or general urticaria, bronchial asthma, orolaryngeal edema, rhinoconjunctivitis, gastrointestinal distress, headache, or an anaphylactic reaction. Any combination of these is subsumed under the expression "syndrome of immediate reactions."

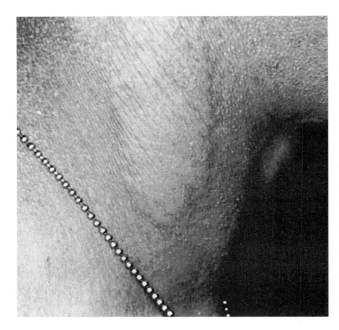

Fig. 6-20 Contact urticaria caused by cobalt chloride used to test for the ability to sweat.

It may be nonimmunologic (no prior sensitization), immunologic, or of unknown mechanism. The nonimmunologic type is the commonest, and may be caused by direct release of vasoactive substances from mast cells. The allergic type tends to be the most severe, as anaphylaxis is possible. The third type has features of both.

Nonimmunologic Mechanism. This type of reaction occurs most frequently and may produce contact urticaria in almost all exposed individuals. Examples of this type of reaction are seen with nettle rash (plants), dimethyl sulfoxide (DMSO), sorbic acid, benzoic acid, cinnamic aldehyde, cobalt chloride (Fig. 6-20), and Trafuril.

Immunologic Mechanism. This reaction is of the immediate (IgE-mediated) hypersensitivity type. This has been reported to be caused by latex, potatoes, phenylmercuric propionate, and many other allergens.

Uncertain Mechanism. This type of reaction occurs with those agents that produce contact urticaria and a generalized histamine type of reaction but lack a direct or immunologic basis for the reaction.

Contact Urticaria–Causing Substances. There are many different substances that can elicit such a reaction. It is seen in homemakers and food handlers who handle raw vegetables, raw meats and fish, shellfish, and other foods. Raw potatoes have been shown to cause not only contact urticaria but also asthma at the same time. It has been seen in hairdressers who handled bleaches and hair dyes containing ammonium persulfate, in whom the contact urticaria was accompanied by swelling and erythema of the face, followed by unconsciousness. Caterpillars and moths may cause contact urticaria just by touching the skin.

Additional substances inducing this reaction are oatmeal, flour, meat, turkey skin, calf liver, banana, lemon, monoamylamine, benzophenone, nail polish, tetanus antitoxin, streptomycin, cetyl alcohol, stearyl alcohol, estrogenic cream, cinnamic aldehyde, sorbic acid, benzoic acid, castor bean, lindane, carrots, spices, wool, silk, dog and cat saliva, dog hairs, horse serum, ammonia, sulfur dioxide, formaldehyde, acrylic monomers, exotic woods, wheat, cod liver oil, and aspirin.

Bacitracin ointment may cause anaphylactic reactions when applied topically, especially to chronic leg ulcer and dermatitis; however; one of us (WDJ) has observed two cases occurring after acute wounds.

The advent of AIDS caused a reemphasis of the use of glove protection in all medical procedures. This led to a marked increased not only in delayed-type hypersensitivity reaction to rubber additives, but also to a tremendous number of reports of contact urticaria and anaphylaxis to latex. Most of these reactions occur in health professionals. It is characterized by itching and swelling of the hands within a few minutes after donning the gloves, and will usually resolve within an hour after removing them. In patients with continued exposures the eruption may eventually appear as chronic eczema. Glove powder may aerosolize the allergen and produce more generalized reactions. While these reactions may occur on the job, many cases present as death or near-death events when sensitized individuals undergo operations or procedures especially when mucosal exposure exists (dental care, barium enemas, childbirth).

In addition to health care workers, with a reported incidence of between 3% and 10%, atopics and spina bifida patients are other risk groups for the development of type I allergy to latex protein. The sensitized individual should also be aware that up to 50% will have a concomitant fruit allergy to such foods as banana, avocado, kiwi, chestnut, and passion fruit.

Testing. The usual closed patch tests do not show sensitivity reactions. Instead, open patch tests are performed for eliciting immediate type hypersensitivity. The substance is applied to a 1-cm square area on the forearm and observed for 20 to 30 minutes for erythema that can evolve into a wheal and flare response. When foods are tested, a small piece of the actual food is placed on the skin. Rubber glove testing can be done by applying one finger of a latex glove to a moistened hand for 15 minutes and if no reaction is observed then wearing the entire glove for another 15 to 20 minutes. RAST testing detects 75% of latex-allergic individuals. There is no standard allergen available for prick testing.

Prick, scratch or intradermal testing is resorted to only when there are problems of interpretation of the open patch

tests. These tests have produced anaphylactic reactions and should only be attempted when support for this complication is available.

Amin S, et al: Contact urticaria syndrome: 1997. *Am J Contact Dermat* 1997, 8:15.

Berky ZT, et al: Latex glove allergy. *JAMA* 1992, 268:2695.

Elpern DJ: The syndrome of immediate reactivities (contact urticaria syndrome). *Hawaii Med J* 1985, 44:426.

Farley M, et al: Bacitracin anaphylaxis. *Am J Contact Dermat* 1995, 6:28.

Okano M, et al: Anaphylactic symptoms due to chlorhexidine gluconate. *Arch Dermatol* 1989, 125:50.

Ownby DR, et al: Anaphylaxis associated with latex allergy during barium enema examinations. *Am J Roentgenol* 1991, 156:903.

Skinner SL, et al: Contact anaphylaxis. *Am J Contact Dermat* 1995, 6:133.

Sussman GL, et al: Allergy to latex rubber. *Ann Intern Med* 1995, 122:43.

Taylor JS, et al: Latex allergy. *Arch Dermatol* 1996, 132:265.

Tuer W, et al: Contact urticaria to sodium-o-phenyl phenol. *Ann Allergy* 1986, 56:19.

Turjanmaak K, et al: Condoms as a source of latex allergen and cause of contact urticaria. *Contact Dermatitis* 1989, 20:360.

Warshaw EM: Latex allergy. *J Am Acad Dermatol* 1998, 39:1.

▲

DRUG REACTIONS
Epidemiology

Adverse reactions to most medications occur at very low rates (about 1/1000 exposures). However, certain commonly used medications (e.g., semisynthetic penicillins and sulfamethoxazole/trimethoprim) have much higher rates of adverse reactions (30 to 50/1000). The presence of HIV disease or EBV infection substantially increases the rate of adverse reactions to certain medications. All these factors result in adverse drug reactions being one of the most common reasons that a patient is seen for a dermatologic evaluation.

Evaluation of the Patient

There are three basic rules that should always be applied in evaluating the patient with suspected drug reactions. First, the patient is probably on unnecessary medications, and all these should be stopped. Pare down the medication list to the bare essentials. Secondly, the patient must be asked about nonprescription medications and pharmaceuticals delivered by other means (eye drops, suppositories, implants, injections, and patches). Thirdly, no matter how atypical the patient's cutaneous reaction, always consider the patient's medication as a possible cause. In patients with unusual reactions, searching the medical literature and calling the manufacturer for prior reports may be very useful.

The first step in evaluating a patient with a potential drug reaction is to diagnose the cutaneous eruption by clinical pattern (e.g., urticaria, exanthem, vasculitis, erythema multiforme, etc.). In determining whether the patient's current eruption could be related to a specific medication, two basic question should be asked: Which of this patient's medications cause this pattern of reaction? How commonly does this medication cause this reaction pattern?

Bruinsma's regularly updated manual or similar databases on the worldwide web are strongly recommended as ready reference sources for this information. Kramer et al developed an algorithm by which one could evaluate the likelihood of a certain medication causing a particular reaction. This algorithm can be used as a framework for the evaluation of a given patient:

1. Previous general experience with the drug: Has the suspected medication been reported to cause the reaction the patient is experiencing? If so, how commonly? Also ask the patient if they have had a previous reaction to any medications, as the current eruption may represent a cross-reaction from a prior exposure.

2. Alternative etiologic candidates: What are other possible causes of the patient's eruption? An exanthem, for instance, could be related to an associated viral illness, not the medication.

3. Timing of events: When did the eruption appear relative to the administration of the suspected medication? A detailed history from the patient and a careful review of the patient record, including the nursing notes are useful to establish the chronologic sequence of all drug therapy.

4. Drug levels and evidence of overdose: Certain reactions are known to be related to rate of administration (vancomycin red-man syndrome) or cumulative dose (lichenoid reactions to gold).

5. Response to discontinuation (dechallenge): Does the eruption clear when the suspected medication is stopped? Because certain eruptions may clear in the face of continuation, this is a useful, but not irrefutable criterion to ascribe a specific reaction to a medication.

6. Rechallenge: If the offending medication reproduces the reaction on readministration, this is strong evidence that the medication did indeed cause the reaction. Reactions associated with an increase in dosage may also be considered in this category. In certain reaction patterns (e.g., exanthems) even a fraction of the original dose may reproduce the reaction. It may be impossible to rechallenge if the reaction was severe, and may not be possible in dose-dependent cases.

In addition to the clinical evaluations noted above, complete evaluation may include special testing for confirmation. Skin testing is most useful in evaluating type I (immediate) hypersensitivity. It is most frequently used in evaluating adverse reactions to penicillin, local anesthetics, insulin, and vaccines. Radioallergosorbent (RAST) tests have a 20% false-negative rate in penicillin type I allergy, so they must be followed by skin testing. In their current form, RAST tests cannot replace skin testing. Intradermal and prick skin testing and patch testing are also reported to be beneficial in some cases of morbilliform reactions or fixed drug reaction. The patient's metabolism of certain drugs in lymphocytotoxicity assays may be associated with an adverse reaction. Such testing is commercially available, but is expensive, time consuming and its value limited to certain situations such as anticonvulsant or sulfonamide hypersensitivity reactions. Lymphocyte transformation tests, basophil degranulation, and determination of drug-specific antibodies are not currently clinically useful in evaluating adverse drug reactions.

The patient should be given concrete advice about his or her reaction. What was the probability the patient's reaction was caused by the medication? Can the patient take the medication again, and if so, what may occur? What cross-reactions are known? What other medications must the patient avoid? Unusual reactions should be reported to regulatory agencies and the manufacturer.

Pathogenesis

In most patterns of drug reactions, the pathogenesis is unknown. Drug reactions are often nonimmunologic in basis. They may result from normal pharmacologic effects of the medication (for instance urticaria worsening with aspirin ingestion). Reactions may be truly immunologic, based on an immune response by the patient to the medication or a metabolite. Studies have shown that the patient's metabolism of the medication may determine the likelihood of a reaction occurring. Specifically, in the case of anticonvulsant and sulfonamide reactions, the P-450 system of affected individuals generate toxic metabolites of the medication that bind to proteins and stimulate an immunologic reaction. This type of defect can be found in family members of affected individuals and are linked to HLA subtypes. In addition, the patient's immune status and clinical condition may influence the rate of adverse reactions, for example the increased rate of drug reactions in AIDS patients, which may be related to glutathione deficiency. Drug reactions are not simply drug allergy, but may result from variations in drug metabolism, immune status, coexistent diseases, and other medications simultaneously administered.

Kramer MS, et al: An algorithm for the operational assessment of adverse drug reactions. *JAMA* 1979, 242:623.

Rieder MJ: In vivo and in vitro testing for adverse drug reactions. *Pediatr Clin North Am* 1997, 44:93.

Rieder MJ: Mechanisms of unpredictable adverse drug reactions. *Drug Safety* 1994, 11:196.

Shear NH: Diagnosing cutaneous adverse reactions to drugs. *Arch Dermatol* 1990, 126:94.

Wolkenstein P, et al: Metabolic predisposition to cutaneous adverse drug reactions. *Arch Dermatol* 1995, 131:544. _____ ▲

Clinical Morphology of Drug Reactions

Adverse drug reactions will initially be discussed by their morphologic pattern. In addition to the cutaneous eruption, some reaction patterns may be associated with other systemic symptoms or findings. Shear et al use the modifier "simple" to describe reactions without systemic symptoms or internal organ involvement and "complex" to describe those reactions with these findings. Complex reactions are also called "hypersensitivity syndromes," since the ancillary features of "complex" reactions are often a characteristic syndrome of findings (e.g., an infectious mononucleosis–like picture with anticonvulsant hypersensitivity reactions).

Drug reactions may cause cutaneous lesions and findings identical to a known disease or disorder. These may be of similar or disparate pathogenesis. For example, true serum sickness caused by the injection of foreign proteins such as antithymocyte globulin is associated with circulating immune complexes. Medications, notably cefaclor, induce a serum sickness–like illness, clinically extremely similar, but not associated with circulating immune complexes. The suffix "-like" is used to describe these syndromes with different or unknown pathogenesis but similar clinical features.

Exanthems (Morbilliform or Scarlatiniform Reactions)

These are the commonest form of adverse cutaneous eruption. They are characterized by erythema, often with small papules throughout. They tend to occur within the first 2 weeks of treatment but may appear later, or even within 10 days after the medication has been stopped. Lesions tend to appear first proximally, especially in the groin and axilla, generalizing within 1 or 2 days. Pruritus is usually prominent, helping to distinguish a drug eruption from a viral exanthem. Antibiotics, especially semisynthetic penicillins and sulfamethoxazole/trimethoprim, are the most common causes of this reaction pattern (Fig. 6-21). Ampicillin given during infectious mononucleosis and sulfamethoxazole/trimethoprim given to AIDS patients cause exanthems in a large proportion of patients treated.

Morbilliform reactions to amoxicillin appear to be mediated by helper T cells in a manner similar to allergic contact dermatitis and tuberculin reactions. Delayed readings (longer than 24 hours) of patch tests, prick tests, and intradermal tests may yield positive results, whereas immediate skin test readings and RAST tests are negative.

In the case of simple exanthems, treatment is supportive. The eruption may clear, even if the offending medication is continued. Topical steroidal medications and antihistamines may benefit and allow the course of therapy to be completed. Rechallenge may or may not result in the reappearance of the eruption. In HIV infection, and rarely, in persons with normal immune function, rechallenge may result in a more severe blistering reaction (erythema multiforme).

Complex exanthems or hypersensitivity syndromes are seen most commonly with anticonvulsants, and long-acting sulfonamides; less commonly with allopurinol, gold, dap-

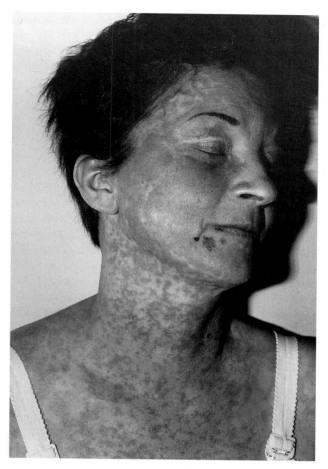

Fig. 6-21 Morbilliform drug eruption caused by sulfonamide.

sone, and sorbinil. They present with fever, rash, and variably, with eosinophilia, lymphadenopathy, hepatitis, nephritis, and rarely, involvement of the heart, lungs, or brain. The hepatitis may be life-threatening. As opposed to simple exanthems, in complex exanthems the inciting agent should be stopped. Their management is discussed in the following section.

Barbaud AM, et al: Role of delayed cellular hypersensitivity and adhesion molecules in amoxicillin-induced morbilliform rashes. *Arch Dermatol* 1997, 133:481.

de Shazo RD, et al: Allergic reactions to drugs and biological agents. *JAMA* 1997, 28:1895.

Prussick R, et al; Dapsone hypersensitivity syndrome. *J Am Acad Dermatol* 1996, 35:346.

Roujeau JC, et al: Severe adverse cutaneous reactions to drugs. *N Engl J Med* 1994, 331, 1272.

Wolverton SE: Update on cutaneous drug eruptions. *Adv Dermatol* 1997, 13:65. ▲

Anticonvulsant Hypersensitivity Syndrome

Anticonvulsant hypersensitivity syndrome can be seen with diphenylhydantoin, phenobarbital, carbamazepine, and other anticonvulsants, so the general term "anticonvulsant hypersensitivity syndrome" is preferred to the original descriptive terms such as "dilantin hypersensitivity syndrome" "phenobarbital hypersensitivity syndrome," etc. This eruption may occur in as many as 1 of 5000 patients treated with these medications. The frequent use of anticonvulsants such as carbamazepine to treat depression has greatly expanded the at-risk pool for these reactions.

The skin eruption is typically initially morbilliform, but may have variable morphologies in different patients or at various times in the same patient. There may be an eczema bullae, purpura, atypical targets, extensive skin sloughing and mucous membrane involvement resembling Stevens-Johnson syndrome or toxic epidermal necrolysis. The histologic picture of each type of eruption is compatible with the clinical morphology, and all are possible in this syndrome. The syndrome begins with fever between 2 and 6 weeks (average 3 weeks) after the offending medication is started. The eruption then appears, often with prominent facial swelling and sometimes with an acral accentuation. Associated with the eruption are findings similar to acute infectious mononucleosis. On physical examination, the patient usually appears quite ill with pharyngitis, lymphadenopathy (75% of cases) and sometimes hepatosplenomegaly. Laboratory evaluation reveals various combinations of eosinophilia (30% of cases), atypical lymphocytosis, elevated liver function tests (51% of cases), and less commonly nephritis (11% of cases). More sophisticated testing may demonstrate various immune abnormalities such as hyperglobulinemia, elevated suppressor T cells, defective cell-mediated immune function on skin testing, and various autoantibodies. Lymph node biopsies usually demonstrate reactive hyperplasia, but pseudolymphoma may also occur.

As the eruption evolves, it is typical for widespread pinpoint pustules to appear on the trunk and extremities, especially in dark skinned patients. Untreated the syndrome continues to progress, and the hepatitis can be life threatening.

The pathogenesis of this syndrome is related to the inability of affected individuals to detoxify arene oxide metabolites of these medications. These metabolites then apparently bind to proteins and elicit in susceptible individuals an immune response leading to an adverse drug reaction. The presence of this defect does not predict the severity of the skin reaction affecting the patient. This explains why there is a marked racial predilection for these cases to occur in blacks, and why the eruption typically occurs with the first exposure to the medication, as opposed to after several exposures in more typical morbilliform reactions. In addition, because many of the anticonvulsants are metabolized through the same pathway, cross-reactions are frequent, making selection of an alternative agent quite difficult. In vitro tests are commercially available and may aid in selecting an agent to which the patient will not cross-react. Generally, diphenylhydantoin, phenobarbital, and carbamazepine cross-react, whereas valproic acid does not.

The management of this syndrome begins with considering it in the appropriate setting and ruling out other infectious possibilities. The offending medication is immediately discontinued. Because cross-reactivity among these drugs is high, therapeutic value of a medication from this class must be carefully reconsidered. If the treatment is for depression, prophylaxis after closed head injury, or for atypical pain syndromes, medications from another class can often be substituted. Treatment is initially supportive until the extent and severity of the syndrome are assessed. Some patients clear with simply discontinuing the medication. If there is liver or renal involvement, or if the patient is ill appearing or requires hospitalization, and there is no contraindication, systemic steroids are given. This syndrome, independent of the skin eruption with which it presents, improves with systemic administration of steroids. Steroid therapy is continued at doses required for control and gradually tapered. It may require months of steroid therapy. If steroids are tapered too rapidly, the syndrome may recur.

Sulfonamide Hypersensitivity Syndrome

Sulfonamide hypersensitivity clinical syndrome is similar to that seen with the anticonvulsants. More commonly the patients develop a severe bullous reaction like Stevens-Johnson syndrome or toxic epidermal necrolysis. Patients with this syndrome are almost always slow acetylators who produce toxic hydroxylamine metabolites during metabolism of the sulfonamides.

Allopurinol Hypersensitivity Syndrome

Allopurinol hypersensitivity syndrome typically occurs in persons with preexisting renal failure, whose allopurinol dose is not adjusted for their renal function. Most commonly they are being treated for asymptomatic hyperuricemia. Weeks to months (average 7 weeks) after the allopurinol is begun, the patient develops a morbilliform eruption (50% of cases) that often evolves to an exfoliative erythroderma (20% of cases) (Fig. 6-22). Bullous eruptions including TEN (25% of cases) may also occur. Associated with the dermatitis is fever, eosinophilia, sometimes hepatitis, and typically worsening of the renal function. This syndrome may be steroid responsive, but is extremely slow to resolve, frequently lasting for months after the allopurinol has been stopped. About 25% of the patients die as a consequence of this syndrome. Dialysis does not appear to accelerate the resolution of the eruption, suggesting that if a drug metabolite is responsible, it is not dialyzable.

Arellano F, et al: Allopurinol hypersensitivity syndrome: a review. *Ann Pharmacother* 1993, 27:337.

Chang DKM, et al: Cutaneous reactions to anticonvulsants. *Semin Neurol* 1992, 12:329.

Handfield-Jones SE, et al: The anticonvulsant hypersensitivity syndrome. *Br J Dermatol* 1993, 129:175.

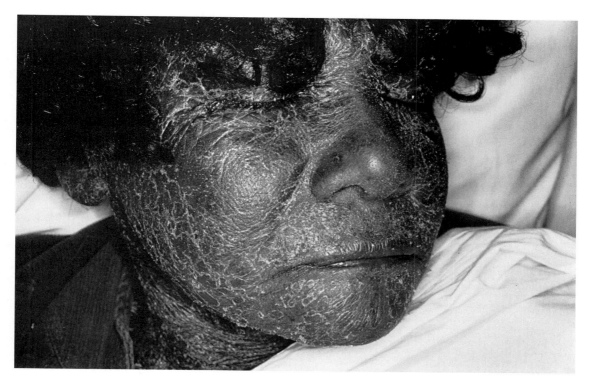

Fig. 6-22 Exfoliative dermatitis caused by allopurinol.

Knutsen AP, et al: Graft versus host-like illness in an child with phenobarbital hypersensitivity. *Pediatrics* 1968, 78:581.

Rieder MJ, et al: Diagnosis of sulfonamide hypersensitivity reactions in-vitro "rechallenge" with hydroxylamine metabolites. *Ann Intern Med* 1989, 110:286.

Silverman AK, et al: Cutaneous and immunologic reactions to phenytoin. *J Am Acad Dermatol* 1988, 18:721.

Travin M, et al: Reversible common variable immunodeficiency syndrome induced by phenytoin. *Arch Intern Med* 1989, 149:1421. ▲

Drug-Induced Pseudolymphoma

At times, exposure to medication may result in cutaneous inflammatory patterns that resemble lymphoma, most frequently mycosis fungoides. The finding of atypical lymphocytes within inflammatory infiltrates is common in many inflammatory dermatoses, including drug reactions, and this alone is insufficient to diagnose pseudolymphoma. The overall histology must be consistent with the diagnosis of lymphoma. These true pseudolymphoma reactions are uncommon or rare. The most frequent setting in which they occur is that of a hypersensitivity syndrome as described above, in which, uncommonly, the histology may resemble cutaneous T-cell lymphoma. Usually, other features such as keratinocyte necrosis and dermal edema help to distinguish these reactions from true lymphoma. Importantly, T-cell receptor gene rearrangements in the skin and blood may be positive in these drug-induced cases, representing a potential pitfall for the unwary physician. More rarely, medications may induce plaques or nodules, usually in elderly

white men after months of treatment. Lymphadenopathy and circulating Sézary cells may also be present. Pseudolymphoma resolves with discontinuation of the medication. The medication groups primarily responsible are anticonvulsants, sulfa drugs (including thiazide diuretics), dapsone, and antidepressants.

Aguilar JL, et al: Generalized cutaneous B-cell pseudolymphoma induced by neuroleptics. *Arch Dermatol* 1992, 128:121.

Braddock SW, et al: Generalized nodular cutaneous pseudolymphoma associated with phenytoin therapy. *J Am Acad Dermatol* 1992, 27:337.

Callot V, et al: Drug-induced pseudolymphoma and hypersensitivity syndrome. *Arch Dermatol* 1996, 132:1315.

De Ponti F, et al: Immunological adverse effects of anticonvulsants. *Drug Safety* 1993, 8:235.

D'Incan M, et al: Hydantoin-induced cutaneous pseudolymphoma with clinical, pathologic, and immunologic aspects of Sézary syndrome. *Arch Dermatol* 1992, 128:1371.

Harris DWS, et al: Phenytoin-induced pseudolymphoma. *Br J Dermatol* 1992, 127:403. ▲

Urticaria/Angioedema

Medications may induce urticaria by immunologic and nonimmunologic mechanisms. In either case, clinically the lesions are pruritic wheals or angioedema. Urticaria may be a part of a more severe anaphylactic reaction with bronchospasm, laryngospasm, or hypotension. Immediate hypersensitivity skin testing and sometimes RAST tests are useful in evaluating risk for these patterns of reaction.

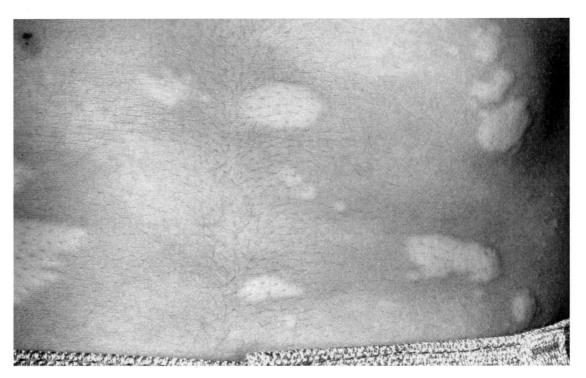

Fig. 6-23 Urticaria caused by amoxicillin.

Aspirin and the nonsteroidal antiinflammatory drugs (NSAIDs) are the most common causes of nonimmunologic urticarial reactions. They alter prostaglandin metabolism, enhancing degranulation of mast cells. They may therefore also exacerbate chronic urticaria of other causes. The nonacetylated salicylates (Trilisate and salsalate) do not cross-react with aspirin in patients experiencing bronchospasm and may be safe alternatives. Other agents causing nonimmunologic urticaria include radiocontrast material, opiates, tubocurarine, and polymyxin B. Pretesting does not exclude the possibility of anaphylactoid reaction to radiocontrast material. The use of low-osmolarity radiocontrast material and pretreatment with antihistamines, systemic steroids, and in those with a history of asthma, theophylline, may reduce the likelihood of reaction to radiocontrast material.

Immunologic urticaria is most commonly associated with penicillin and related beta-lactam antibiotics. It is associated with IgE antibodies to penicillin or its metabolites. Skin testing with penicillin and its major and minor determinants is useful in evaluating patients with a history of urticaria associated with penicillin exposure. If the patient is skin test positive, an alternative antibiotic must be considered, or the patient be given penicillin in a desensitization protocol. Most patients with a history of penicillin "allergy" are skin test negative. These patients can be treated with penicillin with a low likelihood of a severe adverse event. If a semisynthetic penicillin was associated with the initial reaction, the patient may be skin test negative to the standard penicillin-derived reagents and still suffer anaphylaxis. This may be caused by IgE antibodies directed against the acyl side-chain, in the case of amoxicillin (Fig. 6-23). Patients with penicillin allergy have an increased rate of reaction to cephalosporins. In the case of cefaclor, half of anaphylactic reactions occur in patients with a history of penicillin allergy. Third-generation cephalosporins are much less likely to induce a reaction in a penicillin allergic patient than are first- or second-generation ones.

Angioedema is a known complication of the use of angiotensin-converting enzyme (ACE) inhibitors (Fig. 6-24). Blacks are at nearly five times greater risk than whites. Lisinopril and enalapril produce angioedema more commonly than captopril. The episodes may be severe, requiring hospitalization in up to 45% of patients, intensive care in up to 27%, and intubation in up to 18%. One quarter of patients affected give a history of previous angioedema. Captopril enhances the flare reaction around wheals. The angioedema appears to be dose dependent, as it may resolve with decreased dose. All these factors suggest that the angioedema may represent a consequence of a normal pharmacologic effect of the ACE inhibitors. The blocking of kininase II by ACE inhibitors may increase tissue kinin levels, enhancing urticarial reactions and angio-

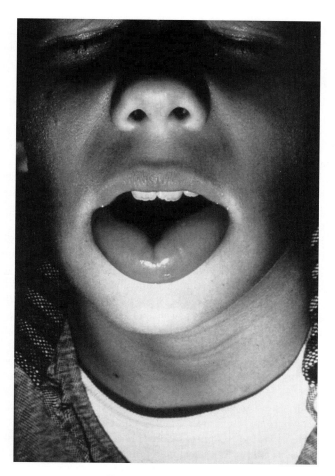

Fig. 6-24 Angioedema.

edema. Although this is dose dependent, ACE inhibitor users with one episode of angioedema have a tenfold risk of a second episode, and the recurrent episodes may be more severe.

Red Man Syndrome

The intravenous infusion of vancomycin is frequently complicated by a characteristic reaction called "red man syndrome." At any time during the infusion, a macular eruption appears initially on the back of the neck, sometimes spreading to the upper trunk, face and arms. Angioedema has been described. There is associated pruritus and "heat" as well as hypotension. The hypotension may be severe enough to cause cardiac arrest. The reaction is caused by elevated blood histamine. Red man syndrome can be prevented in most patients by reducing the rate of infusion of the antibiotic, or by pretreatment with H_1 antihistamines.

Brown NJ, et al: Recurrent angiotensin-converting enzyme inhibitor-associated angioedema. *JAMA* 1997, 278:232.

Israili ZH, et al: Cough and angioneurotic edema associated with angiotensin-converting enzyme inhibitor therapy. *Ann Intern Med* 1992, 117:234.

Lin RY: A perspective on penicillin allergy. *Arch Intern Med* 1992, 152:930.

Martin JA, et al: Allergy to amoxicillin in patients who tolerated benzylpenicillin, aztreonam, and ceftazidime. *Clin Infect Dis* 1992, 14:592.

Sogn DD, et al: Results of the National Institute of Allergy and Infectious Diseases collaborative clinical trial to test the predictive value of skin testing with major and minor penicillin derivatives in hospitalized adults. *Arch Intern Med* 1992, 152:1025.

Wallace MR, et al: Red man syndrome: incidence, etiology, and prophylaxis. *J Infect Dis* 1991, 164:1180. _____ ▲

Photosensitivity Reactions (Photosensitive Drug Reactions)

Medications may cause phototoxic (sunburnlike) reactions, photoallergic reactions, lichenoid reactions, as well as pseudoporphyria. The mechanisms of photosensitivity are discussed in Chapter 3. In many cases the mechanism for drug-induced photosensitivity is unknown. Most medication-related photosensitivity is triggered by radiation in the UVA range, partly for two reasons. First, most photosensitizing drugs have absorption spectra in the UVA range, and second, UVA penetrates into the dermis where the photosensitizing drug is present. The most common causes of photosensitivity are NSAIDs, sulfamethoxazole/ trimethoprim, thiazide diuretics and related sulfonylureas, quinine and quinidine, and certain tetracyclines.

Phototoxic reactions are related to the dose of both the medication and the ultraviolet irradiation. It potentially could occur in anyone if sufficient thresholds are reached, and does not require prior exposure or participation by the immune system. Reactions can appear from hours to days after to exposure. Tetracyclines (especially demeclocycline), amiodarone, and the NSAIDs are common culprits. Treatment may include dose reduction and photoprotection.

Photoallergic reactions are typically eczematous, pruritic, and occur after some period of drug exposure. They involve the immune system, and are confirmed by positive photopatch testing. In general, photoallergic reactions are not as drug dose dependent as phototoxic reactions. Photosensitivity both of the phototoxic and photoallergic types may persist for some period after the medication has been stopped. Photosensitivity reactions to various drugs are discussed individually below, emphasizing the characteristic patterns seen with that medication group.

Amiodarone photosensitivity develops in 75% of treated patients, and occurs after a cumulative dose of 40 g. A reduced MED to UVA, but not UVB occurs, and gradually returns to normal between 12 and 24 months after stopping the medication. Stinging and burning may occur as soon as a half hour after sun exposure. Clinically a dusky, blue-red erythema of the face and dorsa of the hands is most common, but papular reactions are also seen. Desquamation, as seen following sunburn, is not observed following amiodarone photosensitivity reactions.

NSAIDs, especially piroxicam, are frequently associated with photosensitivity. The characteristic reaction is a vesicular eruption of the dorsa of the hands, sometimes associated with a dyshidrosiform pattern on the lateral aspects of the hands and fingers. In severe cases even the palms may be involved. Histologically, this reaction pattern shows intraepidermal spongiosis, exocytosis, and perivascular inflammatory cells—a pattern typical of photoallergy. However, this reaction may occur on the initial exposure to the medication, and phototoxicity tests in animals and man have been negative. Patients with photosensitivity to piroxicam may also react to thiosalicylic acid, a common sensitizer in thimerosal. Half of patients having a positive patch test result to thimerosal with no prior exposure to piroxicam are photopatch test positive to piroxicam. This suggests that piroxicam reactions seen on initial exposure to the medication may be related to sensitization during prior thimerosal exposure.

Sulfonamide antibiotics, related hypoglycemic agents, and the sulfonylurea diuretics may all be associated with photoallergic reactions. These agents may all cross-react. In addition, patients may tolerate one of the medications from this group, but when additional members of the group are added, clinical photosensitivity occurs. The typical pattern is erythema, scale, and in chronic cases, lichenification and hyperpigmentation.

Photodistributed lichenoid reactions have been reported most commonly from thiazide diuretics, quinidine, and NSAIDs. They present as erythematous patches and plaques. Sometimes, typical Wickham's stria are observed in the lesions. Histologically, photodistributed lichenoid reactions are often indistinguishable from idiopathic lichen planus.

Pseudoporphyria is a photodistributed bullous reaction clinically and histologically resembling porphyria cutanea tarda. Hypertrichosis, skin fragility, dyspigmentation, and sclerodermoid changes are not seen. Porphyrin studies are normal and the reaction resolves on discontinuation of the provoking medication. Naproxen is the most commonly reported cause, but similar bullous reactions have been reported to tetracycline, furosemide, nalidixic acid, dapsone, nabumetone, and pyridoxine. Histologically, a pauci-inflammatory subepidermal vesicle is seen. Direct immunofluorescence may show IgG and complement deposition at the dermoepidermal junction and perivascularly, as seen in porphyria cutanea tarda. This histologic resemblance to "cell-poor" pemphigoid has resulted in these reactions being reported as drug induced bullous pemphigoid.

Gould JW, et al: Cutaneous photosensitivity diseases induced by exogenous agents. *J Am Acad Dermatol* 1995, 33:551.

West AD, et al: A comparative histopathologic study of photodistributed and nonphotodistributed lichenoid drug eruptions. *J Am Acad Dermatol* 1990, 23:689. _____ ▲

Anticoagulant-Induced Skin Necrosis

Both warfarin and heparin induce lesions of cutaneous necrosis, albeit by different mechanisms. Obese, postmenopausal women are predisposed, and lesions tend to occur in areas with abundant subcutaneous fat such as the breast, abdomen, or buttocks.

Warfarin necrosis occurs 3 to 5 days after therapy is begun, and higher initial dose increases the risk. It occurs in 1 in 10, 000 persons treated with warfarin. Lesions begin as red, painful plaques that become necrotic (Fig. 6-25). Hereditary or acquired deficiency of protein C and less commonly protein S is associated. Persons are usually asymptomatic heterozygotes with protein C deficiency. Early in warfarin treatment the hepatically produced antithrombotic factors fall to lower levels, especially if already low, leading to a transient hypercoagulable state. This explains why the syndrome is not always reproducible and has been reported to resolve with continued treatment. Histologically, noninflammatory thrombosis with fibrin in the subcutaneous vessels is seen. Treatment is to stop the warfarin, administer vitamin K to reverse the warfarin, and to administer purified protein C, which will rapidly reverse the syndrome. Untreated, the reaction can be fatal.

Heparin induces necrosis both at the sites of local injections and in a widespread pattern when infused intravenously. Local reactions are the most common. Heparin can also induce local allergic reactions at injection sites, which are distinct from the necrosis syndrome. Independent of its method of delivery lesions present as tender red plaques that undergo necrosis, usually 6 to 12 days after the heparin treatments are started. Bovine heparin appears to be more likely to cause the reaction, but it can occur with porcine heparin, and even fractionated low–molecular-weight heparin. Both low- and high-dose heparin therapy can produce the syndrome. Even the heparin used for dialysis may be associated with cutaneous necrosis, simulating calciphylaxis. Some necrotic reactions to local injections, and most disseminated reactions occurring with intravenous heparin are associated with heparin-induced thrombocytopenia. A heparin-dependent anti-platelet antibody is often found, which aggregates platelets. This causes both the thrombocytopenia and aggregation of platelets in vessels, causing thrombosis (white clot syndrome). Histologically, fibrin thrombi are less reproducibly found in affected tissues, since the vascular thrombosis is the result of platelet aggregation, not protein deposition. The process may produce not only infarcts in the skin but may also cause arterial thrombosis of the limbs, heart, lung, and brain resulting in significant morbidity or mortality. The syndrome must be recognized immediately in anyone receiving heparin with late-developing thrombocytopenia. The treat-

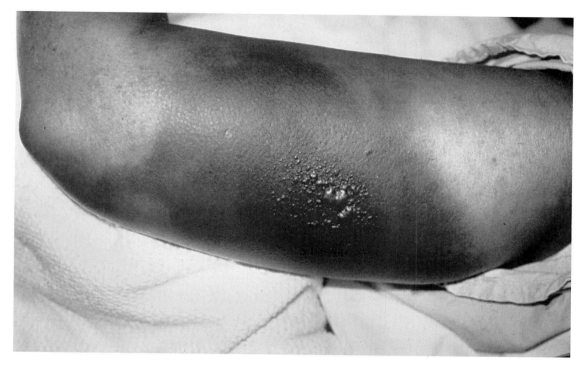

Fig. 6-25 Warfarin-induced necrosis.

ment is to stop the heparin and treat with warfarin if anticoagulation is still required.

Vitamin K Reactions

One to 2 weeks after injection of vitamin K, an allergic reaction at the site of injection may occur (Fig. 6-26). Most affected persons have liver disease and are being treated for elevated prothrombin times. The lesions are pruritic, red plaques that are deep-seated involving the dermis and subcutaneous tissue. There may be superficial vesiculation. Lesions occur most commonly on the posterior arm and over the hip or buttocks. Plaques on the hip tend to progress around the waist and down the thigh, forming a "cowboy gunbelt and holster" pattern. Generalized eczematous small papules may occur on other skin sites in severe reactions. These reactions usually persist for 1 to 3 weeks, but may persist longer, or resolve only to spontaneously recur. On testing, patients with this pattern of reaction are positive on intradermal testing to the pure vitamin K, not to the components of the material.

In Europe, a second pattern of vitamin K reaction has been reported. Subcutaneous sclerosis with or without fasciitis appears at the site of injections many months after vitamin K treatment. There may have been a preceding acute reaction as described above. Peripheral eosinophilia may be found. These pseudoscleroedermatous reactions have been termed *Texier's disease*, and last several years.

Injection Site Reactions

In addition to allergic reactions, as described with vitamin K, cutaneous necrosis may occur at sites of medication injections. These are of two typical forms—those associated with intravenous infusions and those related to intramuscular injections. Pharmacologic agents that extravasate into tissue during intravenous infusion may cause local tissue necrosis resulting from inherent tissue-toxic properties (Fig. 6-27). These include chemotherapeutic agents, calcium salts, radiocontrast material, and nafcillin.

Intramuscular injections may produce a syndrome called *embolia cutis medicamentosa* or *Nicolau syndrome*. Immediately after injection there is local intense pain, and the overlying skin blanches (ischemic pallor). Within minutes to hours the site develops an erythematous macule that evolves into a livedoid violaceous patch with dendrites. This becomes hemorrhagic, then ulcerates, and eventually (over weeks to months) heals with an atrophic scar. Muscle and liver enzymes may be elevated, and neurologic symptoms and sequela occur in a third of patients. The circulation of the limb may be affected, rarely leading to amputation. This syndrome has been described with many unrelated agents. It appears to be caused by periarterial injection leading to arterial thrombosis. Treatment is conservative: dressing changes, debridement, bed rest, and pain control. Surgical intervention is rarely required.

Brunskill NJ, et al: Pseudosclerodermatous reaction to phytomenadione injection (Texier's syndrome). *Clin Exp Dermatol* 1988, 13:276.

Chang JC: White clot syndrome associated with heparin-induced thrombocytopenia: a review of 23 cases. *Heart Lung* 1987, 16:403.

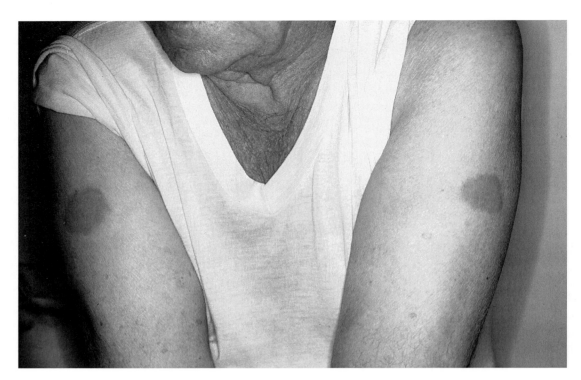

Fig. 6-26 Allergic reaction at site of vitamin K injection.

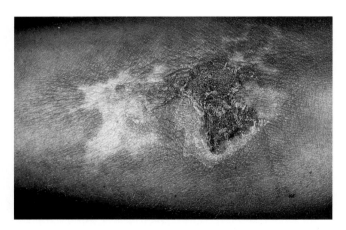

Fig. 6-27 Cutaneous reaction to intravenous infusion and extravasation of chemotherapeutic agent.

Hermes B, et al: Immunopathological events of adverse cutaneous reactions to coumarin and heparin. *Acta Derm Venereol* (Stockh) 1997, 77:35.

Mallory SB, et al: Nicolau syndrome. *Pediatr Dermatol* 1995, 12:187.

Sanders MN, et al: Cutaneous reactions to vitamin K. *J Am Acad Dermatol* 1988, 19:699.

Tonn ME, et al: Enoxaparin-associated dermal necrosis: a consequence of cross-reactivity with heparin-mediated antibodies. *Ann Pharmacother* 1997, 31:323. ───────────────── ▲

Acute Generalized Exanthematous Pustulosis

Acute generalized exanthematous pustulosis (AGEP, toxic pustuloderma, pustular drug eruption) is a not uncommon cutaneous reaction pattern that in 90% of cases are related to medication administration. The eruption is of sudden onset and appears an average of 5 days (2.5 days in antibiotic-induced cases) after the medication is started—in 50% of cases within the first 24 hours. Mercury is the sole cause in 13% of cases in France, beta-lactams in 44%, and macrolides in 17%. Sulfonamides have not been reported to cause this reaction. AGEP should also be distinguished from the generalized pustulation that occurs in the evolution of anticonvulsant hypersensitivity syndrome. Seventeen percent of patients have a prior history of psoriasis, and similar cases have been reported as acute psoriasis induced by medications. The course and evolution are different from true pustular psoriasis, although patients with psoriasis may be at increased risk for this form of drug reaction.

Initially there is a scarlatiniform erythema. The eruption evolves and disseminates rapidly, consisting of usually more than 100 nonfollicular pustules less than 5 mm in diameter. The Nikolsky sign may be positive, and widespread superficial desquamation occurs after a few days. Edema of the face, purpura, and target lesions as in erythema multiforme (EM) may appear in the background. Mucous membranes, usually the oral mucosa, are involved in 22%. Fever is universal, with neutrophilia in 90% and eosinophilia in 30%. Liver function tests are usually normal. Once the inciting agent is discontinued or removed, the eruption resolves within 15 days without sequelae. Patch testing with the suspected agent may reproduce a pustular eruption on an erythematous base at 48 hours. Histologically, early lesions show marked papillary edema, neutrophil clusters in the dermal papillae, and perivascular eosinophils. There may be an associated leukocytoclastic vasculitis. Well-developed lesions show intraepidermal or subcorneal spongiform pustules. If there is a background of EM clinically, the histologic features of EM may be superimposed. The presence of eosinophils, and the marked papillary edema help to distinguish this eruption from pustular psoriasis.

Burrows NP, et al: Pustular drug eruptions: a histopathological spectrum. *Histopathology* 1993, 22:593.

Moreau A, et al: Drug-induced acute generalized exanthematous pustulosis with positive patch tests. *Int J Dermatol* 1995, 34:263.

Roujeau JC, et al: Acute generalized exanthematous pustulosis. *Arch Dermatol* 1991, 127:1333.

Watsky KL: AGEP induced by metronidazole. *Arch Dermatol* 1999, 135:93. ▲

Drug-Induced Pigmentation

Pigmentation of the skin may occur as a consequence of drug administration. The mechanism may be postinflammatory hyperpigmentation in some cases but frequently is related to actual deposition of the offending drug in the skin.

Minocycline induces many types of hyperpigmentation, which may occur in various combinations in the affected patient. Classically, three types of pigmentation are described. The most common is a blue-black discoloration appearing in areas of prior inflammation, often acne or surgical scars. It does not appear to be related to the total dose or daily dose of exposure. In all other types of pigmentation resulting from minocycline the incidence increases with total dose, with approximately 4% of treated patients experiencing hyperpigmentation at a cumulative dose of 100 g. The second type is the appearance of a similar-colored pigmentation on the normal skin of the anterior shins, analogous to that seen in antimalaria-induced hyperpigmentation. It is initially mistaken for ecchymoses but does not fade quickly. In these two types of pigmentation, histologic evaluation reveals pigment granules within macrophages in the dermis, very similar to a tattoo. These granules usually stain positively for both iron and melanin, the usual method for confirming the diagnosis. In unusual cases electron microscopy or sophisticated chemical analysis can confirm the presence of minocycline in the granules. The least common pattern is generalized, muddy brown hyperpigmentation, accentuated in sun-exposed areas. Histologic examination reveals only increased epidermal and dermal melanin. This may represent the consequence of a low-grade photosensitivity reaction. In addition to the skin, minocycline may deposit in the sclera, conjunctiva, bone, thyroid, ear cartilage, nail bed, oral mucosa, and permanent teeth. Contrasted with tetracycline staining of the teeth, which is usually related to childhood or fetal exposure, is brown, and is accentuated on the gingival third, minocycline hyperpigmentation occurs in adults, is gray or gray-green,

and is most marked in the midportion of the tooth. Most patients with affected teeth do not have hyperpigmentation elsewhere. Cutaneous hyperpigmentation from minocycline fades slowly, and the teeth may remain pigmented for years. The blue-gray pigmentation of the skin may be improved with the Q-switched ruby laser.

Chloroquine, hydroxychloroquine, and quinacrine all may cause a blue-black pigmentation of the face, extremities, ear cartilage, oral mucosa, and nails. Pretibial hyperpigmentation is the most common pattern, and is very similar to that induced by minocycline. The gingiva or hard palate may also be discolored. Quinidine may also rarely cause such a pattern of hyperpigmentation. Quinacrine is yellow and is concentrated in the epidermis. Generalized yellow discoloration of the skin and sclera (mimicking jaundice) occurs reproducibly in patients but fades within 4 months after stopping the drug. In dark-skinned patients this color is masked and not so significant cosmetically. Histologically, in both forms of pigmentation, pigment granules are present within macrophages in the dermis.

Amiodarone after 3 to 6 months causes photosensitivity in 30% to 57% of treated patients. In 1% to 10% of patients, a slate-gray hyperpigmentation develops in the areas of photosensitivity. The pigmentation gradually fades after the medication is discontinued. Histologically, periodic acid–Schiff positive yellow-brown granules are seen within the cytoplasm of macrophages in the dermis. Electron microscopy reveals membrane-bound structures resembling lipid-containing lysosomes. It responds to treatment with the Q-switched ruby laser.

Clofazimine treatment is reproducibly complicated by the appearance of a pink discoloration that gradually becomes reddish blue or brown and is concentrated in the lesions of patients with Hansen's disease. This pigmentation may be very disfiguring and is a major cause of noncompliance with this drug in the treatment of Hansen's disease. Histologically, a periodic acid–Schiff positive brown, granular pigment is variably seen within foamy macrophages in the dermis. This has been called "drug-induced lipofuscinosis."

Zidovudine causes a blue or brown hyperpigmentation that is most frequently observed in the nails. The lunula may be blue, or the whole nail plate may become dark brown. Diffuse hyperpigmentation of the skin, pigmentation of the lateral tongue, and increased tanning are less common. It occurs in darkly pigmented persons, is dose dependent, and clears after the medication is discontinued.

Chlorpromazine, thioridazine, imipramine, and clomipramine may cause a slate-gray hyperpigmentation in sun-exposed areas after long periods of ingestion (Fig. 6-28). Frequently, corneal and lens opacities are also present, so all patients with hyperpigmentation from these medications should have an ophthalmologic evaluation. The pigmentation from the phenothiazines fades gradually over years, even if the patient is treated with another phenothiazine.

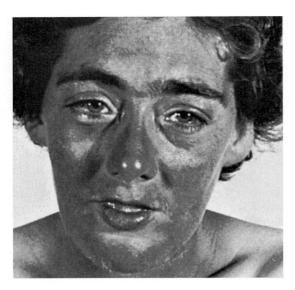

Fig. 6-28 Purple pigmentation in patient who had been on high doses of chlorpromazine. Note sparing of deep creases of the face. (From Satanove A: *JAMA* 191:263, 1965.)

The corneal, but not the lenticular, changes also resolve. Imipramine hyperpigmentation has been reported to disappear within a year. Histologically, in sun-exposed but not sun-protected skin, numerous refractile golden-brown granules are present within macrophages in the dermis along with increased dermal melanin. The slate-gray color comes from a mixture of the golden-brown pigment of the drug and the black color of the melanin viewed in the dermis.

The heavy metals gold, silver, and bismuth produce blue to slate-gray hyperpigmentation. Pigmentation occurs after years of exposure, predominantly in sun-exposed areas, and is permanent. Bismuth also pigments the gingival margin. Histologically, granules of the metals are seen in the dermis and around blood vessels. Arsenical melanosis is characterized by black, generalized pigmentation or by a pronounced truncal hyperpigmentation that spares the face, with depigmented scattered macules that resemble raindrops.

Pigmentary changes induced by chemotherapeutic agents are discussed later is this chapter.

Fitzpatrick JE: New histopathologic findings in drug eruptions. *Dermatol Clin* 1992, 10:19.

Hashimoto K, et al: Imipramine hyperpigmentation: a slate-gray discoloration caused by long-term imipramine administration. *J Am Acad Dermatol* 1991, 25:357.

Hendrix JD, et al: Cutaneous hyperpigmentation caused by systemic drugs. *Int J Dermatol* 1992, 31:458.

Karrer S, et al: Amiodarone-induced pigmentation resolves after treatment with the Q-switched ruby laser. *Arch Dermatol* 1999, 135:251.

Knoell KA, et al: Treatment of minocycline-induced hyperpigmentation with the Q-switched ruby laser. *Arch Dermatol* 1996, 132:1250.

Sicari MC, et al: Photoinduced dermal pigmentation in patients taking tricyclic antidepressants. *J Am Acad Dermatol* 1999, 40:290. ▲

Vasculitis and Serum Sickness–Like Reactions

True leukocytoclastic vasculitis can be induced by many medications, but these events are rare, except in the case of propylthiouracil. True serum sickness is caused by foreign proteins such as antithymocyte globulin. They are caused by circulating immune complexes. In the case of true serum sickness there is a tendency for purpuric lesions to be accentuated along the junction between palmoplantar and glabrous skin (Wallace's line).

Serum sickness–like reactions refer to adverse reactions that have similar symptoms to serum sickness, but in which immune complexes are not found. The use of cefaclor for the treatment of an upper respiratory infection or otitis media in children under age 5 is complicated by a specific hypersensitivity reaction in 3.4% of cases beginning about 1 week into cefaclor therapy. This reaction presents in the skin with urticarial plaques that progress to have dusky centers (misdiagnosed as erythema multiforme). Pruritus is common, as well as acral edema and swollen, painful joints of the hands and feet. The mucous membranes are spared. The eruption rapidly resolves without sequelae once the cefaclor is discontinued. In vitro testing may document enhanced lymphocyte toxicity in affected patients, suggesting a metabolic basis similar to anticonvulsant hypersensitivity syndrome.

Stricker BH, et al: Serum sickness-like reactions to cefaclor. *J Clin Epidemiol* 1992, 45:1177.

Vial T, et al: Cefaclor-associated serum sickness–like disease. *Ann Pharmacother* 1992, 26:910. ▲

Fixed Drug Reactions

Fixed drug reactions are common, being as frequent as exanthems in some large series. Fixed eruptions are so named because they recur at the same site with each exposure to the medication. Six or fewer lesions occur, frequently only one. They may present anywhere on the body, but half of fixed eruptions occur on the oral and genital mucosa. Fixed eruptions represent 2% of all genital ulcers evaluated at clinics for sexually transmitted diseases.

Clinically, a fixed eruption begins as a red patch that soon evolves to an iris or target lesion identical to erythema multiforme, and may eventually blister and erode (Fig. 6-29). Lesions of the genital and oral mucosa usually present as erosions. Characteristically, prolonged or permanent postinflammatory hyperpigmention results. With repeated or continued ingestion of the offending medication, new lesions may be added, sometimes eventuating in a clinical picture similar to drug induced erythema multiforme major. Histologically, an interface dermatitis occurs with intraepidermal and subepidermal vesicle formation, necrosis of keratinocytes, and a mixed superficial and deep infiltrate of neutrophils, eosinophils, and mononuclear cells.

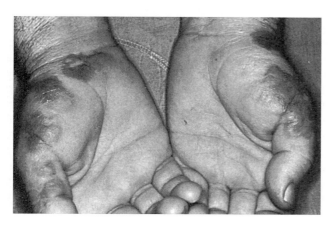

Fig. 6-29 Fixed eruption caused by phenolphthalein.

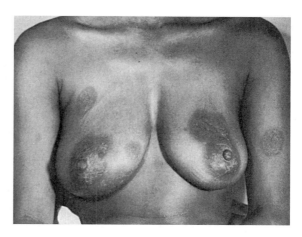

Fig. 6-31 Fixed eruption caused by phenolphthalein.

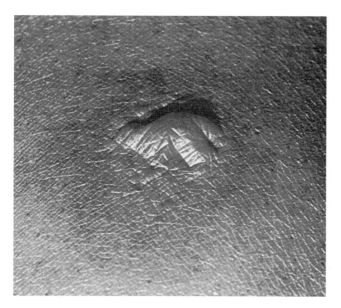

Fig. 6-30 Fixed eruption caused by sulfamethoxazole (Septra).

Pigment incontinence is usually marked, correlating with the pigmentation resulting from fixed drug eruptions.

Medications inducing fixed drug eruptions are usually those taken intermittently. Many of the NSAIDs, especially pyrazolone derivatives, naproxen, and mefenamic acid; and sulfonamides, trimethoprim, or the combination are now responsible for the majority of fixed drug eruptions (Fig. 6-30). Barbiturates, tetracyclines, phenolphthalein (in laxatives), and erythromycin are other possible causes (Fig. 6-31). The pathogenesis is unknown, but persons with fixed eruptions to pyrazolone derivatives are much more likely to be HLA-B22 positive. Inadomi et al modified the topical provocation method of Alanko by tape stripping the skin before applying the suspected medication in various vehicles to the sites of previous reactions. Previously

unaffected skin does not react. This technique appears to be most useful in pyrazolone derivative related reactions that are reproduced in 85% or more of cases.

Occasionally, fixed drug reactions do not result in long-lasting hyperpigmentation. The so-called nonpigmenting fixed drug eruption is distinctive. It is characterized by large, tender, often symmetrical erythematous plaques that resolve completely within weeks, only to recur on reingestion of the offending drug. Pseudoephedrine hydrochloride is by far the most common culprit. Krivda et al list others. Helmbold et al classify the baboon syndrome, where the buttocks, groin, and axilla are preferentially involved in this category.

Alanko K, et al: Topical provocation of fixed drug eruption. *Br J Dermatol* 1987, 116:561.

Helmbold P, et al: Symmetric ptychotropic and nonpigmenting fixed drug eruption due to cimetidine (so-called baboon syndrome). *Dermatology* 1998, 197:402.

Inadomi T, et al: Application of tape-stripping patch test for allopurinol-induced fixed drug eruption. *Eur J Dermatol* 1995, 5:28.

Korkij W, et al: Fixed drug reaction. *Arch Dermatol* 1984, 120:520.

Krivda SJ, et al: Nonpigmenting fixed drug eruption. *J Am Acad Dermatol* 1994, 31:291.

Pellicano R, et al: Genetic susceptibility to fixed drug eruption: evidence for link with HLA-B22. *J Am Acad Dermatol* 1994, 30:52.

Sowden JM, et al: Multifocal fixed drug eruption mimicking erythema multiforme. *Clin Exp Dermatol* 1990, 15:387.

Teraki Y, et al: Drug-induced expression of intercellular adhesion molecule-1 on lesional keratinocytes in fixed drug eruption. *Am J Pathol* 1994, 145:550. ▲

Lichenoid Reactions

Lichenoid reactions can be seen with many medications, but are commonly induced by gold, hydrochlorothiazide, NSAIDs, d-penicillamine, captopril, quinidine and the antimalarials. They may be photodistributed (lichenoid photoeruption) or generalized, and those drugs causing lichenoid photoeruptions may also induce more generalized ones. In either case, the lesions may be plaques (occasionally with Wickham's striae), small papules, or exfoliative erythema. Photolichenoid reactions favor the extensor extremities including the dorsa of the hands. Oral involvement is less common in lichenoid drug reactions than in idiopathic lichen planus but can occur. It appears as either plaques or erosions. The lower lip is frequently involved in photolichenoid reactions. Histologically, there is inflammation along the dermoepidermal junction, with necrosis of keratinocytes and a dermal infiltrate composed primarily of lymphocytes. Eosinophils are useful if present, but are not common in photolichenoid reactions. The histology is often very similar to idiopathic lichen planus, and a clinical correlation is required to determine if the lichenoid eruption is drug induced.

Lichenoid reactions may be restricted to the oral mucosa, especially if induced by dental amalgam. In these cases the lesions are topographically related to the dental fillings or to metal prostheses, and mercury or gold will produce positive patch test results. An unusual form of eruption is the "drug-induced ulceration of the lower lip." Patients present with a persistent erosion of the lower lip that is tender but not indurated. It is induced by diuretics and resolves slowly once they are discontinued.

Laine J, et al: Contact allergy to dental restoration materials in patients with oral lichenoid lesions. *Contact Dermatitis* 1997, 36:141.

McCartan BE, et al: Oral lichenoid drug eruptions. *Oral Dis* 1997, 3:58.

Van den Haute V, et al: Histopathological discriminant criteria between lichenoid drug eruption and idiopathic lichen planus. *Dermatologica* 1989, 179:10.

West AD, et al: A comparative histopathologic study of photodistributed and nonphotodistributed lichenoid drug eruptions. *J Am Acad Dermatol* 1990, 23:689. ▲

Bullous Drug Reactions (Erythema Multiforme, Stevens-Johnson Syndrome, and Toxic Epidermal Necrolysis)

Skin blistering may complicate drug reactions in many ways. Medications may induce known autoimmune bullous diseases such as pemphigus (penicillamine) or linear IgA disease (vancomycin). Acute generalized exanthematous pustulosis may be so extensive as to cause a positive Nikolsky sign, and have a background of purpura and targetoid lesions, simulating erythema multiforme. Pseudoporphyria and other photodermatoses from drugs may form bullae. Cytokines may produce widespread bullous eruptions perhaps through physiologic mechanisms. Rarely, medications may induce subepidermal bullous eruptions with cleavage in the upper dermis by unknown cause. The term *bullous drug reaction*, however, most commonly refers to a drug reaction in the erythema multiforme (EM) group. (For a complete discussion of EM minor, see Chapter 7.)

These are fortunately uncommon reactions to medications, with an incidence of 0.4 to 1.2 per million person-years for toxic epidermal necrolysis (TEN) and 1.2 to 6.0 per million person years for Stevens-Johnson syndrome (SJS). Drug-induced EM is usually more extensive than that induced by infectious agents (except for *Mycoplasma*), but at times the distinction may be difficult. The more severe the reaction, the more likely it is to be definitely drug-induced (50% of cases of SJS and 80% of cases of TEN). The exact definitions of SJS and TEN remain arbitrary as a result of overlap in some cases. One group has proposed the following definitions: SJS has less than 10% body surface area involved, cases with 10% to 30% are overlap cases, and more than 30% is called TEN. Others call cases SJS if they begin with atypical purpuric targetoid lesions, whereas they are called TEN if they begin with skin pain and simple erythema that is rapidly followed by skin loss. Although definitions remain controversial, SJS and TEN probably represent parts of a disease spectrum based on the following: they are most commonly induced by the same medications; patients initially presenting with SJS may progress to extensive skin loss resembling TEN; the histologic findings are indistinguishable; both are increased by the same magnitude in HIV infection; and identical metabolic abnormalities are identified in cases induced by sulfonamides or anticonvulsants.

More than 100 medications have been reported to cause SJS and TEN. The most common are trimethoprim/sulfamethoxazole (1-3/100,000), Fansidar-R, sulfadoxine plus pyrimethamine, (10/100,000), and carbamazepine (14/100,000). Antibiotics (especially long-acting sulfa drugs and penicillins), other anticonvulsants, antiinflammatories (NSAIDs), and allopurinol are also common causes.

Fever and influenza-like symptoms often precede the eruption by a few days. Skin lesions appear on the face and trunk and rapidly spread (usually within 4 days) to their maximum extent (Fig. 6-32). Initial lesions are macular and may remain so, followed by desquamation, or may form atypical targets with purpuric centers that coalesce, form bullae, then slough (Figs. 6-33 and 6-34). Virtually always more than two mucosal surfaces are also eroded, the oral mucosa and conjunctiva being most frequently affected (Fig. 6-35). There may be difficulty with swallowing, photophobia, painful urination, and extensive respiratory and alimentary tract involvement.

A skin biopsy is usually performed. This is to exclude other diseases, and to confirm the diagnosis. Independent of the extent of the slough, the clinical morphology (atypical targets versus simple erythema), or the clinical diagnosis (SJS versus TEN), the histology is similar. There is a lymphocytic infiltrate at the dermoepidermal junction with necrosis of keratinocytes that at times may be full thickness. The infiltrate may be marked or very scant. Paraneoplastic pemphigus also shows changes of erythema multiforme and may be excluded with direct immunofluorescence. Patients with graft-versus host disease may also demonstrate a toxic epidermal necrolysis–like picture with identical histology.

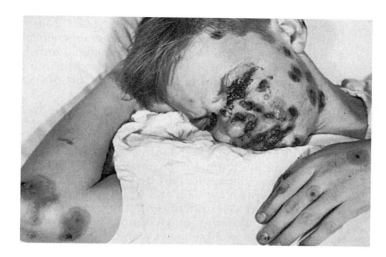

Fig. 6-32 Stevens-Johnson syndrome. Severe involvement of orifices is characteristic.

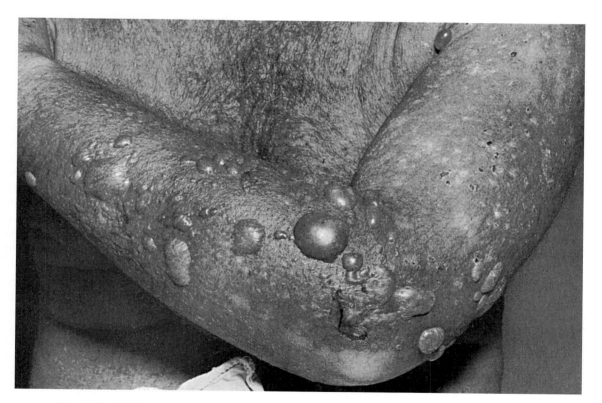

Fig. 6-33 Erythema multiforme bullosum. Note predilection for the arms, sparing the trunk unlike pemphigus.

Management of these patients is similar to an extensive burn. They suffer fluid and electrolyte imbalances, bacteremia from loss of protective skin barrier, hypercatabolism, and sometimes acute respiratory distress syndrome. Survival is improved if the patients are cared for in a specialized "burn unit." Patients who are very ill or with more than 30% to 50% loss of epidermis should be transferred for such care.

A recent report by Viard et al may help to solve the dilemma of treatment of these sick patients. They reported that intravenous immunoglobulin (IVIG) administered to 10 patients in doses up to 0.75 g/kg/day for 4 days led to response in 48 hours and skin healing within 1 week. No adverse reactions were observed. Because this response is dramatically better than that obtained with immunosuppressives, this will likely be the treatment of choice if subsequent reports verify this early experience. The mechanism of action of IVIG in this condition was block-

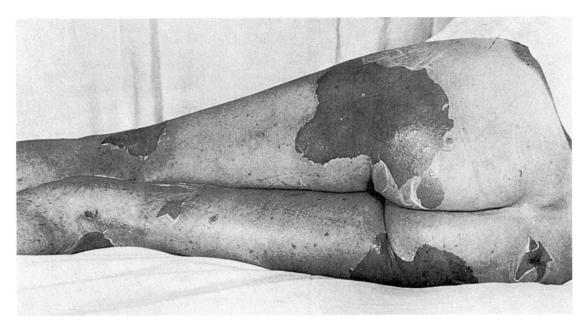

Fig. 6-34　Toxic epidermal necrolysis showing desquamation in sheets, leaving raw, red surface. (Courtesy Dr. A. Lyell.)

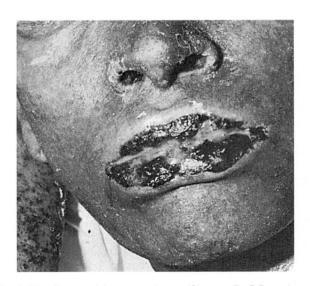

Fig. 6-35　Stevens-Johnson syndrome. (Courtesy Dr. F. Rosenberg.)

ing apoptosis through blockade of the death receptor FAS (CD 95).

The role of immunosuppressive therapy is very controversial in severe bullous drug eruptions. The benefit of immunosuppressives would be to stop the process very quickly to reduce the ultimate amount of skin lost. Once most of the skin loss has occurred, immunosuppressives only add to the morbidity and perhaps mortality of the disorder. In children, this adverse effect has been documented, probably since their mortality from severe bullous

drug eruptions is low. Because the condition evolves rapidly (average 4 days to maximum extent) very early treatment would be required to observe benefit. Patients have developed TEN while undergoing systemic corticosteroid therapy in moderate to high doses (40 to 60 mg of prednisone equivalent daily). Perhaps the therapeutic benefit is not seen at this range, but at higher doses, as is suggested by anecdotal reports of benefit with more potent immunosuppressive regimens. If immunosuppressive treatment is considered, it should be used as soon as possible, in adequate doses, given a short trial to see if the process may be arrested, and then tapered rapidly to avoid the risk of immunosuppression in a host with substantial loss of skin. As with burns, the host's age, severity of underlying disease, and extent of skin loss are the most important factors determining the outcome rather than the use of immunosuppressive agents.

In patients who survive, the average time for epidermal regrowth is 3 weeks. The most common sequelae are ocular scarring and vision loss. A siccalike syndrome may also result. Rarely, complications include cutaneous scarring, eruptive melanocytic lesions, and nail abnormalities. Mortality averages about 5% for patients with SJS and 30% for patients with TEN.

Radiation-Induced EM

If phenytoin is given prophylactically in neurosurgical patients who are receiving whole-brain radiation therapy and systemic steroids, an unusual reaction occurs. As the dose of steroids is being reduced, erythema and edema initially appear on the head in the radiation ports. This evolves over 1 or 2 days to lesions with the clinical appearance and histology of EM. The eruption spreads caudad and mucosal involvement may occur, eventuating in full-blown SJS. This syndrome can rarely be seen with radiation therapy alone, but is much more common if phenytoin is also administered.

Urticarial EM

Urticarial EM is an unusual reaction virtually always associated with antibiotic ingestion. The skin lesions consist of urticarial papules and plaques, some of which clear centrally forming annular lesions, but no true iris lesions. Lesions can be distinguished from true urticaria in that they are fixed for days. Pruritus is common. In contrast to true EM, the annular lesions are not dusky in the center, but rather clear to normal skin. Bullae are absent, and mucous membranes are not involved. Rarely, hypotension may occur, suggesting mast cell products are important in the production of this eruption. Histologically, there is a superficial and deep dermal infiltrate containing eosinophils with dermal edema. The epidermis is uninvolved. Response to systemic steroids is usually dramatic, with clearing in 48 to 72 hours.

Assler H, et al: EM with mucous membrane involvement and SJS are clinically different disorders with distinct causes. *Arch Dermatol* 1995, 131:539.

Bialy-Golan A, et al: Penicillamine-induced bullous dermatoses. *J Am Acad Dermatol* 1996, 35:732.

Breathnach SM, et al: Epidemiology of bullous drug eruptions. *Clin Dermatol* 1993, 11:441.

Chan HL, et al: The incidence of EM, SJS, and TEN. *Arch Dermatol* 1990, 126:43.

Delattre JV, et al: EM and SJS in patients receiving cranial irradiation and phenytoin. *Neurology* 1988, 38:194.

Dietrich A, et al: Low *N*-acetylating capacity in patients with Stevens-Johnson syndrome and toxic epidermal necrolysis. *Exp Dermatol* 1995, 4:313.

Duncan KO, et al: SJS limited to multiple sites of radiation therapy in a patient receiving phenobarbital. *J Am Acad Dermatol* 1999, 40:493.

Giannetti A, et al: Vesiculobullous drug eruptions in children. *Clin Dermatol* 1993, 11:551.

Krischer J, et al: Pseudoporphyria induced by nabumetone. *J Am Acad Dermatol* 1999, 40:492.

Laurencin CT, et al: SJS reaction with vancomycin treatment. *Ann Pharmacother* 1992, 26:1520.

Levy M, et al: Mycoplasma pneumoniae infections and SJS. *Clin Pediatr* 1991, 30:42.

Parsons JM: Toxic epidermal necrolysis. *Int J Dermatol* 1992, 31:749.

Roholt NS, et al: A nonscarring sublamina densa bullous drug eruption. *J Am Acad Dermatol* 1995, 32:367.

Roujeau JC: Drug-induced TEN. *Clin Dermatol* 1993, 11:493.

Roujeau JC: The spectrum of SJS and TEN. *J Invest Dermatol* 1994, 102:28S.

Roujeau JC, et al: Medication use and the risk of SJS or TEN. *N Engl J Med* 1995, 333:1600.

Roujeau JC, et al: Toxic epidermal necrolysis (Lyell syndrome). *J Am Acad Dermatol* 1990, 23:1039.

Rzany B, et al: Toxic epidermal necrolysis in patients receiving glucocorticosteroids. *Acta Derm Venereol* (Stockh) 1991, 71:171.

Viard I, et al: Inhibition of toxic epidermal necrolysis by blockade of CD95 with human intravenous immunoglobulin. *Science* 1998, 282:490. ▲

HIV Disease and Drug Reactions

HIV-infected patients, especially those with helper T-cell counts between 25 and 200, are at increased risk for the development of adverse reactions to medications. Morbilliform reactions to trimethoprim/sulfamethoxazole occur in 45% or more of AIDS patients being treated for *Pneumocystis carinii* pneumonia. Systemic corticosteroid administration reduces this reaction rate to less than 20%. In two of three patients without life-threatening reactions, trimethoprim/sulfamethoxazole treatment can be continued with simple conservative support, and the eruption may resolve. Associated hepatitis or neutropenia may require discontinuation of the drug. A similar increased rate of reaction to amoxicillin-clavulanate in HIV is also seen. If the dermatitis is treatment limiting, but the eruption is not life threatening, low-dose rechallenge/ desensitization may be attempted. It is successful in 65% to 85% of patients in the short term, and higher than 50% in the long term. In fact, initial introduction of trimethoprim/sulfamethoxazole for prophylaxis by dose escalation will reduce the rate of adverse reactions as well. Although low-dose rechallenge is usually safe, severe, acute reactions including marked hypotension may occur. Although most adverse reactions occur in the first few days of rechallenge, adverse reactions may appear months after restarting trimethoprim/sulfamethoxazole, and may be atypical in appearance. The mechanism of this increased adverse reaction to trimethoprim/sulfamethoxazole is unknown, but may be related to the fact that many AIDS patients are slow acetylators.

Severe bullous reactions, SJS, and TEN are between 100 and 1000 times more common per drug exposure in patients with AIDS. These reactions are usually caused by sulfa drugs, especially long acting ones, but may be caused by many agents. Fixed drug eruptions are also frequently seen in patients with HIV infection.

Acyclovir, nucleoside and nonnucleoside reverse transcriptase inhibitors, and protease inhibitors are uncommon causes of adverse drug reactions. Many reactions attributed to these agents may actually be coexistent HIV-associated pruritic disorders, especially folliculitis, which are very common in patients with AIDS.

Caumes E, et al: Efficacy and safety of desensitization with sulfamethoxazole and trimethoprim in 48 previously hypersensitive patients infected with HIV. *Arch Dermatol* 1997, 133:465.

Jung AC, et al: Management of adverse reactions to trimethoprim-sulfamethoxazole in HIV-infected patients. *Arch Intern Med* 1994, 154:2402.

Roudier C, et al: Adverse cutaneous reactions to trimethoprim-sulfamethoxazole in patients with AIDS and *Pneumocystis carinii* pneumonia. *Arch Dermatol* 1994, 130:1383. ▲

Adverse Reactions to Chemotherapeutic Agents

Chemotherapeutic agents can cause adverse reactions by multiple potential mechanisms. Adverse reactions may be related to toxicity either directly to the mucocutaneous surfaces (alopecia) or to some other organ system and reflected in the skin such as purpura resulting from thrombocytopenia. Being organic molecules in many cases, they can act as allergens inducing classic immunologic reactions. In addition, since they are inherently immunosuppressive, they can cause skin reactions associated with alterations of immune function. Some of these patterns may be overlapping and clinically difficult to distinguish. For example oral erosions may occur as a toxic effect of chemotherapy and also by immunosuppression-associated activation of herpes simplex virus.

Dermatologists are rarely confronted with the relatively common acute hypersensitivity reactions seen during infusion of chemotherapeutic agents. These reactions resemble type I allergic reactions, with urticaria and hypotension. Although in only some cases are the type I reactions IgE mediated, they can be prevented with premedication with systemic steroids and antihistamines in most cases.

Numerous macular and papular eruptions have been described with chemotherapeutic agents as well. Many of these occur at the time of the earliest recovery of the bone marrow, as lymphocytes return to the peripheral circulation. They are associated with fever. Horn et al have termed this phenomenon *cutaneous eruptions of lymphocyte recovery*. Histologically, these reactions demonstrate a nonspecific superficial perivascular mononuclear cell infiltrate, composed primarily of T lymphocytes. Treatment is not required, and the eruption spontaneously resolves.

Radiation Enhancement and Recall Reactions.
Radiation dermatitis, in the form of intense erythema and vesiculation of the skin may be observed in radiation ports. Administration of many chemotherapeutic agents, during or in close proximity to the time of radiation therapy, may induce an enhanced radiation reaction. Because it may occur a week or more after the radiation therapy has been completed, it has been termed "radiation recall." A similar reaction of reactivation of a sunburn after methotrexate therapy also occurs. These probably represent synergistic toxicity reactions.

Chemotherapy-Induced Acral Erythema (Palmoplantar Erythrodysesthesia Syndrome).
This is a relatively common syndrome induced by many chemotherapeutic agents, most frequently 5-fluorouracil, doxorubicin, and cytosine arabinoside. The reaction may occur in as many as 40% of treated patients. The reaction is dose dependent, and may appear with bolus short-term infusions or low-dose, long-term infusions. It may present days to months after the treatments are started. It is probably a direct toxic effect of the chemotherapeutic agents on the skin. The large number of sweat glands on the palms and soles that may concentrate the chemotherapeutic agents may explain the localization of the toxicity.

The initial manifestation is often dysesthesia or tingling of the palms and soles. This is followed in a few days by painful, symmetric erythema and edema most pronounced over the distal pads of the digits. The reaction may spread to the dorsal hands and feet, and can be accompanied by a morbilliform eruption of the trunk, neck, scalp and extremities. Over the next several days the erythema becomes dusky, develops areas of pallor, blisters, desquamates, then reepithelializes. The desquamation is often the most prominent part of the syndrome. Blisters developing over pressure areas of the hands and feet are a variant of this syndrome most commonly seen with high dose methotrexate therapy. The patient usually recovers without complication, although rarely full thickness ischemic necrosis occurs in the areas of blistering.

The histopathology is nonspecific, with necrotic keratinocytes and vacuolar changes along the basal cell layer. Acute graft-versus-host disease is in the differential diagnosis. Histologic evaluation may not be useful in the acute setting to distinguish these syndromes. Most helpful are gastrointestinal or liver findings of graft-versus-host disease.

Most cases require only local supportive care. Cold compresses and elevation are helpful, and cooling the hands during treatment may reduce the severity of the reaction. Modification of the dose schedule can be beneficial. Pyridoxine decreases the pain of fluorouracil induced acral erythema.

Neutrophilic Eccrine Hidradenitis.
The majority of cases of neutrophilic eccrine hidradenitis (NEH) occur in neutropenic patients with malignancies, usually acute myelogenous leukemia. It occurs in adults and children, and is most commonly associated with chemotherapy, especially cytarabine. On average, it appears after 7 to 10 days of treatment. The patients are frequently febrile. Skin lesions consist of erythematous papules, plaques or nodules that are usually localized to the trunk, extremities, axillae, or pubic area, but may be generalized. The pinna may also be involved. Purpura may be present, probably related to associated thrombocytopenia. The clinical lesions are nonspecific, and a biopsy is usually performed to exclude infection. Histologically, there is a neutrophilic infiltrate involving the glandular and ductal portions of the eccrine gland. There may be associated necrosis of the eccrine unit, and in later biopsies syringometaplasia. In some cases the infiltrate is scant or absent. The skin lesions resolve spontaneously in 10 days, but in severe cases may be treated with systemic corticosteroids. The pathogenesis of this condition is unknown. Chemotherapy-induced toxicity of the eccrine units is suggested in the majority of cases. A neutrophilic reaction similar to acute febrile neutrophilic dermatosis has

been reported in cancer cases in which no chemotherapy was given. Similar histologic findings may be seen in plantar eruptions in healthy women and children (idiopathic plantar hidradenitis), and those rare cases unassociated with cancer may represent a bacterial infection.

Chemotherapy-Induced Hyperpigmentation. Many chemotherapeutic agents (especially the antibiotics bleomycin, doxorubicin, and daunorubicin) and the alkylating agents (cyclophosphamide and busulfan) cause various patterns of cutaneous hyperpigmentation. Adriamycin (doxorubicin) causes marked hyperpigmentation of the nails, skin and tongue. This is most common in black patients and appears in locations where constitutional hyperpigmentation is sometimes seen. It is very similar to Zidovudine-associated pigmentation seen in pigmented persons. Cyclophosphamide causes transverse banding of the nails or diffuse nail hyperpigmentation beginning proximally. Bleomycin and 5FU causes similar transverse bands. Busulfan and 5FU induce diffuse hyperpigmentation that may be photoaccentuated.

Bleomycin induces characteristic flagellate erythematous urticarial wheals associated with pruritus within hours or days of infusion. Lesions continue to appear for days to weeks. While investigators have not always been able to induce lesions, the pattern strongly suggests scratching is the cause of the erythematous lesions. A similar characteristic pattern of flagellate hyperpigmentation occurs following bleomycin treatment. It may have been preceded by the erythematous reaction or simply pruritus.

Fluorouracil causes a serpentine hyperpigmentation overlying the veins proximal to its infusion site. It represents postinflammatory hyperpigmentation from a chemical phlebitis.

Adverse Reactions to Cytokines

Cytokines, which are normal mediators of inflammation or cell growth, are increasingly used in the management of malignancies and to ameliorate the hematologic complications of disease or its treatment. They have been reviewed by Asnis et al. Skin toxicity is a common complication of the use of these agents. Many of these agents cause local inflammation and/or ulceration at the injection sites in a large number of the patients treated. More widespread papular eruptions are also frequently reported, but these have been poorly studied in most cases and are of unclear pathogenesis.

Granulocyte colony–stimulating factor (G-CSF) has been associated with the induction of several neutrophil mediated disorders, most commonly Sweet's syndrome or bullous pyoderma gangrenosum. These occur about a week after cytokine therapy is initiated and are present despite persistent neutropenia in peripheral blood. Both G-CSF and GM-CSF may exacerbate leukocytoclastic vasculitis. Alpha interferon, gamma interferon and G-CSF have been associated with the exacerbation of psoriasis.

Interleukin-2 (IL-2) commonly causes diffuse erythema followed by desquamation, pruritus, mucositis (resembling aphthosis), glossitis, and flushing. While the majority of erythema reactions with IL-2 treatment are mild to moderate, some may be quite severe. Erythroderma with blistering or toxic epidermal necrolysis–like reactions can occur, and be dose limiting. Administration of iodinated contrast material within 2 weeks of IL-2 therapy will be associated with a hypersensitivity reaction in 30% of cases. Fever, chills, angioedema, urticaria, and hypotension may occur. Subcutaneous injections of IL-2 can lead to injection-site nodules or necrosis. Histologically, a diffuse panniculitis with noninflammatory necrosis of the involved tissue is present.

Asnis LA, et al: Cutaneous reactions to recombinant cytokine therapy. *J Am Acad Dermatol* 1995, 33:393.

Baack BR, et al: Chemotherapy-induced acral erythema. *J Am Acad Dermatol* 1991, 24:457.

Bernstein EF, et al: Recurrent neutrophilic eccrine hidradenitis. *Br J Dermatol* 1992, 127:529.

Dhuhra P, et al: Bleomycin-induced flagellate erythema. *Clin Exp Dermatol* 1991, 16:216.

Horn TD, et al: Cutaneous eruptions of lymphocyte recovery. *Arch Dermatol* 1989, 125:1512.

Johnson ML, et al: Leukocyte colony-stimulating factors. *Arch Dermatol* 1994, 130:77.

Manganoni AM, et al: Neutrophilic eccrine hidradenitis in a healthy woman. *Dermatology* 1994, 189:211.

Ostlere LS, et al: Neutrophilic eccrine hidradenitis with an unusual presentation. *Br J Dermatol* 1993, 128:696.

Stahr BJ, et al: Idiopathic plantar hidradenitis. *J Cutan Pathol* 1994, 21:289.

Stelzer KJ, et al: Radiation recall skin toxicity with bleomycin in a patient with Kaposi sarcoma related to acquired immune deficiency syndrome. *Cancer* 1993, 71:1322.

Susser WS, et al: Mucocutaneous reactions to chemotherapy. *J Am Acad Dermatol* 1999, 40:367.

Vukelja SJ, et al: Unusual serpentine hyperpigmentation associated with 5-fluorouracil. *J Am Acad Dermatol* 1991, 25:905. _____ ▲

Acrodynia

Also known as *calomel disease, pink disease,* and *erythredemic polyneuropathy,* acrodynia is caused by mercury poisoning, usually in infancy. The skin changes are characteristic and almost pathognomonic. They consist of painful swelling of the hands and feet, sometimes associated with considerable itching of these parts. The hands and feet are also cold, clammy, and pink or dusky red. The erythema is usually blotchy but may be diffuse. Hemorrhagic puncta are frequently evident. Over the trunk a blotchy macular or papular erythema is usually present. Stomatitis and loss of teeth may occur. Constitutional symptoms consist of moderate fever, irritability, marked photophobia, increased perspiration, and a tendency to cry most of the time. There is always moderate upper respiratory inflammation with soreness of the throat. There may be hypertension, hypertonia, anorexia, and insomnia. Albuminuria and

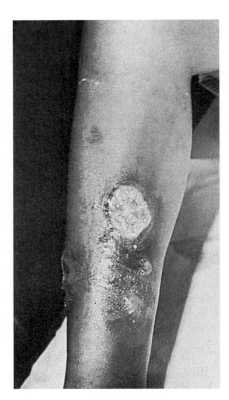

Fig. 6-36 Bromide eruption on shin; bullae and granulomas.

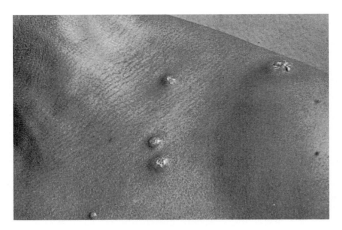

Fig. 6-37 Iododerma.

hematuria are usually present. The diagnosis is made by finding mercury in the urine.

Dinehart SM, et al: Cutaneous manifestations of acrodynia (pink disease). *Arch Dermatol* 1988, 124:107. ▲

Bromoderma

Bromides commonly produce distinctive follicular eruptions. The most common eruption is acneiform, with inflammatory pustules in the hairy parts of the body as well as on the butterfly area of the face, where it must be differentiated from rosacea. Vesicular lesions and bullae are common in bromoderma (Fig. 6-36). Nodular lesions with a violaceous color not infrequently are mistaken for a malignant lymphoma of the skin. A thick inflammatory plaque, with pustules in its border, resembling blastomycosis, may also occur. There is rapid involution of the lesions on cessation of bromide ingestion.

Bromoderma may occur after a small dose or after protracted use of bromides. A small child suffered fatal bromoderma as a result of one 50-mg dose of methacholine bromide by injection. Bromides are excreted in breast milk. No correlation seems to exist between plasma levels and the severity of cutaneous lesions. Treatment of bromoderma is simply cessation of bromide ingestion. In acute intoxication 2 to 4 g of sodium chloride by mouth, taken daily, rapidly replaces the bromide in body fluids. Ammonium chloride is also helpful. In severe cases of intoxication in which the patient is badly confused, ethacrynic acid rapidly decreases the bromide level, with clearing of the lesions.

Burnett JW: Iodides and bromides. *Cutis* 1989, 43:130. ▲

Iododerma

Iodides cause a wide variety of skin eruptions. The most common type is the acneiform eruption with numerous acutely inflamed follicular pustules, each surrounded by a ring of hyperemia (Fig. 6-37). Bullous lesions are also common and may become ulcerated and crusted (Figs. 6-38 and 6-39). Pruritus and urticaria may be the only manifestations of mild iodism. Purpura, furuncles, erythema multiforme, erythema nodosum, and polyarteritis nodosa may also occur. Swelling, redness, and scaling of the eyelids are frequently encountered. Acne vulgaris and rosacea are unfavorably affected by iodides. Treatment is the same as for bromoderma.

Boudonlas O, et al: Iododerma occurring after orally administered topanic acid. *Arch Dermatol* 1987, 123:387. ▲

Adverse Reactions to Corticosteroids

Cutaneous reactions may result from topical, intralesional, subcutaneous, or systemic delivery of corticosteroids.

Topical Application. The prolonged topical use of corticosteroid preparations may produce distinctive changes in the skin. The appearance of these side effects is dependent on three factors: the strength of the steroid, the area to which it is applied, and the individual's predisposition to certain side effects. Atrophy, striae, telangiectasia, skin fragility, and purpura are the most frequent changes seen (Figs. 6-40 and 6-41). The most striking changes of telangiectasia are seen

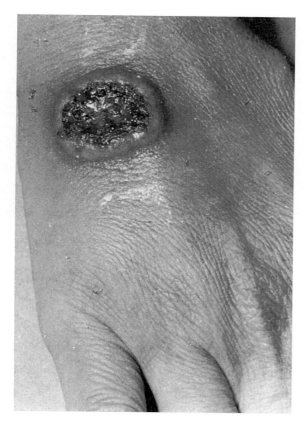

Fig. 6-38 Iododerma. Only brief duration distinguishes it clinically from basal cell carcinoma.

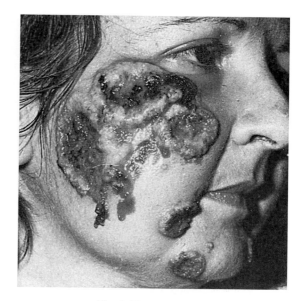

Fig. 6-39 Iododerma.

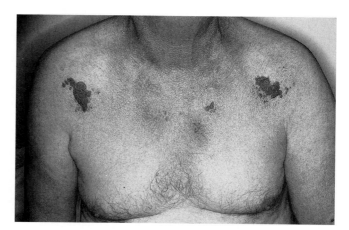

Fig. 6-40 Atrophy and purpura caused by prolonged applications of corticosteroid preparations.

in fair-skinned individuals who use fluorinated corticosteroids on the face. The changes in the skin are enhanced by occlusion. When these side effects occur, the strength of the steroid should be reduced, and adjunctive measures initiated to reduce steroid requirement (addition of topical doxepin, pramoxine, or menthol and camphor to the regimen). Usually the telangiectases disappear in a few months after corticosteroid applications are stopped.

When corticosteroid preparations are applied to the face over a period of weeks or months, persistent erythema with telangiectases, and often small pustules, may occur. Perioral dermatitis and rosacea are in some cases caused by the use of topical corticosteroids. Steroid rosacea has been reported from long-term use of 1% hydrocortisone cream. For this reason, the authors do not recommend chronic topical steroid preparations of any strength in the adjunctive treatment of rosacea or perioral dermatitis.

Repeated application of corticosteroids to the face, scrotum or vulva may lead to marked atrophy of these tissues. These tissues become "addicted" to the topical steroid, so that withdrawing the topical steroid treatment results in severe itching or burning. This syndrome is most difficult to manage, and is best avoided by the most judicious use of topical steroid preparations in these areas.

Topical application of corticosteroids can produce epidermal atrophy with hypopigmentation. If used over large areas, sufficient topical steroids may be absorbed to suppress the hypothalamic pituitary axis. This may affect the growth of children with atopic dermatitis and has led to Addisonian steroid dependency and also Cushing's syndrome. Atopic children with more than 50% body surface area involvement have short stature. This may be related to their increased use of potent topical steroids. In addition, bone mineral density is reduced in adults with chronic atopic dermatitis severe enough to require corticosteroid preparations stronger than hydrocortisone.

Paradoxically, topical corticosteroid preparations may induce allergic contact dermatitis. This complication should be considered in any patient with an eczematous dermatitis

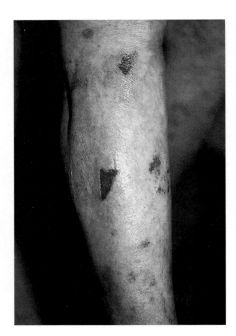

Fig. 6-41 Atrophy and fragility caused by chronic corticosteroid applications.

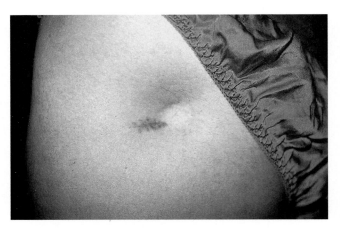

Fig. 6-42 Lipoatrophy of the buttock resulting from a corticosteroid injection.

who becomes worse or is refractory to topical steroid treatment. Systemic corticosteroid administration may be tolerated, but in some patients, there is a cross reaction manifested by whole-body allergic dermatitis.

Injected Corticosteroids. Intralesional injection of corticosteroids is valuable in the management of many dermatoses. The injection of corticosteroids may produce subcutaneous atrophy at the site of injection (Fig. 6-42). The injected corticosteroid may also migrate along lymphatics, causing not only local side effects but also linear atrophic hypopigmented hairless streaks. These may take years to resolve. These complications are best avoided by injecting directly into the lesion, not into the fat, and using only the minimal concentration and volume required.

Intramuscular steroid injections should always be given into the buttocks with a long needle (at least 1½ inches in adults). Injection of corticosteroids into the deltoid muscle sometimes causes subcutaneous atrophy. The patient becomes aware of the reaction by noticing depression and depigmentation at the site of injection. There is no pain, but it is bothersome cosmetically. The patient may be assured that this will fill in but may take several years.

Systemic Corticosteroids. The prolonged use of corticosteroids may produce numerous changes of the skin. In addition, they have a profound effect on the metabolism of many tissues, leading to predictable, and sometimes preventable, complications. Intramuscular injections are not a safer delivery method than oral administration.

PURPURA OR ECCHYMOSES. The skin may become thin and fragile. Spontaneous tearing may occur from trivial trauma. Purpura and ecchymoses are especially seen over the dorsal forearms in many patients over age 50. It is aggravation of actinic purpura.

CUSHINGOID CHANGES. The most common change is probably the alteration in the fat distribution. Buffalo hump, facial and neck fullness, increased supraclavicular and suprasternal fat, gynecomastia, protuberant or pendulous abdomen, and flattening of the buttocks may occur. Aggressive dietary management with reduction in carbohydrate and caloric intake may ameliorate these changes.

STEROID ACNE. Small, firm follicular papules on the forehead, cheeks, and chest may occur. Even inhaled corticosteroids for pulmonary disease can cause acne. Steroid acne can persist as long as the corticosteroids are continued. The management is similar to acne vulgaris with topical preparations and oral antibiotics.

STRIAE. These may be widely distributed, especially over the abdomen, buttocks, and thighs.

OTHER SKIN CHANGES. There may be generalized skin dryness (xerosis); the skin may become thin and fragile; keratosis pilaris may develop; persistent erythema of the skin in sun-exposed areas may occur, and erythromelanosis may rarely occur.

HAIR CHANGES. Hair loss occurs in about half of the patients on long-term corticosteroids in large doses. There may be thinning and brittle fracturing along the hair shaft. There may be increased hair growth on the bearded area and on the arms and back with fine vellus hairs.

SYTEMIC COMPLICATIONS OF SYSTEMIC STEROIDS. Hypertension, cataracts, aseptic necrosis of the hip, and osteoporosis are potential consequences of therapy with systemic steroids. Bone loss can occur early in the course of corticosteroid therapy, so it should be managed preemptively. Effective management can reduce steroid-induced osteoporosis. All patients with anticipated treatment courses longer than 1 month should be supplemented with calcium and vitamin D (1.0 to 1.5 g calcium and 400 to 800 U of cholecalciferol daily). Smoking should be stopped and alcohol consumption minimized. Bone mineral density can be accurately measured at baseline via DEXA scan, and followed during corticosteroid therapy. Hypogonadism, which contributes to osteoporosis, can be treated in men and women with testosterone or estrogen, respectively. Calcitonin and bisphosphonates may be added to the management if necessary.

Aalto-Korte K, et al: Bone mineral density in patients with atopic dermatitis. *Br J Dermatol* 1997, 136:172.

Frauman AG: An overview of the adverse reactions to adrenal corticosteroids. *Adverse Drug React Toxicol Rev* 1996, 15:203.

Lutz ME, et al: Allergic contact dermatitis to topical application of corticosteroids. *Mayo Clin Proc* 1997, 72:1141.

Massarano AA, et al: Growth in atopic eczema. *Arch Dis Child* 1993, 68:677.

Monk, et al: Acne induced by inhaled corticosteroids. *Clin Exp Dermatol* 1993, 18:48.

Murata Y, et al: Systemic contact dermatitis caused by systemic corticosteroid use. *Arch Dermatol* 1997, 133:1053.

Picado C, et al: Corticosteroid-induced bone loss. *Drug Safety* 1996, 15:347.

Rapaport MJ, et al: Eyelid dermatitis to red face syndrome to cure. *J Am Acad Dermatol* 1999, 41:435.

Werth VP: Management and treatment with systemic glucocorticoids. *Adv Dermatol* 1993, 8:81. ▲

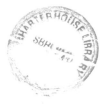

CHAPTER 7

Erythema and Urticaria

FLUSHING

Flushing is a transient, diffuse redness of the face and neck or adjacent trunk. If it is intense and frequent it may eventuate in rosacea. Flushing may be classified as neurally mediated or direct vasodilator mediated. Neurally mediated flushing is usually associated with eccrine sweating at the time of the flush. The most common neurally mediated flushing reactions are to heat—either external (high ambient temperature), internal (fever), or in the oral cavity (orally/thermally induced flushing).

Flushing associated with menopause in women may be either age related or induced by surgery (oophorectomy) or medications (tamoxifen, leuprolide acetate). Menopausal flushing may occur in women who are still having menses in their thirties. Men may also develop climacteric flushing, but rarely during normal aging; rather this occurs in association with surgery or antiandrogen therapy (flutamide).

Blushing, or emotional flushing, may be either emotionally or physiologically induced. Simple facial redness may occur in individuals with translucent skin and who have many dilated vessels near the surface; this may be called *anatomically predisposed blushing*.

Either endogenous or exogenous circulating vasodilating agents may produce flushing. Exogenous agents include niacin, calcium channel blockers, cyclosporine, chemotherapeutic agents, vancomycin, bromocriptine, intravenous contrast material, and high-dose methylprednisolone. Food-associated flushing may be caused by capsaicin (red pepper), sodium nitrate, sulfites, or alcohol or by food poisoning (ciguatera, scombroid). Vasoactive endogenous substances are associated with flushing in carcinoid syndrome, mastocytosis, and pheochromocytoma.

Wilkin JK: The red face: flushing disorders. *Clin Dermatol* 1993, 11:211. ▲

The term *erythema* means redness (hyperemia) of the skin, either localized or widespread. Erythema is caused by dilation of the superficial blood vessels near the surface of the skin. It may be transient or persistent, but in both cases the skin blanches momentarily under the pressure of a finger or when pressed by a diascope. Erythema is the commonest and often the first objective skin reaction produced by inflammatory processes in the skin.

For dermatologists, the word *erythema* may also be used to name reactive conditions in the skin. These conditions are either known or hypothesized to be manifestations of underlying systemic conditions, often infections. These include toxic erythemas related to viral and bacterial infections, erythema multiforme resulting from herpes simplex virus (HSV), erythema nodosum, and the gyrate erythemas.

In this chapter we will address other related conditions that are signs of underlying conditions, including acute febrile neutrophilic dermatitis and pyoderma gangrenosum. These have many clinical characteristics that are also seen in the erythemas, or they may be seen simultaneously or in different persons from the same antigenic exposure. For example, streptococcal infection may induce erythema nodosum or Sweet's syndrome, and patients with Sweet's syndrome may have lesions identical to erythema nodosum on their shins.

Erythema Palmare

Erythema palmare is distinctive localized persistent erythema, is usually most marked on the hypothenar areas, and is associated with an elevated level of circulating estrogen. Cirrhosis, metastatic cancer to the liver, and pregnancy are causes.

Generalized Erythemas

Generalized erythemas vary greatly in their appearance, extent, and distribution; they are most notable on the chest, upper arms, thighs, and face. The eruption consists of pinhead-sized red macules blending into the surrounding macules to produce a diffuse rash that may cover the entire body. Nearly always the follicles are involved. These erythemas may be caused by medications, bacterial toxins, or viral infection. If the etiologic factors are not known or not found, the term *toxic erythema* may be used. In general, these reactions are self-limited and clear either when the offending medication is stopped or when the associated infection is treated or resolves. Specific erythemas associated with bacterial or viral infections are discussed in Chapters 14 and 19.

Erythema Toxicum Neonatorum

Erythema toxicum neonatorum occurs in the majority of healthy full-term newborns, usually on the second or third day. Because it is so common, dermatologists are usually consulted only for the most florid or atypical cases. There are multiple papules that evolve rapidly to pustules each on a broad erythematous macule. The number of lesions may be so large that there is confluent erythema, especially on the face. Lesions involve the face, trunk, and proximal extremities and appear only rarely on the soles or palms. There is no fever. The eruption generally disappears by the tenth day. It must be distinguished from miliaria, bacterial folliculitis, neonatal herpes, and rarely, scabies. Smears of the pustules demonstrating eosinophils are usually adequate in the typical patient to confirm the diagnosis. Rarely, a biopsy will be required, demonstrating a folliculitis containing eosinophils and neutrophils.

ERYTHEMA MULTIFORME

In 1860, von Hebra first described erythema exudativum multiforme. Following his original description, many diseases were initially lumped into the diagnostic category "erythema multiforme," since they were clinically or histologically similar. These included drug-induced bullous eruptions (Stevens-Johnson syndrome and toxic epidermal necrolysis) and annular urticarial reactions (urticarial erythema multiforme). In the last decade, however, classification schemes have been proposed that reaffirm von Hebra's original observation and clearly distinguish subsets within this disease group. The value of this new classification scheme has been confirmed, since it correlates with the pathogenic cause—erythema multiforme of von Hebra being due to herpes simplex and Stevens-Johnson syndrome and toxic epidermal necrolysis representing adverse reactions to medications (see Chapter 6). The original disease described by von Hebra is now called *erythema multiforme minor* or *herpes simplex-associated erythema multiforme* (HAEM). Some patients with this reaction pattern may have more severe disease, which has been called *erythema multiforme with mucous membrane involvement*. About 20% of cases cannot be clinically classified. Eventually, when more accurate methods are available for determining the cause of each case, there will be less need for these classification schemes. Until then, however, management is guided in most cases by an accurate clinical diagnosis.

Clinical Features

True erythema multiforme, including EM minor and EM with mucosal involvement, usually has characteristic clinical features. It is a self-limited, recurrent disease, usually of young adults, occurring seasonally in the spring and fall. There is no or only a mild prodrome; it lasts 1 to 4 weeks. The individual clinical lesions are most helpful in establishing the diagnosis. They begin as sharply marginated, erythematous macules, which become raised, edematous papules over 24 to 48 hours. The lesions may reach several centimeters in diameter. Typically, a ring of erythema forms around the periphery, and centrally the lesions become flatter, more purpuric, and dusky. This lesion is the classic "target" or "iris" lesion with three zones—central dusky purpura; an elevated, edematous, pale ring; and surrounding macular erythema (Figs. 7-1 and 7-2). The central area may blister. Such typical targets are best observed on the palms and soles (Fig. 7-3). Lesions typically appear symmetrically and acrally, initially most frequently on the dorsal hands. The dorsal feet, extensor limbs, elbows and knees, and palms and soles are typically involved. In about 10% of cases more widespread involvement of the trunk may occur. Koebner's phenomenon or photoaccentuation may be observed. Mucosal involvement occurs 25% of the time and is usually limited to the oral mucosa. If more severe classic EM cases are evaluated, however, two or more mucous membranes may be involved in up to 45% of cases (Fig. 7-4). Assier et al suggested that lesion morphology and distribution are better predictors of pathogenesis than is the extent of mucosal involvement. An atypical variant of

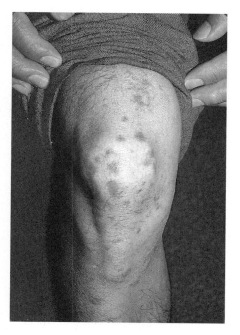

Fig. 7-1 Erythema multiforme as a result of HSV. Accentuated on knees.

HAEM has been described in four women. It consists of outbreaks of unilateral or segmental papules and plaques that may be few in number or solitary. Lesions may be up to 20 cm in diameter. The plaques are erythematous and evolve to have a dusky center, which desquamates. Subcutaneous nodules resembling erythema nodosum may be simultaneously present. Histologic examination shows features of EM, and herpes simplex virus DNA is identified in the lesions by polymerase chain reaction (PCR). Acyclovir sup-

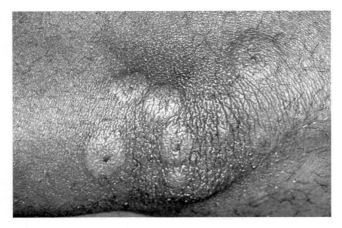

Fig. 7-2 Erythema multiforme as a result of HSV. Accentuated on elbows.

pression prevents the lesions, and prednisone therapy seems to increase the frequency of attacks.

Stevens-Johnson syndrome (less ideally called *erythema multiforme major*) is clinically different in most cases from classic EM minor. It is frequently accompanied by a febrile prodrome. The eruption occurs at all ages; it begins diffusely or on the trunk and mucous membranes. The individual lesions are flat, erythematous, or purpuric macules that form incomplete "atypical targets" that may blister centrally. Lesions tend to be larger and more commonly confluent than in EM minor. Mucous membrane disease is prominent, and more than two mucous membranes are involved in 70% or more of cases (Fig. 7-5). About 20% of cases do not fit into these ideal classifications, emphasizing the need for pathogenically rather than morphologically based diagnostic methods.

Etiologic Factors

The value of the morphologic classification system is that it predicts the cause in most cases. Typical EM minor is usually associated with herpes simplex infection, typically orolabial. HAEM lesions appear 1 to 3 weeks (average, 10 days) after the herpes lesion. Episodes of EM minor may or may not follow every outbreak of herpes, and some EM outbreaks will not be preceded by a clinically recognized herpetic lesion. Using polymerase chain reaction and in situ hybridization techniques, herpes simplex DNA and antigens have been

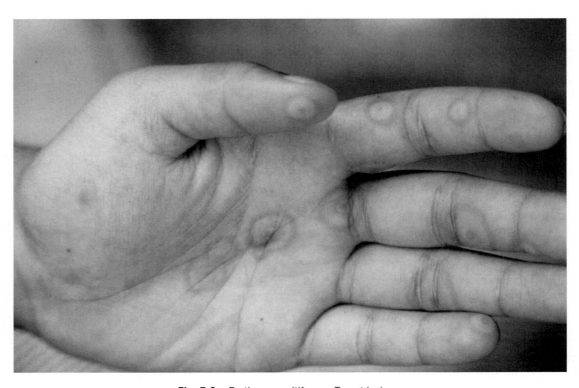

Fig. 7-3 Erythema multiforme. Target lesions.

found in the lesions of EM minor (but not nonlesional skin) and localized to the epidermis. This apparently represents the target of the inflammatory reaction. The majority of "idiopathic" cases of EM, especially when mild and acrally distributed, are also associated with recurrent HSV.

Stevens-Johnson syndrome and most centrally accentuated eruptions with atypical targets are caused by medications. The most common agents are sulfonamides, other antibiotics, NSAIDs, allopurinol, and anticonvulsants. Abnormal metabolism of these medications may be associated with the development of this adverse reaction.

Although there is an extensive list of other agents that have been reported to induce erythema multiforme major, only *Mycoplasma pneumoniae* and radiation therapy have been reproducibly associated. Most cases of *Mycoplasma*-induced EM have prominent mucosal involvement and bullous skin lesions, which are not classic iris or target lesions. They resemble cases of Stevens-Johnson syndrome. Radiation therapy, especially if given with phenytoin and tapering corticosteroids for brain cancers, induces EM that often starts in the radiation port, then generalizes.

Pathogenesis

Activated T lymphocytes are present in lesions of EM, with cytotoxic or suppressor cells more prominent in the epidermis and helper T cells in the dermis. EM minor is linked to specific HLA types (HLA-DQ3) and Stevens-

Johnson syndrome to abnormalities of drug metabolism. Thus there is a genetic component in both diseases.

Histopathology

The histologic features of erythema multiforme are identical across the spectrum from EM minor to toxic epidermal necrolysis (TEN) and are not predictive of etiology. The extent of epidermal involvement depends on where in the lesion the biopsy is taken. Early lesions on the periphery of typical targets will demonstrate more dermal inflammation and less epidermal change. Epidermal changes are more prominent in the central necrotic area of typical targets or in areas of dusky purpura or incipient necrosis in more extensive cases. The previous concept of dermal versus epidermal EM is based on the various areas of the individual lesion rather than two "types" of EM. Erythema multiforme has a vacuolar interface reaction pattern. Within the epidermis necrotic keratinocytes are identified, initially at the dermal-epidermal junction, but at times throughout the epidermis. Necrosis may be confluent. Basal keratinocytes are vacuolated, forming microscopic and macroscopic subepidermal vesicles. The dermal infiltrate is largely mononuclear and tends to be primarily around the upper dermal vessels and along the dermal-epidermal junction. Leukocytoclastic vasculitis is not observed. Eosinophils are often present, and prominent in 10% of cases. The presence of eosinophils is not predictive of the etiology (drug versus

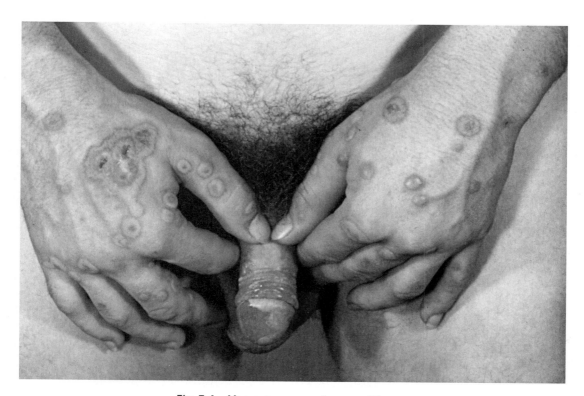

Fig. 7-4 Mucocutaneous erythema multiforme.

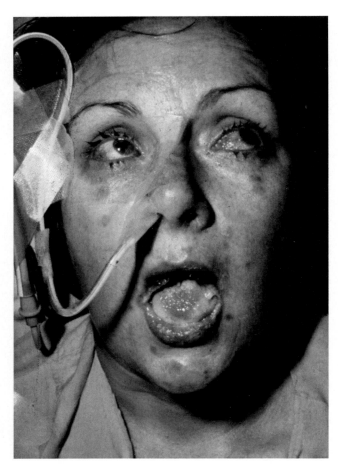

Fig. 7-5 Stevens-Johnson syndrome. Severe involvement of orifices is common.

herpes). Histologically, EM must be distinguished from fixed drug eruption (which tends to have a deeper and more prominent infiltrate), graft-versus-host disease, and lupus erythematosus.

Differential Diagnosis

EM, when characteristic lesions are present, is usually not a difficult clinical diagnosis. When bullae are prominent, EM must be distinguished from the autoimmune bullous diseases, especially pemphigus if mucous membrane involvement is prominent, and bullous pemphigoid if lesions are small and erythema prominent at the periphery of the bulla. Specifically, paraneoplastic pemphigus may histologically demonstrate a vacuolar interface dermatitis, identical to EM. Use of direct immunofluorescence is helpful in excluding this possibility.

Treatment

The treatment of EM is determined by its cause and extent. If HSV can be demonstrated as the trigger, prevention is the cornerstone of treatment. Sunblock creams on the face and lip balm with sunblock should be used daily to prevent UVB-induced outbreaks of HSV. If this does not prevent

recurrences or if genital HSV is the cause, chronic suppressive doses of an antiherpetic antibiotic (acyclovir, valacyclovir, or famciclovir) may be used. This will prevent recurrences in up to 90% of HSV-related cases. Intermittent treatment with systemic antivirals or the use of topical antivirals is of *no* benefit in preventing HSV-associated EM.

Most cases of EM minor (HAEM) are self-limited and require only supportive care. In severe cases, systemic steroids may be used, but because they theoretically may reactivate HSV, the most common trigger of EM minor, they are best avoided if possible. Specifically in HAEM, systemic steroid treatment may be associated with increased frequency and severity of outbreaks. In patients whose condition fails to respond adequately to antiviral antibiotic suppression, dapsone and antimalarials may occasionally be helpful. When all other measures fail, azathioprine will control the disease, but it recurs when the immunosuppressive measures are stopped.

If the extent of cutaneous involvement exceeds 10% to 30% of the body surface area (depending on the age of the patient and associated medical conditions), management in a burn unit will reduce mortality and morbidity. Ophthalmic consultation is critical if ocular involvement is present, because visual loss is the most common complication of severe EM. The use of immunosuppressive agents, specifically systemic corticosteroid drugs, is very controversial. Once the skin loss has occurred, immunosuppressive agents only add to morbidity. Their value may be—if used early and in adequate doses—to stop the evolution of the eruption, reducing the eventual extent of skin loss. Because severe EM often reaches its full extent in only a few days, whether to use immunosuppressive medications should be decided early, the treatment must be adequate and aggressive, and the immunosuppressive agents must be stopped as quickly as possible (even after only a few days).

Assier H, et al: EM with mucous membrane involvement and SJS are clinically different disorders with distinct causes. *Arch Dermatol* 1995, 131:539.

Bastuji-Garin S, et al: Clinical classification of cases of TEN, SJS, and EM. *Arch Dermatol* 1993, 129:92.

Darragh T, et al: Identification of herpes simplex virus DNA in cutaneous lesions of EM. *J Invest Dermatol* 1989, 93:183.

Delattre JY, et al: EM and SJS in patients receiving cranial irradiation and phenytoin. *Neurology* 1988, 38:194.

Fitzpatrick JE, et al: Photosensitive recurrent EM. *J Am Acad Dermatol* 1983, 9:419.

Revuz J, et al: Treatment of TEN. *Arch Dermatol* 1987, 123:1156.

Rzany B, et al: Histopathological and epidemiological characteristics of patients with erythema exudativum multiforme major, SJS and TEN. *Br J Dermatol* 1996, 135:6.

Schofield JK, et al: Recurrent EM. *Br J Dermatol* 1993, 128:542.

Weston WL, et al: Atypical forms of herpes simplex-associated erythema multiforme. *J Am Acad Dermatol* 1998, 39:124.

Wilkins J, et al: Oculocutaneous manifestations of the EM/SJS/TEN spectrum. *Dermatol Clin* 1992, 10:571.

Yong-Kwang Tay, et al: Mycoplasma pneumoniae infection is associated with SJS, not EM (von Hebra). *J Am Acad Dermatol* 1996, 35:757.

▲

Oral Erythema Multiforme

A unique subset of EM patients is seen mostly by oral medicine specialists. These patients have involvement that is limited to or most prominent in the oral cavity. "Oral erythema multiforme" is a not uncommon and difficult to treat disorder. The histology is typical for erythema multiforme. Clinically, the patients are otherwise well, 60% are female, with a mean age of 43 years (range, 17 to 77 years). The minority (about one quarter) have recurrent, self-limited, cyclical disease. The oral cavity is the only site of involvement in 45%, in 30% there is oral and lip involvement, and in 25% the skin is also involved. All portions of the oral cavity may be involved, but the tongue, gingiva, and buccal mucosa are usually most severely affected. Lesions are almost universally eroded, with or without a pseudomembrane, so histology and direct immunofluorescence examination is imperative in this group of patients to establish a diagnosis. In addition, examination for *Candida* infection is critical. Oral and topical antifungal treatment may lead to improvement in about 40% of cases in which *Candida* is identified, with one quarter having a complete remission. Otherwise, treatment is administration of systemic steroidal medications, which are almost always effective but usually do not induce a durable remission. Levamisole and azathioprine may be used in patients whose condition is refractory.

Lozada-Nur F, et al: Oral EM. *Oral Surg Oral Med Oral Pathol* 1989, 67:36. _____ ▲

THE GYRATE ERYTHEMAS: FIGURATE, ANNULAR, AND REACTIVE

The gyrate erythemas are characterized by clinical lesions that are annular or arcuate. The primary lesions are erythematous and slightly elevated. There may be a trailing scale, as in erythema annulare centrifugum. In some of these diseases the lesions are transient and migratory and in some cases they are fixed. Gyrate erythemas may represent the cutaneous manifestations of various infectious and malignant diseases or drug reactions. Certain diseases in this group are now recognized to be of other causes and are discussed in those chapters (erythema marginatum of rheumatic fever; the carrier state of chronic granulomatous disease; and erythema migrans, which is cutaneous borreliosis).

Erythema Annulare Centrifugum

Erythema annulare centrifugum (EAC) is the most common gyrate erythema. It is characterized by polycyclic, erythematous lesions that grow eccentrically and slowly (2 to 3 mm/day), rarely reaching more than 10 cm in diameter. Over several weeks lesions break up, disappear, and are replaced by new elements that follow a similar course. It is minimally symptomatic but is often chronic and recurrent.

Lesions occur on the trunk and especially on the buttocks and inner thighs, where pink rings or partial rings form, with elevated borders in festoons or arcs. Concentric lesions may be seen. Characteristically, there is a trailing scale at the inner border of the annular erythema (Fig. 7-6). Rarely, it is steep, with a firm rubberlike induration, whereas the internal border presents a gentle slope. The surface is typically devoid of crusts or vesicles, although atypical cases with telangiectasia and purpuric spots have been described. Mucosal lesions do not occur.

Histologically, the epidermis may show mild spongiosis or parakeratosis focally but is generally normal. Within the superficial dermis and at times the deep dermis, lymphocytes are tightly associated with the blood vessels in a pattern described as a "coat-sleeve" arrangement. Based on this histology, the gyrate erythemas are divided into the superficial and deep types, but this does not predict the cause.

The pathogenesis of EAC is unknown. Although it is presumed that this condition represents a cutaneous reaction to some underlying disease, it is frequently not discovered. Some cases are associated with dermatophytosis and much more rarely, internal cancer. The initial investigation should be to look carefully for dermatophytosis on the feet and in the groin. An extensive workup beyond a good history and physical examination and perhaps some limited routine laboratory tests (complete blood cell count, liver function tests, urinalysis, and chest x-ray evaluation) is not warranted. The association with drugs, especially the antimalarial medications, is questionable, since reports of such association preceded the description of the annular form of lupus erythematosus (LE) known as *subacute cutaneous LE*.

EAC tends to be persistent over several months to a few years, waxing and waning in severity. Most cases eventually subside spontaneously. While active, the eruption is responsive to topical steroids.

The differential diagnosis includes those conditions that can have annular configuration, including granuloma annulare, secondary syphilis, tinea corporis or cruris, subacute cutaneous LE, sarcoidosis, Hansen's disease, erythema marginatum, erythema migrans, annular urticarial drug reaction, and mycosis fungoides. Histologic examination, clinical features, and basic laboratory examinations will usually allow these diseases to be excluded.

Erythema Gyratum Repens

Erythema gyratum repens (EGR) is a rare disease that is striking and unique in appearance. Lesions consist of undulating wavy bands of slightly elevated erythema over the entire body (Fig. 7-7). Lesions migrate rapidly (up to 1 cm/day) and are characteristically concentric, giving the person a "wood grain" appearance. Trailing scale is present (Fig. 7-8).

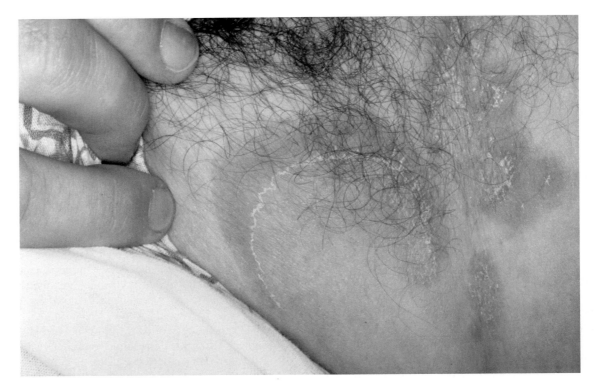

Fig. 7-6 Erythema annulare centrifugum.

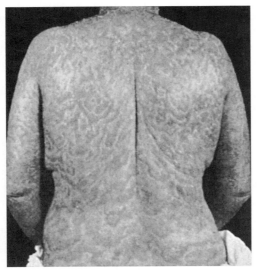

Fig. 7-7 Erythema gyratum repens in association with bronchiogenic carcinoma. (Courtesy Dr. John A. Gammel.)

Pruritus may be severe, and blood eosinophilia is often found. In more than 80% of cases this is a manifestation of an underlying malignant disease of virtually any type, but most commonly it is lung cancer. The skin eruption may precede the detection of the malignancy by an average of 9 months. Given the high frequency of malignant disease, patients with EGR should have extensive evaluations to exclude internal malignancy. If the carcinoma is removed, the lesions clear. Otherwise, the lesions are resistant to treatment. Rarely, EGR may be associated with pulmonary tuberculosis.

Annular Erythema Of Infancy

Peterson and Jarratt reported a case of 3 months' duration in a 6-month-old boy; lesions were transitory (36 to 48 hours), and the eruption stopped without treatment at age 11 months. They called it *annular erythema of infancy*. A similar case, with more persistent lesions, was reported in a 6-month-old girl; it lasted 11 months, without treatment. Cox et al reviewed this syndrome and thought that their cases and some earlier reported ones represented a separate entity.

Boyd AS, et al: EGR. *J Am Acad Dermatol* 1992, 26:757.

Cox NH, et al: Annular erythema of infancy. *Arch Dermatol* 1987, 123:510.

Garcaia-Doval I, et al: Amitriptyline-rendered erythema annulare centrifugum. *Cutis* 1999, 63:35.

Hebert AA, et al: Annular erythema of infancy. *J Am Acad Dermatol* 1986, 14:339.

Langlois JL, et al: EGR unassociated with internal malignancy. *J Am Acad Dermatol* 1985, 12:911.

Shaperio D, et al: EAC as the presenting sign of Hodgkin's disease. *Int J Dermatol* 1993, 32:59.

Tyring SK: Reactive erythemas: EAC and EGR. *Clin Dermatol* 1993, 11:135.

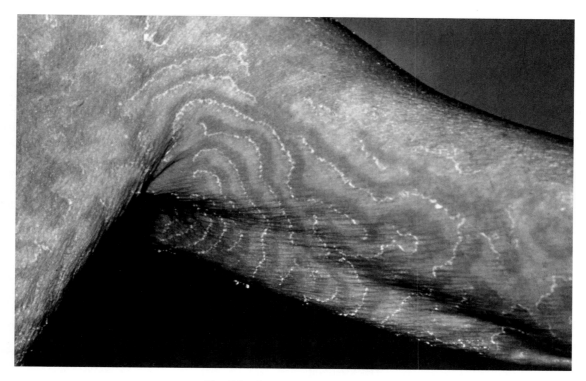

Fig. 7-8 Erythema gyratum repens.

Necrolytic Migratory Erythema (Glucagonoma Syndrome)

Necrolytic migratory erythema is a rare syndrome that is usually associated with an amino precursor uptake and decarboxylation (APUD) cell tumor of the pancreas. These tumors may produce various hormones, but the characteristic syndrome is usually seen if the tumor secretes glucagon. The tumor is frequently silent at the time the eruption appears and is most frequently found in the tail of the pancreas.

The eruption usually occurs in periorificial, flexural, and acral areas and closely resembles the lesions associated with a zinc deficiency. Papulovesicular lesions coalesce to form large plaques with superficial vesiculation and pustulation, followed by erosion or crusting. There are active erythematous gyrate or circinate borders with central confluence. Repeated episodes of inflammation lead to hyperpigmentation. The condition is poorly responsive to topical therapy with corticosteroid and antifungal medications.

Histologically, findings identical to zinc deficiency and certain other metabolic disorders are seen. There is irregular acanthosis with parakeratosis and crust. The characteristic changes include pallor of the keratinocytes in the granular cell layer, which undergo lysis, forming a superficial vesicle.

Most patients are ill at the presentation of the eruption with hyperglycemia, anemia, weight loss, diarrhea, atrophic glossitis, and angular cheilitis (Fig. 7-9). Additional labora-

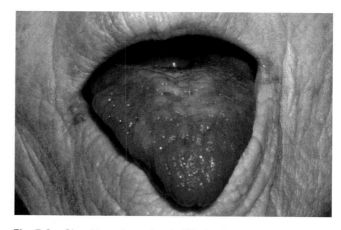

Fig. 7-9 Glossitis and angular cheilitis in glucagonoma syndrome.

tory findings are a low serum zinc level and hypoaminoacidemia. Glucagon levels are elevated. Standard scans of the pancreas may be normal, but angiography will usually detect the neoplasm. Radiolabeled octreotide scans may be useful if the tumor has somatostatin receptors.

The cause of the syndrome is unknown, since some cases are not associated with glucagon-secreting tumors. Amino acid, zinc, and essential fatty acid supplementation has improved the eruption without lowering glucagon levels, suggesting these secondary consequences of hyperglucagonemia are the actual cause of the eruption.

Removal of the tumor leads to resolution. Unfortunately, in half the cases, metastases have already occurred at the time of diagnosis. In these patients streptozotocin or octreotide may be used.

Bewley AP, et al: Successful treatment of a patient with octreotide-resistant necrolytic migratory erythema. *Br J Dermatol* 1996, 134:1101.

Hashizume T, et al: Glucagonoma syndrome. *J Am Acad Dermatol* 1988, 19:377.

Kvols LK, et al: Evaluation of a radiolabeled somatostatin analog (I-123 octreotide) in the detection and localization of carcinoid and islet cell tumors. *Radiology* 1993, 187:129.

Marinkovich MP, et al: Necrolytic migratory erythema without glucagonoma in patients with liver disease. *J Am Acad Dermatol* 1995, 32:604.

Thorisdottir K, et al: Necrolytic migratory erythema. *J Am Acad Dermatol* 1994, 30:324.

van der Loos TLJM, et al: Successful treatment of glucagonoma-related necrolytic migratory erythema with dacarbazine. *J Am Acad Dermatol* 1987, 16:468. ▲

Erythema Brucellum (Contact Brucellosis)

Erythema brucellum is an erythematous eruption that usually occurs in veterinary surgeons and cattlemen after attending cows infected with brucellosis. The eruption begins with itching and erythema of the upper extremities and sometimes also of the face and neck within a few hours after exposure. Soon the skin becomes thickened and covered with conical follicular papules, pustules, and brownish crusts; it heals in about 2 weeks. *Brucella* has not been demonstrated in the lesions, suggesting that the disease is caused by sensitization rather than infection.

White PC, et al: Brucellosis in a Virginia meat-packing plant. *Arch Environ Health* 1974, 28:263. ▲

RECURRENT GRANULOMATOUS DERMATITIS WITH EOSINOPHILIA (EOSINOPHILIC CELLULITIS, WELLS' SYNDROME)

In 1971, Wells described the cases of four patients with acute onset of plaques resembling cellulitis that evolved in a few days to form indolent, infiltrative, dermal, and subcutaneous masses, which persisted for many weeks and finally involuted. The clinical morphology of Wells' syndrome can be thought of as a hybrid between a bacterial cellulitis and urticaria. In unusual cases, lesions may develop subepidermal vesiculation. Wells' syndrome occurs at all ages but is less common in children. Pruritus is common. The condition is typically recurrent, and rarely, the duration of individual episodes may be prolonged. In the well-formed lesions, histologically, dermal eosinophils and histiocytes are seen surrounding central masses of brightly pink collagen that has lost its fibrillar appearance and is more amorphous. This formation has been call a *flame*

figure. Eosinophilic panniculitis may also be present. Flame figures represent extracellular granules of eosinophils (largely eosinophil major basic protein) adherent to and altering the staining of collagen fibers. They are not specific for Wells' syndrome, and can occur in arthropod bites and other disorders with large numbers of degranulating dermal eosinophils. Therefore it is unclear whether Wells' syndrome is a distinct disorder sui generis, or a reaction pattern to many possible allergic stimuli. It has been associated with insect bites, onchocerciasis, intestinal parasites, varicella, mumps, tetanus immunization, drug reactions, myeloproliferative diseases, atopic diathesis, hypereosinophilic syndrome, and fungal infection. Treatment includes oral antihistamines, minocycline, UVB, PUVA, dapsone, and low-dose prednisone. Any triggering factor, such as arthropod bites, should be eliminated.

Amderspom CR, et al: Wells' syndrome in childhood. *J Am Acad Dermatol* 1995, 33:857.

Burket JM, et al: Eosinophilic panniculitis. *J Am Acad Dermatol* 1985, 12:161.

Diridl E, et al: Wells' syndrome responsive to PUVA. *Br J Dermatol* 1997, 137:479.

Friedman IS, et al: Well's syndrome triggered by a centipede bite. *Int J Dermatol* 1998, 37:602.

Hurni MA, et al: Toxocariasis and Wells' syndrome. *Dermatology* 1997, 195:325.

Moreno M, et al: Wells' syndrome related to tetanus vaccine. *Int J Dermatol* 1997, 36:518.

Stam-Westerveld EB, et al: Eosinophilic cellulitis. *Acta Derm Venereol* 1998, 78:159.

Tsuda S, et al: Eosinophilic cellulitis (Wells' syndrome) associated with ascariasis. *Acta Derm Venereol* 1994, 74:292.

Yagi H, et al: Wells' syndrome. *Br J Dermatol* 1997, 136:918. ▲

REACTIVE NEUTROPHILIC DERMATOSES

Erythema nodosum, Sweet's syndrome (acute febrile neutrophilic dermatosis), and pyoderma gangrenosum are discussed as a group. The primary feature that unifies these diseases is that they all contain neutrophils as the predominant inflammatory cell in at least some stage of their evolution. In addition, some or all follow certain stimuli (acute upper respiratory infections), are associated with certain underlying diseases (inflammatory bowel disease, hematologic malignancy), and respond to corticosteroid medications and potassium iodide. Also patients are described with the simultaneous or sequential appearance of two of the conditions, or have lesions that are described as overlaps between two of the conditions. In fact, in some cases, it may be difficult to firmly establish the diagnosis as one or the other of these disorders. For these reasons, it is clinically useful to think of these diseases as forming a constellation of conditions expressed in certain individuals by a group of stimuli and with various overlapping morphologies.

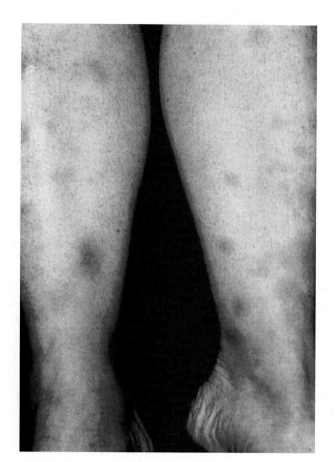

Fig. 7-10 Erythema nodosum in sarcoidosis. (Courtesy Dr. Axel W. Hoke.)

Erythema Nodosum

Erythema nodosum (EN) is the most commonly diagnosed form of inflammatory panniculitis with most cases occurring in young adult women. The eruption consists of bilateral, symmetrical, deep, tender nodules 1 to 10 cm in diameter located pretibially (Fig. 7-10). Initially the skin over the nodules is red, smooth, slightly elevated, and shiny. The onset is acute, frequently associated with malaise, leg edema, and arthritis or arthralgias. Over a few days, the lesions flatten, leaving a purple or blue-green color resembling a deep bruise. The natural history is for the nodules to last a few days or weeks, appearing in crops, and then slowly involute.

Erythema nodosum is a reactive process. It is commonly associated with a streptococcal infection. Tuberculosis was at one time an important causative factor, especially in children. Intestinal infection with *Yersinia, Salmonella,* or *Shigella* may precipitate EN. In endemic areas, systemic fungal infections (coccidioidomycosis, histoplasmosis, sporotrichosis, and blastomycosis) should be considered. Toxoplasmosis is a potential association.

Other noninfectious causes of EN include sarcoidosis, hematologic malignancies (less commonly than Sweet's), pregnancy, and medications including oral contraceptives. The histopathology and other features of erythema nodosum are discussed in Chapter 23.

Sweet's Syndrome (Acute Febrile Neutrophilic Dermatosis)

Since its first description in 1964 by Dr. Robert Sweet, the spectrum of this syndrome has expanded. It is seen throughout the world, and by the size of the series published is recognized as a not uncommon condition.

Sweet's syndrome affects primarily adults. Overall, females outnumber males by about 3 to 1. In younger adults, women are predominantly affected, but in persons older than 50 years of age, the sex ratio is more equal, since cases associated with malignancy have a sex ratio of 1:1. In children, males and females are equally affected. In Europe, cases are more common in the spring and fall. Four subtypes of Sweet's have been described, based on their pathogenesis: the classic type (71%), associated with neoplasia (11%), associated with inflammatory disease (16%), and associated with pregnancy (2%).

The clinical features of all four subtypes are very similar. Where certain subtypes are clinically different, specific mention will be made. The primary skin lesion is a sharply marginated, rapidly extending, tender, erythematous or violaceous, painful, elevated plaque 2 to 10 cm in diameter (Fig. 7-11). Lesions appear typically on the face, neck, upper trunk, and extremities. They may burn but do not itch. The surface of the plaques may develop vesiculation or pustulation as a result of an intense dermal inflammatory infiltrate and accompanying dermal edema. This feature is more common in Sweet's syndrome associated with hematologic malignancy. Localized Sweet's syndrome has been used to describe cases in which lesions are present only on the face, usually the cheeks. Pathergy and Koebnerization after trauma or UVB uncommonly do occur.

More than three quarters of the patients have systemic findings. The most common is fever, occurring in 50% to 80% of patients. Arthritis, arthralgias, or myalgias occur in between one third and two thirds of cases. Conjunctivitis or episcleritis occurs in about a third of cases. Oral lesions resembling aphthae occur in 2% or 3% of classic cases but in 10% or more of cases associated with hematologic malignancy. Cough, dyspnea, and pleuritis may represent pulmonary involvement. Pulmonary infiltrates and effusions are seen on chest x-ray evaluation. Rarely, there may be cardiac, renal, hepatic, intestinal, and neurologic involvement. Multifocal sterile osteomyelitis may occur.

Laboratory findings include an elevated sedimentation rate (90%), neutrophilia (70%), leukocytosis (60%), and a left shift (increased bands) (50%). Antineutrophilic cytoplasmic antigens have been reported by some groups and not by others, suggesting ANCA is not a serologic marker for Sweet's syndrome.

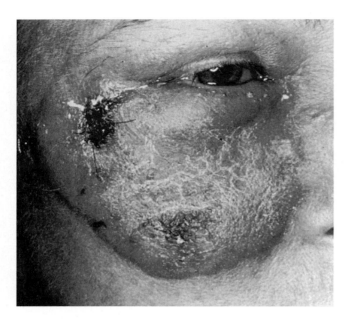

Fig. 7-11 Sweet's syndrome. (Courtesy Dr. Lewis Shapiro.)

In most cases, an attack lasts 3 to 6 weeks and resolves. Recurrences may be seen with the same precipitating cause (e.g., pregnancy). Recurrent Sweet's syndrome is more common in cases associated with underlying malignancy. Chronic or relapsing idiopathic cases do occur.

The hallmark of Sweet's syndrome is a dermal infiltrate of mononuclear cells and many neutrophils with leukocytoclasis, resulting in nuclear dust. Although dermal vessels are dilated, primary leukocytoclastic vasculitis is not seen. Upper dermal edema may be so intense as to form subepidermal vesicles or pustules. Exocytosis of neutrophils through the lower epidermis may result in small subcorneal pustules in 20% of cases.

The majority of cases of Sweet's syndrome follow an upper respiratory tract infection and are therefore acute and self-limited. Other associated inflammatory states are also infectious diseases (*Yersinia,* toxoplasmosis, histoplasmosis, salmonellosis, tuberculosis, and tonsillitis or vulvovaginal infections). The association with various connective tissue diseases must be viewed with caution, as these cases might actually be rheumatoid neutrophilic dermatosis. Sweet's syndrome has been reported with inflammatory bowel disease, peripheral ulcerative keratitis, and Behçet's syndrome.

Hematologic malignancies or solid tumors are present in about 10% of reported cases. Sweet's syndrome often presents early in the course of the cancer, when therapy is more efficacious. Associated malignancies are usually hemoproliferative and may be various leukemias (usually acute myelogenous), lymphomas, anemias, or polycythemias. Solid tumors are of any type but are most commonly genitourinary, breast (in women), or gastrointestinal (in men). Malignancy-associated Sweet's syndrome is more frequently without neutrophilia and is recurrent. It occurs in the older age group; the male-to-female ratio is 1:1. Anemia is found in 93% of men and 71% of women with malignancy-associated Sweet's syndrome. Thrombocytopenia is seen in half. Oral lesions occur in more than 10% of hematopoietic malignancy-associated Sweet's syndrome and about 2% of other cases. Solitary or ulcerative lesions are more frequently associated with malignancy.

Pregnancy-associated Sweet's syndrome typically presents in the first or second trimester with lesions on the head, neck, and trunk, and less commonly on the upper extremities. Lower extremity lesions resembling EN may occur. The condition may resolve spontaneously or clear with topical or systemic steroids. There does not seem to be any fetal risk. It may recur with subsequent pregnancies.

Medications have been associated with Sweet's-like reactions in the skin. The most common cause is granulocyte colony–stimulating factor. This may represent a pharmacologic complication of this agent in the skin. All-transretinoic acid that causes terminal differentiation of leukemic clones is used to treat promyelocytic leukemia. As this effect occurs, after about 2 weeks of treatment, Sweet's-like syndrome lesions may appear. Initially these skin lesions may contain immature blasts, making it difficult to distinguish this condition from leukemia cutis. Later on, the lesions contain more mature neutrophils. The induction of the skin lesions appears to be related to the desired pharmacologic effect of the medication. Oral contraceptives have also been implicated, in parallel with an increased female risk and an association with pregnancy. There are reports of trimethoprim/sulfamethoxazole and minocycline inducing Sweet's syndrome.

Su et al have proposed diagnostic criteria for Sweet's syndrome. Patients must have both of the major and two of the minor criteria for diagnosis (Box 7-1). The two major criteria are the clinical and histologic features of the skin lesions. The minor criteria are the associated symptoms or conditions, laboratory findings, and response to therapy. EM can be distinguished by its typical morphology and histologic features. Clinically, both diseases have annular plaques as the primary lesion, and central vesiculation can rarely occur in Sweet's syndrome. True iris lesions are not seen in Sweet's syndrome. Both Sweet's syndrome and Behçet's syndrome may have oral aphthous like lesions, and EM-like skin lesions. The other features of Behçet's, such as thrombophlebitis and uveitis, are not seen in Sweet's. Reports of neurologic involvement with Sweet's syndrome suggest that there may be some overlap cases. Bowel-bypass syndrome has primarily pustular lesions that on histologic examination demonstrate a neutrophilic dermatosis; fever and arthritis also accompany this condition. The history of prior gastrointestinal surgery or disease may allow for differentiation.

Although it is easy to distinguish classic EN from Sweet's syndrome, these two conditions share many features. They occur most often in young adult women and

BOX 7-1

Revised Version of the Diagnostic Criteria Initiated by Su and Liu for the Diagnosis of Sweet's Syndrome*

MAJOR CRITERIA
1. Abrupt onset of tender or painful erythematous plaques or nodules occasionally with vesicles, pustules, or bullae
2. Predominantly neutrophilic infiltration in the dermis *without* leukocytoclastic vasculitis

MINOR CRITERIA
1. Preceded by a nonspecific respiratory *or* gastrointestinal tract infection *or* vaccination *or* associated with:
   - Inflammatory diseases such as chronic autoimmune disorders, infections
   - Hemoproliferative disorders or solid malignant tumors
   - Pregnancy
2. Accompanied by periods of general malaise and fever (>38° C)
3. Laboratory values during onset: ESR >20 mm; C-reactive protein positive; segmented-nuclear neutrophils and stabs >70% in peripheral blood smear; leukocytosis >8000 (three of four of these values necessary)
4. Excellent response to treatment with systemic corticosteroids or potassium iodide

(From von den Driesch P: *J Am Acad Dermatol* 1994, 31:535.)
*Both major and two minor criteria are needed for diagnosis.

frequently follow upper respiratory infections. They may be associated with pregnancy, underlying malignancy, and inflammatory bowel disease. In both, during the acute episode fever and arthritis may occur, along with leukocytosis with neutrophilia. The lesions on the trunk and face in patients with otherwise classic EN may clinically and histologically resemble Sweet's syndrome. Likewise, there are many reports of simultaneous or sequential erythema nodosum and Sweet's syndrome in the same patient. The relationship of these two conditions has yet to be clarified, but clinicians should not be surprised if they see combination or overlap cases that they have difficulty classifying.

Sweet's syndrome also has considerable overlap with pyoderma gangrenosum. Both are associated with similar diseases, especially inflammatory bowel disease and hematologic malignancy. In early lesions their histologies are virtually identical. In general, pyoderma gangrenosum lesions are chronic and ulcerative; they begin as papulopustules rather than papules and plaques. Patients with pyoderma gangrenosum usually do not have the associated systemic symptoms or abnormal laboratory findings that are seen with Sweet's syndrome. Solitary lesions that begin like Sweet's syndrome may vesiculate and form superficial ulcerations—so-called bullous Sweet's or bullous pyoderma gangrenosum. Similarly, disseminated vesiculopustular forms of pyoderma gangrenosum with systemic

symptoms may closely resemble Sweet's syndrome. Various overlap cases may be seen.

As with other reactive conditions, a search for an underlying cause should be undertaken. This is especially true in persons over the age of 50 and those with anemia, thrombocytopenia, and bullous lesions. The standard treatment is systemic corticosteroids in doses of 40 to 60 mg equivalent of oral prednisone daily. This will result in resolution of fever and skin lesions within days. Potassium iodide in the same doses used to treated erythema nodosum has been reported to be effective. Colchicine, dapsone, doxycycline, clofazimine, indomethacin, and NSAIDs may also be tried. Medication should be continued over an adequate length of time (2 to 4 weeks at least) to prevent relapse, which occurs with some frequency.

Marshall's Syndrome

This rare syndrome is characterized by skin lesions resembling Sweet's syndrome, which are followed by acquired cutis laxa. These cases occur primarily in children. Small red papules develop that expand to urticarial, targetoid plaques with hypopigmented centers. Histologic evaluation of the skin lesions usually shows a neutrophilic dermatosis that is virtually identical to that of Sweet's syndrome. Occasionally, an eosinophilic infiltrate will be found. The lesions resolve with destruction of the elastic tissue at the site, producing soft, wrinkled, skin-colored, protuberant, plaques that can be pushed into the dermis. Biopsies demonstrate loss of elastic tissue. Elastic tissue in other organs may also be affected, especially the heart and lungs. Hwang et al's case was associated with alpha$_1$-antitrypsin deficiency, suggesting that the lack of natural protease inhibitors may allow inflammatory processes to produce the elastic tissue destruction. It may represent a process similar to the panniculitis affecting persons deficient in that enzyme.

Cohen PR, et al: Concurrent Sweet's syndrome and EN. *J Rheumatol* 1992, 19:814.

Cohen PR, et al: Sweet's syndrome and cancer. *Clin Dermatol* 1993, 11:149.

Cohen PR, et al: Sweet's syndrome in patients with solid tumors. *Cancer* 1993, 72:2723.

Cribien B, et al: Erythema nodosum and associated diseases. *Int J Dermatol* 1998, 37:667.

Fain O, et al: Intestinal involvement in Sweet's syndrome. *J Am Acad Dermatol* 1996, 35:989.

Fett DL, et al: Sweet's syndrome. *Mayo Clin Proc* 1995, 70:234.

Goette DK: Sweet's syndrome in subacute cutaneous lupus erythematosus. *Arch Dermatol* 1985, 121:789.

Guia JM, et al: Cardiovascular involvement in a boy with Sweet's syndrome. *Pediatr Cardiol* 1999, 20:295.

Hwang ST, et al: Sweet's syndrome leading to acquired cutis laxa (Marshall's syndrome) in an infant with alpha 1-antitrypsin deficiency. *Arch Dermatol* 1995, 131:1175.

Joshi RK, et al: Successful treatment of Sweet's syndrome with doxycycline. *Br J Dermatol* 1993, 128:584.

Nurre LD, et al: Neutrophilic dermatosis-associated sterile chronic multifocal osteomyelitis in pediatric patients. *Pediatr Dermatol* 1999, 16:214.

Piette WW, et al: Acute neutrophilic dermatosis with myeloblastic infiltrate in a leukemia patient receiving all-*trans*-retinoic acid therapy. *J Am Acad Dermatol* 1994, 30:293.

Satra K, et al: Sweet's syndrome and pregnancy. *J Am Acad Dermatol* 1994, 30:297.

Su WPD, et al: Sweet syndrome. *Semin Dermatol* 1995, 14:173.

Urano Y, et al: Sweet's syndrome associated with chronic myelogenous leukemia. *J Am Acad Dermatol* 1999, 40:275.

Uysal H, et al: Acute febrile neutrophilic dermatosis (Sweet's syndrome) in neuro-Behçet's disease. *Clin Neurol Neurosurg* 1993, 95:319.

von den Driesch P: Sweet's syndrome (acute febrile neutrophilic dermatosis). *J Am Acad Dermatol* 1994, 31:535.

Walker DC, et al: Trimethoprim-sulfamethoxazole-associated acute febrile neutrophilic dermatosis. *J Am Acad Dermatol* 1996, 34:918.

Waltz KM, et al: Sweet's syndrome and erythema nodosum. *Arch Dermatol* 1999, 535:62.

Wilson DM, et al: Peripheral ulcerative keratitis. *J Am Acad Dermatol* 1999, 40:331. _____ ▲

Pyoderma Gangrenosum

Brunsting is credited with the initial clinical description of pyoderma gangrenosum (PG) in 1930. It has recently been classified into four different types; this classification in part predicts the presence of underlying disease and treatment requirements. The "ulcerative" type is the classic PG lesion. It begins as an inflammatory pustule with a surrounding halo that over days enlarges and begins to ulcerate (Fig. 7-12). A primary lesion may not always be seen, as a substantial proportion of lesions appear at sites of trauma (pathergy). The ulcers have distinct rolled edges and may show satellite violaceous papules just peripheral to the border of the ulcer that break down to fuse with the central ulcer. Fully developed lesions are ulcers with sharply marginated, undermined, blue to purple borders (Fig. 7-13). These lesions are typically extremely painful. Lesions most commonly occur in adults 40 to 60 years of age and are most typically present on the lower extremities and trunk but may occur anywhere (Fig. 7-14). They heal with characteristic thin, atrophic scars. "Malignant pyoderma" is no longer to be used as a diagnosis, according to the investigators at the Mayo Clinic who originally described it. Although ulcerative PG may occur on the head and neck, most cases described originally as malignant pyoderma are cANCA positive and represent cutaneous presentations of Wegener's granulomatosis. Pustular PG describes the primary pustular lesions that may or may not progress on to

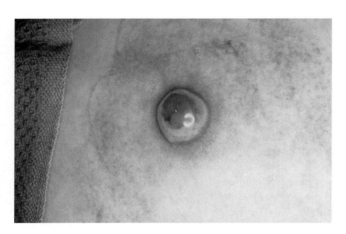

Fig. 7-12 Early lesion of pyoderma gangrenosum.

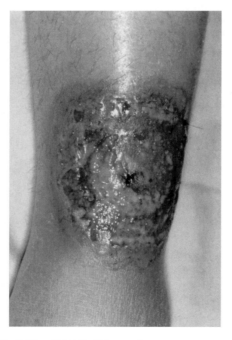

Fig. 7-13 Characteristic pyoderma gangrenosum.

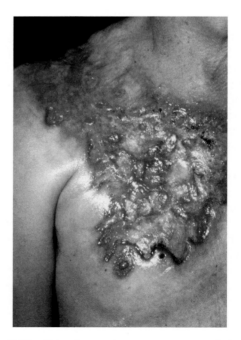

Fig. 7-14 Extensive pyoderma gangrenosum of chest.

ulcerative lesions. They are the forme fruste of PG and are often seen in patients with inflammatory bowel disease. Pyostomatitis vegetans and subcorneal pustular dermatosis are two other pustular neutrophilic diseases reported in association with PG, sometimes in patients with IgA gammopathy.

"Bullous" PG is more superficial and less destructive than the ulcerative type. These lesions have considerable overlap with what has been called *atypical Sweet's syndrome* and are usually seen in patients with leukemia or polycythemia vera. Lesions are red inflammatory plaques that become dusky and develop superficial erosion of the epidermis. They are not deep, usually not undermining, and less painful than ulcerative PG.

"Vegetative" PG is the least aggressive form of PG. It is synonymous with "superficial granulomatous pyoderma." The clinical lesions are cribriform chronic superficial ulcerations usually of the trunk. The lesions enlarge slowly and have elevated, granulomatous borders and clean bases. They are not painful. They respond to relatively conservative treatments and are often not associated with underlying systemic disease. They heal with scarring.

PG is rare in children. More than 40% have underlying inflammatory bowel disease. Another 18% have leukemia. Two children with AIDS and PG have been documented. About one quarter of children with PG have no underlying disease. Genital and head and neck lesions are not uncommon in children.

Overall, approximately 50% of patients have an associated disease. The most common is inflammatory bowel disease, both Crohn's and ulcerative colitis. Between 1.5% and 5% of patients with inflammatory bowel disease develop pyoderma gangrenosum. The two diseases may run an independent course. Surgical removal of the diseased intestine may lead to complete remission, or lesions may persist or first appear after removal of the affected bowel. Most patients with PG and inflammatory bowel disease have involvement of the colon. The ulcerative and pustular types of PG are most commonly seen in patients with associated inflammatory bowel disease.

Many other associated conditions have been reported. Leukemia (chiefly acute or chronic myelogenous leukemia), myeloma, monoclonal gammopathy (chiefly IgA), polycythemia vera, myeloid metaplasia, chronic active hepatitis, hepatitis C, HIV infection, systemic lupus erythematosus, pregnancy, and Takaysu's arteritis are among the many diseases seen in conjunction with pyoderma gangrenosum. It has been associated with an autosomal dominant disorder, PAPA syndrome, which consists of pyogenic arthritis, pyoderma gangrenosum, and severe cystic acne. One case of pyoderma gangrenosum with massive cranial osteolysis demonstrates the ulcerative, destructive nature of this inflammatory disease.

More than one third of PG patients have arthritis, most commonly an asymmetrical, seronegative, monarticular arthritis of the large joints. Monoclonal gammopathy, usually IgA, is found in 10% of PG patients. Children with congenital deficiency of leukocyte-adherence glycoproteins (LAD) develop PG-like lesions.

An early lesion of PG, the papulopustule, shows a deep suppurative folliculitis. The affected follicle is often ruptured. As the lesions evolve, they demonstrate a suppurative inflammation in the dermis and subcutaneous fat. Massive dermal edema and epidermal neutrophilic abscesses are present at the violaceous undermined border. These features are not diagnostic, and infectious causes must still be excluded.

The clinical picture of PG, in the classic ulcerative form, is very characteristic. Because there are no diagnostic serologic or histologic features, however, PG remains a diagnosis of exclusion. Multiple infections, including mycobacteria, deep fungi, gummatous syphilis, synergistic gangrene, and amebiasis must be excluded with cultures and special studies.

Patients and physicians frequently initially diagnose PG as a spider bite if there is only a solitary lesion on an extremity. Spider bites tend to evolve more rapidly and may be associated with other systemic symptoms or findings. Various forms of cutaneous large-vessel vasculitis may produce similar clinical lesions and are excluded by histologic evaluation and ancillary studies, such as antibodies to neutrophilic cytoplasmic antigens (ANCA) and antiphospholipid antibodies tests.

The most difficult diagnosis to exclude is factitial ulcerations. The clinical lesions may be strikingly similar, evolving from small papulopustules to form ulcerations that do not heal. Histologic evaluation will often simply show suppurative dermatitis, since the injected substance may be a toxin that is not identifiable (urine, disinfectants). Even the most experienced clinician may misdiagnose factitial disease as PG.

Management of PG is challenging. The initial step is to attempt to classify the lesion by type, as described earlier. Underlying conditions should be sought, even if no symptoms are found. If the lesions are pustular, treatment of underlying inflammatory bowel disease may lead to improvement. In general, the vegetative type will respond to less aggressive topical or local measures. The aggressiveness of the treatment is determined by the severity of the disease and by its rate of progression. In rapidly progressive cases, aggressive early management may reduce morbidity.

Local treatment includes initially compresses or whirlpool baths, followed by the use of ointment or hydrophilic occlusive dressings. In mild cases application of potent topical steroidal medications, intralesional steroid injections, or topical 4% cromolyn or topical tacrolimus may be beneficial. Hyperbaric oxygen therapy has been successful in many patients but requires special facilities. Its distinct advantage is the rapid relief of pain.

Systemic steroidal medications have been the treatment of choice for several decades. Initial doses are in the range of 1 mg/kg or higher. If control is achieved, the dose may be rapidly tapered. If steroid reduction is not possible, a steroid-sparing agent, as discussed below, may be added. In cases that are unresponsive to oral corticosteroid medications, the use of pulse methylprednisolone may be beneficial.

Sulfapyridine, sulfasalazine, salicylazosulfapyridine, and dapsone have been found helpful, either as a single agents or in combination with corticosteroids. Clofazimine in doses of 200 to 400 mg daily, perhaps by its affect on neutrophils, has been useful in some patients. Minocycline and rarely other antibiotics have anecdotally treated pyoderma gangrenosum.

In general, when the disease is aggressive and use of steroidal medications does not lead to rapid resolution, an immunosuppressive agent is added. Although in the past azathioprine, cyclophosphamide, and chlorambucil have been effectively used, cyclosporine is becoming the immunosuppressive of choice for PG. About 85% of reported cases treated with cyclosporine have responded dramatically, including many that had had not responded adequately to corticosteroid therapy and other treatments, including standard immunosuppressive medications. Initial doses of approximately 5 mg/kg daily are effective in most cases. In failures, the dose can be raised to 10 mg/kg daily. The response is independent of any underlying cause. In very aggressive, rapidly progressive cases, consideration should be given to starting cyclosporin A treatment early to gain control of the disease. FK-506 and mycophenolate mofetil seem to be equally effective, but experience with these agents is much more limited.

Other systemic agents that have been reported as beneficial include thalidomide, potassium iodide, cyproheptadine, and nicotine gum. Such measures as plasma exchange and intravenous human immune globulin are best reserved for cases that have failed more conventional treatments.

Epidermal allografts or autografts may be applied soon after the disease is controlled. Pathergy at the donor site, which is small, has not been reported, probably because the patients were on adequate immunosuppressive therapy.

Abu-Elmagd K, et al: Efficacy of FK 506 in the treatment of recalcitrant PG. *Transplant Proc* 1991, 23:3328.

Anderson LL, et al: Treatment of PG with 4% cromolyn. *Arch Dermatol* 1994, 130:1117.

Bedlow AJ, et al: PG in a child with congenital partial deficiency of leukocyte adherence glycoproteins. *Br J Dermatol* 1998, 139:1064.

Burruss JB, et al: Chlorambucil is an effective corticosteroid-sparing agent for recalcitrant PG. *J Am Acad Dermatol* 1996, 35:720.

Chow RKP, et al: Treatment of PG. *J Am Acad Dermatol* 1996, 34:1047.

Dean SJ, et al: The use of cultured epithelial autograft in a patient with idiopathic PG. *Ann Plast Surg* 1991, 26:1194.

Elgart G, et al: Treatment of PG with cyclosporine. *J Am Acad Dermatol* 1991, 24:83.

Gibson LE, et al: Malignant pyodermas revisited. *Mayo Clin Proc* 1997, 72:734.

Graham JA, et al: PG in infants and children. *Pediatr Dermatol* 1994, 11:10.

Heng MCY: Hyperbaric oxygen therapy for PG. *Aust NZ J Med* 1984, 14:618.

Hurwitz RM, et al: The evolution of PG. *Am J Dermatopathol* 1993, 15:28.

Koester G, et al: Bullous PG. *J Am Acad Dermatol* 1993, 29:875.

Kohl PK, et al: PG followed by subcorneal pustular dermatosis in a patient with IgA paraproteinemia. *J Am Acad Dermatol* 1991, 24:325.

Levitt MD, et al: PG in inflammatory bowel disease. *Br J Surg* 1991, 78:676.

Lichter MD, et al: Superficial granulomatous pyoderma. *Int J Dermatol* 1991, 30:418.

Magid ML, et al: Treatment of recalcitrant PG with cyclosporine. *J Am Acad Dermatol* 1989, 20:293.

Nousari HC, et al: The effectiveness of mycophenolate mofetil in refractory PG. *Arch Dermatol* 1998, 134:1509.

Powell, FC, et al: PG. *J Am Acad Dermatol* 1996, 34:395.

Quimby SR, et al: Superficial granulomatous pyoderma. *Mayo Clin Proc* 1989, 64:37.

Reich U, et al: Topical tacrolimus for pyoderma gangrenosum. *Br J Dermatol* 1998, 139:755.

Rustin MHA, et al: Hairy cell leukemia and PG. *J Am Acad Dermatol* 1985, 13:300.

Rustin MHA, et al: PG associated with Behçet's disease. *J Am Acad Dermatol* 1990, 23:941.

Stone MS, et al: PG and subcorneal pustular dermatosis. *Am J Med* 1996, 100:663.

Van de Kerkhof PCM, et al: Skin manifestations in congenital deficiency of leukocyte-adherence glycoproteins (CDLG). *Br J Dermatol* 1990, 123:395.

Wyrick WJ, et al: Hyperbaric oxygen treatment of PG. *Arch Dermatol* 1978, 114:1232. _____ ▲

URTICARIA (HIVES)

Urticaria is extremely common; it is estimated that approximately 15% to 25% of the population experiences an urticarial illness at some time in their life. Of these, up to 40% will experience urticaria alone, 10% angioedema alone, and 50% will have urticaria and angioedema.

Urticaria is a vascular reaction of the skin characterized by the appearance of wheals, white or red evanescent plaques, generally surrounded by a red halo or flare and associated with severe itching, stinging, or pricking sensations (Fig. 7-15). These wheals are caused by localized edema. Clearing of the central region may occur, producing an annular pattern. The eruption may also consist of macular erythema or papules and may be localized or generalized, the latter being the more common. Their size can vary from 0.5 to more than 10 cm. The eruption usually favors the covered areas, such as the trunk, buttocks, or chest.

Subcutaneous swellings (angioedema), especially of eyelids or lips, may accompany the wheals (50% of urticaria patients) or occur alone. Angioedema may target the gastrointestinal and respiratory tracts, resulting in ab-

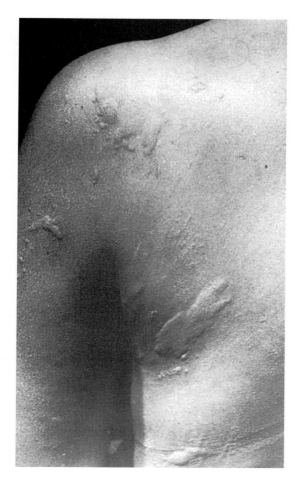

Fig. 7-15 Urticaria. (Courtesy Dr. I. Abrahams.)

dominal pain, coryza, asthma, and respiratory problems. Respiratory tract involvement can produce airway
obstruction. Anaphylaxis and hypotension may also occur.
The number of hives or the presence of angioedema have
not been shown to correlate with the risk of systemic
reactions.

Classification

Acute urticaria evolves over days to weeks, producing
evanescent wheals that individually rarely last more than 12
hours, with complete resolution of the urticaria within 6
weeks of onset. Daily episodes of urticaria and/or angioedema lasting more than 6 weeks is designated chronic
urticaria, which predominantly affects adults and is twice as
common in women as in men.

Urticaria can also be classified by pathogenesis: immunologic, nonimmunologic, and idiopathic. Immunologic
urticaria is subdivided into IgE-dependent, type I hypersensitivity (specific antigen sensitivities and physical urticarias)
and complement-mediated forms (serum sickness, C1
inhibitor deficiencies, and urticarial vasculitis). Nonimmu-

nologic mechanisms produce direct (opiates, polymyxin,
tubocurarine, radiocontrast dye) and indirect (aspirin, other
NSAIDs, tartrazine, and benzoate) mast cell degranulation.
More than 75% of chronic urticaria is idiopathic.

Physical stimuli may produce urticarial reactions and
represent 7% to 17% of chronic urticarias. The physical
urticarias include dermatographic, cold, heat, cholinergic,
aquagenic, solar, vibratory, and exercise-induced cases.

Etiologic Factors

There are many purported causes of urticaria; drugs, food,
and infections are the most common.

Drugs. Drugs are probably the most frequent causes of
urticaria and angioedema. Penicillin and related antibiotics
are the most frequent offenders (see Chapter 6). A frequently overlooked factor is that penicillin sensitivity may
become so exquisite that reactions can occur from
penicillin-contaminated milk (penicillin is sometimes used
for treating mastitis in cows, although this is forbidden by
law). Beer may also produce hives because of penicillin in
the fermentation products.

Aspirin. The incidence of aspirin-induced urticaria has
fallen, most likely related to the availability of alternative
antiinflammatory agents for high-risk patients. Aspirin-
sensitized persons tend to have cross-sensitivity with
tartrazine, the yellow azo-benzone dye, and other azo dyes,
as well as benzoic acid and its derivatives. These are
common food additives and preservatives. Aspirin exacer-
bates chronic urticaria in at least 30% of patients. Aspirin,
salicylates, NSAIDs, opiates, x-ray contrast media, and
angiotensin-converting enzyme inhibitors commonly cause
urticaria by nonimmunologic mechanisms.

Patients may have the triad of allergic rhinitis or asthma,
episodes of food-induced anaphylaxis, and increased frequency of sensitivity to aspirin and other NSAIDs.
Mite-contaminated wheat flour is implicated as an allergen.
The patients manifest episodes of urticaria, angioedema,
and/or anaphylaxis. The nature of the association between
aspirin intolerance and mite-induced respiratory allergies is
unknown.

Food. Foods are a frequent cause of acute urticaria, whereas
in chronic urticaria food is a less frequent factor. The most
allergenic foods are chocolate, shellfish, nuts, peanuts,
tomatoes, strawberries, melons, pork, cheese, garlic, onions,
and spices. Eggs and milk cause urticaria in children.

If the urticaria is acute and recurrent, food allergy may at
times be diagnosed through the use of a food diary kept by
the patient, recording everything ingested within 24 hours
before each attack. The best method of determining a food
allergy in chronic urticaria is by an elimination diet that
allows only bland, nonallergenic foods. Such a diet usually

permits use of the following: lamb, beef, rice, potatoes, carrots, string beans, peas, squash, applesauce, tapioca, preserved pears, peaches, or cherries, Ry-Krisp crackers, butter, sugar, tea without milk or lemon, and coffee without cream. This diet is followed for 3 weeks. If urticaria does not occur, then suspected foods are added one by one and reactions observed.

Food allergens may cross-react with other allergens. Some patients with latex allergies, for example, have been shown to be sensitized to chestnuts, bananas, passion fruit, avocados, and kiwi. Moreno-Ancillo et al have shown that exposure to safely cooked fish and shellfish parasitized by Anisakis simplex can result in angioedema and urticaria, suggesting that some of the seafood allergies may be related to exposure to parasite antigens in the absence of true parasitosis.

The use of scratch and intradermal tests can be misleading. If all food tests are negative, the patient is probably not food allergic. If some tests yield positive results, blind food challenges may need to be undertaken to determine the cause. An offending food may give a negative prick or intradermal test result. Moreover, food additives and preservatives may be responsible.

Food Additives. Although foods may cause urticaria, additives are also important etiologic factors. Greaves reported that less than 10% of cases of chronic urticaria are caused by food additives. Routine challenge testing of such patients may be justified. Natural food additives include yeasts, salicylates, citric acid, egg, and fish albumin. In addition to these, there are the synthetic additives, the most important of which are azo dyes, benzoic acid derivatives, and penicillin.

Yeast is widely used in foods. When suspected as the causative agent, bread and breadstuffs, sausages, wine, beer, grapes, cheese, vinegar, pickled foods, catsup, and yeast tablets should be avoided.

Azo dyes, particularly the yellow dye tartrazine, and the related green and red dyes should be avoided. Foods containing azo dyes and benzoic acid include candy, soft drinks, jelly, marmalade, custards, puddings, various cake and pancake mixes, mayonnaise, ready-made salad dressings and sauces, packaged soups, anchovies, and colored toothpastes. There are undoubtedly many more, and only by constant vigilance regarding ingesting a food with these substances can one be reasonably sure that they are being avoided.

Infections. The possibility of localized infection in the tonsils, a tooth, the sinuses, gallbladder, prostate, bladder, or kidney should be considered as a possible cause in cases of acute or chronic urticaria. In some patients treatment with antibiotics for *Helicobacter pylori* has led to resolution of the urticaria.

Acute urticaria in children may be associated with upper respiratory infections, especially streptococcal infections. Schuller found evidence of streptococcal infection in 40% of pediatric cases of acute urticaria. By contrast, Volonakis found only 4.4% of chronic urticaria in children to be caused by infection.

Emotional Stress. Persons under severe emotional stress may have more marked urticaria, no matter what the primary cause may be. In cholinergic urticaria emotional stress is a particularly well-documented inciting stimulus.

Menthol. Rarely, menthol may cause urticaria; however, when it does occur, a number of different substances into which menthol is incorporated may elicit an urticarial response. Mentholated cigarettes, candy and mints, cough drops, aerosol sprays, and topical medications are among these.

Neoplasms. Urticaria has been associated with carcinomas and Hodgkin's disease. Cold urticaria with cryoglobulinemia has been reported associated with chronic lymphocytic leukemia. Cancers are an infrequent cause of chronic urticaria in adults.

Inhalants. Grass pollens, house dust mites, feathers, formaldehyde, acrolein (produced when frying with lard or by smoking cigarettes containing glycerin as a hygroscopic agent), castor bean or soybean dust, cooked lentils, cottonseed, animal dander, cosmetics, aerosols, pyrethrum, orris, and molds have been known to cause urticaria. Inhalation of latex-laden powder by health professionals is a serious cause of occupational latex asthma and chronic urticaria.

Viruses. Chronic systemic infections such as hepatitis B and hepatitis C may cause urticaria. Acute infectious mononucleosis and psittacosis may also be triggering conditions.

Parasites. Many of the helminthic infestations may cause urticaria. Among these are ascaris, ankylostoma, strongyloides, filaria, echinococcus, schistosoma, trichinella, toxocara, and liver fluke. Witkowski and Parish reported a case of scabies in which urticaria was the presenting complaint. Exposure to parasitic antigens, even cooked parasitized foods, have also been implicated. Parasitic infestations as a cause of chronic urticaria in developed nations, however, is uncommon.

Alcohol. Elphinstone et al recorded a case in which urticaria was induced by the ingestion of ethyl alcohol in any form. The reaction could not be blocked by administration of sodium cromoglycate, indomethacin, chlorpheniramine, cimetidine, or naloxone. Sticherling et al reported three cases, each patient developing generalized urticaria within minutes of consuming small amounts of alcohol. The mechanism of alcohol-induced indirect mast cell stimulation is unknown.

Pathogenesis/Histopathology

The urticarial wheal results from increased capillary permeability, which allows proteins and fluids to extravasate. Capillary permeability results from the increased release of histamine from the mast cells situated around the capillaries. The mast cell is the primary effector cell in urticarial reactions. The mast cell granules containing heparin and histamine disappear or almost disappear during whealing, and the mast cells are said to be "degranulated." Mast cell mediators can cause activation and recruitment of eosinophils, neutrophils, and possibly basophils.

Other substances besides histamine may cause vasodilation and capillary permeability and thereby may possibly become mediators of urticaria and angioedema. These are serotonin, slow-reacting substances (leukotrienes), prostaglandins, proteases, bradykinin, and various other kinins. The role of these substances in the pathogenesis of human urticaria is still speculative. The major basic protein of eosinophil granules is abnormally high in the blood of more than 40% of patients with chronic urticaria, even when peripheral blood eosinophil counts are normal, and there are extracellular deposits of it in the skin in about the same proportion of patients.

Reports by Hide, Greaves, and others have shown that one third of patients with chronic idiopathic urticaria have circulating functional histamine-releasing autoantibodies that bind to the high-affinity IgE receptor (Fc epsilon RI), producing mast cell–specific histamine-releasing activity.

The histopathologic changes in urticaria are not dramatic. The epidermis is normal. Collagen bundles in the reticular dermis are separated by edema, and there is a perivascular lymphocytic inflammatory infiltrate.

Diagnosis

The diagnosis of urticaria and angioedema is usually made on clinical grounds. The differential diagnosis includes urticarial vasculitis, bullous pemphigoid, erythema multiforme, granuloma annulare, sarcoidosis, and cutaneous T-cell lymphoma, most of which have cutaneous findings that are longer lasting than urticaria. If the patient experiences individual wheals that last for longer than 24 hours, a skin biopsy should be performed. Although the diagnosis is often straightforward, determining the cause is frequently difficult.

Clinical Evaluation

Numerous series have been published evaluating the causes of chronic urticaria found in hospitalized patients in specialized centers. They report finding the cause in 75% of cases. This is much higher than the experience of most practicing physicians. If the physical urticarias were to be set aside, about 20% of cases are caused by medications, about 10% by infection, 3% or 4% by inhalants, and up to 10% by food or food additives. The role of *Helicobacter pylori* is questioned. When carefully evaluated, the only cost-effective screening tests of value in elucidating the cause of chronic urticaria are sinus and dental x-ray films, which identify occult infections. These data strongly suggest that evaluation should be history driven, and undirected screening tests should be limited. Kozel et al demonstrated the effectiveness of such a detailed history.

Ghosh et al studied infants and children with acute and chronic urticaria; a definitive cause was found in 40%, the vast majority (34%) having physical urticarias, 5% with food urticaria, and 2% with medication-induced urticaria. Probable causal factors were found in 43%, 11% with more than one factor. In 25%, no cause could be determined. This suggests that causal factors of urticaria may be more readily identifiable in children than in adults. One major problem in studying childhood and infant urticarias is the tendency for health care providers who are not dermatologists to misdiagnose and treat the patients as having erythema multiforme, as Tamayo-Sanchez points out.

Based on these studies, a practical evaluation is limited to a detailed history (foods, drugs, aspirin, physical causes) and challenge tests. If the history and clinical findings suggest a specific cause, such as angioedema in the absence of urticaria (hereditary angioedema), then appropriate evaluation to exclude the suspected disorder is warranted. If there is a history of sinus difficulties, particularly if there is palpable tenderness over the maxillary or ethmoid sinuses, radiologic sinus evaluation is recommended.

In patients with chronic urticaria a review of medications, including aspirin and other nonsteroidal antiinflammatory drugs should be obtained. If the history suggests a physical urticaria then the appropriate challenge test should be used to confirm the diagnosis (see below). Lesions that resolve with purpura or that last longer than 24 hours should prompt a biopsy to exclude urticarial vasculitis. Evaluation beyond this point will rarely lead to identifying the cause of the chronic urticaria. Rather than large, blanket laboratory searches, the patient should be seen regularly, and depending on the severity and response of the hives to treatment and any additional history elicited on the follow-up visits, tests should be ordered selectively.

The laboratory examinations should elucidate any abnormalities elicited in the history and might include tests of thyroid function, thyroid antibodies, liver function, hepatitis B and C serology, antinuclear antibody, and complete blood cell count. Eosinophilia should prompt a search for intestinal parasites, especially if there is a travel history.

Depending on the individual case, the next step is either a restriction diet or a search for an occult underlying infection. Additive-free, salicylate-free food and, in women, a yeast-free diet are initial dietary trials, or a more restricted diet can be attempted for a week with gradual addition of foods if the hives resolve. If a specific food is implicated by a reproduced history, prick and skin testing is strongly suggestive if there is a positive result. The food is eliminated as a cause if the result is negative. However, if there is no supportive history, positive food skin tests are not useful, and their clinical relevance must be confirmed by elimination diet. Such blind allergy testing is usually fruitless.

Sinus x-ray films, a Panorex dental film, a streptococcal throat culture, abdominal ultrasonography, and urinalysis with urine culture (in men, with prostatic massage) may reveal the most common occult infections triggering urticaria. In patients with chronic angioedema, without classic wheals or symptoms of pruritus, an evaluation of C4 level should be ordered. If C4 is low, an evaluation of C1 esterase inhibitor level should be ordered.

Anaphylaxis

Anaphylaxis is an acute and often life-threatening immunologic reaction with features of diffuse erythema, pruritus, urticaria, angioedema, bronchospasm, laryngeal edema, hyperperistalsis, hypotension, and cardiac arrhythmia. Symptoms may range widely in severity from mild pruritus and urticaria to shock and death. The most frequent symptoms are urticaria and/or angioedema (90%) and respiratory complaints of shortness of breath, dyspnea, and/or wheezing (60%). Anaphylaxis usually develops rapidly, with peak severity within 5 to 30 minutes. Antibiotics, especially penicillins and NSAIDs, and radiographic contrast agents are the most common causes of serious anaphylactic reactions, occurring in 1 of every 5000 of the later exposures. Despite a mortality rate of less than 10%, they still account for the vast majority of fatal reactions. One of every 2700 hospitalized patients in the United States experiences anaphylaxis during hospitalization, resulting in 500 annual fatalities.

Hymenoptera stings are the next most frequent cause, followed by ingestion of crustaceans and other food allergens. Atopic dermatitis is commonly associated with anaphylaxis regardless of origin. Causative agents can be identified in up to two thirds of the subjects, and recurrent attacks are the rule.

Although the presentation of severe acute urticaria can be both frightening and debilitating, it is rarely life threatening. However, at times, emergency room physicians need to eliminate the possibility of an allergic or anaphylactic reaction, which is often excluded after 1 or 2 hours of observation. In a patient with significant angioedema involving the upper airway, the patient should be treated with oxygen therapy and a nebulized 5% solution of metaproterenol. A 0.3- to 0.5-ml dose of a 1:1000 dilution of epinephrine is administered subcutaneously every 10 to 20 minutes. In rapidly progressive cases, intubation or tracheotomy may be required. Second-line therapy includes intramuscular antihistamines (25 to 50 mg of hydroxyzine or diphenhydramine every 6 hours as needed), systemic steroidal medication (250 mg of hydrocortisone or 50 mg of methylprednisolone intravenously every 6 hours for 2 to 4 doses), and aminophylline (a 6-mg/kg intravenous loading dose over 30 minutes, then 0.3 to 0.9 mg/kg/hr intravenously for maintenance). Cardiovascular reactions require intravenous administration of fluids (saline solution or colloid) and subcutaneous epinephrine. If the patient is unresponsive, norepinephrine, antihistamines, and/or glucagon may be used as secondary therapy.

Treatment

The mainstay of treatment of acute urticaria is administration of antihistamines. If the cause of the acute episode can be identified, avoiding that trigger should be stressed. Pollack et al reported favorable results in patients treated with antihistamines and 40 mg of prednisone for 4 days following acute onset. The potential benefit from use of such a short course of prednisone outweighs the potential short-term risks and is a reasonable consideration as adjunctive therapy.

The mainstay for treating chronic urticaria is, again, administration of antihistamines. These should be taken on a daily basis; they should not be prescribed to be taken as needed. The patient should be warned about driving an automobile because of the tendency for drowsiness following use of first-generation antihistamines, such as diphenhydramine (Benadryl) or hydroxyzine (Atarax).

The second-generation H_1 antihistamines (cetirizine, famotidine, loratadine, acrivastine, and azelastine) are large, lipophilic molecules with charged side chains that bind extensively to proteins, preventing the drugs from crossing the blood-brain barrier; thus they produce less sedation in most patients. Cetirizine (Zyrtec), however, can cause drowsiness in some individuals, particularly when combined with other antihistamines. The long half-life of these antihistamines and reduced sedation result in improved compliance and efficacy. If a particular antihistamine is ineffective, it is reasonable to switch to another agent, but in general the results are the same. Doxepin, a tricyclic antidepressant with H_1 antihistaminic activity, administered orally (Sinequan or Adapin) may be useful and can be added to the existing antihistamine.

In stubborn cases the combination of H_1 and H_2 antihistamines, such as hydroxyzine and cimetidine or ranitidine, may be effective. Cimetidine or ranitidine should not be used alone for treatment of urticaria. Harvey et al compared a placebo, terbutaline (Brethine), cyproheptadine (Periactin), chlorpheniramine (Chlor-Trimeton), cimetidine (Tagamet), and a combination of the last two. In 23 refractory cases, 58% of patients preferred the H_1-H_2 combination, and it gave the greatest wheal suppression. In a randomized, double-blind, parallel series by Simons et al of patients with chronic urticaria treated with cimetidine and hydroxyzine compared with cimetidine and cetirizine, there was no significant improvement observed in clinical symptoms or findings in the cimetidine-cetirizine group. However, administration of cimetidine and hydroxyzine together produced significantly increased serum hydroxyzine concentrations and increased wheal and flare suppression.

Other second-lines agents include acupuncture, calcium channel antagonists (nifedipine), antimalarial medications, dapsone, gold, azathioprine, and methotrexate. Kennes et al reported success with terbutaline (Brethine), a beta$_2$-adrenergic agent, in urticaria, giving 1.25 mg three times daily, with an extra 2.5 mg when an attack occurred. Our experience (along with Greaves) with terbutaline has been less rewarding.

In general, use of systemic corticosteroid medications should be avoided for the management of chronic urticaria. Unfortunately, although systemic corticosteroids in doses of 0.5 to 1.0 mg/kg/day are effective in suppressing most cases of chronic urticaria, their long-term side effects at these doses make their extended use impractical. In addition, if an infection is the trigger, this could be exacerbated by long-term steroid therapy. Systemic corticosteroids may be used as an initial 3-week trial, then tapered to see if a remission can be induced. If the hives immediately recur, the lowest suppressive dose should be determined, and if low-dose, alternate-day therapy is possible, this may be an alternative. Every 3 months the steroid should be tapered to see if the hives have resolved. A steroid-sparing agent, usually azathioprine or methotrexate, may be used in severe cases, but the long-term consequences of such treatment should be considered.

For local treatment, tepid or cold tub baths or showers may be freely advocated. Their efficacy is increased by the addition of starch, sodium bicarbonate, menthol, or magnesium sulfate. For soothing colloid baths, Aveeno Colloidal Oatmeal or Aveeno Oilated may be used for relief. Sarna lotion contains menthol, phenol, and camphor, and Prax lotion contains pramoxine hydrochloride, an antipruritic.

In patients with chronic urticaria, angiotensin-converting enzyme inhibitors, aspirin and other NSAIDs should be avoided. Topical corticosteroids, topical antihistamines, and topical anesthetics have no role in the management of chronic urticaria.

In chronic urticaria, determination of an offending food is often difficult. When a specific food is suggested by history, the patient should avoid it and be treated supportively. When a food allergy is suspected but not clearly defined, certain foods should be avoided, particularly fish, shellfish (shrimp, lobster, crab, scallops, oysters, clams), turtle, pork, garlic, onions, mushrooms, tomatoes, pickles and relishes, melons, strawberries, citrus fruits, nuts, peanuts, and cheese. Depending on the response, further elimination of foods that may be causative can be instituted as necessary. If a food substance is implicated as a possible cause, suspected foods are eliminated from the diet for 3 weeks and then resumed one by one. In this manner it may be possible to determine the offending substance. Such an approach can be therapeutic as well as diagnostic.

In about one third of cases of chronic idiopathic urticaria, the patients have autoantibodies that bind to high-affinity IgE receptors. Such patients may require more aggressive management to include plasmapheresis, intravenous administration of immunoglobulin (IVIG), or cyclosporine therapy.

Other Variants of Urticaria

Angioedema. *Angioedema* was previously known as angioneurotic edema. Other synonyms are Quincke's edema (hereditary angioedema), Caldwell's syndrome (acquired angioedema I), and giant urticaria.

Angioedema is an acute, evanescent, circumscribed edema that usually affects the most distensible tissues, such as the eyelids, lips, lobes of the ears, and external genitals (the prepuce is a frequent site), or the mucous membranes of the mouth, tongue, or larynx (Fig. 7-16). The swelling occurs in the deeper parts of the skin or in the subcutaneous tissues and as a rule is only slightly tender, with the overlying skin unaltered, edematous, or, rarely, ecchymotic. There may be a diffuse swelling on the hands, forearms, feet, and ankles. Frequently the condition begins during the night and is found on awakening.

There are two distinct subsets of angioedema. The first is considered a deep form of urticaria and may be observed as solitary or multiple sites of angioedema alone or in combination with urticaria. The action of histamine or similar substances creates vasomotor lability, and pruritus is a significant feature. Angioedema associated with C1 esterase inhibitor deficiency is not found in association with

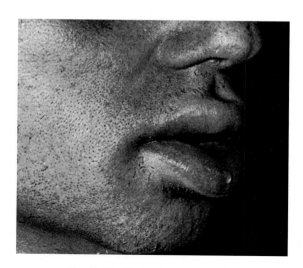

Fig. 7-16 Angioedema of the lips.

lesions of urticaria, and there is no pruritus. Symptoms of pain predominate.

Hereditary Angioedema.

Also known as *chronic familial giant urticaria,* hereditary angioedema was originally described and named by Osler in 1888. Hereditary angioedema characteristically appears in the second to the fourth decade. Sudden attacks of angioedema occur as frequently as every 2 weeks throughout the patient's life, lasting for 2 to 5 days. Swelling is typically asymmetrical, and urticaria or itching does not occur.

A typical feature is the absence of inflammatory signs, although transient and mild eruptions can occasionally precede overt swelling. Perioral and periorbital involvements, which are typically seen in allergic forms of angioedema, are not found in hereditary angioedema. The presence of urticaria in association with angioedema virtually always suggests a diagnosis other than hereditary angioedema.

Patients may experience local swelling in subcutaneous tissues (face, hands, arms, legs, genitals, and buttocks); abdominal organs (stomach, intestines, bladder) mimicking surgical emergencies; and the upper airway (larynx) that can be life threatening. There is little response to antihistamines, epinephrine, or steroids. The mortality rate is high; death is often caused by laryngeal edema. It is important to note that the pulmonary tree is never involved in attacks of hereditary angioedema. The respiratory complications are localized purely to the upper airway. Gastrointestinal edema is manifested by nausea, vomiting, and severe colic, and it may simulate appendicitis so closely that appendectomy is mistakenly performed. The factors that trigger attacks are minor trauma, surgery, sudden changes of temperature, or sudden emotional stress.

Inherited in an autosomal dominant fashion, hereditary angioedema is estimated to occur in 1 in 50,000 to 150,000 persons. There are two phenotypic forms of the disease. Type I is characterized by low antigenic and functional plasma levels of a normal C1 esterase inhibitor protein; type II is characterized by the presence of normal or elevated antigenic levels of a dysfunctional mutant protein with concomitant reduced levels of the functional protein.

The screening test of choice is a C4 level test; C4 will be low as a result of continuous activation and consumption. In addition to depressed C4 levels, these patients also have low C1, C1q, and C2 levels. If the clinical picture and screening tests are positive, a titer of C1 esterase inhibitor should be ordered.

In 25% of deaths from this condition, patients die as a result of laryngeal edema, which is a medical emergency. The treatment of choice for acute hereditary angioedema is replacement therapy with concentrates or fresh frozen plasma. Short-term prophylaxis (for example, for patients undergoing dental care, endoscopy, or intubation for surgery) can be obtained from stanozolol. The anti-

fibrinolytic tranexamic acid, a drug related to epsilon-aminocaproic acid, is given in smaller doses with fewer side effects and has been used to treat acute and chronic disease.

Acquired Angioedema.

Patients with acquired angioedema present with symptoms that are indistinguishable from the hereditary form, but with the onset after the fourth decade of life and lacking a family history. As in hereditary angioedema, there is no associated pruritus or urticaria. This condition is subdivided into acquired angioedema-I, acquired angioedema-II, and an idiopathic form. Acquired angioedema-I is a rare disorder associated with lymphoproliferative diseases. These associations include lymphomas (usually B-cell type), chronic lymphocytic leukemia, undefined lymphoproliferative diseases, myeloma, myelofibrosis, Waldenstrom's macroglobulinemia, monoclonal gammopathies, and one case of T-cell lymphoma.

Acquired angioedema-II is an extremely rare disease defined by the presence of autoantibodies to C1 esterase inhibitor. It is important to realize that autoantibodies directed against C1 esterase inhibitor may also be found in acquired angioedema-I, particularly in patients with B-cell lymphomas, so the diagnosis of acquired angioedema-II is made only when no such underlying condition exists.

The pathophysiology of acquired angioedema-I is unknown but may be related to increased catabolism of C1 esterase inhibitor, since many patients with the disorder have been shown to produce normal amounts of C1 esterase inhibitor. In acquired angioedema-II, hepatocytes and monocytes are able to synthesize normal C1 esterase inhibitor; however, a subpopulation of B cells secretes autoantibodies to the functional region of the C1 esterase inhibitor molecule.

Management of acute attacks in acquired angioedema-I is directed toward replacement of C1 esterase inhibitor through commercial sources, as concentrates or fresh-frozen plasma. For patients with severe or recurrent episodes, danazol or stanozolol, synthetic androgens, are the treatments of choice. Heymann points out, however, that androgens are ineffective in treating patients with acquired angioedema-II, stressing the importance of identifying these patients. Prophylaxis with antifibrinolytic agents such as aminocaproic acid (Amicar) or tranexamic acid may be beneficial. Withdrawal of tranexamic acid maintenance therapy may result in relapse. Immunosuppressive therapy has been shown to be therapeutic in the treatment of acquired angioedema-II by decreasing autoantibody production. Systemic corticosteroids are temporarily effective. Plasmapheresis is another consideration.

Episodic Angioedema with Eosinophilia.

Gleich reported four cases with fever, weight gain, and eosinophilia, and elevated eosinophil major basic protein. There was no underlying disease. Many authors have subsequently confirmed these findings. The disorder is not uncommon. Okubo et al demonstrated increased levels of interleukin-5 during periods of attack. Treatment options include administration of systemic steroidal medications (to which the condition responds quickly at low doses) and antihistamines.

Facial Edema and Eosinophilia.
Songsiridej et al reported on two patients with episodic facial edema and eosinophilia, in whom the eosinophil major basic protein was deposited in the tissue. Both responded well to oral prednisone 30 mg daily.

Schnitzler's Syndrome.
A rare disorder (26 published cases), Schnitzler's syndrome is a combination of chronic, nonpruritic urticaria, fever of unknown origin, disabling bone pain, hyperostosis, increased erythrocyte sedimentation rate, and macroglobulinemia (usually IgM kappa). Pruritus is not a feature (reported in only three cases). The age of onset ranges from 29 to 77 years, without gender predilection. Effective therapy has not been determined, although the bone pain and urticarial lesions responded to systemic corticosteroids in some patients.

Physical Urticarias.
Specific physical stimuli are the cause of approximately 20% of all urticarias. They occur most frequently in persons between ages 17 and 40. The most common form is dermatographism followed by cholinergic and cold urticaria. Several forms of physical urticaria may occur in the same patient. Physical urticarias, particularly dermatographism, delayed pressure, cholinergic, and cold urticaria, are frequently found in patients with chronic idiopathic urticarias. Barlow's series emphasizes the importance of physical urticarias in patients with chronic urticaria. Physical urticarias were present in 71% of patients 22% had immediate dermatographism 37% had delayed pressure urticaria 11% had cholinergic urticaria and 2% had cold urticaria.

DERMATOGRAPHIA (FACTITIOUS URTICARIA). Also known as *dermatographism,* dermatographia is a sharply localized edema or wheal with a surrounding erythematous flare occurring within seconds to minutes after the skin has been stroked (Fig. 7-17). It affects 2% to 5% of the population. This differs from the normal physiologic reaction by an exaggerated response to a much less intense stimulus. When this hypersensitive state is present, a scratch may provoke a linear, raised, pale streak bordered on each side by a hyperemic line, so that it is possible to write on the skin by scratching it with a dull instrument. Minor trauma or pressure, such as that produced by tight belts or brassieres, may also produce urticaria. Dermatographism may also arise spontaneously after drug (penicillin)-induced urticaria and persist for months. Dermatographism has also been reported to be associated with use of the H_2 blocker famotidine (Pepcid). It may occur in hypothyroidism and

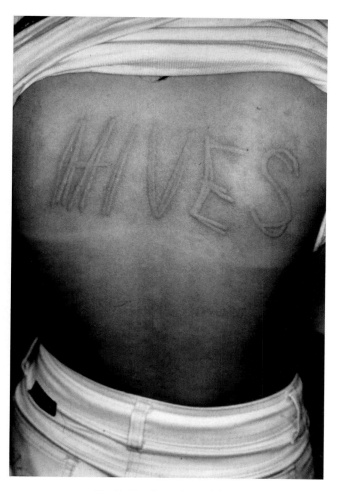

Fig. 7-17 Dermatographism.

hyperthyroidism, infectious diseases, diabetes mellitus, and during onset of menopause. It may be a cause of localized or generalized pruritus.

Standard and second-generation antihistamines suppress this reaction. In this form of physical urticaria, the addition of an H_2 antihistamine may be of benefit. A provocative test is performed with a blunt-tipped object by stroking the skin and observing for a linear wheal.

CHOLINERGIC URTICARIA. Cholinergic urticaria, produced by the action of acetylcholine on the mast cell, is characterized by minute, highly pruritic, punctate wheals or papules 1 to 3 mm in diameter surrounded by areas of erythema (Fig. 7-18). These lesions occur primarily on the trunk and face. The condition spares the palms and soles. Lesions persist from 30 to 90 minutes and are followed by a refractory period up to 24 hours. Bronchospasm may occur. Familial cases have been reported.

The lesions may be induced in the susceptible patient by exercise, emotional stress, increased environmental temperature, or intradermal injection of nicotine picrate or methacholine. Sometimes an attack may be aborted by rapid

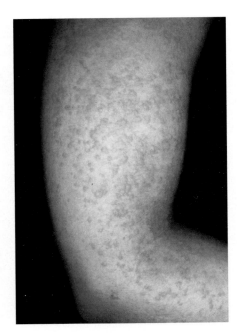

Fig. 7-18 Cholinergic urticaria.

cooling of the body, as by taking a cold shower. A refractory period with no lesions occurs for approximately 24 hours after an attack.

Treatment with antihistamines is effective if dosage is adequate. Cetirizine (Zyrtec), 20 mg/day, and loratadine (Claritin), in doses of 10 to 20 mg daily, have been shown to be effective in controlling symptoms. Hydroxyzine is standard therapy; an initial higher dose of hydroxyzine may be necessary to control symptoms, but later only a low maintenance dose is required. There is no cure, but spontaneous recovery in a few months or years is the rule. Provocative tests include exercise, a warm bath to raise core temperature by 0.7° to 1.0° C (1.2° to 1.8° F), or a methacholine skin test.

ADRENERGIC URTICARIA. In 1985, the Shelleys reported two cases of urticaria that was attributable to norepinephrine. Both were characterized by an eruption of small (1 to 5 mm) red macules and papules with or without a pale halo, appearing within 10 to 15 minutes after emotional upset, or coffee or chocolate, in one case. Serum catecholamines, noradrenalin and adrenalin, rose markedly during attacks, whereas histamine, dopamine, and serotonin levels remained normal. Haustein reported two cases, one of which had elevations in dopamine levels. Propranolol (Inderal) in a dosage of 10 mg four times a day was effective; atenolol (Tenormin) was ineffective. A provocative test consists of intradermal administration of 3 to 10 ng of noradrenalin.

COLD URTICARIA AND ANGIOEDEMA. Exposure to cold may result in edema and whealing on the exposed areas, usually the face and hands. The urticaria does not develop during the chilling but on rewarming. This heterogenous group of disorders is classified into primary (essential), secondary, and familial cold urticaria.

In patients with cold urticaria, one third also have other types of physical urticaria. One fourth of the patients are atopic.

Primary (essential) cold urticaria is not associated with underlying systemic diseases or cold reactive proteins. Symptoms are usually localized to the areas of cold exposure although respiratory and cardiovascular compromise may develop. Fatal shock may occur when these persons go swimming in cold water or take cold showers. This type of cold urticaria usually begins in adulthood. It is usually ice cube test positive (Fig. 7-19).

The treatment of cold urticaria is with cyproheptadine (Periactin) in a dose of 4 mg three times daily. Good therapeutic responses to the second-generation antihistamines acrivastine (Semprex) and cetirizine (Zyrtec) have been reported. Ketotifen may also be effective. Corticosteroid medications are ineffective.

Desensitization by repeated, increased exposures to cold has been effective in some cases. In one report successful desensitization was induced in an 18-year-old patient with severe cold urticaria. Tolerance in a small area of the skin occurred by repeated applications of an ice cube at 30-minute intervals for 7 hours, followed by forearm immersion in cold water hourly for 4 hours. The other limbs were then treated one at a time, and finally the trunk. After a week, the patient was able to tolerate whole-body immersion in cold water for 5 minutes without urticaria. He maintained this "desensitization" by a 5-minute cold shower every 12 hours. He was free from urticaria for 6 months, continuing his daily cold showers.

There is a tendency for cold urticaria to disappear after months or years. As a provocative test, a plastic-wrapped ice cube is applied to the skin for 5 to 20 minutes. If no wheal develops, the area should be fanned for an additional 10 minutes. The use of a combination of cold and moving air is, in some cases, more effective in reproducing lesions than is cold alone. The provocative test is not performed if secondary cold urticaria is being considered.

Secondary cold urticaria is associated with an underlying systemic disease, such as cryoglobulinemia. Other associations include cryofibrinogenemia, multiple myeloma, secondary syphilis, hepatitis, and infectious mononucleosis. Patients may have headache, hypotension, laryngeal edema, and syncope. An ice cube test is not recommended, since it can precipitate vascular occlusion and tissue ischemia.

Familial cold urticaria is observed by the fourth month of life and has an autosomal dominant inheritance pattern. The lesions produce a burning sensation rather than itching. They may have cyanotic centers and surrounding white halos. The lesions last for 24 to 48 hours and may be accompanied by fever, chills, headache, arthralgia, myalgia, and abdominal pain. A prominent feature is leukocytosis,

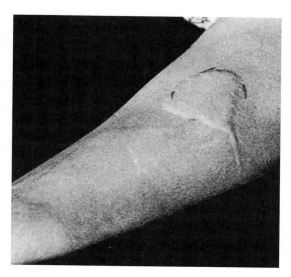

Fig. 7-19 Cold urticaria after ice cube had been applied to site for 3 minutes.

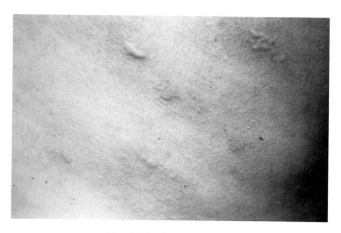

Fig. 7-20 Solar urticaria.

which is the first observable response to cold. Familial cold urticaria will yield a negative result to an ice cube test; patients have been reported to develop urticaria 30 minutes to hours after a more generalized exposure to cold. Biopsies of skin demonstrate features of leukocytoclastic vasculitis. Kalogeromitros et al believe the features are distinct from acquired forms in that there is an absence of serum protein findings and an absence of symptoms of anaphylaxis. Stanozolol therapy has been shown to be effective in treating three of eight patients.

HEAT URTICARIA. Within 5 minutes after the skin has been exposed to heat above 43° C (109.4° F), the exposed area begins to burn and sting and becomes red, swollen, and indurated. This rare type of urticaria may also be generalized and is accompanied by cramps, weakness, flushing, salivation, and collapse. Heat desensitization may be effective. As a provocative test, apply a heated cylinder, 50° to 55° C (122° to 131° F), to a small area of skin of the upper body for 30 minutes.

SOLAR URTICARIA. Solar urticaria appears soon after unshielded skin is exposed to sunlight (Fig. 7-20). It is classified by the wavelengths of light that precipitate the reaction. Visible light can trigger solar urticaria, and sunblocks may not prevent it. Treatment is sun avoidance, sunscreens, antihistamines, repetitive phototherapy, and PUVA. (Solar urticaria is reviewed more extensively in Chapter 3.)

PRESSURE URTICARIA (DELAYED PRESSURE URTICARIA). Pressure urticaria is characterized by the development of swelling with pain that occurs 3 to 12 hours after local pressure has been applied. It occurs most frequently on the feet after walking and on the buttocks after sitting. It is unique in that there may be a latent period of as much as 24 hours before lesions develop. Arthralgias, fever, chills, and leukocytosis

can occur. The pain and swelling last for 8 to 24 hours. Pressure urticaria may be seen in combination with other physical urticarias.

Severe bullous angioedema of one arm 18 hours after a pressure test with progression to generalized urticaria and severe bronchoobstruction requiring intensive management has occurred. Systemic corticosteroids are often therapeutic. Ketotifen may be useful. In general, antihistamines are ineffective. Cetirizine (Zyrtec) and superpotent topical steroid application can be effective in combination. As a provocative test, a 15-pound weight is applied to the skin for 20 minutes and the area inspected in 4 to 8 hours.

EXERCISE-INDUCED URTICARIA. Although both cholinergic urticaria and exercise urticaria are precipitated by exercise, they are distinct entities. Raising the body temperature will not induce exercise urticaria, and the lesions of exercise urticaria are larger than the tiny wheals of cholinergic urticaria (Fig. 7-21). Urticarial lesions appear 5 to 30 minutes after the start of exercise. Anaphylaxis may be associated. Bronchospasm tends not to occur unless associated with a predisposing factor. Of interest is exacerbation of exercise-induced urticaria associated with certain food allergies (ingestion followed by exercise), such as celery. Atopy is common in these patients, and some have documented food allergy, especially to gliadin. Avoiding these allergens may improve symptoms.

Therapy with H_1 and H_2 antihistamines and ketotifen may be partially effective. Self-injectable epinephrine kits are recommended for those rare patients with episodes of anaphylaxis manifesting respiratory symptoms. Exercise is a provocative test.

VIBRATORY ANGIOEDEMA. Vibratory angioedema, a form of physical urticaria, may be an inherited autosomal dominant trait, or it may be acquired, in some cases after prolonged

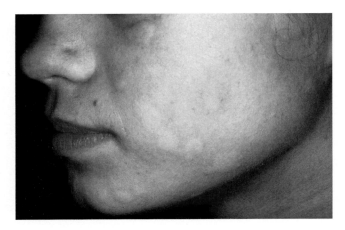

Fig. 7-21 Exercise urticaria.

occupational vibration exposure. Dermatographism, pressure urticaria, and cholinergic urticaria may occur in affected patients. Plasma histamine levels are elevated during attacks. The appearance of the angioedema is usually not delayed. The treatment is antihistamines. As a provocative test, laboratory vortex vibration is applied to the forearm for 5 minutes.

AQUAGENIC URTICARIA. In 1964, Shelley and Rawnsley first described urticaria elicited by water or seawater at any temperature. Pruritic wheals develop immediately or within minutes at the sites of contact of the skin with water, irrespective of temperature or source, and clear within 30 to 60 minutes. Sweat, saliva, and even tears can precipitate a reaction. Aquagenic urticaria may be familial in some cases or associated with atopy or cholinergic urticaria. Systemic symptoms have been reported to include wheezing, dysphagia, and respiratory distress. The pathogenesis is unknown but may be associated with water-soluble antigens that diffuse into the dermis and cause histamine release from sensitized mast cells.

Whealing may be prevented by pretreatment of the skin with petrolatum. Many antihistamines have been effective. There may be a good clinical response to the combination of antihistamines and PUVA. PUVA appears to prevent skin lesions but may not prevent the symptoms of pruritus. Provocative test; apply water compresses (35° C [95° F]) to the skin of the upper body for 30 minutes.

Agostoni A, et al: Hereditary and acquired C1-inhibitor deficiency: biological and clinical characteristics in 235 patients. *Medicine* 1992, 71:206.

Andri L, et al: A comparison of the efficacy of cetirizine and terfenadine: a double-blind, controlled study of chronic idiopathic urticaria. *Allergy* 1993, 48:358.

Barlow RJ, et al: Diagnosis and incidence of delayed pressure urticaria in patients with chronic urticaria. *J Am Acad Dermatol* 1993, 29:954.

Baty V, et al: Schnitzler's syndrome. *Mayo Clin Proc* 1995, 70:572.

Baxter DL, et al: Localized, perifollicular cold urticaria. *J Am Acad Dermatol* 1992, 26:306.

Belaich S, et al: Comparative effects of loratadine and terfenadine in the treatment of chronic idiopathic urticaria. *Ann Allergy* 1990, 64:191.

Blanco C, et al: Anaphylaxis after ingestion of wheat flour contaminated with mites. *J Allergy Clin Immunol* 1997, 99:308.

Bochner BS, et al: Anaphylaxis. *N Engl J Med* 1991, 324:1785.

Borum ML: Hereditary angioedema: an unusual case in an African-American woman. *J Natl Med Assoc* 1998, 90:115.

Breneman D, et al: Cetirizine and astemizole therapy for chronic idiopathic urticaria: a double-blind, placebo controlled, comparative trial. *J Am Acad Dermatol* 1995, 33:192.

Brugnami G, et al: Work-related late asthmatic response induced by latex allergy. *J Allergy Clin Dermatol* 1995, 96:457.

Casale TB, et al: Guide to physical urticarias. *J Allergy Clin Dermatol* 1988, 82:758.

Chang A: Localized heat urticaria. *J Am Acad Dermatol* 1999, 41:354.

Chung HS, et al: Heat urticaria: a case report. *Yonsei Med J* 1996, 37:230.

Crippa M, et al: Allergic reactions to glove-lubricant-powder in health-care workers. *Int Arch Occup Environ Health* 1997, 70:399.

Cugno M, et al: Activation of the coagulation cascade in C1-inhibitor deficiencies. *Blood* 1997, 89:3213.

Deutsch PH: Dermographism treated with hydroxyzine and cimetidine and Ranitidine. *Ann Intern Med* 1984, 101:524.

Dover JS, et al: Delayed pressure urticaria. *J Am Acad Dermatol* 1988, 18:1289.

Dreyfus DH, et al: Steroid-resistant chronic urticaria associated with anti-thyroid microsomal antibodies in a nine-year-old boy. *J Pediatr* 1996, 128:576.

Elphinstone PE, et al: Alcohol-induced urticaria. *J R Soc Med* 1985, 78:340.

Fernandez de Corres L, et al: Sensitization from chestnuts and bananas with urticaria and anaphylaxis from contact with latex. *Ann Allergy* 1993, 70:35.

Fremont S, et al: Prevalence of lysozyme sensitization in a egg-allergic population. *Allergy* 1997, 52:224.

Fujimoto S, et al: Successful prophylaxis of wheat-dependent exercise-induced anaphylaxis with terfenadine. *Intern Med* 1995, 34:654.

Ghosh S, et al: Urticaria in children. *Pediatr Dermatol* 1993, 10:107.

Grant JA, et al: Familial exercise-induced anaphylaxis. *Ann Allergy* 1985, 54:35.

Greaves MW: Chronic urticaria. *N Engl J Med* 1995, 332:1767.

Haustein UF. Adrenergic urticaria and adrenergic pruritus. *Acta Derm Venereol* 1990, 70:82.

Henz BM, et al: Differential effects of new-generation H_1-receptor antagonists in pruritic dermatoses. *Allergy* 1998, 53:180.

Heymann WR: Acquired angioedema. *J Am Acad Dermatol* 1997, 36:611.

Heymann WR: Chronic urticaria and angioedema associated with thyroid autoimmunity. *J Am Acad Dermatol* 1999, 40:229.

Hide M, et al: Autoantibodies against the high-affinity IgE receptor as a cause of histamine release in chronic urticaria. *N Engl J Med* 1993, 328:1599.

Higgins EM, et al: Clinical report and investigation of a patient with localized heat urticaria. *Acta Derm Venereol* (Sweden) 1991, 71:343.

Hirschmann JV, et al: Cholinergic urticaria. *Arch Dermatol* 1987, 123:462.

Humphreys E, et al: The characteristics of urticaria in 390 patients. *Br J Dermatol* 1998, 38:635.

Huston DP, et al: Urticaria and angioedema. *Clin Allergy* 1992, 76:805.

Israili ZH, et al: Cough and angioneurotic edema associated with angiotensin-converting enzyme inhibitor therapy. *JAMA* 1992, 117:1224.

Jorizzo JL: Cholinergic urticaria. *Arch Dermatol* 1987, 123:455.

Juhlin L: Dermatographism and cold-induced urticaria. *J Am Acad Dermatol* 1991, 24:1087.

Kalogeromitros D, et al: Familial cold urticaria. *Ann Allergy Asthma Immunol* 1995, 74:295.

Kanazawa K, et al: Hepatitis C virus infection in patients with urticaria. *J Am Acad Dermatol* 1996, 35:195.

Kanazawa K, et al: Identification of a new physically induced urticaria: cold-induced cholinergic urticaria. *J Allergy Clin Dermatol* 1981, 68:438.

Kaul-Shorten CL, et al: Urticaria, angioedema, and rheumatologic disease. *Clin Immun Rheum* 1996, 22:95.

Kemp SF, et al: Anaphylaxis. *Arch Intern Med* 1995, 155:1749.

Kozel MM, et al: The effectiveness of a history-based diagnostic approach in chronic urticaria and angioedema. *Arch Dermatol* 1998, 134:1575.

Krause LB, et al: A comparison of astemizole and chlorpheniramine in dermographic urticaria. *Br J Dermatol* 1985, 112:447.

Kushimoto H, et al: Masked type I wheat allergy: relation to exercise-induced anaphylaxis. *Arch Dermatol* 1985, 121:355.

Lawlor F, et al: Vibratory angioedema: lesion induction, clinical features, laboratory and ultrastructural findings and response to therapy. *Br J Dermatol* 1989, 120:93.

Ledo A, et al: Doxepin in treatment of chronic urticaria. *J Am Acad Dermatol* 1985, 13:1058.

Lewis FM, et al: Contact sensitivity to food additives can cause oral and perioral symptoms. *Contact Dermatitis* 1995, 33:429.

McLelland J: Mechanism of morphine-induced urticaria. *Arch Dermatol* 1986, 122:138.

Meltzer EO: Comparative safety of H1 antihistamines. *Ann Allergy* 1991, 67:625.

Moneret-Vautrin DA, et al: Food-induced anaphylaxis: a new French multicenter survey. *Ann Gastroenterol Hepatol* (Paris) 1995, 31:256.

Moreno-Ancillo A, et al: Allergic reactions to Anisakis simplex parasitizing seafood. *Ann Allergy Asthma Immunol* 1997, 97:246.

Negro-Alvarez JM, et al: Pharmacologic therapy for urticaria. *Allergol Immunopathol* (Madr) 1997, 25:36.

Neittaanmaki H, et al: Cold urticaria: clinical findings in 220 patients. *J Am Acad Dermatol* 1985, 13:636.

Okubo Y, et al: Periodic angioedema with eosinophilia: increased serum level of interleukin 5. *Intern Med* (Japan) 1995, 34:108.

Onn A, et al: Familial cholinergic urticaria. *J Allergy Clin Dermatol* 1996, 98:847.

Ormerod AD, et al: Familial cold urticaria: investigation of a family and response to stanozolol. *Arch Dermatol* 1993, 129:343.

Panconesi E, et al: Psychophysiology of stress in dermatology. *Dermatol Clin* 1996, 14:399.

Pollack CV, et al: Outpatient management of acute urticaria: a role of prednisone. *Ann Emerg Med* 1995, 26:547.

Sabroe RA, et al: The pathogenesis of chronic idiopathic urticaria. *Arch Dermatol* 1997, 133:1003.

Sanchez-Borges M, et al: A new triad: sensitivity to aspirin, allergic rhinitis, and severe allergic reaction to ingested aeroallergens. *Cutis* 1997, 59:311.

Schuller DE, et al: Acute urticaria associated with streptococcal infection. *Pediatrics* 1980, 65:592.

Sharma JK, et al: Chronic urticaria. *J Cutan Med Surg* 1999, 63:221.

Shelley WB, et al: Adrenergic urticaria: a new form of stress-induced hives. *Lancet* 1985, 1:1031.

Sherertz EF: Clinical pearl: symptomatic dermatographism as a cause of genital pruritus. *J Am Acad Dermatol* 1994, 31:1040.

Silverstein SR, et al: Celery-dependent exercise-induced anaphylaxis. *J Emerg Med* 1986, 4:195.

Simons FE, et al: Effect of the H_2-antagonist cimetidine on the pharmacokinetics and pharmacodynamics of the H_1-antagonists hydroxyzine and cetirizine in patients with chronic urticaria. *J Allergy Clin Immunol* 1995, 95:685.

Songsiridej V, et al: Facial edema and eosinophilia. *Ann Intern Med* 1985, 103:503.

Soter NA: Acute and chronic urticaria and angioedema. *J Am Acad Dermatol* 1991, 25:146.

Sticherling M, et al: Urticarial and anaphylactoid reactions following ethanol intake. *Br J Dermatol* 1995, 132:464.

Sussman G, et al: Controlled trial of H1 antagonists in the treatment of chronic idiopathic urticaria. *Ann Allergy* 1991, 67:433.

Tamayo-Sanchez L, et al: Acute annular urticaria in infants and children. *Pediatr Dermatol* 1997, 14:231.

Taylor JS, et al: Latex allergy: review of 44 cases including outcome and frequent association with allergic hand eczema. *Arch Dermatol* 1996, 132:265.

Ting S, et al: Nonfamilial, vibration-induced angioedema. *J Allergy Clin Immunol* 1983, 71:546.

Torok L, et al: Waldenstrom's macroglobulinemia presenting with cold urticaria and cold purpura. *Clin Exp Dermatol* 1993, 18:277.

Valsecchi R, et al: Autoimmune C1 inhibitor deficiency and angioedema. *Dermatology* 1997, 195:169.

Varjonen E, et al: Life-threatening, recurrent anaphylaxis caused by allergy to gliadin and exercise. *Clin Exp Allergy* 1997, 27:162.

Veraldi S, et al: Acute urticaria caused by pigeon ticks (Argas refleus). *Int J Dermatol* 1996, 35:34.

Volcheck GW, et al: Exercise-induced urticaria and anaphylaxis. *Mayo Clin Proc* 1997, 72:140.

Volonakis M, et al: Etiologic factors in childhood chronic urticaria. *Ann Allergy* 1992, 69:61.

Warner DM, et al: Famotidine (Pepcid)-induced symptomatic dermatographism. *J Am Acad Dermatol* 1994, 31:677.

Weiner MJ: Methotrexate in corticosteroid-resistant urticaria. *Ann Intern Med* 1989, 110:848.

Wener MH, et al: Occupationally acquired vibratory angioedema with secondary carpal tunnel syndrome. *Ann Intern Med* 1983, 98:44.

Wolf C, et al: Episodic angioedema with eosinophilia. *J Am Acad Dermatol* 1989, 20:21.

Wong RC, et al: Dermographism: a review. *J Am Acad Dermatol* 1984, 11:643.

Zuberbier T, et al: Double-blind crossover study of high-dose cetirizine in cholinergic urticaria. *Dermatology* 1996, 193:324. _____ ▲

CHAPTER 8

Connective Tissue Diseases

Lupus erythematosus, dermatomyositis, scleroderma, rheumatoid arthritis, Sjögren's syndrome, eosinophilic fasciitis, mixed connective tissue disease (MCTD), and relapsing polychondritis are classified as connective tissue diseases. Basic to them all is a complex array of autoimmune responses.

Callen JP, et al: Periodic synopsis on collagen vascular disease. *J Am Acad Dermatol* 1993, 28:477.

Condem JJ: The autoimmune diseases. *JAMA* 1992, 268:2882. ▲

LUPUS ERYTHEMATOSUS

Lupus erythematosus (LE) is manifested in many forms and may involve any organ of the body. We classify the specific eruptions of LE in the following way:
  I. Chronic cutaneous LE
     A. Discoid LE, localized (head and neck) or generalized (disseminated) discoid LE
     B. Verrucous (hypertrophic) LE (Behçet)
     C. Lupus erythematosus–lichen planus overlap
     D. Chilblain LE
     E. Lupus panniculitis (LE profundus)
        1. With discoid LE
        2. With systemic LE
 II. Subacute cutaneous LE
     A. Papulosquamous
     B. Annular
     C. Syndromes commonly exhibiting similar morphology
        1. Neonatal LE
        2. Complement deficiency syndromes
III. Acute cutaneous LE (systemic LE with skin lesions) localized or generalized erythema or bullae

Chronic Cutaneous Lupus Erythematosus

Discoid Lupus Erythematosus

Discoid lupus erythematosus (DLE) generally occurs in young adults, with women outnumbering men 2:1. The findings in DLE are characterized by dull red macules with adherent scales extending into patulous follicles. The macule may be 1 cm or more in diameter. Removal of the scale shows its undersurface to be covered with the horny plugs that filled the follicles, resembling carpet tacks or *langue au chat* (cat's tongue). The patches tend to heal centrally first, with atrophy, scarring, dyspigmentation, and telangiectasia (Figs. 8-1 and 8-2).

Some discoid lesions are very superficial, resembling mild seborrheic dermatitis. Others may be brightly erythematous or even urticarial, suggesting dermatitis caused by a drug or contactant, or even erythema multiforme. On the other hand, erythema may be minimal, and the patch merely hyperkeratotic, dark gray, and centrally depressed, suggestive of a solitary lesion of lichen planus or a carcinoma. Very small lesions of discoid LE may be mistaken for actinic keratoses.

LOCALIZED DLE. Discoid lesions are usually localized above the neck. Favored sites are the scalp, bridge of the nose, malar areas, lower lip, and ears. Cyran et al reported two patients who presented with periorbital edema and erythema. In some cases of DLE on the face hyperkeratosis may be severe (Fig. 8-3).

On the scalp the scars are more sclerotic and depressed than on other areas, with scarring alopecia the result. Dilated follicles, with or without horny plugs, are usually seen (Fig. 8-4). Itching and tenderness are common and may rarely be severe.

On the lips (Fig. 8-5) or in the mouth the patches are grayish and hyperkeratotic; they may be eroded and are usually surrounded by a narrow, red inflammatory zone (Fig. 8-6). Burge et al found that 16 of 68 (24%) DLE patients had mucosal involvement of the mouth, nose, eye, or vulva.

GENERALIZED DLE. Generalized DLE is less common than localized DLE and is usually superimposed on a localized discoid case. All degrees of severity are encountered. Most often the thorax and upper extremities are affected (Figs. 8-7 and 8-8), in addition to the usual sites for localized DLE. The scalp may become quite bald, and diffuse scarring may involve the face and upper extremities. In Callen's series, laboratory abnormalities, such as an elevated sedimentation rate, elevated antinuclear antibodies, or

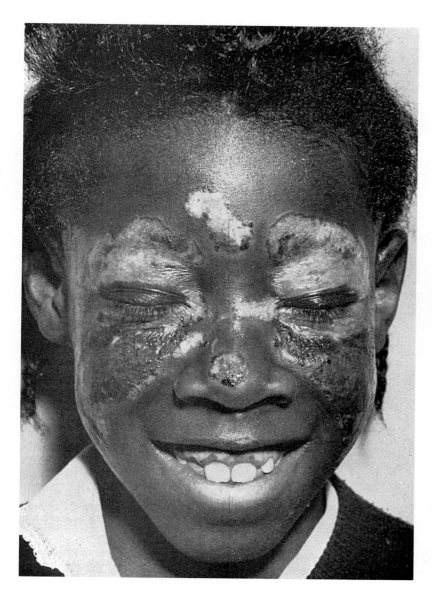

Fig. 8-1 Discoid lupus erythematosus with typical butterfly distribution, atrophy, and depigmentation of skin. (Courtesy Dr. L. Schweich.)

leukopenia, were more common with this form of LE than with localized DLE.

The course of DLE is variable, but 95% of cases confined to the skin at the outset will remain so. Progression from DLE to systemic lupus erythematosus (SLE) is uncommon. Fever may signal its occurrence. Abnormal laboratory tests, such as elevation of antinuclear antibodies (ANA), leukopenia, hematuria, or albuminuria, often identify patients who may progress to SLE. If no abnormalities are found, reassurance is advised; if two or three of the criteria for SLE (see discussion later in this chapter) are present, careful reevaluation should be carried out at regular intervals. If four or more criteria for SLE are met, one may make the diagnosis of SLE.

Spontaneous involution, with scarring, is common. Calcific nodules may develop in affected sites. Deposits of mucin may occur. Relapses are common. Rarely, basal or squamous cell carcinoma, which may be aggressive, may occur in scars (Fig. 8-9). The lower lip of black patients with hypopigmented scars of DLE is a favored site.

CHILDHOOD DLE. There is nothing distinctive about the presentation and clinical course of the skin lesions in DLE in childhood. George et al reviewed the 16 reported cases and found in contrast to adult DLE a lack of female predominance, a low frequency of photosensitivity, and 50% progression to SLE.

HISTOLOGY. The epidermis is usually thin, and there is loss of the normal rete ridge pattern. Hyperorthokeratosis and parakeratosis, with follicular plugging, occur. Hydropic degeneration of the basal layer results in pigmentary incontinence. A primarily lymphocytic perivascular and perifollicular inflammatory infiltrate occurs in the superficial and deep dermis. The superficial dermis may be edematous, and increased mucin is often present.

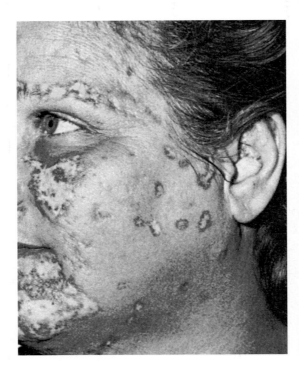

Fig. 8-2 Disseminated discoid lupus erythematosus.

Chronic, inactive lesions show atrophy, with postinflammatory pigmentation. Dermal fibrosis may be present. The basement membrane zone is generally thickened. Inflammatory infiltrate is sparse to absent. Pilosebaceous units, except for arrector muscles, are destroyed.

Direct immunofluorescence test of lesional skin is positive in more than 75% of cases, with immunoglobulin and complement located at the dermoepidermal junction, usually in a granular or particulate pattern. Early lesions (under 8 weeks) may have negative immunofluorescence, especially if on covered skin areas, and uninvolved skin is negative.

DIFFERENTIAL DIAGNOSIS. Chronic cutaneous LE (DLE) must often be differentiated from seborrheic dermatitis, rosacea, lupus vulgaris, sarcoid, drug eruptions, Bowen's disease, lichen planus, tertiary syphilis, polymorphous light eruption, actinic keratosis, and lymphocytic infiltration (Jessner). Immunoglobulin deposits distinguish DLE from the latter condition. Seborrheic dermatitis does not show atrophy, alopecia, or dilated follicles and has greasy, yellowish scale without follicular plugs, and involvement of other sites of election for seborrheic dermatitis.

In rosacea, atrophy does not occur and pustules are nearly always found. Apple-jelly nodules are seen in lupus vulgaris. Sunlight-sensitizing agents, such as sulfonamides, may produce lesions similar to lupus erythematosus. It may be necessary to differentiate syphilis and sarcoid by biopsy and serologic testing. It is difficult to exclude LE in cicatricial alopecia of the scalp; indeed, many such cases are

due to LE. Direct immunofluorescence is especially useful in diagnosing these cases. Polymorphous light eruption offers considerable difficulties. The absence of scarring and the presence of edematous plaques may help in the diagnosis, as does histology, serologic testing, and direct immunofluorescence in selected cases.

Treatment

Certain general measures are important. Exposure to sunlight should be avoided, and a high SPF sunscreen lotion should be used daily. Photosensitivity is frequently present even if the patient denies it, and all patients must be educated about sun avoidance and sunscreen use. The patient should also avoid exposure to excessive cold, to heat, and to localized trauma.

LOCAL. The application of potent or superpotent topical corticosteroids is beneficial. Occlusion may be necessary and may be enhanced by customized vinyl appliances. Tape containing corticosteroid is sometimes helpful. The single most effective local treatment is the injection of corticosteroids into the lesions. Triamcinolone acetonide, 2.5 to 10 mg/ml, is infiltrated into the lesion through a 30-gauge needle at intervals of 4 to 6 weeks. No more than 40 mg of triamcinolone should be used at one time.

SYSTEMIC. The safest and most beneficial systemic therapy is antimalarials. Hydroxychloroquine (Plaquenil), at a dose equal to or less than 6.5 mg/kg/day, is used first because of its safety. If no response occurs after 3 months, a switch to chloroquine (Aralen) is advised, in a dose of 250 mg a day. If response is still incomplete, quinacrine (Atabrine), 100 mg a day, may be added, since this adds no increased risk of retinal toxicity. Systemic treatment may be necessary during the summer, but often can be reduced or stopped during the winter.

Relapses are common even with the antimalarials, and long-term therapy is frequently necessary. Patients should be watched closely for possible side effects, especially ocular toxicity. Ophthalmologic consultation should be obtained before, and at 4- to 6-month intervals during, treatment. In a review of 99 patients taking hydroxychloroquine over a 7-year period, Tobin found only one instance of side effects: a constriction of visual fields to a red object in a man who had taken 444 g of chloroquine in 36 months. Vision was 20/20 throughout, and he was normal 18 months later. In 99 patients taking 400 mg of hydroxychloroquine a day for more than 1 year, Rynes found two with paracentral scotomas, two with slight visual-field constrictions, and one with pigmentation of the retina; all changes were transitory. There were no cataracts. The finding of any visual field defect or pigmentary abnormality is an indication to stop antimalarial therapy.

There may be eruptions of erythema multiforme, purpura, urticaria, nausea, vomiting, nervousness, tinnitus, abducens nerve paralysis, toxic psychoses, leukopenia, and thrombocytopenia. Antimalarials, except in very small

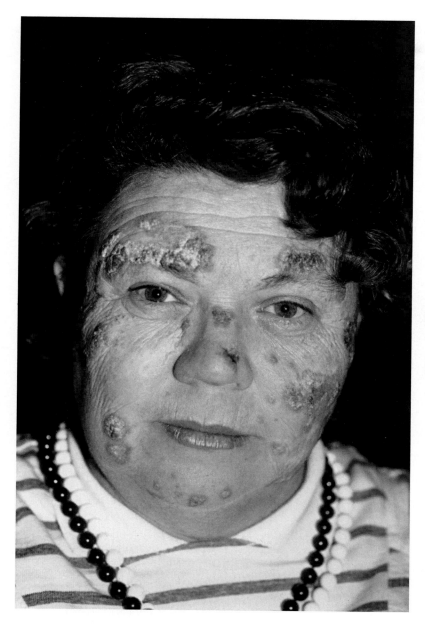

Fig. 8-3 Discoid lupus erythematosus with hyperkeratosis.

doses, will exacerbate porphyria cutanea tarda and may worsen or induce psoriasis. They may also produce maculopapular and light-sensitivity eruptions, and bleach the hair. Chloroquine toxicity may be explained by its tendency to bind to melanin for long periods.

Quinacrine produces a yellow discoloration of the skin, and conjunctivae become yellow. Bullous erythema multiforme, lichen planus–like lesions, and gastrointestinal symptoms of nausea, vomiting, anorexia, and diarrhea may develop. Aplastic anemia has also been noted in long-term therapy. Patients with brown or red hair may turn light blond. Quinacrine has been known to produce blue-black pigmentation of the hard palate, nail beds, cartilage of the ears, alae nasi, and sclerae.

Systemic corticosteroids for widespread or disfiguring lesions are effective; however, treatment should be limited. It may be utilized to obtain initial quick control while antimalarial therapy is being initiated.

Newton et al reported nine patients with chronic or subacute cutaneous LE who responded to 16 weeks of isotretinoin therapy. Shornick et al confirmed this; however, he noted rapid relapse on discontinuance. Dapsone, clofazimine, etretinate, acitretin, azathioprine, interferon alfa-2a, auranofin (oral gold), and thalidomide have all been reported to favorably affect DLE. However, the therapeutic impact of these agents has not been assessed in prospective trials. Rattner et al reported successful treatment of a patient with cribriform scarring with dermabrasion. Because

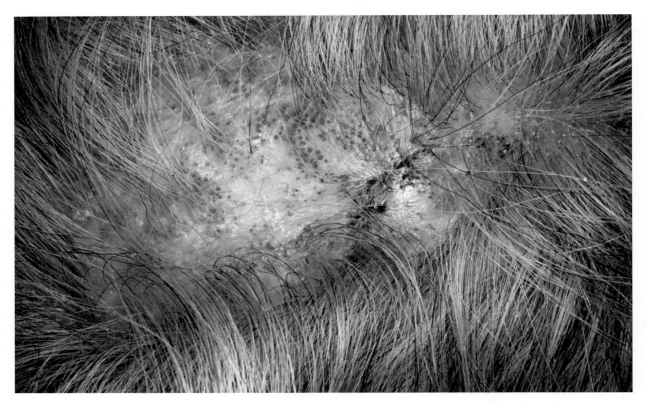

Fig. 8-4 Discoid lupus erythematosus on the scalp, a typical site. Note follicular plugging.

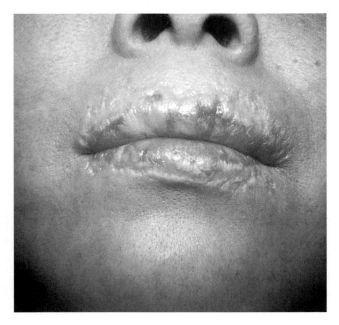

Fig. 8-5 Discoid lupus erythematosus of lips.

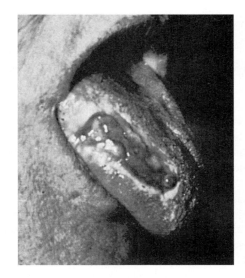

Fig. 8-6 Lupus erythematosus of tongue.

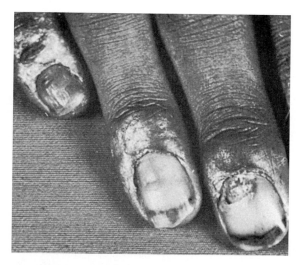

Fig. 8-7 Lupus erythematosus affecting distal phalanges of fingers. (Courtesy Dr. A. Bensel.)

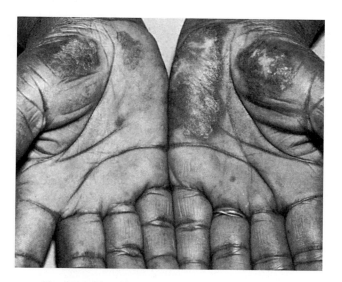

Fig. 8-8 Discoid lupus erythematosus of the palms.

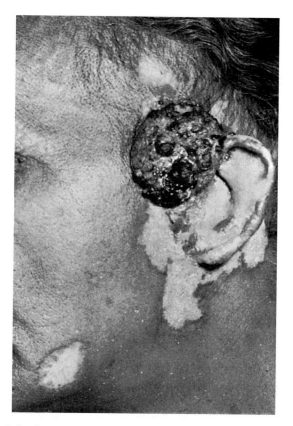

Fig. 8-9 Squamous cell carcinoma in discoid lupus erythematosus. (Courtesy Dr. F. Kerdel-Vegas.)

surgery may flare quiescent lesions, cosmetic procedures must be undertaken cautiously. This is emphasized by two reports on the use of lasers to treat telangiectasias. Nunez et al reported that the pulsed dye laser was successful in treating telangiectatic erythema in four cutaneous lupus patients; however, soon afterward Wolfe et al reported the induction of DLE in a patient whose nasal bridge telangiectasias were treated with this modality.

Verrucous (Hypertrophic) LE. Nonpruritic papulo-nodular lesions may occur on the arms and hands, resembling keratoacanthoma or hypertrophic lichen planus. Spann et al reported nine patients with these lesions and found no characteristic serologic or HLA correlates.

Treatment with intralesional injections of triamcinolone acetonide is usually effective. Success has also been reported with isotretinoin alone or in combination with hydroxychloroquine.

LE–Lichen Planus Overlap Syndrome. The lesions are usually large, atrophic, hypopigmented, bluish-red patches and plaques. Fine telangiectasia and scaling are usually present. The extensor aspects of the extremities are typically affected, and palmoplantar involvement is common (Fig. 8-10). The histology has features of either lichen planus or LE, or both. Direct immunofluorescence usually suggests the former. The lupus band test may be positive. Response to treatment is poor, though dapsone or isotretinoin may be effective.

Chilblain Lupus Erythematosus. Chilblain LE (Hutchinson) is a chronic, unremitting form of LE with the fingertips, rims of ears, calves, and heels affected, especially in women. It is usually preceded by DLE on the face. Systemic involvement is sometimes seen. Mimicry of sarcoidosis may be striking. The chilblain lesions themselves are due to cold. The usual LE treatment modalities are utilized. Allegue et al reported a case associated with

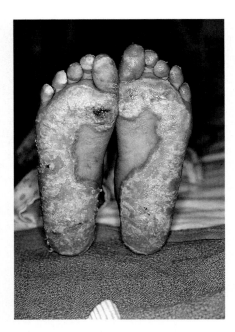

Fig. 8-10 LE–lichen planus overlap syndrome.

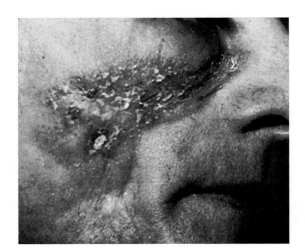

Fig. 8-11 LE panniculitis.

antiphospholipid antibody. A cryoglobulin should also be sought.

LE Panniculitis (LE Profundus). In this type of LE, deep dermal and subcutaneous nodules 1 to 3 or 4 cm in diameter, rubbery-firm, sharply defined, and nontender, occur most often beneath normal skin of the head, face, or upper arms. The chest, buttocks, and thighs may also be involved. This form of LE is characteristically chronic and occurs most often in women between ages 20 and 45. Partly because the diagnosis is more likely to be made if it is known that the patients have LE, many patients have DLE at other sites, or less typically in the overlying skin (Fig. 8-11). The lesions may heal with deep depressions from loss of the panniculus, which may take years to fill in (Fig. 8-12).

The histology shows lymphocytic panniculitis, hyaline degeneration of the fat, hyaline papillary bodies, and dense, sharply circumscribed lymphocytic nodules in the lower dermis and fat. The overlying epidermis may show basal liquefaction and follicular plugging, or may be normal. Seven of nine cases reviewed by Izumi direct immunofluorescence showed granular deposition of immunoglobulin and C3 at the dermoepidermal junction.

Treatment with antimalarials is usually successful, but may take several months to be observed. Hydroxychloroquine given at a dose of less than or equal to 6.5 mg/kg/day is recommended. Intralesional triamcinolone acetonide may also be extremely effective.

Subacute Cutaneous Lupus Erythematosus

Sontheimer, Thomas, and Gilliam in 1979 described a clinically distinct subset of cases of LE to which they gave the name subacute cutaneous lupus erythematosus (SCLE).

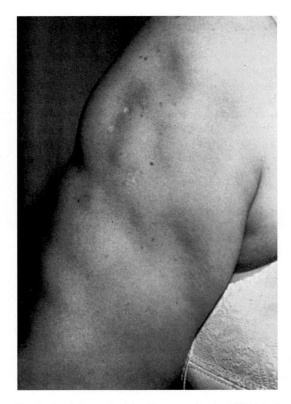

Fig. 8-12 LE panniculitis. (Courtesy Dr. Axel W. Hoke.)

Patients are most often white women aged 15 to 40. SCLE patients make up approximately 10% to 15% of the LE population. Lesions are scaly papules, which evolve into either psoriasiform (Fig. 8-13), more commonly, or polycyclic annular lesions (Fig. 8-14). The scale is thin and easily

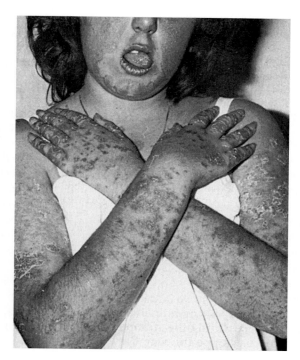

Fig. 8-13 Subacute cutaneous lupus erythematosus, psoriasiform. (Courtesy Dr. J. Kroll.)

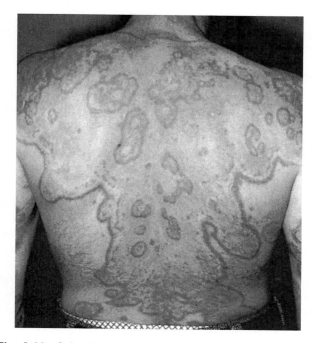

Fig. 8-14 Subacute cutaneous lupus erythematosus, polycyclic lesions.

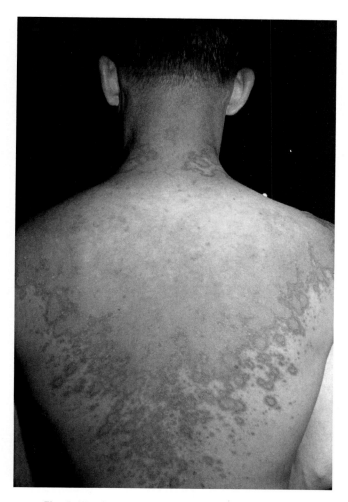

Fig. 8-15 Subacute cutaneous lupus erythematosus.

detached, and telangiectasia and dyspigmentation are nearly always present. Follicles are not involved, and there is no scarring. Lesions tend to occur on sun-exposed surfaces of the face and neck, the V-portion of the chest and back, and the upper outer arms (shawl distribution) (Fig. 8-15); inner arms, axillae and flanks, and knuckles are spared. Photosensitivity occurs in about half, as does alopecia. The hard palate is involved in 40% of cases, and concomitant DLE is present in 20%.

Given these cutaneous parameters, and considering that three fourths of these patients have arthralgia or arthritis, 20% have leukopenia, and 80% have a positive ANA, it is not surprising that (despite the name) at least half meet the American Rheumatism Association criteria for a diagnosis of systemic LE (SLE). The majority of cases have antibodies to Ro/SSA antigen, and a comparable number are HLA-DR3-positive. The disease generally runs a mild course, however, and renal, central nervous system (CNS), or vascular complications are unusual. Hydrochlorothiazide has been reported to have induced this type of LE. David-Bajar lists piroxicam, penicillamine, glyburide, griseofulvin, and Aldactone as other treatments that may produce these lesions.

Histopathology

Histologic changes are similar to those of DLE, except that follicular plugging, hyperkeratosis, and lymphocytic infiltration are less marked. Bielsa et al found that severe epidermal damage with eosinophilic necrosis and/or vacuolization of all epidermal layers occurred in some Ro-positive patients. Direct immunofluorescence is positive in lesions in 60% of cases. A dustlike particulate deposition of IgG in epidermal nuclei of Ro-positive patients may be present. Norris has found that Ro antigen is expressed on the cell membranes of keratinocytes after ultraviolet light exposure. This could lead to autoantibody formation with resultant cell damage by the mechanism of antibody-dependent cellular cytotoxicity.

Treatment

Treatment is primarily with antimalarials (see previous discussion under DLE). Low-dose systemic steroids and photoprotection are helpful. All of the medications listed under DLE have been reported to be beneficial in SCLE. Additionally, methotrexate, cyclophosphamide, plasmapheresis, thalidomide, and pulse methylprednisolone have been used in severe refractory cases. As with DLE careful consideration of risks and benefits need be given, since these two types of lupus are generally benign.

Neonatal Lupus Erythematosus

Annular scaling erythematosus macules and plaques may appear on the head and extremities (Fig. 8-16) within the first few months of life in babies born to mothers with LE, rheumatic disease, or other connective tissue disorders. Half of the mothers are asymptomatic at the time of delivery. McCune et al, however, reported that 18 of 21 mothers of children with neonatal LE developed LE or more commonly Sjögren's syndrome during a follow-up period of 0.25 to 9.5 years. The children's lesions usually resolve spontane-

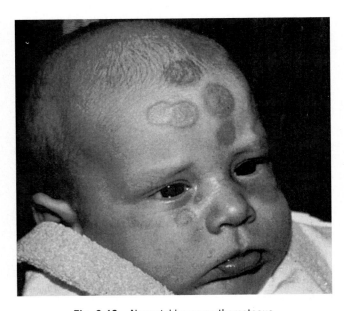

Fig. 8-16 Neonatal lupus erythematosus.

ously by 6 months of age, and usually heal without scarring. Dyspigmentation and persistent telangiectasias may remain for months to years. Telangiectatic macules or angiomatous papules may also be an early feature of neonatal lupus. They may be found in sun-protected sites such as the diaper area, may occur independent of active lupus skin lesions, and may be persistent. Photosensitivity may be prominent. Histopathology and immunopathology are characteristic of SCLE. Seventy-five percent of cases are girls.

Although the skin lesions are transient, half of the patients have an associated isolated congenital heart block, usually third degree, which is permanent. Some infants have only this manifestation of LE, and for cardiac lesions alone, there is no female predominance. In children with cutaneous involvement, thrombocytopenia and hepatic disease occurred as frequently as cardiac disease in the 18 patients reported by Weston et al.

As with other forms of SCLE, there is a strong Ro/SSA autoantibody association. Nearly all mothers, and hence nearly all infants, are positive for this antibody. There is also a linkage to HLA-Dr3 in the mother. Lee has reported that the risk that a second child will have neonatal LE is approximately 25%, and that the outlook for the infants is good. Japanese infants apparently differ in that they may express anti-ds DNA antibodies and 8% progress to SLE. In unselected women with anti-Ro antibodies only 1% to 2% will have an infant with neonatal LE. Occasional cases have been associated with U1RNP antibodies. These infants have not developed heart block.

Complement Deficiency Syndromes

Although deficiency of many complement components may be associated with LE-like conditions, deficiencies of the early components, especially C2 and C4, are most characteristic. Many such cases are found to have photosensitivity, annular SCLE lesions, and Ro/SSA antibody formation.

Systemic Lupus Erythematosus

Young to middle-aged women are predominantly affected with systemic lupus erythematosus (SLE), manifesting a wide range of symptoms and signs. Skin involvement occurs in 80% of cases and is likely to be helpful in arriving at a diagnosis. Its importance is suggested by the fact that four of the American Rheumatism Association's 11 criteria for the diagnosis of SLE are cutaneous findings. The diagnostic criteria are as follows:

1. Malar erythema
2. Discoid LE
3. Photosensitivity
4. Oral ulcer(s)
5. Nonerosive arthritis
6. Serositis (pericarditis or pleurisy)
7. Nephropathy (albuminuria or cellular casts)
8. CNS disorder (unexplained seizures or psychosis)
9. Hematologic disorder (hemolytic anemia with reticulo-

cytosis, or leukopenia below 4000/mm³ on two occasions, or lymphopenia below 1500/mm³ on two occasions)
10. Immunologic disorder: positive LE-cell preparation, or antibody to native DNA or SM antigen, or false-positive serologic test for syphilis (STS)
11. Antinuclear antibody in abnormal titer, unexplained

For identification of patients in clinical studies, a patient may be said to have SLE if four or more criteria are satisfied, serially or simultaneously.

Cutaneous Manifestations

The characteristic butterfly facial erythema seen in patients with SLE is a common manifestation of acute cutaneous LE. The eruption usually begins on the malar area and the bridge of the nose (Fig. 8-17). There may be associated edema (Fig. 8-18). The ears and chest may also be the site of early lesions (Fig. 8-19). The eruption may last from a day to several weeks, and resolves without scarring. There may be more widespread erythema in some cases.

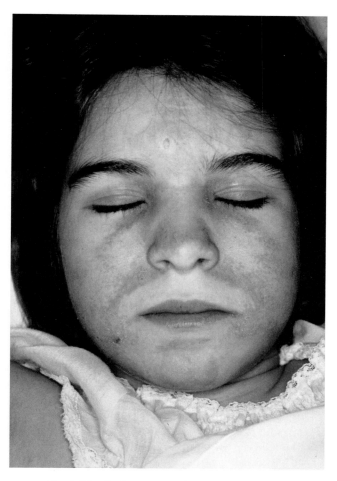

Fig. 8-18 Acute cutaneous lupus erythematosus.

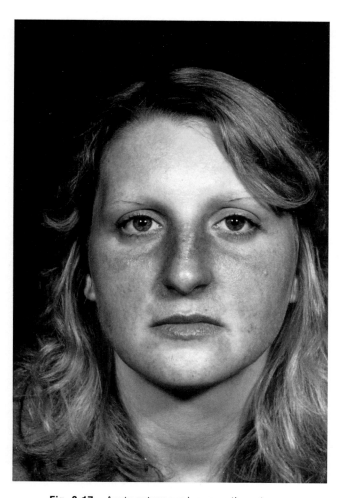

Fig. 8-17 Acute cutaneous lupus erythematosus.

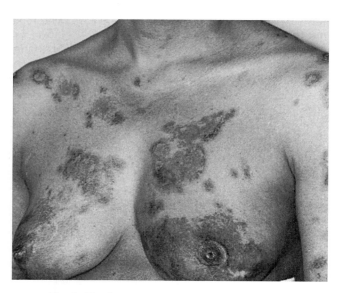

Fig. 8-19 Acute cutaneous lupus erythematosus.

Bullous lesions occur as single or grouped vesicles or bullae, often widespread, with a predilection for sun-exposed areas. Rarely, they may itch. Histologically, there is a subepidermal bulla containing neutrophils. Fluorescence with IgG, IgM, IgA, or C3 is present in a granular or linear pattern at the BMZ on DIF testing. They are found in or below the lamina densa on immunoelectron microscopy. Epidermolysis bullosa acquisita is histopathologically and immunopathologically identical since both diseases are mediated by circulating antibodies against Type VII collagen. Most of these patients are HLA-DR2 positive. The separation of this subset as a distinct one is perhaps made clear, however, by its often dramatic therapeutic response to dapsone, which is ineffective in epidermolysis bullosa acquisita.

A variety of vascular lesions occur in 50% of cases, which, although not specific for SLE, suggest underlying connective tissue disease. Often the fingertips or toe tips show suggestive puffiness, erythema, or telangiectasis. In addition to periungual telangiectasias, red lunulae may be present. The palms, soles, elbows, knees, or buttocks may become persistently erythematous or purplish, sometimes with overlying scale (Fig. 8-20). Minute telangiectases appear in time on the face or elsewhere, and commonly appear about the nail folds. Petechiae may occur in the mouth.

Diffuse, nonscarring hair loss is common. Short, broken-off hairs in the frontal region as a result of increased fragility are referred to as *lupus hairs.*

Mucous membrane lesions are seen in 20% to 30% of SLE patients. Conjunctivitis, episcleritis, and nasal and vaginal ulcerations may occur. Oral mucosal hemorrhages, erosions, shallow ulcerations with surrounding erythema, and gingivitis occur commonly. Erythema, petechiae, and erosions may occur on the hard palate.

Lin et al reported three cases of SLE in which multiple dermatofibromas supervened, 120 in one case. They suggest that 15 should be the lower limit of "multiple."

Leg ulcers, typically deeply punched out, very indolent, and with very little inflammation, may be seen on the pretibial or malleolar areas particularly. Vasculitis or thrombosis caused by the presence of an antiphospholipid antibody may cause them. Cryoglobulinemia, livedo reticularis, thrombophlebitis, and cutaneous infarction may also be present. Gangrene of the digits is a rare event. Erythema multiforme–like lesions may predominate; this has been termed *Rowell's syndrome.*

Cutaneous angiitis manifested by petechiae, papulo-nodules, livedo reticularis, and superficial ulceration may be an initial manifestation of SLE.

Calcinosis cutis is uncommon but may be dramatic as Rothe et al and Nomura et al document. Also seen infrequently are plaquelike or papulo-nodular depositions of mucin. These reddish-purple to skin-colored lesions are often present on the trunk and arms or head and neck. They

may be present as part of the skin findings in SLE or as an isolated chronic cutaneous form of LE (lupus tumidus or tumid lupus). Finally, a symmetrical papular eruption of the extremities may occur. These skin-colored to erythematous lesions with a smooth, ulcerated, or umbilicated surface may show vasculitis or, in older lesions, a palisaded granulomatous inflammation. These occur in patients with SLE, rheumatoid arthritis, or other immune-complex–mediated disease. Chu et al propose calling this palisaded neutrophilic and granulomatous dermatitis of immune complex disease.

Systemic Manifestations

Most organs can be involved; the symptoms and findings are often due to vasculitis. The earliest changes noted may be transitory or migratory arthralgia, often with periarticular inflammation. Fever, weight loss, pleuritis, adenopathy, or acute abdominal pain may occur.

Arthralgia is often the earliest abnormality and may remain the sole symptom for some time at the onset of SLE. Ninety-five percent of SLE patients will manifest

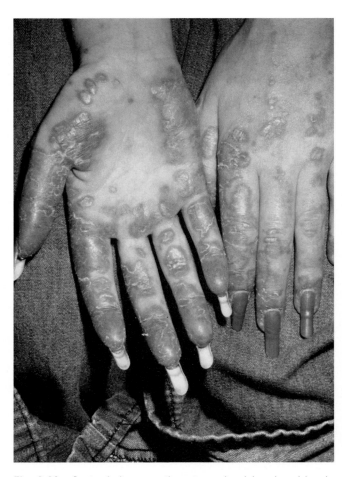

Fig. 8-20 Systemic lupus erythematosus involving dorsal hands and palms.

this symptom. Arthralgia, deforming arthropathy, and acute migratory polyarthritis resembling rheumatoid arthritis may all occur as manifestations of SLE. Avascular necrosis of the femoral head has been observed. Although this has been known to occur during corticosteroid therapy, it has occurred also in patients with SLE who never have had corticosteroids.

Thrombosis in vessels of various sizes and thromboembolism may be a recurring event. It may be attributed to a plasma constituent paradoxically called *lupus anticoagulant (LA)*. Thrombocytopenia, a false-positive STS, livedo reticularis, neurologic disorders, and a high risk of spontaneous abortions further characterize these patients. Asherton et al offer an excellent review.

Renal involvement may be of either nephritic or nephrotic type, leading in either case to chronic renal insufficiency with proteinuria and azotemia. Hypercholesterolemia and hypoalbuminemia may occur. Immunoglobulin and complement components have been found localized to the basement membrane of glomeruli, where vasculitis produces the characteristic "wire-loop" lesion.

Myocarditis is indicated by cardiomegaly and gallop rhythm, but the electrocardiographic changes are usually not specific. Pericarditis (the most frequent cardiac manifestation) and endocarditis also occur. Raynaud's phenomenon occurs in about 15% of patients; these individuals have less renal disease and consequently lower mortality.

The CNS may be involved with vasculitis, manifested by hemiparesis, convulsions, epilepsy, diplopia, retinitis, choroiditis, psychosis, and other personality disorders. Livedo reticularis is a marker for patients at risk for CNS lesions. The combined involvement of the CNS and skin is frequently due to pathogenic antiphospholipid antibodies. In this case only noninflammatory thromboses account for the vascular compromise. Mental depression, cephalalgia, peripheral neuritis, mental confusion, and loss of memory may also be present.

Idiopathic thrombocytopenic purpura is occasionally the forerunner of SLE. Coombs-positive hemolytic anemia, neutropenia, and lymphopenia are other hematologic findings. Gastrointestinal involvement may produce symptoms of nausea, vomiting, and diarrhea. Frequently the intestinal wall and the mesenteric vessels show vasculitis. Pulmonary involvement with pleural effusions, interstitial lung disease, and acute lupus pneumonitis may be present. Sjögren's syndrome (keratoconjunctivitis sicca) and Hashimoto's thyroiditis are associated with SLE with some frequency. Overlap with any of the connective tissue diseases may be seen. Muscular atrophy may accompany extreme weakness so that dermatomyositis may be suspected. Myopathy of the vacuolar type may produce muscular weakness, myocardial disease, dysphagia, and achalasia of the esophagus. Tsokos et al at the National Institutes of Health (NIH) reported 17 women and 1 man with myositis, among 228 patients with SLE (8%), and found the myositis mild and the serum aldolase level (but not creatine phosphokinase) frequently elevated.

A history of exposure to excessive sunlight before the onset of the disease or before an exacerbation is sometimes obtained. Some patients may suffer only mild constitutional symptoms for weeks or months, but immediately after exposure to strong sunlight may develop the facial eruption and severe disease complications.

Childhood SLE. The onset of childhood SLE occurs between ages 3 and 15, with girls outnumbering boys by a ratio of 4:1. The skin manifestations may be the typical butterfly eruption on the face and photosensitivity (Fig. 8-21). In addition, there may be morbilliform, bullous, purpuric, ulcerating, or nodose lesions. The oral mucosa is frequently involved.

The skin eruptions may be associated with joint, renal, neurologic, and gastrointestinal disease. Weight loss, fatigue, hepatosplenomegaly, lymphadenopathy, and fever are other manifestations.

Familial SLE. Familial SLE, a rare subset of SLE, has been found to be associated with hereditary hyperglobulinemia and a high incidence of other connective tissue diseases in family members of those with SLE. Concordance in monozygotic twins is 70%. Lahits et al reported 4 kindreds with 22 members, of whom 10 had clear-cut SLE; 9 of the 10 were male. Several other family members had intermittent symptoms, including tenosynovitis and positive ANA tests.

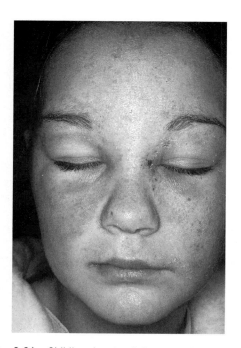

Fig. 8-21 Childhood systemic lupus erythematosus.

Pregnancy and SLE. Women with LE may have successful pregnancies, although there might be difficulty in becoming pregnant, and miscarriages occur with greater frequency. The course of pregnancy may be entirely normal, with remission of the LE, or the symptoms of LE may become worse. Risk of fetal death is increased in women with a previous history of fetal loss and anticardiolipin or anti-Ro antibodies. Low-dose aspirin is often used in the former instance. For the patient with these antibodies but without a history of previous fetal loss, the risk of fetal loss or neonatal lupus is low.

It is in the postpartum period that the risk to the patient is highest; the pregnancy itself is usually well tolerated. A flare of SLE and obstetric complications are risks to the mother.

Evidence that estrogen-containing contraceptives can aggravate SLE is scanty and unconvincing. Jungers et al have shown that progesterone does not have this effect.

Etiology

Genetic factors play a role in the development of SLE. The prevalence of SLE in first-degree relatives of SLE patients is 1.5%. SLE occurs predominantly in females in the reproductive years. Multiple abnormal immune responses are present, which may be responsible for many of the manifestations. An abnormal response to sunlight, both UVB and UVA, exists as reviewed by Hruza et al, Kind et al, and Norris. UV upregulates cytokines, causes release or translocation of sequestered antigens, and causes free radical damage.

Several aspects of the altered immune response are worth particular attention. T-suppressor-cell function is reduced. Overproduction of gamma globulins by B cells causes overresponsiveness to endogenous antigens. The immune complexes thus produced may induce complement-mediated tissue damage. Reduced clearance of immune complexes by the reticuloendothelial system aggravates matters. Also, as just mentioned, there is evidence for externalization of cellular antigens, such as Ro/SSA, in response to sunlight. This may lead to cell injury by way of antibody-dependent cellular cytotoxicity.

Drugs such as hydralazine, procainamide, the sulfonamides, penicillin, anticonvulsants, minocycline, and isoniazid have precipitated or unmasked SLE. Although many such cases run a relatively benign course, with clearing and recovery within a few weeks or months after discontinuation of the drug, some patients continue to be gravely ill, or have repeated relapses, and seem to develop true SLE.

Hydralazine induces a positive ANA in 14% of treated patients. HLA-Dr4 individuals who are slow acetylators, taking 300 mg/day for 3 months or more, are predisposed to develop a drug-induced SLE syndrome. The risk is even higher with procainamide, which induces a positive ANA in about 50% of treated patients who frequently develop symptomatic LE. Antibody to the histone complex H2A-H2B is closely associated with symptomatic disease. There is a 15% incidence of a positive ANA developing with isoniazid taken for a year or more; however, disease is uncommon and generally mild if it does occur. In all these, more than 90% of the positive ANAs are directed against histone. An exception is penicillamine-induced cases, which seem to induce native disease, with anti-dsDNA antibodies. Hydrochlorothiazide has been implicated in production of SCLE as have other drugs listed earlier in this chapter. Drug-induced SLE is typically mild, with skin, renal, and CNS manifestations being unusual compared with naturally occurring disease. Skin lesions occur in about 18% of cases.

Laboratory Findings

Many varied findings are found in SLE. There may be hemolytic anemia, thrombocytopenia, lymphopenia, or leukopenia; the erythrocyte sedimentation rate is usually markedly elevated, Coombs test may be positive, and there is a biologic false-positive test for syphilis in about 20%; and the rheumatoid factor may be present. Levels of IgG may be high, the albumin-globulin ratio is reversed, and the serum globulin is increased, especially the gamma globulin or α_2 fraction. The LE factor is a gamma globulin protein. Albumin, red blood cells, and casts are the most frequent findings in the urine. The specific frequencies of each of these findings, and those that follow, are listed in Tan's article defining these criteria. Similar listings from the study of 140 LE patients are reviewed by Beutner et al.

Immunologic Findings

1. *ANA test.* Positive in about a third of all connective tissue disorders, but in 95% of cases of SLE. Hep-2 tumor cell line is the most sensitive substrate.
2. *LE cell test.* Specific but not very sensitive.
3. *dsDNA:* Anti-double-stranded DNA, anti-native DNA. Specific, not very sensitive. Indicates high risk of renal disease.
4. *Anti-SM antibody.* Sensitivity only 20% to 30% but has highest specificity of any test for SLE.
5. *Antinuclear ribonucleic acid protein (anti-nRNP).* Indicates low risk of renal disease and a good prognosis. Seen in mixed connective tissue disease as well as in SLE.
6. *Anti-La antibodies.* Found in only 10% to 15% of SLE cases and 30% of cases of Sjögren's syndrome.
7. *Anti-Ro antibodies.* Found in about 25% of SLE and 40% of Sjögren's cases. In patients with SCLE (70%), neonatal LE (95%), C2- and C4-deficient LE (50% to 75%), late-onset LE (75%), and in Asian patients with LE (50% to 60%), this antibody is more frequently present. Photosensitivity may be striking.
8. *Serum complement.* Low levels indicate active disease, often renal.
9. *Lupus band test.* Direct cutaneous immunofluorescence. Granular deposits of immunoglobulins and

complement along the dermoepidermal junction occur in more than 75% of lesions of DLE and SLE, and in normal skin in SLE only (where it is twice as common in sun-exposed as in protected skin). A positive test in protected skin correlates well with the presence of anti-dsDNA antibodies and renal disease, and hence with a poor prognosis.

10. *Anti-ssDNA antibody.* Sensitive but not specific. Many are photosensitive. An IgM isotope seen in DLE may identify a subset of patients at risk for developing systemic symptoms.

11. *ANA patterns.* Peripheral, SLE-specific (anti-DNA); in some patients, antibodies to lamin B may be present when this pattern is present. Homogeneous (histone determinants) and particulate patterns are not specific for LE.

12. *Antiphospholipid antibodies.* Both the anticardiolipin antibody and the lupus anticoagulant are subtypes of these. They are associated with a syndrome that includes venous thrombosis, arterial thrombosis, spontaneous abortions, and thrombocytopenia. Livedo reticularis is a frequent skin finding and unfading acral microlivedo, small cyanotic pink lesions on the hands and feet, is a subtle clue to the presence of these antibodies. Antiphospholipid antibodies may occur in association with lupus, other connective tissue disease, or as a solitary event. In the latter case it is referred to as the *primary antiphospholipid syndrome.*

Differential Diagnosis

SLE must be differentiated from dermatomyositis, toxic erythema multiforme, polyarteritis nodosa, acute rheumatic fever, rheumatoid arthritis, pellagra, pemphigus erythematosus (Senear-Usher syndrome), drug eruptions, hyperglobulinemic purpura, Sjögren's syndrome, necrotizing angiitis, and myasthenia gravis. SLE may be differentiated by several factors. In SLE there may be fever, arthralgia, weakness, lassitude, skin lesions suggestive of LE, an increased sedimentation rate, cytopenias, proteinuria, band immunoglobulin deposition at the dermal-epidermal junction, and positive ANA tests. Biopsies of skin lesions and involved kidney are also useful adjuncts.

Treatment

Many cases run a relatively benign course, with mild rheumatoid arthritis–like symptoms requiring only bed rest and salicylates. Salicylates may produce dramatic relief of musculoskeletal symptoms. If salicylates are not tolerated, ibuprofen (Motrin, Advil), 1200 to 3200 mg daily, or other nonsteroidal antiinflammatory medications may be substituted. The importance of daily sunscreen use and sun avoidance cannot be overemphasized.

ANTIMALARIALS. The various antimalarials (Atabrine, chloroquine, and hydroxychloroquine) are effective in the treatment of SLE. These may be used also in conjunction with the corticosteroids. Dosage and side effects of the antimalarials are discussed earlier in this chapter in the treatment section of DLE. A Canadian cooperative study has shown that hydroxychloroquine reduces the likelihood of clinical flare-ups in patients with quiescent SLE. Occasionally, porphyria cutanea tarda may coexist with all forms of LE. If this is the case, standard doses of antimalarials are toxic.

CORTICOSTEROIDS. In moderately severe cases corticosteroids have proved to be effective and to prolong survival. In cases with renal or neurologic involvement, corticosteroids should be administered. Corticosteroid dose should be optimized to the lowest possible dose that controls symptoms and laboratory abnormalities.

Urman and Rothfield reported a group of 156 patients in which corticosteroid dosage was determined by the disease activity as measured by the serum C3 complement levels and the antibody to native DNA titers determined at each patient visit to the clinic. They believe that this is a more exact control of dosage, and it may be an important factor in achieving a longer survival rate in these patients. Their 5- and 10-year survival rates were 93% and 84%, respectively.

Treatment with 1000 mg of methylprednisolone intravenously daily for 3 days, followed by oral prednisone, 0.5 to 1 mg/kg/daily, is effective in quickly reversing most clinical and serologic signs of activity of lupus nephritis.

Mucocutaneous lesions may benefit from additional topical corticosteroid therapy. Lee et al reported that oral ulcers in a patient with LE dramatically responded to fluocinonide gel under occlusion provided by a vinyl prosthetic device.

IMMUNOSUPPRESSIVE THERAPY. Azathioprine, methotrexate, and cyclophosphamide are often employed as steroid-sparing agents.

Other Treatment Modalities

Thalidomide, ultraviolet light A1 (340-400 nm), photopheresis, dihydroepiandrosterone, and high-dose IV gamma globulin have been used to treat some patients.

Ahmed AR, et al: Coexistence of lichen planus and SLE. *J Am Acad Dermatol* 1982, 7:478.

Alegre VA, et al: The Sneddon syndrome. *Int J Dermatol* 1990, 29:45.

Allegue F, et al: Chilblain LE and antiphospholipid antibody syndrome. *J Am Acad Dermatol* 1988, 19:908.

Asherton RA, et al: Antiphospholipid syndrome. *J Invest Dermatol* 1993, 100:21S.

Beaufils M, et al: Clinical significance of anti-Sm antibodies in SLE. *Am J Med* 1983, 74:201.

Beutner EH, et al: Studies on criteria of the EADV for the classification of cutaneous LE. *Int J Dermatol* 1991, 30:411.

Bielsa I, et al: Histopathologic findings in cutaneous LE. *Arch Dermatol* 1994, 130:54.

Brown MM, et al: Skin immunopathology in SLE. *JAMA* 1980, 243:38.

Burge SM, et al: Mucosal involvement in systemic and chronic cutaneous LE. *Br J Dermatol* 1984, 121:727.

Callen JP: Chronic cutaneous lupus erythematosus. *Arch Dermatol* 1982, 118:412.

Callen JP: Serologic and clinical features of patients with DLE. *J Am Acad Dermatol* 1985, 13:748.

Callen JP: SLE in patients with chronic cutaneous (discoid) lupus erythematosus. *J Am Acad Dermatol* 1985, 12:278.

Callen JP, et al: Azathioprine. *Arch Dermatol* 1991, 127:515.

Callen JP, et al: Subacute cutaneous LE. *Arthritis Rheum* 1988, 31:1007.

Canadian Hydroxychloroquine Study Group: A randomized study of the effect of withdrawing hydroxychloroquine sulfate in SLE. *N Engl J Med* 1991, 324:150.

Caruso WR, et al: Skin cancer in black patients with DLE. *J Rheumatol* 1987, 14:156.

Cervera R, et al: SLE: clinical and immunologic patterns of disease expression in a cohort of 1000 patients. *Medicine* 1993, 72:113.

Chalmers A, et al: SLE during penicillamine therapy for rheumatoid arthritis. *Ann Intern Med* 1982, 97:659.

Chlebus E, et al: SCLE versus SLE. *J Am Acad Dermatol* 1998, 38:405.

Chu P, et al: The histopathologic spectrum of palisaded neutrophilic and granulomatous dermatitis in patients with collagen vascular disease. *Arch Dermatol* 1994, 130:1278.

Cryan S, et al: Chronic cutaneous LE presenting as periorbital edema and erythema. *J Am Acad Dermatol* 1992, 26:334.

Dahl MV: Usefulness of direct immunofluorescence in patients with LE. *Arch Dermatol* 1983, 119:1010.

Dalziel K, et al: Oral gold in DLE. *Br J Dermatol* 1986, 45:211.

David-Bajar KM: SCLE. *J Invest Dermatol* 1993, 100:2S.

Davis BM, et al: Prognostic significance of the lupus band test in SLE. *J Invest Dermatol* 1982, 78:360.

Dekle CL, et al: Lupus tumidus. *J Am Acad Dermatol* 1999, 41:250.

Dugan EM, et al: Pregnancy and lupus. *Q J Med* 1988, 66:125.

Dugan EM, et al: U1 RNP Antibody-positive neonatal lupus. *Arch Dermatol* 1992, 128:1490.

Duong DJ, et al: American experience with low-dose thalidomide therapy for severe cutaneous LE. *Arch Dermatol* 1999, 135:1079.

Englert HJ, et al: Clinical and immunologic features of livedo reticularis in LE. *Am J Med* 1989, 87:408.

Felson DT, et al: Evidence for the superiority of immunosuppressive drugs and prednisone over prednisone alone in lupus nephritis. *N Engl J Med* 1984, 309:1528.

Fitzgerald EA, et al: Rowell's syndrome. *J Am Acad Dermatol* 1996, 35:801.

Fox JN, et al: Lupus profundus in children. *J Am Acad Dermatol* 1987, 16:389.

Gammon WR, et al: Bullous SLE. *J Invest Dermatol* 1993, 100:28S.

Garcia-Patos V, et al: Systemic lupus erythematosus presenting with red lunulae. *J Am Acad Dermatol* 1997, 36:834.

Genuereau T, et al: High-dose IVIG in cutaneous LE. *Arch Dermatol* 1999, 135:1124.

George PM, et al: Childhood DLE. *Arch Dermatol* 1993, 129:613.

Gibson GE, et al: Coexistence of LE and PCT in fifteen patients. *J Am Acad Dermatol* 1998, 38:569.

Green SG, et al: Successful treatment of hypertrophic LE with isotretinoin. *J Am Acad Dermatol* 1987, 17:364.

Grob JJ, et al: Cutaneous manifestations associated with the presence of the lupus anticoagulant. *J Am Acad Dermatol* 1986, 15:211.

Grob JJ, et al: Unfading acral microlivedo. *J Am Acad Dermatol* 1991, 24:53.

Herrero C, et al: SCLE. *J Am Acad Dermatol* 1988, 19:1057.

Hess E: Drug related lupus. *N Engl J Med* 1988, 318:1460.

Hruza LL, et al: Mechanisms of UV-induced inflammation. *J Invest Dermatol* 1993, 100:35S.

Hymes SR, et al: The anti-Ro antibody system. *Int J Dermatol* 1986, 25:1.

Izumi AK, et al: LE panniculitis. *Arch Dermatol* 1983, 119:61.

Jonsson H, et al: Outcome in SLE. *Medicine* 1989, 68:141.

Jorizzo JL, et al: Oral lesions in SLE. *J Am Acad Dermatol* 1992, 27:389.

Jungers P, et al: Influence of oral contraceptive therapy on the activity of SLE. *Arthritis Rheum* 1982, 25:618.

Kaneko F, et al: Neonatal LE in Japan. *J Am Acad Dermatol* 1992, 26:397.

Kind P, et al: Phototesting in LE. *J Invest Dermatol* 1993, 100:53S.

Kluher J, et al: Acetylprocainamide therapy in patients with previous procainamide-induced lupus syndrome. *Ann Intern Med* 1981, 95:18.

Kobayashi T, et al: Plaquelike cutaneous lupus mucinosis. *Arch Dermatol* 1993, 129:383.

Lahits RG, et al: Familial SLE in males. *Arthritis Rheum* 1983, 26:39.

Lassoued K, et al: Antinuclear autoantibodies specific for lamins. *Ann Intern Med* 1988, 108:829.

Lee LA: AntiRo (SSA) and AntiLa (SSB) antibodies in LE and in Sjögren's syndrome. *Arch Dermatol* 1988, 124:61.

Lee LA: Neonatal LE. *J Invest Dermatol* 1993, 100:9S.

Lee MS, et al: Oral insertable prosthetic device as an aid in treating oral ulcers. *Arch Dermatol* 1991, 127:479.

Lin RY, et al: Multiple dermatofibromas and SLE. *Cutis* 1986, 37:45.

Lindskov R, et al: Dapsone in the treatment of chronic LE. *Dermatologica* 1986, 172:214.

Lowe L, et al: Papulonodular dermal mucinosis in LE. *J Am Acad Dermatol* 1992, 27:312.

Maggio KL, et al: Discoid lupus erythematosus-treatment with occlusive compression. *J Am Acad Dermatol* 1996, 35:627.

Martinez J, et al: Low-dose intralesional interferon alpha for DLE. *J Am Acad Dermatol* 1992, 26:494.

McCormack LS, et al: Annular subacute cutaneous LE responsive to dapsone. *J Am Acad Dermatol* 1984, 11:397.

McCune AB, et al: Maternal and fetal outcome in neonatal LE. *Ann Intern Med* 1987, 106:518.

McCune WJ, et al: Clinical and immunological effects of monthly administration of IV cyclophosphamide in severe SLE. *N Engl J Med* 1988, 318:1423.

McGrath H, et al: Ultraviolet-A1 (340-400 nm) irradiation therapy in systemic lupus erythematosus. *Lupus* 1996, 5:269.

Millard LE, et al: Chilblain LE (Hutchinson). *Br J Dermatol* 1978, 98:497.

Mills JA: SLE. *N Engl J Med* 1994, 330:1871.

Nomura M, et al: Large subcutaneous calcification in SLE. *Arch Dermatol* 1990, 126:1057.

Norris DA: Pathomechanisms of photosensitive LE. *J Invest Dermatol* 1993, 100:58S.

Norris DG, et al: SLE in children. *Clin Pediatr* 1977, 16:774.

Nunez M, et al: Pulsed dye laser treatment of telangiectatic chronic erythema of cutaneous LE. *Arch Dermatol* 1996, 132:354.

Petri M: Antiphospholipid antibodies. *Curr Prob Dermatol* 1992, 5:171.

Plotnick H, et al: Lichen planus and coexisting LE versus lichen-planus-like LE. *J Am Acad Dermatol* 1986, 14:931.

Provost TT, et al: Anti-Ro HLA-DR3-positive women. *J Invest Dermatol* 1993, 100:14S.

Provost TT, et al: The neonatal lupus syndrome associated with U1RNP (nRNP) antibodies. *N Engl J Med* 1987, 316:1135.

Provost TT, et al: The relationship between anti-Ro(SSA) antibody positive Sjögren's syndrome and anti-Ro(SSA) antibody positive LE. *Arch Dermatol* 1988, 124:63.

Prystowky S, et al: Chronic cutaneous LE (DLE). *Medicine* 1976, 55:183.

Rattner D, et al: DLE scarring and dermabrasion. *J Am Acad Dermatol* 1990, 22:314.

Reed BR, et al: SCLE associated with hydrochlorothiazide therapy. *Ann Intern Med* 1985, 103:49.

Rothe M, et al: Extensive calcinosis cutis with SLE. *Arch Dermatol* 1990, 126:1060.

Ruzicka T, et al: Efficiency of acitretin in the treatment of cutaneous LE. *Arch Dermatol* 1988, 124:897.

Rynes RI: Ophthalmologic safety of long-term hydroxychloroquine sulfate treatment. *Am J Med* 1983, 75(IA):35.

Santa Cruz DJ, et al: Verrucous LE. *J Am Acad Dermatol* 1983, 9:82.

Shornick JK, et al: Isotretinoin for refractory LE. *J Am Acad Dermatol* 1991, 24:49.

Spann CR, et al: Clinical, serologic, and immunogenetic studies in patients with chronic cutaneous LE who have verrucous and/or hypertrophic skin lesions. *J Rheumatol* 1988, 15:256.

Stevens CJM: The antiphospholipid syndrome. *Br J Dermatol* 1991, 125:199.

Stevens RJ, et al: Thalidomide in the treatment of the cutaneous manifestations of lupus erythematosus. *Br J Rheumatol* 1997, 36:353.

Tan M: Autoantibodies to nuclear antigens. *Adv Immunol* 1982, 33:167.

Tan M, et al: The 1982 revised criteria for the classification of SLE. *Arthritis Rheum* 1982, 25:1271.

Thivolet J, et al: Recombinant interferon alpha 2a in the treatment of discoid and subacute cutaneous LE. *Br J Dermatol* 1990, 122:405.

Thorton CM, et al: Cutaneous telangiectases in neonatal LE. *J Am Acad Dermatol* 1995, 33:19.

Tobin DR, et al: Hydroxychloroquine. *Arch Ophthalmol* 1982, 100:81.

Topper SF, et al: Neonatal lupus. *Arch Dermatol* 1994, 130:105.

Triplett DA, et al: The relationship between lupus anticoagulants and autoantibodies to phospholipid. *JAMA* 1988, 259:550.

Tsokos GC, et al: Muscle involvement in SLE. *JAMA* 1981, 246:766.

Tuffanelli DL: LE. *J Am Acad Dermatol* 1981, 4:127.

Urman JD et al: Corticosteroid treatment on SLE. *JAMA* 1977, 238:2272.

Valeski JE, et al: A characteristic cutaneous direct immunofluorescent pattern associated with Ro (SSA) antibodies in SCLE. *J Am Acad Dermatol* 1992, 27:194.

Vandersteen PR, et al: C2-deficient SLE. *Arch Dermatol* 1982, 118:584.

Varner NW, et al: Pregnancy in patients with SLE. *Am J Obstet Gynecol* 1983, 145:1025.

Wallace DJ: Dubois' Lupus erythematosus, ed 3, Philadelphia, 1987, Lea and Febiger.

Wechsler HL, et al: SLE with anti-Ro antibodies. *J Am Acad Dermatol* 1982, 6:73.

Weigand DA: Lupus band test. *J Am Acad Dermatol* 1986, 14:426.

Weinstein CL, et al: Severe visceral disease in SCLE. *Arch Dermatol* 1987, 123:638.

Werth VP, et al: Incidence of alopecia areata in LE. *Arch Dermatol* 1992, 128:368.

Weston WL, et al: The clinical spectrum of anti-Ro-positive cutaneous neonatal LE. *J Am Acad Dermatol* 1999, 40:675.

Wilson CL, et al: Scarring alopecia in DLE. *Br J Dermatol* 1992, 126:307.

Winkelmann RL: Panniculitis in connective tissue disease. *Arch Dermatol* 1983, 119:336.

Wolfe JT, et al: Cutaneous LE following laser-induced thermal injury. *Arch Dermatol* 1997, 133:392.

Wollina U, et al: LE-associated red lunula. *J Am Acad Dermatol* 1999, 41:419.

Yasue T: Livedo vasculitis and central nervous system involvement in SLE. *Arch Dermatol* 1986, 122:66. ▲

DERMATOMYOSITIS

Dermatomyositis (DM) is an inflammatory myositis characterized by vague prodromata, edema, dermatitis, and muscular inflammation and degeneration. Erythema, telangiectasia, pigmentation, and interstitial calcinosis may also be present. Acute, subacute, and chronic forms occur. Muscle involvement without skin changes is called *polymyositis*. With or without skin lesions, weakness of proximal muscle groups is characteristic.

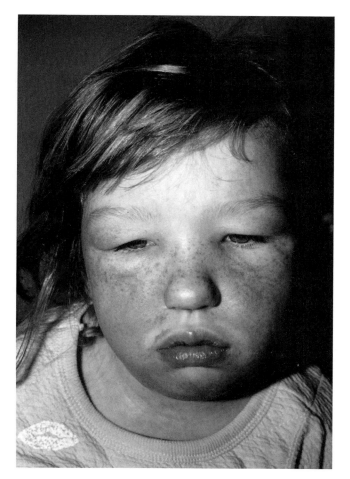

Fig. 8-22 Swelling of the eyelids typical of dermatomyositis.

Skin Findings

Usually the disease begins with erythema and swelling of the face and eyelids, sometimes extending to other regions (Fig. 8-22). The eyelids are often first involved. They become swollen and pinkish violet (heliotrope) and may be tender to the touch, owing to involvement of the orbicularis oculi. Minute telangiectases on the eyelids may be seen with a magnifying glass.

Other skin changes include erythematous or urticarial patches and plaques on the upper portion of the face and the extremities. Firm, slightly pitting edema occurs, especially over the shoulder girdle, arms, and neck. Photosensitivity is common. Pruritus may be severe in some cases. Kasteler et al reported 14 of 17 patients had scalp involvement characterized by atrophic, erythematous scaly plaques. Alopecia occurred in 6 of the 14 patients.

This phase may last for months but is typically succeeded by more widespread skin changes, spreading from the face to the neck, thorax, shoulders, arms, and elsewhere. Characteristic patterns include base of neck and upper chest (V) pattern; an upper back, neck, and shoulder (shawl) pattern;

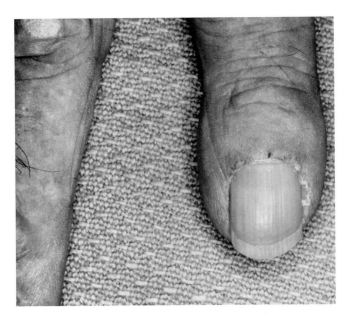

Fig. 8-23 Periungual changes of dermatomyositis.

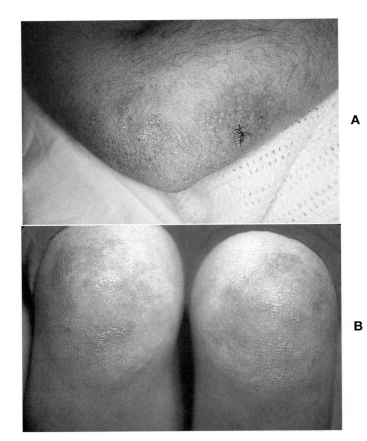

Fig. 8-24 **A** and **B**, Psoriasiform changes of dermatomyositis.

occasionally a flagellate pattern mimicking bleomycin-induced linear edematous streaks, or an erythroderma.

Telangiectatic vessels cause an erythematous line or spots on the proximal fingernail folds (Fig. 8-23). Enlarged capillaries of the nail fold appear as sausage-shaped loops, similar to those changes observed in scleroderma. There may be cuticular overgrowth with an irregular frayed appearance. A reddish purple scaling eruption occurs over the knuckles and over the knees and elbows (Gottron's sign) (Fig. 8-24). Ulceration of the fingertips may occur. Flat-topped, violaceous papules over the knuckles (Gottron's papules) are thought to be pathognomonic of dermatomyositis (Fig. 8-25). Hyperkeratosis, scaling, fissuring, and hyperpigmentation over the fingertips, sides of the thumb, and fingers with occasional involvement of the palms is referred to as *mechanic's hands* and has been reported in 70% of patients with antisynthetase antibodies. Intermittent fever, malaise, anorexia, arthralgia, and marked weight loss are commonly present at this stage.

Other lesions, seen less frequently, include Raynaud's phenomenon and hypertrichosis of the body. Localized deposits of mucin, as seen in SLE, may occur. When there is regression of the disease, a hyperpigmentation develops that simulates the bronze discoloration of Addison's disease. Telangiectasia and erythematous patches on the face and upper chest may persist for months or years, with periodic flare-ups, eventually being replaced by brown pigmentation. In some cases the pigmentation may include areas of hypopigmentation, atrophy, and telangiectasia so that poikiloderma eventually develops. Rarely, large, persistent ulcerations in flexural areas or over pressure points may develop.

Basset-Sequin found this to be a possible marker for malignancy, but it may be seen in patients who do not have cancer.

Calcium deposits in the skin and muscles occur in more than half of children with DM; this occurs rather infrequently in adults. Calcification is related to duration of disease activity and its severity. Calcinosis of the dermis, subcutaneous tissue, and muscle occurs mostly on the upper half of the body around the shoulder girdle, elbows, and hands. Ulcerations and cellulitis are frequently associated with this debilitating and disabling complication of dermatomyositis.

Muscle Changes

In severe cases early and extensive muscular weakness occurs, with acute swelling and pain. The muscle weakness is seen symmetrically, most frequently involving the shoulder girdle and sometimes the pelvic region, as well as the hands. The patients may notice difficulty in lifting even the lightest objects. They may be unable to raise their arms to comb their hair. Patients often complain of pain in the legs when standing barefoot or being unable to climb stairs. Difficulty in swallowing, talking, and breathing, caused by

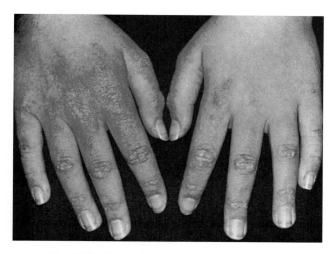

Fig. 8-25 Gottron's papules of dermatomyositis.

weakness of the involved muscles, may be noted early in the disease. The voice may be nasal. Later there are atrophy and arthritic changes leading to ankylosis. Cardiac involvement with cardiac failure may be present in the terminal phase of the disease.

Some patients have typical skin findings of DM but have no muscle involvement. It is typical that the eruption of DM precedes muscle symptoms by 2 to 3 months. Occasionally, patients may not manifest muscle inflammation for a year or longer, and rarely, complete absence of myositis with long-term follow-up has been reported. These cases have been termed *amyopathic dermatomyositis* or *dermatomyositis sine myositis*. It is common, however, for muscle inflammation to be present but not symptomatic. Work-up to include muscle enzymes, electromyogram (EMG), and magnetic resonance imaging (MRI), in addition to a detailed physical examination, should be performed to detect subtle involvement, since early therapy may then be initiated.

Diagnostic Criteria

The following criteria are used to define dermatomyositis/polymyositis:
1. Symmetrical weakness of limb girdle muscles and anterior flexors of the neck
2. Elevated muscle enzymes: creatine phosphokinase, transaminases, lactic dehydrogenase, and aldolase
3. Abnormal EMG
4. Characteristic myositis on muscle biopsy
5. The typical dermatologic features

Two of these criteria (in addition to dermatologic features) make dermatomyositis probable; three permit a diagnosis.

Associated Diseases

Dermatomyositis may be associated with or complicated by other diseases. Sclerodermatous changes are the most frequently observed. This is called *sclerodermatomyositis.*

Antibodies such as anti-Ku and anti-PM/sc1 may be present in this subgroup. Mixed connective tissue disease, and uncommonly, rheumatoid arthritis, lupus erythematosus, and Sjögren's syndrome may occur concomitantly. Dermatomyositis may be associated with interstitial lung disease. The presence of anti-Jo-1 antibody, as well as other anti-synthetase antibodies such as anti-PL-7, anti-PL-12, anti-DJ, and anti-EJ, correlates well with the development of pulmonary disease.

Neoplasia with Dermatomyositis

In adults malignant neoplastic disease is frequently associated with dermatomyositis. In a study of 392 Swedish dermatomyositis patients, 15% developed cancer at the same time or after the diagnosis of DM. In 57 DM patients with 67 malignancies, Callen found that cancer preceded dermatomyositis in 26 cases, occurred simultaneously in 18, and followed it in 23.

In dermatomyositis, malignancy is most frequently seen in patients in the fifth and sixth decades of life. The two entities occur together more often in women than in men. A search for malignancy, directed by historical and physical findings and routine laboratory testing, is warranted in adults (especially those over age 40) with dermatomyositis. Whereas ovarian cancer is present in more than 20% of women over age 40 who have DM and cancer, studies directed at adequate evaluation for this malignancy are indicated.

Childhood Dermatomyositis

Several features of childhood dermatomyositis differ from the adult form. Two childhood variants exist. The more common *Brunsting type* has a slow course, progressive weakness, calcinosis, and steroid responsiveness. Calcinosis may be subcutaneous and acral (elbows, knees, fingers) as in adults, or the classic form, involving intermuscular fascial planes. The second type, the *Banker type,* is characterized by a vasculitis of the muscles and gastrointestinal tract, a rapid onset of severe weakness, steroid unresponsiveness, and death. This type is uncommon. Internal malignancy is seldom seen in children with either type.

Treatment is with systemic corticosteroids until remission has been achieved, then long-term low-dose therapy. Methotrexate, azathioprine, or other steroid-sparing agents may also be used.

Etiology

There is mounting evidence that humoral immunity and a vasculopathy mediated by complement deposition is primarily responsible for the muscle findings in DM, whereas cell-mediated cytotoxicity causes muscle disease in polymyositis (PM). Many autoantibodies may be present in DM, some of which are disease-specific and can identify specific subgroups. In addition to the anti-synthetase antibodies previously discussed, the anti–Mi-2 antibody is present in some patients with the acute onset of classic DM with a good prognosis. Reviews by both Targoff and Miller are recommended. The possible role of viral infections in initiating these diseases is under active investigation. Cukier et al suggested patients who have received bovine collagen dermal implants may have an elevated risk of developing DM.

Incidence

Dermatomyositis is relatively rare. It is twice as prevalent in women as in men and four times as common in black as in white patients. There is a bimodal peak, the smaller one seen in children and a larger peak in adults between ages 40 and 65.

Histopathology

The histologic changes in dermatomyositis are identical to those of lupus erythematosus: thinning of the epidermis, hydropic degeneration of the basal layer, edema in the papillary dermis, and a perivascular and periadnexal lymphocytic infiltrate in the superficial and deep dermis with increased dermal mucin. Scattered melanophages are present. Characteristic changes are found in the muscles. The deltoid, trapezius, and quadriceps muscles seem to be almost always involved, and are good biopsy sites. Muscle biopsy is directed to those areas found to be most tender or in which EMG demonstrates myopathy. MRI is a most useful aid in identifying active sites for muscle biopsy. The MRI short TI interval recovery (STIR) images are best. They can be used to localize disease and longitudinally assess results of treatment.

Laboratory Findings

The serum levels of creatinine kinase are elevated in most patients. Aldolase, lactic dehydrogenase, and transaminases are other indicators of active muscle disease. There may be leukocytosis, anemia with low serum iron, and an increased sedimentation rate. Positive ANAs are seen in 60% to 80% of patients, with 35% to 40% having myositis-specific antibodies.

Cutaneous direct immunofluorescence is positive in at least one third of the cases. Cytoid body staining is the usual type of reaction, with deposition of IgM, IgA, and C3 in large globules in the upper dermis.

X-ray studies with barium swallow may show weak pharyngeal muscles and a collection of barium in the pyriform sinuses and valleculae. MRI of the muscles is an excellent way to assess activity of disease noninvasively.

Electromyographic studies for diagnosis show spontaneous fibrillation, polyphasic potential with voluntary contraction, short duration potential with decreased amplitude, and salvos of muscle stimulation.

Differential Diagnosis

Dermatomyositis must be differentiated from erysipelas, SLE, angioedema, and erythema multiforme. Aldosteronism, with adenoma of adrenal glands and hypokalemia, may also cause puffy heliotrope eyelids and face.

Treatment

Prednisone is the mainstay of treatment given in doses beginning with 60 mg daily until the severity decreases and muscle enzymes are almost normal. The dosage is reduced in line with clinical response. Dawkins et al recommend high-dose daily prednisone initially followed by a slow taper with a target treatment period of 24 to 36 months. The SGOT and creatinine phosphokinase assume normal levels as remission occurs. Dalakas and Targoff both give excellent, concise guidelines for the management of the muscular disease, including indications to utilize immunosuppressives such as azathioprine and methotrexate. Exercise is avoided in the acute period; however, passive range of motion should be begun early. Cyclosporine and intravenous immunoglobulin therapy both show promise in early reports.

The skin lesions may respond to systemic therapy; however, its response is unpredictable and skin disease may persist despite involution of the myositis. Because DM is photosensitive, sunscreens with high SPF (greater than 30) should be used daily. Topical steroids may be helpful in such cases. Antimalarials, such as hydroxychloroquine given in doses of 200 to 400 mg/day, or in doses of 2 to 5 mg/kg/day in children, has been shown to be useful in abating the eruption of DM. Low-dose weekly methotrexate may also be effective. Euwer et al treated five patients with amyopathic DM with systemic steroids for symptomatic skin disease. Although some amyopathic patients treated with systemic steroids have not developed myositis, there is no proof that this treatment prevented progression and we do not endorse their use prophylactically. Only in the most severe symptomatic cases of DM sine myositis should systemic steroids be considered. Calcinosis related to DM has been treated with aluminum hydroxide, diphosphonates, diltiazem, probenecid, colchicine, low doses of warfarin, and surgery with variable, but usually poor, results.

Prognosis

Benvassat et al reviewed the course of 72 cases (and 20 possible cases) over age 20; major causes of death were cancer, ischemic heart disease, and lung disease. Independent risk factors were failure to induce clinical remission, white blood cell count above 10,000/mm^3, temperature greater than 38° C at diagnosis, older age, shorter disease history, and dysphagia. The 5-year survival rate of 80% generally reflects improvements in prognosis related to steroid therapy. Bowyer et al found a good functional outcome in 78% of juvenile cases and state that early treatment with high doses of steroids is important.

Dermatomyositis and pregnancy affect each other adversely. In half the patients who become pregnant, the facial lesions and muscle weakness worsen, and fetal loss occurs in more than half the patients.

Basset-Sequin N, et al: Prognostic factors and predictive signs of malignancy in adult DM. *Arch Dermatol* 1990, 126:633.

Benvassat J, et al: Prognostic factors in PM/DM: a computer-assisted analysis of 92 cases. *Arthritis Rheum* 1985, 28:249.

Bernard P, et al: DM and malignancy. *J Invest Dermatol* 1993, 100:128S.

Bohan A, et al: Polymyositis and DM. *N Engl J Med* 1975, 292:344, 403.

Bowles NE, et al: DM, polymyositis, and Coxsackie-B virus infection. *Lancet* 1987, 1:1004.

Callen JP: The value of malignancy evaluation in DM. *J Am Acad Dermatol* 1982, 6:253.

Cherin P, et al: DM and ovarian cancer. *J Rheumatol* 1993, 20:1897.

Cox NH, et al: DM. *Arch Dermatol* 1990, 126:61.

Cukier J, et al: Association between bovine collagen dermal implants and DM or a polymyositis-like syndrome. *Ann Intern Med* 1993, 118:920.

Dalakas MC: PM, DM and inclusion-body myositis. *N Engl J Med* 1991, 325:1487.

Dalakas MC, et al: A controlled trial of high-dose intravenous immune globulin infusions as treatment for DM. *N Engl J Med* 1993, 329:1993.

Dawkins MA, et al: DM. *J Am Acad Dermatol* 1998, 38:397.

Dunn CL, et al: The role of MRI in the diagnostic evaluation of DM. *Arch Dermatol* 1993, 129:1104.

Euwer RL, et al: Amyopathic DM. *J Am Acad Dermatol* 1991, 24:959.

Franks AG: Important cutaneous markers of DM. *J Musculoskeletal Med* 1988, 5:39.

Grau JM, et al: Amyopathic DM. *J Am Acad Dermatol* 1992, 26:505.

Hochberg MC, et al: Adult-onset PM/DM. *Semin Arthritis Rheum* 1986, 15:168.

James WD, et al: Plaquenil therapy for DM. *J Rheumatol* 1985, 12:1214.

Jara M, et al: Dermatomyositis and flagellate erythema. *Clin Exp Dermatol* 1996, 21:440.

Kasteler JS, et al: Low-dose methotrexate administered weekly is an effective corticosteroid-sparing agent for the treatment of the cutaneous manifestations of dermatomyositis. *J Am Acad Dermatol* 1997, 36:67.

Kasteler JS, et al: Scalp involvement in DM. *JAMA* 1993, 272:1939.

King LE Jr, et al: Evaluation of muscles in a patient with suspected amyopathic DM by MRI and phosphorus 31-spectroscopy. *J Am Acad Dermatol* 1994, 34:137.

Knoell KA, et al: DM associated with bronchiolitis obliterans organizing pneumonia. *J Am Acad Dermatol* 1999, 40:328.

Kovacs SO, et al: DM. *J Am Acad Dermatol* 1998, 39:899.

Lang BA, et al: Treatment of dermatomyositis with intravenous immunoglobulin. *Am J Med* 1991, 91:169.

Malleson P: Juvenile DM: a review. *J R Soc Med* 1982, 75:33.

Miller FW: Myositis-specific antibodies. *JAMA* 1993, 270:1847.

Miller LC, et al: Childhood DM. *Clin Pediatr* (Phila) 1987, 26:561.

Minkin W, et al: Office nailfold capillary microscopy using an ophthalmoscope. *J Am Acad Dermatol* 1982, 7:190.

Miyagawa S, et al: DM presenting as erythroderma. *J Am Acad Dermatol* 1992, 26:489.

Oliveri MB, et al: Regression of calcinosis during diltiazem treatment in juvenile dermatomyositis. *J Rheumatol* 1996, 23:2152.

Olson NY, et al: Adjunctive use of hydroxychloroquine in childhood DM. *J Rheumatol* 1989, 16:1547.

Philips TS, et al: DM and pulmonary fibrosis associated with anti-Jo-1 antibody. *J Am Acad Dermatol* 1987, 17:381.

Rockerbie NR, et al: Cutaneous changes of DM precede muscle weakness. *J Am Acad Dermatol* 1989, 20:629.

Sigurgiersson B, et al: Risk of cancer in patients with DM or PM. *N Engl J Med* 1992, 326:363.

Stonecipher MR, et al: Cutaneous changes of DM in patients with normal muscle enzymes. *J Am Acad Dermatol* 1993, 28:951.

Stonecipher MR, et al: DM with normal muscle enzyme concentrations. *Arch Dermatol* 1994, 130:1294.

Targoff IN: Humoral immunity in PM/DM. *J Invest Dermatol* 1993, 100:116S

Tsao H, et al: Lesions resembling malignant atrophic papulosis in a patient with dermatomyositis. *J Am Acad Dermatol* 1997, 36:317.

Tymms KE, et al: Dermatomyositis and other connective tissue diseases. *J Rheumatol* 1985, 12:1140.

Weng WJ, et al: Calcinosis cutis in juvenile DM. *Arch Dermatol* 1988, 124:1721.

Whitmore SE; et al: Dermatomyositis sine myositis. *J Rheumatol* 1996, 23:101.

Whitmore SE, et al: Serum CA-125 screening for ovarian cancer in patients with dermatomyositis. *Gynecol Oncol* 1997, 65:241.

Winton GB: Skin diseases aggravated by pregnancy. *J Am Acad Dermatol* 1989, 20:1.

Yosipovitch G, et al: STIR magnetic resonance imaging. *Arch Dermatol* 1999, 135:721. _____ ▲

SCLERODERMA

Scleroderma is sclerosis of the skin characterized by the appearance of circumscribed or diffuse, hard, smooth, ivory-colored areas that are immobile and give the appearance of hidebound skin.

Scleroderma occurs in both localized and systemic forms. Cutaneous types may be categorized as morphea (localized, generalized, profunda, and pansclerotic forms) or linear scleroderma (with or without melorheostosis or hemiatrophy). Progressive systemic sclerosis and the Thibierge-Weissenbach syndrome (commonly referred to as the *CREST syndrome*) are the two types of systemic scleroderma.

Cutaneous Types
Localized Morphea

This form of scleroderma is twice as common in women as in men. It occurs in childhood as well as in adult life. It occurs most often as macules or plaques a few centimeters in diameter but also may occur as bands or in guttate lesions (Fig. 8-26). Rose or violaceous macules may appear first, followed by smooth, hard, somewhat depressed, yellowish white or ivory-colored lesions (Fig. 8-27). They are most common on the trunk but also occur on the extremities.

The margins of the areas are generally surrounded by a light violaceous zone or by telangiectases. Within the patch the elasticity of the skin is lost, and when it is picked up between the thumb and index finger it feels rigid. The follicular orifices may be unusually prominent, leading to a condition that resembles pigskin. Such localized lesions generally spread a little but remain circumscribed.

In guttate morphea multiple small, chalk-white, and flat or slightly depressed macules may occur in large numbers over the chest, neck, shoulders, or upper back. These are not very firm or sclerotic and are difficult to separate with confidence from lichen sclerosus et atrophicus.

This type of scleroderma tends to slowly involute over a 3- to 5-year period, leaving only atrophy or normal-appearing skin behind.

Morphea–Lichen Sclerosus et Atrophicus Overlap

There are patients who present with both lesions of morphea and lichen sclerosus et atrophicus (LS+A). They are

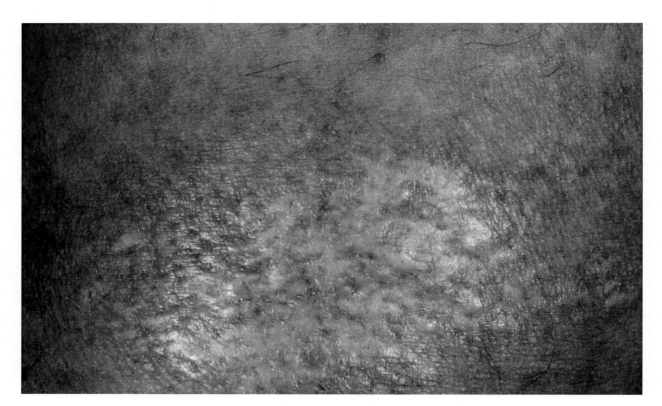

Fig. 8-26 Morphea.

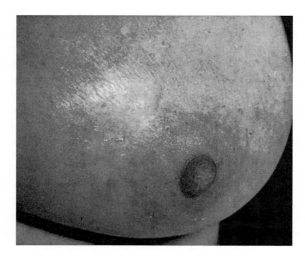

Fig. 8-27 Morphea. Note fine crinkling of skin on the upper part of the lesion.

commonly women with widespread morphea who have typical LS+A lesions either separated from morphea or overlying morphea (Fig. 8-28). These patients should be viewed as having morphea as their primary disease process.

Generalized Morphea
Widespread involvement by indurated plaques with hypo- or hyperpigmentation characterizes this variety. Muscle

atrophy may be associated. There is no systemic involvement. Patients may look young because of the firmness to the skin and absence of wrinkles (Fig. 8-29). Spontaneous involution is less common than in localized lesions.

Atrophoderma of Pasini and Pierini
In 1923, Pasini described a peculiar form of atrophoderma now thought to be in the spectrum of morphea. The disease consists of brownish, oval, round or irregular, smooth atrophic lesions depressed below the level of the skin with a well demarcated, sharply sloping border (Fig. 8-30). It occurs mainly on the trunk of young individuals, predominately females. The lesions are usually asymptomatic. The singly occurring or multiple lesions measure from several to 20 or more centimeters in diameter.

Buechner et al in a review distinguished two clinical subsets. In 23 of the 34 patients the classic variety was observed; however, in the remaining 11 a localized superficial variant was seen. There were solitary lesions on the trunk that were irregular in outline, with satellite brown macules at the periphery. The most common location was the upper back or lumbosacral area.

The histopathologic picture shows reduction in the thickness of the dermal connective tissue. Because of the minimal changes noted, a biopsy should include normal-appearing skin so that a comparison may be made.

The course of the atrophoderma is benign, terminating

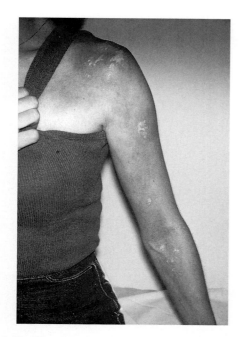

Fig. 8-28 Morphea–lichen sclerosus et atrophicus overlap.

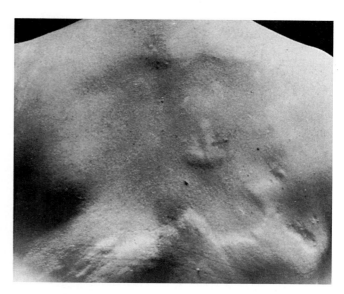

Fig. 8-30 Atrophoderma of Pasini and Pierini.

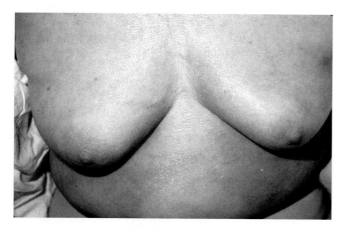

Fig. 8-29 Generalized morphea.

spontaneously after several months or a few years although some cases have persisted indefinitely. There is no known effective treatment.

Pansclerotic Morphea of Children

This variant, described by Diaz-Perez et al, is manifested by sclerosis of the dermis, panniculus, fascia, muscle, and at times, bone. There is disabling limitation of motion of joints. It is also called *morphea profunda.*

Linear Scleroderma

These linear lesions may extend the length of the arm or leg, beginning most often in the first decade of life (Fig. 8-31). They may also occur parasagittally on the frontal scalp and

extend part way down the forehead (en coup de sabre) (Fig. 8-32). The Parry-Romberg syndrome, which manifests progressive facial hemiatrophy, epilepsy, exophthalmos, and alopecia, may be a form of linear scleroderma (Fig. 8-33). When the lower extremity is involved, there may be spina bifida, or faulty limb development, hemiatrophy, or flexion contractures. Melorheostosis, seen in roentgenograms as a dense linear cortical hyperostosis, may occur. At times linear lesions of the trunk merge into more generalized involvement (Fig. 8-34). Generally the only type that shows spontaneous improvement is the childhood type involving the extremities. Physical therapy of the involved limb or limbs is of paramount importance to prevent contractures and frozen joints.

Systemic Types
CREST Syndrome

Systemic sclerosis may be limited to the hands, or sometimes the hands and lower face, for months to years. During this time it is often called *acrosclerosis.* If it is associated with calcinosis (Fig. 8-35), Raynaud's phenomenon, esophageal dysmotility, sclerodactyly (always present), and telangiectasia (Fig. 8-36), it is called *CREST syndrome.* This form of scleroderma is not as severe as PSS. Immunologically, anticentromere antibody appears to be highly specific for the CREST syndrome, being positive in 50% to 90% of cases and in only 2% to 10% of patients with progressive sclerosis.

This variant of systemic scleroderma has the most favorable prognosis, owing to the usually limited systemic involvement.

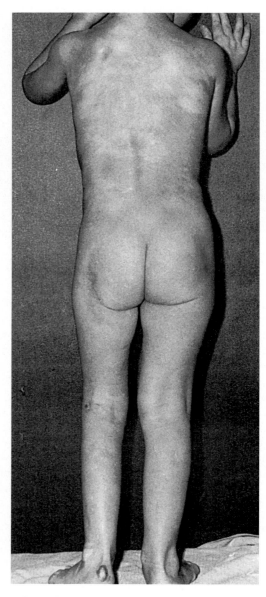

Fig. 8-31 Linear morphea in a 3-year-old boy.

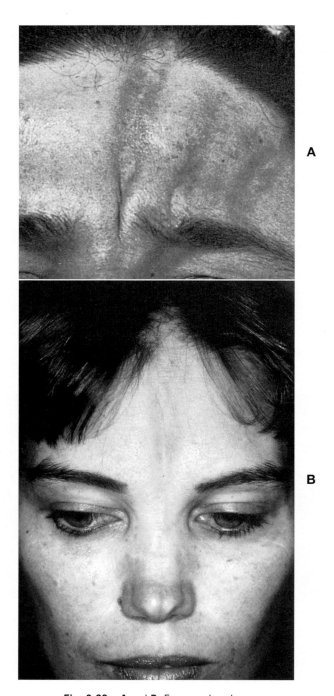

Fig. 8-32 **A** and **B**, En coup de sabre.

Progressive Systemic Sclerosis

Progressive systemic sclerosis (PSS) is a generalized disorder of connective tissue in which there is fibrous thickening of the skin combined with fibrosis and vascular abnormalities in certain internal organs. Raynaud's phenomenon is the first manifestation of PSS in more than half the cases and eventually is nearly always present. The heart, lungs, gastrointestinal tract, kidney, and other organs may be involved. Women are affected three times more commonly than men, with the peak age onset between the third and fifth decade.

SKIN FINDINGS. In the earlier phases of scleroderma the affected areas are erythematous and swollen. Patients are frequently misdiagnosed as having carpal tunnel syndrome and may even have positive EMGs. Raynaud's phenomenon is often present. Sclerosis supervenes. The skin becomes

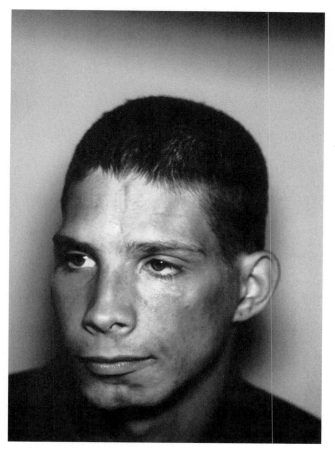

Fig. 8-33 Parry-Romberg syndrome.

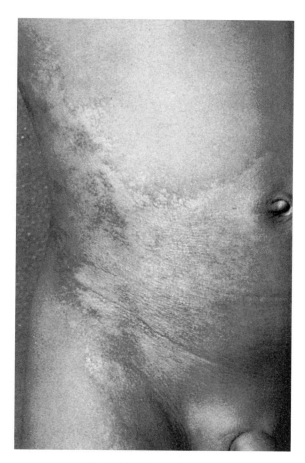

Fig. 8-34 Linear morphea.

smooth, yellowish, and firm and shrinks so that the underlying structures are bound down (Fig. 8-37). The earliest changes often occur insidiously on the face and hands, and in more advanced stages these parts become hidebound, so that the face is expressionless and the hands are clawlike (sclerodactylia) (Fig. 8-38). The skin of the face appears drawn, stretched, and taut, but not hard, with loss of lines or expression. There is difficulty in opening the mouth. The lips are thin, contracted, and radially furrowed, the nose appears sharp and pinched, and the chin may be puckered. Barnett described the "neck sign" as a ridging and tightening of the neck on extension, which occurs in 90% of patients with scleroderma.

The disease may remain localized to the hands and feet for long periods (acrosclerosis). The fingers become semiflexed, immobile, and useless, the skin over them being hard, inelastic, incompressible, and pallid. The terminal phalanges are boardlike and indurated. Mizutani et al have described the "round fingerpad sign." The fingers were found to lose the normal peaked contour, but rather appear as a rounded hemisphere when viewed from the side. This

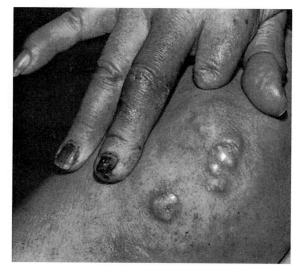

Fig. 8-35 CREST syndrome on the knee and fingers of a 60-year-old woman. Note calcium nodules over the patella, telangiectasia over the upper knuckles, amputation of the forefinger as a result of gangrene, and Raynaud's phenomenon of the fingertips.

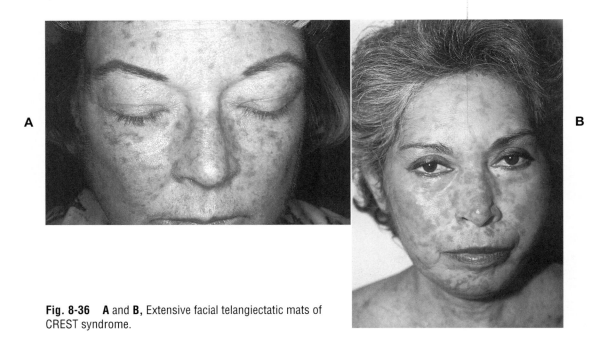

A

B

Fig. 8-36 **A** and **B,** Extensive facial telangiectatic mats of CREST syndrome.

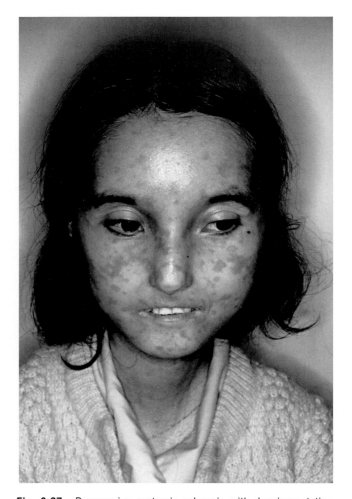

Fig. 8-37 Progressive systemic sclerosis with dyspigmentation.

process may lead to loss of pulp on the distal digit. Trophic ulcerations and gangrene may occur on the tips of the fingers and knuckles, which may be painful or insensitive, usually the latter. Focal mucinosis-type lesions may be present. Pterygium inversum unguis, in which the distal part of the nail bed remains adherent to the ventral surface of the nail plate, may be seen in scleroderma, lupus erythematosus, or may be idiopathic or congenital. Dilated, irregular, nail fold capillary loops are present in 75% of systemic scleroderma patients. In active PSS there is also capillary loss leading to avascular areas. Sato et al found nail fold capillary bleeding an easily observed finding that, when present on two or more fingers, was 90% specific for scleroderma and correlated with the anticentromere antibody. Sclerosis is more marked distally than proximally. Although similar changes occur in the feet and toes, they are seldom as severe as in the hands.

Keloidlike nodules may develop on the extremities or the chest, and there may be a widespread diffuse calcification of the skin as shown by radiographs. A diffuse involvement of the chest may lead to a cuirasslike restraint of respiration. Late in the course of the disorder, hyperpigmented or depigmented spots or a diffuse bronzing may be present. The most characteristic pigmentary change is a loss of pigment in a large patch with perifollicular pigment retention within it (Fig. 8-39). The affected areas become hairless. Jawitz et al reported the finding of pigment retention over superficial blood vessels of the forehead within a wider field of depigmentation. Atrophy may be associated with telangiectasia. Bullae and ulcerations may develop, especially on the distal parts of the extremities. Partial alopecia and decreased sweat gland activity are frequently found.

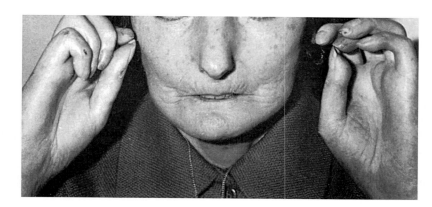

Fig. 8-38 Scleroderma.

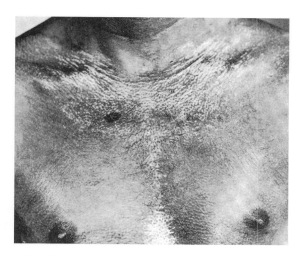

Fig. 8-39 Dermatomyositis with scleroderma in a 37-year-old man. (Courtesy Dr. H. Shatin.)

INTERNAL INVOLVEMENT. Progressive systemic sclerosis may involve most of the internal organs. Fibrosis, loss of smooth muscle of the internal organs, and progressive loss of visceral function characterize this disorder. Most frequently the gastrointestinal tract is involved, followed by the lungs, then the cardiovascular and renal systems. The CNS and the musculoskeletal system are less frequently involved. Esophageal involvement (chiefly atony) is seen in more than 90% of patients. The distal two thirds is affected, leading to dysphagia and reflux esophagitis. Small intestinal atonia may lead to constipation, malabsorption, or diarrhea.

Pulmonary fibrosis with arterial hypoxia, dyspnea, and productive cough may be present. Progressive nonspecific interstitial fibrosis, with bronchiectasis and cyst formation, is the most frequent pathologic change. Pulmonary hypertension and right-sided heart failure are ominous signs, occurring in 5% to 10% of patients. The cardiac involvement produces dyspnea, palpitation, and other symptoms of congestive heart failure. Sclerosis of the myocardium produces conduction changes. Pericarditis may also be present. Death usually occurs from cardiac or renal failure.

Renal disease produces azotemia and proteinuria. Hypertension and retinopathy may be present.

The skeletal manifestations are initially articular pain, swelling, and inflammation. Polyarthritis may be the first symptom in systemic sclerosis. There is limitation of motion, as a result of skin tautness, followed by ankylosis, which may eventually lead to severe contractual deformities. The hand joints are involved most frequently. There may be resorption and shortening of the phalanges, and narrowing of the joint spaces. Osteoporosis and sclerosis of the bones of the hands and feet may occur, as well as decalcification of the vault of the skull. Muscular involvement, with myosclerosis and calcium deposits in the muscles, may occur.

Childhood PSS has identical cutaneous manifestations. Raynaud's phenomenon is less frequent, while cardiac wall involvement is more common and is responsible for half the deaths. Renal disease is unusual. Familial scleroderma rarely occurs. Systemic sclerosis may be associated with Hashimoto's thyroiditis, Sjögren's syndrome, or dermatomyositis.

PROGNOSIS. The course of PSS is variable. Barnett et al found that by simply dividing patients into three groups by extent of skin involvement within 1 year of diagnosis helped predict survival. Patients with sclerodactyly alone had a 71% 10-year survival rate, those with skin stiffness above the metacarpal-phalangeal joints but not involving the trunk had a 58% survival, and those patients with truncal involvement only survived 21% of the time. Others have found older age of onset, male sex, black race, anemia, and, of course, kidney, lung, or cardiac sclerosis to be adverse predictors. ANA patterns predict different subsets of disease with varying prognosis.

Laboratory Findings

ANA testing is positive in more than 90% of patients with systemic scleroderma. Several of these antibodies identify specific clinical subsets of patients. The antinucleolar pattern is considered most specific for scleroderma, and when present as the only pattern, it is highly specific for scleroderma. When antibodies to such nucleolar antigens as

RNA polymerase t and fibrillarin are present, diffuse sclerosis, generalized telangiectasia, and internal organ involvement are often seen. The homogeneous ANA pattern is seen in those patients with PM-Scl antibodies, the marker for polymyositis-scleroderma overlap. The true speckled or anticentromere pattern is sensitive and specific for the CREST variant. Patients may have antibodies to Sc1-70. They tend to have diffuse truncal involvement, pulmonary fibrosis, and digital pitted scars, but a low incidence of renal disease. Antibodies to nuclear RNP are found in patients with Raynaud's phenomenon, polyarthralgia, arthritis, and swollen hands who, more than 80% of the time, eventually develop scleroderma or remain in an "undifferentiated state." Therefore, this group has been referred to as having an *undifferentiated connective tissue syndrome* rather than the old "mixed connective tissue disease" designation. Anti-single stranded DNA antibodies are common in linear scleroderma.

Radiographic Findings

The gastrointestinal tract is commonly involved. The esophagus may have decreased peristalsis and dilation. Esophagogram with cine studies should be performed in these cases; however, scleroderma is most easily recognized by esophageal manometry. In early esophageal involvement, a barium swallow in the usual upright position may be reported as normal. If the patient is supine, however, barium will often be seen to pool in the flaccid esophagus. The stomach may be dilated and atonic, resulting in delayed emptying time. Involvement of the small intestine may cause extreme dilation of the duodenum and jejunum, producing a characteristic roentgenographic picture of persistently dilated intestinal loops long after the barium has passed through. The colon is only rarely involved.

Histology

Systemic and localized forms of scleroderma show identical histologic changes. In the acute phase there is a perivascular lymphocytic infiltrate with plasma cells around the vessels of the junction of the dermis and subcutaneous fat. The epidermis is normal except for increased pigmentation. Collagen is increased and individual bundles less distinct. The whole dermis is uniformly pink with loss of spaces between the collagen bundles. The total thickness of the dermis is increased. Eccrine glands and coiled ducts, instead of being located at the junction of the dermis and subcutaneous tissue, are found in the midportion of the thickened dermis. The subcutaneous fat is quantitatively reduced.

In more advanced lesions, the inflammatory infiltrate may be minimal. Pilosebaceous units are absent, and eccrine glands and ducts are compressed by surrounding collagen. Because the thickness of the dermis normally depends on the anatomic site, biopsy specimens from suspected cases of scleroderma (or morphea) must include the subcutaneous tissue.

On direct immunofluorescent testing of skin the nucleolus may be stained in the keratinocytes if antinucleolar circulating antibodies are present, and a "pepper-dot" epidermal nuclear reaction pattern may be seen in CREST patients who have anticentromere antibodies in their serum.

Differential Diagnosis

The diffuse variety of scleroderma must be distinguished from myxedema, scleredema, and scleromyxedema, in which the parts are softer, edematous, and not atrophic. Sclerodactylia may be confused with leprosy and syringomyelia. Eosinophilic fasciitis is a benign, steroid- responsive disorder simulating some features of scleroderma. The skin is thickened, edematous, and erythematous, and has a coarse peau d'orange appearance, as opposed to its sclerotic, taut appearance in scleroderma. The hands and face are usually spared in eosinophilic fasciitis.

In vitiligo the depigmentation is the sole change in the skin, other features present in scleroderma being absent. Scleroderma in the atrophic stage may so closely resemble acrodermatitis chronica atrophicans that differentiation is impossible. The subject is discussed at greater length under the latter disease. Morphea may resemble vitiligo, lichen sclerosus et atrophicus, and cicatrix, but careful examination can easily establish its identity.

Dermal fibrosis is a major feature in a vast array of diseases. Besides the scleroderma variants just discussed, it may be seen in certain metabolic, genetic, and immunologic disorders such as chronic graft-versus-host disease, porphyria cutanea tarda, phenylketonuria, carcinoid syndrome, paraproteinemia, juvenile-onset diabetes, progeria, Werner's syndrome, Huriez syndrome, human adjuvant disease after injection of silicone and paraffin into the skin, and the Crow-Fukase (POEMS) syndrome. Occupational exposure to silica, epoxy resins, polyvinyl chloride, and vibratory stimuli (jackhammer or chain saw) may produce sclerodermoid conditions. Chemicals such as polyvinyl chloride, bleomycin, isoniazid, pentazocine, valproate sodium, epoxy resin vapor, vitamin K (after injection), Spanish rapeseed oil (toxic oil syndrome), tryptophan (eosinophilia-myalgia syndrome), nitrofurantoin, and hydantoin may also induce various patterns of fibrosis. Augmentation mammoplasty with silicone gel implants have been reported to cause systemic scleroderma and morphea. Collagen-type hamartoma also feature dermal sclerosis. Although collagenomas, scars, and keloids are not a problem in differential diagnosis, pachydermadactyly may be. It is a rare form of digital fibromatosis that is characterized by acquired, asymptomatic, protracted connective tissue swelling on the backs and sides of a few proximal phalanges or proximal interphalangeal joints. Draluck et al have recently reported the tenth case, the first woman. Tompkins et al have reported a distal variant in an older woman. While associated with a thinned rather than thickened dermis, the recently defined disease restrictive dermopathy leads to tight skin, generalized joint contractures, distinct facies, and pulmonary hypoplasia. This is a lethal, autosomal recessive disease. Another genetically determined disease to consider is the "stiff skin syndrome." Also known as *congenital fascial dystrophy,* there is a stony-hard induration of the skin and deeper tissues of the buttocks, thighs, and legs, with joint limitation and limb contractures. The disease begins in infancy.

Pathogenesis

The pathogenesis of scleroderma and morphea is not understood. The theories center on primary vascular damage, autoimmune mechanisms, and microchimerism resulting in fetal antimaternal graft-versus-host reactions. *Borrelia burgdorferi* infection is not associated with morphea in the United States; however, in European and Japanese cases *Borrelia afzelli* and *B. garinii* are related to the development of morphea in some cases.

Treatment

In all varieties treatment is unsatisfactory, but spontaneous recovery may occur, especially in children and in the localized types. Also in localized scleroderma an end point may be reached beyond which the disease does not progress. Well-planned daily general exercise and daily physical therapy emphasizing full range of motion for all joints are important therapeutic measures. Regular massage, warmth, and protection from trauma are advised. Exposure to cold is to be avoided, and smoking is forbidden.

Vasospasm resulting in Raynaud's phenomenon may be treated in a variety of ways. Several studies have documented the usefulness of the calcium-channel blocker nifedipine (Procardia), 10 mg four times daily, in reducing the frequency of vasospastic episodes. Dibenzyline, 10 mg three times daily, then decreased to tolerance; Prazosin (Minipress) 1 mg three times daily; and alpha-methyl dopa, 1 to 2 mg daily, have also been helpful. Intravenous iloprost may arrest acute digital gangrene and treat digital ischemic ulcerations. Topical nitroglycerin and simple hand warming on a regular basis may be effective also. Goodfield et al reported that immersing the hands in warm water for 5 minutes every four hours increased blood flow and decreased the number of episodes. Soaking in DMSO has been found to be beneficial for hands with ulceration secondary to Raynaud's syndrome. Dressing these ulcers with Duoderm and changing them once weekly has led to success in healing and pain reduction.

Hulshot et al reported three patients with extensive morphea who were treated with oral calcitriol. They report clinical improvement after several months. This follows an earlier report of beneficial effect of this therapy in systemic sclerosis and morphea. Subcutaneous calcinosis with ulceration has been successfully treated with intralesional injections of triamcinolone acetonide, 20 mg/ml every 4 to 8 weeks. Colchicine, aluminum hydroxide, and other therapies listed as for dermatomyositis may be tried but are usually to no avail. Malabsorption, a common occurrence in

gastrointestinal sclerosis, is usually effectively controlled with tetracyclines. Reversal of vascular and renal crises by oral angiotensin-converting-enzyme blockade, with captopril (Capoten) and other antihypertensive agents, has dramatically improved the outlook in this situation.

Antiinflammatory therapy has relied mostly on immunosuppressives or corticosteroids, or both. Some improvement in several severe cases with azathioprine or cyclophosphamide has been reported anecdotally. Corticosteroid therapy does not offer any lasting benefit; however, the patient feels better and the joint symptoms may be ameliorated when prednisone is taken, 10 to 15 mg every other day. Corticosteroids are beneficial when there is real evidence of inflammatory myositis. Extracorporeal chemotherapy and D-penicillamine are the subject of much debate. The potential adverse effects, cost, and relative efficacy have limited their use to date. Isotretinoin was reported to improve nine patients in an open trial. Interferon gamma and cyclosporin have also had similar reports in open trials; however, more extensive trials with interferon did not reveal a reversal of the fibrosis. Low-dose UVA1 is being investigated in Europe for a variety of disorders, including scleroderma variants and lichen planus. Kerscher et al reported that 18 of 20 patients with localized scleroderma improved after 12 weeks of treatment. Varga et al warn that patients receiving ionizing radiation who have scleroderma may develop exaggerated fibrosis.

Altman RD, et al: Predictors of survival in SS. *Arthritis Rheum* 1991, 34:403.

Artlett CM, et al: Identification of fetal DNA and cell in skin lesions from women with systemic sclerosis. *N Engl J Med* 1998, 338:1186.

Asboe-Hansen G: Scleroderma. *J Am Acad Dermatol* 1987, 17:102.

Barnett AJ: The neck sign in scleroderma. *Arthritis Rheum* 1989, 32:209.

Barnett AJ, et al: A survival study of patients with scleroderma diagnosed over 30 years. *J Rheumatol* 1988, 15:276.

Blaszczyk M, et al: Autoantibodies to nucleolar antigen in SS. *Br J Dermatol* 1990, 123:421.

Brozena SJ, et al: Human adjuvant disease following augmentation mammoplasty. *Arch Dermatol* 1988, 124:1383.

Buechner SA, et al: Atrophoderma of Pasini and Pierini. *J Am Acad Dermatol* 1994, 30:441.

Bulpitt KJ, et al: Early undifferentiated connective tissue disease. *Ann Intern Med* 1993, 118:602.

Burge KM, et al: Familial scleroderma. *Arch Dermatol* 1969, 99:681.

Caputo R, et al: Pterygium inversum unguis. *Arch Dermatol* 1993, 129:1307.

Clements PJ, et al: Skin score. *Arthritis Rheum* 1990, 30:1256.

Diaz-Perez JL, et al: Disabling pansclerotic morphea in children. *Arch Dermatol* 1980, 116:169.

Draluck JC et al: Pachydermodactyly. *J Am Acad Dermatol* 1992, 27:303.

Falanga V, et al: Antinuclear and anti-single-stranded DNA antibodies in morphea and generalized morphea. *Arch Dermatol* 1987, 123:350.

Falanga V, et al: D-penicillamine in the treatment of localized scleroderma. *Arch Dermatol* 1990, 126:609.

Fenske NA, et al: Silicone-associated connective-tissue disease. *Arch Dermatol* 1993, 129:97.

Fisman SJ, et al: The toxic pseudosclerodermas. *Int J Dermatol* 1991, 30:837.

Frank JM, et al: Atrophoderma of Pasini and Pierini. *J Am Acad Dermatol* 1995, 32:122.

Fujiwara H, et al: Detection of *B. burgdorferi* DNA in morphea and lichen sclerosis et atrophicus tissues of German and Japanese but not of US patients. *Arch Dermatol* 1997, 133:41.

Goodfield MJD, et al: Handwarming as a treatment for Raynaud's phenomenon in SS. *Br J Dermatol* 1988, 119:643.

Gordon ML, et al: Eosinophilic fasciitis associated with tryptophan ingestion. *Arch Dermatol* 1991, 127:217.

Greger RE: Familial progressive systemic scleroderma. *Arch Dermatol* 1976, 111:81.

Gruss C, et al: Low dose UVA1 phototherapy in disabling pansclerotic morphea of childhood. *Br J Dermatol* 1997, 136:293.

Happle R, et al: Restrictive dermopathy in two brothers. *Arch Dermatol* 1992, 128:232.

Haustein UF, et al: Silica-induced scleroderma. *J Am Acad Dermatol* 1990, 22:444.

Hulshot MM, et al: Oral calcitriol as a new therapeutic modality for generalized morphea. *Arch Dermatol* 1994, 130:1290.

Hunzelmann N, et al: Systemic scleroderma: multicenter trial of 1 year of treatment with recombinant interferon gamma. *Arch Dermatol* 1997, 133:609.

Jablonska S, et al: Congenital fascial dystrophy. *J Am Acad Dermatol* 1989, 21:943.

James WD, et al: Nodular (keloidal) scleroderma. *J Am Acad Dermatol* 1984, 11:1111.

Jawitz JC, et al: A new skin manifestation of progressive systemic sclerosis. *J Am Acad Dermatol* 1984, 11:625.

Kasper CS, et al: Talc deposition in skin and tissues surrounding silicone gel-containing prosthetic devices. *Arch Dermatol* 1994, 130:41.

Kerscher M, et al: Low dose UVA1 phototherapy for treatment of localized scleroderma. *J Am Acad Dermatol* 1998, 38:21.

Khan A, et al: Recombinant interferon gamma in the treatment of systemic sclerosis. *Am J Med* 1989, 87:273.

Krieg T, et al: Systemic scleroderma. *J Am Acad Dermatol* 1988, 18:457.

Larrgue M, et al: Systemic scleroderma in childhood. *Ann Dermatol Venereol* 1983, 110:317.

Marzano AV, et al: Unique digital skin lesions associated with systemic sclerosis. *Br J Dermatol* 1997, 136:598.

Mauch C, et al: Control of fibrosis in SS. *J Invest Dermatol* 1993, 100:92S.

Maurice PDL, et al: Isotretinoin in the treatment of SS. *Br J Dermatol* 1989, 121:317.

McGregor AR, et al: Familial clustering of scleroderma spectrum disease. *Am J Med* 1988, 84:1023.

Milburn PB, et al: Treatment of scleroderma skin ulcers with a hydrocolloid membrane. *J Am Acad Dermatol* 1989, 21:200.

Mitchell H, et al: Scleroderma and related conditions. *Med Clin North Am* 1997, 81:129.

Mizutani H, et al: Round fingerpad sign. *J Am Acad Dermatol* 1991, 24:67.

Nelson JL, et al: Microchimerism and HLA-compatible relationships of pregnancy in scleroderma. *Lancet* 1998, 351:559.

Patriz A, et al: Hurriez syndrome. *J Am Acad Dermatol* 1992, 26:855.

Perez MI, et al: Systemic sclerosis. *J Am Acad Dermatol* 1993, 28:525.

Phelps RG, et al: Clinical, pathologic, and immunologic manifestations of the toxic oil syndrome. *J Am Acad Dermatol* 1988, 18:313.

Powell C, et al: The anticentromere antibody: disease specificity and clinical significance. *Mayo Clin Proc* 1984, 59:700.

Rodeheffer RJ, et al: Controlled double-blind trial of nifedipine in Raynaud's phenomenon. *N Engl J Med* 1983, 308:880.

Rook AH, et al: Treatment of SS with extracorporeal photochemotherapy. *Arch Dermatol* 1992, 128:357.

Ruffatti A, et al: Prevalence and characteristics of anti-SS DNA antibodies in localized scleroderma. *Arch Dermatol* 1991, 127:1180.

Sahn EE, et al: Scleroderma following augmentation mammaplasty. *Arch Dermatol* 1990, 126:1198.

Sato S, et al: Diagnostic significance of nailfold capillary bleeding in scleroderma spectrum disorders. *J Am Acad Dermatol* 1993, 28:198.

Silver RM: Unraveling the eosinophilic-myalgia syndrome. *Arch Dermatol* 1991, 127:1214.

Spiera H: Scleroderma after silicone augmentation mammaplasty. *JAMA* 1988, 260:236.

Steen VD, et al: D-penicillamine therapy in progressive systemic sclerosis: a retrospective analysis. *Ann Intern Med* 1982, 97:652.

Stoner MF, et al: Atrophoderma of Pasini and Pierini. *Arch Dermatol* 1990, 126:1639.

Tompkins SD, et al: Distal pachydermodactyly. *J Am Acad Dermatol* 1998, 38:359.

Tork E, et al: Morphea in children. *Am Exp Dermatol* 1986, 11:607.

Trentham DE, et al: Photochemotherapy in SS. *Arch Dermatol* 1992, 128:389.

Tuffanelli DL: Systemic scleroderma. *Med Clin North Am* 1989, 73:1167.

Tuffanelli DL, et al: Anticentromere and anticentriole antibodies in the scleroderma spectrum. *Arch Dermatol* 1983, 119:560.

Varga J, et al: Augmentation mammaplasty and scleroderma. *Arch Dermatol* 1990, 126:1220.

Varga J, et al: Chemical exposure-induced cutaneous fibrosis. *Arch Dermatol* 1994, 130:97.

Varga J, et al: Exaggerated radiation-induced fibrosis in patients with SS. *JAMA* 1991, 265:3292.

Varga J, et al: L-tryptophan and eosinophilia-myalgia syndrome. *J Invest Dermatol* 1993, 100:97S.

Velayos EE, et al: The CREST syndrome. *Ann Intern Med* 1979, 139:240.

Voleski JE, et al: Significance of in vivo pepper-dot epidermal nuclear reactions. *J Am Acad Dermatol* 1994, 30:280.

Welsh KM, et al: Restrictive dermopathy. *Arch Dermatol* 1992, 128:228.

Zachariae H, et al: Treatment of ischaemic digital ulcers and prevention of gangrene with intravenous iloprost in systemic sclerosis. *Acta Derm Venereol* 1996, 76:236. ————————————— ▲

EOSINOPHILIC FASCIITIS

Lawrence Shulman described in 1974 a disorder that he called *diffuse eosinophilic fasciitis*. Classically, patients have been engaging in strenuous muscular effort for a few days or weeks before the acute onset of weakness, fatigability, and pain and swelling of the extremities, soon followed by severe induration of the skin and subcutaneous tissues of the forearms and legs. Both flexion and extension of the limbs are soon limited. The skin is edematous and erythematous, with a coarse peau d'orange appearance, most noticeable inside the upper arms or thighs, or in the flanks. When the patient holds the arms laterally or vertically linear depressions occur within the thickened skin. This "groove sign" follows the course of underlying vessels. The contrast to scleroderma, in which the skin is smooth and taut, is quite striking. The hands and face are usually, but not always, spared. Patients are often unable to stand fully erect. Raynaud's phenomenon is usually absent.

Biopsy shows patchy lymphocytic and plasma cell infiltrate in the fascia and subfascial muscle and great thickening, 10 to 50 times normal, of the fascia. Eosinophils may or may not be present in the affected fascia. Blood eosinophilia of 10% to 40% is usual. The sedimentation rate is increased. Hypergammaglobulinemia is common, and serum eosinophilic chemotactic activity is increased. Patients have been reported to develop pancytopenia, anemia, thrombocytopenia, lymphadenopathy, and pernicious anemia. Two cases have had antibody-mediated hemolytic anemia. Sjögren's syndrome has occurred, and cardiac involvement, usually pericardial effusion, has been reported.

Some consider this disease to be a variant of scleroderma. Patients who developed eosinophilia-myalgia syndrome after ingesting L-tryptophan contaminated with l,l'-ethylidenebis often manifested skin changes similar to eosinophilic fasciitis. Chan et al suggested this may be a paraneoplastic syndrome of hematologic malignant neoplasms, after reporting one patient and reviewing five others from the literature. Reports of eosinophilic fasciitis resulting from *Borrelia burgdorferi* infection suggest this as a possible cause in some cases.

The response to systemic corticosteroids may be excellent. In responders, complete recovery is usual within 1 to 3 years. Patients with a prolonged course unresponsive to systemic steroids are being recognized with increasing frequency.

Blauvelt A, et al: Idiopathic and L-tryptophan-associated eosinophilic fasciitis. *Arch Dermatol* 1991, 126:1159.

Botet MV, et al: The fascia in systemic scleroderma. *J Am Acad Dermatol* 1980, 3:36.

Case records of the Massachusetts General Hospital (Case 4-1990). *N Engl J Med* 1990, 322:252.

Chan LS, et al: Concurrent eosinophilic fasciitis and cutaneous T-cell lymphoma. *Arch Dermatol* 1991, 127:862.

Doyle JA: Eosinophilic fasciitis: extracutaneous manifestations and associations. *Cutis* 1984, 34:259.

Doyle JA, et al: Cutaneous and subcutaneous inflammatory sclerosis syndromes. *Arch Dermatol* 1982, 118:886.

Falanga V, et al: Frequency, levels, and significance of blood eosinophilia in systemic sclerosis, scleroderma, and eosinophilic fasciitis. *J Am Acad Dermatol* 1987, 17:648.

Feldman SR, et al: A histopathologic comparison of Shulman's syndrome and fasciitis associated with the eosinophilia-myalgia syndrome. *J Am Acad Dermatol* 1992, 26:95.

Granter SR, et al: Borrelial fasciitis. *Am J Dermatopathol* 1996, 18:465.

Jarratt M, et al: Eosinophilic fasciitis: an early variant of scleroderma. *J Am Acad Dermatol* 1979, 1:221.

Michet Jr, et al: Eosinophilic fasciitis: report of 15 cases. *Mayo Clin Proc* 1981, 56:27.

Rosenthal J, et al: Diffuse fasciitis and eosinophilia with symmetric polyarthritis. *Ann Intern Med* 1980, 92:507. _____ ▲

MIXED CONNECTIVE TISSUE DISEASE

Sharp et al described a disease, mixed connective tissue disease (MCTD), that has overlapping features of scleroderma, SLE, and dermatomyositis. Twenty-five patients, 21 women, who had severe arthralgia, swelling of the hands and tapered fingers, Raynaud's phenomenon, abnormal esophageal motility, pulmonary fibrosis, muscle pain and tenderness, and weakness of the muscles were reported. Hyperglobulinemia and lymphadenopathy were present in some cases.

The ANA test is an important diagnostic procedure in MCTD. The particulate pattern reflects high titers of nuclear ribonucleoprotein antibodies (anti-RNP antibodies), which persist through periods of remission. In addition, particulate epidermal nuclear IgG deposition on direct immunofluorescence study of skin is a distinctive finding in MCTD. Gratifying improvement has been achieved by the use of a corticosteroid (prednisone) at a daily dose of 1 mg/kg for inflammatory features such as arthritis and myositis.

Sharp and Anderson found that the LE features of MCTD were the most likely, and the scleroderma features the least likely, to improve with time. In a long-term evaluation of Sharp's original study patients, Nimelstein et al found that the inflammatory components became less frequent, while the sclerodermatous features persisted. Some consider this disease to be a subset of scleroderma. Generally the prognosis is good.

Frandsen PB, et al: Follow-up of 151 patients with high-titer U1RNP antibodies. *Clin Rheumatol* 1996, 15:254.

Gilliam JN, et al: Mixed connective tissue disease syndrome. *Arch Dermatol* 1977, 113:583.

Gladman DD: So you suspect mixed connective tissue disease (MCTD): which tests to perform? *Int J Dermatol* 1985, 24:392.

Grant KD, et al: Mixed connective tissue disease: a subset with sequential clinical and laboratory features. *J Rheum* 1982, 8:587.

Nimelstein SH, et al: Mixed connective tissue disease: a subsequent evaluation of the original 25 patients. *Medicine* 1980, 59:239.

Rasmussen EK, et al: Clinical implications of ribonucleoprotein antibody. *Arch Dermatol* 1987, 123:601.

Sharp GC, et al: Current concepts in the classification of connective tissue diseases: overlap syndrome and mixed connective tissue disease (MCTD). *J Am Acad Dermatol* 1980, 2:269. _____ ▲

SJÖGREN'S SYNDROME (SICCA SYNDROME)

Sjögren in 1933 described a triad of keratoconjunctivitis sicca, xerostomia, and rheumatoid arthritis. Dry eyes and dry mouth may occur as *primary Sjögren's syndrome (SS)*, or if a connective tissue disease, such as scleroderma, rheumatoid arthritis, SLE, or polymyositis, is associated it is referred to as *secondary SS*. Most patients are age 50 or older, and more than 90% are women.

Xerostomia (dryness of the mouth) may produce difficulty in speech and eating, increased tooth decay, thrush, and decreased taste (hypogeusia). Rhinitis sicca (dryness of the nasal mucous membranes) may induce nasal crusting and decreased olfactory acuity (hyposmia). Vaginal dryness and dyspareunia may develop. Dry eyes are painful, feel gritty or scratchy, and produce discharge and blurry vision. Fatigue is a prominent symptom.

Skin manifestations of SS include vasculitis, xerosis, and annular erythema of SS. Vasculitis may present as purpura of the legs, which may be palpable or nonpalpable. It may be indistinguishable from Waldenström's benign hypergammaglobulinemic purpura. Approximately 30% of benign hypergammaglobulinemic purpura patients will have or will develop SS. Other cutaneous vascular manifestations are urticarial vasculitis, digital ulcers, and petechiae. Histologically, leukocytoclastic vasculitis, or less often mononuclear vasculitis, is found. Patients with cutaneous vasculitis also have a high prevalence of peripheral or CNS vasculitis.

Xerosis with pruritus is common. Decreased sweating occurs. Asian patients have been described who develop erythematous, indurated, annular dermal plaques primarily on the face. This is different than the annular lesions of SCLE, which show epidermal change and histologic changes of lupus. Provost et al reported 10 patients with an overlap of SS and LE. A common finding is Ro antibody positivity. SCLE patients with SS have a worse prognosis than patients with SCLE unassociated with SS. In addition there may be laryngitis, gastric achlorhydria, thyroid enlargement resembling Hashimoto's thyroiditis, malignant lymphoma, thrombotic thrombocytopenic purpura, and splenomegaly.

Labial salivary gland biopsy from inside the lower lip is regarded by many as the most definitive test for SS. Typically, there is a dense lymphocytic infiltrate with many plasma cells and fewer histiocytes in aggregates around minor salivary glands. More than one focus should be present per 4 mm^2 of the tissue biopsy. Xerostomia is diagnosed by the Schirmer test and reflects diminished glandular secretion from the lacrimal glands.

The diagnosis is made when there is objective evidence for two of the following three major criteria:

1. Xerophthalmia
2. Xerostomia
3. An associated autoimmune, rheumatic, or lymphoproliferative disorder

Numerous serologic abnormalities are frequently found associated with SS. The rheumatoid factor is usually positive, with elevated serum globulin and C-reactive proteins, and high titers of IgG, IgA, and IgM. Cryoglobulins may be demonstrated at times. Eighty percent of patients have anti-Ro/SSA antibodies; half as many have anti-La/SSB antibodies. Antibodies to fodrin, a major component of the membrane cytoskeleton of most eukaryotic cells, is present in patients with primary and secondary SS, with a 93% specificity.

Patients with SS appear predisposed to the development of lymphoreticular malignancies such as non-Hodgkin's lymphoma. These are nearly always B-cell in nature. A nonmalignant, extraglandular lymphoproliferative process may also occur. This produces pseudolymphoma, with a potential for regression.

The differential diagnosis includes sarcoidosis, lymphoma, amyloidosis, and HIV disease. The latter produces diffuse infiltrative lymphocytosis syndrome (DILS), which is characterized by massive parotid enlargement; prominent renal, lung, and gastrointestinal manifestations; and a low frequency of autoantibodies.

Specific treatment is not yet available for Sjögren's syndrome. Any therapy should be directed against the various manifestations of connective tissue disease. Artificial lubricants for oral, nasal, and vaginal dryness may be used, as may artificial tears for eye symptoms and topical lubricants for xerosis.

Alexander E, et al: SS. *Arch Dermatol* 1987, 123:801.

Chudwin DS, et al: Spectrum of SS in children. *J Pediatr* 1981, 98:213.

Fox RI, et al: Primary SS: clinical and immunologic features. *Semin Arthritis Rheum* 1984, 14:77.

Itescu S, et al: Diffuse infiltrative lymphocytosis syndrome. *Rheum Dis Clin North Am* 1992, 18:683.

Katayama I, et al: Annular erythema associated with primary SS. *J Am Acad Dermatol* 1989, 21:1218.

Lee LA: AntiRo(SSA) and antiLa(SSB) antibodies in lupus erythematosus and in SS. *Arch Dermatol* 1988, 124:61.

Provost TT, et al: Cutaneous manifestations of SS. *Rheum Dis Clin North Am* 1992, 18:609.

Provost TT, et al: The relationship between antiRo(SSA) and antibody-positive SS and antiRo(SSA)-antibody-positive lupus erythematosus. *Arch Dermatol* 1988, 124:63.

Ruzicka T, et al: Annular erythema associated with SS. *J Am Acad Dermatol* 1991, 25:557.

Talal N: SS. *Rheum Dis Clin North Am* 1992, 18:507.

Teramoto N, et al: Annular erythema. *J Am Acad Dermatol* 1989, 20:596.

Watanabe T, et al: Anti-α-fodrin antibodies in SS and LE. *Arch Dermatol* 1999, 135:535. ▲

RHEUMATOID ARTHRITIS

The majority of skin manifestations of rheumatoid arthritis (RA) are consequences of the cutaneous vasculitis associated with RA. There may be annular erythemas, purpura, bullae, shallow ulcers, and gangrene of the extremities. Many diseases have been reported to occur in association with RA, such as erythema elevatum diutinum, pyoderma gangrenosum, Felty's syndrome, IgA vasculitis, linear IgA disease, Sjögren's syndrome, bullous pemphigoid, and yellow nail syndrome.

Rheumatoid Nodules

Subcutaneous nodules are seen in 20% to 30% of the patients. They may arise anywhere on the body but most frequently are found over the bony prominences, especially on the extensor surface of the forearm just below the elbow and the dorsal hands (Fig. 8-40). These are 2 mm to 2.5 cm, nontender, firm, skin-colored, round nodules, which may or may not be attached to the underlying tissue. Frequently they are attached to the fibrous portions of the periarticular capsule, or they may be free in the subcutaneous tissue. Rheumatoid nodules can easily be mistaken for xanthomas because of a yellow color (pseudoxanthomatous variant). Rheumatoid nodules also occur in 5% to 7% of patients with SLE, especially around small joints of the hands; rheumatoid factor may or may not be present.

Rare patients present with multiple ulcerated nodules and high rheumatoid factors, but no active joint disease. This variant of rheumatoid disease without destructive joint disease is designated *rheumatoid nodulosis*. Linear, slightly red or skin-colored cords extending from the upper back to

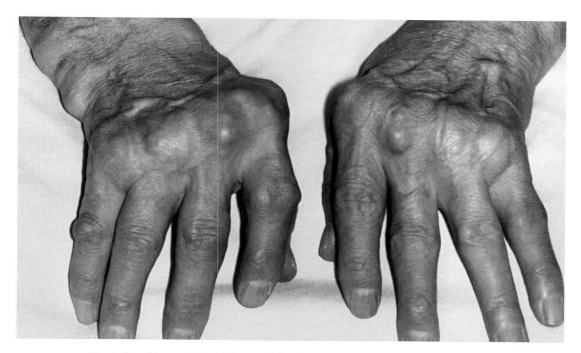

Fig. 8-40 Rheumatoid nodules on the hands over the metacarpal-phalangeal joints.

the axilla that reveal interstitial granulomatous findings histologically may occur. The presence of these linear bands has been called the *rope sign*. Goerttler et al described erythematous indurated papules, usually located on the proximal extremities, that appeared in four patients with rheumatic diseases during treatment with methotrexate. They consider this granulomatous reaction to be a characteristic medication-related phenomenon limited to this population.

Rheumatoid nodules are differentiated from Heberden's nodes, which are tender, hard, bony proliferations on the dorsolateral aspects of the distal interphalangeal joints. Nodules or tophi of gout are characterized by masses of crystals of urates surrounded by a chronic inflammatory cellular infiltrate containing foreign body giant cells. They are difficult to clinically differentiate from rheumatoid nodules and may require biopsy.

Histologic examination of the rheumatoid nodule shows dense foci of fibrinoid necrosis surrounded by histiocytes in palisade arrangement. The upper dermis may show a perivascular inflammation.

Rheumatoid Vasculitis

Peripheral vascular lesions appear as typical features of RA. These are localized purpura (Fig. 8-41), cutaneous ulceration, and gangrene of the distal parts of the extremities. Additionally, papular lesions located primarily on the hands have been described as rheumatoid papules, which show a combination of vasculitis and palisading granuloma formation. Chu et al reviewed all reports (see the previous discussion of SLE). The majority of patients with vasculitis

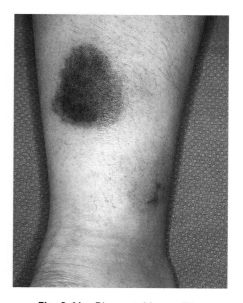

Fig. 8-41 Rheumatoid vasculitis.

have rheumatoid nodules. The rheumatoid factor is present. Peripheral neuropathy is frequently associated with the vasculitis. The presence of rheumatoid nodules may help to distinguish these lesions of vasculitis from SLE, polyarteritis nodosa, Buerger's disease, and the dysproteinemias.

Therapy for these lesions consists of the salicylates, nonsteroidal antiinflammatory agents, dapsone, colchicine, methotrexate, and antimalarials. Corticosteroids should be used in severe cases only.

Rheumatoid Neutrophilic Dermatosis

Chronic urticaria-like plaques characterized histologically by a dense neutrophilic infiltrate, occurring in patients with debilitating rheumatoid arthritis, were described by Ackerman. This disorder is clearly separable from erythema elevatum diutinum and Sweet's syndrome as delineated by Scherbenske et al.

Juvenile Rheumatoid Arthritis

Juvenile rheumatoid arthritis is not a single disease but a group of disorders characterized by arthritis and young age of onset. The subset called *Still's disease* accounts for only 20% of the patients. It shows skin manifestations in some 40% of young patients ranging in age from 7 to 25 years. An eruption consisting of evanescent, nonpruritic, salmon-pink, macular or papular lesions on the trunk and extremities may precede the onset of joint manifestations by many months. The systemic symptoms of fever and serositis usually recur over weeks each afternoon. Most remit permanently by adulthood.

Bossar H, et al: Familial form of rheumatoid nodulosis. *Ann Dermatol Venereol* 1993, 120:369.

Chu P, et al: The histopathologic spectrum of palisaded neutrophilic and granulomatous dermatitis in patients with collagen vascular disease. *Arch Dermatol* 1994, 130:1278.

Goerttler E, et al: Methotrexate-induced papular eruption in patients with rheumatic diseases. *J Am Acad Dermatol* 1999, 40:702.

Higaki Y, et al: Rheumatoid papules. *J Am Acad Dermatol* 1993, 28:406.

Jorizzo JL, et al: Dermatologic conditions reported in patients with RA. *J Am Acad Dermatol* 1983, 8:439.

Nousari HC, et al: Purple toes in a patient with end-stage RA. *Arch Dermatol* 1999, 135:648.

Sanchez JL, et al: Rheumatoid neutrophilic dermatitis. *J Am Acad Dermatol* 1990, 22:922.

Scherbenske JM, et al: Rheumatoid neutrophilic dermatitis. *Arch Dermatol* 1989, 125:1105.

Sibbitt WL Jr, et al: Cutaneous manifestations of RA. *Int J Dermatol* 1982, 21:563.

Smith ML, et al: Rheumatoid papules. *J Am Acad Dermatol* 1989, 20:348.

Upchurch KS, et al: Low-dose methotrexate therapy for cutaneous vasculitis of RA. *J Am Acad Dermatol* 1987, 17:355.

Vollersten RS, et al: Rheumatoid vasculitis. *Medicine* (Baltimore) 1986, 65:365. ▲

RELAPSING POLYCHONDRITIS

Relapsing polychondritis is characterized by intermittent episodes of inflammation of the articular and nonarticular cartilage eventuating in chondrolysis, dystrophy, and atrophy of the involved cartilage. Both sexes are equally affected, with the usual age at onset being in the fourth to fifth decade. There may be dissolution of the cartilage of the ears and nose and of the respiratory tract. The beefy red involvement of the ears is confined to the cartilaginous portion while the ear lobes remain conspicuously normal (Fig. 8-42). The affected areas are swollen and tender. There may be conductive deafness as a result of the obstruction produced by the swollen cartilage. The nasal septal carti-

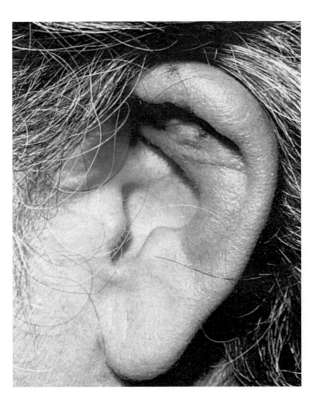

Fig. 8-42 Relapsing polychondritis. (Courtesy Dr. Axel W. Hoke.)

lage is similarly involved to produce rhinitis, with crusting and bleeding and saddle-nose. The involvement of the bronchi produces hoarseness, coughing, and dyspnea. Migratory arthralgia is often present. Ocular disease most often presents as conjunctivitis, scleritis, or iritis.

The MAGIC syndrome is a combination of Behçet's disease and relapsing polychondritis (mouth and genital ulcers with inflamed cartilage). Orme et al reported a patient and reviewed the previously reported 12 cases.

Autoimmune mechanisms appear to be responsible for this disease. Cell-mediated immunity to cartilage has been demonstrated in vitro, with a degree of response correlated with disease activity. IgG anti-type-II-collagen antibodies have been documented in these patients, again in titers corresponding with disease activity. Steroid therapy lowers them. The course of the disease is chronic and variable, with episodic flares.

Histologically, chondrolysis with associated perichondritis occurs. Dapsone, 100 mg once or twice a day, may clear the condition in a couple of weeks. A maintenance dose is usually continued for 4 to 6 asymptomatic months. Systemic corticosteroids have also been effective, as have indomethacin and salicylates.

Cohen PR, et al: Relapsing polychondritis. *Int J Dermatol* 1986, 25:280.

Helm TN, et al: Relapsing polychondritis. *J Am Acad Dermatol* 1992, 26:315.

Orme RL, et al: The MAGIC syndrome. *Arch Dermatol* 1990, 126:940. ▲

CHAPTER 9

Mucinoses

Within the dermis is fibrillar matrix termed *ground substance,* which is composed of proteoglycans and glycosaminoglycans. These acid mucopolysaccharides, produced by fibroblasts, are highly hygroscopic, binding about 1000 times their own volume in water. They are critical in holding water in the dermis and are responsible for dermal volume and texture. Normally, the sulfated acid mucopolysaccharide chondroitin sulfate and heparin are the primary dermal mucins. In certain diseases, fibroblasts produce abnormally large amounts of acid mucopolysaccharides, usually hyaluronic acid. These acid mucopolysaccharides (mucin) accumulate in large amounts in the dermis. They are not routinely visualized with hematoxylin eosin stains, since the water they bind is removed in processing, so the presence of increased mucin is suspected by the presence of large empty spaces between the collagen bundles. They can be detected by special stains such as colloidal iron, alcian blue, and toluidine blue. Incubation of the tissue with hyaluronidase eliminates the staining, confirming the presence of mucin.

Increased dermal mucin may result from many diseases and is a normal component of wound healing. The mucinoses are those diseases in which the production of increased amounts of mucin is the primary process. Mucin may also accumulate in the skin as a secondary phenomenon, such as when it is present in lupus erythematosus, Degos' disease, granuloma annulare, cutaneous tumors, or after therapies such as PUVA or retinoids. Mucin deposits in the skin are also prominent features of eosinophilia-myalgia syndrome and toxic oil syndrome. The genetic diseases in which mucin accumulates as a result of inherited metabolic abnormalities are termed the *mucopolysaccharidoses,* and are discussed in Chapter 25. Myxedema and pretibial myxedema are reviewed in Chapter 24.

Rongioletti F, et al: The new cutaneous mucinoses. *J Am Acad Dermatol* 1991, 24:265.
Truhan AP, et al: The cutaneous mucinoses. *J Am Acad Dermatol* 1986, 14:1. ━━━━━━━━━━━━━━━━ ▲

LICHEN MYXEDEMATOSUS

The terminology used to describe disorders in the disease group known as *lichen myxedematosus* is confusing. Within this group are localized cases involving one area; disseminated cases; and generalized, confluent papular forms with sclerosis, called *scleromyxedema. Papular mucinosis* is used by some as a synonym for all these cases, or is restricted to more mild cases. Because *acral persistent papular mucinosis* is now considered a separate entity, to avoid confusion the term *papular mucinosis* will not be used to describe cases in the lichen myxedematosus group.

Lichen myxedematosus affects adults of both sexes and appears from ages 30 to 80. It is chronic and may be progressive. The primary lesions in all forms of lichen myxedematosus are multiple waxy, 2 to 4 mm, dome-shaped or flat-topped papules (Fig. 9-1). They may coalesce into plaques or be arranged in linear array. Less commonly, urticarial, nodular, or even annular lesions are seen. The dorsal hands, face, elbows, and extensor extremities are most frequently affected. Mucosal lesions are absent. On the glabella and forehead, coalescence of lesions leads to the prominent furrowing of a "leonine facies." Pruritus may occur.

Scleromyxedema is characterized by diffuse or limited infiltration of the skin in addition to the papules or nodules (Figs. 9-2 and 9-3). A leonine facies develops (Fig. 9-4). Woody, fibrous sclerosis of the skin is characteristic and may lead to reduced range of motion of the hands, lips, and extremities. Scleromyxedema not infrequently is associated with visceral disease. Gastrointestinal involvement is most frequent. Dysphagia resulting from involvement of the esophagus is most common, but the stomach or intestine may also be affected. Pulmonary complications with dyspnea caused by restrictive or obstructive disease are the second most common visceral problem. Proximal muscle weakness with an inflammatory myopathy may occur. Carpal tunnel syndrome occurs in 10% of patients, as well as other peripheral neuropathies. Additionally, severe neurologic manifestations, including confusion, dizziness, dysarthria, ascending paralysis, seizures, syncope, and coma, can occur. Visceral disease can be fatal.

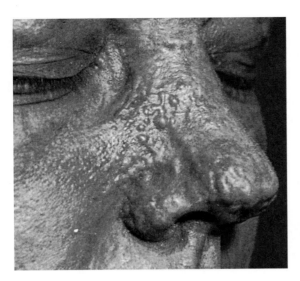

Fig. 9-1 Early papular lesions of lichen myxedematosus.

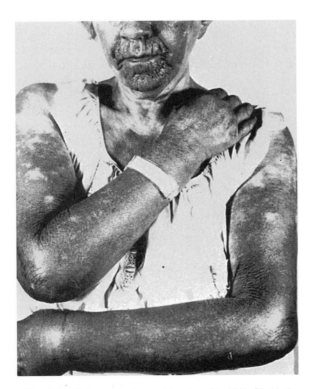

Fig. 9-2 Scleromyxedema. (Courtesy Dr. M.H. Slatkin.)

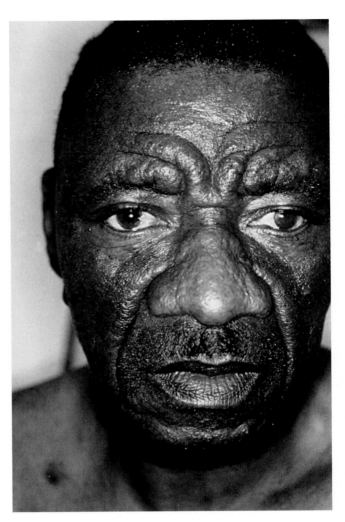

Fig. 9-3 Scleromyxedema.

Thyroid function tests are normal. An abnormal paraprotein is found in 90% of cases, usually an IgG lambda type, suggesting an underlying plasma cell dyscrasia. Bone marrow may be normal or reveal increased numbers of plasma cells or frank myeloma.

The histologic features are increased numbers of fibroblasts and increased mucin in the reticular dermis. There

may be haphazard increased collagen bundles in cases of scleromyxedema. In one case an inflammatory infiltrate with monotypic plasma cells was present, suggesting that local plasma cell dyscrasia is also capable of producing the clinical lesions.

Clinical and histologic features are usually diagnostic. Many of the findings seen in scleromyxedema are also found in systemic scleroderma, including cutaneous sclerosis, Raynaud's phenomenon, dysphagia, and carpal tunnel syndrome. This distinction in some cases may be difficult. Other infiltrative disorders, such as amyloidosis, must be excluded.

Treatment of lichen myxedematosus is difficult. Moderate doses of systemic steroids are not usually helpful, but high doses may temporarily arrest progressive visceral disease. Both isotretinoin and etretinate have been associated with improvement of the skin lesions. These reports did not provide long-term follow-up, nor were they able to prove whether the retinoids had benefit for the systemic

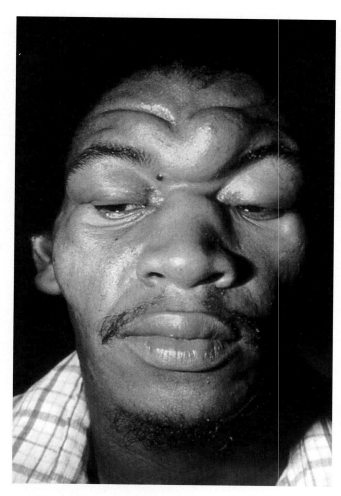

Fig. 9-4 Scleromyxedema.

disease. Alfa interferon, cyclosporine, PUVA treatment, electron beam treatment, and dermabrasion may be attempted for the skin disease as well. Extracorporeal photochemotherapy may be potentially useful. Many patients with scleromyxedema have been treated with immunosuppressive agents, especially melphalan or cyclophosphamide with or without plasma exchange. Temporary remission of progressive visceral disease may occur. These short-term benefits must be weighed against the increase in malignancies and septic complications that commonly lead to death in melphalan-treated patients. One patient has responded to 2-chlorodeoxyadenosine, but had severe, short-term, neurologic complications from the treatment. Lichen myxedematosus, and especially scleromyxedema, remains a therapeutic challenge, and the overall prognosis in scleromyxedema is poor.

Papular Mucinosis and AIDS

Many patients with acquired immunodeficiency syndrome (AIDS) have been reported with mucinous papules, usually widespread, unassociated with a paraprotein. It is virtually always seen in advanced HIV disease in patients with multiple infectious complications of HIV disease. These lesions may occur in association with an eczematous dermatitis or on normal skin. If associated with an eczematous dermatitis, the lesions often clear if the eczema is controlled. Those cases occurring on normal skin may respond to systemic retinoid therapy. The authors have also seen one case of true scleromyxedema with visceral involvement in AIDS.

Acral Persistent Papular Mucinosis

Acral persistent papular mucinosis is similar to the discrete papular form of lichen myxedematosus, from which it may be difficult to absolutely distinguish. Patients with this diagnosis typically are women and have few to 100, bilaterally symmetrical, 2- to 5-mm, flesh-colored papules always on the hands and wrists (Fig. 9-5). The knees and elbows may also be involved in a minority of patients. The face and trunk are spared. A paraprotein is uncommonly present, sclerosis and visceral disease are absent, and the course is of persistence and slow progression. Two involved sisters have been reported. Histologically there is a collection of upper dermal mucin with minimal or no increase in fibroblasts, in contrast to lichen myxedematosus.

Bata-Csorgo Z, et al: Scleromyxedema. *J Am Acad Dermatol* 1999, 40:343.

Bonnetblanc JM, et al: Regression of scleromyxedema with topical betamethasone and dimethyl sulfoxide. *Arch Dermatol* 1991, 127:1733.

Brenner S, et al: Treatment of scleromyxedema with etretinate. *J Am Acad Dermatol* 1984, 10:295.

Clark BJ, et al: Papular mucinosis. *Br J Dermatol* 1996, 135:467.

Davis LS, et al: Treatment of scleromyxedema with 2-chlorodeoxyadenosine. *J Am Acad Dermatol* 1996, 35:288.

Dinneen AM, et al: Scleromyxedema. *J Am Acad Dermatol* 1995, 33:37.

Farr PM, et al: PUVA treatment of scleromyxedema. *Br J Dermatol* 1984, 110:347.

Godby A, et al: Fatal scleromyxedema. *J Am Acad Dermatol* 1998, 38:289.

Hisler BM, et al: Improvement of scleromyxedema associated with isotretinoin therapy. *J Am Acad Dermatol* 1991, 24:854.

Lowe NJ, et al: Electron-beam treatment of scleromyxedema. *Br J Dermatol* 1982, 106:449.

Menni S, et al: Acral persistent papular mucinosis in two sisters. *Clin Exp Dermatol* 1995, 20:431.

Rongioletti F, et al: Cutaneous mucinoses in HIV infection. *Br J Dermatol* 1998, 139:1077.

Tschen JA, et al: Scleromyxedema. *J Am Acad Dermatol* 1999, 40:303.

Webster GF, et al: The association of potentially lethal neurologic syndromes with scleromyxedema (papular mucinosis). *J Am Acad Dermatol* 1993, 28:105.

Yen A, et al: Papular mucinosis associated with AIDS. *J Am Acad Dermatol* 1997, 37:127. ▲

SCLEREDEMA

Scleredema is a skin disease characterized by a stiffening and hardening of the subcutaneous tissues, as if they were infiltrated with paraffin. It occurs in two forms—with and without diabetes mellitus. In a large series of 33 patients,

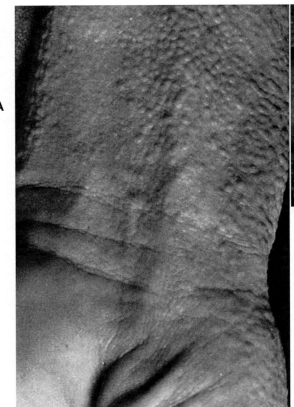

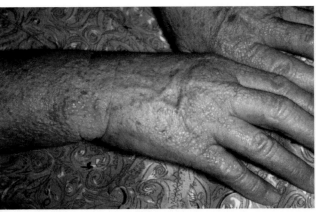

Fig. 9-5   **A** and **B**, Acral persistent papular mucinosis. (**A**, Courtesy Dr. J.R. Haserick.)

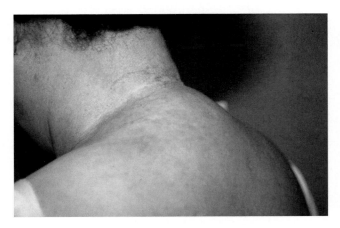

Fig. 9-6   Scleredema.

one quarter of the patients had a sudden onset following an upper respiratory infection, typically caused by streptococcus. In one third, the patients had clinically identical lesions, but the onset was more insidious and there was no documented preceding infection. In 35% the disease is associated with diabetes mellitus and has a different clinical pattern.

In those cases not associated with diabetes, females outnumber males 2:1. The age of onset is from childhood through adulthood. Skin tightness and induration begins on the neck or face (or both), spreading symmetrically to involve the arms, shoulders, back, and chest (Fig. 9-6). The distal extremities are spared. There may be difficulty opening the mouth or eyes, and a masklike expression as a result of the infiltration. The involved skin, which is waxy white and of woodlike consistency, gradually transitions into the normal skin with no clear demarcation. Associated findings occur in variable numbers of patients and can include dysphagia caused by tongue and upper esophageal involvement, cardiac arrhythmias, and sometimes an associated paraprotein, usually an IgG. Myeloma may be present. There may be pleural, pericardial, or peritoneal effusion. In about half the patients in whom the condition follows an infection, spontaneous resolution will occur in months to a few years. The others have a prolonged course. Therapy is of no benefit, but patients may live with the disease for many years. Cyclosporine has been reported as beneficial in two patients.

In the second group, which in most dermatologists' experience is the more common, there is an association with late onset, insulin-dependent diabetes. Men outnumber women 10:1. The affected men tend to be obese. The lesions are of insidious onset and long duration, presenting as woody induration and thickening of the skin of the mid upper back, neck, and shoulders. There is a sharp step-off from the involved to the normal skin. Persistent erythema and folliculitis may involve the affected areas. The associated diabetes is of long duration and is difficult to control. Further, the patients have frequently suffered complications of their diabetes such as nephropathy, atherosclerotic disease, retinopathy, and neuropathy. Control of the diabetes does not affect the course of the scleredema. No paraprotein is detected, and visceral involvement is not seen. Lesions are persistent and unresponsive to treatment. Intravenous penicillin, electron beam, and bath-PUVA have been effective in separate case reports.

The histology of both forms is identical. The skin is dramatically thickened, with the dermis often expanded by twofold to threefold. There is marked fibrosis without the hyalinization seen in scleroderma. The thickened dermal collagen may be separated by clear spaces that contain hyaluronic acid. The amount of mucin is variable and usually only prominent in early lesions. In late lesions, fibrosis is the sole finding, and the amount of mucin is scant.

Hager CM, et al: Bath-PUVA therapy in three patients with scleredema adultorum. *J Am Acad Dermatol* 1998, 38:240.

Kranagakis K, et al: Persistent scleredema of Buschke in a diabetic. *Br J Dermatol* 1996, 134:597.

Mattheou-Vakali G, et al: Cyclosporine in scleredema. *J Am Acad Dermatol* 1996, 35:990.

McFadden N, et al: Scleredema adultorum associated with a monoclonal gammopathy and generalized hyperpigmentation. *Arch Dermatol* 1987, 123:629.

Olita A, et al: Paraproteinemia in patients with scleredema. *J Am Acad Dermatol* 1987, 16:96.

Tamburin LM, et al: Scleredema of Buschke successfully treated with electron beam therapy. *Arch Dermatol* 1998, 134:419.

Venencie PY, et al: Scleredema: review of 33 cases. *J Am Acad Dermatol* 1984, 11:128. _____ ▲

PLAQUELIKE CUTANEOUS MUCINOSIS (RETICULAR ERYTHEMATOUS MUCINOSIS, REM SYNDROME)

Plaquelike cutaneous mucinosis favors women in the third and fourth decades of life. The eruption frequently appears after intense sun exposure. Clinical lesions are large erythematous plaques that are several centimeters in diameter, and are most common in the midline of the chest and back. The face, arms, abdomen, and groin may also be involved (Fig. 9-7). Lesions may have a reticulate or plaquelike appearance. Evolution is gradual. Photosensitivity is common; lesions have rarely been induced with UVB. Onset with oral contraceptives, menses, and pregnancy are other features. Serologic tests for lupus erythematosus are negative. A wide variety of common disorders have been associated, perhaps coincidentally.

Histologically, there are varying degrees of lymphocytic infiltration around dermal vessels, and deposits of mucin in the dermis. Direct immunofluorescence is negative. Treatment with antimalarials is successful in most cases.

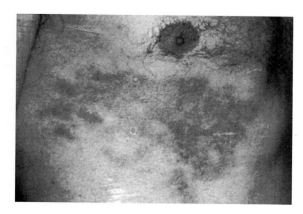

Fig. 9-7   REM syndrome. (Courtesy Dr. E. Kocsard, Australia.)

Braddock SW, et al: Reticular erythematosus mucinosis and thrombocytopenic purpura. *J Am Acad Dermatol* 1988, 19:859.

Quimby SR, et al: Plaque-like cutaneous mucinosis. *J Am Acad Dermatol* 1982, 6:856. _____ ▲

CUTANEOUS FOCAL MUCINOSIS

Focal mucinosis is characterized by a solitary nodule or papule. Lesions are asymptomatic and usually occur on the face, neck, trunk, or extremities. They appear in adulthood. Histologically, the lesion is characterized by a loose dermal stroma containing large quantities of mucin together with numerous dendritic-shaped fibroblasts. The clinical appearance is not distinctive and may at times be suggestive of a cyst, a basal cell carcinoma, or a neurofibroma. The treatment is surgical excision.

Wilk M, et al: Cutaneous focal mucinosis. *J Cutan Pathol* 1994, 21:446 _____ ▲

SELF-HEALING JUVENILE CUTANEOUS MUCINOSIS

Self-healing juvenile cutaneous mucinosis is a rare, but distinct disorder, and is characterized by the sudden onset of skin lesions and polyarthritis, which spontaneously resolves without sequelae over a few months. Children ages 5 to 15 are affected. Skin lesions are ivory white papules of the head, neck, trunk, and typically the periarticular regions; deep nodules on the face and periarticular sites; and hard edema of the periorbital area and face. An acute arthritis affects the knees, elbows, and hand joints. Thyroid tests are normal, and there is no paraprotein. Histology of the skin lesions reveals dermal mucin. Although the initial presentation is worrisome, the prognosis has been excellent.

Caputo R, et al: Self-healing juvenile cutaneous mucinosis. *Arch Dermatol* 1995, 131:459. _____ ▲

CUTANEOUS MUCINOSIS OF INFANCY

Three cases in girls of cutaneous mucinosis of infancy, a rare syndrome, have been reported. At birth or within the first few months of life, skin-colored or translucent, grouped or discrete, 2- to 8-mm papules develop on the trunk or upper extremities, especially the back of the hands. Biopsies show very superficial upper dermal mucin without proliferation of fibroblasts. The condition is unassociated with a paraprotein or thyroid disease. Existing lesions remain static; new lesions continue to gradually accumulate, but visceral involvement has not been detected.

Stokes KS, et al: Cutaneous mucinosis of infancy. *Pediatr Dermatol* 1994, 11:246. _____ ▲

FOLLICULAR MUCINOSIS (ALOPECIA MUCINOSA)

In 1957, Pinkus applied the name *alopecia mucinosa* to a series of cases with inflammatory plaques with alopecia characterized histologically by mucinous deposits in the outer root sheaths of the hair follicles. The plaques may be simply hypopigmented or erythematous and scaly (Fig. 9-8), eczematous, or composed of flesh-colored, follicular papules (Fig. 9-9). There may be only one lesion (Fig. 9-10), especially on the head and neck, or multiple lesions may be present (Fig. 9-11). The plaques are firm and coarsely rough to the palpating finger. They are distributed mostly on the face, neck, and scalp but may appear on any parts of the body. Itching may or may not be present. Alopecia occurs regularly in lesions on the scalp and frequently in lesions located elsewhere. Some papules show a black central dot that corresponds to a hair broken off at the skin surface. These may cause the surface of a patch to look like keratosis pilaris. Sensory dissociation, with hot-cold perception difficulties or anesthesia to light touch,

has been reported in some lesions, with a resultant misdiagnosis of leprosy.

The term *alopecia mucinosa* may be used to describe the disease process, and follicular mucinosis to describe the histologic features. Three categories of alopecia mucinosa have been identified. One comprises younger patients, with few lesions usually confined to the head and neck or upper arms. This group, which is the most common, resolves

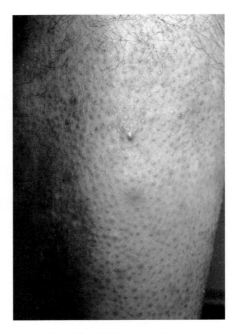

Fig. 9-9 Follicular mucinosis.

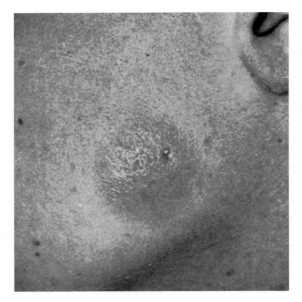

Fig. 9-10 Follicular mucinosis. Cleared entirely within 1 year. (Courtesy Dr. J. Bembenista.)

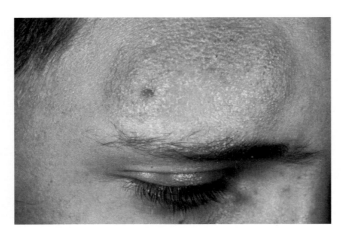

Fig. 9-8 Follicular mucinosis.

spontaneously in 2 months to 2 years. The second group, somewhat older, has larger, more numerous, and more widespread lesions, and resolution may take several years. Hodgkin's disease is associated with alopecia mucinosa in some childhood and adult cases. The third group is older and has cutaneous T-cell lymphoma with follicular mucinosis histologically. Lesions are more numerous and widespread. Approximately 30% of patients with follicular mucinosis have associated mycosis fungoides (Fig. 9-12). If associated with cutaneous T-cell lymphoma, the lymphoma

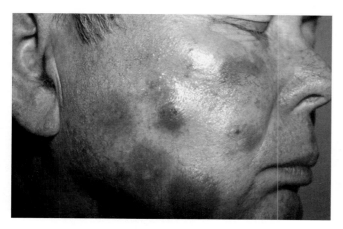

Fig. 9-11 Multiple facial lesions of follicular mucinosis.

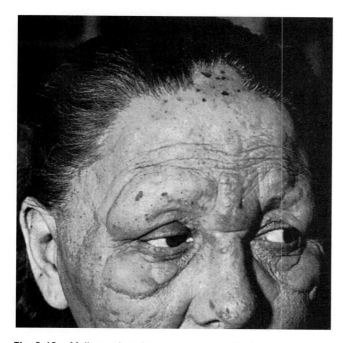

Fig. 9-12 Malignant lymphoma of the skin, with alopecia mucinosa on the anterior scalp line for 1 year. Note alopecia of eyebrows and plaques of infiltration around eyes, glabella, and forehead, producing a leonine facies and accompanied by universal intensely pruritic, excoriated nodules.

is probably present at the onset; however, as with mycosis fungoides, the initial histology may not be diagnostic. In any person over age 30, the finding of follicular mucinosis histologically should result in careful evaluation of the histologic material for features of mycosis fungoides.

Histologically, follicular mucinosis demonstrates large collections of mucin within cells of the sebaceous gland and outer root sheath. A mixed dermal infiltrate is present. When the condition occurs in association with mycosis fungoides (cutaneous T-cell lymphoma), the dermal infiltrate is atypical and other diagnostic features of mycosis fungoides are present.

Spontaneous involution may occur, especially in young children. Corticosteroids externally and internally have produced varying degrees of improvement. Dapsone, PUVA, radiation therapy, interferon alfa-2b, mepacrine, and indomethacin have been reported to be effective in individual cases.

Gibson LE, et al: Follicular mucinosis. *J Am Acad Dermatol* 1989, 20:441.
Mehregan DA, et al: Follicular mucinosis. *Mayo Clin Proc* 1991, 66:387.
Pinkus H: Alopecia mucinosa. *Arch Dermatol* 1983, 119:698.
Wittenberg GP, et al: Follicular mucinosis presenting as an acneiform eruption. *J Am Acad Dermatol* 1998, 38:849. _____ ▲

MYXOID CYSTS

These lesions occur most commonly on the dorsal or lateral terminal digits of the hands (Fig. 9-13) but may also occur on the toes (Fig. 9-14). They present as solitary, 5- to 7-mm, opalescent or skin-colored, usually asymptomatic swellings of the proximal nail fold or over the distal interphalangeal joint. A characteristic groove may be formed in the nail plate by pressure of the lesion on the nail matrix (Fig. 9-15). They contain a clear, viscous, sticky fluid that may spontaneously drain, often from below the proximal nail fold. Women are more frequently affected, and osteoarthritis is frequently present in the adjacent distal interphalangeal joint.

These lesions are called "cysts" but are actually focal accumulations of mucin in the dermis without a defined lining—thus, the terminology *digital mucinous pseudocyst* or *myxoid pseudocyst*. There are conflicting theories about their pathogenesis. One theory is that the mucin accumulates in this area independently of the joint space and is not connected to it. The other theory is that these represent extrusion of mucin from the joint space into the adjacent tissue. Proponents of this second theory might use the term *synovial cysts* to describe these lesions. Support for the second theory are reports of stalks attached to the joint space, injection of dye into the joint space appearing in the cyst, and surgical treatment involving removal of the osteophytes of the associated degenerative joint disease of the adjacent, involved joint being associated with lower recurrence rates postoperatively. Support for the first theory

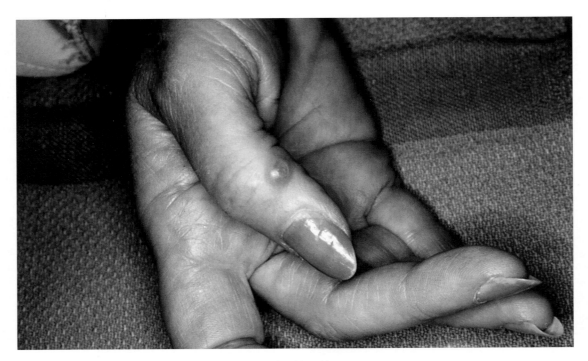

Fig. 9-13   Myxoid cyst.

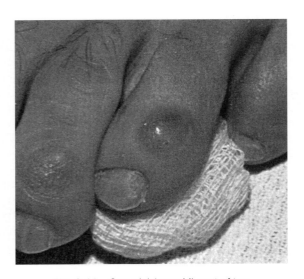

Fig. 9-14   Synovial (myxoid) cyst of toe.

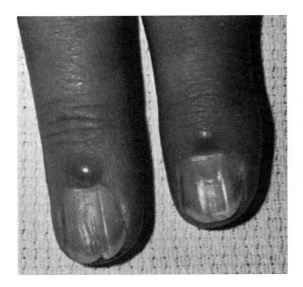

Fig. 9-15   Distortion of nails distal to synovial cysts on two fingers.

are that simple injections, draining, or removal of the lesion may lead to resolution.

Treatment of these lesions is disappointing since they frequently recur regardless of the method of therapy. The repeated puncture technique may achieve up to a 70% cure rate, but multiple punctures (more than 40) may be required. This may be complicated by local tissue or joint infection.

Intralesional steroids may be injected into the tissue after draining the cyst. The base of the lesion may be fulgurated after draining. Salasche reported a method of excision for these cysts that is simple and may be effective. Meticulous excision of the cyst and its "stalk" was successful in 11 cases reported by Nasca et al; there were no recurrences.

A recently recognized association of multiple myxoid cysts is with connective tissue disease. Young children, even infants, may present with multiple myxoid cysts as the initial manifestation of juvenile rheumatoid arthritis. An adult with systemic sclerosis also developed multiple myxoid cysts.

Epstein E: A simple technique for managing digital mucous cysts. *Arch Dermatol* 1979, 115:1315.

Marzano AV, et al: Unique digital skin lesions associated with systemic sclerosis. *Br J Dermatol* 1997, 136:598.

Nasca RJ, et al: Mucous cysts of the digits. *Southern Med J* 1983, 76(9):1142.

Salasche SJ: Myxoid cysts of the proximal nail fold: a surgical approach. *J Dermatol Surg Oncol* 1984, 10:35. ▲

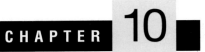

Seborrheic Dermatitis, Psoriasis, Recalcitrant Palmoplantar Eruptions, Pustular Dermatitis, and Erythroderma

SEBORRHEIC DERMATITIS

Synonyms: Seborrheic eczema

Clinical Features

Seborrheic dermatitis is common, occurring from 2% to 5% of the population. It is a chronic, superficial, inflammatory disease of the skin, with a predilection for the scalp, eyebrows, eyelids, nasolabial creases, lips, ears, sternal area, axillae, submammary folds, umbilicus, groins, and gluteal crease (Fig. 10-1). The disease is characterized by scanty, loose, dry, moist, or greasy scales, and by crusted, pink or yellow patches of various shapes and sizes; remissions and exacerbations; and no to mild itching.

On the scalp the least severe but by far the most common form—pityriasis sicca, or dandruff—manifests itself as a dry, flaky, branny desquamation, beginning in small patches and rapidly involving the entire scalp, with a profuse amount of fine, powdery scales. An oily type, pityriasis steatoides, is accompanied by erythema and an accumulation of thick crusts.

Other types of seborrheic dermatitis on the scalp are more severe and are manifested by greasy, scaling, configurate patches or psoriasiform plaques, exudation, and thick crusting. The disease frequently spreads beyond the hairy scalp to the forehead, ears, postauricular regions, and neck. On these areas the patches have convex borders and are reddish yellow or yellowish. In extreme cases the entire scalp is covered by a greasy, dirty crust with an offensive odor. In infants yellow or brown scaling lesions on the scalp with accumulated adherent epithelial debris is called *cradle cap*.

On the supraorbital regions, flaky scales are seen in the eyebrows, and the underlying skin is erythematous and pruritic or may show yellowish scaling patches. The edges of the lids may be erythematous and granular (marginal blepharitis). The conjunctivae are at times injected (Fig. 10-2). The lids may show yellowish pink, fine scales, the borders of which are usually indistinct. Pruritus may be present. If the glabella is involved, there may be cracks in the skin in the wrinkles at the inner end of the eyebrow accompanying the fine scaling on an erythematous base. In the nasolabial creases and on the alae nasi, there may be yellowish or reddish yellow scaling macules, sometimes with fissures. In men folliculitis of the upper lip may occur (Fig. 10-3).

On and in the ears, seborrheic dermatitis is frequently mistaken for otitis externa caused by fungal infection (otomycosis). There is scaling in the aural canals, around the auditory meatus, and in the postauricular region, or under the lobe. In these areas the skin often becomes red, fissured, and swollen. Serous exudation, puffiness of the ears and surrounding parts, and regional adenopathy occur less frequently. Examination for fungus is negative.

In the axillae the eruption begins in the apices, bilaterally, and later progresses to neighboring skin (Fig. 10-4). The involvement may vary from simple erythema and scaling to more pronounced petaloid or discoid patches with fissures. The inframammary folds, especially when the breasts are pendulous, and the umbilicus may be involved. The presternal area is a favored site on the trunk.

Seborrheic dermatitis is common in the groin and gluteal crease, where its appearance may closely simulate tinea cruris, psoriasis, or candidiasis. The patches, however, are more finely scaly with less definite borders and are more likely to be bilateral and symmetrical and of the typical color. In these locations fissures often occur and there may be psoriasiform patches with thick scales in severe cases.

The lesions may be generalized, with erythema, scaling, oozing, and pruritus. Often, however, the eruption remains localized in one area, such as the scalp, ears, sternal region, or umbilicus. In the acute stages the inflammation may be intense, with moist exudation from the scalp and ears and papulovesicles on the palms and soles. Secondary infections, impetiginization, or furunculosis may ensue.

Seborrheic dermatitis may progress to a generalized exfoliative state. In the newborn this type of severe and generalized seborrheic dermatitis is known as *erythroderma desquamativum* (Fig. 10-5). Generalized eruptions may be accompanied by adenopathy and may simulate mycosis fungoides and leukemic or psoriatic erythroderma.

Seborrheic dermatitis may be associated with or accentuated by several internal diseases. In Parkinson's disease a

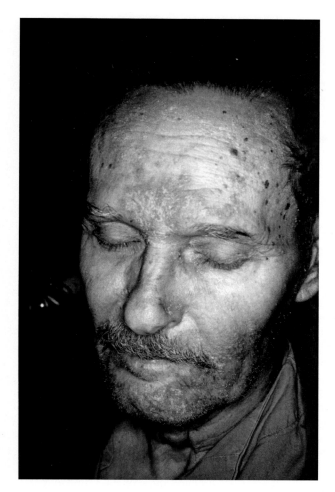

Fig. 10-1   Seborrheic dermatitis.

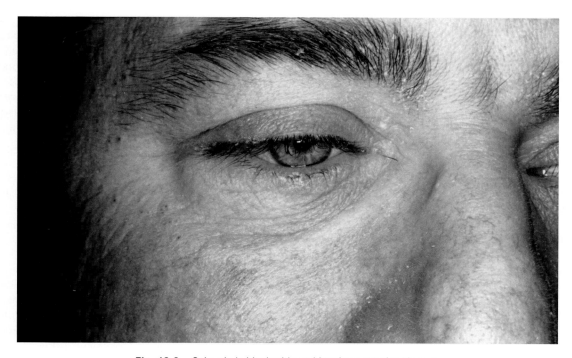

Fig. 10-2   Seborrheic blepharitis and involvement of eyebrows.

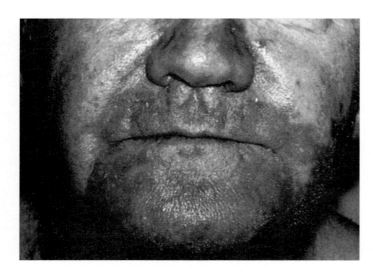

Fig. 10-3 Seborrheic dermatitis of the face.

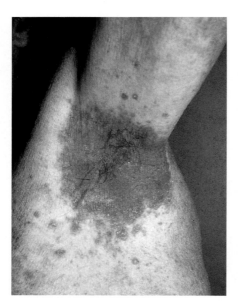

Fig. 10-4 Seborrheic dermatitis affecting the axilla in an HIV-infected patient.

severe seborrheic dermatitis involving the scalp and face, with waxy, profuse scaling, is sometimes seen. A unilateral injury to the innervation of the face may lead to an ipsilateral localized seborrheic dermatitis. Patients infected with the human immunodeficiency virus (HIV) have a markedly increased incidence of seborrheic dermatitis (see Fig. 10-4). Diabetes mellitus, especially in obese persons; sprue; malabsorption disorders; epilepsy; neuroleptic drugs that may induce parkinsonism, such as haloperidol; and reactions to arsenic and gold have all produced seborrheic dermatitis–like lesions.

Etiology and Pathogenesis

The etiology of this common disorder remains unresolved. Investigations have confirmed the presence of the lipophilic yeast *Pityrosporum ovale* in profuse numbers in the scalp lesions. The argument that the yeast is the cause of the dermatitis is a persuasive one. However, others have demonstrated that *P. ovale* may be abundant on the scalps of patients who have no clinical signs of the disease.

Skin flora and skin lipids in individuals with seborrheic dermatitis are significantly higher compared with control subjects. Healthy individuals have been found to have higher IgG antibodies to the organism. Other studies showed decreased lymphocyte stimulation in patients with seborrheic dermatitis when exposed to *P. ovale* extract. All of these mechanisms may promote the propagation of lipophilic organisms, produce inflammation, and possibly precipitate the condition.

The significance of *P. ovale* in infantile seborrheic dermatitis has not been fully evaluated. Tollesson et al have shown 20 of 30 infants with cradle cap had transient impaired function of delta-6-desaturase, an enzyme required for the metabolism of essential fatty acids. The altered essential fatty acid metabolism may be important in the pathogenesis of infantile disease. In a study of 191 children by Mimouni et al a familial tendency toward infantile and adult seborrheic dermatitis was found.

Histology

The epidermis is acanthotic. There is overlying focal scale crust often adjacent to follicular ostia. Slight spongiosis is frequently present. The dermis contains a perivascular mixed cell inflammatory infiltrate.

Differential Diagnosis

Some cases of seborrheic dermatitis bear a close clinical resemblance to psoriasis. Favoring psoriasis are erythema; heavy scales, whose removal discloses bleeding points; strong predilection for involvement of the frontal scalp margin; and resistance to treatment. Absence of itching is also suggestive. Characteristic psoriasis elsewhere (nail pitting, balanitis) may resolve the question. Impetigo of the

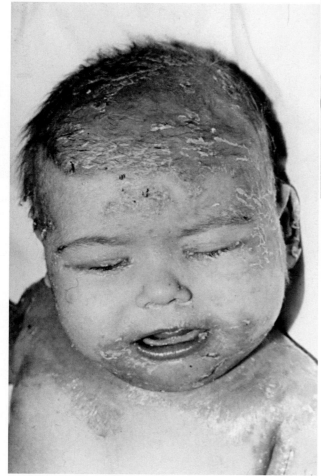

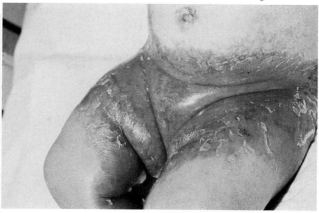

Fig. 10-5 A and **B,** Erythroderma desquamativum in a 10-week-old infant.

scalp, especially when associated with pediculosis and even more so when the eyelashes and eyebrows are involved, may cause difficulty in differentiation. Inverse psoriasis of the intertriginous areas is also frequently mistaken for seborrheic dermatitis. The terminology *sebopsoriasis* sometimes seems more appropriate than either psoriasis or seborrheic dermatitis. In immunodeficiency syndromes crusted scabies of the scalp may be confused with seborrheic dermatitis. Other diseases to be differentiated are otitis externa, blepharitis, tinea corporis, pityriasis rosea, and keratosis lichenoides chronica.

Treatment

Selenium sulfide, tar, zinc pyrithionate, and resorcin shampoos are all excellent. Application at least two to three times weekly is usually necessary. Nizoral (ketoconazole) shampoo may be effective when used as little as twice a week. Corticosteroid solutions or corticosteroids in combination with crude coal tar or with iodochlorhydroxyquin are all effective. In the treatment of the scalp, the ointment forms are preferred by many black patients.

The most efficacious agents on glabrous skin are the corticosteroid creams. In severe cases in which bacterial infection is prominent, the corticosteroids combined with antimicrobial preparations are extremely beneficial. Generally, nonfluorinated topical steroid preparations are adequate. Ketoconazole cream is effective, and there is lower relapse rates after its use. It is frequently used in combination with topical corticoids. In patients infected with HIV lithium succinate ointment (Efalith) has provided excellent results in treating severe facial disease. Bifonazole shampoo has been shown effective in treating infants and small children.

Cortisporin otic suspension, a polymyxin B-hydrocortisone suspension, 4 drops in the auditory meatus, usually brings about prompt clearing. Desonide Otic Lotion, 0.05% desonide and 2% acetic acid, is also effective. Sodium sulfacetamide, which may be applied in 10% strength in any convenient cream such as desonide, works well for dyssebacea. Topical steroids should not be used for blepharitis, since steroid preparations used in this area may induce glaucoma and cataracts. Daily debridement with a cotton-tipped applicator and baby shampoo, sometimes combined with a topical antibiotic ointment, is recommended. In generalized or severe cases, systemic corticosteroids, and antibiotics, for secondary infection, may be necessary and are effective.

Binder RL, et al: Seborrheic dermatitis in neuroleptic-induced parkinsonism. *Arch Dermatol* 1983, 119:473.

Burton JL, et al: Seborrhea is not a feature of seborrheic dermatitis. *Br Med J* 1983, 286:1169.

Faergemann J: Pityrosporum infections. *J Am Acad Dermatol* 1994, 31:S18.

Faergemann J: Pityrosporum yeasts: what's new? *Mycoses* 1997, 40(Suppl):29.

Green CA, et al: Treatment of seborrheic dermatitis with ketoconazole. *Br J Dermatol* 1987, 116:217.

Langtry JA, et al: Topical lithium succinate ointment (Efalith) in the treatment of AIDS-related seborrheic dermatitis. *Clin Exp Dermatol* 1997, 22:216

Levine N: Red, dry skin on the face and scalp. *Geriatrics* 1999, 54:19.

Lewis EJ, et al: Localized scabies of the scalp and feet. *Cutis* 1998, 61:87.

Mathes BM, et al: Seborrheic dermatitis in patients with AIDS. *J Am Acad Dermatol* 1985, 13:947.

Mimouni K, et al: Prognosis of infantile seborrheic dermatitis. *J Pediatr* 1995, 127:744.

Odom RB: Common superficial fungal infections in immunosuppressed patients. *J Am Acad Dermatol* 1994, 31:S56.

Peter RU, et al: Successful treatment and prophylaxis of scalp seborrhoeic dermatitis and dandruff with 2% ketoconazole shampoo. *Br J Dermatol* 1995, 132:441.

Tollesson A, et al: Essential fatty acids in infantile seborrheic dermatitis. *J Am Acad Dermatol* 1993, 28:957.

Yates VM, et al: Early diagnosis of infantile seborrheic dermatitis and atopic dermatitis: clinical features. *Br J Dermatol* 1983, 108:633.

Zeharia A, et al: Treatment with Bifonazole shampoo for scalp seborrhea in infants and young children. *Pediatr Dermatol* 1996, 13:151.

PSORIASIS
Clinical Features

Psoriasis is a common, chronic, recurrent, inflammatory disease of the skin characterized by round, circumscribed, erythematous, dry, scaling plaques of various sizes, covered by grayish white or silvery white, imbricated, and lamellar scales (Fig. 10-6). The lesions have a predilection for the scalp, nails, extensor surfaces of the limbs (especially the shins), elbows, knees, umbilical, and sacral region (Fig. 10-7). The eruption is usually symmetrical and may vary from a solitary macule to more than 100. The eruption usually develops slowly but may be exanthematous, with the sudden onset of numerous guttate lesions, or may consist of a few inveterate patches. Subjective symptoms, such as itching or burning, may be present and may cause extreme discomfort.

The early lesions are guttate erythematous macules, which from the beginning are covered with dry, silvery scales, which typically do not extend all the way to the edge of the erythematous area. By peripheral extension and by

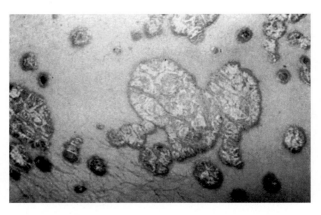

Fig. 10-6 Psoriasis. The silvery scaling, serpiginous outlines, confluence, erythema beyond the scaling area, and varied size of lesions are well illustrated.

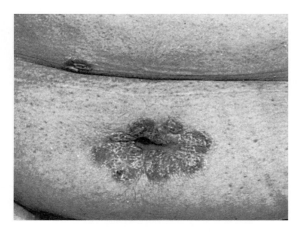

Fig. 10-7 Psoriasis of the umbilicus.

coalescence, the patches increase in size and, through the accumulation of scales, become thicker. The scales are micaceous and are looser toward the periphery of the patch, although adherent at its center; on removal of the scales, bleeding points appear (Auspitz's sign). When the patches reach a diameter of about 5 cm, they may cease spreading and undergo involution in the center, so that annular, lobulated, and gyrate figures are produced.

Old patches may be thickened and tough, and covered with lamellar scales like the outside of an oyster shell (*psoriasis ostracea*) (Fig. 10-8). Various other descriptive terms have in the past been applied to the diverse appearances of the lesions: *psoriasis guttata,* in which the lesions are the size of water drops; *psoriasis follicularis,* in which tiny, scaly lesions are located at the orifices of the pilosebaceous follicles; *psoriasis figurata, psoriasis annulata,* and *psoriasis gyrata,* in which curved linear patterns are produced by central involution; *psoriasis discoidea,* in which central involution does not occur and solid patches

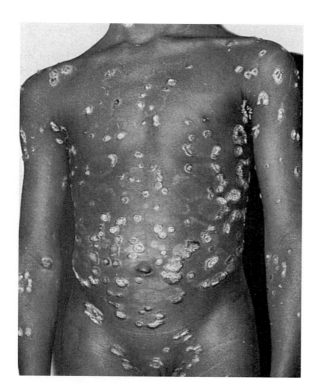

Fig. 10-8 Ostraceous psoriasis.

persist; *psoriasis rupioides,* in which crustaceous lesions occur, resembling syphilitic rupia. The term *plaque psoriasis* is often applied to other than guttate or inverse varieties (Fig. 10-9). Inverse psoriasis is found in intertriginous areas (Fig. 10-10).

Types

Seborrheic-Like Psoriasis. In some cases of psoriasis prominent features of seborrheic dermatitis may occur not only in the typical sites of psoriasis vulgaris but also in the flexural areas such as the antecubital areas, axillae, under the breasts, groins, umbilicus, and intergluteal areas (see Fig. 10-7). The lesions are moist and erythematous, with a minimal amount of greasy and soft, rather than dry and micaceous, scales. This pattern of eruption is also known as *inverse psoriasis* (see the following discussion). Terms such as *sebopsoriasis* and *seborrheic psoriasis* may be used.

Inverse Psoriasis. Also known as *flexural psoriasis* or (on palms or soles) *volar psoriasis,* this form is so called because it selectively and often exclusively involves folds, recesses, and flexor surfaces: ears, axillae, groins, inframammary folds, navel, intergluteal crease, glans penis, lips, and above all, the palms, soles, and nails (Figs. 10-11 and 10-12). The scalp quite often participates as well. In the

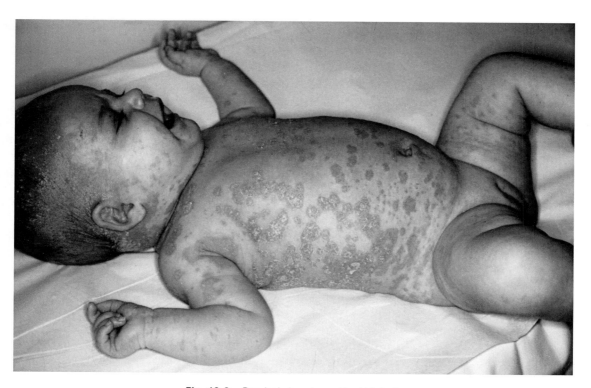

Fig. 10-9 Psoriasis in a 4-month-old infant.

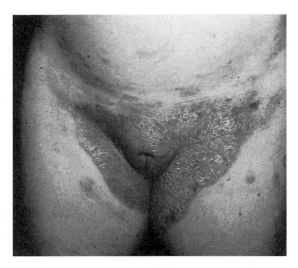

Fig. 10-11 Inverse psoriasis in inguinal region of a 5-year-old girl.

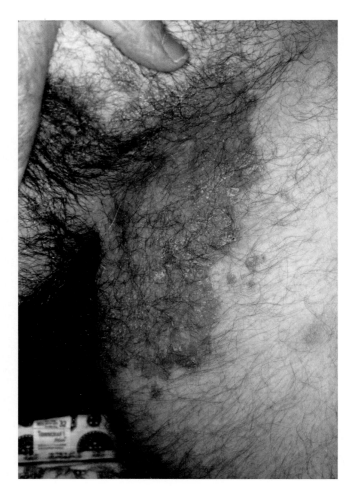

Fig. 10-10 Inverse psoriasis.

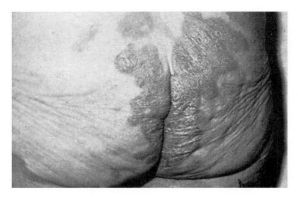

Fig. 10-12 Intertriginous psoriasis (inverse psoriasis) extending onto buttocks.

involved nail simple onycholysis may be seen, or there may be more diagnostic pitting. "Oil spots," round or oval areas of onycholysis 2 to 6 mm in diameter in the nail bed, not extending to the free distal border, are more characteristic and diagnostic than the more commonly seen distal onycholysis. Nail pitting is even more common. In such cases, a characteristic lesion elsewhere or a positive family history may help confirm the diagnosis.

"Napkin" Psoriasis. Diaper dermatitis, caused by the irritative effects of urine in the wet diaper area, may imitate a psoriasiform eruption. In addition, there is commonly infection with *Candida albicans*. On the other hand, napkin psoriasis, or psoriasis in the diaper area, may also be seen in infants between 2 and 8 months of age. Lesions typically clear with mild therapy, but these infants may be at increased risk for psoriasis in adulthood.

Psoriatic Arthritis. The incidence of psoriasis is 10 times greater in persons with seronegative arthritis than in persons

without arthritis (Figs. 10-13 and 10-14). Five clinical patterns of arthritis occur. They are as follows:

1. Asymmetrical distal interphalangeal joint involvement with nail damage (16%)
2. Arthritis mutilans with osteolysis of phalanges and metacarpals (5%)
3. Symmetrical polyarthritis-like rheumatoid arthritis, with claw hands (15%)
4. Oligoarthritis with swelling and tenosynovitis of one or a few hand joints (70%)
5. Ankylosing spondylitis alone or with peripheral arthritis (5%)

In most cases radiographic findings are the same as in rheumatoid arthritis. Suggestive of psoriasis, however, are erosion of terminal phalangeal tufts (acrosteolysis), tapering or "whittling" of phalanges or metacarpals, "cupping" of proximal ends of phalanges, bony ankylosis, osteolysis of metatarsals, predilection for distal interphalangeal and

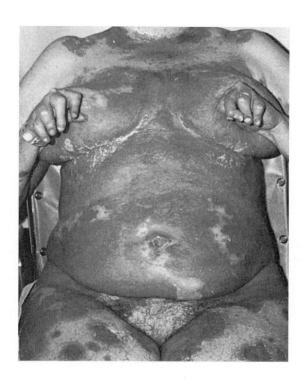

Fig. 10-13 Psoriatic arthritis. Notice the claw hands.

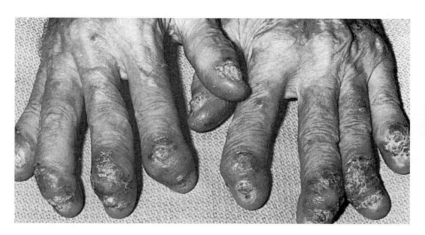

Fig. 10-14 Psoriatic arthritis. (Courtesy Dr. R. Hochman.)

proximal interphalangeal joints, and relative sparing of metacarpal phalangeal and metatarsal phalangeal joints, paravertebral ossification, asymmetrical sacroiliitis, and rarity of "bamboo spine" when the spine is involved. Nearly half the patients with psoriatic arthritis have HLA-B27.

Rest, splinting, passive motion, and aspirin or nonsteroidal antiinflammatory agents are appropriate. Methotrexate, cyclosporine (Neoral), oral retinoids, sulfasalazine, tacrolimus (FK 506), and PUVA are all likely to help both the psoriasis and the arthritis. Systemic steroids are effective in managing arthritis; however, the long-term complications and potential for rebound in cutaneous disease restricts their use.

Guttate Psoriasis. In this distinctive form of psoriasis typical lesions are the size of water drops, 2 to 5 mm in diameter (Fig. 10-15). This type usually occurs as an abrupt eruption following some acute infection, such as a streptococcal pharyngitis. In one series antistreptolysin (ASO) titers were abnormal in 17 of 20 patients with acute guttate psoriasis. In all 20 patients, severe upper respiratory infection preceded the onset of the psoriasis by 1 to 2 weeks.

Guttate psoriasis occurs mostly in patients under age 30. Recurrent episodes are likely, because of pharyngeal carriage of the responsible streptococcus. If penicillin or cephalosporin fail to eradicate it, rifampin should be tried.

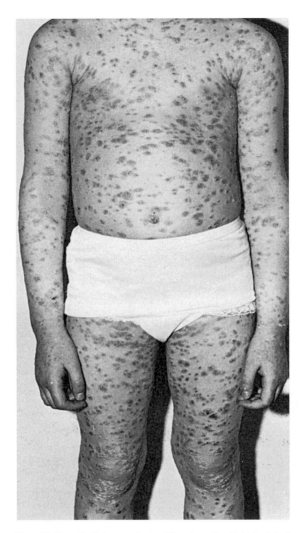

Fig. 10-15 Guttate psoriasis. (Courtesy Dr. R. Feinstein.)

This type of psoriasis is also usually rapidly responsive to topical steroids or UVB.

Generalized Pustular Psoriasis (von Zumbusch). Typical patients have had plaque psoriasis and often psoriatic arthritis. The onset is sudden, with formation of lakes of pus periungually, on the palms, and at the edge of psoriatic plaques. Erythema occurs in the flexures before the generalized eruption appears. This is followed by a generalized erythema and more pustules (Fig. 10-16). Pruritus and intense burning cause extreme discomfort. There is fever, and a fetid odor develops. The pustules dry up to form yellow-brown crusts over a reddish brown, shiny surface.

Mucous membrane lesions are common on the tongue and in the mouth. The lips are red and scaly, and superficial ulcerations of the tongue and mouth occur. Hubler has reported three families in which five examples of geographic tongue and fissured tongue, along with pustular psoriasis, occurred.

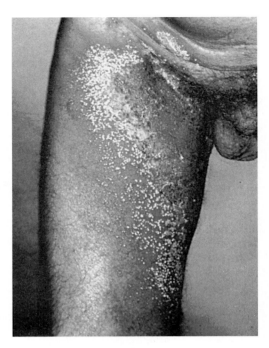

Fig. 10-16 Pustular psoriasis.

Zumbusch's psoriasis may go through several stages. There is the exanthematous febrile eruption of pustules, then there are flare-ups of fever and pustules, and finally continuous fever, erythroderma, and cachexia (Fig. 10-17). A number of cases of acute respiratory distress syndrome associated with pustular and erythrodermic psoriasis have been reported. Other systemic complications include pneumonia, congestive heart failure, and hepatitis. Erythrodermic psoriasis is covered in greater detail under exfoliative dermatitis.

Although the etiology of this type is not any better known than that of psoriasis vulgaris, iodides, coal tar, steroid withdrawal, terbinafine, minocycline, hydroxychloroquine, acetazolamide, and salicylates may trigger the attacks. There is usually a strong familial history of psoriasis.

Generalized pustular psoriasis may occur in infants and children. It may occur as an episodic event punctuating the course of localized acral pustular psoriasis. Rarely, it may be familial. Hubler reported such a kindred, in which three siblings had chronic localized acral-pustular psoriasis with episodes of generalized pustular psoriasis. Takematsu et al reported juvenile generalized pustular psoriasis in a pair of monozygotic twins presenting strikingly similar clinical courses, both having onset 48 days after birth.

Histologic examination shows a characteristic spongiform pustule in the upper epidermis. The pustule is lined with swollen epidermal cells and contains polymorphonuclear leukocytes. Identical pustules are also seen in acrodermatitis continua of Hallopeau, impetigo

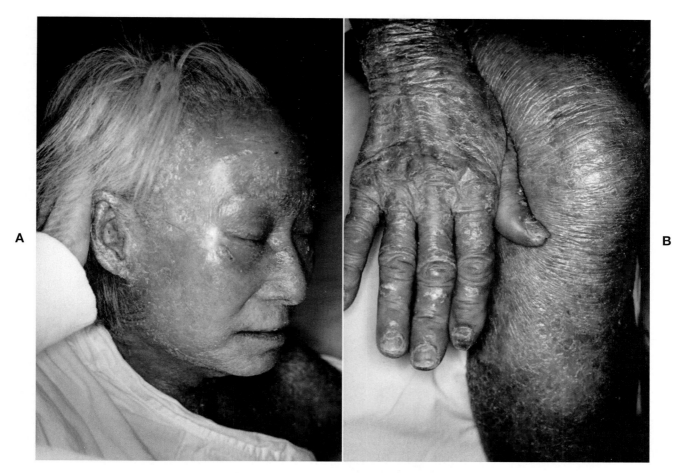

Fig. 10-17 A and **B,** Psoriatic erythroderma.

herpetiformis, and keratoderma blennorrhagica (Reiter's syndrome).

Acitretin is the drug of choice in this severe disease. Response is rapid and predictable. Isotretinoin is also effective. Cyclosporine and methotrexate are alternatives. Sometimes dapsone is effective in doses of 50 mg daily initially, and then increased.

Course

The course of psoriasis is unpredictable. It usually begins on the scalp or on the elbows, and may remain localized in the original region for an indefinite period, or completely disappear, recur, or spread to other parts. It may first be seen over the sacrum, where it may easily be confused with tinea. At other times the onset is more sudden and widespread (Fig. 10-18). The first lesions may be limited to the fingernails (Fig. 10-19).

Two of the chief features of psoriasis are its tendency to recur and its persistence. Rarely, however, patients with psoriasis may remain completely free of the disease for years. On the scalp it rarely causes loss of hair. The lesions—even the chronic ones—are sometimes easily irritated, and when this takes place they are liable to spread by the development of satellites, or new spots in other regions. In acute guttate or spreading nummular eruptions, if irritating remedies or physical agents are applied, a generalized exfoliative dermatitis may result.

The isomorphic response, commonly known as *Koebner's phenomenon,* is the appearance of typical lesions of psoriasis at sites of even trivial injuries (Fig. 10-20). This characteristic feature of the disease accounts for the frequent appearance of typical psoriatic patches on scars and at sites of scratches, eruptions, and burns. The Koebner response occurs in many other skin diseases such as lichen planus and lichen nitidus.

Auspitz's sign is pinpoint bleeding when a psoriatic scale is forcibly removed. It occurs because of the severe thinning of the epidermis over the tips of the dermal papillae. The Woronoff ring is concentric blanching of the erythematous skin at or near the periphery of a healing psoriatic plaque. It does not redden with ultraviolet-induced erythema or under anthralin therapy.

On the scalp the lesions are often nummular plaques, but at times there is a bandlike patch along the anterior hair line,

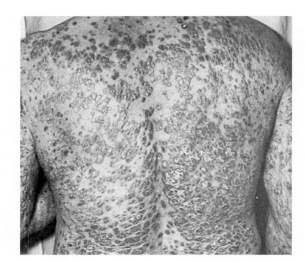

Fig. 10-18 Generalized plaque psoriasis.

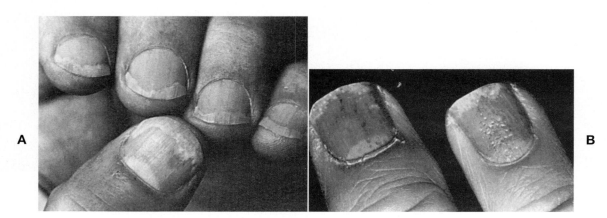

A

B

Fig. 10-19 **A,** Onycholysis with psoriatic nails. Note the "oil spot" on thumb. **B,** Pitting, distal, onycholysis and "oil spots" in psoriatic nails. (Courtesy Dr. Axel W. Hoke.)

or a palm-sized plaque on the occiput, which may be thickened and pruritic, with lichenification (Fig. 10-21). In other cases, profuse scaling may be the only sign. Absence of itching or hair loss, marked predilection for the frontal scalp margin, deep erythema, and resistance to effective therapy for seborrheic dermatitis all suggest psoriasis. In psoriasis the lesions are well demarcated. Associated with the scalp involvement, there are often fissuring of the superior and posterior auricular folds and erythematous scaling plaques about the external auditory meatus. Nail pitting and hyperkeratotic plaques on the glans penis may be early or isolated findings (Fig. 10-22).

On the face (which is generally entirely spared except for the upper edge of the forehead) chiefly guttate lesions are seen, especially in acute, widespread eruptions, although some patients with inveterate patches of the trunk may develop a few on the face. Larger lesions commonly

have the appearance of seborrheic dermatitis or lupus erythematosus.

The palms and soles are often, sometimes exclusively, affected, showing discrete erythematous, dry, scaling patches, or circumscribed verrucous thickenings, which are sometimes linear (Fig. 10-23). Pustular psoriasis of the palms and soles is considered in detail on p. 240. Briefly, the patches begin on the middle portions of the palms or on the soles, and, with recurring crops of small pustules, eventually form exfoliative areas in which the pustules, though more evident at the edges, are often observed throughout (Fig. 10-24). The pustules sometimes fuse to form so-called lakes of pus. The condition is extremely resistant to treatment.

The axillae, submammary folds, pubis, genitalia, groins, and gluteal crease may be affected. "Flexural" or inverse psoriasis shows salmon-red, demarcated plaques that frequently become eczematized, moist, and fissured. There is

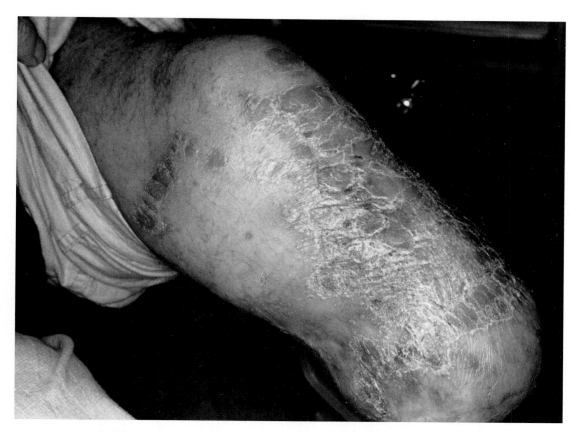

Fig. 10-20   Psoriasis of amputation stump. Koebner reaction induced by prosthesis.

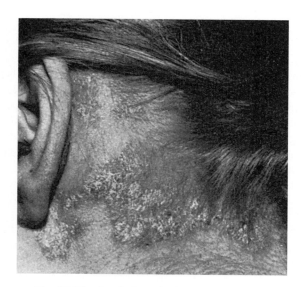

Fig. 10-21   Psoriasis on back of neck and scalp.

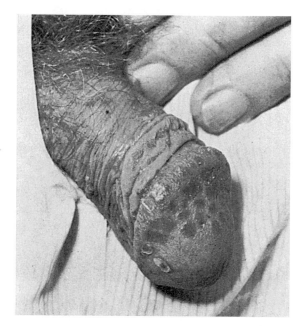

Fig. 10-22   Psoriasis of penis. Predilection for the glans is characteristic, as is scantiness of scale.

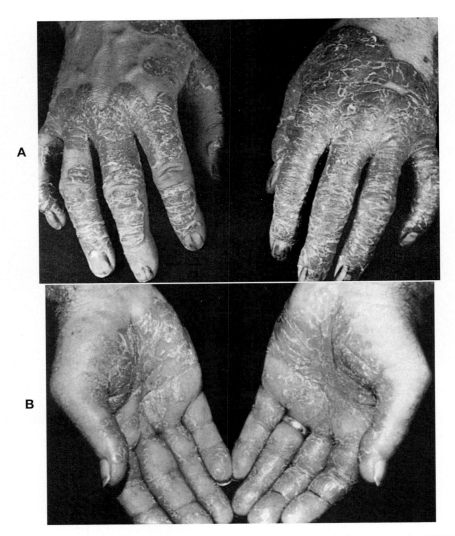

Fig. 10-23 **A,** Psoriasis of backs of hands. **B,** Psoriasis of palms. (**B,** Courtesy Dr. Axel W. Hoke.)

little scaling. Lesions in these locations, owing to perspiration, maceration, and friction, may become extensive, sodden patches that burn and itch.

Numerous cases of psoriasis of the mucous membranes have been reported. The buccal mucosa, the tongue, and especially the lips may be involved. Geographic tongue and fissured tongue may occur in generalized pustular psoriasis (Fig. 10-25). Hietanen et al studied the oral mucosa in 200 consecutive patients with psoriasis. They found histologically proven oral psoriasis in 2% of patients.

Both the fingernails and toenails may be involved. The characteristic changes are numerous pits 1 mm or so in diameter, like dents made with a ball-point pen; tan, oval spots 2 to 4 mm in diameter (oil "spots"); onycholysis (uplifting of the distal portion from the nail bed); cracking of the free edges; and heaped-up crusts accumulated beneath them (see Fig. 10-19).

Many studies report an association of hepatitis C and psoriasis, and some authors have suggested that hepatitis C infection might be one of the triggering factors of psoriasis. Hepatitis C has also been implicated in psoriatic arthritis. If treatment of psoriasis is to include a potentially hepatotoxic drug, such as methotrexate, a hepatitis C serology should be obtained. It should also be noted that interferon-alfa, an agent frequently used to treat patients with hepatitis C, can further exacerbate or induce psoriasis.

Etiology

The cause of psoriasis is still unknown. It is apparent that heredity is of significance in some cases. In a large study of psoriasis in monozygotic twins heritability was high and environmental influence low. In one study some 36% of 2144 patients knew of relatives who also had psoriasis. A multifactorial inheritance is thought to be operating.

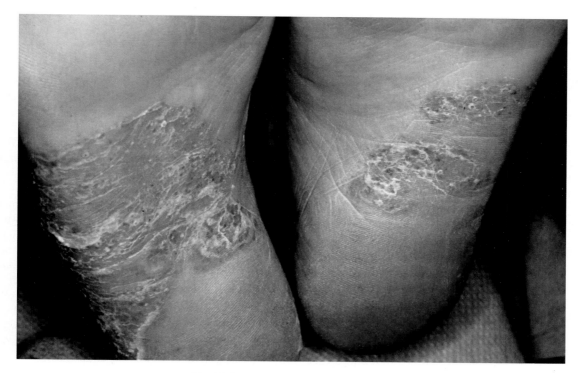

Fig. 10-24 Psoriasis of plantar surfaces.

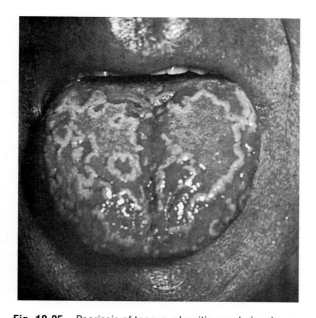

Fig. 10-25 Psoriasis of tongue, glossitis annularis migrans.

Analysis of population-specific human leukocyte antigen (HLA) haplotypes has provided evidence that susceptibility to psoriasis is linked to the class I and II major histocompatibility complex on human chromosome 6 (17q). It has also been shown that there are two subsets that differ

in age of onset and in the frequency of HLA associations. Early onset is type I psoriasis and is associated with mostly -Cw6, -B57, and -DR7. Late onset is type II, which predominantly features -Cw2.

A variety of other HLA associations have been reported by various authors. It is believed that any individual who has -B13 or -B17 has a fivefold risk of developing psoriasis. In pustular psoriasis HLA-B27 may be seen, whereas -B13 and -B17 are increased in guttate and erythrodermic psoriasis. In palmoplantar pustulosis, there is an increased proportion of persons having HLA-B8, -Bw35, -Cw7, and -DR3. HLA typing, however, is of no value in assessing the individual patient.

Epidemiology

Psoriasis occurs with equal frequency in both sexes. The onset of psoriasis is at a mean age of 27 years, but the range is wide, from a few months to the seventies. In one study hot weather improved psoriasis in 77%, cold weather in 12%, and sunlight in 78% of patients. Severe emotional stress tended to aggravate psoriasis in 40%, and worry made psoriasis worse in 37%; there was no definitive reaction in 42%. There was arthritic involvement in 25% of the patients. Complete periodic disappearance of psoriasis during its course was experienced by 39%.

In another series of 5395 individuals in an urban practice the point prevalence was 1.48%, and there was no difference in sexes. The mean age was 33 years. At some stage 60% of individuals required referral to a consultant, and 25% were in remission during their treatment course. Thirty-seven percent thought stress was an exacerbating factor.

One percent to 2% of the U.S. population has psoriasis. It occurs less frequently in the tropics. It is less common in North American and West African blacks. Native Americans and native Fijians do not have psoriasis.

In pregnancy there is a distinct tendency for improvement or even temporary disappearance. After childbirth there is a tendency for exacerbation of lesions. However, the psoriasis may behave differently from one pregnancy to another in the same patient. During menopause lesions may change for better or worse, with no set pattern of behavior.

Pathogenesis

Psoriasis is characterized by three main pathogenic features: abnormal differentiation, keratinocyte hyperproliferation, and inflammation. Accelerated epidermopoiesis has been considered to be the fundamental pathologic event in psoriasis. The transit rate of psoriatic keratinocytes is increased, and the deoxyribonucleic acid synthesis time is decreased. It has been suggested that it is the heightened proportion of epidermal cells participating in the proliferative process, rather than the actual rate of epidermopoiesis, that is the basic fault in psoriatic lesions. The result in either case is greatly increased production of keratin. Whether this is a primary or secondary response to inflammation is yet to be elucidated.

In histologic studies of changes from the earliest erythematous macule through the mature hyperkeratotic plaque, the earliest change is an inflammatory, perivascular, upper dermal infiltrate. Epidermal acanthosis and parakeratosis occur only after the transformation of the lesion into a scaly papule.

Early lesions are infiltrated predominantly by lymphocytes in the papillary dermis. Therapeutic agents such as corticosteroids, cyclosporine, and hydroxyurea affect the inflammatory response, confirming the importance of inflammatory cells and inflammatory mediators in the pathogenesis of psoriasis. The cause of T-lymphocyte activation and the role of these cell populations remains unclear. T-cell activation can subsequently result in the production of a variety of cytokines, some of which have been shown to precipitate or induce psoriasis when used as therapy for other disorders.

Overexpression of proinflammatory, type 1 cytokines has been demonstrated and is believed to be of pathogenic significance in psoriasis. IL-10 is a type 2 cytokine with major influences on immunoregulation, inhibiting type 1 proinflammatory cytokine production. Asadullah et al have shown that patients on established traditional therapies show rising levels of IL-10 mRNA expression, suggesting that IL-10 may have antipsoriatic capacity. These results

suggest that depressed levels of IL-10 may play a role in the pathogenesis of psoriasis, and IL-10 could eventually become an effective therapeutic option.

Stress. Various questionnaires, such as the Psoriasis Life Stress Inventory (PLSI) developed by Gupta et al, have attempted to measure the degree of stress. Other questionnaires have been designed assessing somatization, depression, life change units, and general health. All of these studies have shown a positive correlation between stress and severity of disease.

Drug-Induced Psoriasis. Psoriasis may be induced by many drugs: beta blockers, lithium, and antimalarials, among others. More recent additions include terbinafine, calcium channel blockers (nicardipine, nifedipine, nisoldipine, verapamil, and diltiazem), captopril, glyburide, and the lipid-lowering drugs such as gemfibrozil. It has long been known that systemic steroids may cause rebound in patients with psoriasis. Demitsu et al reported a case of dexamethasone-induced, widespread exanthemous pustulosis, which was patch-test positive to dexamethasone.

Because cytokines have been implicated in the pathogenesis of psoriasis, it is not surprising that cytokine therapies may induce or exacerbate psoriasis. G-CSF, interleukin therapy, and more than 20 cases of interferon-alfa and 1 case of interferon-beta induction or exacerbations of psoriasis have been reported.

Pathology

Skin biopsy is rarely necessary in the evaluation of psoriasis. Clinically characteristic lesions have diagnostic histology. Atypical (nondiagnostic) lesions often demonstrate nondiagnostic features histologically and are often interpreted as "psoriasiform dermatitis." There is regular epidermal hyperplasia with long, test-tube-shaped rete ridges. There is thinning over the dermal papillae, thus explaining Auspitz's sign. The granular layer is thin or absent, and there is overlying parakeratosis. Small collections of neutrophils (Munro microabscesses) may be present in the stratum corneum. The dermal papillae are prominent and contain ectatic vessels. There is a perivascular mononuclear cell infiltrate. In guttate lesions the epidermal hyperplasia may be less marked.

Psoriasis may be distinguished from dermatitis by the paucity of edema, the absence of spongiosis and vesicle formation, the clubbing of the papillary bodies, and the tortuosity of the capillary loops. In psoriasiform syphilis the panarteritis and the plasma cell infiltration are characteristic, and in psoriasiform lesions of mycosis fungoides there is epidermotropism of lymphocytes without spongiosis. The microabscesses in mycosis fungoides contain lymphocytes and monocytes, whereas the microabscesses of Munro in psoriasis contain polymorphonuclear leukocytes.

Differential Diagnosis

Psoriasis must be differentiated from seborrheic dermatitis, pityriasis rosea, lichen planus, eczema, the psoriasiform syphilid, and lupus erythematosus. The distribution in psoriasis is on the extensor surfaces, especially of the elbows and knees, and on the scalp, whereas in seborrheic dermatitis, although the scalp is involved, there is a predilection for the eyebrows, nasolabial angle, ears, sternal region, and flexures. The scales in psoriasis are dry, white, and shiny, whereas those in seborrheic dermatitis are greasy and lusterless. On removal of the scales in psoriasis there is an oozing of blood from the capillaries (Auspitz's sign), whereas this does not occur in seborrheic dermatitis.

In pityriasis rosea the eruption is located on the upper arms, trunk, and thighs, and the duration is a matter of weeks. There are oval, fawn-colored patches that centrally show a crinkling of the epidermis and collarette scaling. The onset with the herald patch, and the tendency of the subsequent lesions to arrange themselves so that their long diameters are parallel to skin tension lines, helps to distinguish between pityriasis rosea and psoriasis.

Lichen planus affects chiefly the flexor surfaces of the forearms and wrists, and the shins and ankles. The patches are pruritic and thickened. Often the violaceous color is pronounced, but at other times the patches are a dirty brown color and are then only distinguished from psoriasis by scale that is not at all micaceous, but scanty and tightly adherent. The scalp is much less frequently involved, and the nails are not pitted as in psoriasis, but longitudinally ridged and thickened, with pterygium a characteristic finding.

In atopic dermatitis the distribution is usually not on the extensor surfaces of the elbows and knees, and exudation and a slight grayish scaling, accompanied by severe itching, are present.

The psoriasiform syphilid has infiltrated patches of copper-colored papules, often arranged in a configurate manner. The scales are brownish and sparse. Serologic tests for syphilis are positive; a general adenopathy, and often mucous patches, condylomata, and other symptoms of secondary syphilis are present. Itching is usually absent.

In lupus erythematosus (LE) the lesions are discrete plaques, usually on the face and scalp, associated with atrophy, scaling, and alopecia. The face is rarely affected by psoriasis. The scales of lupus erythematosus are grayish and adherent. On removal of the scale the undersurface is seen to be papillose as a result of the projecting follicular plugs. There is a psoriasiform subset of subacute cutaneous LE that may be distinguished by its location on the upper trunk, arms, and face and by other signs of LE such as photosensitivity.

Patients with psoriasis may develop other skin diseases. Psoriasis, elicited by a Koebner response, may accompany other diseases, or follow them when they subside. This is of great practical importance in relation to drug eruptions, scarlatina, and other exanthems.

Psoriasis and Skin Cancer. For years it was believed that patients with psoriasis enjoyed particular freedom from skin cancer. However, Halprin et al in 1982 found in 150 patients with psoriasis who had never been treated with PUVA that the incidence of skin cancer (basal and squamous cell combined) was 1.96 per year—three times that of a control group of patients with diabetes. Studniberg et al wrote an extensive review and meticulously analyzed studies correlating PUVA, UVB, and nonmelanoma skin cancer. The authors concluded that (1) PUVA is an independent carcinogen; (2) the risk is not simply dose related; (3) history of arsenic exposure, ionizing radiation therapy, and prior skin cancer is important; (4) factors that appear to be associated with little or no risk of increased PUVA-induced carcinogenesis are prior exposure to methotrexate, UVB, or concomitant use of topical tar; (5) dose-related risk of PUVA-induced squamous cell carcinoma is independent of skin type (although the absolute risk is much higher in skin types I and II); (6) men treated without genital protection are at an increased risk of developing squamous cell carcinomas of the penis and scrotum; (7) PUVA-induced squamous cell carcinomas do not appear to be aggressive; (8) there is no definitive level of cumulative PUVA exposure above which carcinogenicity can be predicted; and (9) therapeutic UVB is associated with minimal risk of cutaneous carcinogenesis. High doses of methotrexate exposure or combination treatment with both methotrexate and PUVA has been shown to increase the risk for the development of cutaneous squamous cell carcinomas. In 1997 Stern et al reported the results of 1380 patients with psoriasis treated with PUVA. The authors concluded that approximately 15 years after the first treatment with PUVA the risk of malignant melanoma increases, especially among patients who received 250 treatments or more.

Treatment

The lesions may disappear spontaneously or as the result of therapy, but recurrences are almost certain, and there is a tendency for each remedy to lose its effectiveness gradually. Treatment methods will vary according to the site, severity, duration, previous treatment, and the age of the patient. In some instances treatment may be solely topical, may be systemic, or may be a combination of both. Rotating therapeutic approaches, especially with systemic agents that have varying toxicities, has a conceptual appeal.

Topical Treatment

In many patients topical applications alone will suffice to keep psoriasis under control. Numerous local medications are available.

CORTICOSTEROIDS. Topical application of corticosteroids in creams, ointments, lotions, and sprays is the most frequent therapy, prescribed in 70% of visits to dermatologists. The class I steroids are the strongest and should be used on more severe disease. On the scalp corticosteroids in propylene glycol or a gel base are used, except in blacks, who often prefer ointments. Corticosteroids may be incorporated into oils. The creams are preferred in the intertriginous areas and in exposed areas. With all corticosteroids, ointments are more effective than creams of the same strength.

To augment effectiveness of the topical corticosteroids, application is followed by an occlusive dressing of a polyethylene film (Saran Wrap), which may remain in place for 12 to 24 hours at a time. A prompt response is usually noted. Unfortunately there is recurrence of the lesions within a short time with this type of therapy. Side effects (miliaria, pyoderma, epidermal atrophy) may be troublesome and even serious. Clobetasol lotion applied under Duofilm and left in place for several days will clear many recalcitrant plaques.

Intralesional corticosteroid injections of triamcinolone are frequently used. Triamcinolone acetonide (Kenalog) suspension 10 mg/ml may be diluted with sterile saline to make a concentration of 5 mg/ml or even 2.5 mg. This is an excellent method for treating small lesions of psoriasis. Usually one injection produces clearing locally. Good results are also obtained in the treatment of psoriatic nails by injecting triamcinolone into the region of the matrix and the lateral nail folds. Injections are given once a month. It should be remembered that intralesional therapy may cause atrophy of the subcutaneous tissue at the site of injection. Usually the depression will disappear in a few months. Of all localized methods, intralesional steroid therapy is the most ideal because of its prompt and effective action, and because of its long-acting benefit.

TARS. The staining property and odor of the tars may hinder the use of these otherwise effective topical medications. Several tar ointments in which the staining properties have been reduced are available. Coal tar solution or liquor carbonis detergens is applied to the lesions before ultraviolet treatment in the Goeckerman method. It is also incorporated into liquid solutions to be used for a tar bath. Oil of cade (pine tar) or birch tar in concentrations of 5% to 10% may be incorporated into ointments.

DIHYDROXYANTHRALIN. Dihydroxyanthralin has been used extensively for more than 50 years and is of unquestionable effectiveness, but it is highly irritating and stains skin, clothing, and bedding. To avoid these drawbacks, lower concentrations (0.01% to 1%) have been used. Micanol, dithranol microencapsulated in crystalline monoglycerides, is easier to wash off, causes less staining, and is less irritating than standard preparations. Short-contact treatment (SCAT) may be effective and reduce staining, irritation, and inconvenience. Anthralin exerts a direct effect on keratinocytes and leukocytes by suppressing neu-

trophil superoxide generation and inhibition of monocyte-derived IL-6, IL-8, and TNF-alpha. Contact sensitization may occur.

TAZAROTENE. Tazarotene is a novel, nonisomerizable class of retinoic acid receptor-specific retinoid developed for the treatment of psoriasis. It appears to treat psoriasis by modulating keratinocyte differentiation and hyperproliferation, as well as suppressing inflammation. Once-daily tazarotene 0.05% and 0.1% gels demonstrated more prolonged therapeutic effect after discontinuation than twice-daily fluocinonide cream. The medication produces local irritation. Combining its use with topical corticosteroids aids in patient acceptance.

VITAMIN D. Vitamin D_3 affects keratinocyte differentiation partly through its regulation of epidermal responsiveness to calcium. Treatment with the vitamin D analogue calcipotriene (Dovonex) in ointment, cream, or solution form has been shown to be very effective in the treatment of plaque-type and scalp psoriasis. Combination therapy with calcipotriene and high-potency steroids may provide greater response rates, fewer side effects, and steroid sparing, allowing a shift to a less potent topical steroid or less frequent use of a class I steroid. Tacalcitol, another vitamin D analogue, has also been shown to be very effective with minimal side effects. Monitoring of serum calcium levels in adults is not required.

SALICYLIC ACID. Usually a 3% to 5% concentration is incorporated into cold cream or hydrophilic ointment. This aids in removing the scale and promoting the efficacy of other topical agents. Widespread application may lead to salicylate toxicity manifesting with tinnitus, acute confusion, and refractory hypoglycemia, especially in patients with diabetes and those with compromised renal function.

ULTRAVIOLET LIGHT. In most instances sunlight improves psoriasis remarkably. However, burning of the skin may cause Koebner's phenomenon and an exacerbation. Artificial ultraviolet light (UVB) is frequently used as a substitute. Daily exposures should be regulated so as not to produce burns but only a mild transient erythema. The time of exposure can be slowly increased by a few seconds daily. Although tar applications or baths before UVB exposure have been credited with enhancing its effects, studies indicate that an emollient followed by suberythemogenic doses of UVB gives results comparable to those with the use of a tar followed by UVB. Maintenance UVB phototherapy after clearing contributes to the duration of remission and is justified for many patients.

Using a monochromator, it has been shown that wavelengths of 254, 280, and 290 nm are ineffective; at 296, 300, 304, and 313 nm there is clearing, with the lowest total dose achieved by fixed daily doses, not by an incrementally increased daily dose. Narrowband UVB has been shown to be more effective in treating psoriasis than broadband. In a study by Oakley et al comparisons between patients treated with UVB versus PUVA showed 73% versus 87.5% improvement, respectively.

Hecker et al in a controlled, investigator-blinded, right-left study comparing topical calcipotriene with mineral oil combined with UVB showed 11 of 20 patients (55%) had a greater decrease in the severity of their psoriasis with UVB plus calcipotriene compared with UVB and mineral oil.

GOECKERMAN TECHNIQUE. The Goeckerman technique is an effective and frequently gratifying method of treatment, and despite the popularity of PUVA treatment, this technique, with its many modifications, continues to be popular. The technique has been modified, simplified, and changed, but basically the principles are the same as originally described. Essentially, a 2% to 5% tar preparation is applied to the skin, and a tar bath is taken at least once daily. The excess tar is removed with mineral or vegetable oil, and ultraviolet light is given.

Menter et al reported the results of Goeckerman therapy in two day-care centers, in a population of 300 severe, resistant cases; they cleared in an average of 18 days, and 75% remained free of disease for more than 1 year. Horwitz showed that the addition of a topical hydrocortisone cream to the Goeckerman regimen shortened the time required for remission.

INGRAM TECHNIQUE. The Ingram technique consists of a daily coal tar bath in a solution such as 120 ml liquor carbonis detergens to 80 L of warm water. This is followed by exposure to an ultraviolet light for daily increasing periods. An anthralin paste is then applied to each psoriatic plaque. Talcum powder is sprinkled over the lesions, and stockinette dressings are applied. The method requires close attention to details and personal supervision. If properly used, it is very effective; however, the availability of many other more easily applied and effective topicals make this more of a historic footnote.

PUVA THERAPY. Parrish et al reported that high-intensity longwave ultraviolet radiation (UVA) given 2 hours after ingestion of 8-methoxypsoralen (Oxsoralen), and given two or three times a week, would completely clear almost every patient with severe psoriasis in 20 to 25 treatments. Maintenance treatment is needed. A new dosage form of methoxsalen with greater bioavailability, Oxsoralen-Ultra, is now standard. The risk of enhanced carcinogenesis is now proved, with a reversal of the usual ratio of squamous cell carcinomas to basal cell carcinomas. Accelerated actinic elastosis, melanocyte dysplasia, and the possible increased incidence of melanoma should be considered when recommending this treatment. In addition, the potential for eye damage and the deleterious effects to lymphocytes remain areas of concern when deciding to recommend this treatment to any patient.

Boer et al compared UVB and PUVA and found that, in patients with less than 50% of the skin surface affected, UVB was as good as PUVA or better. In more extensive cases, PUVA required less frequent maintenance therapy. Psoralen-311 nm UVB therapy is as effective as conventional PUVA. Polyethylene sheet bath PUVA is another therapeutic alternative to oral psoralen-PUVA.

Surgical Treatment

Although no one seriously embraces it as an acceptable therapy, denervation by surgery has long been known to abolish psoriatic plaques. Kiil et al reported that surgical excision in 24 patients of a psoriatic plaque to the depth of the reticular dermis, with a dermatome, completely abolished the lesion for 3 to 36 months in 17 and required only reexcision of minor recurrences in the other 7.

In a group of 14 patients with pharyngeal colonization by streptococci unresponsive to antibiotic therapy, Skinner et al reported an excellent response (9 cleared their psoriatic plaques) after tonsillectomy.

Lasers in Psoriasis

Psoriatic plaques can be cleared by destruction of the upper dermis. Dilated blood vessels are prominent in the psoriatic dermal papillae, which can be selectively destroyed with yellow light lasers. Numerous authors have shown the therapeutic effectiveness and long-term responses of plaque-type psoriasis treated with a flashlamp pulsed dye laser. Only practical considerations limit the use of this therapeutic modality, including the small spot size, the lack of cost effectiveness, and prolonged postoperative healing. There has also been some success using a CO_2 resurfacing laser.

Hyperthermia

Twenty-two chronic psoriatic plaques in 9 patients were heated to 42° to 45° C with ultrasound for 30 minutes 3 times a week for 4 to 10 treatments, by Orenberg et al, and 15 completely cleared; only 2 remained unchanged. Most patients relapsed within 3 months. Urabe et al carried out various conventional therapies on one side of the body in 22 patients with plaque psoriasis and heated the opposite half of the body with exothermal pads continuously for 5 weeks. Skin lesions disappeared from the heated side in 19 patients. Microwave hyperthermia may produce significant complications such as pain over bony prominences and hypotension.

Occlusive Treatment

Shore reported clearing of psoriatic lesions by occluding them with tape. Friedman showed that hydrocolloid occlusion (with Actiderm) had a similar effect on small lesions.

Systemic Treatment

In some instances psoriatic involvement may be so extensive and recalcitrant that systemic treatment is necessary.

CORTICOSTEROIDS. The hazards of the injudicious use of systemic corticosteroids must be emphasized. The side effects of orally administered prednisone are so dangerous that its use should be limited to patients with unusual individual circumstances. There is great risk of "rebound" or induction of pustular psoriasis when it is stopped.

METHOTREXATE. This folic acid antagonist was the first effective systemic drug for psoriasis and is the standard for systemic therapy. Methotrexate has a greater affinity for dihydrofolic acid reductase than has folic acid. The synthesis of deoxyribonucleic acid is blocked when dihydrofolic acid reductase is bound and thereby cell division is thwarted; in psoriasis the greatly increased epidermal cell turnover rate is slowed. Like cyclosporine, methotrexate may also affect the inflammatory element of psoriasis, producing a decrease in CD8+ cells and other T-cell functions or through suppressed neutrophil chemotaxis.

The indications for the use of methotrexate are psoriatic erythroderma, moderate to severe psoriatic arthritis, acute pustular psoriasis (von Zumbusch type), more than 20% total body surface involvement, localized pustular psoriasis, psoriasis that affects certain areas of the body so that normal function and employment are prevented (such as hands), and lack of response to phototherapy, PUVA, or retinoids.

Before treatment is started it is important to make sure that the patient has no history of liver or kidney disease. Other important factors to consider are whether alcohol abuse, cirrhosis, severe illness, debility, pregnancy (or nursing), male or female fertility, leukopenia, thrombocytopenia, active infectious disease, immunodeficiency, anemia, colitis, or noncompliance is present. Serum glutamic oxaloacetic transaminase (SGOT or AST), serum glutamic pyruvic transaminase (SGPT or ALT), bilirubin, serum albumin, creatinine, alkaline phosphatase, complete blood count (CBC), platelet count, hepatitis serology (B and C), and urinalysis should all be done before starting treatment. Patients with hypoalbuminemia have the highest risk of developing pulmonary complications. HIV antibody determination should be obtained.

The need for baseline liver biopsy in patients with psoriasis has always been controversial and is not without risks. According to the 1998 guidelines (Roenigk et al) in most patients with no risk factors for liver disease the first liver biopsy should be obtained at approximately 1.0 to 1.5 g of cumulative methotrexate and repeated every subsequent 1.5 g until a total of 4.0 g is reached. The frequency then changes to every 1.0 to 1.5 g cumulative intervals.

Numerous treatment schedules have evolved. Of these the ones recommended are either three divided oral doses (12 hours apart) weekly, once weekly doses orally, or single weekly subcutaneous injections. The weekly dose varies from 5 mg to more than 50 mg. Once the dose exceeds 25 mg at a time oral absorption is unpredictable and subcutaneous injections are recommended.

CYCLOSPORINE. The therapeutic benefit of the immunosuppressive features of cyclosporine in psoriatic disease may be related to down modulation of proinflammatory epidermal cytokines, but the exact mechanisms are not fully understood. Many studies have shown the beneficial effects of cyclosporine in the treatment of recalcitrant psoriasis, and the new microemulsion formulation Neoral has provided even greater efficacy and bioavailability. However, there are serious long-term complications with its use, even with low-dose therapy.

Zachariae performed renal biopsies in 30 patients with psoriasis during long-term cyclosporine therapy ranging from 2.5 to 6 mg/kg/day with treatment durations ranging from 6 months to 8 years. After 2 years all biopsies shared features consistent with cyclosporine-induced nephrotoxicity. The authors conclude that other forms of treatment should be used after 2 years of cyclosporine therapy. In a study performed by Powles et al the authors measured glomerular filtration rate (GFR) in 2 groups, the original cohort of 9 patients (7 of whom were treated from 9.5 to 10 years on cyclosporine) and a second group of 20 patients treated an average of 6 years (range from 5 to 8 years). In the original group treated more than 9.5 years, all 7 had decreased GFR greater than 30%, and 2 patients (29%) had decreased GFR greater than 50%. In the second group, 9 out of 20 had decreased GFR greater than 30% (45%) and 5 (25%) were greater than 50%. These authors state that patient variation regarding commencement of nephrotoxicity and speed of progression is unpredictable; therefore, they concluded that cyclosporine may be used long-term (5 to 10 years) in severe, recalcitrant psoriasis if renal function is closely monitored.

Induction therapy with cyclosporine is 2.5 to 3.0 mg/kg given as a divided dose twice daily and can be increased to 5.0 mg/kg/day until a clinical response is noted. The dose is then tapered. On discontinuation of cyclosporine a severe flare may occur, suggesting an alternative treatment (such as phototherapy or Acitretin) should be instituted as the cyclosporine dose is reduced.

DIET. Ever since psoriasis became known as an entity, dietary restrictions frequently have been imposed on the patient. Dietary fads have come and gone. Controlled studies evaluating various dietary restrictions, especially those of low protein intake, showed no appreciable difference in the course of psoriasis.

Fleischer et al evaluated 371 university-affiliated dermatology clinic patients with psoriasis in relation to alternative therapy. Excluding sunlight and nonprescription tanning, 51% used one or more alternative modalities. Psoriasis was more severe in patients trying herbal remedies, vitamin therapy, and dietary manipulation. Controlled clinical trials are needed to answer the question of the effectiveness of alternative treatments in psoriasis.

The most recent such trials have demonstrated the antiinflammatory effects of fish oils rich in n-3 polyunsaturated fatty acids in rheumatoid arthritis, inflammatory bowel disease, psoriasis, and asthma. It has been shown that n-3 and n-6 polyunsaturated fatty acids affect a variety of cytokines, including IL-1, IL-6, and tumor necrosis factor. Through changes in cell membrane fluidity there may be alterations in the binding of cytokines to receptors, G protein activity, alteration in eicosanoid production, and activation of protein kinase C. Mayser et al reported a study analyzing 83 chronic plaque-type psoriasis patients treated with infusions of omega-3 or omega-6 fatty acids and showed improvement in 16 of 43 patients (37%) in the omega-3-treated group compared with 9 of 40 (23%) treated with omega-6. In the omega-3-treated group there were significant elevations in neutrophil leukotriene B5 and platelet thromboxane B3 generation. These results suggest that dietary manipulation of free fatty acids may be effective in treating chronic plaque-type psoriasis, mediated through alterations in inflammatory eicosanoid generation.

ORAL ANTIMICROBIAL THERAPY. The association of streptococcal pharyngitis with initiation or exacerbations of guttate psoriasis is well established, but the mechanism is unknown. Recent evidence suggests that *Staphylococcus aureus* and streptococci secrete a large family of exotoxins that are superantigens, producing massive T-cell activation. Oral antibiotic therapy for psoriasis patients infected with these organisms is imperative and may require extended treatment in those with generalized plaque-type psoriasis infected with staphylococci.

Rosenberg et al has published extensively on the aggravation of psoriasis by activation of the alternate pathway of complement by *Malassezia ovalis,* or by intestinal yeasts, or by endotoxins produced by gram-negative bacteria in the gut. He believed this helps to explain the following:

1. Seborrheic localization (*M. ovalis* effect)
2. Poststreptococcal flares
3. Diaper area lesions *(Candida albicans)*
4. Precipitation by typhoid vaccine (which contains endotoxin)
5. Improvement during imprisonment and relapse when *Enterobacteriaceae* return to the gut on resumption of a "good" Western diet
6. Severity of psoriasis in alcoholics, who are not well protected against release of endotoxins into the circulation by their damaged Kupffer cells

Rosenberg et al has achieved good results with oral ketoconazole. Palmoplantar pustulosis responds positively to itraconazole. There have also been reports of the beneficial action of metronidazole (Flagyl) in acute flares of plaque psoriasis.

RETINOIDS. Treatment internally with 13-cis-retinoic acid can produce good results, especially in pustular psoriasis in dosages of 0.5 to 0.74 mg/kg/day. Side effects are cheilitis, conjunctivitis sicca, facial dermatitis, xerosis, rhinitis sicca with nose bleed, and skin fragility. It is a potent teratogen. Combinations of retinoic acids with photochemotherapy for chronic plaque psoriasis may also be very effective. In this manner it is possible to reduce the amount of UVA given during the course of treatment by up to 75%.

The aromatic retinoid ethylester, etretinate, appears to be far more effective in generalized pustular psoriasis than chronic plaque lesions. It is given at a dose level of 0.5 to 1.0 mg/kg/day. Its effects in psoriatic erythroderma are also impressive. Psoriatic arthritis may also improve significantly. Side effects include dry lips, skin, and nasal mucosa; hair loss; and skin fragility. Triglycerides can be elevated. Remission averages 8 weeks, and maintenance therapy is required, usually 20 to 60 mg/day.

Acitretin was found by Gollnick to be as effective as etretinate and has replaced it. It has a very much shorter half-life in the body. Acitretin is teratogenic, and women of child-bearing years are strongly advised to avoid pregnancy for up to 3 years following cessation of therapy. Alcohol ingestion is strongly discouraged in women of child-bearing potential on Acitretin.

DAPSONE. Dapsone use is limited largely to palmoplantar pustulosis.

Combination Therapy. In more severe forms of psoriasis a combination of treatment modalities may be employed. In treating patients with methotrexate, for example, concomitant topical steroids may be used to minimize the dose. Good results with methotrexate and PUVA have been obtained, but the risk of developing squamous cell carcinomas limits this regimen. Methotrexate with etretinate (Acitretin) has been very effective in managing patients with severe, generalized pustular psoriasis. Combination systemic therapy should be used with caution because the potential complication rates are a function of the agents used. Experience with each treatment modality is imperative. Concomitant cyclosporine and methotrexate use, even for a short term, is not recommended.

Combination therapy offers enhanced efficacy with reduced individual drug toxicity, and multiple combinations have been studied. PUVA with Acitretin (etretinate), PUVA and cyclosporine, and PUVA and methotrexate have been used with good results. The use of PUVA and retinoids is called Re-PUVA. Likewise, cyclosporine and Acitretin have shown promise in treating severe, recalcitrant disease; however, this combination may cause additive hyperlipidemia. Cyclosporine and sulfasalazine may result in nephrotoxicity. Topical calcipotriene ointment (Dovonex) has been used in combination with Acitretin, cyclosporine, methotrexate, and phototherapy, demonstrating enhanced efficacy while improving the risk/benefit ratio. The principle behind combination therapy is the use of agents in which the side effects profile is different or partly opposing.

Hydroxyurea and sulfasalazine have been used in severe cases and in combination with other modalities, such as PUVA. Hydroxyurea can cause pain in psoriatic lesions or psoriatic flares during administration of phototherapy. Sulfasalazine can result in photosensitivity and should be used with caution with phototherapy. These agents are usually adjunctive to other methods to which the patient is only partially responding, such as phototherapy.

Combined agents are particularly useful in topical therapy, where the risk profiles are considerably less. Calcipotriene together with superpotent steroids can result in greater improvement and fewer long-term side effects. Similar results have been seen when tazarotene is used with topical steroids.

Alora MB, et al: CO_2 laser resurfacing of psoriatic plaques. *Lasers Surg Med* 1998, 22:165.

Asadullah K, et al: Interleukin 10 treatment of psoriasis. *Arch Dermatol* 1999, 135:187.

Boer J, et al: Comparison of phototherapy (UV-B) and photochemotherapy (PUVA) for clearing and maintenance therapy of psoriasis. *Arch Dermatol* 1984, 120:52.

Boffa MJ, et al: Methotrexate for psoriasis. *Clin Exp Dermatol* 1996, 21:399.

Brechtel B, et al: Combination of etretinate with cyclosporine in the treatment of severe recalcitrant psoriasis. *J Am Acad Dermatol* 1994, 30:1023.

Breuer-McHam J, et al: Alterations in HIV expression in AIDS patients with psoriasis or pruritus treated with phototherapy. *J Am Acad Dermatol* 1999, 40:48.

Chouela E, et al: Hepatitis C virus antibody (anti-HCV): prevalence in psoriasis. *Int J Dermatol* 1996, 35:797.

Coven TR, et al: Narrowband UVB produces superior clinical and histopathological resolution of moderate-to-severe psoriasis in patients compared with broadband UVB. *Arch Dermatol* 1997, 133:1514.

Cuellar ML, et al: Management of spondyloarthropathies. *Curr Opin Rheumatol* 1996, 8:288.

de Berker DA, et al: Comparison of psoralen-UVB and psoralen-UVA photochemotherapy in the treatment of psoriasis. *J Am Acad Dermatol* 1997, 36:577.

Demitsu T, et al: Acute generalized exanthematous pustulosis induced by dexamethasone injection. *Dermatology* 1996, 193:56.

Duvic M, et al: AIDS-associated psoriasis and Reiter's syndrome. *Arch Dermatol* 1988, 123:1622.

Duvic M, et al: Molecular mechanisms of tazarotene action in psoriasis. *J Am Acad Dermatol* 1997, 37:S18.

Eells LD, et al: Comparison of euerythemogenic and maximally aggressive ultraviolet therapy for psoriasis. *J Am Acad Dermatol* 1984, 11:105.

Enlund F, et al: Analysis of three suggested psoriasis susceptibility loci in a large Swedish set of families: confirmation of linkage to chromosome 6 (HLA region), and to 17q, but not to 4q. *Hum Hered* 1999, 49:2.

Farber EM, et al: Psoriasis: questionnaire survey of 2,144 patients. *Arch Dermatol* 1968, 98:248.

Feliu J, et al: Worsening psoriasis after treatment with G-CSF in a patient with small-cell lung cancer. *J Natl Cancer Inst* 1997, 89:1315.

Fleischer AB Jr, et al: Alternative therapies commonly used within a population of patients with psoriasis. *Cutis* 1996, 58:216.

Friedman SJ: Management of psoriasis with a hydrocolloid dressing. *Arch Dermatol* 1987, 123:1046.

Gold MH, et al: Beta blockers and psoriasis. *J Am Acad Dermatol* 1988, 19:458.

Gollnick H: Oral retinoids: efficacy and toxicity in psoriasis. *Br J Dermatol* 1996, 135:6.

Grimble RF, et al: Modulation of pro-inflammatory cytokine biology by unsaturated fatty acids. *Z Ernahrungswiss* 1998, 37(Suppl):57.

Gupta AK, et al: Woronoff ring during anthralin therapy for psoriasis. *Arch Dermatol* 1986, 122:248.

Gupta AK, et al: Cutaneous adverse effects associated with terbinafine therapy: 10 case reports and a review of the literature. *Br J Dermatol* 1998, 138:529.

Gupta AK, et al: The Psoriasis Life Stress Inventory: a preliminary index of psoriasis-related stress. *Acta Derm Venereol* 1995, 75:240.

Guzzo C: Recent advances in the treatment of psoriasis. *Dermatol Clin* 1997, 15:59.

Harvima RJ, et al: Association of psychic stress with clinical severity and symptoms of psoriatic patients. *Acta Derm Venereol* 1996, 76:467.

Hecker D, et al: Topical calcipotriene in combination with UVB phototherapy for psoriasis. *Int J Dermatol* 1997, 36:302.

Heng MCY, et al: Beta-adrenoceptor-antagonist-induced psoriasiform eruption. *Int J Dermatol* 1988, 27:619.

Henseler T: The genetics of psoriasis. *J Am Acad Dermatol* 1997, 37:S1.

Hietanen J, et al: Study of oral mucosa in 200 consecutive patients with psoriasis. *Scand J Dent Res* 1984, 92:50.

Horwitz SN: Addition of topically applied corticosteroid to a modified Goeckerman regimen. *J Am Acad Dermatol* 1985, 13:784.

Hubler WR Jr: Familial juvenile generalized pustular psoriasis. *Arch Dermatol* 1984, 120:1174.

Hubler WR Jr: Lingual lesions of generalized pustular psoriasis. *J Am Acad Dermatol* 1984, 11:1069.

Jenisch S, et al: Linkage disequilibrium analysis of familial psoriasis: identification of multiple disease-associated MHC haplotypes. *Tissue Antigens* 1999, 53:135.

Kanazawa K, et al: Hepatitis C virus infection in patients with psoriasis. *Arch Dermatol* 1996, 132:1391.

Katz HI: Combination topical calcipotriene ointment 0.005% and various systemic therapies in the treatment of plaque-type psoriasis vulgaris. *J Am Acad Dermatol* 1997, 37:S62.

Kavanagh GM, et al: Effects of dithranol on neutrophil superoxide generation in patients with psoriasis. *Br J Dermatol* 1996, 134:234.

Keddy-Grant J, et al: Complications of microwave hyperthermia treatment of psoriasis. *J Am Acad Dermatol* 1990, 22:651.

Kiil J, et al: Surgical treatment of psoriasis. *Lancet* 1985, 2:116.

Kitamura K, et al: Cutaneous reactions induced by calcium channel blocker. *J Dermatol* 1993, 20:279.

Lanse SB, et al: Low incidence of hepatotoxicity associated with long-term, low-dose oral methotrexate in treatment of refractory psoriasis, psoriatic arthritis, and rheumatoid arthritis: an acceptable risk-benefit ratio. *Dig Dis Sci* 1985, 30:104.

Lassus A, et al: The effect of etretinate compared with different regimens of PUVA in treatment of persistent palmoplantar pustulosis. *Br J Dermatol* 1985, 112:455.

Lauharanta J, et al: A double-blind comparison of Acitretin and etretinate in combination with bath PUVA in the treatment of psoriasis. *Br J Dermatol* 1989, 121:107.

Lebwohl M: The role of salicylic acid in the treatment of psoriasis. *Int J Dermatol* 1999, 38:16.

Lebwohl M: Topical application of calcipotriene and corticosteroids: combination regimens. *J Am Acad Dermatol* 1997, 37:S55.

Lee RE, et al: Interleukin-2 and psoriasis. *Arch Dermatol* 1988, 124:1811.

Leung DY, et al: The role of superantigens in skin disease. *J Invest Dermatol* 1995, 105:37S.

Lowe NJ, et al: Long-term low-dose cyclosporine therapy for severe psoriasis. *J Am Acad Dermatol* 1996, 35:710.

Marks R: Surgery for psoriasis (letter). *Lancet* 1985, 2:335.

Mayser P, et al: Omega-3 fatty acid-based lipid infusion in patients with chronic plaque psoriasis. *J Am Acad Dermatol* 1998, 38:539.

Melski JW: The Koebner (isomorphic) response in psoriasis. *Arch Dermatol* 1983, 119:655.

Menter MA, et al: The Goeckerman regimen in two psoriasis day-care centers. *J Am Acad Dermatol* 1983, 9:59.

Morimoto S, et al: Psoriasis and vitamin D_3. *Arch Dermatol* 1989, 125:231.

Morison WL, et al: Combined methotrexate-PUVA therapy in the treatment of psoriasis. *J Am Acad Dermatol* 1982, 6:46.

Mrowietz U, et al: Anthralin (dithranol) in vitro inhibits human monocytes to secrete IL-6, IL-8, and TNF-alpha, but not IL-1. *Br J Dermatol* 1997, 136:542.

Nevitt GJ, et al: Psoriasis in the community: severity and patients' beliefs and attitudes towards the disease. *Br J Dermatol* 1996, 135:533.

Nikaein A, et al: Characterization of T-cell clones generated from skin of patients with psoriasis. *J Am Acad Dermatol* 1993, 28:551.

Oakley AM, et al: A review of ultraviolet treatment for psoriasis at Waikato Hospital. *Australas J Dermatol* 1996, 37:132.

Orenberg EK, et al: Response of chronic psoriatic plaques to localized heating induced by ultrasound. *Arch Dermatol* 1980, 116:893.

Ortonne JP: Aetiology and pathogenesis of psoriasis. *Br J Dermatol* 1996, 135(Suppl):1.

Park BS, et al: Factors influencing psoriasis. *J Dermatol* 1998, 25:97.

Parrish JA, et al: Photochemotherapy of psoriasis with oral methoxalen and long-wave UVL. *N Engl J Med* 1974, 291:1207.

Pearlman DL, et al: Paper-tape occlusion of anthralin paste. *Arch Dermatol* 1984, 120:625.

Pearlman DL, et al: Weekly psoriasis therapy using fluorouracil. *J Am Acad Dermatol* 1987, 17:78.

Petzelbauer P, et al: Cyclosporin A in combination with photochemotherapy (PUVA) in the treatment of psoriasis. *Br J Dermatol* 1990, 123:641.

Poulin YP: Tazarotene 0.1% gel in combination with mometasone furoate cream in plaque psoriasis. *Cutis* 1999, 63:41.

Powles AV, et al: Renal function after 10 years' treatment with cyclosporine for psoriasis. *Br J Dermatol* 1998, 138:443.

Proksch E: Antilipemid drug-induced skin manifestations. *Hautarzt* 1995, 46:76.

Ramsay CA: Management of psoriasis with calcipotriol used as monotherapy. *J Am Acad Dermatol* 1997, 37:S53.

Roenigk HH Jr, et al: Methotrexate in psoriasis: consensus conference. *J Am Acad Dermatol* 1998, 38:478.

Roenigk HH Jr, et al: Serial liver biopsies in psoriatic patients receiving long-term etretinate. *Br J Dermatol* 1985, 112:77.

Rosenberg EW, et al: Koebner phenomenon and the microbial basis of psoriasis. *Arch Dermatol* 1987, 123:151.

Rosenberg EW, et al: Microbial factors in psoriasis (letter). *Arch Dermatol* 1982, 118:143.

Ruzicka T: Psoriatic arthritis. *Arch Dermatol* 1996, 132:215.

Sadeh JS, et al: Pustular and erythrodermic psoriasis complicated by acute respiratory distress syndrome. *Arch Dermatol* 1997, 133:747.

Shore RN: Clearing psoriasis lesions under tape. *N Engl J Med* 1985, 312:246.

Shupack J, et al: Cyclosporine as maintenance therapy in patients with severe psoriasis. *J Am Acad Dermatol* 1997, 36:423.

Silverman A, et al: Tars and anthralins. *Dermatol Clin* 1995, 13:817.

Skinner RB, et al: Antimicrobial treatment of psoriasis. *Dermatol Clin* 1995, 13:909.

Steck WD: Contribution of topical tar oil to UVB phototherapy of psoriasis. *J Am Acad Dermatol* 1986, 14:742.

Steck WD: Nonmelanoma skin cancer after PUVA. *J Invest Dermatol* 1988, 91:120.

Steck WD: The effect of continued UVB therapy on the duration of remission of psoriasis. *J Am Acad Dermatol* 1986, 115:546.

Stern RS, et al: Malignant melanoma in patients treated for psoriasis with methoxsalen (psoralen) and ultraviolet A radiation (PUVA): the PUVA follow-up study. *N Engl J Med* 1997, 336:1090.

Stern RS, et al: The safety of etretinate as long-term therapy for psoriasis. *J Am Acad Dermatol* 1995, 33:44.

Streit V, et al: Treatment of psoriasis with polyethylene sheet bath PUVA. *J Am Acad Dermatol* 1996, 35:208.

Studniberg HM, et al: PUVA, UVB, and nonmelanoma skin cancer. *J Am Acad Dermatol* 1993, 29:1013.

Taglione E, et al: Hepatitis C virus infection: prevalence in psoriasis and psoriatic arthritis. *J Rheumatol* 1999, 26:370.

Takematsu H, et al: Juvenile generalized pustular psoriasis in a pair of monozygotic twins presenting strikingly similar clinical courses. *Acta Derm Venereol* (Stockh) 1992, 72:443.

Urabe H, et al: Hyperthermia in the treatment of psoriasis. *Arch Dermatol* 1981, 117:770.

Van de Kerkhof PC, et al: Tacalcitol ointment in the treatment of psoriasis vulgaris. *Br J Dermatol* 1996, 135:758.

Van der Vleuten CJ, et al: A novel dithranol formulation (Micanol). *Acta Derm Venereol* 1996, 76:387.

Webster GF, et al: Cutaneous ulcerations and pustular psoriasis flare caused by recombinant interferon beta injections in patients with multiple sclerosis. *J Am Acad Dermatol* 1996, 34:365.

Weinstein GD: Tazarotene gel. *J Am Acad Dermatol* 1997, 37:S33.

Weinstein GD, et al: Cytotoxic and immunologic effects of methotrexate in psoriasis. *J Invest Dermatol* 1990, 95:49S.

White SW: Palmoplantar pustular psoriasis provoked by lithium therapy. *J Am Acad Dermatol* 1982, 7:660.

Wolfer LU, et al: Interferon-alpha-induced psoriasis vulgaris. *Hautarzt* 1996, 47:124.

Wolska H, et al: Etretinate in severe psoriasis. *J Am Acad Dermatol* 1983, 9:883.

Wong KC, et al: Low dose cyclosporin A and methotrexate in the treatment of psoriasis. *Acta Derm Venereol* 1999, 79:87.

Yamamoto T, et al: Psoriasis and hepatitis C virus. *Acta Derm Venereol* 1995, 75:482.

Zachariae H: Renal toxicity of long-term cyclosporin. *Scand J Rheumatol* 1999, 28:65.

Zelickson BD, et al: Clinical and histologic evaluation of psoriatic plaques treated with a flashlamp pulsed dye laser. *J Am Acad Dermatol* 1996, 35:64.

Ziboh VA: Implication of dietary aids and polyunsaturated fatty acids in management of cutaneous disorders. *Arch Dermatol* 1989, 125:241. ▲

REITER'S SYNDROME

Reiter's syndrome is a characteristic clinical triad consisting of urethritis, conjunctivitis, and arthritis. There may also be other features that involve the skin, mucous membranes, gastrointestinal tract, and cardiovascular system. Realizing that few patients present with the classic triad, the American Rheumatism Association adopted criterion of peripheral arthritis of more than 1 month's duration in association with urethritis and/or cervicitis. The disease occurs chiefly in young men of HLA-B27 genotype, although it may also occur in children and older men, but rarely in women.

Clinical Features

Any one of the triad of urethritis, conjunctivitis, or arthritis may occur first, accompanied by fever, weakness, and weight loss. A nonbacterial urethritis may develop with painful and bloody urination and pyuria. Cystitis, prostatitis, and seminal vesiculitis may be accompaniments. About a third of the patients develop conjunctivitis, which may be bulbar, tarsal, or angular. Keratitis is usually superficial and extremely painful and may lead to corneal ulceration. Iritis is common, especially in recurrent cases. Infrequently optic neuritis may occur. An asymmetric arthritis afflicts synovial joints, especially those that are weight-bearing. Its onset is sudden, with heat, tenderness, and swelling, with a predilection for the knees, ankles, foot joints, and wrists. Pain in one or both heels is a frequent symptom. Sacroiliitis may develop in up to two thirds of patients, most of whom are of HLA-B27 type.

The skin lesions start as multiple, small, yellowish vesicles that break, become confluent, and form superficial erosions. They develop frequently on the genitals and palms. Eruption on the glans penis occurs in 25% of patients. Those on the soles are different; they start as pustules, which become very crusted or hyperkeratotic and are suggestive of rupial psoriasis (Fig. 10-26). These are painless, occur approximately 1 month after the urethritis, and are present in about 10% of patients. The eruption is known as *keratoderma blennorrhagicum* (Fig. 10-27). The lesions may ulcerate.

The penile lesions, which are frequent, are characterized by perimeatal balanitis, which becomes crusted and forms circinate lesions. Similar lesions are present in the vaginal mucosa of affected women. The buccal, palatal, and lingual mucosa may show painless, shallow, red erosions, and severe stomatitis may ensue. The nails become thick and brittle, and heavy keratotic deposits develop under them (subungual keratosis) not unlike those seen in severe nail involvement of psoriasis (Fig. 10-28).

There is usually a thick, dry, horny crusting about the toes that spreads over the soles. This is the result of coalescence of the individual crusted lesions, so that the new plaques have the appearance of a relief map. Ultimately, the crusts and horny masses become detached and are shed, often leaving residual pigmentation.

Endocarditis, pericarditis, and myocarditis, as well as aortic insufficiency, occur in some patients. Coronary artery stenosis and cardiac conduction defects have also been shown.

In children conjunctivitis is the most frequent complaint, and young children are much more likely to have the postdysenteric form of Reiter's syndrome than the posturethritic form seen in adults. Arthritis is often the most prominent physical sign involving the large, weight-bearing joints of the lower extremity.

Etiology

Reiter's syndrome has been attributed to many different agents such as *Shigella flexneri, Salmonella* spp., *Yersinia*

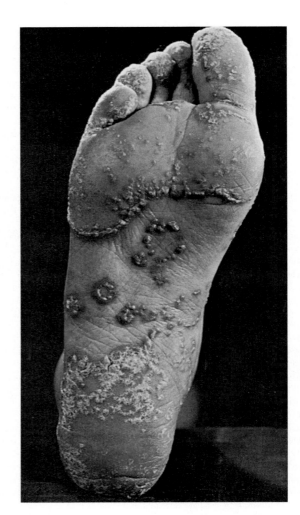

Fig. 10-26 Reiter's syndrome. Note resemblance to volar psoriasis. (Courtesy Dr. H. Shatin.)

spp., *Ureaplasma urealyticum, Borrelia burgdorferi, Cryptosporidia,* and *Campylobacter fetus,* which may be responsible for the infectious enteritis that precedes onset in a small percentage of patients (Fig. 10-29). Reiter's syndrome has also been observed in HIV disease, but it is unknown if the virus itself produces the susceptibility, causes the disease, or is unrelated. In cases that follow infection of the genitourinary tract, *Chlamydia trachomatis* may be associated. The exact causative role of these or other infectious agents is still unclear.

Immunologically mediated tissue injury in a genetically predisposed patient is believed to be important. HLA-B27 positivity is present in 80% of cases of Reiter's syndrome, rising to 90% to 100% in patients with accompanying sacroiliitis, uveitis, or aortitis. Because of this, some have linked psoriasis (pustular and spondylitic arthritis forms) and ankylosing spondylitis to Reiter's disease. The relationship of these disorders to one another is still unclear.

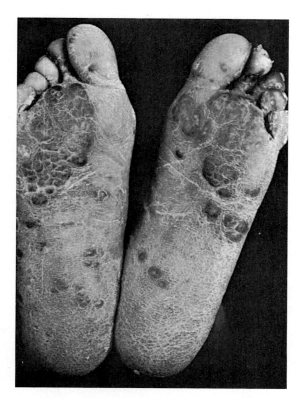

Fig. 10-27 Keratoderma blennorrhagicum. (Courtesy Dr. H. Shatin.)

Psoriasis and Reiter's disease may be caused by abnormalities in the production and elicitation of immune mediators or T cells. Further proof for the involvement of cytokines is that, like in psoriasis, treatments with interferon have been reported to induce Reiter's syndrome. Other immune-modulating agents, such as bacille Calmette-Guérin (BCG) and hepatitis B vaccines, have also been implicated. It has been suggested that an amino acid sequence within the HLA-B27 molecule allows microbial peptides to bind and be presented to T cells (CD8).

Laboratory Findings

No specific changes are characteristic of this syndrome. A leukocytosis of 10,000 to 20,000/mm^3 and elevated sedimentation rate, depending on the severity of the disease, are the most consistent findings. There is no specific test for Reiter's syndrome.

Histopathology

The histopathology of Reiter's is identical to psoriasis.

Differential Diagnosis

Reiter's disease may be confused with rheumatoid arthritis, ankylosing spondylitis, gout, psoriatic arthritis, gonococcal arthritis, acute rheumatic fever, chronic mucocutaneous candidiasis, and serum sickness. Edwards et al reported a woman with vulvar Reiter's syndrome that was mistakenly treated for mucocutaneous candidiasis for 4 years.

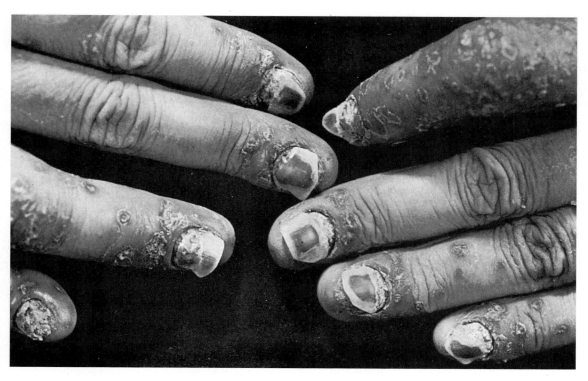

Fig. 10-28 Reiter's syndrome. (Courtesy Dr. H. Shatin.)

Treatment

Usually the mucocutaneous lesions are self limited and clear within a few months. Topical steroids are helpful. For the joint disease, rest and nonsteroidal antiinflammatory agents should be used first. Methotrexate, 7.5 to 20 mg/week, may be tried in patients with severe, refractory joint disease. Acitretin may be used in treating HIV-infected persons with Reiter's. Cyclosporine therapy has also been shown to be effective in treating severe recurrent disease. Once the acute arthritis is controlled it is important to begin physical therapy to maintain joint mobility.

The course of Reiter's disease is characterized by exacerbations and remission in about one third of patients. A chronic deforming arthritis occurs in about 20% of patients, with significant disability resulting, chiefly from foot deformities.

Altman EM: AIDS-associated Reiter's syndrome. *Ann Allergy* 1994, 72:307.
Blanche P: Acitretin and AIDS-related Reiter's disease. *Clin Exp Rheumatol* 1999, 17:105.

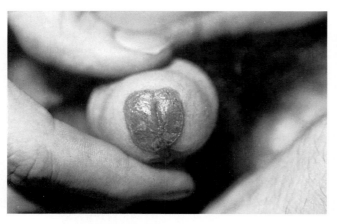

Fig. 10-29 Reiter's syndrome: balanitis.

Cleveland MG, et al: Incomplete Reiter's syndrome induced by systemic interferon alpha treatment. *J Am Acad Dermatol* 1993, 29:788.
Cron RQ, et al: Reiter's syndrome associated with cryptosporidial gastroenteritis. *J Rheumatol* 1995, 22:1962.
Deer T, et al: Cardiac conduction manifestations of Reiter's syndrome. *South Med J* 1991, 84:799.
Edwards L, et al: Reiter's syndrome of the vulva. *Arch Dermatol* 1992, 128:811.
Fraser PA, et al: Reiter's syndrome attributed to hepatitis B immunization. *BMJ* 1994, 309:94.
Hoogland YT, et al: Coronary artery stenosis in Reiter's syndrome. *J Rheumatol* 1994, 21:757.
Huff R, et al: Penile erythematous eruption in a man with diabetes. *Arch Dermatol* 1999, 135:845.
Kiyohara A, et al: Successful treatment of severe recurrent Reiter's syndrome with cyclosporine. *J Am Acad Dermatol* 1997, 36:482.
Miller KA, et al: Family studies with HLA typing in Reiter's syndrome. *Am J Med* 1981, 70:1210.
Rothe MJ, et al: Reiter syndrome. *Int J Dermatol* 1991, 30:173.

SUBCORNEAL PUSTULAR DERMATOSIS (SNEDDON-WILKINSON DISEASE)

Sneddon and Wilkinson in 1956 described this chronic pustular disease, which occurs chiefly in middle-aged women. The pustules are as superficial as those of impetigo and are arranged in annular and serpiginous patterns, especially on the abdomen, axillae, and groins (Fig. 10-30). Sometimes vesicles are present, but these usually change into pustular blebs. Cultures from the pustules are sterile. Oral lesions are rare. Some cases occur in association with an IgA (or infrequently another) monoclonal gammopathy.

Histologically, the pustules form below the stratum corneum, as in impetigo and in pemphigus foliaceus. Acantholysis is absent. The cavity contains many neutrophils. Spongiosis occurs subjacent to the blister, and a perivascular mantle composed of neutrophils and some eosinophils is present in the upper dermis. The histologic differential diagnosis includes pustular psoriasis, subcorneal pustular dermatosis, intraepidermal neutrophilic IgA derma-

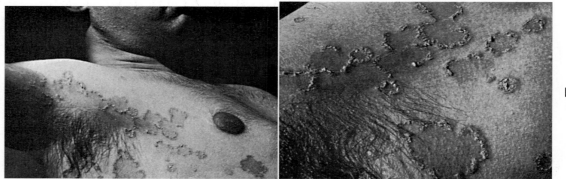

Fig. 10-30 **A,** Subcorneal pustular dermatosis of Sneddon and Wilkinson. Note peripheral pustulation of lesions. **B,** Close view. (Courtesy Dr. A. Kaminsky.)

tosis, and superficial fungal and bacterial infections. Some cases will show upper epidermal intercellular IgA staining.

IgA pemphigus showing IgA antikeratinocyte cell surface autoantibodies is divided into subcorneal pustular dermatosis and intraepidermal neutrophilic IgA dermatosis types. Using immunoblotting techniques, Hashimoto et al have shown that human desmocollin 1 is an autoantigen for the subcorneal pustular dermatosis type of IgA pemphigus.

Dapsone, 50 to 200 mg daily, appears to be effective in most cases; however, some patients have responded better to sulfapyridine therapy. Acitretin has been helpful in several cases. Narrowband UVB phototherapy may also be effective. Corticosteroids, colchicine, and tetracycline with niacinamide are all possible treatment considerations. Without treatment this is a chronic condition with remissions of variable duration.

Atukorala DN, et al: Subcorneal pustular dermatosis and IgA myeloma. *Dermatology* (Basel) 1993, 187:124.

Boyd AS, et al: Vesiculopustules of the thigh and abdomen. *Arch Dermatol* 1991, 127:1571.

Cameron H, et al: Subcorneal pustular dermatosis (Sneddon-Wilkinson disease) treated with narrowband (TL-01) UVB. *Br J Dermatol* 1997, 137:150.

Hashimoto T, et al: Human desmocollin 1 is an autoantigen for subcorneal pustular dermatosis type of IgA pemphigus. *J Invest Dermatol* 1997, 109:127.

Hashimoto T, et al: Intercellular IgA dermatosis with clinical features of subcorneal pustular dermatosis. *Arch Dermatol* 1987, 123:1062.

Kasha EE, et al: Subcorneal pustular dermatosis (Sneddon-Wilkinson disease) in association with a monoclonal gammopathy. *J Am Acad Dermatol* 1988, 19:854.

Kohl PK, et al: Pyoderma gangrenosum followed by subcorneal pustular dermatosis in a patient with IgA paraproteinemia. *J Am Acad Dermatol* 1991, 24:325. _____ ▲

EOSINOPHILIC PUSTULAR FOLLICULITIS

Eosinophilic pustular folliculitis (EPF) was first described in 1970 by Ofuji but is also referred to as *sterile eosinophilic pustulosis*. It occurs in males five times more commonly than in females and has its peak age of onset in the third decade, although a number of pediatric cases have been reported. It is characterized by pruritic, follicular papulopustules that measure 1 to 2 mm. The lesions tend to be grouped; plaques may form. New lesions may form at the edges of the plaques, leading to peripheral extension, while central clearing takes place. Distribution is usually asymmetrical, with the face, trunk, and upper extremities most often afflicted. Twenty percent have palmoplantar pustules. The condition is to be distinguished from HIV-associated EF, which presents in a different manner, and will be discussed in HIV-associated dermatoses (Chapter 19).

Histologically, there is spongiosis and vesiculation of the follicular infundibula, with infiltration with eosinophils. There is a peripheral eosinophilia in half the cases. The cause is unknown; however, numerous studies have implicated chemotactic substances, ICAM-1, and cyclooxygenase-generated metabolites. Indomethacin treatment of three patients by Teraki et al demonstrated increased interferon gamma, which correlated with an improved clinical status, suggesting that indomethacin may provide remission by altering cytokine production.

The typical course is one of spontaneous remissions and exacerbations lasting from a few months to several years. Dapsone or systemic steroids are the treatments of choice. Others have described success with intralesional steroids, clofazimine, minocycline, isotretinoin, UVB therapy, indomethacin, colchicine, cyclosporine, and cetirizine. Itraconazole, reported to be effective in HIV-associated EF, may be tried.

Lucky et al described another variant, which occurs in early childhood. These patients develop sterile pustules and papules preferentially over the scalp; however, scattered clusters of pustules may occur over the trunk and extremities. Leukocytosis and eosinophilia are often present. High-potency topical steroids are the treatment of choice. Recurrent exacerbations and remissions usually occur with spontaneous resolution.

Blume-Peytavi U, et al: Eosinophilic pustular folliculitis (Ofuji's disease). *J Am Acad Dermatol* 1997, 37:259.

Darmstadt GL, et al: Eosinophilic pustular folliculitis. *Pediatrics* 1992, 89:1095.

Giard F, et al: Eosinophilic pustular folliculitis (Ofuji disease) in childhood: a review of four cases. *Pediatr Dermatol* 1991, 8:189.

Larralde M, et al: Eosinophilic pustular folliculitis in infancy: report of two new cases. *Pediatr Dermatol* 1999, 16:118.

Lucky AW, et al: Eosinophilic pustular folliculitis in infancy. *Pediatr Dermatol* 1984, 1:202.

Moritz DL, et al: Eosinophilic pustular dermatosis. *J Am Acad Dermatol* 1991, 24:903.

Steffen CS: Eosinophilic pustular folliculitis (Ofuji's disease) with response to dapsone therapy. *Arch Dermatol* 1985, 121:921.

Taieb A, et al: Eosinophilic pustulosis of the scalp in childhood. *J Am Acad Dermatol* 1992, 27:55.

Takematsu H, et al: Eosinophilic pustular folliculitis. *Arch Dermatol* 1985, 121:917.

Teraki Y, et al: Ofuji's disease and cytokines. *Dermatology* 1996, 192:16.

Veraldi S, et al: Evidence of retroviral involvement in an Italian patient with Ofuji's disease. *Dermatology* 1999, 198:86. _____ ▲

RECALCITRANT PALMOPLANTAR ERUPTIONS

Recalcitrant pustular eruptions of the hands and feet are often examples of psoriasis, and a search for lesions elsewhere (e.g., scalp, ears, nails, glans penis) or for a positive family history will many times confirm this suspicion.

Dermatitis Repens

Dermatitis repens, also known as *acrodermatitis continua* and *acrodermatitis perstans,* is a chronic inflammatory disease of the hands and feet (Fig. 10-31). It usually involves the extremities but in rare cases may become generalized. The disease usually begins distally on a digit, either as a pustule or as a paronychia. Thus, at the beginning it is unilateral and localized. At the edge of the pustules the epidermis is cast off, leaving a red surface, from which a clear or slightly turbid fluid oozes. An irregular ring of loose, sodden epidermis remains about the denuded areas. Extension takes place by the further detachment of the epidermis as the result of continued exudation, or there may be fresh pustules just beyond the border, which break down and add another denuded area to the original adjacent one. Crusted, eczematoid, and psoriasiform lesions may be observed, and there may be moderate itching. The disease is essentially unilateral in its beginning and asymmetrical throughout its entire course. Although new foci may thus be formed locally, the disease seldom becomes generalized or spreads to distant parts.

The involved areas are the hands and feet and occasionally the mucous membranes, particularly of the mouth. The nails are often affected. As the disease progresses, one or more of the nails may become dystrophic or be destroyed. The lesions cause atrophy of the skin. Involvement of the mucous membranes may occur even when the eruption of the skin is localized. Painful, circular, white plaques surrounded by inflammatory areolae are found on the tongue and may form a diphtheritic membrane; fissures have been described.

Histologically, the primary lesion is found in the epidermis, where the intraepithelial spongiform pustule is formed by infiltration with vast numbers of polymorphonu-

clear leukocytes. This abscess dries up and is exfoliated together with the overlying parakeratotic horny layer.

The histologic changes are similar to those seen in psoriasis. Pustular psoriasis of Zumbusch, acrodermatitis continua (Hallopeau), and impetigo herpetiformis represent the same features. The characteristic spongiform pustule of Kogoj is present in all three diseases.

Numerous treatment options have been used to include sulfapyridine, topical mechlorethamine, topical steroids, PUVA, and fluorouracil. Treatment successes have also been obtained with Acitretin, low-dose cyclosporine, combination Acitretin and calcipotriol, and topical calcipotriol alone. Harland et al reported a case of recalcitrant acrodermatitis continua that was refractory to high-dose methotrexate but responded well to low-dose cyclosporine. The decision regarding which agent to use for treatment should take into consideration the severity of disease, age, and general physical well-being of the patient, and the patient's desires.

Palmoplantar Pustulosis (Pustular Psoriasis of the Extremities)

Pustular psoriasis of the extremities, in contradistinction to dermatitis repens, is essentially a bilateral and symmetrical dermatosis. The favorite locations are the thenar or hypothenar eminences or the central portion of the palms and soles (Figs. 10-32 and 10-33). The patches begin as erythematous areas in which minute intraepidermal pustules form. At the beginning these are pinhead-sized; then they may enlarge and coalesce to form small lakes of pus that are not at all or only slightly elevated above the skin surface

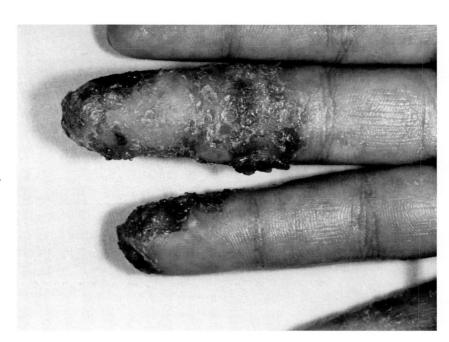

Fig. 10-31 Dermatitis repens.

(Fig. 10-34). As a rule these pustules do not rupture but in the course of a week or two tend to dry up, leaving punctate brown scabs that eventually are exfoliated (Fig. 10-35). Stages of quiescence and exacerbation characterize the condition. Medications, such as lithium, which aggravate psoriasis, have also been reported to induce palmoplantar pustular psoriasis. Before the brown scabs of preceding

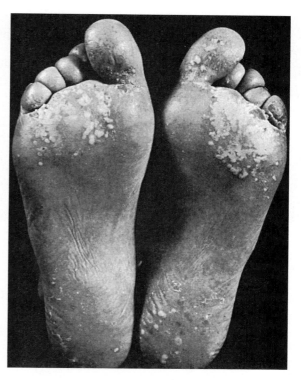

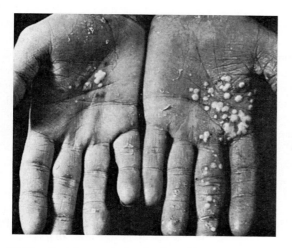

Fig. 10-32 Pustular psoriasis of palms. (Courtesy Dr. H. Shatin.)

Fig. 10-33 Pustular psoriasis of soles. (Courtesy Dr. H. Shatin.)

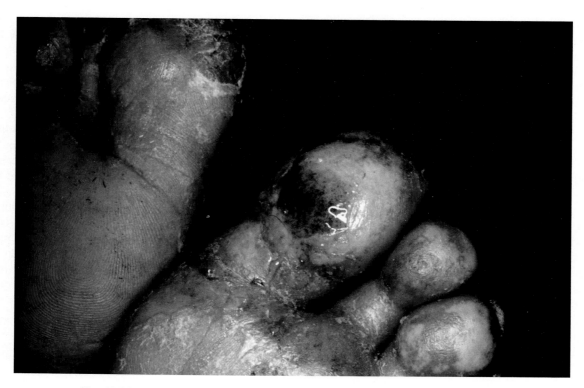

Fig. 10-34 "Lakes of pus" on plantar surfaces of toes in patient with pustular psoriasis.

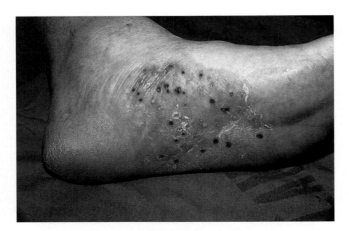

Fig. 10-35 Pustular psoriasis of soles.

lesions are gone, crops of fresh pustules often appear either within the scaly patch or beyond its edge.

Through the repetition of these attacks, in the course of time a patch is produced that is deeply erythematous and markedly exfoliative and in which the pustules are more evident at the edges but also are observed throughout. The scales are large and tenacious, usually being adherent at one edge so that it is difficult or impossible to pull them off without causing pain and bleeding.

The fully developed patches clinically resemble psoriasis. The nails are often affected, becoming malformed, ridged, stippled, pitted, and discolored. Both generalized eruptions of pustular psoriasis and pustular psoriasis limited to the hands and feet may be associated with typical psoriasis vulgaris. Indeed, some authors regard palmoplantar pustulosis as a form of psoriasis, while others consider it a separate disease entity because of (1) higher age at onset, (2) a female predominance, (3) lack of seasonal variation, (4) different histopathologic features, and (5) no increased frequency of psoriasis-linked alloantigens. A possible sixth feature is a unique form of arthrosteitis.

In 1968 Kato et al described the first case of bilateral clavicular osteomyelitis with palmar and plantar pustulosis. Sonozaki et al from Japan in 1974 subsequently described persistent palmoplantar pustulosis and seronegative rheumatoid syndrome, referred to as *sternoclavicular hyperostosis*. It manifests as pain and swelling of one or both sternoclavicular joints and often the sternomanubrial and upper costochondral junctions as well. There is shoulder, neck, and back pain, and limitation of motion of the shoulders and neck is common. Brachial plexus neuropathy and subclavian vein occlusion may occur. The lumbar spine and sacroiliac joints are usually spared. Chronic multifocal osteomyelitis in children may be a pediatric variant. Sternoclavicular hyperostosis is most likely the same disorder as the recently described SAPHO syndrome.

Since Kato's original description numerous investigators

have noted similar cases and referred to them by different names (sternoclavicular hyperostosis, arthrites pseudoseptiques et bacterides d'Andrews, arthrosteitis with pustulosis palmoplantaris, chronic recurrent multifocal osteomyelitis, and pustulotic arthrosteitis). Kahn et al noted that sterile arthrosteitis was the common denominator in a series of patients with chest wall pain or other musculoskeletal symptoms in the setting of palmoplantar pustulosis and/or acne fulminans. They coined the term *SAPHO syndrome,* which stands for *s*ynovitis, *a*cne, *p*ustulosis, *h*yperostosis, and *o*steitis. Others have described an association between palmoplantar pustulosis and osteoarthritis. Costner et al point out that it is not osteoarthritis, but more correctly referred to as arthrosteitis. Torii et al reported 84 Japanese patients with palmoplantar pustulosis and associated arthrosteitis involving the knees, spine, ankles, and the anterior aspect of the chest wall. There was no identifiable HLA alloantigen pattern. The authors believe this disorder is unique, with joint involvement that is distinct from psoriatic arthritis and ankylosing spondylitis.

It is clear that these authors have been writing about the same disease, which should be considered to be a form of palmoplantar pustulosis, a defining feature of the SAPHO syndrome. Kahn et al reported a case of SAPHO syndrome that developed 20 years after the cutaneous lesions. With such a latent onset as a possibility, any patient with palmoplantar pustulosis may be predisposed to joint disease.

Palmoplantar pustulosis has also been associated with thyroid disorders and cigarette smoking.

The disease is resistant to most treatments. Acitretin is reported to be extremely effective, in a dose of 1 mg/kg/day, although rebound may occur. Low-dose cyclosporine in doses ranging from 1.25 mg/kg/day to 3.75 mg/kg/day has also been very effective. Intramuscular Kenalog, 40 to 60 mg, may be useful for short-term relief. Oral 8-methoxypsoralen and high-intensity UVA irradiation is effective and is superior to topical psoralen applications followed by UVA light. Occlusive polyethylene gloves under which fluocinolone or another corticosteroid has been placed are also helpful; however, the beneficial effects are usually short lived. Colchicine has been used with success in some cases. The dose is 0.6 to 2.4 mg daily, reduced to 0.6 to 1.2 mg daily for maintenance. Nausea or diarrhea may occur. Itraconazole 100 mg/day for 2 weeks stopped new pustules in 7 patients treated by Mihara et al. Maintenance kept them clear, but recurrence developed after discontinuation.

Costner MI, et al: Osteoarthritis in 84 Japanese patients with palmoplantar pustulosis (letter). *J Am Acad Dermatol* 1995, 33:543.

Emtestam L, et al: Successful treatment for acrodermatitis continua of Hallopeau using topical calcipotriol. *Br J Dermatol* 1996, 135:644.

Harland CC, et al: Acrodermatitis continua responding to cyclosporin therapy. *Clin Exp Dermatol* 1992, 17:376.

Jurik AG, et al: Arthro-osteitis in pustulosis palmoplantaris. *J Am Acad Dermatol* 1988, 18:666.

Kahn MF, et al: SAPHO syndrome. *Rheum Dis Clin North Am* 1992, 1:225.

Kuijpers AL, et al: Acrodermatitis continua of Hallopeau: response to combined treatment with Acitretin and calcipotriol ointment. *J Am Acad Dermatol* 1996, 192:357.

Mihara M, et al: Itraconazole as a new treatment for pustulosis palmaris et plantaris. *Arch Dermatol* 1998, 134:639.

Miyagawa S, et al: Generalization of palmoplantar pustulosis after withdrawal of etretinate. *J Am Acad Dermatol* 1991, 24:305.

Reitamo S, et al: Cyclosporine in the treatment of palmoplantar pustulosis. *Arch Dermatol* 1993, 129:1273.

Rosen K, et al: PUVA, etretinate, and PUVA-etretinate for pustulosis palmoplantaris. *Arch Dermatol* 1987, 123:885.

Slawsky LD, et al: Successful treatment of acrodermatitis continua of Hallopeau with etretinate. *J Am Acad Dermatol* 1990, 23:1176.

Sonozaki H, et al: Four cases with symmetrical ossifications between the clavicles and first ribs of both sides. *Kanto J Orthop Trauma* 1974, 5:244.

Takigawa M, et al: Pustulosis palmaris et plantaris treated with oral colchicine. *Arch Dermatol* 1982, 118:458.

Torii H, et al: Osteoarthritis in 84 Japanese patients with palmoplantar pustulosis. *J Am Acad Dermatol* 1994, 31:732.

Tsuji T, et al: Topically administered fluorouracil in acrodermatitis continua of Hallopeau. *Arch Dermatol* 1991, 127:27. _____ ▲

Pustular Bacterid

Pustular bacterid was first described by George Andrews. It is characterized by a symmetric, grouped, vesicular or pustular eruption on the palms and soles marked by exacerbations and remissions over long periods. The basic lesions are pustules. At the beginning it is possible that they are vesicles that become rapidly purulent. Tiny hemorrhagic puncta intermingled with the pustules are frequently seen. When lesions are so numerous as to coalesce, they form a honeycomblike structure in the epidermis. The disease usually begins on the midportions of the palms or soles, from which it spreads outwardly until it may eventually cover the entire flexor aspects of the hands and feet. There has been no involvement of the webs of the fingers or toes, or in the flexion creases of the toes, as in tinea pedis.

When the eruption is fully developed, both palms and soles are completely covered, and the symmetry is pronounced. During fresh outbreaks, the white blood count may show a leukocytosis that ranges from 12,000 to 19,000/mm^3 with 65% to 80% of them polymorphonuclears. As a rule scaling is present and the scales are adherent, tough, and dry. During exacerbations, crops of pustules or vesicles make their appearance, and there is often severe itching of the areas and sometimes swelling, pain, and infiltration. From day to day fresh crops of lesions appear. Then the number of new lesions gradually diminishes, and the condition subsides to a quiescent stage. Andrews regarded the discovery of a remote focus of infection, and cure on its elimination, as crucial to the diagnosis.

The existence of this entity as a distinctive disease is questioned by many. The occasional observation of typical cases that respond to antibiotics or removal of a focus of

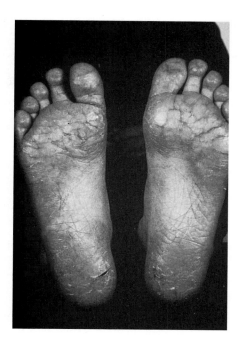

Fig. 10-36 Juvenile plantar dermatosis.

infection leads us to include this entity as a distinct disease. We suspect, however, that it is a variant of psoriasis triggered by infection.

Bacharach-Buhles M, et al: The pustular bacterid (Andrews): are there clinical criteria for differentiating from psoriasis pustulosa palmaris et plantaris? *Hautarzt* (Germany) 1993, 44:221. _____ ▲

Juvenile Plantar Dermatosis

This plantar disorder of children, first described by Enta and Moller in 1972, and named juvenile plantar dermatosis by Mackie in 1976, was reviewed by Ashton et al in 1985 in a study of 56 cases. It usually begins as a patchy, symmetrical, smooth, red, glazed macule on the great toes, sometimes with fissuring and desquamation (Fig. 10-36), in children aged 3 to 13. Toe webs are rarely involved; fingers may be. In a study by Svensson following patients over a 10-year period 52% with juvenile plantar dermatosis had atopic dermatitis and 26% developed hand eczema as adults, suggesting that patients with this disease may be more prone to eczematous difficulties as adults.

Histologically, there is psoriasiform acanthosis and a sparse, largely lymphocytic infiltrate in the upper dermis. Spongiosis is commonly present.

The diagnosis may be apparent on inspection, especially if there is a family or personal history of atopy and the toe webs are spared. Shoe dermatitis and dermatophytosis should be considered in the differential diagnosis. Patch testing should be seriously considered when entertaining the diagnosis of juvenile plantar dermatosis because patients with atopic dermatitis have been shown to be more sensitive to contact allergens.

Bed rest may be needed in the most severe cases. Cotton socks may be helpful. Topical steroids are of value as are urea preparations. Because repetitive drying and wetting plays a role (toxic shock syndrome), cotton socks and ointment protection may be helpful. Spontaneous clearing within 4 years of diagnosis is the rule.

Ashton RE, et al: Juvenile plantar dermatosis: a clinicopathologic study. *Arch Dermatol* 1985, 121:225.

Jones SK, et al: Juvenile plantar dermatosis. *Clin Exp Dermatol* 1987, 12:5.

Stables GI, et al: Patch testing in children. *Contact Dermatitis* 1996, 34:341.

Svensson A: Prognosis and atopic background of juvenile plantar dermatosis and gluteo-femoral eczema. *Acta Derm Venereol* 1988, 68:336. ▲

Infantile Acropustulosis

Jarratt and Ramsdell, and Kahn and Rywlin, in 1979, simultaneously described infantile acropustulosis (acropustulosis of infancy), an intensely itchy vesicopustular eruption of the hands and feet, beginning at any age up to 10 months, clearing in a few weeks, and recurring repeatedly until final subsidence at 6 to 36 months of age (Fig. 10-37). Dapsone at 2 mg/kg/day may be helpful. Potent topical steroids are reported to afford symptomatic relief.

The identification of pustular dermatosis during the first months of life may promote an extensive clinical evaluation to eliminate potentially serious infectious causes. Van Praag et al suggest a systematic approach to such patients consisting of (1) Tzanck prep, (2) Gram stain, and (3) potassium hydroxide preparations of the pustules as the most important quick diagnostic tests.

There is speculation that in some cases this condition may be a persistent reaction to prior scabies. Dromy et al reported on 25 children, noting that siblings were also afflicted, suggesting an infectious etiology. Humeau et al reported six immigrant children with the disease that had been recently treated for scabies. Infantile acropustulosis could be a hypersensitivity reaction to *Sarcoptes scabiei* in some cases.

Dromy R, et al: Infantile acropustulosis. *Pediatr Dermatol* 1991, 8:284.

Humeau S, et al: Infantile acropustulosis in six immigrant children. *Pediatr Dermatol* 1995, 12:275.

Van Praag MC, et al: Diagnosis and treatment of pustular disorders in the neonate. *Pediatr Dermatol* 1997, 14:131. ▲

Pompholyx (Dyshidrosis)

Clinical Features

Pompholyx (meaning *bubble*) is also known as *dyshidrosis* and was once called *cheiropompholyx*. It is a vesicular eruption of the palms and soles characterized by spongiotic intraepidermal vesicles, and often by burning or itching.

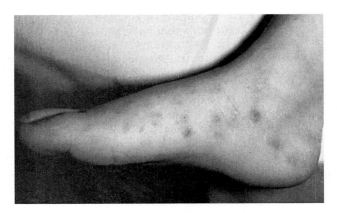

Fig. 10-37 Infantile acropustulosis.

Hyperhidrosis may be present. The application of the term *pompholyx* is at present limited to those typical eruptions that have small, deep-seated vesicles resembling tapioca occurring only on the palms, soles, and interdigits, accompanied by itching or burning, in which examination fails to reveal fungi or external chemical cause.

As a rule distribution of the lesions is bilateral and roughly symmetrical. Sometimes the vesicles are arranged in groups. By coalescence of several contiguous vesicles, bullae may be formed. The contents are clear and colorless but may later become straw-colored or purulent. Attacks generally last a few weeks, but, because of the tendency to relapse, the condition may persist for long periods. The lesions involute by drying up and desquamating rather than by rupturing.

Etiology

The literature emphasizes three major considerations: stress, atopy, and topical as well as ingested contactants. In 104 patients studied by Lodi et al, 50% were found to have familial and personal atopic diathesis compared with 11.5% of controls. Nickel was the most frequent patch-test positive agent at 20%. An additional 6% were positive to oral provocative tests for nickel. The authors found no correlation between age, sex, grading of pompholyx, and the allergologic parameters investigated. Veien et al found that a diet low in nickel provided long-term benefit to 40 of 216 patients with nickel allergy, many of whom had recurrent symmetrical vesicular hand dermatitis. These studies emphasize the difficulty physicians may have in eliminating a contactant, or proving a true contact dermatitis association for chronic blistering disorders of the hand.

Histopathology

The sweat ducts are not involved. Spongiotic vesicles are found in the epidermis.

Differential Diagnosis

Vesicular eruptions of the palms and soles closely resemble each other, so that the clinical features may not be enough to arrive at a diagnosis. Dermatophytid, contact dermatitis (allergic), atopic dermatitis, drug eruption (NSAID), pustular psoriasis of the palms and soles, acrodermatitis continua, and pustular bacterid are some dermatoses to be kept in mind. Localized bullous pemphigoid has been reported to initially manifest in this way. Rarely, T-cell lymphoma can present with similar clinical findings, but biopsy of the vesicles will be diagnostic.

Treatment

Topical application of high-potency corticosteroid creams is the major form of therapy. Triamcinolone acetonide intramuscularly or a short course of oral prednisone is rapidly effective, often inducing remissions of a month or two. In patients with refractory disease and documented nickel allergies a diet low in nickel may be worth trying.

Previously, radiation therapy had been widely used, but advances in topical management have eliminated radiation therapy as a practical option. Oral or topical psoralen plus ultraviolet A light (PUVA) is effective, but in view of its cost and inconvenience, and potential for side effects it is not often used. The immunosuppressive agent mycophenolate mofetil has been effective but should be considered only in the most severe forms of the disease.

Jakob T, et al: Dyshidrotic cutaneous T-cell lymphoma. *J Am Acad Dermatol* 1996, 34:295.

Landow K: Hand dermatitis: the perennial scourge. *Postgrad Med* 1998, 103:141.

Lodi A, et al: Epidemiological, clinical and allergological observations on pompholyx. *Contact Dermatitis* 1992, 26:17.

Niels K, et al: Low nickel diet. *J Am Acad Dermatol* 1993, 29:1002.

Pickenacker A, et al: Dyshidrotic eczema treated with mycophenolate mofetil. *Arch Dermatol* 1998, 134:378.

Veien NK, et al: Nickel, cobalt and chromium sensitivity in patients with pompholyx (dyshidrotic eczema). *Contact Dermatitis* 1979, 5:371. ▲

Lamellar Dyshidrosis (Keratolysis Exfoliativa, Recurrent Palmar Peeling)

Lamellar dyshidrosis (dyshidrosis lamellosa) is a superficial exfoliative dermatosis of the palms and sometimes soles characterized by the absence of inflammatory changes and by pinhead-sized white spots that gradually extend peripherally. Also referred to as *recurrent palmar peeling,* the disorder spreads; new desquamating areas develop and eventually by coalescence the entire part may show flaky scales (Fig. 10-38). The involvement is bilateral, and it can occur in association with dyshidrosis, although at times no cause can be ascertained. It is often exacerbated by environmental factors. Some authors believe it is a disorder of cohesion of the stratum corneum.

The condition must be differentiated from dermatophytosis. It frequently is misdiagnosed as chronic contact dermatitis. The diagnosis is supported by negative patch tests. It is likely to be a common disorder that rarely presents to dermatologists because it is largely asymptomatic.

Treatment is difficult for this mild malady, but spontaneous involution can occur in a few weeks for some. For most it tends to be a chronic, recurring condition. Tar creams (Zetone cream) usually produce satisfactory results. Five percent tar in gel (Estar Gel) is an excellent preparation to use. A mild emollient, however, may suffice. Lac-Hydrin lotion and urea preparations such as Carmol 10 or 20 are often effective.

PALMOPLANTAR KERATODERMA

Keratoderma is frequently used synonymously with hyperkeratosis, keratosis, and tylosis. Palmoplantar keratoderma is characterized by excessive formation of keratin on the palms and soles. The acquired and congenital varieties may be present alone, or they may accompany other diseases or be a part of a syndrome.

The most important features in classification of the palmoplantar keratodermas include the specific morphology

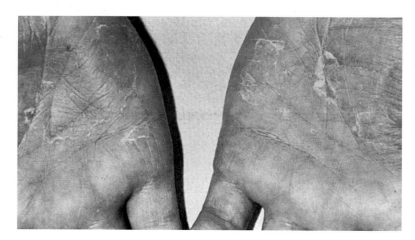

Fig. 10-38 Keratolysis exfoliativa; dry desquamation of horny layer of palm (or sole) in thin sheets.

and distribution of the hyperkeratosis, evidence for genetic transmission and particular inheritance pattern, presence of skin lesions on areas other than palms and soles, other ectodermal or systemic abnormalities, age at onset of the keratoderma, severity and prognosis of the disease process, and histopathologic findings.

The acquired types include keratoderma climactericum, arsenical keratoses, corns, calluses, porokeratosis plantaris discreta, porokeratotic eccrine ostial and dermal duct nevus, glucan-induced keratoderma in acquired immunodeficiency syndrome (AIDS), keratosis punctata of the palmar creases, and many skin disorders that are associated with palmoplantar keratoderma such as psoriasis, cancer-associated paraneoplastic disorders, pityriasis rubra pilaris, lichen planus, and syphilis.

The hereditary types include hereditary palmoplantar keratoderma (Unna-Thost), punctate palmoplantar keratosis, Papillon-Lefèvre syndrome, mal de Meleda, familial keratoderma with carcinoma of the esophagus (Howell-Evans), acrokeratoelastoidosis, focal acral hyperkeratosis, and several inherited disorders that have palmoplantar keratoderma as an associated finding, such as pachyonychia congenita, tyrosinemia II (Richner-Hanhart), basal-cell nevus syndrome, Darier's disease, and dyskeratosis congenita. A number of mutations in keratin genes have been found for some of these disorders. American patients with nonepidermolytic palmoplantar keratoderma associated with malignancy were linked to abnormalities of 17q24 distal to the keratin cluster. Pachyonychia congenita is associated with mutations in the helical initiation peptide of K6a, K16, or K17. A classification of keratodermas by means of a number system has been proposed.

The acquired types will be reviewed first. Four diseases will be discussed here: keratosis punctata of the palmar creases, punctate keratoses of the palms and soles, porokeratosis plantaris discreta, and keratoderma climactericum. Malignancies associated with acquired palmoplantar keratosis are reviewed along with Howell-Evans syndrome.

Acquired Syndromes

Keratosis Punctata of the Palmar Creases.
Keratosis punctata of the palmar creases has also been referred to as *keratotic pits of the palmar creases, punctate keratosis of the palmar creases, keratosis punctata, keratodermia punctata, hyperkeratosis penetrans, lenticular atrophia of the palmar creases,* and *hyperkeratosis punctata of the palmar creases.* This common disorder occurs most often in black patients. The primary lesion is a 1- to 5-mm depression filled with a conical keratinous plug, primarily in the creases of the palms or fingers, and occasionally on the soles (Fig. 10-39). Lesions are multiple. Friction aggravates the lesions and often causes them to become verrucoid or surrounded by callus. At times only conical depressions are

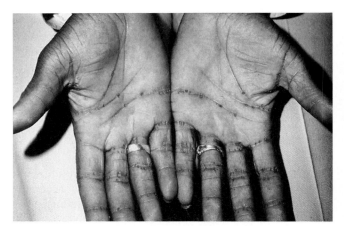

Fig. 10-39 Keratosis punctata of the palmar creases.

noted. An autosomal dominant inheritance pattern has been suggested.

Rustad et al studied 283 consecutive patients for the presence of palmar and plantar pits. Eleven percent were found to have punctate keratosis of the palms and soles, and 3% had keratotic pits of the palmar creases (5% had both). Black men were more commonly found to have palmar crease involvement, although it was seen in whites. The age of onset was between 15 to 40 years. The histology demonstrates hyperkeratosis and parakeratosis. Keratosis punctata of the palmar creases has been reported to be associated with Dupuytren's contractures, pterygium inversum unguis, dermatitis herpetiformis, knuckle pads, striate keratoderma, and psoriasis.

For most patients the pits are an annoyance, but the pain and tenderness in some can be so severe that surgical intervention is required. Keratolytic agents and topical retinoids have provided temporary relief. Tazarotene, a nonisomerizable retinoid used to treat psoriasis, should be another consideration.

Punctate Keratoses of the Palms and Soles.
Punctate keratoses of the palms and soles has also been referred to as *punctate keratoderma, keratodermia punctata, keratosis punctata palmaris et plantaris, keratoma hereditarium dissipatum palmare et plantare, keratoderma disseminatum palmaris et plantaris, palmar keratoses, palmar* and *plantar seed dermatoses,* and other terms (Fig. 10-40). The spiny keratoderma of the palms and soles known as "music box spines" is most likely another variant.

The primary lesion is a 1- to 5-mm round to oval, dome-shaped papule distributed primarily over the left hand and hypothenar eminence. There may be from 1 to more than 40 papules, with an average in one series of 8.3. The main symptom is pruritus. The onset is between ages 15 to 68. Blacks predominate, and it most frequently afflicts men. There have been reports of sporadic autosomal dominant

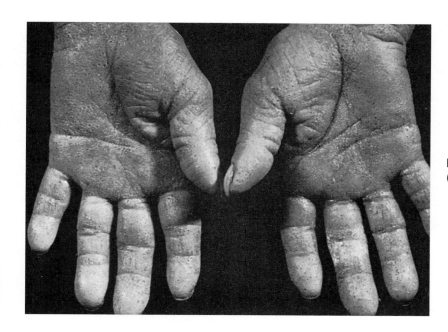

Fig. 10-40 Keratosis punctata palmoplantaris. (Courtesy Dr. H. Shatin.)

inheritance. The histology demonstrates hyperkeratosis and parakeratosis, pyknotic, vacuolated epithelium, basal layer spongiosis and dilated, occluded sweat ducts, blood vessels, and lymph vessels. There appears to be a potential risk of developing malignancies such as lung and colon. Only mechanical debridement and excision have achieved any permanent results.

Porokeratosis Plantaris Discreta. Porokeratosis plantaris discreta occurs in adults, with a 4:1 female preponderance. It is characterized by a sharply marginated, rubbery, wide-based papule that on blunt dissection reveals an opaque plug without bleeding on removal. Lesions are multiple, painful, and usually 7 to 10 mm in diameter. They are usually confined to the weight-bearing area of the sole, beneath the metatarsal heads. Treatment may be begun with fitted foot pads to redistribute the weight. Surgical excision or blunt dissection by electrocautery may be done. Limmer found cryotherapy successful in a high percentage of cases.

Keratoderma Climactericum. Keratoderma climactericum is characterized by hyperkeratosis of the palms and soles (especially the heels) beginning at about the time of the menopause. The discrete, thickened, hyperkeratotic patches are most pronounced at sites of pressure such as around the rim of the sole (Fig. 10-41). Fissuring of the thickened patches may be present. There is a striking resemblance to plantar psoriasis, and indeed, keratoderma climacterium may represent a form of psoriasis. Therapy consists of keratolytics such as 10% salicylic acid ointment, lactic acid creams, or 20% to 30% urea mixtures. Acitretin is more effective than isotretinoin.

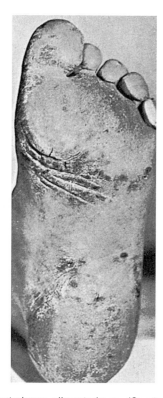

Fig. 10-41 Keratoderma climactericum. (Courtesy Dr. P. Gross.)

Hereditary Syndromes

Discussion of the hereditary syndromes follows. Many disorders that have palmoplantar keratoderma as a feature, such as pachyonychia congenita, Darier's disease, and tyrosinemia II, will be discussed in other chapters.

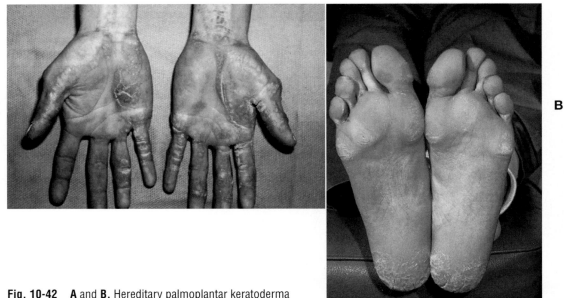

Fig. 10-42 **A** and **B,** Hereditary palmoplantar keratoderma (Unna Thost).

Hereditary Palmoplantar Keratoderma.

Hereditary palmoplantar keratoderma (Unna Thost) is characterized by a dominantly inherited, marked, congenital thickening of the epidermal horny layer of the palms and soles, usually symmetrical and affecting all parts equally (Fig. 10-42). At times the thickening extends to the lateral or dorsal surfaces, especially over the knuckles. When the keratoderma is on the soles, the arches are generally not involved. The epidermis becomes thick, yellowish, verrucous, and horny. Striate and punctate forms occur. In the ordinary variety the uniform thickening forms a rigid plate, which ends with characteristic abruptness at the periphery of the palm, usually without any contiguous inflammatory margin. There is frequently hyperhidrosis, which causes a sodden appearance. Occasionally there are associated changes in the nails, which become thickened.

Local medications are rarely of value. Five percent salicylic acid is helpful. Twelve percent ammonium lactate lotion (Lac-Hydrin) may be tried. Acitretin or isotretinoin may be considered; however, the need for lifetime treatment makes them impractical because of bone toxicity.

Palmoplantar Keratodermas and Malignancy.

Howell-Evans reported a diffuse, waxy keratoderma of the palms and soles occurring as an autosomal dominant trait associated with esophageal carcinoma. Other related features are oral leukoplakia, esophageal strictures, squamous cell carcinoma of tylotic skin, and carcinoma of the larynx and stomach. Acquired forms of palmoplantar keratodermas have also been associated with cancers of the esophagus, lung, breast, urinary bladder, and stomach.

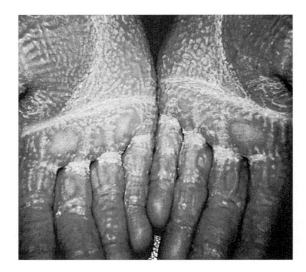

Fig. 10-43 Mutilating keratoderma of Vohwinkel: diffuse honeycomb hyperkeratosis of the palms. (From Gibbs RC, Frank SB: *Arch Dermatol* 1966, 94:619.)

Mutilating Keratoderma of Vohwinkel.

Vohwinkel described this palmoplantar hyperkeratosis of the honeycomb type, associated with starfishlike keratoses on the backs of the hands and feet, linear keratoses of the elbows and knees, and annular constriction (pseudo-ainhum) of the digits, which may progress to autoamputation (Figs. 10-43 and 10-44).

More than 30 cases have been reported in the world literature inherited mostly in an autosomal dominant fashion

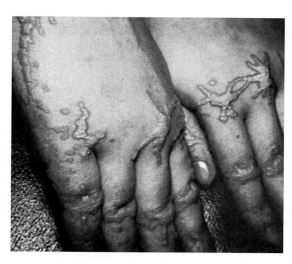

Fig. 10-44 Mutilating keratoderma of Vohwinkel: "starfish" hyperkeratosis on backs of hands. (From Gibbs RC, Frank SB: *Arch Dermatol* 1966, 94:619.)

although a recessive type also exists. The disease is more frequent in women and in whites, with onset in infancy or early childhood. Reported associations include deafness, deaf-mutism, high-tone acoustic impairment, congenital alopecia universalis, pseudopelade-type alopecia, acanthosis nigricans, ichthyosiform dermatoses, spastic paraplegia, myopathy, nail changes, mental retardation, and bullous lesions on the soles. Vohwinkel's keratoderma maps to chromosome 1q21 and represents a mutation of loricrin.

Rivers et al reported four cases, all family members, spanning three generations. There was marked improvement of the hyperkeratosis, as well as the pseudo-ainhum, with Acitretin (etretinate) therapy. The effectiveness of Acitretin has been confirmed by Peris et al.

Olmstead syndrome should be included in the differential diagnosis, a rare disorder characterized by a mutilating palmoplantar keratoderma and periorificial keratotic plaques. The distinctive features of this syndrome include a congenital, sharply marginated palmoplantar keratoderma; constriction of the digits; linear keratotic streaks on the flexural aspects of the wrists; onychodystrophy; and periorificial keratoses. The latter feature may cause confusion with acrodermatitis enteropathica.

Acrokeratoelastoidosis of Costa.

This autosomal dominantly inherited condition is more common in women. Costa described small, round, firm papules occurring over the dorsal hands, knuckles, and lateral margins of the palms and soles. The lesions appear in early childhood and progress slowly. They are most often asymptomatic. A significant histologic feature is dermal elastorrhexis. The differential diagnosis includes focal acral hyperkeratosis, verruca plana, acrokeratosis verruciformis of Hopf, colloid milium, xanthoma, and punctate keratoderma of the palms

and soles. Multiple therapies, such as liquid nitrogen, salicylic acid, tretinoin, and prednisone, have been tried, with minimal success. Treatment should only be attempted if there are symptoms.

Dowd et al described focal acral hyperkeratosis, which, while it closely resembles acrokeratoelastoidosis, shows no elastorrhexis on biopsy. Twelve of 15 patients were female, and 14 were black. All had papules on the medial and lateral edges of the hands and feet, developing at about age 20, and half had a family history of the disorder. Generally treatment is not necessary, but Acitretin and cryotherapy have been used successfully. Patients tend to develop recurrence after discontinuing Acitretin (etretinate).

Papillon-Lefèvre Syndrome.

Papillon-Lefèvre syndrome manifests with palmoplantar hyperkeratosis and periodontosis. It usually develops within the first few months of life but may occur in childhood after the eruption of the deciduous teeth. Common cutaneous changes include well-demarcated, erythematous, hyperkeratotic lesions on the palms and soles, which may extend to the dorsal hands and feet (Fig. 10-45). These changes often start in early childhood and may also be present on the elbows, knees, and Achilles tendon areas. Transverse grooves of the fingernails may occur. In most cases the cutaneous changes appear concomitantly with the odontal change; however, in some cases, skin changes precede the dental change. It is believed that this is an autosomal recessive disorder.

The early onset of periodontal disease has been attributed to damage and alteration in polymorphonuclear leukocyte function caused by *Actinomyces actinomycetemcomitans*. Disease associations include acroosteolysis and pyogenic liver abscesses. There are asymptomatic ectopic calcifications in the choroid plexus and tentorium. Therapy may retard both the dental and skin abnormalities. Nazzaro et al reported such a response in four siblings treated with Acitretin.

The stocking-glove distribution of the hyperkeratosis is similar to that seen in *mal de Meleda,* an autosomal recessive disorder seen in individuals from the island of Meleda (Fig. 10-46). No dental abnormalities are present in mal de Meleda syndrome, and there are often associated keratotic lesions of the groin and axilla. The disorder has been reported from other areas of the world to include the United Arab Emirates, Chile, and possibly Japan. Lio et al reported a 38-year-old Japanese male with possible Papillon-Lefèvre syndrome and an aggressive squamous cell carcinoma of the right sole, necessitating amputation of the lower leg. Effective responses have been achieved with Acitretin (etretinate) and isotretinoin.

Anderson WA, et al: Keratosis punctata and atopy. *Arch Dermatol* 1984, 12:884.

Atherton DJ, et al: Mutilating palmoplantar keratoderma with periorifacial keratotic plaques (Olmstead syndrome). *Br J Dermatol* 1990, 122:245.

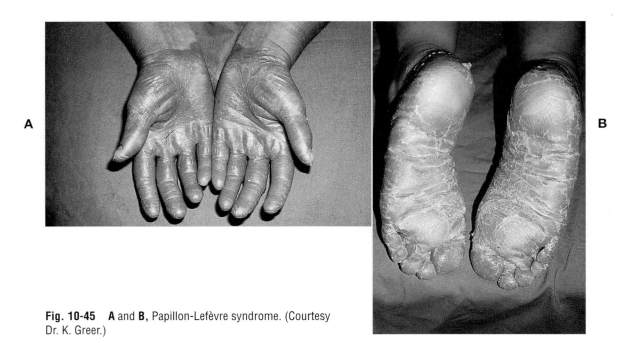

Fig. 10-45 **A** and **B**, Papillon-Lefèvre syndrome. (Courtesy Dr. K. Greer.)

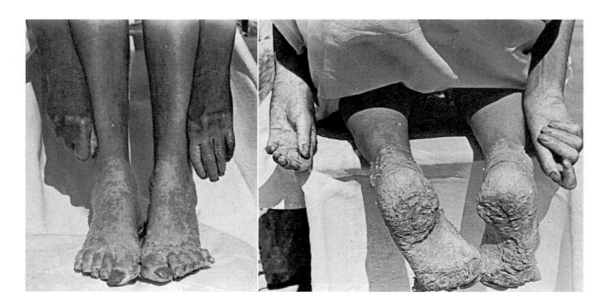

Fig. 10-46 Mal de Meleda. (Courtesy Dr. Mladen Filiporic, Split, Yugoslavia.)

Bergfeld WF, et al: The treatment of keratosis palmaris et plantaris with isotretinoin. *J Am Acad Dermatol* 1982, 6:727.

Bhatia KK, et al: Keratoma hereditaria mutilans (Vohwinkel's disease) with congenital alopecia universalis (atrichia congenita). *J Dermatol* 1989, 16:231.

Blanchet-Bardon C, et al: Acitretin in the treatment of severe disorders of keratinization. *J Am Acad Dermatol* 1991, 24:982.

Blum SL, et al: Hyperkeratosis papular in the hands and feet. *Arch Dermatol* 1987, 123:1225.

Boutsi EA, et al: Follow-up of two cases of Papillon-Lefèvre syndrome and presentation of two new cases. *Int J Periodontics Restorative Dent* 1997, 17:334.

DeSchamps P, et al: Keratoderma climactericum (Haxthausen's disease). *Dermatologica* 1986, 172:258.

Dowd PM, et al: Focal acral hyperkeratosis. *Br J Dermatol* 1983, 109:97.

Duvic M, et al: Glucan-induced keratoderma in AIDS. *Arch Dermatol* 1987, 123:751.

El Darouti MA, et al: Papillon-Lefèvre. *Int J Dermatol* 1988, 27:63.

Friedman SJ, et al: Punctate porokeratotic keratoderma. *Arch Dermatol* 1988, 124:1678.

Gonzalez JR, et al: Papillon-Lefèvre syndrome. *P R Health Sci J* 1997, 16:279.

Khanna SK, et al: Nonfamilial diffuse palmoplantar keratoderma associated with bronchial carcinoma. *J Am Acad Dermatol* 1993, 28:295.

Kore A, et al: Acrokeratoelastoidosis of Costa in North America. *J Am Acad Dermatol* 1985, 12:832.

Kress DW, et al: Olmstead syndrome. *Arch Dermatol* 1996, 132:797.

Lee YC, et al: Recurrent focal palmar peeling. *Australas J Dermatol* 1996, 37:143.

Lestringant GG, et al: Mal de Meleda. *Pediatr Dermatol* 1997, 14:186.

Limmer B: Cryotherapy of porokeratosis plantaris discreta. *Arch Dermatol* 1979, 115:582.

Lio T, et al: Mal de Meleda-like palmoplantar keratoderma. *J Dermatol* 1991, 18:43.

Mallory SB, et al: Acrokeratoelastoidosis of Costa. *Int J Dermatol* 1995, 34:431.

Margo CM, et al: A novel nonepidermolytic palmoplantar keratoderma. *J Am Acad Dermatol* 1997, 37:27.

Moreno A, et al: Porokeratotic eccrine ostial and dermal duct nevus. *J Cutan Pathol* 1988, 15:43.

Murrata Y, et al: Acquired diffuse keratoderma of the palms and soles with bronchial carcinoma. *Arch Dermatol* 1988, 124:497.

Nazzaro V, et al: Papillon-Lefèvre syndrome: ultrastructural study and successful treatment with Acitretin. *Arch Dermatol* 1988, 124:533.

Oguzkurt P, et al: Increased risk of pyogenic liver abscess in children with Papillon-Lefèvre syndrome. *J Pediatr Surg* 1996, 31:955.

Ortega M, et al: Keratosis punctata of the palmar creases. *J Am Acad Dermatol* 1985, 13:381.

Osman Y, et al: Spiny keratoderma of the palms and soles. *J Am Acad Dermatol* 1992, 26:879.

Parker CM: Tender linear lesions of the fingers: acrokeratoelastoidosis (acquired type) or degenerative collagenous plaques of the hands. *Arch Dermatol* 1991, 127:114.

Peris K, et al: Keratoderma hereditarium mutilans (Vohwinkel's syndrome) associated with congenital deaf-mutism. *Br J Dermatol* 1995, 132:617.

Rajashekhar N, et al: Palmoplantar keratoderma: Mal de Meleda syndrome. *Int J Dermatol* 1997, 36:854.

Richey TK, et al: Yellowish papules on lateral aspect of palms: focal acral hyperkeratosis. *Arch Dermatol* 1996, 132:1365.

Rivers JK, et al: Etretinate: management of keratoma hereditaria mutilans in four family members. *J Am Acad Dermatol* 1985, 13:43.

Rustad OJ, et al: Punctate keratoses of the palms and soles and keratotic pits of the palmar creases. *J Am Acad Dermatol* 1990, 22:468.

Shbaklo Z, et al: Acrokeratoelastoidosis. *Int J Dermatol* 1990, 29:333.

Simon M, et al: The Clark-Howel-Evans-McConnell syndrome: observations in one family over 5 generations. *Hautarzt* 1997, 48:800.

Sybert VP, et al: Palmo-plantar keratoderma. *J Am Acad Dermatol* 1988, 18:75.

Trattner A, et al: Papillon-Lefèvre syndrome with acroosteolysis. *J Am Acad Dermatol* 1991, 24:835.

Urbina F, et al: Mal de Meleda. *Cutis* 1995, 56:235. ▲

EXFOLIATIVE DERMATITIS (Erythroderma)

Synonyms: Dermatitis exfoliativa, pityriasis rubra (Hebra), erythroderma (Wilson-Brocq)

Clinical Features

Although the clinical picture is similar in most patients, there are many etiologic factors in exfoliative dermatitis. This disease is characterized by a universal or very extensive obstinate scaling and itching erythroderma, often associated with loss of hair (Fig. 10-47). The disease starts with erythematous plaques, which spread rapidly until the whole integument is involved. The onset is often accompanied by symptoms of general toxicity. The skin becomes

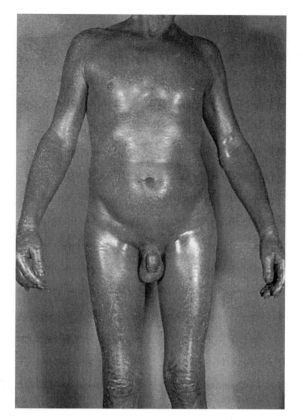

Fig. 10-47 Universal erythroderma.

scarlet and swollen and may ooze a straw-colored exudate. Desquamation is evident after a few days.

The scales are of various kinds, in some cases being small and thin and, in others, large sheets. The latter are often seen on the palms and soles. On the scalp thick crusts are formed, combined with sebum and products of secondary infection. The conjunctivae and the mucous membrane of the upper respiratory tract may be affected by desquamation. Secondary infections by pyogenic organisms often complicate the course of the disease in the absence of treatment.

There is a vivid, widespread erythema, particularly on the face and extremities, and ultimately the entire body surface is dull scarlet and covered by small, laminated scales that exfoliate profusely. Vesiculation and pustulation are usually absent. Pruritus is usually present and may be almost intolerable. Chilliness is a constant complaint owing to the patients' inability to constrict cutaneous blood vessels; there is severe heat loss.

One attack may follow another. The course of the disease may be very protracted, lasting over a period of years, or it may simply persist and resist therapy.

Etiology

The original picture of exfoliative dermatitis may be considerably influenced by the causative factor. Both benign and malignant forms occur.

In a series of 102 patients reported by Sigurdsson et al the largest group was preexisting dermatoses (53%; atopic dermatitis, chronic actinic dermatitis, psoriasis, seborrheic dermatitis, vesicular palmoplantar eczema, pityriasis rubra pilaris, and contact dermatitis, in order of prevalence), drug eruptions (5%; allopurinol, gold, carbamazepine, phenytoin, and quinidine), cutaneous T-cell lymphoma (13%; Sézary syndrome and mycosis fungoides), paraneoplastic (2%; carcinoma of the lung and carcinoma of the stomach), and leukemia cutis (1%). Twenty-six percent were idiopathic. The mortality rate at a mean follow-up interval of 51 months was 43%.

In another series of 56 cases reported by Botella-Estrada et al the mortality rate was 19%, but only 7% were directly attributed to the erythroderma. The breakdown of causes was similar to other series except for a larger number of patients with lymphomas (62.5% from dermatoses, 16% from drugs, and 19% from T-cell lymphomas).

Psoriasis. Psoriatic erythroderma is one of the most common precursors of exfoliative dermatitis (Fig. 10-48). Pruritus and lymphadenopathy are usually minor features in this type of exfoliative dermatitis.

Eczema, Neurodermatitis. Exfoliative dermatitis is often preceded by the typical lesions of atopic dermatitis or other forms of eczema. Pruritus is intense, with great discomfort.

Drug Allergy. Among the drugs that may cause a generalized erythroderma are allopurinol, sulfa drugs, gold, phenytoin, phenobarbital, isoniazid, carbamazepine, cisplatin, dapsone, mefloquine, tobramycin, minocycline, nifedipine, and iodine (Fig. 10-49).

Pityriasis Rubra Pilaris. Even the most severe or generalized pityriasis rubra pilaris (PRP) will at some time have clear and normal-appearing "islands" of skin. These are characteristic of PRP. The thickened, hyperkeratotic, and shiny palms and the "nutmeg grater" follicular papules on the dorsum of the fingers are helpful in differentiating this from the other forms of erythroderma.

Seborrheic Dermatitis. Only rarely does generalized seborrheic dermatitis occur. It resembles psoriatic erythroderma. Usually, seborrheic dermatitis has typical sites of predilection such as the scalp, ears, backs of the ears, alae nasi, midline of the chest, axillae, and inguinal regions.

Other Dermatoses. Internal malignancies, pemphigus foliaceus, generalized dermatophytosis, and even Norwegian scabies may show the picture of generalized exfoliative dermatitis. There have been reports of inadequate intake of branched-chain amino acids in infants with maple syrup urine disease producing exfoliative erythroderma.

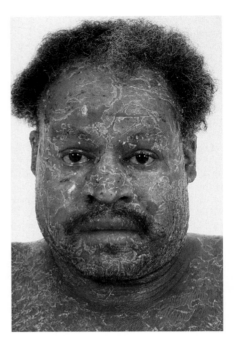

Fig. 10-48   Psoriatic erythroderma.

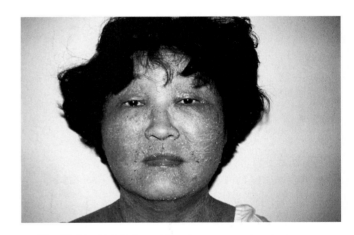

Fig. 10-49   Exfoliative erythroderma secondary to dapsone.

Malignant Lymphoma. Mycosis fungoides may have several cutaneous forms. A generalized exfoliative dermatitis may be present with poikiloderma as a part of the erythrodermic eruption. With it pigmentation and even infiltrated tumors may be present. Sézary syndrome consists of generalized exfoliative dermatitis with intense pruritus, leonine facies, alopecia, palmoplantar hyperkeratosis, and onychodystrophy.

Hodgkin's disease may show generalized exfoliative dermatitis. Lymphadenopathy, splenomegaly, and hepatomegaly are frequently present. The erythrocyte sedimentation rate is elevated in most of these patients.

Leukemia may also present with generalized exfoliative dermatitis. Erythroderma occurs most frequently in lymphocytic leukemia, in both the acute and chronic forms. Splenomegaly and lymph node enlargement are early signs in leukemia.

Histopathology

Exfoliative dermatitis, regardless of its cause, often retains the histologic features of the original disease process. Exfoliative dermatitis may at times retain the histology of the underlying disease process. More commonly, however, the histology is nonspecific. The epidermis on a punch biopsy will show abnormalities across its whole surface. There is hyperkeratosis with focal parakeratosis. The epidermis shows mild acanthosis, and there is a scant superficial upper dermal infiltrate of mononuclear cells. There may be small areas of spongiosis. Chronic dermatitis, psoriasis, and pityriasis rubra pilaris may not be distinguishable histologically in erythrodermic patients.

Treatment

Topical steroids, soaks, and compresses are nonspecific treatments but benefit most cases. Acitretin and cyclosporine are useful in psoriatic erythroderma, and isotretinoin in erythroderma caused by PRP. Systemic corticosteroids may be life saving in severe involvement. Immunosuppressives such as azathioprine, methotrexate, and cyclophosphamide may occasionally be necessary. Specific modes of therapy useful for the lymphomas and leukemias are indicated in those disorders. Discontinuance of the offending drug in drug-induced cases is, of course, mandatory.

Adam JE: Exfoliative dermatitis (erythroderma). *Curr Prob Dermatol* 1971, 4:1.

Botella-Estrada R, et al: Erythroderma: a clinicopathological study of 56 cases. *Arch Dermatol* 1994, 130:1503.

King LE, et al: Erythroderma. *South Med J* 1986, 79:1210.

Northrup H, et al: Exfoliative erythroderma resulting from inadequate intake of branched-chain amino acids in infants with maple syrup urine disease (letter). *Arch Dermatol* 1993, 129:384.

Sehgal VN, et al: Exfoliative dermatitis. *Dermatologica* 1986, 173:278.

Sigurdsson V, et al: Erythroderma: a clinical and follow-up study of 102 patients, with special emphasis on survival. *J Am Acad Dermatol* 1996, 35:53.

Thestrup-Pedersen K, et al: The red man syndrome. *J Am Acad Dermatol* 1988, 18:1307.

Van der Vleuten CJ, et al: A therapeutic approach to erythrodermic psoriasis. *Acta Derm Venereol* 1996, 76:65. _____ ▲

CHAPTER 11

Parapsoriasis, Pityriasis Rosea, Pityriasis Rubra Pilaris

PARAPSORIASIS

The term *parapsoriasis* was applied by Brocq (1902) to a group of maculopapular scaly eruptions of slow evolution, whose marked chronicity, resistance to treatment, and absence of subjective symptoms are characteristic features. Although the eruptions are psoriasiform and lichenoid, the diseases do not correspond to psoriasis, lichen planus, or other recognized dermatoses, and although the details of the eruptions do not harmonize, there is sufficient essential conformity to justify placing them in a distinct group. Now we divide them into pityriasis lichenoides chronica, pityriasis lichenoides et varioliformis acuta, and parapsoriasis en plaques.

Pityriasis Lichenoides Chronica

In pityriasis lichenoides chronica (Fig. 11-1), erythematous, yellowish, scaly macules and lichenoid papules appear insidiously. They persist indefinitely with little change, chiefly on the sides of trunk, thighs, and upper arms. From time to time the eruption may be augmented by the development of a few new lesions. Several patients have been reported to have scaly, hypopigmented, guttate macules, which on biopsy revealed the findings of pityriasis lichenoides chronica. The disease may be confused with psoriasis and secondary syphilis.

The histologic features of pityriasis lichenoides chronica are not specific. Focal parakeratosis, acanthosis, and even spongiosis may be present. There is an infiltrate of lymphocytes in the superficial dermis. These findings may be difficult to distinguish from those of guttate psoriasis, pityriasis rosea, and certain types of drug eruptions.

Treatment with ultraviolet light is beneficial; however, intensive doses may be necessary for good results. PUVA has also been reported to be effective, but should be limited in use owing to adverse long-term effects. Piamphongsant treated 13 cases with oral tetracycline. Five were completely cured. The addition of an antihistamine enhanced the beneficial effects in one case.

Pityriasis lichenoides chronica is a benign disease that clears spontaneously in a few months or years.

Pityriasis Lichenoides et Varioliformis Acuta

Pityriasis lichenoides et varioliformis acuta (PLEVA) (Figs. 11-2 to 11-4) has also been known as *parapsoriasis lichenoides, Habermann's disease, Mucha-Habermann disease,* and *parapsoriasis varioliformis acuta.* It is a self-limited disease that favors children.

This form occurs with the sudden appearance of a polymorphous eruption composed of macules, papules, and occasional vesicles. It may run an acute, subacute, or chronic course. The papules are usually yellowish or brownish red rounded lesions, which tend to crusting, necrosis, and hemorrhage. Vesicular lesions are not common but are of great diagnostic importance. On close examination the vesicles are found to be deep-seated and varicelliform. Papulonecrotic lesions with blackish brown crusts and hemorrhagic excoriations are evident. The exanthem then heals, leaving smooth, pigmented, depressed, varioliform scars. By this time, however, a new crop of lesions has usually appeared.

Almost the entire integument may be involved, favorite sites being the anterior trunk, the flexor surfaces of the upper extremities, and the axillary regions (see Fig. 11-3). The palms and soles are infrequently involved but the mucous membranes are not. The general health in most cases is not affected, but generalized lymphadenopathy has been noted. The manifestations of the exanthem vary considerably. Although originally thought to be a benign, self-limited disorder, more recent evidence confirms that there are more chronic and severe forms.

An unusually severe form was first described by Degos in 1966 and is characterized by the acute onset of diffuse, coalescent, large, ulceronecrotic skin lesions associated with high fever and constitutional symptoms. More than 17 cases of ulceronecrotic Mucha-Habermann disease have been reported, and 2 deaths have been attributed to this variant. Treatment is aggressive; PUVA, methotrexate, systemic steroids, antibiotics, and a variety of topical agents have been used.

Fortson et al reported two cases of PLEVA that developed into cutaneous T-cell lymphoma. The authors

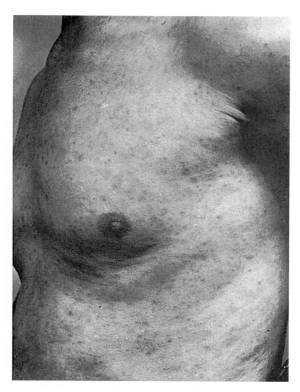

Fig. 11-1 Pityriasis lichenoides chronica. (Courtesy Dr. R. Clayton, London.)

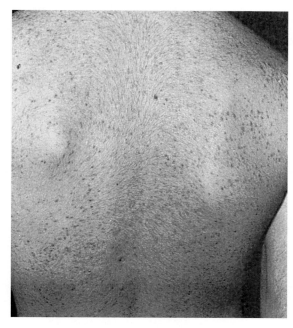

Fig. 11-2 Pityriasis lichenoides et varioliformis acuta.

suggest that pityriasis lichenoides may be part of a spectrum of cutaneous T-cell lymphoma. Still others argue that such cases were misdiagnosed lymphomatoid papulosis. Knowing that there may be difficulty in confirming a specific diagnosis it is prudent to perform repeat biopsies for histology and gene rearrangement studies in those cases that do not appear to follow a typical clinical course.

The disorder must be differentiated from leukocytoclastic angiitis, papulonecrotic tuberculid, psoriasis, lichen planus, varicella, pityriasis rosea, drug eruptions, maculopapular syphilid, some forms of viral and rickettsial diseases, and most of all, lymphomatoid papulosis.

In a study by Gelmetti et al of 89 children with PLEVA, they found that the prognosis correlated with lesion distribution. Fifty-four had a diffuse pattern, with an average course of 11 months. A second group of 19 had a central pattern with a course of 17 months, and a third group of 16 had a peripheral pattern whose disease averaged 31 months before spontaneous involution. The etiology has not been determined. Many authors have suggested an infectious cause but none has been proved.

Histologically, PLEVA is characterized by epidermal necrosis, together with prominent hemorrhage and primarily a dense perivascular infiltrate of lymphocytes in the superficial dermis. The absence of neutrophils simplifies the

distinction from leukocytoclastic angiitis, which PLEVA may clinically resemble. Lymphomatoid papulosis differs histologically by the presence of large, atypical mononuclear cells in the dermal infiltrate.

No one treatment is reliably effective. Tetracycline and erythromycin have both been reported to be effective and are worth trying. UVB and PUVA are additional options. Methotrexate, 2.5 to 7.5 mg every 12 hours for 3 doses 1 day each week, has been shown effective. Several serious reactions, a few of them fatal, have been reported from the simultaneous administration of methotrexate and nonsteroidal antiinflammatory drugs. Dapsone and pentoxifylline (Trental), 400 mg twice daily, have been used successfully in individual cases.

Parapsoriasis en Plaques

The division of parapsoriasis en plaques into small-plaque and large-plaque types, as proposed by Lambert et al, has clinical and prognostic utility. Small-plaque parapsoriasis is characterized by nonindurated, brownish, hypopigmented, or yellowish red scaling patches, round to oval, with sharply defined, regular borders (Fig. 11-5). Most lesions occur on the trunk, and most are between 1 and 5 cm in diameter. The eruption may be mildly itchy or asymptomatic. The patches may persist for years to decades and do not progress to lymphoma.

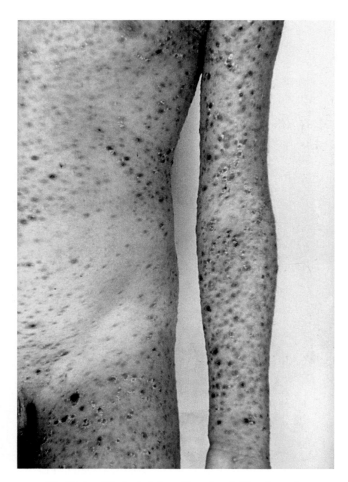

Fig. 11-3 Pityriasis lichenoides et varioliformis acuta.

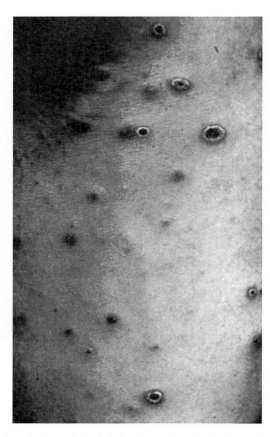

Fig. 11-4 Pityriasis lichenoides et varioliformis acuta.

Large-plaque parapsoriasis has patches 5 to 15 cm in diameter, but is similar in other respects to those of the small-plaque type (Fig. 11-6). The prognosis, especially if pruritus is severe, is less benign: 10% may eventuate in T-cell lymphoma. Ominous signs are the development of indurated areas within the patches and at times the development of intense erythema.

Some degree of epidermal atrophy is present in many cases of either type, and poikiloderma is common in the large-plaque type. This change is particularly prominent in the retiform subtype, which is characterized by a netlike distribution of red to brownish red, flat-topped, scaling papules over the trunk and proximal extremities. This subtype carries the poorest prognosis: many cases progress to mycosis fungoides.

The histologic findings of small-plaque parapsoriasis are characterized by a dense infiltrate in the superficial dermis composed predominantly of lymphocytes. Lymphocytes are also found within the epidermis, which is otherwise unremarkable except for focal parakeratosis, edema, and mild acanthosis. Small-plaque parapsoriasis is considered a type of chronic, spongiotic dermatitis. Large-plaque para-

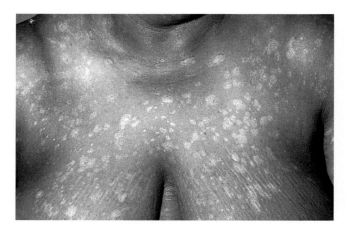

Fig. 11-5 Small-plaque parapsoriasis.

psoriasis may be indistinguishable from small-plaque parapsoriasis. Large-plaque parapsoriasis is distinguished from mycosis fungoides by the absence of cytologically atypical lymphocytes and the absence of Pautrier microabscess formation (i.e., collections of atypical lymphocytes in the

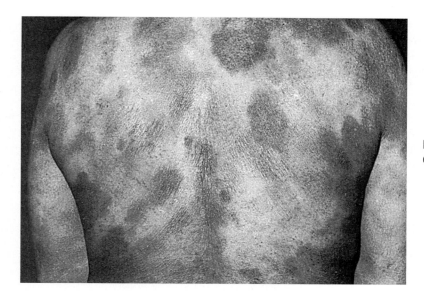

Fig. 11-6   Large-plaque parapsoriasis of 35 years' duration in a 64-year-old man.

epidermis). Atypical lymphocytes, however, may appear (particularly within the epidermis) in those lesions that progress to lymphoma.

The pathology is not pathognomonic, and in questionable cases it is beneficial to send tissue for the detection of DNA rearrangement for the T-cell receptor gene to investigate further the diagnosis of cutaneous T-cell lymphoma. Clonality has been detected in PLEVA, follicular mucinosis, lymphomatoid papulosis, and even small-plaque parapsoriasis, all of which are considered benign disorders. The lack of detecting clonality does have clinical and prognostic significance and will support the prediction of a benign course. As Haeffner et al point out, it remains to be determined if the dominant T-cell clones detected in some cases of small-plaque parapsoriasis can ever be the direct precursors of overt cutaneous T-cell lymphomas.

The treatment of choice is ultraviolet radiation, either natural or in UVB units. Lubricants are helpful. Topical steroids are useful. UVA—long-wave ultraviolet radiation—with or without preliminary 8-methoxy psoralen is effective but should be used only if UVB is ineffective. The use of PUVA or high-potency topical steroids in the small-plaque type should be restricted, owing to their adverse, long-term effects. The large-plaque variant's potential to develop lymphoma justifies more intense therapeutic endeavors. Vitamin D_2 in a single daily dose of 250,000 units over a 2- to 4-month course has been shown effective.

Burg G, et al: Small plaque (digitate) parapsoriasis is an "abortive cutaneous T-cell lymphoma" and is not mycosis fungoides (editorial). *Arch Dermatol* 1995, 131:336.

Cerroni L: Lymphomatoid papulosis, pityriasis lichenoides et varioliformis acuta, and anaplastic large-cell (Ki-1+) lymphoma (letter). *J Am Acad Dermatol* 1997, 37:287.

Clayton R, et al: An immunofluorescence study of pityriasis lichenoides. *Br J Dermatol* 1978, 99:491.

De Cuyper C, et al: Febrile ulceronecrotic pityriasis lichenoides et varioliformis acuta. *Dermatology (Basel)* 1994, 189:50.

Fortson JS, et al: Cutaneous T-cell lymphoma (parapsoriasis en plaque). *Arch Dermatol* 1990, 126:1449.

Gelmetti C, et al: Pityriasis lichenoides in children. *J Am Acad Dermatol* 1990, 23:473.

Haeffner AC, et al: Differentiation and clonality of lesional lymphocytes in small plaque parapsoriasis. *Arch Dermatol* 1995, 131:321.

Hood AF, et al: Histopathologic diagnosis of pityriasis lichenoides et varioliformis acuta and its clinical correlation. *Arch Dermatol* 1982, 118:478.

Kikuchi A, et al: Parapsoriasis en plaques. *J Am Acad Dermatol* 1993, 29:419.

Lambert WC, et al: The nosology of parapsoriasis. *J Am Acad Dermatol* 1981, 5:373.

Lindae ML, et al: Poikilodermatous mycosis fungoides and atrophic large-plaque parapsoriasis exhibit similar abnormalities of T-cell antigen expression. *Arch Dermatol* 1988, 124:366.

Longley J, et al: Clinical and histologic features of pityriasis lichenoides et varioliformis in children. *Arch Dermatol* 1987, 123:1335.

Piamphongsant T: Tetracycline for pityriasis lichenoides. *Br J Dermatol* 1974, 91:319.

Powell FC, et al: PUVA therapy of pityriasis lichenoides. *J Am Acad Dermatol* 1984, 10:59.

Puddu P, et al: Febrile ulceronecrotic Mucha-Habermann's disease with fatal outcome. *Int J Dermatol* 1997, 36:691.

Romani J, et al: Pityriasis lichenoides in children. *Pediatr Dermatol* 1998, 15:1.

Rongioletti F, et al: Pityriasis lichenoides and acquired toxoplasmosis. *Int J Dermatol* 1999, 38:372.

Sauer GC: Pentoxifylline (Trental) therapy for vasculitis of pityriasis lichenoides et varioliformis. *Arch Dermatol* 1985, 121:487.

Shavin JS, et al: Mucha-Habermann disease in children. *Arch Dermatol* 1978, 114:1679.

Tham SN: UVB phototherapy for pityriasis lichenoides. *Austral J Dermatol* 1985, 26:9.

Truhan AP, et al: Pityriasis lichenoides in children: therapeutic response to erythromycin. *J Am Acad Dermatol* 1986, 15:66.

Tsuji T, et al: Mucha-Habermann disease and its febrile ulceronecrotic variant. *Cutis* 1996, 58:123.

Warshauer BL, et al: Febrile ulceronecrotic Mucha-Habermann disease. *Arch Dermatol* 1983, 119:597. _____ ▲

PITYRIASIS ALBA

Pityriasis alba (Fig. 11-7) is known by a plethora of names: *pityriasis streptogenes, furfuraceous impetigo, pityriasis simplex, pityriasis sicca faciei,* and *erythema streptogenes.*

Pityriasis alba is characterized by hypopigmented, round to oval, scaling patches on the face, upper arms, neck, or shoulders. The patches vary in size, being usually a few centimeters in diameter. The color is white (but never actually depigmented) or light pink. The scales are fine and adherent. Usually the patches are sharply demarcated; the edges may be erythematous and slightly elevated. The lack of any early specifically follicular localization helps greatly to distinguish the lesions from those of follicular mucinosis. Vellus hairs are not lost in pityriasis alba, nor does hypesthesia to cold occur, as often happens in follicular mucinosis. As a rule. pityriasis alba is asymptomatic; however, there may be mild pruritus. The disease occurs chiefly in children and teenagers. It is particularly a cosmetic problem in dark-skinned individuals.

The cause is unknown. Excessively dry skin appears to be contributory. The patches are more visible in contrast to dark skin or a suntan, so sunlight makes them more apparent. Efforts to isolate an infectious agent, either bacterial, viral, or fungal, have been unsuccessful.

Most lesions tend to disappear with time, but repigmentation can be accelerated with treatment. Emollients and bland lubricants should be encouraged. We have found low-strength corticosteroid creams alone or in combination with Lac-Hydrin to be helpful. Others have recommended oral PUVA in severe cases.

The prognosis is good. Healing usually occurs spontaneously within several months to a few years.

Galan EB, et al: Pityriasis alba. *Cutis* 1998, 61:11.

Laude TA: Approach to dermatologic disorders in black children. *Semin Dermatol* 1995, 14:15.

Wells BY, et al: Pityriasis alba: 10-year survey and review. *Arch Dermatol* 1960, 82:183.

Zaynoun ST: Oral methoxsalen photochemotherapy for extensive pityriasis alba. *J Am Acad Dermatol* 1986, 15:61.

Zaynoun ST, et al: Extensive pityriasis alba. *Br J Dermatol* 1983, 108:83.

▲

PITYRIASIS ROSEA
Clinical Features

Pityriasis rosea is a mild inflammatory exanthem of unknown origin, characterized by salmon-colored papular and macular lesions that are at first discrete but may become confluent. The individual patches are oval or circinate and covered with finely crinkled, dry epidermis, which often desquamates, leaving a collarette of scaling. The disease most frequently begins with a single herald or mother patch (Figs. 11-8 and 11-9), usually larger than succeeding

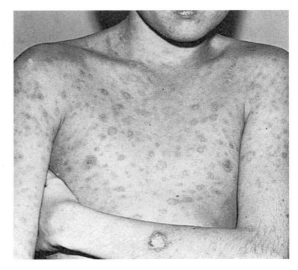

Fig. 11-8 Pityriasis rosea with the herald patch on the forearm. (Courtesy Dr. C.F. Burgoon, Jr.)

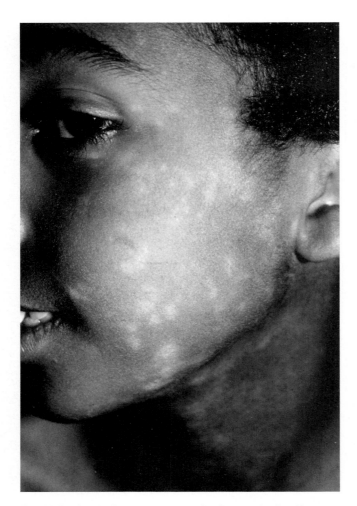

Fig. 11-7 Atypically extensive example of pityriasis alba. (Courtesy Dr. F. Kerdel-Vegas.)

lesions, which may persist a week or more before others appear. By that time involution of the herald patch has begun, the efflorescence of new lesions spreads rapidly, and after 3 to 8 weeks they usually disappear spontaneously.

The incidence is highest between the ages of 15 and 40, and the disease is most prevalent in the spring and autumn. Women are more frequently affected.

The fully developed eruption has a striking appearance because of the distribution and definite characteristics of the individual lesions. These are arranged so that the long axis of the macules runs parallel to the lines of cleavage (Fig. 11-10). The eruption is usually generalized, affecting chiefly the trunk, and sparing sun-exposed surfaces. At times it is localized to a certain area, such as the neck, thighs, groins, or axillae. In these regions confluent circinate patches with gyrate borders may be formed; these may strongly resemble

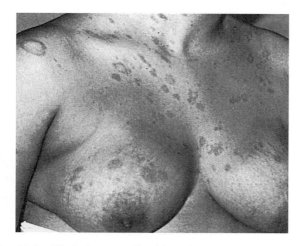

Fig. 11-9 Pityriasis rosea. Herald patch on right shoulder with central clearing.

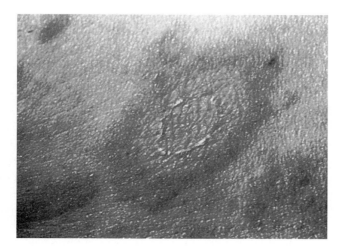

Fig. 11-10 Pityriasis rosea. Note orientation of lesions along cleavage lines. (Courtesy Dr. Axel W. Hoke.)

tinea corporis (tinea circinata). Rarely, the eyelids, scalp, or penis may be involved. Sometimes involvement of the scalp is encountered. Purpuric pityriasis rosea may manifest with petechiae and ecchymoses along Langer's lines of the neck, trunk, and proximal extremities. Oral lesions are relatively uncommon. They are asymptomatic, erythematous macules with raised borders and clearing centers or aphthous, ulcerlike lesions. They involve simultaneously with the skin lesions.

Moderate pruritus may be present, particularly during the outbreak, and there may be mild constitutional symptoms before the onset. Variations in the mode of onset, course, and clinical manifestations are extremely common. An unusual form, common in children under age 5, is that of papular pityriasis rosea, occurring in the typical sites and running a course similar to that of the common form of pityriasis rosea. Black children are particularly predisposed to this papular variant. An inverse distribution, sparing covered areas, is unusual but not rare (Fig. 11-11). It is common in papular cases. Relapses and recurrences are observed infrequently.

Etiology

The etiology of pityriasis rosea remains unknown. A viral infection is most frequently suggested but remains unproved. It does not occur in epidemic forms. The formation of a herald patch, the self-limited course, the seasonal preponderance, and rare recurrence are all suggestive of a viral infection. On the other hand, cases only rarely occur either together or consecutively in the same household.

A pityriasis rosea–like eruption may occur as a reaction to captopril, arsenicals, gold, bismuth, clonidine, methoxypromazine, tripelennamine hydrochloride, or barbiturates.

Histology

The histologic features of pityriasis rosea include mild acanthosis, focal parakeratosis, and extravasation of erythrocytes into the epidermis. Spongiosis may be present in acute cases. A mild perivascular infiltrate of lymphocytes is found in the dermis. Histologic evaluation is especially helpful in excluding the conditions with which pityriasis rosea may be confused.

Differential Diagnosis

Pityriasis rosea may closely mimic seborrheic dermatitis, tinea circinata, the macular syphilid, drug eruption, viral exanthema, and psoriasis. In seborrheic dermatitis the scalp and eyebrows are usually scaly and there is a predilection for the sternal and interscapular regions, and the flexor surfaces of the articulations, where the patches are covered with greasy scales. Tinea corporis is rarely so widespread. Tinea versicolor may also closely simulate pityriasis rosea. A positive KOH examination serves well to differentiate these last two. In the macular syphilid the lesions are of a uniform size and soon assume a brownish tint. Scaling and

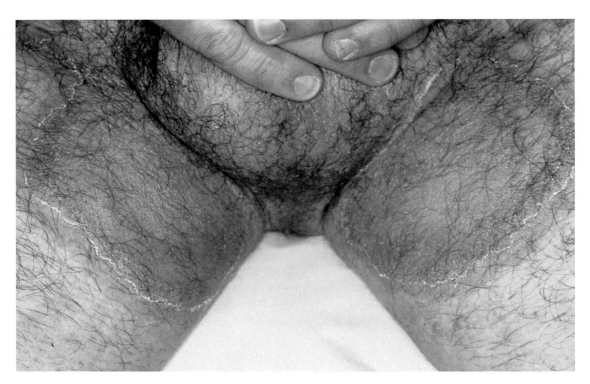

Fig. 11-11 Inverse pityriasis rosea. (Courtesy Dr. Axel W. Hoke.)

itching are absent or slight, and there are generalized adenopathy, mucous membrane lesions, palmoplantar lesions, positive nontreponemal and treponemal tests, and often the remains of a chancre. Scabies and lichen planus may be confused with the papular type.

Treatment

Treatment is symptomatic. The duration may be notably reduced by appropriate therapy.

Ultraviolet B in erythema exposures should be used to expedite the involution of the lesions after the acute inflammatory stage has passed. The erythema produced by ultraviolet treatment is succeeded by superficial exfoliation. In a comparison study by Leenutaphong et al using a "placebo" of 1 joule UVA on the untreated side compared with the UVB-treated side, there was significant improvement in the severity of the disease on the treated side. However, there was no difference in the symptoms of itching or the course of the disease. Addition of topical steroids should be used for symptomatic relief.

Pruritus may uncommonly be intense and lead to eczematization and secondary infection as a result of scratching. Corticosteroid lotions, creams, or sprays give immediate relief. Antihistamines by mouth are also beneficial. For severe generalized forms a short course of systemic corticosteroids or one intramuscular injection of triamcino-

lone diacetate or acetonide, 20 to 40 mg, may be in order. For dryness and irritation, simple emollients are advised.

Allen RA, et al: Pityriasis rosea. *Cutis* 1995, 56:198.
Drago F, et al: Human herpesvirus 7 in patients with pityriasis rosea: electron microscopy investigations and polymerase chain reaction in mononuclear cells, plasma and skin. *Dermatology* 1997, 195:374.
Hartley A: Pityriasis rosea. *Pediatr Rev* 1999, 20:266.
Kempf W, et al: Pityriasis rosea is not associated with human herpesvirus 7. *Arch Dermatol* 1999, 135:1070.
Leenutaphong V, et al: UVB phototherapy for pityriasis rosea: a bilateral comparison study. *J Am Acad Dermatol* 1995, 33:996.
Pierson JC, et al: Purpuric pityriasis rosea. *J Am Acad Dermatol* 1993, 28:1021. ▲

PITYRIASIS RUBRA PILARIS
Clinical Features

Pityriasis rubra pilaris (PRP) is a chronic skin disease characterized by small follicular papules, disseminated yellowish pink scaling patches, and, often, solid confluent palmoplantar hyperkeratosis (Fig. 11-12). The papules are the most important diagnostic feature, being more or less acuminate, reddish brown, about pinhead size, and topped by a central horny plug (Fig. 11-13). In the horny center a hair, or part of one, is usually embedded. The disease

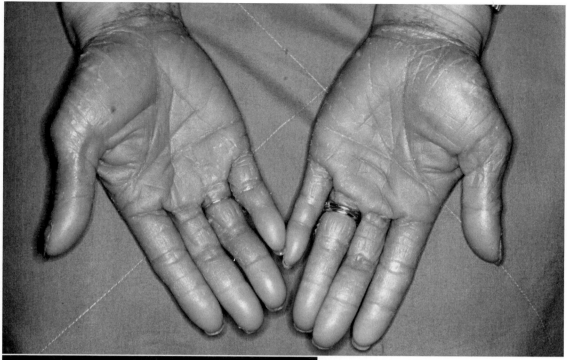

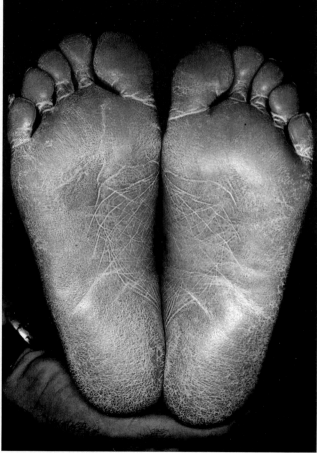

Fig. 11-12 Palms and soles of a woman with pityriasis rubra pilaris. (Courtesy Dr. L. Dantzig.)

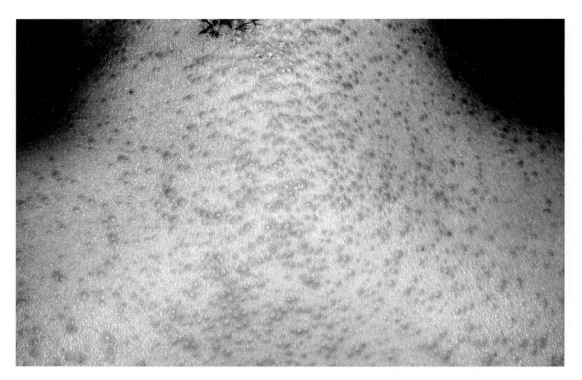

Fig. 11-13 Follicular keratotic papules characterize pityriasis rubra pilaris.

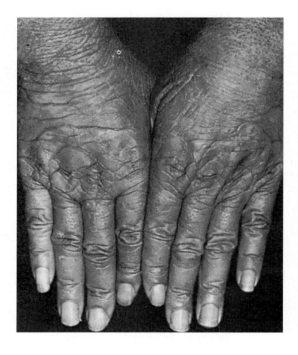

Fig. 11-14 Pityriasis rubra pilaris. Note the horny plugs on the backs of proximal phalanges and on the wrists. (Courtesy Dr. L. Fragola.)

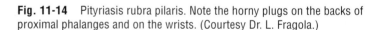

generally manifests itself first by scaliness and erythema of the scalp. The eruption is limited in the beginning, having a predilection for the sides of the neck and trunk and the extensor surfaces of the extremities, especially the backs of the first and second phalanges. Then, as new lesions occur, extensive areas are converted into sharply marginated patches of various sizes, which look like exaggerated goose-flesh and feel like a nutmeg grater. Any portion of the body area or the entire surface may be affected (Figs. 11-14 to 11-16).

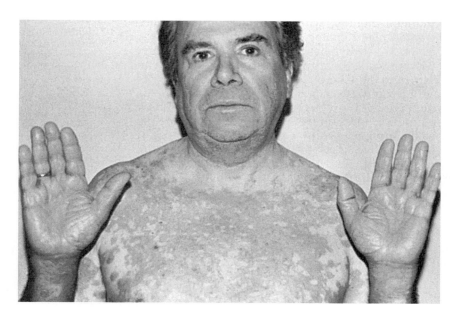

Fig. 11-15 Pityriasis rubra pilaris. Note sparing of islands of normal skin. (Courtesy Dr. Axel W. Hoke.)

The involvement is generally symmetrical and diffuse, with, however, characteristic small islands of normal skin within the affected areas. There is a hyperkeratosis of the palms and soles, with a tendency to fissures. On the soles especially, the hyperkeratosis typically extends up the sides, and is so solid that it has been called a "sandal." The nails may be dull, rough, thickened, brittle, and striated, and are apt to crack and break (Fig. 11-17). They are rarely, if ever, pitted. In the study by Sonnex et al, no pits were seen in the nails of 24 adult patients with PRP, but pits were found in 97% of patients with psoriasis. The exfoliation may become generalized and the follicular lesions less noticeable, finally disappearing and leaving a widespread dry, scaly erythroderma. The skin becomes dull red, glazed, and atrophic, sensitive to slight changes in temperature, and, over the bony prominences, subject to ulcerations.

There are no subjective symptoms except itching in some cases. Koebner's phenomenon may be present. The general health in most patients is not affected. A number of cases of associated malignancy have recently been reported, to include Kaposi's sarcoma, leukemia, and basal cell, lung, unknown primary metastatic and hepatocellular carcinoma. It remains to be established whether these are true associations or chance findings. Castanet et al reported a case of juvenile PRP associated with *Staphylococcus aureus* folliculitis, furunculosis, and sepsis that was subsequently found to have hypogammaglobulinemia.

PRP may be classified in respect to familial or acquired types and in respect to the onset of the disease in childhood or in adulthood. Griffith's classification is useful in this regard. Type I, the classic adult type, is seen most commonly and carries the best prognosis, with 80%

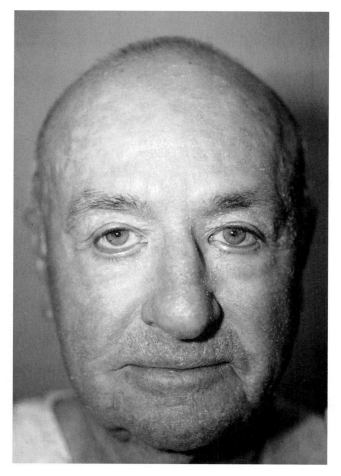

Fig. 11-16 Pityriasis rubra pilaris.

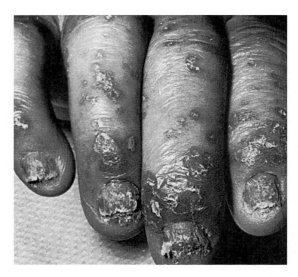

Fig. 11-17 Nail changes in pityriasis rubra pilaris. (Courtesy Dr. L. Dantzig.)

involuting over a 3-year period. Three types of juvenile-onset forms account for up to 40% of cases, with a poor prognosis for involution. Accordingly, the highest incidence is during the first 5 years of life or between ages 51 and 55.

Etiology

The etiology is unknown. The tendency to this disease is usually transmitted as an autosomal dominant characteristic in juvenile-onset PRP. Either sex may be affected, with equal frequency. Both clinically and histologically, the disease has many features that suggest it is a vitamin deficiency disorder, particularly of vitamin A. Some reports of patients with low serum levels of retinol-binding protein have appeared, but this is not a reproducible finding.

Histology

There is hyperkeratosis, follicular plugging, and focal parakeratosis at the follicular orifice. The inflammatory infiltrate in the dermis is composed of mononuclear cells and is generally mild. Specimens should be obtained from skin sites where hair follicles are numerous. Although there may be difficulty in making an unequivocal histologic diagnosis of pityriasis rubra pilaris, one can at least rule out the diagnosis of psoriasis, which is the most common clinical entity in the differential diagnosis.

Diagnosis

The diagnosis of fully developed PRP is rarely difficult because of its distinctive features, such as the peculiar orange or salmon-yellow color of the follicular papules, containing a horny center, on the backs of the fingers, sides of the neck, and extensor surfaces of the limbs; the thickened, rough, and slightly or moderately scaly, harsh

skin; the sandal-like palmoplantar hyperkeratosis; and the islands of normal skin in the midst of the eruption (see Fig. 11-15). It is distinguished from psoriasis by the scales, which in the latter are silvery, light, and overlap like shingles, and by the papules, which extend peripherally to form patches. Lichen planus has characteristics such as shiny plaques of a violaceous or dark red hue and flattened, angular, shiny papules that rarely involve the face, scalp, and palms. Phrynoderma caused by vitamin A deficiency gives a somewhat similar appearance to the skin, as may also eczematous eruptions caused by vitamin B deficiency. Rheumatologic disorders such as subacute cutaneous lupus erythematosus and dermatomyositis may present with similar cutaneous findings.

Treatment

The management of pityriasis rubra pilaris has changed markedly in recent years; however, symptomatic treatment is still important. Topical applications of bland emollients are recommended. Lac-Hydrin is particularly helpful.

Systemic retinoids are effective. A several-month course of isotretinoin in doses of 0.5 to 2 mg/kg/day may induce prolonged remissions or cures. Vitamin A in doses of 300,000 to 500,000 units daily, with the possible addition of vitamin E, 400 units two or three times daily, is often effective, but the synthetic retinoids are preferable.

Response to topical corticosteroids are variable, and as a rule not very effective. Systemic steroids are beneficial for acute short-term management, but are not recommended on a regular basis.

Methotrexate therapy has been used with good results in doses of 2.5 mg orally alternating one day with 5 mg the next. A continuous daily regimen has been purported to be superior to the one-day-a-week approach that many utilize. Clayton et al reported a series of 24 patients, 22 of whom were treated with a combination of isotretinoin or acitretin and low-dose methotrexate (weekly doses ranging from 5 to 30 mg). Seventeen patients showed 25% to 75% response rates after 16 weeks of therapy. Azathioprine has also been reported to be effective in a small series of patients. Extracorporeal photochemotherapy has been used successfully in combination with systemic retinoids and cyclosporine in the most severe cases.

Monitoring and treatment for secondary infections with antibiotics is important with any generalized cutaneous disorder, particularly PRP or psoriasis.

Albert MR, et al: Pityriasis rubra pilaris. *Int J Dermatol* 1999, 38:1.

Boyd AS, et al: PRP presenting as subacute cutaneous lupus erythematosus. *Cutis* 1993, 52:177.

Castanet J, et al: Juvenile PRP associated with hypogammaglobulinemia and furunculosis. *Br J Dermatol* 1994, 131:717.

Clayton BD, et al: Adult PRP: A 10-year case series. *J Am Acad Dermatol* 1997, 36:959.

Dicken CH: Treatment of classic PRP. *J Am Acad Dermatol* 1994, 31:997.

Goldsmith LA, et al: PRP: Response to 13-cis retinoic acid. *J Am Acad Dermatol* 1982, 6:710.

Griffiths WAD: PRP: clinical features and natural history in a study of 93 patients. *Br J Dermatol* 1977, 97(Suppl 15):18.

Hofer A, et al: Extracorporeal photochemotherapy for treatment of erythrodermic pityriasis rubra pilaris. *Arch Dermatol* 1999, 135:475.

Requena L, et al: Dermatomyositis with a pityriasis rubra-like eruption. *Br J Dermatol* 1997, 136:768.

Sanchez-Regana M, et al: PRP as the initial manifestation of internal neoplasia. *Clin Exp Dermatol* 1995, 20:436.

Sharma S, et al: PRP as an initial presentation of hepatocellular carcinoma. *Dermatology* 1997, 194:166.

Sonnex TS, et al: The nails in adult type 1 PRP. *J Am Acad Dermatol* 1986, 15:956.

Tannenbaum CB, et al: Multiple cutaneous malignancies in a patient with PRP and focal acantholytic dyskeratosis. *J Am Acad Dermatol* 1996, 35:781.

Vanderhooft SL, et al: Familial pityriasis rubra pilaris. *Arch Dermatol* 1995, 131:448.

CHAPTER 12

Lichen Planus and Related Conditions

LICHEN PLANUS

Lichen planus is a common, pruritic, inflammatory disease of the skin, hair follicles, and mucous membranes. It occurs throughout the world, in all races. It may be familial in 1% to 2% of cases. It appears in men at a constant rate from the early twenties through the sixties, whereas in women the rate of new cases continues to increase with increasing age, reaching a peak in the sixties. The primary lesions of lichen planus are characteristic, almost pathognomonic, small, violaceous, flat-topped, polygonal papules. The color of the lesions initially is erythematous, but well developed lesions are violaceous. Older and resolving lesions are often hyperpigmented. The surface is glistening, dry, with scant, adherent scales. On the surface, gray or white puncta or streaks (Wickham's striae) (Fig. 12-1) cross the lesions. Lesions begin as pinpoint papules and expand to 0.5- to 1.0-cm plaques. Infrequently, larger lesions are seen. There is a predilection for the flexor wrists (Fig. 12-2), trunk, medial thighs (Fig. 12-3), shins, dorsal hands (Fig. 12-4, *A*), and glans penis. The face is only rarely involved, and when it is, lesions are usually confined to the eyelids or lips, or both. The palms and soles may be affected with plaques or small papules (Fig. 12-4, *B*). Koebner's phenomenon occurs in lichen planus.

Pruritus is often prominent in lichen planus. The pruritus may precede the appearance of the skin lesions, and, as with scabies, the intensity of the itch may seem out of proportion to the amount of skin disease. It may be almost intolerable in acute cases. The pruritus occurs in spasms and causes frenzied itching that lasts for minutes to hours and then gradually subsides. Most patients react to the itching of lichen planus by rubbing rather than scratching and consequently scratch marks are usually not discernible.

The natural history of lichen planus is highly variable, and dependent on the site of involvement and the clinical pattern. Two thirds of patients with skin lesions will have lichen planus less than 1 year, and many patients spontaneously clear in the second year. Mucous membrane disease is much more chronic. Recurrences are not uncommon, occurring in up to half of patients.

Lichen planus is uncommon in children. Children represent only 4% of cases of lichen planus, and their lesions are often atypical. Linear or zosteriform patterning, prominent follicular involvement, significant nail changes with deformities, and a long course are common in children. Classic lesions are uncommon. Children with lichen planus often have affected family members. Children from the Indian subcontinent appear to have lichen planus more frequently.

Nail changes are present in approximately 5% to 10% of patients. Subungual papules may cause thickening and malformation of the nails with tumefaction of the matrix region (Fig. 12-5, *A*). Pterygium formation is characteristic of lichen planus of the nails (Fig. 12-5, *B*). The nail matrix is destroyed by the inflammation and replaced by fibrosis. The proximal nail fold fuses with the proximal portion of the nail bed. Involvement of the entire matrix may lead to obliteration of the whole nail. Longitudinal grooving, proximal and distal onycholysis, ridging, and splitting and a peculiar midline fissure are some of the manifestations of lichen planus of the nails. Some cases of twenty-nail dystrophy of childhood may represent lichen planus involving only the nails.

The mucous membranes, especially the oral mucosa, are frequently affected. Twenty percent of patients with oral lichen planus will also have skin lesions. Oral lesions may be reticulate, atrophic, or ulcerative (erosive). Patients may simultaneously have several patterns. The most common pattern in oral lichen planus is the ulcerative form, occurring in just under half of patients. In oral lichen planus the "classic" reticulate lesions represent about a third of cases, and about one fifth have atrophic lesions. Reticulate lesions are usually located on the inner sides of the cheeks, but any site may be involved (Fig. 12-6). Lesions consist of pinhead-sized, silvery-white papules that form annular or linear patterns, appear as discrete puncta, or, most commonly, form irregular reticulated or lacelike patterns. Similar lesions may occur on the palate, lips (Fig. 12-7), and tongue (Fig. 12-8). In the last two locations they are less characteristic and may be mistaken for leukoplakia. On the

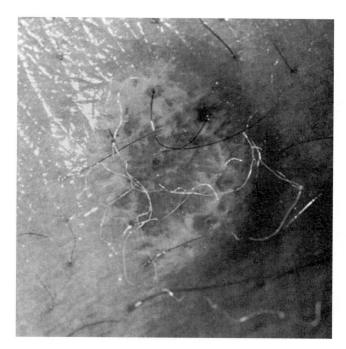

Fig. 12-1 Wickham's striae in lichen planus. (Courtesy Dr. Axel W. Hoke.)

lips the papules are often annular, but may be erosive. Oral lichen planus is stable but chronic, with less than 3% having a spontaneous remission in an average 5-year follow-up.

Involvement of the genitalia, with or without lesions at other sites, is common. On the glans penis the lesions consist of flat, polygonal papules, or may be arranged in rings. On the labia and anus similar lesions are observed; they are generally whitish, owing to maceration. In the vulvovaginal areas, erosive or ulcerative disease is common, and may coexist with typical reticulate lesions.

There are many clinical variants of lichen planus. Whether these represent separate diseases or part of the lichen planus spectrum is unknown. They all demonstrate typical lichen planus histologically. They are described separately, since their clinical features are distinct from classic lichen planus. Some patients with these clinical variants may have typical skin lesions of classic lichen planus as well. The more common or well known variants are described below.

Linear Lichen Planus (Zosteriform Lichen Planus)

Small linear lesions caused by Koebner's phenomenon often occur in classic lichen planus. Limitation of lichen planus to one band or streak has also been described in less than 1% of patients, except in Japan, where up to 10% of reported cases are linear (Fig. 12-9). Although originally suspected as following dermatomes (zosteri-

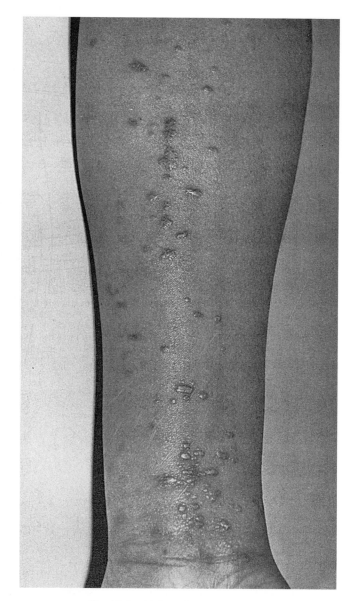

Fig. 12-2 Lichen planus on forearm.

form), recent reports suggest the lesions actually follow Blaschko's lines.

Annular Lichen Planus

Most frequently, annular configurations of lichen planus are located on the lips or penis (Fig. 12-10), although they may be found scattered on the skin, especially in the axilla or groin. The ringed lesions are composed of small papules and measure about 1 cm in diameter. Central hyperpigmentation may be the dominant feature. They may coalesce to form polycyclic figures. Annular lesions may also result from central involution of flat papules or plaques, forming lesions with violaceous, elevated borders and central hyperpigmented macules.

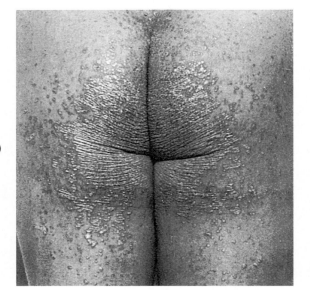

Fig. 12-3 Acute widespread lichen planus. (Courtesy Dr. L. Schweich.)

A

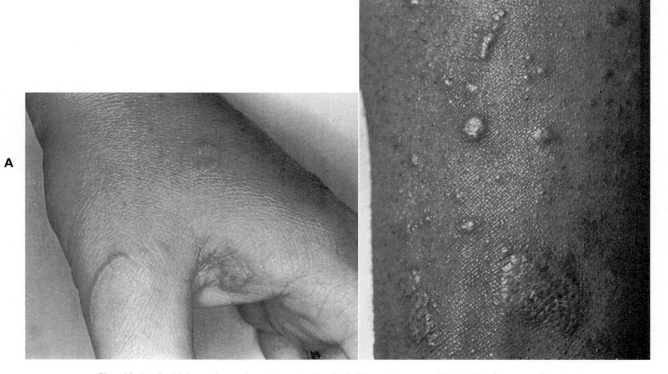

Fig. 12-4 **A,** Lichen planus involving the hand *(left)* and forearm *(right).* (**A,** Courtesy Dr. Axel W. Hoke.)

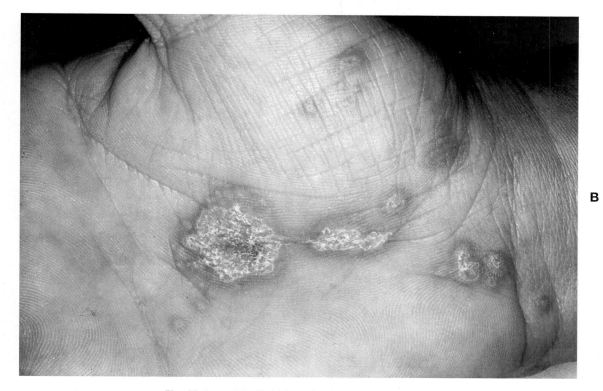

Fig. 12-4, cont'd B, Lichen planus of palmar surfaces.

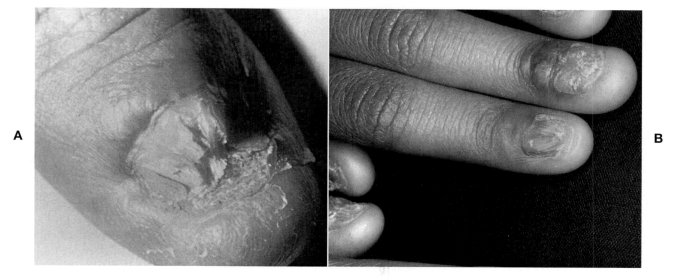

Fig. 12-5 A, Lichen planus of the nails. Note pterygium formation. **B,** Lichen planus of the nails.
(**A,** Courtesy Dr. Axel W. Hoke.)

Hypertrophic Lichen Planus (Lichen Planus Verrucosus)

Hypertrophic lichen planus occurs most commonly on the shins, although it may be situated anywhere. The typical lesions are verrucous plaques with variable amounts of scale, from minimal to very marked (Fig. 12-11). At the edges of the plaques, small, flat-topped, polygonal papules may be discovered on careful search. Superficial inspection of the lesion often suggests psoriasis rather than lichen planus. The lesions are of variable size, but frequently larger than the lesions of classic lichen planus. The clinical diagnosis is made from the violaceous color of the lesions,

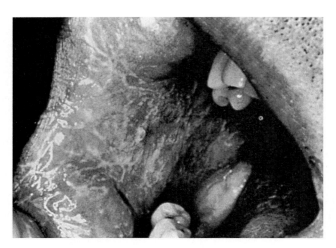

Fig. 12-6 Lichen planus of the buccal mucosa. (Courtesy Dr. Axel W. Hoke.)

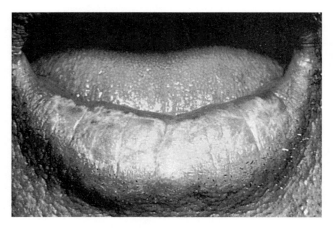

Fig. 12-7 Lichen planus of the lips. (Courtesy Dr. Axel W. Hoke.)

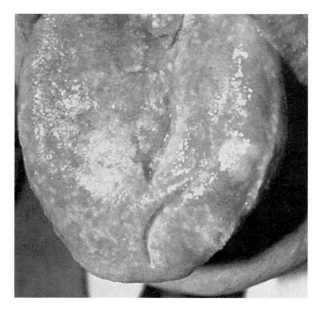

Fig. 12-8 Lichen planus of the tongue.

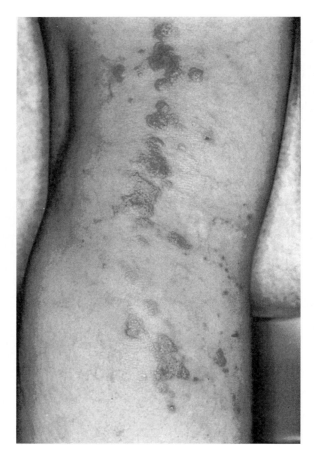

Fig. 12-9 Linear lichen planus.

their thickening and scales, the itching, and the symmetric location on the shins, usually without any other skin lesions. Hypertrophic lichen planus represents lichen planus with simultaneous changes of lichen simplex chronicus.

Ulcerative Lichen Planus

Ulcerative lichen planus is rare on the skin but common on the mucous membranes. Typical skin lesions of lichen planus rarely ulcerate. A rare ulcerative variant of cutaneous lichen planus affects the feet and toes, causing bullae, ulcerations, and permanent loss of the toenails. These chronic ulcerations on the feet are painful and disabling. Cicatricial alopecia may be present on the scalp, and the buccal mucosa may also be affected. Skin grafting of the soles has produced successful results.

Although erosion or ulceration is rare in cutaneous lichen planus, in the oral mucosa this is the most common form, and it is usually chronic. Lesions appear on any portion of the mouth, and multisite involvement is common. The buccal mucosa is involved in 90%, the gingiva in more than half, and the tongue in about 40%. On the gingiva, lichen planus may produce desquamative gingivitis. Erosive lichen planus commonly causes discomfort or pain.

Involvement of the vulva and vagina with lichen planus, along with gingivitis, has been described as the

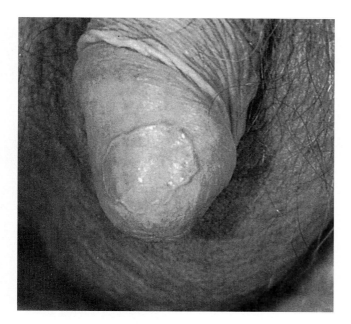

Fig. 12-10 Annular lichen planus on glans penis.

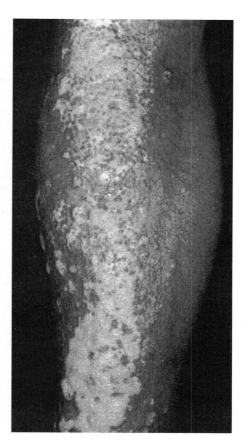

Fig. 12-11 Hypertrophic lichen planus.

vulvovaginal-gingival syndrome. Although all three of these mucous membranes may be involved, the disease may begin on one and later appear on another, or appearance on the various mucous membranes may be simultaneous. This characteristic has resulted in expansion of the spectrum of lichen planus and demonstrates that erosive disease of the female genitalia is more frequently present than previously appreciated (Fig. 12-12). These women have vulvar pain or burning; however, many women with lichen planus will not volunteer their vulvovaginal complaints unless specifically asked. The vulva has lesions very similar to oral lichen planus, with erythema, leukokeratosis, and erosion. Surrounding the red or eroded lesions is a narrow rim of white reticulation. This rim is the most fruitful area to biopsy to confirm the diagnosis. The vaginal mucosa is involved in two thirds of the patients. Scarring of the vagina and vulva with adhesions, vestibular bands, and atrophy of the labia minora or prepuce occur, making the morphology similar to vulvar lichen sclerosus. In one third, typical reticulate buccal lichen planus is seen, and 10% have cutaneous lichen planus.

Cancer Risk and Lichen Planus

Rare cases of squamous cell carcinoma of the skin occurring on the lower leg in lesions of hypertrophic lichen planus have been reported. These patients had also received agents known to be carcinogenic (arsenic and radiation therapy). There is no statistical increase in cutaneous or visceral carcinoma in patients with lichen planus. Oral lichen planus does appear, however, to increase the risk of developing oral squamous cell carcinoma. Overall, about 1 in 200 patients with cutaneous lichen planus will develop oral squamous cell carcinoma. If only patients with oral lichen planus are considered, the risk may be as high as 1% over a 3-year period. Most cases of oral squamous cell carcinoma occur in patients with erosive oral lichen planus. Similarly, squamous cell carcinoma may develop in erosive lichen planus of the vagina or anus. Erosive mucosal lichen planus is thus best considered a potentially premalignant condition, and clinicians should have a low threshold to biopsy fixed erosive or leukokeratotic lesions.

Hepatitis-Associated Lichen Planus

Hepatitis C virus infection is found in proportionately more patients with lichen planus than in controls. Depending on the background rate of hepatitis C virus infection in the region, between 4% and 38% of lichen planus patients may have coexistent hepatitis C infection. In northern Japan, where the seroprevalence of hepatitis C virus infection is 8%, 60% of patients with oral lichen planus had hepatitis C virus infection. One group has reported that 5% of all hepatitis C-virus–infected patients have lichen planus. The clinical features of lichen planus are identical in patients with and without hepatitis C infection, but lichen planus patients with hepatitis C infection are more likely to have erosive mucous membrane disease. The existence of underlying hepatitis cannot be predicted by clinical pattern or the results of liver function tests. Treatment of hepatitis C

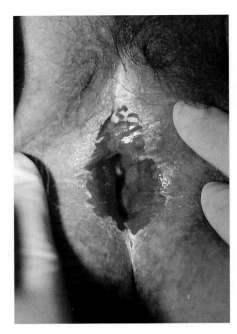

Fig. 12-12 Erosive vulvar lichen planus. (Courtesy Dr. E. Klemperer.)

with alfa interferon may be associated with initial appearance of the lichen planus or exacerbate it. Lichen planus may also clear or not change with this treatment. Primary biliary cirrhosis and lichen planus may coexist. Patients with this liver abnormality, in addition, have a marked propensity to develop a lichenoid eruption while on D-penicillamine therapy.

Lichen Planus–Lupus Erythematosus Overlap

This unusual variant of lichen planus presents with discoid lesions with central atrophy and hypopigmentation outlined by a reddish purple periphery. They typically are atrophic centrally. Lesions are fixed, have a predilection for acral areas, especially the dorsal hands and feet, and digits, but may be widespread. Palm and sole involvement is common. Nail dystrophy is frequent, often resulting in anonychia. Scarring scalp lesions and oral lesions can occur. The course is chronic. The histologic and immunopathologic features are most consistent with the diagnosis of lichen planus, but in some cases coexistent features of lupus erythematosus are found.

Bullous Lichen Planus

Two forms of lichen planus may be accompanied by bullae. In classic lichen planus, usually on the lower extremities, individual lesions will vesiculate centrally. This represents macroscopic exaggeration of the subepidermal space formed by the lichenoid interface reaction destroying the basal keratinocytes. These lesions often spontaneously resolve.

Lichen planus pemphigoides describes a rare subset of patients who usually have typical lichen planus, then develop blistering on their lichen planus lesions and on normal skin. Less commonly the blistering antedates the lichen planus. They clinically appear to be a combination of lichen planus and bullous pemphigoid. Oral disease may occur and resemble either lichen planus or pemphigoid. Histologically, the lichen planus lesions show lichen planus and the bullous lesions the features of bullous pemphigoid. On direct immunofluorescence the features of bullous pemphigoid are found. The antigen targeted by the autoantibody is located in the same region as the bullous pemphigoid antigens (at the basal hemidesmosomes). Antibodies from patients with lichen planus pemphigoides bind the 180 Kd bullous pemphigoid antigen (BPAg2) and, in some cases, perhaps other less well-defined molecules. Treatment is similar to bullous pemphigoid, with potent topical steroids, systemic steroids, tetracycline, and nicotinamide, isotretinoin, and immunosuppressives all being variably effective.

Pathogenesis and Histology

Lichen planus is characterized by an immunologic reaction of primarily helper T cells along the basal cell layer. The cause of this reaction is unknown. Although human papilloma virus (HPV) was reported in oral lichen planus lesions by polymerase chain reaction (PCR), studies on cutaneous lichen planus have been negative, making HPV unlikely as the antigenic target of this attack. The association of hepatitis C virus with lichen planus is well documented, but how this results in clinical lesions is unknown. Increased sensitivity of mast cells from lichen planus to substance P suggests neuropeptides may be important.

The histologic features of lichen planus are distinctive and vary with the stage of the lesion. In early lesions there is an interface dermatitis along the dermoepidermal junction. As the lesion evolves, the epidermis takes on a characteristic appearance. There is a "saw-tooth" pattern of epidermal hyperplasia together with orthokeratosis and hypergranulosis. There is vacuolar alteration of the basal layer of the epidermis. The basal cells are lost, so the basal layer is described as "squamatized." Necrotic keratinocytes are present in the basal layer. In the superficial dermis there is a dense, bandlike infiltrate composed of lymphocytes, histiocytes, and melanophages. "Civatte bodies" represent necrotic keratinocytes in the dermis. In idiopathic lichen planus, the necrotic keratinocytes rarely are eliminated through the epidermis, in contrast to other lichenoid interface reactions, especially lichenoid drug eruptions. Hypertrophic lichen planus shows the histologic features of lichen simplex chronicus superimposed on those of lichen planus.

Lichen planopilaris and Graham Little–Piccardi-Lassueur syndrome show the findings of lichen planus, centered on the superficial follicular epithelium. On direct immunofluorescence, clumps of IgM and less frequently IgA, IgG, and C3 are commonly present subepidermally, corresponding to the colloid bodies. A lichenoid drug eruption may be difficult to differentiate histologically from lichen planus. The presence of eosinophils supports drug as a cause, but these are not universally present, especially if the drug eruption is photodistributed. Graft-versus-host disease tends to have a sparser infiltrate and may show satellite cell necrosis. In lupus erythematosus, there is a greater tendency for epidermal atrophy with parakeratosis, dermal mucin is found, and follicular plugging may be seen. The infiltrate in lupus tends to surround and involve the appendageal structures.

Differential Diagnosis

Classic lichen planus displays lesions that are so characteristic that clinical examination is often adequate to suspect the diagnosis. Lichenoid drug eruptions may be difficult to distinguish. A lichenoid drug reaction should be suspected if the eruption is photodistributed, scaly but not hypertrophic, or confluent or widespread—clinical features that are unusual for idiopathic lichen planus. The presence of oral mucosa involvement may help one to suspect lichen planus, but oral lesions may occur in lichenoid drug eruptions as well. As with other common diseases, atypical cases are not rare, and lichen planus may thus mimic many diseases. Pityriasis rosea (Fig. 12-13), psoriasis guttata, the small-papular or lichenoid syphilid, and pityriasis lichenoides et varioliformis acuta are dermatoses that may resemble generalized lichen planus. Mucous membrane lesions may be confused with leukoplakia, lupus erythematosus, mucous patches of syphilis, candidiasis, cancer, and the oral lesions of autoimmune bullous diseases such as pemphigus or cicatricial pemphigoid. On the scalp the atrophic lesions may be mistaken for other cicatricial alopecias such as lupus erythematosus, folliculitis decalvans, and pseudopelade of Brocq. Hypertrophic lichen planus type may simulate psoriasis, Kaposi's sarcoma, and squamous cell carcinoma in situ. Isolated patches of lichen planus may resemble lichen simplex chronicus or, if heavily pigmented, may suggest a fixed drug eruption.

Treatment

Treatment of lichen planus is difficult. Limited lesions may be treated with super potent topical steroids or intralesional steroid injections. In patients with widespread disease, these treatments are usually unsatisfactory. Widespread lesions respond well to systemic corticosteroids but tend to relapse as the dose is reduced. PUVA may be used. Isotretinoin and acetretin in doses similar to or slightly lower than used for psoriasis may also be useful and avoid the long-term complications of systemic steroids. Low–molecular-weight heparin (enoxaparin), 3 mg injected subcutaneously once weekly, was highly efficacious for cutaneous, but not oral, lichen planus in one study. Cyclosporine in typical psoriasis

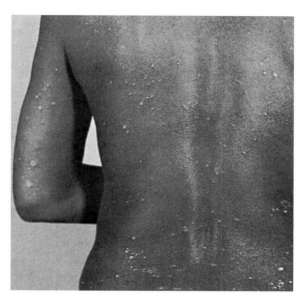

Fig. 12-13 Acute widespread lichen planus resembling pityriasis rosea. (Courtesy J.L. Miller.)

doses is very beneficial, but because of its potential toxicities, its use is reserved for only the most severe cases. A durable remission is sometimes achieved with cyclosporine therapy. Dapsone, metronidazole, and griseofulvin have been anecdotally successful but are frequently ineffective.

For oral lesions, mixtures of superpotent steroids in Orabase may be useful. Vinyl dental trays may be used to apply steroid ointments to the gingiva. Begin with 30-minute applications three times daily and reduce to maintenance of 20 minutes every evening. Topical tretinoin may be added to the topical steroids. Intralesional injections may be used for focal unresponsive lesions. Topical tetracycline can be tried. In refractory oral cases, cyclosporine mouthwash may be beneficial. Hydroxychloroquine, 200 to 400 mg daily for 6 months, was reported to produce an excellent response in 9 of 10 patients with oral lichen planus. The systemic agents recommended above to treat cutaneous lichen planus may also improve oral disease. For vulvovaginal-gingival syndrome, corticosteroids topically and systemically are beneficial. Topical therapy with corticosteroids may be enhanced by mixing the steroid in vaginal bioadhesive moisturizer (Replens). Iontophoresis may improve delivery. Retinoids may also be used. Cyclosporine is virtually always beneficial.

Boyd AS, et al: Absence of human papillomavirus infection in cutaneous lichen planus. *J Am Acad Dermatol* 1997, 36:267.

Clover GB, et al: Is childhood idiopathic atrophy of the nails due to lichen planus? *Br J Dermatol* 1987, 116:709.

Daoud MS, et al: Chronic hepatitis C and skin diseases. *Mayo Clin Proc* 1995, 70:559.

Duschet P, et al: Effect of anatomic location on immunofluorescence in lichen planus. *J Am Acad Dermatol* 1985, 13:1057.

Eisen D: Hydroxychloroquine sulfate (Plaquenil) improves oral lichen planus. *J Am Acad Dermatol* 1993, 28:609.

Eisen D: The vulvovaginal-gingival syndrome of lichen planus. *Arch Dermatol* 1994, 130:1379.

Falk DK, et al: Dapsone in the treatment of erosive lichen planus. *J Am Acad Dermatol* 1985, 12:567.

Fivenson DP, et al: Lichen planus pemphigoides. *J Am Acad Dermatol* 1997, 36:638.

Franck JM, et al: Squamous cell carcinoma in situ arising within lichen planus of the vulva. *Dermatol Surg* 1995, 21:890.

Giustina TA, et al: Isotretinoin gel improves oral lichen planus. *Arch Dermatol* 1986, 122:534.

Gonzalez E, et al: Bilateral comparison of generalized lichen planus treated with psoralens and ultraviolet A. *J Am Acad Dermatol* 1984, 10:958.

Hodak E, et al: Low-dose low-molecular-weight heparin (enoxaparin) is beneficial in lichen planus. *J Am Acad Dermatol* 1998, 38:564.

Holmstrup P, et al: The controversy of a premalignant potential of oral lichen planus is over. *Oral Surg Oral Med Oral Pathol* 1992, 73:704.

Irvine C, et al: Long-term follow-up of lichen planus. *Acta Derm Venereol (Stockh)* 1991, 71:242.

Itin P, et al: Lack of effect after local treatment with a new cyclosporin formulation in recalcitrant erosive oral lichen planus. *Dermatology* 1992, 185:262.

Jubert C, et al: Lichen planus and hepatitis C virus-related chronic active hepatitis. *Arch Dermatol* 1994, 130:73.

Karvonen J, et al: Topical trioxsalen PUVA in lichen planus and nodular prurigo. *Acta Dermatol Venereol (Stockh)* 1985, 120:53.

Kechijian P: Twenty-nail dystrophy of childhood: a reappraisal. *Cutis* 1985, 35:38.

Levy A, et al: Treatment of lichen planus with griseofulvin. *Int J Dermatol* 1986, 25:405.

Lewis FM: Vulval lichen planus. *Br J Dermatol* 1998, 138:569.

Liden C: Lichen planus in relation to occupational and non-occupational exposure to chemicals. *Br J Dermatol* 1986, 115:23.

Long CC, et al: Multiple linear lichen planus in the lines of Blaschko. *Br J Dermatol* 1996, 135:275.

Maceyko RF, et al: Oral and cutaneous lichen planus pemphigoides. *J Am Acad Dermatol* 1992, 27:889.

Milligan A, et al: Lichen planus in children: a review of six cases. *Clin Exp Dermatol* 1990, 15:340.

Moss ALH, et al: Surgery for painful lichen planus of the hand and foot. *Br J Plast Surg* 1986, 39:402.

Nagao Y, et al: Lichen planus and hepatitis C virus in the Northern Kyushu region of Japan. *Eur J Clin Invest* 1995, 25:910.

Pawlotsky JC, et al: Lichen planus and hepatitis C virus-related chronic active hepatitis. *Arch Dermatol* 1994, 130:73.

Pelisse M, The vulvo-vaginal-gingival syndrome. *Int J Dermatol* 1989, 28:381.

Plotnick H, et al: Lichen planus and coexisting LE vs. lichen planus-like LE. *J Am Acad Dermatol* 1986, 14:931.

Powell FC, et al: Primary biliary cirrhosis and lichen planus. *J Am Acad Dermatol* 1983, 9:540.

Protzer U, et al: Exacerbation of lichen planus during interferon alfa-2 therapy for chronic active hepatitis C. *Gastroenterology* 1993, 104:903.

Sanchez-Perez J, et al: Lichen planus and hepatitis C virus: prevalence and clinical presentation of patients with lichen planus and hepatitis C virus infection. *Br J Dermatol* 1996, 134:715.

Schafer JR, et al: Lichen planus-like lesions caused by penicillamine in primary biliary cirrhosis. *Arch Dermatol* 1981, 117:140.

Schlesinger TE, et al: Oral erosive lichen planus with epidermolytic hyperkeratosis during interferon alfa-2b therapy for chronic hepatitis C virus infection. *J Am Acad Dermatol* 1997, 36:1023.

Silverman S, et al: A prospective follow-up study of 570 patients with oral lichen planus. *Oral Surg Oral Med Oral Pathol* 1985, 60:30.

Staus ME, et al: Treatment of lichen planus with low-dose isotretinoin (letter). *J Am Acad Dermatol* 1984, 11:527.

Walchner M, et al: Topical tetracycline treatment of erosive oral lichen planus. *Arch Dermatol* 1999, 135:92.

Walsh DS, et al: A vaginal prosthetic device as an aid in treating ulcerative lichen planus of the mucous membrane. *Arch Dermatol* 1995, 131:265.

Zijdenbos LM, et al: Ulcerative lichen planus with associated sicca syndrome and good therapeutic result of skin grafting. *J Acad Am Dermatol* 1985, 13:667.

Zillikens D, et al: Autoantibodies in lichen planus pemphigoides react to a novel epitope within the C-terminal NC16A domain of BP180. *J Invest Dermatol* 1999, 113:117. _____ ▲

FOLLICULAR LICHEN PLANUS (Lichen Planopilaris)

Follicular lichen planus may involve only the scalp or involve the scalp and other hair-bearing body sites (Graham Little syndrome). It is four times more common in women and appears between ages 30 and 70 in most cases. The hallmark of follicular involvement on the scalp is polygonal patches of scarring alopecia. One or more residual tufts of normal-appearing hair in the areas of cicatricial alopecia is characteristic (Fig. 12-14). Rarely, only nonscalp sites are involved (Fig. 12-15). Initially there is mild erythema around involved follicles. Follicular hyperkeratosis leads to keratotic, sometimes spiny papules. The eruption may not be pruritic. Gradually, hair is lost, and is replaced by smooth skin with loss of follicular markings. A pull test will yield anagen hairs. Clinically, the end-stage lesions are indistinguishable from pseudopelade of Brocq. Kossard has

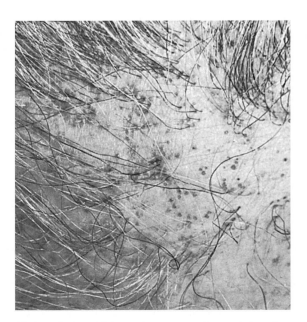

Fig. 12-14 Graham Little syndrome on scalp consisting of acuminate follicular papules, alopecia, and lichen planus. (Courtesy Dr. D. Torre.)

described a series of postmenopausal women with progressive, frontal, cicatricial alopecia that histologically shows features of lichen planopilaris. The eyebrows are also involved. The involvement of the frontal hairline and loss of eyebrows distinguishes these women from patients with pure androgenetic alopecia.

Typical cutaneous and oral lesions of lichen planus may be found in more than half the cases, or there may be a history of prior lichen planus. Histologically, there is lichenoid interface inflammation involving the upper half of the outer root sheath and lower infundibular epithelium. Cytoid bodies may be seen, and follicular fusion is present. Later lesions show marked lamellar perifollicular fibrosis, naked hair shafts in the dermis, and eventually simply scarring along previous follicular tracts.

Graham Little–Piccardi-Lassueur syndrome is characterized by patchy cicatricial alopecia of the scalp and by patches of follicular spinous papules involving the trunk, the upper parts of the arms and legs, and the scalp. There may be typical oral or cutaneous lichen planus. In addition, there may be patches of noncicatricial alopecia in the axillae and pubic areas.

The treatment of localized and generalized lichen planopilaris is very difficult. Topical, intralesional, and systemic steroids are beneficial but have limitations. Antimalarials for a 6-month trial may be attempted. Once hair is lost, the alopecia is permanent.

Headington JT: Cicatricial alopecia. *Dermatol Clin* 1996, 14:773.

Ioannides D, et al: Immunofluorescence abnormalities in lichen planopilaris. *Arch Dermatol* 1992, 128:214.

Kossard S, et al: Postmenopausal frontal fibrosing alopecia. *J Am Acad Dermatol* 1997, 36:59.

Matta M, et al: Lichen planopilaris. *J Am Acad Dermatol* 1990, 22:594.

Mehregan DA, et al: Lichen planopilaris. *J Am Acad Dermatol* 1992, 27:935. ▲

THE "TROPICAL" DYSCHROMIC LICHENOID DISORDERS

This section discusses a disease group that is very common in tropical countries and Japan, and not commonly recognized in Europe and North America. They are all lichenoid dermatoses, but the predominant clinical feature is marked dyschromia, usually hyperpigmentation. Numerous names have been applied to these diseases. In Central America these cases are diagnosed as either lichen planus pigmentosus or erythema dyschromicum perstans, considered there as two distinct entities. In the Middle East and the Indian subcontinent, lichen planus actinicus is the more frequent diagnosis. In Japan, lichen planus pigmentosus is typically seen. Whether these represent variations of one disease or several diseases is unknown.

Lichen Planus Actinicus

Lichen planus actinicus has been variously named *lichen planus actinicus, actinic lichen planus, lichenoid melanodermatitis,* and *summertime actinic lichenoid eruption.* It is a disorder seen most frequently in Africa, the Middle East, and the Indian subcontinent, favoring Asians. Cases are diagnosed clinically and are regionally reasonably uniform. There seems to be a genetic predilection, since Europeans who move into areas of endemicity are not affected by this disorder but regularly develop typical lichen planus. Most cases occur in childhood through young adulthood. It represents a substantial proportion of cases diagnosed as lichen planus in endemic regions.

The disease presents in the spring or summer and is frequently quiescent during the winter. The third decade of life is the primary age of appearance. Lesions favor the sun-exposed parts of the body, especially the face, which is almost always most severely affected. Most lesions occur on the forehead, cheeks, and lips. Outside the face, the V area of the chest, the neck, the backs of the hands, and the lower extensor forearms are involved. Associated pruritus, the hallmark of lichen planus, is usually described as mild or nonexistent. Lesions are usually annular but may be reticulate or diffuse. Individual lesions are often macular but may be plaques with peripheral violaceous papules (Fig. 12-16). Characteristically, lesions are hyperpigmented, sometimes with the blue-gray tinge of dermal melanin. Lesions may resemble melasma.

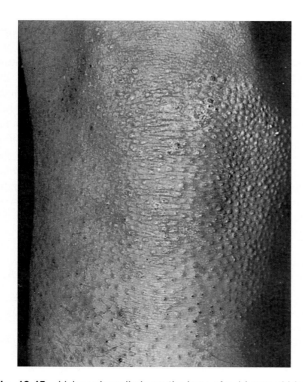

Fig. 12-15 Lichen planopilaris on the knee of a 14-year-old boy.

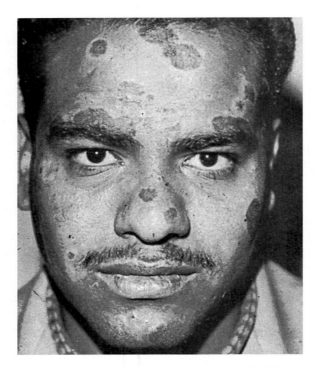

Fig. 12-16 Lichen planus tropicus. (Courtesy Dr. M. El-Zawahry, U.A.R.)

Actinic lichen planus is hypothesized to be elicited by long exposure to sun, particularly in the cases of adolescents and young adults who work all day in the fields. Photo-testing with UVB has not uniformly reproduced the lesions. In cases seen in the United States, blacks have been preferentially affected. Intense sun exposure may be required to elicit the lesions. In one case six times the minimal erythema dose (MED) was applied to reproduce the lesions. Typical lichenoid papules, eczematous-appearing plaques with a lichenoid histology, or lesions with the clinical and histologic features of lichen nitidus (lichen nitidus actinicus) appearing on the dorsal hands may be seen.

Histologically, there are variable degrees of vacuolar alteration along the basal cell layer. Cytoid bodies are sometimes seen. The epidermis is overall thinned, with squamatization of the basal cell layer. An inflammatory infiltrate is found if an infiltrated papule or plaque is biopsied. It will show an inflammatory infiltrate composed of lymphocytes and macrophages along the dermoepidermal junction or around the superficial blood vessels. Some authors describe cases that also have histologic features of dermatitis, with spongiosis. In all cases, incontinence of pigment is prominent, correlating with the prominent dyspigmentation observed clinically.

In summary, sun-induced lichenoid eruptions seem to be common in tropical countries and are not related to medication ingestion. They affect primarily young natives and result in annular hyperpigmented lesions of the face. These cases may represent lichen planus that is sun induced.

The histologic features may be that of lichen planus, but some cases have features of both a lichenoid tissue reaction and a dermatitis, leading some authors to suggest this is a subtype of polymorphous light eruption.

Lichen Planus Pigmentosus

Lichen planus pigmentosus is seen in Central America, the Indian subcontinent, and Japan. These patients may be older, have associated pruritus, lesions in the skin flexors, and sometimes classic lichen planus papules at other sites or at the periphery of their lesions. Facial involvement is still common, and dyspigmentation marked. This appears to represent lichen planus, which resolves with marked hyperpigmentation, probably related to the racial background of the affected patients.

Erythema Dyschromicum Perstans

Erythema dyschromicum perstans is also known as *ashy dermatosis* or *dermatosis cinecienta*. The age of onset is virtually always before 40, but since it is a chronic disease, patients of all ages are seen. Lesions are usually symmetrical and generalized, involving the face, neck, trunk, and proximal extremities. Lesions are of various sizes and shapes, ashy-gray, and macular (Fig. 12-17). Sometimes a characteristic, very fine (several millimeters), erythematous, palpable, nonscaling border is seen at the periphery of the lesions. This is described as feeling like a small cord. Pruritus is not reported, and typical lichenoid papules are said not to occur. Nail and mucosal involvement is not found.

At the active border the characteristic histologic features are those of a lichenoid dermatitis with disruption of the basal layer of the epidermis and a bandlike inflammatory infiltrate in the superficial dermis. In the centers of the lesions, the histologic changes are those of postinflammatory pigmentation; the characteristic gray-blue skin hue reflecting the presence of melanin-laden macrophages in the dermis. Immunofluorescence microscopy reveals numerous cytoid bodies. Because of the active border, this disease was originally considered a form of persistent gyrate erythema. The lichenoid histology clearly confirms it as a lichenoid tissue reaction. Therapeutically, clofazimine appears to benefit virtually all patients, after 3 to 8 months of treatment, with half the patients clearing completely.

Arenas R, et al: Ashy dermatosis and lichen planus pigmentosus. *Int J Dermatol* 1992, 31:90.

Baranda L, et al: Involvement of cell adhesion and activation molecules in the pathogenesis of erythema dyschromicum perstans (ashy dermatitis). *Arch Dermatol* 1997, 133:325.

Berger RS, et al: Erythema dyschromicum perstans and lichen planus? *J Am Acad Dermatol* 1989, 21:438.

Isaacson D, et al: Summertime actinic lichenoid eruption (lichen planus actinicus). *J Am Acad Dermatol* 1981, 4:404.

Piquero-Martin J, et al: Clinical trial with clofazimine for treating erythema dyschromicum perstans. *Int J Dermatol* 1989, 28:198.

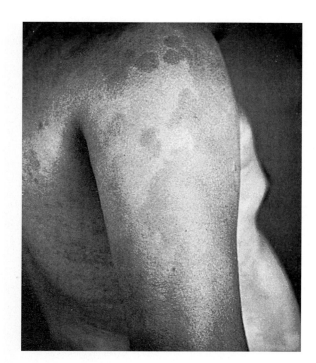

Fig. 12-17 Erythema dyschromicum perstans. (Courtesy Dr. F. Kerdel-Vegas.)

Salmon SM, et al: Actinic lichen planus. *J Am Acad Dermatol* 1989, 20:226.

Verhagen ARHB, et al: Lichenoid melanodermatitis. *Br J Dermatol* 1979, 101:651. ▲

LICHENOID CONTACT DERMATITIS

Lichenoid reactions with histology similar to idiopathic lichen planus may be produced by contact to certain allergens. Derivatives of paraphenylenediamine used in color film developing may result in lichenoid lesions, usually on the dorsal hands. These cases are rare, and patch testing is only recommended in patients with a clear history of such exposure.

Lichenoid reactions of the oral mucosa may be seen adjacent to amalgam fillings. Some of these patients may have widespread lichenoid lesions in the mouth and even on the body. About half of these patients are patch-test positive for mercury compounds. Patients with oral complaints but no lichenoid lesions are rarely patch-test positive. Replacement of the amalgam fillings leads to resolution of the lichenoid lesions and the oral symptoms in more than half the patients with positive patch tests and lichenoid lesions, with partial improvement in the majority. The widespread lichenoid lesions may also clear.

Lane J, et al: Resolution of oral lichenoid lesions after replacement of amalgam restorations in patients allergic to mercury compounds. *Br J Dermatol* 1992, 126:10. ▲

KERATOSIS LICHENOIDES CHRONICA

This very rare dermatosis is characterized by its chronicity. It may begin in childhood or even near birth. The typical lesions are violaceous papulonodular, hyperkeratotic lesions covered with gray scales. These lesions favor the extremities and buttocks. Although initially discrete, the lesions frequently coalesce to form linear and reticulate arrays of warty lichenoid lesions. Keratotic plugs and prominent telangiectasia may be present. The palms and soles may be diffusely thickened or have discrete hyperkeratotic papules. There is an associated sharply marginated erythema, scaling, and telangiectasia of the face superficially resembling seborrheic dermatitis or rosacea. Nail changes, including thickening of the nail plate, yellowing, longitudinal ridging, onycholysis, hyperkeratosis of the nail bed, paronychia, and warty lesions of the periungual areas, have been described. In addition, painful oral aphthaelike lesions often occur. Other findings include keratoconjunctivitis resembling ocular pemphigoid and hoarseness.

Histologically, there is irregular acanthosis, a lichenoid infiltrate consisting of lymphocytes, histiocytes, and plasma cells with foci of vacuolar alteration at the basal cell layer. This condition is usually unresponsive to corticosteroid therapy but may respond to either PUVA or systemic retinoid (etretinate or isotretinoin) therapy.

Baran R, et al: The nails in keratosis lichenoides chronica. *Arch Dermatol* 1984, 120:1471.

David M, et al: Keratosis lichenoides chronica with prominent telangiectasia: response of etretinate. *J Am Acad Dermatol* 1989, 21:1112.

Konstantinov K, et al: Keratosis lichenoides chronica. *J Am Acad Dermatol* 1998, 38:306.

Torrelo A, et al: Keratosis lichenoides chronica in a child. *Pediatr Dermatol* 1994, 11:46. ▲

LICHEN NITIDUS
Clinical Features

Lichen nitidus is a chronic inflammatory disease characterized by minute, shiny, flat-topped, pale, exquisitely discrete, uniform papules, rarely larger than the head of a pin (Fig. 12-18). Usually there is no itching. Linear arrays of papules (Koebner's phenomenon) are common, especially on the forearms. Initially, lesions are localized and often remain so, in such cases being limited to a few areas, chiefly the penis and lower abdomen (Figs. 12-19 and 12-20), the inner surfaces of the thighs, and the flexor aspects of the wrists and forearms. In other cases the disease assumes a more widespread distribution, and the papules fuse into erythematous, finely scaly plaques. The reddish color varies with tints of yellow, brown, or violet. This generalized type of lichen nitidus affects chiefly the groins and thighs, ankles and wrists, feet and hands, the submammary region in women, the folds of the neck, and the extensor surfaces of the elbows.

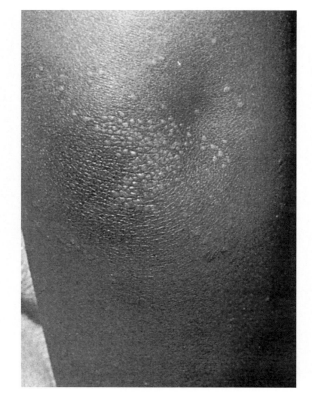

Fig. 12-18 Lichen nitidus on knee. Note coalescence of lesions from Koebner's phenomenon.

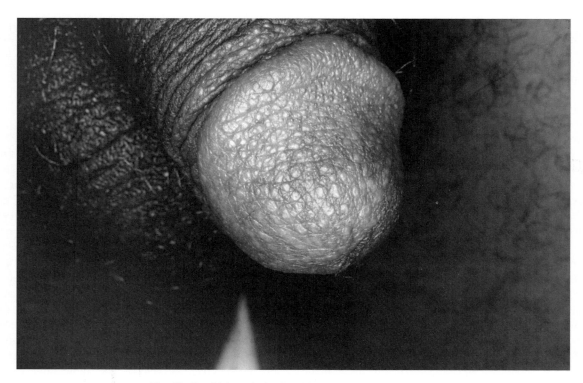

Fig. 12-19 Lichen nitidus involving the penis, a typical site.

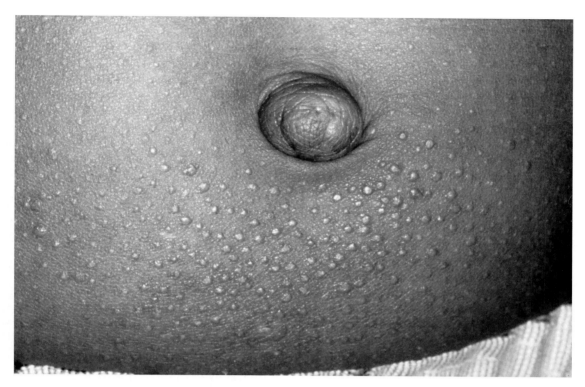

Fig. 12-20 Lichen nitidus on a child's abdomen.

Palm and sole involvement by lichen nitidus may occur, and the disease may be restricted to these areas. It may present with multiple, tiny, hyperkeratotic papules. The papules may coalesce to form diffuse hyperkeratotic plaques that fissure. The differentiation from hyperkeratotic hand eczema may be quite difficult if discrete individual lesions are not present. Nail involvement with pitting, beaded, longitudinal ridging, and nail fold inflammation has been reported.

A variant of lichen nitidus, termed *actinic lichen nitidus,* has been reported in black, Middle Eastern, and Indian subcontinent patients. These patients are identical to some patients reported as having summertime actinic lichenoid eruption. They have lesions clinically and histologically identical to lichen nitidus that are limited to the sun-exposed areas of the dorsal hands, brachioradial area, and posterior neck. They usually respond to sun protection with or without topical steroids.

The course of lichen nitidus is slowly progressive, with a tendency to remissions. The lesions may remain stationary for years but sometimes disappear spontaneously and entirely. The cause of lichen nitidus is unknown. Rare familial cases do occur. It is clinically and histologically distinct from lichen planus. Immunohistochemical studies also suggest they are distinct disorders. However, patients have been reported who have had both disorders, suggesting some pathogenic relationship. Lichen nitidus has a charac-

teristic histologic appearance. Dermal papillae are widened and contain a dense infiltrate composed of lymphocytes, histiocytes, and melanophages. Multinucleate giant cells are often present, imparting a granulomatous appearance to the infiltrate. The epidermal rete ridges on either side of the papilla form a clawlike collarette. The overlying epidermis is attenuated, and there is usually vacuolar alteration of its basal layer.

Differential Diagnosis

The discrete, hypopigmented or red papules of lichen nitidus are very characteristic. The lesions of lichen nitidus are differentiated from flat warts by their smaller size, greater number, and distribution. Micropapular lichen planus is usually accompanied by larger papules or plaques; lesions are violaceous, usually pruritic, and have a different histology. Lesions of lichen nitidus that form hyperkeratotic plaques on the palms and soles may be impossible to differentiate from chronic eczema if there are no lesions on other areas of the body. Histology is still diagnostic, however.

Treatment

Because lichen nitidus is usually asymptomatic, treatment is often not necessary. Topical application of potent or superpotent corticosteroids is helpful if pruritus is severe. PUVA, systemic steroids with UVA/UVB phototherapy, DNCB, and retinoids (etretinate and acitretin) have been effective.

Chen W, et al: Generalized lichen nitidus. *J Am Acad Dermatol* 1997, 36:630.

Hussain K: Summertime actinic lichenoid eruption, a distinct entity, should be termed actinic lichen nitidus. *Arch Dermatol* 1998, 134:1302.

Kano Y, et al: Improvement of lichen nitidus after topical DNCB application. *J Am Acad Dermatol* 1998, 39:305.

Kanwar AJ, et al: Lichen nitidus actinicus. *Pediatr Dermatol* 1991, 8:94.

Kato N: Familial lichen nitidus. *Clin Exp Dermatol* 1995, 20:336.

Kawakami T, et al: Generalized lichen nitidus appearing subsequent to lichen planus. *J Dermatol* 1995, 22:434.

Lucker GPH, et al: Treatment of palmoplantar lichen nitidus with acitretin. *Br J Dermatol* 1994, 130:791.

Munro CS, et al: Lichen nitidus presenting as palmoplantar hyperkeratosis and nail dystrophy. *Clin Exp Dermatol* 1993, 18:381.

Natarajan S, et al: Lichen nitidus: nail changes. *Int J Dermatol* 1986, 25:461.

Randle HW, et al: Treatment of generalized lichen nitidus with PUVA. *Int J Dermatol* 1986, 25:330.

Smoller BR, et al: Immunohistochemical examination of lichen nitidus suggests that it is not a localized papular variant of lichen planus. *J Am Acad Dermatol* 1992, 27:232. ▲

LICHEN STRIATUS

Lichen striatus is a fairly common linear, self-limited eruption that is seen primarily in children. Girls outnumber boys in most series by 2 to 1. The average age is 3 years, but young adults may also be affected. Lesions begin as small papules that are erythematous and slightly scaly. In more darkly pigmented persons, hypopigmentation is prominent. The 1- to 3-mm papules form a band 1 to 3 cm wide, either continuous or interrupted, that over a few weeks progresses down the extremity or around the trunk, following Blaschko's lines (Fig. 12-21). An extremity is more commonly involved, but trunk lesions, or lesions extending from the trunk onto an extremity, can also occur. About 10% of cases occur on the face. Multiple bands can rarely occur. Lesions are usually asymptomatic.

Nail involvement can occur if the process extends down the digit to the nail. Only the nail may be involved for months, with later appearance of the band on the skin, or the nail may remain the sole area of involvement throughout the course of the disease. Nail plate thinning, longitudinal ridging, splitting, and nail bed hyperkeratosis may be seen. Often only a part of the nail is involved.

The active lesions of lichen striatus last for months and spontaneously resolve. Hypopigmentation may persist for several years. The nails also spontaneously improve, usually within a year. Recovery is complete.

The histologic features of lichen striatus vary somewhat, probably depending on the stage of evolution of the lesion. There may be a spongiotic dermatitis, but most frequently some lichenoid component is present. There is a bandlike infiltrate with necrotic keratinocytes at the dermoepidermal junction and at all layers of the epidermis. Granulomatous inflammation may be present. Typically there is a dense infiltrate around the eccrine sweat glands and ducts. This helps to distinguish lichen striatus from lichen planus.

Multiple reports exist of simultaneous cases in siblings. There is also a seasonal variation, with most cases occurring in the spring and summer. Epidemic outbreaks have been reported. All these features and the young age at which patients usually are affected strongly suggest a viral etiology for this condition.

Usually the diagnosis is straightforward in the setting of a young child, with the sudden onset of a linear eruption. The differential diagnosis could include linear lichen planus, linear psoriasis, inflammatory linear verrucous epidermal nevus, epidermal nevus, and verruca plana. Histologic evaluation will usually distinguish these entities, but it is rarely required.

Treatment is usually not necessary. Parents may be reassured of the uniformly excellent prognosis. Topical steroids may accelerate the resolution of lesions.

Gianotti R, et al: Lichen striatus. *J Cutan Pathol* 1995, 22:18.

Kennedy D, et al: Lichen striatus. *Pediatr Dermatol* 1996, 13:95.

Smith SB, et al: Lichen striatus. *Pediatr Dermatol* 1997, 14:43.

Tosti A, et al: Nail lichen striatus. *J Am Acad Dermatol* 1997, 36:908. ▲

LICHEN SCLEROSUS (LICHEN SCLEROSUS ET ATROPHICUS—LS&A)

Lichen sclerosus is a chronic disease of the skin and mucosae encompassing the disorders lichen sclerosus et atrophicus, kraurosis vulvae, and balanitis xerotica obliterans. It can present from childhood to old age, and occurs in all races. Both sexes are affected both before and after puberty, with females predominating at all ages.

The initial lesions of lichen sclerosus are white, polygonal, and flat-topped papules or plaques. Follicular, black, horny plugs resembling comedos are evenly spaced on the plaques. Lesions are surrounded by an erythematous to violaceous halo. Later the lesions may coalesce into large atrophic patches, leaving the skin smooth, slightly wrinkled, soft, and white. Bullae, often hemorrhagic, may occur on the patches. Itching is frequently severe, especially in the anogenital area. In the genital area fissuring and erosion may occur. This may result in dysuria, urethral and vaginal discharge, dyspareunia, and burning pain. Normal anatomic structures may be obliterated with loss of the labia minora, clitoral hood, and urethral meatus. In women, this perineal involvement typically involves the vulvar and perianal areas, forming a "figure-eight" or "hourglass" appearance (Fig. 12-22). Labial stenosis or fusion may occur. In men lesions are atrophic and may be markedly hypopigmented or depigmented. Lesions may involve only the glans penis (balanitis xerotica obliterans) (Fig. 12-23) or also involve the penile shaft and scrotum (Fig. 12-24). If the glans is involved, hemorrhage is common, and shallow erosions may occur. Unlike in women, however, lichen sclerosus

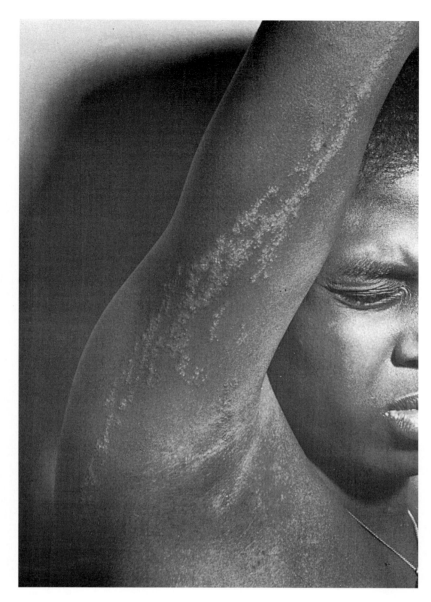

Fig. 12-21 Lichen striatus. (Courtesy Dr. E. Johlin.)

of the glans does not usually lead to nonhealing erosions of the glans, but rather simply skin fragility.

Extragenital lesions are most frequent on the upper back, chest, and breasts, and are usually asymptomatic (Fig. 12-25). The tongue and oral mucosa may also be involved, either alone or with lesions elsewhere. There are patients with only extragenital lesions with histologic features of both lichen sclerosus and morphea. They may also have other cutaneous lesions of morphea or atrophoderma of Pasini and Perini. These patients are best viewed as having morphea.

Lichen Sclerosus and Cancer

Although not as high as was proposed early in this century, lichen sclerosus of the genitalia is a condition with increased risk for genital squamous cell carcinoma in both women and men. The lifetime risk for women who are carefully followed appears to be less than 5%, but clearly increased over the general population. Human papilloma virus (HPV) infection, the most common cause of genital squamous cell carcinoma, is not found in the majority of cancers arising in genital lichen sclerosus.

Etiology

In Europe and Japan infection with *Borrelia burgdorferi* has been linked to lichen sclerosus by finding *Borrelia* DNA in the lesions of lichen sclerosus by polymerase chain reaction. Similar studies in the United States have not found this association. Autoimmune phenomena seem to be more common in patients with lichen sclerosus, with about 20% of both men and women having at least one autoimmune disease (usually vitiligo, alopecia areata, or thyroid disease),

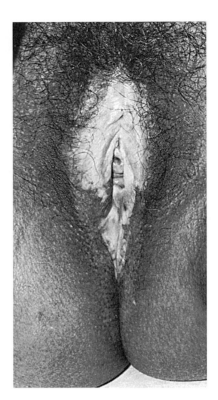

Fig. 12-22   Vulvar lichen sclerosus et atrophicus.

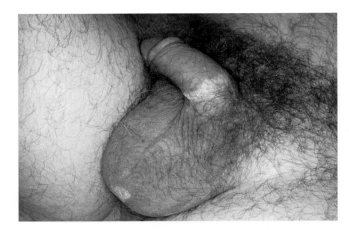

Fig. 12-24   Lichen sclerosus of the penile shaft and scrotum.

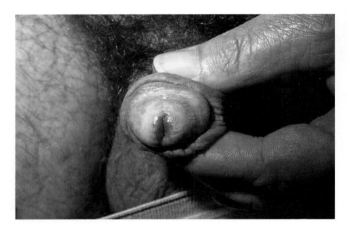

Fig. 12-23   Balanitis xerotica obliterans (lichen sclerosus of the glans penis).

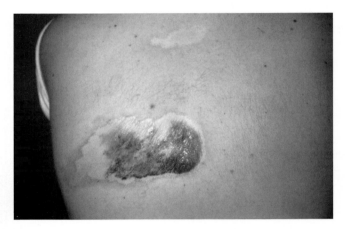

Fig. 12-25   Extragenital lichen sclerosus. Hemorrhagic bullous lesion on the back.

and a larger proportion having circulating autoantibodies. Trauma can induce lesions and may explain the improvement in boys after circumcision, and the frequent appearance of lesions after surgical removal.

Childhood Lichen Sclerosus

Childhood onset of lichen sclerosus occurs in 10% to 15% of cases. Girls outnumber boys about 10 to 1 (Fig. 12-26). Genital disease represents 90% of childhood lichen sclero-

sus. In girls presenting symptoms include difficulty with defecation (especially constipation), dysuria, perineal pruritus, and perineal skin lesions. In boys phimosis is the most common presentation. Acquired phimosis of a previously retractable foreskin, or phimosis after age 6 suggests lichen sclerosus. Constipation may also occur in boys with lichen sclerosus. Childhood lichen sclerosus may involute spontaneously, sometimes around the time of puberty. In boys circumcision for phimosis may lead to resolution or improvement. In girls spontaneous resolution is supposed to occur in 50% of cases, but many women with lichen sclerosus report symptoms initially in childhood.

Histopathology

Early lesions are characterized by an interface dermatitis with vacuolar alteration of keratinocytes. With evolution the epidermis is thinned and the rete ridges are effaced. Hyperkeratosis and follicular and eccrine plugging are present. Hydropic degeneration of the basal keratinocytes

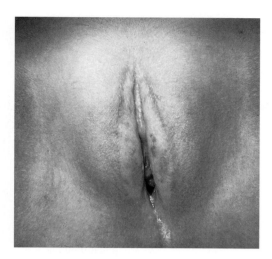

Fig. 12-26 Lichen sclerosus in a 6-year-old girl.

and histologic reversal of the epidermal atrophy. Coexistent candidiasis may be present or appear with this treatment and can be managed with topical or oral agents.

Recent controlled trials have shown that 2% testosterone ointment and 2% progesterone cream have limited efficacy compared with superpotent topical steroids. Maintenance testosterone ointment after achieving control with steroids actually had a negative effect and was less efficacious than a bland emollient. These agents and topical isotretinoin may be considered in patients inadequately controlled with superpotent steroids.

Oral retinoid therapy and topical tretinoin may be useful in anogenital lichen sclerosus in both men and women. Antimalarial agents may also be beneficial. Surgical modalities are rarely indicated, except for dysplasia or correction of adhesions.

persists in later lesions, which are characterized by typical changes in the papillary dermis. The upper dermis is edematous, the upper dermal collagen sclerotic, and upper dermal vessels telangiectatic. Immediately beneath the altered papillary dermis there is a bandlike and perivascular cellular infiltrate composed primarily of lymphocytes but with occasional plasma cells and even eosinophils. In very late lesions, the inflammatory cells are sparse or absent. In pruritic lesions, coexistent changes of lichen simplex chronicus may be seen.

Differential Diagnosis

Extragenital lichen sclerosus must be differentiated from guttate morphea and lichen planus, especially of the atrophic type. Anogenital lichen sclerosus must be distinguished from genital lichen planus, lichen simplex chronicus, vulvar intraepithelial neoplasia (Bowen's disease), and extramammary Paget's disease. The white color and atrophic surface are characteristic, and such areas are most fruitful for biopsy to confirm the diagnosis.

Treatment

The use of superpotent topical steroids has dramatically changed the management of anogenital lichen sclerosus. Most patients will respond to twice-daily applications of these agents and can subsequently be tapered to less frequent applications (once or twice weekly) or to lower-strength steroids. Although the lesions are already atrophic, potent topical steroid treatment is associated with clinical

Bornstein J, et al: Clobetasol dipropionate 0.05% versus testosterone propionate 2% topical application for severe vulvar lichen sclerosus. *Am J Obstet Gynecol* 1998, 178:80.

Bousema MT, et al: Acitretin in the treatment of severe lichen sclerosus et atrophicus of the vulva. *J Am Acad Dermatol* 1994, 30:225.

Cattaneo A, et al: Testosterone maintenance therapy: effects of vulvar lichen sclerosus treated with clobetasol propionate. *J Reprod Med* 1996, 41:99.

Dahlman-Ghozlan K, et al: Penile lichen sclerosus et atrophicus treated with clobetasol dipropionate 0.05% cream. *J Am Acad Dermatol* 1999, 40:451.

Dalziel KL, et al: Long-term control of vulval lichen sclerosus after treatment with a potent topical steroid cream. *J Reprod Med* 1993, 38:25.

Fischer G, et al: Treatment of childhood vulvar lichen sclerosus with potent topical corticosteroid. *Pediatr Dermatol* 1997, 14:235.

Fujiwara H, et al: Detection of *Borrelia burgdorferi* DNA in morphea and lichen sclerosus et atrophicus tissues of German and Japanese but not of US patients. *Arch Dermatol* 1997, 133:41.

Garzon MC, et al: Ultrapotent topical corticosteroid treatment of childhood genital lichen sclerosus. *Arch Dermatol* 1999, 135:525.

Ledwig PA, et al: Late circumcision and lichen sclerosus et atrophicus of the penis. *J Am Acad Dermatol* 1989, 20:211.

Liatsikos EN, et al: Lichen sclerosus et atrophicus: findings after complete circumcision. *Scand J Urol Neph* 1997, 31:453.

Lindhagen T: Topical clobetasol propionate compared with placebo in the treatment of unretractable foreskin. *Eur J Surg* 1996, 162:969.

Meffert JJ, et al: Lichen sclerosus. *J Am Acad Dermatol* 1995, 32:393.

Meuli M, et al: Lichen sclerosus et atrophicus causing phimosis in boys. *J Urol* 1994, 152:987.

Ridley CM: Genital lichen sclerosus in childhood and adolescence. *J Royal Soc Med* 1993, 86:69.

Virgili A, et al: Open study of topical 0.025% tretinoin in the treatment of vulvar lichen sclerosus. *J Reprod Med* 1995, 40:614.

Wakelin SH, et al: Lichen sclerosus in women. *Clin Dermatol* 1997, 15:155. ▲

CHAPTER 13

Acne

ACNE VULGARIS
Clinical Features

Acne vulgaris is a chronic inflammatory disease of the pilosebaceous follicles, characterized by comedones, papules, pustules, cysts, nodules, and often scars. Sites of predilection are the face, neck, upper trunk, and upper arms. It is a disease of the adolescent, with 90% of all teenagers being affected to some degree. It may begin in the twenties or thirties, or may persist in adults for many years. As a rule, there is involution of the disease before age 25.

Acne vulgaris occurs primarily in the oily (seborrheic) areas of the skin. On the face it occurs most frequently on the cheeks, and to a lesser degree on the nose, forehead, and chin. The ears are frequently involved, with large comedones in the concha, cysts in the lobes, and sometimes retroauricular comedones and cysts. On the neck, especially in the nuchal area, large cystic lesions may predominate. These may later become keloidal.

The comedo, commonly known as the *blackhead,* is the basic lesion in acne (Fig. 13-1). It is produced by hyperkeratosis of the lining of the follicles, with retention of keratin and sebum. The plugging produced by the comedo dilates the mouth of the follicle, and papules are formed by inflammation around the comedones.

In typical mild acne vulgaris the comedones predominate, with but occasional pustules. In more severe cases pustules and papules may predominate (Figs. 13-2 and 13-3). These heal with scar formation, if the lesions are deep seated. In moderately severe cases, cystic lesions occur (Fig. 13-4). In acne conglobata the suppurating cystic lesions predominate (Fig. 13-5), and severe scarring results.

Some patients present with a monomorphous appearance. In the mild case the eruption is composed almost entirely of comedones on an oily skin: acne comedo. Papular acne has numerous inflammatory papules (Fig. 13-6); this is the type most common in young men with coarse, oily skin. Atrophic acne is characterized by residual atrophic pits and scars (Fig. 13-7). Quite the opposite of these are the elevated hypertrophic or sometimes keloidal scars seen not only in blacks but also, to a lesser extent, in whites. They frequently appear in adult black men on the bearded region.

Acne vulgaris is mostly a disease of the adolescent; it occurs with greatest frequency between the ages of 15 and 18 in both sexes. Nevertheless, acne may occur in prepubertal youngsters. It is also true that acne may first appear in women over age 21 and persist for many years. When acne persists in men after age 21, it is often acne conglobata. The back is the usual major site of involvement in such cases. In reviewing the National Health and Nutrition Examination Survey (HANES) data, Stern found that 27% of women and 34% of men ages 15 to 44 had active acne.

Etiology

Multiple factors cause acne vulgaris. There is undoubtedly a hereditary factor. Several members of the same family may be affected with severe scarring acne.

The primary defect in acne is the formation of a keratinous plug in the lower infundibulum of the hair follicle. Other major factors contributing to the formation of acne lesions are androgenic stimulation of sebaceous glands and proliferation of a resident anaerobic organism, *Propionibacterium acnes,* which metabolizes sebum to produce free fatty acids. The occurrence of androgen secretion at the onset of puberty explains the usual onset of acne at that age. Much evidence suggests that liberation of free fatty acids by the metabolic activity of *P. acnes* is a major factor in the genesis of acne papules and pustules.

Pathogenesis

Acne vulgaris is exclusively a follicular disease, with comedo formation produced by the impaction and distension of the follicles with tightly packed horny cells. Disruption of the follicular epithelium permits discharge of the follicular contents into the dermis. This, in turn, causes the formation of inflammatory papules, pustules, and nodulocystic lesions (Fig. 13-8).

As mentioned, comedo formation is caused by "stickiness" of the horny cells, which fail to be properly

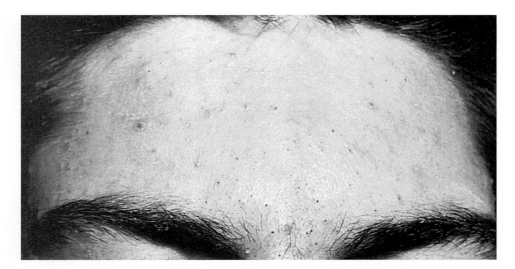

Fig. 13-1 Acne vulgaris with comedones on the forehead.

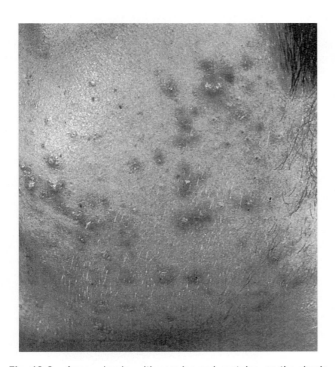

Fig. 13-2 Acne vulgaris, with papules and pustules, on the cheek.

discharged at the follicular orifice. As the retained cells block the follicular opening, the lower portion of the follicle is dilated by entrapped sebum. Bacterial lipase acts on the sebum to produce free fatty acids. Largely because it is so abundant, the bacterium most responsible for this enzymatic reaction is *P. acnes*. Leyden et al showed that the ratio of *P. acnes* counts in patients with acne, compared with those without acne, is very high—15,000:0 from ages 11 to 15, and 85,000:590 from ages 16 to 20. Above age 21 the ratio

is 1:1; that is, there is no difference between those with acne and those without.

Free fatty acids are chemotactic to the components of inflammation; if the follicle dilates sufficiently to rupture, these and other irritants are released into the dermis, where inflammation ensues. The beneficial effects of tetracycline are chiefly obtained by the reduction of the free fatty acids.

Tetracyclines, clindamycin, benzoyl peroxide, or erythromycin applied topically can reduce the number of *P. acnes*. Kligman stresses that antibiotics do not produce involution of the inflammatory lesions present but rather inhibit the formation of new lesions. Topical retinoic acid acts by its influence on keratinization, causing horny cells to lose their stickiness.

Androgens (such as testosterone) enlarge the sebaceous glands and thereby increase sebum production. Several studies demonstrate that women with acne can show biochemical hyperandrogenism. In one such study by Marynick et al, 91 patients with resistant cystic acne were found to have dehydroepiandrosterone sulfate elevated in both men and women, testosterone and luteinizing hormone elevated in women, and higher 17-hydroxyprogesterone levels in men; sex-hormone–binding globulin was decreased in both sexes. Other studies confirm increases in various androgen blood levels in acne patients, especially older women; however, the exact androgenic substances reported to be elevated vary from study to study. Also, a role of increased peripheral metabolic conversion of testosterone to dihydrotestosterone at the level of the skin in acne patients remains unproven.

In all women with acne the possibility of a hyperandrogenic state should be considered. The presence of irregular menses and hirsutism increase the likelihood of finding clinically significant hyperandrogenism (Fig. 13-9). Gynecologic endocrine evaluation of such patients is indicated.

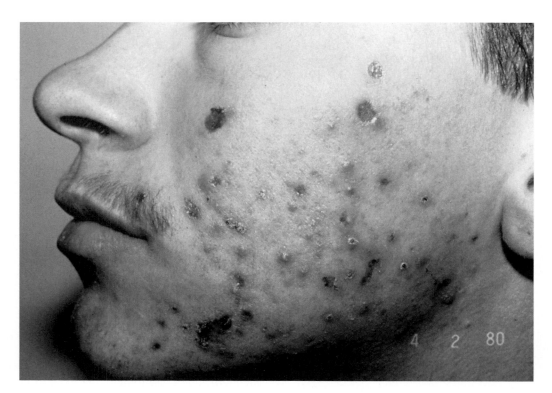

Fig. 13-3 Inflammatory acne. Note excoriations.

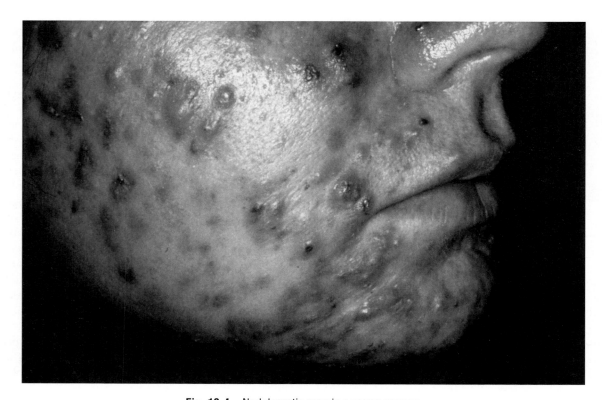

Fig. 13-4 Nodulocystic acne in a young woman.

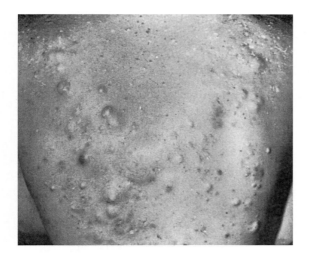

Fig. 13-5 Acne conglobata in a 17-year-old boy.

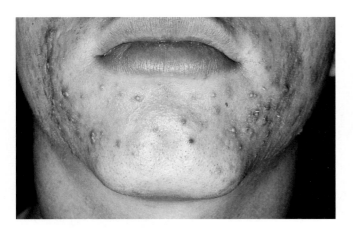

Fig. 13-6 Inflammatory acne with papules and pustules.

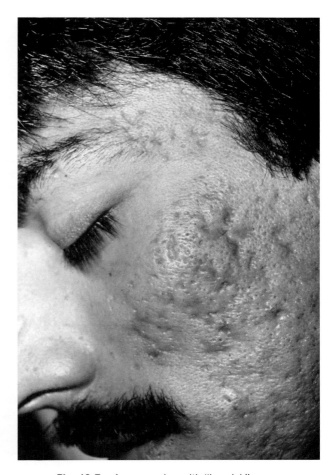

Fig. 13-7 Acne scarring with "ice pick" scars.

Pathology

Acne is characterized by perifollicular inflammation around comedones In pustular cases there are folliculocentric abscesses surrounded by a dense inflammatory exudate of lymphocytes and polymorphonuclear leukocytes. Indolent lesions frequently show, in addition to these findings, plasma cells, foreign body giant cells, and proliferation of fibroblasts. In the larger lesions the sebaceous gland is partly or completely destroyed, sometimes with the formation of large cysts. Epithelial-lined sinus tracts may form.

Treatment

Depending on the severity and extent of involvement, treatment varies from application of topical medications to systemic therapy with antibiotics or retinoids. Treatment in pregnancy is a special situation reviewed by Rothman et al.

Diet

There is no evidence that dietary habits influence acne; therefore, elimination diets are not indicated, and no foods are explicitly forbidden.

Antibacterials

TETRACYCLINE. Tetracycline has been the preferred antibiotic since 1951, when Andrews and Domonkos first reported the use of tetracyclines in the treatment of acne vulgaris. It is the safest and cheapest choice, and is usually very effective. The usual dosage of tetracycline is 250 to 500 mg one to four times daily initially, with gradual reduction of the dose, depending on clinical response. It is best to take tetracycline on an empty stomach, at least a half hour before meals, so that it will be absorbed. Calcium or iron in food combine with tetracycline, reducing absorption by as much as half.

Tetracycline acts by killing *P. acnes* and thus reducing the concentration of fatty acids in the sebaceous follicles. Constant or intermittent therapy may sometimes be necessary for several months or years. Tetracyclines as sole treatment will give a positive response in approximately

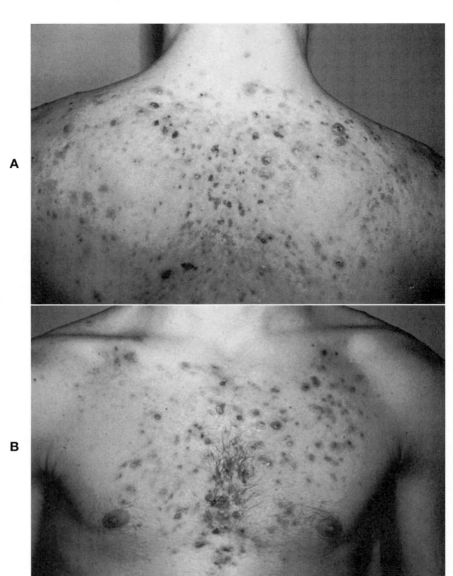

Fig. 13-8   A and **B**, Severe pustulocystic acne. (Courtesy Dr. Axel W. Hoke.)

70% of patients. It may take 4 to 6 weeks of tetracycline therapy before a response is noted. This is because its action is preventive, and lesions present at the outset of therapy require their usual time to resolve.

Vaginitis or perianal itching may result from the tetracycline therapy in about 5% of patients, with *Candida albicans* usually present in the involved site. The only other common side effects are gastrointestinal symptoms such as nausea, and staining of growing teeth, which precludes its use in pregnant women and in children under age 9 or 10. Miller et al have reviewed reports that raise concern that tetracycline may reduce the effectiveness of oral birth control pills. A table in this article may be used to help educate the patient. It is appropriate for this as yet unproved association to be discussed with patients and a second form

of birth control offered. Tetracycline should also be avoided when renal function is impaired.

Although phototoxicity and other reactions may occur infrequently, an ad hoc committee of the American Academy of Dermatology found it almost as safe as erythromycin, not requiring monitoring of laboratory parameters during long-term use. Sauer found no deleterious effects in 325 patients who took tetracyclines for 3 years or longer, except for one instance of transient hyperbilirubinemia with mild jaundice while taking 500 mg tetracycline daily. Tanzman in 1988 reported that routine monitoring of laboratory parameters was not done by nearly two thirds of college health services and found that only four instances of significant side effects had been reported in 70,297 treated patients. She advised such tests only on symptomatic

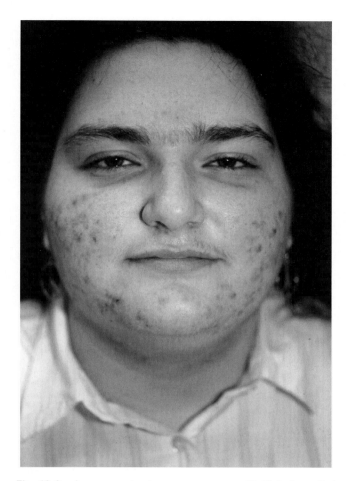

Fig. 13-9 Acne occurring in a young woman with Stein-Leventhal syndrome (polycystic ovary disease).

or high-risk patients. Driscoll et al's conclusion was the same in their 1993 study.

MINOCYCLINE. Minocycline is more effective than tetracycline in treating acne vulgaris. Hubbell et al, in a randomized double-blind prospective study, showed that 100 mg a day of minocycline was superior to 500 mg of tetracycline. In patients whose *P. acnes* develop tetracycline resistance, minocycline is an excellent choice for alternative oral antibiotic therapy. The usual dose is 50 to 100 mg once or twice daily depending on the severity of disease. Its absorption is less affected by milk and food than is that of tetracycline. Vertigo may occur, and beginning therapy with a single dose in the evening may be prudent. Staining of teeth and pigmentation in some areas of inflammation of oral tissues, in postacne osteoma cutis, in a photo-distributed pattern, on the shins, in the sclera, the nail bed, and the ear cartilage, or in a generalized pattern may also be seen. These pigmentary changes are discussed in detail in Chapter 6. Additionally, lupuslike syndromes, a hypersensitivity syndrome consisting of fever, hepatitis, and eosinophilia, serum sickness, pneumonitis, and hepatitis are uncommon but potentially serious adverse effects of minocycline.

DOXYCYCLINE. Harrison reported 50 mg of doxycycline once daily to be as effective as 50 mg of minocycline twice daily. Photosensitivity reactions can occur. In patients who develop *P. acnes* resistant to erythromycin, doxycycline is an excellent choice for alternative oral antibiotic therapy.

ERYTHROMYCIN. For those who cannot take tetracyclines because of side effects or in pregnant women requiring oral antibiotic therapy erythromycin may be considered. Side effects are mostly gastrointestinal upset; vaginal itching is a rare occurrence. The dose is 250 to 500 mg two to four times a day initially, reduced gradually after control is achieved. Because of increasing antibiotic resistance of *P. acnes* to erythromycin, combining its administration with benzoyl peroxide when possible is recommended.

CLINDAMYCIN. Past experience has shown clindamycin to give an excellent response in the treatment of acne; however, the potential for the development of pseudomembranous colitis and the availability of retinoids has limited its use. The dose is 150 mg three times a day initially, reduced gradually as control is achieved.

SULFONAMIDES. Sulfonamides are occasionally prescribed; however, the potential for severe drug eruptions limits their use. Sulfisoxazole or sulfamethoxazole is taken in 2-g doses daily until a good response is elicited; then 1-g maintenance dosage is followed. Trimethoprim-sulfamethoxazole (Bactrim, Septra) is also effective in many cases unresponsive to other antibiotics. Dapsone may be used in severe acne conglobata, but isotretinoin is favored.

Bacterial resistance. Although it had long been believed that antibiotic resistance was rare, Leyden et al were able to show a close correlation between an unchanging or worsening clinical condition and a high mean minimum inhibitory concentration (MIC) requirement for both erythromycin and tetracycline against *P. acnes*. The antibiotic resistance was lost over a period of 1 or 2 months after withdrawal of the antibiotic. This problem is growing in clinical importance. Means by which to address this are to prescribe antibiotics only when non-antibiotic therapy will not suffice, discontinue antibiotics during maintenance, use benzoyl peroxide with antibiotics, and avoid the use of different oral and topical antibiotics at the same time.

Hormonal Therapy

ORAL CONTRACEPTIVES. Andrews and Domonkos first reported the efficacy of estrogen in 1951; Strauss and Pochi believe that stimulation of sebum secretion in women is due mostly to the secretion of androgens from the ovary and that estrogen inhibits the activity of the ovarian androgen. They also found that with estrogen therapy the sebum production is markedly decreased (sometimes as much as 40%) by the end of 3 months of oral contraceptive medication. Estradiol suppresses the uptake of testosterone by the sebaceous glands; it also inhibits its conversion into dihydrotestosterone.

Oral contraceptives containing androgenic progesterones may trigger or exacerbate acne in women. Low-dose oral contraceptives containing a nonandrogenic progestin can be effective. One oral birth control pill containing ethinyl estradiol and norgestimate is approved as a treatment for acne, and others are currently being studied and will likely receive the same indication. Beneficial effects may be noted only after several months of therapy and in general prolonged treatment is needed for control. Both the physician and the patient should be familiar with the adverse reactions associated with oral contraceptives.

Spironolactone

Antiandrogenic substances may be utilized to counteract sebum overproduction in women practicing effective birth control. Spironolactone may be effective in doses from 25 to 300 mg/day. Several months of therapy are usually required to see benefit. Cyproterone acetate is a potent antiandrogen available in Europe.

Dexamethasone

Marynick et al found dexamethasone in doses from 0.125 to 0.5 mg given once at night reduced androgen excess and alleviated cystic acne.

Prednisone

Although steroids may produce steroid acne, they are also effective antiinflammatory agents in severe and intractable acne vulgaris. In severe acne cystica and acne conglobata, corticosteroid treatment is effective; however, the side effects of this medication restrict its use. It is generally only given to patients with severe inflammatory acne during the first few weeks of treatment with isotretinoin to prevent flares.

Vitamin A

With the availability of isotretinoin, the use of vitamin A in acne therapy is largely of historical interest.

Isotretinoin (Accutane)

Although no comparison studies have been done, this retinoid exerts much the same effects as large doses of vitamin A, and is a reliable remedy in all forms of acne. The dose is 0.5 to 1 mg/kg/day in one or two doses, for 15 to 20 weeks. For severe truncal acne in patients who tolerate higher doses treatment may be given at 2 mg/kg/day. In practice, most patients (because of the high cost) are given 40 or 80 mg daily. Doses as low as 0.1 mg/kg/day are very nearly as effective as the larger; the disadvantage is that it is less likely to produce a prolonged remission even after 20 weeks of treatment. To obtain the greatest chance of a prolonged remission patients should receive at least 120 mg/kg over the 5-month treatment course. An easy way to calculate the total dose needed is to multiply the weight in kilograms by 3. The product is the total number of 40-mg capsules needed. The major advantage of isotretinoin (Accutane) is that it is the only acne therapy that is not open-ended (i.e., that leads to a remission, which may last many months or years). Approximately 40% to 60% of patients remain acne-free after a single course of isotretinoin. White et al's experience is that 39% remain clear without treatment 3 years after stopping isotretinoin, 17% will need additional topical medication, 25% will need additional oral antibiotics, and 19% will need additional isotretinoin. In adult acne patients, who frequently tolerate the side effects of isotretinoin less well, lower doses and/or intermittent therapy are being explored. Goulden et al studied 80 adult acne patients whom they treated with 0.5 mg/kg/day for 1 week out of every 4 during a period of 6 months. Acne resolved in 88%, and 39% relapsed after 1 year. Seukeran and Cunliffe treated 9 patients aged 56 to 75 with 0.25 mg/kg/day for 6 months. All patients cleared, and all but one remained clear 36 months later.

Patient education is critical in isotretinoin therapy. Its most serious side effect is the virtual certainty that it will severely damage a fetus if it is given during pregnancy; it is of the utmost importance that a woman of child-bearing potential follow closely the recommendations clearly outlined in the patient package insert. The use of consent forms, contraception education, documentation of the absence of pregnancy by a negative blood test and a normal menstrual period after the negative test are important components of a program to prevent pregnancy during treatment.

Apart from fetal damage, the side effects of isotretinoin are dose dependent and generally not serious. One of the most common is progressive hypertriglyceridemia. It may be controlled by avoidance of smoking and alcohol, and by following a diet that is low in fat. Dry skin, lips, eyes, and nose occur in up to 90% of patients. This dryness of the nasal mucosa leads to colonization by *Staphylococcus aureus* in 80% to 90% of treated subjects. Skin abscesses, staphylococcal conjunctivitis, impetigo, facial cellulitis, and folliculitis may result. Such colonization may be avoided by the use of bacitracin ointment applied to the anterior nares twice daily during isotretinoin therapy. Williams et al could show no benefit with pulsed mupirocin.

The drug is approved only for severe cystic acne; however, it is now common practice to use it in less severe forms of acne, so as to prevent the need for continuous treatment and the repeated office visits that many patients require. It was a consensus of experts in the field that acne conditions that warrant oral isotretinoin treatment include severe acne and poorly responsive acne that improves less than 50% after 6 months of therapy with combined oral and topical antibiotics, and acne that relapses, scars, or induces consequential psychologic distress. Additionally, other agreed-on indications were gram-negative folliculitis, inflammatory rosacea, pyoderma faciale, acne fulminans, and hidradenitis suppurativa.

Many patients experience worsening of the acne some time in the first month of treatment. Continuing oral antibiotics, or occasionally giving prednisone, helps to prevent this. Arthralgias may occur, but like other side effects, it does not require interruption of therapy, unless severe.

Monthly serum pregnancy tests are taken before, after, and monthly during treatment in women of child-bearing potential. Monitoring for serum lipid elevations, liver function abnormalities, and hematologic abnormalities should be checked at regular intervals depending on patient risk factors, the dose utilized, and community standards.

Hoffman-LaRoche will furnish patient-information brochures; write to them at Nutley, 340 Kingsland Street, New Jersey 07110.

Topical Treatment

As with oral antibiotics, topical treatments are solely preventative. Therefore, use for 4 to 6 weeks is required to judge efficacy. The entire acne-affected area is treated, not just the lesions, and long-term usage is the rule. Many times topical therapy may be effective as maintenance therapy after initial control is achieved by combination oral and topical treatment.

BENZOYL PEROXIDE. Benzoyl peroxide is available as gels, creams, lotions, washes, and bars. It is used in 2.5% to 10% concentrations. The water-based formulation is less irritating. A combination 5% benzoyl peroxide and 3% erythromycin is often effective and well tolerated. Treatment is usually once or twice daily.

Benzoyl peroxide has a potent antibacterial effect, suppressing *P. acnes* and consequently reducing free fatty acids in the follicles. Some studies have shown it to be comedolytic also. Its concomitant use during treatment with antibiotics will limit resistance development. Benzoyl peroxide may irritate the skin and produce peeling. In that case the frequency of application should be lessened to once daily or every other day.

TOPICAL RETINOIDS. Tretinoin (Retin-A) may be used as a solution, cream, or gel. It is available in 0.01%, 0.025%, 0.05%, and 0.1% concentrations. Popular forms are 0.025% and 0.05% tretinoin in a cream base because these are less irritating than the gels and liquids. Therapy is generally started with nightly application of the 0.05% cream. It may take 8 to 12 weeks before improvement occurs. In cases slow to respond to topical retinoic acid cream, retinoic acid gel or solution may be necessary. Its ability to profoundly affect follicular keratinization makes this an excellent comedolytic medication.

To reduce irritancy additional vehicles, delivery methods, and retinoid molecules have been developed. These include tretinoin in a microsponge, tretinoin in a polyolprepolymer, adapalene, and tazarotene. Topical retinoids are especially effective against comedones too small to express.

They may produce severe irritation or erythema at the onset of treatment; if this occurs they should be used only every other day until the skin becomes tolerant.

TOPICAL ANTIBACTERIALS. In addition to benzoyl peroxide, topical antibiotics are effective in reducing the levels of *P. acnes* and free fatty acids in the follicle.

Clindamycin. A 1% concentration of clindamycin is available as a solution, gel, pledgets, or lotion. Clindamycin is effective in decreasing the counts of *P. acnes*. It is most effective against pustules and small papulopustular lesions. It is used once or twice daily alone or in combination with other topical therapies.

Erythromycin. Two percent solutions, gels, and swabs, and a 3% concentration combined with 5% benzoyl peroxide in a gel form are available. Thomas et al conducted a double-blind study comparing topical erythromycin 1.5% with topical clindamycin 1.0% and found the two equally effective; two thirds of the patients had a good or excellent response in 12 weeks. Use of topical erythromycin alone is not recommended because of increasing antibiotic resistance. Concurrent therapy with benzoyl peroxide is recommended.

SULFUR, RESORCIN, AND SALICYLIC ACID. Although benzoyl peroxide, the retinoids, and antibiotic topical lotions have largely supplanted the older medications, sulfur, resorcin, and salicylic acid preparations are still useful and moderately helpful if the newer medications are not tolerated.

AZELEIC ACID. This dicarboxylic acid is remarkably free from adverse actions and is reported to have some efficacy.

Abrasive Cleansers

Despite the therapeutic claims made for abrasive cleansers, Fulghum et al were able to show no difference between lesion counts using a cleanser with and without abrasives, over an 8-week period. In general, their use, as well as the use of astringents and drying soaps, only makes the skin dry and more susceptible to the irritant effects of the truly effective topical preparations and are therefore discouraged.

Surgical Treatment

Local surgical treatment is helpful in bringing about quick resolution of the comedones and pustules as well as the cysts. The edge of the follicle is nicked with a sharp, pointed No. 11 Bard-Parker scalpel blade, and the contents of the comedo are expressed with a comedo extractor. Scarring is not produced by this procedure. In isotretinoin-treated patients, macrocomedones present at week 10 to 15 may be expressed, since they tend to persist throughout therapy.

Intralesional Corticosteroids

Intralesional corticosteroids are especially effective in reducing inflammatory papules, pustules, and smaller cysts. Kenalog-10 (triamcinolone acetonide 10 mg/ml) is best diluted with sterile normal saline solution to 5 or 2.5 mg/ml (or even, as Levine et al showed, 1.5 or 0.75 mg/ml) to safeguard against atrophy and hypopigmentation at the site of injection.

Complications

Even with the excellent treatment options available, scarring may occur. This may be quite prominent and often results from the cystic type of acne, although even smaller lesions may produce scarring in some individuals. Pitted scars, and wide-mouthed depressions and keloids, primarily seen along the jawline, are common types of scarring. These may improve spontaneously over the course of a year or more. Many treatment options are available. Chemical peeling, ultrapulsed laser resurfacing, dermabrasion, scar excision, punch grafts alone or followed by dermabrasion, and collagen injections are among the procedures effective in improving the appearance. On the trunk 1- to 6-mm hypopigmented follicular papules may result. Wilson et al called them *papular acne scars,* whereas others refer to them as *postacne anetoderma-like scars.* They occurred in 28% of the 133 general dermatology patients Wilson et al screened, and 57% of patients with a history of acne vulgaris.

Other complications from acne are prominent residual hyperpigmentation, which is especially a problem in darker-skinned patients; pyogenic granuloma formation, which is more common in isotretinoin-treated patients; osteoma cutis, which are small, firm papules resulting from long-standing acne vulgaris; and solid facial edema. The latter is a persistent, firm facial swelling that is an uncommon, though distressing, result of acne vulgaris or acne rosacea. Both corticosteroids and isotretinoin have been reported to be effective treatment.

Alster TS, et al: Treatment of scars. *Ann Plast Surg* 1997, 39:418.

Bigby M, et al: Adverse reactions to isotretinoin. *J Am Acad Dermatol* 1988, 18:543.

Boffa MW, et al: Facial cellulitis during oral isotretinoin treatment for acne. *J Am Acad Dermatol* 1994, 31:800.

Camacho-Martinez F, et al: Solid facial edema as a manifestation of acne vulgaris. *J Am Acad Dermatol* 1990, 22:129.

Camera G, et al: Ear malformation baby born to mother using tretinoin cream. *Lancet* 1992, 339:687.

Campbell JP, et al: Retinoid therapy is associated with excess granulation tissue responses. *J Am Acad Dermatol* 1983, 9:708.

Cunliffe WJ: Evolution of a strategy for treatment of acne. *J Am Acad Dermatol* 1987, 16:591.

Cunningham WJ, et al: Clinical aspects of the retinoids. *Semin Dermatol* 1983, 2:145.

Driscoll MS, et al: Long-term oral antibiotics for acne. *J Am Acad Dermatol* 1993, 28:595.

Exner JH, et al: Pyogenic granuloma-like acne lesions during isotretinoin therapy. *Arch Dermatol* 1983, 119:808.

Friedman SJ, et al: Solid facial edema as a complication of acne vulgaris. *J Am Acad Dermatol* 1986, 15:286.

Fulghum DD, et al: Abrasive cleansing in the management of acne vulgaris. *Arch Dermatol* 1982, 118:658.

Gammon WR, et al: Comparative efficacy of oral erythromycin versus oral tetracycline in the treatment of acne vulgaris: a double-blind study. *J Am Acad Dermatol* 1986, 14:183.

Goulden V, et al: Treatment of acne with intermittent isotretinoin. *Br J Dermatol* 1997, 137:106.

Harrison DV: A comparison of doxycycline and minocycline in the treatment of acne vulgaris. *Clin Exp Dermatol* 1989, 23:242.

Helander I, et al: Solid facial edema as a complication of acne vulgaris. *Acta Derm Venereol* (Stockh) 1987, 67:535.

Hjurth N, et al: Azelaic acid for the treatment of acne. *Acta Derm Venereol* (Stockh) 1989, 143:45.

Hubbell CG, et al: Efficacy of minocycline compared with tetracycline in the treatment of acne vulgaris. *Arch Dermatol* 1982, 118:989.

Hughes BR, et al: Strategy of acne therapy with long-term antibiotics. *Br J Dermatol* 1989, 121:623.

Humbert P, et al: The tetracyclines in dermatology. *J Am Acad Dermatol* 1991, 25:691.

Lammer EJ, et al: Retinoic acid embryopathy. *N Engl J Med* 1985, 313:834.

Lasek RJ, et al: Acne vulgaris and the quality of life of adult dermatology patients. *Arch Dermatol* 1998, 134:454.

Layton AM, et al: Guidelines for optimal use of isotretinoin in acne. *J Am Acad Dermatol* 1992, 27:52.

Levine RM, et al: Intralesional corticosteroids in the treatment of nodulocystic acne. *Arch Dermatol* 1983, 119:480.

Leyden JJ: Absorption of minocycline hydrochloride: effect of milk, food, and iron. *J Am Acad Dermatol* 1985, 12:308.

Leyden JJ: Retinoids in acne. *J Am Acad Dermatol* 1988, 19:164.

Leyden JJ: Therapy for acne vulgaris. *N Engl J Med* 1997, 336:1156.

Leyden JJ, et al: Erythromycin gel compared with clindamycin solution in acne vulgaris. *J Am Acad Dermatol* 1987, 16:822.

Leyden JJ, et al: *Propionibacterium acnes* resistance to antibiotics in acne patients. *J Am Acad Dermatol* 1983, 8:41.

Leyden JJ, et al: Staphylococcus complicating isotretinoin therapy. *Arch Dermatol* 1987, 123:606.

Leyden JJ, et al: Tetracycline and minocycline treatment: effects on skin-surface lipid levels and *Propionibacterium acnes. Arch Dermatol* 1982, 118:19.

Lucky AW, et al: Acne vulgaris in premenarchal girls. *Arch Dermatol* 1994, 130:308.

Lucky AW, et al: Effectiveness of norgestimate and ethinyl estradiol in treating moderate acne vulgaris. *J Am Acad Dermatol* 1997, 37:746.

Marynick SP, et al: Androgen excess in cystic acne. *N Engl J Med* 1983, 308:981.

Miller DM, et al: A practical approach to antibiotic treatment in women taking oral contraceptives. *J Am Acad Dermatol* 1994, 30:1008.

Mills OH, et al: Comparing 2.5%, 5%, and 10% benzoyl peroxide on inflammatory acne vulgaris. *Int J Dermatol* 1986, 25:664.

Moritz DP, et al: Oral spironolactone. *Br J Dermatol* 1986, 115:227.

Muhlemann MF, et al: Oral spironolactone. *Br J Dermatol* 1986, 115:227.

Ortonne JP: Oral isotretinoin treatment policy. *Dermatology* 1997, 195S1:34.

Pochi PE: Endocrinology of acne (editorial). *J Invest Dermatol* 1983, 81:1.

Pochi PE: Hormones, retinoids, and acne. *N Engl J Med* 1983, 308:1024.

Rothman KF, et al: Use of oral and topical agents for acne in pregnancy. *J Am Acad Dermatol* 1988, 19:431.

Sauer G: Prospective study on the safety of long-term tetracycline therapy for acne. *Cutis* 1981, 27:492.

Schachner L, et al: A clinical trial comparing the safety and efficacy of a topical erythromycin-zinc formulation with a topical clindamycin formulation. *J Am Acad Dermatol* 1991, 22:489.

Seukeran DC, Cunliffe WJ: Acne in the elderly. *Br J Dermatol* 1998, 139:99.

Shalita AR: Acne revisited. *Arch Dermatol* 1994, 130:363.

Shalita AR, et al: Acne vulgaris. *J Am Acad Dermatol* 1987, 16:410.

Shalita AR et al: Isotretinoin revisited. *Cutis* 1988, 42:1.

Shalita AR, et al: Topical erythromycin vs clindamycin therapy for acne: a multicenter double-blind comparison. *Arch Dermatol* 1984, 120:351.

Solotoff SA: Pitted scars. *J Dermatol Surg* 1986, 12:1079.

Stern RS: The prevalence of acne on the basis of physical examination. *J Am Acad Dermatol* 1992, 26:931.

Stern RS, et al: Isotretinoin and pregnancy. *J Am Acad Dermatol* 1984, 10:851.

Strauss JS, et al: Isotretinoin therapy for acne: results of a multicenter dose-response study. *J Am Acad Dermatol* 1984, 10:490.

Swinyer LJ, et al: A comparative study of benzoyl peroxide and clindamycin phosphate for treating acne vulgaris. *Br J Dermatol* 1988, 119:615.

Tanzman ES: Long-term tetracycline use in treatment of acne: the role of routine laboratory monitoring. *J Am Coll Health* 1988, 36:272.

Thiboutot D, et al: Androgen metabolism in sebaceous glands from subjects with and without acne. *Arch Dermatol* 1999, 135:1041.

Valentic JP, et al: Inflammatory neovascular nodules associated with oral isotretinoin treatment of severe acne. *Arch Dermatol* 1983, 119:871.

Weiss JS: Current options for the topical treatment of acne vulgaris. *Pediatr Dermatol* 1997, 14: 480.

Whang K-K, et al: The principle of a three-staged operation in the surgery of acne scars. *J Am Acad Dermatol* 1999, 40:95.

White GM: Acne therapy. *Adv Dermatol* 1999, 14:29.

White GM, et al: Recurrence rates after the first course of isotretinoin. *Arch Dermatol* 1998, 134:376.

Wilson BB, et al: Papular acne scars. *Arch Dermatol* 1990, 126:797.

Wong RC, et al: Oral ibuprofen and tetracycline for the treatment of acne vulgaris. *J Am Acad Dermatol* 1984, 11:1076. _____ ▲

ACNE CONGLOBATA

Cystic acne is the mildest form of acne conglobata (*conglobate:* shaped in a rounded mass or ball), an unusually severe form of acne. This form is characterized by numerous comedones (many of which are double or triple), large abscesses with interconnecting sinuses, cysts containing a viscid fluid, and grouped inflammatory nodules. Suppuration is characteristic of acne conglobata.

Pronounced scars remain after healing and produce an unsightly appearance. The cysts are distinctive since they occur most frequently on the forehead, cheeks, and anterior neck (Fig. 13-10). They contain a thick, yellowish, viscid, stringy, blood-tinged fluid. After incision and drainage of the cyst there is frequently prompt refilling with the same type of material. These cysts are suggestive of the type found in hidradenitis suppurativa (Fig. 13-11). Hidradenitis suppurativa and dissecting cellulitis of the scalp may be seen with acne conglobata, an association known as the follicular occlusion triad.

This severe and distinctive disease occurs most frequently in young men around age 16; it may extend and persist into adulthood and even into the fifth decade of life, especially on the posterior neck and back. Women have this severe and painful disease less frequently. Resnick et al reported late-onset acne conglobata with accompanying widespread, filiform, keratotic lesions to be a sign of HIV infection.

The therapy of choice in all but the earliest lesions is isotretinoin, 1 to 2 mg/kg/day for 5 months, with a second course if resolution does not occur after a rest period of 2 months.

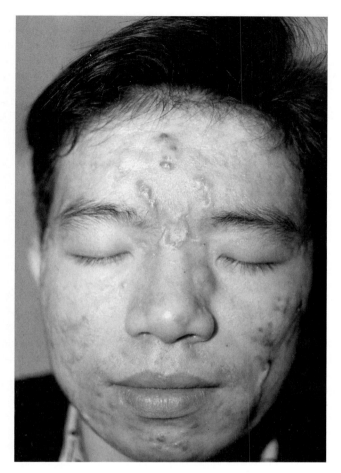

Fig. 13-10 Acne conglobata.

Resnick SD, et al: Acne conglobata and a generalized lichen spinulosa-like eruption in a man seropositive for HIV. *J Am Acad Dermatol* 1991, 26:1013.

Warshaw T: Conglobate acne vulgaris. *J Med Soc New Jersey* 1967, 64:218. _____ ▲

ACNE FULMINANS

Acne fulminans is a rare form of extremely severe cystic acne occurring in teenage boys. It is characterized by highly inflammatory nodules and plaques that undergo swift suppurative degeneration, leaving ragged ulcerations, mostly on the chest and back (Fig. 13-12). The face is usually less severely involved. Fever and leukocytosis are common. Polyarthralgia and polymyalgia, destructive arthritis, and myopathy have been reported in association with it. Focal lytic bone lesions may be seen. Karvonen reported abnormal bone scans in 14 of 17 cases studied and abnormal radiographs in 11 of 22 patients.

Karvonen showed 40 to 60 mg of oral prednisone to be effective therapy. The addition of isotretinoin after initially calming the dramatic inflammatory responses is recom-

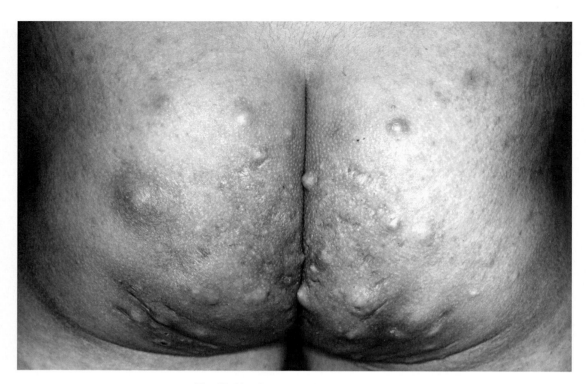

Fig. 13-11 Acne conglobata of buttocks.

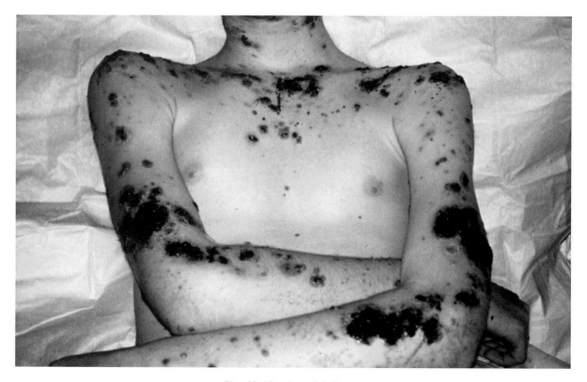

Fig. 13-12 Acne fulminans.

mended. Large cysts may be opened, and the contents expressed. Intralesional corticosteroids will aid their resolution. Success has been reported with dapsone but only in toxic doses—100 mg three or four times daily—so retinoids are the treatment of choice.

Hault P, et al: Acne fulminans with osteolytic lesions. *Arch Dermatol* 1965, 121:662.

Jemec GBE, et al: Bone lesions of acne fulminans. *J Am Acad Dermatol* 1989, 20:353.

Karvonen SL: Acne fulminans. *J Am Acad Dermatol* 1993, 28:572.

Traupe H, et al: Acne of fulminans type following testosterone therapy in 3 excessively tall boys. *Arch Dermatol* 1988, 124:414. _____ ▲

SAPHO SYNDROME

SAPHO syndrome is characterized by *s*ynovitis, *a*cne, *p*ustulosis, *h*yperostosis, and *o*steomyelitis. Skin findings include acne fulminans, acne conglobata, pustular psoriasis, and palmoplantar pustulosis. The chest wall is the most common site for musculoskeletal complaints. Others report similar findings as the acquired hyperostosis syndrome (AHYS) and in a familial setting of a dominantly inherited disorder of pyogenic sterile arthritis, pyoderma gangrenosum, and acne (PAPA syndrome).

Boutin RD, Resnick D: The SAPHO syndrome. *Am J Roentgenol* 1998, 170:585.

Dihlmann W, et al: Acquired hyperostosis syndrome (AHYS). *Clin Rheumatol* 1997, 16:13.

Lindor NM, et al: A new autosomal dominant disorder of pyogenic sterile arthritis, pyoderma gangrenosum, and acne: PAPA syndrome. *Mayo Clin Proc* 1997, 72: 611. _____ ▲

OTHER ACNE VARIANTS
Tropical Acne

Tropical acne is unusually severe acne occurring in the tropics during the seasons when the weather is hot and humid. Nodular, cystic, and pustular lesions occur chiefly on the back, buttocks, and thighs. Characteristically, the face is spared from lesions. Conglobate abscesses occur often, especially on the back. Comedones are sparse. Acne tropicalis usually occurs in young adult patients who may have had acne vulgaris at an earlier age. This is especially true of those in the armed forces stationed in the tropics and carrying backpacks. Treatment is that of cystic acne, but acne tropicalis may persist until the patient moves to a cooler and less humid climate.

Premenstrual Acne

Many women with acne note a premenstrual exacerbation of papulopustular lesions. Usually 5 to 10 lesions will appear a week or so before menstruation. There is some evidence that progesterone mediates premenstrual acne. Frequently, estrogen-dominant contraceptive pills will diminish or prevent premenstrual flares of acne.

Preadolescent Acne

Preadolescent acne can be subdivided into neonatal, infantile, and childhood acne. Neonatal acne (acne neonatorum) is a common condition that by definition is limited to the neonatal period or the first 4 weeks of life. It develops a few days after birth, has a male sex preponderance, and is characterized by transient facial papules or pustules, which usually clear spontaneously in a few days or weeks. Infantile acne includes those cases that persist beyond the neonatal period or have an onset after the first 4 weeks of life. The acne process can extend into childhood, puberty, or adult life.

Childhood acne may evolve from persistent infantile acne or begin after age 2. It is uncommon and has a male predominance. Grouped comedones, papules, pustules, and cysts can occur alone or in any combination, usually limited to the face. The duration is variable, from a few weeks to several years, and occasionally extends into a more severe pubertal acne. Often there is a strong family history of moderately severe acne.

Preadolescent acne is a syndrome of multifactorial etiology. Acne neonatorum results from circulating maternal hormones, whereas acne extending or developing after the neonatal period may be a form of acne cosmetica, acne venenata, drug-induced acne, or part of an endocrinologic disorder. In the absence of any of the mentioned etiologies, one could postulate qualitative or quantitative alterations of cutaneous androgen synthesis or metabolism or increased end-organ sensitivity as pathogenetic mechanisms for preadolescent acne.

Acne Venenata

Contact with a great variety of acnegenic chemicals can produce comedones and result in acne venenata. The most extensive and worst cases are seen in the industrial setting. The better known acnegens of occupational acne venenata are chlorinated hydrocarbons (chloracne), cutting oils, petroleum oil, and coal tar and pitches. Treatment consists of stopping the exposure to causative chemicals and topical application of tretinoin. Several patients have been reported to develop acne in sites of radiation therapy given for malignancy. We have seen such cases also. These respond to topical acne therapy.

Acne Cosmetica

A persistent low-grade acne manifested by closed comedones and papulopustules occurring on the chin and cheeks of adult women, presumably from acnegenic cosmetics, has been described. Avoidance of comedogenic cosmetics is curative, but it may take several months for complete clearing. Many cosmetic companies now test their products for comedogenicity so this type of acne has become uncommon. Avoidance is possible because of the wide variety of acceptable alternatives.

Pomade Acne

Pomade acne is a variety of acne cosmetica occurring almost exclusively in blacks, especially males, who apply various greases and oils to scalp hair or the face as a grooming aid. The lesions are usually closed comedones on the forehead, temples, cheeks, and chin. Comedogenicity of various pomades has been documented. Mineral oil is a very weak comedogenic agent and can be recommended for those who do not wish to avoid pomades altogether.

Acne Detergicans

This type of acne may develop in acne patients who overwash with soaps that contain comedogenic substances. These patients face-wash at least four times daily. Closed comedones are the principal lesions seen. Few ordinary soaps are comedogenic. Unsaturated fatty acids, bacteriostatic substances, and friction probably contribute to the comedogenicity of soap.

Acne Aestivalis

Also known as *Mallorca acne,* this rare form of acne starts in the spring, progresses during the summer, and resolves completely in the fall. It affects almost exclusively women between ages 25 and 40. Dull red, dome-shaped, hard, small papules, usually not more than 3 to 4 mm, develop on the cheeks and commonly extend onto the sides of the neck, chest, shoulders, and characteristically the upper arms. Comedones and pustules are notably absent or sparse. Acne aestivalis does not respond to antibiotics but is benefited by application of retinoic acid.

Acne Mechanica

Many types of mechanical forces, including various pressures, tensions, frictions, stretchings, rubbings, pinchings, and pullings, can aggravate existing acne. The key feature is an unusual distribution pattern of the acne lesions. Provocative factors include chin straps, violins, hats, collars, surgical tape, orthopedic casts, chairs, and seats. Prophylactic measures against various mechanical forces are beneficial.

Excoriated Acne

Also known as *picker's acne* and *acne excorie des jeunes filles,* excoriated acne is seen primarily in girls with a superficial type of acne in which the primary lesions are trivial or even nonexistent, but in which the compulsive neurotic habit of picking the face and squeezing minute comedones produces secondary lesions that may leave scars. Often the lesions are too small to be seen by the naked eye, and the patient resorts to the use of a magnifying

mirror. Eventually, crusts form, and scarring with atrophy results.

Practical assistance to such patients includes suggestions to refrain from unreasonable efforts at cleanliness, to eliminate the use of a magnifying mirror for close observation of the skin, and to forego long fingernails. Acne excorie may be a sign of depression.

Adriaans B, et al: Acne in an irradiated site. *Arch Dermatol* 1989, 125:1005.
Albrecht H, et al: Acne excorie des jeunes filles: psychiatrically considered. *Arch Klin Exp Dermatol* 1965, 223:509.
Hjorth N, et al: Acne aestivalis: Mallorca acne. *Acta Derm Venereol* 1972, 52:61.
Kligman AM, et al: Acne cosmetica. *Arch Dermatol* 1972, 106:843.
Lucky AW, et al: Acne vulgaris in early adolescent boys. *Arch Dermatol* 1991, 127:210.
Mills OH, et al: Acne aestivalis. *Arch Dermatol* 1975, 111:891.
Mills OH, et al: Acne detergicans. *Arch Dermatol* 1975, 111:65.
Mills OH, et al: Acne mechanica. *Arch Dermatol* 1975, 111:481.
Plewig G, et al: Pomade acne. *Arch Dermatol* 1970, 101:580.
Stevanovic DV: Acne in infancy. *Australas J Dermatol* 1960, 5:224.
Tindall JP: Chloracne and chloracnegens. *J Am Acad Dermatol* 1985, 13:539.
Tromovitch TA, et al: Acne in infancy. *Am J Dis Child* 1963, 106:230.

ACNEIFORM ERUPTIONS

Acneiform eruptions are characterized by papules and pustules resembling acne lesions, not necessarily confined to the usual sites of acne vulgaris. The eruptions are distinguished by their sudden onset, usually in a patient well past adolescence.

Most of the acneiform eruptions originate from skin exposure to various industrial chemicals. Acneiform eruptions may be induced by exposure of the skin to the fumes generated in the manufacture of chlorine and its byproducts. These chlorinated hydrocarbons may cause chloracne, consisting of cysts, pustules, folliculitis, and comedones. The most potent acneiform-inducing agents are the polyhalogenated hydrocarbons, notably dioxin (2,3,7,8 tetrachlorobenzodioxin). Cutting oils, lubricating oils, crude coal tar applied to the skin for medicinal purposes, heavy tar distillates, coal tar pitch, and asbestos are known substances that may produce acneiform eruptions. Although commonly called *trade acne, bromine acne,* and *chloracne,* they are not a true acne, even though they are often ushered in by open comedones.

Some of the acneiform eruptions are induced by oral medications such as iodides in vitamins with mineral supplements, and bromides in drugs such as propantheline bromide (Pro-Banthine), testosterone, cyclosporine, antiepileptic medications, lithium, and systemic corticosteroids. When medium or high doses of corticosteroids are taken for as short a time as 3 to 5 days a distinctive eruption may occur, known as *steroid acne.* It is a sudden out-cropping of inflamed papules, most numerous on the upper trunk and arms, but also seen on the face. The lesions typically present as papules rather than comedones; however, Hurwitz's histologic study clearly showed them to be follicular with microcomedon formation. Tretinoin (Retin-A), 0.05% in a vanishing cream applied once or twice daily, may clear the lesions within 1 to 3 months despite the continuation of high doses of corticosteroid. Oral antibiotics and other typical acne medications are also effective. Topical steroids, especially of the fluorinated types, or when applied under occlusion, may also induce an acneiform eruption.

Finkelstein E, et al: Oil acne. *J Am Acad Dermatol* 1994, 30:491.
Fuchs E, et al: Dialysis acne. *J Am Acad Dermatol* 1990, 23:125.
Hitch JM: Acneiform eruptions induced by drugs and chemicals. *JAMA* 1967, 200:879.
Hurwitz, RM: Steroid acne. *J Am Acad Dermatol* 1989, 21:1179.
Tindall JP: Chloracne and chloracnegens. *J Am Acad Dermatol* 1985, 13:539. ⎯⎯⎯⎯⎯⎯⎯⎯⎯⎯⎯⎯⎯⎯⎯⎯ ▲

GRAM-NEGATIVE FOLLICULITIS

Gram-negative folliculitis occurs in patients who have had moderately inflammatory acne for long periods and have been treated with long-term antibiotics, mainly tetracyclines. While on antibiotic treatment, patients develop either superficial pustules 3 to 6 mm in diameter flaring out from the anterior nares, or fluctuant, deep-seated nodules (Fig. 13-13). Culture of these lesions usually reveals a species of *Enterobacter, Klebsiella,* or, from the deep cystic lesions, *Proteus.*

With long-term, broad-spectrum antibiotic therapy the anterior nares may become colonized with these gram-negative organisms. As the use of long-term antibiotic therapy declines (as it has done since the introduction of isotretinoin) this disease is becoming less common.

Isotretinoin is marvelously effective and is the treatment of choice in this disease. James and Leyden have shown that this treatment not only clears the acne component of the disease but also eliminates the colonization of the anterior nares with gram-negative organisms. If isotretinoin cannot be tolerated or is contraindicated, amoxicillin (Augmentin) or trimethoprim-sulfamethoxazole may be effective in suppressing the disease.

James WD, et al: Treatment of gram-negative folliculitis with isotretinoin. *J Am Acad Dermatol* 1985, 12:319.
Leyden JJ, et al: Gram-negative folliculitis: a complication of antibiotic therapy in acne vulgaris. *Br J Dermatol* 1973, 88:533. ⎯⎯⎯⎯⎯ ▲

ACNE KELOIDALIS

Acne keloidalis is also known as *keloidal acne* and *folliculitis keloidalis.* An older, obsolete name was dermatitis papillaris capillitii, the capillitium being the suboccipital portion of the scalp.

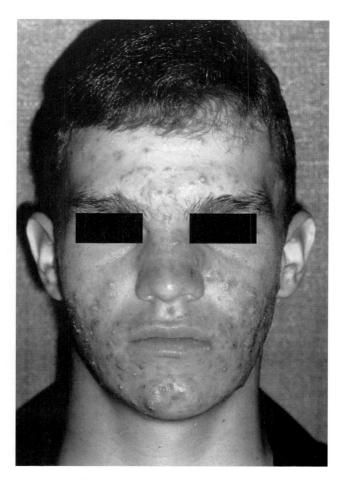

Fig. 13-13 Gram-negative folliculitis.

Acne keloidalis nuchae is most frequently encountered in young adult black or Asian men who otherwise are in excellent health. It is unassociated with acne vulgaris. It is a persistent folliculitis and perifolliculitis of the back of the neck that presents as inflammatory papules and pustules (Fig. 13-14). Over time fibrosis ensues with coalescence of firm papules into keloidal plaques. At times sinus tract formation results.

Histologically, acne keloidalis is a folliculitis of the deep levels of the hair follicle that progresses into a perifolliculitis with an infiltrate consisting of polymorphonuclears, lymphocytes, plasma cells, mast cells, and even foreign-body giant cells. The normal connective tissue is eventually replaced by hypertrophic connective tissue that becomes sclerotic, forming hypertrophic scars or keloids. Persistent free hairs in the dermis may be responsible for the prolonged inflammation and eventual scarring.

Triamcinolone acetonide by intralesional injection, using Kenalog-10 diluted as described under acne vulgaris, into the inflammatory follicular lesions and Kenalog-40 into the hypertrophic scars and keloids is useful in reducing inflammation and fibrosis. This may be combined with surgical treatments.

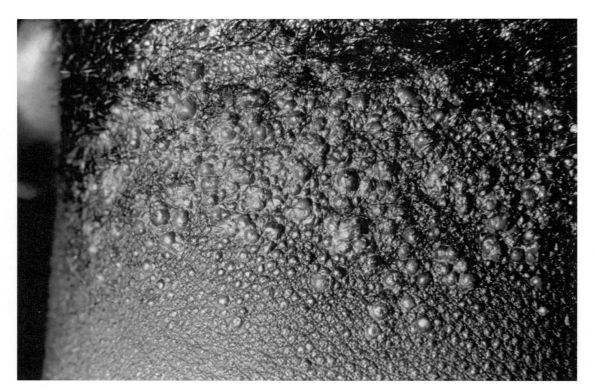

Fig. 13-14 Acne keloidalis.

Kantor et al reported gratifying results in eight consecutive cases using the CO_2 laser to excise the involved plaques. Two of three patients in whom vaporization of lesions was employed experienced recurrences within 8 and 9 months, respectively, and they consider this method to be contraindicated.

Treatment aims are to arrest the active inflammatory component and to reduce or surgically remove the fibrous lesions.

Antibacterials such as the tetracyclines are taken on a long-term basis. Topical steroid ointments in addition to oral antibiotics will be helpful in the majority of patients.

Dinehart SM, et al: Acne keloidalis. *J Dermatol Surg Oncol* 1989, 15:642.
Halder RM: Hair and scalp disorder in blacks. *Cutis* 1983, 32:378.
Herzberg AJ, et al: Acne keloidalis. *Am J Dermatopathol* 1990, 12:109.
Kantor GR, et al: Treatment of acne keloidalis nuchae with carbon dioxide laser. *J Am Acad Dermatol* 1986, 14:263.
Knable AL Jr., et al: Prevalence of acne keloidalis nuchae in football players. *J Am Acad Dermatol* 1997, 37:570. _____ ▲

HIDRADENITIS SUPPURATIVA
Clinical Features

Hidradenitis suppurativa is a disease of the apocrine gland-bearing areas, which occur in the axillae and groin and on the buttocks. The abscesses may also occur around the areolae of the breasts. Obesity and a genetic tendency to acne, especially acne conglobata, seem to be predisposing factors.

The disease is characterized by the development of tender, red nodules, which at first are firm but later become fluctuant and painful. A helpful clinical sign to differentiate early hidradenitis from furunculosis is the presence of comedones in the apocrine areas in the former. Rupture of the lesion, suppuration, and the formation of sinus tracts are distinctive for this process. As these heal, recurrent lesions form, so that the course of the disease is often protracted. It may eventually lead to the formation of honeycombed, fistulous tracts with chronic infection. The individual lesions contain a thick, viscous, mucoid, suppurative material. When a probe is used to explore the suppurating nodule a burrowing sinus tract is usually detected that may extend for many centimeters, running horizontally just underneath the skin surface.

Hidradenitis suppurativa occurs most frequently in the axillae of young women. Men also are affected, but more frequently the groin and perianal area are the sites of involvement (Fig. 13-15). In its severest form, hidradenitis suppurativa is associated with acne conglobata, pilonidal sinus, and dissecting cellulitis of the scalp. Squamous cell carcinoma; interstitial keratitis; spondyloarthropathy; urethral, vesical, and rectal fistulas; anemia; hypoproteinemia; amyloidosis; and eventual renal failure and death have been reported to be associated with hidradenitis suppurativa, but they are extremely rare.

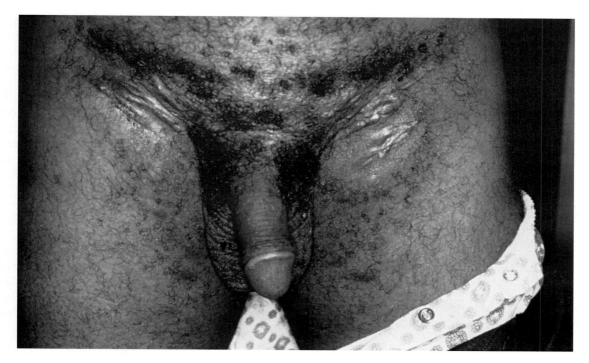

Fig. 13-15 Hidradenitis suppurativa.

Etiology

Hidradenitis suppurativa represents a poral occlusion disease with secondary bacterial infection of the apocrine glands. The initial event is follicular keratinization with resultant plugging of the apocrine duct, followed by dilation and a severe inflammatory response in the apocrine gland. If the glandular inflammation persists, the overlying skin may rupture, and considerable fibrosis and sinus tract formation results. As the disease becomes chronic, ulcers evolve, sinus tracts enlarge, fistulas develop, and fibrosis and scarring become more evident. The process smolders, and acute episodic eruptions intervene indefinitely. The cause of the initiating events remains unknown, but hormonal mechanisms are suspected. Many consider it an axillary cystic acne.

Differential Diagnosis

Hidradenitis is to be differentiated from common furuncles, which are typically unilateral and not associated with comedones as hidradenitis is. Hidradenitis must also be differentiated from Bartholin abscess, scrofuloderma, actinomycosis, and granuloma inguinale.

Treatment

Despite the numerous forms of treatment available, the possibilities for a permanent cure are elusive. The earliest lesions often heal quickly with intralesional steroid therapy, and this should be tried initially in combination with oral antibiotics. Oral tetracycline, minocycline, and erythromycin are useful. Topical daily cleansing with an antibacterial soap or topical clindamycin is an important preventative measure. In cases with draining sinuses, culture of the pus may reveal *Staphylococcus aureus* or gram-negative organisms. The latter are usually cultured in chronic cases. Antibiotics should be selected based on sensitivities of the cultured organism.

Once chronic suppuration and fistulous tracts have become established, incision, drainage, and exteriorization of sinus tracts is helpful. The chances for permanent cure are best when excision of the affected areas is done. Surgical extirpation of cyst-bearing tissues is curative at that site. It is effective but has moderate morbidity, especially in the groin and perianal areas.

Isotretinoin is effective in some cases, but a remission seldom follows its use. In the largest study to date Boer et al treated 68 patients with a mean dose of 0.56 mg/kg of isotretinoin for 4 to 6 months. Clearing was obtained in 23.5%, and long-term remission resulted in 16.2%. Secondary infection with *S. aureus* usually occurs, if it has not already.

Banerjee AK: Surgical treatment of hidradenitis suppurativa. *Br J Surg* 1992, 79:863.

Boer J, et al: Hidradenitis suppurativa or acne inversa. *Br J Dermatol* 1996, 135:721.

Boer J, et al: Long-term results of isotretinoin in the treatment of 68 patients with hidradenitis suppurativa. *J Am Acad Dermatol* 1999, 40:73.

Dicken CH, et al: Evaluation of isotretinoin treatment of hidradenitis suppurativa. *J Am Acad Dermatol* 1984, 11:500.

Dufresne RG Jr, et al: Squamous cell carcinoma arising from the follicular occlusion triad. *J Am Acad Dermatol* 1996, 35:475.

Finley EM, et al: Treatment of hidradenitis suppurativa with carbon dioxide laser excision and second-intention healing. *J Am Acad Dermatol* 1996, 34:465.

Jemec GB, et al: Hidradenitis suppurativa: characteristics and consequences. *Clin Exp Dermatol* 1996, 21:419.

Jemec GB, et al: Ultrasound examination of hair follicles in hidradenitis suppurativa. *Arch Dermatol* 1997, 133:967.

Jemec GB, et al: Histology of hidradenitis suppurativa. *J Am Acad Dermatol* 1996, 34:994.

Jemec GB, et al: The prevalence of hidradenitis suppurativa and its potential precursor lesions. *J Am Acad Dermatol* 1996, 34:191.

Mortimer PS, et al: Androgens in hidradenitis. *Br Med J* 1986, 292:245.

Parks RW, et al: Pathogenesis, clinical features and management of hidradenitis suppurativa. *Ann R Coll Surg Engl* 1997, 79:83.

Rubin RJ, et al: Perianal hidradenitis suppurativa. *Surg Clin North Am* 1994, 74:1317. ▲

PERIFOLLICULITIS CAPITIS ABSCEDENS ET SUFFODIENS

Also known as *dissecting cellulitis of the scalp,* perifolliculitis capitis abscedens et suffodiens is an uncommon chronic suppurative disease of the scalp characterized by numerous follicular and perifollicular inflammatory nodules (Fig. 13-16). These nodules suppurate and undermine to form intercommunicating sinuses. These sinuses, as long as 5 cm, can be easily traced by a probe. Scarring and alopecia ensue, although seropurulent drainage may last indefinitely. Adult black men are most commonly affected, and the vertex and occiput of the scalp are the sites of predilection.

The primary lesions are follicular and perifollicular erythematous papules about which the abscesses develop as a reaction of the tissues against foreign bodies. It is believed that this disease process is a variant of acne vulgaris; it closely resembles acne conglobata and hidradenitis suppurativa. Coagulase-positive *Staphylococcus aureus* and hemolytic *S. albus* may be found in the lesions.

Histologically, the disease is an occluded folliculitis with keratinous debris and a perifolliculitis. The usual inflammatory reaction is similar to that of acne keloidalis.

Treatment is varied and generally unsuccessful unless the most vigorous procedures are followed. The combination of intralesional steroid injections, as described in acne vulgaris, and isotretinoin at a dose of 0.5 to 1.5 mg/kg/day for 6 months may be successful. The length of remission with isotretinoin is variable. Oral antibiotics as given in acne vulgaris and oral zinc have occasionally produced good results.

A surgical approach may be employed if medical treatment fails. The lesions are incised and drained. It is often possible to pass a probe through burrows of intercon-

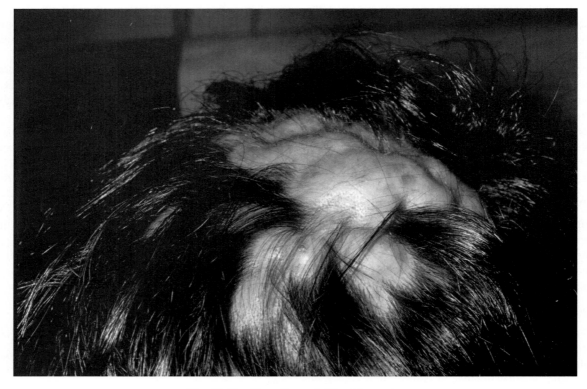

Fig. 13-16 Dissecting cellulitis of the scalp.

necting pustular nodules. These intercommunicating sinuses should be marsupialized. The surface is cauterized to destroy the epithelium lining the sinuses. A similar situation is frequently encountered in hidradenitis suppurativa. Moschella et al have reported successful results from removal of the entire scalp with subsequent grafting.

We have seen excellent results using x-ray epilation. This is also effective in acne keloidalis. Despite this positive experience, radiation therapy for benign conditions is rarely, if ever, utilized today because of potential long-term adverse effects.

Benvenuto ME, et al: Fluctuant nodules and alopecia of the scalp. *Arch Dermatol* 1992, 128:1115.

Berne B, et al: Perifolliculitis capitis abscedens et suffodiens (Hoffman). *Arch Dermatol* 1985, 121:1028.

Moschella SL, et al: Perifolliculitis capitis abscedens et suffodiens. *Arch Dermatol* 1967, 96:195.

Shaffer N, et al: Perifolliculitis capitis abscedens et suffodiens. *Arch Dermatol* 1992, 128:1329.

Taylor AEM: Dissecting cellulitis of the scalp: response to isotretinoin. *Lancet* 1987, 2:225. ▲

ROSACEA

Clinical Features

Rosacea is a chronic inflammatory eruption of the flush areas of the face. It is characterized by erythema, papules, pustules, telangiectasia, and hypertrophy of the sebaceous glands. The latter condition, known as *rhinophyma,* will be discussed subsequently.

Usually the mid-face is involved and most frequently the nose and cheeks, with the brow and chin also affected at times (Figs. 13-17 and 13-18). The eyelids and eyes may be involved (ocular rosacea). Rosacea may be superimposed on seborrhea. Rosacea occurs most often in women between ages 30 and 50; however, the most severe cases are seen in men.

In the mild form of rosacea there is but slight flushing of the nose and cheeks and possibly the forehead and chin. As the process becomes more severe, the lesions become a deeper red or purplish red with chronic dilation of the superficial capillaries (telangiectasia) and inflammatory acneiform pustules.

In the most severe form lesions develop. These are deep-seated, indolent pustules, furuncles, or cystic nodules that may resemble acne conglobata with large abscesses, discharging sinuses, and keloidal scarring. The eyelids may become involved, with blepharitis and conjunctivitis. The eye itself may be affected, with keratitis, iritis, and episcleritis. Gundmundsen et al found an abnormal Schirmer's test in 40% of rosacea patients. Complaints are often of a gritty, stinging, or burning sensation in the eye. Ocular rosacea occurs equally in men and women.

Vin-Christian et al reported acne rosacea as an intensely erythematous pustular eruption in a photosensitive distribution in three HIV-positive patients.

Granulomatous Rosacea

Mullanax and Kierland have called attention to a distinctive form of papular rosacea designated as granulomatous rosacea. This type of rosacea is found not only on the butterfly areas but also on the lateral areas below the mandible, and periorally. The discrete papules appear as yellowish brown nodules on diascopy and as noncaseating epithelioid cell granulomas resembling sarcoidosis, tuberculosis, or other granulomas histologically.

Two other granulomatous papular facial diseases that are considered to be variants of acne rosacea should be mentioned. Lupus miliaris disseminatus faciei consists of multiple, smooth- surfaced, brownish red, 1- to 3-mm papules that occur over the face, including the eyelids and upper lip. It develops rapidly, has a self-limited course of several months to 2 years, and may leave behind pitted scars. Tetracycline may be helpful, but response usually takes 3 to 6 months. A second condition now considered to be a variant of rosacea is a granulomatous perioral dermatitis in children, reported earlier by Williams et al as FACE (Facial Afro-Caribbean Childhood Eruption) syndrome. There is a profusion of grouped papules on the perioral, periocular, and perinasal areas. Black children are

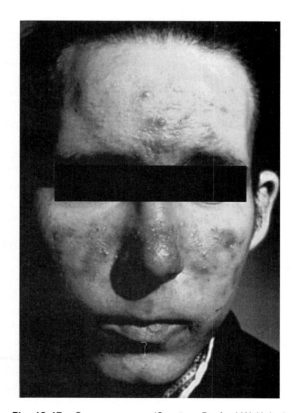

Fig. 13-17 Severe rosacea. (Courtesy Dr. Axel W. Hoke.)

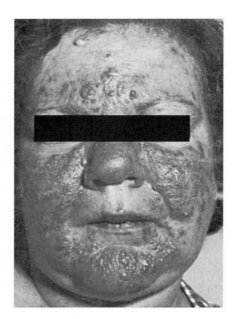

Fig. 13-18   Severe rosacea, with acnelike pustules in typical butterfly distribution on cheeks. (Courtesy Dr. A. Silva.)

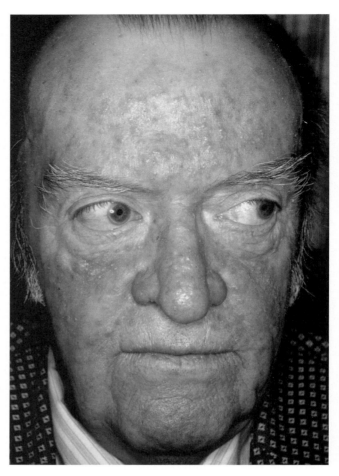

Fig. 13-19   Steroid rosacea.

usually affected, and because the histologic appearance is granulomatous, sarcoidosis is often considered. Topical steroids, however, may worsen the condition and many patients response to topical metronidazole.

Etiology

Vasomotor lability may be closely connected with the pathogenesis of rosacea. Traditionally, caffeine-containing beverages—tea and coffee—have been proscribed on the grounds that, since both cause flushing and both contain caffeine, caffeine must be responsible. Wilkin showed that this is not the case; it is heat that is the common and responsible cause. Hot water, even if merely held in the mouth and not swallowed, causes the same degree of flushing as does hot coffee; cold coffee and caffeine (200 mg) cause no flushing. Alcohol is also well known as an inducer of facial flushing.

The lengthy application of fluorinated corticosteroids may induce a rosacea-like syndrome consisting of severe erythema with telangiectases and often pustules (Fig. 13-19). This may also be seen in perioral dermatitis.

Demodex folliculorum is frequently found in the expressed contents of an inflamed pustular follicle of the nose in cases of rosacea. Its pathogenicity has been controversial for many years. Two recent, large histologic studies of rosacea, with a combined total of 128 patients, revealed *D. folliculorum* in the follicles of only 9 patients. It does not appear to be an etiologic factor in common or granulomatous rosacea, but the possibility that *Demodex* folliculitis exists as an uncommon acne rosacea simulator exists.

Differential Diagnosis

Rosacea is simulated by acne vulgaris, lupus erythematosus, bromoderma, iododerma, and papular syphilid. Haber's syndrome is a genodermatosis characterized by a rosacea-like facial dermatosis and multiple verrucous lesions on non–sun-exposed skin. The onset of the facial lesions is in the first two decades of life, in contrast to the later onset of rosacea. A papulo-nodular eruption of the face that may simulate acne rosacea occurs in patients with AIDS that, on expressing the contents of hair follicles with a comedo extractor, reveals numerous *Demodex* mites. In this case success with permethrin cream and lindane have been reported. We find a lotion containing 5% benzoyl peroxide and 5% precipitated sulfur (Sulfoxyl) is helpful.

Treatment

Long-term oral administration of tetracycline, on a minimum maintenance dose basis, is highly effective, although it is only suppressive, not curative. It has excellent effects on the papulo-pustular component, and systemic therapy is needed for ocular rosacea. Metronidazole, 200 mg twice a day, was reported to be as effective as tetracycline, 250 mg twice a day. It is, however, not as safe when given on a chronic basis. Topical metronidazole is both safe and effective, and metronidazole-containing creams, gels, and lotions are excellent topical choices.

Topical therapy is helpful; however, like other forms of treatment for rosacea (with the occasional exception of isotretinoin) it is only suppressive and must be used on a long-term, daily basis. Sunscreens daily and avoidance of flushing triggers if possible are helpful long-term interventions. Topical medications similar to those used in acne vulgaris may be employed. Topical antibiotics and benzoyl peroxide preparations may control the disease although the skin of patients with rosacea is easily irritated and has a low tolerance for many acne preparations.

Isotretinoin produces dramatic improvement even in cases resistant to other forms of therapy, but relapse in a few weeks or months often occurs. In the menopausal age estrogens have been found to be effective in some women with severe rosacea. The flash lamp pumped dye laser offers adjunctive therapy to the telangiectatic component.

In patients with topical steroid-induced red faces, treatment is to discontinue the corticosteroid usage. Flares of redness and swelling will occur, but cure will not be obtained until topical steroids are ceased.

Bleicher PA, et al: Topical metronidazole therapy for rosacea. *Arch Dermatol* 1987, 123:609.

Ertl GA, et al: A comparison of the efficacy of topical tretinoin and low-dose isotretinoin in rosacea. *Arch Dermatol* 1994, 130:319.

Frieden, IJ, et al: Granulomatous perioral dermatitis in children. *Arch Dermatol* 1989, 125:369.

Frieden IJ, et al: You say potato, we say potatoe (reply). *Arch Dermatol* 1994, 130:114.

Gundmundsen KJ, et al: Schirmer testing for dry eyes in patients with rosacea. *J Am Acad Dermatol* 1992, 26:211.

Helm KF, et al: A clinical and histologic study of granulomatous rosacea. *J Am Acad Dermatol* 1991, 25:1038.

Hoting E, et al: Treatment of rosacea with isotretinoin. *Int J Dermatol* 1986, 25:660.

Kikuchi I, et al: Haber's syndrome. *Arch Dermatol* 1981, 117:321.

Lowe NJ, et al: Flash lamp pumped dye laser for rosacea-associated telangiectasia and erythema. *J Dermatol Surg Oncol* 1991, 17:522.

Lowe NJ, et al: Topical metronidazole for severe and recalcitrant rosacea. *Cutis* 1989, 43:283.

Martin DL, et al: Recent onset of smooth, shiny, erythematous papules of the face. *Arch Dermatol* 1989, 125:827.

Montes LF, et al: Topical treatment of acne rosacea with benzoyl peroxide acetone gel. *Cutis* 1983, 32:185.

Mullanax MG, et al: Granulomatous rosacea. *Arch Dermatol* 1970, 101:206.

Puppin D Jr, et al: Lupus miliaris faciei. *Arch Dermatol* 1994, 130:369.

Ramelet AA, et al: Rosacea: a histopathologic study of 75 cases. *Ann Dermatol Venereol* 1988, 115:801.

Rapaport MJ, Rapaport V: Eyelid dermatitis to red face syndrome to cure. *J Am Acad Dermatol* 1999, 41:435.

Rosen T, et al: Acne rosacea in blacks. *J Am Acad Dermatol* 1987, 17:70.

Saihan EM, et al: A double-blind trial of metronidazole vs oxytetracycline treatment for rosacea. *Br J Dermatol* 1980, 102:443.

Schewach-Millet M, et al: Granulomatous rosacea. *J Am Acad Dermatol* 1988, 18:1362.

Schmidt JB, et al: 13-cis-retinoic acid in rosacea. *Acta Derm Venereol* (Stockh) 1984, 64:15.

Shitara A: Lupus miliaris disseminatus faciei. *Int. J Dermatol* 1984; 23:542.

Vin-Christian K, et al: Acne rosacea as a cutaneous manifestation of HIV infection. *J Am Acad Dermatol* 1994, 30:139.

Wilkin JK: Rosacea. *Arch Dermatol* 1994, 130:359.

Wilkin JK: Use of topical products for maintaining remission in rosacea. *Arch Dermatol* 1999, 135:79.

Williams HC, et al: FACE: facial Afro-Caribbean childhood eruption. *Clin Exp Dermatol* 1990, 15:163. ▲

RHINOPHYMA

Rhinophyma consists of hypertrophic, hyperemic, large nodular masses centered on the distal half of the nose. Rhinophyma is seen almost exclusively in men over age 40. The tip and wings of the nose are usually involved by large lobulated masses, which may even be pendulous. The hugely dilated follicles contain long vermicular plugs of sebum and keratin. The cause of rhinophyma is unknown. It is usually associated with a long history of rosacea. The histologic features are pilosebaceous gland hyperplasia with fibrosis, inflammation, and telangiectasia.

Treatment of this disfigurement is simple and most effective. Isotretinoin, though surprisingly helpful, is hardly worth giving because the benefit is so temporary. Rhinophyma is best treated by surgical ablation, electrosurgery (surgical cutting current) (Fig. 13-20), laser surgery, or wire-brush surgery.

For anesthesia a bilateral infraorbital nerve block just below the notch in the maxilla on both sides and a ring of 1% lidocaine (Xylocaine) in the skin around the nose produce complete anesthesia. Often the latter is sufficient. The needle is introduced opposite each ala and the injection is made upward toward the bridge of the nose. If a needle 1½ inches long is used, the two injections will meet on the bridge of the nose. If the needle is partially withdrawn and then reintroduced along the upper lip horizontally, a complete ring of anesthesia is given through the same puncture wound. In addition, it is advisable to withdraw the needle partially again and then to make an injection downward toward the corner of the mouth.

Surgical ablation of redundant grapelike masses and of the bulbous swollen tip of the nose is easily done with a razor blade or Shaw scalpel. This instrument has a copper- and Teflon-coated standard scalpel blade with a thermostatically controlled heating element that heats it to 110° to 270° C, which provides hemostasis. The excessive tissue is shaved off in successive layers until the desired amount has been removed. Bleeding is minimal. A hydrogel dressing such as Vigilon may be utilized. Dermabrasion is useful for

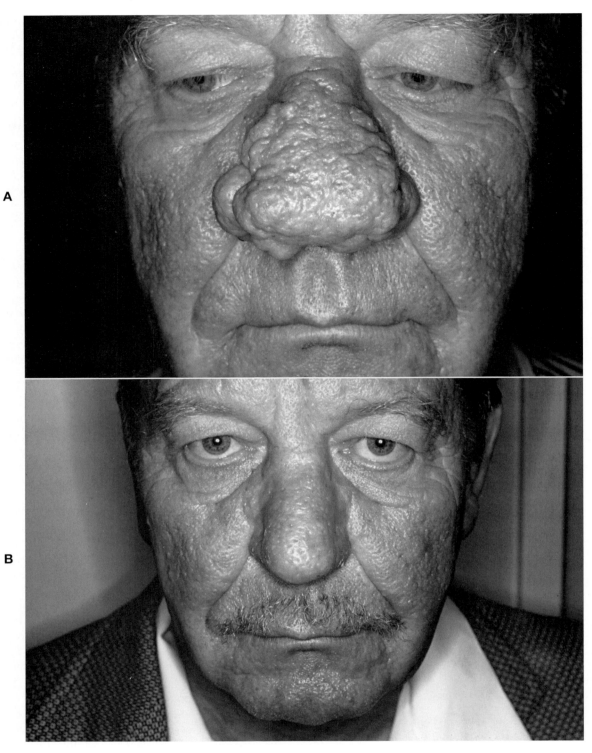

Fig. 13-20 **A** and **B**, Rhinophyma before and after electrosurgical ablation.

mild cases. If there are pendulous redundant masses, these should first be cut off with a scalpel or with surgical cutting current. Dermabrasion may then be used to remove any objectionable remnants. The CO_2 laser may also be used to excise redundant tissue, and the argon laser may ameliorate the vascular component of rosacea.

Eisen RF, et al: Surgical treatment of rhinophyma with the Shaw scalpel. *Arch Dermatol* 1986, 122:307.

Fisher WJ: Rhinophyma: its surgical treatment. *Plast Reconstr Surg* 1970, 45:466.

Greenbaum SS, et al: Comparison of CO_2 laser and electrosurgery in the treatment of rhinophyma. *J Am Acad Dermatol* 1988, 18:363.

Simpson GT, et al: Rhinologic laser surgery. *Otolaryngol Clin North Am* 1983, 16:829.

Tromovitch TA, et al: The Shaw scalpel. *J Dermatol Surg Oncol* 1983, 9:316. ▲

PYODERMA FACIALE

O'Leary and Kierland described pyoderma faciale, which occurs on the face. It consists of an intense reddish or cyanotic erythema, combined with superficial and deep abscesses and cystic lesions (Fig. 13-21). Some cysts are connected by communicating channels or sinus tracts. Some contain greenish or yellowish purulent material. Older cysts contain an oily substance. The condition occurs mostly in postadolescent girls and is distinguished from acne by the absence of comedones, the rapid onset, the fulminating course, and the absence of acne on the back and chest.

A Mayo Clinic series of 29 patients, all women, ranged in age from 19 to 59 years old; only 2 were over age 40. Late-onset acne preceded pyoderma faciale by from 7 to 20 years. None had gram-negative organisms; only two had *Staphylococcus*. Most had the usual acne pathogens. Plewig et al reported 20 women with a mean age of 25. All were flushers and blushers. They consider it a variant of severe rosacea and suggest the name *rosacea fulminans.*

Treatment is similar to that of acne fulminans. Oral steroids given for several weeks followed by the addition of isotretinoin is recommended. Oral steroids may usually be discontinued after an additional 2 weeks; however, isotretinoin should be maintained for a full 5-month course. Whereas the patients are predominately women of childbearing age, pregnancy issues require full discussion. Indeed, four of Plewig et al's patients were pregnant and thus could only use erythromycin.

Markson VJ, et al: Pyoderma faciale. *J Am Acad Dermatol* 1987, 17:1062.

Massa MC, et al: Pyoderma faciale: a clinical study of 29 patients. *J Am Acad Dermatol* 1982, 6:84.

Plewig G, et al: Pyoderma faciale. *Arch Dermatol* 1992, 128:1611. ▲

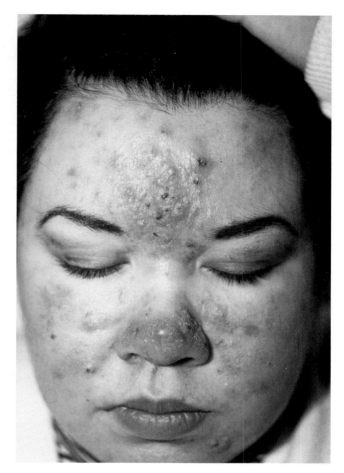

Fig. 13-21 Pyoderma faciale.

PERIORAL DERMATITIS

This common perioral papulosquamous eruption consists of discrete papules and vesicopustules on an erythematous and scaling base (Fig. 13-22). It is a distinctive dermatitis confined symmetrically around the mouth, with a clear zone of some 5 mm between the vermilion border and the affected skin. There is no itching; however, an uncomfortable burning sensation may be present. It occurs almost exclusively in women between ages 23 and 35. Frieden et al described granulomatous perioral dermatitis in children. This entity is discussed earlier in this chapter under acne rosacea.

Wilkinson espouses the English view that since only 5% to 8% of patients deny using strong corticosteroid creams, these creams must be the cause. Fluoridated dentifrices have been suspected but not incriminated conclusively. *Demodex* has been suspected, and when it has been found, benzoyl peroxide lotion has often been effective.

Tetracycline, 250 to 1000 mg by mouth daily, should be used for pustular lesions, with dosages decreased as control is attained.

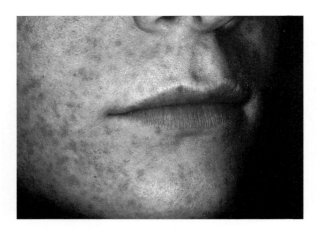

Fig. 13-22 Perioral dermatitis.

Periorbital Dermatitis

Periorbital (periocular) dermatitis is a variant of perioral dermatitis occurring in a distribution around the lower eyelids and skin adjacent to the upper and lower eyelids. Fluorinated topical steroid cream has been implicated as the cause. Prompt response to 250 mg of tetracycline four times a day with hydrocortisone topically has been reported.

Fisher AA: Periocular dermatitis akin to the perioral variety. *J Am Acad Dermatol* 1986, 15:642.
Frieden IJ, et al: Granulomatous perioral dermatitis in children. *Arch Dermatol* 1989, 125:369.
Wilkinson D: What is perioral dermatitis? *Int J Dermatol* 1981, 20:485. ▲

ACNE MILIARIS NECROTICA (ACNE VARIOLIFORMIS)

Acne miliaris necrotica consists of follicular vesicopustules, sometimes occurring as solitary lesions that are usually very itchy. They appear anywhere in the scalp or adjacent areas, rupture early, and dry up after a few days. In some patients, especially those who manipulate the lesions, *Staphylococcus aureus* may be cultured. If they leave large scars the name *acne varioliformis* is used; they are probably not separate diseases. This is probably closely aligned to the scalp folliculitis reported by Maibach to be caused by *Propionibacterium acnes*.

Treatment is with culture-directed antibiotics, or if the culture is negative, tetracycline. Fisher also feels doxepin is helpful if patients manipulate their lesions.

Fisher DA: Acne necroticans and *Staphylococcus aureus*. *J Am Acad Dermatol* 1988, 18:1136.
Kossard S, et al: Necrotizing lymphocytic folliculitis: the early lesion of acne necrotica. *J Am Acad Dermatol* 1987, 16:1007.
Maibach HI: Scalp pustules due to *Corynebacterium acnes*. *Arch Dermatol* 1967, 96:453. _____ ▲

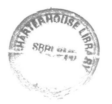

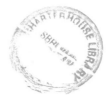

CHAPTER 14

Bacterial Infections

Bacterial infections in the skin often have distinct morphologic characteristics that should alert the clinician that a potentially treatable and reversible condition exists. These cutaneous signs may be an indication of a generalized systemic process or simply an isolated superficial event.

Immunodeficiencies with low immunoglobulins, neutropenia, reduced neutrophil migration or killing, and disease caused by the human immunodeficiency virus (HIV) may be associated with severe or refractory pyogenic infections. Atopic dermatitis and syndromes with atopic-like dermatitis are also predisposed to bacterial infections.

The categorization of these infections will be first those diseases caused by gram-positive bacteria, then those caused by gram-negative bacteria, and finally several miscellaneous diseases caused by the rickettsiae, mycoplasmas, chlamydiae, and spirochetes.

1998 STD Treatment Guidelines. *MMWR* 1998, 47:1.

Epstein ME, et al: Antimicrobial agents for the dermatologist. Part I. *J Am Acad Dermatol* 1997, 37:149.

Epstein ME, et al: Antimicrobial agents for the dermatologist. Part II. *J Am Acad Dermatol* 1997, 37:365.

Feingold DS: Bacterial adherence, colonization, and pathogenicity. *Arch Dermatol* 1986, 122:161.

Feingold DS, et al: Bacterial infections of the skin. *J Am Acad Dermatol* 1989, 20:469.

Hauser C, et al: Superantigens and their role in immune-mediated disease. *J Invest Dermatol* 1993, 101:503.

Hirschmann JV: Topical antibiotics in dermatology. *Arch Dermatol* 1988, 124:1691.

Kovacs A, et al: Bacterial infections. *Med Clin North Am* 1997, 81:319.

Leyden JJ: Infections in the immunocompromised host. *Arch Dermatol* 1985, 121:854.

Roth RR, James WD: Microbiology of the skin: resident flora, ecology, infection. *J Am Acad Dermatol* 1989, 20:367.

Sadick NS: Current aspects of bacterial infections of the skin. *Dermatol Clin* 1997, 15:341. ▲

Infections caused by gram-positive organisms

STAPHYLOCOCCAL INFECTIONS

The skin lesions induced by this gram-positive coccus appear usually as simply pustules, furuncles, or erosions with honey-colored crusts; however, bullae, widespread erythema and desquamation, or vegetating pyodermas may also be indicators of *Staphylococcus aureus* infection. Purulent purpura may indicate bacteremia or endocarditis caused by *S. aureus,* or, in immunocompromised patients, *S. epidermidis.* Two distinctive cutaneous lesions that occur with endocarditis are the Osler's node and Janeway lesion, or spot. The former is a painful, erythematous nodule with a pale center located on the fingertips. The latter is a nontender, hemorrhagic lesion of the palms and soles. Cardullo et al present evidence that Janeway lesions are septic emboli. Osler's nodes probably have a similar pathomechanism.

S. aureus is a normal inhabitant of the anterior nares in approximately 20% of adults. These nasal carriers are particularly prone to infections with this bacterium because of its continuous presence on the skin and nasal mucosa. HIV-infected patients are at least twice as commonly nasal carriers, predisposing them to skin and systemic infection.

Superficial Pustular Folliculitis (Impetigo of Bockhart)

Bockhart's impetigo is a superficial folliculitis with thin-walled pustules at the follicle orifices. Favorite locations are the extremities and scalp, although it is also seen on the face, especially periorally (Fig. 14-1). These fragile, yellowish white, domed pustules develop in crops and heal in a few days. *S. aureus* is the most frequent cause. The infection may secondarily arise in scratches, insect bites, or other skin injuries.

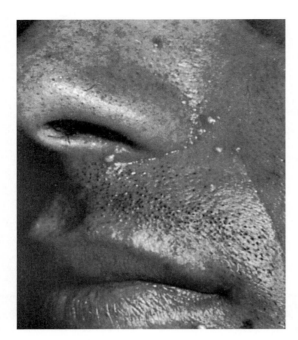

Fig. 14-1 Impetigo of Bockhart (note superficial, persistent pustules).

Sycosis Vulgaris (Sycosis Barbae)

Sycosis vulgaris, formerly known as barber's itch, is a perifollicular, chronic, pustular staphylococcal infection of the bearded region, characterized by the presence of inflammatory papules and pustules, and a tendency to recurrence (Fig. 14-2). The disease begins with erythema and a burning or itching, usually on the upper lip near the nose. In a day or two one or more pinhead-sized pustules, pierced by hairs, develop. These rupture after shaving or washing and leave an erythematous spot, which is later the site of a fresh crop of pustules. In this manner the infection persists and gradually spreads. With the formation of pus about the hairs they become loose and can be readily epilated. Marginal blepharitis with conjunctivitis usually is present in severe cases of sycosis.

Sycosis vulgaris is to be distinguished from tinea, acne vulgaris, pseudofolliculitis barbae, and herpetic sycosis. Tinea barbae rarely affects the upper lip, which is a common location for sycosis. In tinea barbae the involvement usually is in the submaxillary region or on the chin, and spores and hyphae are found in the hairs. Pseudofolliculitis barbae manifests torpid papules at the sites of ingrowing beard hairs, in black men. In herpes simplex the duration is usually only a few days and even in persistent cases there are vesicles, which help to differentiate the disease from sycosis vulgaris.

Folliculitis

Staphylococcal folliculitis may affect other areas, such as the eyelashes, axillae, pubis, and thighs. On the pubis it may be transmitted among sexual partners, and mini-epidemics

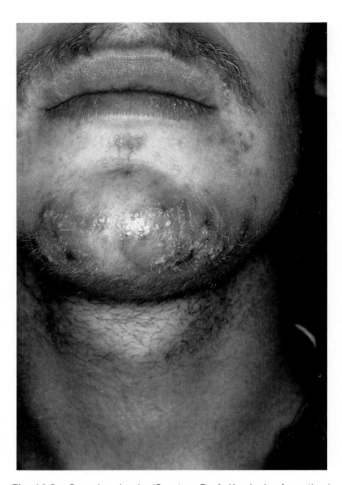

Fig. 14-2 Sycosis vulgaris. (Courtesy Dr. A. Kaminsky, Argentina.)

of folliculitis and furunculosis of the genital and gluteal areas may be considered a sexually transmitted disease. Staphylococcal folliculitis has also been reported frequently among patients with acquired immunodeficiency syndrome (AIDS) and may be a cause of pruritus. An atypical, plaquelike form has been reported.

Sycosis Lupoides

Sycosis lupoides is a staphylococcal infection that, by peripheral extension and central scar formation, forms a patch somewhat resembling lupus vulgaris; hence the name. The hairless atrophic area is usually bordered by pustules and crusts. *S. aureus* from the nasal cavity or from colonized skin often acts as a reservoir. Direct inoculation from shaving may cause the disease. It is a pyogenic folliculitis and perifolliculitis, with the infection extending deep into the follicles. Inflammatory changes with vascular dilation and cellular infiltration are present, with edema and infiltration of neutrophils and plasma cells.

Treatment of All Forms of Folliculitis

A thorough cleansing of the affected areas with antibacterial soap and water three times daily is recommended. Bac-

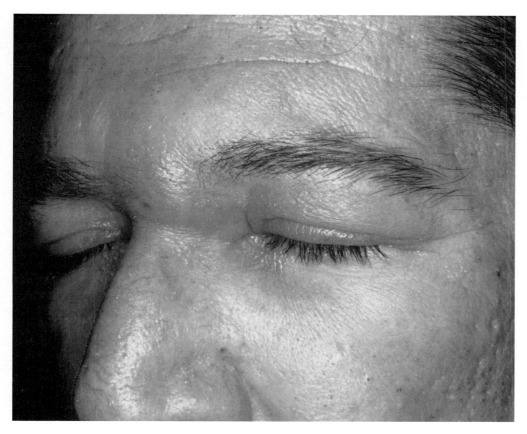

Fig. 14-3 Furuncle of glabella.

troban (mupirocin) ointment topically is advised. If it fails, a first-generation cephalosporin, or a penicillinase-resistant penicillin such as oxacillin, cloxacillin, or dicloxacillin, is indicated. When the inflammation is acute, hot, wet soaks with Burow's solution diluted 1:20 (Domeboro) are beneficial. An anhydrous formulation of aluminum chloride (Drysol, Xerac-AC) has been reported by Shelley and Hurley to be effective when used once nightly for chronic folliculitis, especially of the buttocks. Antibiotic ophthalmic ointments are used for blepharitis.

Furunculosis

A furuncle, or boil, is an acute, round, tender, circumscribed, perifollicular staphylococcal abscess that generally ends in central suppuration (Fig. 14-3). A carbuncle is merely two or more confluent furuncles, with separate heads (Fig. 14-4).

The lesions begin in hair follicles, and often continue for a prolonged period by autoinoculation. Some lesions disappear before rupture, but most undergo central necrosis and rupture through the skin, discharging purulent, necrotic debris. Sites of predilection are the nape, axillae, and buttocks, but boils may occur anywhere.

The integrity of the skin surface may be impaired by irritation, pressure, friction, hyperhidrosis, dermatitis, dermatophytosis, or shaving, among other factors. This may provide a portal of entry for the ubiquitous *S. aureus*. Compromised local integrity predisposes to infection. The proximate cause is either contagion, or autoinoculation from a carrier focus, usually in the nose or groin.

Certain systemic disorders may predispose to furunculosis: alcoholism; malnutrition; blood dyscrasias; disorders of neutrophil function; iatrogenic or other immunosuppression, including AIDS; and diabetes. Patients with several of the diseases just mentioned, as well as those receiving renal dialysis or under treatment with isotretinoin or etretinate, are often nasal carriers of *S. aureus*. Additionally, atopic dermatitis also predisposes to the *S. aureus* carrier state. This fact helps explain the observed increases in the incidence of infections in these diseases.

Hospital Furunculosis. Epidemics of staphylococcal infections occur in hospitals. Marked resistance to antibacterial agents in these cases is commonplace. Attempts to control these outbreaks center on meticulous handwashing. In nurseries, a fall in neonatal colonization and infections with *S. aureus* and non-group A streptococci by using a 4% solution of chlorhexidine for skin and umbilical cord care may be achieved.

The histopathologic appearance is of a deep abscess with both lymphocytes and neutrophils, and in long-standing cases, plasma cells and foreign-body giant cells.

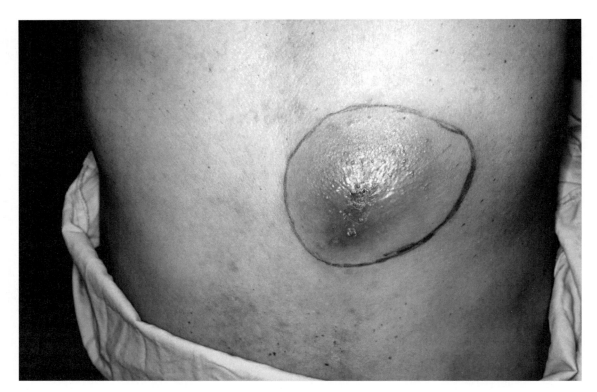

Fig. 14-4 Carbuncle.

Treatment

Warm compresses and antibiotics taken internally may arrest early furuncles. A penicillinase-resistant penicillin or a first-generation cephalosporin should be given orally in a dose of 1 to 2 g/day according to the severity of the case. Methicillin-resistant and even vancomycin-resistant strains occur. In cases of staphylococcal infections that are unresponsive to these usual measures, antibiotic-resistant strains should be suspected and sensitivities checked. Bactroban applied to the anterior nares daily for 5 days may help prevent recurrence.

When the lesions are incipient and acutely inflamed, incision should be strictly avoided and moist heat employed. When the furuncle has become localized and shows definite fluctuation, incision, with drainage, is indicated. The cavity should be packed with iodoform or Vaseline gauze.

SPECIAL LOCATIONS. In boils of the external auditory canal, irrigations and early incisions should not be attempted. An antibiotic ointment (Bactroban) should be applied, and antibiotics should be given internally. Heat should be applied to the auricle and side of the face.

Nasal furuncles should be treated in the early stages by application of hot, saline-solution compresses inside and outside the nostril, until softening occurs. They should not be incised but steamed. Antibiotics should be given internally and applied locally.

On the upper lip and nose, energetic treatment should be instituted because of the dangers of sinus thrombosis, meningitis, and septicemia developing from boils on these parts. Trauma must be prevented by the use of an adequate dressing. Local and general treatment should be followed in accordance with the principles already described. Adequate doses of systemic antibiotics are essential. Incision should not be made unless all other treatments fail.

Chronic Furunculosis.

Despite treatment, recurrences of some boils may be anticipated. Usually no underlying disease is present to predispose to this; rather, autoinoculation and intrafamilial spread among colonized individuals is responsible.

One of the most important factors in prevention is to avoid autoinoculation. It is important to emphasize that the nasal carrier state predisposes to chronic furunculosis. In addition, the hazard of contamination from the perianal and intertriginous areas is to be considered. Routine precautions to be taken in attempting to break the cycle of recurrent furunculosis should be the daily use of an antibacterial soap or chlorhexidine, with special attention to the axillae, groin, and perianal area; laundering of bedding and clothing daily initially; and frequent handwashing. Additionally, the daily application of Bactroban ointment twice daily to the nares of patients and family members every fourth week has been found to be effective. Rifampin, 600 mg daily for 10 days,

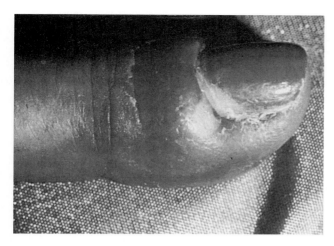

Fig. 14-5 Paronychia caused by *Staphylococcus aureus.*

combined with cloxacillin, 500 mg four times daily, or low-dose (150 mg/day) clindamycin for 3 months are other options that are effective in eradicating the nasal carriage state. The use of bacitracin ointment inside the nares twice daily throughout the course of isotretinoin therapy eliminates, or markedly reduces, the risk of inducing nasal carriage of *S. aureus,* and hence staphylococcal infections.

Pyogenic Paronychia

Paronychia is an inflammatory reaction involving the folds of the skin surrounding the fingernail. It is characterized by acute or chronic purulent, tender, and painful swellings of the tissues around the nail, caused by an abscess in the nail fold (Fig. 14-5). When the infection becomes chronic, horizontal ridges appear at the base of the nail. With recurrent bouts new ridges appear.

The primary predisposing factor that is identifiable is separation of the eponychium from the nail plate. The separation is usually caused by trauma as a result of moisture-induced maceration of the nail folds from frequent wetting of the hands. The relationship is close enough to justify treating chronic paronychia as work-related in bartenders, food servers, nurses, and others who often wet their hands. The moist grooves of the nail and nail fold become secondarily invaded by pyogenic cocci and yeasts. The causative bacteria are usually *Staphylococcus aureus, Streptococcus pyogenes, Pseudomonas* species, *Proteus* species, or anaerobes. The pathogenic yeast is most frequently *Candida albicans.*

The bacteria usually cause acute abscess formation *(Staphylococcus)* or erythema and swelling *(Streptococcus)* (Fig. 14-6), and *C. albicans* most frequently cause a chronic swelling. There may be overlap, as reported by Montemarano et al. Smears of purulent material will help confirm the clinical impression. Additionally, myremecial warts may at times mimic paronychia, as reported by Holland et al. Boiko et al reported the appearance of sub-

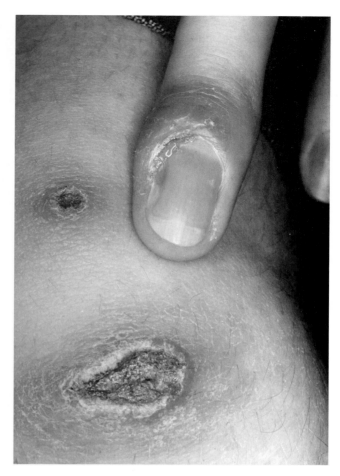

Fig. 14-6 Streptococcal paronychia and impetigo.

ungual black macules followed by edema, pain, and swelling in three children with atopic dermatitis. This was a sign of osteomyelitis caused by *S. aureus* in two and *Streptococcus viridans* in the third.

Treatment of pyogenic paronychia consists mostly of protection against trauma and studious, concentrated efforts to keep the affected fingernails meticulously dry. Rubber or plastic gloves over cotton gloves should be used whenever the hand must be placed in water. Incision and drainage should be done on the acutely inflamed pyogenic abscesses. The abscess may often be opened by pushing the nail fold away from the nail plate. In acute suppurative paronychia, especially if stains show pyogenic cocci, a semisynthetic penicillin or a first-generation cephalosporin should be given orally. If these are ineffective, Brook reported the recovery of anaerobic bacteria frequently and suggested Augmentin may improve cure rates. Rarely, long-term antibiotic therapy may be required.

For chronic paronychia a fungicide and bactericide such as Neosporin solution, Vioform, or 2% thymol in acetone may be used. Castellani paint, which should be applied several times daily regularly for several months, is effective, and with the omission of the acid fuchsin, the colorless preparation does not stain the lesions or clothing. Oral azole antifungals will clear the soft-tissue infection if topical care is ineffective.

Botryomycosis

Botryomycosis is an uncommon, chronic, indolent disorder characterized by nodular, crusted, purulent lesions. Sinuses that discharge sulfur granules are present. These heal with atrophic scars. The granules yield most commonly *S. aureus* on culture, although cases caused by *Pseudomonas aeruginosa, Escherichia coli, Proteus, Bacteroides,* and *Streptococcus* have been reported. It occurs frequently in patients with altered immune function, such as in patients with neutrophilic defects. Other predisposing factors include diabetes, alcoholism, and Job's syndrome. Appropriate antibiotics, surgical drainage, and surgical excision are methods used to treat botryomycosis.

Blastomycosis-Like Pyoderma

Large verrucous plaques with elevated borders and multiple pustules may occur as a chronic vegetating infection. Most patients have some underlying systemic or local host compromise. Bacteria such as *S. aureus, P. aeruginosa, Proteus, E. coli,* or streptococci may be isolated. Antibiotics appropriate for the organism isolated are curative; however, response may be delayed and prolonged therapy required.

Pyomyositis

S. aureus abscess formation within the deep, large, striated muscles usually presents with fever and muscle pain. It is more common in the tropics, where it occurs in adults and children. In temperate climates it occurs in children and patients with AIDS. The most frequent site is the thigh. Maddox et al reported a case that presented with a purplish discoloration of the lower extremity. Occasionally, erythema or yellow discoloration develops, but these are late findings. Magnetic resonance imaging (MRI) will help delineate the extent of disease. Drainage of the abscess and appropriate systemic antibiotics are required.

Impetigo Contagiosa

Impetigo contagiosa is staphylococcal, streptococcal, or combined infection characterized by discrete, thin-walled vesicles that rapidly become pustular and then rupture (Figs. 14-7 and 14-8). Impetigo occurs most frequently on the exposed parts of the body: the face, hands, neck, and extremities. Impetigo on the scalp is a frequent complication of pediculosis capitis.

The disease begins with 2-mm erythematous macules, which may shortly develop into vesicles or bullae. As soon as these lesions rupture, a thin, straw-colored, seropurulent discharge is noticed. The exudate dries to form loosely stratified golden yellow crusts, which accumulate layer upon layer until they are thick and friable.

The crusts can usually be removed readily, leaving a smooth, red, moist surface that soon collects droplets of fresh exudate again; these are spread to other parts of the body by fingers or towels. As the lesions spread peripherally and the skin clears centrally, large circles are formed by fusion of the spreading lesions to produce gyrate patterns. In streptococcal-induced impetigo, regional lymphadenopathy is common, but not serious.

Although two decades ago streptococci caused the majority of cases of impetigo, by the end of the 1970s it became apparent that the predominant pathogen was *Staphylococcus aureus*. Most studies now find 50% to 70% of cases are due to *S. aureus,* with the remainder either being due to *Streptococcus pyogenes* or a combination of these two organisms. Group B streptococci are associated with newborn impetigo and groups C and G are rarely isolated from impetigo, as opposed to the usual group A.

Impetigo occurs most frequently in early childhood, although all ages may be affected. It occurs in the temperate zone, mostly during the summer in hot, humid weather. Common sources of infection for children are pets, dirty fingernails, and other children in schools, day-care centers, or crowded housing areas; for adults, common sources include barber shops, beauty parlors, meat-packing plants, swimming pools, and infected children. Impetigo often complicates pediculosis capitis, scabies, herpes simplex, insect bites, poison ivy, eczema, and other exudative, pustular or itching skin diseases.

Group A beta-hemolytic streptococcal skin infections are sometimes followed by acute glomerulonephritis (AGN). Some types of nephritogenic streptococci are associated with impetigo rather than with upper respiratory infections. There is no evidence that AGN occurs with staphylococcal impetigo. The important factor predisposing to AGN is the serotype of the streptococcus producing the impetigo. Type 49, 55, 57, and 60 strains and strain M-type 2 are related to nephritis.

The incidence of AGN with impetigo varies from about 2% to 5% (10% to 15% with nephritogenic strains of streptococcus) and occurs most frequently in childhood, generally under age 6. The prognosis in children is mostly excellent; however, in adults the prognosis is not as good. Treatment, however early and however appropriate, is not believed to reduce the risk of occurrence of AGN.

The histopathology is that of an extremely superficial inflammation about the funnel-shaped upper portion of the pilosebaceous follicles. A subcorneal vesicopustule is formed, containing a few scattered cocci, together with debris of polymorphonuclear leukocytes and epidermal cells. In the dermis there is a mild inflammatory reaction—vascular dilation, edema, and infiltration of polymorphonuclear leukocytes.

Impetigo may simulate several diseases. The circinate patches are frequently mistaken for ringworm, but clinically are quite different. Impetigo is characterized by superficial,

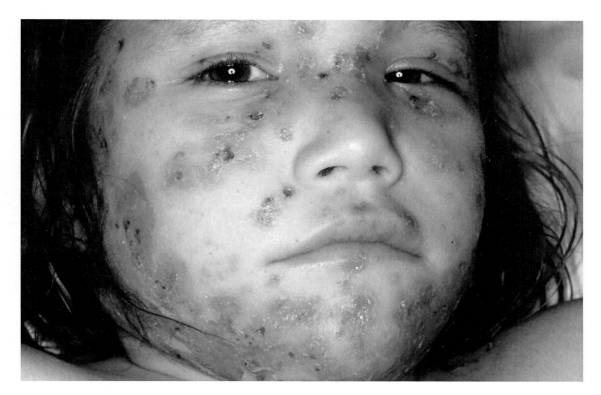

Fig. 14-7 Impetigo contagiosa.

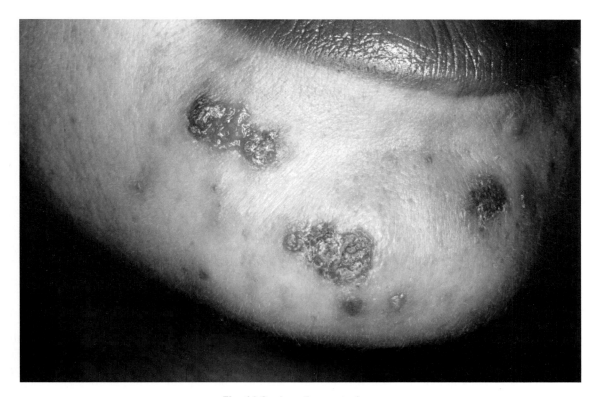

Fig. 14-8 Impetigo contagiosa.

very weepy lesions covered by thick, bright yellow or orange crusts with loose edges, which do not resemble the scaling patches with peripheral erythema seen in tinea. Impetigo may be mistaken for *Toxicodendron* dermatitis, but it is more crusted and pustular, and more liable to involve the nostrils, corners of the mouth, and ears; not associated with it is puffing of the eyelids and the linear lesions, or the itchiness, that are so often present in dermatitis caused by poison ivy or oak. In varicella the lesions are small, widely distributed, discrete, umbilicated vesicles that are usually also present in the mouth, a site not involved by impetigo. In ecthyma the lesions are crusted ulcers, not erosions.

Treatment

Systemic antibiotics combined with topical therapy are advised. Because most cases are caused by *Staphylococcus*, a semisynthetic penicillin or a first-generation cephalosporin is recommended. All treatment should be given for 7 to 10 days. It is necessary to soak off the crusts frequently, after which bacitracin or mupirocin ointment should be applied. If the lesions are localized, especially if facial, such topical therapy may be effective as the sole treatment.

Maddox et al studied the effect of applying antibiotic ointment as a prophylactic to sites of skin trauma to prevent impetigo in a group of children at a rural day-care center. Streptococci were frequently cultured from normal skin throughout the study and were regularly available to infect a traumatized site. Infections were reduced by 47% with antibiotic ointment compared with 15% with a placebo. Additionally, if recurrent staphylococcal impetigo develops, a culture of the anterior nares may yield this organism. Such carrier states may be treated by application of mupirocin ointment to the anterior nares twice daily or rifampin, 600 mg daily for 5 days.

Bullous Impetigo

This variety of impetigo occurs characteristically in newborn infants, though it may occur at any age. The neonatal type is highly contagious and is a threat in nurseries. In most cases the disease begins between the fourth and tenth days of life with the appearance of bullae, which may appear on any part of the body (Fig. 14-9). Common early sites are the face and hands. Constitutional symptoms are at first absent, but later weakness and fever or a subnormal temperature may be present. Diarrhea with green stools frequently occurs. Bacteremia, pneumonia, or meningitis may develop rapidly, with fatal termination.

In warm climates particularly, adults may have bullous impetigo, most often in the axillae or groins, or on the hands. Usually no scalp lesions are present. The lesions are strikingly large, fragile bullae, suggestive of pemphigus (Fig. 14-10). When these rupture they leave circinate, weepy, or crusted lesions, and in this stage it may be called *impetigo circinata* (Fig. 14-11). Children with bullous

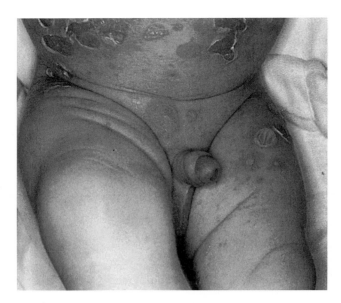

Fig. 14-9   Bullous impetigo in a neonate.

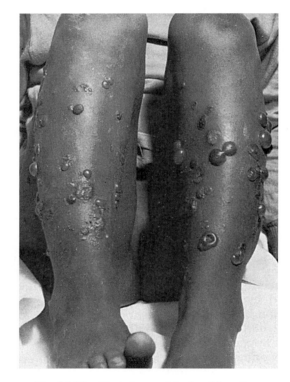

Fig. 14-10   Staphylococcal (bullous) impetigo.

impetigo may give a history of an insect bite at the site of onset of lesions. Dillon found in a study of 31 patients, that the majority were caused by phage type 71 coagulase-positive *S. aureus* or a related group 2 phage type. Bullous impetigo may be an early manifestation of HIV infection.

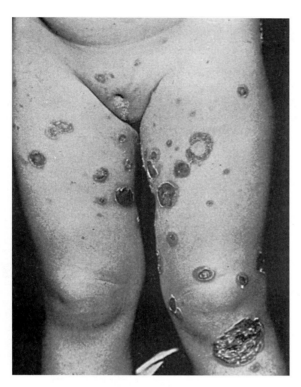

Fig. 14-11 Staphylococcal (bullous) impetigo. Annular lesions are characteristic. Note collarette scale.

Staphylococcal Scalded Skin Syndrome

Staphylococcal scalded skin syndrome (SSSS) is a generalized, confluent, superficially exfoliative disease, occurring most commonly in neonates and young children. It was known in the past as Ritter's disease or dermatitis exfoliativa neonatorum. It has been reported to occur rarely in adults. When it does occur in an adult, usually either renal compromise or immunosuppression is a predisposing factor.

SSSS is a febrile, rapidly evolving, generalized, desquamative infectious disease, in which the skin exfoliates in sheets. It does not separate at the dermoepidermal junction, as in toxic (drug-induced) epidermal necrolysis (TEN), but immediately below the granular layer. The lesions are thus much more superficial and less severe than in TEN, and healing is much more rapid. They also extend far beyond areas of actual staphylococcal infection, by action of the epidermolytic exotoxin elaborated by the staphylococcus in remote sites. Usually the staphylococci are present at a distant focus such as the pharynx, nose, ear, or conjunctiva. Septicemia or a cutaneous infection may also be the causative focus.

Its clinical manifestations begin abruptly with fever, skin tenderness, and erythema involving the neck, groins, and axillae. There is sparing of the palms, soles, and mucous membranes. Nikolsky's sign is positive. Generalized exfoliation follows within the next hours to days, with large sheets of epidermis separating (Fig. 14-12).

Group 2 *Staphylococcus aureus,* most commonly phage type 71, has been the causative agent in most cases. If cultures are taken they should be obtained from the mucous membranes because the skin erythema and desquamation is due to the distant effects of the exfoliative toxin, unlike the situation in bullous impetigo, where *S. aureus* is present in the lesions.

Rapid diagnosis can be made by examining frozen sections of a blister roof and observing that the full thickness of the epidermis is not necrotic as in TEN but rather is cleaved below the granular layer. Treatment of choice is a penicillinase-resistant penicillin such as cloxacillin or dicloxacillin combined with fluid therapy and general supportive measures. The prognosis is good.

Toxic Shock Syndrome

Toxic shock syndrome (TSS), an acute, febrile, multisystem illness, has as one of its major diagnostic criteria a widespread macular erythematous eruption. It is usually caused by toxin-producing strains of *S. aureus,* most of which were initially isolated from the cervical mucosa in menstruating young women. Recent cases are most often due to infections in wounds, catheters, contraceptive diaphragms, or nasal packing. The mortality of these nonmenstrual cases is higher (12%) versus menstrual-related cases (5%), probably as a result of delayed diagnoses. Additionally, a very similar syndrome in which the cause is group A streptococci has been defined. This multiorgan disease has systemic components similar to classic staphylococcal TSS; however, the infection is usually a rapidly progressive, destructive soft-tissue infection such as necrotizing fasciitis. It has a case fatality rate of 30%. The streptococci are usually of M-types 1 and 3, with 80% of the isolates producing pyrogenic exotoxin A.

The Center for Communicable Diseases (CDC) case definition of TSS includes the following: a temperature of 38.9° C or higher, an erythematous eruption, desquamation of the palms and soles 1 to 2 weeks after onset, hypotension, and involvement of three or more other systems—gastrointestinal (vomiting, diarrhea), muscular (myalgias, increased creatinine phosphokinase level), mucous membrane (hyperemia), renal (pyuria without infection or raised creatinine or blood urea nitrogen levels), hepatic (increased bilirubin, SGOT, or SGPT), hematologic (platelets less than 100,000/mm^3), or central nervous system (disorientation). In addition, serologic tests for Rocky Mountain spotted fever, leptospirosis, and rubeola, and cultures of blood, urine, and cerebrospinal fluid should be negative. Bach emphasized bulbar conjunctival hyperemia and palmar edema as two additional clinical clues.

Ninety percent of the early cases occurred in young women between the first and sixth days of a menstrual period. During the initial outbreak, between 1979 and 1982, the majority were using a superabsorbent tampon. Cases have been reported in women using contraceptive sponges,

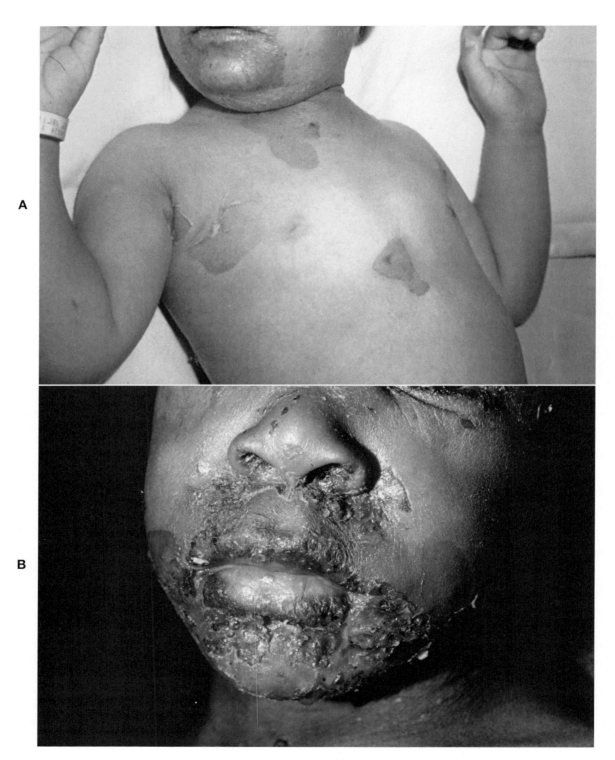

Fig. 14-12 Staphylococcal scalded skin syndrome (SSSS). **A,** Young boy with exfoliation. **B,** Young boy with early periorificial crusting and desquamation.

in patients with nasal packing after rhinoplasty, and in patients with staphylococcal infections of bone, lung, or soft tissue. Huntley et al reported a case that occurred as a complication of dermatologic surgery. The offending *S. aureus* strain produces one or more exotoxins.

Histologic findings are spongiosis, neutrophils scattered throughout the epidermis, individual necrotic keratinocytes, perivascular and interstitial infiltrates composed of lymphocytes and neutrophils, and edema of the papillary dermis. TSS must be differentiated from other diseases that can closely mimic its cutaneous presentation, such as viral exanthems, Kawasaki's disease, scarlet fever, drug eruptions, Rocky Mountain spotted fever, systemic lupus erythematosus, toxic epidermal necrolysis, and staphylococcal scalded skin syndrome. Leung et al reported 16 patients with Kawasaki's disease; 11 had TSS-toxin–producing staphylococcus recovered and 2 had streptococci that produced pyrogenic exotoxin B and C. They suggested Kawasaki's is caused by toxin-secreting bacteria. Manders et al reported two patients with recurrent perineal erysipelas-like erythema that resolved with desquamation, a staphylococcal or streptococcal pharyngitis, and a marked tendency to recurrence. They termed this *recurrent toxin-mediated perianal erythema.*

Treatment consists of systemic antibiotics such as nafcillin, 1 to 1.5 g intravenously every 4 hours, vigorous fluid therapy to treat shock, and drainage of the *S. aureus*-infected site.

Bach MC: Dermatologic signs of toxic shock syndrome. *J Am Acad Dermatol* 1983, 8:343.

Barton LL, et al: Impetigo. *Pediatr Dermatol* 1987, 4:185.

Becker BA, et al: Atypical plaquelike staphylococcal folliculitis in HIV-infected persons. *J Am Acad Dermatol* 1989, 21:1024.

Bellman B, et al: Infection with methicillin-resistant *Staphylococcus aureus* after carbon dioxide resurfacing of the face: successful treatment with minocycline, rifampin, and mupirocin ointment. *Dermatol Surg* 1998, 24:279.

Boiko S, et al: Osteomyelitis of the distal phalanges in three children with atopic dermatitis. *Arch Dermatol* 1988, 124:418.

Brook I: Aerobic and anaerobic microbiology of paronychia. *Ann Emerg Med* 1990, 19:994.

Bulengo-Ransby SM, et al: Staphylococcal botryomycosis and Job's syndrome in an infant. *J Am Acad Dermatol* 1993, 28:109.

Cardullo AC, et al: Janeway lesions and Osler's nodes. *J Am Acad Dermatol* 1990, 22:1088.

Cone LA, et al: Clinical and bacteriologic observations of a toxic shock-like syndrome due to *S. pyogenes. N Engl J Med* 1987, 317:146.

Coskey RJ, et al: Diagnosis and treatment of impetigo. *J Am Acad Dermatol* 1987, 17:62.

Cribier B, et al: Staphylococcal scalded skin syndrome in adults. *J Am Acad Dermatol* 1994, 30:319.

David TJ, et al: Bacterial infection of atopic eczema. *Arch Dis Child* 1986, 61:20.

Demidovitch CW, et al: Impetigo. *Am J Dis Child* 1990, 44:1313.

Dillon HC: Treatment of staphylococcal skin infections. *J Am Acad Dermatol* 1983, 8:177.

Duvic M: Staphylococcal infections and the pruritus of AIDS-related complex. *Arch Dermatol* 1987, 123:1599.

Eykyn SJ: Staphylococcal sepsis. *Lancet* 1988, 1:100.

Faich G, et al: Toxic shock syndrome and the vaginal contraceptive sponge. *JAMA* 1986, 255:216.

Garbe PL, et al: *S. aureus* isolation from patients with nonmenstrual toxic shock syndrome. *JAMA* 1985, 253:25.

Gorden DM, et al: Staphylococcal folliculitis of the nose. *JAMA* 1988, 260:2915.

Graham ML, et al: Isotretinoin and *S. aureus* infection. *Arch Dermatol* 1986, 122:815.

Herzog JL, et al: Desquamative rash in an immunocompromised adult. *Arch Dermatol* 1990, 126:815.

Hoge CW, et al: The changing epidemiology of invasive group A streptococcal infections and the emergence of streptococcal toxic shock-like syndrome. *JAMA* 1993, 269:384.

Holland TT, et al: Tender periungual nodules. *Arch Dermatol* 1992, 128:105.

Howe RA, et al: Vancomycin-resistant *Staphylococcus aureus. Lancet* 1997, 351:602.

Huntley AC, et al: Toxic shock syndrome as a complication of dermatologic surgery. *J Am Acad Dermatol* 1987, 16:227.

James WD: *S. aureus* and etretinate. *Arch Dermatol* 1986, 122:976.

Kain KC, et al: Clinical spectrum of nonmenstrual TSS. *Clin Infect Dis* 1993, 16:100.

Klempner MS, et al: Prevention of recurrent staphylococcal skin infection with low-dose oral clindamycin therapy. *JAMA* 1988, 260:2682.

Laber H, et al: Mupirocin and the eradication of *S. aureus* in atopic dermatitis. *Arch Dermatol* 1988, 124:853.

Leung DYM, et al: Toxic-shock syndrome toxin-secreting *Staphylococcus aureus* on Kawasaki syndrome. *Lancet* 1993, 342:1385.

Leyden JJ, et al: *S. aureus* infection as a complication of isotretinoin therapy. *Arch Dermatol* 1987, 123:60s.

Maddox JS, et al: Pyomyositis in a neonate. *J Am Acad Dermatol* 1984, 10:391.

Manders SM, et al: Recurrent toxin-mediated perianal erythema. *Arch Dermatol* 1996, 132:57.

Mehregan DA, et al: Cutaneous botryomycosis. *J Am Acad Dermatol* 1991, 24:393.

Mertz PM et al: Topical mupirocin treatment of impetigo is equal to oral erythromycin therapy. *Arch Dermatol* 1989, 125:1069.

Montemarano AD, et al: Acute paronychia apparently caused by *Candida albicans* in a healthy female. *Arch Dermatol* 1993, 129:786.

Reagan DR, et al: Elimination of coincident *S. aureus* nasal and hand carriage with intranasal application of mupirocin calcium ointment. *Ann Int Med* 1991, 114:101.

Saiag P, et al: MRI in adults presenting with severe acute infectious cellulitis. *Arch Dermatol* 1994, 130:1150.

Scully M, et al: Pruritus, *S. aureus* and HIV infection. *Arch Dermatol* 1990, 126:684.

Smith KJ, et al: *S. aureus* carriage and HIV disease. *Arch Dermatol* 1994, 130:521.

Steele RW: Recurrent staphylococcal infection in families. *Arch Dermatol* 1980, 116:189.

Tanner MH, et al: Toxic shock syndrome from *S. aureus* infection at insulin pump infusion sites. *JAMA* 1988, 259:394.

Taub DD: Superantigens and microbial pathogenesis. *Ann Intern Med* 1993, 119:89.

Wheat LJ, et al: Prevention of infections of the skin and skin structure. *Am J Med* 1984, 76(5A):187.

Working Group: Defining of group A streptococcal toxic shock syndrome. *JAMA* 1993, 263:390. _____ ▲

STREPTOCOCCAL SKIN INFECTIONS
Ecthyma

Ecthyma is an ulcerative staphylococcal or streptococcal pyoderma, nearly always of the shins or dorsal feet. The disease begins with a vesicle or vesicopustule, which enlarges and in a few days becomes thickly crusted. When the crust is removed there is a superficial saucer-shaped ulcer with a raw base and elevated edges (Fig. 14-13). In urban areas these lesions are due to *S. aureus* and are seen in intravenous drug users and HIV-infected patients.

The lesions tend to heal after a few weeks, leaving scars, but rarely may proceed to gangrene when resistance is low. In fact, a debilitated condition and a focus of pyogenic infection precede the onset of ecthyma in many cases. Local adenopathy may be present. Uncleanliness, malnutrition, and trauma are predisposing causes.

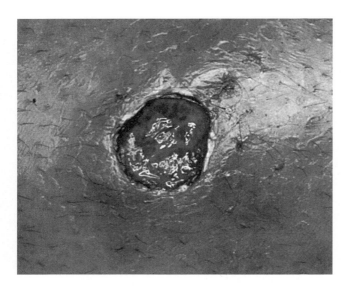

Fig. 14-13 Ecthyma. (Courtesy Dr. Axel W. Hoke.)

Treatment is cleansing with soap and water, followed by the application of mupirocin or bacitracin ointment, twice daily. Cloxacillin or a first-generation cephalosporin must be given orally or parenterally.

Scarlet Fever

Scarlet fever is a diffuse erythematous exanthem that occurs during the course of streptococcal pharyngitis. It affects primarily children, who develop the eruption 24 to 48 hours after the onset of pharyngeal symptoms. The tonsils are red, edematous, and covered with exudate. The tongue has a white coating through which reddened, hypertrophied papillae project, giving the so-called white strawberry tongue appearance. By the fourth or fifth day the coating disappears, the tongue is bright red, and the red strawberry tongue remains.

The cutaneous eruption begins on the neck, spreads to the trunk, and finally the extremities. Within the widespread erythema are 1- to 2-mm papules, which give the skin a rough sandpaper quality. There is accentuation over the skin folds, and a linear petechial eruption, called *Pastia's lines,* is often present in the antecubital and axillary folds. There is facial flushing and circumoral pallor. A branny desquamation occurs as the eruption fades, with peeling of the palms and soles taking place about 2 weeks after the acute illness. The latter may be the only evidence that the disease has occurred.

The eruption is produced by erythrogenic exotoxin-producing group A streptococci. Cultures of the pharynx, or rarely a surgical wound or burn, will recover this organism. An elevated antistreptolysin O titer may provide evidence of recent infection if cultures are not taken early. A condition known as *staphylococcal scarlatina* has been described that mimics scarlet fever; however, the strawberry tongue is not seen.

Penicillin, erythromycin, or cloxacillin treatment is curative, and the prognosis is excellent.

Erysipelas

Also once known as *St. Anthony's fire* and *ignis sacer,* erysipelas is an acute beta-hemolytic group A streptococcal infection of the skin involving the superficial dermal lymphatics. Occasional cases caused by streptococci of group C or G are reported in adults. Group B streptococcus is often responsible in the newborn and may be the cause of abdominal or perineal erysipelas in postpartum women. It is characterized by local redness, heat, swelling, and a highly characteristic raised, indurated border (Fig. 14-14). The onset is often preceded by prodromal symptoms of malaise for several hours, which may be accompanied by a severe constitutional reaction with chills, high fever, headache, vomiting, and joint pains. There is commonly a polymorphonuclear leukocytosis of 20,000/mm^3 or more. However, many cases present solely as an erythematous lesion without associated systemic complaints.

The skin lesions may vary from transient hyperemia followed by slight desquamation to intense inflammation with vesiculation and phlegmon. The eruption begins at any one point as an erythematous patch and spreads by peripheral extension. In the early stages the affected skin is scarlet, hot to the touch, brawny, and swollen. A distinctive feature of the inflammation is the advancing edge of the patch. This is raised and sharply demarcated, and feels like a wall to the palpating finger. In some cases vesicles or bullae that contain seropurulent fluid occur and may result in local gangrene.

The face and the legs are the most frequent sites affected. When on the face the inflammation generally begins on the cheek near the nose or in front of the lobe of the ear and spreads upward to the scalp, the hairline acting in some instances as a barrier against further extension. In severe cases the head, particularly the ears, may be tremendously swollen and distorted, and there may be associated delirium. Septicemia or deep cellulitis may occur as complications. These are more common in the newborn and following operations on the elderly.

Predisposing causes are operative wounds, or fissures in the nares, in the auditory meatus, under the lobes of the ears, on the anus or penis, and between or under the toes, usually the little toe. Any inflammation of the skin, especially if fissured or ulcerative, may provide an entrance for the causative streptococcus. Slight abrasions or scratches, accidental scalp wounds, unclean tying of the umbilical cord, vaccination, and chronic leg ulcers may lead to the disease.

Recognition of the disease is generally not difficult. It may be confused with contact dermatitis from plants, drugs, or dyes and with angioneurotic edema; however, with each of these fever, pain, and tenderness are absent and itching is severe. In scarlet fever, there is a widespread punctate erythema, never localized and edematous as in erysipelas. A

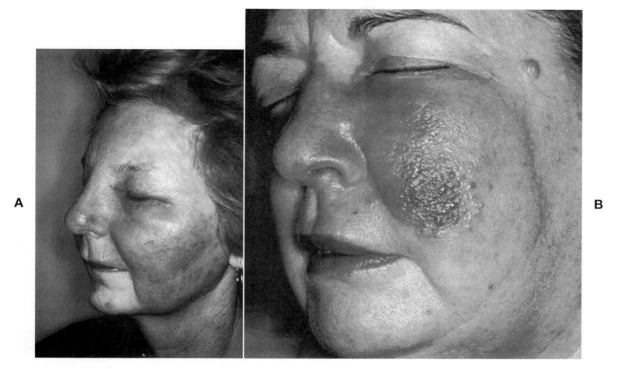

Fig. 14-14 **A** and **B**, Erysipelas.

butterfly pattern on the face may mimic lupus erythematosus, and ear involvement may suggest relapsing polychondritis. Acute tuberculoid leprosy of the face may look exactly like erysipelas, but the absence of fever, pain, or leukocytosis is distinctive.

Systemic penicillin is rapidly effective. Improvement in the general condition occurs in 24 to 48 hours, but resolution of the cutaneous lesion may require several days. Vigorous treatment with antibiotics should be continued for at least 10 days. Erythromycin is also efficacious. Locally, ice bags and cold compresses may be used.

Cellulitis

Cellulitis (Fig. 14-15) is a suppurative inflammation involving particularly the subcutaneous tissue, caused most frequently by *Streptococcus pyogenes* or *S. aureus*. Usually, but not always, this follows some discernible wound. On the leg tinea pedis is the most common portal of entry. Mild local erythema and tenderness, malaise, and chilly sensations, or a sudden chill and fever may be present at the onset. The erythema rapidly becomes intense and spreads. The area becomes infiltrated and pits on pressure. Sometimes the central part becomes nodular and surmounted by a vesicle that ruptures and discharges pus and necrotic material. Streaks of lymphangitis may spread from the area to the neighboring lymph glands. Gangrene, metastatic abscesses, and grave sepsis may follow. These complications are unusual in immunocompetent adults, but children and compromised adults are at higher risk.

Hook evaluated 50 patients with cellulitis prospectively by culture of the primary site of infection (when one was present), and also by aspiration of the advancing edge, by skin biopsy, and by blood culture. In 24 patients the primary site was identified and in 17 beta-hemolytic streptococci were isolated, with *S. aureus* being present in 13. Kielhofner et al also evaluated needle aspirates in cellulitis. Of 87 patients, 33 were culture positive. Of significance is that 26 of 46 (57%) were positive if there was coexistent underlying disease such as hematologic malignancy, diabetes mellitus, intravenous drug abuse, or cardiovascular disorders. *S. aureus* was present in 33% and group A streptococci in 27%. Other cultures were seldom positive and yielded no additional information.

Initial empiric therapy should cover both staphylococci and streptococci. Intravenous penicillinase-resistant penicillins or a first-generation cephalosporin are usually effective.

Chronic Recurrent Erysipelas, Chronic Lymphangitis

Recurrence of erysipelas or cellulitis may cause local persistent lymphedema. This type of chronic lymphedema is the end result of recurrent bouts of bacterial lymphangitis and obstruction of the major lymphatic channels of the skin. The final result is a permanent hypertrophic fibrosis to which the term *elephantiasis nostras* has been given. It must be differentiated from lymphangioma, acquired lymphangiectasia, and from other causes such as neoplasms, syphilis, filariasis, and tuberculous lymphangitis.

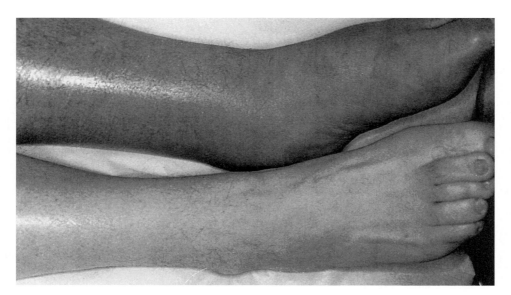

Fig. 14-15 Cellulitis.

Bacterial infection may complicate any acquired lymphangiectasias. During periods of active lymphangitis, antibiotics in large doses are beneficial and their use must be continued intermittently in smaller maintenance doses for long periods to achieve their full benefits. Plastic surgery is recommended for persistent solid edema that does not respond to the measures just mentioned. Compression therapy to decrease lymphedema will aid in the prevention of recurrence. Landthaler et al reported the use of the CO_2 laser in preventing recurrent infections.

Necrotizing Fasciitis

Necrotizing fasciitis (Fig. 14-16) is an acute necrotizing infection involving the fascia. It may follow surgery or perforating trauma or may occur de novo. Within 24 to 48 hours redness, pain, and edema quickly progress to central patches of dusky blue discoloration, with or without serosanguineous blisters. Anesthesia of the involved skin is very characteristic. By the fourth or fifth day, these purple areas become gangrenous. Many forms of virulent bacteria have been cultured from necrotizing fasciitis, including microaerophilic beta-hemolytic streptococci, hemolytic staphylococcus, coliforms, enterococci, *Pseudomonas,* and *Bacteroides.* Both aerobic and anaerobic cultures should always be taken. The presence of anesthesia should suggest a deeper component. MRI may aid in delineating the extent of deep involvement. Treatment should include early surgical debridement, intravenously administered appropriate antibiotics and supportive care. There may be a 20% mortality even in the best of circumstances. Poor prognostic factors are age over 50, underlying diabetes, or atherosclerosis; delay of more than 7 days in diagnosis and surgical intervention, and infection on or near the trunk rather than the more commonly involved extremities.

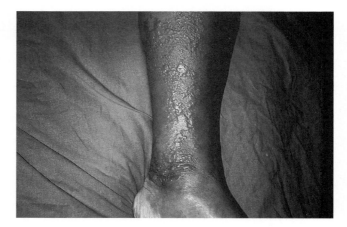

Fig. 14-16 Necrotizing fasciitis. Note characteristic blistering.

Blistering Distal Dactylitis

Blistering distal dactylitis is characterized by tense superficial blisters on a tender erythematous base over the volar fat pad of the phalanx of a finger or thumb or occasionally a toe (Fig. 14-17). The typical patient is between ages 2 and 16. Group A beta-hemolytic streptococcus or *Staphylococcus aureus* are the most common causes. They may be cultured from blister fluid and occasionally from clinically inapparent infections of the nasopharynx or conjunctiva. Benson et al reported this clinical entity caused by group B streptococcus in an adult patient with diabetes.

Perianal Dermatitis

Clinically, this entity presents as a superficial perianal, well-demarcated rim of erythema; sometimes fissuring may also be seen. Pain or tenderness, especially prominent on defecation, may lead to fecal retention in affected patients, who are usually between ages 1 and 8. It may not resemble

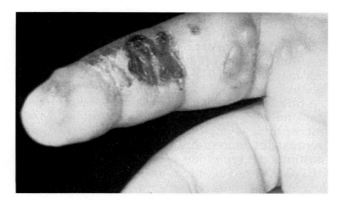

Fig. 14-17   Blistering dactylitis.

a cellulitis, but rather a dermatitis. Group A streptococci are most often the cause, and oral penicillin will cure it. However, Montemarano and James reported a case caused by *Staphylococcus aureus*. Mostafa et al confirmed the occasional association with *S. aureus* and non-group A streptococci. The most frequent cause was hemolytic group A streptococcus in their study of a large number of affected children, and they documented simultaneous pharyngeal colonization with the recovered organism.

Group B Streptococcal Infection

Streptococcus agalactiae is the major cause of bacterial sepsis and meningitis in neonates. It may cause orbital cellulitis or facial erysipelas in these patients. Up to 25% of healthy adults harbor group B streptococcus in the genital or gastrointestinal tract. It has been reported by James and others to cause balanitis. It may also cause cellulitis, perianal dermatitis, recurrent erysipelas, or blistering dactylitis in adults. Diabetes mellitus and peripheral vascular disease predispose patients to infection with this organism. In the postpartum period abdominal or perineal erysipelas may be due to this organism. Both Farley et al and Schwartz et al document that invasive disease caused by this organism is becoming more common.

Streptococcus Iniae Infections

In 1997 cellulitis of the hands was reported to be caused by this fish pathogen. All patients had handled freshly killed fish, usually tilapia (also known as St. Peter's fish or Hawaiian sunfish). In Asian cuisine this fish is often purchased live from aquariums in retail stores. In cleaning the fish before cooking puncture wounds of the skin were sustained from the dorsal fin, a fish bone, or a knife. Within 24 hours fever, lymphangitis, and cellulitis without skin necrosis or bulla formation occurred. This is a newly recognized cause of human infection, so that cultured organisms may be misidentified. Treatment with penicillin is curative.

Benson PM, et al: Group B streptococcal blistering distal dactylitis in an adult diabetic. *J Am Acad Dermatol* 1987, 17:310.

Binnick AN, et al: Recurrent erysipelas caused by group B streptococcus organism. *Arch Dermatol* 1980, 116:798.

Bisno AL: Group A streptococcal infections and acute rheumatic fever. *New Engl J Med* 1991, 325:783.

Chartier C, et al: Erysipelas. *Int J Dermatol* 1990, 29:459.

Farley MM, et al: A population-based assessment of invasive disease due to group B streptococcus in nonpregnant adults. *New Engl J Med* 1993, 328:1807.

Fehrs LJ, et al: Group A beta-hemolytic streptococcal skin infections in US meat-packing plants. *JAMA* 1987, 258:3131.

Feingold DS, et al: Group A streptococcal infections. *Arch Dermatol* 1996, 132:67.

Frieden IJ, et al: Blistering dactylitis caused by group B streptococci. *Pediatr Dermatol* 1989, 6:300.

Gentry RH, et al: A peculiar purple bruise. *Arch Dermatol* 1990, 126:815.

Hook EW III: Acute cellulitis. *Arch Dermatol* 1987, 123:460.

James WD: Cutaneous group B streptococcal infection. *Arch Dermatol* 1984, 120:85.

Janssen F, et al: Group A streptococcal cellulitis-adenitis in a patient with AIDS. *J Am Acad Dermatol* 1991, 24:363.

Kaul R, et al: Population-based surveillance for group A streptococcal necrotizing fasciitis. *Am J Med* 1997, 103:18.

Kielhofner MA, et al: Influence of underlying disease process on the utility of cellulitis needle aspirates. *Arch Intern Med* 1988, 148:2451.

Kranz DR, et al: Necrotizing fasciitis associated with porphyria cutanea tarda. *J Am Acad Dermatol* 1986, 14:361.

Krol AL: Perianal streptococcal dermatitis. *Pediatr Dermatol* 1990, 7:97.

Landthaler M, et al: Acquired lymphangioma of the vulva. *Arch Dermatol* 1990, 126:967.

Manders SM, et al: Recurrent toxin-mediated perineal erythema. *Arch Dermatol* 1996, 132:57.

Mastro TD, et al: An outbreak of surgical-wound infections due to group A streptococcus carried on the scalp. *New Engl J Med* 1990, 323:968.

McCray MU, et al: Blistering distal dactylitis. *J Am Acad Dermatol* 1981, 5:592.

Montemarano AD, et al: Staphylococcus aureus as a cause of perianal dermatitis. *Pediatr Dermatol* 1993, 10:259.

Mostafa WZ, et al: An epidemiologic study of perianal dermatitis among children in Egypt. *Pediatr Dermatol* 1997, 14:351.

Rehder PA, et al: Perianal cellulitis. *Arch Dermatol* 1988, 124:702.

Sachs MK: Cutaneous cellulitis. *Arch Dermatol* 1991, 127:481.

Saiag P, et al: MRI in adults presenting with severe acute infections cellulitis. *Arch Dermatol* 1994, 13:1150.

Schwartz B, et al: Invasive group B streptococcal disease in adults. *JAMA* 1991, 266:1112.

Semel JD, et al: Association of athlete's foot with cellulitis of the lower extremities. *Clin Infect Dis* 1996, 23:1162.

Shaunak S, et al: Septic scarlet fever due to *S. pyogenes* cellulitis. *Q J Med* 1988, 69:921.

Weinstein MR, et al: Invasive infections due to a fish pathogen, *Streptococcus iniae*. *N Engl J Med* 1997, 337:589.

Wessels MR, et al: The changing spectrum of group B streptococcal disease. *New Engl J Med* 1993, 328:1843.

Zemtsov A, et al: *S. aureus*-induced blistering distal dactylitis in an adult immunosuppressed patient. *J Am Acad Dermatol* 1992, 26:784. ▲

MISCELLANEOUS GRAM-POSITIVE SKIN INFECTIONS
Erysipeloid of Rosenbach

The most frequent form of erysipeloid is a purplish marginated swelling on the hands. The first symptom is pain at the site of inoculation; this is followed by swelling and erythema. The most distinctive feature is the sharply

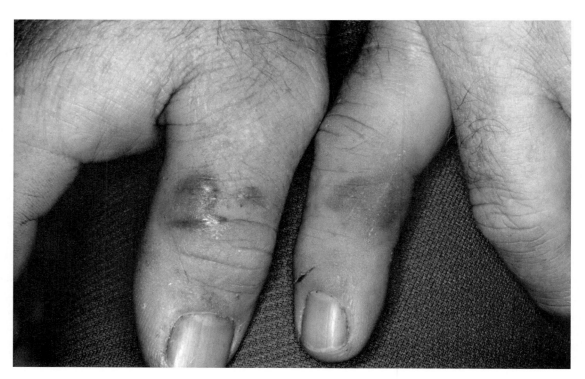

Fig. 14-18 Erysipeloid.

marginated and often polygonal patches of bluish erythema (Fig. 14-18). The erythema slowly spreads to produce a sharply defined, slightly elevated zone that extends peripherally as the central portion fades away. If the finger is involved the swelling and tenseness make movement difficult. Vesicles frequently occur.

Another characteristic of the disease is its migratory nature; new purplish red patches appear at nearby areas. If the infection originally involved one finger, eventually all of the fingers and the dorsum of the hand, palm, or both may become infected, the erythema appearing and disappearing; or extension may take place by continuity. The disease involutes without desquamation or suppuration.

A diffuse or generalized eruption in regions remote from the site of inoculation may occur, with fever and arthritic symptoms. Rarely, septicemia may eventuate in endocarditis, with prolonged fever and constitutional symptoms.

The infection is caused by *Erysipelothrix rhusiopathiae*. *E. rhusiopathiae* is present on dead matter of animal origin. Swine are more frequently infected than any other animal. A large percentage of healthy swine are carriers of the organism. Turkeys are also often infected, and the disease may arise from handling contaminated dressed turkeys. It is also present in the slime of saltwater fish, on crabs, and on other shellfish.

The disease is widespread along the entire Atlantic seacoast among commercial fishermen who handle live fish, crabs, and shellfish. The infection also occurs among veterinarians, and in the meat-packing industry, principally from handling pork products.

E. rhusiopathiae is a rod-shaped, nonmotile, gram-positive organism that tends to form long-branching filaments. The organism is cultured best on media fortified with serum, at room temperature.

Treatment

The majority of the mild cases of erysipeloid run a self-limited course of about 3 weeks. In some patients, after a short period of apparent cure, the eruption reappears either at the same area or, more likely, at an adjacent previously uninvolved area. Penicillin, 1 g/day for 5 to 10 days, is the best treatment for localized disease. If penicillin cannot be used, erythromycin, 250 mg every 6 hours for 7 to 10 days, in combination with rifampin is effective. For systemic forms 12 to 20 million units of intravenous penicillin daily for up to 4 weeks may be necessary.

Barnett JH: Erysipeloid. *J Am Acad Dermatol* 1983, 9:116.
Razsi L, et al: Progressively enlarging painful annular plaque on the hand: erysipeloid. *Arch Dermatol* 1994, 130:1311. _____ ▲

Pneumococcal Cellulitis

Reports have documented cases of periorbital cellulitis with fever in infants, caused by *Streptococcus pneumoniae*. These children presented with violaceous discoloration of the skin identical to that in cellulitis of *Haemophilus influenzae.* Sometimes bullae may be present. Most patients have been chronically ill or immunosuppressed. This emphasizes the importance of obtaining cultures of the blood and soft-tissue aspirate.

Lawlor MT, et al: Cellulitis due to *S. pneumoniae. Clin Infect Dis* 1992, 14:247.

Rusonis PA, et al: Livedo reticularis and purpura. *J Am Acad Dermatol* 1986, 15:1120. _____ ▲

Anthrax

Anthrax is an acute infectious disease characterized by a rapidly necrosing, painless carbuncle with suppurative regional adenitis. Three forms of the disease occur in humans: cutaneous, accounting for 95% of cases worldwide but nearly all U.S. cases; inhalation, known as *woolsorter's disease;* and gastrointestinal, not yet reported in the United States. The first clinical manifestation of the cutaneous form is an inflammatory papule, which begins a few hours or days after infection. The inflammation develops rapidly so that there is a bulla surrounded by intense edema and infiltration. It then ruptures spontaneously, the contents being purulent or sanguineous. A dark brown eschar is then visible surrounded by vesicles and pustules situated on a red, hot, swollen, and indurated area (Fig. 14-19). The regional lymph glands become enlarged and frequently suppurate.

In severe cases the inflammatory signs increase; there is extensive edematous swelling and other bullae and necrotic lesions develop, accompanied by a high temperature and prostration, terminating in death in a few days or weeks. This may occur in up to 20% of untreated cases. In mild cases the constitutional symptoms are sometimes slight; the gangrenous skin sloughs, and the resulting ulcer heals. The lesion is neither tender nor painful. This is of diagnostic importance.

Internally, inhalation anthrax is manifested as a necrotizing, hemorrhagic mediastinal infection. Anthrax spores involve the alveoli, then the hilar and tracheobronchial nodes. Bacteremia followed by hemorrhagic meningitis is the usual sequence of events, almost always ending in death. Gastrointestinal anthrax results when spores are ingested and multiply in the intestinal submucosa. A necrotic ulcerative lesion in the terminal ileum or cecum may lead to hemorrhage.

The disease is produced by *Bacillus anthracis,* a large, square-ended, rod-shaped, gram-positive organism, which occurs singly or in pairs in smears from the blood or in material from the local lesion, or in long chains on artificial media, where it tends to form spores. The bacillus possesses three virulence factors: a polyglutamate acid capsule inhibits phagocytosis; an edema toxin, composed of edema factor and a transport protein termed *protective factor;* and lethal toxin, composed of lethal factor plus protective factor.

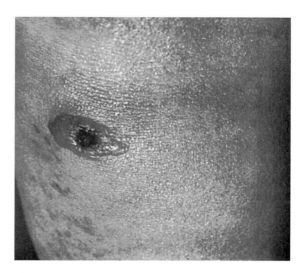

Fig. 14-19 Anthrax on thigh. (Courtesy Dr. A. Johnson, Australia.)

Human infection generally results from infected animals or the handling of hides or other animal products from stock that has died from splenic fever. Cattlemen, woolsorters, tanners, butchers, and workers in the goat-hair industry are most liable to infection. Human-to-human transmission has occurred from contact with dressings from lesions.

Histologically, there is loss of the epidermis at the site of the ulcer, with surrounding spongiosis and intraepidermal vesicles. Leukocytes are abundant in the epidermis. The dermis is edematous and is infiltrated with abundant erythrocytes and neutrophils. Vasodilation is marked. The causative organisms are numerous and are easily seen, especially with Gram stain.

The diagnosis is made by the demonstration of the causative agent in smears and cultures of the local material. Because aerobic nonpathogenic bacilli may be confused with *B. anthracis,* a specific gamma bacteriophage may be used to identify the organism. All virulent strains are pathogenic to mice. A fourfold rise in the indirect hemagglutination titer in paired serum specimens confirms the diagnosis. Electrophoretic-immunoblots to detect antibodies to protective antigen or enzyme-linked immunosorbent assay for the presence of antibodies to the capsule were specific and sensitive in making the retrospective diagnosis of anthrax. The characteristic gangrenous lesion, surrounded by vesiculation, intense swelling and redness, lack of pain, and the occupation of the victim are accessory factors. Staphylococcal carbuncle is the most easily confused entity, but here tenderness is prominent.

Early diagnosis and prompt treatment with penicillin G, 2 million units intravenously every 6 hours for 4 to 6 days, followed by a 7- to 10-day course of oral penicillin, is curative in the cutaneous form. Tetracycline is the preferred alternative treatment for patients who are allergic to penicillin.

Burnett JW: Anthrax. *Cutis* 1991, 48:113.

Franz DR, et al: Clinical recognition and management of patients exposed to biological warfare agents. *JAMA* 1997, 278:399.

Human cutaneous anthrax. *Arch Dermatol* 1988, 124:1324.

Mallon E, et al: Extraordinary case report: cutaneous anthrax. *Am J Dermatopathol* 1997, 19:79.

McGovern TW, et al: Cutaneous manifestations of biologic warfare and related threat agents. *Arch Dermatol* 1999, 135:311.

Smego RA Jr, et al: Cutaneous manifestations of anthrax in rural Haiti. *Clin Infect Dis* 1998, 26:97. ▲

LISTERIOSIS

Listeria monocytogenes is a gram-positive bacillus with rounded ends that may be isolated from soil, water, animals, and asymptomatic individuals. Human infection probably occurs via the gastrointestinal tract; however, in the majority of patients the portal of entry is unknown. Infections in man usually produce meningitis or encephalitis with monocytosis.

Cutaneous listeriosis is a rare disease. Owens reported a veterinarian who contracted cutaneous listeriosis from an aborting cow. The organism in the skin lesions was identical with that isolated from the fetus. The eruption consisted of erythematous tender papules and pustules scattered over the hands and arms. There were axillary lymphadenopathy, fever, malaise, and headache. Treatment with sulfonamides caused the disease to disappear within a few days.

Risk factors include alcoholism, advanced age, pregnancy, and immunosuppression. Neonates are also at risk. Smith et al reported a newborn of an HIV-infected mother who died with a diffuse papular, petechial, and pustular eruption secondary to disseminated listeriosis. *Listeria* may cause a granulomatous disease of infants (granulomatosis infanta peptica). The endocarditis, meningitis, and encephalitis caused by listeria may be accompanied by petechiae and papules in the skin.

Cases of listeriosis may easily be missed on bacteriologic examination, because the organism produces few colonies on original culture and may be dismissed as a streptococcus or as a contaminant diphtheroid because of the similarity in Gram-stained specimens. Serologic tests help to make the diagnosis.

L. monocytogenes is sensitive to most antibiotics. Ampicillin is probably the most effective, but tetracycline, penicillin, and erythromycin are also effective.

Owens CR, et al: Case of primary listeriosis. *N Engl J Med* 1960, 262:1026.

Smith KJ, et al: Diffuse petechial pustular lesions in a newborn. *Arch Dermatol* 1994, 130:243.

Van Praag MC, et al: Diagnosis and treatment of pustular disorders in the neonate. *Pediatr Dermatol* 1997, 14:131. ▲

Cutaneous Diphtheria

The skin may become infected by the Klebs-Loeffler bacillus, *Corynebacterium diphtheriae,* in the form of

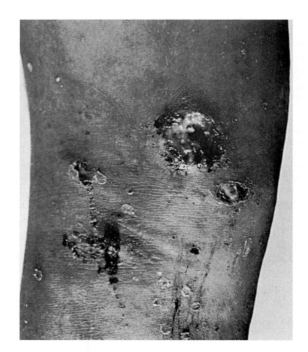

Fig. 14-20 Cutaneous diphtheria on the popliteal space. (Courtesy Armed Forces Institute of Pathology.)

ulcerations (Fig. 14-20). The ulcer is punched-out and has hard, rolled, elevated edges with a pale blue tinge. Often the lesion is covered with a leathery, grayish membrane. Regional lymph nodes may be affected. Another type of skin involvement is that occurring in eczematous, impetiginous, vesicular, or pustular scratches, from which *C. diphtheriae* may be recovered (Fig. 14-21). Postdiphtherial paralysis and potentially fatal cardiac complications may occur. These are mediated by a potent exotoxin, which stops protein production at the ribosome level.

Cutaneous diphtheria is common in tropical areas. Most of the cases occurring in the United States are in unimmunized migrant farm worker families and in elderly alcoholics. Travelers to Third World countries may also import disease.

Treatment consists of intramuscular injections of diphtheria antitoxin, 20,000 to 100,000 units, after a conjunctival test has been performed to rule out hypersensitivity to horse serum. One drop of antitoxin diluted 1:10 is placed in one eye and a drop of saline is placed in the other eye. If after 30 minutes there is no reaction 20,000 to 40,000 units of antitoxin is given. Erythromycin, 2 g/day, is the drug of choice, unless large proportions of resistant organism are known in the area. Rifampin, 600 mg/day for 7 days, will eliminate the carrier state. In severe cases IV penicillin G, 600,000 units/day for 14 days is indicated.

Hart PE, et al: Cutaneous and pharyngeal diphtheria imported from the Indian subcontinent. *Postgrad Med J* 1996, 72:619.

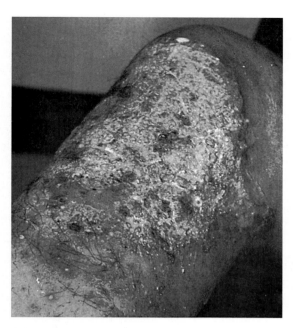

Fig. 14-21 Cutaneous diphtheria on knee. (Courtesy Dr. F. Reiss.)

Karzon DT, et al: Diphtheria outbreaks in immunized populations. *N Engl J Med* 1988, 318:41.

Thomann U, et al: Cutaneous diphtheria imported from tropical countries. *Schweiz Med Wochenschr* 1988; 118:676. _____ ▲

Group JK *Corynebacterium* Sepsis

Group JK *Corynebacterium (C. jeikeium)* colonize the skin of healthy individuals, with highest concentration being in the axillary and perineal areas. Hospitalized patients are more heavily colonized. Patients with granulocytopenia, indwelling catheters, prosthetic devices, and valvular defects are at highest risk for the development of sepsis or endocarditis. A papular eruption, cellulitis, tissue necrosis, and palpable purpura may be seen on the skin. Vancomycin is the drug of choice.

Jerdan et al in 1987 reported a case of group JK *Corynebacterium* sepsis occurring in an immunosuppressed teenage boy. There was an extensive papular eruption, with effacement of eccrine glands by numerous pleomorphic bacilli, morphologically consistent with *Corynebacterium,* on biopsy. Ticarcillin, nafcillin, and gentamicin (later changed to tobramycin) were ineffective; so was a combination of tobramycin, clindamycin, and trimethoprim-sulfamethoxazole. On the day the eruption appeared, vancomycin was begun, and from the fourth day on, no new lesions appeared.

Dan M, et al: Cutaneous manifestation of infection with *Corynebacterium* group JK. *Rev Infect Dis* 1988, 10:1204.

Jerdan MS, et al: Cutaneous manifestations of *Corynebacterium* group JK sepsis. *J Am Acad Dermatol* 1987, 16:444.

Spach DH, et al: Palpable purpura associated with *Corynebacterium* JK endocarditis. *Arch Dermatol* 1991; 127:1071. _____ ▲

Desert Sore

Also known as *veldt sore, septic sore, diphtheric desert sore,* and *Barcoo rot,* desert sore is an ulcerative disease that is endemic among bushmen and soldiers in Australia and Burma. The disease is characterized by the occurrence of grouped vesicles on the extremities, chiefly on the shins, knees, and backs of the hands. These rupture and form superficial indolent ulcers.

The ulcers enlarge and may attain a diameter of 2 cm. The floor of the ulcer may be covered by a diphtheritic membrane. The original lesions may start as insect bites. Cultures show staphylococci, streptococci, and *Corynebacterium diphtheriae.* Treatment of the desert sore is with diphtheria antitoxin if *C. diphtheriae* is present. Antibiotic ointments are used topically, and oral penicillin or erythromycin is the treatment of choice.

Bailey H: Ulcers of the leg and their differential diagnosis. *Dermatol Trop* 1962, 1:45. _____ ▲

Tropical Ulcer

Synonyms: Tropical phagedena, Aden ulcer, Malabar ulcer, jungle rot; also various native terms

Tropical ulcer occurs on exposed parts of the body, chiefly the legs and arms, frequently on preexisting abrasions or sores, sometimes beginning from a mere scratch. As a rule, only one extremity is affected and usually there is a single lesion, although it is not uncommon to find multiple ulcers on both legs (Fig. 14-22). Satellite lesions ordinarily occur as a result of autoinoculation.

The lesions begin with inflammatory papules that progress into vesicles and rupture with the formation of an ulcer. The ulcers vary in diameter and may, through coalescence, form extensive lesions. The lesions of some varieties are elevated or deeply depressed and generally the edges are undermined and either smooth or ragged.

At times the ulcers are covered by thick, dirty crusts or by whitish pseudomembranes. The edges are flat, without thickening, and around them there is a zone of inflammation characterized by redness, swelling, and some tenderness. Other than a slight itching, there is usually no distress.

The disease is most common in native laborers and in schoolchildren during the rainy season; it is probably caused in many instances by the bites of insects, filth, and pyogenic infection.

Under the term *tropical ulcer* a variety of skin conditions have been described. Many of these have been due to yaws or to the infection of abrasions by pyogenic organisms. Vincent has demonstrated the *Bacteroides fusiformis,* a fusiform bacillus, and *Borrelia vincentii,* the spirillum better known in connection with Vincent's angina, in smears from tropical ulcers, and in other lesions spirochetes of various forms have been found. Adriaans et al reviewed the infectious etiology with special reference to the role of

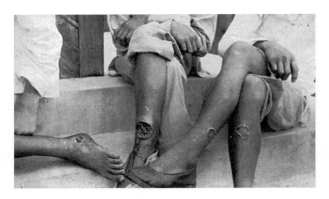

Fig. 14-22 Tropical ulcer. (Courtesy Dr. T. Corpus.)

anaerobic bacteria, especially fusobacteria and spirochetes, in 1987. They found that anaerobic bacteria together with aerobes, some of them facultative anaerobes, were always present, especially in early lesions, suggesting that they were important in the pathogenesis of the lesions. Malnutrition appears to be a predisposing factor.

Because the concept of tropical ulcer is tenuous at best, various ulcers of known etiologies must be kept in mind. Discussions of some of these follow. The septic desert ulcer is superficial and shows *C. diphtheriae*. The gummatous ulcer is punched out, with a sinking floor. Other signs of syphilis are present, and the serologic test for syphilis is positive. The tuberculous ulcer is undermined and usually not found on the leg. The mycobacterium can be isolated from the lesion. The mycotic ulcer is nodulo-ulcerative, with demonstrable fungi both by direct microscopic examination and by culture. The frambesia ulcer grows rapidly and yields *Treponema pertenue.*

The Buruli ulcer shows abundant *Mycobacterium ulcerans* in biopsies. The leishmanial ulcer contains *Leishmania tropica;* it is not usually found on the leg. Carcinoma must be considered in any leg ulcer of long duration. A biopsy is indicated.

The arteriosclerotic ulcer is seen in older people at sites of frequent trauma; it is deep and penetrates through the deep fascia to expose tendons. The hypertensive ischemic ulcer is caused by thrombosis of the cutaneous arterioles. These painful ulcers are extremely shallow and usually bilateral and are seen most frequently on the mid and lower parts of the leg. Varicosities are usually absent. The varicose or venous ulcer is shallow and has irregularly shaped edges. It is located typically on the lower half of the shins, mostly above and anterior to the medial malleolus along the course of the long saphenous vein.

The ulcers of blood dyscrasias are frequent in sickle-cell anemia, in hereditary spherocytosis, Mediterranean anemia, and Felty's syndrome. The diagnosis is aided by the fact that there is hypersplenism in each of these diseases. The ulcer of rheumatoid arthritis occurs frequently in patients who have abundant concomitant subcutaneous nodules. The

ulcer of Kaposi's sarcoma frequently occurs on the lower extremities and is accompanied by a purpuric discoloration of the skin and by other violaceous nodules that may occur anywhere on the body. In the tropics it is endemic among the South African Bantus.

Treatment

Prevention of the disease is aided by protection from insect bites and from predisposing causes, such as debility, malnutrition, and filth. Topical and systemic antibiotic treatment is indicated in most patients.

Adriaans B, et al: The infectious aetiology of tropical ulcer: a study of the role of anaerobic bacteria. *Br J Dermatol* 1986, 116:31.

Erythrasma

Erythrasma is characterized by sharply delineated, dry, brown, slightly scaling patches (Figs. 14-23 and 14-24) occurring in the intertriginous areas, especially the axillae, the genitocrural crease, and the webs between the fourth and fifth toes and, less commonly, between the third and fourth toes. There may also be patches in the intergluteal cleft, perianal skin, and in the inframammary area. Rarely, widespread eruptions with lamellated plaques occur. Even the nails may be involved.

The lesions are asymptomatic except in the groins, where there may be some itching and burning. Patients with extensive erythrasma have been found to have diabetes mellitus or other debilitating diseases.

Erythrasma is caused by the diphtheroid *Corynebacterium minutissimum.* Two other diseases caused by a corynebacterium, pitted keratolysis and trichomycosis axillaris, were reported to occur as a triad in two patients reported by Shelley et al. The Wood's light is the diagnostic medium for erythrasma. The affected areas show a coral red fluorescence, which results from the presence of a porphyrin. Washing of the affected area before examination may eliminate the fluorescence. In the differential diagnosis, tinea cruris caused by fungi, intertrigo, seborrheic dermatitis, inverse psoriasis, candidiasis, and lichen simplex chronicus must be considered.

Treatment

Treatment of choice is erythromycin, 250 mg four times daily for 1 week. Tolnaftate solution applied twice daily for 2 to 3 weeks or topical miconazole is equally effective. Topical erythromycin solution or topical clindamycin is easily applied and rapidly effective.

Mattox TF, et al: Nonfluorescent erythrasma of the vulva. *Obstet Gynecol* 1993, 81:862.
Shelley WB, et al: Coexistent erythrasma, trichomycosis axillaris, and pitted keratolysis. *J Am Acad Dermatol* 1982, 7:752.

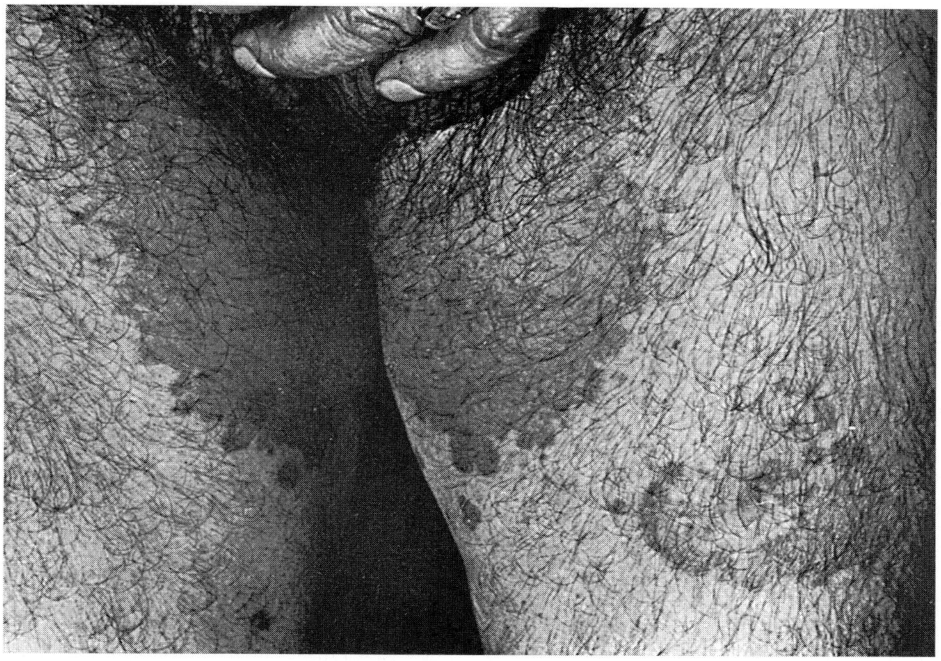

Fig. 14-23   Erythrasma. (Courtesy Dr. E. Florian, Budapest.)

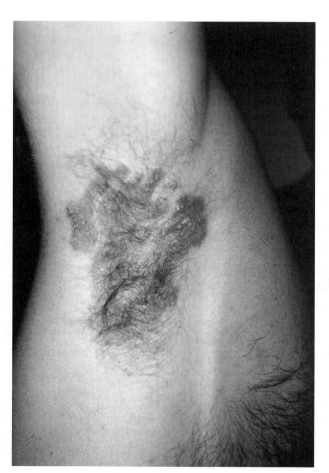

Fig. 14-24   Erythrasma. (Courtesy Dr. H. Shatin.)

Sindhuphak W, et al: Erythrasma. *Int J Dermatol* 1985, 24:95.
Svejgaard E, et al: Tinea pedis and erythrasma in Danish recruits. *J Am Acad Dermatol* 1986, 14:993. ▲

Arcanobacterium Haemolyticum Infection

This pleomorphic, nonmotile, non–spore-forming, beta-hemolytic, gram-positive bacillus causes pharyngitis and an exanthem in young adults. Acute pharyngitis in the 10- to 30-year-old age group is only due to group A streptococci 10% to 25% of the time. A proportion of the remainder will be caused by *Arcanobacterium haemolyticum.*

The exanthem is an erythematous morbilliform or scarlatiniform eruption involving the trunk and extremities. Although it usually spares the face, palms, and soles, atypical acral involvement was reported by Gaston and Zurowski. The general clinical presentation may include a mild pharyngitis, a severe diphtheria-like illness, or even a septicemia.

Cultures for this organism should be done on 5% blood agar plates and observed for 48 hours. The diagnostic features are enhanced by a 5% to 8% carbon dioxide atmosphere during incubation at 37° C. Routine pharyngeal specimens are done on sheep blood agar and will miss the growth of this organism because of its slow hemolytic rate and growth of normal throat flora. Treatment of choice is erythromycin, or in the case of severe infection, high-dose penicillin G.

Gaston DA, Zurowski SM: *Arcanobacterium haemolyticum* pharyngitis and exanthem. *Arch Dermatol* 1996;132:61. ▲

Intertrigo

Intertrigo is a superficial inflammatory dermatitis occurring where two skin surfaces are in apposition. It is discussed here because of its clinical association with several diseases in this chapter. As a result of friction (skin rubbing skin), heat, and moisture, the affected fold becomes erythematous, macerated, and secondarily infected. There may be erosions, fissures, and exudation, with symptoms of burning and itching. Intertrigo is most frequently seen during hot and humid weather, chiefly in obese persons. This type of dermatitis may involve the retroauricular areas; the folds of the upper eyelids; the creases of the neck, axillae, antecubital areas; finger webs; inframammary area; umbilicus; inguinal, perineal, and intergluteal areas; popliteal spaces; and toe webs.

As a result of the maceration, a secondary infection by bacteria (or fungi) is induced. The inframammary area in obese women is most frequently the site of intertriginous candidiasis. The groins are also frequently affected by fungal (yeast or dermatophyte) infection. Bacterial infection may be caused by streptococci, staphylococci, pseudomonas, or corynebacteria.

In the differential diagnosis, seborrheic dermatitis typically involves the skinfolds. Intertriginous psoriasis and erythrasma are frequently overlooked, especially when the inguinal and intergluteal areas or fourth toe webs are involved, as in erythrasma.

Treatment is directed toward the elimination of the maceration. Appropriate antibiotics or fungicides are applied locally. The apposing skin surfaces may be separated with gauze or other appropriate dressings. Castellani paint is also useful, as is Polysporin ointment.

Guitart J, et al: Intertrigo. *Compr Ther* 1994, 20:402. ▲

Pitted Keratolysis

This bacterial infection of the plantar stratum corneum was first named keratoma plantare sulcatum by Castellani in 1910, but was given its present name, *pitted keratolysis,* by Taplin and Zaias in 1967. The thick, weight-bearing portions of the soles become gradually covered with shallow asymptomatic discrete round pits 1 to 3 mm in diameter, some of which become confluent, forming furrows (Fig. 14-25). Men with very sweaty feet, during hot, humid weather, are most susceptible. Rarely, palmar lesions may occur. No discomfort is produced, though the lesions are often malodorous.

The causative organism is still debated; however, a synergistic role of corynebacteria and *Micrococcus sedentarius* is hypothesized. Clinical diagnosis is not difficult, based on its unique appearance.

Topical antibiotics, such as erythromycin or clindamycin, are curative. Miconazole or clotrimazole cream and Whitfeld's ointment are effective alternatives. Both 5% benzoyl peroxide gel and a 10% to 20% solution of aluminum chloride may be used.

Nordstrom KM , et al: Pitted keratolysis. *Arch Dermatol* 1987, 123:1320.
Shah AS, et al: Painful, plaque-like, pitted keratolysis occurring in childhood. *Pediatr Dermatol* 1992, 9:251.
Takama H, et al: Pitted keratolysis. *Br J Dermatol* 1997, 137:282.
Zaias N: Pitted and ringed keratolysis. *J Am Acad Dermatol* 1982, 7:787. ▲

Clostridial Infections and Gangrene of the Skin (Dermatitis Gangrenosa)

Gangrene of the skin results from loss of the blood supply of a particular area and, in some instances, from bacterial invasion that promotes necrosis and sloughing of the skin. Various forms of bacterial infections causing gangrene will be discussed here. The infectious causes are often severe and acute in nature. These may involve deep tissues, and MRI may delineate the depth of involvement. Vascular gangrene, purpura fulminans, and diabetic gangrene are covered in Chapter 35; vaccinia gangrenosa in Chapter 19; and gangrenous balanitis and necrotizing fasciitis in other areas of this chapter.

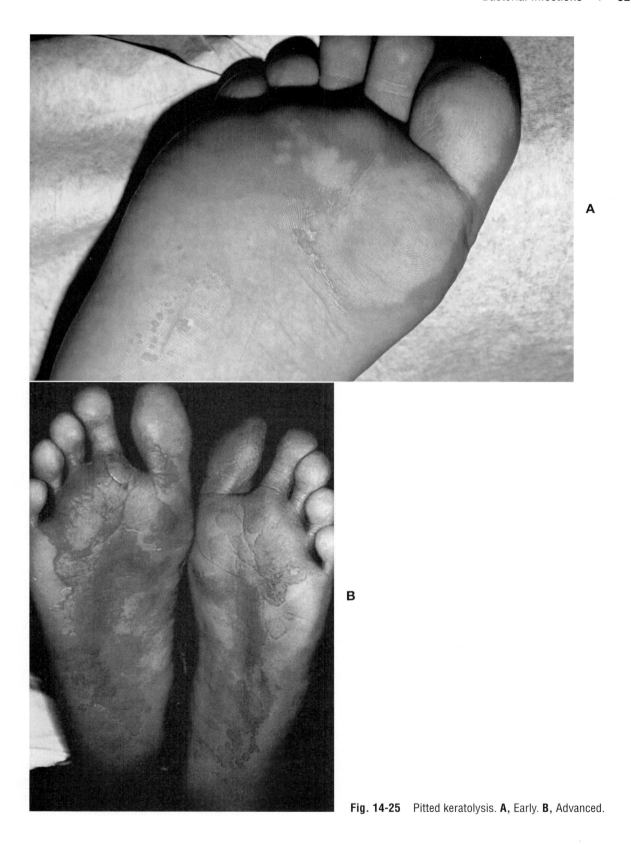

Fig. 14-25 Pitted keratolysis. **A,** Early. **B,** Advanced.

Gas Gangrene (Clostridial Myonecrosis). Gas gangrene is the most severe form of infectious gangrene; it develops in deep lacerated wounds of muscle tissue. The incubation period is only a few hours. The onset is usually sudden and is characterized by a chill, a rise in temperature, marked prostration, and severe local pain. Gas bubbles (chiefly hydrogen) produced by the infection cause crepitation when the area is palpated. A mousy odor is characteristic. Gas gangrene is caused by a variety of species of the genus *Clostridium,* most frequently *C. perfringens, C. oedematiens, C. septicum,* and *C. haemolyticum.* These are thick, gram-positive rods. Khavari et al reported an immunocompromised adult who presented with a large necrotic bulla and fever. The Gram stain revealed thick, gram-positive rods, but culture proved the organism to be *Bacillus cereus.* This is important, since it produces a beta-lactamase and is resistant to penicillin.

A subacute variety occurs, which is due to an anaerobic streptococcus (peptostreptococcus). This nonclostridial myositis may be clinically similar, but with delayed onset (several days). The purulent exudate has a foul odor, and gram-positive cocci in chains are present. It is important to distinguish these two entities, since involved muscle may recover in nonclostridial myositis, and debridement may safely be limited to removal of grossly necrotic muscle. Infections with both clostridia and nonclostridial organisms such as *Streptococcus faecalis, S. anginosus, Proteus, Escherichia coli, Bacteroides,* and *Klebsiella* species may also cause crepitant cellulitis, when the infection is limited to the subcutaneous tissue. Treatment of all clostridial infections is wide surgical debridement and intensive antibiotic therapy with intravenous penicillin G. Hyperbaric oxygen therapy may be of value if immediately available.

Chronic Undermining Burrowing Ulcers (Meleney's Gangrene). This entity was first described by Meleney as postoperative progressive bacterial synergetic gangrene. It usually follows drainage of peritoneal abscess, lung abscess, or chronic empyema. After 1 or 2 weeks the wound markings or retention suture holes assume a carbunculoid appearance, finally differentiating into three skin zones: outer, bright red; middle, dusky purple; and inner, gangrenous with a central area of granulation tissue. The pain is excruciating. In Meleney's postoperative progressive gangrene, the essential organism is a microaerophilic, nonhemolytic streptococcus (peptostreptococcus) in the spreading periphery of the lesion, associated with *Staphylococcus aureus* or *Enterobacteriaceae* in the zone of gangrene. This disease is differentiated from gangrenous ecthyma, which begins as vesicles rapidly progressing to pustulation and gangrenous ulceration in debilitated subjects, and is due to *Pseudomonas aeruginosa.* It is differentiated from fusospirochetal gangrene, which occurs from human bites. Amebic infection with gangrene usually follows amebic abscess of the liver. The margins of the ulcer are raised and everted,

and the granulations have the appearance of raw beef covered with shreds of necrotic material. Glairy pus can be expressed from the margins. Pyoderma gangrenosum occurs in a different setting, lacks the bacterial findings, and does not respond to antibiotic therapy.

Wide excision and grafting are primary therapy. Antimicrobial agents, penicillin, and an aminoglycoside should be given as adjunctive therapy.

Fournier's Gangrene of the Penis or Scrotum. Fournier's syndrome is a malignant gangrenous infection of the penis, scrotum, or perineum, which may be due to infection with group A streptococci or a mixed infection with enteric bacilli and anaerobes. This is usually considered a form of necrotizing fasciitis, as it spreads along fascial planes. Peak incidence is between 20 and 50 years, but cases have been reported in children. Culture for aerobic and anaerobic organisms should be done, and appropriate antibiotics started; surgical debridement and general support should be instituted.

Feingold DS: Gangrenous and crepitant cellulitis. *J Am Acad Dermatol* 1982, 6:289.

Jones DJ, et al: Diagnosis of Meleney's synergistic gangrene. *Br J Surg* 1988, 75:267.

Khavari PA, et al: Periodic acid-Schiff positive organisms in primary cutaneous *Bacillus cereus* infection. *Arch Dermatol* 1991, 127:543.

Saiag P, et al: MRI in adults presenting with severe acute infectious cellulitis. *Arch Dermatol* 1994, 130:1150.

Samlaska CP, et al: Subcutaneous emphysema. *Adv Dermatol* 1996, 11:117.

Shimizu T, et al: Nonclostridial gas gangrene due to *Streptococcus anginosus. J Am Acad Dermatol* 1999, 40:347.

van der Meer JB, et al: Fournier's gangrene. *Arch Dermatol* 1990, 126:1377. _____ ▲

Infections caused by gram-negative organisms

PSEUDOMONAS INFECTIONS
Ecthyma Gangrenosum

In the gravely ill patient opalescent, tense vesicles or pustules are surrounded by narrow pink to violaceous halos. These lesions quickly become hemorrhagic and violaceous and rupture to become round ulcers with necrotic black centers (Fig. 14-26). They are usually on the buttocks and extremities and are often grouped closely together.

Ecthyma gangrenosum occurs in debilitated persons who may be suffering from leukemia, in the severely burned patient, in pancytopenia or neutropenia, in patients with a functional neutrophilic defect, terminal carcinoma, or other severe chronic disease. Healthy infants may develop lesions in the perineal area after antibiotic therapy in conjunction with maceration of the diaper area.

The classic vesicle suggests the diagnosis. The contents

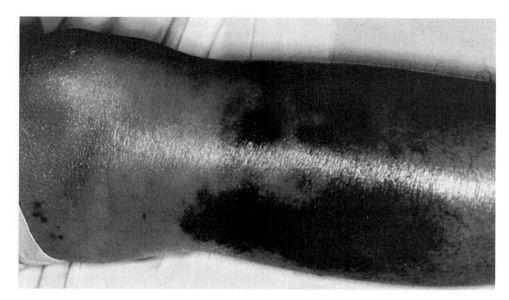

Fig. 14-26 Ecthyma gangrenosum.

of the vesicles or hemorrhagic pustules will show gram-negative bacilli on Gram stain and cultures will be positive for *Pseudomonas aeruginosa.* As this is usually a manifestation of sepsis, the blood culture will show *P. aeruginosa.* However, in healthy infants with diaper area lesions, in patients with HIV infection, and in other occasional cases early lesions may occur at the portal of entry, allowing for diagnosis and treatment before evolution into sepsis occurs.

Treatment is the immediate institution of intravenous anti-*Pseudomonas* medications. An aminoglycoside in combination with an antpseudomonal penicillin, such as piperacillin, is recommended. The addition of granulocyte-macrophage colony-stimulating factor to stimulate both proliferation and differentiation of myeloid precursors was reported by Becherel et al to be a helpful adjunct in a patient with myelodysplastic syndrome. Greene et al found patients had a poor prognosis if there were multiple lesions, if there was a delay in diagnosis and institution of appropriate therapy, and if neutropenia did not resolve by the end of a course of antibiotics. Instrumentation or catheterization increased the risk of this infection.

Other lesions are also seen with *Pseudomonas* septicemia. These may be sharply demarcated areas of cellulitis, macules, papules, plaques, and nodules, characteristically found on the trunk. *Pseudomonas mesophilica* and *Stenotrophomonas* (formerly *Xanthomonas* and *Pseudomonas*) *maltophilia* may also produce such skin lesions in immunocompromised individuals.

Several patients with AIDS have been reported who developed nodular skin lesions or abscesses secondary to *P. aeruginosa.* Generally these patients are systemically ill; however, blood cultures are negative.

Green Nail Syndrome

Green nail syndrome is characterized by onycholysis of the distal portion of the nail and a striking greenish discoloration in the separated areas. It is frequently associated with paronychia in persons whose hands are often in water. Soaking the affected finger in a 1% acetic acid solution twice daily for an hour has been found to be helpful. Trimming the onycholytic nail plate followed by twice-daily application of Neosporin solution is also effective.

Gram-Negative Toe Web Infection

This type of infection often begins with dermatophytosis. Dermatophytosis may progress to a condition referred to by Leyden et al as *dermatophytosis complex,* where many types of gram-negative organisms may be recovered, and as inflammation, maceration, and inflammation progress, it is less often possible to culture dermatophytes. Prolonged immersion may also cause hydration and maceration of the interdigital spaces, with overgrowth of gram-negative organisms. *Pseudomonas aeruginosa* is the most prominent among them, but commonly a mixture of other gram-negative organisms, such as *Escherichia coli* and *Proteus* are present.

Finally, denudation with purulent or serous discharge and marked edema and erythema of the surrounding tissue may be seen. One of the authors (WDJ) has seen two patients with chronic, recurrent gram-negative abscesses of the leg associated with gram-negative toe web infection. These middle-aged men suffered from red, painful nodules of the calf that did not drain to the surface but would involute spontaneously only to reappear 1 to 2 weeks later. The origin of the *Pseudomonas* cultured from one and *Serratia* from the other was thought to be due to the toe web infection.

Early dermatophytosis, dermatophytosis simplex, may simply be treated with topical antifungals. However, once the scaling and peeling progress to white maceration, soggy scaling, bad odor, edema, and fissuring, treatment must also include topical antibiotics or acetic acid compresses. Full-blown gram-negative toe web infection with widespread denudation and erythema, purulence, and edema requires systemic antibiotics. A third-generation cephalosporin or a fluoroquinolone such as ciprofloxacin or ofloxacin is recommended.

Blastomycosis-Like Pyoderma

Large verrucous plaques with elevated borders and multiple pustules may occur as a chronic vegetating infection. Most patients have an underlying systemic or local host compromise. Bacteria such as *P. aeruginosa, S. aureus, Proteus, E. coli,* or streptococci may be isolated. Trygg et al reported a case that responded to 500 mg of ciprofloxacin twice daily.

Pseudomonas Aeruginosa Folliculitis (Hot Tub Folliculitis)

Pseudomonas folliculitis is characterized by pruritic follicular, maculopapular, vesicular, or pustular lesions occurring within 1 to 4 days after bathing in a hot tub, whirlpool, or public swimming pool. Lacour et al reported two cases in which *P. aeruginosa* folliculitis was acquired from diving suits that were apparently colonized from the wash water. Most lesions occur on the sides of the trunk, axillae, buttocks, and proximal extremities (Fig. 14-27). The apocrine areas of the breasts and axilla are often involved. Associated complaints may include earache, sore throat, headache, fever, and malaise. Rarely, systemic infection may result; breast abscess and bacteremia have been reported. Large outbreaks have occurred.

The folliculitis involutes usually within 7 to 14 days without therapy, although on occasion multiple prolonged recurrent episodes have been reported. In patients with fever, constitutional symptoms, or prolonged disease a third-generation oral cephalosporin or a fluoroquinolone such as ciprofloxacin or ofloxacin may be useful. Preventive measures have been water filtration, automatic chlorination to maintain a free chlorine level of 1 ppm, maintenance of water at pH 7.2 to 7.8, and frequent changing of the water.

External Otitis

Swelling, maceration, and pain may be present. In up to 70% of cases *P. aeruginosa* may be cultured. This is especially common in swimmers. Local applications of antipseudomonal Cortisporin Otic Solution or Suspension or 2% acetic acid compresses will help clear this infection.

There is also a threat of external otitis occurring after ear surgery. If the patient is a swimmer or has diabetes, acetic acid compresses for a day or two before surgery may prevent this complication.

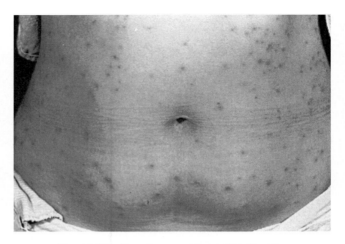

Fig. 14-27 Pseudomonas "hot tub" folliculitis.

A more severe type, referred to as *malignant external otitis,* occurs in elderly patients with diabetes. The swelling, pain, and erythema are more pronounced, with purulence and a foul odor. Facial nerve palsy develops in 30% of cases, and cartilage necrosis may occur. This is a life-threatening infection in these older, compromised individuals, and requires swift institution of appropriate systemic antibiotics.

Gram-Negative Folliculitis

Although this is usually due to *Enterobacteriaceae, Klebsiella, Escherichia, Proteus,* or *Serratia,* occasional cases caused by *Pseudomonas* have been seen, as reported by Leyden et al. They differed from the other types of gram-negative infection in patients with acne in that the site of colonization of *Pseudomonas* was the external ear, and topical therapy alone to the face and ears was sufficient for cure. Finally, an outbreak of gram-negative pustular dermatitis on the legs, arms, torso, and buttocks occurred in a group of college students who hosted a mud-wrestling social event.

Adler AI, et al: An outbreak of mud wrestling-induced pustular dermatitis in college students. *JAMA* 1993, 269:502.

Baze PE, et al: *P. aeruginosa* 0-11 folliculitis. *Arch Dermatol* 1985, 121:873.

Becherel PA, et al: Granulocyte-macrophage colony-stimulating factor in the management of severe ecthyma gangrenosum related to myelodysplastic syndrome. *Arch Dermatol* 1995, 131:892.

Blumenthal NC, et al: Ecthyma gangrenosum. *Arch Dermatol* 1990, 126:527.

Boisseau AM, et al: Perineal ecthyma gangrenosum in infancy and early childhood. *J Am Acad Dermatol* 1992, 27:415.

Chandrasekar PH, et al: Hot tub-associated dermatitis due to *P. aeruginosa. Arch Dermatol* 1984, 120:1337.

Eaglstein NF, et al: Gram-negative bacterial toe web infection. *J Am Acad Dermatol* 1983, 8:225.

Fox AB, et al: Recreationally associated *P. aeruginosa* folliculitis. *Arch Dermatol* 1984, 120:1304.

Greene SL, et al: Ecthyma gangrenosum. *J Am Acad Dermatol* 1984, 11:781.

King DF, et al: Importance of debridement in the treatment of gram-negative toe web infection. *J Am Acad Dermatol* 1986, 14:278.

Lacour JP, et al: Diving suit dermatitis caused by *Pseudomonas aeruginosa*. *J Am Acad Dermatol* 1994; 31:1055.

Leyden JJ, et al: Interdigital athletes foot. *Arch Dermatol* 1978, 114:1466.

Leyden JJ, et al: *P. aeruginosa* gram-negative folliculitis. *Arch Dermatol* 1979, 115:1203.

Merritt WT, et al: Malignant external otitis in an adolescent with diabetes. *J Pediatr* 1980, 96:872.

Nieves D, et al: Smoldering gram-negative cellulitis. *J Am Acad Dermatol* 1999, 41:319.

Pham BN, et al: *Xanthomonas* (formerly *Pseudomonas*) *maltophilia*-induced cellulitis in a neutropenic patient. *Arch Dermatol* 1992; 128:702.

Roberts R, et al: Erysipelas-like lesions and hyperesthesia as manifestations of *P. aeruginosa* septicemia. *JAMA* 1982, 248:2156.

Sangeorzan JA, et al: Cutaneous manifestations of *Pseudomonas* infection in AIDS. *Arch Dermatol* 1990, 126:832.

Scherbenske JM, et al: Acute *Pseudomonas* infection of the external ear. *J Dermatol Surg Oncol* 1988, 14:165.

Sevinsky LD, et al: Ecthyma gangrenosum. *J Am Acad Dermatol* 1993, 29:104.

Strazzi SR, et al: *P. mesophilica* cutaneous infection in an immunocompetent host. *Arch Dermatol* 1992, 128:273.

Trygg KJ, et al: Blastomycosis-like pyoderma caused by *P. aeruginosa*. *J Am Acad Dermatol* 1990, 23:750. ▲

MALACOPLAKIA (MALAKOPLAKIA)

This rare granuloma, originally reported only in the genitourinary tract of immunosuppressed renal transplant recipients, may also occur in the skin and subcutaneous tissues of other patients with deficient immune responsiveness such as is present in HIV infection. Patients are unable to resist infections with *S. aureus, P. aeruginosa,* and *E. coli.* There is defective intracellular digestion of the bacteria once they have been phagocytized.

The granulomas may arise as yellowish red papules in the natal cleft, as draining sinuses in the vicinity of the urethra, as perianal ulcers, as a painful draining abscess on the thigh, or as lesions on the vulva.

Histologically, there are foamy eosinophilic Hansemann macrophages containing calcified, concentrically laminated, intracytoplasmic bodies called *Michaelis-Gutmann bodies.* Scattered immunoblasts, neutrophils, and lymphocytes are found in the dermis.

Successful treatment depends on the isolated organism; a fluoroquinolone such as ciprofloxacin or ofloxacin is usually useful.

Almagro UA, et al: Cutaneous malakoplakia: report of a case and review of the literature. *Am J Dermatopathol* 1981, 3:295.

Helander I, et al: Lupus vulgaris with Michaelis-Gutmann–like bodies in an immunologically compromised patient. *J Am Acad Dermatol* 1988, 18:577.

Herrero C, et al: Successful treatment of a patient with cutaneous malacoplakia with clofazimine and trimethoprim sulfamethoxazole. *J Am Acad Dermatol* 1990, 23:947.

Wittenberg GP, et al: Cutaneous malacoplakia in a patient with AIDS. *Arch Dermatol* 1998, 134:244. ▲

HAEMOPHILUS INFLUENZAE CELLULITIS

Haemophilus influenzae type B causes a distinctive bluish or purplish red cellulitis of the face accompanied by fever in children below age 2. The importance of recognizing the entity is related to the bacteremia that often accompanies the cellulitis. The bacteremia may lead to meningitis, orbital cellulitis, osteomyelitis, or pyarthrosis. Cultures of the blood and needle aspirates of the cellulitis should yield the organism.

In a series of 72 cases reported by Ginsburg, 86% had bacteremia, 68% had had otitis media, and 8% had meningitis. Cefuroxime intravenously, or a third-generation cephalosporin, or ampicillin with chloramphenicol is effective. In a family with children under age 4, the index case, both parents, and children at risk (unvaccinated) should be given rifampin to clear the nasal carriage state and prevent secondary cases. A vaccine is available and is given at 2, 4, and 6 months of age. This has led to a marked diminution of infections with this organism as Barone et al document.

Barone SR, et al: Periorbital and orbital cellulitis in the *Haemophilus influenzae* vaccine era. *J Pediatr Ophthalmol Strabismus* 1997, 34:293.

Carter S, et al: Etiology and treatment of facial cellulitis in pediatric patients. *Pediatr Infect Dis J* 1983, 2:222.

Ginsburg CM: *H. influenzae* type B buccal cellulitis. *J Am Acad Dermatol* 1981, 4:661.

Prevention of secondary cases of *H. influenzae* type B disease. *MMWR* 1982, 31:672. ▲

CHANCROID

Chancroid (soft chancre), is an infectious, contagious, ulcerative, sexually transmitted disease caused by the gram-negative bacillus *Haemophilus ducreyi* (the Ducrey bacillus). One or more deep or superficial tender ulcers on the genitalia, and painful inguinal adenitis in 50%, which may suppurate, are characteristic of the disease. Men outnumber women manyfold.

Chancroid begins as an inflammatory macule or pustule 1 to 5 days—or rarely, as long as 2 weeks—after intercourse. It generally appears on the distal penis (or perianal area) in men, or on the vulva, cervix, or perianal area in women. However, many cases of extragenital infection on hands, eyelids, lips, or breasts have been reported. Autoinoculation frequently forms kissing lesions on the genitalia, and women are apt to have more numerous lesions.

The pustule ruptures early with the formation of a ragged ulcer that lacks the induration of a chancre, usually being soft with an indefinite inflammatory thickening. The ulcers appear punched-out or have undermined irregular edges surrounded by mild hyperemia (Figs. 14-28 and 14-29). The base is covered with a purulent, dirty exudate. The ulcers bleed easily and are very tender.

A number of clinical variants have been described, including granuloma inguinale–like, giant ulcers, serpigi-

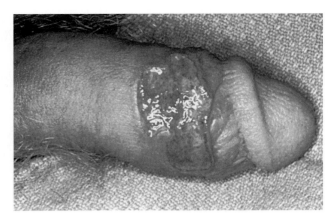

Fig. 14-28 Chancroid with painful perforation of frenum, a common location.

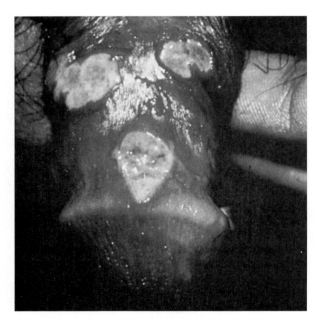

Fig. 14-29 Chancroid.

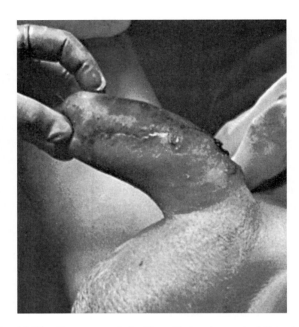

Fig. 14-30 Gangrenous balanitis, with involvement of the whole penis.

penis (Fig. 14-30), sometimes attacking the scrotum or pubes. The edges of the ulcer are likely to be elevated, firm, and undermined. The granulating base, which bleeds easily, is covered with a thick, purulent exudate and dirty, necrotic detritus. The neighboring skin may be edematous and dusky red, and the regional lymph glands may be swollen, although this is not necessarily a marked feature. There is severe mutilation as a result of sloughing, without any evidence of spontaneous healing.

This type of phagedena (spreading and sloughing ulceration) is a rare complication of chancre and chancroidal infections together with another secondary bacterial infection. Treatment is by the use of antibiotics locally and internally, directed against secondary bacteria, as well as the primary process, such as chancroid, syphilis, or granuloma inguinale, if present.

Chancroid is caused by the gram-negative bacillus *Haemophilus ducreyi* and is sexually transmitted.

On histologic investigation the ulcer may include a superficial necrotic zone with an infiltrate consisting of neutrophils, lymphocytes, and red blood cells. Deep to this, new vessel formation is present, with vascular proliferation. Deeper still is an infiltrate of lymphocytes and plasma cells. Ducrey's bacilli may or may not be seen in the sections.

The diagnosis of chancroid was, in the past, a clinical diagnosis, by exclusion of other clinically similar conditions. Solid-media culture techniques now make definitive diagnosis possible, and permit sensitivity testing. Specimens for culture should be taken from the purulent ulcer base and active border without extensive cleaning. They

nous ulcers, transient chancroid, and follicular and papular variants.

Only about half the cases of genital chancroid manifest inguinal adenitis. Suppuration of the bubo (inguinal lymph node) may occur despite early antibiotic therapy. The lymphadenitis of chancroid, mostly unilateral, is tender and may rupture spontaneously. Left untreated, the site of perforation of the broken-down bubo may assume the features of a soft chancre (chancrous bubo).

As a result of mixed infection, phagedenic and gangrenous features may develop. Gangrenous balanitis is a form of phagedena. Clinically, the disease is characterized by chronic, painful, destructive ulcers that begin on the prepuce or glans and spread by direct extension along the shaft of the should be inoculated in the clinic, as transport systems have not been evaluated. The selective medium contains vancomycin, and cultures are done in a water-saturated environment with 1% to 5% carbon dioxide, at a temperature of 33° C. Occasional outbreaks are due to vancomycin-sensitive strains. In these cases, culture will only be successful using vancomycin-free media.

Smears are only diagnostic in 50% of cases in the best hands. A recent combined polymerase chain reaction (PCR) technique allows the diagnosis of syphilis, herpes simplex, and chancroid from a single swab. Probably the disease for which chancroid is most frequently mistaken is herpes progenitalis. A history of recurrent grouped vesicles at the same site should help eliminate the chance of a misdiagnosis. Traumatic ulcerations should also be ruled out. These occur mostly along the frenulum or as multiple erosions on the prepuce. Adenopathy is absent, and some degree of phimosis is present.

The clinical features that differentiate chancroid from syphilitic chancre are given in Chapter 18. However, the diagnosis of chancroid does not rule out syphilis. Either the lesion may be already a mixed sore or the subsequent development of syphilis should be anticipated, since the incubation period of the chancre is much longer than that of chancroid. Repeated darkfield examinations for *Treponema pallidum* are necessary even in a sore where the diagnosis of chancroid has been established. Serologic tests for syphilis should be obtained initially, and monthly for the next 3 months, and serologic testing for HIV infection should also be done. Chancroidal genital ulcer disease facilitates the transmission of HIV infection.

Treatment

The treatment of choice for chancroid is azithromycin, 1 g orally in a single dose. Erythromycin, 500 mg four times daily for 7 days; ceftriaxone, 250 mg intramuscularly in a single dose; or ciprofloxacin, 500 mg orally twice daily for 3 days, are also recommended treatments. Ciprofloxacin should not be used for pregnant or lactating women or in children less than 17 years of age. Partners who have had sexual contact with the patient within the 10 days before the onset of symptoms should be treated with a recommended regimen.

Phimosis that does not subside following irrigation of the preputial cavity may have to be relieved by a dorsal slit. Circumcision should be deferred for at least 2 or 3 months. If frank pus is already present, repeated aspirations (not incisions) may be necessary.

Abeck D, et al: Chancroid. *Curr Probl Dermatol* 1996, 24:90.

Jones CC, et al: Cultural diagnosis of chancroid. *Arch Dermatol* 1991, 127:1823.

Kraus SJ, et al: Pseudogranuloma inguinale caused by *H. ducreyi. Arch Dermatol* 1982, 118:494.

McCurley ME, et al: Chancroid. *J Am Acad Dermatol* 1988, 19:330.

1998 STD Guidelines. *MMWR* 1998, 47:1.

Salzman RS, et al: Chancroidal ulcers that are not chancroid. *Arch Dermatol* 1984, 120:636.

Schmid GP, et al: Chancroid in the US. *JAMA* 1987, 258:3265. ▲

GRANULOMA INGUINALE (GRANULOMA VENEREUM, DONOVANOSIS)

Granuloma inguinale is a mildly contagious, chronic, granulomatous, locally destructive disease characterized by progressive, indolent, serpiginous ulcerations of the groins, pubes, genitalia, and anus.

The disease begins as single or multiple subcutaneous nodules, which erode through the skin to produce clean, sharply defined lesions, which are usually painless. More than 80% of cases demonstrate hypertrophic, vegetative granulation tissue, which is soft, has a beefy-red appearance, and bleeds readily (Fig. 14-31). Approximately 10% of cases have ulcerative lesions with overhanging edges and a dry or moist floor. A membranous exudate may cover the floor of fine granulations, and the lesions are moderately painful. Occasional cases are misdiagnosed as carcinoma of the penis. The lesions enlarge by autoinoculation and peripheral extension with satellite lesions, and by gradual undermining of tissue at the advancing edge.

The genitalia are involved in 90% of cases, the inguinal region in 10% (Fig. 14-32), the anal region in 5% to 10%, and distal sites in 1% to 5%. Lesions are limited to the genitalia in approximately 80% of cases and to the inguinal region in less than 5%. In men, the lesions most commonly occur on the prepuce or glans, and in women, lesions on the labia are most common (Fig. 14-33).

The incubation period is unknown; it may vary between 8 and 80 days, with a 2- to 3-week period being most common.

Persisting sinuses and hypertrophic scars, devoid of pigment, are fairly characteristic of the disease. The regional lymph nodes are usually not enlarged. The lesions are not painful and produce only mild subjective symptoms. In later stages, as a result of cicatrization, the lymph channels are sometimes blocked and pseudoelephantiasis of the genitals (esthiomene) may occur. Mutilation of the genitals and destruction of deeper tissues are observed in some instances.

Dissemination from the inguinal region may be by hematogenous or lymphatic routes. There may be involvement of liver, other organs, eyes, face, lips, larynx, chest, and, rarely, bones. Hematogenous spread is believed to occur after pregnancy. During childbearing the cervical lesions may extend to the internal genital organs. Squamous cell carcinoma may rarely supervene.

Granuloma inguinale is caused by the gram-negative bacterium *Calymmatobacterium granulomatis*. The exact mode of transmission of infection is undetermined. The role

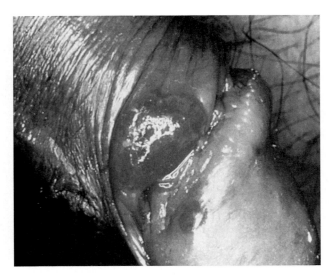

Fig. 14-31 Early granuloma inguinale, showing beefy granulations.

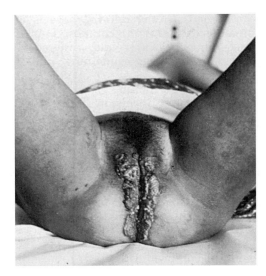

Fig. 14-33 Granuloma inguinale. (Courtesy Dr. Arturo L. Carrion.)

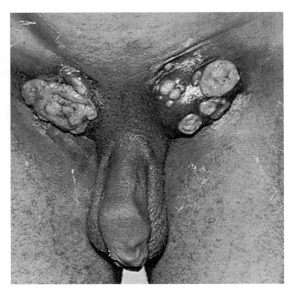

Fig. 14-32 Granuloma inguinale. (Courtesy Dr. H. Shatin.)

of sexual transmission is controversial, but several factors, including the genital location of the initial lesion in the majority of cases, the relationship of the first lesion to an incubation period following coitus, and the occurrence of conjugal infection in 12% to 52% of marital or steady sexual partners, strongly favor sexual transmission. An unusual American epidemic reported by Rosen et al supports the venereal transmission of this disorder. Also, it has been speculated that *C. granulomatis* is an intestinal inhabitant that leads to granuloma inguinale through autoinoculation, or sexually through vaginal intercourse if the vagina is contaminated by enteric bacteria, or through rectal intercourse, heterosexual or homosexual. *C. granulo-*

matis probably requires direct inoculation through a break in the skin or mucosa to cause infection. Those affected are generally young adults.

On histologic investigation in the center of the lesion the epidermis is replaced by serum, fibrin, and polymorphonuclear leukocytes. At the periphery the epidermis is thickened. In the dermis there is a dense granulomatous infiltration composed chiefly of plasma cells and histiocytes, and scattered throughout are small abscesses containing polymorphonuclear leukocytes.

Characteristic pale-staining macrophages that have intracytoplasmic inclusion bodies are found. The parasitized histiocytes may measure 20 µm or more in diameter. The ovoid Donovan bodies measure 1 to 2 µm and may be visualized by using Giemsa or silver stains. The best method, however, is toluidine blue staining of semi-thin, plastic-embedded sections. Crushed smears of fresh biopsy material stained with Wright or Giemsa stain permit the demonstration of Donovan bodies and provide rapid diagnosis.

Granuloma inguinale may be confused with ulcerations of the groin caused by syphilis or carcinoma, but it is differentiated from these diseases by its long duration and slow course, by the absence of lymphatic involvement, and, in the case of syphilis, by a negative test for syphilis and failure to respond to antisyphilitic treatment. It should not be overlooked that other venereal diseases, especially syphilis, often coexist with granuloma inguinale. Additionally, all patients presenting with sexually transmitted diseases should be tested for HIV infection. Lymphogranuloma venereum at an early stage would most likely be accompanied by inguinal adenitis. In later stages when stasis, excoriations, and enlargement of the outer genitalia are common to granuloma inguinale and lymphogranuloma venereum, the absence of a positive lymphogranuloma venereum complement-fixation test and the presence of Donovan bodies in the lesions permit the diagnosis of granuloma inguinale.

Treatment

Trimethoprim-sulfamethoxazole, one double-strength tablet orally twice daily for a minimum of 3 weeks, or doxy-cycline, 100 mg orally twice a day for a minimum of 3 weeks, are the recommended regimens. Therapy should be continued until all lesions have healed completely. Alternative regimens are ciprofloxacin, 750 mg orally twice a day for a minimum of 3 weeks, or erythromycin base, 500 mg orally four times a day for a minimum of 3 weeks. The addition of an aminoglycoside (gentamicin), 1 mg/kg IV every 8 hours, should be considered if lesions do no respond within the first few days.

Hart G: Donovanosis. *Clin Infect Dis* 1997, 25:24.

Manders SM, et al: Granuloma inguinale and HIV. *J Am Acad Dermatol* 1997, 37:494.

1998 STD Guidelines. *MMWR* 1998, 47:1.

Richens J: The diagnosis and treatment of donovanosis. *Genitourin Med* 1991, 67:441.

Rosen T, et al: Granuloma inguinale. *J Am Acad Dermatol* 1984, 11:433. ▲

GONOCOCCAL DERMATITIS

Primary gonococcal dermatitis is a rare infection that occurs mostly as erosions that may be 2 to 20 mm in diameter; however, several unusual presentations have been reported.

A physician attending a patient with gonorrhea received a wound on his thumb followed 30 hours later by lymphangitis of the arm, with two small nodules on the thumb. The pus from the incised nodules showed grouped intracellular diplococci. The physician became severely ill and developed polyarticular gonococcal arthritis. Gonococcal dermatitis has been reported as occurring on the median raphe without urethritis, as extragenital gonococcal ecthyma, as grouped pustules on an erythematous base on the finger that simulates herpetic whitlow, and as scalp abscesses in infants secondary to direct fetal monitoring in mothers with gonorrhea.

Treatment is the same as that of gonorrheal urethritis. Ciprofloxacin as a 500-mg single oral dose, cefixime as a single 400-mg oral dose, or ofloxacin as a single 400-mg oral dose are all effective.

Gonococcemia

Gonococcemia is characterized by a hemorrhagic vesiculopustular eruption (Fig. 14-34), bouts of fever, and arthralgia or actual arthritis of one or several joints.

The skin lesions begin as tiny erythematous macules that evolve into vesicopustules on a deeply erythematous base or into purpuric macules that may be as much as 2 cm in diameter. These purpuric lesions occur acrally, mostly on

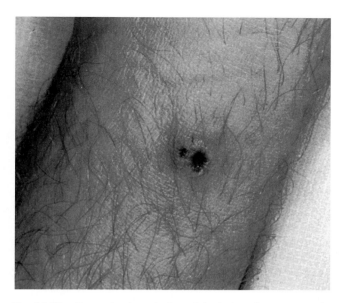

Fig. 14-34 Hemorrhagic vesiculopustular lesion of gonococcemia.

the palms and soles and over joints. These lesions are accompanied by fever, chills, malaise, migratory polyarthralgia, myalgia, and tenosynovitis. The vesicopustules are usually tender and sparse, and occur principally on the extremities. Involution of the lesions takes place in about 4 days.

Many patients seen are women with asymptomatic anogenital infections in whom dissemination occurs during pregnancy or menstruation. Liver function abnormalities, myocarditis, pericarditis, endocarditis, and meningitis may complicate this infection. In severe or recurrent cases complement deficiency, especially of the late (C5, C6, C7, or C8) components, should be investigated.

The causative organism is *Neisseria gonorrhoeae*. These organisms can at times be demonstrated in the early skin lesion histologically, by smears, and by cultures. Gonococci may be found in the blood, genitourinary tract, joints, and skin.

The skin lesions of gonococcemia may be identical to those seen in meningococcemia, nongonococcal bacterial endocarditis, rheumatoid arthritis, the rickettsial diseases, systemic lupus erythematosus, periarteritis nodosa, Haverhill fever, and typhoid fever.

The treatment of choice is ceftriaxone, 1 g IV daily for 24 to 48 hours after improvement begins. Then therapy may be switched to either cefixime, 400 mg orally twice daily, or ciprofloxacin, 500 mg orally twice daily, or ofloxacin, 400 mg orally twice a day. Treatment with these should continue for a full week. An alternative initial IV drug is cefotaxime, 1 g every 8 hours. Spectinomycin, 2 g intramuscularly (IM) every 12 hours, may be used for persons allergic to beta-lactam drugs. Ciprofloxacin is contraindicated for children under age 17 and in pregnant and lactating women. If a cephalosporin is used, doxycycline should be given l00 mg twice daily for 7 days to treat coexisting chlamydial infection. Serologic testing for HIV infection should also be done.

Geelhoed-Duyrestiyir PHLM, et al: Disseminated gonococcal infection in elderly patients. *Arch Intern Med* 1986, 146:1739.

Lind I: Gonorrhea. *Curr Probl Dermatol* 1996, 24:12.

1998 STD Guidelines. *MMWR*, 47:1.

Osttere LS, et al: Gastrointestinal and cutaneous vasculitis associated with gonococcal infection in an HIV-seropositive patient. *J Am Acad Dermatol* 1993, 29:276.

Rosen T: Unusual presentations of gonorrhea. *J Am Acad Dermatol* 1982, 6:369. _____ ▲

MENINGOCOCCEMIA

Acute meningococcemia presents with fever, chills, hypotension, and meningitis. Half to two thirds of patients develop a petechial eruption, most frequently on the trunk and lower extremities, which may progress to ecchymoses, bullous hemorrhagic lesions, and ischemic necrosis. Occasionally a transient, blanchable, morbilliform eruption is the only cutaneous finding. The oral and conjunctival mucous membranes may be affected.

Meningococcemia primarily affects young children, males more frequently than females. Patients with inherited or acquired deficiencies of the terminal components of complement or properdin are predisposed to infection.

A rare variant is chronic meningococcemia. There are recurrent episodes of fever, arthralgias, and erythematous macules that may evolve into lesions with central hemorrhage. Patients are generally young adults with fevers lasting 12 hours interspersed with 1 to 4 days of well-being.

The disease is caused by the fastidious gram-negative diplococcus *Neisseria meningitides*. It has a polysaccharide capsule that is important in its virulence and serotyping. The human nasopharynx is the only known reservoir, with carriage rates in the general population estimated to be 5% to 10%.

Treatment is with penicillin G, 300,000 units/kg/day intravenously up to 24 million units/day for 7 days. Chloramphenicol is used in penicillin-allergic patients although ceftriaxone and other newer cephalosporins are gaining acceptance as experience grows. Rifampin, 600 mg every 12 hours for 2 days (or 10 mg/kg every 12 hours for children), is given after the initial course of antibiotics to clear nasal carriage. Household members, and day-care and close school contacts should receive prophylactic therapy. A polyvalent vaccine is effective against groups A, C, Y, and W-135, and is recommended for high-risk groups.

Assier H, et al: Chronic meningococcemia in AIDS. *J Am Acad Dermatol* 1993; 29:793.

Frank M: Complement in the pathophysiology of human disease. *New Engl J Med* 1987, 316:1525.

Giraud T, et al: Adult overwhelming meningococcal purpura. *Arch Intern Med* 1991, 151:300.

Gregory B, et al: Cyclic fever and rash in a 66-year-old woman. *Arch Dermatol* 1992, 128:1643.

Ploysangam T, et al: Chronic meningococcemia in childhood. *Pediatr Dermatol* 1996, 13:483. _____ ▲

VIBRIO VULNIFICUS INFECTION

Infection with *Vibrio vulnificus,* a gram-negative rod of the noncholera group of vibrios, produces a rapidly expanding cellulitis or septicemia in patients who have been exposed to the organism, which occurs mainly along the Atlantic seacoast. It may be acquired via the gastrointestinal tract, where, after being ingested with raw oysters or other seafood, the bacterium enters the bloodstream at the level of the duodenum. Pulmonary infection by the aspiration of seawater has been reported. Localized skin infection may result after exposure of an open wound to seawater.

Skin lesions characteristically begin within 24 to 48 hours of exposure, with localized tenderness followed by erythema, edema, and indurated plaques. They occur in nearly 90% of patients and are most common on the lower extremities. A purplish discoloration develops centrally, then undergoes necrosis, forming hemorrhagic bullae or ulcers. Other reported lesions include hemorrhagic bullae, pustules, petechiae, generalized macules or papules, and gangrene.

If the skin is invaded primarily, septicemia may not develop, but the lesions may be progressive and at times limb amputation may be necessary. With septicemia, cellulitic lesions are the result of seeding of the subcutaneous tissue during bacteremia. Patients with advanced liver disease are at particular risk for developing septicemia. Other predisposing disorders are immunosuppression, alcoholism, diabetes, renal failure, and iron-overload states such as hemochromatosis. The virulence of the bacterium is related to the production of exotoxin and various other factors. The mortality in patients with septicemia is greater than 50%.

Treatment of this fulminant infection, which rapidly produces septic shock, includes antibiotics, surgical debridement, and appropriate resuscitative therapy. *V. vulnificus* is sensitive to penicillins, cephalosporins, tetracyclines, cotrimoxazole, and chloramphenicol. Doxycycline together with ceftazidime is the treatment of choice. Surgical debridement of necrotizing tissue is recommended.

Chan HC, et al: Cutaneous manifestations of non-01 *V. cholerae* septicemia with gastroenteritis and meningitis. *J Am Acad Dermatol* 1994, 30:626.

Halow KD, et al: Primary skin infection due to *Vibrio vulnificus*. *J Am Coll Surg* 1996, 183:329.

Hlady WG, et al: *V. vulnificus* infection associated with raw oyster consumption. *Arch Dermatol* 1993, 129:957.

Klontz KC, et al: Syndromes of *V. vulnificus* infections. *Ann Intern Med* 1988, 109:318.

Morris JG Jr: *V. vulnificus:* a new monster of the deep. *Ann Intern Med* 1988, 109:318.

Newman C, et al: Fatal septicemia and bullae caused by non-01 *V. cholerae. J Am Acad Dermatol* 1993, 29:909. _____ ▲

CHROMOBACTERIOSIS AND *AEROMONAS* INFECTIONS

Chromobacteria are a genus of gram-negative rods that produce various discolorations on gelatin broth. They have been shown to be common water and soil saprophytes of the southeastern United States. Several types of cutaneous lesions are caused by chromobacteria, ranging from fluctuating abscesses and local cellulitis to anthraxlike carbuncular lesions with lymphangitis and lymphadenopathy and fatal septicemia. *Chromobacterium violaceum,* the most common organism in this genus, produces a violet pigment.

Macher et al reviewed the 12 known cases of *C. violaceum* infection and found that all had been infected in Louisiana or Florida between June and September. Eight had had soil or groundwater contact before the onset, and 10 were seen with skin lesions. Sepsis, liver abscess, and death are frequent. Patients with chronic granulomatous disease may be at particular risk. Aminoglycosides systemically are indicated.

A gram-negative bacterium, *Aeromonas hydrophilia,* another typical soil and water saprophyte, may cause similar skin infections manifesting as cellulitis, pustules, furuncles, gas gangrene, or ecthyma gangrenosum–like lesions, after water-related trauma and abrasions. Such a case was reported by Young et al. The treatment of choice for cellulitis is ciprofloxacin.

Bodey GP: Dermatologic manifestations of infections in neutropenic patients. *Infect Dis Clin North Am* 1994, 8:655.

Macher AM, et al: Chronic granulomatous disease of childhood and *Chromobacterium violaceum* infections in the southeastern United States. *Ann Intern Med* 1982, 97:51.

Young DF, et al: *Aeromonas hydrophila* infection of the skin. *Arch Dermatol* 1981, 117:244. _____ ▲

SALMONELLOSIS

Salmonellae are a genus of gram-negative rods that exist in humans either in a carrier state or as a cause of active enteric or systemic infection. Most cases are acquired by ingestion of contaminated food or water. Poultry and poultry products are the most important sources and are believed to be the cause in about half of common-source epidemics.

After an incubation period of 1 to 2 weeks, there is usually an acute onset of fever, chills, headache, constipation, and bronchitis. After 7 to 10 days of fever, diarrhea, and skin lesions, rose-colored macules or papules ("rose spots") 2 to 5 mm in diameter appear on the anterior trunk, between the umbilicus and the nipples. They occur in crops, each group of 10 to 20 lesions lasting 3 to 4 days, the total duration of the exanthem being 2 to 3 weeks in untreated cases. Rose spots occur in 50% to 60% of cases. A more extensive erythematous eruption occurring early in the course, erythema typhosum, is rarely reported, as are erythema nodosum, urticaria, and ulcers or abscesses.

The diagnosis is confirmed by culturing the organism from blood, stool, skin, or bone marrow. If the organism is not grown on *Shigella-Salmonella* medium, or not analyzed correctly, it may be erroneously reported as a coliform. The antibiotic of choice is a fluoroquinolone or ceftriaxone.

Goldberg MB, et al: The spectrum of *Salmonella* infection. *Infect Dis Clin North Am* 1988, 2:571.

Kovacs A, et al: Bacterial infections. *Med Clin North Am* 1997, 81:319. ▲

SHIGELLOSIS

Shigellae are small gram-negative rods that cause bacillary dysentery, an acute diarrheal illness. Most cases are a result of person-to-person transmission; however, widespread epidemics have resulted from contaminated food and water. Small, blanchable, erythematous macules on the extremities, as well as petechial or morbilliform eruptions, may occur. Stoll reported a male homosexual who developed a 1-cm furuncle on the dorsal penile shaft from which a pure culture of *Shigella flexneri* was grown. Shigellosis may then occur as a purely cutaneous form of sexually transmitted disease. *Shigella* and *Salmonella* are among the infections reported to induce the postdysenteric form of Reiter's syndrome. Therapy with a fluoroquinolone is curative.

Stoll DM: Cutaneous shigellosis. *Arch Dermatol* 1986, 122:22. _____ ▲

HELICOBACTER CELLULITIS

Fever, bacteremia, cellulitis, and arthritis may all be caused by *Helicobacter cinaedi*. Generally, these manifestations occur in HIV-infected patients; however, malignancy, diabetes, and alcoholism are other predisposing conditions. The cellulitis may be multifocal and recurrent, and have a distinctive red-brown or copper color with minimal warmth. Ciprofloxacin is generally effective.

Burman WJ, et al: Multifocal cellulitis and monoarticular arthritis as manifestations of *Helicobacter cinaedi* bacteremia. *Clin Infect Dis* 1995, 20:564.

Sullivan AK, et al: Recurrent *Helicobacter cinaedi* cellulitis and bacteremia in a patient with HIV infection. *Int J STD-AIDS* 1997, 8:59. ▲

RHINOSCLEROMA

Rhinoscleroma is a chronic, inflammatory, granulomatous disease of the upper respiratory tract characterized by sclerosis, deformity, remission, and eventual debility. Death resulting from obstructive sequelae may occur. The infection is limited to the nose, pharynx, and adjacent structures.

The disease begins insidiously with nasal catarrh, increased nasal secretion, and subsequent crusting. Gradually there ensues a nodular or rather diffuse sclerotic enlargement of the nose, upper lip, palate, or neighboring structures. The nodules at first are small, hard, subepidermal, and freely movable, but they gradually fuse to form sclerotic plaques that adhere to the underlying parts (Fig. 14-35). Ulceration is common (Figs. 14-36 and 14-37). The lesions have a distinctive stony hardness, are insensitive, and are of a dusky purple or ivory color. Hyperpigmentation can be expected in dark-complexioned individuals.

In the more advanced stages of rhinoscleroma, the reactive growth produces extensive mutilation of the face and marked disfigurement. Complete obstruction of the nares, superficial erosions, and seropurulent exudation may occur.

A microorganism, *Klebsiella pneumoniae,* ssp. *rhinoscleromatis,* first isolated by von Frisch, is the causative agent. The rhinoscleroma bacillus is a gram-negative rod, short, nonmotile, round at the ends, always encapsulated in a gelatinous capsule, and measuring 2.0 to 3.0 μm. It is found in the throats of scleroma patients only.

The disease occurs in both sexes, and is most common during the third and fourth decades of life. Although endemic in Austria and southern Russia and occasionally found in Brazil, Argentina, Chile, Spain, Italy, Sweden, and the United States, it is especially prevalent in El Salvador, where many workers in the dye industry have been affected. It was first described by Hebra in 1870 and later by von Mikulicz, von Frisch, and others.

In the primary stage of nasal catarrh, the histologic picture is that of a mild, nonspecific inflammation. When proliferation and tumefaction develop, the granulomatous tumor is made up largely of plasma cells, Mikulicz's cells, an occasional hyaline degenerated plasma cell (Russell body), a few spindle cells, and hypertrophic collagenous tissue.

The bacilli of rhinoscleroma are found within foamy macrophages known as *Mikulicz's cells*. They are best visualized with the Warthin-Starry silver stain. It is fibrosis that is responsible for the hardness of rhinoscleroma.

Rhinoscleroma has such distinctive features that its diagnosis should not be difficult. The diagnosis depends on bacteriologic, histopathologic, and serologic tests. Heat-

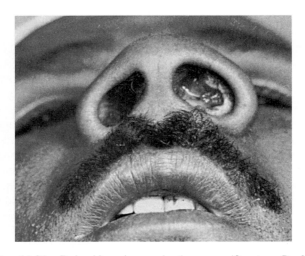

Fig. 14-35 Early rhinoscleroma in the nose. (Courtesy Dr. M. El-Zawahry, Egypt.)

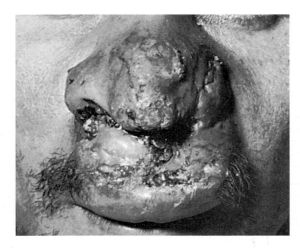

Fig. 14-36 Rhinoscleroma. (Courtesy Dr. F. Kerdel-Vegas.)

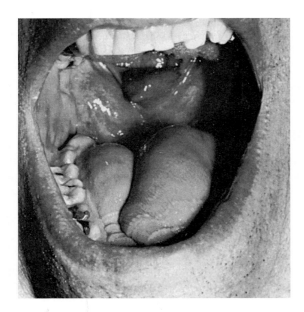

Fig. 14-37 Rhinoscleroma on the palate and nasopharynx.

killed antigen gives a positive complement-fixation reaction with scleroma patients' serum. Titers run as high as 1:1280. Clinically, it can be confused with syphilitic gumma, sarcoid, leishmaniasis, frambesia, keloid, lepra, hypertrophic forms of tuberculosis, and rhinosporidiosis.

Treatment

This disease is usually progressive and extremely resistant to therapy; however, it appears that the fluoroquinolones will prove to be the best therapy. Corticosteroids are useful in the acute phase. Surgical intervention or CO_2 laser treatments may be needed to prevent airway obstruction or to correct deformities.

Andraca R, et al: Rhinoscleroma. *Mayo Clin Proc* 1993, 68:1151.
Avery RK, et al: Rhinoscleroma treated with ciprofloxacin. *Laryngoscope* 1995, 105:854.
Lenis A, et al: Rhinoscleroma. *South Med J* 1988, 81:1580.
Maher AI, et al: Rhinoscleroma. *Laryngoscope* 1990; 100:783. _____ ▲

PASTEURELLOSIS

Primary cutaneous (ulceroglandular) infection caused by *Pasteurella hemolytica* occurred in a woman who acquired numerous lacerations on the hands from berry bushes while hunting and later dressed a deer. The lacerations became inflamed, lymphangitis developed, and her axillary lymph nodes were enlarged. There was moderate fever. From the exudate of a papular lesion of the finger *P. hemolytica* was isolated in pure culture. *P. hemolytica* is a common pathogen of domestic animals, being associated with shipping fever in cattle and septicemia in lambs and newborn pigs.

Pasteurella Multocida Infections

Pasteurella multocida is a small, nonmotile, gram-negative, bipolar-staining bacterium. It is known to be part of the normal oral and nasal flora of cats and dogs, but may also be an animal pathogen. The most common type of human infection follows injuries from animal bites, principally cat and dog bites, but also cat scratches. Following animal trauma, erythema, swelling, pain, and tenderness develop within a few hours of the bite, with a gray-colored serous or sanguinopurulent drainage from the puncture wounds. There may or may not be regional lymphadenopathy or evidence of systemic toxicity such as chills and fever. Septicemia may follow the local infection in rare cases, and tenosynovitis and osteomyelitis appear with some frequency. It is recommended that all cat bites and scratches, all sutured wounds of any animal source, and any other animal injuries of an unusual type or source be treated with systemic penicillin or tetracycline in addition to careful cleansing and tetanus prophylaxis.

Though a gram-negative bacillus, *P. multocida* is highly sensitive to penicillin.

Brue C, et al: *Pasteurella multocida* wound infection and cellulitis. *Int J Dermatol* 1994, 33:471.
Griego RD, et al: Dog, cat, and human bites. *J Am Acad Dermatol* 1995, 33:1019.
Weber DJ, et al: *P. multocida* infections: report of 34 cases and review of the literature. *Medicine* 1984; 63:133. _____ ▲

DOG AND HUMAN BITE PATHOGENS

Capnocytophaga canimorsus, formerly referred to as *DF-2,* is a gram-negative rod that is part of the normal oral flora of dogs and cats. It is associated with severe septicemia after dog bites. Patients who have undergone splenectomy are at particular risk. Alcoholism, chronic respiratory disease, and other medical conditions also predispose to infection; only one quarter of the 52 cases reviewed by Herbst et al were healthy before infection with *C. canimorsus.* A characteristic finding is a necrotizing eschar at the site of the bite. Fever, nausea, and vomiting occur abruptly within 1 to 3 days, and the eschar develops soon thereafter. Disseminated intravascular coagulation and extensive dry gangrene may complicate the course. Sepsis after a dog bite is another hazard splenectomized patients face in addition to their particular problems with pneumococcus, *Haemophilus influenzae* group B, babesiosis, *Neisseria meningitides,* and group A streptococcus.

C. canimorsus is difficult to identify by conventional cultures. Laboratory personnel need to be aware of the clinical suspicion of infection with this organism. A false-positive latex agglutination test for cryptococcal antigen in the spinal fluid may occur.

Treatment is with intensive intravenous antibiotics. In less severely affected patients amoxicillin clavulanate may be effective.

Grob et al reported an HIV-infected patient who developed extensive skin ulcerations resulting from eugonic fermenting bacteria (EF-4). This is another oral and nasal commensal in dogs, thus most reports of human disease follow animal bites. Datar et al reported the case of a woman who stepped on a used toothpick and developed cellulitis of the foot caused by *Eikenella corrodens,* a facultative gram-negative bacillus. This is a normal inhabitant of the human mouth. Most infections are caused by human bites or fist fights. Amoxicillin clavulanate or penicillin G are effective.

Datar S, et al: Cellulitis of the foot due to *Eikenella corrodens. Arch Dermatol* 1989, 123: 849.
Goldstein EJL: Management of human and animal bite wounds. *J Am Acad Dermatol* 1989, 21:1275.
Griego RD, et al: Dog, cat, and human bites. *J Am Acad Dermatol* 1995, 33:1019.
Grob JJ, et al: Extensive skin ulceration due to EF-4 bacterial infection in a patient with AIDS. *Br J Dermatol* 1989, 121:507.
Herbst JS, et al: Dysgonic fermenter type 2 septicemia with purpura fulminans. *Arch Dermatol* 1989, 125:1380. _____ ▲

GLANDERS

Once known as *equinia, farcy,* and *malleus,* glanders is a rare, usually fatal, infectious disease that occurs in humans by inoculation with *Pseudomonas mallei.* It is encountered in those who handle horses, mules, or donkeys.

The distinctive skin lesion is an inflammatory papule or vesicle that arises at the site of inoculation, rapidly becomes nodular, pustular, and ulcerative, and forms an irregular excavation with undermined edges and a base covered with a purulent and sanguineous exudate (Fig. 14-38). In a few days or weeks other nodules (called "farcy buds") develop along the lymphatics in the adjacent skin or subcutaneous tissues; subsequently these break down. In the acute form the skin involvement may be severe and accompanied by grave diarrhea. In the chronic form there are few skin lesions and milder constitutional symptoms, but repeated cycles of healing and breakdown of nodules may occur for weeks.

The respiratory mucous membranes are especially susceptible to the disease. After accidental inhalation, first catarrhal symptoms are present and there may be epistaxis or a mucoid nasal discharge. The nasal discharge is a characteristic feature of the disease.

The diagnosis is established by finding the gram-negative *P. mallei* in this discharge or in the skin ulcers, and should be confirmed by serum agglutination. This organism has been fatal to many laboratory workers, but it is now rare in this country.

Treatment is chiefly by immediate surgical excision of the inoculated lesions and by streptomycin plus a tetracycline.

Bovine farcy also occurs and is caused by *Nocardia farcinica.* Schiff et al reported a nonimmunocompromised patient with an infected facial laceration. Osteomyelitis complicated the course. Amikacin treatment after surgical debridement resulted in complete cure.

Howe C, et al: Human glanders. *Ann Intern Med* 1947, 26:93.
Schiff TA, et al: Cutaneous *Nocardia farcinica* infection in a nonimmuno-compromised patient. *Clin Infect Dis* 1993, 16:756. _____ ▲

MELIOIDOSIS

Melioidosis (Whitmore's disease) is a specific infection caused by a glanderslike bacillus, *Burkholderia* (formerly *Pseudomonas*) *pseudomallei.* The disease has an acute pulmonary and septicemic form with multiple miliary abscesses in the viscera and ends in early death. Less often it runs a chronic course, with subcutaneous abscesses and multiple sinuses of the soft tissues (Fig. 14-39). Its clinical characteristics are similar to glanders, disseminated fungal infections, and tuberculosis. Severe urticaria may occur with pulmonary melioidosis and may disappear after 1 week of tetracycline therapy.

Melioidosis is endemic in Southeast Asia and should be suspected in military and other personnel who have characteristic symptoms of a febrile illness and have been in that region. Koponen et al emphasize that recrudescence of disease after a long latency period may occur. They saw a Vietnam veteran with melioidosis of the bone present 18 years after exposure.

Diagnosis is made from the recovery of the bacillus from the skin lesions or sputum, and by serologic tests.

Effective therapy is guided by the antibiotic sensitivity of the specific strain although at times clinical efficacy does not necessarily follow in vitro results. The majority of

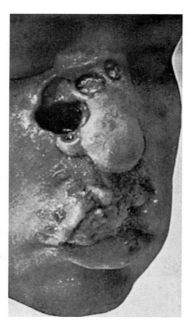

Fig. 14-38 Human glanders; duration, 4 months. Note carbuncular lesion on upper lip and farcy buds. Patient was a groom. (Courtesy Army Medical Museum.)

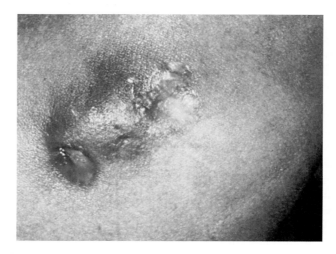

Fig. 14-39 Draining subcutaneous abscesses and sinuses caused by melioidosis. (Courtesy Dr. Axel W. Hoke.)

infections respond well to tetracyclines in doses of 2 to 3 g daily for at least 30 days. Trimethoprim-sulfamethoxazole and many third-generation cephalosporins are also effective.

Chodimella U, et al: Septicemia and suppuration in a Vietnam veteran. *Hosp Pract (Off Ed)* 1997, 32:219.

Koponen MA, et al: Melioidosis. *Arch Intern Med* 1991, 151:605.

McGovern TW, et al: Cutaneous manifestations of biologic warfare and related threat agents. *Arch Dermatol* 1999, 135:311. _____ ▲

INFECTIONS CAUSED BY *BARTONELLA*

Bartonella are aerobic, fastidious, gram-negative bacilli. Several species cause human diseases, including *B. henselae* (cat scratch disease and bacillary angiomatosis), *B. quintana* (trench fever and bacillary angiomatosis), *B. bacilliformis* (verruga peruana and Oroya fever), and *B. clarridgeiae* (a possible cause of cat-scratch disease). These agents are transmitted by arthropod vectors in some cases. Unique to this genus is the ability to cause vascular proliferation as is seen in bacillary angiomatosis and verruga peruana. The bartonellae in affected tissue stain poorly with tissue Gram stain, and are usually identified in tissue using modified silver stains such as Warthin-Starry. They are difficult to culture, making tissue identification of characteristic bacilli an important diagnostic test. Electron microscopy and polymerase chain reaction (PCR) can be used if routine staining is negative.

Cat-Scratch Disease

Cat-scratch disease is relatively common. About 22,000 cases are reported annually in the United States, with between 60% and 90% of cases occurring in children and young adults. Cat-scratch disease is the most frequent cause of chronic lymphadenopathy in children and young adults.

B. henselae causes the vast majority of cases of cat-scratch disease. The infectious agent is transmitted from cat to cat by fleas, and from cats to humans by cat scratches or bites. The organism can be found in the primary skin and conjunctival lesions, lymph nodes, and other affected tissues. In geographic areas where cat fleas are present, about 40% of cats are asymptomatically bacteremic with this organism.

The primary skin lesion appears within 3 to 5 days after the cat scratch, and may last for several weeks. It is present in 50% to 90% of patients. The primary lesion is not crusted, and lymphangitis does not extend from it (Fig. 14-40). The primary lesion may resemble an insect bite but is not pruritic. The primary lesion heals within a few weeks, usually with no scarring.

Lymphadenopathy, the hallmark of the disease, appears within a week or two, after the primary lesions or between 10 and 50 days (average 17 days) after inoculation. Usually the lymphadenopathy is regional and unilateral. Because most inoculations occur on the upper extremities, epitrochlear and axillary lymphadenopathy is most common (50%),

followed by cervical (25%) or inguinal (18%). Generalized lymphadenopathy does not occur, but systemic symptoms such as fever, malaise, and anorexia may be present. Without treatment the adenopathy resolves over a few weeks to months, with spontaneous suppuration occurring in between 10% and 50% of cases. If the primary inoculation is in the conjunctiva, there is chronic granulomatous conjunctivitis and preauricular adenopathy—the so-called oculoglandular syndrome of Parinaud. Uncommonly, acute encephalopathy, osteolytic lesions, hepatic and splenic abscesses, hypercalcemia, and pulmonary manifestations have been reported. In addition, erythema nodosum and a diffuse exanthem may accompany cat-scratch disease.

Diagnosis of is made largely on clinical features. The primary skin lesion or lymph node may be biopsied, and the infectious agent identified. Involved lymph nodes and skin lesions demonstrate granulomatous inflammation with central "stellate" necrosis. A serologic test is available but is not reproducibly positive early in the disease, limiting its usefulness. Cat-scratch skin testing (Hanger and Rose test) can be used but is rarely required if the history and clinical features are characteristic. Other infectious and neoplastic causes of localized lymphadenopathy, such as tularemia, sporotrichosis, atypical mycobacterial infection, and Hodgkin's disease, may need to be excluded.

The vast majority of cases of cat-scratch disease resolve spontaneously without antibiotic therapy. Such therapy has not been demonstrated to shorten the duration of the disease in most typical cases. Fluctuant lymph nodes should be aspirated, not incised and drained. In patients with severe visceral disease, erythromycin, tetracycline, or doxycycline may be used.

Trench Fever

Trench fever affected more than 1 million soldiers in World War I. It is caused by *B. quintana,* which is spread from

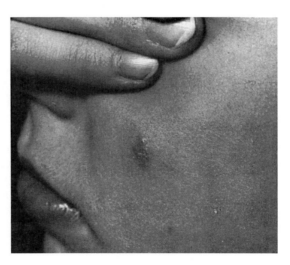

Fig. 14-40 Cat-scratch disease.

person to person by the body louse. Urban cases of trench fever caused by this agent have been reported in the United States and Europe in the 1990s in homeless, alcoholic persons, also associated with body louse infestation.

Patients present with fever that initially lasts about a week, then recurs about every 5 days. Other symptoms are headache, neck, shin, and back pain. Endocarditis may occur. There are no skin lesions.

Treatment has not been studied systematically. Ceftriaxone for 7 days, followed by erythromycin or another macrolide, is one effective regimen.

Bacillary Angiomatosis

Bacillary angiomatosis (BA) describes a clinical condition characterized by vascular skin lesions resembling pyogenic granulomas. Only two organisms have been proven to cause BA: *B. henselae* (the cause of cat-scratch disease) and *B. quintana* (the cause of trench fever). The skin lesions caused by these two agents are identical. If the BA is caused by *B. henselae,* there is usually a history of cat exposure, and the same *Bartonella* can also be isolated from the blood of the source cat. BA caused by *B. quintana* is associated with homelessness and louse infestation. The incubation period is unknown but may be years.

BA occurs primarily in the setting of immunosuppression, especially AIDS. The helper T-cell count is usually less than 50/ml. Other immunosuppressed hosts, such as those with leukemia, have been reported. Rarely, BA can occur in HIV-negative persons with no apparent immune impairment. In immunoincompetent hosts, the bacteria proliferate locally and are frequently bloodborne. The local proliferation of bacteria apparently produces angiogenic factors leading to the characteristic skin lesions. Immunocompetent hosts resist this bacterial proliferation, resulting in granulomatous and necrotic, rather than angiomatous, lesions.

Several different forms of cutaneous lesions occur. The most common form is lesions resembling pyogenic granulomas. Less commonly, subcutaneous masses, plaques, and ulcerations may occur. A single patient may exhibit several of these morphologies. The pyogenic granuloma–like lesions range from minute to large tumors. The smaller lesions typically have a surrounding collarette. Lesions are tender and bleed easily. Subcutaneous nodules are also tender and may be poorly marginated. Lesions may number from one to thousands, usually with the number gradually increasing over time if the patient is untreated.

In the setting of bacillary angiomatosis, the infection must be considered as multisystem. Bacteremia is detected in about 50% of AIDS patients with BA. This leads to dissemination of organisms to many visceral sites, but most frequently the lymph node, liver and spleen, and bone are involved. Less commonly pulmonary, gastrointestinal, muscle, oral, and brain lesions can occur. *B. henselae* is associated with lymph node and liver and spleen involve-

ment, whereas *B. quintana* causes bone disease and subcutaneous masses. Thus, the source of infection and pattern of visceral disease can predict the infecting agent. Visceral disease can be confirmed by appropriate radiologic or imaging studies. Bone lesions are typically lytic, resembling osteomyelitis. In the liver and spleen "peliosis" occurs. Liver function tests characteristically demonstrate a very elevated lactic dehydrogenase level, an elevated alkaline phosphatase level, slight elevation of the levels of hepatocellular enzymes, and a normal bilirubin level. Lesions on other epithelial surfaces, in muscle, and in lymph nodes are usually angiomatous.

Biopsies of BA skin lesions have the same low-power appearance as a pyogenic granuloma, with the proliferation of endothelial cells, forming normal small blood vessels. BA is distinguished from pyogenic granuloma by the presence of neutrophils throughout the lesion, not just on the surface as is seen in a pyogenic granuloma. The neutrophils are sometimes aggregated around granular material that stains slightly purple. This purple material represents clusters of organisms, which can at times be confirmed by modified silver stain such as Warthin-Starry. Tissue Gram stain and Warthin-Starry stain used for syphilis do not routinely stain the bacteria in BA lesions. Electron microscopy may identify bacteria in cases in which special stains are negative. BA is easily distinguished histologically from Kaposi's sarcoma (KS). In patch or plaque lesions of KS the new blood vessels are abnormal in appearance, being angulated. Endothelial proliferation in KS is seen in the dermis around the eccrine units, follicular structures, and existing normal vessels. Nodular KS is a spindle cell tumor with slits rather than well-formed blood vessels. Neutrophils and purple granular material are not found in KS, but intracellular hyaline globules are present.

The natural history of BA is extremely variable. In most patients, however, lesions either remain stable, or most commonly, the size or number of lesions gradually increases over time. The initial lesions are usually the largest, and multiple satellite or disseminated smaller lesions occur, representing miliary spread. Untreated BA can be fatal, with patients dying of visceral disease or respiratory compromise from obstructing lesions.

The diagnosis of BA is virtually always made by identifying the infectious agent in affected tissue. The organisms can also be cultured from the lesions and about half the time from the patient's blood. However, these organisms grow very slowly, so cultures may not be positive for more than 1 month. Thus, tissue and blood cultures are usually confirmatory, rather than primary, diagnostic procedures in most cases. Antibodies to *Bartonella* can be detected in most BA cases by an indirect fluorescence assay. Because of its limited availability and background positivity in the general population of cat owners, this test is not generally useful in establishing the diagnosis of BA.

Treatment

Bacillary angiomatosis is dramatically responsive to treatment. Erythromycin, 500 mg four times daily, or doxycycline, 100 mg twice daily, are the treatments of choice. Minocycline, tetracycline, clarithromycin, azithromycin, roxithromycin, and chloramphenicol may also be effective. Trimethoprim-sulfamethoxazole, ciprofloxacin, penicillins, and cephalosporins are not effective. Prophylactic regimens containing a macrolide antibiotic or rifampin appear to prevent the development of bacillary angiomatosis. Treatment duration depends on the extent of visceral involvement. In cases with skin lesions or bacteremia only, at least 8 weeks of treatment are required. For liver and spleen involvement 3 to 6 months of treatment are recommended, and for bone disease, at least 6 months of treatment should be considered. Once treatment is begun, symptoms begin to resolve within hours to days. A Jarisch-Herxheimer reaction may occur with the first dose of antibiotic. If patients relapse after an apparent adequate course of treatment, chronic suppressive antibiotic therapy should be considered.

Oroya Fever and Verruga Peruana

Oroya fever and verruga peruana represent two stages of the same infection. Oroya fever (Carrion's disease) is the acute febrile stage, and verruga peruana the chronic delayed stage. These conditions are limited to and endemic in Peru and a few neighboring countries in the Andes, and restricted to valleys between 500 and 3200 meters above sea level. Both of these conditions are caused by *B. bacilliformis*, which is transmitted by a sandfly, usually *Lutzomyia verrucarum*. Humans represent the only known reservoir. Men represent about three quarters of cases, and all ages may be affected.

After an incubation period averaging 3 weeks, the acute infection, Oroya fever, develops. Symptomatology is highly variable. Some patients have very mild symptoms. Others may have high fevers, headache, and arthralgias. Severe hemolytic anemia can develop, sometimes with leukopenia, and thrombocytopenia. Untreated the fatality rate is 40% to 88%, and with antibiotic treatment is still 8%. After the acute infection resolves, a latency period follows, lasting from weeks to months. The eruptive verruga peruana then occur. They are angiomatous, pyogenic granuloma–like lesions, clinically and histologically virtually identical to the lesions of bacillary angiomatosis. They may be large and few in number (mular form), small and disseminate (miliary form), or nodular and deep (Figs. 14-41 and 14-42). Visceral disease has not been found in verruga peruana, which is rarely fatal. Lesions usually spontaneously heal over several weeks to months without scarring. A lasting immunity results from infection.

The diagnosis of Oroya fever is made by identifying the bacteria within or attached to circulating erythrocytes using a Giemsa stain. Verruga peruana can be diagnosed by skin biopsy, showing the same features as BA, but with the organisms staining with Giemsa stain.

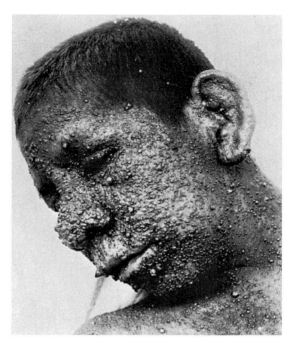

Fig. 14-41 Verruga peruana showing small nodules that cover face and body. (Courtesy Dr. P. Weiss.)

The antibiotic treatment of choice for Oroya fever is chloramphenicol, since *Salmonella* coinfection is the most frequent cause of death. Protection from sandfly bites is all-important.

Amano Y, et al: Bartonellosis in Ecuador. *Am J Trop Med Hyg* 1997, 57:174.

Bosch X: Hypercalcemia due to endogenous overproduction of active vitamin D in identical twins with cat-scratch disease. *JAMA* 1998, 279:532.

Caceres-Rios H, et al: Verruga peruana. *Crit Rev Oncog* 1995, 6:47.

Carither HA, et al: Cat-scratch disease. *Am J Dis Child* 1991, 145:98.

Holmes AH, et al: *Bartonella henselae*: endocarditis in an immunocompetent adult. *Clin Infect Dis* 1995, 21:1004.

Koehler JE, et al: Molecular epidemiology of *Bartonella* infections in patients with bacillary angiomatosis-peliosis. *N Engl J Med* 1997, 337:1876.

Koehler JE, et al: *Rochalimaea henselae* infection. *JAMA* 1994, 271:531.

Kordick DL, et al: *Bartonella clarridgeiae*: a newly recognized zoonotic pathogen causing inoculation papules, fever, and lymphadenopathy (cat scratch disease). *J Clin Microbiol* 1997, 35:1813.

Nosal JM: Bacillary angiomatosis, cat-scratch disease, and bartonellosis. *Int J Dermatol* 1997, 36:405.

Spach DH, et al: *Bartonella*-associated infections. *Infect Dis Clin North Am* 1998, 12:137.

Spach DH, et al: *Bartonella quintana*: bacteremia in inner-city patients with chronic alcoholism. *N Engl J Med* 1995, 332:424.

Wong R, et al: Bacillary angiomatosis and other *Bartonella* species infections. *Semin Cutan Med Surg* 1997, 16:188.

Zangwill KM, et al: Cat scratch disease in Connecticut. *N Engl J Med* 1993, 329:8. ▲

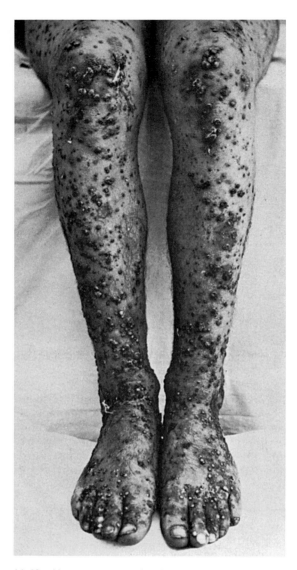

Fig. 14-42 Verruga peruana showing verrucous nodules on legs. (Courtesy Drs. O. Canizares and H. Fox.)

PLAGUE

Plague normally involves an interaction among *Yersinia pestis,* wild rodents, and fleas parasitic on the rodents. Infection in humans with *Y. pestis* is accidental and presents usually as bubonic plague. Other clinical forms include pneumonic and septicemic plague.

In the milder form, the initial manifestations are general malaise, fever, and pain or tenderness in areas of regional lymph nodes, most often in the inguinal or axillary regions. In more severe infections, findings of toxicity, prostration, shock, and, occasionally, hemorrhagic phenomena prevail. Less common symptoms include abdominal pain, nausea, vomiting, constipation followed by diarrhea, generalized macular erythema, and petechiae. Rarely, vesicular and pustular skin lesions occur.

Plague is caused by *Y. pestis,* a pleomorphic, gram-negative bacillus. The principal animal hosts involved have been rock squirrels, prairie dogs, chipmunks, marmots, skunks, deer mice, wood rats, rabbits, and hares. Transmission occurs through contact with infected rodent fleas or rodents, pneumonic spread, or infected exudates. *Xenopsylla cheopis* (Oriental rat flea) has traditionally been considered the vector in human outbreaks, but *Diamanus montanus, Chrassis bacchi,* and *Opisocrostis hirsutus* are species of fleas on wild animals responsible for spreading sylvatic plague in the United States. Rodents carried home by dogs or cats are a potential source—and an important one in veterinarians—of infection. In the United States, 89% of cases since 1945 have occurred in the Rocky Mountain states.

Blood, bubo or parabubo aspirates, exudates, and sputum should be examined by smears stained with Gram stain or specific fluorescent antibody techniques, culture, and animal inoculation. A retrospective diagnosis can be made by serologic analysis.

The most effective drug against *Y. pestis* is streptomycin. It should be given in doses of 2 g daily intramuscularly for 10 days. Other effective drugs include kanamycin, chloramphenicol, the tetracyclines, and certain sulfonamides. Nearly all cases are fatal if not treated promptly.

Hull HF, et al: Septicemic plague in New Mexico. *J Infect Dis* 1987, 155:113.

Fatal human plague: Arizona and Colorado, 1996. *JAMA* 1997, 278:380.

Franz DR, et al: Clinical recognition and management of patients exposed to biological warfare agents. *JAMA* 1997, 278:399.

McGovern TW, et al: Cutaneous manifestations of biological warfare and related threat agents. *Arch Dermatol* 1999, 135:311.

Scott DW, et al: Zoonotic dermatoses of dogs and cats. *Vet Clin North Am* 1987, 17:117.

RAT-BITE FEVER

This febrile, systemic illness is usually acquired by direct contact with rats or other small rodents, which carry the gram-negative organisms *Spirillum minor* and *Streptobacillus moniliformis* among their oropharyngeal flora. *S. moniliformis* is the principal cause in the United States, and bites of laboratory rats are an increasing source of infection. Although it usually follows a rat bite, it may follow the bites of squirrels, cats, weasels, pigs, and a variety of other carnivores that feed on rats.

There are at least two distinct forms of rat-bite fever: (1) "sodoku," caused by *S. minus,* and (2) septicemia, produced by *S. moniliformis,* otherwise known as *epidemic arthritic erythema* or *Haverhill fever.* The latter usually follows the bite of a rat, but some cases have been caused by contaminated milk. The clinical manifestations of these two infections are similar in that both produce a systemic illness characterized by fever, rash, and constitutional symptoms. However, clinical differentiation is possible.

In the streptobacillary form, incubation is brief, usually lasting 10 days after the bite, when chills and fever occur. Within 2 to 4 more days the generalized morbilliform eruption appears and spreads to include the palms and soles. It may become petechial. Arthralgia is prominent, and pleural effusion may occur. Endocarditis, pneumonia, and septic infarcts may occur, and 10% of untreated cases may die from these causes.

Although infection with *S. minor* also begins abruptly with chills and fever, the incubation period is longer, ranging from 1 to 4 weeks. The bite site is often inflamed and may become ulcerated. Lymphangitis may be present. The eruption begins with erythematous macules on the abdomen, resembling rose spots, which enlarge, become purplish red, and form extensive indurated plaques. Arthritis may rarely occur. Endocarditis, nephritis, meningitis, and hepatitis are potential complications. Six percent of untreated cases die.

In both types of disease a leukocytosis of 15,000 to 30,000/mm³ is present, sometimes with eosinophilia. A biologic false-positive VDRL is found in 25% to 50% of cases. The course without treatment is generally from 1 to 2 weeks, though relapses may occur for months.

The diagnosis is confirmed by culturing the causative organism from the blood or joint aspirate, or demonstration of an antibody response in the streptobacillary form.

S. minus is demonstrable by animal inoculation with the patient's blood, usually in the guinea pig or mouse. Their blood will show large numbers of organisms in Wright-stained smears. Demonstration of *S. minus* in a darkfield preparation of exudate from an infected site establishes the diagnosis.

Rat-bite fever must be differentiated from erysipelas, pyogenic cellulitis, viral exanthems, gonococcemia, meningococcemia, and Rocky Mountain spotted fever.

Prompt cauterization of bites by nitric acid may prevent the disease. Cleansing of the wound, tetanus prophylaxis, and 3 days of penicillin (2 g/day) are recommended for patients seen shortly after a bite. Both types respond readily to penicillin, tetracycline, or second- or third-generation cephalosporin therapy.

Cunningham BB, et al: Rat bite fever. *J Am Acad Dermatol* 1998, 38:330.

Holroyd KJ, et al: *Streptobacillus moniliformis* polyarthritis mimicking rheumatoid arthritis. *Am J Med* 1988, 85:711.

Vasseur E, et al: Cutaneous abscess: a rare complication of *S. moniliformis* infection. *Br J Dermatol* 1993, 129:95. _____ ▲

TULAREMIA

Synonyms: Ohara's disease, deer fly fever

Tularemia is a febrile disease produced by *Francisella tularensis;* it is characterized by sudden onset, with chills, headache, and leukocytosis, after an incubation period of 2 to 7 days. Its clinical course is divided into several general types.

The large majority are the ulceroglandular type, which begins with a primary papule or nodule that rapidly ulcerates at the site of infection. This occurs usually through contact with tissues or body fluid of infected mammals, via an abrasion or scratch, usually on the fingers, neck, or conjunctiva. The bites of a tick, *Dermacentor andersoni* or *Amblyomma americanum,* and of a deer fly, *Chrysops discalis,* transmit this disease also, in which case primary lesions are usually found on the legs or the perineum. The primary ulcer is tender, firm, indolent, and punched-out, with a necrotic base that heals with scar formation in about 6 weeks (Fig. 14-43). A lymphangitis spreads from the primary lesion; the regional lymph glands become swollen, painful, and inflamed, and tend to break down, forming subcutaneous suppurative nodules resembling those of sporotrichosis (Fig. 14-44). The ulcers extend in a chain from the ulcer to the enlarged lymphatic glands.

The course of the ulceroglandular type is marked in the early stages by headache, anorexia, and vomiting, and by articular and muscular pains. The fever is at first continuous, varying between 102° and 104° F, and later shows morning remissions, then falls by lysis to normal. Other skin lesions are encountered in the course of the disease, which are in no way characteristic and are probably of a toxic nature. A macular, papular, vesicular, or petechial exanthem may occur. Erythema multiforme and erythema nodosum often occur. The clinical similarity of the primary ulcer of tularemia to a chancre of sporotrichosis, or *Pasteurella* infections is important in the differential diagnosis.

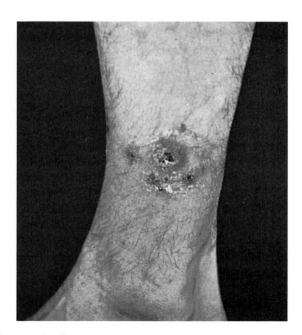

Fig. 14-43 Tularemia above ankle; primary lesion. (Courtesy Armed Forces Institute of Pathology.)

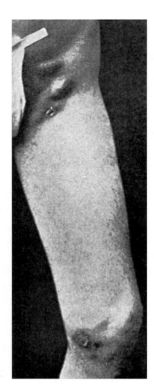

Fig. 14-44 Tularemia following tick bite on left knee. Note enlargement of left inguinal glands. (Courtesy Drs. T.B. Magath and W.M. Yater.)

In the typhoidal type the site of inoculation is not known and there is no local sore or adenopathy. This form of the disease is characterized by persistent fever, malaise, gastrointestinal symptoms, and the presence of specific agglutinins in the blood serum after the first week.

In addition to these two types, there is the oculoglandular type, in which primary conjunctivitis is accompanied by enlargement of the regional lymph nodes. The pneumonic form occurs rarely in laboratory workers and is most severe. The oropharyngeal form may occur after ingestion of infected and inadequately cooked meat. In the glandular type there is no primary lesion at the site of infection, but there is enlargement of regional lymph glands followed by generalized involvement. Several cases, mostly in children, have been acquired from cat bites, the cats having previously bitten infected rabbits.

Tularemia is caused by *F. tularensis,* a short, nonmotile, non–spore-forming, gram-negative coccobacillus.

The most frequent sources of human infection are the handling of wild rabbits and the bite of deer flies or ticks. No instance of the spread of the infection from person to person by contact has been reported. Outbreaks of the disease occur chiefly at those times of the year when contact with these sources of infection is likely.

The disease occurs most often in the western and southern United States, although cases have been reported

in almost all parts of the United States and in Japan. In Russia and other countries in the northern hemisphere it may be contracted from polluted water contaminated by infected rodent carcasses.

A definite diagnosis is made by staining the exudate smears with specific fluorescent antibody. *F. tularensis* can be cultured only on special media containing cystine glucose blood agar or other selective media. Routine culture media do not support growth. The bacilli can be identified by inoculating guinea pigs intraperitoneally with sputum or with bronchial or gastric washings, exudate from draining lymph nodes, or blood.

The agglutination test is the most reliable diagnostic procedure. The titer becomes positive in the majority of patients after 2 weeks of illness. A fourfold rise in titer is diagnostic; a single convalescent titer of 1:160 or greater is diagnostic of past or current infection.

The main histologic feature of tularemia is that of a granuloma; the tissue reaction consists primarily of a massing of endothelial cells and the formation of giant cells. Central necrosis and liquefaction occurs accompanied by polymorphonuclear leukocytic infiltration. Surrounding this is a tuberculoid granulomatous zone, and peripherally lymphocytes form a third zone. Small secondary lesions may develop. These pass through the same stages and tend to fuse with the primary one.

All butchers, hunters, cooks, and others who dress rabbits should wear protective gloves when doing so. Thorough cooking destroys the infection in a rabbit, thus rendering an infected animal harmless as food. Ticks should be removed promptly, and tick repellents may be of value for people with occupations that require frequent exposure to them.

Streptomycin, 0.5 g intramuscularly every 12 hours for 10 days, is the treatment of choice. Obvious clinical improvement occurs after 48 hours, although the fever may persist for as long as a week after treatment is begun. Gentamicin is also effective, but the tetracyclines are useful only if given in doses of 2 g daily for 15 days.

Cerny Z: Skin manifestations of tularemia. *Int J Dermatol* 1994, 33:468.
Kodama B, et al: Tularemia. *Cutis* 1994, 54:279.
McGovern TW, et al: Cutaneous manifestations of biological warfare and related threat agents. *Arch Dermatol* 1999, 135:311.
Myers SA, et al: Dermatologic manifestations of arthropod-borne diseases. *Infect Dis Clin North Am* 1994, 8:689.
Sanford JP: Tularemia. *JAMA* 1983, 250:3225.
Spach DH, et al: Tick-borne diseases in the US. *New Engl J Med* 1993, 329:936. ▲

BRUCELLOSIS
Synonym: Undulant fever

Brucellae are gram-negative rods that produce an acute febrile illness with headache, or at times an indolent chronic disease characterized by weakness, malaise, and low-grade fever. It is acquired primarily by contact with infected animals or animal products. Primarily, workers in the meat-packing industry are at risk; however, veterinarians, pet owners, and travelers who consume unpasteurized milk or cheese may also acquire the disease.

Approximately 5% to 10% of patients develop skin lesions. The variety of cutaneous manifestations reported is large and has been reviewed by Ariza et al. Erythematous papules, diffuse erythema, abscesses, erysipelas-like lesions, and erythema nodosum–like lesions are some possible findings. Biopsy may reveal noncaseating granulomas.

Diagnosis is by culture of blood, bone marrow, or granulomas, and may be confirmed by a rising serum agglutination titer. Treatment is with doxycycline and rifampin in combination for 6 weeks.

Ariza J, et al: Characteristic cutaneous lesions of brucellosis. *Arch Dermatol* 1989, 125:380.

Berger TG, et al: Cutaneous lesions in brucellosis. *Arch Dermatol* 1981, 117:40.

Colmenero JD, et al: Complications associated with *Brucella melitensis* infection. *Medicine* (Baltimore) 1996, 75:195. _____ ▲

Rickettsial diseases

Rickettsiae are obligate, intracellular, gram-negative bacteria. The natural reservoirs of these organisms are the blood-sucking arthropods; when transmitted to humans through insect inoculation, the rickettsiae may produce disease. Most of the human diseases incurred are characterized by skin eruptions, fever, headache, malaise, and prostration. In addition to those discussed in the following sections, Sennetsu fever, caused by *Ehrlichia sennetsu,* and Q fever, caused by *Coxiella burnetii,* are acute, febrile illnesses from this general class that uncommonly have skin manifestations, but these are nonspecific and nondiagnostic in nature.

TYPHUS GROUP

Louse-borne epidemic typhus, caused by *Rickettsia prowazekii,* and murine or cat or rat flea-borne endemic typhus, caused by *R. typhi* (formerly *R. mooseri*), constitute this group.

Epidemic Typhus

Humans contract epidemic typhus from an infestation by body lice *(Pediculus humanus var. corporis),* which harbor the rickettsiae. *R. prowazekii* is not transmitted transovarially, since it kills the louse 1 to 3 weeks after infection. For many years humans were the only known vector, but several cases of sporadic disease have been reported in which there was direct or indirect contact with the flying squirrel, and a reservoir apparently exists in this animal. While the louse feeds on the person's skin, it defecates. The organisms in the feces are scratched into the skin. Some 2 weeks after infection the prodromal symptoms of chills, fever, aches, and pains appear. After 5 days a pink macular eruption appears on the trunk and axillary folds and rapidly spreads to the rest of the body, but usually spares the face, palms, and soles. These macules may later become hemorrhagic, and gangrene of the fingers, toes, nose, and ear lobes may occur. Mortality is from 6% to 30% in epidemics, with the highest death and complication rates occurring in patients over age 60.

Agglutinins for OX-19 and complement-fixing antibodies are demonstrable after the eighth to twelfth day of illness.

Treatment is with tetracyclines. Doxycycline in a single dose of 100 mg orally is effective. Alternatively, 25 mg/kg of oral tetracycline is given daily until 3 to 4 days after defervescence. Prophylaxis is by vaccination and delousing; people who succumb are usually living under miserable sanitary conditions such as occur during war and following natural disasters. Vaccination is suggested for only special high-risk groups.

Brill-Zinsser disease may occur as a recrudescence of previous infection, with a similar but milder course of illness, which more closely resembles murine typhus.

Endemic Typhus

Endemic (murine) typhus is a natural infection of rats (and mice), sporadically transmitted to humans by the rat flea, *Xenopsylla cheopis.* It has the same skin manifestations as epidemic typhus, but they are less severe, and petechiae and gangrene do not supervene. Dumler et al found that 54% of 80 patients with murine typhus had a skin eruption. The OX-19 test is also positive, and the complement fixation test helps in making the diagnosis. Fever and severe headache are suggestive early symptoms.

This disease occurs worldwide. In the United States the southeastern states and those bordering the Gulf of Mexico have been the most common sites of incidence. It most often occurs in urban settings, with peak incidence in the summer and fall.

Treatment is the same as that of louse-borne (epidemic) typhus.

SPOTTED FEVER GROUP

To this group belong Rocky Mountain spotted fever, caused by *Rickettsia rickettsii;* tick typhus such as Mediterranean (boutonneuse) fever and South African tick-bite fever, caused by *R. conorii;* North Asian tick-borne rickettsiosis, caused by *R. sibirica;* Queensland tick typhus, caused by *R. australis;* and rickettsialpox and Russian vesicular rickettsiosis, caused by *R. akari.*

Rocky Mountain Spotted Fever

One to 2 weeks after the tick bite, there will be chills, fever, and weakness. An eruption appears, unlike typhus in that it begins on the ankles, wrists, and forehead rather than on the trunk. The initial lesions are small, red macules, which blanch on pressure and rapidly become papular in untreated patients. Spread to the trunk occurs over 6 to 18 hours, and the lesions become petechial and hemorrhagic over a period of 2 to 4 days.

A vasculitis of the skin is the pathologic process, and *R. rickettsii* can be found in these initial macules by applying a fluorescent antibody technique to frozen sections. This a very specific, but not very sensitive, method.

In the 10% to 20% of cases without a rash, the risk of a delay in diagnosis and a fatal outcome is greatest, with the case fatality rate rising precipitously if antibiotics are not initiated before the fifth day. Mortality in older persons approaches 60%; it is far lower in younger patients. Tetracycline or chloramphenicol, given early, is almost always effective. In all of the 10 fatal cases in the series reported by Walker et al, multifocal, perivascular, interstitial nephritis was the principal pathologic lesion.

The causative organism, *R. rickettsii*, is spread by ixodid ticks, one or another species of which is found in all parts of the United States and in scattered pockets in Canada and Mexico. Principal offenders are the wood tick *(Dermacentor andersoni)*, the dog tick *(D. variabilis)*, and the Lone Star tick *(Amblyomma americanum)*.

Antibodies to Proteus OX-2 and OX-19 become positive in the second or third week of illness, too late to be of help when the decision to institute therapy is necessary. This decision is usually made by clinical considerations.

The treatment is high doses of tetracycline, 25 to 50 mg/kg/day, or chloramphenicol, 50 mg/kg/day, with tetracycline being preferred. Medication should be continued for 2 to 3 days after the temperature returns to normal, the usual course being 5 to 7 days.

Tick Typhus

Tick typhus is a collective name for the varieties of spotted fever transmitted by ticks. Boutonneuse fever, or Mediterranean fever, is an acute febrile disease endemic in southern Europe and northern Africa, and is the prototype of these diseases. It affects children mostly and is characterized by a sudden onset with chills, high fever, headache, and lassitude. The tick bite produces a small, indurated papule known as *tache noir*, which becomes a necrotic ulcer. A macular or maculopapular eruption develops on the trunk, palms, and soles.

The causative organism is *R. conorii*, transmitted by the dog tick, *Rhipicephalus sanguineus*.

Similar clinical manifestations are seen with the other diseases in this group. All have type-specific antigens and can be identified by complement fixation and neutralization tests. The OX-19 and OX-2 Weil-Felix reactions are positive.

Treatment with tetracycline or chloramphenicol is effective. Even without therapy the prognosis is good, and complications are rare.

MITE-BORNE DISEASES
Rickettsialpox

First recognized in New York in 1946, rickettsialpox has been found in other cities of the United States and in Russia.

Rickettsialpox is an acute febrile disease characterized by the appearance of an initial lesion at the site of the mite bite about a week before the onset of the fever and by the appearance of a rash resembling varicella 3 or 4 days after the development of fever. The fever is accompanied by chills, sweats, headache, and backache. The fever is remittent and lasts for about 5 days. The initial lesions are firm, 5- to 15-mm round or oval vesicles (Fig. 14-45). They are accompanied by a regional lymphadenitis. This initial lesion persists 3 to 4 weeks and leaves a small pigmented scar. The secondary eruption appears 24 to 96 hours after the fever begins and fades in about 1 week. Generalized lymphadenopathy and enlargement of the spleen may occur but are rarely encountered.

The causative organism, *Rickettsia akari,* is transmitted by the rodent mite, *Allodermanyssus sanguineus*. The house mouse *(Mus musculus)* is the reservoir. All cases have occurred in neighborhoods infested by mice, on which the rodent mite has been found.

Complement fixation tests demonstrate the antibodies of

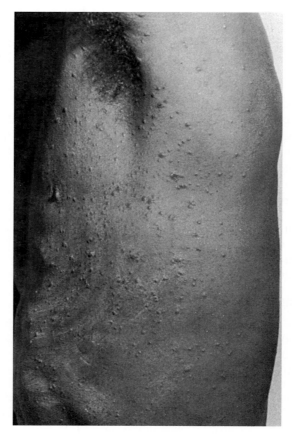

Fig. 14-45 Rickettsialpox. (Courtesy Dr. M. Liebman.)

this disease. The Weil-Felix test is negative. Kass et al have reported on the utility of a direct fluorescent antibody test of the eschar in making the diagnosis.

The disease is self limited, and complete involution occurs in at most 2 weeks. Tetracyclines are the agents of choice for treatment.

Scrub Typhus

Also known as *tsutsugamushi fever,* scrub typhus is characterized by fever, chills, intense headache, skin lesions, and pneumonitis. The primary lesion is an erythematous papule at the site of the mite bite, most commonly on the scrotum, groin, or ankle. It becomes indurated, and a multilocular vesicle rests on top of the papule. Eventually a necrotic ulcer with eschar and surrounding indurated erythema develops and there is regional lymphadenopathy. Some 10 days after a mite bite, fever, chills, and prostration develop and within 5 days thereafter pneumonitis and the skin eruption evolve. The erythematous macular eruption begins on the trunk, extends peripherally, and fades in a few days. Deafness and tinnitus occur in about a fifth of untreated cases.

Scrub typhus is caused by *Rickettsia tsutsugamushi*. The vector is the trombiculid red mite (chigger), which infests wild rodents in scrub or secondary vegetation in transitional terrain between forests and clearings in Far Eastern countries such as Japan, Korea, Southeast Asia, and Australia.

Antibodies to OX-K proteus antigen occur in 50% of patients by the second week and are rather specific for this disease, although cross reactivity does occur in leptospirosis.

Treatment is as for other forms of rickettsias.

EHRLICHIOSIS

An illness similar to spotted fever is caused by a closely related rickettsia, *Ehrlichia chaffeensis*. Only 30% of adults manifest an eruption. The lesions are reported as being of many types. A generalized mottled or diffuse erythema, a fine petechial eruption or a macular, papular or urticarial morphology have all been seen. It appears to be tickborne and is most common in men between ages 30 and 60. The predominant regions reporting the disease are the south central, southeastern, and mid-Atlantic states. It is responsive to tetracycline.

Anderson BE, et al: *Ehrlichia chaffeensis:* a new species associated with human ehrlichiosis. *J Clin Microbiol* 1991, 29:2838.
Baxter JD: The typhus group. *Dermatol Clin* 1996, 14:271.
Bhattacharya S, et al: Rickettsialpox. *Arch Dermatol* 1998, 134:365.
Blemker AL, et al: Petechial eruption in a toxic-appearing young man. *Arch Dermatol* 1991, 127:1049.
Burnett JW: Rickettsioses. *J Am Acad Dermatol* 1980, 2:359.
Dumler JS et al: Clinical and laboratory features of marine typhus in South Texas, 1980 through 1987. *JAMA* 1991, 266:1365.
Everett ED, et al: Human ehrlichiosis in adults after tick exposure. *Ann Intern Med* 1994, 120:730.
Fishbein DB, et al: Human ehrlichiosis in the US. *Ann Intern Med* 1994, 120:736.
Harkness JR, et al: Ehrlichiosis in children. *Pediatrics* 1991, 87:199.
Human ehrlichiosis. *Arch Dermatol* 1988, 124:993.
Jayaseelan E, et al: Cutaneous eruptions in Indian tick typhus. *Int J Dermatol* 1991, 30:790.
Kass EM, et al: Rickettsial pox in NYC hospital. *New Engl J Med* 1994, 331:1612.
McDonald JC, et al: Imported rickettsial disease. *Am J Med* 1988, 85:795.
Raoult D, et al: Mediterranean spotted fever. *Ann Dermatol Venereol* 1983, 110:909.
Salgo MP, et al: A form of Rocky Mountain spotted fever within New York City. *N Engl J Med* 1988, 318:1345.
Spach DH et al: Tick-borne diseases in the US. *New Engl J Med* 1993, 329:936.
Stewart RS. Flinders Island spotted fever. *Med J Aust* 1991, 143:94.
Supont HT, et al: Epidemiologic features and clinical presentation of acute Q fever in hospitalized patients. *Ann J Med* 1992, 93:427.
Walker DH, et al: Emerging and reemerging rickettsial diseases. *New Engl J Med* 1994, 331:1651.
Walker DH, et al: The occurrence of eschars in Rocky Mountain spotted fever. *J Am Acad Dermatol* 1981, 4:571. _____ ▲

LEPTOSPIROSIS

Leptospirosis is also known as *Weil's disease, pretibial fever,* and *Fort Bragg fever*. This is a systemic disease caused by many strains of the genus *Leptospira*. After an incubation period of 8 to 12 days, Weil's disease (icteric leptospirosis) starts with an abrupt onset of chills, followed by high fever, intense jaundice, petechiae, and purpura on both skin and mucous membranes, and renal disease, manifested by proteinuria, hematuria, and azotemia. Death may occur in 5% to 10% of cases, as a result of renal failure, vascular collapse, or hemorrhage. Leukocytosis of 15,000 to 30,000/mm^3 and lymphocytosis in the spinal fluid are commonly present.

Pretibial fever ("Fort Bragg fever," anicteric leptospirosis) has an associated acute exanthematous infectious erythema, generally most marked on the shins. High fever, conjunctival suffusion, nausea, vomiting, and headache characterize the septicemic first stage. This lasts 3 to 7 days, followed by a 1- to 3-day absence of fever. During the second stage, when IgM antibody develops, headache is intense, fever returns, and ocular manifestations, such as conjunctival hemorrhage and suffusion, ocular pain, and photophobia, are prominent. At this time the eruption occurs. It consists of 1- to 5-cm erythematous patches or plaques that histologically show only edema and nonspecific perivascular infiltrate. The skin lesions resolve spontaneously after 4 to 7 days. There may be different clinical manifestations from identical strains of leptospira.

Leptospira interrogans, serotype *icterohaemorrhagiae,* has been the most common cause of Weil's disease, whereas pretibial fever is most commonly associated with serotype *autumnalis*. Humans acquire both types accidentally from urine or tissues of infected animals, or indirectly from contaminated soil or from drinking or swimming in contaminated water. In the continental United States dogs are the most common animal source; worldwide, rats are more often responsible. *Leptospira* enter the body through abraded or diseased skin, and the gastrointestinal or upper respiratory tract.

Leptospirosis may be diagnosed by finding the causative spirochetes in the blood by darkfield microscopy during the first week of illness, and by blood cultures, guinea pig inoculation, and the demonstration of rising antibodies during the second week of the disease. The genus-specific HA serologic test permits relatively early diagnosis.

Treatment with tetracyclines and penicillin shorten the disease duration if given early. Doxycycline, 100 mg daily for a week, has been shown by McClain et al to be effective in a controlled trial in anicteric patients. A dose of 200 mg once weekly will prevent infection while visiting a hyperendemic area.

McClain JBL, et al: Doxycycline treatment of leptospirosis. *Ann Intern Med* 1984, 100:696.

Takafuji ET, et al: An efficacy trial of doxycycline chemoprophylaxis against leptospirosis. *N Engl J Med* 1984, 310:497.

Vinetz JM, et al: Sporadic urban leptospirosis. *Ann Intern Med* 1996, 125:794.

Watt G, et al: Placebo-controlled trial of intravenous penicillin for severe and late leptospirosis. *Lancet* 1988, 1:433. _____ ▲

BORRELIOSIS

The spirochetes in the genus *Borrelia* are important, since much work is focused on Lyme disease. These microorganisms are also the cause of relapsing fever, an acute illness characterized by paroxysms of fever. The more common type is tickborne, occasionally being reported in the United States. An unknown louseborne type is endemic only in Ethiopia. The nonspecific macular or petechial eruption occurs near the end of the 3- to 5-day febrile crisis.

Lyme Disease

Borrelia burgdorferi sensu lato, a tickborne spirochete, is the agent responsible for inducing Lyme disease. The characteristic cutaneous eruption that is the early manifestation of this systemic illness is erythema migrans (EM). A late sequel of chronic infection is acrodermatitis chronica atrophicans (ACA).

The clinical features typically begin with EM and are often accompanied by an acute flulike illness. If it is untreated, chronic arthritis and neurologic and cardiac complications frequently develop.

As Shrestha et al have shown, diagnosing early Lyme disease depends on recognition of the skin eruption, which occurs in 75% of adults but only about 25% of children.

Twenty percent to 30% of patients recall a tick bite, which leaves a small red macule or papule at the site. The areas most often involved are the thighs, groins, and axilla. Three to 32 (median: 7) days after the bite, there is gradual expansion of the redness around the papule. The advancing border is usually slightly raised, warm, red to bluish red, and free of any scale. Centrally, the site of the bite may clear, leaving only a ring of peripheral erythema, or it may become indurated, vesicular or necrotic. The annular erythema usually grows to a median diameter of 15 cm, but may range from 3 to 68 cm. It is accompanied by a burning sensation in half the patients; rarely is it pruritic or painful. Localized alopecia may result at the site of EM.

Twenty-five percent to 50% of patients will develop multiple secondary annular lesions, similar in appearance to the primary lesion, but without indurated centers, and generally of smaller size (Fig. 14-46). They spare the palms and soles. Their number ranges from 2 to 100. Without treatment, EM and the secondary lesions fade in a median of 28 days, although some may be present for months. Of untreated cases, 10% experience recurrences of EM over the following months. European cases of *Borrelia*-induced lymphocytoma occur generally early, from the time of EM until 10 months later.

Diffuse urticaria, malar erythema, and conjunctivitis may be present during this early period. Malaise, fever, fatigue, headaches, stiff neck, arthralgia, myalgia, lymphadenopathy, anorexia, and nausea and vomiting may accompany early signs and symptoms of infection. These are more

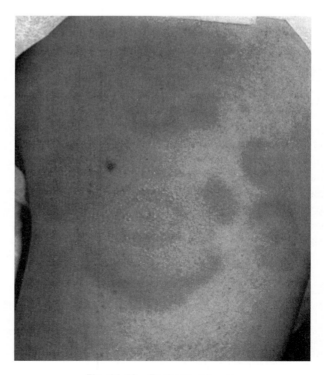

Fig. 14-46 Erythema migrans.

common in patients coinfected with babesiosis, as is the case in approximately 10% of cases in southern New England.

Ten percent of patients eventually develop a chronic arthritis of the knees, which in half of these leads to severe disability. Cardiac involvement occurs most often in young men, with fluctuating degrees of atrioventricular block or complete heart block occurring over a brief time (3 days to 6 weeks) early in the course of the illness. Neurologic findings include stiff neck, headache, meningitis, Bell's palsy, and cranial and peripheral neuropathies.

Nonspecific findings include an elevated sedimentation rate in 50%, and an elevated IgM level, mild anemia, and elevated liver function tests in 20%.

Burgdorfer et al in 1982 isolated a spirochete from adult *Ixodes dammini* ticks, which were a known vector for Lyme disease. The spirochete was then identified by Warthin-Starry silver stain in skin biopsy specimens of EM. Subsequently the spirochete, now designated *Borrelia burgdorferi sensu lato,* has been cultured on artificial (modified Kelly's) medium from the blood, skin, and cerebrospinal fluid of patients with Lyme disease. Three subtypes are now recognized. *B. burgdorferi sensu stricto* is commonly the cause of Lyme disease in the United States. *B. garinii* and *B. afzelii* are also present in Europe, with early data indicating the latter to be associated with acrodermatitis chronica atrophicans.

Males and females are equally affected, and the age range most commonly affected is 20 to 50. Onset of this illness is generally between May and November, with more than 80% of cases identified in June, July, or August, in the northern hemisphere. In the United States, Lyme disease occurs primarily in three geographic areas: the Northeast, Midwest, and West. Tick transmission has been proved, with large studies documenting spirochetes present in various members of the family of hard ticks, Ixodidae. Specifically, *Ixodes scapularis* is the vector in the Northeast and Midwest and *I. pacificus* is incriminated in the West. *I. dammini,* previously classified as a separate species, is the same as *I. scapularis.*

Afzelius in Sweden described EM in 1909. European cases are transmitted by the tick *I. ricinus.* The different subtypes of *Borrelia* present in Europe may account for the fact that the clinical illness resulting from infection is somewhat different from that seen in the United States. European EM occurs more often in females. It is less likely to have multiple lesions; untreated lesions last longer; there are more laboratory abnormalities in Lyme disease; the arthritis symptoms are prominent in the United States but unusual in Europe; and the neurologic manifestations differ. In Europe, infection may lead to Bannwarth's syndrome, which is characterized by focal, severe, radicular pains; lymphocytic meningitis; and cranial nerve paralysis. Finally, acrodermatitis chronica atrophicans and possibly morphea, lymphocytoma cutis, benign lymphocytic infil-

trates, atrophoderma of Pasini and Pierini, anetoderma, and lichen sclerosus et atrophicus may eventuate as late cutaneous sequelae of *Borrelia afzelii* or *B. garinii* infection in Europe.

Transplacental transmission of *Borrelia,* resulting in infant death, has been reported in several cases. However, studies of Lyme disease in pregnancy have generally failed to directly implicate an association with fetal malformations.

On histologic investigation there is a superficial and deep perivascular and interstitial mixed-cell infiltrate. Lymphocytes, plasma cells, and eosinophils may be seen, the latter especially prominent when the center of the lesion is biopsied. Warthin-Starry staining may reveal spirochetes in the upper dermis.

The clinical finding of EM is the most sensitive evidence of early infection. Serologic tests are still considered unreliable. A newly developed flow cytometry test may be more accurate and specific for serodiagnosis. The most frequently ordered test is the enzyme-linked immunosorbent assay (ELISA). When EM is present alone, 67% of patients have a positive ELISA. Patients with rheumatologic, neurologic, or cardiac complications should have at least one positive test result, although Dattwyler et al have reported seronegative Lyme disease, in which there is a specific T-cell blastogenic response but no antibody response. False-positive tests occur in syphilis, pinta, yaws, leptospirosis, relapsing fever, infectious mononucleosis, and disease associated with autoantibody formation. The VDRL is negative in *Borrelia burgdorferi* infection. The organism may be cultured in modified Kelly's medium.

Treatment

The treatment of choice in adults is doxycycline, 100 mg twice daily for 10 to 30 days. Amoxicillin, 500 mg three times daily for 10 to 30 days, is also effective. Children under age 9 should be treated with amoxicillin, 20 mg/kg daily in divided doses for 10 to 30 days. Pregnant women with localized early Lyme disease should take amoxicillin; however, if disseminated disease is present, penicillin G, 20 million units daily for 14 to 21 days, is used. Penicillin-allergic children may be given erythromycin, 30 mg/kg/day in divided doses for 10 to 30 days, although this is less effective. The shorter courses are for patients with a single skin lesion only. These recommendations are for early Lyme disease such as those patients with EM.

More aggressive regimens are necessary for carditis and neurologic and arthritic involvement, and often require IV penicillin or IM ceftriaxone. For example, in established Lyme arthritis and Lyme meningitis, ceftriaxone, 2 g once daily IV or IM for 2 weeks, is the treatment of choice. Intravenous penicillin G, 20 million units/day for 10 days, is an alternative. Of patients with arthritis, 50% will not respond to penicillin therapy.

Inspecting for ticks after returning from outdoor activity is a good preventative. The tick needs to be attached for more than 24 hours to transmit disease. Nymphs are small; they may be hard to see. Beware of the freckle that moves. Prophylactic antibiotic therapy after known tick bite is not recommended.

Acrodermatitis Chronica Atrophicans

Also known as *primary diffuse atrophy,* acrodermatitis chronica atrophicans (ACA) is characterized by the appearance on the extremities of diffuse reddish or bluish red, paper-thin skin. The underlying blood vessels are easily seen through the epidermis. It occurs almost exclusively in Europe.

The disease begins on the backs of the hands and feet, then gradually spreads to involve the forearms, then the arms, and on the lower extremities, knees and shins. Occasionally, even the trunk may become involved.

In the beginning the areas may be slightly edematous and scaly, but generally they are level with the skin and smooth. After several weeks to months the skin has a smooth, soft, thin, velvety feel and may easily be lifted into fine folds. It may have a peculiar pinkish gray color and a crumpled cigarette-paper appearance (Fig. 14-47).

Well-defined, smooth, edematous, bandlike thickenings may extend from a finger to the elbow (ulnar bands) (Fig. 14-48) or develop in the skin over the shins. With progression of the disease, marked atrophy of the skin occurs (Fig. 14-49).

Subcutaneous fibrous nodules may form, chiefly over the elbows, wrists, and knees. They may be single or multiple, and are firm and painless. Diffuse extensive calcification of the soft tissues may be revealed by radiographic examination. Xanthomatous tumors may occur in the skin. Hypertrophic osteoarthritis of the hands is frequently observed. Occasionally, atrophy of the bones of the involved extremities is encountered.

Ulcerations and carcinoma may supervene on the atrophic patches. The disease is slowly progressive but may remain stationary for long periods. Patches may change slightly from time to time, but complete involution never occurs.

ACA is a spirochetosis, a late sequel of infection with *Borrelia afzelii.* It is tick-transmitted by *Ixodes ricinus.* Nearly all patients with ACA have a positive test for antibodies to the spirochete, and Warthin-Starry stains demonstrate the organism in tissue in some cases. The organism has been cultured from skin lesions of ACA.

Histologically, there is marked atrophy of the epidermis and dermis without fibrosis. The elastic tissue is absent, and the cutaneous appendages are atrophic. In the dermis a bandlike lymphocytic infiltration is seen, which varies in abundance according to the stage of the disease. The epidermis is slightly hyperkeratotic and flattened, and beneath it there is a distinctive narrow zone of connective tissue in which the elastic tissue is intact.

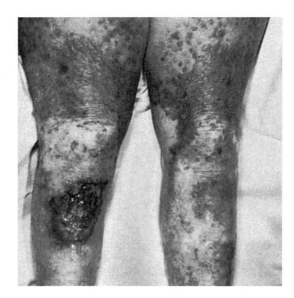

Fig. 14-47 Acrodermatitis chronica atrophicans with severe ulceration. Note crinkled cigarette paper appearance of the skin at the knee. (Courtesy Dr. R. Ames.)

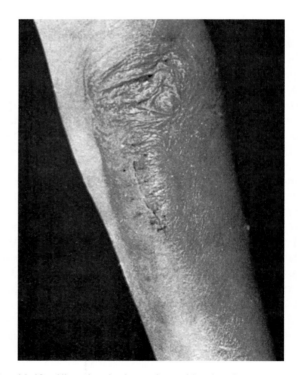

Fig. 14-48 Ulnar band of acrodermatitis chronica atrophicans. (Courtesy Dr. F. Daniels, Jr.)

Penicillin G, 1.5 million units three times daily, or doxycycline, 100 mg twice daily, cures most patients with ACA.

Abele DC, et al: The many faces and phases of borreliosis. I. *J Am Acad Dermatol* 1990, 23:167.

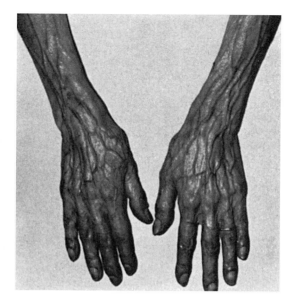

Fig. 14-49 Acrodermatitis chronica atrophicans.

Abele DC, et al: The many faces and phases of borreliosis. II. *J Am Acad Dermatol* 1990, 23:401.

Aberer E, et al: Success and failure in the treatment of acrodermatitis chronica atrophicans. *Infection* 1996, 24:85.

Albrecht S, et al: Lymphadenosis benigna cutis resulting from *Borrelia* infection. *J Am Acad Dermatol* 1991, 29:621.

Berg D, et al: The laboratory diagnosis of Lyme disease. *Arch Dermatol* 1991, 127:866.

Berger BW: Current aspects of Lyme disease and other *Borrelia burgdorferi* infections. *Dermatol Clin* 1997, 15:247.

Berger BW: ECM of Lyme disease. *Arch Dermatol* 1984, 120:1017.

Berger BW, et al: Cultivation of *B. burgdorferi* from the blood of two patients with ECM lacking extracutaneous signs and symptoms of Lyme disease. *J Am Acad Dermatol* 1994, 30:48.

Berger BW, et al: Isolation and characterization of the Lyme disease spirochete from the skin of patients with ECM. *J Am Acad Dermatol* 1985, 13:444.

Buechner SA, et al: Acrodermatitis chronica atrophicans. *J Am Acad Dermatol* 1993, 28:399.

Burgdorfer W, et al: Lyme disease: a tick-borne spirochetosis? *Science* 1982, 216:1317.

Callister SM, et al: Detection of borreliacidal antibodies by flow cytometry. *Arch Intern Med* 1994, 154:1625.

Costello CM, et al: A prospective study of tick bite in an endemic area for Lyme disease. *J Infect Dis* 1989, 159:136.

Dattwyler RJ, et al: Seronegative Lyme disease. *N Engl J Med* 1988, 319:1441.

Edwards L, et al: Acrodermatitis chronica atrophicans. *Arch Dermatol* 1992, 128:858.

Fujiwara H, et al: Detection of *Borrelia burgdorferi* DNA (*B garinii* or *B afzelii*) in morphea and lichen sclerosus et atrophicus tissues of German and Japanese but not of US patients. *Arch Dermatol* 1997, 133:41.

Goldberg NW, et al: Vesicular erythema migrans. *Arch Dermatol* 1992, 128:1495.

Krause PJ, et al: Concurrent Lyme disease and babesiosis. *JAMA* 1996, 275:1657.

Lastavica CC, et al: Rapid emergence of a focal epidemic of Lyme disease in coastal Massachusetts. *N Engl J Med* 1989, 320:133.

Malane MS, et al: Diagnosis of Lyme disease based on dermatologic manifestations. *Ann Intern Med* 1991, 114:490.

Melski JW, et al: Primary and secondary erythema migrans in central Wisconsin. *Arch Dermatol* 1993, 29:709.

Ohlenbusch A, et al: Etiology of the acrodermatitis chronica atrophicans lesion in Lyme disease. *J Infect Dis* 1996, 174:421.

Piesman J, et al: Duration of tick attachment and *B. burgdorferi* transmission. *J Clin Microbiol* 1987, 25:557.

Rabb DC, et al: Polymerase chain reaction conformation of *B. burgdorferi* in benign lymphocytic infiltrate of dermis. *J Am Acad Dermatol* 1992, 26:267.

Rahn DW, et al: Lyme disease: recommendations for diagnosis and treatment. *Ann Intern Med* 1991, 114:472.

Schlesinger PA, et al: Maternal-fetal transmission of the Lyme disease spirochete. *Ann Intern Med* 1985, 103:67.

Shrestha M, et al: Diagnosing early Lyme disease. *Am J Med* 1988, 18:235.

Spach DH, et al: Localized alopecia at the site of erythema migrans. *J Am Acad Dermatol* 1992, 27:1023.

Spach DH, et al: Tick-borne diseases in the US. *New Engl J Med* 1993, 329:936.

Steere AC, et al: Lyme disease. *New Engl J Med* 1989, 321:586.

Trevisan G, et al: Lyme disease. *Int J Dermatol* 1990, 20:1.

Wrenecke R, et al: Molecular subtyping of *Borrelia burgdorferi* in erythema migrans and ACA. *J Invest Dermatol* 1994, 103:19.

▲

MYCOPLASMA

Mycoplasmas are distinct from true bacteria in that they lack a cell wall and differ from viruses in that they grow on cell-free media. *Mycoplasma pneumoniae* (Eaton agent) is an important cause of acute respiratory disease in children and young adults. It has been estimated that in the summer it may account for 50% of pneumonias.

Skin eruptions occur during the course of infection in 17% of patients. The most frequently reported dermatologic manifestation is Stevens-Johnson syndrome. Erythema nodosum has been occasionally reported. Of the various exanthems documented, they include urticarial, vesicular, vesiculopustular, maculopapular, scarlatiniform, and mor-billiform lesions, distributed primarily on the trunk, arms, and legs. Ulcerative stomatitis and conjunctivitis may be present. Ramilo et al reported a 9-year-old boy with fever and a petechial and purpuric eruption that resembled acute meningococcemia. Goodyear et al found 5 of 100 children evaluated for fever and widespread erythema to have *M. pneumoniae* infection.

The diagnosis of *M. pneumoniae* infection is made in the acute situation by clinical means, but definitive diagnosis is made either by culture of the organism or by a rise in the specific antibody titer. The serologic procedures used are a complement fixation test and a sensitive ELISA test. Cold agglutinins with a titer of 1:128 or more are usually due to *M. pneumoniae* infection. Occasionally, acrocyanosis may occur secondary to cold agglutinin disease, which clears with antibiotic therapy.

Treatment is with erythromycin, 500 mg three times daily, or tetracycline, 250 mg four times daily, both courses lasting a total of 6 to 8 days.

Goodyear HM, et al: Acute infectious erythema in children. *Br J Dermatol* 1991, 145:433.

Ramilo AL, et al: *Mycoplasma* infection simulating acute meningococcemia. *Arch Dermatol* 1983, 119:786.

Shelley WB, et al: Acrocyanosis of cold agglutinin disease successfully treated with antibiotics. *Cutis* 1984, 33:556.

Tay YK, et al: *Mycoplasma pneumoniae* infection is associated with Stevens-Johnson syndrome, not erythema multiforme (von Hebra). *J Am Acad Dermatol* 1996, 35:757. _____ ▲

CHLAMYDIAL INFECTIONS

Two species of chlamydias, *Chlamydia trachomatis* and *C. psittaci,* have been recognized. The two species share a major common antigen, and there are numerous serotypes within each species. In humans, *Chlamydia* cause trachoma, inclusion conjunctivitis, nongonococcal urethritis, cervicitis, epididymitis, proctitis, endometritis, salpingitis, pneumonia in the newborn, psittacosis (ornithosis), and lymphogranuloma venereum.

LYMPHOGRANULOMA VENEREUM

Lymphogranuloma venereum (LGV) was formerly called lymphopathia venerea, climatic bubo, or lymphogranuloma inguinale. It is a sexually transmitted disease that is characterized by suppurative inguinal adenitis with matted lymph nodes, inguinal bubo with secondary ulceration, and constitutional symptoms.

After an incubation period of 3 to 20 days, a primary lesion consisting of a 2- to 3-mm herpetiform vesicle or erosion develops on the glans penis, prepuce, or coronal sulcus, or at the meatus (Fig. 14-50, *A*). In women it occurs on the vulva, vagina, or cervix. The lesion is painless and soon becomes a shallow ulceration. The primary lesion may also be a urethritis.

Extragenital primary infections of LGV are rare. An ulcerating lesion may appear at the site of infection on the fingers, lips, or tongue. Primary lesions heal in a few days.

About 2 weeks after the appearance of the primary lesion, enlargement of the regional lymph nodes occurs. In one third of cases, the lymphadenopathy is bilateral (Fig. 14-50, *B*). In the rather characteristic inguinal adenitis of LGV, in men the nodes in a chain fuse together into a large mass. The color of the skin overlying the mass usually becomes violaceous, the swelling is tender, and the bubo may break down, forming multiple fistulous openings.

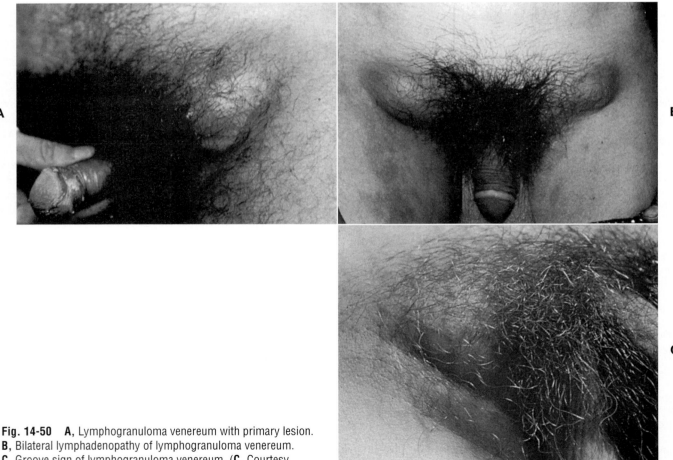

Fig. 14-50 A, Lymphogranuloma venereum with primary lesion. **B,** Bilateral lymphadenopathy of lymphogranuloma venereum. **C,** Groove sign of lymphogranuloma venereum. (**C,** Courtesy Dr. Axel W. Hoke.)

Adenopathy above and below Poupart's ligament produces the characteristic, but not diagnostic, groove sign (Fig. 14-50, *C*). Along with the local adenitis there may be systemic symptoms of malaise, joint pains, conjunctivitis, loss of appetite, weight loss, and fever, which may persist for several weeks. Cases with septic temperatures, enlarged liver and spleen, and even encephalitis have occasionally been observed.

Primary lesions of LGV are rarely observed in female patients; women also have a lower incidence of inguinal buboes. Their bubo is typically pararectal in location. The diagnosis is recognized only much later when the patient presents an increasingly pronounced inflammatory stricture, which may be annular or tubular, of the lower rectal wall. Because most of the lymph channels running from the vulva drain into the nodes around the lower part of the rectum, an inflammatory reaction in these nodes results in secondary involvement of the rectal wall. The iliac nodes may also be involved.

LGV may start in the rectum as proctitis, which may then progress to the formation of a stricture. The clinical hallmark is bloody, mucopurulent rectal discharge. The stricture can usually be felt with the examining finger 4 to 6 cm above the anus. Untreated rectal strictures of men and women may eventually require colostomy. With or without rectal strictures, women may in later stages of the disease show elephantiasis of the genitals with chronic ulcerations and scarring of the vulva (esthiomene). Such a reaction is rare in men.

Cutaneous eruptions take the form of erythema nodosum, erythema multiforme, photosensitivity, and scarlatiniform eruptions. Arthritis associated with LGV involves finger, wrist, ankle, knee, or shoulder joints. Marked weight loss, pronounced secondary anemia, weakness, and mental depression are often encountered in the course of the anorectal syndrome. Colitis resulting from LGV is limited to the rectum and rectosigmoid structures. Perianal fistulas or sinuses are often seen in cases of anorectal LGV.

Among the various extragenital manifestations that occur are glossitis with regional adenitis, unilateral conjunctivitis with edema of the lids caused by lymphatic blockage with lymphadenopathy, acute meningitis, meningoencephalitis, and pneumonia.

The complement fixation test is the most feasible and the simplest serologic test for detecting antibodies, which become detectable some 4 weeks after onset of illness. A titer of 1:64 is highly suggestive. Microhemagglutination inhibition assays are also available and not only confirm the diagnosis but also identify the strain.

LGV is a sexually transmitted disease caused by microorganisms of the *Chlamydia trachomatis* group. Three serotypes, designated L1, L2, and L3, are known for the LGV chlamydia. Characteristic surface antigens allow separation of the LGV chlamydias from the agents that cause trachoma, inclusion conjunctivitis, urethritis, and cervicitis, which also belong to the *C. trachomatis* group.

LGV is contracted by heterosexual or homosexual sexual contact. It occurs in all races and is more common among the sexually active. The highest incidence is found in the 20- to 40-year-old group. Asymptomatic female contacts who shed the organism from the cervix are an important reservoir of infection. The classic disease in men is declining in the United States, whereas anorectal LGV has been increasing in the homosexual population.

The characteristic changes in the lymph nodes consist of an infectious granuloma with the formation of stellate abscesses. There is an outer zone of epithelioid cells with a central necrotic core composed of debris of lymphocytes, and leukocytes. In lesions of long duration plasma cells may be present.

As opposed to LGV, with chancroid a primary chancre or multiple chancroidal ulcers are present and may permit the demonstration of *Haemophilus ducreyi*. The skin lesions are characteristic and usually much larger and more persistent than the primary lesion of LGV. Donovan bodies are demonstrable in granuloma inguinale; however, inguinal adenitis is not characteristic. Esthiomene may also be seen in both diseases.

If the primary lesion of LGV is well developed, it may be confused with the primary lesion of syphilis. In any genital lesion, darkfield examination for *Treponema pallidum* should be made. Syphilitic inguinal adenitis shows small, hard, nontender glands. It should be emphasized again that all venereal infections may be mixed infections and that observation for simultaneous or subsequent development of another venereal disease should be unrelenting. This includes serologic testing for HIV disease. Late stages of LGV esthiomene with ulcerating and cicatrizing lesions have to be differentiated from syphilis by search for spirochetes, the serologic tests for syphilis, and complement fixation tests.

Treatment

The recommended treatment is doxycycline, 100 mg twice daily for 3 weeks. An alternative is erythromycin, 500 mg four times daily for 21 days. Sexual partners should also be treated. The fluctuant nodules are aspirated through healthy adjacent normal skin to prevent rupture.

Dan M, et al: A case of LGV of 20 years' duration. *Br J Venereal Dis* 1980, 56:344.

Ellis RE: Chlamydial genital infections. *South Med J* 1981, 74:109.

Goens JL, et al: Mucocutaneous manifestations of chancroid, lymphogranuloma venereum and granuloma inguinale. *Am Fam Physician* 1994, 49:415.

Joseph AK, et al: Laboratory techniques used in the diagnosis of chancroid, granuloma inguinale, and lymphogranuloma venereum. *Dermatol Clin* 1994, 12:1.

1998 STD Guidelines: *MMWR* 1998, 47:1.

CHAPTER 15

Diseases Resulting from Fungi and Yeasts

The superficial mycoses

The skin constitutes the main site of recognizable fungal infections in humans, and these infections can be divided into superficial and deep mycoses. When restricted to the skin, most mycotic infections are superficial and are limited to a depth of 1 or 2 mm. The fungi that usually cause only superficial infection on the skin are called *dermatophytes*. They are classified in three genera: *Microsporum, Trichophyton,* and *Epidermophyton*. Each species of dermatophyte tends to produce its own clinical picture, although several species may provoke identical eruptions. At other times the eruptions are so distinctive and characteristic that the species may be identified from the clinical findings. The skin appendages, namely, the hair and nails, are also vitally involved in these infections.

The mycoses caused by dermatophytes are called *dermatophytosis, tinea,* or *ringworm*. On certain parts of the body tinea has certain distinctive features characteristic of that particular site. For this reason the tineas are divided into (1) tinea capitis (ringworm of the scalp and kerion), (2) tinea barbae (ringworm of the beard), (3) tinea faciei, (4) tinea corporis, (5) tinea manus, (6) tinea pedis, (7) tinea cruris, and (8) onychomycosis (fungus infection of the nails).

Superficial mycoses are also classified according to the causative dermatophyte. However, this is of largely epidemiologic interest. The management of such infections is only rarely assisted by the identification of the genus and species of the causative organism.

SUSCEPTIBILITY

The dermatophytes are soil saprophytes that have acquired the ability to digest keratinous debris in soil, thus becoming "keratinophilic fungi." Some of these organisms evolved to parasitize keratinous tissues of animals frequently in contact with soil, classified as zoophilic, and lost their ability to survive in soil. The anthropophilic dermatophytes are believed to have evolved from zoophilic fungi, adapting to human keratin and losing their ability to digest animal

keratin. Environmental conditions help promote the propagation of many opportunistic fungi; however, host factors are also significant.

The best example of host factors that promote dermatophytosis is the immunosuppressed patient. Dermatophytes are eliminated from the skin by a cell-mediated immune reaction. The combination of an inflammatory response coupled with increased proliferative activity of keratinocytes helps to minimize progression and slough the fungus from the skin surface. Immunocompromised states, such as with acquired immunodeficiency syndrome (AIDS), may result in severe forms of dermatophyte infections.

Other host factors have been implicated. Genetic susceptibility to certain forms of fungal infections may be related to the types of keratin or degree or mix of cutaneous lipids produced. Others have shown that surface antigens, such as the ABO system, can be important. Balajee et al studied 108 culture-proven dermatophytosis patients and noted that patients with A blood groups were more prone to chronic disease. Others have shown that human steroid hormones can inhibit the growth of dermatophytes, particularly androgens such as androstenedione. Brasch et al believe that the high susceptibility of *Trichophyton rubrum* and *Epidermophyton floccosum* to intrafollicular androstenedione could be one reason why these two species are unable to cause tinea capitis. The degree to which some of these factors contribute to the progression of dermatophyte infections remains to be elucidated.

ANTIFUNGAL THERAPY

When considering use of an oral antifungal agent there are three considerations: (1) the spectrum of activity of the antifungal agent, (2) pharmacokinetic profile of the agent, and (3) the clinical type of infection. Additional considerations should be safety, compliance, and cost. Griseofulvin is still a viable therapeutic option in many cases; however, in study after study the newer antifungals are being shown to be more efficacious.

The imidazoles comprise clotrimazole, miconazole, econazole, sulconazole, oxiconazole, and ketoconazole and are used mostly for topical therapy. They work by inhibition of the cytochrome P450 14-α-demethylase, an essential enzyme in ergosterol synthesis. Nystatin is a polyene that works by irreversibly binding to ergosterol, an essential component of fungal cell membranes. Naftifine, terbinafine, and butenafine are allylamines, and their mode of action is similar to the thiocarbamates, inhibiting squalene epoxydation. The triazoles include itraconazole and fluconazole, which affect the cytochrome P450 system. As such numerous drug interactions occur, some of which may be life threatening. A thorough knowledge of the patient's concurrent medications and the potential for alterations of drug levels is required when prescribing these two agents. The triazoles have the broadest in vitro spectrum of activity, including dermatophytes, *Candida* species, and *Malassezia furfur*. Itraconazole is fungistatic; food increases its absorption, antacids and gastric acid secretion suppressors produce erratic or lowered absorption, pulse dosing limits concern over laboratory abnormalities. Fluconazole's absorption is not affected by food. Terbinafine is less active against *Candida* species in in vitro studies; however, clinically it is usually effective. It has been shown ineffective in the oral treatment of tinea versicolor but is effective topically. Although few drug interactions have been reported and the bioavailability is unchanged in food, hepatotoxicity, leukopenia, severe exanthems, and taste disturbances occur uncommonly but should be monitored for clinically and by laboratory testing if continuous dosing over 6 weeks is given. Ketoconazole has a wide spectrum against dermatophytes, yeasts, and some systemic mycoses. It has the potential for serious drug interactions and a higher incidence of hepatotoxicity during long-term daily therapy.

Aly R: Ecology and epidemiology of dermatophyte infections. *J Am Acad Dermatol* 1994, 31:S21.

Aly R, et al: Common superficial fungal infections in patients with AIDS. *Clin Infect Dis* 1996, 22:S128.

Babel DE: How to identify fungi. *J Am Acad Dermatol* 1994, 31:S108.

Balajee SA, et al: ABO blood groups in relation to the infection rate of dermatophytosis. *Mycoses* 1996, 39:475.

Bicks DR: Antifungal therapy: potential interactions with other classes of drugs. *J Am Acad Dermatol* 1994, 31:S87.

Brasch J: Hormones, fungi, and skin. *Mycoses* 1997, 40(Suppl 1):11.

Brasch J, et al: The effect of selected human steroid hormones upon the growth of dermatophytes with different adaptation to man. *Mycopathologia* 1992, 120:87.

Brennan B, et al: Overview of topical therapy for common superficial fungal infections and the role of new topical agents. *J Am Acad Dermatol* 1997, 36:S3.

Degreef HJ, et al: Current therapy of dermatophytosis. *J Am Acad Dermatol* 1994, 31:S25.

Elewski BE, Hay RJ: Novel treatment strategies for superficial mycoses. *J Am Acad Dermatol* 1999, 40:S1.

Elmets CA: Management of common superficial fungal infections in patients with AIDS. *J Am Acad Dermatol* 1994, 31:S60.

Graybill JR: Therapeutic agents. *Infect Dis Clin North Am* 1988, 2:805.

Greer DL: An overview of common dermatophytes. *J Am Acad Dermatol* 1994, 31:S112.

Greer DL: Differentiating yeasts from bacteria in the physician's office. *J Am Acad Dermatol* 1994, 31:S111.

Gupta AK, et al: Drug interactions with itraconazole, fluconazole, and terbinafine and their management. *J Am Acad Dermatol* 1999, 41:237.

Odom RB: Common superficial fungal infections in immunosuppressed patients. *J Am Acad Dermatol* 1994, 31:S56.

Roberts DT, et al: Oral therapeutic agents in fungal nail disease. *J Am Acad Dermatol* 1994, 31:S78.

Roderick JH: Antifungal drugs on the horizon. *J Am Acad Dermatol* 1994, 31:S82.

Stevens DA: Management of systemic manifestations of fungal disease in patients with AIDS. *J Am Acad Dermatol* 1994, 31:S64. ▲

TINEA CAPITIS

Synonym: Scalp ringworm

Ringworm of the scalp is an infectious disease occurring chiefly in schoolchildren and less commonly in infants and adults (Fig. 15-1). Boys have tinea capitis more frequently than girls; however, in epidemics caused by *Trichophyton tonsurans* there is often equal frequency in the sexes. The clinical types of infections can be conveniently divided into inflammatory and noninflammatory lesions. Tinea capitis can be caused by all the pathogenic dermatophytes except for *Epidermophyton floccosum* and *T. concentricum*. In the United States, most cases are caused by *T. tonsurans* (which has removed *Microsporum audouinii* from first place) and *M. canis*.

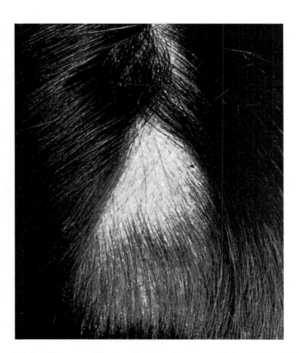

Fig. 15-1 Tinea capitis, localized patch, caused by *Trichophyton tonsurans*.

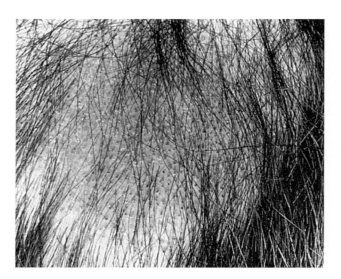

Fig. 15-2 Tinea capitis. "Black dot" ringworm caused by *Trichophyton tonsurans.*

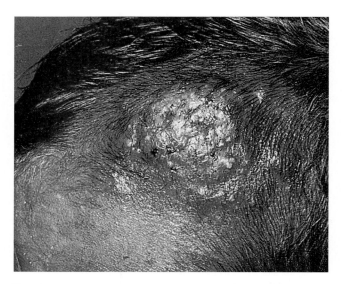

Fig. 15-3 Kerion. Inflammatory reaction of tinea capitis frequently caused by *Microsporum canis* or *Trichophyton mentagrophytes.* (Courtesy Dr. J. Penner.)

M. audouinii infections present as the classic form of noninflammatory tinea capitis, characterized by multiple scaly lesions ("gray-patch"), stubs of broken hair, and a minimal inflammatory response. Occasionally the glabrous skin, eyelids, and eyelashes are involved. This infection sometimes is observed in epidemics in schools and orphanages. Over the past 30 years, *M. audouinii* infections gradually have been replaced by increasing numbers of cases of "black-dot" ringworm, caused primarily by *T. tonsurans* but occasionally by *T. violaceum. T. tonsurans* is the preponderant cause of tinea capitis in the United States. Whereas the incidence of *T. tonsurans* has increased tremendously, that of *M. audouinii* has decreased. "Black dot" ringworm, caused by *T. tonsurans* and occasionally, *T. violaceum,* presents as multiple areas of alopecia studded with black dots representing infected hairs broken off at or below the surface of the scalp (Fig. 15-2).

Inflammatory tinea capitis is usually caused by *M. canis* but can be caused by *T. mentagrophytes, T. tonsurans, M. gypseum,* or *T. verrucosum. M. canis* infections begin as scaly, erythematous, papular eruptions with loose and broken-off hairs, followed by varying degrees of inflammation, but in many cases it suddenly becomes severe (Fig. 15-3). At times, a localized spot is accompanied by pronounced swelling, developing into boggy and indurated areas exuding pus, known as *kerion celsii* (Fig. 15-4). This inflammatory reaction is felt to be a delayed type hypersensitivity reaction to fungal elements. If extensive lesions form, fever, pain, and regional lymphadenopathy may be present. Widespread "id" eruptions may appear concomitantly on the trunk and extremities. These are vesicular, lichenoid, or pustular. Kerion may be followed by scarring and permanent alopecia in the areas of inflammation and

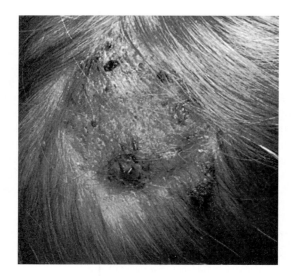

Fig. 15-4 Kerion caused by *Microsporum canis.*

suppuration. Systemic steroids for a short period will greatly diminish the inflammatory response and reduce the risk of scarring.

Favus. Favus, which is very rare in the United States, appears chiefly on the scalp but may affect the glabrous skin and nails. On the scalp, concave sulfur-yellow crusts form around loose, wiry hairs (Fig. 15-5). Atrophy ensues, leaving a smooth, glossy, thin, paper-white patch (Fig. 15-6). On the glabrous skin the lesions are pinhead to 2 cm in diameter with cup-shaped crusts called *scutulae,* usually pierced by a hair as on the scalp. The scutula have a distinctive mousy odor. When the nails are affected they

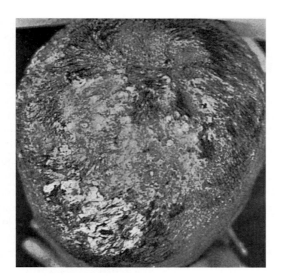

Fig. 15-5 Favus of scalp, showing scutulae.

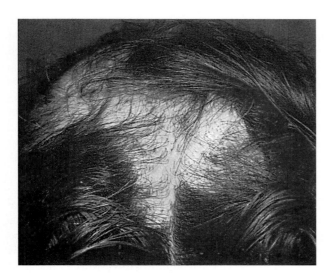

Fig. 15-6 Scarring after favus infection.

become brittle, irregularly thickened, and crusted under the free margins.

Favus is not often seen in North America, although it has been reported in Kentucky and in Canada. Favus among the Bantus in South Africa is called, in Afrikaans, *witkop* (whitehead). It is also prevalent in the Middle East, southeastern Europe, and the countries bordering the Mediterranean Sea.

Etiology

Tinea capitis can be caused by any one of several of the dermatophytes. The most frequent causative fungi are *T. tonsurans, M. audouinii,* and *M. canis.* The first two spread from human to human, whereas the latter is caught from animals such as kittens or dogs. *M. ferrugineum* and

M. gypseum species may occasionally cause ringworm of the scalp.

Among the trichophytons, endothrix types, such as *T. tonsurans* (black-dot ringworm) and *T. violaceum,* are the most frequent invaders of the scalp. It is noteworthy that *T. tonsurans* alone affects adults (chiefly women) regularly; the others are almost always confined to children. The ectothrix fungi found most frequently on the scalp are *T. verrucosum* and *T. mentagrophytes;* less frequently seen is *T. megninii,* which is probably restricted to southwest Europe.

Incidence and Epidemiology

Both *M. audouinii* and *M. canis* are endemic and infect mostly city children. *T. tonsurans* in 1978 was the major cause of tinea capitis in urban areas with a large Latin-American population. In the succeeding two decades it has consolidated and extended its territory. It is difficult to diagnose clinically so it is probably far more widespread than is reported. *M. audouinii* is a human pathogen and can occur in epidemic proportions. The fungus has been found in barbers' brushes, on the backs of theater seats, and in caps and hats; however, transmission is probably from child to child. The same statements apply to *T. tonsurans. M. canis* is acquired from infected kittens or dogs; *T. mentagrophytes* is also transmitted by animals. *T. schoenleinii* and *T. violaceum* appear to be transmitted from human to human. In children up to 18 years of age, the latter occurs more frequently in boys than in girls; however, among adults women greatly outnumber men.

In Kansas City, random cultures showed an overall infection rate of 4%. Of all girls in the study, 12.7% had positive cultures. In another study by Vargo et al 15% of black children who used the outpatient services at a Baltimore hospital had positive cultures. In a series of 1057 children examined in London schools, the infection rate ranged from 0% to 12%, with a mean of 2.5%. Scalp carriers of dermatophytes numbered 4.9%, and *T. tonsurans* was the predominant organism detected.

Geographic locations are important factors in the types of infection seen. *M. audouinii* and *M. canis* have been frequently noted fungi in the New York area; however, as noted previously there has been a steady increase in *T. tonsurans.* This organism is now endemic in Latin and South America and Mexico. *T. violaceum* is prevalent in the former Soviet Union, Yugoslavia, and Spain. *T. schoenleinii* is rarely seen in the United States and usually only in immigrants, whereas it is predominant in the Middle East. In Africa, large-scale epidemics are associated with other trichophytons *(T. soudanense, T. violaceum, T. schoenleinii)* and *Microsporum* species.

Pathogenesis

The incubation period lasts 2 to 4 days. The hyphae grow downward into the follicle, on the hair's surface, and the intrafollicular hyphae break up into chains of spores. There is a period of spread (4 days to 4 months) during which the lesions enlarge and new lesions appear. At about 3 weeks hairs break off a few millimeters above the surface. Intrapilary hyphae descend to the exact upper limit of the keratogenous zone and here form Adamson's "fringe" on about the twelfth day. The external portions of the intrapilary hyphae segment into chains of ectothrix spores. No new lesions develop during the refractory period (4 months to several years). The clinical appearance is constant, with the host and parasite at equilibrium. This is followed by a period of involution in which the formation of ectothrix spores and intrapilary hyphae gradually diminishes.

Asymptomatic carrier states among young black children may occur. In a large series of 1404 inner-city children cultured by Williams et al, there were 3% index cases and 14% asymptomatic carriers. Of interest was the lack of correlation between the number of asymptomatic carriers and index cases, suggesting that carrier cases of *T. tonsurans* are not the primary mode of transmission.

Diagnosis

Wood's Light

Ultraviolet of 365 nm wavelength is obtained by passing the beam through a Wood's filter composed of nickel oxide-containing glass. This apparatus, commonly known as the *Wood's light,* is available commercially. A simple form is the 125-volt purple bulb.

In a dark room the skin under this light fluoresces faintly blue; however, the infected hair fluoresces bright green, beads on the hairs contrasting strongly with the dark field. Bare, scaly areas show a turquoise blue color. Fluorescent-positive infections are caused by *M. audouinii, M. canis, M. ferrugineum, M. distortum,* and *T. schoenleinii;* hairs infected with *T. tonsurans* and *T. violaceum* and others of the endothrix type do not fluoresce. The fluorescent substance is a pteridine.

Microscopic Examination

For demonstration of the fungus, two or three loose hairs are removed with epilating forceps from the suspected areas. When the hairs are all broken off at the surface ("black-dot" ringworm), it is usually possible to tease a few out with a needle point. If fluoresence occurs it is important to choose these hairs. Bear in mind that hairs infected with *T. tonsurans* do not fluoresce. The hairs are placed on a slide and covered with a drop of a 10% to 20% solution of potassium hydroxide (KOH). Then a coverslip is applied, and the specimen is warmed over a flame until the hairs are macerated. They are examined first with a low-power objective and then with a high-power objective for detail. Xylol is as satisfactory as KOH and need not be warmed. Scales or hairs cleared with it can still be cultured.

The fungus invades the hair shaft two ways, one being ectothrix involvement in which the hair is surrounded with a sheath of tiny spores (Fig. 15-7, *A*). *Microsporum* species, as well as *T. mentagrophytes* and *T. verrucosum,* are ectothrix fungi. *T. verrucosum* is the fungus most frequently acquired by humans from cattle and causes a severe inflammatory tinea barbae in men or tinea capitis in children. The other mode of fungus infection is the endothrix type in which the arthrospores are formed inside the hair shaft (Fig. 15-7, *B* and *C*). This type is seen with *T. tonsurans, T. violaceum,* and *T. schoenleinii* infections.

The final and exact identification of the causative fungus may be determined by culture. It should be acknowledged, however, that such identification is of largely epidemiologic and academic interest; it makes little or no difference to the treatment of the patient. Several of the infected hairs are planted on Sabouraud's glucose agar or Dermatophyte Test Medium (DTM). On the former a distinctive growth appears within 1 to 2 weeks. Most frequently the diagnosis is made by the gross appearance of the culture growth. In the case of an atypical growth and questionable identification the culture is examined under the microscope for characteristic morphologic forms. DTM not only contains antibiotics to reduce growth of contaminants but also contains a colored pH indicator to denote the alkali-producing dermatophytes. A few nonpathogenic saprophytes will also produce alkalinization and in the occasional case of onychomycosis of toenails caused by airborne molds, a culture medium containing an antibiotic may inhibit growth of the true pathogen. Cultures are best taken by rubbing the lesion vigorously with a sterile cotton swab moistened with sterile water and then streaked over the agar surface.

T. tonsurans. This microorganism grows slowly in culture to produce a granular or powdery yellow to red, brown, or buff colony. Crater formation with radial grooves may be produced. Microconidia may be seen regularly. Diagnosis is confirmed by the fact that cultures grow poorly or not at all without thiamine.

T. mentagrophytes. Cultural growth is velvety or granular or fluffy, flat or furrowed, light buff, white, or sometimes pink. The back of the culture can vary from buff to dark red. Round microconidia borne laterally and in clusters confirm the diagnosis within 2 weeks. Spirals are sometimes present, and macroconidia may be seen.

T. verrucosum. Growth is slow and cannot be observed well for at least 3 weeks. The colony is compact, glassy, velvety, heaped or furrowed, and usually white, but may be yellow or gray. Chlamydospores are present in early cultures, and microconidia may be seen.

M. audouinii. The gross appearance of the culture shows a slowly growing, matted, velvety, light brown colony, the back of which is reddish brown to orange. Under the

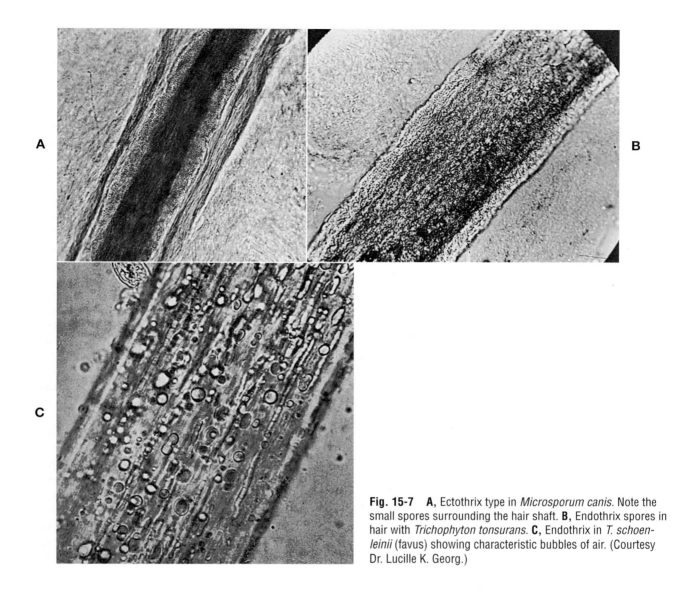

Fig. 15-7 A, Ectothrix type in *Microsporum canis.* Note the small spores surrounding the hair shaft. **B,** Endothrix spores in hair with *Trichophyton tonsurans.* **C,** Endothrix in *T. schoenleinii* (favus) showing characteristic bubbles of air. (Courtesy Dr. Lucille K. Georg.)

microscope a few large multiseptate macroconidia (macroaleuriospores) are seen. Microconidia (microaleuriospores) in a lateral position on the hyphae are clavate. Racquet mycelium, chlamydospores, and pectinate hyphae are sometimes seen.

M. canis. The culture grossly shows profuse, fuzzy, cottony, aerial mycelia tending to become powdery in the center. The color is buff to light brown. The back of the colony is lemon to orange-yellow. There are numerous spindle-shaped multiseptate microconidia and thick-walled macroconidia. Clavate microconidia are found along with chlamydospores and pectinate bodies.

Differential Diagnosis

Tinea capitis must at times be differentiated clinically from impetigo, pediculosis capitis, alopecia areata, atopic derma-

titis, psoriasis, seborrheic dermatitis, secondary syphilis, trichotillomania, lupus erythematosus, lichen planus, lichen simplex chronicus, and various inflammatory follicular conditions. Only uncommonly is ringworm of the scalp observed in patients older than age 15, and although favus can occur in adult life, it is more frequent in childhood. Alopecia areata, seborrheic dermatitis, atopic dermatitis, psoriasis, lichen planus, and other inflammatory follicular conditions can occur at any age. The distinctive clinical features of tinea capitis are broken-off stumps of hairs, usually in rounded erythematous patches in which there are crusts or pustules and few hairs. The broken-off hairs are loose and when examined are found to be surrounded by, or contain, the fungus.

In alopecia areata the affected patches are bald, and the skin is smooth and shiny without any signs of inflammation or scaling. Stumps of broken-off hairs are infrequently found, and no fungi are demonstrable. In seborrheic dermatitis the involved areas are covered by fine, dry, or greasy scales. Atopic dermatitis is rarely associated with localized scalp involvement, and clinical examination frequently reveals more typical generalized findings. In psoriasis, well-demarcated, sometimes diffuse, areas of erythema and white or silver scaling are noted. Lichen simplex chronicus frequently is localized to the inferior margin of the occipital scalp. In trichotillomania, as in alopecia areata, inflammation and scaling are absent. Circumscribed lesions are very rare. Serologic testing, scalp biopsies, and immunofluorescent studies may be indicated if the alopecia of secondary syphilis or lupus erythematosus is a serious consideration.

Treatment

Griseofulvin of ultramicronized form, 10 mg/kg/day, is the daily dose recommended for children. Grifulvin V is the only oral suspension available for children unable to swallow tablets. The dose is 20 mg/kg/day. Treatment should continue for 2 to 4 months, or for at least 2 weeks after negative microscopic and culture examinations are obtained. Griseofulvin does not primarily affect the delayed type hypersensitivity reaction responsible for the inflammation in kerion. For this, systemic steroids, to minimize scarring, can be given concomitantly with the griseofulvin.

Numerous clinical trials exist that demonstrate the effectiveness of other oral agents, such as itraconazole, terbinafine, and fluconazole. These studies show them to be excellent alternatives, but the total reported experience to date is low. As little as 20 days of fluconazole, 6 mg/kg/day in liquid or tablet form, produced a cure in one study. Krafchik et al showed that 2 weeks of terbinafine, 3 to 6 mg/kg/day, cured nearly all children with *Trichophyton* infections. Those with *Microsporum* species required an additional 2 weeks of therapy. Selenium sulfide shampoo or ketoconazole shampoo left on the scalp for 5 minutes three times weekly can be used as adjunctive therapy to oral antifungal agents.

Herbert recommends culture of family members, caution regarding the sharing of potentially contaminated fomites, and simultaneous treatment of all persons infected clinically or by culture. Drake et al recommend treating family members with ketoconazole shampoo, selenium sulfide shampoo, or povidone-iodine even if they are asymptomatic. Some advise keeping children out of school for a week or two, but we are not among them.

Prognosis

Recurrence usually does not take place when adequate amounts of griseofulvin, fluconazole, or terbinafine have been taken. As Herbert points out, exposure to infected persons, asymptomatic carriers, or contaminated fomites will increase the relapse rate. Without medication there is spontaneous clearing at about age 15, except with *T. tonsurans*, which persists into adult life.

DERMATOPHYTID

A generalized or localized skin reaction to fungal antigen is an "id" reaction, associated with some of the common dermatophytoses of the scalp, feet, and other sites. The primary site of infection is usually acutely inflamed, manifesting such lesions as kerion or bullous tinea pedis. The most common type of "id" reaction is seen on the hands and sides of the fingers when there is an acute fungus infection of the feet. These lesions are mostly vesicular and are extremely pruritic and even tender (Fig. 15-8). Secondary bacterial infection may occur; however, fungus is not demonstrable and should not be if it is a true dermatophytid. The onset is at times accompanied by fever, anorexia, generalized adenopathy, spleen enlargement, and leukocytosis. The dermatophytid may be an acute widespread eruption, usually follicular and lichenoid or decidedly scaly. The lesions are chiefly on the trunk, where there are pinhead-sized acuminate or flat-topped lichenoid papules, which are often grouped to form rings or scaly patches. Rarely, the eruption may be morbilliform or scarlatiniform. This type of reaction is seen occasionally in tinea capitis with or without kerion reactions.

The histologic picture is characterized by spongiotic vesicles and a superficial, perivascular, predominantly lymphohistiocytic infiltrate. Eosinophils may be present.

Other reactive patterns have been noted, with speculation as to their true nature. These reactions may be in the form of erythema nodosum; erythema annulare centrifugum; migratory thrombophlebitis; erysipelas-like reaction, especially of the shin; and urticaria. However, very few of these eruptions occur secondary to a dermatophytosis. More commonly they are either idiopathic, or are reactions to drugs, carcinoma, or bacterial infections.

The erysipelas-like dermatophytid is most commonly seen on the shin, where it appears as an elevated, sharply defined, erysipelas-like plaque about the size of the hand, usually with toe web tinea on the same side. It responds promptly to systemic steroids.

Diagnosis of a dermatophytid reaction is dependent on the demonstration of a fungus at some site remote from the suspect lesions of the dermatophytid, the absence of fungus in the "id" lesion, and involution of the lesion as the fungal infection subsides.

TINEA BARBAE

Synonyms: Tinea sycosis, barber's itch

Ringworm of the beard is not a common disease. It occurs chiefly among those in agricultural pursuits, especially those in contact with farm animals. The involve-

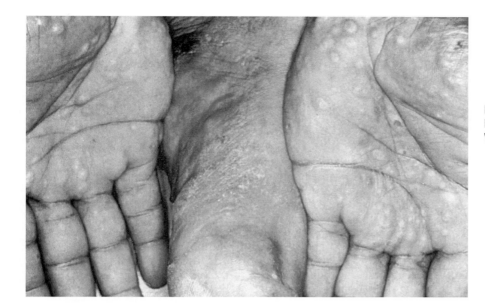

Fig. 15-8 Dermatophytid caused by bullous tinea pedis. (Courtesy Dr. Axel W. Hoke.)

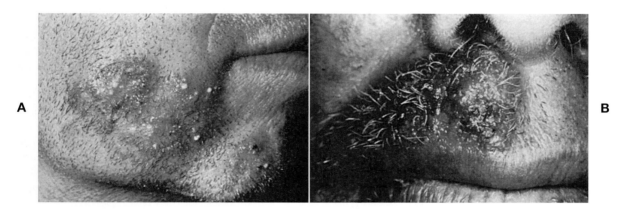

A   B

Fig. 15-9 **A** and **B,** Tinea barbae caused by *Trichophyton mentagrophytes.*

ment is mostly one-sided on the neck or face. Two clinical types are distinguished: deep, nodular, suppurative lesions; and superficial, crusted, partially bald patches with folliculitis.

The deep type develops slowly and produces nodular thickenings and kerion-like swellings, usually caused by *T. mentagrophytes* or *T. verrucosum.* As a rule the swellings are confluent and form diffuse boggy infiltrations with abscesses (Fig. 15-9). The overlying skin is inflamed, the hairs are loose or absent, and pus may be expressed through the remaining follicular openings. Generally, the lesions are limited to one part of the face or neck in men. The upper lip is not usually involved, although the mustache area may occasionally be the site of tinea barbae. The superficial crusted type causes mild pustular folliculitis with broken-off hairs *(T. violaceum)* or without broken-off hairs *(T. rubrum)* (Fig. 15-10). The

hairs affected are generally loose, dry, and brittle, and when extracted the bulb appears intact.

Diagnosis

The clinical diagnosis is confirmed by the microscopic findings of the fungus and by standard culture techniques for dermatophyte infections. Rarely, *Epidermophyton floccosum* may cause widespread verrucous lesions known as *verrucous epidermophytosis* (Fig. 15-11).

Differential Diagnosis

Tinea barbae differs from sycosis vulgaris by usually sparing the upper lip, and by often being unilateral. In sycosis vulgaris the lesions are pustules and papules, pierced in the center by a hair, which is loose and easily extracted after suppuration has occurred. Contact dermatitis and herpes infections are important differential diagnostic

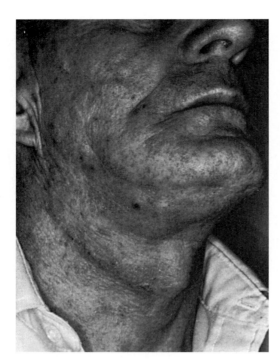

Fig. 15-10 Tinea on the face and neck. Note arcuate margin.

considerations. Careful history, patch testing, and appropriate cultures will resolve such possibilities.

Treatment

Like tinea capitis, oral antifungal agents are required to cure tinea barbae. Topical agents may be used for adjunctive therapy. Micronized or ultramicronized griseofulvin orally in a dosage of 500 to 1000 mg or 350 to 700 mg, respectively, daily for adults will usually cure tinea barbae in 4 to 6 weeks. Oral ketoconazole, fluconazole, itraconazole, and terbinafine have also been effective. Topical antifungals, such as miconazole, clotrimazole, oxiconazole, sulconazole, econazole, ketoconazole, naftifine, terbinafine, or ciclopirox olamine, should be applied from the beginning of treatment. The affected parts should be bathed thoroughly in soap and water, and the healthy areas that are not epilated may be shaved or clipped. When kerion is present a short course of systemic steroid therapy may help reduce inflammation and the risk of scarring.

TINEA FACIEI

Fungal infection of the face (apart from the beard) is frequently misdiagnosed, since the typical ringworm is only uncommonly seen on the face. Instead, erythematous, slightly scaling, indistinct borders are usually seen. The diagnosis is easily established by direct microscopic examination.

Most frequently tinea of the face is mistaken for seborrheic dermatitis, contact dermatitis, lupus erythemato-

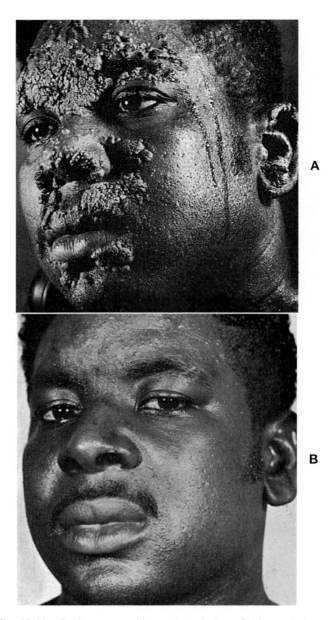

Fig. 15-11 **A,** Verrucous epidermophytosis from *Epidermophyton floccosum*. **B,** Complete involution after 48 days of griseofulvin therapy. (Courtesy Department of Dermatology, University of Miami Medical School.)

sus, or a photosensitive dermatosis, until the lack of response to various medication makes one think of fungal infection. Usually the infection is caused by *T. rubrum*, *T. mentagrophytes*, or *M. canis* (Fig. 15-12). Tinea faciei caused by *M. nanum* has been described in hog farmers and should be considered an occupational source.

Topical applications of clotrimazole, naftifine, miconazole, ciclopirox olamine cream, econazole, oxiconazole, ketoconazole, sulconazole, or terbinafine usually bring about a prompt response. Oral griseofulvin administered for

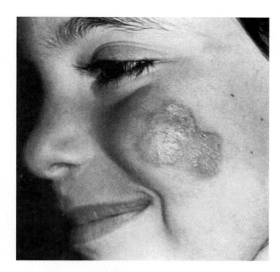

Fig. 15-12   Tinea faciei *(Microsporum canis)* in a child.

2 to 4 weeks, as well as fluconazole, itraconazole, or terbinafine, are all effective particularly in combination with topical therapy.

TINEA CORPORIS (TINEA CIRCINATA)

Tinea corporis includes all superficial dermatophyte infections of the skin other than those involving the scalp, beard, face, hands, feet, and groin. Sites of predilection are the neck, upper and lower extremities, and trunk. It can be caused by any of the dermatophytes. This form of ringworm is characterized by one or more circular, sharply circumscribed, slightly erythematous, dry, scaly, usually hypopigmented patches (Fig. 15-13). These lesions may be slightly elevated, particularly at the border, where they are more inflamed and scaly than at the central part (Fig. 15-14). Progressive central clearing produces annular outlines that give them the name "ringworm." These lesions may widen to form rings many centimeters in diameter. In some cases concentric circles form rings on one another, making intricate patterns (tinea imbricata). Multiple disseminated patches of both dry (macular) (Fig. 15-15) and moist (vesicular) types of tinea circinata are encountered in which most of the skin surface may be involved. Widespread tinea corporis may be the presenting sign of AIDS.

Histopathology

Rarely, the question of microscopic pathology may arise—rarely, because there are better ways to make the diagnosis than by histopathology. But if compact orthokeratosis is found in a section, a search should be made for fungal hyphae stained with hematoxylin. This is diagnostic.

Etiology

Various organisms may cause this type of fungal infection. *Microsporum canis, T. rubrum,* and *T. mentagrophytes* are

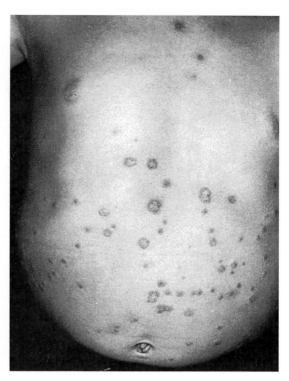

Fig. 15-13   Tinea corporis in a child, caused by *Microsporum canis.*

frequently the causative organisms. *T. tonsurans* has experienced a dramatic rise as a cause of tinea corporis, as it has done for tinea capitis. *T. rubrum* is the most common dermatophyte in the United States and worldwide. In children, *M. canis* is the cause of the moist type of tinea circinata. Other causative organisms and their characteristic skin manifestations will be discussed under other forms of tinea corporis

Epidemiology

Tinea corporis is frequently seen in children, particularly those who are exposed to animals with ringworm *(M. canis),* especially cats, dogs, and less commonly, horses and cattle. In adults, excessive perspiration is the most common predisposing factor. The incidence is especially high in hot, humid areas of the world.

Diagnosis

The diagnosis is relatively easily made by finding the fungus under the microscope in skin scrapings. In addition, skin scrapings can be cultured on a suitable medium. Growth of the fungus on culture medium is apparent within a week or two at most and, in most instances, is identifiable by the gross appearance of the culture. Identification of the fungus is of epidemiologic interest, and is not helpful in managing the infection.

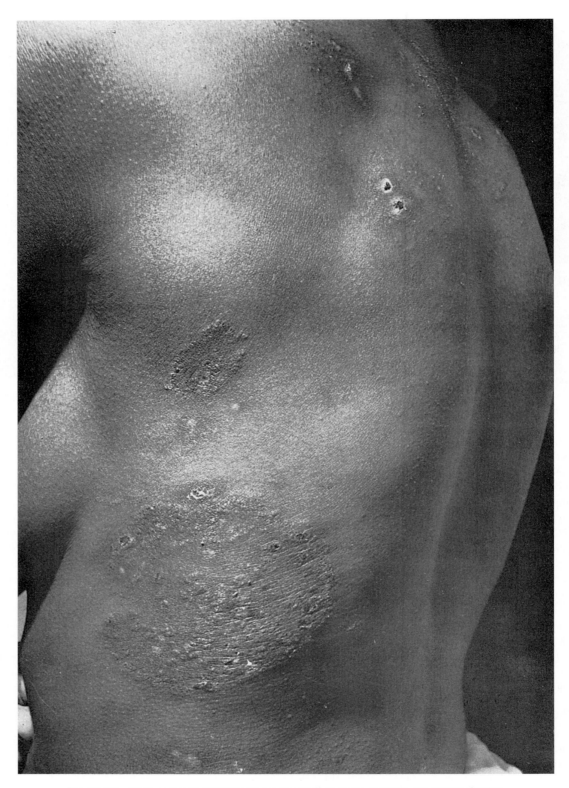

Fig. 15-14 Tinea corporis *(Trichophyton rubrum).* Note sharp margins and central clearing.

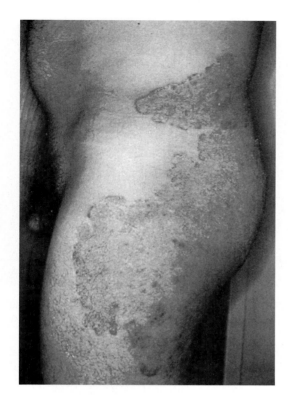

Fig. 15-15 *Trichophyton rubrum* infection of an American soldier in Vietnam.

It is best not to rely solely on cultures. Indeed, cultures are most useful when, having been performed on lesions thought surely to be nonfungal, they surprise the physician by being positive. Sterile cultures are frequently found in fungal lesions. Other diseases that may closely resemble tinea corporis are pityriasis rosea, impetigo, nummular dermatitis, secondary and tertiary syphilids, seborrheic dermatitis, and psoriasis.

Treatment

Extensive disease may require systemic antifungal treatment. When tinea corporis is caused by *T. tonsurans, M. canis, T. mentagrophytes,* or *T. rubrum,* griseofulvin, terbinafine, itraconazole, and fluconazole are all effective. The ultra-micronized form (Fulvicin P/G, Grisactin Ultra, or GrisPEG) is standard therapy, and the usual dose is 350 to 750 mg once daily for 4 to 6 weeks. This dose may be increased to twice daily if necessary. Approximately 10% of individuals will experience nausea with griseofulvin. These persons should stop therapy for 3 or 4 days and then resume to ascertain whether this pause will circumvent the unfavorable reactions. Other toxic reactions to griseofulvin are rare. However, headache, gastric upset, and infrequent and unusual skin eruptions with photosensitivity, glossitis, and stomatitis have been reported.

Absorption of griseofulvin in children is improved when given with milk. Effective blood levels occur at doses of 20 mg/kg/day, with milk.

Terbinafine, itraconazole, and fluconazole are systemic therapies for which published experience is less; however, they appear to be effective, with a shorter course of treatment. Their safety profiles are reviewed on p. 359. Terbinafine at 250 mg daily for 2 weeks; itraconazole, 200 mg twice daily for 1 week; and fluconazole, 150 mg once a week for 4 weeks, seem to be effective doses.

When only one or two patches occur, topical treatment is sufficient. Sulconazole (Exelderm), oxiconazole (Oxistat), miconazole (Monistat cream or lotion, or Micatin cream), clotrimazole (Lotrimin or Mycelex cream), econazole (Spectazole), naftifine (Naftin), ketoconazole (Nizoral), ciclopirox olamine (Loprox), terbinafine (Lamisil), and butenafine (Mentax) are currently available and effective. Most treatment times are between 2 to 4 weeks with twice daily use. Econazole, ketoconazole, oxiconazole, and terbinafine may be used once daily. With terbinafine the course can be shortened to 1 week. Creams are more effective than lotions. Sulconazole may be less irritating in folded areas. Castellani paint (which is colorless if made without fuchsin) is very effective. Salicylic acid 3% to 5% with precipitated sulfur 5%, or half-strength Whitfield's ointment, both standbys 30 years ago, are little used today. The addition of a low-potency steroid cream during the initial 3 to 5 days of therapy will decrease irritation rapidly without compromising the effectiveness of the antifungal.

OTHER FORMS OF TINEA CORPORIS
Trichophytic Granuloma (Perifollicular Granuloma, Majocchi's Granuloma, Tinea Incognito)

Occasionally a deep, pustular type of tinea circinata resembling a carbuncle or kerion is observed on the glabrous skin. It is a circumscribed, annular, raised, crusty, and boggy granuloma in which the follicles are distended with viscid purulent material (Fig. 15-16). These occur most frequently on the shins or wrists. This type of lesion is a perifollicular granuloma caused most often by *T. rubrum* or *T. mentagrophytes* infecting hairs at the site of involvement, but other dermatophytes have been reported (*T. epilans, T. violaceum, M. audouinii, M. gypseum, M. ferrugineum,* and *M. canis*). In immunosuppressed patients the lesions may be deep and nodular. Early in its course, such a deep lesion may be a pale, circular edematous plaque, often KOH- and culture-negative.

Majocchi's granuloma occurs naturally in situations of occlusion or may be related to superficial trauma, such as shaving. Diagnosis is made by demonstration of the fungus by direct microscopic potassium hydroxide slide and by culture or by clinical suspicion. Occasionally the diagnosis is made on a biopsy specimen.

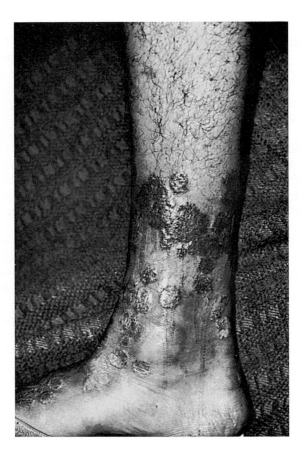

Fig. 15-16 *Trichophyton mentagrophytes* infection on lower leg of American soldier in Vietnam. (Courtesy Profs. H. Blank, D. Taplin and N. Zaias.)

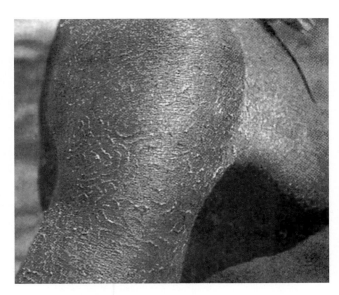

Fig. 15-17 Tinea imbricata in New Guinea native. (Courtesy Dr. J.C. Belisario.)

filaments that branch dichotomously. Polyhedral spores are also present.

The treatment of choice is griseofulvin, given in the same manner as for tinea corporis; terbinafine, fluconazole, and itraconazole should also be effective. There is a tendency for recurrence or reinfection when treatment is stopped. It may be necessary to give several courses of therapy and to remove the patient from the hot, humid environment.

TINEA CRURIS
Synonyms: Jock itch, crotch itch

Tinea cruris occurs most frequently in men on the upper and inner surfaces of the thighs, especially during the hot summer if the humidity is high (Fig. 15-18). It begins as a small erythematous and scaling or vesicular and crusted patch that spreads peripherally and partly clears in the center, so that the patch is characterized chiefly by its curved, well-defined border, particularly on its lower edge. The border may have vesicles, pustules, or papules. It may extend downward on the thighs and backward on the perineum or about the anus. The penoscrotal fold or sides of the scrotum are seldom involved, and we have never seen involvement of the penis.

Etiology

Ringworm of the groin usually is caused by *T. rubrum*, *T. mentagrophytes*, or *E. floccosum*. Infection with *Candida albicans* may closely mimic tinea cruris; the most useful distinguishing features it possesses are the regular occur-

Treatment is the same as for tinea corporis, except that even for localized lesions oral therapy is necessary.

Tinea Imbricata (Tokelau)

Tinea imbricata is a superficial fungal infection limited to southwest Polynesia, Melanesia, Southeast Asia, India, and Central America. It is characterized by concentric rings of scales forming extensive patches with polycyclic borders. The eruption begins with one or several small, rounded macules on the trunk and arms. The small macular patch splits in the center and forms large, flaky scales attached at the periphery. As the resultant ring spreads peripherally, another brownish macule appears in the center and undergoes the process of splitting and peripheral extension. This is repeated over and over again. When fully developed the eruption is characterized by concentrically arranged rings or parallel undulating lines of scales overlapping each other like shingles on a roof (*imbrex* means shingle) (Fig. 15-17).

The causative fungus is *T. concentricum*. Microscopically, the scrapings show interlacing, septate, mycelial

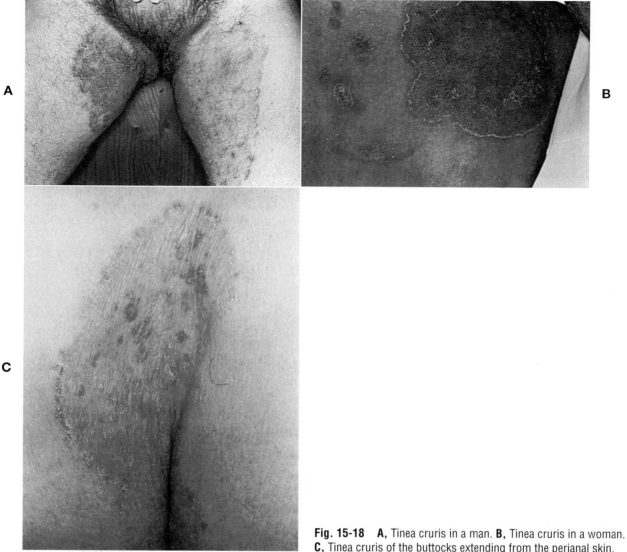

Fig. 15-18 **A,** Tinea cruris in a man. **B,** Tinea cruris in a woman. **C,** Tinea cruris of the buttocks extending from the perianal skin.

rence of small "daughter" macules, centrally desquamating to form collarette scales, and satellite pustules, scattered along the periphery of the main macule.

Epidemiology

Heat and high humidity are the predisposing factors for the development of tinea cruris. Tight jockey shorts, which prevent evaporation of the increased perspiration produced during warm weather, may be an additional predisposing factor.

Differential Diagnosis

The crural region is not only a common site for tinea cruris infections but also for erythrasma, seborrheic dermatitis, pemphigus vegetans, and intertriginous psoriasis. Erythrasma is diagnosed by the Wood's light examination,

which produces coral red fluorescence. When this fluorescence is found in the groin, examination should also be made of the axillae and the interdigital spaces of the toes, especially the fourth interspace. Demonstration of fungus by potassium hydroxide microscopic examination and culture establishes the diagnosis. As with dermatophytosis elsewhere, however, failure to demonstrate the fungus does not mean it is not there, and treatment should never be withheld in typical cases merely on this account.

Treatment

The reduction of perspiration and enhancement of evaporation from the crural area are important prophylactic measures. The area should be kept as dry as possible by the wearing of loose underclothing and trousers. Plain talcum powder or antifungal powders are helpful. Specific topical and oral treatment is the same as that described earlier for tinea corporis.

TINEA OF HANDS AND FEET

Dermatophytosis of the feet, long popularly called *athlete's foot,* is by far the most common fungal disease. The primary lesions often consist of maceration, slight scaling (Fig. 15-19), and occasional vesiculation (Fig. 15-20) and fissures between and under the toes. Any or all of the toe webs may be thus affected, although most often the third toe web is involved. The patient usually seeks relief because of itching or painful fissuring. If this condition is allowed to progress, there may be an overgrowth of gram-negative organisms.

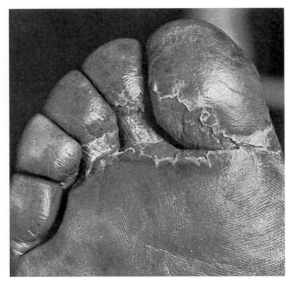

Fig. 15-19 Tinea pedis showing interdigital scalping *(Trichophyton mentagrophytes).*

This may eventuate in an ulcerative, exudative process involving the toe webs, and at times the entire soles. It is discussed in Chapter 14.

Trichophyton mentagrophytes produces an acutely inflammatory condition. If the fungus invades the skin of the toes or of the soles, an acute vesicular or bullous eruption may occur. The vesicular eruption tends to spread by extension and unless checked, may involve the entire sole (Fig. 15-21). The vesicles are usually about 2 or 3 mm in diameter. They sometimes coalesce to form bullae of various sizes (Fig. 15-22). They are firm to the touch and sometimes of a bluish tint. They do not rupture spontaneously but dry up as the acute stage subsides, leaving yellowish brown crusts. The burning and itching that accompany the formation of the vesicles may cause great discomfort, which is relieved by opening the tense vesicles. They contain a clear tenacious fluid of the consistency of glycerin. Extensive or acute eruptions on the soles may be incapacitating. The fissures between the toes, as well as the vesicles, may become secondarily infected with pyogenic cocci, which may lead to recurrent attacks of lymphangitis and inguinal adenitis.

Hyperhidrosis is frequently present in this type of dermatophytosis. The sweat between the toes and on the soles has a high pH, and keratin damp with it is a good culture medium for the fungi.

T. rubrum, which causes the majority of cases, produces a relatively noninflammatory type of dermatophytosis characterized by a dull erythema and pronounced scaling that may involve the entire sole and sides of the foot, giving a moccasin or sandal appearance (Fig. 15-23). The eruption may, however, be limited to a small patch adjacent to a fungus-infected toenail, or to a patch between or under the toes, on a hand, or other part. Most frequently the involvement is bilateral, but it may be limited to one hand and both feet, an observation that is still awaiting an

Fig. 15-20 Interdigital scaling with vesiculation caused by *Trichophyton mentagrophytes.*

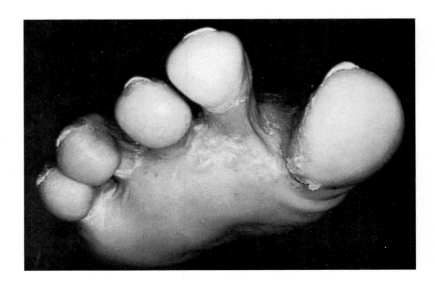

explanation. Sometimes an extensive, patchy, scaly eruption covers most of the trunk, buttocks, and extremities (Fig. 15-24). Rarely, there is a patchy hyperkeratosis resembling verrucous epidermal nevus.

Generally, tinea infection of the hands is of the dry, scaly,

and erythematous type that is suggestive of *T. rubrum* infection (Figs. 15-25 and 15-26). Other areas are frequently affected at the same time. However, the moist, vesicular, and eczematous type caused by *T. mentagrophytes,* which is seen more often on the feet, may at times occur on the hand. These two are the types of fungus involvement most frequently seen. Verrucous lesions on the hands resembling tuberculosis verrucosa cutis and caused by *T. rubrum* have been reported.

Occurring more frequently perhaps than true fungal infections, dermatophytid of the hands commonly begins with the appearance of groups of minute, clear vesicles on the palms and fingers. The itching may be intense. As a rule, both hands are involved and the eruption tends to be symmetrical; however, there are cases in which only one hand is affected.

Dermatophytosis of the hands is frequently difficult to differentiate from allergic contact or irritant dermatitis, especially occupational, or from pompholyx, atopic dermatitis, or psoriasis. It may also resemble lamellar dyshidrosis. Eczematoid or dyshidrotic lesions of unknown cause on the hands call for careful search for clinical evidence of dermatophytosis of the feet and microscopic or cultural study of suspected skin from the toe webs or nails. Although positive findings on the feet do not alone prove that the condition on the hands is dermatophytid, they do suggest a probable cause if no other findings are apparent. Negative findings do not rule out fungal causes. If the feet get well but the hands do not, the condition may be pompholyx, or psoriasis and therapeutic trials should be implemented with this in mind.

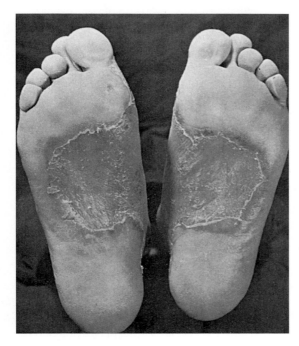

Fig. 15-21 Dermatophytosis of the soles *(Trichophyton mentagrophytes).* (Courtesy Dr. H. Shatin.)

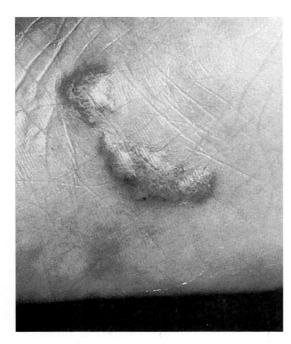

Fig. 15-22 Acute vesiculobullous eruption on sole caused by *Trichophyton mentagrophytes.*

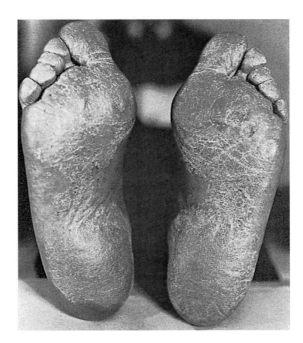

Fig. 15-23 Tinea pedis *(Trichophyton rubrum).* (Courtesy Dr. E. Florian, Budapest.)

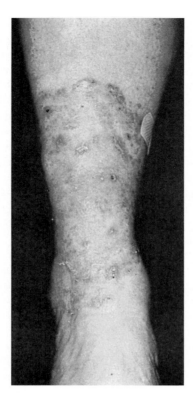

Fig. 15-24 *Trichophyton rubrum* infection of the lower leg.

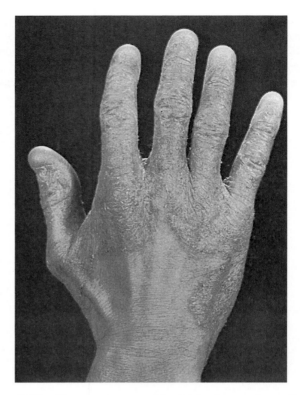

Fig. 15-26 Tinea manus caused by *Trichophyton rubrum*. Note severe involvement of nail beds and sharp, arcuate margins. (Courtesy Dr. H. Shatin.)

Etiology

T. rubrum is the most frequent causative fungus. Cultures of this organism are usually fluffy, but they can be granular or folded. The backside of the culture is usually deep red; sometimes no color is produced. Microconidia are found in clusters and singly on the hyphae. Macroconidia, chlamydospores, coils, and racquet hyphae are rarely seen. Less frequent causes are *T. mentagrophytes* and *E. floccosum*.

Diagnosis

Demonstration of the fungus by microscopic examination of the scrapings taken from the involved site establishes the diagnosis. In addition, cultures made from the affected skin establish the identity of the fungus. However, failure to find the fungus does not rule out a fungal cause.

Tissue for examination is scraped off and placed on a glass slide. When the lesion is a vesicle, it is clipped off close to the margin by small, pointed scissors; when dry or scaly, the material is scraped off with a scalpel or curet, an effort being made especially to obtain material from deep beneath the surface of chronic eruptions. A drop of a 10% to 20% solution of potassium hydroxide is added to the material on the glass slide. A coverslip is placed over the specimen and pressed down firmly. Gentle heat is applied until the scales are thoroughly macerated. It is then ready for

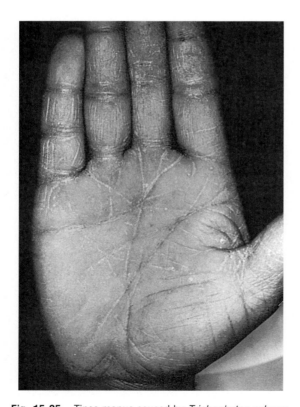

Fig. 15-25 Tinea manus caused by *Trichophyton rubrum*.

a thorough microscopic study. The mycelium may be seen under low power, but better observation of both hyphae and spores is obtained by the use of the high dry objective with reduced illumination (Fig. 15-27). The lines of juncture of normal epidermal cells are hyaloid and greenish, and may easily be mistaken for fungus structures. If you wonder whether it is really mycelium or not, it is not.

A rapid staining method using 100 mg of chlorazol black E dye in 10 ml of dimethyl sulfoxide (DMSO) and adding it to 5% aqueous solution of potassium hydroxide (KOH) can be helpful. The solution is then used in the same way as ordinary KOH solution, pressing coverglass and slide between pieces of filter paper. It is viewed under bright illumination; hyphae and spores are green against a gray background.

The other portion of the material is planted on Sabouraud's glucose agar or Mycosel agar, and cultured at room temperature. Adequate growth for identification occurs in 5 to 14 days, depending on the kind of fungus. Taplin et al have devised a culture medium, Dermatophyte Test Medium (DTM), for the diagnosis of dermatophytosis. The medium inhibits growth of bacterial and saprophytic contaminants. The alkaline metabolites of the dermatophytes change the color of the pH indicator in the medium from yellow to red, which distinguishes them from fungal contaminants and *Candida albicans*. If a dermatophyte is present, the medium will turn red. Saprophytes turn the medium green. *C. albicans* does not cause color changes, but produces a typical yeast colony.

Mosaic Fungus. In microscopic examination of the skin for fungi, one often finds the so-called mosaic fungus, which may closely resemble true hyphae. It is caused by overlapping cell borders (Fig. 15-28). A positive KOH preparation should reveal definite hyphal elements traversing several epidermal cells.

Prophylaxis

Hyperhidrosis is a predisposing factor. Because the disease often starts on the feet, the patient should be advised to dry the toes thoroughly after bathing. Dryness of the parts is essential if reinfection is to be avoided.

The use of a good antiseptic powder on the feet after bathing, particularly between the toes, is strongly advised for susceptible persons. Tolnaftate powder (Tinactin powder) or Zeasorb medicated powder are excellent dusting powders for the feet. Plain talc, cornstarch, or rice powder may be dusted into socks and shoes to keep the feet dry.

Treatment

Clotrimazole, miconazole, sulconazole, oxiconazole, ciclopirox, econazole, ketoconazole, naftifine, terbinafine, and butenafine are effective fungicides and pleasant to use. In severe disease with significant maceration wet dressings or soaks with solutions such as aluminum acetate, one part

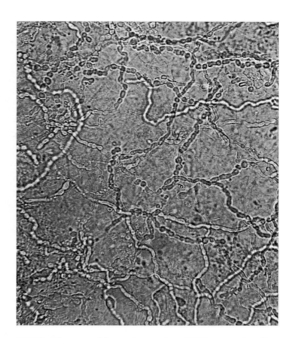

Fig. 15-27 Fungus filaments under KOH mount, direct examination.

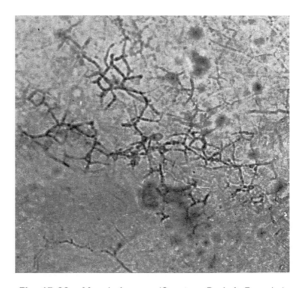

Fig. 15-28 Mosaic fungus. (Courtesy Dr. L.A. Fragola.)

to 20 parts of water are beneficial. The antiinflammatory effects of the corticosteroids are markedly beneficial. Topical antibiotic ointments, such as gentamicin (Garamycin), which are effective against gram-negative organisms, are helpful additions in the treatment of the moist type of interdigital lesions. In the ulcerative type of gram-negative toe web infections, systemic floxins are necessary. See Chapter 14 for a discussion on gram-negative toe web infections. Keratolytic agents, such as salicylic acid, lactic acid lotions, and Carmol are therapeutic when the fungus is

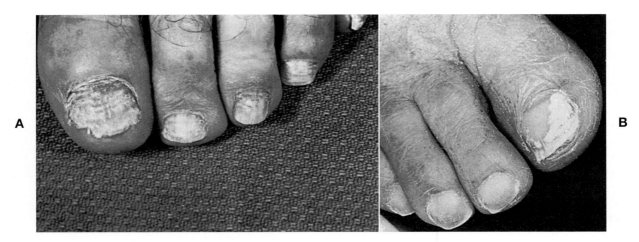

Fig. 15-29 A, Onychomycosis caused by *Trichophyton rubrum.* **B,** White superficial onychomycosis caused by *Trichophyton mentagrophytes.*

protected by a thick layer of overlying skin, such as that on the soles.

Treatment of fungal infection of the feet and hands with griseofulvin is effective when infection is caused by pathogens such as *T. mentagrophytes, T. rubrum, E. floccosum,* and others. However, it is not effective in the treatment of *C. albicans* infections. Griseofulvin is only effective against dermatophytes. When the infection is due to *T. mentagrophytes* the acute inflammatory reaction is not decreased by griseofulvin; addition of a potent topical steroid will help. Griseofulvin in ultramicronized particles is taken orally in doses of 350 to 750 mg daily. Dosage for children is 10 mg/kg/day. The period of therapy depends on the response of the lesions. Repeated KOH scrapings and cultures should be negative.

Recommended adult dosing for the newer oral antifungals is terbinafine, 250 mg/day for 2 weeks; itraconazole, 200 mg twice daily for 1 week; or fluconazole, 150 mg once weekly for 4 weeks.

Onychomycosis (Tinea Unguium). Onychomycosis is defined as the infection of the nail by fungus and represents up to 30% of diagnosed superficial fungal infections. Universally recognized as etiologic agents are species of *Epidermophyton, Microsporum,* and *Trichophyton* fungi, but it may also be caused by other dermatophytes, yeasts, and nondermatophytic molds. Nondermatophytic molds usually involve toenails and are rarely seen in fingernails.

Frequently, the clinical appearance of onychomycosis caused by one species of fungus is indistinguishable from that caused by any other species; however, there are various clinical clues that could allow one to speculate that an organism of a certain species is probably not responsible for a particular case of onychomycosis.

There are four classic types of onychomycosis. They are as follows:

1. Distal subungual onychomycosis: primarily involves the distal nail bed and the hyponychium, with secondary involvement of the underside of the nail plate of fingernails and toenails (Fig. 15-29, *A*).
2. White superficial onychomycosis (leukonychia trichophytica): this is an invasion of the toenail plate on the surface of the nail (Fig. 15-29, *B*). It is produced by *T. mentagrophytes,* species of *Cephalosporium* and *Aspergillus,* and *Fusarium oxysporum* fungi.
3. Proximal subungual onychomycosis: involves the nail plate mainly from the proximal nail fold, producing a specific clinical picture. It is produced by *T. rubrum* and *T. megninii,* and may be an indication of HIV infection.
4. Candidaonychomycosis involves all the nail plate. It is due to *Candida albicans* and is seen in patients with chronic mucocutaneous candidiasis (Fig. 15-30).

Onychomycosis caused by *T. rubrum* is usually a deep infection. The onset is slow and insidious, with little inflammatory reaction. The disease usually starts at the distal corner of the nail and involves the junction of the nail and its bed (Fig. 15-31). First a yellowish discoloration occurs, which may spread until the entire nail is affected. Beneath this discoloration the nail plate comes loose from the nail bed. Gradually the entire nail becomes brittle and separated from its bed as a result of the piling up of subungual keratin; it may break off, leaving an undermined remnant that is black and yellow from the dead nail and fungi that are present (Fig. 15-32). Fingernails and toenails present a similar appearance, and the skin of the toes or soles is likely also to be involved, with characteristic branny, scaling, erythematous, well-defined patches.

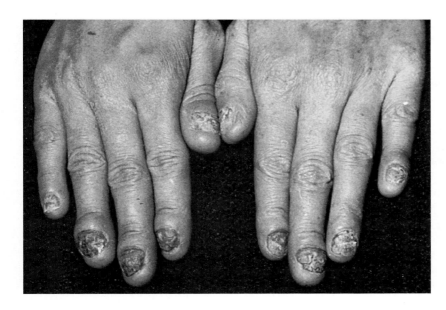

Fig. 15-30 Onychomycosis caused by *Candida albicans* in mucocutaneous candidiasis.

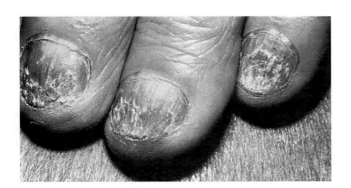

Fig. 15-31 Onychomycosis.

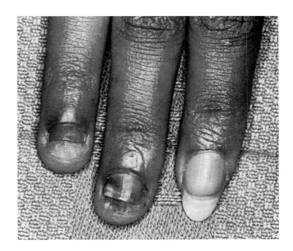

Fig. 15-32 Onychomycosis caused by *Trichophyton rubrum*.

Onychomycosis caused by *T. mentagrophytes* is usually superficial, and there is no paronychial inflammation. The infection generally begins with scaling of the nail under the overhanging cuticle and remains localized to a portion of the nail. In time, however, the entire nail plate may be involved. Leukonychia trichophytica is the name given to one type of superficial nail infection caused by this fungus in which small, chalky white spots appear on or in the nail plate. These may be multiple and variously shaped or just a single spot. They are so superficial that they may be easily shaved off.

However, white spots that resemble ordinary leukonychia may also occur, as Shelley and Wood showed, and they are an excellent "hunting ground" for hyphae lying well within the nail plate, so that overlying normal nail plate must be shaved away before a shaving of fungus-bearing nail plate can be removed.

In nail lesions caused by *C. albicans* there is usually paronychia. The disease begins under the lateral or proximal nail fold, and a small amount of pus may be expressed. The adjacent cuticle is pink, swollen, and tender on pressure. The neighboring portion of the nail becomes dark, ridged, and separated from its bed. Later the entire nail plate may separate. The fingernails are more commonly infected than the toenails; and it is encountered mostly in homemakers, canners, and others who have their hands in water a great deal. In a candidal infection the nail plate does not become friable, yellow, or white as in trichophyton infections, but remains hard and glossy as a normal nail plate unless immunocompromise is present. Associated paronychia is a characteristic feature.

Scopulariopsis brevicaulis has been infrequently isolated from onychomycosis. Infection usually begins at the lateral edge of the nail, burrows beneath the plate, and produces large quantities of cheesy debris.

Hendersonula toruloidea and *Scytalidium hyalinum* have been reported to cause onychomycosis, as well as a moccasin-type tinea pedis. In addition to the more common features of onychomycosis, such as nail plate thickening, opacification, and onycholysis, features of infection with these fungi include lateral nail invasion alone, paronychia, and transverse fracture of the proximal nail plate. When these agents are suspected, culture must be done with a medium that does not contain cycloheximide. Oral ketoconazole and griseofulvin are not effective in treatment.

In addition to the already mentioned causative fungi, *T. violaceum, T. schoenleinii,* and *T. tonsurans* occasionally invade the nails.

In an inexplicable way, fungal infection may affect only some of the nails and leave the others completely free of involvement. One hypothesis is that slower growing nails are more easily infected. Usually, onychomycosis is accompanied by infection in other sites. In tinea pedis, especially when the toe webs are affected, the nails may act as a reservoir from which reinfection may occur under proper environmental conditions. Infection of the great toenails is frequent in adults. Generally, there is only slight, or no, discomfort.

Diagnosis

The demonstration of fungus is made by microscopic examination and by culture. Immediate examination may be made if very thin shavings are taken from the diseased portion of the nail and heated gently for a minute or so in a drop of KOH solution—with or without chlorazol black E—under a coverglass. As the pieces of nail soften they may be pressed thin under the glass. The excess fluid should be removed by touching the sides of the coverglass with small squares of blotting paper. Similar thin shavings are inoculated into culture media such as Mycosel agar or DTM.

Differential Diagnosis

Numerous afflictions of the nails make a firm diagnosis of onychomycosis difficult unless fungi are actually demonstrated; therefore, great care should be exercised in the performance of the microscopic fungus examination. One is confronted most frequently with the fingernail problems of women. Allergic contact dermatitis caused by nail polish is exceedingly difficult to distinguish from onychomycosis; one must resort to repeated fungus examination. Recurrent contact urticaria to foods or other sensitizers among kitchen workers may give a clinical picture similar to chronic candidal paronychia. Psoriasis may involve one nail by only a slight pitting, or onycholysis, or by heaped-up subungual keratinization that eventually produces a moist, oozing mass that separates the nail from its bed. Psoriasis, however, typically begins in the middle of the free edge of the nail rather than in a corner, and may, pathognomonically, begin proximal to the free edge ("oil spots"). Lichen planus is exceedingly difficult to differentiate, and again demonstration of the fungus is essential. Both psoriasis and lichen planus usually show other areas of skin involvement. Various nail dystrophies, such as those seen in Darier's disease, Reiter's disease, and hyperkeratotic ("Norwegian") scabies, should also be kept in mind.

Treatment

Until the past few years pedal onychomycosis was considered by many to be incurable. The advent of new agents such as itraconazole, terbinafine, and fluconazole has revolutionized the approach to therapy. In addition to providing a broad spectrum of antifungal activity, these drugs appear in the nail plate within days of starting oral therapy and are incorporated within the nail matrix and nail bed. The duration of therapy has been reduced and the efficacy increased compared with older medications such as griseofulvin. Another truly remarkable achievement is the low risk-to-benefit ratio. These agents are much safer to use than ketoconazole and much more effective. Studies abound with treatment successes.

Terbinafine should be given at 250 mg/day for 6 weeks if treating the fingernails and for 12 weeks at the same dose when treating toenails. Itraconazole, 200 mg twice daily for 1 week of each month for 2 months when treating fingernails and for 3 months when treating toenails, appears effective. The experience with fluconazole is less well published to date, but 150 to 300 mg once weekly for 6 to 12 months appears to be effective dosing. The potential for drug interactions and monitoring is reviewed on p. 359.

For treatment with griseofulvin the therapy should be continued until the nails become clinically normal. For griseofulvin the recommended dose is 330 mg three times a day, with meals, for 4 to 6 months for fingernails and 10 to 18 months for toenails. Success rates are low, being 15% to 30% for toenails and 50% to 70% for fingernails. Griseofulvin does not treat nail disease caused by candida.

Assaf RR, et al: Intermittent fluconazole dosing in patients with onychomycosis. *J Am Acad Dermatol* 1996, 35:216.

Bronson DM, et al: An epidemic of infection with *Trichophyton tonsurans* revealed in a 20-year survey of fungal infections in Chicago. *J Am Acad Dermatol* 1983, 8:332.

Budimulja U, et al: A double-blind, randomized, stratified controlled study of the treatment of tinea imbricata with oral terbinafine or itraconazole. *Br J Dermatol* 1994, 130(Suppl):29.

Burke WA, et al: A simple stain for rapid office diagnosis of fungus infections of the skin. *Arch Dermatol* 1984, 120:1519.

Daniel CR III: Traditional management of onychomycosis. *J Am Acad Dermatol* 1996, 35:S21.

Drake LA, et al: Guidelines of care for superficial mycotic infections of the skin: onychomycosis. *J Am Acad Dermatol* 1996, 34:116.

Drake LA, et al: Guidelines of care for superficial mycotic infections of the skin: tinea capitis and tinea barbae. *J Am Acad Dermatol* 1996, 34:290.

Drake LA, et al: Guidelines of care for superficial mycotic infections of the skin: tinea corporis, tinea cruris, tinea faciei, tinea manuum, and pedis. *J Am Acad Dermatol* 1996, 34:282.

Eaglstein NF, et al: Gram-negative toeweb infection. *J Am Acad Dermatol* 1983, 8:225.

Elewski BE: Diagnostic techniques for confirming onychomycosis. *J Am Acad Dermatol* 1996, 35:S6.

Elewski BE: Treatment of tinea capitis. *J Am Acad Dermatol* 1999, 40:S27.

Elgart ML: Tinea incognito: an update on Majocchi granuloma. *Dermatol Clin* 1996, 14:51.

Galimberti R, et al: Onychomycosis treated with a short course of oral terbinafine. *Int J Dermatol* 1996, 35:374.

Gan VH, et al: Epidemiology and treatment of tinea capitis: ketoconazole vs. griseofulvin. *Pediatr Infect Dis J* 1987, 6:46.

Greenberg J, et al: Vein-donor-leg cellulitis after coronary artery bypass surgery. *Ann Intern Med* 1982, 97:565.

Greer DL, et al: A randomized trial to assess once-daily topical treatment of tinea corporis with butenafine, a new antifungal agent. *J Am Acad Dermatol* 1997, 37:231.

Greer DL, et al: Tinea pedis caused by *Hendersonula toruloidea*. *J Am Acad Dermatol* 1987, 16:1111.

Gupta AK, et al: Current management of onychomycosis. *Dermatol Clin* 1997, 15:121.

Gupta AK, et al: Itraconazole for the treatment of tinea pedis: a dosage of 400 mg/day given for 1 week is similar in efficacy to 100 or 200 mg/day given for 2 to 4 weeks. *J Am Acad Dermatol* 1997, 36:789.

Hanifin JM, et al: Itraconazole therapy for recalcitrant dermatophyte infections. *J Am Acad Dermatol* 1988, 18:1077.

Hay RJ, et al: Clinical features of superficial fungus infections caused by *Hendersonula toruloidea* and *Scytalidium hyalinum*. *Br J Dermatol* 1984, 110:677.

Hay RJ, et al: Tinea capitis in south-east London: a new pattern of infection with public health implications. *Br J Dermatol* 1996, 135:955.

Head ES, et al: The cotton swab technique for the culture of dermatophyte infections: its efficacy and merit. *J Am Acad Dermatol* 1984, 11:797.

Herbert AA: Tinea capitis. *Arch Dermatol* 1988, 124:1559.

Jacobs AH, et al: Tinea in tiny tots. *Am J Dis Child* 1986, 140:1034.

Jolly HW Jr, et al: A multicenter double-blind evaluation of ketoconazole in the treatment of dermatomycoses. *Cutis* 1983, 31:208.

Joly J, et al: Favus. *Arch Dermatol* 1978, 114:1647.

Kearse HL, et al: Tinea pedis in prepubertal children. *J Am Acad Dermatol* 1988, 19:619.

Keipert JA: Beneficial effect of corticosteroid therapy in *Microsporum canis* kerion. *Australas J Dermatol* 1984, 25:127.

Kemna ME, et al: A US epidemiologic survey of superficial fungal diseases. *J Am Acad Dermatol* 1996, 35:539.

Kligman AM, et al: Evaluation of ciclopirox olamine cream for tinea pedis. *Clin Ther* 1985, 7:409.

Krafchik B, et al: An open study of tinea capitis in 50 children treated with a 2-week course of oral terbinafine. *J Am Acad Dermatol* 1999, 41:60.

Lesher JL, et al: Oral therapy of common superficial fungal infections of the skin. *J Am Acad Dermatol* 1999, 40:S31.

Lewis JH, et al: Hepatic injury from ketoconazole. *Gastroenterology* 1984, 86:503.

McNeely W, et al: Butenafine. *Drugs* 1998, 55:405.

Mercurio MG, et al: Tinea capitis. *Pediatr Dermatol* 1998, 15:229.

Midgley G, et al: Mycology of nail disorders. *J Am Acad Dermatol* 1994, 31:S68.

Odom RB: New therapies for onychomycosis. *J Am Acad Dermatol* 1996, 35:S26.

Odom RB: Update on topical therapy for superficial fungal infections: focus on butenafine. *J Am Acad Dermatol* 1997, 36:S1.

Odom RB, et al: A multicenter, placebo-controlled, double-blind study of intermittent therapy with itraconazole for the treatment of onychomycosis of the fingernail. *J Am Acad Dermatol* 1997, 36:231.

Radentz WH, et al: Papular lesions in an immunocompromised patient: *Trichophyton rubrum* granulomas (Majocchi's granuloma). *Arch Dermatol* 1993, 129:1189.

Roberts DT: Oral therapeutic agents in fungal nail disease. *J Am Acad Dermatol* 1994, 31:S78.

Roller JA, et al: *Microsporum nanum* infection in hog farmers. *J Am Acad Dermatol* 1986, 15:935.

Rosen T, et al: Radiation port dermatophytosis. *J Am Acad Dermatol* 1988, 19:1053.

Rudolph AH: Diagnosis and treatment of tinea capitis due to *Trichophyton tonsurans*. *Int J Dermatol* 1985, 24:426.

Scher RR: Onychomyosis. *J Am Acad Dermatol* 1999, 40:S21.

Shelley WB, Wood MG: The white spot target for microscopic examination of the nails for fungi. *J Am Acad Dermatol* 1982, 6:92.

Smith KJ, et al: Majocchi's granuloma. *J Cutan Pathol* 1991, 18:28.

Taplin D, et al: Isolation and recognition of dermatophytes on a new medium (DTM). *Arch Dermatol* 1969, 99:203.

Tosti A, et al: Treatment of dermatophyte nail infections. *J Am Acad Dermatol* 1996, 34:595.

Vargo K, et al: Prevalence of undetected tinea capitis in household members of children with disease. *Pediatrics* 1993, 92:155.

Williams JV, et al: Semiquantitative study of tinea capitis and the asymptomatic carrier state in inner-city school children. *Pediatrics* 1995, 96:265. _____ ▲

CANDIDIASIS

Synonyms: Candidosis, moniliasis, thrush, oidiomycosis

Candida albicans may cause different types of lesions of the skin, nails, mucous membranes, and viscera. It may be a normal inhabitant at various sites until there is some change in the state of the area; then it becomes a pathogen.

The intertriginous areas are frequently affected. Here warmth, moisture, and maceration of the skin permit the organism to thrive. The areas most often involved are the perianal and inguinal folds, interdigital areas, nail folds, and axillae. There may be a generalized type in which not only most of the skin surface is involved but also the mucous membranes of the mouth and the gastrointestinal tract. Systemic forms may be superimposed on cutaneous candidiasis.

Candida proliferates in both budding and mycelial forms in the outer layers of the stratum corneum where the horny cells are desquamating. The organism usually is found outside the living portion of the epidermis. It does not attack the hair, rarely involves the nail, and is incapable of breaking up the stratum corneum.

It is important to remember that *C. albicans* is very largely an opportunistic organism, able to behave as a pathogen for the most part only in the presence of impaired immune response, or in body folds (inframammary, axillary, nail, intercrural-inguinal, preputial, or vulvovaginal). Moisture also promotes its growth, as in moist lip corners (perlèche).

Diagnosis

The demonstration of the pathogenic yeast *C. albicans* establishes the diagnosis. Under the microscope the KOH preparation may show spores and pseudomycelium (Fig. 15-33). On Gram stain the yeast forms are dense, gram-positive, ovoid bodies, 2 to 5 μm in diameter. In culture *C. albicans* should be differentiated from other forms of *Candida* that are only rarely pathogenic, such as *C. krusei, C. stellatoidea, C. tropicalis, C. pseudotropicalis,* and *C. guilliermondii.*

Culture on Sabouraud's glucose agar shows a growth of creamy, grayish, moist colonies in about 4 days. In time the colonies form small, rootlike penetrations into the agar. Microscopic examination of the colony shows clusters of budding cells. When inoculated into cornmeal agar culture, thick-walled, round chlamydospores characteristic of *C. albicans* are produced.

Topical Anticandidal Agents

Throughout this section references will be made to anticandidal topical therapy. These agents include, but are not limited to: clotrimazole (Lotrimin, Mycelex), econazole (Spectazole), ketoconazole (Nizoral), miconazole (Monistat-Derm Lotion, Micatin), oxiconazole (Oxistat), sulconazole (Exelderm), naftifine (Naftin), terconazole (vaginal candidiasis only), ciclopirox olamine (Loprox), butenafine (Mentax), nystatin, and topical amphotericin B lotion. Terbinafine (Lamisil) has been reported to be less active against *Candida* species by some authors. Studies have, however, confirmed the effectiveness of systemic terbinafine in the treatment of candidal nail infections and cutaneous candidosis. Zaias reported that topical terbinafine appeared to be as effective, if not more effective, than other anticandidal agents based on clinical outcomes.

Oral Candidiasis (Thrush). The mucous membrane of the mouth may be involved in the healthy newborn or the marasmic infant. In the newborn the infection may be acquired from contact with the vaginal tract of the mother. Grayish white membranous plaques are found on the surface of the mucous membrane. The base of these plaques is moist, reddish, and macerated. In its spread the angles of the mouth may become involved, and lesions in the intertriginous areas may occur, especially in marasmic infants. The diaper area is especially susceptible to this infection. Most of the intertriginous areas and even the exposed skin may be involved, with small pustules that quickly turn into macerated and erythematous scaling patches.

In adults the buccal mucosa (Fig. 15-34), lips (Fig. 15-35), and tongue may become involved. The papillae of the tongue are atrophied, the surface is smooth, glazed, and bright red. Sometimes there are small erosions on the edges. Frequently the infection extends onto the angles of the mouth to form perlèche. This is seen in elderly, debilitated,

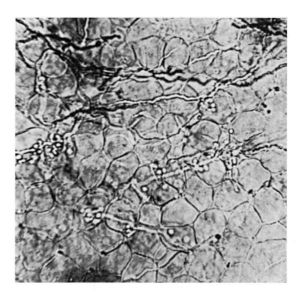

Fig. 15-33 Mycelium and spores of *Candida albicans* in a KOH mount of skin scrapings.

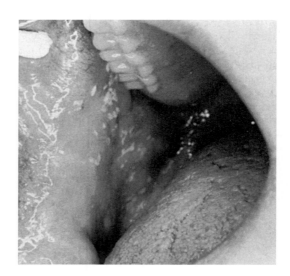

Fig. 15-34 Thrush.

and malnourished patients, and in patients with diabetes. It is often the first manifestation of AIDS, and is present in nearly all untreated patients with full-blown AIDS. The observation of oral "thrush" in an adult with no known predisposing factors warrants a search for other evidence of infection with the human immunodeficiency virus (HIV), such as lymphadenopathy, leukopenia, or HIV antibodies in the serum. One predisposing factor to oral thrush is broad-spectrum antibiotics.

During the 1980s there was a dramatic increase in the number and severity of cases of oropharyngeal candidiasis. According to the National Center for Health Statistics there was an increase of 4.7 times, from 0.34 to 1.6 cases per

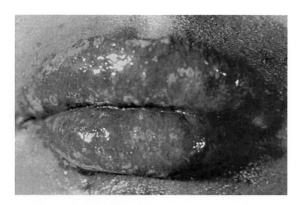

Fig. 15-35 Candidiasis of the lips.

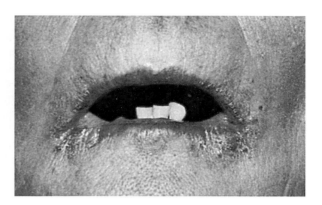

Fig. 15-36 Perlèche. *Candida albicans* was present.

1000 pediatric admissions, and the number of deaths among patients with oropharyngeal candidiasis increased fivefold. The greatest rate of increases, however, was among 15- to 44-year-old patients at thirteenfold. The rate of increase between 1985 and 1989 among patients with HIV infection was tenfold, compared with a twofold rate of increase among patients with malignancies or transplants. Oropharyngeal candidiasis is a modern disease with potentially life-threatening consequences.

Various treatment options are available. A baby with thrush may be allowed to suck on a clotrimazole suppository inserted into the slit tip of a pacifier four times a day for 2 or 3 days. An adult can let tablets of clotrimazole or Mycelex troches dissolve in the mouth. In immunocompromised patients, the goal is to reduce symptoms since continuous oral systemic therapy has led to a clinically relevant problem of drug resistance. Fluconazole, 100 to 200 mg/day for 5 to 10 days with doubling of the dose if it fails, or itraconazole, 200 mg daily for 5 to 10 days with doubling of the dose if it fails, are usually effective in reducing symptoms. Both are available in liquid forms.

Perlèche. Perlèche or, more aptly, angular cheilitis, is a maceration with transverse fissuring of the oral commissures. The earliest lesions are ill-defined, grayish white, thickened areas with slight erythema of the mucous membrane at the oral commissure (Fig. 15-36). When more fully developed this thickening has a bluish white or mother-of-pearl color and may be contiguous with a wedge-shaped erythematous scaling dermatitis of the skin portion of the commissure. Fissures, maceration, and crust formation ensue. Soft, pinhead-sized papules may appear. Involvement usually is bilateral. Perlèche is regarded as a symptom, analogous to intertrigo elsewhere, that may come from infection by *C. albicans* (the patient may also have paronychia or interdigital erosions), by coagulase-positive *Staphylococcus aureus,* or from manifold other causes. Although it has been regarded as an infectious disease,

similar changes may occur in riboflavin deficiency. Iron deficiency anemia may be present.

Identical fissuring occurs at the mucocutaneous junction from drooling in persons with malocclusion caused by ill-fitting dentures and in the aged in whom atrophy of the alveolar ridges, "closing" the bite, has caused the upper lip to overhang the lower at the commissures. There is sometimes a vertical shortening of the lower third of the face. Chernosky gives detailed instructions for measuring the face in the office to determine the degree of this shortening. Perlèche may commonly be seen also in children who lick their lips, drool, or suck their thumbs.

Treatment of perlèche depends on its cause. If due to *C. albicans,* anticandidal creams and lotions (see under topical anticandidal agents listed previously) are effective. Occasionally, diabetes complicates this disease, which will persist unless the diabetes is brought under control. It may be seen in AIDS patients with or without thrush. Antibiotic topical medications are used when there is bacterial infection. If the perlèche is due to vertical shortening of the lower third of the face, dental or oral surgical intervention may be helpful. Injection of collagen into the depressed sulcus at the oral commissure may be beneficial. Softform (Collagen Corporation) implants are a more permanent solution. In severe chronicity vegetative lesions with fissuring develop. These are best handled by the removal of the hyperkeratotic tissue by electrosurgery or a vaporizing laser.

Candidal Vulvovaginitis. *C. albicans* is a common inhabitant of the vaginal tract, and in some cases it may cause severe pruritus, irritation, and extreme burning. The labia may be erythematous, moist, and macerated and the cervix hyperemic, swollen, and eroded, showing small vesicles on its surface. The vaginal discharge is not usually profuse but is frequently thick and tenacious. Extreme hyperemia of the introitus is often present.

This type of infection may develop during pregnancy, in diabetes, or secondary to therapy with broad-spectrum antibiotics. Recurrent vulvovaginal candidiasis has also been associated with long-term tamoxifen treatment. Candidal balanitis may be present in an uncircumcised sexual partner (Fig. 15-37). If this is not recognized, repeated reinfection of a partner may result. Diagnosis is established by the clinical symptoms and findings as well as the demonstration of the fungus by KOH microscopic examination and culture.

Treatment for this common vulvovaginitis is often disappointing because of frequent recurrences. The male partner should be examined if recurrent disease is a problem. Oral fluconazole, 150 mg given once, is easy and effective. Fluconazole, 100 mg/day for 5 to 7 days, and itraconazole, 200 mg/day for 3 to 5 days, are alternatives. Topical options include miconazole (Monistat cream), nystatin vaginal suppositories or tablets (Mycostatin), or clotrimazole (Gyne-Lotrimin or Mycelex G) vaginal tablets inserted once daily for 7 days. The clotrimazole vaginal tablets may be used successfully by inserting 2 tablets at bedtime for 3 consecutive days. The anticandidal topicals (see earlier discussion) can be used if there is involvement of the introitus.

Candidal Intertrigo. The pruritic intertriginous eruptions caused by *C. albicans* may arise between the folds of the genitals; in groins or armpits; between the buttocks; under large, pendulous breasts; under overhanging abdominal folds; or in the umbilicus. The pinkish intertriginous moist patches are surrounded by a thin, overhanging fringe of somewhat macerated epidermis ("collarette" scale). Some eruptions in the inguinal region may resemble tinea cruris, but usually there is less scaliness and a greater tendency to fissuring. Persistent excoriation and subsequent lichenification and drying may, in the course of time, modify the original appearance. Often, tiny, superficial, white pustules are observed closely adjacent to the patches. Topical anticandidal preparations (see earlier discussion) are usually effective, but recurrence is common.

Pseudo Diaper Rash. In infants, *C. albicans* infection may gain a foothold on the skin in the diaper area, usually starting in the perianal region and spreading over the entire area. The dermatitis is enhanced by the maceration produced by the wet diapers. Scaly macules and vesicles with maceration in the involved areas cause burning, pruritus, and extreme discomfort. Diaper friction may also contribute to skin irritation and compromised function of the stratum corneum.

The diagnosis of candidiasis may be suspected by the finding of involvement of the folds and occurrence of many small erythematous desquamating "satellite" or "daughter" lesions scattered along the edges of the larger macules (Fig. 15-38), and is usually easily confirmed by direct KOH microscopic and culture examinations. *C. albicans* is more consistently demonstrable by culture than by direct exami-

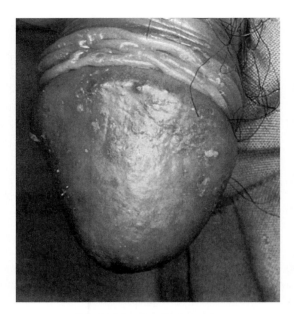

Fig. 15-37 *Candida* balanitis.

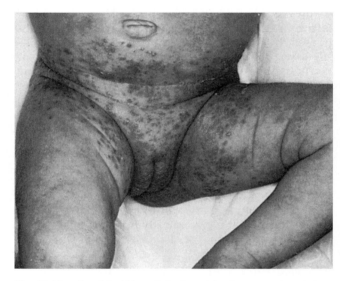

Fig. 15-38 *Candida albicans* infection of the diaper area in an infant. Note characteristic "satellite pustules" and involvement of the folds.

nation of smears. Swabbing is inadequate for making smears; one must scrape the surface to remove the horny material. The floor of opened pustules may be similarly scraped for specimens. However, such examinations are rarely needed.

Pierard-Franchimont et al showed a decrease in candidal cultures and skin irritation after use of a miconazole nitrate-containing paste for the prevention of diaper dermatitis. Pseudo diaper rash also responds well to topical antifungals (see earlier discussion) that cover *Candida* species.

Congenital Cutaneous Candidiasis. Infection of an infant during passage through a birth canal infected with *C. albicans* may lead to congenital cutaneous candidiasis. The eruption is usually noted within a few hours of delivery. Erythematous macules progress to thin-walled pustules, which rupture, dry, and desquamate within a week or so. Lesions are usually widespread, involving the trunk, neck, and head, and at times the palms and soles, including the nail folds. The oral cavity and diaper area are spared, in contrast to the usual type of acquired neonatal infection. The differential diagnosis includes other neonatal vesiculopustular disorders, such as listeriosis, syphilis, staphylococcal and herpes infections, erythema toxicum neonatorum, transient neonatal pustular melanosis, miliaria rubra, drug eruption, and congenital icthyosiform erythroderma. If suspected early the amniotic fluid, placenta, and cord should be examined for evidence of infection.

Infants with candidiasis limited to the skin have favorable outcomes; however, systemic involvement may occur. Disseminated infection is suggested by (1) evidence of respiratory distress or other laboratory or clinical signs of neonatal sepsis, (2) birth weight less than 1500 g, (3) treatment with broad-spectrum antibiotics, (4) extensive instrumentation during delivery or invasive procedures in the neonatal period, (5) positive systemic cultures, or (6) evidence of an altered immune response. Infants with congenital cutaneous candidiasis meeting any of these six criteria may be considered for systemic antifungal therapy. More than 16 cases of systemic disease have been reported, resulting in two deaths. Most did well with a combination of topical and oral antifungal therapy. For uncomplicated congenital cutaneous candidiasis topical anticandidal agents (see earlier discussion) are effective.

Perianal Candidiasis. When pruritus ani is present, *C. albicans* infection should be suspected. Frequently, the entire gastrointestinal tract is involved. This type of infection can be precipitated by oral antibiotic therapy. Perianal dermatitis with erythema, oozing, and maceration is present (Fig. 15-39). Pruritus and burning can be extremely severe.

A psychogenic component is more frequent as a cause of pruritus ani than is candidiasis. Furthermore, psoriasis, seborrheic dermatitis, streptococcal and staphylococcal infections, and contact dermatitis need to be considered in any form of perianal dermatitis. Extramammary Paget's disease has also been mistaken for a chronic fungal infection.

In addition to the use of fungicides, other measures are essential. Meticulous cleansing of the perianal region after bowel movement must be practiced. The use of topical corticosteroids and antipruritic medications such as hydroxyzine (Atarax) is helpful and may be indicated. The usual anticandidal imidazoles (see earlier discussion) are recommended for this infection.

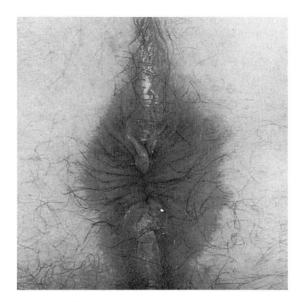

Fig. 15-39 Perianal candidiasis.

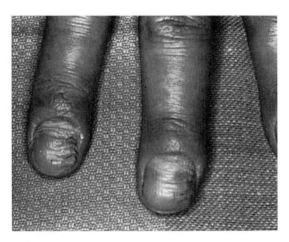

Fig. 15-40 Paronychial infection and onychodystrophy caused by *Candida albicans.*

Candidal Paronychia. Chronic inflammation of the nail fold produces occasional discharge of thin pus, cushionlike thickening of the paronychial tissue, slow erosion of the lateral borders of the nails, gradual thickening and brownish discoloration of the nail plates, and development of pronounced transverse ridges (Fig. 15-40). Mostly the fingernails only are affected, and frequently only one nail. Although usually a chronic disease, candida causing acute paronychia has been reported.

Chronic paronychia is caused by *C. albicans,* but at times there may be secondary mixed bacterial infection as well. Those whose hands are frequently in water or who handle moist objects are the prime sufferers from this type of disease; among them are food handlers; cooks; dishwashers; bartenders; nurses; canners, especially fruit canners using sugar syrup; and laundry workers. Repetitive contact urticaria to foods and spices may mimic candidal paronychia. Manicuring the nails sometimes is responsible for mechanical or chemical injuries that lead to this infection. Candidiasis is often present in chronic paronychia caused by an ingrown toenail.

Candidal paronychia is frequently seen in patients with diabetes, and one aspect of the treatment consists of bringing the diabetes under control. The avoidance of chronic exposure to moisture is also an important prophylactic measure. Oral fluconazole once weekly or itraconazole in pulse dosing should be effective, but published dosing recommendations are not available. Anticandidal lotions are probably preferable to creams and may also be effective, but therapy should be continued for 2 to 3 months to prevent recurrence.

Erosio Interdigitalis Blastomycetica.
This form of candidiasis is seen as an oval-shaped area of macerated white skin on the web between and extending onto the sides of the fingers. Usually at the center of the lesion there are one or more fissures with raw, red bases; as the condition progresses the macerated skin peels off, leaving a painful, raw, denuded area surrounded by a collar of overhanging white epidermis (Fig. 15-41). It is nearly always the third web, between the middle and ring fingers, that is affected. The moisture beneath the rings macerates the skin and predisposes to infection. The disease is also seen in patients

with diabetes, those who do housework, launderers, and others whose skin is exposed to the macerating effects of water and strong alkalis.

Intertriginous lesions between the toes are similar. Usually the white, sodden epidermis is thick and does not peel off freely. On the feet it is the fourth interspace that is most often involved, but the areas are apt to be multiple. Clinically, this may be indistinguishable from tinea pedis. Diagnosis is made by culture. Shroff et al reported 150 patients with cutaneous candidiasis in Bombay. The most common presentations were intertrigo (75), vulvovaginitis (19), and paronychia (17). Of interest was that 94 had histories of chronic water exposure, all of which had either erosio interdigitalis blastomycetica and/or paronychia. Diabetes was a predisposing factor in 22 patients. Treatment with topical anticandidal preparations (see earlier discussion) in cream or lotion is effective.

Chronic Mucocutaneous Candidiasis.
The term *chronic mucocutaneous candidiasis* designates a heterogeneous group of patients whose infection with *Candida* is chronic but superficial (Fig. 15-42). Onset is before age 6 as a rule; onset in adult life may herald the occurrence of thymoma. These cases may be either inherited or sporadic; in the inherited types endocrinopathy is often found. Most cases have well-defined limited defects of cell-mediated immunity. Oral lesions are diffuse (Fig. 15-43), and perlèche and lip fissures are common. The entire thickness of the nail

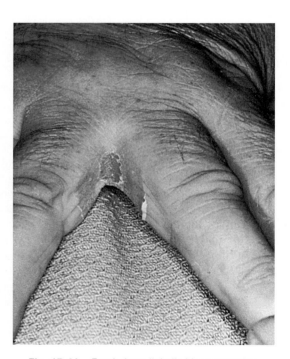

Fig. 15-41 Erosio interdigitalis blastomycetica.

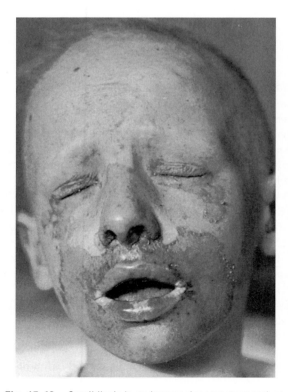

Fig. 15-42 Candidiasis in an immunoincompetent patient.

plates is invaded, and they become thickened and dystrophic. There is associated paronychia. Hyperkeratotic, horn-like, or granulomatous lesions are often seen (Figs. 15-44 and 15-45).

Systemic fluconazole, itraconazole, or ketoconazole is necessary and may need to be prolonged, repeated, and given at higher than the usual recommended dose. The management protocols vary, and experience is limited. In addition, cimetidine is worth trying. Using it, Jorizzo et al

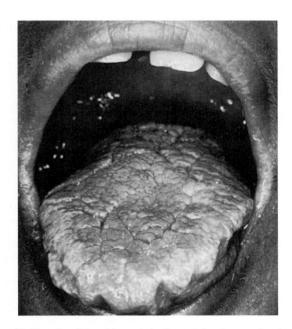

Fig. 15-43 *Candida albicans* infection of the tongue in chronic mucocutaneous candidiasis.

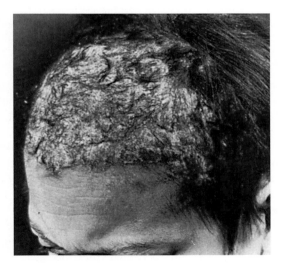

Fig. 15-44 Candidiasis of the scalp. The patient has generalized mucocutaneous candidiasis. Nevertheless, note the striking resemblance to rupial psoriasis.

restored deficient cell-mediated immunity in four adults from one family, at a dose of 300 mg four times a day.

Systemic Candidiasis. *Candida albicans* is capable of causing a severe, destructive, disseminated disease, invariably when host defenses are compromised. Those who are at high risk include patients with malignancies, especially leukemias and lymphomas, in which there may be impaired immune defenses; patients with AIDS; debilitated and malnourished patients; patients with transplants requiring immunosuppressive drugs for prolonged periods; patients receiving oral cortisone; patients who have had multiple surgical operations, especially cardiac surgery; patients with indwelling intravenous catheters; and heroin addicts.

The initial sign of systemic candidiasis may be any of a number of clinical findings such as fever of unknown origin, pulmonary infiltration, gastrointestinal bleeding, endocarditis, renal failure, meningitis, osteomyelitis, endophthalmitis, peritonitis, or a disseminated maculopapular exanthema. The cutaneous findings are erythematous macules that become papular, pustular, and hemorrhagic, and may progress to necrotic, ulcerating lesions resembling ecthyma gangrenosum. Deep abscesses may occur. The trunk and extremities are the usual sites of involvement. Proximal muscle tenderness is a common finding and may be a valuable clue to the correct diagnosis.

The demonstration of microorganisms or a positive culture will substantiate a diagnosis of candidiasis only if the microorganism is found in tissues or fluids ordinarily sterile for *Candida* and if the clinical picture is compatible. *Candida* colonization of endotracheal tubes used in supporting low–birth-weight neonates predisposes to systemic disease. If candida is cultured within the first week of life there is a high rate of systemic disease. There is a 50% chance of systemic disease if one or more cultures is positive.

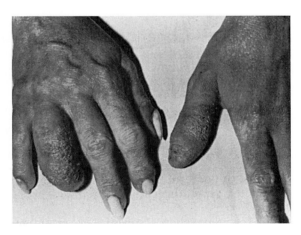

Fig. 15-45 Candidal granulomas on fingers and candidal onychomycosis in a 34-year-old woman with generalized candidiasis for 30 years. Successfully treated with amphotericin B.

The mortality attributed to systemic candidosis has declined from 80% in the 1970s to 40% in the 1990s, mainly because of early empiric antifungal treatment and better prophylaxis. Although amphotericin B is considered the mainstay of treatment in systemic candidiasis, other potentially safer options are available. Amphotericin B is now available in various lipid forms, which appear to be less toxic. Pahls et al have shown that these newer liposomal formulations, such as AmBisome (available in some countries), in in vitro studies has four to eight times less antifungal activity compared with the standard form. The therapeutic index of such agents must be tested clinically before their use can be recommended solely on toxicity data. Fluconazole has been shown effective as prophylaxis of bone marrow transplantation as well as in treatment of oropharyngeal candidosis and candidemia in nonneutropenic patients. More limited data are available for itraconazole, but preliminary reports are encouraging. Ketoconazole (Nizoral) is fungistatic, rather than fungicidal like amphotericin B, and though it is effective in mucocutaneous candidiasis, it is not effective in systemic candidiasis in immunocompromised hosts.

Candidid. As in dermatophytosis with trichophytid, immunologically mediated lesions called *candidids* may develop secondary to *C. albicans* infection. They are much less common than the reactions seen with acute inflammatory dermatophytosis. The reactions, which have been reported to clear with treatment of candidal infection, are usually of the erythema annulare centrifugum or chronic urticaria type.

Antibiotic (Iatrogenic) Candidiasis. The use of oral antibiotics, such as the tetracyclines and their related products, may induce clinical candidiasis involving the mouth, gastrointestinal tract, or perianal area. In addition, vulvovaginitis may occur. The most frequent complaint is severe pruritus ani.

It has been suggested that perhaps the bacterial flora in the gastrointestinal system is changed by suppression of some of the antibiotic-sensitive bacteria, thereby permitting other organisms such as *Candida* to flourish. Fluconazole, 150 mg once, will treat this adequately if antibiotic therapy is given for a limited time.

Bielsu I, et al: Systemic candidiasis in heroin abusers. *Int J Dermatol* 1987, 26:314.

Brennan B, et al: Overview of topical therapy for common superficial fungal infections and the role of new topical agents. *J Am Acad Dermatol* 1997, 36:S3.

Chapel TA, et al: Congenital cutaneous candidiasis. *J Am Acad Dermatol* 1982, 6:926.

Chernosky ME: Collagen implant in the management of perlèche. *J Am Acad Dermatol* 1985, 12:493.

Cosgrove BF, et al: Congenital cutaneous candidiasis associated with respiratory distress and elevation of liver function tests. *J Am Acad Dermatol* 1997, 37:817.

Crislip MA, et al: Candidiasis. *Infect Dis Clin North Am* 1989, 3:103.

Drake LA, et al: Guidelines of care for superficial mycotic infections of the skin: mucocutaneous candidiasis. *J Am Acad Dermatol* 1996, 34:110.

Epstein JB, et al: Oropharyngeal candidiasis. *Clin Ther* 1998, 20:40.

Fisher-Hoch SP, et al: Opportunistic candidiasis: an epidemic of the 1980s. *Clin Infect Dis* 1995, 21:897.

Gibney MD, et al: Cutaneous congenital candidiasis: a case report. *Pediatr Dermatol* 1995, 12:359.

Hay RJ: The management of superficial candidiasis. *J Am Acad Dermatol* 1999, 40:S35.

Held JL, et al: Use of touch preparation for rapid diagnosis of disseminated candidiasis. *J Am Acad Dermatol* 1988, 19:1063.

Honig P, et al: Amoxicillin and diaper dermatitis. *J Am Acad Dermatol* 1988, 19:275.

Jorizzo JC, et al: Cimetidine as an immunomodulator: chronic mucocutaneous candidiasis as a model. *Ann Intern Med* 1980, 92:192.

Jung EG, et al: Systemic treatment of skin candidosis: a randomized comparison of terbinafine and ketoconazole. *Mycoses* (Germany) 1994, 37:361.

Meunier F: Therapy of systemic candidiasis. *Mycoses* 1994, 34(Suppl):52.

Mobacken H, et al: Ketoconazole treatment of 13 patients with chronic mucocutaneous candidiasis. *Dermatologica* 1986, 173:229.

Montemarano AD, et al: Acute paronychia apparently caused by *Candida albicans* in a healthy female. *Arch Dermatol* 1993, 129:786.

Odds FC: Pathogenesis of *Candida* infections. *J Am Acad Dermatol* 1994, 31:S2.

Odom RB: Update on topical therapy for superficial fungal infections: focus on butenafine. *J Am Acad Dermatol* 1997, 36:S1.

Pahls S, et al: Comparison of the activity of free and liposomal amphotericin B in vitro and in a model of systemic and localized candidiasis. *J Infect Dis* 1994, 169:1057.

Pierard-Franchimont C, et al: Tribological and mycological consequences of the use of a miconazole nitrate-containing paste for the prevention of diaper dermatitis. *Eur J Pediatr* 1996, 155:756.

Segal R, et al: Treatment of *Candida* nail infection with terbinafine. *J Am Acad Dermatol* 1996, 35:958.

Shroff PS, et al: Clinical and mycological spectrum of cutaneous candidiasis in Bombay. *J Postgrad Med* (India) 1990, 36:83.

Tanenbaum L, et al: A new treatment for cutaneous candidiasis: sulconazole nitrate cream 1%. *Int J Dermatol* 1983, 22:318.

Waquespack-LaBiche J, et al: Disseminated congenital candidiasis in a premature infant. *Arch Dermatol* 1999, 135:510.

Zaias N: *Candida*: a review of clinical experience with Lamisil. *Dermatology* 1997, 194(Suppl):10. _____ ▲

GEOTRICHOSIS

Geotrichosis may produce symptoms of oral lesions of erythema, pseudomembranes, and mucopurulent sputum similar to that seen in thrush. The intestinal, bronchial, and pulmonary forms are similar to candidal infection. The etiologic agent, *Geotrichum candidum*, is considered to be a pathogen only when it is repeatedly found at a diseased site. Its mere presence in undiseased sites is probably only as a saprophyte. In nature it is frequently found on fruit, tomatoes, in soil, and in similar locations.

The diagnosis is made by the demonstration of the organism by KOH microscopic examination and by its culture from sputum on Sabouraud's dextrose agar. Direct examination shows branching septate mycelium and chains of rectangular cells. In culture there is a mealy growth at room temperature. The hyphae form rectangular arthrospores.

Treatment is with oral nystatin, potassium iodide, or mycostatin suspension in uncomplicated cases. For more severe or disseminated disease intravenous or colloidal amphotericin B or itraconazole have been effective in some cases.

Cofrancesco E, et al: Treatment of chronic disseminated *Geotrichum capitatum* infection with high cumulative dose of colloidal amphotericin B and itraconazole in a leukemia patient. *Mycoses* (Germany) 1995, 38:377.

Heinic GS, et al: Oral *Geotrichum candidum* infection associated with HIV infection: a case report. *Oral Surg Oral Med Oral Pathol* 1992, 73:726.

Mahul P, et al: Disseminated *Geotrichum capitatum* infection in a patient with acute myeloid leukemia. *Mycoses* (Germany) 1989, 32:573. ▲

TINEA NIGRA

This characteristic disorder manifests itself as one or several brown or black spots that resemble junction type nevi, melanoma, or silver nitrate or India ink stains, most frequently on the palms but also on the soles (Fig. 15-46). The patches are not elevated or scaly. The fungus can easily be demonstrated and cultured. In appearance young colonies are glossy, black, and yeastlike, but older colonies are filamentous and grayish. Groups or chains of conidia, resulting from sporulation of the saprophyte *Exophiala phaeoannellomyces* (formerly *werneckii*), produce a melanin-like pigment.

Topical imidazoles such as clotrimazole, miconazole, ketoconazole, sulconazole, and econazole are effective; griseofulvin is not. Simply shaving away the superficial epidermis with a No. 15 Bard-Parker blade is frequently beneficial.

Burke WA: Tinea nigra: treatment with topical ketoconazole. *Cutis* 1993, 52:209.

Sayegh-Carreno R, et al: Therapy of tinea nigra plantaris. *Int J Dermatol* 1989, 28:46. ▲

PIEDRA (TRICHOSPOROSIS)

In piedra, dark, pinhead-sized, gritty formations occur on the hairs of the scalp, brows, lashes, or beard. Minute, round or ovoid, hard nodules develop on the shaft of the hairs, not on the root (Figs. 15-47 and 15-48). These nodules are distributed irregularly along the length of the shaft and are easily felt by palpation when too small to be recognized without close scrutiny.

Two varieties exist. White piedra, caused by *Trichosporon beigelii* (transiently named *T. cutaneum*), occurs commonly in temperate climates. The nodes are composed of hyphae and arthrospores. The culture shows cream-colored, soft colonies composed of blastospores and septate hyphae, which fragment into arthrospores. Black piedra,

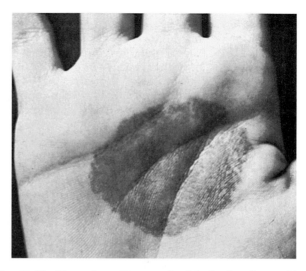

Fig. 15-46 Tinea nigra. (Courtesy Dr. A.L. Carrion, Puerto Rico.)

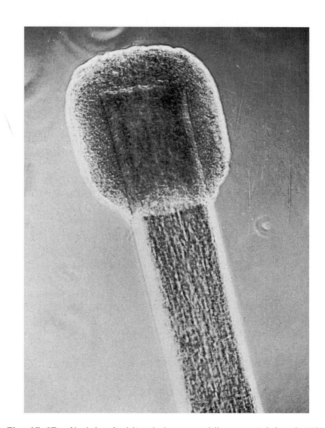

Fig. 15-47 Nodule of white piedra resembling a match head at the end of the hair shaft. (Courtesy Dr. A.T. Londero, Brazil.)

caused by *Piedraia hortai,* occurs mostly in the tropics. It is frequently found in Brazil, Colombia, and other South American countries and in the Orient, or wherever the climate combines high temperature with high humidity. The nodelike masses in KOH preparations show numerous oval

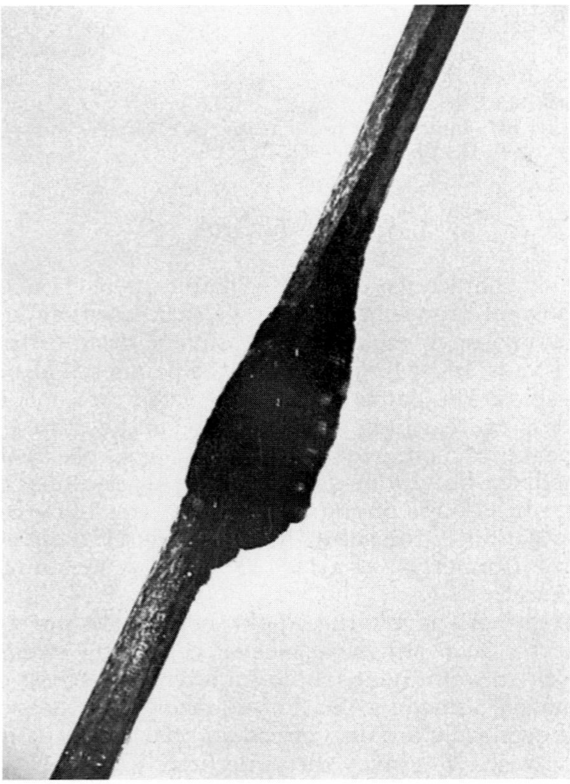

Fig. 15-48 Nodule of black piedra on hair shaft. (Courtesy Dr. A.T. Londero, Brazil.)

asci containing two to eight ascospores and mycelium. Cultures produce black colonies composed of hyphae and chlamydospores.

Treatment is by cutting the hair. Oral terbinafine (Lamisil), 250 mg daily for 6 weeks, has been shown effective against black piedra. For white piedra a variety of treatment options are available to include, but not excluding, imidazoles, ciclopirox olamine, 2% selenium sulfide, 6% precipitated sulfur in petrolatum, chlorhexidine solutions, castellani's paint, zinc pyrithione, amphotericin B lotion, and 2% to 10% glutaraldehyde. Spontaneous remissions were observed in some patients by Kalter et al. Rarely, deep invasion and systemic dissemination may occur in patients with leukemia or other forms of immunocompromise.

Drake LA, et al: Guidelines of care for superficial mycotic infections of the skin: piedra. *J Am Acad Dermatol* 1996, 34:122.

Gip L: Black piedra: the first case treated with terbinafine (Lamisil). *Br J Dermatol* 1994, 130:26.

Kalter DC, et al: Genital white piedra: epidemiology, microbiology, and therapy. *J Am Acad Dermatol* 1986, 14:982.

LeBlond V, et al: Systemic infections with *Trichosporon beigelii (cutaneum)*. *Cancer* 1986, 58:2399.

Otsuka F, et al: Facial granuloma associated with *Trichosporon cutaneum* infection. *Arch Dermatol* 1986, 122:1176.

Walsh TJ: Trichosporonosis. *Infect Dis Clin North Am* 1989, 3:43.

TINEA VERSICOLOR (PITYRIASIS VERSICOLOR)

On the upper trunk and extending onto the upper arms, finely scaling, guttate or nummular patches appear, particularly on young adults who perspire freely. The individual patches are yellowish or brownish macules in pale skin (Fig. 15-49), or hypopigmented macules in dark skin, with delicate scaling (Fig. 15-50). Mild itching and inflammation about the patches may be present. In other instances a follicular tendency is a marked feature of the eruption. Sites of predilection are the sternal region and the sides of the chest, the abdomen, back, pubis, neck, and intertriginous areas. The disease may even occur on the scalp, palms, and soles. Rarely, the face is involved, in which event the lesions resemble either chloasma or pityriasis alba. Facial lesions occur fairly commonly in infants and immunocompromised patients. In the latter, penile lesions may occur as well.

In hypopigmented tinea versicolor, the fungus apparently compels the production of abnormally small melanosomes, which are not transferred to keratinocytes properly. This becomes conspicuous in dark-skinned people, on whom the white spots look almost as pale as vitiligo. This hypopigmentation may persist for weeks or months after the fungal disease is cured unless an effort is made to regain the lost pigmentation through ultraviolet exposure. This common disease is most prevalent in the tropics, where there are high humidity and high temperatures and frequent exposure to sunlight.

Etiology

Tinea versicolor is due to *Malassezia furfur*. The yeast phase of this organism is classified as *Pityrosporum orbiculare*.

Diagnosis

Lesions that are imperceptible or doubtful may be brought readily into view in a darkened room by use of the Wood's light. This causes fluorescence of the lesions, which appear yellowish or brownish; it also assists in determining the extent of involvement or the achievement of a cure.

Brown hyperpigmentation in tinea versicolor appears to arise from an increase in size of the melanosomes and a change in their epidermal distribution pattern. Occasionally, it is difficult to be certain whether the lighter or darker skin is the affected tissue. Generally, the skin involved by the fungus will produce moderate scaling when scratched with the fingernails or scraped with a blade, whereas uninvolved skin yields little or no scale if gently abraded. If the lesions have a convex border, the involved skin is usually inside the arc.

The fungus is easily demonstrated in scrapings of the scales that have been soaked in 15% solution of KOH. Scales may also be removed by Scotch tape, which is examined directly. Microscopically, there are short, thick fungal hyphae and large numbers of variously sized spores. This combination of strands of mycelium and numerous spores is commonly referred to as "spaghetti and meatballs" (Fig. 15-51). Identification by culture is impractical and is not done to establish the diagnosis.

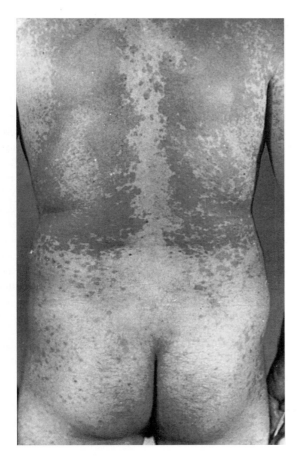

Fig. 15-49 Hyperpigmented tinea versicolor. Tan lesions on pale skin.

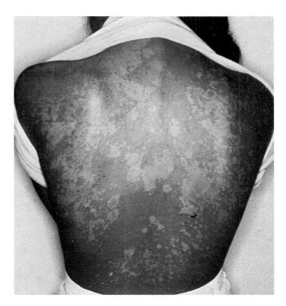

Fig. 15-50 Tinea versicolor on the back of a 20-year-old man. Pale lesions on tan skin.

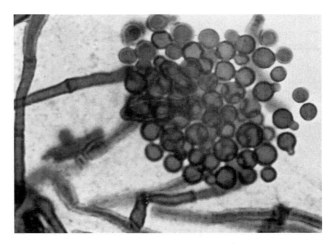

Fig. 15-51 *Malassezia furfur.* Note blunt-ended hyphae and clusters of spores that form "spaghetti and meat balls" pattern. KOH mount.

Differential Diagnosis

Tinea versicolor must be differentiated from seborrheic dermatitis, pityriasis rosea, pityriasis alba, leprosy, syphilis, and vitiligo. The diagnosis is generally easy because of the typical fawn color of the patches in tinea versicolor and their distribution on the upper trunk without involvement of the face or scalp, except occasionally by extension from the sides of the neck. The scalp is not visibly involved, but it usually is affected and provides a locus from which the upper back and shoulders can be rapidly reinfected. In seborrheic dermatitis the patches have an erythematous yellowish tint and the scales are soft and greasy, whereas in tinea versicolor the scales are furfuraceous. The macular syphilid consists of faint pink lesions, less than 1 cm in diameter, irregularly round or oval, which are distributed principally on the nape, sides of the trunk, and flexor aspects of the extremities. There may be general adenopathy. Serologic tests are positive in this phase of syphilis. The demonstration of this fungus also differentiates this disease from vitiligo and leprosy. It may be clinically indistinguishable from the latter.

Treatment

Imidazoles, selenium sulfide shampoos and lotions, ciclopirox olamine, zinc pyrithione shampoos, sulfur preparations, salicylic acid preparations, propylene glycol lotions, and benzoyl peroxide have been used successfully as topical agents. In a multicenter, randomized, double-blind, placebo-controlled series reported by Lange et al using ketoconazole 2% shampoo applied to damp skin and left on for 5 minutes, followed by rinsing, patients were evaluated in weekly treatment groups of 3-day, 1-day, and placebo controls. Thirty-one days later the cure rates were 73%, 69%, and 5%, respectively. There was no statistical difference between the 3-day and 1-day treatment groups. In a study by Katsambas et al, econazole 1% shampoo applied to the whole wet body, rubbed in and left on overnight for 6 consecutive days, with a maintenance application 30 and 60 days later, had 93% cure rates compared with 91% for selenium sulfide (2.5% concentration). Econazole shampoo showed better tolerance rates (98%) compared with selenium sulfide (84%).

Ketoconazole in 400-mg doses repeated in weekly or monthly intervals is very effective. Oral fluconazole and itraconazole are evolving treatment options, but 200 mg of itraconazole for 5 to 7 days or fluconazole, 400 mg once, may be effective. The use of terbinafine has been shown to be ineffective via the oral route but useful as a 1% topical solution.

Patients should be informed that the hypo- and hyperpigmentation will take time to resolve and is not a sign of treatment failure. Relapse after 2 to 12 months is likely if prophylactic doses are not given occasionally, but the question of maintenance therapy is unsettled. In view of the results reported by Katsambas et al and Lange et al, a single overnight application of selenium sulfide, ketoconazole, or econazole shampoo every 30 to 60 days during predisposed periods seems prudent.

Bamford JTM: Treatment of tinea versicolor with sulfur-salicylic shampoo. *J Am Acad Dermatol* 1983, 8:211.

Daneshvar SA, et al: An unusual presentation of tinea versicolor in an immunosuppressed patient. *J Am Acad Dermatol* 1987, 17:304.

Drake LA, et al: Guidelines of care for superficial mycotic infections of the skin: pityriasis (tinea) versicolor. *J Am Acad Dermatol* 1996, 34:287.

Gomez Urcuyo F, et al: Successful treatment of pityriasis versicolor by systemic ketoconazole. *J Am Acad Dermatol* 1982, 6:24.

Hickman JG: A double-blind, randomized, placebo-controlled evaluation of short-term treatment with oral itraconazole in patients with tinea versicolor. *J Am Acad Dermatol* 1996, 34:785.

Katsambas A, et al: Econazole 1% shampoo versus selenium in the treatment of tinea versicolor: a single-blind randomized clinical study. *Int J Dermatol* 1996, 35:667.

Lange DS, et al: Ketoconazole 2% shampoo in the treatment of tinea versicolor. *J Am Acad Dermatol* 1998, 39:944.

Lesher JL: Oral therapy of common superficial fungal infections of the skin. *J Am Acad Dermatol* 1999, 40:S31.

Rausch LJ, et al: Tinea versicolor: treatment and prophylaxis with monthly administration of ketoconazole. *Cutis* 1984, 34:470.

Savin RC: Systemic ketoconazole in tinea versicolor: a double blind evaluation and 1-year follow-up. *J Am Acad Dermatol* 1984, 10:824.

Vermeer BJ, et al: The efficacy of a topical application of terbinafine 1% solution in subjects with pityriasis versicolor: a placebo-controlled study. *Dermatology* 1997, 194(Suppl):22.

Wurtz RM, et al: *Malassezia furfur* fungemia in a patient without the usual risk factors. *Ann Intern Med* 1988, 109:432.

Zimney ML, et al: Tinea versicolor. *Arch Dermatol* 1988, 124:492. ▲

Pityrosporum Folliculitis. What used to be called a "follicular seborrheide" is apparently finding its place as pityrosporum folliculitis, a chronic, moderately itchy eruption of dome-shaped papules and tiny pustules involving the upper back and adjacent areas as far distant as the forearms, lower legs, face, and scalp, sometimes in association with either tinea versicolor or seborrheic dermatitis. Back et al collected 39 women and 12 men with the disease and established it as an entity by biopsy, skin scrapings, and the response to selenium sulfide shampoo, 50% propylene glycol in water, and topical econazole cream. Bufill et al described this occurring in marrow transplant patients. *M. furfur* may occasionally even cause fungemia in patients who have central arterial or venous catheters in place. Jillson has suggested that pityrosporum folliculitis may emerge when *Corynebacterium acnes* is suppressed by tetracycline therapy, and that it may be the same disorder as "acne estivalis." He suggested that it should respond well to ketoconazole. Jacinto-Jamora evaluated 68 patients for a variety of treatment options: selenium sulfide shampoo, 200 mg ketoconazole once daily with topical econazole, ketoconazole cream in tretinoin (0.025%), miconazole cream in tretinoin, and econazole lotion for various periods and various combinations. Treatment successes did occur, but relapses were common except for those patients on maintenance doses of topical econazole. Fluconazole, 400 mg once, or itraconazole, 200 mg daily for 5 to 7 days, are other options to try.

Back O, et al: Pityrosporum folliculitis: a common disease of the young and middle-aged. *J Am Acad Dermatol* 1985, 12:56.

Bufill JA, et al: Pityrosporum folliculitis after bone marrow transplantation. *Ann Intern Med* 1988, 108:560.

Faergemann J: Pityrosporum infections. *J Am Acad Dermatol* 1994, 31:S18.

Jacinto-Jamora S, et al: Pityrosporum folliculitis in the Philippines: diagnosis, prevalence, and management. *J Am Acad Dermatol* 1991, 24:693.

Jillson OF: Pityrosporum folliculitis. *Cutis* 1985, 33:226.

Lesher JL: Oral therapy of common superficial fungal infections of the skin. *J Am Acad Dermatol* 1999, 40:S31. _____ ▲

CONFLUENT AND RETICULATED PAPILLOMATOSIS

Gougerot and Carteaud in 1932 described three forms of papillomatosis, as follows: punctate pigmented verrucous papillomatosis, confluent and reticulated papillomatosis, and nummular and confluent papillomatosis. This disease begins in the intermammary region as punctate, verrucous, pigmented papules, which become generalized over the trunk. There may be severe itching and great discomfort. In time one can distinguish pale red macules and papules, reticulation, isolated circinate disks, and confluent, brownish, papillomatous surfaces. The changes show greatest intensity between the breasts and around the umbilicus.

Histologically, hyperkeratosis with thinning of the granular layer is seen. Acanthosis is a regular finding. The dermis shows edema and a perivascular infiltrate. The principal differential diagnosis occurs between cutaneous papillomatosis and tinea versicolor, seborrheic keratoses, keratosis follicularis, and acanthosis nigricans.

Odom has experienced success with minocycline, 100 mg twice daily given for 3 to 6 weeks, which has been supported by the series reported by Montemarano et al. This is the treatment of choice. Bruynzeel-Koomen et al reported a patient who was cleared by 50 mg of etretinate (Tigason) daily for 4 weeks. Nagy et al reported two cases in which they obtained moderate improvement from the use of topical Retin-A 0.01% gel in one case, and keratolytic agents and 10% urea cream in the other.

Pseudo-atrophoderma colli occurs on the neck as a papillomatous and pigmented dermatosis with glossy lesions that produce a delicate wrinkling that can be obliterated by stretching the skin. The lesions tend to be arranged vertically. The light areas may suggest the appearance of vitiligo. Minocycline should be tried here also.

Bruynzeel-Koomen CAFM, et al: Confluent and reticulated papillomatosis successfully treated with the aromatic retinoid etretinate. *Arch Dermatol* 1984, 120:1236.

Friedman SJ, et al: Confluent and reticulated papillomatosis of Gougerot and Carteaud: treatment with selenium sulfide lotion. *J Am Acad Dermatol* 1986, 14:280.

Kellet JK, et al: Confluent and reticulated papillomatosis (letter). *Arch Dermatol* 1985, 121:587.

Lee MP, et al: Confluent and reticulated papillomatosis: response to high-dose oral isotretinoin therapy and reassessment of epidemiologic data. *J Am Acad Dermatol* 1994, 31:327.

Montemarano AD, et al: Confluent and reticulated papillomatosis: response to minocycline. *J Am Acad Dermatol* 1996, 34:253.

Nagy R, et al: Confluent and reticulated papillomatosis. *Cutis* 1982, 29:48.

Nordby CA, et al: Confluent and reticulated papillomatosis. *Int J Dermatol* 1986, 25:194.

Sau P, et al: Reticulated truncal pigmentation. *Arch Dermatol* 1988, 124:1271. _____ ▲

The deep mycoses

Most of the deep or systemic fungal infections come from inhalation of dust contaminated with fungus, from droppings of animals, or from contamination from other sources. When primary infection is into the skin from puncture wounds, abrasions, or other trauma, a chancriform lesion is often produced and a secondary lymphangitis follows. Nodules and ulcerations that are not chancriform, particularly bilateral ones, should be considered to arise from an internal focus, usually in the lungs or upper respiratory tract.

The outlook for spontaneous recovery is good when a chancriform lesion denotes primary cutaneous infection. On the other hand, the prognosis is grave when the skin lesions result from dissemination of the disease from one or more visceral foci. Chest radiographs should be taken when investigating patients with deep mycoses except for the

classic inoculation types such as sporotrichosis, mycetoma, chromoblastomycosis, and phaeohyphomycosis.

The fungi will be presented in the following order: systemic infection, primarily inoculation disease, and those affecting the immunocompromised patient.

Body BA: Cutaneous manifestations of systemic mycoses. *Dermatol Clin* 1996, 14:125.

Como, JA, et al: Oral azole drugs as systemic antifungal therapy. *New Engl J Med* 1994, 330:263.

Gupta AK, et al: Antifungal agents. Part I. *J Am Acad Dermatol* 1994, 30:677.

Gupta AK, et al: Antifungal agents. Part II. *J Am Acad Dermatol* 1994, 30:911.

Minamoto GY, et al: Fungal infections in patients with acquired immunodeficiency syndrome. *Med Clin North Am* 1997, 81:381.

Myskowski PL, et al: Fungal disease in the immunocompromised host. *Dermatol Clin* 1997, 15:295.

Radentz WH: Opportunistic fungal infections in immunocompromised hosts. *J Am Acad Dermatol* 1989, 20:989. _____ ▲

COCCIDIOIDOMYCOSIS
Synonyms: Coccidioidal granuloma, valley fever, San Joaquin valley fever

Primary pulmonary, disseminated (coccidioidal granuloma), and primary cutaneous coccidioidomycosis forms exist.

Primary Pulmonary Coccidioidomycosis. Inhalation of *Coccidioides immitis,* followed by an incubation period of 10 days to several weeks, produces a respiratory infection that may be mild, with only a low-grade fever resembling a flulike illness. Approximately 60% of infected persons are entirely asymptomatic. Severe symptoms of chills, high fever, night sweats, severe headache, backache, and malaise may ensue in a small minority. A large percentage of patients show lung changes on roentgenographic examination. These may be due to a peribronchial infiltration or an infiltrate compatible with bronchopneumonia. At the time of onset a generalized maculopapular eruption may be present, which may be confused with a drug eruption, measles, or scarlet fever.

Within a few weeks the pulmonary symptoms subside. In about 30% of women and in 15% of men, allergic skin manifestations appear in the form of erythema nodosum over the shins and sometimes over the thighs, hips, and buttocks. These tender lesions may become confluent, gradually turn from purple to brown, and then disappear in about 3 weeks. This rarely occurs in blacks. Erythema nodosum is a favorable prognostic sign. Sometimes erythema multiforme may develop in a similar clinical setting.

Although valley fever is usually self-limited and patients recover spontaneously, a small percentage steadily progress into the chronic, progressive, disseminated form, which carries a high mortality. The propensity for severe disease is severalfold higher in Mexicans and Native Americans and

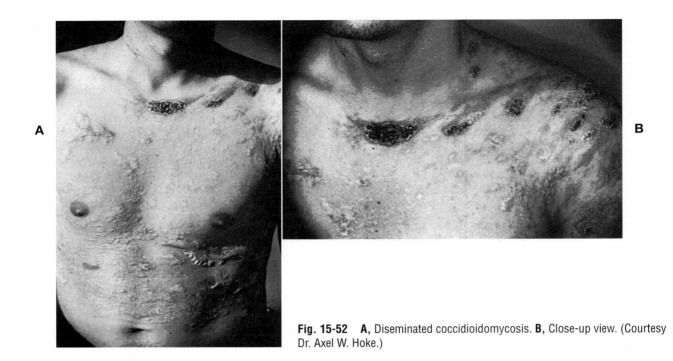

Fig. 15-52 **A,** Diseminated coccidioidomycosis. **B,** Close-up view. (Courtesy Dr. Axel W. Hoke.)

considerably more so for blacks and Filipinos. It is more often self-limited in women than men, except that pregnancy may predispose to systemic disease. Infants, the elderly, persons with blood types B or AB, and immunosuppressed patients, including patients with AIDS, are at increased risk for severe disease.

Disseminated Coccidioidomycosis (Coccidioidal Granuloma).
From the localized pulmonary lesion dissemination may occur in less than 1% of infections. Target organs include the bones, joints, viscera, brain, meninges, and skin. A single organ or multiple organs may be involved.

Skin lesions occur in 15% to 20% of patients with disseminated disease. They appear mostly as subcutaneous abscesses that may remain localized for several years. They are indolent and eventually suppurate, with the formation of numerous sinuses that are similar to the more acute forms of cutaneous tuberculosis. Some resemble mycosis fungoides, whereas other lesions, such as the verrucous nodules and plaques (Fig. 15-52), simulate North American blastomycosis, and umbilicated papules, seen especially in patients with AIDS, may mimic molluscum contagiosum. The face (Fig. 15-53), especially the nasolabial fold, and the scalp are sites commonly involved, although skin lesions may develop at any part of the body. The disease spreads slowly and causes considerable scarring.

Primary Cutaneous Coccidioidomycosis.
This form rarely occurs as most often the disease is attributable to dissemination from a primary lesion in the lung. One to 3 weeks following inoculation an indurated nodule develops that

may ulcerate. Later nodules appear along the lymphatic vessels. Spontaneous recovery may result after several weeks.

Etiology

The causative organism is *Coccidioides immitis.* This fungus has been isolated from the soil and from vegetation, especially fruit.

Some believe that the disease is endemic in rodents, especially those common to the southwestern states. Most infections are thought to occur through inhalation of dust laden with the organisms. A large outbreak occurred in 1994 in Ventura County, California, after the Northridge earthquake. It may occur in laboratory workers; therefore, caution should be exercised when handling cultures.

C. immitis is dimorphous, reproducing in tissue in an entirely different form from that seen in culture media. The parasite appears in tissues as a nonbudding, spherical, thick-walled structure 5 to 200 μm in diameter. This spherule contains numerous small endospores. These small, rounded bodies are usually capsulated and range from 2 to 5 μm in diameter. At maturity the spherule ruptures, with release of the endospores.

Culture

The colonies appear on Sabouraud's dextrose agar within 2 to 7 days as small, slightly raised disks penetrating the medium. Older cultures become covered with a dusty layer of aerial hyphae and assume a brownish color with age. In culture, spherical bodies throw out filaments of arthrospores that are branched and septate, 2 to 8 μm in diameter. Beard

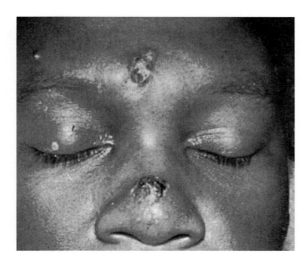

Fig. 15-53 Disseminated coccidioidomycosis. (Courtesy Dr. N. Levan.)

et al reported the use of a commercially available DNA probe to ribosomal RNA that rapidly confirmed that *C. immitis* was growing on 2-day-old culture material.

Epidemiology

It is interesting to note that this disease occurs in limited areas in the Western Hemisphere. The original diagnosis was in a soldier from Argentina, where the disease is endemic in the Gran Chaco area. It is also endemic in northern Mexico, Venezuela, and in southwest United States, especially California (the lower Sonoran Life Zone). In the endemic areas most of the residents are infected, and new residents have a good chance of becoming infected within 6 months.

Pathology

The histopathology is that of infectious granulomas. The essential lesions occur in the deep dermis, especially about the hair follicles and sweat glands, where there is a collection of neutrophils, plasma cells, and varying numbers of epithelioid and giant cells. The spherules occur free among the localized cellular collections and within the giant cells.

Differential Diagnosis

Clinically, it is extremely difficult to differentiate this disease from blastomycosis, which it closely resembles. Definite diagnosis depends on the demonstration of *C. immitis* microscopically, culturally, or by animal inoculation. Guinea pigs inoculated with *C. immitis* die from the systemic infection, whereas no evidence of infection is apparent after inoculation with *Blastomyces*. Intradermal testing with coccidioidin is of value. A positive reaction of the delayed tuberculin type develops early and remains high in those who resist the disease well. A negative skin test does not exclude active disease. Negative tests may be the result of anergy, tolerance, impotent antigen, or administration before development of cell-mediated immunity.

Evaluation of skin lesions should include potassium hydroxide (KOH) preparation and culture of available exudate. Tissue sections obtained by skin biopsy may reveal microorganisms when stained with hematoxylin-eosin; however, confirmation should be obtained by the use of special stains, such as the Gridley or Gomori methenamine silver stain.

Immunology

An extract prepared from a culture of *C. immitis* is used to perform the coccidioidin skin test. A tuberculin type of delayed response indicates present or past infection. A positive reaction usually appears several days after symptoms have developed. From date of exposure a positive reaction may occur within 1 to 6 weeks. Cross reactions with histoplasmin, blastomycin, and paracoccidioidin antigens may result in a false-positive reaction.

In addition, the precipitin, latex agglutination, immunodiffusion, and complement fixation serologic tests have been developed. The precipitin and latex agglutination tests indicate a very recent infection, since a maximum titer is reached in 1 to 2 weeks and then gradually falls and finally disappears. In later infections, the immunodiffusion test can be used for screening purposes. The complement fixation test is useful in diagnosing disseminated coccidioidomycosis since in primary coccidioidomycosis the titer is low, whereas in subsequent dissemination there is a rapid rise in titer.

Treatment

The treatment of choice is fluconazole at a dose of 400 to 800 mg/day orally. In pulmonary and extrapulmonary, nonmeningeal cases the duration of therapy is uncertain; however, 12 to 18 months is usually given. In patients infected with HIV, lifetime suppressive doses of 200 mg daily are advised. In coccidioidomycotic meningitis, fluconazole 400 to 600 mg is given daily indefinitely. The alternative treatments for nonmeningeal disease are itraconazole, 200 mg twice daily for 12 to 18 months, or amphotericin B IV for a total dose of 2.5 g or more. In meningeal disease itraconazole is not effective and amphotericin needs to be given intrathecally in addition to intravenously.

Beard JS, et al: Rapid diagnosis of coccidioidomycosis with a DNA probe to ribosomal RNA. *Arch Dermatol* 1993, 129:1589.

Catanzaro A, et al: Fluconazole in the treatment of persistent coccidioidomycosis. *Chest* 1990, 97:666.

Coccidioidomycosis: Arizona, 1990-1995. *Arch Dermatol* 1997, 133:403.

Ingelman JD, et al: Persistent facial plaque. *Arch Dermatol* 1987, 123:937.

Knoper SR, et al: Coccidioidomycosis. *Infect Dis Clin North Am* 1988, 2:861.

Marrero GM, et al: Nonhealing neck ulcers. *Arch Dermatol* 1998, 134:365.

Pappagianis D, et al: Coccidioidomycosis following the Northridge earthquake. *Arch Dermatol* 1994, 130:555.

Quimby SR, et al: Clinicopathologic spectrum of specific cutaneous lesions of disseminated coccidioidomycosis. *J Am Acad Dermatol* 1992, 26:79.

Schneider E, et al: A coccidioidomycosis outbreak following the Northridge, Calif, earthquake. *JAMA* 1997, 277:904. _____ ▲

HISTOPLASMOSIS

Histoplasmosis is caused by inhalation of airborne spores. It may be asymptomatic or cause limited lung disease. Dissemination to other organs, including the skin, occurs in about 1 in 2000 acute infections. Immunodeficiency and old age predispose to widespread disease. The primary lesion can rarely be in the skin.

Primary Pulmonary Histoplasmosis. Primary pulmonary histoplasmosis is usually a benign form of acute pneumonitis characterized by fever, malaise, night sweats, chest pain, cough, adenopathy, and weight loss. Resolution of the pneumonitis occurs rapidly, and the only residua may be calcifications in the lung and a positive skin test to histoplasmin. However, acute fatal pneumonitis caused by histoplasmosis does occur. Such cases have been reported among the workers in guano caves in Mexico. Also, a chronic pulmonary form in patients with emphysema occurs.

Approximately 10% of patients with acute symptomatic infection develop arthritis and erythema nodosum. Erythema multiforme and a reactive panniculitis have also been described.

Progressive, Disseminated Histoplasmosis. Patients who develop this severe form are usually immunocompromised. Leukemia, lymphoma, lupus erythematosus, renal transplantation, or AIDS are frequent predisposing diseases. Witty et al reported three patients receiving low-dose methotrexate for psoriasis. Approximately 20% have no identifiable risk factor.

The reticuloendothelial system, genitourinary tract, adrenals, gastrointestinal tract, and heart may be involved. Ulcerations and granulomas of the oronasopharynx are the most common mucocutaneous lesions, occurring in about 20% of patients with disseminated disease. Beginning as solid, indurated plaques, they ulcerate and become deep-seated, painful, and secondarily infected.

Skin lesions are present in approximately 6% of patients with dissemination and may be more common in patients with AIDS and in renal transplant recipients. The morphologic patterns are nonspecific and protean. Umbilicated nodules, papules, and ulcers appear on the skin (Fig. 15-54). The ulcers have a punched-out appearance. They appear in crops and are extremely sensitive. Abscesses, pyoderma, pustules, and furuncles may be the first lesions on the skin. Demonstration of the organisms is readily made in the

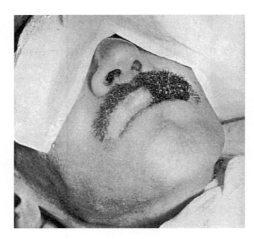

Fig. 15-54 Histoplasmosis.

histologic sections and cultures of the exudate. The most common manifestation in children is purpura. Usually it appears a few days before death and is probably caused by severe involvement of the reticuloendothelial system, with emaciation, chronic fever, and severe gastrointestinal symptoms. Erythema, eczematous dermatitis, panniculitis, psoriasiform dermatitis, and cellulitis may be other forms (Fig. 15-55).

Primary Cutaneous Histoplasmosis. This rare entity is characterized by a chancre-type lesion with regional adenopathy. This type has been reported as occurring on the penis.

African Histoplasmosis. This type is caused by *Histoplasma duboisii*. Its cutaneous manifestations are superficial cutaneous granulomas, subcutaneous granulomas, and osteomyelitic lesions with secondary involvement of the skin (cold abscesses). In addition, papular, nodular, circinate, eczematoid, and psoriasiform lesions may be seen. The granulomas are dome-shaped nodules, painless but slightly pruritic. There may be skin and mucous membrane manifestations such as ulcerations of the nose, mouth, pharynx, genitals, and anus. These ulcers are chronic, superficial lesions with no induration or noticeable inflammatory reaction. Erythema nodosum occurs frequently. Purpuric eruptions may also occur. Emaciation and chronic fevers are common systemic signs.

Etiology

Histoplasmosis was first discovered in Panama by S.T. Darling in 1906. It is caused by *Histoplasma capsulatum*. It is a dimorphic fungus that exists as a saprophyte in the soil; there are also tissue (yeast) and mycelial phases. In tissue there are 1- to 5-μm oval bodies in large macrophages. Budding forms may be present. In direct examination the organism may be demonstrated in the peripheral blood,

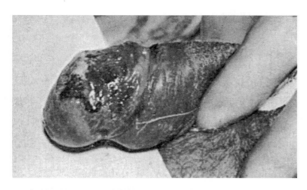

Fig. 15-55 Histoplasmosis. (Courtesy Drs. A. Amolsch and A.E. Palmer.)

sputum, bronchial washings, spinal fluid, sternal marrow, lymph node touch smears, or ulcers when stained with Wright's, Giemsa, or periodic acid-Schiff stains. Gomori methenamine silver is the most reliable stain for showing microorganisms. In African histoplasmosis the ovoid bodies are 10 to 13 μm in diameter.

The mycelial phase may be demonstrated on Sabouraud's dextrose agar, Mycosel medium, or brain-heart infusion agar to which blood has been added. A white, fluffy colony is found, with microconidia and macroconidia. One set of cultures should be inoculated at room temperature to demonstrate the mycelial phase and another at 37° C to produce the yeast phase. In disseminated disease the bone marrow is frequently involved. Blood, urine and tissue from oral and skin lesions should also be cultured. A DNA probe is available for rapid culture confirmation.

Epidemiology

Although histoplasmosis occurs throughout the world, it is most frequent in North America, especially in the central states of the United States along the Mississippi River basin. Histoplasmosis is found frequently in river valley areas in the tropical and temperate zones. The Nile River valley seems to be one exception. Besides the Mississippi and Ohio river valleys, it has been found along the Potomac, Delaware, Hudson, and St. Lawrence rivers. It has been reported in the major river valleys of South America, Central Africa, and Southeast Asia.

Transmission of the disease does not occur between individuals; instead, the infection is contracted from the soil by inhalation of the spores, especially in a dusty atmosphere. Feces of birds and bats contain the fungus. The spores have been demonstrated in the excreta of starlings, chickens, and bats. The disease may be contracted by persons who enter caves inhabited by bats or birds. Epidemics have been reported from exposure to silos, abandoned chicken houses, and storm cellars. Infected people throughout the world number in the many millions.

In an outbreak occurring in Indianapolis in 1978, analyzed by Wheat et al, 120,000 residents were infected;

488 clinically recognized cases occurred, and 55 had disseminated disease. Nineteen died. None under age 1 died. Fatal or disseminated infections occurred in 74% of immunosuppressed persons, compared with 6.5% of those without immunosuppression. Age over 54 was a worse prognostic factor than chronic lung disease in nonimmunosuppressed persons.

Disseminated histoplasmosis is seen as an opportunistic infection in HIV-infected individuals, reflecting impaired cellular immune function.

Pathology

Histologic examination shows a chronic granuloma containing innumerable intracellular oval bodies surrounded by a capsule that is an artifact produced by shrinkage of the cytoplasm away from the rigid cell wall. *H. capsulatum* has a predilection for the reticuloendothelial system and probably proliferates within these cells, differentiating it from most fungi. The granulomatous nodule may show chiefly histiocytes, lymphocytes, plasma cells, epithelioid cells, giant cells, and the organism.

Immunology

The best diagnostic test is the urinary enzyme-linked immunosorbent assay (ELISA). Serologic testing for antibodies requires that the patient have normal immune responsiveness and is further limited by a high rate of false-positives and false-negatives. The complement fixation test, when positive at a titer of 1:32 or greater, indicates active or recent infection.

Treatment

Whereas minimal disease heals spontaneously in the majority of cases only moderate to severe disease requires therapy. Amphotericin B is the treatment of choice in severely ill patients without AIDS who have disseminated disease and as initial treatment in all immunocompromised patients. In patients infected with HIV a suppressive dose of 200 mg/day of itraconazole follows the intravenous amphotericin. Itraconazole, 200 mg/day for 9 months, may be given for moderate disease in immunocompetent patients.

Bellman B, et al: Cutaneous disseminated histoplasmosis in AIDS patients in south Florida. *Int J Dermatol* 1997, 36:599.

Bradsher RW: Histoplasmosis and blastomycosis. *Clin Infect Dis* 1996, 22:S102.

Casariego Z, et al: Disseminated histoplasmosis with orofacial involvement in HIV-infected patients with AIDS. *Oral Dis* 1997, 3:184.

Cave-associated histoplasmosis. *Arch Dermatol* 1988, 124:994.

Dismukes WE, et al: Itraconazole therapy for blastomycosis and histoplasmosis. *Am J Med* 1992, 93:489.

Myers SA, et al: Cutaneous cryptococcosis and histoplasmosis coinfection in a patient with AIDS. *J Am Acad Dermatol* 1996, 34:898.

Ozols II, et al: Erythema nodosum in an epidemic of histoplasmosis in Indianapolis. *Arch Dermatol* 1981, 117:709.

Phillips CM, et al: Palpable purpura in an HIV-positive patient. *Arch Dermatol* 1996, 132:341.

Silverman AD, et al: Panniculitis in an immunocompromised patient. *J Am Acad Dermatol* 1991, 24:912.

Wheat J, et al: Histoplasmosis. *Medicine* (Baltimore) 1997, 76:339.

Witty LA, et al: Disseminated histoplasmosis in patients receiving low-dose methotrexate therapy for psoriasis. *Arch Dermatol* 1992, 128:92. ———————————————————— ▲

CRYPTOCOCCOSIS

Cryptococcosis is primarily a pulmonary infection that remains localized to the lung in 90% of cases. In the remaining 10% the organisms hematogenously disseminate to other organs, with the central nervous system (CNS) and the skin the two most common secondary sites. Patients in this latter group are usually immunocompromised or debilitated. The incidence of dissemination is much higher in patients with AIDS, occurring in up to 50% of this population.

Primary pulmonary cryptococcosis infection may be so mild that the symptoms of fever, cough, and pain may be absent or present only mildly. On the other hand, some cases may be severe enough to cause death. Radiographic studies will reveal disease at this stage.

When dissemination occurs the organism has a special affinity for the CNS. It is the most common cause of mycotic meningitis. There may be restlessness, hallucinations, depression, severe headache, vertigo, nausea and vomiting, nuchal rigidity, epileptiform seizures, and symptoms of intraocular hypertension. Other organs, such as the liver, skin, spleen, myocardium, and skeletal system, as well as the lymph nodes, may be involved. Disseminated cryptococcosis can present in many organ systems; hepatitis, osteomyelitis, prostatitis, pyelonephritis, peritonitis, and skin involvement have all been reported as initial manifestations of disease. The incidence of skin involvement in cases of cryptococcosis is between 10% and 15%; however, in patients infected with HIV the frequency of skin lesions is only about 6%. Cutaneous lesions may precede overt systemic disease by 2 to 8 months.

Skin infection with cryptococcosis occurs most frequently on the head and neck. A variety of morphologic lesions have been reported, including subcutaneous swellings, abscesses, blisters, tumorlike masses, molluscum contagiosum–like lesions, draining sinuses, ulcers, eczematous plaques, granulomas, papules, nodules, pustules, acneiform lesions, plaques, and cellulitis (Figs. 15-56 and 15-57). Approximately 50% of patients with HIV will develop molluscum contagiosum–like lesions. In these patients there is often a central hemorrhagic crust.

Primary inoculation of the skin is a very rare disease. For all practical purposes, identification of cryptococci in the skin indicates disseminated disease with a poor prognosis, and it requires a search for other sites of involvement.

Etiology

The causative organism is *Cryptococcus neoformans*.

Epidemiology

Cryptococcosis has a worldwide distribution and affects both humans and animals. The organism has been recovered from human skin, soil, dust, and pigeon droppings. The latter, when deposited on window ledges in large cities, are a source of infection. The patient with disseminated cryptococcosis usually has a concomitant debilitating disease such as AIDS, cancer, leukemia, lymphoma, renal failure, hepatitis, alveolar proteinosis, severe diabetes mellitus, sarcoidosis, tuberculosis, or silicosis. Long-term oral prednisone or immunosuppressive therapy for chronic illnesses, such as renal transplantation or connective tissue disease, may also be a factor. The portal of entry is the lungs. Males outnumber females 2 to 1. Cryptococcosis is most frequent in persons aged 30 to 60 years.

Patients with AIDS are particularly at risk for disseminated disease. Cryptococcosis is the fourth leading cause of opportunistic infection and is the second most common fungal opportunist, with 5% to 9% of patients manifesting symptomatic disease. Dissemination occurs in 50% of patients with AIDS; skin involvement is reported to be present in 6% of patients with AIDS.

Immunology

The latex slide agglutination test is a sensitive and specific test. It may give false-positives in the presence of rheumatoid factor. Porges et al reported the use of latex agglutination in lesional skin scrapings to aid in the rapid diagnosis. The complement fixation test for cryptococcal polysaccharide has also been found to be a sensitive test, and the indirect fluorescence test is also a valuable aid to the diagnosis of cryptococcosis. The enzyme immunoassay (EIA) for cryptococcal antigen detection is capable of detecting the presence of antigen earlier and at a lower concentration than other tests.

Pathology

Two patterns of involvement can be seen microscopically. The gelatinous type demonstrates numerous budding yeasts in a foamy stroma with little or no inflammation. The granulomatous type is characterized by fewer, smaller organisms and a granulomatous inflammatory infiltrate.

Usually the organism is easily demonstrated in histologic sections of the lesion. *Cryptococcus neoformans* is an oval of rounded, thick-walled spherule measuring 5 to 20 μm in diameter. The organism is surrounded by a polysaccharide capsule that can be demonstrated by special staining such as methylene blue, Alcian blue, or mucicarmine stain. The latter method stains the budding cells and capsules brilliant carmine red.

Mycology

For direct examination, a drop of serum or exudate is placed on a slide and then covered with a coverslip. If examination shows yeast, 1 drop of 10% sodium hydroxide is added to half of the coverslip and 1 drop of India ink to the other half

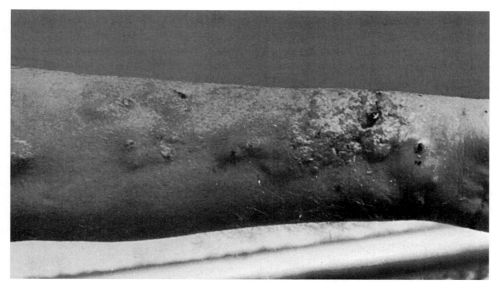

Fig. 15-56 Cryptococcosis on the forearm in 28-year-old man with AV shunt for dialysis. (Courtesy Dr. R.N. Buchanan, Jr.)

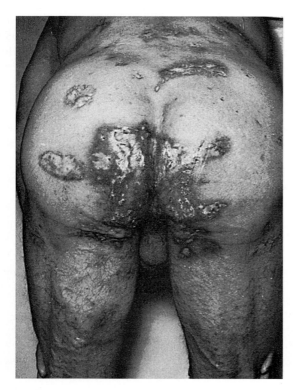

Fig. 15-57 Cryptococcosis of 14 years' duration in a 42-year-old man. (Courtesy Dr. E. Florian, Budapest.)

to demonstrate the capsule. In their article, Porges et al discuss several methods with which to critically examine direct smears.

The organism produces a moist, shiny, white colony on Sabouraud's dextrose agar. With aging the culture may turn to a cream and then a tan color. Subcultures from Sabouraud's may be made onto cornmeal agar, and onto urea medium to aid in distinguishing the yeast from *Candida* and other yeasts. A commercially available DNA probe detection assay allows rapid culture confirmation.

Differential Diagnosis

With regard to skin lesions, it is helpful to know that the lesions are indolent and nonspecific. Smears and cultures will easily demonstrate the causative organism.

Treatment

In all patient populations amphotericin B intravenously initially followed by fluconazole orally is recommended; however, in less severely ill non-AIDS patients, fluconazole 400 mg daily for 8 to 10 weeks may be effective. In non-AIDS meningitis, flucytosine is given in combination with amphotericin B, and in patients infected with HIV fluconazole is given indefinitely at a suppressive dose of 200 mg/day.

Carlson KC, et al: Cryptococcal cellulitis in renal transplant patients. *J Am Acad Dermatol* 1987, 17:469.

Dover JS, et al: Cutaneous manifestations of HIV infection. *Arch Dermatol* 1991, 127:1549.

Durden FM, et al: Cutaneous involvement with *Cryptococcus neoformans* in AIDS. *J Am Acad Dermatol* 1994, 30:844.

Feldman SR, et al: Fluconazole treatment of cutaneous cryptococcosis. *Arch Dermatol* 1992, 128:1045.

Hall JC, et al: Cryptococcal cellulitis with multiple sites of involvement. *J Am Acad Dermatol* 1987, 17:329.

Johnson DS, et al: Symmetrical hemorrhagic bullae in an immunocompromised host. *Arch Dermatol* 1999, 135:983.

Lui H, et al: An ulcerated plaque in a gay man. *Arch Dermatol* 1993, 129:495.

Micalizzi C, et al: Primary cutaneous cryptococcosis in an immunocompetent pigeon keeper. *Clin Exp Dermatol* 1997, 22:195.

Murakawa GJ, et al: Cutaneous cryptococcus infection and AIDS. *Arch Dermatol* 1996, 132:545.

Perfect JR: Cryptococcosis. *Infect Dis Clin North Am* 1989, 3:77.

Porges DY, et al: A noted use of the cryptococcal latex agglutination test for rapid presumptive diagnosis of cutaneous cryptococcosis. *Arch Dermatol* 1992, 128:461.

Sanchez-Albisua B, et al: Cryptococcal cellulitis in an immunocompetent host. *J Am Acad Dermatol* 1997, 36:109.

Tomasini C, et al: Granulomatous ulcerative vulvar cryptococcosis in a patient with advanced HIV disease. *J Am Acad Dermatol* 1997, 37:116. ▲

NORTH AMERICAN BLASTOMYCOSIS

Synonyms: Gilchrist's disease, blastomycosis, blastomycetic dermatitis

Cutaneous North American blastomycosis may appear in two forms. One is the rare primary cutaneous lesion characterized by the formation of a small primary nodule

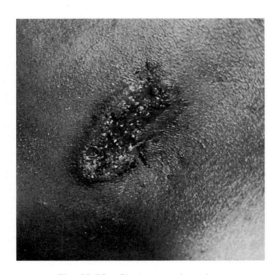

Fig. 15-58   Blastomycosis on jaw.

and subsequent small nodules along the draining lymphatics. This is similar to sporotrichosis. Healing takes place within several months.

The other form consists of chronic, slowly progressive, granulomatous lesions characterized by thick crusts, warty vegetations, discharging sinuses, and unusual vascularity (Fig. 15-58). The lesions are often multiple and are located mostly on exposed parts (Figs. 15-59 and 15-60, *A*), although they may occur anywhere on the integument (Fig. 15-60, *B*). Papillomatous proliferation is most pronounced in lesions on the hands and feet, where the patches become very thick. There is a tendency for the patches to involute centrally and to form white scars while they spread peripherally (Fig. 15-61). The crusts are thick and dirty gray or brown. Beneath them there are exuberant granulations covered with a seropurulent exudate, which oozes out of small sinuses that extend down to indolent subcutaneous abscesses.

In this chronic cutaneous form, the primary infection is almost always in the upper or middle lobes of the lungs, and the cutaneous lesions are disseminations from a primary pulmonary focus. The most frequent site of dissemination is the skin, occurring in at least 80% of cases. It also frequently disseminates to the osseous system, especially the ribs and vertebrae. Other targets are the CNS, the liver and spleen, and the genitourinary system, especially the prostate, but rarely, if ever, the gastrointestinal tract.

Etiology

The fungus *Blastomyces dermatitides* causes North American blastomycosis, which was first described by Gilchrist in 1894.

Epidemiology

North American blastomycosis is prevalent in the southeastern United States and the Ohio and Mississippi river basins, reaching epidemic proportions in Kentucky. There is a

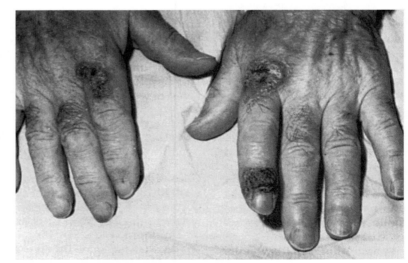

Fig. 15-59   North American blastomycosis.

male-female ratio of approximately 6:1, and most of the patients are over age 60. Often the cutaneous form occurs without a known history of pulmonary lesions.

Blastomycosis has been reported from the bite of a dog suffering from pulmonary blastomycosis. Also, there is a report of transmission occurring between men with prostatic involvement and their sexual partners. Klein et al investigated an outbreak of blastomycosis among children attending summer camp. They were able to culture *B. dermatitides* from the soil in a beaver dam, which they concluded was the reservoir for human infection.

Pathology

Primary cutaneous blastomycosis consists of a polymorphonuclear infiltrate with many budding cells of blastomycetes. The lymph nodes may show marked inflammatory changes, giant cells, giant cells containing the organisms, lymphocytes, and plasma cells. Various manifestations are present in the chronic disseminated type skin lesion. The verrucous lesion shows pseudoepitheliomatous hyperplasia. Microabscesses may abound in the epidermis, with giant cells, epithelioid cells, plasma cells, and lymphocytes in the dermis. A KOH slide preparation containing a smear of pus

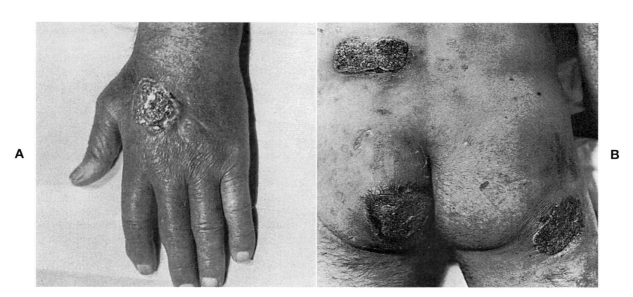

Fig. 15-60 **A** and **B**, Blastomycosis.

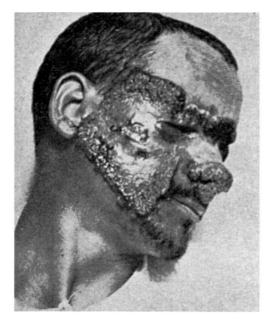

Fig. 15-61 Blastomycosis. Note typical granular appearance.

from the lesion will show single or singly budding spherical cells with refractile walls.

Lung involvement may show many changes that are suggestive of carcinoma or tuberculosis with tubercle formation. Purulent abscesses form not only in the lungs but also elsewhere when dissemination is taking place. The abscesses may break through to form draining abscesses and sinuses on the skin. There may be innumerable organisms in the pus.

Mycology

Blastomyces dermatitides is a dimorphic fungus with a mycelial phase at room temperature and a yeast phase at 37° C. Direct microscopic examination of a KOH slide of the specimen should always be made, since culture of the fungus is difficult. The specimen is cultured on Sabouraud's dextrose agar, Mycosel, and brain-heart infusion agar to which blood has been added. Aerial mycelium will develop in 10 to 14 days, forming a white, cottony growth that turns tan with age. The structures are septate mycelium and characteristic conidia on the sides of hyphae. The conidia are 3 to 5 μm and variously shaped from round to oval forms. Culture at 37° C produces a slow-growing, wrinkled yeast with spherules, single budding cells, and some abortive hyphae. A DNA probe detection assay is commercially available for rapid culture confirmation.

Immunology

Serologic tests are performed by immunodiffusion or ELISA. No reliable skin test reagent is available.

Differential Diagnosis

Blastomycosis may closely resemble tuberculosis verrucosa cutis, syphilis, granuloma inguinale, drug eruptions, trichophytic granuloma, and chronic serpiginous and gangrenous pyoderma. The similarity to tuberculosis verrucosa cutis is sometimes so close that one is unable to differentiate the two diseases by clinical examination without resorting to laboratory procedures. The course of blastomycosis is more rapid; however, suppuration usually occurs early and involvement is more extensive than is common in the verrucous type of tuberculosis. Vegetative lesions of tertiary syphilis usually are accompanied by other signs of the disease and have a predilection for the scalp and mucocutaneous junctions, areas not commonly affected by blastomycosis. Bromide and iodide eruptions are generally more acutely inflammatory and less purulent than blastomycosis.

Examination of the tissue or of smears from the exudate, together with the history, will determine the diagnosis. In deep trichophytic granuloma the duration is, as a rule, less than in blastomycosis, and the lesions are not so papillomatous. Microscopic demonstration of the causative fungi is conclusive.

Treatment

Itraconazole, at a dose of 200 to 400 mg daily for 6 months, is the treatment of choice. Amphotericin B for a total dose of 1.5 g is necessary for very sick patients. Fluconazole, 400 to 800 mg daily for at least 6 months, is effective in 85% of patients in non–life-threatening disease.

Blastomycosis acquired occupationally during prairie dog relocation—Colorado, 1998. *Arch Dermatol* 1999, 48(5):98.

Blastomycosis: Wisconsin, 1986-1995. *MMWR* 1996, 45:601.

Bradsher RW: Histoplasmosis and blastomycosis. *Clin Infect Dis* 1996, 22:S102.

Cohen LM, et al: Widespread papules and nodules in a Ugandan man with acquired immunodeficiency syndrome. *Arch Dermatol* 1996, 132:821.

Gnann JW Jr, et al: Human blastomycosis after a dog bite. *Ann Intern Med* 1983, 98:48.

Klein BS, et al: Isolation of *Blastomyces dermatitides* from soil associated with a large outbreak of blastomycosis in Wisconsin. *N Engl J Med* 1986, 314:529.

Leet NA, et al: Multiple verrucous skin lesions. *Arch Dermatol* 1991, 127:721.

Weil M, et al: Cutaneous lesions provide a clue to mysterious pulmonary process: pulmonary and cutaneous North American blastomycosis infection. *Arch Dermatol* 1996, 132:822.

Yen A, et al: Primary cutaneous blastomycosis. *J Am Acad Dermatol* 1994, 31:277. ▲

SOUTH AMERICAN BLASTOMYCOSIS
Synonyms: Paracoccidioidal granuloma, paracoccidioidomycosis

South American blastomycosis is almost always primary in the lungs. Some cases may arise from inoculation of the mucous membranes of the pharynx or other parts of the gastrointestinal tract. Lymph gland involvement is commonly present. Wide dissemination of the disease occurs to the skin and to all organs of the body, with a fatal termination unless treatment is instituted.

The mucocutaneous type usually begins in the region of the mouth, where small papules and ulcerations appear (Fig. 15-62). These spread, and ultimately extensive ulcerations destroy the nose, lips, and face (Fig. 15-63). The skin lesions may show ulcerations, pseudoepitheliomatous hyperplasia, and microabscesses (Figs. 15-64 and 15-65). In the latter *Paracoccidioides brasiliensis* may be seen. This is a round cell, 10 to 60 μm in diameter, with multiple buds.

The lymphangitic type manifests itself by enlargement of the regional lymph nodes soon after the appearance of the initial lesions about the mouth. The adenopathy may extend to the supraclavicular and axillary regions. Nodes may become greatly enlarged and break down with ulcerations that secondarily involve the skin, causing severe pain and dysphagia with progressive cachexia and death. It may closely simulate Hodgkin's disease, especially when the suprahyoid, preauricular, or retroauricular groups of lymph nodes are involved.

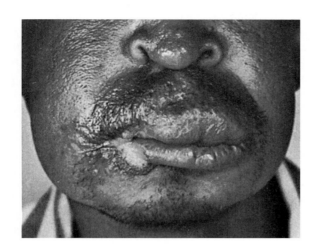

Fig. 15-62 Paracoccidioidomycosis. (Courtesy Dr. J. Convit, Venezuela.)

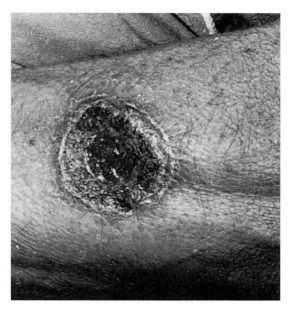

Fig. 15-64 South American blastomycosis on forearm. (Courtesy Dr. J. Kroll.)

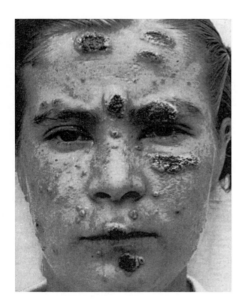

Fig. 15-63 South American blastomycosis. (Courtesy Dr. T.A. Furtado.)

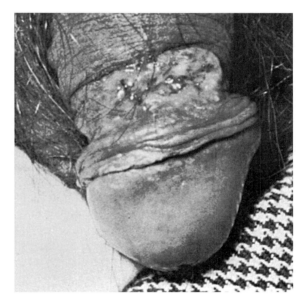

Fig. 15-65 South American blastomycosis. (Courtesy Dr. A.T. Londero, Brazil.)

There is a visceral type, caused probably by hematogenous spread of the disease from the lungs to the liver, spleen, intestines, and other organs. There is also a mixed type that has the combined symptomatology of the mucocutaneous, lymphangitic, and visceral types. The disease may present either as a rapidly progressive, acute disease or follow a subacute course, or occur as a chronic, slowly advancing form.

Etiology

Lutz first described South American blastomycosis in Brazil in 1908. It is caused by the fungus *Paracoccidioides brasiliensis*.

Epidemiology

This chronic granulomatous disease is endemic in Brazil and also occurs in Argentina and Venezuela. Occasional cases have been reported in the United States, Mexico, and Central America. The disease is generally found among laborers, mostly in men, and many are infected by picking the teeth with twigs or from chewing leaves. The fact that the disease is 15 times more common in men is of particular interest, since it has been shown that 17B-estradiol inhibits transition from the mycelial to the tissue-invasive yeast form. *P. brasiliensis* can lodge in periodontal tissues, and some cases start after extraction of teeth. Many cases have been reported in patients with AIDS. The course is usually acute and severe.

Pathology

An infectious granuloma occurs with abscess formation similar to that of blastomycosis.

Mycology

The causative fungus in tissue is a large, thick-walled cell with multiple buds, the "pilot wheel" appearance. In culture the colony is cream-colored, compact, and powdery. Chlamydospores are round or oval. Elongate lateral conidia may be present.

Immunology

Complement fixation tests are positive in 97% of severe cases, and the titer rises as the disease becomes more severe. With improvement, the titer decreases.

Treatment

Itraconazole, 200 mg/day for 6 months, or ketoconazole, 400 mg/day for 6 to 18 months, is the treatment of choice and improves more than 90% of patients. Amphotericin B and the sulfonamides have activity; however, they have largely been replaced by the more effective, less toxic oral azoles. Trimethoprim/sulfamethoxazole retains use as a suppressive dose in patients infected with HIV. It should be given indefinitely once active therapy is completed.

Bakos L, et al: Disseminated paracoccidioidomycosis with skin lesions in a patient with AIDS. *J Am Acad Dermatol* 1989, 20:854.

Gimenez MF, et al: Langerhans cells in paracoccidioidomycosis. *Arch Dermatol* 1987, 123:479.

Manns BJ, et al: Paracoccidioidomycosis: case report and review. *Clin Infect Dis* 1996, 23:1026.

Negroni R: Paracoccidioidomycosis. *Int J Dermatol* 1993, 32:847.

Sugar AM: Paracoccidioidomycosis. *Infect Dis Clin North Am* 1988, 2:913.

▲

SPOROTRICHOSIS

Most common and least serious of the deep mycoses, sporotrichosis is a chronic infectious disease caused by *Sporothrix schenckii,* a dimorphic fungus that grows in a yeast form at 37° C and in a mycelial form at room temperature. Human infection occurs accidentally at the site of some insignificant wound. The earliest manifestation may be a small nodule or ulcer, which may heal and disappear before the advent of further symptoms. In the course of a few weeks nodules generally develop along the draining lymphatics. These lesions are at first small, dusky red, painless, firm infiltrations. In time the overlying skin becomes adherent to them and may ulcerate, and may even show fistulous tracts or papillomatous vegetations. When the lesions occur near the eye, they may be confused with dacryocystitis. Sometimes the lesions heal spontaneously, but more often they progress slowly and persist indefinitely.

The disease, as a rule, is localized in the skin and subcutaneous tissues, and only exceptionally does it become disseminated. Regional lymphangitic sporotrichosis is the common type, accounting for 75% of the cases. It causes first a primary sore, a sporotrichotic chancre (Fig. 15-66), at the site of inoculation and then, in the course of a few days, weeks, or months, an ascending lymphangitis and multiple, subcutaneous, indolent, painless, granulomas, which soften and form cold abscesses and sometimes ulcers (Figs. 15-67 and 15-68).

Fixed cutaneous sporotrichosis is seen in 20% of cases and is characterized by a solitary ulcer or plaque without regional lymphangitis, or a rosacea-like lesion of the face without regional adenopathy. Increased host resistance, a lower magnitude of inoculum, facial location, and variations in strain pathogenicity have all been hypothesized as reasons favoring the fixed cutaneous form.

Factors that predispose to extracutaneous disease include oral prednisone therapy, chronic alcoholism, diabetes mellitus, hematologic malignancies, and AIDS.

Disseminated Sporotrichosis. Systemic invasion by an opportunistic infection with *S. schenckii* may produce cutaneous, pulmonary, gastrointestinal, or articular lesions, and may involve the CNS. This form is strikingly similar to other systemic fungal diseases.

The cutaneous lesions are reddish, tender nodules, which soften, form cold abscesses, and eventually suppurate, leaving chronic ulcers or fistulas. These are usually around arthritic joints and the face and scalp, but may occur anywhere on the skin. At times the primary site may be indiscernible and only internal involvement, such as of the lungs, CNS, or osteomyelitis, is apparent. Arthritis or bone involvement occurs in most cases; lung involvement is much less frequent.

Epidemiology

There seems to be no geographic limitation to the occurrence of sporotrichosis. Most often the primary invasion is seen as an occupational disease in gardeners, florists, and laborers following injuries by thorns of plants or by straw. The pathogen commonly lives as a saprophyte on grasses, shrubs, and other plants. Carnations, rose-

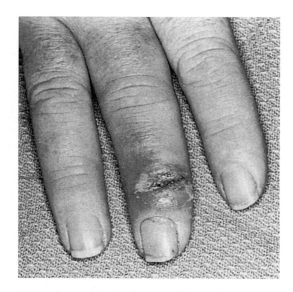

Fig. 15-66 Sporotrichotic chancre. Primary lesion of 3 weeks' duration.

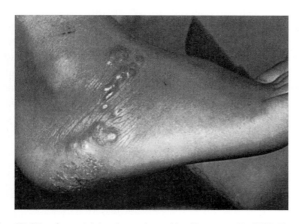

Fig. 15-67 Sporotrichosis on the ankle. (Courtesy Dr. V.M. Torres-Rodriguez.)

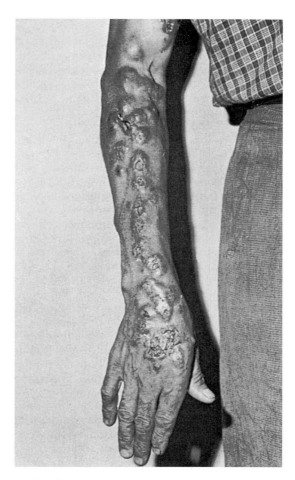

Fig. 15-68 Sporotrichosis of 6 months' duration on arm of 45-year-old farmer. (Courtesy Dr. A.T. Londero, Brazil.)

Mycology

S. schenckii is not often found in histologic tissue taken from the human lesion. Even with special stains it is difficult to recognize; however, when the organism-containing material is injected into a rat or mouse many organisms may be seen. These are small, 3 to 5 µm, oval or elongated, budding cells of cigar shape, often called *cigar bodies*. Fluorescent antibody staining of *S. schenckii* in cultures and clinical materials is a rapid method of identifying the organism. Asteroid bodies and mycelial elements are prevalent in regional lymphangitic sporotrichosis.

On Sabouraud's agar a moist, white colony develops within 3 to 7 days. The surface becomes wrinkled and folded. Later the culture turns tan and, ultimately, black. In slide culture preparations the colony shows septate mycelium that is branched. Conidia are found in clusters or in a sleevelike arrangement on delicate sterigmata. If the culture is grown at 37° C, grayish yellow, velvety colonies are produced. Cigar-shaped, round, oval and budding cells, hyphae, and conidia may be seen microscopically.

bushes, barberry shrubs, and sphagnum moss are some of the sources from which inoculation into the skin takes place. High humidity and high temperature favor infection. An epidemic of sporotrichosis among South African miners was ascribed to inoculation of the organism by rubbing against the supporting wooden beams in the mines. Experimentally, it has been produced in many laboratory animals, and spontaneous cases have been observed in horses, mules, dogs, cats, mice, and rats. Several reports have documented the transmission of sporotrichosis from cats to humans. Dunstan et al reported five such cases.

Pathology

The histologic changes are those of an infectious granuloma, with the formation of deep abscesses, sinuses, and ulcerations. Toward the center of a well-developed lesion are collections of polymorphonuclear leukocytes, eosinophils, and macrophages. Between the central and peripheral zones are numerous epithelioid cells and giant cells of the Langhans type, and the peripheral part is made up of plasma cells, lymphocytes, and connective tissue cells.

Immunology

Culture extracts from *S. schenckii*, known as *sporotrichins*, will produce a delayed tuberculin type reaction in persons who have, or have had, sporotrichosis. The test is fairly reliable, but only indicates previous exposure. Agglutination is the most satisfactory test, and a titer of 1:80 or higher establishes the diagnosis.

Differential Diagnosis

The diagnosis is established by the history of the onset, the indolent character, and the linear distribution of the nodules along the lymphatic drainage of the area. Demonstration by culture clinches the diagnosis. Clinically, atypical mycobacteriosis (swimming pool granuloma), tuberculosis, syphilis, leishmaniasis, furunculosis, *Nocardia brasiliensis,* cat-scratch disease, anthrax, tularemia, and the primary inoculation of several other deep fungal organisms, such as histoplasmosis, coccidioidomycosis, and North American blastomycosis, may resemble sporotrichosis, but differentiation is made without difficulty.

Treatment

Itraconazole is effective at a dose of 100 to 200 mg/day for 6 months followed by 200 mg twice daily long term. For cutaneous and lymphonodular forms potassium iodide in doses of 2 to 6 g daily is effective and should be continued for 1 month after apparent recovery to prevent recurrences. This generally requires 6 to 12 weeks of treatment. It is important to begin with 5 drops of the saturated solution in grapefruit juice or milk three times a day after meals. This dose should be gradually increased until 40 to 50 drops are taken thrice daily. It is not suitable for pregnant women. Adverse effects of iodide therapy include nausea, vomiting, parotid swelling, acneiform rash, coryza, sneezing, swelling of the eyelids, hypothyroidism, a brassy taste, increased lacrimation and salivation, and occasionally, depression. Most of the side effects can be controlled by stopping the drug for a few days and reinstituting therapy at a slightly reduced dosage. Application of local hot compresses, hot packs, or a heating pad twice daily has been advocated as a useful adjunct. *S. schenckii* is intolerant to temperatures above 38.5° C (101° F).

In the disseminated cases itraconazole, 300 mg twice daily for 6 months, followed by 200 mg twice daily long term is the treatment of choice. Amphotericin B, 0.5 mg/kg/day, is the alternative.

Chung G, et al: Fixed cutaneous sporotrichosis. *Arch Dermatol* 1990, 126:399.

Davis BA: Sporotrichosis. *Dermatol Clin* 1996, 14:69.

Dellatorre DL: Fixed cutaneous sporotrichosis of the face. *J Am Acad Dermatol* 1982, 6:97.

Dunstan RW, et al: Feline sporotrichosis: report of 5 cases with transmission to humans. *J Am Acad Dermatol* 1986, 15:37.

Friedman SJ, et al: Extracutaneous sporotrichosis. *Int J Dermatol* 1983, 22:171.

Itoh M, et al: Survey of 200 cases of sporotrichosis. *Dermatologica* 1986, 172:209.

Kwon KS, et al: Verrucous sporotrichosis in an infant treated with itraconazole. *J Am Acad Dermatol* 1998, 38:112.

Purvis RS, et al: Sporotrichosis presenting as arthritis and subcutaneous nodules. *J Am Acad Dermatol* 1993; 28:879.

Sharkey-Mathis PR, et al: Treatment of sporotrichosis with itraconazole. *Ann Intern Med* 1993, 95:279.

Shaw JC, et al: Sporotrichosis in AIDS. *J Am Acad Dermatol* 1989, 21:1145.

Ware AJ, et al: Disseminated sporotrichosis with extensive cutaneous involvement in a patient with AIDS. *J Am Acad Dermatol* 1999, 40:350.

Yalisove BL, et al: Multiple pruritic purple plaques. *Arch Dermatol* 1991, 127:721. ▲

CHROMOBLASTOMYCOSIS

Chromoblastomycosis usually affects one leg or foot. As a rule, it begins as a small, pink, scaly papule or warty growth on some part of the foot, from whence it slowly spreads by the growth of satellite lesions (Fig. 15-69). The extremity is usually swollen and at its distal portion becomes covered with various nodular, tumorous, verrucous lesions that may resemble a cauliflower (Figs. 15-70 and 15-71). The small lesions may resemble common warts. Plaquelike and cicatricial types of lesions also occur (Figs. 15-72 and 15-73).

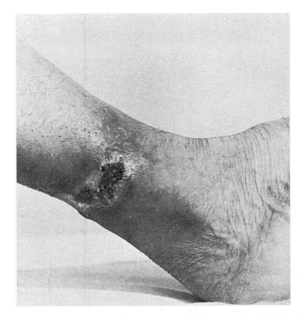

Fig. 15-69 Early chromoblastomycosis. (Courtesy Dr. A.L. Carrion, Puerto Rico.)

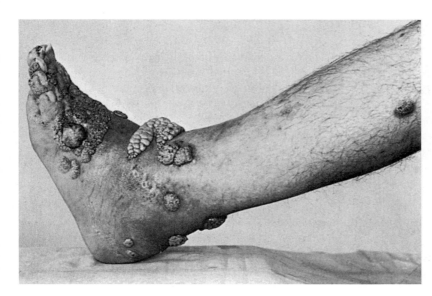

Fig. 15-70 Chromoblastomycosis. (Courtesy Dr. A.L. Carrion, Puerto Rico.)

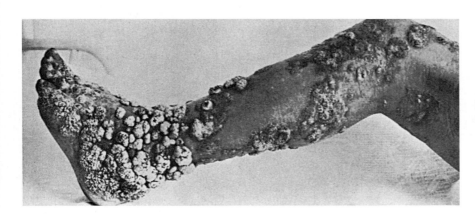

Fig. 15-71 Chromoblastomycosis. (Courtesy Dr. A.L. Carrion, Puerto Rico.)

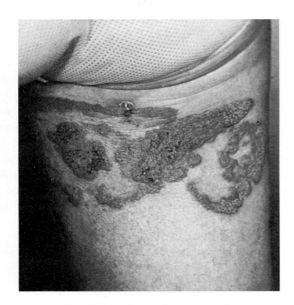

Fig. 15-72 Chromoblastomycosis.

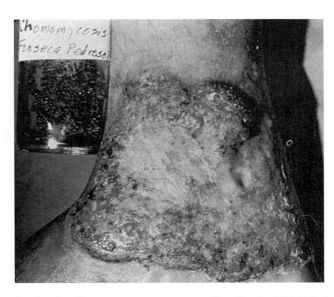

Fig. 15-73 Chromoblastomycosis. (Courtesy Dr. Axel W. Hoke.)

The cicatricial types are formed by nodules and spread peripherally; healing with sclerosis takes place at the center, at times associated with keloid formation. Adenitis as a result of bacterial complications may occur. In rare instances the disease begins on the hand or wrist and involves the entire upper extremity. It may also begin on the nose. There is slow progression; it may take many years to develop fully.

Usually the disease process remains localized to one lower extremity; however, there have been rare reports of CNS involvement both with and without associated skin lesions. Metastases through the blood stream are rare, but there is no doubt that they can occur.

Etiology

Five dematiaceous fungi are the main causative agents: *Cladosporium carrionii, Phialophora verrucosa, Fonsecaea pedrosoi, F. compacta,* and *Rhinocladiella aquaspersa.*

Exophiala spinifera and *E. jeanselmei* have been reported in isolated cases.

Epidemiology

Chromoblastomycosis was first recognized in Brazil by Pedroso in 1911. Since then it has been found in Cuba, West Indies, Madagascar, United States, Russia, and other countries. The distribution is predominantly among barefooted farm laborers. Trauma from wood products and soil exposure results in implantation of the organism. It occurs 20 times more commonly in men than in women, usually in the 20- to 50-year age range.

Pathology

The essential pathologic changes are characterized by a granulomatous reaction, with the formation of pseudotubercles containing giant cells, and a focal round cell infiltration in the superficial portions of the dermis. The fungus occurs in the form of brown, spherical cells with thick, dark cell walls and coarsely granular, pigmented protoplasm. The fungi appear in clusters of spherical cells that reproduce by equatorial splitting, not by budding. Septate forms (Medlar bodies, sclerotic bodies, "copper pennies") are occasionally encountered in the dermis, this being the characteristic tissue morphology of chromoblastomycosis, differentiating it from phaeomycosis.

Mycology

The microorganisms produce black, slowly growing, heaped-up colonies. The three types differ according to the type of conidiophore produced; they are the *Phialophora,* the *Cladosporium,* and the *Acrotheca* types of sporulation.

Treatment

Chromoblastomycosis is best treated by surgical excision and grafting of the affected area if lesions are small or few. If the lesions are chronic, extensive, or burrowing then itraconazole, 100 mg/day for 18 months, is given. Terbinafine, 500 mg/day for 6 to 12 months, has been remarkably effective in patients treated to date. Application of heat has been reported effective, as it has with sporotrichosis and atypical mycobacterial infections. Kuttner et al described a case treated successfully with the carbon dioxide laser. Cryosurgery has also been recommended. Despite these options, some lesions remain resistant, and amputation may be unavoidable.

Artuz F, et al: Purple erythematous plaques on the face and left arm. *Arch Dermatol* 1997, 133:1029.

Barba-Gomez JF, et al: Chromoblastomycosis caused by *Exophiala spinifera. J Am Acad Dermatol* 1992, 26:367.

Bouffard D, et al: Long-standing verrucous lesion. *Arch Dermatol* 1995, 131:1195.

Esterre P, et al: Treatment of chromomycosis with terbinafine. *Br J Dermatol* 1996, 134(Suppl):33.

Fader RC, et al: Infections caused by dematiaceous fungi. *Infect Dis Clin North Am* 1988, 2:925.

Gross DJ, et al: Chromomycosis on the nose. *Arch Dermatol* 1991, 127:1831.

Kuttner BJ, et al: Treatment of chromomycosis with a CO_2 laser. *J Dermatol Surg Oncol* 1986, 12:695.

Rubin HA, et al: Evidence for percutaneous inoculation as the mode of transmission of chromoblastomycosis. *J Am Acad Dermatol* 1991, 25:951.

Smith CH, et al: A case of chromoblastomycosis responding to treatment with itraconazole. *Br J Dermatol* 1993, 128:436. ▲

PHAEOHYPHOMYCOSIS

This heterogeneous group of mycotic infections is caused by dematiaceous fungi whose morphologic characteristics in tissue include yeastlike cells, hyphae, pseudohypha-like elements, or any combination of these. This contrasts with chromomycosis in that the morphology in tissue appears as single, thick-walled, muriform fungal cells.

There are many types of clinical lesions one may see with this histologic picture. They include superficial, cutaneous, subcutaneous, and systemic disease. Black piedra and tinea nigra are examples of superficial infection. Cutaneous disease causes lesions similar to dermatophytosis. Subcutaneous disease occurs most commonly as abscesses at the site of minor trauma, with *Exophiala jeanselmei* being the most common cause in temperate climates, although *Bipolaris* and *Exserohilum* genera are being more commonly recovered as causes of both subcutaneous lesions and systemic infections. Finally, systemic phaeohyphomycosis is more frequently being reported as the population of immunocompromised patients increases.

Etiology

More than 30 agents are capable of causing phaeohyphomycosis. Among them are *E. jeanselmei, Dactylaria gallopava, Phialophora parasitica, Phaeoannellomyces werneckii, Hendersonula toruloidea, Wangiella dermatiti-*

dis, *Exserohilum rostratum*, *Bipolaris spicifera*, *Cladophialophora bantiana*, and *Xylohypha bantiana*. Some fungi, such as *Phialophora verrucosa*, can cause both phaeohyphomycosis and chromoblastomycosis. Some fungi, such as *E. jeanselmei*, may cause mycetoma (characterized by granule formation) in some patients, phaeohyphomycosis in others, and chromoblastomycosis in others.

Treatment

Cutaneous and superficial phaeohyphomycosis may respond to topical antifungal agents. Surgical excision, if feasible, combined with itraconazole, 400 mg/day for 6 months, is recommended for deeper lesions.

Burges GE, et al: Subcutaneous phaeohyphomycosis caused by *Exserohilum rostratum* in an immunocompetent host. *Arch Dermatol* 1987, 123:1346.

Clancy CJ, et al: Subcutaneous phaeohyphomycosis. *Clin Infect Dis* 1997, 25:1065.

Coldiron BM, et al: Cutaneous phaeohyphomycosis caused by a rare fungal pathogen, *Hormonema dermatitides*. *J Am Acad Dermatol* 1990, 23:363.

Duvic M, et al: Superficial phaeohyphomycosis of the scrotum in a patient with AIDS. *Arch Dermatol* 1987, 123:1597.

Hsu MM, et al: Cutaneous and subcutaneous phaeohyphomycosis caused by *Exserohilum rostratum*. *J Am Acad Dermatol* 1993, 28:340.

McCown HF, et al: Subcutaneous phaeohyphomycosis and nocardiosis in a kidney transplant patient. *J Am Acad Dermatol* 1997, 36:863.

McGinnis MR, et al: Infections caused by black fungi. *Arch Dermatol* 1987, 123:1300.

Noel SB, et al: Primary cutaneous phaeohyphomycosis. *J Am Acad Dermatol* 1988, 18:1023.

Patterson JW, et al: Cutaneous phaeohyphomycosis due to *Cladophialophora bantiana*. *J Am Acad Dermatol* 1999, 40:364.

Radentz WH: Opportunistic fungal infections in immunocompromised hosts. *J Am Acad Dermatol* 1989, 20:989.

Rinaldi MG: Phaeohyphomycosis. *Dermatol Clin* 1996, 14:147.

Sharkey PK, et al: Itraconazole treatment of phaeohyphomycosis. *J Am Acad Dermatol* 1990, 23:577.

Straka BF, et al: Cutaneous *Bipolaris spicifera* infection. *Arch Dermatol* 1989, 125:1383.

Vidmar DA: Phaeomycotic cyst. *Arch Dermatol* 1991, 127:721. ▲

MYCETOMA

Synonyms: Madura foot, maduromycosis

Mycetoma is a clinical entity but not an etiologic one. It comprises actinomycetomas caused by *Streptomyces, Nocardia,* or *Actinomyces* species, and eumycetomas caused by true fungi: *Madurella, Cephalosporium,* or *Pseudallescheria.*

Mycetoma generally begins as a subcutaneous swelling, usually occurring on the instep or the toe webs. The tumor is 8 to 10 mm, painless, nontender, firm, and of rubbery texture. The overlying skin may be normal or attached to the underlying tumor. The mature, fully developed lesion is a tumefaction accompanied by the formation of nodules, tubercles, and draining sinuses, usually on the foot or ankle (Fig. 15-74). The draining sinuses secrete microcolonies or

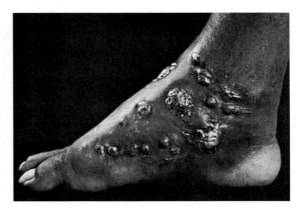

Fig. 15-74 Mycetoma in typical location, caused by *Nocardia brasiliensis.* (Courtesy Dr. F. Latapi, Mexico.)

grains of the causative organism. Not only the skin and subcutaneous tissues but also the underlying fascia and bone are usually involved. There is severe swelling, but pain may not be present. The lesion spreads by local extension, which may go on for decades before it interferes with local function.

Other parts of the body, such as the hands, arms, chest, and buttocks, may also be involved. Extensive osteomyelitis may be present. The progression of the disease is slow. As the foot enlarges, the leg atrophies from disuse. After decades the disease, if untreated, terminates in death caused by sepsis and exhaustion.

Etiology

Mycetoma is divided into eumycetoma, produced by true fungi, and actinomycetoma, produced by actinomycetes. Examples of eumycetomas are those caused by *Pseudallescheria boydii, Acremonium falciforme, A. recifei, Leptosphaeria senegalensis, L. tompkinsii, Madurella grisea, M. mycetomatis, Exophiala jeanselmei, Pyrenochaeta romeri,* and *Phialophora verrucosa.* Examples of actinomycetomas are those caused by *Nocardia asteroides, N. brasiliensis, N. caviae, Actinomadura madurae, A. pelletier, Actinomyces israelii,* and *Streptomyces somaliensis. Actinomyces israelii,* an anaerobic species of Actinomycetales, is placed by some in the actinomycetoma group. Eubacteria, including staphylococcus and streptococcus, and various dermatophytes have also caused mycetoma. Grains and bone involvement are sufficient to justify the diagnosis of mycetoma.

Epidemiology

Mycetoma occurs everywhere. In the Western Hemisphere the incidence is highest in Mexico, followed by Venezuela and Argentina. In Africa it is found most frequently in Senegal, Sudan, and Somalia. It occurs in males five times as often as females, and is most common in the third and fourth decades of life.

Pathogenesis

Mycetoma is probably acquired from the soil by walking barefooted and sustaining some form of injury either by pricking or abrasion.

Mycology

No attempt is made to describe the various culture characteristics of the causative organisms. For true fungi (eumycetoma), cultures are made from the grains on Sabouraud's dextrose agar containing 0.5% yeast extract and suitable antibiotics. Cultures should be incubated at 37° C and room temperature. For actinomycetes grains, culture should be made in brain-heart infusion agar, incubated aerobically and anaerobically at 37° C, and on Sabouraud's dextrose agar with 0.5% yeast extract incubated aerobically at 37° C and room temperature. The specimen for culture should be taken from a deep site, preferably from the base of a biopsy.

Diagnosis

Mycetoma may be diagnosed by keeping in mind a triad of signs, namely: tumefaction, sinuses, and granules. Pus gathered from a deep sinus will show the granules when examined with the microscope. The slide containing the specimen should have a drop of 10% sodium hydroxide added and a coverslip placed on top; the granule with the hyphae will be colored black, white, or red.

Grains may be light-colored (white, pearly, cream, sulfur), red or black, or dark-colored. Light-colored grains are caused by *Actinomyces israelii, Actinomadura madurae, Nocardia* species, *Streptomyces somaliensis, Pseudallescheria boydii, Acremonium* species, *Aspergillus nidulans, Fusarium* species, and *Neotestudina rosatii.* Red grains are produced only by *Actinomadura pelletieri.* Black or dark grains are produced by *Curvularia geniculata, Helminthosporium spiciferum, Leptosphaeria senegalensis, Madurella grisea* and *M. mycetomatis, Exophiala jeanselmei, Phialophora verrucosa,* and *Pyrenochaeta romeri.*

Special stains for demonstration of fungi, such as PAS and Gomori's methenamine silver, will clearly show hyphae and other fungal structures within the grain. Hyphae 2 to 5 µm in thickness suggest true fungus mycetoma. Gram stain of an actinomycotic grain shows gram-positive, thin filaments, 1 to 2 µm thick, embedded in a gram-negative amorphous matrix. Club formation in the periphery of a grain may be seen but is of limited value in the identification of the organism.

Radiographs will show the bone involvement, and mycetoma can be diagnosed readily by expert radiologists.

Treatment

Patients in the early stage of mycetoma are successfully treated by thorough removal of the affected area by cautery. In the more advanced stages, especially of the eumycetomas, amputation is frequently necessary.

In *A. israelii* infection, penicillin in large doses is curative. *Nocardia asteroides* or *N. brasiliensis* should be treated with sulfonamides. Cases caused by the true fungi generally have not responded reliably to systemic antifungal agents; however, surgical excision when possible combined with itraconazole, 200 mg twice daily until clinically well, may be effective in those cases caused by *P. boydii.* This approach, and the use of other newer antifungals if cure does not result, may be tried, for the only alternative is amputation, unfortunately a frequent outcome in the past.

Degavre B, et al: First report of mycetoma caused by *Arthrographis kalrae. J Am Acad Dermatol* 1997, 37:318.

Lee MW, et al: Mycetoma caused by *Acremonium falciforme. J Am Acad Dermatol* 1995, 32:897.

McGinnis MR: Mycetoma. *Dermatol Clin* 1996, 14:97.

Soroush V, et al: A draining tumor in the popliteal fossa. *Arch Dermatol* 1999, 135:983.

Turiansky GW, et al: *Phialophora verrucosa:* a new agent for mycetoma. *J Am Acad Dermatol* 1995, 32:311.

Welsh O: Mycetoma. *Int J Dermatol* 1991; 30:387.

Welsh O, et al: Amikacin alone or in combination with trimethoprim-sulfamethoxazole in the treatment of actinomycotic mycetoma. *J Am Acad Dermatol* 1987, 17:443.

Wortman PD, et al: Treatment of *Nocardia brasiliensis* mycetoma with sulfamethoxazole and trimethoprim, amikacin, and amoxicillin and clavulanate. *Arch Dermatol* 1993, 129:564. ▲

KELOIDAL BLASTOMYCOSIS (LOBOMYCOSIS)

Keloidal blastomycosis was originally described by Jorge Lobo in 1931. All cases reported since then have occurred in countries in Central and South America, except for an aquarium attendant who cared for an infected dolphin in Europe.

The disease may involve any part of the body (Fig. 15-75). As the name implies, the lesions appear characteristically keloidal, with or without fistulas. The nodules increase in size gradually by invasion of the surrounding normal skin or through the superficial lymphatics. Long-standing cases involve the regional lymph nodes. A common location is the ear (Fig. 15-76), which looks like the cauliflower ear of a boxer, with pseudokeloidal nodules and infiltrations of the helix. These are painless, violet to pink, and generally not associated with lymphadenopathy.

The fungus is felt to be present in water, soil, or vegetation in forested areas where the disease is prevalent. Dolphins may harbor this infection. More than 300 cases have been reported, with equal distribution between the sexes. The age of patients is usually between 30 and 80. Agricultural laborers have been most frequently affected.

Histologically, the epidermis is atrophic. Numerous organisms with double-contoured walls are seen in the dermis. Refringent parasites are always conspicuous. The cellular infiltrate is composed of vacuolated histiocytes, giant cells, and parasites. The organisms are thick-walled, refractile spherules larger than those of *Paracoccidioides*

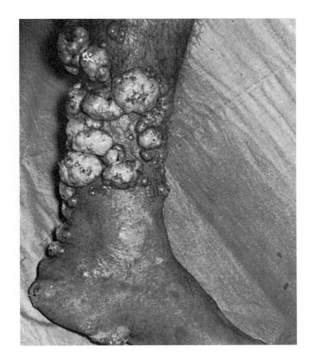

Fig. 15-75 Keloidal blastomycosis. (Courtesy Dr. J. Lobo, Brazil.)

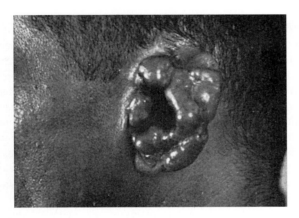

Fig. 15-76 Keloidal blastomycosis in a typical location. (Courtesy Dr. M. de Moraes, Brazil.)

brasiliensis. One or two buds may be seen, but never multiple budding as in *P. brasiliensis.* It has not been cultured. The causative fungus is a blastomyces-like organism called *Loboa loboi.*

Surgical excision of the affected areas is usually unsuccessful, being followed by recurrence. No form of chemotherapy has produced any consistently favorable results, but clofazimine or amphotericin B may be tried.

Elgart ML: Unusual subcutaneous infections. *Dermatol Clin* 1996, 14:105.
Rodriguez-Toro G: Lobomycosis. *Int J Dermatol* 1993, 32:324. _____ ▲

RHINOSPORIDIOSIS

Rhinosporidiosis is a polypoid disease involving the nasal mucosa chiefly. The lesions begin as small papillomas and develop into pedunculated tumors with fissured and warty surfaces, on which there is a myxomatous material containing grayish white flecks or spots, which are large sporangia. The lesions are friable and may resemble a cauliflower (Fig. 15-77). Bleeding occurs easily. Infection of the lacrimal sac, uvula, ears, vulva, vagina, or penis may occur. Conjunctival lesions begin as small, pinkish papillary nodules. Later they become dark and lobulated. Penile lesions resemble venereal warts and may become cauliflower-like vegetative growths. Rectal and vaginal lesions may have a similar appearance or may resemble condylomata or polyps. Widespread dissemination to all the viscera may occur.

Etiology

Rhinosporidium seeberi is the causative organism. In infected tissue the organisms are usually numerous and occupy much of the tissue. They appear as spores 7 to 10 μm in diameter, which are contained within large cystic structures, sporangia, that may be as large as 300 μm in diameter.

Epidemiology

The disease is endemic in Ceylon and India, but it also occurs in Argentina and Brazil. It has been seen in southern United States, England, Italy, Cuba, and Mexico. Young adults and children are most frequently affected. It is more common in men than in women.

Diagnosis

The demonstration of characteristic large sporangia in the polypoid mass is pathognomonic.

Treatment

Destruction of the involved area by electrosurgery is best. Chemotherapy is of no value.

Batsakis JG, et al: Rhinoscleroma and rhinosporidiosis. *Ann Otol Rhinol Laryngol* 1992, 101:879.
Elgart ML: Unusual subcutaneous infections. *Dermatol Clin* 1996, 14:105.
Levy MG, et al: Cultivation of *Rhinosporidium seeberi* in vitro. *Science* 1986, 234:474.
Ramanan C: Giant cutaneous rhinosporidiosis. *Int J Dermatol* 1996, 35:44.
Yesudian P: Cutaneous rhinosporidiosis mimicking verruca vulgaris. *Int J Dermatol* 1988, 27:47. _____ ▲

ACTINOMYCOSIS

Actinomycosis is an anaerobic, gram-positive, bacterial infection, seen most often in the cervicofacial area but also seen commonly on the abdominal region and thoracic area. Although it is bacterial, its clinical manifestations and long

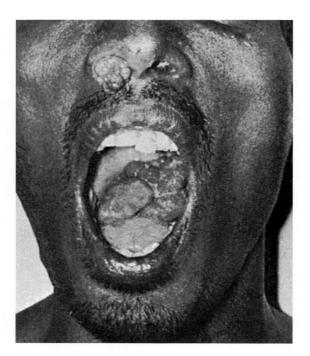

Fig. 15-77 Rhinosporidiosis in the nasal mucosa and soft palate. (Courtesy Dr. Kameswaran, Madurai, India.)

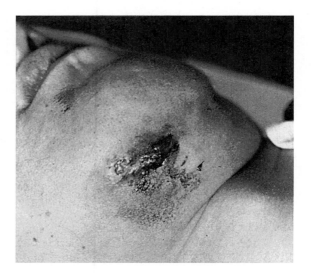

Fig. 15-78 Actinomycosis.

history of grouping with the deep fungi justify its placement here with them. Middle-aged men are affected most often. The lesions are characteristic, being local, dusky red swellings; firm, fluctuating nodules; and sinuses exuding a purulent discharge. In this exudate may be whitish or yellowish granules, commonly known as *sulfur granules,* which are masses of microorganisms. The aggregate is usually surrounded by marked wooden induration, which produces in the cervicofacial region a lumpy jaw (Fig. 15-78). The underlying jaw bone may be involved with periostitis and even osteomyelitis. Mandibular infection is seen four times as often as maxillary involvement (Fig. 15-79). When the gastrointestinal system is involved, the cecum and appendix are the more commonly affected organs, the gallbladder and the stomach less so. Extension into the abdomen and then the abdominal wall may produce draining sinuses on the abdominal skin. Abscesses may occur in the vertebrae, kidneys, ovaries, and urinary bladder.

The third most frequent site of involvement is the thoracic region, as a result of inhalation of the organism and infection of the lungs (Fig. 15-80). Subsequent thoracic wall sinuses may form, and extension into the vertebrae and ribs ensues.

Etiology

Actinomycosis is caused in humans by *Actinomyces israelii* and in animals by *Actinomyces bovis.* Human infections caused by *A. bovis, A. naeslundii,* and *A. viscosus* have been documented.

Diagnosis

On a microscope slide or Petri dish should be placed sputum; bronchial aspirates; pleural, joint, or pericardial fluid; pus; or biopsy specimens, which should be closely examined for sulfur-yellow granules measuring 1 to 5 mm in diameter. Microscopic examination shows lobulated bodies consisting of delicate branching and intertwining filaments suggestive of clubs. These are best seen at the periphery of the sulfur granule body. They resemble rays; hence the name, ray fungus *(Actinomyces).* Gram stain on the crushed sulfur granule will show delicate, branching, intertwined, gram-positive filaments.

The crushed granule is used for inoculating cultures containing brain-heart infusion blood agar, incubated under anaerobic conditions at 37° C. Culture is difficult, with less than 50% of cases being confirmed in this manner. Direct microscopy is of utmost importance.

Pathogenesis

Actinomycosis is believed to be acquired by endogenous implantation into deep tissues where anaerobic conditions prevail. Puncture wounds, dental extractions, or compound fractures are some of the routes of infection. *A. israelii* has been recovered from the normal mouth, from tonsils, and from carious teeth and is thought to be commonly present. The belief that infection is from endogenous sources is further confirmed by the fact that *A. israelii* has never been demonstrated in soil, in plants, or in any other object outside the body.

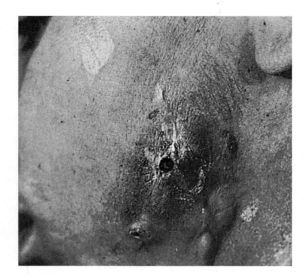

Fig. 15-79 Actinomycosis ("lumpy jaw").

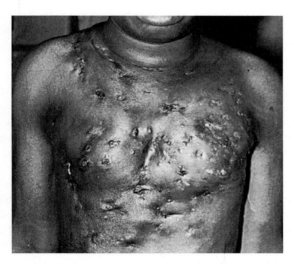

Fig. 15-80 Actinomycosis of the skin with a primary lesion in the lung of a 25-year-old man. (Courtesy Dr. El-Zawahry, U.A.R.)

Pathology

The histologic finding is that of an infective granuloma forming a deep nodular process, with granulation tissue, epithelioid cells, plasma and giant cells, and degenerative changes. Large and deep abscesses and sinuses are found, which contain polymorphonuclear leukocytes and miscellaneous debris, along with the organism and its filaments.

Differential Diagnosis

Actinomycosis must be differentiated from scrofuloderma, which is likely to cause less infiltration and more corded and hypertrophic scars. Superficial examination may suggest sarcoma, carcinoma, blastomycosis, or tertiary syphilis, but these are readily excluded by a close study of the

characteristics of the lesions. Positive diagnosis is made by a demonstration of the organism in the discharge or in scrapings from the edge of the lesions.

Treatment

Penicillin G in large doses, 10 to 20 million units daily for 1 month, followed by 4 to 6 g of oral penicillin daily for another 2 months, may produce successful and lasting results. Other effective medications have been ampicillin, erythromycin, tetracyclines, ceftriaxone, and clindamycin. Surgical incision, drainage, and excision of devitalized tissue is important in the treatment.

Prognosis

Of the three forms described, the cervical type usually responds best to treatment. When surgical treatment is feasible and penicillin therapy can be continued for a long time, a cure may be expected.

Cirillo-Hyland V, et al: Cervicofacial actinomycosis resembling a ruptured cyst. *J Am Acad Dermatol* 1993, 29:308.

Deloach-Banta LJ, et al: Nonhealing masses of the right cheek and submandibular areas. *Arch Dermatol* 1991, 167:1831.

Katz BJ, et al: Subcutaneous nodules in a man diagnosed as having tuberculosis. *Arch Dermatol* 1988, 124:121.

Warren NG: Actinomycosis, nocardiosis, and actinomycetoma. *Dermatol Clin* 1996, 14:85. ——————————————————— ▲

NOCARDIOSIS

Nocardiosis usually begins as a pulmonary infection from which dissemination occurs. The clinical picture is not distinctive; however, weight loss, anorexia, night sweats, and cough symptoms similar to those of tuberculosis are frequently seen. In about one third of the patients there is CNS involvement. Symptoms are usually due to the formation of brain abscesses suggestive of brain tumors. Disseminated lesions may also involve the ribs, femurs, vertebrae, and pelvis. Multiple abscesses may develop in the skin in about 10% of cases. A generalized vesicular or pustular eruption may also occur. The skin lesions may be draining abscesses as an extension of the infective processes in the chest wall and lungs.

Nocardia asteroides, which is responsible for this disseminated form in most cases, occurs most commonly in association with debilitating disease such as Hodgkin's disease, periarteritis nodosa, leukemia, AIDS, organ transplants, or systemic lupus erythematosus. Approximately 20% of disseminated infections occur in immunocompetent patients.

Localized lymphocutaneous lesions in a sporotrichoid pattern occur after trauma to an extremity, usually the hand. A chancriform lesion develops with a proximal chain of nodules. This occurs usually in healthy individuals and is nearly always caused by *N. brasiliensis.* Superficial skin

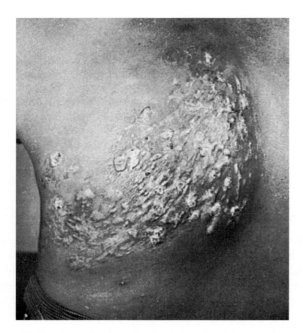

Fig. 15-81 Nocardiosis cutis involving the left scapular area *(Nocardia brasiliensis).* (Courtesy Dr. J. Convit, Venezuela.)

Angelika J, et al: Primary cutaneous nocardiosis in a husband and wife. *J Am Acad Dermatol* 1999, 41:338.

Johnson M, et al: A palmar chancre and multiple proximal erythematous nodules. *Arch Dermatol* 1996, 132:964.

Kannon GA, et al: Superficial cutaneous *Nocardia asteroides* infection in an immunocompetent pregnant woman. *J Am Acad Dermatol* 1996, 35:1000.

Moeller CA, et al: Primary lymphocutaneous *Nocardia brasiliensis* infection. *Arch Dermatol* 1986, 122:1180.

Saff DM, et al: Ulcerative lesions in a gardener. *Arch Dermatol* 1994, 130:243.

Schiff TA, et al: Primary cutaneous nocardiosis caused by an unusual species of nocardia: *Nocardia transvalensis*. *J Am Acad Dermatol* 1993, 28:336.

Soroush V, et al: A draining tumor in the popliteal fossa. *Arch Dermatol* 1999, 135:983.

Tsuboi R, et al: Lymphocutaneous nocardiosis caused by *Nocardia asteroides*. *Arch Dermatol* 1986, 122:1183.

Yang LJ, et al: Lymphocutaneous nocardiosis caused by *Nocardia caviae*. *J Am Acad Dermatol* 1993, 29:639. _____ ▲

infections also occur and present as cellulitis, abscesses, ulcers, or granulomas (Fig. 15-81). Mycetoma caused by *Nocardia* is discussed under that clinical heading.

Etiology

Nocardiosis is caused by *N. asteroides, N. caviae, N. transvalensis,* or *N. brasiliensis,* which are found in soil and may be inhaled in dust. Implantation from contaminated dust directly into the skin may also occur. A thorn prick by a briar on which *N. brasiliensis* was residing has caused infections. The organisms have also been recovered from the noses and throats of normal individuals.

Diagnosis

N. asteroides can be demonstrated in pus or sputum when stained with Gram stain. These are gram-positive, partially acid-fast filaments measuring about 1 μm in diameter. Some are branched. On Sabouraud's dextrose agar, without antibacterial additives, there are creamy or moist, white colonies, which later become chalky and orange-colored.

Clinically, many cases resemble tuberculosis; however, the pulmonary form of nocardiosis should be considered, especially when abscesses and draining sinuses appear on the chest wall.

Treatment

Trimethoprim-sulfamethoxazole (Bactrim, Septra), 4 tablets twice daily for 6 to 12 weeks, is the drug of first choice. Minocycline for *N. asteroides* and Augmentin for *N. brasiliensis* are alternatives. Amikacin combined with ceftriaxone is also effective.

ZYGOMYCOSIS (PHYCOMYCOSIS)

There are a number of important pathogens in the class Zygomycetes. The two orders within this class that cause cutaneous infection most often are the Mucorales and Entomophthorales.

Entomophthoromycosis. Infections caused by the order Entomophthorales have been named entomophthoromycosis, rhinoentomophthoromycosis, conidiobolomycosis, or basidiobolomycosis. They occur usually in healthy individuals, unlike mucormycosis. The infections may be classified as cutaneous, subcutaneous, visceral, and disseminated.

Subcutaneous lesions occur in two basic types, each involving different anatomic sites. Well-circumscribed subcutaneous masses involving the nose, paranasal tissue, and upper lip, as in the case reported by Towersey et al, characterize one type. The second type occurs as indurated, nodular, subcutaneous lesions located on the extremities, buttocks, and trunk.

Etiology

Conidiobolus coronatus typically causes the perinasal disease, whereas *Basidiobolus ranarum* causes the type of subcutaneous disease seen off the face.

Epidemiology

Occurrence is worldwide. It was first reported in Indonesia, where it is prevalent. Since then reports have come from Africa, Asia, and the Americas. Generally, infection occurs in countries situated between 15º latitude North and 15º latitude South.

Diagnosis

Isolation and identification of the causative fungus are fundamental to the diagnosis. Culture on Sabouraud's dextrose agar is made of nasal discharge, abscess fluid, or

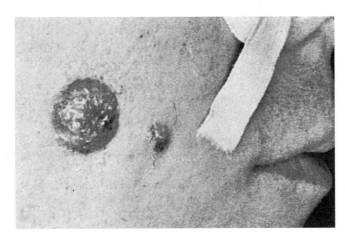

Fig. 15-82 Cutaneous *Mucor* infection of face. (Courtesy Dr. J.L. Wade.)

biopsy specimens. Biopsy specimens will show fibroblastic proliferation and an inflammatory reaction with lymphocytes, plasma cells, histiocytes, eosinophils, and giant cells. Broad, thin-walled hyphae with occasional septa, branched at right angles, are seen. The Splendore-Hoeppli phenomenon may be seen, in which an eosinophilic sleeve surmounts the hyphae. Triscott et al emphasize the histologic similarity of subcutaneous pythiosis, a primitive aquatic hyphal organism. Their report, of two immunocompetent boys with rapidly swelling and inflamed areas on the central face, reviewed this disease. Amphotericin B cured their patients.

Treatment

Potassium iodide has been the drug of choice. Sometimes, combining this with trimethoprim-sulfamethoxazole improves results. Amphotericin B has also been effective in some cases. Several reports, including the one by Towersey et al, document a response to ketoconazole. Excision of small lesions is an alternative method of management.

Mucormycosis. *Mucormycosis* refers to infections caused by the order Mucorales of the class Zygomycetes (Fig. 15-82). They characteristically are acute, rapidly developing, often fatal, opportunistic infections of immunocompromised patients. Most occur in ketoacidotic diabetes, but leukemia, lymphoma, AIDS, iatrogenic immunosuppression, burns, chronic renal failure, and malnourishment all predispose to these infections. Occasionally, healthy individuals have been reported to develop these infections.

The five major clinical forms (rhinocerebral, pulmonary, cutaneous, gastrointestinal, and disseminated) share features that include invasion of blood vessel walls by organisms. This leads to infarction, gangrene, and the formation of black, necrotic pus. Ulceration, cellulitis, ecthyma gangrenosum–like lesions, and necrotic abscesses constitute the usual cutaneous appearance. It may involve

the skin through traumatic implantation or by hematogenous dissemination. An eschar at an IV site, while classically a sign of *Aspergillus* infection, may be caused by *Rhizopus*.

Etiology

The fungi that cause this infection are ubiquitous molds common in the soil, on decomposing plant and animal matter, and in the air. The pathogenic genera include *Absidia, Mucor, Rhizopus, Cunninghamella, Apophysomyces, Rhizomucor, Saksenaea, Mortierella,* and *Cokeromyces.*

Diagnosis

Tissue obtained by biopsy or curettage is cultured. Prompt diagnosis by this method is essential in this rapidly fatal infection.

Treatment

Basic to effective therapy is gaining control of the underlying disease. A combination of excision of affected tissue with amphotericin B is necessary.

Bittencourt AL, et al: Basidiobolomycosis. *Pediatr Dermatol* 1991, 8:325.

Droubet DL, et al: Laboratory and clinical assessment of ketoconazole in deep-seated mycosis. *Am J Med* 1983, 74:30.

Elgart ML: Zygomycosis. *Dermatol Clin* 1996, 14:141.

Geller JD, et al: Cutaneous mucormycosis resembling superficial granulomatous pyoderma in an immunocompetent host. *J Am Acad Dermatol* 1993, 29:462.

Hata TR, et al: Ecthymalike lesions on the leg of an immunocompromised patient. *Arch Dermatol* 1995, 131:833.

Khardori N, et al: Cutaneous *Rhizopus* and *Aspergillus* infections in 5 patients with cancer. *Arch Dermatol* 1989, 125:952.

Lehrer RI, et al: Mucormycosis. *Ann Intern Med* 1980, 93:93.

Prevooe RMA, et al: Primary cutaneous mucormycosis in a healthy young girl. *J Am Acad Dermatol* 1991, 24:882.

Restrepo A: Treatment of tropical mycoses. *J Am Acad Dermatol* 1994, 31:S91.

Rinaldi MG: Zygomycosis. *Infect Dis Clin North Am* 1989, 3:19.

Sanchez MR, et al: Zygomycosis and HIV infection. *J Am Acad Dermatol* 1991, 24:882.

Towersey L, et al: *Conidiobolus coronatus* infection treated with ketoconazole. *Arch Dermatol* 1988, 124:1392.

Triscott JA, et al: Human subcutaneous pythiosis. *J Cutan Pathol* 1993, 20:267.

Umbert IJ, et al: Cutaneous mucormycosis. *J Am Acad Dermatol* 1989, 21:1232.

Weinberg JM, et al: Mucormycosis in a patient with acquired immunodeficiency syndrome. *Arch Dermatol* 1997, 133:249.

Wirth F, et al: Cutaneous mucormycosis with subsequent visceral dissemination in a child with neutropenia. *J Am Acad Dermatol* 1997, 36:336.

Woods SG, et al: Zosteriform zygomycosis. *J Am Acad Dermatol* 1995, 32:357. ⎯⎯⎯⎯⎯⎯⎯⎯⎯⎯⎯ ▲

HYALOHYPHOMYCOSIS

The term *hyalohyphomycosis* complements phaeohyphomycosis and comprises those opportunistic mycotic infections caused by nondematiaceous molds whose basic form consists of hyaline hyphal fragments that are septate, branched or unbranched, or toruloid. It is not intended to replace such well-established names as aspergillosis or candidiasis but rather refers to infections caused by organisms such as *Fusarium, Penicillium,* and *Paecilomyces.*

These organisms are ubiquitous; they occur as saprophytes in soil or water or on decomposing organic debris. They generally do not cause disease except in immunocompromised patients. *Fusarium solani* (keratomycosis) and *F. oxysporum* (white superficial onychomycosis) are exceptions. There is no classic clinical morphology to the lesions, but keratotic masses, ulcerations, ecthyma gangrenosum–like lesions, erythematous nodules, and disseminated erythema have been described. *Penicillium marneffei* infection has emerged as a new potential indicator of HIV disease in Southeast Asia.

Most of the infections are treated with a combination of excision and amphotericin B. Success is generally low.

Arrese JE, et al: Fatal hyalohyphomycosis following *Fusarium onychomycosis* in an immunocompromised patient. *Am J Dermatopathol* 1996, 18:196.

Borradori L, et al: *Penicillium marneffei* infection and AIDS. *J Am Acad Dermatol* 1994, 31:843.

Diven DG, et al: Cutaneous hyalohyphomycosis caused by *Paecilomyces lilacinus* in a patient with lymphoma. *J Am Acad Dermatol* 1996, 35:779.

Helm TM, et al: Case report and review of resolved fusariosis. *J Am Acad Dermatol* 1990, 23:393.

Jade KB, et al: *Paecilomyces lilacinus* cellulitis in an immunocompromised patient. *Arch Dermatol* 1986, 122:1169.

Matsuda T, et al: Disseminated hyalohyphomycosis in a leukemic patient. *Arch Dermatol* 1986, 122:1171.

Repiso T, et al: Disseminated fusariosis. *Pediatr Dermatol* 1996, 13:118.

Rinaldi MG: Emerging opportunists. *Infect Dis Clin North Am* 1989, 3:65.

Sayama K, et al: Squamous cell carcinoma arising in long-standing granulomatous hyalohyphomycosis caused by *Fusarium solani. Arch Dermatol* 1991, 1275:1735.

Veglia KS, et al: *Fusarium* as a pathogen. *J Am Acad Dermatol* 1987, 16:260.

Weitzman I: Saprophytic molds as agents of cutaneous and subcutaneous infection in the immunocompromised host. *Arch Dermatol* 1986, 122:1161. _____ ▲

ASPERGILLOSIS

Aspergillosis is second only to candidiasis in frequency of opportunistic fungal disease in patients with leukemia and other hematologic neoplasia. Renal and heart transplant patients receiving immunosuppressive drugs may show aspergillosis at autopsy. Neonates, burns, patients on long-term corticosteroid therapy, or those on cytotoxic chemotherapy with neutropenia are also predisposed to *Aspergillus* infections. Invasive aspergillosis is difficult to diagnose and is often lethal in the immunosuppressed host. Blood cultures and serologic tests are usually negative. Pulmonary involvement is usually present in invasive

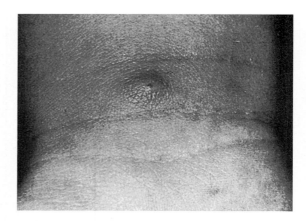

Fig. 15-83 Cutaneous lesion on wrist of young girl with primary disseminated aspergillosis of the lungs. (Courtesy Drs. J. Vedder and W.F. Schorr.)

aspergillus disease, but skin lesions are present in only about 10% of cases.

The skin lesions associated with systemic aspergillosis are grouped into five categories: the solitary necrotizing dermal plaque; the subcutaneous granuloma or abscess; persistent eruptive dermal papules with suppurative (Fig. 15-83), vegetating, or necrobiotic tendencies; miscellaneous erythemas and toxicodermas; and progressive confluent granulomas. *Aspergillus fumigatus* is the most common cause of disseminated aspergillosis with cutaneous involvement. It is imperative to obtain a cutaneous biopsy and culture of skin lesions when the clinical setting suggests the possibility of opportunistic fungal infections. In tissue septate hyphae with 45-degree angle branching are seen. They tend to invade and thrombose vessels, leading to infarction. The organism grows on media without cycloheximide in 24 hours or more.

Amphotericin B has been the drug of choice in invasive aspergillosis and cutaneous infections in immunocompromised patients. Itraconazole is an excellent alternative medication, at a dose of 200 to 400 mg daily for 1 year. Ketoconazole and fluconazole have limited to no efficacy.

Primary Cutaneous Aspergillosis. Primary cutaneous aspergillosis is a rare disease. Grossman et al's report of six children with hematologic malignancies who developed skin lesions at the site of intravenous cannulas typifies these cases. Hemorrhagic bullae, which progressed to necrotic ulcers, were present. *Aspergillus flavus* is most commonly associated with this form of infection. All recovered when treated with intravenous amphotericin B.

Hunt et al described two patients with AIDS who developed molluscum contagiosum–like papules beneath adhesive tape near central venous catheters. The use of nonocclusive dressings and local wound care resulted in involution of several lesions. *Aspergillus* is a frequent contaminant in cultures from thickened, friable, dystrophic nails. Various *Aspergillus* species have been reported to be etiologic agents in onychomycosis. Scher et al report successful treatment of a nail infection with itraconazole.

Otomycosis. A favorite site of infection is the ear canal, although its role as a pathogen has been questioned. Only erythema and scaling are present in the ear canal. *Aspergillus fumigatus, A. flavus,* and *A. niger* are the most prevalent species found. They are composed of compact clusters of branching septate hyphae 4 to 6 µm in diameter. Examination of a KOH wet slide shows densely packed hyphae. On Sabouraud's medium the black mold of *A. niger* grows.

There is always some doubt as to whether *A. niger* is the etiologic agent or is, rather, a contaminant. Pathogenic bacteria, especially *Pseudomonas aeruginosa,* are often found concurrently in otomycosis. Treatment should be directed toward keeping the ear dry. Iodochlorhydroxyquin (Vioform, Ciba) is the treatment of choice. A 3% lotion is applied to the canal three times daily.

Pulmonary Aspergillosis. The lungs are the most common site for aspergillosis, which occurs when there is some underlying disease that impairs the host's defense mechanisms. Bronchitis, pulmonary infiltrations, and pulmonary nodules known as *aspergillomas* may occur.

Aspergillosis of the lung is usually caused by *A. fumigatus,* which can be diagnosed by finding conidiophores in histologic sections. Direct examination of sputum and cultures from sputum and bronchial washings also aid in the diagnosis.

Keratomycosis. Ulceration of the cornea along with penetration into the deep stromal layers with an acute inflammatory reaction that may later progress into mycotic endophthalmitis may be a concomitant infection of the eye. Many different fungi, including *A. flavus,* may be the cause.

Dupont B: Itraconazole therapy in aspergillosis. *J Am Acad Dermatol* 1990, 23:607.

Greenbaum RS, et al: Subcutaneous nodule in a cardiac transplant. *Arch Dermatol* 1993, 129:1189.

Grossman ME, et al: Primary cutaneous aspergillosis in six leukemic children. *J Am Acad Dermatol* 1985, 12:313.

Harmon CB, et al: Cutaneous aspergillosis complicating pyoderma gangrenosum. *J Am Acad Dermatol* 1993, 29:656.

Hunt SJ, et al: Primary cutaneous aspergillosis near central venous catheters in patients with AIDS. *Arch Dermatol* 1992, 128:1229.

Isaac M: Cutaneous aspergillosis. *Dermatol Clin* 1996, 14:137.

Morrison VA, et al: Non-Candida fungal infections after bone marrow transplantation. *Ann J Med* 1994, 96:497.

Papouli M, et al: Primary cutaneous aspergillosis in neonates. *Clin Infect Dis* 1996, 22:1102.

Ricci RM, et al: Primary cutaneous *Aspergillus ustus* infection. *J Am Acad Dermatol* 1998, 38:797.

Romero LS, et al: Hickman catheter-associated primary cutaneous aspergillosis in a patient with the acquired immunodeficiency syndrome. *Int J Dermatol* 1995, 34:551.

Rowen JL, et al: Invasive aspergillosis in neonates. *Pediatr Infect Dis J* 1992, 11:576.

Scher RK, et al: Successful treatment of *Aspergillus flavus* onychomycosis with itraconazole. *J Am Acad Dermatol* 1993, 23:749.

Watsky KL, et al: Unilateral cutaneous emboli of *Aspergillus. Arch Dermatol* 1990, 26:1217.

Weitzman I: Sporophytic molds as agents of cutaneous and subcutaneous infection in the immunocompromised host. *Arch Dermatol* 1986, 122:1161. _____ ▲

ALTERNARIOSIS

Alternaria is a genus of molds recognized as common plant pathogens but very rare causes of human infection. Most reported cases have occurred in immunocompromised patients. Cutaneous alternariosis usually presents as focal ulcerated papules and plaques on exposed skin of the face, forearms and hands, or knees. The course is chronic. Surgical excision, intralesional miconazole, ketoconazole, and itraconazole have been reported to be effective in individual cases.

Del Palacio A, et al: Cutaneous *Alternaria alternata* infection successfully treated with itraconazole. *Clin Exp Dermatol* 1996, 21:241.

Iwatsu T: Cutaneous alternariosis. *Arch Dermatol* 1988, 124:1822.

Junkins JM, et al: Unusual fungal infection in immunocompromised oncology patient: cutaneous alternariosis. *Arch Dermatol* 1988, 124:1421.

Lerner LH, et al: Co-existence of cutaneous and presumptive pulmonary alternariosis. *Int J Dermatol* 1997, 36:285. _____ ▲

DISEASE CAUSED BY ALGAE (PROTOTHECOSIS)

Protothecosis is a verrucous skin disease caused by the *Prototheca* genus of saprophytic, achloric (nonpigmented) algae. These organisms reproduce asexually via internal septation, producing autospores identical to the parent cell. This reproductive method, along with the absence of glucosamine and muramic acid in the cell wall, separates the genus from the bacteria and fungi. Two *Prototheca* species cause disease in humans, *Prototheca wickerhamii* and *P. zopfi.* Stagnant water and soil appear to be the source of infection in most cases.

Skin lesions observed have included papulonodular lesions, crusted papules with umbilication and ulceration, and an extensive granulomatous eruption. Protothecosis of the olecranon bursa is usually seen in healthy individuals, but cutaneous infections have been most often reported in patients receiving immunosuppressive therapy, in renal failure, with widespread carcinomatosis, with AIDS, or with diabetes mellitus.

Prototheca species are easily recognized in PAS-stained tissue specimens when the characteristic endosporulating cells are visible. The organisms are grown on most routine mycologic media; however, cycloheximide, used to inhibit growth of saprophytic fungi, will also suppress growth of *Prototheca* species. Colonies on Sabouraud's agar are smooth, creamy, and yeastlike. The use of fluorescent antibody reagents makes possible the rapid and reliable identification of *Prototheca* species in culture and tissue.

Amphotericin B combined with tetracycline, 250 mg four times a day, has cured several patients. The drugs are effective in vitro and appear to act in synergism. Topical amphotericin B and tetracycline cured Tyring et al's patient with purely cutaneous protothecosis. Fluconazole was effective in Kim et al's patient.

Carey WP, et al: Cutaneous protcthecosis in a patient with AIDS and a severe functional neutrophil defect. *Clin Infect Dis* 1997, 25:1265.

Kim ST, et al: Successful treatment with fluconazole of protothecosis developing at the site of an intralesional corticosteroid injection. *Br J Dermatol* 1996, 135:803.

McAnally T, et al: Cutaneous protothecosis presenting as recurrent chromomycosis. *Arch Dermatol* 1985, 121:1066.

Monopoli A, et al: Cutaneous protothecosis. *Int J Dermatol* 1995, 34:766.

Tejada E, et al: Cutaneous erythematous nodular lesion in a crab fisherman. *Arch Dermatol* 1994, 130:243.

Tyring SK, et al: Papular protothecosis of the chest. *Arch Dermatol* 1989, 125:1249.

Woolrich A, et al: Cutaneous protothecosis and AIDS. *J Am Acad Dermatol* 1994, 51:920. ▲

CHAPTER 16

Mycobacterial Diseases

TUBERCULOSIS

No ideal classification scheme exists for cutaneous tuberculosis, but the system below is logical and takes into account both the mechanism of disease acquisition and the host immunity. There are four major categories of cutaneous tuberculosis:

1. Inoculation from an exogenous source (primary inoculation tuberculosis and tuberculosis verrucosa cutis)
2. Endogenous cutaneous spread contiguously or by autoinoculation (scrofuloderma, tuberculosis cutis oroficialis)
3. Hematogenous spread to the skin (lupus vulgaris; acute miliary tuberculosis; and tuberculosis ulcer, gumma, or abscess)
4. Tuberculids (erythema induratum [Bazin's disease], papulonecrotic tuberculid, and lichen scrofulosorum)

The finding of mycobacterial DNA by polymerase chain reaction in tuberculids suggests that tuberculids also represent hematogenous dissemination of tuberculosis, which is quickly controlled by the host, usually resulting in the absence of detectable organisms.

Epidemiology

Tuberculosis in the United States had declined at a rate of 5% to 6% per year until 1984. From 1985 until 1991, there was an 18% increase in the number of cases of tuberculosis. Similar increases were seen in some European countries. This increase was associated with three phenomena: large numbers of immigrants from high-prevalence countries, the AIDS epidemic, and an increasing number of persons in congregative facilities (shelters for the homeless and prisons). Therefore, Asians, blacks, and Hispanics have the greatest risk for developing tuberculosis in the United States. Tuberculosis is also increasing worldwide, especially in developing countries where 30% to 60% of adults are infected with *Mycobacterium tuberculosis*. The global increase in tuberculosis is related to HIV infection, since many regions of the developing world where tuberculosis is common are also areas of high HIV infection rate. It is estimated that in Africa the number of cases of tuberculosis will increase by at least 50% by the end of the decade. Cutaneous tuberculosis had become quite uncommon in North America. However, with the dramatic increase in the number of cases of tuberculosis globally in both developed and developing countries, an increase in cutaneous tuberculosis may be anticipated.

Tuberculin Testing

The tuberculin test is designed to detect a cell-mediated immune response to *M. tuberculosis*. It remains the most useful method of identifying infected persons. The test becomes positive between 2 and 10 weeks following infection and remains positive for many years, although it may wane with age. Purified protein derivative (PPD) preparations are currently used for testing in the United States and Canada at a dose of 5 TU. The intradermal, or Mantoux, test is the standard, and it offers the highest degree of consistency and reliability. The test is read 48 to 72 hours after intradermal injection. Induration measuring 5 mm or more is considered positive in HIV-infected patients or in those with risk factors, recent close contacts, or those with chest x-ray findings consistent with healed tuberculosis. If it measures more than 10 mm, it is considered positive in injection drug users, low income patients, those born in foreign countries of high prevalence, nursing home patients, and those with medical conditions that predispose to tuberculosis. If induration is more than 15 mm, it is positive in all others; 0 to 4 mm induration is negative. This means that 10 mm or more induration most likely represents specific sensitivity to *M. tuberculosis* (i.e., infection). As the amount of induration become progressively smaller, the likelihood that this represents true infection decreases. Many intermediate responses may represent cross-reaction with atypical mycobacteria. Although tuberculins and PPDs have been prepared for other mycobacteria, they are less sensitive and less specific and are not currently recommended for diagnostic purposes. BCG immunization (see the following discussion) leads to a positive tuberculin result in immunized children, but this reaction usually does not persist beyond 10 years. Therefore, positive reactions in adults should not automatically be attributed to childhood BCG administration.

Reactivity to the tuberculin protein is impaired in certain conditions in which cellular immunity is impaired. Lymphoproliferative disorders, sarcoidosis, corticosteroids and immunosuppressive medications, severe protein deficiency, chronic renal failure, and numerous infectious illnesses, including HIV infection, are capable of diminishing tuberculin reactivity. In overwhelming tuberculosis (miliary disease), more than 50% of patients have a negative skin test before beginning therapy. A negative or doubtful reaction to a PPD preparation does not rule out tuberculosis infection, particularly in the face of suggestive symptoms and signs. Testing with higher concentrations of tuberculin and repeated testing increase false-positive reactions and are not recommended.

Because of the frequent anergy of HIV-infected persons to skin testing, at least two controls should be administered along with the tuberculin. A reaction of larger than 5 mm to standard tuberculin testing is considered positive in an HIV-infected person, and failure to react to all antigens documents anergy. Because children are at increased risk of developing active tuberculosis after exposure, in contact investigations, a 5-mm or larger reaction is considered positive.

BCG Vaccination

Bacillus Calmette-Guérin (BCG) is a living attenuated bovine tubercle bacillus used in many parts of the world to enhance immunity to tuberculosis. Vaccination is given only to tuberculin-negative persons. It is effective in reducing childhood tuberculosis if given to neonates, but its efficacy when given to adults is less clear. Once the patient has been vaccinated, the tuberculin test becomes positive, and remains so for a variable length of time. In an adult who was vaccinated as a child in a foreign country with a high prevalence of tuberculosis, whose tuberculin test measures more than 10 mm, active tuberculosis should be assumed.

Dermatologic complications of BCG vaccination are rarely seen. Dostrowsky et al reported skin reactions in 27 patients among more than 200,000 vaccinated with BCG. Among reactions attributed to the vaccination were exaggerated or persistent regional lymphadenitis, sometimes causing scrofuloderma, lupus vulgaris, and lichen nitidus–like lesions. Excessive ulceration may occur if the BCG is inoculated too deeply. Nonspecific reactions were noted in 33 patients. These included urticaria, erythema nodosum, erythema multiforme, and granuloma annulare.

Occasionally, BCG will cause progressive local, disseminated, or even fatal disease in the immunocompetent host. In the immunodeficient host, however, progressive disease is much more common. BCG should be given only to HIV-infected neonates if they are asymptomatic and live in a region where the risk of acquiring tuberculosis is high. HIV-infected persons living in areas of low tuberculosis prevalence or who are symptomatic from HIV disease should not receive BCG vaccine. The value of vaccinating adult HIV-infected persons is unproven.

Inoculation Cutaneous Tuberculosis from an Exogenous Source

Primary Inoculation Tuberculosis (Primary Tuberculous Complex, Tuberculous Chancre)

Primary inoculation tuberculosis develops at the site of inoculation of tubercle bacilli into a tuberculosis-free individual. Regional lymphadenopathy usually occurs, completing the "complex." It occurs chiefly in children and affects the face or extremities. Usually the inoculation occurs in previously traumatized skin or mucosa, but the trauma may have been relatively minor. Horney et al reported the development of this disease after tattooing. The earliest lesion, appearing 2 to 4 weeks after inoculation, is a painless brown-red papule (Fig. 16-1), which develops into an indurated nodule or plaque that may ulcerate. This is the tuberculous chancre. Prominent regional lymphadenopathy appears 3 to 8 weeks after infection and, occasionally, cold, suppurative, and draining lesions may appear over involved lymph nodes. Primary tuberculous complex occurs on the mucous membranes in about one third of the patients. It also may occur after BCG vaccination in tuberculin-negative children. Spontaneous healing usually occurs within a year or less, with the skin lesion healing first, then the lymph node, which is often persistently enlarged and calcified. Delayed suppuration of the affected lymph node, lupus vulgaris overlying the involved node, and occasionally dissemination may follow this form of cutaneous tuberculosis.

Histologically, there is a marked inflammatory response during the first 2 weeks, with many polymorphonuclear leukocytes and tubercle bacilli. During the next 2 weeks, the

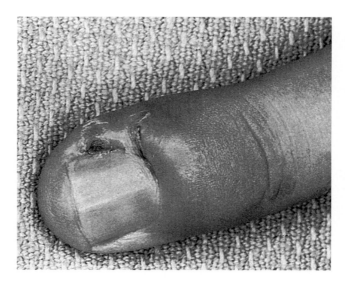

Fig. 16-1 Primary inoculation tuberculosis in a 30-year-old pathologist.

picture changes. Lymphocytes and epithelioid cells appear and replace the polymorphonuclear leukocytes. Distinct tubercles develop not only at the site of inoculation but also in the regional lymph nodes within 3 or 4 weeks after inoculation. Simultaneously, with the appearance of epithelioid cells, the number of tubercle bacilli decreases rapidly.

The differential diagnosis of primary inoculation tuberculosis extends over the spectrum of chancriform conditions of deep fungal or bacterial origin, such as sporotrichosis, blastomycosis, histoplasmosis, coccidioidomycosis, nocardiosis, syphilis, leishmaniasis, yaws, tularemia, and atypical mycobacterial disease. Pyogenic granuloma and cat-scratch disease must also be considered.

Tuberculosis Verrucosa Cutis

Tuberculosis verrucosa cutis occurs from exogenous inoculation of bacilli into the skin of a previously sensitized person with reasonably strong immunity against *M. tuberculosis*. The tuberculin test is strongly positive. It is rare in Western countries and Africa, but it is the most common form of cutaneous tuberculosis in Hong Kong and Vietnam. The prosector's wart resulting from inoculation during an autopsy is the prototype of tuberculosis verrucosa cutis.

Clinically, the lesion begins as a small papule, which becomes hyperkeratotic, resembling a wart. The lesion enlarges by peripheral expansion, with or without central clearing, sometimes reaching several centimeters or more in diameter (Fig. 16-2). Fissuring of the surface may occur, discharging purulent exudate. Lesions are almost always solitary, and regional adenopathy is usually present only if secondary bacterial infection occurs. Frequent locations for tuberculosis verrucosa cutis are on the dorsa of the fingers and hands in adults, and the ankles and buttocks in children.

The lesions are persistent, although usually superficial and limited in their extent. They may be separated by exudative or suppurative areas, but they seldom ulcerate and may heal spontaneously.

Histologically, there is pseudoepitheliomatous hyperplasia of the epidermis and hyperkeratosis. Suppurative and granulomatous inflammation is seen in the upper and mid dermis, sometimes perforating through the epidermis. The number of acid-fast bacilli is usually scant.

DIFFERENTIAL DIAGNOSIS. Tuberculosis verrucosa cutis is differentiated only by culture from atypical mycobacteriosis caused by *M. marinum* (Fig. 16-3). It must also be distinguished from North American blastomycosis, Majocchi's granuloma, chromoblastomycosis, verrucous epidermal nevus, hypertrophic lichen planus, iododerma, bromoderma, and verruca vulgaris.

Cutaneous Tuberculosis from Endogenous Source by Direct Extension or Autoinoculation

Scrofuloderma

Scrofuloderma is tuberculous involvement of the skin by direct extension, usually from underlying tuberculous lymphadenitis. It occurs most frequently over the cervical lymph nodes (Figs. 16-4 and 16-5) but also may occur over bone or around joints if these are involved. Clinically, the lesions begin as subcutaneous masses, which enlarge to form nodules. Suppuration occurs centrally. They may be erythematous or skin colored, and usually the skin temperature is not increased over the mass. Lesions may drain, forming sinuses or ulcerate with reddish granulation at the

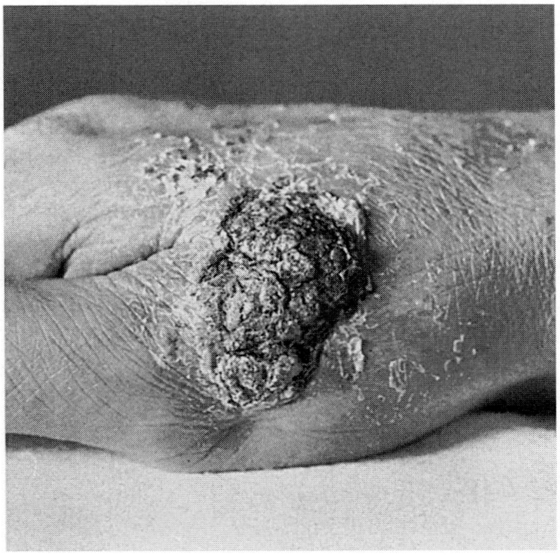

Fig. 16-2 Tuberculosis verrucosa cutis.

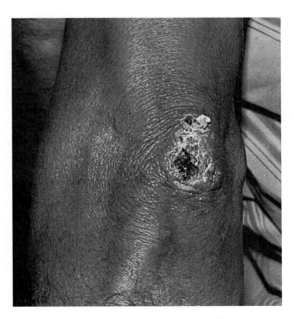

Fig. 16-3 Lesion caused by *M. marinum* on the left elbow of a 40-year-old Puerto Rican man. (Courtesy Dr. V. Torres-Rodriguez.)

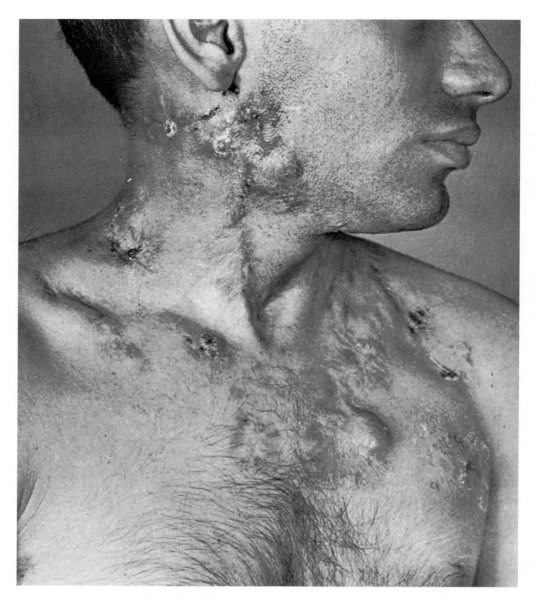

Fig. 16-4 Scrofuloderma. Scrofulous gummas and scarring.

base. Scrofuloderma heals with characteristic cordlike scars, frequently allowing the diagnosis to be made many years later.

Tuberculosis fistulosa subcutanea is characterized by a chronic anal fistula in adults between 30 and 50 years of age. Involvement of the intestinal tract, especially the rectum, is present in most of these cases. Anal strictures and involvement of the scrotum are frequently observed. The lesions consist of one or more fistulas extending into the deep tissue, infiltrated nodules, and swelling of the affected area.

Histologically, in scrofuloderma, the tuberculous process begins in the underlying lymph node or bone and extends through the deep dermis. Necrosis occurs with formation of a cavity filled with liquefied debris and polymorphonuclear leukocytes. At the periphery, more typical granulomatous inflammation is seen, along with acid-fast bacilli.

Scrofuloderma is to be differentiated from atypical mycobacterial infection; sporotrichosis, which is usually along a lymphatic of an extremity; actinomycosis; and coccidioidomycosis. Lymphogranuloma venereum (LGV) favors the inguinal and perineal areas, and has positive serologic tests for LGV.

Tuberculosis Cutis Orificialis

Tuberculosis cutis orificialis is a form of cutaneous tuberculosis that occurs at the mucocutaneous borders of the nose, mouth, anus, urinary meatus, and vagina, and on the mucous membrane of the mouth or tongue. It is caused by

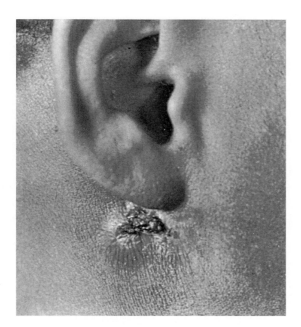

Fig. 16-5   Scrofuloderma.

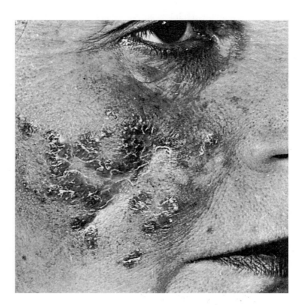

Fig. 16-6   Lupus vulgaris. (Courtesy Dr. G. Wagner, Heidelberg.)

autoinoculation from underlying active visceral tuberculo-sis, particularly of the larynx, lungs, intestines, and genitourinary tract. It indicates failing resistance to the disease. Consequently, tuberculin positivity is variable but usually present. Lesions ulcerate from the beginning and extend rapidly, with no tendency to spontaneous healing. The ulcers are usually soft, punched out, and have under-mined edges.

Histologically, the ulcer base is usually composed largely of granulation tissue infiltrated with polymorphonuclear leukocytes. Deep to the ulcer granulomatous inflammation may be found, and acid-fast bacilli are numerous.

Cutaneous Tuberculosis from Hematogenous Spread

Lupus Vulgaris

Lupus vulgaris may appear at sites of inoculation, in scrofuloderma scars, or most commonly at distant sites from the initial infectious focus. Approximately half of such cases will have evidence of tuberculosis elsewhere, so a complete evaluation is mandatory. Because lupus vulgaris is associ-ated with moderately high immunity to tuberculosis, most patients will have a positive tuberculin test.

Lupus vulgaris typically is a single plaque composed of grouped red-brown papules, which, when blanched by diascopic pressure, have a pale brownish yellow or "apple-jelly" color (Figs. 16-6 to 16-9). The papules tend to heal slowly in one area and progress in another. The papules are minute, translucent, and embedded deeply and diffusely in the infiltrated dermis, expanding by the development of new papules at the periphery, which coalesce with the main plaque. The plaques are slightly elevated and often are

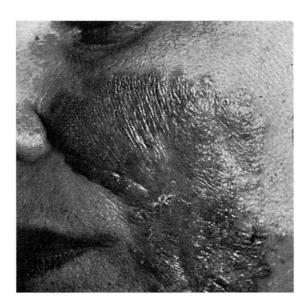

Fig. 16-7   Lupus vulgaris.

covered by adherent scales. The disease is destructive, frequently causes ulceration, and on involution leaves deforming scars as it slowly spreads peripherally over the years. Ninety percent of lupus vulgaris lesions occur on the head and neck. At times there may be associated lymphan-gitis or lymphadenitis. If lesions involve the nose or the lobes of the ears, after involution of the lesions, these structures are shrunken and scarred, as if nibbled away. Atrophy is prominent, and ectropion and eclabion may occur. The tip of the nose may be sharply pointed and beaklike, or the whole nose may be destroyed, and only the

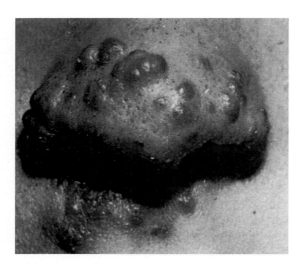

Fig. 16-8 Lupus vulgaris with large apple-jelly nodules on the nose and lip.

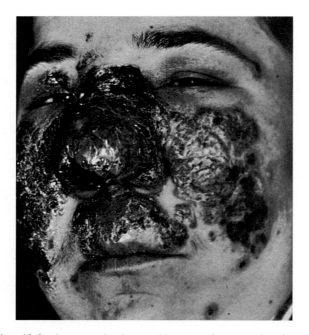

Fig. 16-9 Lupus vulgaris, tumid type. (Courtesy Dr. Simon, Szeged.)

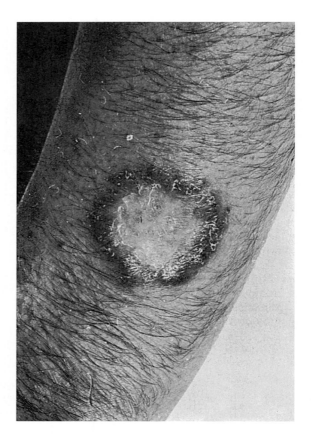

Fig. 16-10 Lupus vulgaris on the forearm. (Courtesy Dr. G. Wagner, Heidelberg.)

orifices and the posterior parts of the septum and turbinates visible. The upper lip, a site of predilection, may become diffusely swollen and thickened, with fissures, adherent thin crusts, and ulcers, or granulations on the mucous aspect. On the trunk and extremities, lesions may be annular or serpiginous or may form gyrate patterns (Fig. 16-10). On the hands and feet and around the genitals or buttocks, lesions may cause mutilation by destruction, scar formation, warty thickenings, and elephantiasic enlargement.

When the mucous membranes are involved, the lesions become papillomatous or ulcerative. They may appear as circumscribed, grayish, macerated, or granulating plaques. On the tongue, irregular, deep, painful fissures occur, sometimes associated with microglossia to the degree that nutrition is compromised.

The rate of progression of lupus vulgaris is slow, and a lesion may remain limited to a small area for several decades. The onset may be in childhood and persist throughout a lifetime. It may slowly spread, and new lesions may develop in other regions. In some instances, the lesions become papillomatous, vegetative, or thickly crusted so that they have a rupioid appearance.

Histologically, classic tubercles are the hallmark of lupus vulgaris. Caseation within the tubercles is seen in about half the cases and is rarely marked. Sarcoidosis may be simulated. The epidermis is affected secondarily, sometimes flattened and at other times hypertrophic. Acid-fast bacilli are found in 10% of cases or less with standard acid-fast stains. Polymerase chain reaction (PCR) may identify mycobacterial DNA in these cases, confirming the diagnosis. Cultures of the skin lesions grow *M. tuberculosis* in about half the cases.

Colloid milia, acne vulgaris, sarcoidosis, or rosacea may simulate lupus vulgaris. Differentiation from tertiary syphilis, chronic discoid lupus erythematosus, leprosy, systemic mycoses, and leishmaniasis may be more difficult, and biopsy and tissue cultures may be required.

Miliary (Disseminated) Tuberculosis

Miliary tuberculosis appears in the setting of fulminant tuberculosis of the lung or meninges. Generally, patients have other unmistakable signs of severe miliary tuberculosis. It is most common in children but may occur in adults. Most reported instances of cutaneous tuberculosis seen in patients with AIDS are of this type. Miliary tuberculosis may also follow infectious illnesses that reduce immunity, especially measles. Because this represents uncontrolled hematogenous infection, the tuberculin test is negative. Lesions are generalized and may appear as erythematous macules or papules, pustules, subcutaneous nodules, and purpuric "vasculitic" lesions. Ulceration may occur, and the pain in the infarctive lesions may be substantial. The prognosis is guarded.

Skin biopsies show diffuse suppurative inflammation of the dermis or subcutis with predominantly polymorphonuclear leukocytes. Vasculitis or abscesses may be seen. Acid-fast bacilli are abundant.

Metastatic Tuberculous Abscess or Ulceration

The hematogenous dissemination of mycobacteria from a primary focus may result in firm, nontender erythematous nodules, which soften, ulcerate, and form sinuses. These are usually seen in children, and most patients have decreased immunity from malnutrition, intercurrent infection, or an immunodeficiency state. Patients presenting with tuberculous skin ulcers may or may not have other foci of tuberculosis identified. Two cases of tuberculous skin ulcers in elderly patients reported by Frampton and Hutton et al are noteworthy because they document a high rate of infection among the surgical and nursing staff treating the ulcers. Apparently, aerosolization of mycobacteria occurred during incision and drainage and dressing changes, leading to secondary cases. Chronic mastitis with abscess and sinus formation is another presentation of tuberculosis. Histologically, abscess formation and numerous acid-fast bacilli are seen.

Tuberculids

Tuberculids are a group of skin eruptions associated with an underlying or silent focus of tuberculosis. They are diagnosed by their characteristic clinical features, histologic findings, a positive tuberculin reaction, sometimes the finding of tuberculosis at some other site, and resolution of the eruption with antituberculous therapy. Tuberculids represent cutaneous lesions induced by hematogenous dissemination of tubercle bacilli to the skin. Lupus vulgaris may develop at the sites of tuberculids, and *M. tuberculosis* DNA may be found in tuberculid lesions. Polymerase chain reaction is a valuable diagnostic technique, especially for physicians who have limited clinical experience with tuberculids. Tuberculids usually occur in persons with a strong immunity to tuberculosis, resulting in rapid destruction of the bacilli and autoinvolution of individual lesions in many cases. New lesions continue to appear, however, since hematogenous dissemination from the underlying focus continues. Tuberculids tend to be bilaterally symmetrical eruptions because they result from hematogenous dissemination.

Papulonecrotic Tuberculid

Papulonecrotic tuberculid is usually an asymptomatic, chronic disorder, presenting in successive crops. Lesions are symmetrically distributed on the extensor extremities, especially on the tips of the elbows, and knees; on the dorsal surfaces of the hands and feet; on the buttocks; on the face and ears; and on the glans penis. Lesions may favor pernio-prone sites and may be worse during winter months. Two thirds of the cases occur before age 30, and females are favored 3:1. Evidence of prior or active tuberculosis is found in between one third and two thirds of patients, especially in the lymph nodes. The tuberculin skin test is positive and may generate a necrotic reaction.

The typical lesions vary in size from 2 to 8 mm, and are firm, inflammatory papules that become pustular or necrotic (Fig. 16-11). Lesions resolve slowly over several weeks, but occasional ulcers persist longer. Varioliform scarring follows the lesions. Crops recur over a course of months to years.

Papulonecrotic tuberculids may appear in association with other cutaneous manifestations of tuberculosis, particularly erythema induratum or scrofuloderma. Associated clinical phenomena have included tuberculous arteritis with gangrene in young adult Africans and the development of lupus vulgaris from lesions of papulonecrotic tuberculid.

Histologically, the epidermis is ulcerated in well-developed lesions. A palisaded collection of histiocytes surrounds an ovoid or wedge-shaped area of dermal necrosis. Well-formed tubercles are not seen, except in nonhealing lesions evolving into lupus vulgaris. Vascular changes are prominent, ranging from a mild lymphocytic vasculitis to fibrinoid necrosis and thrombotic occlusion of vessels. This is not a neutrophilic leukocytoclastic vasculitis, but rather a chronic granulomatous small vessel vasculitis. Capillaries, venules, and arterioles may be involved. By polymerase chain reaction, mycobacterial DNA can be found in 50% of cases of papulonecrotic tuberculid.

Papulopustular secondary syphilis, pityriasis lichenoides et varioliformis acuta, Churg-Strauss granuloma, lymphomatoid papulosis, perforating granuloma annulare, perforating collagenosis, and necrotizing or septic vasculitis share clinical and histologic features with papulonecrotic tuberculid.

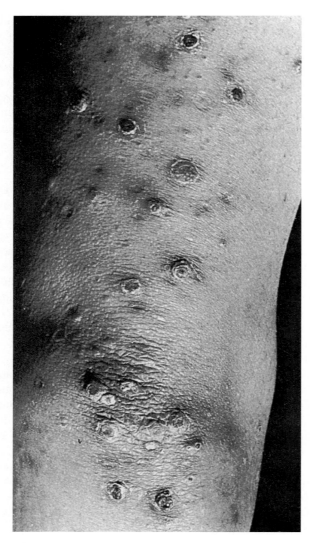

Fig. 16-11 Papulonecrotic tuberculid on elbow and upper arm. Note new, active crusted lesions and scarring of old healed lesions. (Courtesy Dr. A. Kaminsky, Argentina.)

Lichen Scrofulosorum

Also known as *tuberculosis cutis lichenoides*, lichen scrofulosorum (Fig. 16-12) consists of groups of indolent, minute, keratotic, discrete papules, scattered over the trunk. The lesions are 2 to 4 mm and yellow-pink to reddish brown. They are firm and flat-topped, or surmounted by a tiny pustule or thin scale. The lesions are arranged in nummular or discoid groups, where they persist unchanged for months and cause no symptoms. They may slowly undergo spontaneous involution, followed at times by recurrences. As a rule, they appear in children, adolescents, or adults who have tuberculosis of the bones or lymph nodes. In cases of lichen scrofulosorum, the tuberculin test is always positive.

Histologically, lichen scrofulosorum shows noncaseating tuberculoid granulomas, situated just beneath the epidermis,

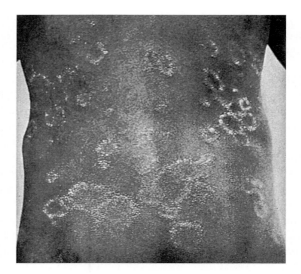

Fig. 16-12 Lichen scrofulosorum.

between and surrounding hair follicles. Normally, tubercle bacilli are not seen in the pathologic specimens, nor can they be cultured from biopsy material.

Lichen nitidus, lichen planus, secondary syphilis, and sarcoidosis should be considered in the differential diagnosis.

Erythema Induratum

Erythema induratum (Bazin's disease) is chronic and occurs predominantly (80%) in women of middle age. Lesions favor the posterior lower calf, which may also show acrocyanosis (Figs. 16-13 and 16-14). Individual lesions are tender, erythematous, 1 to 2 cm subcutaneous nodules. Lesions resolve spontaneously, with or without ulceration, over several months. Ulcerated, and some nonulcerated lesions, may heal with scarring. The tuberculin skin test is positive. Idiopathic nodular vasculitis unassociated with tuberculosis may have identical clinical and histologic features.

The primary pathology occurs in the subcutaneous fat, which shows lobular pannicullitis with fat necrosis. Granulomatous inflammation occurs in two thirds of cases and is noncaseating. In addition, a vasculitis of arterioles is present in the fat and is the apparent cause of the fat necrosis. Acid-fast bacilli are not found on special stains or cultures of the biopsy. Polymerase chain reaction may help to confirm the diagnosis of erythema induratum and distinguish it from idiopathic nodular vasculitis.

Erythema induratum must be distinguished from erythema nodosum, nodular vasculitis, polyarteritis nodosa, tertiary syphilis, and other infectious and inflammatory panniculitides. Erythema nodosum is of relatively short duration and of rapid development and affects chiefly the anterior rather than the posterior calves. It produces tender, painful, scarlet or contusiform nodules that appear simulta-

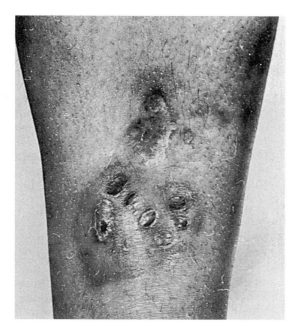

Fig. 16-13 Erythema induratum on the shin. (Courtesy Dr. G. Wagner, Heidelberg.)

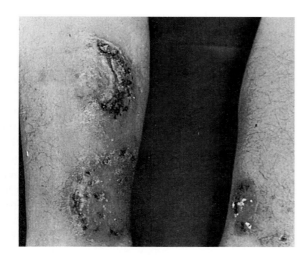

Fig. 16-14 Erythema induratum on the shins. (Courtesy Dr. F. Daniels, Jr.)

neously and do not ulcerate; in erythema induratum, the pain is less, and the lesions tend to evolve serially or in crops. A syphilitic gumma is usually unilateral and single, or may appear as a small, distinct group of lesions. Serologic tests and histology are useful in the differential diagnosis. Nodular vasculitis is clinically and histologically quite similar, but there is no associated tuberculous infection, and it does not respond to antituberculous therapy.

Treatment of Tuberculosis

HIV testing is recommended for all patients diagnosed with tuberculosis, because they may require longer courses of therapy. In addition, every effort should be made to culture the organism for sensitivity testing, since multidrug resistant tuberculosis is common in some communities. For all forms of cutaneous tuberculosis, multidrug chemotherapy is recommended. For disease associated with high degrees of immunity (for example, lupus vulgaris or tuberculosis verrucosa cutis), sometimes two drugs may be used. Three-drug regimens are now the standard in the United States for treating pulmonary tuberculosis. For severe disease, such as miliary tuberculosis, additional agents may be used. Surgical excision is useful for the treatment of isolated lesions of lupus vulgaris and tuberculosis verrucosa cutis, and surgical intervention also may benefit some cases of scrofuloderma.

For isoniazid-sensitive tuberculosis, three drugs are recommended: isoniazid (5 mg/kg, up to 300 mg), rifampin (10 mg/kg, up to 600 mg), and oral pyrazinamide (15 to 30 mg/kg, up to 2 g) daily for 2 months. Isoniazid and rifampin are continued for 4 to 10 additional months. If isoniazid resistance is suspected, ethambutol (15 mg/kg per day) is added to the regimen. If isoniazid resistance is confirmed in an HIV-negative person, rifampin and ethambutol, with or without pyrazinamide, are continued for 12 to 24 months. For an HIV-positive person, triple-drug therapy is given for 18 to 24 months, or 12 months beyond a negative sputum culture. Because the drug resistance patterns for tuberculosis vary by region and vary over time, and because these guidelines will change based on newer drugs, consultation with your local health department is strongly recommended.

Barnes PF, et al: Tuberculosis in the 1990s. *Ann Intern Med* 1993, 119:400.

Baselga E, et al: Detection of *Mycobacterium tuberculosis* DNA in lobular granulomatous panniculitis (erythema induratum-nodular vasculitis). *Arch Dermatol* 1997, 133:457.

Chang MW, et al: Erythema induratum of Bazin in an infant. *Pediatrics* 1999, 103:498.

Chong LY, et al: Cutaneous tuberculosis in Hong Kong. *Int J Dermatol* 1995, 34:26.

Choonhakarn C, et al: Sweet's syndrome associated with non-tuberculous mycobacterial infection. *Br J Dermatol* 1998, 139:107.

Chuang YH, et al: Simultaneous occurrence of papulonecrotic tuberculide and erythema induratum and the identification of *Mycobacterium tuberculosis* DNA by polymerase chain reaction. *Br J Dermatol* 1997, 137:276.

Degitz K: Detection of mycobacterial DNA in the skin. *Arch Dermatol* 1996, 132:71.

Dostrowsky A, et al: Dermatologic complications of BCG vaccination. *Br J Dermatol* 1963, 75:181.

Ellner JJ, et al: Tuberculosis symposium: emerging problems and promise. *J Infect Dis* 1993, 168:537.

Frampton MW: An outbreak of tuberculosis among hospital personnel caring for a patient with a skin ulcer. *Ann Intern Med* 1992, 117:312.

Genne D, et al: Tuberculosis of the thumb following a needlestick injury. *Clin Infect Dis* 1998, 26:210.

Harris A, et al: Cutaneous tuberculous abscess. *Br J Dermatol* 1996, 135:457.

Horney DA, et al: Cutaneous inoculation tuberculosis secondary to jailhouse tattooing. *Arch Dermatol* 1985, 121:648.

Huebner RE, et al: Tuberculosis commentary. The tuberculin skin test. *Clin Infect Dis* 1993, 17:968.

Hutton MD, et al: Nosocomial transmission of tuberculosis associated with a draining abscess. *J Infect Dis* 1990, 161:286.

Kumar B, et al: Cutaneous tuberculosis. *Int J Tuberculosis Lung Dis* 1999, 3:494.

Lantos G, et al: Tuberculous ulcer of the skin. *J Am Acad Dermatol* 1988, 19:1067.

Li VW, et al: BCG vaccination and interpretation of purified protein derivative test results. *Arch Dermatol* 1997, 133:916.

MacGregor RR: Cutaneous tuberculosis. *Clin Dermatol* 1995, 13:245.

Marcoval J, et al: Lupus vulgaris clinical, histopathologic, and bacteriologic study of 10 cases. *J Am Acad Dermatol* 1992, 26:404.

Margall N, et al: Detection of *Mycobacterium tuberculosis* complex DNA by the polymerase chain reaction for rapid diagnosis of cutaneous tuberculosis. *Br J Dermatol* 1996, 135:231.

Panzarelli A: *Tuberculosis cutis orificialis*. *Int J Dermatol* 1996, 35:443.

Penneys NS, et al: Identification of *Mycobacterium tuberculosis* DNA in five different types of cutaneous lesions by the polymerase chain reaction. *Arch Dermatol* 1993, 129:1594.

Rademaker M, et al: Erythema induratum (Bazin's disease). *J Am Acad Dermatol* 1989, 21:740.

Reider HC: *Tuberculosis verrucosa cutis*. *J Am Acad Dermatol* 1988, 18:1367.

Rogioletti F, et al: Papules on lower limbs of a woman with cervical lymphadenopathy, lichen scrofulosorum. *Arch Dermatol* 1988, 124:1421.

Telzak EE: Tuberculosis and human immunodeficiency virus infection. *Med Clin North Am* 1997, 81:345.

Ten Dam HG: BCG vaccination and HIV infection. *Bull Int Union Tuberc Lung Dis* 1990, 65:38.

Visser AJ, et al: Skin tuberculosis as seen at Ga-Rankuwa hospital. *Clin Exp Dermatol* 1993, 18:507.

Wilson Jones E, et al: Papulonecrotic tuberculid: a neglected disease in western countries. *J Am Acad Dermatol* 1986, 14:815.

Yates VM, et al: Cutaneous tuberculosis in Blackburn district (UK). *Br J Dermatol* 1997, 136:483.

Yen A, et al: Erythema induratum of Bazin as a tuberculid. *J Am Acad Dermatol* 1997, 36:99.

Young LS, et al: The resurgence of tuberculosis. *Scand J Infect Dis* 1994, Suprol 93:9. _____ ▲

ATYPICAL MYCOBACTERIOSIS

Approximately 30 facultative pathogens and saprophytes, which are acid-fast mycobacteria but do not cause tuberculosis or leprosy, are grouped under the designation "atypical" mycobacteria. They were recognized as a cause of human disease nearly 70 years ago. They exist in a wide variety of natural sources such as soil, water, and animals; most human disease is acquired from the environment. *M. marinum* is the most common cause of skin mycobacterial infections in the United States. In addition to skin disease, pulmonary infections, adenitis, osteomyelitis, and disseminated involvement may occur. *M. avium-intracellulare* complex is the most common cause of systemic infection.

Classification of Mycobacteria

Runyon has classified the atypical mycobacteria into four groups.

Group I contains photochromogens. A yellow pigment on Löwenstein-Jensen culture medium is produced in 24 hours when exposed to light and cultured at 37º C. This group includes *M. kansasii*, *M. marinum*, and *M. simiae*.

Group II are the scotochromogens, which produce a yellow-orange pigment even when cultured in darkness. The main pathogen in this group is *M. scrofulaceum*. *M. szulgai*, *M. gordonae*, and *M. xenopi* also occasionally cause human disease.

Group III are the nonphotochromogens, which do not produce pigment. In this group are *M. avium-intracellulare* complex, *M. haemophilum*, *M. ulcerans*, and *M. malmoense*.

Group IV, or rapid growers, do not produce identifying pigment but are distinguished by their rapid growth rate of 3 to 5 days. The most important pathogens are *M. fortuitum* and *M. chelonei*.

PPD-S (human tuberculin), PPD-B (Battey strain), PPD-Y (photochromogen), PPD-G (scotochromogen), and PPD-F (rapid growers) are tested in the same manner as PPD. These antigens are of limited availability and are of limited usefulness in diagnostic clinical medicine, since cross-reactivity is frequent. Culture and polymerase chain reaction identification are the only definitive diagnostic procedures.

Swimming Pool Granuloma (Aquarium Granuloma)

Swimming pool granuloma is caused by *M. marinum*, a group I photochromogen, growing optimally at 30º C in Löwenstein-Jensen medium. The usual source is an aquarium, swimming pool, lagoon, or lake. An injury preceding or simultaneous with exposure to contaminated water is usually present. An indolent lesion usually starts about 3 weeks after exposure as a small papule located on the hands, knees, elbows, or feet (Fig. 16-15). More infections in the United States are acquired from home aquariums than from other sources, and in such cases, the fingers and hands are the sites of the lesion. A sporotrichoid pattern with a succession of nodules ascending the arm is common. The lesions may be erosions or verrucous papules or plaques. Multiple primary lesions occur infrequently. Usually there is no ulceration or necrosis. Synovitis, draining sinuses, bursitis, arthritis, and osteomyelitis may be seen, however. The tendon sheaths of the dorsal hands and less commonly the palms may be affected, limiting range of motion and resulting in a thickening and induration. Such cases may require surgical, as well as medical, management. The natural history is for slow progression, and lesions may be relatively indolent for years. Spontaneous resolution may occur in 10% to 20% of patients after a period of many months.

Histopathologically, there is an initial mixed inflammatory reaction with overlying hyperkeratosis and acanthosis.

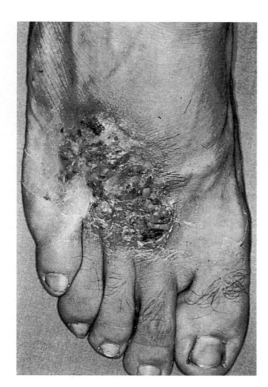

Fig. 16-15 Swimming pool granuloma caused by *Mycobacterium marinum.*

Later, epithelioid cell tubercles with giant cells are present. Central necrosis may occur. Acid-fast organisms occasionally may be seen. The organisms are longer and thicker than *M. tuberculosis.* The tuberculin reaction to *M. tuberculosis* usually becomes positive in those who have had *M. marinum* infection.

Excision of the lesion, when feasible, may be effective. Minocycline, 100 mg twice daily, is curative in the majority of cases. Doxycycline or tetracycline also may be effective, as may trimethoprim-sulfamethoxazole (Bactrim, Septra). Treatment with 600 mg of rifampin and 800 mg of ethambutol daily may be curative in those patients who do not respond to the tetracyclines or sulfa drugs. Clarithromycin, 2 g/day for 50 days, effectively treated this infection as a single drug in one case. It also cured an HIV-infected patient when given in combination with ethambutol. Levofloxacin may be effective in cases resistant to other treatments. The duration of any of these treatments is at least 6 weeks, but a cure may require many months. No current recommendation for a drug of choice is available, and the clinician may choose from a number of effective options.

Other Cutaneous Atypical Mycobacterial Infections

M. kansasii, a group I organism, occasionally involves the skin in a sporotrichoid pattern. Localized granulomatous or cellulitis-like lesions also may be seen. Inoculation is usually by minor trauma, and minocycline, sulfonamides, amikacin, or clarithromycin may be given if the infection is limited to the skin and if excision is impractical. If pulmonary involvement is present, high-dose isoniazid, rifampin, and ethambutol are necessary and are continued until the sputum is clear for 12 to 15 months. This organism may be reisistant to rifampin, and in this case a four-drug regimen is followed.

Group II organisms rarely involve the skin. *M. scrofulaceum* may produce a scrofulodermatous appearance. Shelley et al reported the first isolation of *M. gordonae* from a nodule on the hand; it was sensitive only to rifampin and ethambutol, and was resistant to isoniazid, streptomycin, and aminosalicylic acid. This pattern of multiple drug resistance is common among atypical mycobacteria. Clarithromycin may play a role in such cases. Surgical excision, if practical, is recommended. Cross et al reported a case of *M. szulgai* infection of skin and bone, which began during oral prednisone therapy for desquamative pneumonitis and responded well to combined therapy with isoniazid, ethambutol, and rifampin. For *M. gordonae* and *M. xenopi* treatment is not defined; however, the three-drug antituberculous regimen, excision, or clarithromycin may be used.

Group III organisms were uncommon causes of skin infection before the AIDS epidemic. In patients with AIDS who developed disseminated *M. avium—intracellulare complex* infections, the skin may be involved by hematogenous dissemination and may present as nodules, ulcers, pustules, or a cellulitis-like appearance. Friedman et al reviewed 11 cases of disseminated *M. avium-intracellulare* infection in non-AIDS patients. Most occurred in immunocompromised children with chronic pulmonary infections. Therapy for disseminated infection is undertaken with at least three agents, one of which should be azithromycin or clarithromycin. Ethambutol, clofazimine, and streptomycin or amikacin are given to immunocompetent patients until the culture is negative for 1 year. For patients with AIDS, rifabutin is added to clarithromycin and ethambutol, and, if no response is obtained in 2 to 4 weeks, then one or more drugs may be added. Rifabutin, clarithromycin, or azithromycin are routinely given to severely immunocompromised AIDS patients (helper T cells <50) to prevent infection (primary prophylaxis), and similar treatments are given for posttreatment suppression (secondary prophylaxis).

M. haemophilum may cause multiple ulcers on the extremities, often overlying joints. Straus et al reported 13 patients who had infection with this organism, 12 of whom had skin lesions. Eleven were AIDS patients and two were bone marrow transplant recipients. Renal transplant patients are also at risk. Because *M. haemophilum* has specific growth requirements, isolation is not possible using routine laboratory culture techniques. If acid-fast stains of tissue are positive and cultures are negative, the laboratory should be alerted to utilize appropriate media and culture conditions for this organism. McGovern et al reported successful treatment of an isolated lesion by surgical excision. When systemic infection is present, the best treatment is not defined. Combination therapy including rifabutin and clarithromycin may prove effective.

Group IV organisms usually cause subcutaneous abscesses or cellulitis following trauma in immunocompetent patients. Sporotrichoid or disseminated disease may occur in immunocompromised patients. In renal transplant cases tender, nodular lesions of the legs are most common. Clarithromycin, 500 mg twice daily for 4 to 9 months, is effective and well tolerated in the majority of patients with disseminated cutaneous infection caused by *M. chelonei*. Unfortunately, monotherapy may allow resistance to occur. The combination of clarithromycin with a furoquinolone may be successful. Most isolates are also sensitive to amikacin. The optimal regimen for treatment of *M. fortuitum* likewise has not been defined. This organism is resistant to standard antituberculous therapy, but in vitro sensitivites include doxycycline, minocycline, amikacin, trimethoprim-sulfamethoxazole, ciprofloxacin, ofloxacin, clarithromycin, and azithromycin.

Buruli Ulcer

Buruli ulcer (Fig. 16-16) is also known as *Bairnsdale ulcer* and *Searl ulcer*. The lesion begins as a solitary, hard, painless, subcutaneous nodule that subsequently ulcerates and becomes undermined. There is a predilection for the occurrence of these ulcers on the extremities. Ulcers may become very large, exposing muscle and tendon over a large portion of an affected extremity.

Mycobacterium ulcerans is the cause of Buruli ulcer. It is cultured in Löwenstein-Jensen medium at 33° C. This organism occurs in Australia, Nigeria, Zaire, the Buruli district of Uganda, Mexico, and Malaysia. An environmental source was finally proved with the finding of *M. ulcerans* by PCR in a swamp and irrigation system in an area of a recent epidemic outbreak of disease. *Mycobacterium ulcerans* produces a toxin that may be responsible for the extensive necrosis and ulceration seen in these infections.

Histologically, there is an initial mixed inflammatory reaction with overlying hyperkeratiosis. Effective treatment is not available at present. When feasible, wide and deep excision is probably the best form of therapy. Hayman reported seven cases from Australia; one responded to a combination of rifampin and ethionamide, but two did not; excision of the ulcer was carried out in all cases. A combination of rifampin and amikacin or ethambutol or trimethoprim-sulfamethoxazole for 4 to 6 weeks are other recommeded drug treatments.

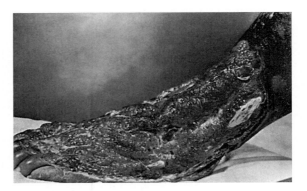

Fig. 16-16 Mycobacterial (Buruli) ulcer on the foot of a 20-year-old man in the Peace Corps, contracted in Nigeria. (Courtesy Dr. E.R. Farber.)

Cross GM, et al: Cutaneous *M. szulgai* infection. *Arch Dermatol* 1985, 121:247.

Curco N, et al: *Mycobacterium kansasii* infection limited to the skin in a patient with AIDS. *Br J Dermatol* 1996, 135:324.

Darling TN, et al: Treatment of *Mycobacterium haemophilum* infection with an antibiotic regimen including clarithromycin. *Br J Dermatol* 1994, 131:376.

Dobas KM, et al: Emergence of a unique group of necrotizing mycobacterial diseases. *Emerg Infect Dis* 1999, 5:367.

Drabic JJ, et al: Disseminated *M. chelonae subspecies chelonae* infection with cutaneous and osseous manifestations. *Arch Dermatol* 1990, 126:1067.

Drabic JJ, et al: Ulcerative perianal lesions due to *M. kansasii*. *J Am Acad Dermatol* 1988, 18:1146.

Driscoll MS, et al: Development of resistance to clarithromycin after treatment of cutaneous *Mycobacterium chelonae* infection. *J Am Acad Dermatol* 1997, 36:495.

Edelstein H: *Mycobacterium marinum* skin infections. *Arch Intern Med* 1994, 154:1359.

Fitzgerald DA, et al: Cutaneous infection with *Mycobacterium abscessus*. *Br J Dermatol* 1995, 132:800.

Fonseca E, et al: Nodular lesions in disseminated *M. fortuitum* infection. *Arch Dermatol* 1987, 123:1603.

Frank N, et al: Treatment of *M. chelonae*-induced skin infection with clarithromycin. *J Am Acad Dermatol* 1993: 28:1019.

Freed JA, et al: Cutaneous mycobacteriosis. *Arch Dermatol* 1987, 123:1601.

French AL, et al: Nontuberculous mycobacterial infections. *Med Clin North Am* 1997, 81:361.

Friedman BF, et al: *M. avium-intracellulare*: Cutaneous presentations of disseminated disease. *Am J Med* 1988, 85:257.

Gluckman SJ: *Mycobacterium marinum*. *Clin Dermatol* 1995, 13:273.

Gutknecht DR: Treatment of *M. chelonae* infection with ciprofloxacin. *J Am Acad Dermatol* 1990, 23:1179.

Hanke CW, et al: *M. kansasii* infection with multiple cutaneous lesions. *J Am Acad Dermatol* 1987, 16:1122.

Hayman J: Clinical features of *M. ulcerans* infection. *Australas J Dermatol* 1985, 26:67.

Hendrick SJ, et al: Giant *M. fortuitum* abscess associated with SLE. *Arch Dermatol* 1986, 122:695.

Huminer D, et al: Aquarium-borne *M. marinum* skin infection. *Arch Dermatol* 1986, 122:698.

Iijima S, et al: *Mycobacterium marinum* skin infection successfully treated with levofloxacin. *Arch Dermatol* 1997, 133:947.

Infection with *Mycobacterium abscessus* associated with intramuscular injection of adrenal cortex extract: Colorado and Wyoming, 1995-1996. *MMWR* 1996, 45:713.

Bonnet E, et al: Clarithromycin. *Clin Infect Dis* 1994, 18:664.

Breathnach A, et al: Cutaneous *Mycobacterium kansasii* infection. *Clin Infect Dis* 1995, 20:812.

Levine N, et al: Treatment of *M. chelonae* infection with controlled heating. *J Am Acad Dermatol* 1991, 24:867.

McBride ME, et al: Diagnostic and therapeutic considerations for cutaneous *M. haemophilum* infections. *Arch Dermatol* 1991, 127:276.

McGovern J, et al: *M. haemophilum* skin disease successfully treated with excision. *J Am Acad Dermatol* 1994, 30:269.

Meyers WM, et al: *Mycobacterium ulcerans* infection (Buruli ulcer). *Br J Dermatol* 1996, 134:1116.

Muelder K, et al: Wounds that will not heal: the Buruli ulcer. *Int J Dermatol* 1992, 128:25.

Murray Leisure KA, et al: Skin lesions caused by *M. scrofulaceum*. *Arch Dermatol* 1987, 123:369.

Nedorost ST, et al: Rosacea-like lesions due to *M. avium-intracellulare* infections. *Int J Dermatol* 1991, 30:991.

Nelson BR, et al: Disseminated *M. chelonae ssp abscessus* in an immunocompetent host and with a known portal of entry. *J Am Acad Dermatol* 1989, 20:909.

Piketty C, et al: Sporotrichosis-like infection caused by *M. avium* in AIDS. *Arch Dermatol* 1993, 129:1343.

Rosenmeier GJ, et al: Latent cutaneous *M. fortuitum* infection in a healthy man. *J Am Acad Dermatol* 1991, 25:898.

Ross BC, et al: Detection of *Mycobacterium ulcerans* in environmental samples during an outbreak of ulcerative disease. *Appl Environ Microbiol* 1997, 63:4135.

Safraneck TJ, et al: *M. chelonae* wound infections after plastic surgery employing contaminated gentian violet skin-marking solution. *N Engl J Med* 1987, 317:197.

Shelley WB, et al: *M. gordonae* infection of the hand. *Arch Dermatol* 1984, 120:1064.

Straus WL, et al: Clinical and epidemiologic characteristics of *M. haemophilum*. *Ann Intern Med* 1994, 120:118.

Street ML, et al: Nontuberculous mycobacterial infections of the skin. *J Am Acad Dermatol* 1991, 24:208.

Wallace RJ, Jr: Clinical trial of clarithromycin for cutaneous infection due to *M. chelonae*. *Ann Intern Med* 1993, 119:482.

Wallace RJ, Jr: Recent clinical advances in knowledge of the nonleprous environmental mycobacteria responsible for cutaneous disease. *Arch Dermatol* 1987, 123:337.

Wallace RJ, Jr: Treatment of nonpulmonary infections due to *M. fortuitum* and *M. chelonei* on the basis of in vitro susceptibilities. *J Infect Dis* 1985, 152:5001.

Wegner JD, et al: Outbreak of *M. chelonae* infection associated with use of jet injectors. *J Am Acad Dermatol* 1990, 264:373. _____ ▲

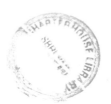

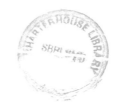

CHAPTER 17

Hansen's Disease (Leprosy)

EPIDEMIOLOGY

It is estimated that there are between 10 and 15 million people in the world with leprosy. The disease is endemic in many areas of Asia, especially the Indian subcontinent, in sub-Saharan Africa, South and Central America, the Pacific Islands, and the Philippines. Although 90% of cases diagnosed in the United States are imported, Hansen's disease is endemic in the coastal southeastern United States and in Hawaii. In the southeastern United States cases may be related to exposure to armadillos, a natural host for the infectious agent.

There is an apparent genetic susceptibility to acquiring infection with Hansen's disease. Immunologic evidence of exposure to the organism is present in 50% or more of potentially exposed persons. Attack rates in this group are only 5%, however, similar to the 6% attack rates in the spouses of patients with Hansen's disease. This suggests that while most persons can be transiently infected, they are able to resist infection. Monozygotic twins have concordant infection in 60% to 85% of cases, and dizygotic twins 15% to 25%.

In adults, cases in men outnumber those in women by twofold to threefold. In children, the gender ratio is 1:1. Although leprosy occurs at all ages, there are two peaks of presentation: in children aged 10 to 20 years, and in adults 30 to 60 years of age. The latency period between exposure and overt signs of the disease is usually from 2 to 5 years, but may be much longer. In children, this may be shorter, as children with leprosy under age 1 have been identified. These may represent cases of vertical transmission, although only half of the mothers of infants diagnosed with leprosy had clinical leprosy. Infected women are likely to present during pregnancy.

The mode of transmission remains controversial. Except for cases associated with armadillo exposure, other Hansen's disease cases are felt to be the only possible source of infection. Multibacillary cases are much more infectious than paucibacillary cases, so that, after genetic susceptibility, the nature of the source case is the most important factor in transmission. There are two recognized potential modes of transmission. Infectious droplets from nasal secretions of active multibacillary cases with nasal erosions are felt by some to spread the disease via the respiratory route. Others hypothesize that ulcerated skin lesions shed organisms into the environment, which can be inoculated into susceptible persons. It is possible that both mechanisms, or some other mode of transmission are operative. Clearly, close contact is associated with acquiring infection, and when identified, family members are the most frequent source of infection. Children are apparently more easily infected than adults. Up to 25% of children living in leprosaria develop initial lesions of leprosy, but without treatment, the durable infection rate in these children is only 6%, even without treatment. In Africa, where decorative tattooing is practiced, this may be a means of transmission. Insects have never been documented as vectors.

Most cases occur in the tropical, developing world, and it has been hypothesized that infection is more common in environments where the people are of low economic status, with inadequate housing, unsuitable sanitation, poor nutrition, and lack of education. This theory is supported by the dramatic disappearance of Hansen's disease from Europe as the standard of living improved through the late nineteenth and early twentieth centuries. This has not been proven, however, and there are clear exceptions to this pattern throughout the world.

The Infectious Agent

All cases of human and animal leprosy are caused by the same organism, *Mycobacterium leprae*. *M. leprae* is a weakly acid-fast organism that has not been successfully cultured reproducibly in vitro. It grows best at temperatures below humans' core body temperature of humans (32° to 35° C [89.6° to 95° F]). The organism may be cultivated in mouse foot pads and most effectively in armadillos, whose lower body temperature is more optimal for growth of *M. leprae*. Phenolic glycolipid-1 (PGL-1) is a surface glycolipid unique to the leprosy bacillus. In infected tissues, the leprosy bacillus favors intracellular locations.

Diagnosis

A diagnosis of leprosy must be considered in any patient with neurologic and cutaneous lesions. The diagnosis is frequently delayed in the developed world; clinicians do not readily think of Hansen's disease, since they may not have seen the disease. In the United States, this diagnostic delay averages 1½ to 2 years.

Leprosy is diagnosed, as with other infectious diseases, by identifying the infectious organism in affected tissue. Because the organism cannot be cultured, this may be very difficult. Skin biopsies from skin or nerve lesions, stained for the bacillus with Fite-Faraco stain, are usually performed in the developed world. In some Hansen's disease clinics, and in the developing world where disease is endemic, organisms are identified in slit smears of the skin. Smears are taken from lesions and cooler areas of the skin, such as the earlobes, elbows, and knees, and stained with acid-fast stains. Organisms are counted per high-power field, and a bacillary index (BI) is determined. This BI is the "bacterial load" of infection. The staining characteristics are also determined, called the morphologic index (MI). Because the MI changes sooner than the BI, it can be an early indicator of efficacy of treatment, and can help detect dapsone resistance. If organisms are found on skin smears, the patients are said to be *multibacillary*. If the results of skin smears are negative, they are called *paucibacillary*. To detect early nerve damage, a histamine test (to detect the loss of the normal flare response accompanying a histamine-induced wheal), or a methacholine sweat test (to detect anhidrosis) may be used.

Newer diagnostic tests are being developed. The florescent lepromin antibody–absorbed (FLA-ABS), which is analogous to the FTA-ABS for the diagnosis of syphilis, unfortunately has a low specificity. Specific antibodies to phenolic glycolipid-1 are found in many multibacillary cases, but false-negative results occur in many paucibacillary patients, making it less than ideal for diagnosis. PGL-1 itself may be detected in the urine of multibacillary patients,

and may be used to follow treatment. False negatives in paucibacillary cases make it useless in diagnosis. Polymerase chain reaction (PCR) is being developed, and may be used in some settings. The high sensitivity and sophistication make PCR impractical for use in the developing world.

The lepromin skin test is not useful in the diagnosis of leprosy; it may be used to determine the immunologic status of the patient with respect to the leprosy bacillus and thus may help to classify a given case. Lepromin skin test reagent is currently produced from armadillo-cultivated organisms. It is a classic test for cell-mediated immunity, with an early reading at 24 to 48 hours called the *Fernandez reaction,* or at 4 weeks, the *late reaction of Mitsuda.*

Classification of Leprosy

Leprosy may present with a broad spectrum of clinical diseases. The Ridley and Jopling classification or modifications to it have classified cases based on clinical, bacteriologic, immunologic, and histopathologic features (Table 17-1). In many infected patients the infection apparently spontaneously clears and no clinical lesions develop. Patients who do develop clinical disease are broadly classified into two groups: a patient with few organisms in his or her tissue is said to have a *paucibacillary* case, and a patient with large number of organisms in his or her tissue is said to have a *multibacillary* case. In the developing world this determination is made by skin smears. The individual's cell-mediated immune response to the organism determines the form Hansen's disease will take in the individual. If the cell-mediated immune response against *M. leprae* is strong, the number of organisms will be low (paucibacillary), and conversely if CMI is inadequate, the number of organisms will be high (multibacillary).

The initial clinical lesion may be a single hypopigmented patch, perhaps with slight anesthesia. This is called *indeterminate* disease, since the course of the disease cannot be predicted. The lesion may clear or may progress to any other form of leprosy.

TABLE 17-1

Spectrum of Host-Parasite Resistance

	High Resistance		Unstable Resistance		No Resistance
	Tuberculoid TT	**Borderline Tuberculoid BT**	**Borderline BB**	**Borderline Lepromatous BL**	**Lepromatous LL**
Lesions	One to three	Few	Few or many asymmetrical	Many	Numerous and symmetrical
Smear for bacilli	0	1 +	2 +	3 +	4 +
Lepromin test	3 +	2 +	+	±	0
Histology	Epithelioid cells decreasing ⟶ Nerve destruction, sarcoidlike granuloma			Increasing histiocytes, foam cells granuloma, xanthoma-like	

Adapted from Dr. J.H. Pettit.

The spectrum of leprosy has two stable poles, the tuberculoid and lepromatous forms (see Table 17-1). These so-called polar forms do not change; the patient remains in one or the other form throughout the course of the disease. The polar tuberculoid form (called TT), the form of high cell-mediated immunity, is characterized by less than three lesions and few organisms (paucibacillary disease). The lepromin skin test result will be positive. The polar lepromatous form (called LL) has very limited cell-mediated immunity against the organism, lesions are numerous, and they contain many organisms (multibacillary). The lepromin skin test yields a negative result. Between these two poles are every possible grade of infection, forming the borderline spectrum. Cases near the tuberculoid pole are called *borderline tuberculoid* (BT), those near the lepromatous pole are called *borderline lepromatous* (BL), and those in the middle are called *borderline borderline* (BB). Borderline disease is characteristically unstable, and with time cases move from the tuberculoid to the lepromatous pole, a process called *downgrading*. Leprosy may involve only the nerves. This pure neural disease may be indeterminate, tuberculoid, or lepromatous and is so classified.

Early and Indeterminate Leprosy. Usually the onset of leprosy is insidious. Prodromal symptoms are generally so slight that the disease is not recognized until the appearance of a cutaneous eruption. Actually, the first clinical manifestation in 90% of patients is numbness, and years may elapse before skin lesions or other signs are identified. The earliest sensory changes are loss of the senses of cold and light touch, most often in the feet or hands. The light touch of a wisp of cotton or even a fingertip may not elicit a response, although a pinprick may be discerned. The bony prominences, the knuckles, elbows, patellae, and malleoli, have a raised threshold of reaction. The sense of cold may be lost before pinprick sensibility. Such dissociation of sensibility is especially suspicious. The distribution of these neural signs and their intensity will depend on the type of disease that is evolving.

Often the first lesion noted is a solitary, ill-defined, hypopigmented macule that merges into the surrounding normal skin. Less often, erythematous macules may be present. Such lesions are most likely to occur on the cheeks, upper arms, thighs, and buttocks. Examination reveals that sensory functions are either normal or minimally altered. Peripheral nerves are not enlarged, and plaques and nodules do not occur. Histologically, a variable lymphocytic infiltrate (without granulomas) is seen, sometimes with involvement of the cutaneous nerves. Usually no bacilli, or only a few, are seen on biopsy of this indeterminate form. It is the classification, not the diagnosis that is indeterminate. Few cases remain in this state; they evolve into lepromatous, tuberculoid, or borderline types, or (if immunity is good) may spontaneously resolve and never develop other signs or symptoms of leprosy.

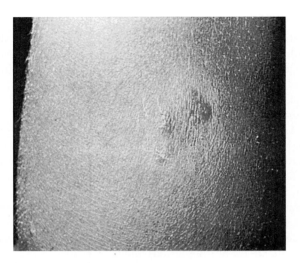

Fig. 17-1 Early lesion of tuberculoid leprosy just below the popliteal space. (Courtesy Dr. J. Convit, Venezuela.)

Tuberculoid Leprosy. Tuberculoid lesions are solitary or few in number (usually three or less) and asymmetrically distributed. Lesions may be hypopigmented or erythematous and are usually dry, scaly, and hairless (Fig. 17-1). The typical lesion of tuberculoid leprosy is the large, erythematous plaque with a sharply defined and elevated border that slopes down to a flattened atrophic center (Fig. 17-2). This has been described as having the appearance of "a saucer right side up." Lesions may also be macular and hypopigmented or erythematous, resembling clinically indeterminate lesions. The presence of palpable induration and neurologic findings distinguishes indeterminate lesions from tuberculoid lesions clinically. The most common locations are the face, limbs, or trunk; the scalp, axillae, groin, and perineum are not involved. As the lesions clear, they tend to become annular, arciform, or circinate, with borders of variable thickness.

A tuberculoid lesion is anesthetic or hypesthetic and anhidrotic, and superficial peripheral nerves serving or proximal to the lesion are enlarged, tender, or both. The greater auricular nerve and the superficial peroneal nerve may be visibly enlarged. Nerve involvement is early and prominent in tuberculoid leprosy, leading to characteristic changes in the muscle groups served. There may be atrophy of the interosseous muscles of the hand, with wasting of the thenar and hypothenar eminences, contracture of the fingers, paralysis of the facial muscles, and foot drop.

The evolution of the lesions is generally slow. There is often spontaneous remission of the lesions in about 3 years, or remission may result sooner with treatment. Spontaneous involution may leave pigmentary disturbances.

Borderline Tuberculoid Leprosy. Borderline tuberculoid (BT) lesions are similar to TT lesions, except that they are smaller and more numerous (usually three to ten). Satellite

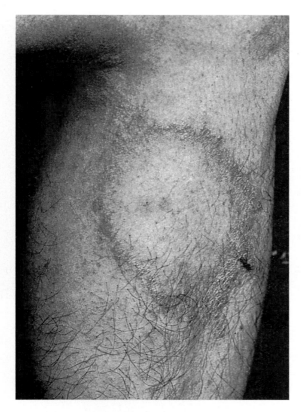

Fig. 17-2 Tuberculoid (TT) leprosy on inner calf. (Courtesy Dr. F. Reiss.)

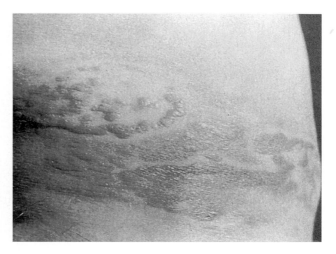

Fig. 17-3 Borderline tuberculoid (BT) leprosy.

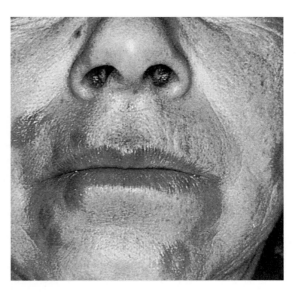

Fig. 17-4 Borderline tuberculoid (BT) leprosy. (Courtesy Dr. F. Latapi, Mexico.)

lesions around large macules or plaques are characteristic (Figs. 17-3 to 17-5).

Borderline Leprosy. In borderline (BB) leprosy, the skin lesions are numerous (but countable) and consist of red, irregularly shaped plaques (Fig. 17-6). Small satellite lesions may surround larger plaques (Fig. 17-7). Lesions are generalized but asymmetrical. The edges of lesions are not so well defined as the ones seen in the tuberculoid pole. Nerves may be thickened and tender, but anesthesia is only moderate in the lesions.

Borderline Lepromatous Leprosy. In borderline lepromatous (BL) leprosy, the lesions are symmetrical, numerous (too many to count), and may include macules, papules, plaques, and nodules (Figs. 17-8 and 17-9). The number of small lepromatous lesions outnumbers the larger borderline-type lesions (Fig. 17-10). Nerve involvement appears later; nerves are enlarged, tender, or both; it is important to note that involvement is symmetrical. Sensation and sweating over individual lesions is normal. Patients usually do not show the features of full-blown lepromatous leprosy, such as madarosis, keratitis, nasal ulceration, and leonine facies.

Lepromatous Leprosy. Lepromatous leprosy (LL) may begin as such or develop following indeterminate leprosy or

from downgrading of borderline leprosy. The cutaneous lesions of lepromatous leprosy consist mainly of pale lepromatous macules or lepromatous infiltrations, with numerous bacilli in the lesions. There is a negative reaction to lepromin, a typical histopathology, and a tendency for the disease to become progressively worse without treatment. Lepromatous leprosy may be divided into a polar form (LL_p) and subpolar form (LL_s); these forms may behave differently.

Macular lepromatous leprosy lesions are diffusely and symmetrically distributed over the body. Tuberculoid macules are large and few in number, whereas lepromatous macules are small and numerous. Lepromatous macules are ill defined, show no change in skin texture, and blend

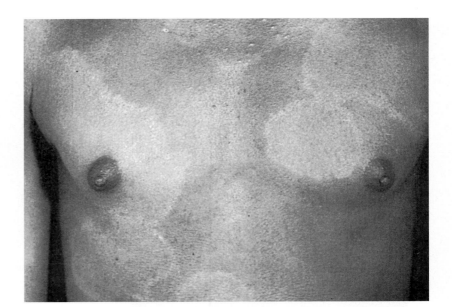

Fig. 17-5 Borderline tuberculoid (BT) leprosy. Hypopigmented, anesthetic, anhidrotic patches on chest. (Courtesy Dr. F. Kerdel-Vegas, Venezuela.)

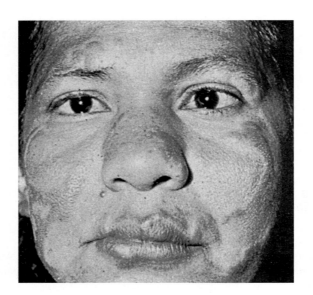

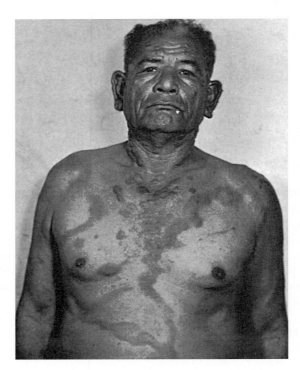

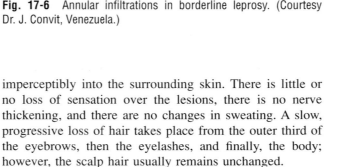

Fig. 17-6 Annular infiltrations in borderline leprosy. (Courtesy Dr. J. Convit, Venezuela.)

Fig. 17-7 Borderline leprosy, showing nodules and bizarre erythematous-bordered plaques on chest. (Courtesy Dr. J. Convit, Venezuela.)

imperceptibly into the surrounding skin. There is little or no loss of sensation over the lesions, there is no nerve thickening, and there are no changes in sweating. A slow, progressive loss of hair takes place from the outer third of the eyebrows, then the eyelashes, and finally, the body; however, the scalp hair usually remains unchanged.

Lepromatous infiltrations may be divided into the diffuse, plaque, and nodular types (Figs. 17-11 and 17-12). The diffuse type is characterized by the development of a diffuse infiltration of the face, especially the forehead, loss of the eyebrows (madarosis), and a waxy and shiny appearance of the skin, sometimes described as a "var-

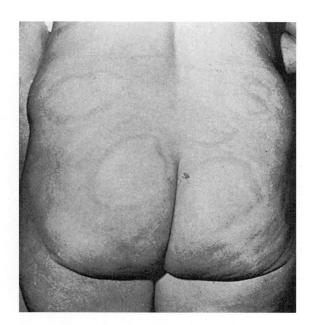

Fig. 17-8 Annular macules clearing in the center in borderline (BL) leprosy. (Courtesy Dr. J. Convit, Venezuela.)

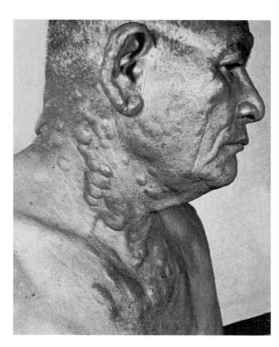

Fig. 17-9 Nodular lesions of borderline leprosy. (Courtesy Dr. J. Convit, Venezuela.)

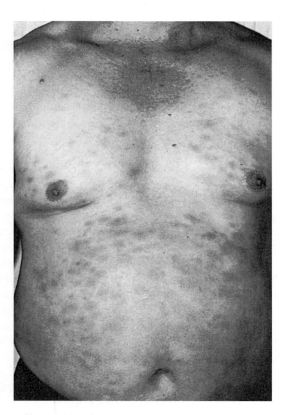

Fig. 17-10 Borderline lepromatous leprosy (BL).

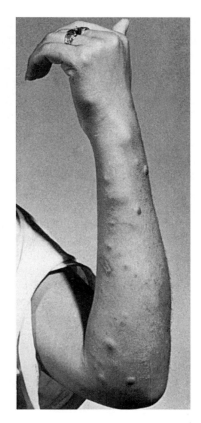

Fig. 17-11 Nodules of lepromatous leprosy.

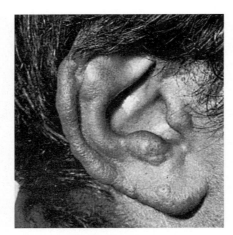

Fig. 17-12 Leprosy, lepromatous. Note nodules in ear. (Courtesy Dr. G. Salinger.)

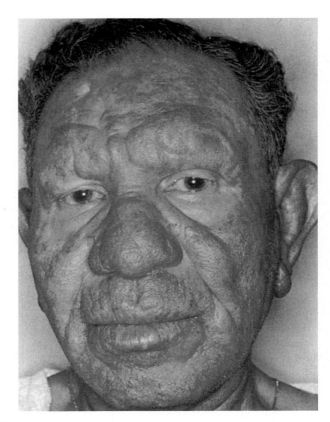

Fig. 17-13 Lepromatous leprosy. Note loss of the eyebrows and eyelashes (madarosis).

nished" appearance (Fig. 17-13). Diffuse leprosy of Lucio is a striking form, uncommon except in western Mexico and certain other Latin American areas, where nearly one third of lepromatous cases may be of this type. This form of lepromatous leprosy is characterized by diffuse lepromatous infiltration of the skin: localized lepromas do not form. A unique complication of this subtype is the reactional state referred to as *Lucio's phenomenon* (erythema necroticans) (Fig. 17-14).

The infiltrations may be manifested by the development of nodules called *lepromas.* The early nodules are ill defined and occur most often in acral parts: ears, brows, nose, chin, elbows, hands, buttocks, or knees. Nerve involvement invariably occurs, but develops very slowly. Like the skin lesions, nerve disease is bilaterally symmetrical, usually in a stocking-glove pattern. This is frequently misdiagnosed as diabetic neuropathy in the United States if it is the presenting manifestation.

Histoid Leprosy. Histoid leprosy is an uncommon form of multibacillary leprosy in which skin lesions appear as yellow-red, shiny, large papules and nodules in the dermis or subcutaneous tissue. Lesions appear on a background of normal skin. They vary in size from 1 to 15 mm in diameter and may appear anywhere on the body but favor the buttocks, lower back, face, and bony prominences. This pattern may appear de novo or in patients with dapsone resistance.

Nerve Involvement

Nerve involvement is a hallmark of leprosy. Nerve enlargement is rare in other diseases, so the finding of skin lesions with enlarged nerves should raise the possibility of leprosy. Nerve involvement tends to occur with skin lesions, and the pattern of nerve involvement parallels the skin disease. Tuberculoid leprosy is characterized by asymmet-

rical nerve involvement localized to the skin lesions. Lepromatous nerve involvement is symmetrical and not associated with skin lesions. Nerve involvement without skin lesions, called *pure neural leprosy,* can occur and may be either tuberculoid or lepromatous. In tuberculoid leprosy, neural lesions are caused by the inflammatory infiltrate in the nerves, and these lesions occur early in the disease. In the lepromatous pole, nerve involvement is by massive bacillary infiltration of the nerves with compression and eventual fibrosis. It occurs later in the course of the disease.

The neural signs in leprosy are dysesthesia, nerve enlargement, muscular weakness and wasting, and trophic changes. The lesions of the vasomotor nerves accompany the sensory disturbances or may precede them. Dysesthesia develops in a progressive manner. The first symptom is usually an inability to distinguish hot and cold. Subsequently, the perception of light touch is lost, then that of pain, and lastly the sense of deep touch. At times the sensory changes in large leprosy lesions are not uniform because of the variation in the involvement of the individual neural filaments supplying the area. Therefore the areas of dysesthesia may not conform to the distribution of any particular nerve, nor (except in lepromatous cases) are they symmetrical.

Nerve involvement affects chiefly (and is most easily

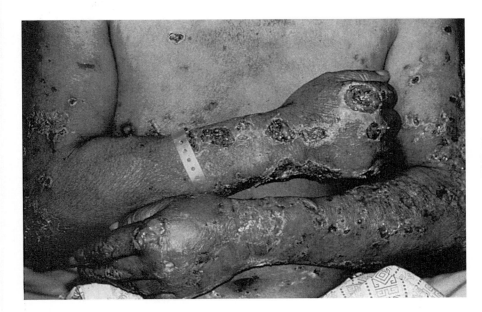

Fig. 17-14 Diffuse leprosy, Lucio's phenomenon (erythema necroticans). (Courtesy Dr. Axel W. Hoke.)

observed in) the more superficial nerve trunks, such as the ulnar, median, radial, peroneal, posterior tibial, fifth and seventh cranial nerves, and especially the great auricular nerve (Fig. 17-15). Beaded enlargements, nodules, or spindle-shaped swellings may be found, which at first may be tender. Neural abscesses may form. The ulnar nerve near the internal condyle of the humerus may be as thick as the little finger, round and stiff, and often easily felt several centimeters above the elbow.

As a result of the nerve damage, areas of anesthesia, paralysis, and trophic disorders in the peripheral parts of the extremities gradually develop. Muscular paralysis and atrophy generally affect the small muscles of the hands and feet or some of the facial muscles, producing weakness and progressive atrophy. Deeper motor nerves are only rarely involved. The fingers develop contractures, with the formation of a claw hand (Fig. 17-16), and, as the result of resorption of phalangeal bones, fingers, and toes become shorter (Fig. 17-17). Ptosis, ectropion, and a masklike appearance occur from damage to the fifth and seventh cranial nerves.

Subsequent to nerve damage ulceration, hyperkeratosis, bullae, alopecia, anhidrosis, and malum perforans pedis can develop. Trophic ulceration usually manifests as a perforating ulcer on the ball or heel of the foot (Fig. 17-18).

Ocular Involvement

Corneal erosions, exposure keratitis, and ulcerations may occur as a result of involvement of the seventh nerve. Specific changes may include corneal opacity, avascular keratitis, pannus formation, interstitial keratitis, and corneal lepromas (Fig. 17-19). The corneal opacities enlarge and finally form visible white flecks called pearls. When (in BL or LL cases only) the iris and the ciliary body become

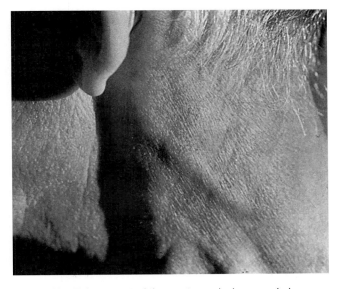

Fig. 17-15 Enlargement of the greater auricular nerve in lepromatous leprosy. (Courtesy Dr. Axel W. Hoke.)

involved, miliary lepromata (iris pearls), nodular lepromata, chronic granulomatous iritis, and acute diffuse iridocyclitis may result.

Mucous Membrane Involvement

The mucous membranes may also be affected, especially in the nose, mouth, and larynx. The nasal mucosa is most commonly involved, and lepromatous patients, if queried, frequently complain of chronic nasal congestion. By far the most common lesions in the nose are infiltrations and nodules. Perforation of the nasal septum may occur in advanced cases, with collapse of the nasal bridge. Nodules

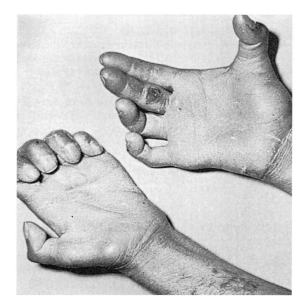

Fig. 17-16 Muscle atrophy and claw hand with polyneuritis in tuberculoid leprosy. Note external rotation of thumbs ("ape" hand). (Courtesy Dr. J. Convit, Venezuela.)

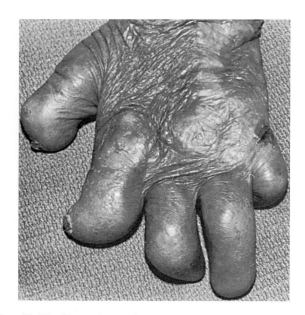

Fig. 17-17 Shortening and contractures of the phalanges in a 60-year-old woman with lepromatous leprosy. (Courtesy Dr. V.M. Torres-Rodriguez, Puerto Rico.)

occurring on the vocal cords will produce hoarseness. Saddle-nose deformities and loss of the upper incisor teeth can occur.

Visceral Involvement

In lepromatous leprosy the body is diffusely involved and bacteremia occurs. Except for the gastrointestinal tract,

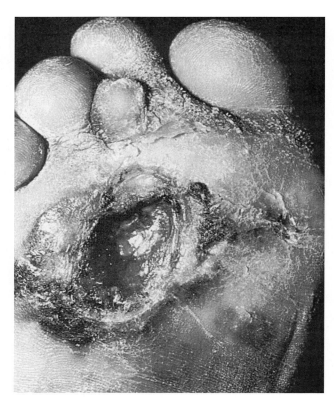

Fig. 17-18 Trophic ulcer (malum perforans) caused by lepromatous leprosy. (Courtesy Dr. Axel W. Hoke.)

lungs, and brain, virtually every organ can contain leprosy bacilli. The lymph nodes, bone marrow, liver, spleen, and testicles are most heavily infected. Visceral infection is restricted mostly to the reticuloendothelial system, that despite extensive involvement, rarely produce symptoms or findings. Testicular atrophy with resultant gynecomastia or premature osteoporosis is an exception. Secondary amyloidosis may complicate multibacillary leprosy.

PREGNANCY AND HANSEN'S DISEASE

Hansen's disease may be complicated in several ways by pregnancy. As a state of relative immunosuppression, pregnancy may lead to an exacerbation or reactivation after apparent cure. In addition, pregnancy may induce reactional states in patients with Hansen's disease. Pregnant patients with Hansen's disease cannot be given certain medications used to treat Hansen's disease such as thalidomide, quinolones, and minocycline. In general dapsone monotherapy is used during pregnancy, and reactions controlled with systemic corticosteroids as needed.

HIV DISEASE AND HANSEN'S DISEASE

HIV infection, while a cause of profound immunosuppression of the cell-mediated immune system, does not seem to

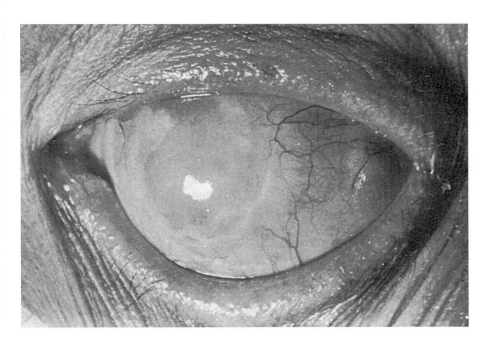

Fig. 17-19 Leproma and a complete pannus in lepromatous leprosy. (Courtesy Dr. J. Convit, Venezuela.)

adversely affect the course of Hansen's disease. Patients are treated with the same agents and can be expected to have similar outcomes in general. Duration of treatment with multidrug therapy may need to be extended in patients with HIV infection.

PATHOGENESIS OF HANSEN'S DISEASE

The host's immune reaction to the leprosy bacillus is a critical element in determining the outcome of infection. Most patients apparently resist disease, but may show immunologic evidence of prior exposure by activation of their lymphocytes when exposed to leprosy antigens. In those who become infected, self healing occurs in those in the tuberculoid pole. Borderline and lepromatous disease is progressive. This spectrum of disease and outcome correlates with the host's cell-mediated immune function against the leprosy bacillus, in that tuberculoid patients have positive lepromin skin tests and lepromatous patients negative ones. Tuberculoid patients make well-formed granulomas that contain helper T cells, where as lepromatous patients have poorly formed granulomas, and suppressor T cells predominate. The cytokine profile in tuberculoid lesions is that of good cell-mediated immunity with gamma interferon and interleukin-2 being present. In lepromatous patients these cytokines are reduced and interleukin-4, -5, and -10, cytokines that downregulate cell-mediated immunity and enhance suppressor function and antibody production are prominent. Lepromatous patients have polyclonal hypergammaglobulinemia, and may have false-positive syphilis serology, rheumatoid factor, and antinuclear antibodies, as a result. Lepromatous leprosy thus represents a classic helper T cell type 2 (Th-2) response to *M. leprae.*

Although the cell-mediated immune response of lepromatous patients to *M. leprae* is reduced, these patients are not immune suppressed for other infectious agents. Tuberculosis behaves normally in patients with lepromatous leprosy. Macrophages of patients with lepromatous leprosy phagocytose *M. leprae* poorly but other infectious agents normally. Phenolic glycolipid-1 and lipoarabinomannan impair monocyte and immune function against *M. leprae* in lepromatous patients. The underlying defect, which may be genetically determined and programs how the host will react to *M. leprae,* is unknown. All the immunologic events described above may be a consequence of this underlying defect.

HISTOPATHOLOGY OF HANSEN'S DISEASE

Ideally, biopsies should be performed from the active border of typical lesions and should extend into the subcutaneous tissue. Punch biopsies are usually adequate. Fite-Faraco stain is optimal for demonstrating *M. leprae.* Because the diagnosis of leprosy is associated with significant social implications, evaluation must be complete, to include evaluation of multiple sections in paucibacillary cases, and consultation if the diagnosis is suspected, but organisms cannot be identified in the affected tissue.

The histologic features of Hansen's disease correlate with the clinical pattern of disease. Nerve involvement is characteristic of leprosy, and perineural and neural involvement should raise the possibility of leprosy.

Tuberculoid Leprosy (TT)

Dermal tuberculoid granulomas, consisting of groups of epithelioid cells with giant cells are found. The epithelioid cells are not vacuolated or lipidized. The granulomas extend up to the epidermis, with no grenz zone. Lymphocytes are found at the periphery of the granulomas. Acid-fast bacilli are rare. The most important specific diagnostic feature, next to finding a bacillus, is selective destruction of nerve trunks. An S-100 stain may demonstrate this selective neural destruction by demonstrating unrecognizable nerve remnants in the inflammatory foci. Bacilli are most frequently found in nerves, but the subepidermal zone and the arrector pili muscles are other fruitful areas.

Borderline Tuberculoid Leprosy

The histopathology of the borderline tuberculoid (BT) type is similar to that seen in the tuberculoid variety, but epithelioid cells may show some vacuolation, bacilli are more abundant, and a grenz zone separates the inflammatory infiltrate from the overlying epidermis.

Borderline Leprosy

In borderline (BB) leprosy granulomas are less well organized, giant cells are not seen, the macrophages have some foamy cytoplasm, and organisms are abundant.

Borderline Lepromatous Leprosy

In borderline lepromatous (BL) lesions, foamy histiocytes, rather than epithelioid cells, make up the majority of the granuloma. Lymphocytes are still present and may be numerous in the granulomas, but are dispersed diffusely within them, not organized at the periphery. Perineural involvement with lymphocyte infiltration may be present. Organisms are abundant, and may be found in clumps.

Lepromatous Leprosy

In lepromatous leprosy (LL), granulomas are composed primarily of bacilli- and lipid-laden histiocytes. These are the so-called lepra cells or foam cells of Virchow. The infiltrate is localized in the dermis and is always separated from the epidermis by a well-defined grenz zone. Acid-fast bacilli are typically abundant. Pure polar lepromatous leprosy differs from the subpolar type primarily by the paucity of lymphocytes in the pure polar form.

REACTIONAL STATES

Reactions are a characteristic and clinically important aspect of Hansen's disease. Fifty percent of patients will experience a reaction after the institution of antibiotic therapy. In addition to antibiotic therapy, intercurrent infections, vaccination, pregnancy, vitamin A, iodides, and bromide may trigger reactions. Reactions can be severe, and are an important cause of permanent nerve damage in borderline patients. Reactional states are frequently abrupt in their appearance, as opposed to Hansen's disease itself, which changes slowly. It is therefore a common reason for patients to seek consultation. In addition, if the patient feels

that the chemotherapy is triggering the reaction, he or she will tend to discontinue the treatment, leading to treatment failure and secondary drug resistance.

Reactional states are divided into two forms, called type 1 and type 2 reactions. Type 1 reactions are caused by cell-mediated immune inflammation within existing skin lesions. They generally occur in patients with borderline leprosy (BT, BB, BL). Type 2 reactions are mediated by immune complexes and occur in lepromatous patients (BL, LL).

Type 1 Reactions (Lepra, Reversal, and Downgrading Reactions)

Type 1 reactions represent an enhanced cell-mediated immune response to *M. leprae*. If the reactions occur with antibiotic chemotherapy, they are called *reversal reactions*, and if they occur as borderline disease shifts toward the lepromatous pole (downgrading), they are called *downgrading reactions*. These two reaction types are clinically identical. Patients in all parts of the borderline spectrum may be affected by type 1 reactions, but these are most severe in patients with borderline lepromatous leprosy who have a large amount of *M. leprae* antigen and therefore have prolonged and repeated reactions during treatment.

Type 1 reactions clinically present with inflammation of existing lesions (Fig. 17-20). There are no systemic symptoms (such as fever, chills, and arthralgias). Lesions swell, become erythematous, and are sometimes tender, simulating cellulitis. In severe cases, ulceration can occur. Patients may state that new lesions appeared with the reaction, but these probably represent subclinical lesions that were highlighted by the reaction. The major complication of type 1 reactions is nerve damage. As the cell-mediated inflammation attacks *M. leprae* antigen, any infected tissue compartment can be

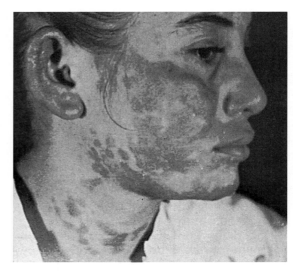

Fig. 17-20 Acute erythema in lepra reaction in borderline (BL) leprosy.

damaged. Because bacilli are preferentially in nerves, neural symptoms and findings are often present. Swelling of the peripheral nerve within its sheath may lead to sudden loss of function, making type 1 reactions an emergency. In this setting, affected nerves are enlarged and tender. In other patients the neuritis may be subacute or chronic and of limited acute symptomatology, but may still result in severe nerve damage.

Histologically, skin lesions show perivascular and perineural edema and large numbers of lymphocytes. Severe reactions may demonstrate tissue necrosis. Bacilli are reduced.

Type 2 Reactions (Erythema Nodosum Leprosum)

Erythema nodosum leprosum (ENL) occurs in half of patients with borderline lepromatous or lepromatous leprosy, 90% of the time, within a few years of institution of antibiotic treatment for Hansen's disease. ENL is a circulating immune complex–mediated disease. As such, in contrast to type 1 reactions, it can result in multisystem involvement and is usually accompanied by systemic symptoms (fever, myalgias, arthralgias, anorexia). Skin lesions are characteristically erythematous subcutaneous and dermal nodules that are widely distributed (Fig. 17-21). They do not occur at the sites of existing skin lesions. Severe skin lesions can ulcerate. Unlike classic erythema nodosum, lesions are generalized and favor the extensor arms and medial thighs.

ENL is a multisystem disease and can produce conjunctivitis, neuritis, keratitis, iritis, synovitis, nephritis, hepatosplenomegaly, orchitis, and lymphadenopathy (Fig. 17-22). The intensity of the reaction may vary from mild to severe and it may last from a few days to weeks, months, or even years. Histologically, ENL demonstrates a leukocytoclastic vasculitis.

Lucio's Phenomenon

Lucio's phenomenon is an uncommon and unusual reaction that occurs in patients with diffuse lepromatous leprosy of the "la bonita" type, most commonly in western Mexico. Some persons consider it a subset of ENL, but it differs in that it lacks neutrophilia and systemic symptoms. It is not associated with institution of antibiotic treatment as is ENL, but it is commonly the reason for initial presentation in affected patients. Bullous lesions appear that rapidly ulcerate, especially below the knees. They may be painful, but may also be relatively asymptomatic. Histologically, bacilli are seen within blood vessel walls, and thrombosis of middermal vessels occurs, resulting in cutaneous infarcts.

TREATMENT

Before 1982, dapsone monotherapy was the standard treatment for Hansen's disease, and while it was effective in many patients, primary and secondary dapsone-resistant cases had occurred. In addition, multibacillary patients required lifelong treatment, which had inherent compliance problems. To circumvent these problems and shorten therapeutic courses, the World Health Organization (WHO) proposed multidrug therapy (MDT). MDT has been very effective in treating active cases of Hansen's disease. Relapse rates are low with this treatment, ranging from 2%

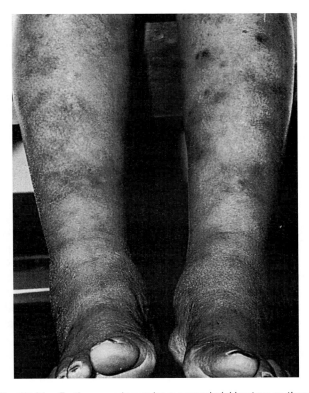

Fig. 17-21 Erythema nodosum leprosum mimicking true erythema nodosum.

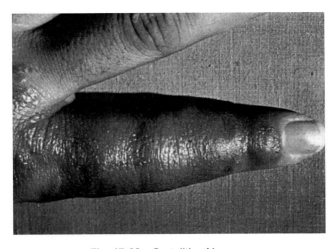

Fig. 17-22 Dactylitis of leprosy.

to 6% if patients are followed for many years. A common cause of failure is initial misdiagnosis; that is, diagnosing multibacillary patients as having paucibacillary disease through failure or inability to do a skin biopsy. Failure may also result from drug resistance, relapse after apparent clinical and bacteriologic cure, and persistence. *Persisters* are viable organisms that by mouse foot pad testing are sensitive to the antimicrobial agents given but persist in tissue despite bactericidal tissue levels in the patient.

There are several different MDT recommendations, but only two will be given here—those recommended by the Gillis W. Long Hansen's Disease Center in Carville for patients in the United States and those recommended by the WHO. Because dapsone resistance is less common in the United States, and effective compliance programs can be developed, enhancing monotherapy, dapsone monotherapy is still used after MDT in the United States. For paucibacillary cases (no organisms found on skin smears; indeterminate and TT leprosy) in the United States, the recommendation is 600 mg of rifampin and 100 mg of dapsone daily for 6 months. Dapsone monotherapy at a dose of 100 mg daily is continued for 3 years. BT patients are treated with this same regimen, but the dapsone monotherapy is continued for 5 years. In the United States, multibacillary cases receive 100 mg of dapsone and 600 mg of rifampin daily for 3 years. BB cases then receive dapsone monotherapy for 10 years, and BL and LL patients for life. Clofazimine may be added to this regimen at a dose of 50 mg daily, especially if there is suspicion of dapsone resistance. For known dapsone resistance, patients should receive rifampin 600 mg and clofazimine 50 mg for 3 years followed by clofazimine monotherapy indefinitely, or ethionamide 250 mg daily plus rifampin 600 mg daily for life (Table 17-2).

The WHO-recommended protocol is shorter and cheaper than those recommended in the United States. The recommendation for paucibacillary disease (abacillary disease; indeterminate and TT patients) is 600 mg of rifampin under supervision once a month for 6 months and 100 mg of dapsone daily for 6 months. For single-lesion paucibacillary disease a single dose of 600 mg rifampin, 400 mg ofloxacin, and 100 mg minocycline (ROM) all at one time has been recommended. Multibacillary patients (BT, BB, BL, and LL) are treated with three drugs. Rifampin 600 mg and clofazimine 300 mg once a month under supervision is taken with dapsone 100 mg and clofazimine 50 mg daily. Treatment is for 12 months or until the findings on smear are negative, whichever is longer.

Minocycline and ofloxacin are now regularly used for treating Hansen's disease, especially in patients in whom clofazimine pigmentation is problematic, and in whom dapsone or rifampin are not tolerated or resistance has been documented or is suspected. For multibacillary patients who cannot for some reason take dapsone and rifampin, the treatment regimen is 6 months of clofazimine 50 mg daily,

TABLE 17-2

Treatment Recommendations for Hansen's Disease: United States

		Dapsone 100 mg Daily after MDT* for:
Paucibacillary (I, TT, BT)	Dapsone 100 mg daily plus rifampin 600 mg daily for 6 mos	3 yr (I and TT) 5 yr (BT)
Multibacillary† (BB, BL, LL)	Dapsone 100 mg daily plus rifampin 600 mg daily for 3 yr	10 yr (BB) Lifelong (BL, LL)

*MDT = Multidrug therapy.
†Clofazimine 50 mg daily may be added to the initial regimen.
BB, Mid borderline; BL, borderline lepromatous; BT, borderline tuberculoid; I, indeterminate; LL, lepromatous leprosy; TT, pure tuberculoid.

ofloxacin 400 mg daily, and minocycline 100 mg daily, followed by 18 months of clofazimine 50 mg daily plus either ofloxacin 400 mg daily or minocycline 100 mg daily. For multibacillary patients who refuse clofazimine, 100 mg of minocycline or 400 mg of ofloxacin daily may be substituted for clofazimine 50 mg daily in the standard treatment regimen outlined in the previous paragraph and given for 12 months. An alternative 24-month regimen to avoid clofazimine is rifampin 600 mg, ofloxacin 400 mg, and minocycline 100 mg, each at the same time once a month. Clarithromycin 500 mg daily may also be used in treatment regimens but is not currently a recommended agent.

At the end of treatment, visible skin lesions may still be present, especially with the WHO short-duration treatments. In the United States, treatment would be continued until skin lesions are clear, even if the recommended duration of treatment has been passed. With short-duration MDT, it is very difficult to distinguish clinical relapse (failure of treatment) from late type 1 lepra reactions causing skin lesions to reappear. Histologic examination is required.

Dapsone (DDS)

Dapsone is the cornerstone of therapy, since it is effective, inexpensive, and relatively free of side effects in the recommended doses. The chief risks of sulfone therapy are methemoglobinemia and anemia (especially in G6PD-deficient patients). Other side effects are exfoliative dermatitis, hepatitis, neuropathy, and agranulocytosis.

Rifampin

Rifampin is highly bactericidal for *M. leprae* but, to avoid resistance, should never be used as monotherapy. It has been shown to render LL cases noninfective for the mouse foot pad by the seventh day of treatment. Untoward side effects are rarely encountered, except in patients receiving concomitant therapy with ethionamide.

Clofazimine (Lamprene)

Clofazimine is a riminophenazine derivative that is bacteriostatic and antiinflammatory; thus it is useful both for treating the disease and managing reactive episodes. Lepromatous lesions in areas exposed to sunlight turn a red-brown to grayish blue color during therapy, and the color persists for months or years after treatment is stopped.

Ethionamide

Ethionamide is intermediate in its bactericidal efficacy between rifampin and dapsone. It is used only as a combination drug, and side effects are common. They include gastrointestinal upset, hepatitis (especially when used with rifampin), peripheral neuropathy, skin eruptions, and thrombocytopenia. Pyridoxine should be given to patients on ethionamide to prevent drug-induced neurologic complications.

Adjunctive Treatments

Once neurologic complications have occurred, patients with Hansen's disease should be offered occupational therapy. This should include training on how to avoid injury to insensitive skin of the hands and feet. Special shoes may be required. Ocular complications are frequent, and an ophthalmologist with specific skill in treating leprosy patients is an invaluable member of the treatment team.

MANAGEMENT OF REACTIONS

Even though reactions may appear after drug treatment is instituted, it is not advisable to discontinue or reduce antileprosy medication because of this. In mild reactions—those without neurologic complications or severe systemic symptoms or findings—treatment may be supportive. Bed rest and administration of aspirin or nonsteroidal antiinflammatory agents may be used.

Type 1 reactions are usually managed with systemic corticosteroids. Prednisone is given orally, starting at a dose of 40 to 60 mg daily. Neuritis and eye lesions are urgent indications for systemic steroid therapy. Nerve abscesses may also need to be surgically drained immediately to preserve and recover nerve function. The corticosteroid dose and duration are determined by the clinical course of the reaction. Once the reaction is controlled, the prednisone may need to be tapered slowly—over months to years. The minimum dose required and alternate day treatment should be used in corticosteroid treatment courses more than 1 month in duration. Clofazimine appears to have some activity against Type 1 reactions and may be added to the treatment in doses of up to 300 mg daily if tolerated. Cyclosporine can be used if steroids fail or as a steroid-sparing agent. The starting dose would be 5 to 10 mg/kg. If during treatment the function of some nerves fails to improve while the function of others normalizes, the possibility of mechanical compression should be evaluated by surgical exploration. Transposition of the ulnar nerve does not seem to be more effective than immunosuppressive treatment for ulnar nerve dysfunction.

Thalidomide has been demonstrated to be uniquely effective against erythema nodosum leprosum and is the treatment of choice. The initial recommended dosage is 400 mg daily in patients weighing more than 50 kg. This dose is highly sedating in some patients, and patients may complain of central nervous system side effects, even at doses of 100 mg daily. For this reason, such a high dose should be used for only a brief period, or in milder cases, treatment may be started at a much lower dose, such as 100 mg to 200 mg daily. In cases in which there is an acute episode of erythema nodosum leprosum, the drug may be discontinued after a few weeks to months. In chronic type 2 reactions, an attempt to discontinue the drug should be made every 6 months. Systemic corticosteroids are also effective in type 2 reactions, but long-term use may lead to complications. Clofazimine in higher doses (up to 300 mg daily) may be used in an effort to reduce corticosteroid or thalidomide doses. *Thalidomide is a potent teratogen and should not be given to women of childbearing potential.*

Lucio's phenomenon is unresponsive to both corticosteroids and thalidomide. Effective antimicrobial chemotherapy for lepromatous leprosy is the only recommended treatment, combined with wound management for leg ulcers.

PREVENTION

Because a defect in CMI is inherent in the development of leprosy, vaccine therapies are being tested. When combined with multidrug therapy, vaccination with killed *M. leprae* appears to accelerate response to treatment, leading to a more rapid decline in BI and a more rapid return to a positive result on the lepromin skin test.

Until an effective vaccine is developed, prevention largely depends on treating active multibacillary patients to prevent transmission. Once an index case is identified, household contacts of lepromatous patients should be examined by an experienced person for 5 years after the diagnosis of the index case.

Arunthathi S, et al: Does clofazimine have a prophylactic role against neuritis? *Leprosy Rev* 1997, 68:233.

Becx-Bleumink M: Duration of multidrug therapy in paucibacillary leprosy patients. *Int J Leprosy* 1992, 68:436.

Becx-Bleumink M: Relapses among leprosy patients treated with multidrug therapy. *Int J Leprosy* 1992, 68:421.

Biedermann T, et al: Leprosy type 1 reaction as the first manifestation of borderline lepromatous leprosy in a young native German. *Br J Dermatol* 1997, 137:1006.

Britton WJ, et al: The management of leprosy reversal reactions. *Leprosy Rev* 1998, 69:225.

de Carsalade G-Y, et al: Daily multidrug therapy for leprosy: results of a fourteen-year experience. *Int J Leprosy* 1997, 65:37.

Dietrich M, et al: An international randomized study with long-term follow-up of singles versus combination chemotherapy of multibacillary leprosy. *Antimicrob Agents Chemother* 1994, 38:2249.

Grosset JH, et al: Workspot on chemotherapy. *Int J Lepr Other Mycobact Dis* 1998, 66:5.

Jacob M, et al: Short-term follow up of patients with multibacillary leprosy and HIV infection. *Int J Leprosy* 1996, 64:392.

Ji B, et al: Bactericidal activity of single dose of clarithromycin plus minocycline, with or without ofloxacin, against *Mycobacterium leprae* in patients. *Antimicrob Agents Chemother* 1996, 40:2137.

Ji B, et al: Powerful bactericidal activities of clarithromycin and minocycline against *Mycobacterium leprae* in lepromatous leprosy. *J Infect Dis* 1993, 168:188.

Kamradt T: T cell unresponsiveness in lepromatous leprosy. *J Rheumatol* 1993, 20:904.

Lyde C: Pregnancy in patients with Hansen disease. *Arch Dermatol* 1997, 133:623.

Meyers WM: Leprosy. *Dermatol Clin* 1992, 10:73.

Meyerson MS: Erythema nodosum leprosum. *Int J Dermatol* 1996, 35:389.

Moran CA, et al: Leprosy in five human immunodeficiency virus-infected patients. *Mod Pathol* 1995, 8:662.

Naafs B: Treatment of reactions and nerve damage. *Int J Leprosy* 1996, 64:S21.

Piscitelli SC, et al: Therapeutic monitoring and pharmacist intervention in a Hansen's disease clinic. *Ann Pharmacother* 1993, 27:1526.

Rea TH, et al: Immunopathology of leprosy skin lesions. *Semin Dermatol* 1991, 10:188.

Saxena U, et al: Giant nerve abscesses in leprosy. *Clin Exp Dermatol* 1990, 15:349.

Saxena U, et al: Treatment of paucibacillary leprosy. *Int J Dermatol* 1993, 32:135.

Schurr E, et al: Genetics of leprosy. *Am J Trop Med Hyg* 1991, 44:4.

Sehgal VN: Leprosy. *Dermatol Clin* 1994, 12:629.

Wathen PI: Hansen's disease. *South Med J* 1996, 89:647.

Zaheer SA: Addition of immunotherapy with *Mycobacterium* w vaccine to multi-drug therapy benefits multibacillary leprosy patients. *Vaccine* 1995, 13:1102. ▲

Syphilis, Yaws, Bejel, and Pinta

SYPHILIS

Syphilis, also known as *lues,* is a contagious, sexually transmitted disease caused by the spirochete *Treponema pallidum.* The spirochete enters through the skin or mucous membranes, on which the primary manifestations are seen. In congenital syphilis the treponeme crosses the placenta and infects the fetus. Syphilis results in multiple patterns of skin and visceral disease and is potentially lifelong.

Treponema pallidum is a delicate spiral spirochete that is actively motile. The number of spirals varies from 4 to 14 and the entire length is 5 to 20 μ. It can be demonstrated in preparations from fresh primary or secondary lesions by darkfield microscopy or by fluorescent antibody techniques. The motility is characteristic, consisting of three movements: a projection in the direction of the long axis, a rotation on its long axis, and a bending or twisting from side to side. The precise uniformity of the spiral coils is not distorted during these movements. *T. pallidum* cannot be distinguished from commensal oral treponemes, so darkfield examination of oral lesions is untrustworthy. The electron microscope shows the organism to have an axial filament with several fibrils, a protoplasmic cylinder, and a thin membranaceous envelope called the *periplast.* The organism is pathogenic for the anthropoid apes and produces a primary sore and secondary skin eruption closely simulating the disease in humans. It is also pathogenic for rabbits.

Syphilis remains a major health problem throughout the world. Using serologic testing, contact tracing, and penicillin treatment, the health departments in the United States reduced the incidence of syphilis dramatically from the turn of the century through the mid-1950s. Then the incidence of syphilis gradually increased through the next two decades and into the 1980s. In the early 1980s, half of the cases of syphilis diagnosed were in homosexual men. Changes in sexual behavioral patterns among gay men in response to the AIDS epidemic reduced the number of these cases, but in the late 1980s syphilis again began to increase dramatically, associated with drug usage, especially crack cocaine. The incidence of syphilis increased disproportionately among socioeconomically disadvantaged minority populations, especially in major cities. Throughout the 1990s the rate of syphilis fell in the United States, so that by 1999 the national rate of 2.6 cases per 100,000 was the lowest level ever recorded. In addition, half of new cases were concentrated in 28 counties mainly in the southeastern United States and in selected urban areas. Elimination of endemic syphilis in the United States may be possible.

Syphilis and other genital ulcer diseases enhance the risk of transmission and acquisition of the human immunodeficiency virus (HIV). HIV testing is recommended in all patients with syphilis. Syphilis is a reportable disease, and contact tracing and treatment of contacts are critical in reducing the incidence of syphilis.

Serologic Tests for Syphilis

Serologic tests for syphilis (STS) reveal the individual's immunologic status, but not (unless in rising titer) whether the patient is currently infected. Serum containing the antibody against *T. pallidum* forms aggregates with a cardiolipin-cholesterol-lecithin antigen that can be viewed directly in tubes or on cards or slides or can be examined in an autoanalyzer. Because these tests use lipoidal antigens rather than *T. pallidum* or components of it, they are called *nontreponemal antigen tests.* Most widely used are the rapid plasma reagin (RPR) and Venereal Disease Research Laboratory (VDRL) tests. Tests yield a positive result, as a rule, within 5 to 6 weeks after infection, shortly before the chancre heals. Tests are invariably strongly positive throughout the secondary phase, except in rare AIDS patients, whose response is less predictable; and results usually become negative during therapy, especially if therapy is begun within the first year. Results may also become negative after a few decades, even without treatment.

By diluting the serum serially, the strength of the reaction can be stated in dilutions, the number given being the highest dilution giving a positive test result. In primary infection the titer may be only 1:2; in secondary syphilis it is regularly high, 1:32 to 1:256 or higher; in late syphilis, much lower as a rule, perhaps 1:4 or 1:8. The rise of titer in early infection is of great potential diagnostic value, as is the fall after proper treatment or the rise again if there is reinfection or relapse.

Patients with very high antibody titers, as occur in secondary syphilis, may have a false negative result when undiluted serum is tested. This "prozone" phenomenon will be overcome by diluting the serum.

To improve sensitivity and specificity, tests have been devised using a specific treponemal antigen. Foremost among these are the microhemagglutination assay for *T. pallidum* (MHA-TP) and the fluorescent treponemal antibody absorption (FTA-ABS) test, which reliably identify seroreactivity caused by treponemal diseases (syphilis, yaws, bejel, or pinta). All positive nontreponemal test results should be confirmed with a specific treponemal test. Treponemal test results may be positive in borreliosis, but Lyme disease is not a common cause of false-positive nontreponemal test results, so it is not clinically important.

The treponemal tests become positive early, before the nontreponemal tests and may be useful in confirming primary syphilis. They usually remain positive for life and are therefore not useful in diagnosing other than the initial episode of syphilis. Because the nontreponemal tests tend to become negative in late syphilis, the specific treponemal tests are useful in diagnosing late disease. Gourevitch et al and Romanowski et al demonstrated that treatment of syphilis leads to loss of the positivity of both the FTA-ABS and MHA-TP in between 13% and 24% of patients, regardless of stage of syphilis and HIV status.

Biologic False-Positive Test Results. The term *biologic false-positive* (BFP) is used to denote a positive STS in persons with no history or clinical evidence of syphilis. Ninety percent of BFP test results are of low titer (less than 1:8). Acute BFP reactions are defined as those that revert to negative in less than 6 months; those that persist for more than 6 months are categorized as chronic. Acute BFP reactions may result from vaccinations, infections (infectious mononucleosis, hepatitis, measles, typhoid, varicella, influenza, lymphogranuloma venereum, malaria), and pregnancy. Chronic BFP reactions are seen in connective tissue diseases, especially systemic lupus erythematosus (SLE) (44%), chronic liver disease, multiple blood transfusions/intravenous drug usage, and advancing age.

False-positive results to specific treponemal tests are less common but have been reported to occur in lupus erythematosus, drug-induced lupus, scleroderma, rheumatoid arthritis, smallpox vaccination, pregnancy, and genital herpes simplex infections. A pattern of beaded fluorescence associated with FTA-ABS testing may be found in the sera of patients without treponemal disease who have systemic lupus erythematosus. The beading phenomenon, however, is not specific for SLE or even for connective tissue diseases.

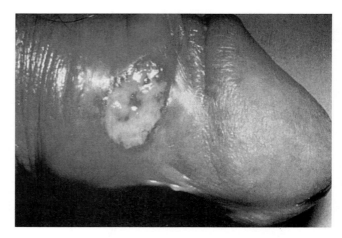

Fig. 18-1 Typical chancre. (Courtesy Dr. Axel W. Hoke.)

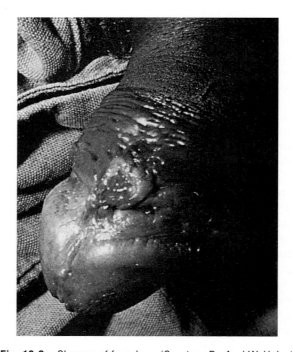

Fig. 18-2 Chancre of frenulum. (Courtesy Dr. Axel W. Hoke.)

Cutaneous Syphilis
Chancre (Primary Stage)

The chancre is usually the first cutaneous lesion, appearing 18 to 21 days after infection. The typical incipient chancre is a small red papule or a crusted superficial erosion. In a few days to weeks it becomes a round or oval, indurated, slightly elevated papule, with an eroded but not ulcerated surface that exudes a serous fluid (Figs. 18-1 to 18-3). On palpation it has a cartilage-like consistency. The lesion is usually, but not invariably, painless. This is the uncomplicated or classic Hunterian chancre. The regional lymph

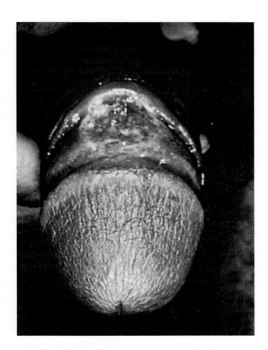

Fig. 18-3 Chancre near coronal sulcus.

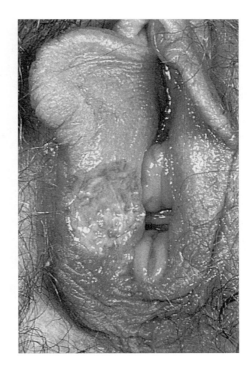

Fig. 18-4 Chancre of labium minus. (Courtesy Dr. Axel W. Hoke.)

nodes on one or both sides are usually enlarged, firm, and nontender and do not suppurate. Adenopathy begins 1 or 2 weeks after the appearance of the chancre. The Hunterian chancre leaves no scar when it heals.

Chancres generally occur singly, although they may be multiple; they vary in diameter from a few millimeters to several centimeters. In women the genital chancre is less often observed because of its location within the vagina or on the cervix (Fig. 18-4). Extensive edema of the labia or cervix may occur. In men the chancre is common in the coronal sulcus or on either side of the frenum. A chancre in the prepuce, being too hard to bend, will flip over all at once when the prepuce is drawn back, a phenomenon called a *dory flop,* from the resemblance to the movement of a broad-beamed skiff or dory as it is being turned upside down. Untreated, the chancre tends to heal spontaneously in 1 to 4 months. About the time of its disappearance, or usually a little before, constitutional symptoms and objective signs of generalized (secondary) syphilis occur.

Extragenital chancres may be larger than those on the genitalia. A frequent location of extragenital primary lesions is the lips, from orogenital sexual contact (Fig. 18-5). They appear rarely in other locations, the most important sites being the tongue, tonsil, female breast, index finger, and, especially in male homosexuals, the anus (Fig. 18-6). The presenting complaints of an anal chancre include an anal sore or fissure and irritation or bleeding on defecation. Anal chancre must be ruled out in any anal fissure not at the 6

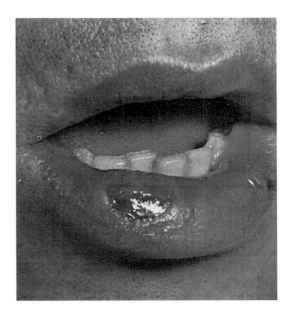

Fig. 18-5 Chancre on lower lip.

o'clock or 12 o'clock positions. When there is a secondary eruption, no evidence of chancre, and the glands below Poupart's ligament are markedly enlarged, anal chancre should be suspected.

Atypical chancres are common. Simultaneous infection by a spirochete and some other microbial agent may

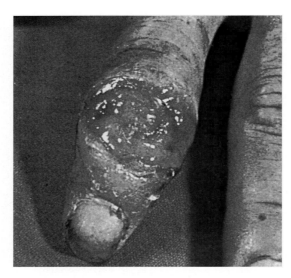

Fig. 18-6　Chancre of finger. (Courtesy Dr. S. Olansky.)

produce an atypical chancre. The mixed chancre caused by infection with *Haemophilus ducreyi* and *T. pallidum* will produce a lesion that runs a course different from either chancroid or primary syphilis alone. Such a sore begins a few days after exposure, since the incubation period for chancroid is short, and later the sore may transform into an indurated syphilitic lesion. A phagedenic chancre results from the combination of a syphilitic chancre and contaminating bacteria that may cause severe tissue destruction and result in scarring. Edema indurativum, or penile venereal edema, is marked solid edema of the labia or the prepuce and glans penis accompanying a chancre. Chancre redux is relapse of a chancre with insufficient treatment. It is accompanied by enlarged lymph nodes. Pseudochancre redux is a gumma occurring at the site of a previous chancre. It is distinguished from relapsing chancre by the absence of lymphadenopathy and a negative darkfield examination.

Histologic evaluation of a syphilitic chancre reveals an ulcer covered by neutrophils and fibrin. Subjacent there is a dense infiltrate of lymphocytes and plasma cells. Blood vessels are prominent with plump endothelial cells, but these vascular changes, while helpful in evaluation, are nonspecific. Spirochetes are numerous in untreated chancres of primary syphilis and can be demonstrated with an appropriate silver stain, such as the Warthin-Starry, Levaditi, or Steiner methods, or by immunoperoxidase staining. They are best found in the overlying epithelium or adjacent or overlying blood vessels in the upper dermis. The direct fluorescent antibody tissue test for *T. pallidum* (DFAT-TP) may be used in combination with histologic stains to demonstrate pathogenic treponemes in formalin-fixed tissues.

In a patient who presents with an acute genital ulceration, a darkfield examination should be performed if this investigation is available. The finding of typical *T. pallidum* in a sore on the cutaneous surface establishes a diagnosis of syphilis. *T. pertenue,* which causes yaws, and *T. carateum,* which causes pinta, are both indistinguishable morphologically from *T. pallidum,* but the diseases that they produce are usually easy to recognize. Commensal spirochetes of the oral mucosa are indistinguishable from *T. pallidum,* making oral darkfield examinations unreliable. If the darkfield examination results are negative, the examination should be repeated daily for several days, especially if the patient has been applying any topical antibacterial agents.

The lesion selected for examination is cleansed with water and dried. It is grasped firmly between the thumb and index finger and abraded sufficiently to cause clear or faintly blood-stained plasma to exude when squeezed. In the case of an eroded chancre, a few vigorous rubs with dry gauze are usually sufficient. If the lesion is made to bleed, it is necessary to wait until free bleeding has stopped to obtain satisfactory plasma. The surface of a clean coverslip is touched to the surface of the lesion so that plasma adheres. Then it is dropped on a slide and pressed down so that the plasma spreads out in as thin a film as possible. The specimen must be examined quickly, before the thin film of plasma dries.

An alternative to darkfield microscopy is the direct fluorescent antibody test (DFAT-TP) for the identification of *T. pallidum* in lesions. Serous exudate from a suspected lesion is collected as described above, placed on a slide, and allowed to dry. Many health departments will examine such specimens with fluorescent antibodies specific to *T. pallidum.* The method, unlike the darkfield examination, can be used for diagnosing oral lesions. Multiplex polymerase chain reaction (PCR) is also an accurate and reproducible method for diagnosing genital ulcerations. It has the advantage of being able to diagnose multiple infectious agents simultaneously. In genital ulcer disease outbreaks it should be made available.

The results of serologic tests for syphilis are positive in 50% (nontreponemal tests) to 90% (treponemal tests) of patients with primary syphilis; these tests should be performed in every patient with suspected syphilis. The likelihood of positivity depends on the duration of infection. If the chancre has been present for several weeks, test results are usually positive.

The chancre must be differentiated from chancroid. The chancre has an incubation period of 3 weeks; is usually a painless erosion, not an ulcer; has no surrounding inflammatory zone; and is round or oval. The edge is not undermined, and the surface is smooth and at the level of the skin. It has a dark, velvety red, lacquered appearance, is without a membrane, and is cartilage-hard on palpation. Lymphadenopathy may be bilateral and is nontender and nonsuppurative. Chancroid, on the other hand, has a short incubation period of 4 to 7 days; the ulcer is acutely inflamed, is extremely painful, and has a surrounding inflammatory zone. The ulcer edge is undermined and extends into the dermis. It has a yellowish red color, is covered by a membrane, and is soft to the touch. Lymphadenopathy is usually unilateral, tender, and suppurative. The lesions are usually multiple and extend into each other. Darkfield examination and cultures for chancroid confirm the diagnosis. However, since a combination of a syphilitic chancre and chancroid (mixed sores) is indistinguishable from chancroid alone, appropriate direct and serologic testing should be performed to investigate the presence of syphilis. Multiplex PCR allows for the simultaneous diagnosis of multiple infectious agents in genital ulcer diseases.

The primary lesion of granuloma inguinale begins as an indurated nodule that erodes to produce hypertrophic, vegetative granulation tissue. It is soft, beefy-red, and bleeds readily. A smear of clean granulation tissue from the lesion stained with Wright's or Giemsa's stain reveals Donovan bodies in the cytoplasm of macrophages.

The primary lesion of lymphogranuloma venereum (LGV) is usually a small, painless, transient papule or a superficial nonindurated ulcer. It most commonly occurs on the coronal sulcus, prepuce, or glans in men, or on the fourchette, vagina, or cervix in women. A primary genital lesion is noticed by about 30% of infected heterosexual men, but less frequently in women. Primary lesions are followed in 7 to 30 days by adenopathy of the regional lymph nodes. LGV is confirmed by serologic tests.

Herpes simplex begins with grouped vesicles, often accompanied or preceded by burning pain. After rupture of the vesicles, irregular, tender, soft erosions form.

Secondary Syphilis

CUTANEOUS LESIONS. The skin manifestations of secondary syphilis are called *syphilids* and occur in 80% of cases. The early eruptions are symmetrical, more or less generalized, superficial, nondestructive, exanthematic, transient, and macular; later they are maculopapular or papular eruptions, which are usually polymorphous, and less often scaly, pustular, or pigmented. The early manifestations are apt to be distributed over the face, shoulders, flanks, palms and soles, and anal or genital regions. The severity varies widely in different cases. The presence of lesions on the palms and soles is strongly suggestive. However, a generalized syphilid can spare the palms and soles. The individual lesions are generally less than 1 cm in diameter, except in the later secondary eruptions or in relapsing secondary eruptions.

Macular eruptions. The earliest form of macular secondary syphilis begins with the appearance of an exanthematic erythema 6 to 8 weeks after the development of the chancre, which may still be present or may have healed. The syphilitic exanthem extends rapidly, so that it is usually pronounced a few days after onset. It may be evanescent, lasting only a few hours or days, or it may last several months, or partially recur after having disappeared. This macular eruption appears first on the sides of the trunk, about the navel, and on the inner surfaces of the extremities. Of special importance is the appearance of slightly scaling ham-colored macules on the palms and soles (Fig. 18-7).

Individual lesions of macular secondary syphilis consist of round indistinct macules that are nonconfluent and may rarely be slightly elevated or urticarial (Fig. 18-8). The color varies from a light pink or rose to brownish red. The macular eruption may not be noticed on black skin and may be so faint that it is not recognized in other skin colors. Pain, burning, and itching are usually absent, although pruritus may be present in 10% to 40% of cases. Simultaneous with the onset of the eruption there is a generalized shotty adenopathy most readily palpable in the posterior cervical, axillary, and epitrochlear areas. Rarely, secondary syphilis may cause livedo reticularis (Fig. 18-9). The macular eruption may disappear spontaneously after a few days or weeks without any residuum, or may result in postinflammatory hyperpigmentation. After a varying interval, macular syphilis may be followed by other eruptions.

Papular eruptions. The papular types of eruption usually arise a little later than the macular. The fully developed lesions are of a raw-ham or coppery shade, round, and from 2 to 5 mm or more in diameter (Fig. 18-10). They are often only slightly raised, but a deep, firm infiltration is palpable. The surface is smooth, sometimes shiny, at other times covered with a thick, adherent scale. When this desquamates, it leaves a characteristic collarette of scales overhanging the border of the papule.

Papules are frequently distributed on the face and flexures of the arms and lower legs but are often distributed all over the trunk (Fig. 18-11). Palmar and plantar involvement characteristically appears as indurated, yellowish red spots (Figs. 18-12 and 18-13). Ollendorf's sign is present: the papule is exquisitely tender to the touch of a blunt probe. Healing lesions frequently leave hyperpigmented spots that, especially on the palms and soles, may persist for weeks or months. Split papules are hypertrophic, fissured papules that form in the creases of the alae nasi and at the oral commissures (Fig. 18-14). These may persist for a long period. The papulosquamous syphilids in which the adherent scales covering the lesions more or less dominate the picture may produce a psoriasiform eruption (Fig. 18-15). Follicular or lichenoid syphilids, which occur much less frequently, appear as minute scale-capped papules. If they are at the ostia of hair follicles, they are likely to be conical; elsewhere on the skin, they are domed. Often they are grouped to form scaling plaques in which the minute component papules are still discernible.

Like the other syphilids, papular eruptions tend to be disseminated but may also be localized, asymmetrical, configurate, hypertrophic, or confluent. Grouping is a diagnostic aid of great value. The arrangement may be corymbose or in patches, rings, or serpiginous patterns.

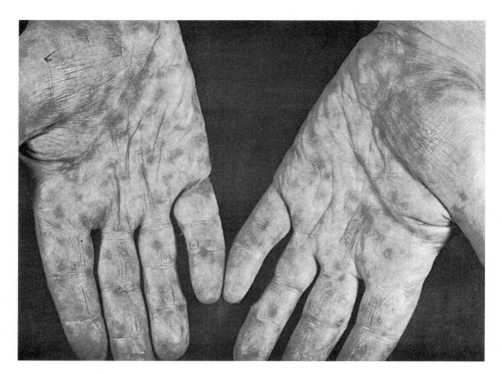

Fig. 18-7 Typical palmar macules of early syphilis. (Courtesy Dr. H. Shatin.)

Fig. 18-8 Early syphilis.

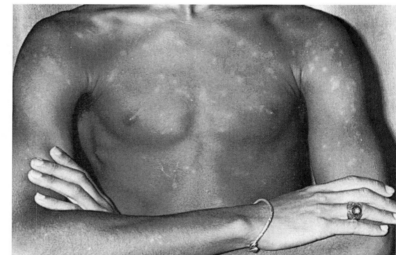

The annular syphilid, like sarcoidosis (which it may mimic), is more common in blacks (Figs. 18-16 to 18-18). It is often located on the cheeks, especially close to the angle of the mouth. Here it may form annular, arcuate, or gyrate patterns of delicate, slightly raised, infiltrated, finely scaling ridges. These ridges are made up of minute, flat-topped papules, and the boundaries between ridges may be difficult to discern. An old term for annular syphilids was *nickels and dimes.*

The corymbose syphilid is another infrequent variant, usually occurring late in the secondary stage, in which a large central papule is surrounded by a group of minute satellite papules. The pustular syphilids are among the rarer manifestations of secondary syphilis. They occur widely scattered over the trunk and extremities, but they usually involve the face, especially the forehead. The pustule usually arises on a red, infiltrated base. Involution is usually slow, resulting in a small, rather persistent, crust-covered,

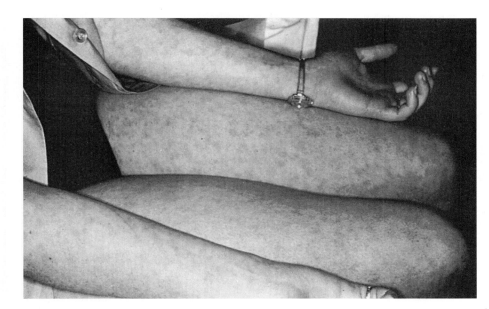

Fig. 18-9 Livedo reticularis as a manifestation of secondary syphilis.

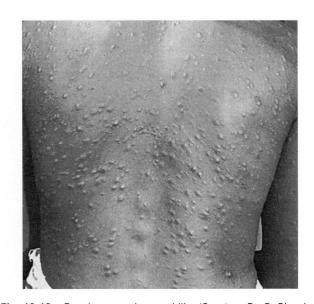

Fig. 18-10 Papular secondary syphilis. (Courtesy Dr. S. Olansky.)

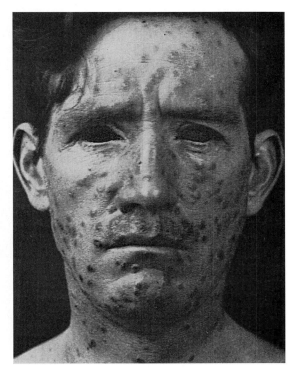

Fig. 18-11 Papular syphiloderm.

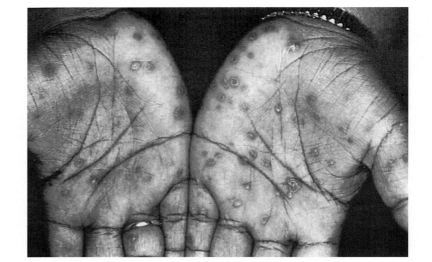

Fig. 18-12 Typical papulosquamous syphilid of the palms.

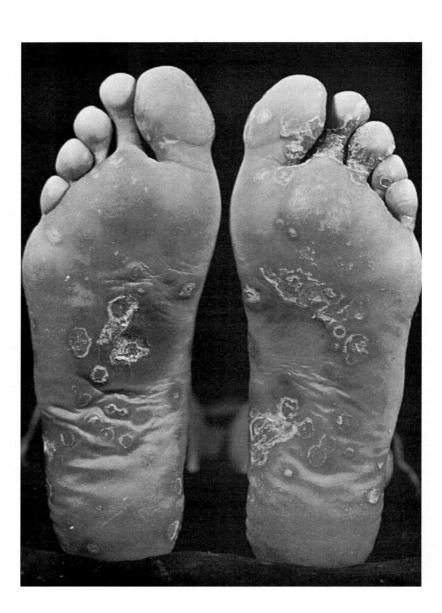

Fig. 18-13 Papulosquamous syphilid in early syphilis. (Courtesy Dr. H. Shatin.)

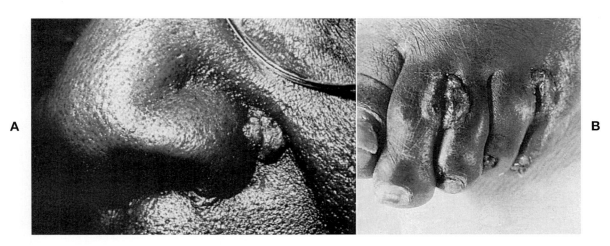

Fig. 18-14 Split papules of secondary syphilis. **A,** Nasolabial fold. **B,** Interdigital lesions.

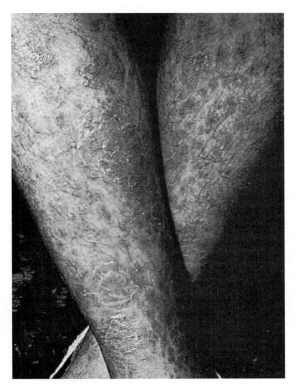

Fig. 18-15 Papulosquamous lesions of early secondary syphilis on the legs of a 26-year-old woman.

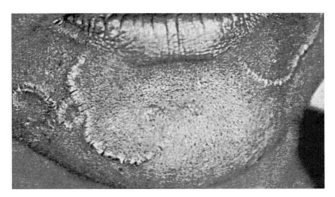

Fig. 18-16 Annular eruption in secondary syphilis.

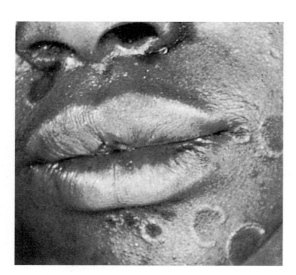

Fig. 18-17 Annular secondary syphilid of the face. Note the dryness and nonscaling nature distinguishing it from impetigo. (Courtesy Dr. S. Olansky.)

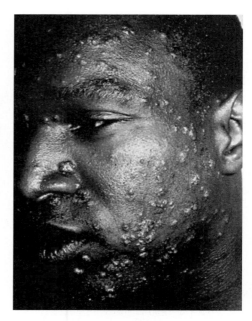

Fig. 18-19 Pustular syphilid.

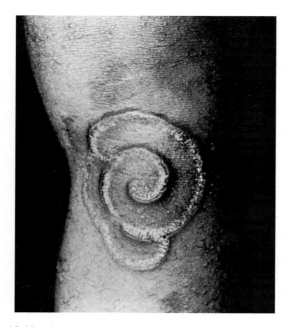

Fig. 18-18 An unusual morphologic lesion of secondary syphilis.

superficial ulceration. Lesions in which the ulceration is deep are called *ecthymatous*. Closely related is the rupial syphilid, a lesion in which a relatively superficial ulceration is covered with a pile of terraced crusts resembling an oyster shell. Lues maligna is a rare form of secondary syphilis with severe ulcerations, pustules, or rupioid lesions, accompanied by severe constitutional symptoms (Fig. 18-19).

Condylomata lata are papular lesions, relatively broad and flat, located on folds of moist skin, especially about the genitalia and anus; they may become hypertrophic and, instead of infiltrating deeply, protrude above the surface, forming a soft, red, often mushroomlike mass 1 to 3 cm in diameter, usually with a smooth, moist, weeping, gray surface (Figs. 18-20 and 18-21). It may be lobulated but is not covered by the digitate elevations characteristic of venereal warts (condylomata acuminata).

Syphilitic alopecia is irregularly distributed so that the scalp has a moth-eaten appearance. It is unusual, occurring in about 5% of patients with secondary syphilis (Figs. 18-22 and 18-23).

Mucous membrane lesions are present in one third of patients with secondary syphilis. The most common mucosal lesion in the early phase is the syphilitic sore throat, a diffuse pharyngitis that may be associated with tonsillitis or laryngitis. Hoarseness and sometimes complete aphonia may be present. On the tongue, smooth, small or large, well-defined patches devoid of papillae may be seen, most frequently on the dorsum near the median raphe. Ulcerations often occur on the tongue and lips during the late secondary period.

Mucous patches are the most characteristic mucous membrane lesions of secondary syphilis. They are macerated, flat, grayish, rounded erosions covered by a delicate, soggy membrane (Figs. 18-24 and 18-25). These highly infectious lesions are about 5 mm in diameter and teem with treponema. They occur on the tonsils, tongue, pharynx, gums, lips, and buccal areas, or on the genitalia, chiefly in women. In the latter they are most common on the labia minora, the vaginal mucosa, and the cervix. Such mucous

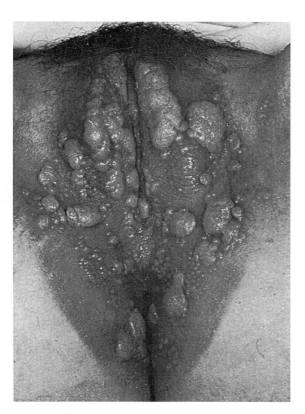

Fig. 18-20 Condylomata lata on the labia. (Courtesy Dr. S. Olansky.)

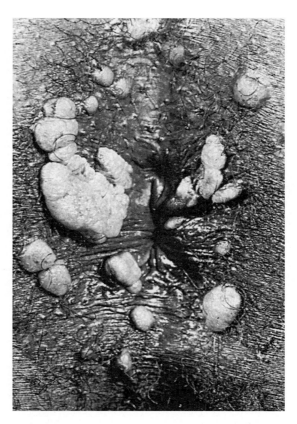

Fig. 18-21 Perianal condylomata lata in early syphilis. (Courtesy Dr. H. Shatin.)

erosions are transitory and change from week to week, or even from day to day.

RELAPSING SECONDARY SYPHILIS. The early lesions of syphilis undergo involution either spontaneously or with treatment. Relapses occur in about 25% of untreated patients, 90% within the first year. Such relapses may take place at the site of previous lesions, on the skin or in the viscera. Recurrent eruptions tend to be more configurate or annular, larger, and asymmetrical.

SYSTEMIC INVOLVEMENT. The lymphatic system in secondary syphilis is characteristically involved. The lymph nodes most frequently affected are the inguinal, posterior cervical, postauricular, and epitrochlear. The nodes are shotty, firm, slightly enlarged, nontender, and discrete.

Acute glomerulonephritis, gastritis or gastric ulceration, proctitis, hepatitis, acute meningitis, sensorineural hearing loss, iritis, anterior uveitis, optic neuritis, Bell's palsy, multiple pulmonary nodular infiltrates, periostitis, osteomyelitis, polyarthritis, or tenosynovitis may all be seen in secondary syphilis.

Histopathology. Macules of secondary syphilis feature superficial and deep perivascular infiltrates of lymphocytes, macrophages and plasma cells without epidermal change, or accompanied by slight vacuolar change at the dermoepidermal junction.

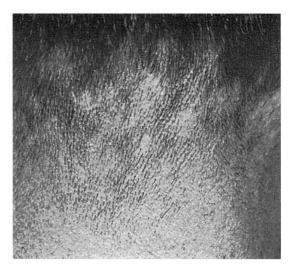

Fig. 18-22 Moth-eaten alopecia of early syphilis. (Courtesy Dr. F. Kerdel-Vegas, Venezuela.)

Papules and plaques of secondary syphilis usually show dense superficial and deep infiltrates of lymphocytes, macrophages, and plasma cells. These cells are usually distributed in a bandlike pattern in the papillary dermis and cuffed around blood vessels, accompanied by psoriasiform

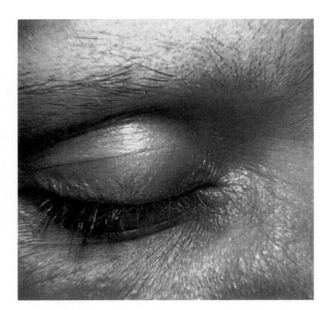

Fig. 18-23 Alopecia of eyebrows in secondary syphilis.

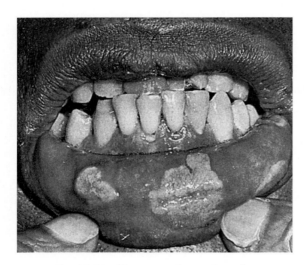

Fig. 18-24 Mucous patches on inner lip.

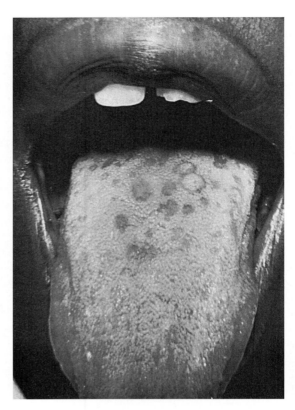

Fig. 18-25 Mucous patches on the tongue. (Courtesy Dr. S. Olansky.)

epidermal hyperplasia and hyperkeratosis. The presence of numerous macrophages often gives the infiltrates a pallid appearance under scanning magnification. Vacuolar degeneration of keratinocytes is often present, giving the lesions a "psoriasiform and lichenoid" histologic pattern. Plasma cells are said to be absent in 10% of cases. As lesions age, macrophages become more numerous, so that in late secondary lues, granulomatous foci are often present, mimicking sarcoidosis. Condylomata lata show spongiform pustules within areas of papillated epithelial hyperplasia, and spirochetes are numerous. Spirochetes are most numerous within the epidermis and around superficial vessels. PCR and immunoperoxidase may identify *T. pallidum* infection when silver stains are negative.

Diagnosis and Differential Diagnosis. The nontreponemal serologic tests for syphilis are almost invariably strongly reactive in secondary syphilis. An exception occurs when very high titers of antibody are present, producing a false-negative result (prozone phenomenon). The true positivity of the serum is detected on dilutional testing. Also, rarely, seronegative secondary syphilis may occur in patients with AIDS. Identification of spirochetes by dark-field examination or histologic examination of affected tissues may be used to confirm the diagnosis, especially in patients who are seronegative.

Syphilis has long been known as the "great imitator," because the various cutaneous manifestations may simulate almost any cutaneous or systemic disease. Pityriasis rosea may be mistaken for secondary syphilis, especially since both begin on the trunk. The herald patch, the oval patches with a fine scale at the edge, patterned in the lines of skin cleavage, the absence of lymphadenopathy, and infrequent mucous membrane lesions help to clinically distinguish pityriasis rosea from secondary syphilis. Drug eruptions may produce a similar picture; however, they tend to be scarlatiniform or morbilliform. Drug eruptions are often pruritic, whereas secondary syphilis usually is not. Lichen planus may resemble papular syphilid. The characteristic papule of lichen planus is flat topped, polygonal, has

Wickham's striae, and exhibits the Koebner's phenomenon. Pruritus is severe in lichen planus and less common and less severe in syphilis. Psoriasis may be distinguished from papulosquamous secondary syphilis by the presence of adenopathy, mucous patches, and alopecia in the latter. Sarcoidosis may produce lesions morphologically identical to secondary syphilis. Histologically, multisystem involvement, adenopathy, and granulomatous inflammation are common to both diseases. Serologic testing and silver staining of biopsy specimens will distinguish these two disorders.

The differential diagnosis of mucous membrane lesions of secondary syphilis is of importance. Infectious mononucleosis may cause a biologic false-positive test for syphilis but is diagnosed by a high heterophile antibody titer. Geographic tongue may be confused with the desquamative patches of syphilis or with mucous patches. Lingua geographica occurs principally near the edges of the tongue in relatively large areas, which are often fused and have lobulated contours; it continues for several months or years and changes in extent and degree of involvement from day to day. Recurrent aphthous ulceration produces one or several painful ulcers 1 to 3 mm in diameter, surrounded by hyperemic edges, with a grayish covering membrane, on nonkeratinized mucosal epithelium, especially in the gingival sulcus. A prolonged, recurrent history is characteristic.

Latent Syphilis

After the lesions of secondary syphilis have involuted, a latent period occurs. This may last for a few months or continue for the remainder of the infected person's life. Sixty percent to 70% of untreated infected patients remain asymptomatic for life. During this latent period there are no clinical signs of syphilis, but the serologic tests for syphilis are reactive. During the early latent period infectivity persists: for at least 2 years a woman with early latent syphilis may infect her unborn child.

Late Syphilis

Late syphilis is defined by the CDC as infection of greater than 1 year's duration, or by the WHO as greater than 2 years' duration.

Tertiary Cutaneous Syphilis

Tertiary syphilids most often occur 3 to 5 years after infection. Sixteen percent of untreated patients will develop tertiary lesions of the skin, mucous membrane, bone, or joints. Skin lesions tend to be localized, to occur in groups, to be destructive, and to heal with scarring. Treponema are usually not found by silver stains or darkfield examination but may be demonstrated by PCR.

Two main types of tertiary syphilids are recognized, the nodular syphilid and the gumma, although the distinction is sometimes difficult to make. The nodular, noduloulcerative, or tubercular type consists of reddish brown or copper-

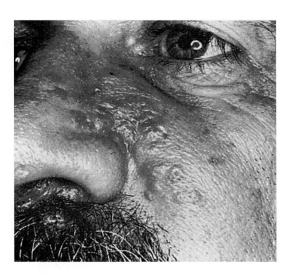

Fig. 18-26 Tertiary syphilis, rosacea-like appearance.

colored firm papules or nodules, 2 mm or larger (Fig. 18-26). The individual lesions are usually covered with adherent scales or crusts. The lesions tend to form rings and to undergo involution as new lesions develop just beyond them, so that characteristic circular or serpiginous patterns are produced (Fig. 18-27). A distinctive and characteristic type is the kidney-shaped lesion (Fig. 18-28). These frequently occur on the extensor surfaces of the arms and on the back of the trunk. Such patches are composed of nodules in different stages of development so that it is common to find scars and pigmentation together with fresh and also ulcerated lesions. On the face the nodular eruption closely resembles lupus vulgaris (Figs. 18-29 and 18-30). When the disease is untreated, the process may last for years, slowly marching across large areas of skin. The nodules may enlarge and eventually break down to form painless, rounded, smooth-bottomed, reddish ulcers a few millimeters deep. These punched-out ulcers arise side by side and form serpiginous syphilitic ulcers, palm-sized in aggregate, enduring for many years.

Gummas may occur as unilateral, isolated, single or disseminated lesions, or in serpiginous patterns resembling those of the nodular syphilid. They may be restricted to the skin or, originating in the deeper tissues, break down and secondarily involve the skin. The individual lesions, which begin as small nodules, slowly enlarge to several centimeters (Fig. 18-31). Central necrosis is extensive and may lead to the formation of a deep punched-out ulcer with steep sides and a gummy base (Fig. 18-32). Again, progression may take place in one area while healing proceeds in another. Perhaps the most frequent site of isolated gummas is the lower legs, where deep punched-out ulcers are formed, often in large infiltrated areas.

Histologically, nodular lesions of late syphilis usually have changes that resemble those of secondary lesions, with the addition of tuberculoid granulomas containing various numbers of multinucleate giant cells. The epidermis is often atrophic rather than hyperplastic. In gummas, there is necrosis within granulomas and fibrosis as lesions resolve. Spirochetes are scant.

In addition to the typical and distinctive morphologic structure of the skin lesions, for diagnosis of late syphilis

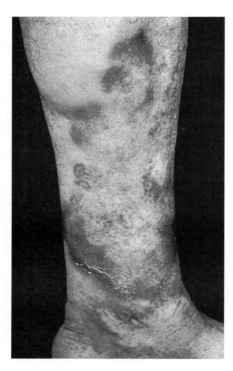

Fig. 18-27 Noduloulcerative tertiary syphilis. (Courtesy Communicable Disease Center.)

clinicians rely heavily on the serologic tests for syphilis. The nontreponemal tests, such as the VDRL and RPR, are positive in approximately 75% of cases. The treponemal tests, such as the FTA-ABS, MHA-TP, and the TPI, are positive in nearly 100% of patients. When there are mucous membrane lesions for which a diagnosis of carcinoma must also be considered, histologic examination is performed. Darkfield examination is not indicated, since it is always negative, but PCR of biopsy material may be positive. In late syphilis the mucous membranes are attacked; the tongue is a frequent site. Gumma of the tongue usually involves the edge, toward the back, and rapidly breaks down to form a punched-out ulcer with irregular, soft edges.

When not ulcerated these syphilids must be distinguished from malignant tumors, leukemids, and sarcoidosis. Glanders and sporotrichosis may be distinguished by demonstration of the causative organisms. The ulcerated syphilids must be differentiated from scrofuloderma, atypical mycobacterial infection, sporotrichosis, and blastomycosis. Mycosis fungoides is accompanied by eczematous changes and pruritus. Carcinoma and sarcoma have distinctive histologic findings. On the lower extremities gummas are frequently mistaken for erythema induratum and the various nonsyphilitic ulcers.

A superficial glossitis may cause irregular ulcers, atrophy of the papillae, and smooth, shiny scarring, a condition known as *smooth atrophy*. In interstitial glossitis there is an underlying induration resulting from sclerosis. In the advanced stages, tertiary syphilis of the tongue may lead to a diffuse enlargement (macroglossia). Perforation of the hard palate from gummatous involvement is a characteristic tertiary manifestation. It generally occurs near the center of

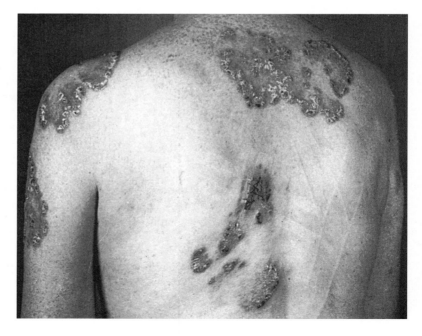

Fig. 18-28 Tertiary noduloulcerative syphilis. Note kidney-shaped lesions. (Courtesy Dr. J. Lowry Miller.)

the hard palate. Destruction of the nasal septum may also occur.

Late Osseous Syphilis

Not infrequently, gummatous lesions involve the periosteum and the bone. Skeletal syphilids occur most commonly on the head and face, then on the tibia. Late manifestations of syphilis may produce periostitis, osteomyelitis, osteitis, and gummatous osteoarthritis. Osteocope—bone pain, most often at night—is a suggestive symptom.

Syphilitic joint lesions also occur, with the Charcot joint being the most prevalent manifestation. They are often associated with tabes dorsalis and occur most frequently in men. Although any joint may be involved, the knees and ankles are the most frequently affected. There is hydrops, then loss of the contours of the joint, hypermobility, and painlessness. It is readily diagnosed by x-ray examination.

Neurosyphilis

Central nervous system (CNS) involvement with syphilis can occur at any stage of syphilis, even the primary stage. Most persons with CNS involvement have no symptoms,

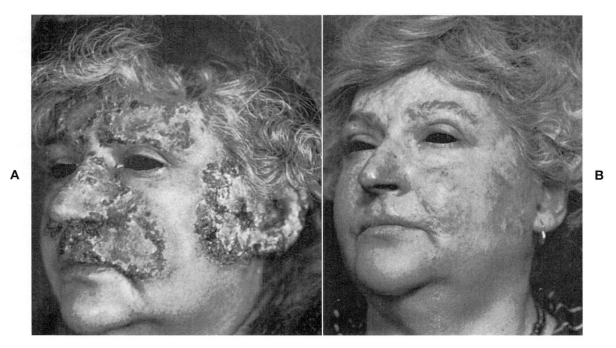

Fig. 18-29　Tertiary syphilis. **A,** Before treatment. **B,** After treatment.

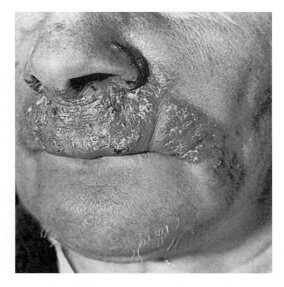

Fig. 18-30　Tubercular tertiary syphilid.

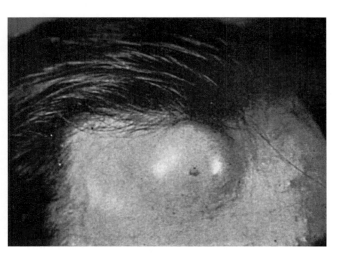

Fig. 18-31　Gumma of forehead.

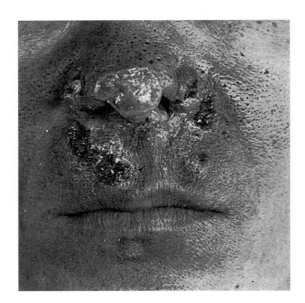

Fig. 18-32 Gumma of tertiary syphilis.

but the disease can be detected by finding cerebrospinal fluid (CSF) pleocytosis or a positive CSF serology. From this group of persons with "asymptomatic" neurosyphilis, symptomatic disease will occur in some. Persons with negative CNS examinations have almost no risk of developing neurosyphilis. Four percent to 9% of persons with untreated syphilis will develop neurosyphilis. Symptomatic neurosyphilis occurs from early in the secondary phase through the tertiary phase. It is divided into early and late forms, which do not directly correlate with early and late syphilis as defined above.

CSF evaluation is recommended in all syphilis patients with any neurologic, auditory, or ophthalmic signs or symptoms, possibly resulting from syphilis, independent of stage. Patients with latent syphilis should have CSF evaluation if they are HIV positive, fail initial therapy, have an RPR or VDRL titer of more than 1:32 and have syphilis of longer than 1 year's duration, or therapy other than penicillin is planned for syphilis of more than 1 year's duration. Patients with tertiary syphilis should have CSF evaluation before treatment to exclude neurosyphilis.

EARLY NEUROSYPHILIS. Early neurosyphilis is mainly meningeal, occurring in the first year of infection, and spinal fluid abnormalities herald the early changes. Spinal fluid examination shows a positive serology and a pleocytosis with lymphocytosis. Meningeal neurosyphilis manifests as meningitis, with headache, stiff neck, cranial nerve disorders (loss of hearing, facial weakness, visual disturbances), seizures, and delirium, with increased intracranial pressure indicated by papilledema.

MENINGOVASCULAR NEUROSYPHILIS. Meningovascular neurosyphilis most frequently occurs 4 to 7 years after infection. It is caused by thrombosis of vessels in the CNS and presents as in other CNS ischemic events. Hemiplegia, aphasia, hemianopsia, transverse myelitis, and progressive muscular atrophy may occur. Cranial nerve palsies may also occur, such as eighth nerve deafness and eye changes. The eyes may show fixed pupils, Argyll Robertson pupils, or anisocoria.

LATE (PARENCHYMATOUS) NEUROSYPHILIS. Parenchymatous neurosyphilis tends to occur more than 10 years after infection. There are two classic clinical patterns: tabes dorsalis and general paresis.

Tabes dorsalis is the degeneration of the dorsal roots of the spinal nerves and of the posterior columns of the spinal cord. The symptoms and signs are so numerous that only a partial listing is feasible here. Gastric crisis with severe pain and vomiting is the most frequent symptom. Some other symptoms are lancinating pains, urination difficulties, paresthesias (numbness, tingling, and burning), spinal ataxia, diplopia, strabismus, vertigo, and deafness. The signs that may be present are Argyll Robertson pupils, absent or reduced lower cord reflexes, Romberg sign, sensory loss (deep tendon tenderness, vibration, and position), atonic bladder, trophic changes, malum perforans pedis, Charcot's joints, and optic atrophy (Fig. 18-33).

Paresis has prodromal manifestations of headache, fatigability, and inability to concentrate. Later, personality changes occur, along with memory loss and apathy. Grandiose ideas, megalomania, delusions, hallucinations, and finally dementia may occur.

Late Cardiovascular Syphilis

Late cardiovascular syphilis occurs in about 10% of untreated patients. Aortitis is the basic lesion of cardiovascular syphilis, resulting in aortic insufficiency, coronary disease, and ultimately aortic aneurysm.

Congenital Syphilis

Prenatal syphilis is acquired in utero from the mother, who usually has early syphilis. Infection through the placenta usually does not occur before the fourth month, so treatment of the mother before this time will almost always prevent infection in the fetus. If the mother has early syphilis and prenatal infection occurs soon after the fourth month, fetal death and miscarriage occur in about 40% of pregnancies. During the remainder of the pregnancy, infection is equally likely to produce characteristic developmental physical stigmata, or, after the eighth month, active, infectious congenital syphilis. Forty percent of pregnancies in women with untreated early syphilis will result in a syphilitic infant. In utero infection of the fetus is rare when the pregnant mother has had syphilis for 2 or more years. Most neonates with congenital syphilis are normal at birth. Lesions occurring within the first 2 years of life are called *early congenital syphilis*, and those developing thereafter are called *late congenital syphilis*. The clinical manifestations of these two syndromes are different.

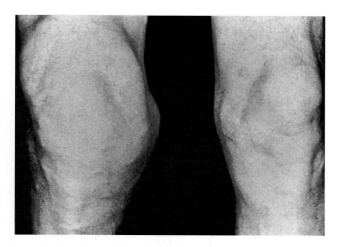

Fig. 18-33 Charcot's joint. (Courtesy Communicable Disease Center.)

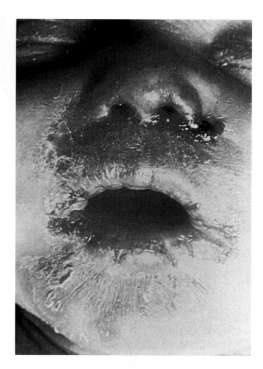

Fig. 18-34 Snuffles.

Early Congenital Syphilis. Early congenital syphilis describes those cases presenting within the first 2 years of life. Most neonates with congenital syphilis are normal at birth. Cutaneous manifestations appear most commonly during the third week of life, but sometimes occur as late as 3 months after birth. Neonates born with findings of congenital syphilis are usually severely affected. They may be premature, are often marasmic, fretful, and dehydrated. The face is pinched and drawn, resembling that of an old man or woman. Multisystem disease is characteristic.

Snuffles, a form of rhinitis, is the most frequent and often the first specific finding (Fig. 18-34). It blocks the nose, often with blood-stained mucus; a copious discharge of mucus runs down over the lips. The nasal obstruction often interferes with the child's nursing. In persistent and progressive cases ulcerations develop that may involve the bones and ultimately cause perforation of the septum or development of saddle nose, which are important stigmata later in the disease.

Cutaneous lesions of congenital syphilis resemble those of acquired secondary syphilis and occur in 30% to 60% of infants with syphilis. The early skin eruptions are usually maculopapular, and more rarely, purely papular (Fig. 18-35). The lesions are at first a bright or violaceous red, later fading to a coppery color. The papules may become large and infiltrated; frequently scaling is pronounced. There is secondary pustule formation with crusting, especially in lesions that appear 1 or more years after birth. The eruption shows a marked predilection for the face, arms, buttocks, legs, palms, and soles.

Syphilitic pemphigus, a bullous eruption, usually on the palms and soles, is a relatively uncommon lesion. The bullae quickly become purulent and rupture, leaving exuding areas. They are found also on the eponychium, wrists, ankles, and, infrequently, other parts of the body. Even in the absence of bullous lesions, desquamation is common, often preceded by edema and erythema, especially on the palms and soles.

Various morphologies of cutaneous lesions occur on the face, perineum, and intertriginous areas. They are usually fissured lesions resembling mucous patches. In these sites radial scarring often results, leading to rhagades. Condylomata lata, large, moist, hypertrophic papules, are found about the anus and in other folds of the body. They are more common around the first year of life than in the newborn period. In the second or third year, recurrent secondary eruptions are likely to take the papulopustular form. Annular lesions similar to those in adults occur. Mucous patches in the mouth or on the vulva are seen infrequently.

Bone lesions occur in 70% to 80% of cases of early congenital syphilis. Epiphysitis is common and apparently causes pain on motion, leading to the infant's refusing to move (Parrot's pseudoparalysis). Radiologic features of the bone lesions in congenital syphilis during the first 6 months after birth are quite characteristic, and x-ray films are an important part of the evaluation of a child suspected of having congenital syphilis. Bone lesions occur chiefly at the epiphyseal ends of the long bones. The changes may be classified as osteochondritis, osteomyelitis, and osteoperiostitis.

A general enlargement of the lymph nodes usually occurs, with enlargement of the spleen. Clinical evidence of involvement of the liver is common, manifested both by hepatomegaly and elevated liver function test results, and interstitial hepatitis is a frequent finding at autopsy. The

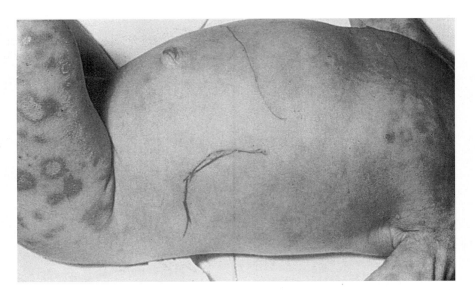

Fig. 18-35 Early congenital syphilis. (Courtesy Dr. Alagil.)

nephrotic syndrome, and less commonly, acute glomerulonephritis have been reported in congenital syphilis.

Symptomatic or asymptomatic neurosyphilis, as demonstrated by a positive spinal fluid serologic test result, may be present. Clinical manifestations do not appear until the third to sixth month of life and are meningeal or meningovascular in origin. Meningitis, obstructive hydrocephalus, cranial nerve palsies, and cerebrovascular accidents may all occur.

Late Congenital Syphilis. Although no sharp line can be drawn between early and late congenital syphilis, children who appear normal at birth and develop the first signs of the disease after the age of 2 years show a different clinical picture. Lesions of late congenital syphilis are of two types: malformations of tissue affected at critical growth periods (stigmata) and persistent inflammatory foci.

INFLAMMATORY LATE CONGENITAL SYPHILIS. Lesions of the cornea, bones, and central nervous system are the most important. Interstitial keratitis, which begins with intense pericorneal inflammation and persists to characteristic diffuse clouding of the cornea without surface ulceration, occurs in 20% to 50% of cases of late congenital syphilis. If persistent, it leads to permanent partial or complete opacity of the cornea. Interstitial keratitis must be differentiated from Cogan's syndrome, consisting of nonsyphilitic interstitial keratitis, usually bilateral, associated with vestibuloauditory symptoms, such as deafness, tinnitus, vertigo, nystagmus, and ataxia. It is congenital.

Perisynovitis (Clutton's joints), which affects the knees, leads to symmetrical, painless swelling. Gummas may also be found in any of the long bones or in the skull. Ulcerating gummas are frequently seen. They probably begin more often in the soft parts or in the underlying bone than in the skin itself, and when they occur in the nasal septum or palate may lead to painless perforation.

The CNS lesions in late congenital syphilis are, as in late adult neurosyphilis, usually parenchymatous (tabes dorsalis or generalized paresis). Seizures are a frequent symptom in congenital cases.

MALFORMATIONS (STIGMATA). The destructive effects of syphilis in young children often leave scars or developmental defects called *stigmata,* which persist throughout life and enable one to make a diagnosis of congenital syphilis. Hutchinson emphasized the diagnostic importance of changes in the incisor teeth, opacities of the cornea, and eighth nerve deafness, which have since become known as the *Hutchinson triad.* Hutchinson's teeth, corneal scars, saber shins, rhagades of the lips, saddle nose, and mulberry molars are of diagnostic importance (Fig. 18-36).

Hutchinson's teeth are a malformation of the central upper incisors that appears in the second or permanent teeth (Fig. 18-37). The characteristic teeth are cylindrical rather than flattened, the cutting edge is narrower than the base, and in the center of the cutting edge a notch may develop. The *mulberry molar* (usually the first molar, appearing about the age of 6 years) is a hyperplastic tooth, the flat occlusal surface of which is covered with a group of little knobs representing abortive cusps. Nasal chondritis in infancy results in flattening of the nasal bones forming a so-called *saddle nose* (Fig. 18-38).

The unilateral thickening of the inner third of one clavicle *(Higouménaki's sign)* is a hyperostosis resulting from syphilitic osteitis in individuals who have had late congenital syphilis. The lesion appears typically on the right side in right-handed persons and on the left side in left-handed persons.

Diagnosis of Congenital Syphilis

Infants of women who meet the following criteria should be evaluated for congenital syphilis:

1. Maternal untreated syphilis, inadequate treatment, or no documentation of adequate treatment
2. Treatment of syphilis with erythromycin
3. Treatment less than 1 month before delivery

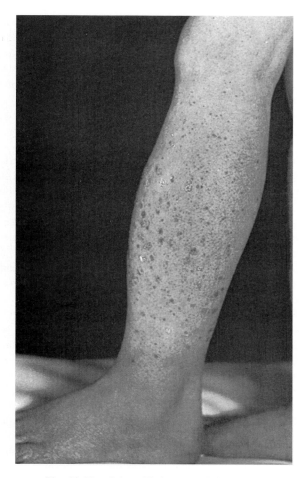

Fig. 18-36   Saber skin in congenital syphilis.

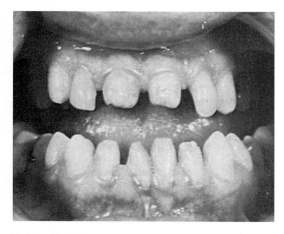

Fig. 18-37   Hutchinson's teeth. Upper central incisors are peg shaped and centrally notched.

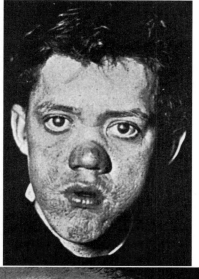

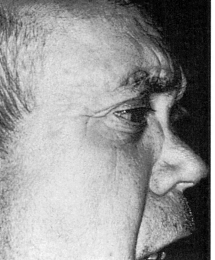

Fig. 18-38   **A,** Saddle nose in congenital syphilis, with interstitial keratitis and prominent rhagades radiating from mouth. **B,** Frontal bossing, interstitial keratitis, and saddle nose in congenital syphilis. (**A,** Courtesy Dr. E.A. Oliver.)

4. Inadequate response to treatment
5. Appropriate treatment before pregnancy, but insufficient serologic follow-up to document adequacy of therapy. The results of serologic tests for syphilis for every woman delivering a baby must be known before the

discharge of that baby from the hospital. Serologic testing of the mother and child at delivery are recommended. Evaluation of the children noted above should include:

A. A complete physical examination for findings of congenital syphilis
B. Nontreponemal serology of the infant's sera (not cord blood)
C. CNS evaluation
D. Long-bone x-ray evaluation
E. Pathologic evaluation of the placenta using specific antitreponemal antibody staining
F. For infants with no evidence of congenital syphilis on the above evaluations, determination of specific antitreponemal IgM should be considered

Treatment of Syphilis

Penicillin remains the drug of choice for treatment of all stages of syphilis. Erythromycin is not recommended for treatment of any stage or form of syphilis. HIV testing is recommended in all patients with syphilis. Treatment for HIV-infected patients is discussed in the section on syphilis and HIV disease (facing page). Patients with primary, secondary, or early latent syphilis known to be of less than 1 year's duration can be treated with a single intramuscular injection of 2.4 million units of benzathine penicillin G. The addition of a second dose 1 week later has been recommended by Fiumara. In nonpregnant, penicillin-allergic, HIV-negative patients, tetracycline 500 mg orally four times daily or doxycycline 100 mg orally twice daily for 2 weeks is recommended.

The recommended treatment of late or late latent syphilis of more than 1 year's duration in an HIV-negative patient is benzathine penicillin G 2.4 million units intramuscularly weekly for 3 weeks. In a penicillin-allergic, nonpregnant, HIV-negative patient tetracycline 500 mg orally four times daily or doxycycline 100 mg orally twice daily for 30 days is recommended. Cerebrospinal fluid evaluation is recommended if neurologic or ophthalmologic findings are present, if there is evidence of active late syphilis, if treatment has previously failed, if the nontreponemal serum titer is 1:32 or higher, or if any regimen not based on penicillin is planned.

Recommended treatment regimens for neurosyphilis include penicillin G crystalline, 2 to 4 million units intravenously every 4 hours for 10 to 14 days; or penicillin G procaine, 2.4 million units intramuscularly daily plus probenecid 500 mg by mouth four times daily, both for 10 to 14 days. These regimens are shorter than for treatment of late syphilis, so they may be followed by benzathine penicillin G, 2.4 million units intramuscularly, weekly for 3 weeks. Patients allergic to penicillin should have their allergy confirmed by skin testing. If allergy exists, desensitization and treatment with penicillin is recommended.

Infants with congenital syphilis should be given 100,000 to 150,000 units/kg/day (administered as 50,000 units/kg intravenously every 12 hours during the first 7 days of life and every 8 hours thereafter) for 10 to 14 days; or procaine penicillin G, 50,000 units intramuscularly daily in a single dose for 10 to 14 days. If more than 1 day of treatment is missed, the course should be restarted. Benzathine penicillin G , 50,000 units/kg intramuscularly in a single dose may be used to treat infants with a completely normal evaluation and whose mother was (1) treated for syphilis with erythromycin, (2) treated for syphilis less than 1 month before delivery, or (3) treated with an appropriate regimen during pregnancy but has not yet had adequate serologic response. Older children with congenital syphilis should have a CSF evaluation and be treated with aqueous crystalline penicillin G, 200,000 to 300,000 units/kg/day intravenously or intramuscularly (50,000 units every 4 to 6 hours) for 10 to 14 days.

Pregnant women with syphilis should be treated with penicillin in doses appropriate for the stage of syphilis, and follow-up quantitative serologic tests should be performed monthly until delivery. Pregnant women who are allergic to penicillin should be skin tested and desensitized if test results are positive. Single-dose azithromycin, as used to treat nongonococcal urethritis, is effective in treating incubating syphilis.

Jarisch-Herxheimer or Herxheimer Reaction. A febrile reaction often occurs after the initial dose of antisyphilitic treatment, especially penicillin, is given. It occurs in about 60% of patients treated for seronegative primary syphilis, 90% of those with seropositive primary or secondary syphilis, and 30% of those with neurosyphilis. The reaction generally occurs 6 to 8 hours after treatment and consists of shaking chills, fever, malaise, sore throat, myalgia, headache, tachycardia, and exacerbation of the inflammatory reaction at sites of localized spirochetal infection.

Rosen et al described a vesicular Herxheimer reaction in four black patients, the mechanism of which is as yet unknown. An increase of inflammation in a vital structure may have serious consequences, as when there is an aneurysm of the aorta or iritis. When the CNS is involved, special importance is attached to avoiding the Herxheimer reaction, even though paralyses that may result are often transitory. It is important to distinguish the Herxheimer reaction from a drug reaction to penicillin or other antibiotics. The reaction has also been described in other spirochetal diseases, such as leptospirosis and louse-borne relapsing fever.

Treatment of Sex Partners. Persons exposed to a patient with early syphilis within the previous 3 months should be treated for early syphilis even if seronegative. Persons exposed to a patient with early syphilis between 3 months and 1 year previously but who may not return for results of serologic tests should be treated for early syphilis immediately. Otherwise, physical examination, serologic evaluation and HIV testing should be performed on the initial visit, and appropriate treatment given at follow-up. Single-dose azithromycin, as used to treat nongonococcal urethritis, is effective in treating incubating syphilis. Therefore, contacts of syphilis cases who have been so treated may be serologically tested and followed, and additional penicillin therapy is not required.

Serologic Testing After Treatment. Before therapy and then regularly thereafter, quantitative VDRL or RPR testing should be performed on patients who are to be treated for syphilis to ensure appropriate response. For primary and secondary syphilis in an HIV-negative nonpregnant patient, testing is repeated every 3 months in the first year, every 6 months in the second year, and yearly thereafter. At least a fourfold decrease in titer should be seen at 6 months. Patients with prior episodes of syphilis may respond more slowly. If response is inadequate, HIV testing (if HIV status is unknown) and CSF evaluation are recommended. For HIV-negative patients who fail to respond and have a normal CSF evaluation, 3 weekly injections of benzathine penicillin G 2.4 million units are recommended.

The response for patients with latent syphilis is slower, but a fourfold decrease in titer should be seen by 12 to 24 months. If no such response occurs, HIV testing and CSF evaluation are recommended. Patients treated for latent or late syphilis may be serofast, so that failure to observe a titer fall in these patients does not in itself indicate a need for retreatment. If the titer is less than 1:32, the possibility of a serofast state exists, and retreatment should be planned on an individual basis.

In 1986, Fiumara reported a series of 588 patients with primary syphilis and 623 patients with secondary syphilis treated with two intramuscular injections of 2.4 million units of penicillin G benzathine a week apart. He found that they became seronegative within 1 and 2 years, respectively. Romanowski et al found that 72% of patients with first-episode primary or secondary syphilis were RPR negative by 36 months. A fourfold reduction in titer was seen at 6 months and an eightfold reduction by 12 months. Early latent syphilis had only a fourfold reduction in titer by 12 months. In this study seroreversion in specific treponemal tests also occurred, so that by 36 months 24% of patients had a negative FTA-ABS and 13% a negative MHA-TP. A fourfold (two dilution) rise in nontreponemal test results strongly suggests reinfection in the serofast individual.

Patients with documented neurosyphilis should also have a repeat CSF evaluation at 6 months and at 6-month intervals thereafter until response can be documented by resolution of pleocytosis and/or fall in the CSF nontreponemal titer.

Syphilis and HIV Disease

Most HIV-infected patients with syphilis exhibit the classic clinical manifestations with appropriate serologic titers for that stage of disease. Response to treatment, both clinical and serologic in HIV-infected patients with syphilis, generally follow the clinical and serologic patterns seen in patients without coexisting HIV infection. In a large study that compared HIV-positive with HIV-negative syphilis patients, patients with HIV were more likely to present with secondary syphilis (53% versus 33%) and were more likely to have a chancre that persisted when they had secondary syphilis (43% versus 15%). Unusual clinical manifestations of syphilis in HIV include florid skin lesions to few atypical ones, but these are exceptions, not the rule.

In general, the nontreponemal tests are of higher titer in HIV-infected persons. Rarely, the serologic response to infection may be impaired or delayed, and seronegative secondary syphilis has been reported. Biopsy of the skin lesions and histopathologic evaluation with silver stains will confirm the diagnosis of syphilis in such cases. This approach, along with darkfield examination of appropriate lesions, should be considered if the clinical eruption is characteristic of syphilis and the serologic tests yield negative results.

Neurosyphilis has been frequently reported in HIV-infected persons, even after appropriate therapy for early syphilis. Manifestations have been those of early neurosyphilis or meningeal or meningovascular syphilis. These have included headache, fever, hemiplegia, and cranial nerve deficits especially deafness (cranial nerve VIII), decreased vision (cranial nerve II), and ocular palsies (cranial nerves III and VI). Whether HIV-infected persons are at increased risk for these complications or whether they occur more quickly is unknown. It is known that spirochetes are no more likely to remain in the CSF after treatment in HIV-infected persons than in HIV-negative persons. Whether the impaired host immunity allows these residual spirochetes to more frequently or more quickly cause clinical relapse in the setting of HIV is unknown.

HIV-infected patients who have primary or secondary syphilis, who are not allergic to penicillin, and who have no neurologic or psychiatric findings should be treated with benzathine penicillin G 2.4 million units intramuscularly each week for a minimum of two doses, preferably three. The third dose, while it may be unnecessary, will not harm the patient and reassures the physician that the patient's treatment was adequate. Patients who are allergic to penicillin should be desensitized and treated with penicillin. Following treatment, the patient should have monthly serologic follow-up with quantitative nontreponemal tests for the first 6 months. Failure of the titer to fall is an indication for reevaluation, including lumbar puncture.

Because of the concerns of neurologic relapse in the setting of HIV disease, more careful CNS evaluation is recommended. Lumbar puncture is recommended in HIV-infected persons with latent syphilis (of any duration), late syphilis (even with a normal neurologic examination), and HIV-infected persons with any neurologic or psychiatric signs or symptoms. Treatment in these patients will be determined by the result of their CSF evaluation. HIV-infected persons with primary and secondary syphilis should be counseled about their possible increased risk of CNS relapse and the possibility of a lumbar puncture should be explored.

Augenbraun MH, et al: Biological false-positive syphilis test results for women infected with human immunodeficiency virus. *Clin Infect Dis* 1994, 19:1040.

Berinstein D, et al: Recently acquired syphilis in the elderly population. *Arch Intern Med* 1992, 152:330.

Berry CD, et al: Neurologic relapse after benzathine penicillin therapy for secondary syphilis in a patient with HIV infection. *N Engl J Med* 1987, 316:1587.

Bromberg K, et al: Diagnosis of congenital syphilis by combining *Treponema pallidum*-specific IgM detection with immunofluorescent antigen detection for *T. pallidum*. *J Infect Dis* 1993, 168:238.

Carey LA, et al: Lumbar puncture for evaluation of latent Syphilis in hospitalized patients. *Arch Intern Med* 1995, 155:1657.

Centers for Disease Control: 1998 Sexually transmitted diseases treatment guidelines. 47:1.

Coles FB, et al: Congenital syphilis surveillance in upstate New York, 1989-1992: implications for prevention and clinical management. *J Infect Dis* 1995, 171:732.

Dorfman DH, et al: Congenital syphilis presenting in infants after the newborn period. *N Engl J Med* 1990, 323:1299.

Duffy J, et al: Serologic testing in Lyme disease. *Ann Intern Med* 1985, 103:458.

Duncan WC: Failure of erythromycin to cure secondary syphilis in a patient infected with HIV. *Arch Dermatol* 1989, 125:82.

Fiumara NJ: Treatment of primary and secondary syphilis: serologic response. *J Am Acad Dermatol* 1986, 14:487.

Gourevitch MN, et al: Effects of HIV infection on the serologic manifestations and response to treatment of syphilis in intravenous drug users. *Ann Intern Med* 1993, 118:350.

Guinan ME: Treatment of primary and secondary syphilis: defining failure at 3- and 6-month follow-up. *JAMA* 1987, 257:359.

Hager WD: Transplacental transmission of spirochetes in congenital syphilis: a new perspective (editorial). *Sex Transm Dis* 1986, 5:122.

Handsfield HH, et al: Demonstration of *Treponema pallidum* in a cutaneous gumma by indirect immunofluorescence. *Arch Dermatol* 1983, 119:677.

Heimberger TS, et al: High prevalence of syphilis detected through a jail screening program. *Arch Intern Med* 1993, 153:1799.

Hicks CB, et al: Seronegative secondary syphilis in a patient infected with the human immunodeficiency virus (HIV) with Kaposi's sarcoma. *Ann Intern Med* 1987, 107:492.

Hook EW: Elimination of syphilis transmission in the United States. *Trans Am Clin Climatol Assoc* 1999, 110:195.

Hook EW, et al: Acquired syphilis in adults. *N Engl J Med* 1992, 326:1060.

Hook EW, et al: Azithromycin compared with penicillin G benzathine for treatment of incubating syphilis. *Ann Int Med* 1999, 131:434.

Hutchinson CM, et al: Altered clinical presentation of early syphilis in patients with human immunodeficiency virus infection. *Ann Intern Med* 1994, 121:94.

Johnson PC, et al: Testing for syphilis. *Dermatol Clin* 1994, 12:1:9.

Jurando RL, et al: Prozone phenomenon in secondary syphilis. *Arch Intern Med* 1993, 153:2496.

Kilmarx PH, et al: The evolving epidemiology of syphilis (editorial). *Am J Publ Health* 1995, 85:1053.

Lukehart SA, et al: Invasion of the central nervous system by *Treponema pallidum. Ann Intern Med* 1988, 109:855.

Malone JL, et al: Syphilis and neurosyphilis in a human immunodeficiency virus type-1 seropositive population: evidence for frequent serologic relapse after therapy. *Am J Med* 1995, 99:55.

Marra CM, et al: Alterations in the course of experimental syphilis associated with concurrent simian immunodeficiency virus infection. *J Infect Dis* 1992, 165:1020.

McPhee SJ, et al: Secondary syphilis: uncommon manifestations of a common disease. *West J Med* 1984, 140:35.

Mertz KJ, et al: An investigation of genital ulcers in Jackson, Mississippi, with use of a multiplex PCR assay. *J Infect Dis* 1998, 178:1060.

Musher DM: Syphilis, neurosyphilis, penicillin and AIDS. *J Infect Dis* 1991, 163:1201.

Perry HO, et al: Secondary and tertiary syphilis presenting as sarcoidal reactions of the skin. *Cutis* 1984, 34:253.

Romanowski B, et al: Serologic response to treatment of infectious syphilis. *Ann Intern Med* 1991, 114:1005.

Rompalo AM, et al: Association of biologic false-positive reactions for syphilis with human immunodeficiency virus infection. *J Infect Dis* 1992, 165:1124.

Rosen T, et al: Vesicular Jarisch-Herxheimer reaction. *Arch Dermatol* 1989, 125:77.

Sanchez PJ, et al: Evaluation of molecular methodologies and rabbit infectivity testing for the diagnosis of congenital syphilis and neonatal central nervous system invasion by *Treponema pallidum. J Infect Dis* 1993, 167:148.

Schmid GP: Approach to the patient with genital ulcer disease. *Med Clin North Am* 1990, 74:559.

Simon RP: Neurosyphilis. *Arch Neurol* 1985, 42:606.

Tikjob G, et al: Seronegative secondary syphilis in a patient with AIDS: identification of *Treponema pallidum* in biopsy specimen. *J Am Acad Dermatol* 1991, 114:521.

Tramont EC: Syphilis in adults: from Christopher Columbus to Sir Alexander Fleming to AIDS. *Clin Infect Dis* 1995, 21:1361.

Wiesel J, et al: Lumbar puncture in asymptomatic late syphilis: an analysis of the benefits and risks. *Arch Intern Med* 1985, 145:464.

Yinnon AM: Serologic response to treatment of syphilis in patients with HIV infection. *Arch Intern Med* 1996, 156:321.

Zenker PN, et al: Congenital syphilis: trends and recommendations for evaluation and management. *Ped Infect Dis J* 1991, 10:516.

Zoechling N, et al: Molecular detection of *Treponema pallidum* in secondary and tertiary syphilis. *Br J Dermatol* 1997, 136:683. ▲

NONVENEREAL TREPONEMATOSES: YAWS, ENDEMIC SYPHILIS, AND PINTA
Yaws (Pian, Frambesia, Bouba)

Yaws is an infectious systemic disease, caused by *T. pallidum* subsp. *pertenue,* which is endemic in some tropical, rural regions. Overcrowding, poverty, and poor hygiene predispose to yaws. It is transmitted nonsexually, by contact with infectious lesions. Yaws predominantly affects children younger than 15 years of age. The disease has a disabling course, affecting the skin, bones, and joints, and is divided into early (primary and secondary) and late (tertiary) disease.

Early Yaws. A primary papule or group of papules appear at the site of inoculation after an incubation period of about 3 weeks, during which there may be headache, malaise, and other mild constitutional symptoms. The initial lesion becomes crusted and larger, and is known as the mother yaw (*maman pian*). The crusts are amber-yellow. They may be knocked off, forming an ulcer with a red, pulpy, granulated surface but quickly reform, so that the typical yaws lesion is crusted. The lesion is not indurated. There may be some regional adenopathy.

Exposed parts are most frequently involved—the extremities, particularly the lower legs (Fig. 18-39), feet, buttocks and the face—although the mother's breasts and trunk may be infected by her child. The lesion is practically always extragenital, and when genital, is a result of accidental contact rather than intercourse. After being present a few months, the mother yaw spontaneously disappears, leaving slight atrophy and depigmentation.

Weeks or months after the primary lesion appears, secondary yaws develops. Secondary lesions resemble the mother yaw, but they are smaller and may appear around the primary lesions or in a generalized pattern (Fig. 18-40). The secondary lesions may clear centrally and coalesce

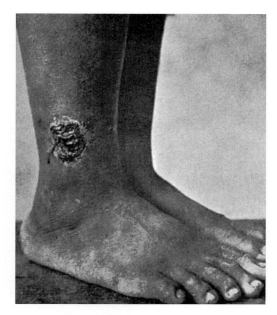

Fig. 18-39 Yaws, primary stage. Note crusts around lesions. (Courtesy Army Medical Museum.)

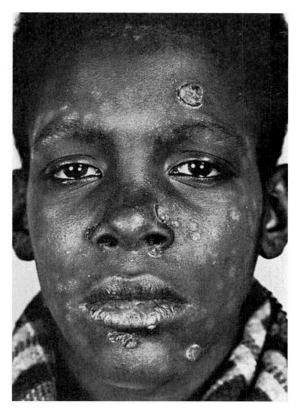

Fig. 18-41 Secondary yaws in a 15-year-old boy.

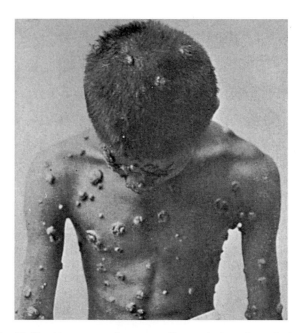

Fig. 18-40 Yaws, secondary stage. Note typical raspberry lesions. (Courtesy Army Medical Museum.)

peripherally, forming annular lesions (ringworm yaws) (Fig. 18-41). The palms and soles may be involved, resembling secondary syphilis (Fig. 18-42). In some sites, especially around the body orifices, and in the armpits, groins, and gluteal crease, condylomatous lesions may arise. On the dorsa of the feet, thick, hyperkeratotic plaques that fissure

may form. They are painful, resulting in a crablike gait (crab yaws). At times there is paronychia.

In the course of a few weeks or months the secondary lesions may undergo spontaneous involution, leaving either no skin changes or hypopigmented macules that later become hyperpigmented. However, the eruption may persist for many months as a result of fresh recurrent outbreaks. The course is slower in adults than in children, in whom the secondary period rarely lasts longer than 6 months.

Painful osteoperiostitis and polydactylitis may present in early yaws as fusiform swelling of the hands, feet, arms and legs.

Late Yaws. The disease usually terminates with the secondary stage, but in about 10% it progresses to the late stage, in which gummatous lesions occur. These present as indolent ulcers with clean-cut or undermined edges, which tend to fuse to form configurate and, occasionally, serpiginous patterns clinically indistinguishable from those of tertiary syphilis. On healing, these sores cause scar tissue, leading to contractures and deformities (Fig. 18-43).

Similar processes may occur in the skeletal system and other deep structures, leading to painful nodes on the bones, or destruction of the palate and nasal bone (gangosa) (Fig. 18-44). There may be periostitis, particularly of the tibia (saber shin), epiphysitis, chronic synovitis, and

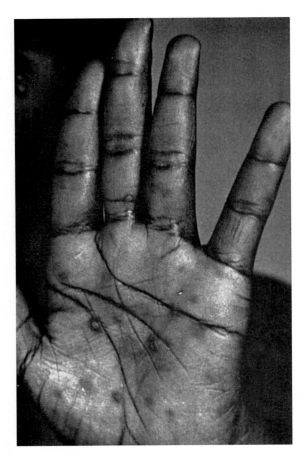

Fig. 18-42 Palmar macules in secondary yaws.

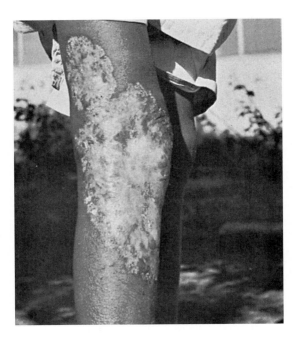

Fig. 18-43 Tertiary yaws (scarring after treatment). (Courtesy Drs. O. Reyes and F. Kerdel-Vegas, Venezuela.)

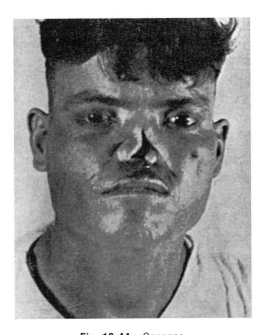

Fig. 18-44 Gangosa.

juxtaarticular nodules. Goundou is bilateral swelling of the external aspects of the maxilla, producing bony masses on either side of the nasal bridge that can cause nasal obstruction. Although classically felt to spare the eye and nervous system, abnormal CSF findings in early yaws and scattered reports of eye and neurologic findings in patients with late yaws suggest that yaws, like syphilis, has the potential to cause neurologic or ophthalmic sequelae.

Histopathology

Early yaws shows epidermal edema, acanthosis, papillomatosis, neutrophilic intraepidermal microabscesses, and a moderate to dense perivascular infiltrate of lymphocytes and plasma cells. Treponema are usually demonstrable in the primary and secondary stages with the use of the same silver stains used in diagnosing syphilis. Tertiary yaws shows features identical to the gumma of tertiary syphilis.

Diagnosis

The diagnosis should be suspected by the typical clinical appearance in a person living in an endemic region. The presence of keratoderma palmaris et plantaris in such a person is highly suggestive of yaws. Darkfield demonstra-

tion of spirochetes in the early lesions and a reactive VDRL or RPR test can be used to confirm primary and secondary yaws.

Endemic Syphilis (Bejel)

Bejel is a Bedouin term for this nonvenereal treponematosis, which occurs primarily in the seminomadic tribes who live in the arid regions of North Africa, Southwest Asia, and the Eastern Mediterranean. The etiologic agent of bejel is considered to be *T. pallidum* subsp. *endemicum*. It occurs primarily in childhood and is spread by skin contact or from mouth to mouth by kissing or use of contaminated drinking vessels. The skin, oral mucosa, and skeletal system are primarily involved.

Primary lesions are rare, probably occurring undetected in the oropharyngeal mucosa. The most common presentation is with secondary oral lesions resembling mucous patches. These are shallow, relatively painless ulcerations, occasionally accompanied by laryngitis. Split papules, condylomatous lesions of the axillae and groin, and a nonpruritic generalized papular eruption may be seen. Generalized lymphadenopathy is common. Osteoperiostitis of the long bones may occur, causing nocturnal leg pains.

Untreated secondary bejel heals in 6 to 9 months. In the tertiary stage, leg pain and gummatous ulcerations of the skin, nasopharynx, and bone occur. Reported neurologic sequelae seem to be restricted to the eye, including uveitis, choroiditis, chorioretinitis, and optic atrophy. The diagnosis of bejel is confirmed by the same means as for venereal syphilis.

Pinta

Pinta is an infectious, nonvenereal, endemic treponematosis caused by *T. carateum*. Only skin lesions occur. By contrast with yaws and bejel, pinta affects persons of all ages. It is found only in scattered areas of the Brazilian rain forest. The manifestations of pinta may be divided into primary, secondary, and tertiary stages, but historically patients may describe continuous evolution from secondary dyspigmented lesions to the characteristic achromic lesions of tertiary pinta.

Primary Stage. It is believed that the initial lesion appears 7 to 60 days after inoculation. The lesion begins as a tiny red papule that becomes an elevated, ill-defined, erythematous, infiltrated plaque up to 10 to 12.5 cm in diameter in the course of 2 to 3 months (Fig. 18-45). Expansion of the primary lesion may occur by fusion with surrounding satellite macules or papules (Figs. 18-46 and 18-47). Ultimately, it becomes impossible to distinguish the primary lesion from the secondary lesions. At no time is there erosion or ulceration such as occurs in the syphilitic chancre. Most initial lesions of pinta develop on the legs and other uncovered parts. The STS is nonreactive in the primary stage. Darkfield examination may be positive.

Secondary Stage. The secondary stage appears from 5 months to 1 year or more after infection. It begins with small, scaling papules that may enlarge and coalesce, simulating psoriasis, ringworm, eczema, syphilis, or leprosy. They are located mostly on the extremities and face and frequently are somewhat circinate (Fig. 18-48). Over

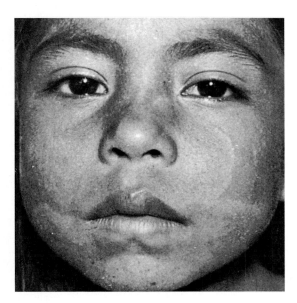

Fig. 18-45 Primary lesion of pinta. (Courtesy Dr. R. Medina, Venezuela.)

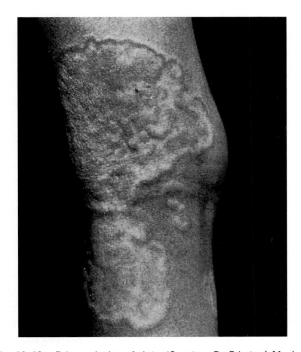

Fig. 18-46 Primary lesion of pinta. (Courtesy Dr. F. Latapí, Mexico.)

time, the initially red to violaceous lesions show postinflammatory hyperpigmentation in shades of gray, blue, brown, or black. Nontreponemal tests for syphilis are reactive in the secondary stage in about 60% of patients. Darkfield examination may show spirochetes.

Late Dyschromic Stage. Until the 1940s, the late pigmentary changes were the only recognized clinical manifesta-

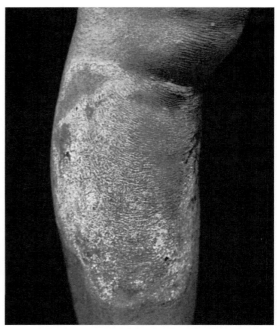

Fig. 18-47 Early pinta on the shin. (Courtesy Dr. B.S. Camacho, Mexico.)

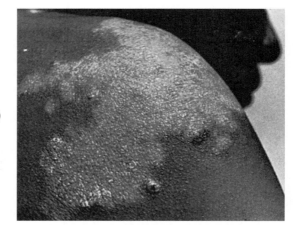

Fig. 18-48 Late pinta on the shoulder. (Courtesy Dr. R. Medina, Venezuela.)

tions of pinta. These have an insidious onset, usually in adolescents or young adults, of hyperpigmented and eventually widespread depigmented macules resembling vitiligo (Figs. 18-49 and 18-50). The lesions are located chiefly on the face, waistline, wrist flexures, and trochanteric region, although at times diffuse involvement occurs, so that large areas on the trunk and extremities are affected. The lesions are symmetrical in more than one third of the patients. Hemipinta is a rare variety of the disease in which the pigmentary disturbances affect only half of the body. In the late dyschromic stage of pinta, the STS is positive in nearly all patients.

Histopathology of Pinta
Skin lesions in early pinta show moderate acanthosis; occasionally, lichenoid changes with basal layer vacuoliza-tion; and an upper dermal perivascular infiltrate of lymphocytes and plasma cells. Melanophages are prominent in the upper dermis. Spirochetes may be demonstrated in the epidermis by special stains in primary, secondary, and hyperpigmented lesions of tertiary pinta. In tertiary pinta the depigmented skin shows a loss of basal pigment, pigmentary incontinence, and virtually no dermal inflammatory infiltrate. Spirochetes are rarely found in depigmented tertiary lesions.

Treatment of Yaws, Bejel, and Pinta
The treatment of choice is benzathine penicillin G, 1.2 to 2.4 million units intramuscularly (0.6 to 1.2 million units for children under 10 years of age). In penicillin-allergic patients, tetracycline 500 mg four times daily for adults (and erythromycin for children, 8 to 10 mg/kg four times daily

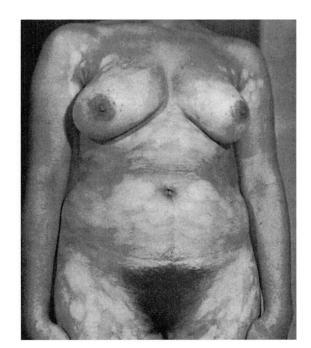

Fig. 18-49 Symmetrical achromic patches in late pinta. (Courtesy Dr. F. Kerdel-Vegas, Venezuela.)

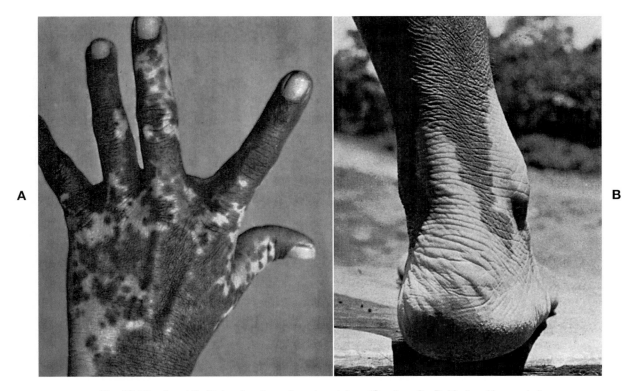

Fig. 18-50 **A** and **B,** Pinta, showing achromic patches. (Courtesy Dr. R. Medina, Venezuela.)

for 15 days) are recommended. In tertiary pinta, the blue color gradually disappears, as do the areas of partial depigmentation. The vitiliginous areas, if present for more than 5 years, are permanent. Because these diseases may reach high prevalence within communities, consideration may be given to mass treatment of households, villages, or endemic regions. Penicillin-resistant yaws has been reported from New Guinea.

Backhouse JL, et al: Failure of penicillin treatment of yaws on Karkar Island, Papua New Guinea. *Am J Trop Med Hyg* 1998, 59:388.

Engelkens HJH, et al: Nonvenereal treponematoses in tropical countries. *Clin Dermatol* 1999, 17:143.

Fuchs J, et al: Tertiary pinta: case reports and overview. *Cutis* 1993, 51:425.

Koff AB, et al: Nonvenereal treponematoses: yaws, endemic syphilis, and pinta. *J Am Acad Dermatol* 1993, 29:519.

Woltsche-Kuhr I, et al: Pinta in Austria (or Cuba). *Arch Dermatol* 1999, 135:685. ▲

CHAPTER 19

Viral Diseases

Viruses are obligatory intracellular parasites. The structural components of a viral particle (virion) consist of a central core of nucleic acid, a protective protein coat (capsid), and (in certain groups of viruses only) an outermost membrane or envelope. The capsid of the simplest viruses is made up of many identical polypeptides (structural units) that fold and interact with one another to form morphologic units (capsomeres). The number of capsomeres is believed to be constant for each virus with cubic symmetry, and it is an important criterion in the classification of viruses. The protein coat determines serologic specificity, protects the nucleic acid from enzymatic degradation in biologic environments, controls host specificity, and increases the efficiency of infection. The outermost membrane of the enveloped viruses is essential for the attachment to, and penetration of, host cells. The envelope also contains important viral antigens.

Two main groups of viruses are distinguished: DNA and RNA. The DNA virus types are parvovirus, papovavirus, adenovirus, herpesvirus, and poxvirus. RNA viruses are picornavirus, togavirus, reovirus, coronavirus, orthomyxovirus, retrovirus, arenavirus, rhabdovirus, and paramyxovirus. Some viruses are distinguished by their mode of transmission: arthropod-borne viruses, respiratory viruses, fecal-oral or intestinal viruses, venereal viruses, and penetrating wound viruses.

HERPESVIRUS GROUP

The herpesviruses are medium-sized viruses that contain double-stranded DNA and replicate in the cell nucleus. They are characterized by the ability to produce latent, but lifelong infection, which may be intermittently clinically apparent. Viruses in this group are varicella zoster virus (VZV); herpes simplex virus (HSV), types 1 and 2; cytomegalovirus (CMV); Epstein-Barr virus (EBV); human herpesviruses-6, -7, and -8 (HHV-6, 7, 8); *Herpesvirus simiae* (B virus); and other viruses of animals.

Herpes Simplex

Infection with the herpes simplex viruses is one of the most prevalent infections worldwide. Because many infected persons have asymptomatic or subclinical infection, serologic testing is used to determine prevalence of infection. HSV-1 infection, the cause of most cases of orolabial herpes simplex, is more common than infection with HSV-2, the cause of genital herpes. Eighty-five percent of adults worldwide are seropositive for HSV-1. Seroprevalence for HSV-2 is lower, and it appears at the age of onset of sexual activity. In Scandinavia, the rate of infection with HSV-2 increases from 2% in 15-year-olds to 25% in 30-year-olds. About 2.4% of adults become infected annually with HSV-2 in their third decade of life. Currently in the United States, about 23% of adults are infected with HSV-2; the seroprevalence has increased by 30% during the AIDS era. In STD clinic patients, the infection rate is between 30% and 50%. In the developing world, infection rates are between 60% and 95%. Worldwide, the seroprevalence is higher in HIV-infected persons. Serologic data have demonstrated that many more people are infected than give a history of clinical disease. For HSV-1, about 50% of infected persons give a history of orolabial lesions. For HSV-2, 20% of infected persons are completely asymptomatic, 20% have recurrent genital herpes they recognize, and 60% have clinical lesions that appear but that they do not recognize as genital herpes (subclinical or unrecognized). Most persons with HSV-2 infection are symptomatic, but the majority do not recognize that their symptoms are caused by HSV. These persons may represent an important reservoir for transmission.

Herpes simplex infections can be classified as true primary infections (Fig. 19-1) (initial exposure to the virus), nonprimary initial episode (the initial clinical lesion from HSV-1 or HSV-2 in a person previously infected with the other virus and with partial cross-immunity), and recurrent infection. Persons with chronic or acute immunosuppression may have prolonged and atypical clinical courses.

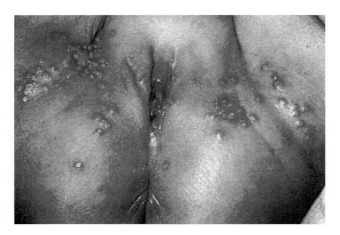

Fig. 19-1 Primary herpes simplex in an infant. Sexual abuse was considered.

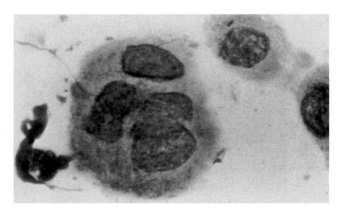

Fig. 19-2 Multinucleate giant cell of herpes simplex (Tzanck smear).

Infections with HSV-1 or HSV-2 are diagnosed by specific and nonspecific methods. The most common procedure used in the office is the Tzanck smear. It is nonspecific, since both HSV and VZV infections result in the formation of multinucleate epidermal giant cells. The multiple nuclei are molded or fit together like pieces of a puzzle (Fig. 19-2). Although the technique is rapid, its success depends heavily on the skill of the interpreter. The accuracy rate is between 60% and 90%, with a false-positive rate of 3% to 13%. The direct fluorescent antibody test is more accurate, will identify virus type, and results can be available in hours if a virology laboratory is nearby. Viral culture is very accurate and rapid, since HSV is stable in transport and grows readily and rapidly in culture. Results are often available in 48 to 72 hours. Polymerase chain reaction (PCR) is as accurate as viral culture and can be performed on dried or fixed tissue. Skin biopsies of lesions can detect viropathic changes caused by HSV, and with specific HSV antibodies, immunoperoxidase techniques can accurately diagnose infection.

The accuracy of various tests is dependent on lesion morphology. Only acute, vesicular lesions are likely to be positive with Tzanck smears. Crusted, eroded, or ulcerative lesions are best diagnosed by viral culture, fluorescent antibody, histologic methods, or PCR.

Serologic tests are generally not used in determining whether a skin lesion is due to HSV infection. A positive result to a serologic test indicates only that the individual is infected with that virus, not that the viral infection is the cause of the current lesion. The background positivity rate is high. Because of cross-reaction of HSV-1 and HSV-2, nonspecific serologic tests can mistype HSV infection. Sera drawn in the acute and convalescent stages can help detect primary infection, but only a small fraction of patients with herpes have primary infection. Specific Western blot serologic tests can detect specific infection with HSV-1 and HSV-2 but cannot determine the duration of that infection.

Serologic tests are most useful in evaluating couples in which one gives a history of genital herpes, in couples at risk for neonatal herpes infection, and for possible herpes simplex vaccination when available.

The treatment of herpes simplex infections has two aims: to shorten the current attack and to prevent recurrences. Oral or intravenous acyclovir (Zovirax) is effective in the treatment of patients with all forms of primary herpes simplex infections and immunocompromised patients and in prevention of recurrences. Topical use is not recommended.

Acyclovir is an acyclic nucleoside analog of guanosine. It is a selective substrate for and inhibitor of herpesvirus DNA polymerase. Its selectivity is determined by its high affinity for the viral enzyme thymidine kinase. Side effects are uncommon. The major route of elimination is through the kidneys; therefore dose reduction is recommended in patients with impaired renal function. Valacyclovir and famciclovir are closely related medications with enhanced absorption when administered orally, allowing for reduction in dosing frequency.

Orolabial Herpes. Most lesions on the lips and face are caused by HSV-1. Initial infection is usually asymptomatic. In 1% or less, herpetic gingivostomatitis develops, chiefly in children and young adults. The onset is often accompanied by high fever, regional lymphadenopathy, and malaise. The herpetic lesions in the mouth are usually broken vesicles that appear as erosions or ulcers covered with a white membrane (Fig. 19-3). The erosions may become widespread on the oral mucosa, tongue, and tonsils and produce pain, foul breath, and loss of appetite (herpetic gingivostomatitis). In young children dehydration may occur. It may cause pharyngitis, with ulcerative or exudative lesions of the posterior pharynx. The duration, untreated, is 1 to 2 weeks.

The most frequent presentation of orolabial herpes is the "cold sore" or "fever blister." This is caused by recurrent HSV-1 95% of the time, and typically presents as grouped

A

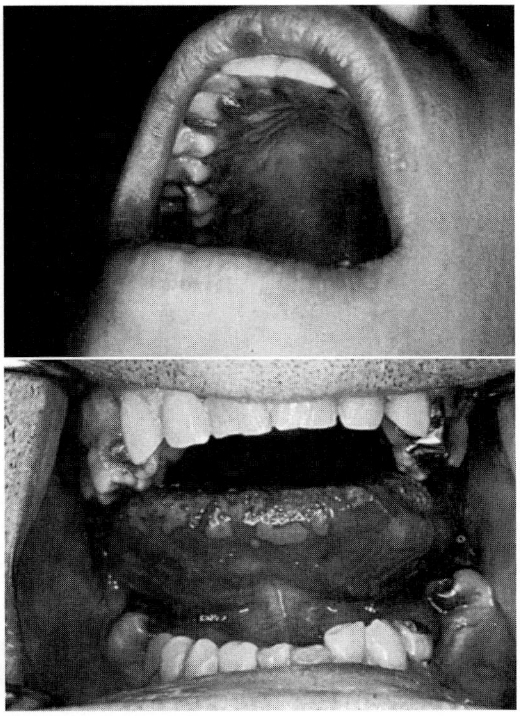

B

Fig. 19-3 Herpetic gingivostomatitis. **A,** A 16-year-old boy. **B,** A 51-year-old man.

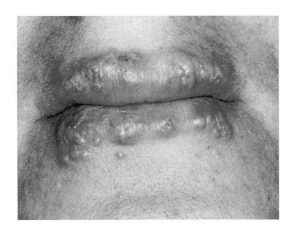

Fig. 19-4 Herpes simplex. Note clusters of grouped vesicles.

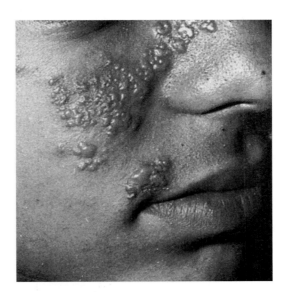

Fig. 19-5 Herpes simplex, unusually extensive.

blisters on an erythematous base. The lips near the vermilion are most frequently involved (Fig. 19-4). Lesions may, however, occur wherever the virus was inoculated or proliferated during the initial episode. Recurrences may be seen on the cheeks, eyelids, and earlobes (Figs. 19-5 to 19-7). Outbreaks are variable in severity, partly related to the trigger of the outbreak. Some outbreaks are small and resolve rapidly, while others may be severe, involving both the upper and lower lips. In severe outbreaks, lip swelling is often present. Patient symptomatology is variable. A prodrome of up to 24 hours of tingling, itching, or burning may precede the outbreak. Local discomfort as well as headache, nasal congestion, or mild flulike symptoms may occur. Ultraviolet exposure, especially UVB, is a frequent trigger of recurrent orolabial HSV, and the severity of the outbreak may correlate with the intensity of the sun exposure. Herpes simplex may also recur intraorally, usually on fixed, keratinized mucosa of the gingiva or hard palate.

In most patients recurrent orolabial herpes represents more of a nuisance than a disease. Because UVB radiation is a common trigger, use of a sunblock daily on the lips and facial skin may reduce recurrences. Topical treatment with drying agents such as benzoyl peroxide or over the counter "cold sore" remedies may accelerate healing. In patients with severe individual outbreaks, or in those whose triggers for outbreaks can be identified, intermittent treatment with

acyclovir 200 mg five times daily for 5 days may be indicated. Treatment should be begun 24 hours before the trigger if possible, or at the first prodromal symptoms. Prophylaxis could be considered before skiing or tropical vacations, and extensive dental procedures. If dermabrasion, laser resurfacing, or a medium to deep chemical peel is to be performed around the lips, prophylactic acyclovir is recommended, especially if there is a history of recurrent orolabial herpes simplex. In persons with frequent recurrences, chronic suppressive acyclovir therapy in a dose of 400 mg twice daily can reduce the number of outbreaks by 50%.

Herpetic Sycosis. Following an attack of facial herpes simplex, the patient who shaves with a blade razor may experience a slowly spreading folliculitis of the beard, with

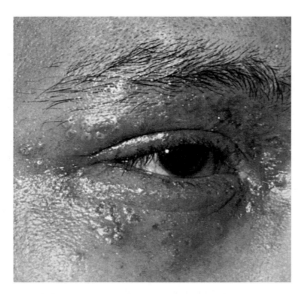

Fig. 19-6   Herpes simplex of eyelids in a 27-year-old man.

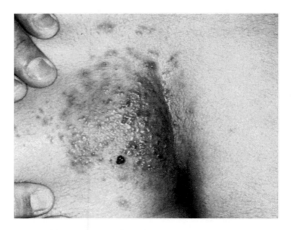

Fig. 19-8   Herpes gladiatorum in a young male wrestler.

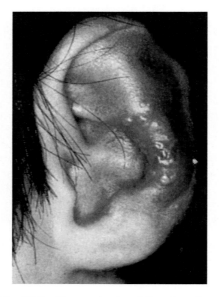

Fig. 19-7   Herpes simplex of the external ear.

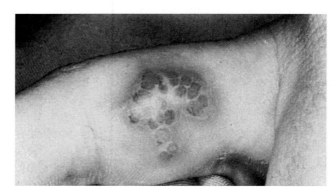

Fig. 19-9   Primary herpes simplex of the finger.

a few isolated vesicles. Only its transient course, lasting 2 or 3 weeks, and the presence of vesicles, indicate that it is not ordinary bacterial sycosis.

Herpes Gladiatorum. HSV-1 infection can occur in epidemic outbreaks among wrestlers via skin-to-skin contact with a wrestler with recurrent orolabial herpes (Fig. 19-8). Rugby players, especially the forwards who participate in the scrums, are also at risk. Lesions tend to occur on the face, sides of the neck and the inner arms.

Herpetic Whitlow. Herpes simplex virus infection may rarely take the form of a felon, or whitlow: infection of the pulp of a fingertip. There is tenderness and erythema usually of the lateral nail fold. Deep-seated blisters develop 24 to 48 hours after symptoms begin (Fig. 19-9). The blisters may be very small, requiring careful inspection to detect. Before the universal use of gloves, such lesions were most often seen in dentists, dental hygienists, and other health care workers. Currently, most cases are seen in persons with herpes elsewhere. Children may be infected while thumbsucking or nailbiting during primary herpes, or by touching an infectious lesion of an adult. Herpetic whitlow is bimodal in distribution, with about 20% of cases occurring in children less than 10 years old, and 55% of cases between the ages of 20 and 40. All cases in the children are caused by HSV-1, but in adults up to three quarters of cases are caused by HSV-2. Among adults, herpetic whitlow is twice as common in females. Herpetic whitlow in health care workers can be transmitted to patients. In patients exposed in their oropharynx, 37% percent develop herpetic pharyngitis.

Herpetic Keratoconjunctivitis. Herpes simplex infection of the eye is a common cause of blindness in the United States. It occurs as a punctate or marginal keratitis, or as a dendritic corneal ulcer, which may cause disciform keratitis and leave scars that impair vision. Topical corticosteroids in this situation may induce perforation of the cornea. Vesicles may appear on the lids, and preauricular nodes may be enlarged and tender. Recurrences are common.

Recurrent Erythema Multiforme Minor. Recurrent erythema multiforme (EM minor) is usually caused by recurrent herpes simplex, most commonly HSV-1 orolabial disease. This is more correctly now called *herpes-associated erythema multiforme* (HAEM). Clinically, it presents with papules, some of which become classic target lesions, of the palms, elbows, knees, and oral mucosa. Atypical lesions occur in 3% of HAEM patients and may present as multiple or solitary large red painful plaques (resembling Sweet's syndrome), subcutaneous nodules (like erythema nodosum), or large asymmetrical targets. In classic and atypical cases the histologic features of erythema multiforme are found. By polymerase chain reaction, HSV DNA is detected in classic and atypical cases. Treatment with suppressive doses of acyclovir chronically will prevent HAEM in the majority of patients. Some patients with no history of herpes simplex as a trigger for their EM are controlled by oral antivirals, suggesting subclinical HSV infection is the trigger for some "idiopathic" cases of recurrent EM.

Genital Herpes (Herpes progenitalis). Genital herpes infection is usually due to HSV-2, causing 85% of initial infections and up to 98% of recurrent lesions. In the mid-1980s, the prevalence of genital herpes caused by HSV-1 began to increase because of changes in sexual habits, so that in some developed countries HSV-1 has caused up to 40% of anogenital herpes in women. HSV-1 in the genital area is much less likely to recur than HSV-2.

Genital herpes is spread by skin to skin contact, usually during sexual activity. The incubation period averages 5 days. Active lesions of HSV-2 contain live virus and are infectious. Persons with recurrent genital herpes shed virus asymptomatically between outbreaks (asymptomatic shedding). Asymptomatic shedding occurs simultaneously from several anatomic sites (vagina, cervix, and rectum), and can occur through normally appearing intact skin and mucosae. In addition, persons with HSV-2 infection may have lesions they do not recognize as being caused by HSV (unrecognized outbreak), or have recurrent lesions that do not cause symptoms (subclinical outbreak). Most transmission of genital herpes occurs during subclinical, or unrecognized outbreaks, or while the infected person is shedding asymptomatically. The risk of transmission in monogamous couples, in which only one is infected, is about 10% annually, with women being infected more commonly than

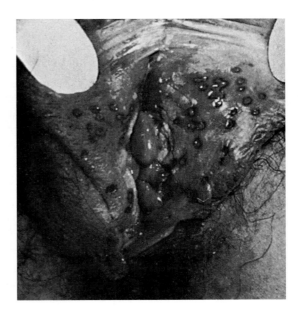

Fig. 19-10 Herpes progenitalis on labia. (Courtesy Dr. W.B. Hurlbut.)

men. Prior HSV-1 infection does not reduce the risk of being infected with HSV-2 but does make it more likely that initial infection will be asymptomatic. Barrier methods of contraception may reduce transmission. Primary infection with HSV-2 has a broad clinical spectrum from totally asymptomatic to severe genital ulcer disease. Only 57% of new HSV-2 infections are symptomatic.

True primary infection in persons with no prior infection with genital HSV-1 or HSV-2 can present as a severe systemic illness. Grouped blisters and erosions appear in the vagina, rectum, or on the penis with continued development of new blisters over 7 to 14 days. Lesions are bilaterally symmetrical, often extensive, and the inguinal lymph nodes can be enlarged bilaterally. Fever and flulike symptoms may be present, but in women the major complaint is vaginal pain and dysuria (herpetic vulvovaginitis) (Fig. 19-10). The whole illness may last 3 weeks or more. Persons with prior infection with HSV-1 have a less severe initial infection that may present as grouped blisters or erosions, resembling recurrent genital herpes, but perhaps lasting a few days longer. If the inoculation occurs in the rectal area, severe proctitis may occur from extensive erosions in the anal canal and on the rectal mucosa. Primary or the initial clinical episode of genital herpes is treated with oral acyclovir 200 to 400 mg five times a day. Famciclovir, 250 mg three times daily, and valacyclovir, 1000 mg twice daily, are alternatives.

Most persons infected with HSV-2 will have recurrences, even if the initial infection was subclinical or asymptomatic. HSV-2 infection results in recurrences six times more frequently than HSV-1. Most patients, however, who are seropositive for HSV-2 have unrecognized infection. Twenty percent of persons with HSV-2 infection are truly asymptomatic. Twenty percent of patients have lesions they recognize as recurrent genital herpes, and 60% have clinical lesions that are culture positive for HSV-2, but that are unrecognized by the patient as being caused by genital herpes. This large group of persons with subclinical or unrecognized genital herpes are infectious, at least intermittently, and represent one factor in the increasing number of new HSV-2 infections.

Typical recurrent genital herpes begins with a prodrome of burning, itching, or tingling. Usually within 24 hours red papules appear at the site, progress to blisters filled with clear fluid over 24 hours, form erosions over the next 24 to 36 hours, and heal in another 2 to 3 days (Fig. 19-11). The total duration of a typical outbreak of genital herpes is 7 days. Lesions are usually grouped blisters, and the coalescent grouped erosions they evolve into characteristically have a scalloped border. Erosions or ulcerations from genital herpes are usually very tender, and not indurated (as opposed to the chancre of primary syphilis). Lesions tend to recur in the same anatomic region, although not in exactly the same site (as opposed to a fixed drug eruption). Less classic clinical manifestations are tiny erosions or linear fissures on the genital skin. Lesions occur on the vulva, vagina, and cervical mucosa as well as the penile and vulval skin. The upper buttocks is a common site for recurrent genital herpes, in both men and women. Recurrent genital herpes heals without scarring unless the lesion is secondarily infected.

The natural history of untreated recurrent genital herpes is not well studied. Over a period of several years, the frequency of recurrences often stays the same. Over longer periods (more than 5 years), especially in those treated with acyclovir suppression, the frequency of outbreaks decreases.

Recurrent genital herpes is a significant disease because of the social stigma associated with it. Because it is not curable, patients frequently demonstrate a significant emotional response when they are diagnosed. These include anger (at the presumed source of the infection), depression, and guilt. This component of the illness must be recognized and managed for the therapy of recurrent genital herpes to be successful.

Management of recurrent genital herpes should be individualized. A careful history, including a sexual history, should be obtained. Examination should include seeing the patient during an active recurrence, so that the infection can be confirmed. The diagnosis of recurrent genital herpes should not be made on clinical appearance alone because of the psychologic impact of the diagnosis.

The treatment given depends on several factors including the frequency of recurrences, the severity of recurrences, the infection status of the sexual partner, and the psychologic impact of the infection on the patient. For patients with few

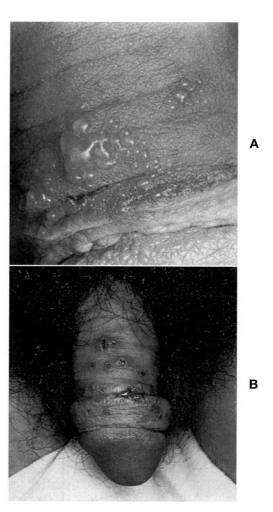

Fig. 19-11   **A,** Early-stage herpes progenitalis. **B,** Late-stage herpes progenitalis.

or mildly symptomatic recurrences, treatment is often not necessary. Counseling regarding transmission risk is required. In patients with severe but infrequent recurrences or in those whom the psychologic complications are severe, intermittent therapy may be useful. To be effective intermittent therapy must be initiated at the earliest sign of an outbreak. The patient must be given the medication before the recurrence, so treatment can be started by the patient when the first symptoms occur. Intermittent therapy only reduces the duration of the average recurrence by less than 1 day. However, it is a powerful tool in the patient who is totally overwhelmed by each outbreak. The dosage is acyclovir, 200 mg five times daily; valacyclovir, 500 mg twice daily; or famciclovir, 125 mg to 250 mg twice daily, all for 5 days.

For patients with frequent recurrences (more than 6 to 12 per year), suppressive therapy is probably more reasonable. Acyclovir, 400 mg twice daily or 200 mg three times daily, will suppress 85% of recurrences, and 20% of patients will be recurrence free during suppressive therapy. Valacyclovir,

500 mg once daily (or 1000 mg once daily for persons with greater than 10 recurrences per year), or famciclovir, 250 mg twice daily, are equally effective alternatives. In addition, chronic suppressive therapy reduces asymptomatic shedding by almost 95%. After 10 years of suppressive therapy a large number of the patients can stop treatment with a substantial reduction in frequency of recurrences. Chronic suppressive therapy is very safe, and laboratory monitoring is not required.

Intrauterine and Neonatal Herpes Simplex. Neonatal herpes infections occurs in approximately one in every 3000 deliveries per year in the United States, resulting in 1500 to 2200 cases of neonatal herpes. Most cases of neonatal infection with herpes simplex occur around the time of delivery. Rarely, herpes simplex infection of the fetus can occur in utero before delivery, usually in mothers who have primary genital herpes during pregnancy. In utero infection may result in fetal anomalies to include skin lesions and scars, microcephaly, microphthalmos, encephalitis, chorioretinitis, and intracerebral calcifications. Affected neonates may die, and if they survive virtually always suffer permanent neurologic sequelae.

Seventy percent of cases of neonatal herpes simplex are caused by HSV-2 and acquired as the child passes through an infected birth canal. Neonatal HSV-1 infections are usually acquired postnatally through contact with a person with orolabial disease. The clinical spectrum of perinatally acquired herpes simplex in the neonate ranges from localized skin infection to severe disseminated disease with encephalitis, hepatitis, pneumonia, and coagulopathy. Extent of involvement at presentation is important prognostically. With treatment, localized disease (skin, eyes, or mouth) is rarely fatal, whereas brain or disseminated disease is fatal in 15% to 50% of neonates so affected. In treated neonates, long-term sequelae occur in 10% of neonates with localized disease. More than 50% of cases of brain or disseminated neonatal herpes suffer neurologic disability.

In 70% of babies, skin vesicles are the presenting sign, and are a good source for virus recovery. Because the incubation period may be as long as 3 weeks, and averages about 1 week, the vesicles may not appear until the child has been discharged from the hospital. Disseminated herpes with central nervous system (CNS) involvement may occur without skin lesions ever having been present; 20% of cases of neonatal herpes never have vesicles. Neonatal herpes infections are treated with IV acyclovir 250 mg/m^2 every 8 hours for 7 days. Acyclovir is easier to administer and has lower toxicity than IV vidarabine.

Seventy percent of mothers of infants with neonatal herpes simplex are asymptomatic at the time of delivery and have no history of genital herpes. Thus extended history taking is of no value in predicting which pregnancies may be complicated by neonatal herpes. The most important predictors of infection appear to be the nature of the mother's infection at delivery (primary versus recurrent), and the presence of active lesions on the cervix, vagina, or vulvar area. The risk of infection for an infant delivered vaginally when the mother has active *recurrent* genital herpes infection is between 2% and 5%, whereas it is 33% to 50% if the maternal infection at delivery is a primary one. All women with active lesions at delivery are delivered by cesarean section, ideally within 4 hours of rupture of the membranes.

The appropriate management of pregnancies complicated by genital herpes is complex and there are still areas of controversy. The review paper by Brown provides guidelines for such cases. Routine prenatal cultures are not recommended for women with recurrent genital herpes, as they do not predict shedding at the time of delivery. Such cultures may be of value in women with primary genital herpes during pregnancy, or in women with an outbreak late in gestation, to document cessation of viral shedding. Scalp electrodes should be avoided in deliveries where cervical shedding of HSV is possible, as they have been documented to increase the risk of infection of the newborn. Genital HSV-1 infection appears to be more frequently transmitted. Because the risk of neonatal herpes is much greater in women with their initial episode during pregnancy, acyclovir suppression has been used in these women to reduce outbreaks during the third trimester and thus prevent the need for cesarean section.

Disseminated Herpes Simplex Infection. A disease of children, usually between 6 months and 3 years of age, disseminated herpes simplex generally starts with a severe herpetic gingivostomatitis. Dissemination to the viscera, especially the liver, follows. Involvement of the lungs and a massive viremia may follow and produce gastroenteritis, encephalitis, and hepatic and adrenal dysfunction. Most deaths occur during the stage of severe viremia.

Severe disseminated herpes simplex occurs in the newborn, especially the premature (see the section on Neonatal herpes simplex), and also in infants and malnourished persons such as those with kwashiorkor; in associated infections, particularly measles; in immunocompromised hosts being treated with immunosuppressive drugs; with Hodgkin's and other related diseases; and in the Wiskott-Aldrich syndrome. The treatment of disseminated herpes simplex is intravenous acyclovir.

Eczema Herpeticum. Infection with herpesvirus in patients with atopic dermatitis may lead to spread of herpes simplex throughout the eczematous areas (Kaposi's varicelliform eruption). The same may occur in severe seborrheic dermatitis, scabies, Darier's disease, benign familial pemphigus, pemphigus (foliaceus or vulgaris), pemphigoid, Wiskott-Aldrich syndrome, or burns. Hundreds of umbilicated vesicles may be present at the onset, with fever and regional adenopathy (Fig. 19-12). Although the cutaneous

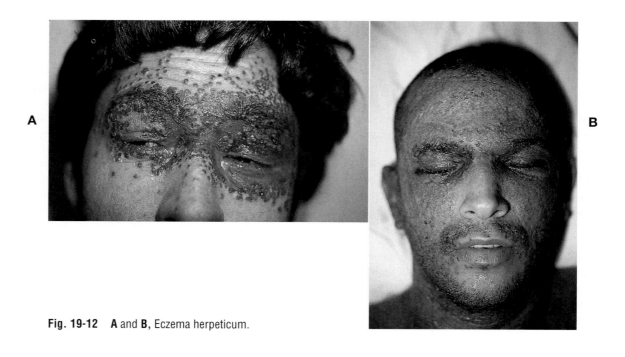

Fig. 19-12 **A** and **B**, Eczema herpeticum.

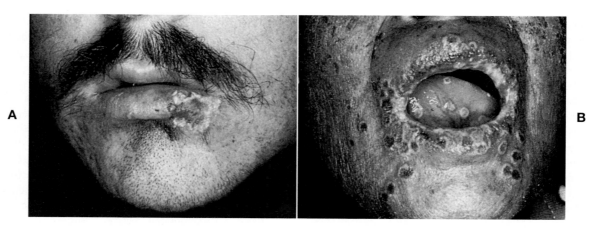

Fig. 19-13 **A**, Chronic herpes simplex in a young man with lymphosarcoma. **B**, Acute orocutaneous herpes simplex in a woman on high doses of prednisone with a severe drug reaction.

eruption is alarming, the disease is often self-limited in healthy individuals. Depending on the severity of the disease, either intravenous or oral acyclovir therapy should be given in all cases of Kaposi's varicelliform eruption.

Herpes Simplex Infection in Immunocompromised Patients. In patients with immunosuppression of the cell-mediated immune system by cytotoxic agents, corticosteroids, or congenital or acquired immunodeficiency, primary and recurrent cases of herpes simplex are more severe, more persistent, and more symptomatic. In some settings (such as in bone marrow transplant recipients), the risk of severe reactivation is so high that prophylactic systemic antivirals are administered. In immunosuppressed patients, any erosive mucocutaneous lesion should be considered herpes simplex until proved otherwise, especially lesions in the genital and orolabial regions. Atypical morphologies are also seen.

Typically, lesions appear as erosions or crusts. The early vesicular lesions may be transient or never seen. The three clinical hallmarks of herpes simplex infection are pain, an active vesicular border, and a scalloped periphery (Fig. 19-13). Untreated erosive lesions may gradually expand. In the oral mucosa numerous erosions may be seen, involving all surfaces (as opposed to only the hard, keratinized surfaces usually involved by recurrent oral herpes simplex in the immunocompetent host). The tongue may be affected with geometric fissures on the central dorsal surface. Symptomatic stomatitis associated with cancer chemotherapy is at times caused or exacerbated by HSV infection.

Rather than gradually expanding, mucocutaneous lesions may also appear and remain fixed and even become papular. Herpetic whitlow presents as a painful paronychia that is initially vesicular and involves the lateral or proximal nail folds. Untreated, it may lead to loss of the nailplate and ulceration of a large portion of the digit.

Despite the frequent and severe skin infections caused by HSV in the immunosuppressed, visceral dissemination is unusual. Extension of oral HSV into the esophagus or trachea may develop spontaneously or as a complication of intubation through an infected oropharynx. Ocular involvement can occur from direct inoculation, and if lesions are present around the eye, careful ophthalmologic evaluation is required.

In an immunosuppressed host, since most lesions are ulcerative and not vesicular, Tzanck smears are of less value. Viral cultures taken from the ulcer margin are positive. Direct fluorescent antibody testing is specific and rapid, and is very useful in immunosuppressed hosts in whom therapeutic decisions need to be made expeditiously.

Therapy often can be instituted on clinical grounds pending confirmatory tests. Acyclovir is effective and very safe. The initial dose is 200 to 400 mg orally five times daily. In severe infection, or in the hospitalized patient with moderate disease, intravenous acyclovir (5 mg/kg) can be given initially to control the disease. In patients with AIDS and those with persistent immunosuppression, consideration should be given to chronic suppressive therapy with acyclovir, 400 mg twice daily; valacyclovir, 500 mg once or twice daily; or famciclovir, 250 mg twice daily.

Long-duration treatment with acyclovir and its analogs, or treatment of large herpetic ulcerations may be complicated by the development of acyclovir resistance. Antiviral resistance is suspected when high doses of acyclovir do not lead to improvement. HSV isolates can be tested for sensitivity to acyclovir and some other antivirals. The standard treatment of acyclovir-resistant herpes simplex is intravenous foscarnet. Smaller lesions can sometimes be treated with topical trifluorothymidine (Viroptic) with or without topical or intralesional interferon alfa.

Histopathology of Herpes Simplex Infection

The vesicles of herpes simplex are intraepidermal. The affected epidermis and the adjacent inflamed dermis are infiltrated with leukocytes, and a serous exudate containing dissociated cells collects to form the vesicle. There is ballooning degeneration of the epidermal cells to produce acantholysis. Minute eosinophilic intranuclear bodies occur in the epithelial cells' nuclei. These small bodies increase in size, coalesce, and finally occupy the majority the nucleus to form the inclusion body.

Differential Diagnosis of Herpes Simplex

Herpes labialis must most frequently be differentiated from impetigo. Herpetic lesions are composed of groups of tense, small vesicles, whereas in bullous impetigo the blisters are unilocular, occur at the periphery of a crust, and are flaccid. A mixed infection is not unusual, and should especially be suspected in immunosuppressed hosts, and when lesions are present in the typical herpetic regions around the mouth. Herpes zoster presents with clusters of lesions along a dermatome, but early on if the number of lesions of zoster is limited, it can be relatively indistinguishable from herpes simplex. In general, herpes zoster will be more painful and over 24 hours will progress to involve more of the affected dermatome. Direct fluorescent antibody testing can rapidly make this distinction.

A genital herpes lesion, especially on the glans or corona, is easily mistaken for a syphilitic chancre or chancroid. Darkfield examination, multiplex PCR, and cultures for *Haemophilus ducreyi* on selective media will aid in making the diagnosis, as will diagnostic tests for HSV (Tzanck, culture, or DFA).

Herpetic gingivostomatitis is often difficult to differentiate from aphthosis, streptococcal infections, diphtheria, coxsackievirus infections, and oral erythema multiforme. Aphthae have a tendency to occur mostly on the buccal and labial mucosae. They usually form shallow, grayish erosions, generally surrounded by a prominent ring of hyperemia. Although aphthae commonly occur on nonattached mucosa, recurrent herpes of the oral cavity primarily affects the attached gingiva and palate.

Arndt KA: Adverse reactions to acyclovir. *J Am Acad Dermatol* 1988, 18:188.

Ashley R, et al: Genital herpes: review of epidemic and potential use of type specific serology. *Clin Microbiol Rev* 1999, 12:1.

Ashley R, et al: Inability of enzyme immunoassays to discriminate between infections with herpes simplex virus types 1 and 2. *Ann Intern Med* 1991, 115:520.

Aslanzadeh JA, et al: Detection of HSV-specific DNA in biopsy tissue of patients with erythema multiforme by polymerase chain reaction. *Br J Dermatology* 1992, 126:19.

Belongia EA, et al: An outbreak of herpes gladiatorum at a high-school wrestling camp. *N Engl J Med* 1991, 13:906.

Bork K, et al: Increasing incidence of eczema herpeticum. *J Am Acad Dermatol* 1988, 19:1024.

Brown ZA: Genital herpes complicating pregnancy. *Dermatol Clin* 1998, 16:805.

Brown ZA, et al: Neonatal herpes simplex virus infection in relation to asymptomatic maternal infection at the time of labor. *N Engl J Med* 1991, 324:1247.

Bryson Y, et al: Risk of acquisition of genital herpes simplex virus type 2 in sex partners of persons with genital herpes: a prospective couple study. *J Infect Dis* 1993, 167:942.

Chatis PA, et al: Successful treatment with foscarnet of an acyclovir-resistant mucocutaneous infection with herpes simplex virus in a patient with AIDS. *N Engl J Med* 1989, 320:279.

Conant MA: Prophylactic and suppressive treatment with acyclovir and the management of herpes in patients with AIDS. *J Am Acad Dermatol* 1988, 18:186.

Conant MA, et al: Genital herpes. *J Am Acad Dermatol* 1996, 35:601.

Cone RW, et al: Frequent detection of genital herpes simplex virus DNA by polymerase chain reaction among pregnant women. *JAMA* 1994, 272:792.

Elder DE, et al: Neonatal herpes simplex infection. *J Pediatr* 1995, 31:307.

Erlich KS, et al: Acyclovir-resistant herpes simplex virus infections in patients with AIDS. *N Engl J Med* 1989, 320:293.

Fife KH, et al: Recurrence and resistance patterns of herpes simplex virus following cessation of >6 years of chronic suppression with acyclovir. *J Infect Dis* 1994, 169:1338.

Gill MJ, et al: Herpes simplex virus infection of the hand. *Am J Med* 1988, 84:89.

Grossman MC, et al: The Tzanck smear: can dermatologists accurately interpret it? *J Am Acad Dermatol* 1992, 27:403.

Husak R, et al: Pseudotumor of the tongue caused by herpes simplex virus type 2 in an HIV-1 infected immunosuppressed patient. *Br J Dermatol* 1998, 139:118.

Jacobs RF: Neonatal herpes simplex infections. *Semin Perinatol* 1998, 22:64.

Jawitz JC, et al: Treatment of eczema herpeticum with systemic acyclovir. *Arch Dermatol* 1985, 121:274.

Kinghorn GR: Genital herpes: natural history and treatment of acute episodes. *J Med Virol* 1993, 1(Suppl):33.

Kohl S: Neonatal herpes simplex virus infection. *Clin Perinatol* 1997, 24:129

Lafferty WE, et al: Recurrences after oral and genital HSV infection. *N Engl J Med* 1987, 316:1444.

Langenberg AGM, et al: A prospective study of new infections with herpes simplex virus type 1 and 2. *N Engl J Med* 1999, 341:1432.

Laskin OL: Acyclovir and suppression of frequently recurring herpetic whitlow. *Ann Intern Med* 1985, 102:494.

Malm G, et al: Neonatal herpes simplex: clinical findings and outcome in relation to type of maternal infection. *Acta Paediatr* 1995, 84:256.

Manzella JP, et al: An outbreak of herpes simplex virus type I gingivostomatitis in a dental hygiene practice. *JAMA* 1984, 252:2019.

Mertz GJ, et al: Risk factors for the sexual transmission of genital herpes. *Ann Intern Med* 1992, 116:197.

Nahass GT, et al: Comparison of Tzanck smear, viral culture, and DNA diagnostic methods in detection of herpes simplex and varicella zoster infection. *JAMA* 1992, 268:2541.

Norris SA, et al: Severe, progressive herpetic whitlow caused by an acyclovir-resistant virus in a patient with AIDS. *J Infect Dis* 1988, 157:209.

Oliver L, et al: seroprevalence of herpes simplex virus infections in a family medicine clinic. *Arch Fam Med* 1995, 4:228.

Pereira FA: Herpes simplex. *J Am Acad Dermatol* 1996, 35:503.

Prober CG, et al: The management of pregnancies complicated by genital infections with herpes simplex virus. *Clin Infect Dis* 1992, 15:1031.

Rand KH, et al: Cancer-chemotherapy–associated symptomatic stomatitis. *Cancer* 1982, 50:1262.

Randolph AG, et al: Cesarean delivery for women presenting with genital herpes lesions. *JAMA* 1993, 270:77.

Rooney JF, et al: Oral acyclovir to suppress frequently recurrent herpes labialis. *Ann Intern Med* 1993, 118:268.

Sacks SL, et al: Patient-initiated, twice-daily oral famciclovir for early recurrent genital herpes. *JAMA* 1996, 276:44.

Salzman RS, et al: Chancroidal ulcers that are not chancroid. *Arch Dermatol* 1984, 120:636.

Sands M, et al: Herpes simplex lymphangitis. *Arch Intern Med* 1988, 148:2066.

Schomogyi M, et al: Herpes simplex virus-2 infection. *Infect Dis Clin North Am* 1998, 12:47.

Scott LL, et al: Prevention of perinatal herpes. *Clin Obstet Gynecol* 1999, 42:134.

Severson JL, et al: Relation between herpes simplex and human immunodeficiency virus. *Arch Dermatol* 1999, 135:1393.

Shaw M, et al: Failure of acyclovir cream in the treatment of recurrent herpes. *Br Med J* 1985, 291:7.

Silverman AK, et al: Activation of herpes simplex following dermabrasion. *J Am Acad Dermatol* 1985, 13:103.

Spruance SL: Prophylactic chemotherapy with acyclovir for recurrent herpes simplex labialis. *J Med Virol* 1993, 1:S27.

Taieb A, et al: Clinical epidemiology of symptomatic primary herpetic infection in children. *Acta Pediatr Scand* 1987, 76:128.

Tatnall FM, et al: A double-blind, placebo-controlled trial of continuous acyclovir therapy in recurrent erythema multiforme. *Br J Dermatol* 1995, 132:267.

Tayal SC, et al: High prevalence of herpes simplex virus type 1 in female anogenital herpes simplex in Newcastle upon Tyne 1983-92. *Int J STD AIDS* 1994, 5:359.

Taylor JR, et al: Interrelation between ultraviolet light and recurrent herpes simplex infections in man. *J Dermatol* 1994, 8:224.

Vonderheid EC, et al: Chronic herpes simplex infection in cutaneous T-cell lymphoma. *Arch Dermatol* 1982, 116:1018.

Wald A: New therapies and prevention strategies for genital herpes. *Clin Infect Dis* 1999, 28:S4.

Westheim AI, et al: Acyclovir resistance in a patient with chronic mucocutaneous herpes simplex infection. *J Am Acad Dermatol* 1987, 17:875.

Weston WL, et al: Atypical forms of herpes simplex-associated erythema multiforme. *J Am Acad Dermatol* 1998, 39:124.

White C, et al: Genital herpes simplex infection in women. *Clin Dermatol* 1997, 15:81.

White WB, et al: Transmission of herpes simplex virus type-1 infection in rugby players. *JAMA* 1984, 252:533.

Whitley R, et al: Predictors of morbidity and mortality in neonates with herpes simplex virus infections. *N Engl J Med* 1991, 324:450.

Yeager AS, et al: Reasons for the absence of a history of recurrent genital infections in mothers of neonates infected with herpes simplex virus. *Pediatrics* 1984, 73:188. ▲

Varicella

Varicella, commonly known as *chickenpox,* is primary infection with the varicella zoster virus. In temperate regions, 90% of cases occur in children less than 10 years of age. In tropical countries, however, varicella tends to be a disease of teenagers. The incubation period is 10 to 21 days (usually 14 to 15 days). Transmission is by direct contact with the lesions and by the respiratory route, with initial viral replication in the nasopharynx and conjunctiva. There is an initial viremia between days 4 and 6 seeding the liver, spleen, lungs, and perhaps other organs. A secondary viremia occurs at days 11 to 20, resulting in infection of the epidermis and the appearance of the characteristic skin lesions. Individuals are infectious for at least 4 days before and 5 days after the appearance of the exanthem. Low-grade fever, malaise, and headache are usually present but slight. The severity of the disease is age dependent, with adults having more severe disease and a greater risk of visceral disease. In healthy children the death rate from varicella is 1.4 per 100,000 cases; in adults, 30.9 deaths per 100,000 cases. As with most viral infections, immunosuppression may worsen the course of the disease (see below). Lifelong immunity follows varicella.

Varicella is characterized by a vesicular eruption consisting of delicate "teardrop" vesicles on an erythematous base. The eruption starts with faint macules that develop rapidly into vesicles within 24 hours. Successive fresh crops of vesicles appear for a few days, mainly on the trunk, face, and on the oral mucosa (Figs. 19-14 and 19-15). Initially, the exanthem may be limited to sun-exposed areas or areas of inflammation (Fig. 19-16).

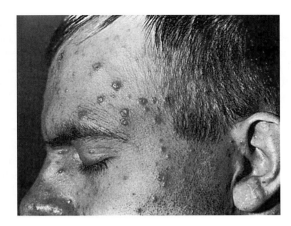

Fig. 19-14   Varicella.

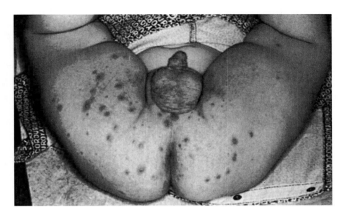

Fig. 19-16   Varicella initially involving the diaper area.

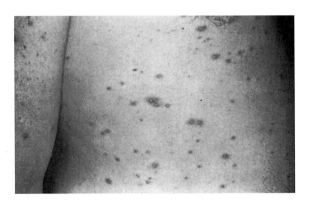

Fig. 19-15   Varicella.

The vesicles quickly become pustular, umbilicated, then crusted. Lesions tend not to scar, but larger lesions and those that become secondarily infected may heal with a characteristic round, depressed scar.

Secondary bacterial infection with *Staphylococcus aureus* or a streptococcal organism is the most common complication of varicella. Rarely, it may be complicated by osteomyelitis. Other complications are rare. Pneumonia is uncommon in normal children but is seen in 1 in 400 adults with varicella. It may be bacterial or be caused by the varicella, a difficult differential diagnosis. Cerebellar ataxia and encephalitis are the most common neurologic complications. Asymptomatic myocarditis and hepatitis are not uncommon in children with varicella, but these conditions are rarely significant and resolve spontaneously with no treatment. Reye's syndrome, a syndrome of hepatitis and acute encephalopathy, is associated with the use of aspirin to treat the symptoms of varicella. Aspirin is absolutely contraindicated in patients with varicella. Any child with varicella and severe vomiting should be referred immediately to exclude Reye's syndrome. Symptomatic thrombocytopenia is a rare manifestation of varicella, which can occur either with the exanthem or several weeks after.

Purpura fulminans, a form of disseminated intravascular coagulation associated with low levels of protein C and S, may complicate varicella.

The diagnosis of varicella is easily made clinically. In atypical cases, a Tzanck smear from a vesicle will usually show characteristic multinucleate giant cells. If needed, the most useful clinical test is a direct fluorescent antibody test, which is rapid and will both confirm the infection and type the virus.

Treatment of Varicella

Both immunocompetent children and adults with varicella are benefited by acyclovir therapy if started early (within 24 hours of the appearance of the eruption). Therapy does not appear to alter the development of adequate immunity to reinfection. Because the complications of varicella are infrequent in children, routine treatment is not recommended; therapeutic decisions are made on a case-by-case basis. Acyclovir therapy seems to benefit most secondary cases within a household, which tend to be more severe than the index case. In this setting, therapy can be instituted earlier. Therapy does not, however, return children to school sooner, and the impact on parental work days missed is not known. The dose is 20 mg/kg (maximum 800 mg per dose) four times daily for 5 days. Aspirin and other salicylates should not be used as antipyretics in varicella, because their use increases the risk of Reye's syndrome. Topical antipruritic lotions, oatmeal baths, and dressing the patient in light, cool clothing and keeping the environment cool may all relieve some of the symptomatology. Children living in warm homes and kept very warm with clothing have anecdotally been observed to have more numerous skin lesions. Children with diabetes, cystic fibrosis, and inborn errors of metabolism should be treated with acyclovir since they may suffer more complications or exacerbations of their underlying illness with varicella.

Because varicella is more severe and complications are more common in adults, treatment is recommended in adolescents and adults (13 and older). The dose is 800 mg four or five times daily for 5 days. Severe, fulminant cutaneous disease and visceral complications are treated with intravenous acyclovir 10 mg/kg every 8 hours, adjusted for creatinine clearance. If the patient is hospitalized for therapy, strict isolation is required. Patients with varicella should not be admitted to wards with immunocompromised hosts or onto pediatric wards, but rather are best placed on wards with healthy patients recovering from acute trauma.

Varicella in Pregnant Women and Neonates.
Maternal infection with the varicella zoster virus during the first 20 weeks of gestation may result in a syndrome of congenital malformations (congenital varicella syndrome) as well as severe illness in the mother. In one study, 4 of 31 women with varicella in pregnancy developed varicella pneumonia. The risk for spontaneous abortion by 20 weeks is 3%; in an additional 0.7% of pregnancies, fetal death occurs after 20 weeks. The risk of preterm labor, as reported in various studies, has varied from no increase to a threefold increase. Severe varicella and varicella pneumonia or disseminated disease in pregnancy should be treated with intravenous acyclovir. The value of oral acyclovir in other patterns of varicella in pregnancy is unknown.

Varicella zoster immune globulin (VZIG) should not be given once the pregnant woman has developed varicella. VZIG should be given for significant exposures (see below) within the first 72 to 96 hours to ameliorate maternal varicella and prevent complications. Its use should be limited to seronegative women because of its cost and the high rate of asymptomatic infection in the United States. The lack of a history of prior varicella is associated with seronegativity in only 20% or fewer of the U.S. population.

Congenital varicella syndrome is characterized by a series of anomalies, including hypoplastic limbs (usually unilateral and lower extremity), cutaneous scars, and ocular and CNS disease. Female fetuses are affected more commonly than males. The overall risk for this syndrome is between 1% and 2% (the former figure from the largest series). The highest risk is from maternal varicella between weeks 13 and 20 where the risk is 2%. Infection of the fetus in utero may result in zoster occurring postnatally, often in the first 2 years of life. This occurs in about 1% of varicella-complicated pregnancies, and the risk for this complication is greatest in varicella occurring in weeks 25 to 36 of gestation. The value of VZIG in preventing or modifying fetal complications of maternal varicella is unknown. In one study, however, of 97 patients with varicella in pregnancy who were treated with VZIG, none had complications of congenital varicella syndrome or infantile zoster, suggesting some efficacy for VZIG. Although apparently safe in pregnancy, acyclovir's efficacy in preventing fetal complications of maternal varicella is unknown.

If the mother develops varicella between 5 days before and 2 days after delivery, neonatal varicella can occur and be severe, as transplacental delivery of antivaricella antibody has been inadequate. These neonates develop varicella at 5 to 10 days of age. In such cases the administration of VZIG is warranted, and acyclovir therapy intravenously should be considered.

Varicella Vaccine.
Live attenuated viral vaccine for varicella is a currently recommended childhood immunization. Complications are uncommon. A mild skin eruption from which virus can usually not be isolated, occurring locally at the injection site within 2 days or generalized 1 to 3 weeks after immunization occurs in 6% of children. In healthy children, the vaccine is very efficacious, with 95% of children remaining free of varicella during a 7-year follow-up. Household exposures resulted in a 12% rate of breakthrough varicella, well below the expected 90%. Many of the breakthrough cases were mild, and many of the skin lesions not vesicular (see modified varicella-like syndrome below). Immunized children with no detectable antibody also have reduced severity of varicella after exposure. Secondary complications of varicella including scarring are virtually eliminated by vaccination. Antibodies appear to persist for many years, but the duration of immunity is unknown, so long-term studies are being performed following immunized children for up to 15 years.

Household exposure of immunosuppressed children to recently immunized siblings does not appear to pose a great risk. Children whose leukemia is in remission are also protected by the vaccine but may require three doses. Leukemic children still receiving chemotherapy have a complication rate from vaccination (usually a varicella-like eruption) approaching 50%. They may require acyclovir therapy. Unprotected close contacts developed varicella 15% of the time. In leukemic children, adequate immunization results in complete immunity in some and partial immunity in the rest, protecting them from severe varicella. Immunization also reduces the attack rate for zoster in leukemic children.

MODIFIED VARICELLA-LIKE SYNDROME. Children immunized with live attenuated varicella vaccine may develop varicella of reduced severity on exposure to natural varicella. This has been called modified varicella-like syndrome or MVLS. The frequency of MVLS is between 2% and 4% per year, and children with lower antibody titers are more likely to develop MVLS. The illness occurs an average of 15 days after exposure to varicella and consists primarily of macules and papules with relatively few vesicles. The average number of lesions is about 35 to 50, compared with natural varicella, which usually has about 300 lesions. The majority of patients are afebrile, and the illness is mild, lasting less than 5 days on the average.

Varicella in Immunocompromised Patients.
Varicella cases can be extremely severe and even fatal in immuno-

suppressed patients, especially in individuals with impaired cell-mediated immunity. Before effective antiviral therapy, nearly one third of children with cancer developed complications of varicella, and 7% died. In this setting, varicella pneumonia, hepatitis, and encephalitis are frequent. Prior varicella does not always protect the immunosuppressed host from multiple episodes. The skin lesions in the immunosuppressed host are usually identical to varicella in the healthy host, however, the number of lesions may be numerous. In an immunosuppressed patient, the lesions more frequently become necrotic and ulceration may occur. Even if the lesions are few, the size of the lesion may be large (up to several centimeters), and necrosis of the full thickness of dermis may occur. In HIV infection, varicella may be severe and fatal. Atypical cases of few scattered lesions but without a dermatomal distribution usually represent reactivation disease with dissemination. Chronic varicella may complicate HIV infection, resulting in ulcerative (ecthymatous) or hyperkeratotic (verrucous) lesions. These patterns of infection may be associated with acyclovir resistance.

The degree of immunosuppression likely to result in severe varicella has been a matter of debate. There are case reports of severe and even fatal varicella in otherwise healthy children given short courses of oral steroids or even using only inhaled steroids. In a case-control study, however, corticosteroid use did not appear to be a risk factor for the development of severe varicella. In the United Kingdom, any patient receiving or having received systemic steroids in the prior 3 months, regardless of dose, is considered at increased risk for severe varicella. Inhaled steroids are not considered an indication for prophylactic VZIG or antiviral treatment. A "high-risk" or significant exposure had been defined as (1) household contact, i.e., living in the same house as a case of chickenpox or zoster, (2) face-to-face contact with a case of chickenpox for at least 5 minutes, (3) contact indoors with a case of chickenpox or herpes zoster for more than 1 hour or, within a hospital setting, a case of chickenpox or herpes zoster in an adjacent bed or in the same open ward. Immunosuppressed children with no prior history of varicella and a high-risk exposure should be treated with VZIG as soon as possible after exposure (within 96 hours). Preengraftment bone marrow transplant patients should be treated the same. VZIG treatment does not reduce the frequency of infection, but it does reduce the severity of infection and reduces complications. The value of prophylactic antivirals is unknown. Parents of immunosuppressed children and their doctors should be aware that severe disease can occur, and the parents counseled to return immediately after significant exposure, or if varicella develops.

Ideally, management of varicella in the immunocompromised patient would involve prevention through the use of varicella vaccination before immunosuppression. Intravenous acyclovir at a dose of 10 mg/kg three times daily (or 500 mg/m^2 in children) is given as soon as the diagnosis is suspected. Intravenous therapy is continued until 2 days after all new vesicles have stopped. Oral antivirals are continued for a minimum of 10 days of treatment. VZIG is of no proven benefit once clinical disease has developed but may be given if the patient has severe life-threatening disease and is not responding to intravenous acyclovir.

In HIV-infected adults, treatment is individualized. Persons with typical varicella should be evaluated for the presence of pneumonia or hepatitis. Valacyclovir, 1 g three times daily; famciclovir, 500 mg three times daily; or acyclovir, 800 mg every 4 hours may be used if no visceral complications are present. The former two agents may be preferable to acyclovir because of their enhanced oral bioavailability. Visceral disease mandates intravenous therapy. If the response to oral antiviral agents is not rapid, intravenous acyclovir therapy should be instituted. Antiviral treatment must be continued until all lesions are completely healed. Most cases of chronic or acyclovir-resistant varicella zoster virus infection are associated with initial inadequate oral doses of acyclovir (either too short in duration, too low a dose, or in patients with gastrointestinal disease, in whom reduced gastrointestinal absorption may be associated with inadequate blood levels of acyclovir). Atypical disseminated cases must be treated aggressively until all lesions resolve. The diagnosis of acyclovir-resistant varicella zoster virus infection may be difficult. Acyclovir-resistant varicella zoster virus strains may be hard to culture, and sensitivity testing is still not standardized or readily available for varicella zoster virus. Acyclovir-resistant varicella is treated with foscarnet.

Abzug MJ, et al: Severe chickenpox after intranasal use of corticosteroids. *J Pediatr* 1993, 123:577.

Alessi E, et al: Unusual varicella zoster virus infection in patients with AIDS. *Arch Dermatol* 1988, 124:1011.

Asano Y, et al: Postexposure prophylaxis of varicella in family contact by oral acyclovir. *Pediatrics* 1993, 92:219.

Baba K, et al: Increased incidence of herpes zoster in normal children infected with varicella zoster virus during infancy. *J Pediatr* 1986, 108:372.

Balfour HH, et al: Acyclovir treatment of varicella in otherwise healthy children. *J Pediatr* 1990, 116:633.

Baxter JD, et al: Relapsing chickenpox in a young man with non-Hodgkin's lymphoma. *Clin Infect Dis* 1994, 18:785.

Boyd K, et al: Acyclovir treatment of varicella in pregnancy. *Br Med J* 1988, 296:393.

Brunell PA: Varicella in pregnancy, the fetus, and the newborn: problems in management. *J Infect Dis* 1992, 166:S42.

Clements DA: Modified varicella-like syndrome. *Infect Dis Clin North Am* 1996, 10:617.

Dowell SF, et al: Severe varicella associated with steroid use. *Pediatrics* 1993, 92 223.

Dunkle LM, et al: A controlled trial of acyclovir for chickenpox in normal children. *N Engl J Med* 1991, 325:1539.

Enders G, et al: Consequences of varicella and herpes zoster in pregnancy: prospective study of 1739 cases. *Lancet* 1994, 343:1548.

Feder HM, et al: Varicella mimicking a vesiculobullous sun eruption. *J Infect Dis* 1988, 158:243.

Felder HM: Treatment of adult chickenpox with oral acyclovir. *Arch Intern Med* 1990, 150:2061.

Gershon AA, et al: Varicella vaccine: the American experience. *J Infect Dis* 1992, 166:S63.

Gershon AA, et al: Persistence of immunity to varicella in children with leukemia immunized with live attenuated varicella vaccine. *N Engl J Med* 1989, 320:893.

Janier M, et al: Chronic varicella zoster infection in AIDS. *J Am Acad Dermatol* 1988, 18:584.

Kasper WJ, et al: Fatal varicella after a single course of corticosteroids. *Pediatr Infect Dis* 1990, 9:729.

Krause PR, et al: Efficacy, immunogenicity, safety, and use of live attenuated chickenpox vaccine. *J Pediatr* 1995, 127:518.

Lawrence R, et al: The risk of zoster after varicella vaccination in children with leukemia. *N Engl J Med* 1988, 318:543.

Lipton SV, et al: Management of varicella exposure in a neonatal intensive care unit. *JAMA* 1989, 261:1782.

Messner J, et al: Accentuated viral exanthems in areas of inflammation. *J Am Acad Dermatol* 1999, 40:345.

Ogilve MM: Antiviral prophylaxis and treatment in chickenpox. *J Infect Dis* 1998, 36:S31.

Pahwa S, et al: Continuous varicella zoster infection associated with acyclovir resistance in a child with AIDS. *JAMA* 1988, 260:2879.

Patel H, et al: Recent corticosteroid use and the risk of complicated varicella in otherwise immunocompetent children. *Arch Pediatr Adolesc Med* 1996, 150:409.

Perrone C, et al: Varicella in patients infected with the human immunodeficiency virus. *Arch Dermatol* 1990, 126:1033.

Prober CG, et al: Consensus: varicella zoster infections in pregnancy and the perinatal period. *Pediatr Infect Dis J* 1990, 9:865.

Tarlow MJ, et al: Chickenpox in childhood. *J Infect Dis* 1998, 36(Suppl):39.

Ventura A: Varicella vaccination guidelines for adolescents and adults. *Am Fam Phys* 1997, 55:1220. ▲

Zoster (Shingles, Herpes Zoster)

Zoster is caused by the varicella zoster virus. Following natural infection or immunization the virus remains latent in the sensory dorsal root ganglion cells. The virus begins to replicate at some later time, traveling down the sensory nerve into the skin. Other than immunosuppression and age, the factors involved in reactivation are unknown.

The incidence of zoster increases with age. Below age 45, the annual incidence is less than 1 in 1000 persons. Among patients older than 75 years of age, the rate is more than four times greater. For white persons more than 80 years of age the lifetime risk of developing zoster is 10% to 30%. For unknown reasons African Americans are four times less likely to develop zoster. Immunosuppression, especially hematologic malignancy and HIV infection dramatically increase the risk for zoster. In HIV-infected persons the annual incidence is 30 of 1000 persons, or an annual risk of 3%.

Herpes zoster classically occurs unilaterally within the distribution of a cranial or spinal sensory nerve, often with some overflow into the dermatomes above and below. The dermatomes most frequently affected are the thoracic (55%) (Fig. 19-17), the cranial (20%, with the trigeminal nerve being the most common single nerve involved) (Fig. 19-18), the lumbar (15%), and the sacral (5%). The cutaneous

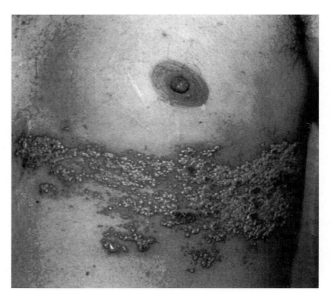

Fig. 19-17 Herpes zoster.

eruption is frequently preceded by several days of pain in the affected area, although the pain may appear simultaneously or even following the skin eruption; or the eruption may be painless. The eruption initially presents as papules and plaques of erythema in the dermatome. Within hours the plaques develop blisters. Lesions continue to appear for several days. The eruption may have few lesions or reach total confluence in the dermatome (Fig. 19-19). Lesions may become hemorrhagic, necrotic, or bullous. Rarely, the patient may have pain, but no skin lesions (zoster sine herpete). There is a correlation with the pain severity and the extent of the skin lesions, and elderly persons tend to have more pain. In patients under 30 years of age, the pain may be minimal. It is not uncommon for there to be scattered lesions outside the dermatome, usually less than 20. In the typical case, new vesicles appear for 1 to 5 days, become pustular, crust, and heal. The total duration of the eruption depends on three factors: patient age, severity of eruption, and presence of underlying immunosuppression. In younger patients, the total duration is 2 to 3 weeks, whereas in elderly patients, the cutaneous lesions of zoster may require 6 weeks or more to heal. Scarring is uncommon, except in elderly and immunosuppressed patients; scarring is also correlated with the severity of the initial eruption. Lesions may develop on the mucous membranes within the mouth in zoster of the maxillary or mandibular division of the facial nerve, or in the vagina in zoster in the S2 or S3 dermatome.

The nature of the pain associated with herpes zoster varies, but three basic types of pain have been described. There is the constant, monotonous, usually burning or deep, aching pain; the shooting, lancinating (neuritic) pain; and triggered pain. The latter is usually allodynia: pain produced

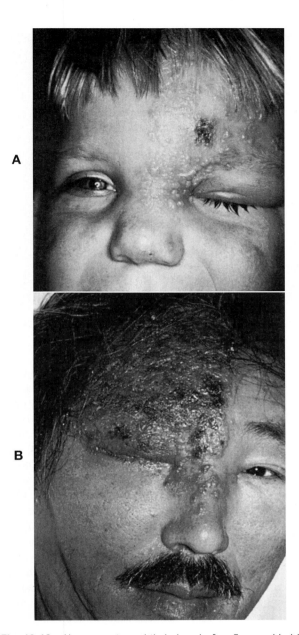

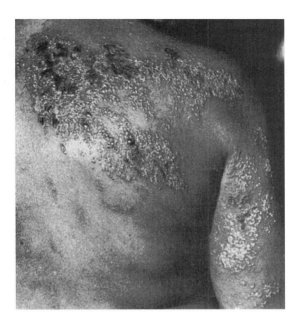

Fig. 19-19 Severe herpes zoster on right first thoracic dermatome, with spillover to C8 and T2 areas.

Fig. 19-18 Herpes zoster ophthalmicus in **A**, a 5-year-old girl and **B**, a man.

by normally innocuous stimuli, such as clothing touching the skin. It is usually impossible to sharply distinguish acute zoster pain from the pain that persists after the skin lesions have healed (postherpetic neuralgia). They are of the same quality. The pain associated with zoster is best viewed as zoster-associated pain, whether the associated skin lesions are still present or not.

Disseminated Herpes Zoster. Herpes zoster generalisatus is a generalized varicelliform eruption accompanying the segmental eruption (Fig. 19-20). It has been defined as more than 20 lesions outside the affected dermatome. It occurs

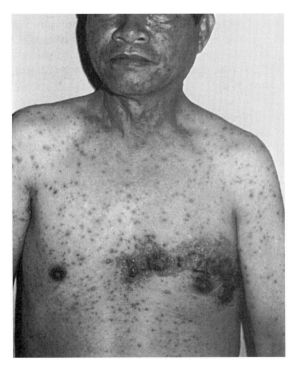

Fig. 19-20 Herpes zoster generalisatus. (Courtesy Dr. Axel W. Hoke.)

chiefly in old or debilitated individuals, especially in patients with lymphoreticular malignancy or AIDS. Mazur et al showed that low levels of serum antibody are a highly significant risk factor in predicting dissemination of disease. The dermatomal lesions are sometimes hemorrhagic or gangrenous. The outlying vesicles or bullae, which are usually not grouped, resemble varicella and are often umbilicated and may be hemorrhagic. Fever, prostration, headache, and signs of meningeal irritation or viral meningitis may be present. Rarely, zoster encephalomyelitis may follow and is often fatal.

Ophthalmic Zoster. In herpes zoster ophthalmicus, the ophthalmic division of the fifth cranial nerve is involved. If the external division of the nasociliary branch is affected, with vesicles on the side and tip of the nose (Hutchinson's sign), the eyeball is involved 76% of the time, as compared with 34% when it is not involved. Vesicles on the lid margin are virtually always associated with ocular involvement. In any case, the patient with ophthalmic zoster should be seen by an ophthalmologist. Ocular involvement is most commonly in the form of uveitis (92%) and keratitis (50%). Less common but severe complications include glaucoma, optic neuritis, encephalitis, hemiplegia, and acute retinal necrosis. Unlike the cutaneous lesions, ocular lesions of zoster and their complications tend to recur, sometimes as long as 10 years after the zoster episode.

Other Complications of Zoster. Motor nerve neuropathy occurs in about 3% of patients with zoster, and is three times more common if zoster is associated with underlying malignancy. Seventy-five percent of cases slowly recover, leaving 25% with some residual motor deficit. If the sacral dermatome S3 or less often S2 or S4 are involved, urinary hesitancy or actual urinary retention may occur. The prognosis is good for complete recovery. Similarly pseudoobstruction, colonic spasm, dilation, obstipation, constipation, and reduced anal sphincter tone can occur with thoracic (T6 to T12), lumbar, or sacral zoster. Recovery is complete.

Ramsay Hunt syndrome results from involvement of the facial and auditory nerves by the varicella zoster virus (Fig. 19-21). Herpetic inflammation of the geniculate ganglion is felt to be the cause of this syndrome. The presenting features include zoster of the external ear or tympanic membrane; herpes auricularis with ipsilateral facial paralysis; or herpes auricularis, facial paralysis, and auditory symptoms. Auditory symptoms include mild to severe tinnitus, deafness, vertigo, nausea and vomiting, and nystagmus.

Treatment of Zoster

Middle-aged and elderly patients are urged to restrict their physical activities or even stay home in bed for a few days. Bed rest may be of paramount importance in the prevention of neuralgia. Younger patients may usually continue with their customary activities. Local applications of heat, as with an electric heating pad or a hot-water bottle, are recommended. Simple local application of gentle pressure with the hand or with an abdominal binder often gives great relief, as reported by Tepperman. Topical anesthetics may be useful.

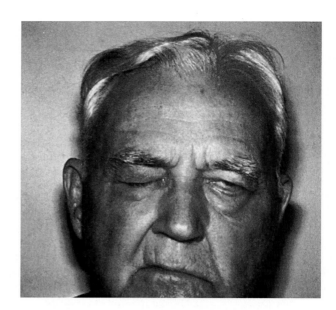

Fig. 19-21 Ramsay Hunt syndrome. (Courtesy Dr. Axel W. Hoke.)

Antiviral therapy has become the cornerstone in the management of herpes zoster. The main benefit of therapy is in reduction of the duration of zoster-associated pain. Therefore, treatment in immunocompetent patients is restricted to those at highest risk for persistent pain—those over 50 years of age. Exceptions are patients with very painful or severe cases of zoster, ophthalmic zoster, Ramsay Hunt syndrome, all immunosuppressed patients, and probably patients with motor nerve involvement. In the most severe cases, especially in ophthalmic zoster and in disseminated zoster, initial intravenous therapy may be considered. Therapy should be started as soon as the diagnosis is confirmed, preferably within the first 3 or 4 days. In immunocompetent patients, the efficacy of starting treatment beyond this time is unknown. Treatment leads to more rapid resolution of the skin lesions and, most importantly, substantially decreases the duration of zoster-associated pain. Initially, acyclovir at a dose of 800 mg five times daily was used. The newer antivirals, valacyclovir (1000 mg) and famciclovir (500 mg), may be given only three times daily. These agents are as effective as or superior to acyclovir, probably because of better absorption and the fact that higher blood levels are achieved. They are as safe as acyclovir. If not contraindicated, they are preferred.

For acyclovir, 7 days of treatment has been shown to be as good as 21 days of treatment. The newer antivirals are recommended for 7 days also. Valacyclovir and famciclovir must be dose adjusted in patients with renal impairment. In an elderly patient, if the renal status in unknown, the newer agents may be started at twice-daily dosing (which is almost as effective) pending laboratory renal evaluation of the patient, or acyclovir can be used. For patients with renal failure (creatinine clearance of less than 25 ml/min), acyclovir is preferable.

In an immunosuppressed patient, an antiviral agent should always be used because of the increased risk of dissemination and zoster-associated complications. The doses are identical to those used in immunocompetent hosts. In immunosuppressed patients with ophthalmic zoster or Ramsay Hunt syndrome, and in patients failing oral therapy, intravenous acyclovir should be used at a dose of 10 mg/kg three times daily, adjusted for renal function.

Zoster-Associated Pain (Postherpetic Neuralgia). The pain associated with herpes zoster and its tendency to persist is the major complication of zoster. Overall, about 10% of patients have pain 1 month after the onset of zoster infection. The tendency to have persistent pain is age dependent, rarely occurring in persons under 40 years of age, but 50% of persons over 60 years of age and 75% of those over 70 years of age continue to have pain beyond 1 month. Although the natural history is for gradual improvement, 10% to 25% of those having pain at 1 month will still have pain at 1 year. In some patients the pain may persist for long periods, and in a still smaller group, the pain may progressively worsen. The cause of this persistent pain is unknown.

Zoster-associated pain, especially that of long duration, is very difficult to manage. As in all pain syndromes, pain control should be achieved as quickly as possible. Adequate medication should be provided to control the pain, because chronic pain may lead to depression, complicating management of the pain. Patients with persistent moderate to severe pain may benefit from referral to a pain clinic. With this background, the importance of early and adequate antiviral therapy to reduce the duration of pain must be stressed.

Capsaicin applied topically every few hours may reduce pain, but the application itself may cause burning, and the benefits are modest. Local anesthetics, such as 10% lidocaine in gel form, 5% lidocaine-prilocaine, or lidocaine patches (Lidoderm), may acutely reduce pain, but long-term results are not available. Topical aspirin dissolved in ether or chloroform (750 mg of acetylsalicylic acid in 20 to 30 ml of liquid) in the form of a poultice or paste is also effective. Nerve blocks are effective for the reduction of acute herpetic pain and may reduce the total duration of pain. For patients with severe or incapacitating acute pain, this option should be offered, because most patients get relief for at least 8 hours, and some for much longer periods. However, the benefit of nerve blocks in preventing persistent zoster-associated pain seems limited. In a series of 26 patients, lidocaine 0.05% with 1:1,000,000 epinephrine (as is used for liposuction tumescent anesthesia), plus 60 to 80 mg of triamcinolone acetonide, was force injected using an infusion pump or syringe into the whole affected area, and marked reduction of both acute and chronic zoster-associated pain was reported by Chiarello.

The value of systemic corticosteroid therapy in the prevention of postherpetic neuralgia is controversial. Corticosteroids would be used in patients at greatest risk for persistent zoster-associated pain—those over 50 years of age. Most recent studies have failed to show reduction in the duration of zoster-associated pain, however, if an antiviral is also given. Systemic steroids do reduce acute pain during the first week. Corticosteroids reduce the overall severity of zoster-associated pain, improve quality of life, and return the patient to full daily activity sooner. Therefore, they should be given if there is no contraindication. Systemic steroidal agents should not be used in immunosuppressed hosts, because they may increase the risk of dissemination. However, steroids do not increase complications in immunocompetent hosts.

Administration of tricyclic antidepressants, such as amitriptyline and desipramine, is the first-line systemic treatment beyond giving simple analgesics, such as aspirin and acetaminophen. Tricyclic medications are given at a dose of 25 to 75 mg in a single nightly dose. Anticonvulsants, such as carbamazepine and valproate, neuroleptics, such as chlorprothixene and phenothiazines, and H_2 blockers, such as cimetidine, have all been advocated but have been not been studied critically. Many of these agents are difficult for the elderly to take because of their frequent side effects. If pain is not controlled with tricyclics, gabapentin (Neurontin) may be added in escalating doses up to 3200 mg daily. Opiate analgesia may be effective if these measures fail.

Zoster and Immunosuppressed Patients. Fueyo and Lookingbill concluded that herpes zoster should not be taken as a marker of malignancy and that screening for underlying malignancy is not indicated in patients with zoster. However, since zoster is 30 times more common in HIV-infected persons, the zoster patient should be questioned about HIV risk factors, and especially in persons under 50 years of age, in whom zoster is normally infrequent, appropriate counseling and testing should be considered. In pediatric patients with HIV infection and in other immunosuppressed children, zoster may rapidly follow primary varicella.

Although it is not cost effective to search for underlying malignancy in patients with zoster, patients with malignancy (especially Hodgkin's disease and leukemia) are five times more likely to develop zoster than are their age-matched counterparts. Other patients who also have a higher incidence of zoster include patients with deficient immune systems, such as individuals who are immunosuppressed for organ transplantation, by connective tissue disease, and by the agents used to treat these conditions (especially corticosteroids).

The clinical appearance is usually identical to typical zoster, but the lesions may be more ulcerative and necrotic and may scar more severely. Dermatomal zoster may appear, progress to involve the dermatome, and persist without resolution. Visceral dissemination and fatal outcome are extremely rare in immunosuppressed patients (about 0.3%), but cutaneous dissemination is not uncommon, occurring in 12% of cancer patients, especially those with hematologic malignancies (Figs. 19-22 and 19-23). Bone marrow transplant patients with zoster develop disseminated zoster 25% of the time, and visceral dissemination 10% to 15% of the time. Mortality in patients with zoster who have undergone bone marrow transplanta-

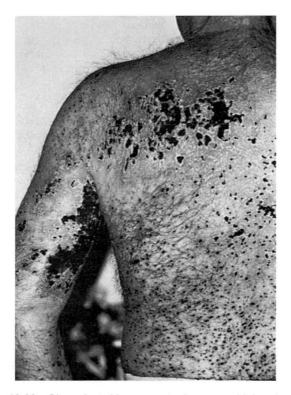

Fig. 19-22 Disseminated herpes zoster in a man with lymphoma.

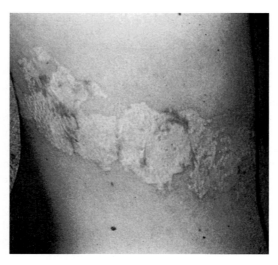

Fig. 19-23 Post-herpes zoster scarring in a young man with Hodgkin's disease.

tion is 5%. Prophylactic antiviral agents are used in this high-risk group. In AIDS patients, ocular and neurologic complications of herpes zoster are increased. Immunosuppressed patients often have recurrences of zoster, up to 25% in patients with AIDS.

Two atypical patterns of zoster have been described in AIDS patients: ecthymatous lesions, which are punched-out ulcerations with a central crust, and verrucous lesions. These patterns were not reported before the AIDS epidemic. Atypical clinical patterns, especially the verrucous pattern, may correlate with acyclovir resistance.

Diagnosis of Herpes Zoster

The same techniques used for the diagnosis of varicella are used to diagnose herpes zoster. The clinical appearance is often adequate to suspect the diagnosis, and an in-office Tzanck smear can rapidly confirm the clinical suspicion. Zosteriform herpes simplex could also produce a positive result to a Tzanck smear, but the number of lesions is usually more limited, and degree of pain substantially less. Beyond Tzanck preparation, direct fluorescent antibody testing is preferred to a viral culture, since it is rapid, types the virus, and has a higher yield than a culture will produce. When compared in documented VZV infections, Tzanck smear was 75% positive (with up to 10% false-positive results and high variability, depending on the skill of the examiner), and culture only was 44% positive. Polymerase chain reaction testing is 97% positive but is not usually immediately available. In atypical lesions, biopsy may be necessary to demonstrate the typical herpes virus cytopathic effects. Immunoperoxidase stain tests can then be performed on paraffin-fixed tissue to specifically identify the varicella zoster virus. In cases in which acyclovir fails clinically, viral culture may be attempted, but acyclovir sensitivity testing is not standardized for the varicella zoster virus, and its availability is limited.

Histopathology of Herpes Zoster

As in the case of herpes simplex, the vesicles in zoster are intraepidermal. Within and at the sides of the vesicle are found large, swollen cells called *balloon cells,* which are degenerated cells of the spinous layer. Acidophilic inclusion bodies similar to those seen in herpes simplex are present in the nuclei of the cells of the vesicle epithelium. In the vicinity of the vesicle there is marked intercellular and intracellular edema. In the upper part of the dermis, vascular dilation, edema, and a perivascular infiltration of lymphocytes and polymorphonuclear leukocytes are present. An underlying lymphocytic or leukocytoclastic vasculitis is not uncommonly seen in the dermis. Inflammatory and degenerative changes are also noted in the posterior root ganglia and in the dorsal nerve roots of the affected nerve. The lesions correspond to the areas of innervation of the affected nerve ganglion, with necrosis of the nerve cells.

Differential Diagnosis of Herpes Zoster

The distinctive clinical picture permits a diagnosis with little difficulty. A unilateral, painful eruption of grouped vesicles along a dermatome, with hyperesthesia and regional lymph node enlargement, is typical. Occasionally, segmental cutaneous paresthesias or pain may precede the eruption by 4 or 5 days. In such patients, prodromal symptoms are easily confused with the pain of angina pectoris, duodenal ulcer, biliary or renal colic, appendicitis, pleurodynia, or early glaucoma. The diagnosis becomes obvious once the cutaneous eruption appears. Herpes simplex infections may occasionally have a similar clinical presentation. Direct fluorescent antibody testing or viral culture will distinguish them.

Inflammatory Skin Lesions Following a Zoster Infection.

Following a zoster infection, inflammatory skin lesions may rarely occur within the affected dermatome, perhaps analogous to the long-standing immunologic ocular and CNS reactions seen in ophthalmic zoster. Lesions usually appear within a month, and rarely, longer than 3 months after the zoster. Clinically, the lesions are usually flat topped or annular papules in the dermatome. Histologically, such papules most frequently demonstrate various patterns of granulomatous inflammation from typical granuloma annulare, to sarcoidal reactions, or even granulomatous vasculitis. Less commonly the lesions may show benign lymphocytic infiltrates. Persistent viral genome has not been detected in these lesions, suggesting that continued antiviral therapy is not indicated. Topical and intralesional therapy with corticosteroid medications is beneficial, but the natural history of these lesions is generally spontaneous resolution.

Alessi E, et al: Unusual varicella zoster virus infection in patients with AIDS. *Arch Dermatol* 1988, 124:1011.

Baba K, et al: Increased incidence of herpes zoster in normal children infected with varicella zoster virus during infancy. *J Pediatr* 1986, 108:372.

Balfour HH: Current management of varicella zoster virus infections. *J Med Virol* 1993, 1(Suppl):74.

Bennett GJ: Hypotheses on the pathogenesis of herpes zoster-associated pain. *Ann Neurol* 1994, 35:S38.

Bernstein JE, et al: Treatment of chronic post-herpetic neuralgia with topical capsaicin. *J Am Acad Dermatol* 1987, 17:93.

Beutner KR, et al: Valacyclovir compared with acyclovir for improved therapy for herpes zoster in immunocompetent adults. *Am Soc Microbiol* 1995, 39:1546.

Buchbinder SP, et al: Herpes zoster and human immunodeficiency virus infection. *J Infect Dis* 1992, 166:1153.

Chiarello SE: Tumescent infiltration of corticosteroids, lidocaine, and epinephrine into dermatomes of acute herpetic pain or postherpetic neuralgia. *Arch Dermatol* 1998, 134:279.

Cohen LM, et al: Urinary retention associated with herpes zoster infection. *Int J Dermatol* 1993, 32:24.

Cohen PR, et al: Disseminated herpes zoster in patients with HIV infection. *Am J Med* 1988, 89:1076.

Elliot KJ: Other neurological complications of herpes zoster and their management. *Ann Neurol* 1994, 35:S57.

Esmann V, et al: Prednisolone does not prevent post-herpetic neuralgia. *Lancet* 1987, 1:126.

Feldman S: Varicella zoster infections in bone marrow transplants. *Recent Results Cancer Res* 1993, 132:175.

Fueyo MA, et al: Herpes zoster and occult malignancy. *J Am Acad Dermatol* 1984, 11:480.

Gilden DH, et al: Varicella zoster virus reactivation without rash. *J Infect Dis* 1992, 166:S30.

Gilden DH, et al: Zoster sine herpete, a clinical variant. *Ann Neurol* 1994, 35:530.

Glesby MJ, et al: Clinical spectrum of herpes zoster in adults infected with human immunodeficiency virus. *Clin Infect Dis* 1995, 21:370.

Harding: Management of ophthalmic zoster. *J Med Virol* 1993, 1(Suppl):97.

Hellinger WC, et al: Varicella zoster virus retinitis in a patient with AIDS-related complex. *Clin Infect Dis* 1993, 16:208.

Hirschmann JV: Herpes zoster. *Semin Neurol* 1992, 12:322.

Hoppenjans WB, et al: Prolonged cutaneous herpes zoster in acquired immunodeficiency syndrome. *Arch Dermatol* 1990, 126:1048.

Hwang SM, et al: The effects of epidural blockade on the acute pain in herpes zoster. *Arch Dermatol* 1999, 135:1359.

Jellinek EH, et al: Herpes zoster with dysfunction of bladder and anus. *Lancet* 1976, 2:1219.

Langenberg A, et al: Granulomatous vasculitis occurring after cutaneous herpes zoster despite absence of viral genome. *J Am Acad Dermatol* 1991:24:429.

Lawrence R, et al: The risk of zoster after varicella vaccination in children with leukemia. *N Engl J Med* 1988, 318:543.

Lee JJ, et al: Postherpetic neuralgia: current concepts and management. *Br J Hosp Med* 1994, 52:565.

Marsch RJ, et al: Ophthalmic herpes zoster. *Eye* 1993, 7:350.

Post BT, et al: Do corticosteroids prevent post-herpetic neuralgia? *J Am Acad Dermatol* 1988, 18:605.

Ragozzino MD, et al: Population-based study of herpes zoster and its sequelae. *Medicine* 1982, 61:310.

Riopelle JM, et al: Chronic neuralgia incidence following local anesthetic therapy for herpes zoster. *Arch Dermatol* 1984, 120:747.

Rowbotham MC: Treatment of postherpetic neuralgia. *Semin Dermatol* 1992, 11:218.

Sadick NS, et al: Comparison of detection of varicella zoster virus by Tzanck smear, direct immunofluorescence with a monoclonal antibody, and virus isolation. *J Am Acad Dermatol* 1987, 17:64.

Schmader K, et al: Racial differences in the occurrence of herpes zoster. *J Infect Dis* 1995, 171:701.

Solomon AR: Comparison of the Tzanck smear and viral isolation in varicella and herpes zoster. *Arch Dermatol* 1986, 122:282.

Straus SE, et al: Varicella zoster virus infections. *Ann Intern Med* 1988, 108:221.

Tepperman J: Symptomatic relief in herpes zoster (letter). *N Engl J Med* 1981, 306:1553.

Thomas CA, et al: Clinical application of PCR amplification to diagnosis of herpes virus infection. *Am J Dermatopathol* 1994, 16:268.

Tribble DR, et al: Gastrointestinal visceral complications of dermatomal herpes zoster: report of two cases and review. *Clin Infect Dis* 1993, 17:431.

Tyring S, et al: Famciclovir for the treatment of acute herpes zoster: effects on acute disease and postherpetic neuralgia. *Ann Intern Med* 1995, 123:89.

Watson CP, et al: Amitriptyline versus placebo in postherpetic neuralgia. *Neurology* 1982, 32:671.

Williams DL, et al: Herpes zoster following varicella vaccine in a child with acute lymphocytic leukemia. *J Pediatr* 1985, 106:259. ▲

Epstein-Barr Virus

Infectious mononucleosis, also known as *glandular fever,* is characterized by fever, adenopathy, splenomegaly, lymphocytosis with atypical lymphocytes, and evidence of acute infection by Epstein-Barr virus (EBV). After an incubation period of 3 to 7 weeks, bilateral enlargement of the cervical lymph nodes and, at times, of the axillary and inguinal nodes develops with accompanying fever as high as 40° C (104° F), malaise, and headache. Pharyngitis is the most frequent sign, with hyperplasia of the pharyngeal lymphoid tissue.

Cutaneous and mucous membrane lesions are present in 3% to 16% of patients with infectious mononucleosis. Edema of the eyelids and a macular or morbilliform rash may occur. The macular eruption is usually on the trunk and upper extremities. Scarlatiniform, herpetiform, erythema multiforme–like or Gianotti-Crosti–like eruptions, urticaria, and purpura are rare manifestations. One case of annular erythema of infancy was temporally related to EBV infection. The mucous membrane lesions consist of distinctive pinhead-sized petechiae, 5 to 20 in number, at the junction of the soft and hard palate (Forsheimer's spots).

Evaluation of blood shows absolute lymphocytosis and monocytosis with abnormally large lymphocytes. Atypical lymphocytes (Downey cells) usually represent at least 10% of the total leukocyte count. The white blood cell count ranges from 10,000 to 40,000/mm^3. Heterophile antibodies will be present in titers of 1:160 or higher. A rise in titer of EBV antibodies points to a diagnosis of infectious mononucleosis. The serologic responses to EBV and their use in clinical diagnosis are complex, as discussed by Straus et al. Treatment is symptomatic; there is no specific therapy. Antimicrobial agents have no effect on uncomplicated cases of infectious mononucleosis. If patients have severe pharyngeal involvement with encroachment on the airway, a short course of corticosteroid therapy is useful to induce a prompt antiinflammatory effect. Most patients recover completely.

Patients with mononucleosis treated with ampicillin or its analogs commonly develop a generalized, erythematous, morbilliform exanthem on the seventh to tenth day of therapy. The eruption lasts about 1 week. The eruption does not recur when these medications are given after the acute mononucleosis has resolved.

Chronic active EBV infection is rare. Two unusual skin eruptions have been described in patients with EBV. Spencer et al described a granuloma annulare–like eruption, and Drago et al reported a case of a chronic erythema multiforme–like eruption.

Oral hairy leukoplakia (OHL) is a distinctive condition strongly associated with EBV. It appears as poorly demarcated, corrugated white plaques seen on the lateral aspects of the tongue. Lesions on the other areas of the oral mucosa are simply white plaques without the typical corrugations. OHL can be distinguished from thrush by the fact that OHL cannot be removed by firm scraping with a tongue blade. More than a third of patients with AIDS have OHL. It is not restricted to patients with HIV infection; it also occurs in other immunosuppressed hosts, especially renal and bone marrow transplant recipients. EBV does not establish infection in the basal cell layer of the oral epithelium but is maintained by repeated direct infection of the epithelium by EBV in the oral cavity; it is not reactivation of EBV at the site. Only chronically immunosuppressed patients continuously shed EBV in their oral secretions; hence the restriction of OHL to immunosuppressed hosts. In normal persons a similar morphologic and histologic picture can be seen (pseudo-OHL), but EBV is not found in these patients' lesions. Thus, the finding of OHL warrants HIV testing. If results are negative, special histologic studies searching for EBV in the OHL biopsy should be performed. If EBV is found, a workup for immunosuppression is recommended.

OHL is usually asymptomatic and requires no treatment. If treatment is requested in immunosuppressed hosts, podophyllin applied for 30 seconds to 1 minute to the lesions once each month is the easiest treatment. Tretinoin gel applied topically twice daily or oral acyclovir, 400 mg five times daily, is also effective. Lesions recur when treatment is discontinued.

In immunosuppressed hosts, EBV may be responsible for lymphoproliferative disorders, which can be fatal. These include X-linked lymphoproliferative disease, as well as B cell proliferations, which may be monoclonal or polyclonal.

In immunocompetent hosts, EBV is associated with lymphoma. EBV is frequently found in patients with Hodgkin's disease, especially the mixed cellularity type. This may be useful in distinguishing Hodgkin's disease in the skin from lymphomatoid papulosis and anaplastic large cell lymphoma, both of which are negative for EBV.

Cosky RJ, et al: Ampicillin sensitivity in infectious mononucleosis. *Arch Dermatol* 1969, 100:717.

Drago F, et al: Epstein-Barr virus-related persistent erythema multiforme in chronic fatigue syndrome. *Arch Dermatol* 1992, 128:217.

Greenspan D, et al: Significance of oral hairy leukoplakia. *Oral Surg Oral Med Oral Pathol* 1992, 73:151.

Itin, PH: Oral hairy leukoplakia: 10 years on. *Dermatology* 1993, 187:159.

Kumar S, et al: Primary cutaneous Hodgkin's disease with evolution to systemic disease. *Am J Surg Pathol* 1996, 20:754.

Labbe A, et al: Gianotti-Crosti syndrome and Epstein-Barr virus infection. *J Pediatr* 1983, 102:1013.

Lowe NJ, et al: Gianotti-Crosti syndrome associated with Epstein-Barr virus infection. *J Am Acad Dermatol* 1989, 20:336.

Lozada-Nur F, et al: Oral hairy leukoplakia in nonimmunosuppressed patients. *Oral Surg Oral Med Oral Pathol* 1994, 78:599.

Naparstek Y, et al: Rash and infectious mononucleosis. *Ann Intern Med* 1982, 97:284.

Spencer SA, et al: Granuloma annulare-like eruption due to chronic Epstein-Barr virus infection. *Arch Dermatol* 1988, 124:250.

Straus SE, et al: Epstein-Barr Virus infections: Biology, pathogenesis, and management. *Ann Intern Med* 1993, 118:45. _____ ▲

Cytomegalic Inclusion Disease

Congenital cytomegalovirus (CMV) infection, as documented by CMV excretion, is found in 1% of newborns. Ninety percent of these children are asymptomatic. Clinical manifestations in infants may include jaundice, hepato-splenomegaly, cerebral calcifications, chorioretinitis, micro-cephaly, mental retardation, and deafness. Cutaneous manifestations may result from anemia and thrombocytopenia, with resultant petechiae, purpura, and ecchymoses. A generalized macular, papular, or nodular purpuric eruption may occur, giving the "blueberry muffin baby" appearance. Most symptomatic cases occur within the first 2 months of life. Neonatal disease is more severe and sequelae more frequent in neonates born of mothers with primary rather than recurrent CMV disease in pregnancy.

Fifty percent to 80% of immunocompetent adults and up to 100% of HIV-infected homosexual men are infected with CMV. Infection in adults may be acquired by exposure to infected children, by sexual transmission, and by transfusion of CMV-infected blood. Symptomatic infection in adults is unusual, resembles infectious mononucleosis caused by EBV, and may be accompanied by an urticarial or morbilliform eruption (especially if ampicillin is given).

CMV infection is very common in AIDS patients, most frequently causing retinitis (20% of patients), colitis (15% of patients), cholangitis, encephalitis, polyradiculomyopathy, and adrenalitis.

CMV infection in the skin, as reviewed by Toome et al, is very uncommon; most cases have occurred in immunosuppressed hosts. CMV is reported to cause painful, superficial ulcerations or fissures of the oral or anal area. Erosive diaper dermatitis is also described in pediatric patients with HIV disease. The lesions are clinically identical to HSV or VZV skin lesions, or appear to be like aphthous ulcerations. Concurrent CMV viremia has been variably present, and CMV retinitis is not often found. When anal ulceration occurs, CMV colitis may or may not coexist. The diagnosis is usually established by histologic identification of a specific "cytopathic CMV" effect in blood vessels in a skin lesion. CMV has not been reproducibly demonstrated in the epithelium of these ulcerative lesions, but only in the dermal vessels. As Garcia-Patos et al observed, determining a pathogenic role for CMV is difficult, since CMV may be expressed in inflamed skin without being the primary pathogen. It may be found in normal skin of CMV infected patients. Polymerase chain reaction and DNA hybridization may identify CMV in the tissue, but these do not prove its pathogenicity. Electron microscopy cannot distinguish among HSV, VZV, and CMV.

CMV ulcerations have resolved with topical therapy not directed at the virus, such as topical steroids. Specific treatment for CMV with ganciclovir or foscarnet may not lead to improvement. Such therapies are also effective against HSV and VZV, making it difficult to conclude that eradication of CMV led to improvement of the ulcerative lesion. Until this situation is further defined, a diagnosis of CMV ulceration should not be made until all other diagnostic possibilities have been excluded. Such ulcer-ations should be managed with antiherpetic agents: initially, high-dose acyclovir (doses effective for VZV) and if this fails, foscarnet. Ganciclovir and cidofovir are alternatives. Lesions that fail to respond to antiviral therapy may be considered aphthous equivalents and can be treated with topical or intralesional corticosteroids. Other described patterns of cutaneous CMV infection include purpura (either palpable or nonpalpable), and one case of a purpuric vesiculobullous eruption has been described. In the latter case, CMV was reported to have been cultured from the skin, but the isolated virus was not identified by specific antisera. Whether these represent true cases of cutaneous CMV disease or expression of CMV in inflamed tissue is unclear.

Garcia-Patos V, et al: Cytomegalovirus-induced cytopathic changes in skin biopsy specimens. *Arch Dermatol* 1992, 128:1552.

Horn TD, et al: Cytomegalovirus is predictably present in perineal ulcers from immunosuppressed patients. *Arch Dermatol* 1990, 126:642.

Jones AC, et al: Cytomegalovirus infections of the oral cavity. *Oral Surg Oral Med Oral Pathol* 1993, 75:76.

Pass RF, et al: Young children as a probable source of maternal and congenital cytomegalovirus infection. *N Engl J Med* 1987, 316:1366.

Puy-Montbrun T, et al: Anal ulcerations due to cytomegalovirus in patients with AIDS. *Dis Colon Rectum* 1990, 33:1041.

Thiboutot DM: Cytomegalovirus diaper dermatitis. *Arch Dermatol* 1991, 127:396.

Toome BK, et al: Diagnosis of cutaneous cytomegalovirus infection. *J Am Acad Dermatol* 1991, 24:857. ▲

Human Herpesviruses 6 and 7 (HHV-6, HHV-7)

Roseola Infantum (Exanthem Subitum, Sixth Disease).

Roseola infantum is a common cause of sudden, unexplained high fever in young children between 6 and 36 months of age. Prodromal fever is usually high; convulsions and lymphadenopathy may accompany it. Suddenly, on about the fourth day, the fever drops. Coincident with the drop in temperature, a morbilliform erythema consisting of rose-colored discrete macules appears on the neck, trunk, and buttocks and sometimes on the face and extremities. Often there is a blanched halo around the lesions. The eruption may also be papular or, rarely, even vesicular. The mucous membranes are spared. Complete resolution of the eruption occurs in 1 to 2 days.

Infection with HHV-6 is almost universal in adults, with seropositivity in the 80% to 85% range in the United States and seroprevalence almost 100% in children. There are intermittent periods of viral reactivation throughout life; persistent infection occurs in several organs, and particularly in the CNS. Acute seroconversion to HHV-6 and HHV-7 appears to be responsible for about one third of roseola cases each; in another third neither is found. HHV-6 infection occurs earlier than HHV-7 does, and second episodes of roseola in HHV-6 seropositive children may be caused by HHV-7. Primary infection with HHV-6 is associated with roseola only 9% of the time, and 18% of children with seroconversion have a rash. Primary infection may occur with only fever and no rash or rash without fever. Other common findings include otitis media, diarrhea, and bulging fontanelles, sometimes with findings of meningo-encephalitis. Uncommonly, hepatitis, intussusception, and even fatal multisystem disease may occur. In adults, acute HHV-6 infection resembles acute mononucleosis. Viral recovery is reduced in patients receiving acyclovir therapy, but ganciclovir is the recommended agent for treatment of severe disease associated with HHV-6.

As with other herpesviruses, the pattern of disease in HHV-6 may be different in immunosuppressed hosts. Chronic macular or papular generalized exanthems have been reported in two patients, one following bone marrow transplantation for severe combined immunodeficiency and one with acute leukemia who was undergoing chemotherapy. In the latter patient, the eruption cleared with recovery of the bone marrow.

Campodelli-Fiume G, et al: HHV-6. *Emerg Infect Dis* 1999, 5:353.
Fujita H, et al: HHV-6-associated exanthema in a patient with acute lymphocytic leukaemia. *Br J Haematol* 1996, 92:947.
Michel D, et al: Human herpesvirus 6 DNA in exanthematous skin in BMT patient. *Lancet* 1994, 344:686.
Pruksananonda P, et al: Primary human herpesvirus 6 infection in young children. *N Engl J Med* 1992, 326:1445.
Suga S, et al: Detection of HHV-6 DNAs in samples from several body sites of patients with exanthem subitum and their mothers by polymerase chain reaction assay. *J Med Virol* 1995, 46:52.
Tanaka K, et al: HHV-7: another causal agent for roseola (exanthem subitum). *J Pediatr* 1994, 125:1.
Torigoe S, et al: Clinical manifestations associated with HHV-7 infection. *Arch Dis Child* 1995, 72:518.
Yoshida M, et al: Exanthem subitum (roseola infantum) with vesicular lesions. *Br J Dermatol* 1995, 132:614. _____ ▲

Human Herpesvirus 8 (HHV-8)

HHV-8, a gamma herpesvirus, is most closely related to EBV and *Herpesvirus saimiri*. It has been found in virtually all patients with Kaposi's sarcoma (KS), including those who have AIDS, in African cases, cases in elderly men from the Mediterranean basin, and in transplant patients with KS. In addition, the seropositivity rate (infection rate) for this virus correlates with the prevalence of KS in a given population. Seroprevalence is high in endemic areas in Africa, in HIV-infected gay men (but not women or children with HIV), and to a lesser degree, in Italians. Finally, infection with HHV-8 precedes and predicts subsequent development of KS in HIV-infected men. HHV-8 can be found in KS lesions, saliva, and in circulating blood cells in infected patients. HHV-8 is also found in the semen of up to 20% of patients with KS, explaining its sexual transmission.

HHV-8 is present in a rare type of B-cell lymphoma called *body cavity–based B-cell lymphoma,* which presents

with pleural, pericardial, and peritoneal malignant effusions. HHV-8 is also found in all cases of Castleman's disease associated with HIV infection and a large proportion of cases in HIV-negative persons.

Gaspari A, et al: Identification of HHV-8 DNA in the skin lesions of Kaposi's sarcoma in an immunocompromised patient with bullous pemphigoid. *J Am Acad Dermatol* 1997, 37:843.
Henghold WB, et al: Kaposi sarcoma-associated herpesvirus/HHV-8 and EBV in iatrogenic Kaposi sarcoma. *Arch Dermatol* 1997, 133:109.
Moore PS, et al: Detection of herpesvirus-like DNA sequences in Kaposi's sarcoma in patients with and those without HIV infection. *N Engl J Med* 1995, 332:1181.
Smith NA, et al: Serologic evidence of HHV-8 transmission by homosexual but not heterosexual sex. *J Infect Dis* 1999, 180:600. _____ ▲

B Virus

B virus (*Herpesvirus simiae*) infects macaques and other monkeys. Vesicular lesions similar to herpes simplex are seen on the oral mucosal surfaces as well as the lips or skin in these animals. Humans become infected after being bitten, scratched, or contaminated by an animal shedding B virus. Usually these patients are animal handlers or researchers. Benson et al reviewed 22 cases of symptomatic human infection. Within a few days after the bite, a vesicular eruption may occur at the site of inoculation. It is the rapid progression to fatal encephalitis that is feared: 15 of 22 reported cases died, and all survivors of encephalitis suffered severe neurologic sequelae. Treatment with acyclovir or ganciclovir has been successful in some cases, but other patients similarly treated have died. Because *H. simiae* infection may recur after a period of latency, lifetime surveillance is required.

Benson PM, et al: B virus (*Herpesvirus simiae*) and human infection. *Arch Dermatol* 1989, 125:1247.
Centers for Disease Control: B virus infections in humans. *MMWR* 1987, 36:289.
Holmes GP, et al: B virus (*Herpesvirus simiae*) infection in humans. *Ann Intern Med* 1990, 112:833. _____ ▲

Gianotti-Crosti Syndrome (Papular Acrodermatitis of Childhood, Papulovesicular Acrolocated Syndrome)

Gianotti-Crosti syndrome includes cases with or without hepatitis B infection that resemble the initial cases described by Gianotti. Other implicated infectious agents have included cytomegalovirus, Epstein-Barr virus, enteroviruses (coxsackie A-16), vaccinia virus, rotavirus, poliovaccine virus, hepatitis A, respiratory syncytial virus, parainfluenza virus, and streptococcus. Most cases in the United States are not associated with hepatitis B infection. The clinical features of the eruption caused by the other agents cannot be distinguished from hepatitis B–associated Gianotti-Crosti syndrome, so the synonymous terms listed above can be used interchangeably, or, as Caputo recommends, the latter terms discarded.

The condition affects children between 6 months and 14 years of age (median age, 2 years). The eruption is characterized by a monomorphous eruption of flat-topped, erythematous, 1- to 5-mm papules or papulovesicles that erupt suddenly and symmetrically, favoring the face, buttocks and extensor limbs, and sparing the trunk (Figs. 19-24 and 19-25). This is in contrast to most viral exanthems which are concentrated on the trunk. The lesions develop over a few days but last longer than most viral exanthems (2 to 4 weeks). Pruritus is variable, and the mucous membranes are spared, except when inflamed by the associated infectious agent.

Depending on the cause, the lymph nodes, mainly inguinal and axillary, are moderately enlarged for 2 to 3 months. Splenomegaly, if present, is slight and rarely lasts long. In cases associated with hepatitis B, acute viral hepatitis occurs, beginning at the same time as or 1 to 2 weeks after onset of the skin eruption. It is generally anicteric, but in some children jaundice may appear about 20 days after onset of the skin eruption. The liver usually remains moderately enlarged, but not tender, for 1 to 2 months. No treatment appears to shorten the course of the disease, which is self-limited. Children with hepatitis B–associated disease may develop chronic active or chronic persistent hepatitis.

Boeck K, et al: Gianotti-Crosti syndrome. *Cutis* 1998, 62:271.

Caputo R, et al: Gianotti-Crosti syndrome. *J Am Acad Dermatol* 1992, 26:207.

Hoffman B, et al: Gianotti-Crosti syndrome associated with EBV infection. *Pediatr Dermatol* 1997, 14:273.

Velangi SS, et al: Gianotti-Crosti after MMR vaccination. *Br J Dermatol* 1998, 139:1122. _____ ▲

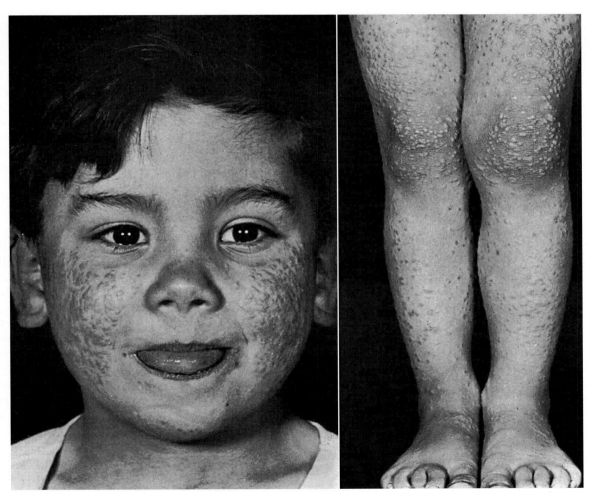

Fig. 19-24   Gianotti-Crosti syndrome. (Courtesy Dr. M. Eiloart.)

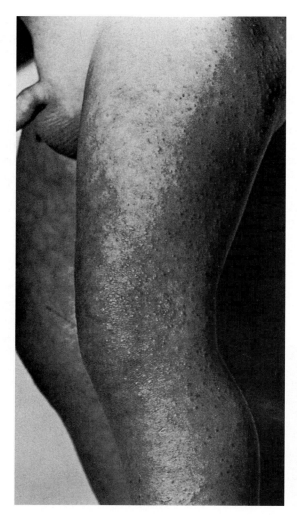

Fig. 19-25 Gianotti-Crosti syndrome. (Courtesy Dr. M.J. Woerdeman, Amsterdam.)

MANIFESTATIONS OF INFECTIOUS HEPATITIS
Hepatitis B Antigenemia

Ten percent to 20% of persons with acute hepatitis B virus (HBV) infection have a serum sickness–like illness with urticaria, arthralgias, and occasionally, arthritis, glomerulonephritis, or vasculitis. These symptoms appear several days to weeks before the onset of clinically apparent liver disease. Immune complexes containing hepatitis B surface antigen and low levels of complement occur in the serum and in joint fluid. The process spontaneously resolves as antigen is cleared from the blood.

Hepatitis B is also associated with polyarteritis nodosa (PAN) in 10% to 50% of cases. This usually occurs within the first 6 months of infection, even during the acute phase, but may occur as long as 12 years after infection. Unlike the urticarial reaction, which is usually associated eventually with the development of clinical hepatitis, hepatitis B infection associated with PAN may be silent. Guillevin et al

reported successful management of hepatitis B–associated PAN: they combined short-duration corticosteroid agents, plasma exchange, and antiviral therapy (vidarabine or interferon-alfa).

Leyden et al reported that in a survey of 593 dermatologists, 15.4% demonstrated evidence of previous infection by HBV, indicating the high risk in this profession for acquisition of HBV infection. All health care workers who have not had a hepatitis B infection should be vaccinated against it.

Hepatitis C

Hepatitis C virus (HCV) is responsible for the majority of non-A, non-B viral hepatitis. Infection is persistent, leading to chronic hepatitis (50% to 70% of cases), cirrhosis (20% to 30% of cases), and hepatocellular carcinoma. Chronic HCV infection is associated with various skin disorders, either by direct effect or as a consequence of the associated hepatic damage. Hepatitis C infection may cause pruritus without evidence of cholestasis.

Cutaneous necrotizing vasculitis, which is usually associated with a circulating type II cryoglobulin, has been frequently reported in association with HCV. In 84% of cases of type II cryoglobulinemia the patients have an HCV infection. Two percent to 5% of HCV-infected patients develop cutaneous vasculitis, and this finding often leads to the discovery of previously undiagnosed HCV infection. The most common clinical presentation is palpable purpura of the lower extremities. Livedo reticularis and urticaria may also occur. Histologically, in all cases a leukocytoclastic vasculitis is seen. Arthropathy, glomerulonephritis, and neuropathy frequently accompany the skin eruption. Interferon alfa treatment may lead to improvement of the vasculitis, but it frequently recurs when the interferon is stopped. In some cases the vasculitis may involve small arteries, giving a histologic pattern, similar to that seen in PAN. In various studies 12% to 31% of patients with PAN were HCV positive, suggesting that both HBV and HCV can cause PAN.

Patients with porphyria cutanea tarda (PCT) often have hepatocellular abnormalities. Depending on the prevalence of HCV infection in the population studied, between 10% and 95% of sporadic (not familial) PCT cases are HCV associated. Treatment of the HCV infection with interferon may lead to improvement of the PCT.

In 4% to 38% of cases of lichen planus, an HCV infection is present. Interferon treatment may or may not improve the lichen planus condition. HCV may also be associated with cutaneous B-cell lymphoma.

Agnello V, et al: A role for hepatitis C virus infection in type II cryoglobulinemia. *N Engl J Med* 1992, 327:1490.

Carson CW, et al: Frequency and significance of antibodies to hepatitis C virus in polyarteritis nodosa. *J Rheumatol* 1993, 20:304.

Cribier B, et al: Systematic cutaneous examination in hepatitis C virus infected patients. *Acta Derm Venereol* 1998, 78:355.

Doutre MS: Hepatitis C virus-related skin diseases. *Arch Dermatol* 1999, 135:1401.

Dupin N, et al: Essential mixed cryoglobulinemia. *Arch Dermatol* 1995, 131:1124.

Guillevin L, et al: Polyarteritis nodosa related to hepatitis B virus. *Medicine* 1995, 74:238.

Karlsberg PL, et al: Cutaneous vasculitis and rheumatoid factor positivity as presenting signs of hepatitis C virus-induced mixed cryoglobulinemia. *Arch Dermatol* 1995, 131:1119.

Levey JM, et al: Mixed cryoglobulinemia in chronic hepatitis C infection. *Medicine* 1994, 73:53.

Leyden JJ, et al: Serologic survey for markers of hepatitis B infection in dermatologists. *J Am Acad Dermatol* 1985, 12:676.

McKiernan S, et al: Primary cutaneous B cell lymphoma. *Eur J Gastro Hepatol* 1999, 11:669.

Misiani R, et al: Interferon alfa-2a therapy in cryoglobulinemia associated with hepatitis C virus. *N Engl J Med* 1994, 330:751.

Pawlotsky JM, et al: Hepatitis C virus in dermatology. *Arch Dermatol* 1995, 131:1185.

Sovfir N, et al: Hepatitis C virus infection in cutaneous PAN. *Arch Dermatol* 1999, 135:1001.

Tsukazaki N, et al: Porphyria cutanea tarda and hepatitis C virus infection. *Br J Dermatol* 1998, 138:1015.

von Kobyletzki G, et al: Severe therapy-resistant necrotizing vasculitis associated with hepatitis C virus infection. *Br J Dermatol* 1998, 138:926. _____ ▲

POXVIRUS GROUP

The poxviruses are DNA viruses of a high molecular weight. The viruses are 200 to 300 nm in diameter.

Variola Major (Smallpox)

Smallpox was eradicated worldwide in 1977. It had an incubation period of 12 days, after which there was a sudden onset of fever and malaise, which ceased abruptly and completely when the exanthem appeared. The lesions were distributed in a centrifugal pattern; the face, arms, and legs more heavily involved than the trunk. Beginning as erythematous macules, the lesions all in synchrony became papular and evolved progressively through the vesicular and pustular stages to crusts in about 2 weeks. The crusts separated, leaving fresh scars, which were permanent in half the survivors. A variety of complications occurred, including pneumonitis, corneal destruction, encephalitis, joint effusions, and osteitis. Immunity is lifelong. The mortality rate was 5% to 40%.

Glickman FS: A ring around the rosie (the rash that was). *J Am Acad Dermatol* 1987, 16:1282. _____ ▲

Vaccinia

The vaccinia virus has been propagated in laboratories for immunization against smallpox. Vaccinia virus–induced dermatoses resulted from complications of vaccination against smallpox.

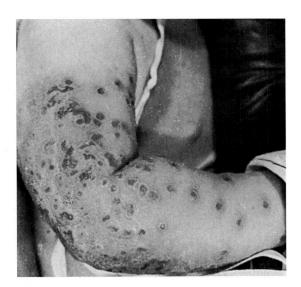

Fig. 19-26   Vaccinia. (Courtesy Dr. F. Daniels, Jr.)

Vaccination. Reactions to vaccination have been divided into three types. Primary response occurred in susceptible persons. On the fifth day a papule appeared that became a vesicle; on the ninth day a maximal reaction appeared, usually as a pustule with regional lymph node enlargement. The accelerated response (in the partially immune patients) consisted of a small vesicle on the fifth day, which involuted by the tenth day. In immune persons, the immune or immediate reaction occurred: a papule appeared that involuted rapidly by the third day after vaccination.

Generalized Vaccinia. Four to 10 days after vaccination, a generalized vaccinia eruption may occur (Fig. 19-26). The lesions are first papulovesicles that become pustules and involute in 3 weeks, although successive crops may occur within that time. Complications are ocular paralysis and postvaccinial retinitis.

Autoinoculation. Accidental inoculation of vaccinia may occur from contact with one's own vaccination or from contact with another person's vaccination site (Fig. 19-27).

Eczema Vaccinatum. Eczema vaccinatum is analogous to eczema herpeticum, representing vaccinia virus infection superimposed on a chronic dermatitis, usually atopic dermatitis (Fig. 19-28). The vesicles appear suddenly, mostly in eczematous areas. The lesions are sometimes umbilicated and appear in crops, resembling smallpox or chickenpox. The onset is sudden, and fresh vesicles appear for several days. Scarring is common. Often there is cervical adenopathy, fever, and prostration, sometimes ending in death. Encephalitis and other neurologic disturbances are not uncommon.

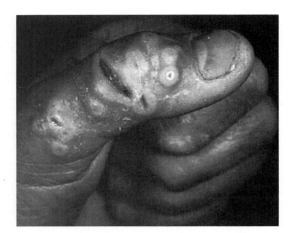

Fig. 19-27 Autoinoculation from vaccinia vaccination.

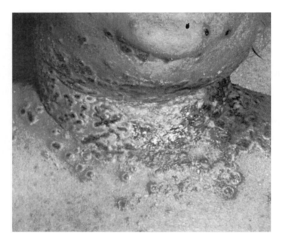

Fig. 19-28 Eczema vaccinatum with multiple umbilicated lesions. (Courtesy Dr. W.B. Muston, Australia.)

Vaccinia Necrosum. Gangrenous vaccinia is rare, occurring principally in infants under 6 months of age who are immunodeficient. The vesicular lesions involve the skin and mucous membranes and persist for months, becoming progressively gangrenous, until death occurs. Necrotic lesions may occur throughout the body. Vaccinia immune globulin, which is available from the American Red Cross, should be used in these severe cases. Such a reaction was observed in a military recruit who had undiagnosed HIV infection.

Vaccination for smallpox should no longer be given, except as determined by the armed forces. Lane reported 68 deaths in the United States from complications of smallpox vaccination from 1959 to 1968: 19 from vaccinia necrosum, 36 from postvaccinial encephalitis, 12 from eczema vaccinatum, and 1 from Stevens-Johnson syndrome.

Roseola Vaccinia. Roseola vaccinia is characterized by an extensive symmetrical eruption of macules and papules

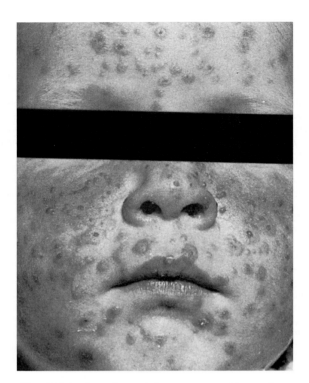

Fig. 19-29 Roseola vaccinia; a monomorphic eruption.

that appears 2 weeks after a primary smallpox vaccination (Fig. 19-29). In addition to the morbilliform eruption, the vaccination site contains a crust and is surrounded by a large erythematous halo. Individual lesions are discrete and do not coalesce to form a scarlatiniform eruption. The patient is afebrile, and no other signs or symptoms are present. Involution takes place in a few days.

Other Skin Lesions in Vaccination Scars. Marmelzat reported 6 cases of melanoma, 13 cases of basal cell carcinomas and 5 cases of squamous cell carcinoma that occurred in vaccination scars. Benign lesions with a tendency to occur in scars, such as sarcoidosis and granuloma annulare, also can occur in vaccination scars.

James WD: Autoinoculation vaccinia. *J Assoc Milit Dermatol* 1984, 10:21.
Lane JM, et al: Complications of smallpox vaccination. *N Engl J Med* 1969, 281:1201.
Marmelzat WL: Malignant tumors in smallpox vaccination scars. *Arch Dermatol* 1968, 94:400.
Reed WB, et al: Malignant tumors as a late complication of vaccination. *Arch Dermatol* 1968, 98:132. _____ ▲

Cowpox

Cowpox is an orthopoxvirus related to smallpox and vaccinia that is geographically restricted to Britain, Europe, Russia, and adjacent states. It is largely a zoonosis that rarely affects cattle. The domestic cat is the usual source of

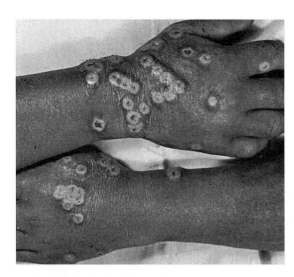

Fig. 19-30 Typical cowpox on hands of an Australian dairyman. Note umbilication. (Courtesy Dr. A. Johnson, Australia.)

human infection, but the animal reservoirs are apparently small wild mammals. Most cases occur in the late summer and in autumn.

Lesions are usually solitary (72%). They occur on the hands and fingers in half the cases and the face in another third. Secondary lesions are uncommon (Fig. 19-30), and generalized disease is rare, occurring usually in patients with atopic dermatitis. The lesion progresses from a macule through a vesicular stage, then a pustule that becomes blue-purple and hemorrhagic. A hard, painful, 1 to 3 cm indurated eschar develops after 2 to 3 weeks. Lesions are always painful, and there is local lymphadenopathy. Patients are systemically ill until the eschar stage. Healing usually takes 6 to 8 weeks. Scarring is common. Acyclovir has no activity against the virus.

The diagnosis is established by viral culture, electron microscopy, or serologies. Histologic evaluation in human cases has not revealed diagnostic cytoplasmic inclusions but has revealed vacuolar degeneration of the epidermis, as is typical of a viral blister. Milker's nodule is not painful, and adenopathy is rare (see discussion below). Anthrax is also painless and develops an eschar by day 6.

Farmyard Pox

Because closely related parapoxviruses of sheep and cattle cause similar disease in humans, orf and milkers' nodules have been collectively called *farmyard pox.* The epidemiologic features are discussed separately, but the clinical and histologic features, which are identical, are discussed jointly. The diagnosis of these infections is based on taking an accurate history. The diagnosis can virtually always be confirmed by routine histologic evaluation.

Milker's Nodules. Also known as *paravaccinia* or *pseudocowpox,* milker's nodule is a worldwide occupational dis-

ease of milkers or veterinarians, most commonly directly transmitted from the udders of infected cows. Lesions are usually solitary or only a few in number and are confined to the hands or forearms. Schuler et al reported four patients who developed numerous lesions in healing first- and second-degree burns. These cases had occurred on farms with infected cattle, but the patients had not had direct contact with the cattle, suggesting indirect viral transmission.

Orf. Also known as *ecthyma contagiosum, contagious pustular dermatosis, sheep pox,* and *infectious labial dermatitis,* orf is a common disease in sheep-farming regions throughout the world. Direct transmission from active lesions on lambs is most common, but infection from fomites is also frequent, since the virus is resistant to heat and dryness. Autoinoculation to the genital area can occur, but human-to-human transmission is rare.

Clinical Features of Farmyard Pox
The incubation period for farmyard pox is about 1 week. Lesions evolve through six stages: (1) The lesion begins as a papule, which then becomes a target lesion with a red center surrounded successively with a white ring and then a red halo (Fig. 19-31); (2) next is the acute stage, in which a red, weeping nodule not unlike pyogenic granuloma appears (Figs. 19-32 and 19-33); (3) in a hairy area, temporary alopecia ensues; (4) during the regenerative stage, the lesion becomes dry with black dots on the surface; (5) the nodule then becomes papillomatous; and (6) finally flattens to form a dry crust, eventually healing. Lesions are usually about 1 cm, except in immunosuppressed patients, in whom giant lesions may occur. Spontaneous resolution occurs in about 6 weeks, leaving minimal scarring. Mild swelling, fever, pain, and lymphadenitis may accompany the lesions, but these symptoms are milder than those seen in cowpox. Orf may be associated with an erythema multiforme–like eruption in about 5% of cases. Treatment is supportive, although shave excision may accelerate healing.

Histologic Features of Farmyard Pox
Histologic features correlate with the clinical stage. Nodules show a characteristic pseudoepitheliomatous hyperplasia covered by a parakeratotic crust. Keratinocytes always demonstrate viropathic changes of nuclear vacuolization and cytoplasmic 3 to 5 μ eosinophilic inclusions surrounded by a pale halo. The papillary dermis is markedly edematous. The dermal infiltrate, which is dense and extends from the interface to the deep dermis, consists of lymphocytes, histiocytes, neutrophils, and eosinophils. Massive capillary proliferation and dilation are present in the upper dermis.

Bovine Papular Stomatitis

Bovine papular stomatitis, a disease of cattle, has a cutaneous form in humans. The incubation period is 5 to 8

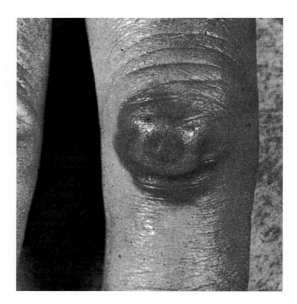

Fig. 19-31 Orf on index finger of a 37-year-old woman, acquired through feeding "Bummer" lambs in Northern California. (Courtesy Dr. R.C. Rucker.)

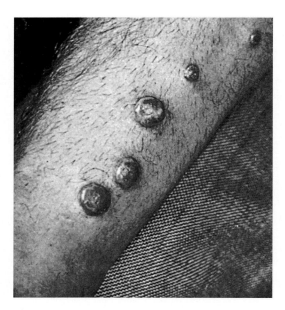

Fig. 19-33 Orf on forearm. (Courtesy Dr. B. Barrack, Australia.)

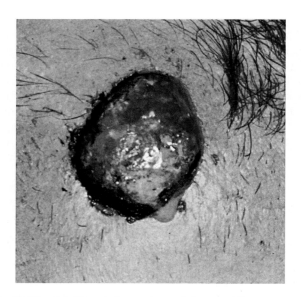

Fig. 19-32 Orf. Ulcerated, weeping nodule resembling a pyogenic granuloma. (From Leavell UW, Jr: *JAMA* 1968, 204:657.)

days. The clinical lesions, which are identical to those of milker's nodule or orf in humans, last about 3 weeks. The affected cattle may not have mucocutaneous lesions, which distinguishes the condition from milker's nodule. The diagnosis is confirmed by isolation of the virus in culture. The disease is self-limited.

Parapoxvirus Infections from Wildlife

Smith et al reported two patients with solitary lesions on the fingers, one following direct inoculation while cleaning a deer and another at the site of a cut sustained on a camping trip in an area with wild deer. Lesions were present for more than 2 months before biopsy. Histologically, there was marked hyperkeratosis, parakeratosis, and pseudoepitheliomatous hyperplasia. The midepidermal cells showed vacuolization with pyknotic nuclei. There was no intraepidermal or subepidermal vesiculation. The dermis had prominent vascular proliferation and a mild mononuclear cell infiltrate. Viral particles were identified by electron microscopy in the keratinocytes.

Bassioukas K, et al: Orf: clinical and epidemiological study. *Australas J Dermatol* 1993, 34:119.

Baxby D, et al: Human cowpox 1969-93: a review based on 54 cases. *Br J Dermatol* 1994, 131:598.

Blackford S, et al: Cowpox infection causing a generalized eruption in a patient with atopic dermatitis. *Br J Dermatol* 1993, 129:628.

Bowman KF, et al: Cutaneous form of bovine papular stomatitis in man. *JAMA* 1981, 246:2813.

Groves RW, et al: Human orf and milkers' nodule: a clinicopathologic study. *J Am Acad Dermatol* 1991, 25:706.

Kennedy CTC, et al: Perianal orf. *J Am Acad Dermatol* 1984, 11:72.

Savage J, et al: Giant orf of finger in a patient with a lymphoma. *Proc R Soc Med* 1972, 65:766.

Schuller G, et al: The syndrome of milker's nodules in burn injury. *J Am Acad Dermatol* 1982, 6:332.

Shelley WB: Surgical treatment of farmyard pox: Orf, milkers' nodules, bovine papular stomatitis pox. *Cutis* 1983, 31:191.

Smith KJ, et al: Parapoxvirus infections acquired after exposure to wildlife. *Arch Dermatol* 1991, 127:79.

Stead JW, et al: Rare case of autoinoculation of orf. *Br J Gen Practice* 1992, 42:395.

Zimmerman JL: Orf. *JAMA* 1991, 266:476. ▲

Molluscum Contagiosum

Molluscum contagiosum is caused by up to four closely related types of poxvirus, MCV-1 to -4, and their variants. Although the proportion of infection caused by the various types varies geographically, throughout the world MCV-1 infections are most common. In small children virtually all infections are caused by MCV-1. There is no difference in the anatomic region of isolation with regard to infecting type (as opposed to herpes simplex virus for example). In patients infected with HIV, however, MCV-2 causes the majority of infections (60%), suggesting that HIV infection–associated molluscum does not represent recrudescence of childhood molluscum.

Infection with MCV is worldwide. Three groups are primarily affected: young children, sexually active adults, and immunosuppressed persons, especially those with HIV infection. Molluscum is most easily transmitted by direct skin to skin contact, especially if the skin is wet. Swimming pools have been associated with infection.

In all forms of infection, the lesions are relatively similar. Individual lesions are smooth surfaced, firm, dome shaped, pearly papules, averaging 3 to 5 mm in diameter (Fig. 19-34). Some "giant" lesions may be up to 1.5 cm in diameter. A central umbilication is characteristic. Irritated lesions may become crusted and even pustular, simulating secondary bacterial infection. This may precede spontaneous resolution. Lesions that rupture into the dermis may elicit a marked suppurative inflammatory reaction that resembles an abscess.

The clinical pattern depends on the risk group affected. In young children the lesions are usually generalized and number from a few to more than 100 (Fig. 19-35). Lesions tend to be on the face, trunk, and extremities. Genital lesions may occur as part of a wider distribution. When molluscum is restricted to only the genital area in a child, the possibility of sexual abuse must be considered.

In adults, molluscum is sexually transmitted, and other sexually transmitted diseases may coexist. There are usually less than 20 lesions; these favor the lower abdomen, upper thighs, and the penile shaft in men (Figs. 19-36 and 19-37). Mucosal involvement is very uncommon.

Immunosuppression, either systemic T-cell immunosuppression (usually HIV, but also sarcoidosis and malignancies) or abnormal cutaneous immunity (as in atopic dermatitis or topical steroid use), predisposes the individual to infection. In atopic dermatitis, lesions tend to be confined to dermatitic skin.

Secondary infection may occur. In addition in about 10% of lesions a surrounding eczematous reaction is present (molluscum dermatitis). Rarely, erythema annulare centrifugum may be associated. Lesions on the eyelid margin or conjunctiva may be associated with a conjunctivitis or keratitis. Rarely, the molluscum lesions may present as a cutaneous horn (molluscum contagiosum cornuatum).

Ten percent to 30% of patients with AIDS have

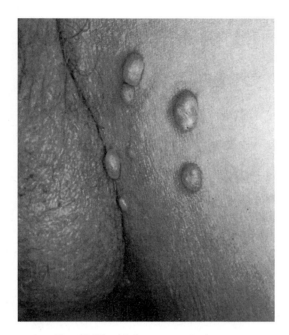

Fig. 19-34   Molluscum contagiosum.

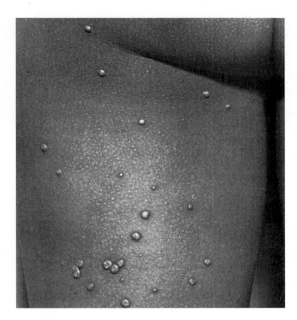

Fig. 19-35   Molluscum contagiosum. (Courtesy Dr. R. Walzer.)

molluscum contagiosum. Virtually all HIV-infected patients with MC have already had an AIDS diagnosis and have a helper T-cell count of less than 100. In HIV disease, lesions favor the face (especially the cheeks, neck, and eyelids) and genitalia (Fig. 19-38). They may be few or numerous, forming confluent plaques. Giant lesions are not uncommon and may be confused with a basal cell carcinoma. Involvement of the oral and genital mucosa may occur,

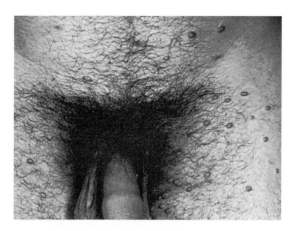

Fig. 19-36 Molluscum contagiosum. Sexual transmission is probable. (Courtesy Dr. H. Shatin.)

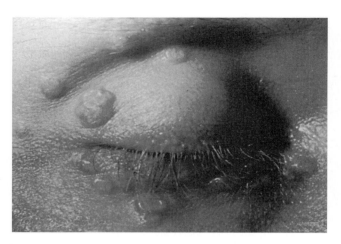

Fig. 19-38 Multiple large molluscum contagiosum lesions in patient with AIDS. (Courtesy Dr. Axel W. Hoke.)

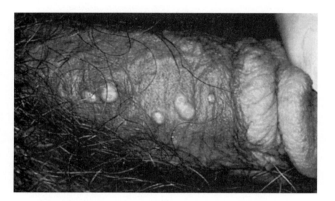

Fig. 19-37 Molluscum contagiosum on penis.

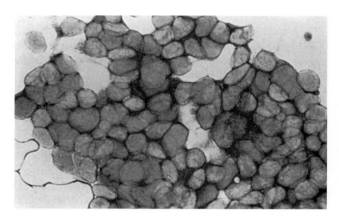

Fig. 19-39 Microscopic appearance of molluscum bodies smeared on a glass slide and stained with methylene blue. (Courtesy Dr. Axel W. Hoke.)

virtually always indicative of advanced AIDS (helper T-cell count less than 50). Facial disfigurement with numerous lesions can occur.

Molluscum contagiosum has a characteristic histopathology. The lesion is acanthotic and cup shaped. In the cytoplasm of the prickle cells, numerous small eosinophilic and later basophilic inclusion bodies, called *molluscum bodies* or *Henderson-Paterson bodies,* are formed. Eventually, their bulk compresses the nucleus to the side of the cell. In the fully developed lesion each lobule empties into a central crater. Inflammatory changes are slight or absent. Characteristic brick-shaped poxvirus particles are seen on electron microscopy in the epidermis. In AIDS patients, even normal-appearing skin may contain viral particles, suggesting that latent infection may occur.

The diagnosis is easily established in most instances because of the distinctive central umbilication of the dome-shaped lesion. This may be enhanced by light cryotherapy that leaves the umbilication appearing clear

against a white (frozen) background. For confirmation, Shelley's method of expressing the pasty core of a lesion can be used, squashing it between two microscope slides (or a slide and a coverglass) and staining it (Fig. 19-39). Firm compression between the slides is required.

The treatment used is determined by the clinical setting. There is no proven systemic antiviral agent. One study using cimetidine at a dose of 40 mg/kg per day for 2 months led to resolution in 90% of children who completed the therapy. These results need to be confirmed in a prospective randomized trial. In young children, especially those with numerous lesions, the most practical course may be to not treat or to use only topical tretinoin or imiquimod cream daily. Aggressive treatment may be emotionally traumatic and cause scarring. Spontaneous resolution is virtually a certainty in this setting, avoiding these sequelae. Individual lesions last 2 to 4 months each; the duration of infection is about 2 years. Continuous application of surgical tape to each lesion daily after bathing for 16 weeks led to cure in

90% of children so treated. If lesions are limited and the child cooperative, nicking the lesions with a blade to express the core (with or without the use of a comedo extractor), light cryotherapy, application of trichloracetic acid (35% to 100%), 10% potassium hydroxide, cantharidin applied for 4 to 8 hours, or removal by curettage are all good options. The application of EMLA for 1 hour before any painful treatments has made the treatment of molluscum in children much easier.

In adults with genital molluscum, removal by cryotherapy or curettage is very effective. In one study, podophyllotoxin 0.5% cream applied twice daily for 3 consecutive days per week for up to 12 weeks led to a 90% cure rate in non–HIV-infected Pakistani males. Sexual partners should be examined; screening for other coexistent sexually transmitted diseases is mandatory.

In patients with atopic dermatitis, application of EMLA followed by curettage or cryotherapy is most practical. Caustic chemicals should not be used on atopic skin. Topical steroid application to the area should be reduced to the minimum strength possible. A brief course of antibiotic therapy should be considered after initial treatment, since dermatitic skin is frequently colonized with *Staphylococcus aureus*.

In immunosuppressed patients, especially those with AIDS, management of molluscum can be very difficult. Aggressive treatment of the HIV infection with combination therapy, including a protease inhibitor, if it leads to improvement of the helper T-cell count, is often associated with a dramatic resolution of the lesions. This response is delayed 6 to 8 months from the institution of the treatment. Molluscum occurs frequently in the beard area, so shaving with a blade razor should be discontinued to prevent its spread. If lesions are few, curettage or core removal with a blade and comedo extractor are most effective. EMLA application may permit treatment without local anesthesia. Cantharone or 100% trichloracetic acid may be applied to individual lesions. Temporary dyspigmentation and slight surface irregularities may occur. Cryotherapy may be effective but must be used in caution in persons of pigment. Subcutaneous interferon alfa has been anecdotally effective. When lesions are numerous or confluent, treatment of the whole affected area may be required because of the possibility of latent infection. Trichloracetic acid peels above 35% concentration (medium depth), or daily applications of 5-fluorouracil to the point of skin erosion may eradicate lesions, at least temporarily. At times removal by curette is required. Electron beam has been effective. In patients with HIV infection, continuous application of tretinoin cream once nightly at the highest concentration tolerated seems to reduce the rate of appearance of new lesions. Topical cidofovir application and systemic infusion of this agent have been reported to lead to dramatic resolution of molluscum in patients with AIDS.

Brandrup F, et al: Molluscum contagiosum–induced comedo and secondary abscess formation. *Pediatr Dermatol* 1989, 6:118.

Castilla MT, et al: Molluscum contagiosum in children and its relationship to attendance at swimming pools. *Dermatology* 1995,191:165.

Charteris DG, et al: Ophthalmic molluscum contagiosum. *Br J Ophthalmol* 1995, 79:476.

Davies EG, et al: Topical cidofovir for severe molluscum contagiosum. *Lancet* 1999, 353:2042.

Dohil M, et al: Treatment of molluscum contagiosum with oral cimetidine. *Pediatr Dermatol* 1996, 13:310.

Epstein E: Cantharidin treatment of molluscum contagiosum. *Acta Derm Venereol* (Stockh) 1989, 69:91.

Garrett SJ, et al: Trichloroacetic acid peel of molluscum contagiosum in immunocompromised patients. *J Dermatol Surg Oncol* 1992, 18:885.

Gottlieb SL, et al: Molluscum contagiosum. *Int J Dermatol* 1994, 33:453.

Harrigan P, et al: Treatment of molluscum contagiosum with hypoallergenic surgical adhesive tape. *Cosmetic Dermatol* 1996, 9:46.

Hourihane J, et al: Interferon alpha treatment of molluscum contagiosum in immunodeficiency. *Arch Dis Child* 1999, 80:77.

Janniger CK, et al: Molluscum contagiosum in children. *Pediatr Dermatol* 1993, 52:194.

Koopman RJJ, et al: Molluscum contagiosum: a marker for advanced HIV infection. *Br J Dermatol* 1992, 126:528.

Meadows KP, et al: Resolution of recalcitrant molluscum contagiosum in HIV-infected patients treated with cidofovir. *Arch Dermatol* 1997, 133:987.

Nakamura J, et al: Analysis of molluscum contagiosum virus genomes isolated in Japan. *J Med Virol* 1995, 46:339.

Romiti R, et al: Treatment of molluscum contagiosum with potassium hydroxide. *Pediatr Dermatol* 1999, 16:228.

Rosdahl I, et al: Curettage of molluscum contagiosum in children. *Acta Derm Venereol* (Stockh) 1988, 68:149.

Schwartz JJ, et al: Molluscum contagiosum in patients with human immunodeficiency virus infection. *J Am Acad Dermatol* 1992, 27:583

Scolaro MJ, et al: Electron beam therapy for AIDS-related molluscum contagiosum lesions. *Radiology* 1999, 210:479.

Smith KJ, et al: Molluscum contagiosum. *Arch Dermatol* 1992, 128:223.

Syed TA, et al: Topical 0.3% and 0.5% podophyllotoxin cream for self-treatment of molluscum contagiosum in males. *Dermatology* 1994, 189:65.

Thompson CH, et al: Clinical and molecular aspects of molluscum contagiosum infection in HIV-1 positive patients. *Int J STD AIDS* 1992, 3:101. ▲

Human Monkeypox

Human monkeypox is a rare, sporadic zoonosis that occurs in remote areas of the tropical rainforests in central and western Africa. More than 90% of cases occur in children under 15 years of age, in whom the fatality rate is 11%. The disease is clinically similar to smallpox, with initial fever followed by a vesiculopustular eruption. The disease is less severe in persons previously vaccinated against smallpox. Most patients develop monkeypox from contact with wildlife sources, although many cases of human-to-human transmission occur. The attack rate among unvaccinated household contacts was 12%. Early lymphadenopathy was the most important sign in differentiating human monkeypox from smallpox and chickenpox.

Jezek Z, et al: Human monkeypox. *J Infect Dis* 1987, 156:293. ▲

PICORNAVIRUS GROUP

Picornavirus designates viruses that were originally called *enteroviruses* (polioviruses, coxsackieviruses, and echoviruses), plus the rhinoviruses. The picornaviruses are small, RNA-containing, icosahedral viruses varying in size from 20 to 30 nm. Only the coxsackieviruses, the echoviruses, and enterovirus type 71 are significant causes of skin disease.

Enterovirus Infections

Person-to-person transmission occurs by the intestinal-oral route and less commonly the respiratory route. Enteroviruses are identified by type-specific antigens. These type-specific antibodies appear in the blood about 1 week after infection has occurred and attain their maximum titer in 3 weeks. Unfortunately, the large number of enteroviruses precludes screening of acute and convalescent sera for all known types. Viral cultures obtained from the rectum, pharynx, eye, and nose may isolate the infecting agent. Usually the diagnosis is by clinical characteristics, and except in specific clinical settings, the causative virus is not identified.

Many nonspecific exanthems and enanthems that occur during the summer and early fall are caused by coxsackievirus or echovirus. The exanthems may be diffuse macular or morbilliform erythemas, vesicular lesions, or petechial or purpuric eruptions. Each type of exanthem has been associated with many subtypes of coxsackievirus or echovirus. Echovirus 9, the most prevalent enterovirus, causes a maculopapular exanthem initially on the face and neck, then the trunk and extremities. Only occasionally is there an eruption on the palms and soles. Small red or white lesions on the soft palate may occur. Rare presentations of enterovirus infection that have been reported include a unilateral vesicular eruption simulating herpes zoster, caused by echovirus 6; a fatal dermatomyositis-like illness in a patient with hypogammaglobulinemia, caused by echovirus 24; and a widespread vesicular eruption in atopic dermatitis that simulated Kaposi's varicelliform eruption, caused by coxsackievirus A-16.

Herpangina. Herpangina, a disease of children worldwide, is caused by multiple types of coxsackieviruses and echoviruses. It begins with acute onset of fever, headache, sore throat, dysphagia, anorexia, and sometimes, stiff neck. The most significant finding, which is present in all cases, is of one or more yellowish white, slightly raised 2 mm vesicles in the throat, usually surrounded by an intense areola. The lesions are found most frequently on the anterior faucial pillars, tonsils, uvula, or soft palate. Only one or two lesions might appear during the course of the illness, or the entire visible pharynx may be studded with them. The lesions often occur in small clusters and later coalesce. Usually the individual or coalescent vesicles ulcerate, leaving a shallow, punched-out, grayish yellow crater 2 to 4 mm in diameter. The lesions disappear in 5 to 10 days.

Treatment is supportive, consisting of topical anesthetics or allopurinol mouthwashes (3g/L).

Herpangina is differentiated from aphthosis and primary herpetic gingivostomatitis by the location of the lesions in the posterior oropharynx and by isolation of an enterovirus. Coxsackievirus A-10 causes acute lymphonodular pharyngitis, a variant of herpangina, characterized by discrete yellow-white papules in the same distribution as herpangina.

Hand-Foot-and-Mouth Disease. Infection begins with a fever and sore mouth. In 90% of cases oral lesions develop; these consist of small, rapidly ulcerating vesicles surrounded by a red areola on the buccal mucosa, tongue, soft palate, and gingiva. Lesions on the hands and feet are red papules that quickly become small, gray, 3 to 7 mm vesicles surrounded by a red halo. They are often oval, linear, or crescentic and run parallel to the skin lines on the fingers and toes (Fig. 19-40). They are distributed sparsely on the dorsa of the fingers and toes and more frequently on the palms and soles. Especially in children who wear diapers, vesicles and erythematous, edematous papules may occur on the buttocks. The infection is usually mild and seldom lasts more than a week. Treatment is supportive, with the use of oral topical anesthetics.

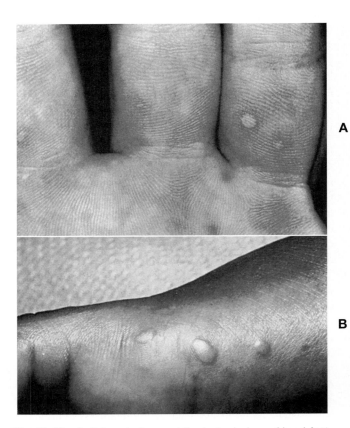

A

B

Fig. 19-40 A, Palmar lesions and **B,** plantar lesions of hand-foot-and-mouth disease. (Courtesy Dr. Axel W. Hoke.)

Hand-foot-and-mouth disease is most frequently caused by coxsackievirus A-16, although many other coxsackie A and B viruses as well as enterovirus 71 can cause it. The virus may be recovered from the skin vesicles. Histopathologic findings are those of an intraepidermal blister forming by vacuolar and reticular degeneration of keratinocytes similar to other viral blisters. Inclusion bodies and multinucleated giant cells are absent. Hand-foot-and-mouth syndrome is distinguished from herpangina by the distribution of the oral lesions and the presence of skin lesions. It is differentiated from erythema multiforme minor by the skin lesions, which are oval and gray, as opposed to targetoid, as in erythema multiforme.

Boston Exanthem Disease. The so-called Boston exanthem disease occurred as an epidemic in Boston and was caused by echovirus 16, a now uncommon cause of viral exanthems. The eruption consisted of sparsely scattered pale red macules and papules. In severe cases, the lesions were morbilliform and even vesicular. The eruption was chiefly on the face, chest, and back and in some cases on the extremities. On the soft palate and tonsils, small ulcerations like those of herpangina were noted. There was little or no adenopathy. The incubation period was 3 to 8 days.

Eruptive Pseudoangiomatosis. Young children during or immediately after a viral illness develop up to ten 2- to 4-mm blanchable red papules that resemble angiomas. These appear on the face, trunk, and extremities and resolve spontaneously within 10 days. Histologically, the lesions are composed of dilated superficial vessels without an increase in vessel number, distinguishing them from true angiomas. Echoviruses 25 and 32 have been implicated.

Boyd AS: Laboratory testing in patients with morbilliform viral eruptions. *Dermatol Clin* 1994, 12:69.

Calza A, et al: Eruptive pseudoangiomatosis: a unique childhood exanthem? *J Am Acad Dermatol* 1994, 31:517.

Dolin R: Enterovirus 71. *N Engl J Med* 1999, 341:984.

Frieden IJ, et al: Childhood exanthems old and new. *Pediatr Dermatol* 1991, 38:859.

Frieden IJ, et al: Viral infections. In Schachner LA, Hansen RC, editors: Pediatric dermatology. New York, 1995, Churchill Livingstone.

Goodyear HM, et al: Acute infectious erythemas in children. *Br J Dermatol* 1991, 124:433.

Messner J, et al: Accentuated viral exanthems in areas of inflammation. *J Am Acad Dermatol* 1999, 40:345.

Prose NS, et al: Eruptive pseudoangiomatosis: a unique childhood exanthem? *J Am Acad Dermatol* 1993, 29:857.

Thomas I, et al: Hand, foot, and mouth disease. *Pediatr Dermatol* 1993, 52:265.

Waldfahrer F, et al: Successful treatment of herpangina with allopurinol mouthwashes. *Laryngoscope* 1995, 105:1405. _____ ▲

PARAMYXOVIRUS GROUP

The paramyxoviruses are RNA viruses that range from 100 to 300 nm in size. In this group, the virus diseases of dermatologic interest are measles (rubeola) and German measles (rubella). Others viruses of this group are mumps virus, parainfluenza virus, Newcastle disease virus, and respiratory syncytial virus.

Measles

Also known as *rubeola* and *morbilli,* measles is a worldwide disease that in developed countries most commonly affects children under 15 months of age. It is spread by respiratory droplets and has an incubation period of 9 to 12 days. Currently available immunizations are highly effective, but in recent urban outbreaks about 20% of cases occurred in immunized children, emphasizing the importance of herd immunity.

The prodrome consists of fever, malaise, conjunctivitis, and prominent upper respiratory symptoms (nasal congestion, sneezing, coryza, and cough). After 1 to 7 days, the exanthem appears, usually as macular or maculopapular lesions on the anterior scalp line and behind the ears. Lesions begin as discrete erythematous papules that gradually coalesce. The rash spreads quickly over the face, then by the second or third day (unlike the more rapid spread of rubella) extends down the trunk to the extremities (Fig. 19-41). By the third day, the whole body is involved. Lesions are most prominent and confluent in the initially involved areas and may be more discrete on the extremities. Purpura may be present, especially on the extremities, and should not be confused with "black measles," a rare, disseminated intravascular coagulation–like complication of measles. Koplik's spots, which are pathognomonic, appear

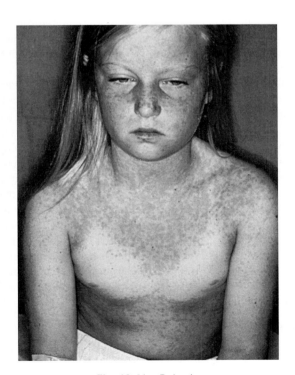

Fig. 19-41 Rubeola.

during the prodrome. They appear first on the buccal mucosa nearest to the lower molars as 1-mm white papules on an erythematous base. They may spread to involve other areas of the buccal mucosa and pharynx. After 6 to 7 days the exanthem clears, with simultaneous subsidence of the fever.

Complications include otitis media, pneumonia, encephalitis, and thrombocytopenic purpura. Infection in pregnant patients is associated with fetal death. Complications and fatalities are more common in malnourished and children with T-cell deficiencies. In HIV-infected children the exanthem may be less prominent.

Modified measles occurs in a partially immune host as a result of prior infection, persistent maternal antibodies, or immunization and is a milder disease. The course is shorter, the exanthem less confluent, and Koplik's spots may be absent. It is difficult to differentiate from other viral exanthems.

Atypical measles was seen in patients who received killed measles vaccine in the early to middle 1960s. The syndrome consists of fever, cough, headache, abdominal pain, myalgia, edema of extremities, pleural effusion, pneumonia, and hilar adenopathy. Morbilliform lesions occur on the skin, occasionally with intermingled petechiae or vesicles or both, beginning on the hands and feet and spreading centripetally. The main differential diagnosis is Rocky Mountain spotted fever.

A diagnosis of measles is established by the presence of a high fever, Koplik's spots, the characteristic conjunctivitis, upper respiratory symptoms, and typical exanthem. Lymphopenia is common, with a decreased white blood cell count. Biopsies of skin lesions may show syncytial keratinocytic giant cells, similar to those seen in respiratory secretions. Laboratory confirmation is usually with acute and convalescent serologic tests. German measles, scarlet fever, secondary syphilis, enterovirus infections, and drug eruptions are in the differential diagnosis. Administration of high doses of vitamin A will reduce the morbidity and mortality of hospitalized children with measles. Two doses of retinyl palmitate 200,000 IU 24 hours apart are recommended for all children 6 months to 24 months of age, for immunodeficient children, children with malnutrition or evidence of vitamin A deficiency, and in recent immigrants from areas of high measles mortality. Otherwise, treatment is symptomatic, with bed rest, analgesics, and antipyretics.

Live virus vaccination is recommended at 15 months with a booster at 5 years. A faint maculopapular exanthem may occur 7 to 10 days after immunization. When given up to 5 days after exposure, vaccination may prevent infection. Children less than 1 year of age who are exposed should be treated with immune serum globulin.

Rubella

Rubella, commonly known as *German measles,* is caused by a togavirus and probably spreads by respiratory secre-

tions. The incubation period is 12 to 23 days (usually 15 to 21). Live virus vaccination is highly effective, providing lifelong immunity.

There is a prodrome of from 1 to 5 days consisting of fever, malaise, sore throat, eye pain, headache, red eyes, runny nose, and adenopathy. Pain on lateral and upward eye movement is characteristic. The exanthem begins on the face and progresses caudad, covering the entire body in 24 hours and resolving by the third day (Fig. 19-42). The lesions are typically pale pink morbilliform macules, smaller than those of rubeola. The eruption may resemble roseola or erythema infectiosum. An enanthem of pinhead-sized red macules or petechiae on the soft palate and uvula (Forscheimer's sign) may be seen. Posterior cervical, suboccipital, and postauricular lymphadenitis occurs in more than half of cases. Rubella is in general a much milder disease than rubeola is. Arthritis and arthralgias are a common complication, especially in adult women. These last a month or longer.

Congenital Rubella Syndrome. Infants born to mothers who have had rubella during the first trimester of pregnancy may have congenital cataracts, cardiac defects, and deafness. Numerous other manifestations, such as glaucoma, microcephaly, and various visceral abnormalities, may emerge. Among the cutaneous expressions are thrombocy-

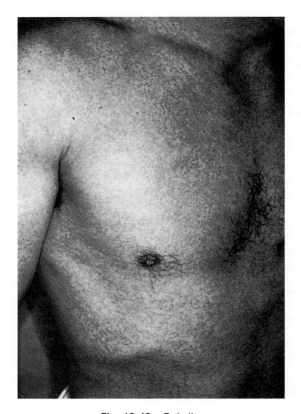

Fig. 19-42 Rubella.

topenic purpura; hyperpigmentation of the navel, forehead, and cheeks; bluish red infiltrated 2 to 8 mm lesions ("blueberry muffin" type), which represent dermal erythropoiesis; chronic urticaria; and reticulated erythema of the face and extremities.

Asymmetric Periflexural Exanthem of Childhood

This clinical syndrome, also known as *unilateral laterothoracic exanthem,* occurs primarily in the late winter and early spring, and affects girls more often than boys (1.2:1 to 2:1). It occurs in children 8 months to 10 years of age, but most cases are between 2 and 3 years of age. Its cause is unknown, but a viral origin has been proposed, since it occurs in young children and is seasonal, and secondary cases in families have been reported. Except for the isolation of parainfluenza virus in four cases and adenovirus in two cases of 26 cases in one study, no confirmation of this theory has been found. Clinically, two thirds to three fourths of affected children have symptoms of a mild upper respiratory or gastrointestinal infection, usually preceding the eruption. The lesions are usually discrete 1-mm erythematous papules that coalesce to poorly marginated morbilliform plaques. Pruritus is usually present, but mild. Lesions begin unilaterally close to a flexural area, usually the axilla. Spread is centrifugal with new lesions appearing on the adjacent trunk and extremity. Normal skin may intervene between lesions. The contralateral side is involved in 70% of cases, but the asymmetrical nature is maintained throughout the illness. Lymphadenopathy occurs in about 70% of cases. The syndrome lasts 2 to 6 weeks on average, but may last more than 2 months, and resolves spontaneously. Topical steroids and oral antibiotics are of no benefit, but oral antihistamines may help associated pruritus. Histologically, a mild to moderate lymphocytic (CD8-positive T cell) infiltrate surrounds and involves the eccrine ducts but not the secretory coils. There may be an accompanying interface dermatitis of the upper eccrine duct and adjacent epidermis.

Bialecki C, et al: The six classic childhood exanthems. *J Am Acad Dermatol* 1989, 21:891.

Bodemer C, et al: Unilateral laterothoracic exanthem in children. *J Am Acad Dermatol* 1992, 27:693.

Caballero B, et al: Low serum retinol is associated with increased severity of measles in New York City children. *Nutr Rev* 1992, 50:291.

Cherry JD: Contemporary infectious exanthems. *Clin Infect Dis* 1993, 16:199.

Coustou D, et al: Asymmetric periflexural exanthem of childhood. *Arch Dermatol* 1999, 135:799.

Current trends in measles—1987. *Arch Dermatol* 1988, 124:1627.

Davis RM, et al: Transmission of measles in medical settings, 1980 through 1984. *JAMA* 1986, 255:1295.

Edmonson MB, et al: Mild measles and secondary vaccine failure during a sustained outbreak in a highly vaccinated population. *JAMA* 1990, 263:2467.

Fine JD, et al: The TORCH syndrome: a clinical review. *J Am Acad Dermatol* 1985, 12:697.

Gelmetti C, et al: Asymmetric periflexural exanthem of childhood. *Pediatr Dermatol* 1994, 11:42.

Harangi F, et al: Asymmetric periflexural exanthem of childhood and viral examinations. *Pediatr Dermatol* 1995, 12:112.

Hussey GD, et al: A randomized, controlled trial of vitamin A in children with severe measles. *N Engl J Med* 1990, 323:160.

Markowitz LE, et al: Patterns of transmission of measles outbreaks in the United States, 1985—1986. *N Engl J Med* 1989, 320:75.

McCuaig CC, et al: Unilateral laterothoracic exanthem. *J Am Acad Dermatol* 1996, 34:979.

Wong RD, et al: Clinical and laboratory features of measles in hospitalized adults. *Am J Med* 1993, 95:377. _____ ▲

PARVOVIRUS GROUP
Erythema Infectiosum (Fifth Disease)

Erythema infectiosum is a worldwide benign infectious exanthem that occurs in epidemics in the late winter and early spring. It is caused by parvovirus B19 and is spread by respiratory droplets. In normal hosts (but not immunosuppressed or sickle cell patients in crisis), viral shedding has stopped by the time the exanthem appears, making isolation unnecessary. Most infections by parvovirus B19 cause either no exanthem or a nonspecific exanthem. The incubation period is 4 to 14 days (average, 7 days). Uncommonly, a mild prodrome of headache, runny nose, and low-grade fever may precede the rash by 1 or 2 days.

Erythema infectiosum has three phases. It begins abruptly with an asymptomatic erythema of the cheeks, referred to as *slapped cheek.* The erythema is typically diffuse and macular, but tiny translucent papules may be present. It is most intense beneath the eyes and may extend over the cheeks in a butterfly-wing pattern (Fig. 19-43). The perioral area, lids, and chin are usually unaffected. After 1 to 4 days the second phase begins, consisting of discrete erythematous macules and papules on the proximal extremities and later the trunk. This evolves into a reticulate or lacy pattern. These two phases typically last 5 to 9 days. A characteristic third phase is the recurring stage. The eruption is markedly reduced or invisible, only to recur after the patient is exposed to heat or sunlight, or in response to crying or exercise.

Papular Purpuric Stocking and Glove Syndrome

This syndrome, which is less common than erythema infectiosum, occurs in teenagers and young adults. Pruritus, edema, and erythema of the hands and feet appear and a fever is present. The lesions are sharply cut off at the wrists and ankles. Over a few days they become purpuric. There is a mild erythema of the cheeks, elbows, knees, and groin folds. Oral erosions or aphthouslike lesions may be seen on the buccal or labial mucosa. Transient lymphocytopenia, a drop in the platelet count, and elevation of liver function tests may be seen. The syndrome resolves within 2 weeks. Evidence of seroconversion for parvovirus B19 has been found in several patients, although similar eruptions have been described with measles, hepatitis B, and

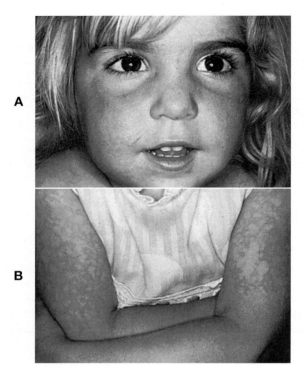

Fig. 19-43 **A,** "Slapped cheek" appearance and **B,** retiform erythema of upper extremities, in erythema infectiosum.

cytomegalovirus. Histologically, there is a dermal infiltrate of CD30+ T lymphocytes surrounding the upper dermal vessels. Parvovirus B19 antigen has been found in the endothelial cells, sweat glands and ducts, and epidermis in three patients.

Complications of parvovirus B19 infection are uncommon and are age dependent. Acute, moderately severe, symmetrical, peripheral arthritis and arthralgias occur in 60% of adult women, 30% of adult men, and 10% of children. This usually lasts less than 2 months but may be chronic and resemble juvenile rheumatoid arthritis or *Borrelia*-associated arthritis. The bone marrow is transiently suppressed by the infection, which in the normal host usually is of no consequence. Purpura from thrombocytopenia may transiently occur. In persons with disorders of reduced red cell survival, especially sickle cell anemia, aplastic crises may result. Chronic bone marrow failure occurs, especially in those with congenital or acquired immunodeficiency. In primarily infected pregnant women, especially women in the first 20 weeks of gestation, fetal death can result from hydrops fetalis as a result of intrauterine anemia.

Aractingi S, et al: Immunohistochemical and virological study of the skin in the papular-purpuric gloves and socks syndrome. *Br J Dermatol* 1996, 135:599.

Halasz CLG, et al: Petechial glove and sock syndrome caused by parvovirus B19. *J Am Acad Dermatol* 1992, 27:835.
Heegaard ED, et al: Parvovirus. *Acta Paediatr* 1995, 84:109.
Kurtzman GJ, et al: Chronic bone marrow failure due to persistent B19 parvovirus infection. *N Engl J Med* 1987, 317:287.
Larralde M, et al: Papular-purpuric "gloves and socks" syndrome due to parvovirus B-19 infection in childhood. *Pediatr Dermatol* 1998, 15:413.
Markenson GR, et al: Parvovirus B19 infections in pregnancy. *Semin Perinatol* 1998, 22:309.
Naides SJ, et al: Human parvovirus B19–induced vesiculopustular skin eruption. *Am J Med* 1988, 84:968.
Nocton JJ, et al: Human parvovirus B19-associated arthritis in children. *J Pediatr* 1993, 122:186.
Perez-Ferriols A, et al: Papular-purpuric "gloves and socks" syndrome caused by measles virus. *J Am Acad Dermatol* 1994, 30:291.
Trattner A, et al: Purpuric "gloves and socks" syndrome. *J Am Acad Dermatol* 1994, 30:267. ▲

ARBOVIRUS GROUP

The arboviruses comprise the numerous arthropod-borne RNA viruses. These viruses multiply in vertebrates as well as in arthropods. The vertebrates usually act as reservoirs and the arthropods as vectors of the various diseases.

West Nile Fever

A maculopapular eruption accompanied by lymphadenopathy and fever characterize this disease. The complement fixation test is the test of choice. The disease is seen in the Middle East, especially in Egypt and Israel. The *Culex* mosquito is the vector, and therefore the disease is most prevalent during the summer.

Sandfly Fever

Sandfly fever is also known as *phlebotomus fever* and *pappataci fever*. The vector, *Phlebotomus papatasii* is found in the Mediterranean area, Russia, China, and India. Small pruritic papules appear on the skin after the sandfly bite and persist for 5 days. After an incubation period of another 5 days, fever, headache, malaise, nausea, conjunctival injection, stiff neck, and abdominal pains suddenly develop. The skin manifestations consist of a scarlatiniform eruption of the face and neck. Recovery is slow, with recurring bouts of fever. No specific treatment is available.

Dengue

Dengue, also known as *break-bone fever,* is a common disease of tropical regions throughout the world, but especially in Southeast Asia. It is spread by the *Aedes aegypti* mosquito. Two to 15 days after the bite of an infected mosquito, the disease begins with a sudden high fever, headache, backache, retroorbital pain, bone and joint pain, weakness, depression, and malaise. A scarlatiniform or morbilliform exanthem, especially on the thorax and joint flexors, may accompany these symptoms. The patient may recover completely at this stage. About the fourth day, after a brief remission of fever, another scarlatiniform exanthem may appear, most vividly over the trunk, face, and extremities. It may be petechial or purpuric.

In 1% to 7% of cases, dengue hemorrhagic fever develops. It usually begins with similar symptoms, but bleeding, thrombocytopenia, and hemoconcentration develop. Fatalities may occur from gastrointestinal bleeding, disseminated intravascular coagulation, and shock. Mortality rates are from 1% to 15%. The disease is not modified by high doses of systemic corticosteroids.

Alphavirus

In Finland, Sindbis virus infection is transmitted by the *Culiseta* mosquito. An eruption of multiple, erythematous, 2- to 4-mm papules with a surrounding halo is associated with fever and prominent arthralgias. The eruption and symptoms resolve over a few weeks. Histologically, the skin lesions show a perivascular lymphocytic infiltrate with large atypical cells, simulating lymphomatoid papulosis. CD30 does not stain the large cells, however, allowing distinction.

Autio P, et al: An eruption associated with alphavirus infection. *Br J Dermatol* 1996, 135:320.

Hayes EB, et al: Dengue and dengue hemorrhagic fever. *Pediatr Infect Dis J* 1992, 11:311.

Tassniyom S, et al: Failure of high-dose methylprednisolone in established dengue shock syndrome. *Pediatrics* 1993, 92:111. ⎯⎯⎯⎯⎯ ▲

PAPOVAVIRUS GROUP

Papovaviruses are double-stranded, naked DNA viruses characterized as slow growing. They replicate inside the nucleus. Because they contain no envelope, they are resistant to drying, freezing, and solvents. In addition to the human papillomaviruses (HPV), which cause warts, papillomaviruses of rabbits and cattle, polyomaviruses of mice, and vacuolating viruses of monkeys are some of the other viruses in this group.

Warts (Verruca)

Human papillomaviruses include more than 80 types. A new type is defined when there is less than 90% DNA homology with any other known type. Most HPV types cause specific types of warts and favor certain anatomic locations, such as plantar warts, common warts, genital warts, and so on. A large proportion of the HPV types are rare and appear to be pathogenic only in immunosuppressed patients with epidermodysplasia verruciformis.

Infection with HPV may be clinical, subclinical, or latent. Clinical lesions are visible by gross inspection. Subclinical lesions may be seen only by aided examination (e.g., the use of acetic acid soaking). Latent infection describes the presence of HPV virus or viral genome in apparently normal skin. Latent infection is thought to be common, especially in genital warts, and explains in part the failure of destructive methods to eradicate warts.

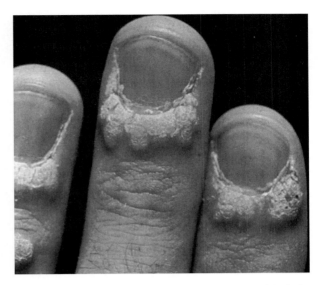

Fig. 19-44 Periungual warts. (Courtesy Dr. Axel W. Hoke.)

Management of warts is based on their clinical appearance, location, and the immune status of the patient. Because warts in some settings are important cofactors in cancer, histologic evaluation of warty lesions in these situations may be important.

Verruca Vulgaris. HPV type 2, and, less frequently, 1, 4, 7, and other HPV types are most frequently responsible for common warts. Common warts occur largely between the ages of 5 and 20 and only 15% occur after the age of 35. The prevalence in children is about 5%. Frequent immersion of hands in water is a risk factor for common warts. Meat handlers (butchers) have a high incidence of common warts of the hands. The natural history of common warts is for them to spontaneously resolve—half by 1 year and two thirds by 2 years.

Common warts are usually located on the hands; they favor the fingers and palms. Periungual warts are more common in nail biters and may be confluent, involving the proximal and lateral nail folds (Fig. 19-44). Fissuring may lead to tenderness. Lesions range in size from pinpoint to more than 1 cm, most averaging about 5 mm. They grow in size for weeks to months and usually present as elevated, rounded papules with a rough, grayish surface so characteristic that it has given us the word *verrucous,* used to describe lesions with similar surface character (e.g., seborrheic keratosis) (Fig. 19-45). In some instances a single wart (mother wart) appears and grows slowly for a long time, and then suddenly many new warts erupt. On the surface of the wart, tiny black dots may be visible, representing thrombosed, dilated capillaries. Trimming the surface keratin makes the capillaries more prominent and may be used as an aid in diagnosis. Warts do not have dermatoglyphics (fingerprint folds), as opposed to callouses, in which these lines are accentuated.

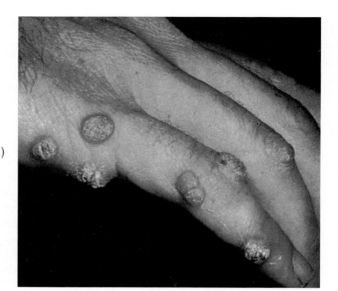

Fig. 19-45 Verrucae vulgares. (Courtesy Dr. Axel W. Hoke.)

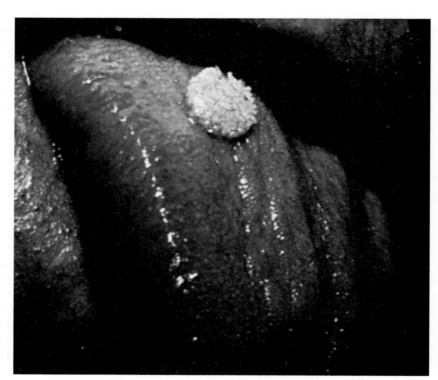

Fig. 19-46 Verruca on tongue.

Common warts may occur any place on the skin, apparently spreading from the hands by autoinoculation. In nail biters, warts may be seen on the lips and tongue, usually in the middle half, and, uncommonly, in the commissures (Fig. 19-46). Digitate or filiform warts tend to occur on the face and scalp and present as single or multiple spikes stuck on the surface of the skin.

Flat Warts (Verruca Plana). HPV type 3 and, less often, types 10, 27, and 41 most often cause flat warts. Children and young adults are primarily affected. This wart pattern presents most typically as 2- to 4-mm flat-topped papules that are slightly erythematous or brown on pale skin and hyperpigmented on darker skin. They are generally multiple and are grouped on the face, neck, dorsa of the hands,

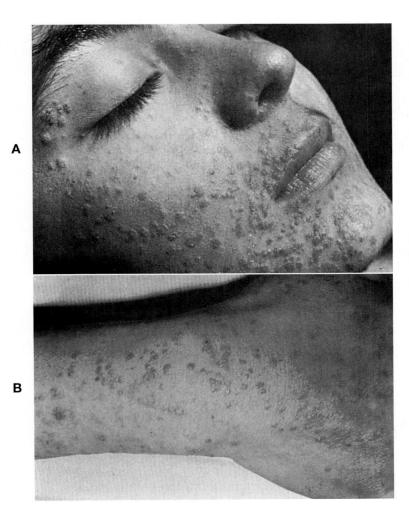

Fig. 19-47 **A**, Verruca plana juvenilis. Unusually florid example. **B**, Verruca plana of forearm and hand. Note "Koebner" streak. (**A**, Courtesy Dr. A. Kaminsky. **B**, Courtesy Dr. Axel W. Hoke.)

wrists, or knees. The forehead, cheeks, and nose and particularly the area around the mouth and the backs of the hands are the favorite locations (Fig. 19-47). In men who shave their beards and in women who shave their legs, numerous flat warts may develop as a result of autoinoculation. A useful finding is the tendency for the warts to koebnerize, forming linear, slightly raised, papular lesions. Hyperpigmented lesions occur, and when scarcely elevated, they may be confused with lentigines or ephelides. Plaquelike lesions may be confused with verrucous nevus, lichen planus, and molluscum contagiosum. When lesions occur only on the central face and are erythematous, they can be easily confused with papular acne vulgaris. Of all clinical HPV infections, flat warts have the highest rate of spontaneous remission.

Plantar Warts (Verruca Plantaris).
HPV type 1 and, less commonly, 2, 4, and other HPV types cause plantar warts. These warts generally appear at pressure points on the ball of the foot, especially over the midmetatarsal area (Fig. 19-48). They may, however, be anywhere on the sole.

Frequently there are several lesions on one foot. Sometimes they are grouped, or several contiguous warts fuse so that they appear as one. Such a plaque is known as a *mosaic wart* (Fig. 19-49). The soft, pulpy cores are surrounded by a firm, horny ring. Over the surface of the plantar wart, most clearly if the top is shaved off, may be seen multiple small black points that represent dilated capillary loops within elongated dermal papillae. Plantar warts may be confused with corns or calluses, but plantar warts have a soft central core and black or bleeding points when pared down, features that calluses do not have.

The myrmecia type of verruca occurs as smooth-surfaced, deep, often inflamed and tender papules or plaques, mostly on the palms or soles, but also beside or beneath the nails, or, less often, on the pulp of the digits. They are distinctively dome shaped and much bulkier beneath the surface than they appear. Myrmecia are caused by HPV-1. They can be mistaken for a paronychia or digital mucinous cyst.

HPV-60 causes a peculiar type of plantar wart called a *ridged wart* because of the persistence of the dermatoglyph-

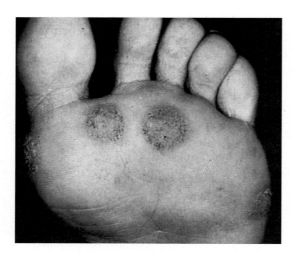

Fig. 19-48   Verrucae plantaris.

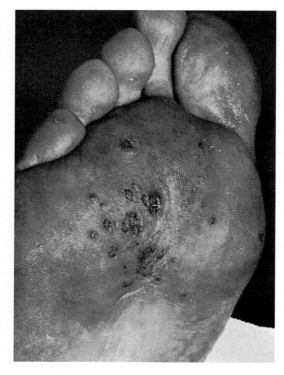

Fig. 19-49   Multiple plantar verrucae.

ics across the surface of the lesion. Typically, the warts are slightly elevated, skin colored, 3- to 5-mm papules. They occur on non–weight-bearing areas and lack the typical features of plantar warts. HPV-60 also causes plantar verrucous cysts, 1.5 to 2 cm epithelium-lined cysts on the plantar surface. The cysts tend to occur on weight-bearing areas, suggesting that HPV-infected epidermis is implanted into the dermis, forming the cyst. It is common to see ridged warts near plantar verrucous cysts.

Histologic Features of HPV Infection

Typical nongenital warts rarely require histologic confirmation. A biopsy may be useful in several settings, however. Histology can be used to distinguish warts from corns and other keratotic lesions that they resemble. This is enhanced by immunoperoxidase staining for HPV capsid antigen. Cytologic atypia and penetration into the dermis suggest the diagnosis of an HPV-induced squamous cell carcinoma. There is a correlation between HPV type and the histologic features of the wart, allowing identification of the HPV types that cause specific lesions, a useful feature in the diagnosis of epidermodysplasia verruciformis, for example.

Treatment of Warts

The form of therapy used depends on the type of wart being treated, the age of the patient, and previous therapies used and their success or failure. With any treatment modality, at least 2 or 3 months of sustained management by that method is considered a reasonable therapeutic trial. Do not abandon any treatment too quickly.

FLAT WARTS. Flat warts frequently undergo spontaneous remission, so therapy should be as mild as possible, and potentially scarring therapies should be avoided. If lesions are few, light cryotherapy is recommended. Topical salicylic acid products can also be used. If the lesions are more extensive, treatment is often with topical tretinoin once or twice daily in the highest concentration tolerated to produce mild erythema of the warts without frank dermatitis. Should this fail, 5-fluorouracil (5-FU) cream 5% applied twice daily may be very effective. On the legs, topical formalin 8 ml in 30 g of Aquaphor, applied twice daily, can be used to treat extensive flat warts that have spread by shaving. Anthralin, although staining, could be similarly used for its irritant effect. For refractory lesions, pulse dye laser therapy might be considered before electrodesiccation because of the reduced risk of scarring.

COMMON WARTS. Treatments for common warts involve two basic approaches: those based on destruction of the wart slowly or quickly, and those based on induction of local immune reactions (immunotherapy). Destructive methods are most commonly used as initial therapy by most practitioners. Cryotherapy is a reasonable first-line therapy for most common warts. The wart should be frozen adequately to produce a blister after 1 or 2 days. This correlates with a thaw time of 30 to 45 seconds for most common warts. Berth-Jones et al found that a single treatment was as effective as two freeze-thaw cycles. The ideal frequency of treatment is every 2 or 3 weeks, just as the old blister peels off. A spray device, while more costly, is quicker, avoids potential explosions of glass thermoses, and cannot spread infectious diseases (especially viral hepatitis) from one patient to the next. Children may be frightened by such a device, so a cotton-tipped swab is preferred for them. Complications of cryotherapy include hypopigmentation, uncommonly scarring, and rarely, damage to the digital nerve from freezing too deeply on the side of the digit. Patients with cryoglobulinemia, poor peripheral circulation, and Raynaud's may develop severe blisters when cryotherapy is used to treat their warts.

Products containing salicylic acid with or without lactic acid are effective patient-applied treatments; these have an efficacy comparable to that of cryotherapy. After the wart-affected area is soaked in water for 5 to 10 minutes, the topical medication is applied, allowed to dry, and covered with a strip bandage for 24 hours. This is repeated daily. The superficial keratinous debris may be removed by scraping with a table knife, pumice stone, or an emery board.

A small amount of cantharone (0.7% cantharidin) is applied to the wart, allowed to dry, and covered for 24 hours. A blister, similar to that produced by cryotherapy, develops in 24 to 72 hours. These blisters may be as painful as or more painful than those following cryotherapy. Treatment is repeated every 2 to 3 weeks. Perhaps more than any other method, there is a tendency for cantharidin to produce doughnut warts, a round wart with a central clear zone at the site of the original wart (Fig. 19-50). Nonetheless, this agent is a very useful adjunct in the management of difficult-to-treat verrucae.

Bleomycin has high efficacy and is now an important form of treatment for recalcitrant common warts. It is used at a concentration of 1 unit/ml, which is injected into and immediately beneath the wart until it blanches. The multiple-puncture technique of Shelley—delivering the medication into the wart by multiple punctures of the wart with a needle through a drop of bleomycin—may also be used. For small warts (less than 5 mm), 0.1 ml is used, and 0.2 ml for larger warts. The injection is painful enough to require local anesthesia in some patients. Pain for 24 to 72 hours can occur. The wart becomes black, and the black eschar separates in 2 to 3 weeks. Treatment may be repeated every 3 weeks, but it is unusual for common warts to require more than one or two treatments. Systemic side effects are not reported. Scarring is rare. Response rates vary by location but average 90% with two treatments for most common, nonplantar warts, even periungual ones. Treatment of finger warts with bleomycin may uncommonly be complicated by localized Raynaud's phenomenon of treated fingers. Bleomycin treatment of digital warts may rarely result in digital necrosis and permanent nail dystrophy, so extreme caution should be used in treating warts around the nailfolds.

Surgical ablation of warts can be effective treatment, but even complete destruction of a wart and the surrounding skin does not guarantee the wart will not recur. Surgical methods should be reserved for warts that are refractory to more conservative approaches. The two most commonly used surgical techniques are curettage alone or curettage combined with electrodesiccation. Local anesthesia is required, and scarring usually results. Carbon dioxide laser destruction requires local anesthesia, causes scarring, and

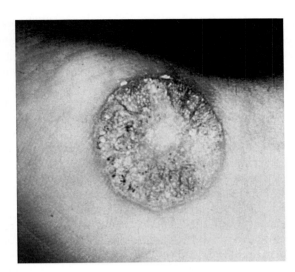

Fig. 19-50 Development of a "doughnut" wart after liquid nitrogen treatment.

may lead to nail dystrophy. Its efficacy is between 56% and 81% in refractory warts. A potentially infectious plume is produced. Pulsed dye laser therapy appears to have high efficacy, less plume is produced, and the treatment can be performed in two thirds of patients without anesthesia, although some pain occurs. The energy is 7 J/cm^2 for thinner lesions, and up to 9.5 J/cm^2 for more hyperkeratotic ones. Five or 7 mm spot-size is used, and treatment is extended 2 mm beyond the visible wart. Immediately after treatment, the skin has a gray-black discoloration, which evolves to an eschar over 10 to 14 days. Treatment is repeated every 2 to 4 weeks, and up to five treatments may be required. In immunocompetent patients, response rates for refractory warts were 95% for hand warts and 83% for periungual warts.

Oral cimetidine, 30 to 40 mg/kg/day, has been anecdotally reported to lead to resolution of common warts, perhaps because of its immunomodulatory effects. When used as a single agent, however, in both children and adults, the efficacy is low (30%), comparable with a placebo. It may be beneficial as an adjunct to other methods, however, or for treatment of refractory warts. Heat treatment, either localized to the wart and delivered by radiofrequency or by application to the affected part by soaking it in a hot bath, have been reported to be effective. Temperatures of 43° to 50° C (107.6° to 122° F) for from 15 minutes at the lower temperatures to as little as 30 seconds at the higher ones have been used. Oral administration of acitretin or isotretinoin may also provide activity against HPV and may be used in refractory cases. Hypnotic suggestion and hypnoanalysis for warts has been reviewed by Ewin, who found these methods to be 80% effective.

Application of dinitrochlorobenzene (DNCB) to warts is associated with resolution in about 85% of cases. Patients may be initially sensitized at a distant site, or the DNCB may be applied initially to the warts directly biweekly, weekly, or twice weekly. The DNCB may dissolved in acetone, collodion, or petrolatum. The treated wart should be kept covered for 24 hours after application. Initial treatment strength may be from 2% to 5% and the dose decreased by one log (to 0.2% to 0.5%) if the reaction is overly severe. Wart tenderness may indicate the need to reduce treatment concentration. Warts begin to resolve in from one to 20 treatments, but on the average, 2 to 3 months of treatment are required. Side effects of treatment include local pruritus, local pain, and a mild eczematous dermatitis. Scarring has not been reported.

PLANTAR WARTS. In general, plantar warts are more refractory to any form of treatment than are common warts. Initial treatment usually involves daily application of salicylic acid in liquid, film, or plaster form after soaking. In failures, cryotherapy or cantharidin application may be attempted, alone or in combination. A second freeze-thaw cycle is beneficial in the treatment of plantar warts. Bleomycin injections, laser therapy, or DNCB sensitization, as discussed earlier, may be used in refractory cases. Surgical destruction with cautery or blunt dissection should be reserved for failures with nonscarring techniques, since a plantar scar may be persistently painful.

Genital Warts. Genital warts are the most common sexually transmitted disease. Among sexually active young adults in the United States and Europe, infection rates as high as 50% in some cohorts have been found using sensitive polymerase chain-reaction techniques. It is estimated that the lifetime risk for infection in sexually active young adults may be as high as 80%. The number of new cases of genital wart infection diagnosed in the United States yearly may approach 1 million. In the vast majority of couples in whom one has evidence of HPV infection, the partner will be found to be concordantly infected. The risk of transmission is not known, however. A large portion of genital HPV infection is either subclinical or latent. Unfortunately, the infectivity of subclinical and latent infection is unknown. Subclinical and latent infection are probably responsible for most "recurrences" following treatment of genital warts.

Genital HPV infection is closely linked with cancer of the cervix, glans penis, anus, vulvovaginal area, and periungual skin. In most persons, genital wart infection appears to be transient and results in no sequelae. In a small proportion, infection persists and may progress to cancer. The exact reason for this is unknown, but certain cofactors such as HPV type causing the infection, location of infection, cigarette smoking, and immunosuppressed status are associated with progression to cancer. The transition zones of the cervix and anus are at highest risk for the development of cancer.

Numerous HPV types are associated with genital warts. The HPV types producing genital infection are divided into

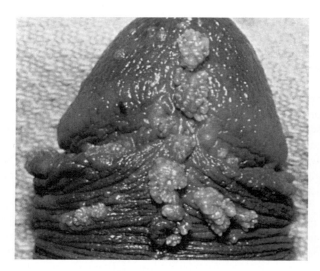

Fig. 19-51 Penile warts. (Courtesy Dr. John Reeves.)

two broad categories—those that produce benign lesions, or low-risk types, and those associated with cancer, the so-called high-risk or oncogenic types. The most common low-risk genital HPV types are HPV-6 and HPV-11, and most HPV-induced genital dysplasias are caused by HPV types 16 and 18. There is a strong correlation between the HPV type and the clinical appearance of HPV induced genital lesions. Virtually all condylomata acuminata are caused by "benign" HPV types 6 and 11. High-risk HPV types 16 and 18 produce flat, often hyperpigmented lesions. For this reason, biopsy of genital warts is rarely necessary.

CONDYLOMATA ACUMINATA. Condylomata appear as lobulated papules that average 2 to 5 mm in size, but they may range from microscopic to several centimeters in diameter and height. Lesions are frequently multifocal. They occur in men anywhere on the penis (Fig. 19-51) or about the anus (Figs. 19-52 and 19-53). Scrotal condylomata occur in only 1% of immunocompetent male patients with warts. Intraurethral condylomata may present with terminal hematuria, altered urinary stream, or urethral bleeding. In women, lesions appear on the mucosal surfaces of the vulva, cervix, on the perineum, or about the anus. Cauliflower-like masses may develop in moist, occluded areas such as the perianal skin, vulva, and inguinal folds (Fig. 19-54). As a result of accumulation of purulent material in the clefts, these may be malodorous. Their color is generally gray, pale yellow, or pink. When perianal lesions occur, a prior history of receptive anal intercourse will usually predict whether intraanal warts are present and will help to determine the need for anoscopy. Numerous genital warts may appear during pregnancy.

Genital warts are sexually transmitted, and other sexually transmitted diseases may be found in patients with genital warts. A complete history should be taken and the patient screened for other sexually transmitted diseases as appro-

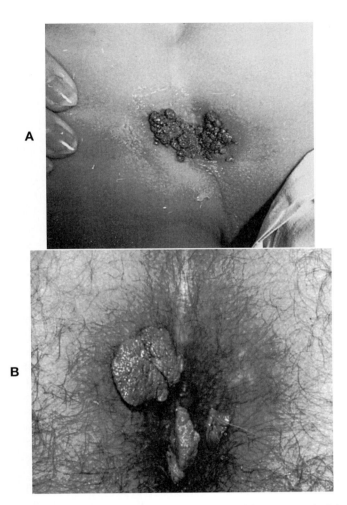

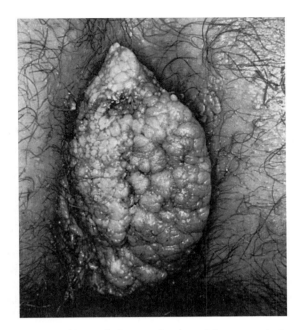

Fig. 19-53 Unusually large perianal condyloma acuminatum.

Fig. 19-52 **A** and **B,** Perianal verrucae (condylomata acuminata). (**B,** Courtesy Dr. Axel W. Hoke.)

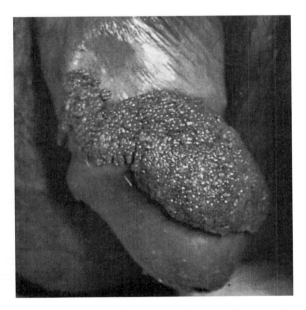

Fig. 19-54 Giant condyloma acuminatum. (Courtesy Dr. V. Beltrani.)

priate. Women with genital HPV infection should have a routine cervical cytologic screening (Papanicolaou smear) to detect cervical dysplasia.

BOWENOID PAPULOSIS AND HPV-INDUCED GENITAL DYSPLASIAS. Bowenoid papulosis is characterized by flat, often hyperpigmented papules a few millimeters to several centimeters in diameter. These occur singly, or, more often, may be found in multiples on the penis, near the vulva, or perianally. Histologically, they demonstrate abnormal epithelial maturation and cellular atypia closely resembling Bowen's disease. They are usually caused by HPV-16. On the glabrous external genitalia, bowenoid papulosis usually behaves similar to other external genital warts. On the glans penis of an uncircumcised male and on the cervical, vaginal, or rectal mucosa, progression to invasive squamous cell carcinoma may occur. The female partners of men with bowenoid papulosis and women with bowenoid papulosis have a risk of cervical dysplasia.

GIANT CONDYLOMA ACUMINATUM (BUSCHKE-LOWENSTEIN TUMOR). Giant condyloma acuminatum is a rare, aggressive, wart-

like growth that is a verrucous carcinoma. Unlike other HPV-induced genital carcinomas, this tumor is caused by HPV-6. It occurs most often on the glans or prepuce of an uncircumcised male; less often it may occur on perianal skin or the vulva. Despite its bland histologic picture, it may invade deeply, and uncommonly it may metastasize to regional lymph nodes. Treatment is by complete surgical excision. Recurrence after radiation therapy may be associated with a more aggressive course.

DIAGNOSIS OF GENITAL WARTS. Virtually all condylomata can be diagnosed by inspection. Bright lighting and magnification should be used when examining for genital HPV infection. Bowenoid papulosis is more difficult and may require a biopsy. Subclinical and latent infections are no longer sought or investigated, because they are very common and there is no management strategy known to eradicate these forms of HPV infection. Soaking with acetic acid is not recommended, except in unusual circumstances. In patients with multiple recurrences, acetic acid soaking may determine the extent of infection, helping to define the area for application of topical therapies. Acetowhitening may also help in the differentiating certain genital papules from genital warts. Subclinical infection is detected by soaking the external genitalia in men, and the vagina and cervix in women with 3% to 5% acetic acid for up to 10 minutes. Genital warts turn white (acetowhitening), making them easily identifiable. Any process that alters the epidermal barrier will be acetowhite, however (dermatitis, for example), so only typical acetowhite lesions should be treated as warts. In atypical cases, a 2-week trial is attempted with a 1% hydrocortisone preparation plus a topical anticandidal imidazole cream. If the acetowhitening persists, a biopsy is performed and histologic evidence of HPV infection sought. Immunoperoxidase or in situ hybridization methods may aid in evaluation. Polymerase chain reaction should probably not be performed on such biopsied specimens, except possibly in childhood cases. The high background rate of latent infection (up to 50%) makes interpretation of a positive PCR result impossible.

TREATMENT OF GENITAL WARTS. Because no effective virus-specific agent exists for the treatment of genital warts, their recurrence is frequent. Treatment is not proven to reduce transmission to sexual partners nor to prevent progression to dysplasia or cancer. Specifically the treatment of male sexual partners of women with genital warts does not reduce the recurrence rate of warts in these women. Subclinical infection on the external genitalia should not be sought or treated. Therefore, the goals of treatment must first be discussed with the patient, and perhaps with his or her sexual partner. Observation represents an acceptable option for some patients with typical condylomata acuminata. In some patients, only wart-free periods are achieved. Because genital warts may cause discomfort, genital pruritus, malodor, bleeding, and substantial emotional distress, treatment is indicated if the patient desires it. Bleeding genital warts may increase the sexual transmission of HIV and hepatitis B and C.

The method of treatment chosen is in part dictated by the size of the warts and their location. Podophyllin is more effective in treating warts on occluded or moist surfaces, such as mucosa or under the prepuce. It is available as a crude extract, usually in 25% concentration in tincture of benzoin. It is applied weekly by the physician and is washed off 4 to 8 hours later by the patient, depending on the

severity of the reaction. After six consecutive weekly treatments, approximately 40% of patients are free of warts, and 17% are free of warts at 3 months after treatment. Purified podophyllotoxin 0.5% solution is applied by the patient twice daily for 3 consecutive days of each week in 4- to 6-week treatment cycles. Efficacy approaches 60% for typical condylomata, and side effects are less than with standard, physician-applied podophyllin preparations. Therefore, use of podophyllotoxin is preferred to use of classic podophyllin in most cases.

Imiquimod, a local interferon inducer, has an efficacy similar to cryotherapy and yields a low recurrence rate. It is more effective than podophyllotoxin in treating women with external genital warts, but it is only equally or less effective in men, especially for warts on the penile shaft. Response is slow, requiring 10 or more weeks in some patients to see a response. It is patient applied, once daily for 3 alternate days per week (usually Monday, Wednesday, and Friday). Treatment results in mild to moderate irritation (less than with podophyllin or cryotherapy in men, but with a similar side effect profile in women). Initial trials suggest that the recurrence rate is about 20%, which is lower than with other nonsurgical methods. It may be used alone as treatment or in cases in which recurrence has been frequent after other forms of treatment were attempted.

Bichloroacetic or trichloroacetic acid (TCA) 35% to 85% can be applied to condylomata weekly or biweekly. When compared with cryotherapy, TCA has the same or lower efficacy and causes more ulcerations and pain. TCA is safe for use in pregnant patients.

Cryotherapy with liquid nitrogen is more effective than podophyllin, approaching 80% resolution during treatment and 55% 3 months after treatment. One or two freeze-thaw cycles are applied to each wart every 1 to 3 weeks. A zone of 2 mm beyond the lesion is frozen. Cryotherapy is effective in dry as well as moist areas. Perianal lesions are more difficult to treat than other genital sites, and two freeze-thaw cycles are recommended in this location. Cryotherapy is safe to use in pregnant patients.

Electrofulguration or electrocauterization with or without snip removal of the condyloma is more effective than TCA, cryotherapy, or podophyllin. Wart clearance during therapy is nearly 95%, and wart cure at 3 months exceeds 70%. Local anesthesia is required, and scarring may occur. A minor surgical removal procedure is ideal for large exophytic warts that might require multiple treatments with other methods. It has high acceptance in patients who have had recurrences from other methods, because results are immediate and cure rates higher.

The use of CO_2 laser in the treatment of genital warts has not been demonstrated to be more effective than simpler surgical methods. Although visible warts are eradicated by the laser, HPV DNA can still be detected at the previous site of the wart. The CO_2 laser has the advantage of being bloodless, but it is costlier and requires more technical skill on the part of the surgeon to avoid complications. It should be reserved for treatment of extensive lesions in which more cost-effective methods have been attempted and failed.

Any surgical method that generates a smoke plume is potentially infectious to the surgeon. HPV DNA is detected in the plumes generated during CO_2 laser or electrocoagulation treatment of genital warts. The laser-generated plume results in longer duration HPV aerosol contamination and wider spread of detectable HPV DNA. If these methods of wart treatment are used, an approved face mask should be worn, a smoke evacuator should be operated at the surgical site during the procedure to remove the plume, and decontamination of the equipment after the surgery should be carried out.

5-FU 5% cream applied twice daily may be effective, especially in the treatment of flat, hyperpigmented lesions, such as those in bowenoid papulosis. Twice-daily instillation of 5-FU into the urethra with a syringe can be used to treat intraurethral condylomata. It may also be used to treat intravaginal warts by instillation in the vagina. Intermittent therapy (twice weekly for 10 weeks) is better tolerated than daily therapy. An injectable form of 5-FU in a protein matrix has an efficacy similar to that of standard methods but requires weekly injection and is more expensive. Its role in the management of genital warts has not yet been defined.

The efficacy of systemic and intralesional interferon alfa therapy has been found to be relatively low in eradicating genital warts. Intralesional therapy eradicates 40% to 60% of warts, and systemic interferon treatment will eradicate warts in only about 20% of patients. Interferon treatment of genital warts in patients with AIDS has lower efficacy rates than those listed above. However, response rates to interferon have never reached the levels achieved with electrosurgical methods. Because of the high cost, frequent side effects, and low efficacy associated with interferon therapy, the CDC no longer recommends the use of interferon for the treatment of genital warts.

GENITAL WARTS IN CHILDREN. Children can acquire genital warts through vertical transmission perinatally, digital inoculation or autoinoculation, fomite or social nonsexual contact, and through sexual abuse. The proportion of genital warts in children acquired by each of these methods is extremely controversial. HPV typing has demonstrated that most warts in the genital area of children are "genital" HPV types, and most children with genital warts have family members with a genital HPV infection. HPV typing may be useful in determining the source of infection.

However, a finding of a nongenital HPV type, such as HPV-2, does not exclude the possibility of transmission through sexual abuse. In children younger than 1 year of age, vertical transmission is possible and is probably the most common means of acquisition. The risk for sexual abuse is highest in children older than 3 years of age, and all such children should be referred to child protective services

if the practitioner is not skilled in evaluating children for sexual abuse. Children between 1 and 3 years of age are primarily nonverbal and are most difficult to evaluate. Management of such patients is on a case-by-case basis. Other sexually transmitted diseases should be screened for in children who have a genital HPV infection. Genital warts in children usually respond quickly to topical therapy, such as podophyllotoxin, imiquimod, or light cryotherapy. In refractory cases, surgical removal or electrocautery may be used. The use of EMLA before treatment is recommended.

Recurrent Respiratory (Laryngeal) Papillomatosis. HPV-associated papillomas may occur throughout the respiratory tract, from the nose to the lungs. Recurrent respiratory papillomatosis has a bimodal distribution—in children under 5, and after the age of 15. Affected young children were born to mothers with genital condylomata, and they present with hoarseness. The HPV types found in these lesions, HPV-6 and -11, are the types seen in genital condylomata. Treatment is with CO_2 laser surgery and interferon. Carcinoma that is often fatal develops in 14% of patients, even in young children. The incidence of carcinoma is higher in those treated with radiation therapy.

Heck's Disease. Small white to pinkish papules occur diffusely in the oral cavity in this disease, also known as *focal epithelial hyperplasia*. It occurs most commonly in Native Americans. HPV-13 has been linked to this condition.

Epidermodysplasia Verruciformis

Epidermodysplasia verruciformis (EV) is a rare, inherited disorder characterized by widespread HPV infection and cutaneous squamous cell carcinomas. Most commonly it is inherited as an autosomal recessive trait. HPV types associated with this syndrome include types infecting normal hosts such as HPV-3 and -10, as well as many "unique" HPV types found only rarely in patients who do not have EV. These HPV types are called *EV HPVs* and include HPV-5, -8, -9, -12, -14, -15, -17, -19 through -25, and -36 through -38. The pathogenesis of this syndrome is unknown but is felt to be a specific defect of cell-mediated immunity. EV patients cannot be sensitized to DNCB.

The condition presents in childhood and continues throughout life. Skin lesions include flat, wartlike lesions of the dorsal hands, extremities, and face. These are flatter than typical flat warts, and may be quite abundant, growing to confluence (Fig. 19-55). Typical HPV-3 and -10 induced flat warts may be admixed. In addition, on the trunk are lesions which are red plaques or hypopigmented, very slightly scaly plaques resembling tinea versicolor.

The histologic features of an EV-specific HPV infection are very characteristic. The cells of the upper epidermis have a clear, smoky or light-blue pale cytoplasm and a central pyknotic nucleus.

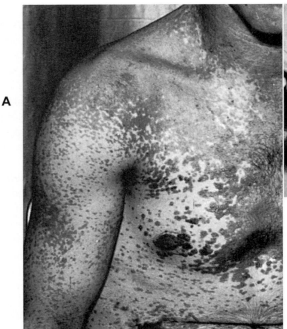

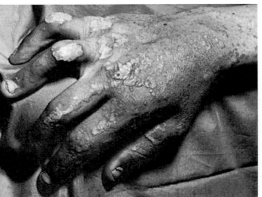

Fig. 19-55 **A,** Epidermodysplasia verruciformis. Verrucous plaques can be seen, especially on the sternum. **B,** Lesions consist of flat papules and hyperkeratotic scaly patches, especially over the knuckles. (Courtesy Drs. M. Ruiter and P.J. Van Mullen.)

Squamous cell carcinomas develop in 30% to 60% of patients. Most often skin cancers appear on sun-exposed surfaces, but they can appear on any part of the body. They begin to appear at ages 20 to 40. Skin cancers are less common in African patients, suggesting a protective effect of skin pigmentation. HPV-5, -8, and -47 are found in the more than 90% of EV skin cancers. The squamous cell carcinomas may appear de novo but usually appear on the background of numerous actinic keratoses and lesions of Bowen's disease. Surgical treatment is curative. Radiation therapy is contraindicated. If skin grafting is required, the grafts should be taken from sun-protected skin, such as the buttocks or inner upper arm.

Aside from surgical intervention for skin cancer, the treatment for EV consists largely of preventive measures. Strict sun avoidance and protection should be started as soon as the syndrome is diagnosed. An approach similar to that for children with xeroderma pigmentosa could be instituted.

Warts in Immunosuppressed Patients. Patients with defects in their cell-mediated immunity may have an increased frequency of HPV infection. Predisposing conditions include organ transplantation, immunosuppressive medications, congenital immunodeficiency diseases, lymphoma, and HIV infection.

Organ transplant recipients begin to develop warts soon after transplantation, and by 5 years up to 90% of transplant patients have warts. Initially these are common and plantar warts, but later numerous flat warts appear, particularly in sun-exposed areas. Depending on the background level of ultraviolet radiation, the lifetime risk for cutaneous carcinomas may exceed 40%. Skin cancers begin to appear 5 years or more after transplantation, occur in sun-exposed sites, and are more common in persons with skin types I and II. The duration and intensity of immunosuppression appear more important in causing the skin cancers than are the specific immunosuppressive agents used. Malignant lesions may resemble Bowen's disease, keratoacanthomas, squamous cell carcinomas, or warts. Genital warts are also increased, and especially in women, genital dysplasias are more frequent.

EV types and some unique HPV types are frequently found in the nongenital dysplasias among organ transplant recipients. The skin of organ transplant patients should be examined closely, and once skin cancers begin to appear, regular dermatologic examinations should be performed.

In HIV disease, common, plantar, flat, and genital warts are all very common. Genital warts are increased fifteenfold among HIV-infected women. Fifty percent or more of HIV-infected homosexual men have evidence of anal HPV infection. Genital neoplasia associated with HPV-16 and -18 occurs much more frequently in HIV-infected women and homosexual men. Uncommonly, HIV-infected patients develop HPV-5 and -8 induced EV-like lesions. Although nongenital skin cancers are also common in some fair-skinned HIV-infected patients, HPV has not been demonstrated in the nongenital squamous cell carcinomas of these patients.

The treatment of warts in immunosuppressed hosts is very difficult. Although standard methods are used, their efficacy may be reduced. It is especially important in these patients to regularly monitor the genital and anal areas for changing lesions and to have a low threshold for performing a biopsy.

Ambrose DN: Treatment vs nontreatment of asymptomatic genital warts. *Am Fam Physician* 1996, 54:59.

Amer M, et al: Therapeutic evaluation for intralesional injection of bleomycin sulfate in 143 resistant warts. *J Am Acad Dermatol* 1988, 18:1313.

Arends MJ, et al: Renal allograft recipients with high susceptibility to cutaneous malignancy have an increased prevalence of HPV DNA in skin tumors and a greater risk of anogenital malignancy. *Br J Cancer* 1997, 75:722.

Armstrong DKB, et al: Combined therapy trial with interferon alpha-2a and ablative therapy in the treatment of anogenital warts. *Genitourin Med* 1996, 72:103.

Baken LA, et al: Genital human papillomavirus infection among male and female sex partners: prevalence and type-specific concordance. *J Infect Dis* 1995, 171:429.

Barrasso R, et al: High prevalence of papillomavirus-associated penile intraepithelial neoplasia in sexual partners of women with cervical intraepithelial neoplasia. *N Engl J Med* 1987, 317:916.

Baruch K: Blunt dissection for the treatment of plantar verrucae. *Cutis* 1990, 46:145.

Barzegar C, et al: Epidemodysplasia verrucformis-like eruption complicating HIV infection. *Br J Dermatol* 1998, 139:122.

Bauer HM, et al: Genital human papillomavirus infection in female university students as determined by a PCR-based method. *JAMA* 1991, 265:472.

Bauman C, et al: Cimetidine therapy for multiple viral warts in children. *J Am Acad Dermatol* 1996, 35:271.

Bergbrant IM, et al: Polymerase chain reaction for monitoring human papillomavirus contamination of medical personnel during treatment of genital warts with CO_2 laser and electrocoagulation. *Acta Derm Venereol* (Stockh) 1994, 74:393.

Berth-Jones J, et al: Value of a second freeze-thaw cycle in cryotherapy of common warts. *Br J Dermatol* 1994, 131:883.

Beutner KR, et al: Genital warts and their treatment. *Clin Infect Dis* 1999, 28:S37.

Beutner KR, et al: Human papillomavirus and human disease. *Am J Med* 1997, 102:9.

Beutner KR, et al: Treatment of genital warts with an immune-response modifier (imiquimod). *J Am Acad Dermatol* 1998, 38:230.

Bonnez W, et al: Therapeutic efficacy and complications of excisional biopsy of condyloma acuminatum. *Sex Transm Dis* 1996, 23:273.

Christophersen J, et al: Recurrent condylomata acuminata treated with recombinant interferon alpha-2a. *Acta Derm Venereol* (Stockh) 1993, 73:223.

Claire-Benton E: Therapy of cutaneous warts. *Clin Dermatol* 1997, 15:449.

De Pablo, et al: Raynaud's phenomenon and intralesional bleomycin. *Acta Derm Venereol* (Stockh) 1992, 72:465.

de Villiers EM, et al: Prevailing papillomavirus types in non-melanoma carcinomas of the skin in renal allograft recipients. *Int J Cancer* 1997, 73:356.

Dunagin WG, et al: Dinitrochlorobenzene immunotherapy for verrucae resistant to standard treatment modalities. *J Am Acad Dermatol* 1982, 6:40.

Edwards L, et al: Self administered topical 5% imiquimod cream for external anogenital warts. *Arch Dermatol* 1998, 134:25.

Epstein E: Persisting Raynaud's phenomenon following intralesional bleomycin treatment of finger warts. *J Am Acad Dermatol* 1985, 13:469.

Euvrard S, et al: External anogenital lesions in organ transplant recipients. *Arch Dermatol* 1997, 133:175.

Evander M, et al: Human papillomavirus infection is transient in young women. *J Infect Dis* 1995, 171:1026.

Ewin DM: Hypnotherapy for warts (verruca vulgaris). *Am J Clin Hypn* 1992, 35:1.

Feldman JG, et al: Association of smoking and risk of condyloma acuminatum in women. *Obstet Gynecol* 1997, 89:346.

Ferenczy A, et al: Latent papillomavirus and recurring genital warts. *N Engl J Med* 1985, 313:784.

Glass AT, at al: Cimetidine therapy for recalcitrant warts in adults. *Arch Dermatol* 1996, 132:680.

Gutman LT, et al: Transmission of human genital papillomavirus disease. *Pediatrics* 1993, 91:31.

Handley JM, et al: Anogenital warts in children. *Clin Exp Dermatol* 1993, 18:241.

Handsfield HH: Clinical presentation and natural course of anogenital warts. *Am J Med* 1997, 102:16.

Happle R: The potential hazards of dinitrochlorobenzene. *Arch Dermatol* 1985, 121:330.

Hellberg D, et al: Self-treatment of female external genital warts with 0.5% podophyllotoxin cream (condyline) vs weekly applications of 20% podophyllin solution. *Int J STD AIDS* 1995, 6:257.

Hjorth N, et al: Anthralin stick (Anthra-Derm) in the treatment of mosaic warts. *Acta Derm Venereol* (Stockh) 1986, 66:181.

Ho GYF, et al: Natural history of cervicovaginal papillomavirus infection in young women. *N Engl J Med* 1998, 338:423.

Honda A, et al: Human papillomavirus type 60–associated plantar wart. *Arch Dermatol* 1994, 130:1413.

Jacyk WK, et al: Epidermodysplasia verruciformis in Africans. *Int J Dermatol* 1993, 32:806.

Kauvar ANB, et al: Pulsed dye laser treatment of warts. *Arch Fam Med* 1995, 4:1035.

Kiviat NB, et al: Association of anal dysplasia and human papillomavirus with immunosuppression and HIV infection among homosexual men. *AIDS* 1993, 7:43.

Koutsky L: Epidemiology of genital human papillomavirus infection. *Am J Med* 1997, 102:3.

Krebs HB, et al: Treatment failure of genital condylomata acuminata in women: role of the male sexual partner. *Am J Obstet Gynecol* 1991, 165:337.

Kundu A, et al: Warts in the oral cavity. *Genitourin Med* 1995, 71:194.

Lassus J, et al: Carbon dioxide (CO_2) laser therapy cures macroscopic lesions, but viral genome is not eradicated in men with therapy-resistant HPV infection. *Sex Transm Dis* 1994, 21:297.

Leigh IM, et al: Cutaneous warts and tumors in immunosuppressed patients. *J Royal Soc Med* 1995, 88:61.

Leventhal BG, et al: Long-term response of recurrent respiratory papillomatosis to treatment with lymphoblastoid interferon alfa-n1. *N Engl J Med* 1991, 325:613.

Majewski S, et al: Epidermodysplasia verruciformis as a model of human papillomavirus-induced genetic cancer of the skin. *Arch Dermatol* 1995, 131:1312.

Mendelson J, et al: Randomized placebo-controlled double-blind combined therapy with laser surgery and systemic interferon alfa-2a in the treatment of anogenital condylomata acuminatum. *J Infect Dis* 1993, 167:824.

Menter A, et al: The use of EMLA cream and 1% lidocaine infiltration in men for relief of pain associated with the removal of genital warts by cryotherapy. *J Am Acad Dermatol* 1997, 37:96

Orlow SJ, et al: Cimetidine therapy for multiple viral warts in children. *J Am Acad Dermatol* 1993, 28:794.

Palefsky JM, et al: Anal intraepithelial neoplasia and anal papillomavirus infection among homosexual males with group IV HIV disease. *JAMA* 1990, 263:2911.

Penn I: Cancers of the anogenital region in renal transplant recipients. *Cancer* 1986, 58:611.

Pfister H, et al: Characterization of HPV-13 from focal epithelial hypoplasia. *J Virol* 1983, 47:363.

Schafer A, et al: The increased frequency of cervical dysplasia-neoplasia in women infected with the human immunodeficiency virus is related to the degree of immunosuppression. *Am J Obstet Gynecol* 1991, 164:593.

Shamanin V, et al: Human papillomavirus infections in nonmelanoma skin cancers from renal transplant recipients and nonimmunosuppressed patients. *J Nat Cancer Inst* 1996, 88:802.

Shelley WB, et al: Intralesional bleomycin sulfate therapy for warts. *Arch Dermatol* 1991, 127:234.

Simma B, et al: Squamous-cell carcinoma arising in a non-irradiated child with recurrent respiratory papillomatosis. *Eur J Pediatr* 1993, 152:776.

Spinillo A, et al: Prevalence, diagnosis and treatment of lower genital neoplasia in women with human immunodeficiency virus infection. *Eur J Obstet Gynecol* 1992, 43:235.

Stern P, et al: Controlled localized heat therapy in cutaneous warts. *Arch Dermatol* 1992, 128:945.

Stone KM: Human papillomavirus infection and genital warts: update on epidemiology and treatment. *Clin Infect Dis* 1995, 20:S91.

Tyring S, et al: Safety and efficacy of 0.5% podofilox gel in the treatment of anogenital warts. *Arch Dermatol* 1998, 134:33.

von Krogh G, et al: Anogenital warts. *Clin Dermatol* 1997, 15:355.

Webster GF, et al: Treatment of recalcitrant warts using the pulsed dye laser. *Cutis* 1995 56:230.

Yilmaz E, et al: Cimetidine therapy for warts: a placebo-controlled, double-blind study. *J Am Acad Dermatol* 1996, 34:1005. _____ ▲

RETROVIRUSES

These oncoviruses are unique in that they contain RNA, which is converted by a virally coded reverse transcriptase to DNA in the host cell. The target cell population is primarily CD4+ lymphocytes (primarily helper T cells) but also, in some cases, macrophages. For this reason they are called human T-lymphotropic viruses (HTLV). Transmission may be by sexual intercourse, blood products/intravenous drug use, and from mother to child during childbirth and breast-feeding. There is often a very long "latent" period from the time of infection until presentation with clinical disease.

HTLV-1

HTLV-1 is endemic in Japan, the Caribbean, sub-Saharan Africa, and the southeastern United States. In endemic areas infection rates may be quite high, with only a small percentage of infected patients ever developing clinical disease. HTLV-1 is responsible for several clinical syndromes. About 1% of persons who are infected will develop adult T-cell leukemia-lymphoma (ATLL). HTLV-1–associated myelopathy or tropical spastic paraparesis (HAM/TSP) is a less common degenerative neurologic syndrome.

There are four forms of ATLL: smoldering, chronic, acute, and lymphomatous, usually progressing in that order. ATLL is characterized by lymphadenopathy, hepatosplenomegaly, hypercalcemia, and skin lesions. Skin lesions in ATLL include erythematous papules or nodules. Prurigo may be a prodrome to the development of ATLL. Histologically, the cutaneous infiltrates are pleomorphic, atypical lymphocytes with characteristic "flower cells"

representing HTLV-1 infected lymphocytes. Epidermotropism may be present, mimicking mycosis fungoides.

HTLV-1 infected patients may also develop various forms of dermatitis mimicking other skin diseases, and in infected children "infective dermatitis." Infective dermatitis occurs in Jamaican children infected with HTLV-1. It is diagnosed by major and minor criteria as delineated by La Grenade et al. Clinically, the children present at an early age (on average, about 7 years) with a chronic eczema of the scalp, axilla, groin, external auditory canal, retroauricular area, eyelid margins, paranasal areas, and neck. There is a chronic nasal discharge. Cultures from the skin and nares are positive for *Staphylococcus aureus* or beta-hemolytic streptococcus and the condition responds rapidly to antibiotics. However, the condition, is relapsing and recurrent. Skin biopsies show a nonspecific dermatitis.

La Grenade L, et al: Clinical, pathologic, and immunologic features of human T-lymphotrophic virus type 1-associated infective dermatitis in children. *Arch Dermatol* 1998, 134:439.

Setoyama M, et al: Prurigo as a clinical prodrome to adult T-cell leukemia/lymphoma. *Br J Dermatol* 1998, 138:137. _____ ▲

Human Immunodeficiency Virus (HIV, HTLV III)

HIV infects human helper T cells, leading to a progressive immunodeficiency disease. In its end stages it is called *acquired immunodeficiency syndrome* (AIDS). Cutaneous manifestations are prominent, affecting up to 90% of HIV-infected persons. Many patients have multiple skin lesions of different kinds. The skin lesions or combinations of skin conditions are so unique that the diagnosis of HIV infection or AIDS can often be suspected from the skin examination only. The skin findings can be classified into three broad categories: infections, inflammatory dermatoses, and neoplasms. The skin conditions also tend to appear at a specific stage in the progression of HIV disease, making them useful markers of the stage of HIV disease.

The natural history of HIV infection is a gradual loss of helper T cells in the vast majority of patients. The rate of this decline is variable, with some patients progressing rapidly and others very slowly or not at all (long term non-progressors). Soon after infection there is a seroconversion syndrome called primary HIV infection, or acute infection (group I). Patients recover from this syndrome and enter a relatively long latent period (asymptomatic infection or group II), which averages about 10 years. During this period patients may have persistent generalized lymphadenopathy (group III). When symptoms begin to appear they are often nonspecific and include fever, weight loss, chronic diarrhea, and mucocutaneous disease (group IV A). Helper T-cell counts in group II, III, and IV A patients usually range from 200 to 500. The skin findings at this stage (originally called ARC [AIDS-related complex]) include seborrheic dermatitis (Fig. 19-56), pruritus ani, psoriasis, Reiter's

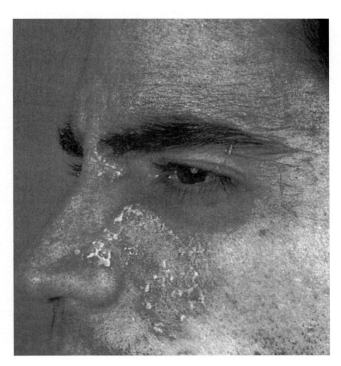

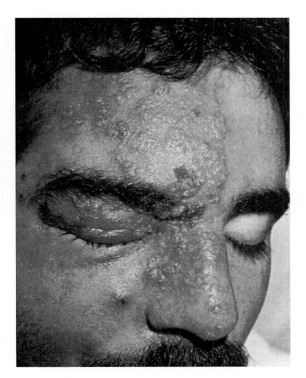

Fig. 19-56 Seborrheic dermatitis. Pinkish-red scaly and crusted plaques are seen in the malar areas but also in other locations. (From Friedman-Kien AE: Color atlas of AIDS, International edition, 1989, Philadelphia, WB Saunders.)

Fig. 19-57 Herpes zoster in AIDS.

syndrome, atopic dermatitis, herpes zoster (Fig. 19-57), acne rosacea, oral hairy leukoplakia (Fig. 19-58), onychomycosis, warts, recurrent *S. aureus* folliculitis, and mucocutaneous candidiasis.

Once the helper T-cell count is 200 or less the patient is defined as having AIDS. In this stage of HIV disease the skin lesions are more characteristic of immunodeficiency and include characteristic opportunistic infections: chronic herpes simplex (Fig. 19-59), molluscum contagiosum, bartonellosis (bacillary angiomatosis), systemic fungal infections (cryptococcosis, histoplasmosis, coccidioidomycosis, and penicilliosis), and mycobacterial infection. Paradoxically, patients at this stage also have hyperreactive skin and frequently have inflammatory, often pruritic skin diseases. These skin conditions include eosinophilic folliculitis, granuloma annulare, drug reactions, and photodermatitis.

When the T-cell count falls below 50, the patient is often said to have "advanced AIDS." These patients may have very unusual presentations of their opportunistic infections. These include multicentric, refractory molluscum contagiosum (Fig. 19-60); chronic herpes simplex; chronic cutaneous varicella zoster infection; cutaneous acanthamebiasis, cutaneous atypical mycobacterial infections (including *Mycobacterium avium* complex and *M. haemophilum*), and crusted scabies. Treatment of their infections is of-

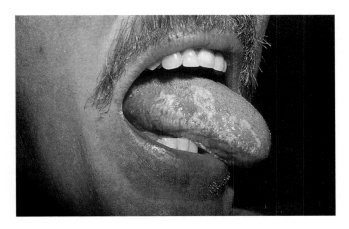

Fig. 19-58 Oral hairy leukoplakia.

ten very difficult because of the significant chronic immunosuppression.

It is now clear that HIV itself is the cause of the loss of helper T cells and that effective treatment of HIV infection may halt or reverse the natural history of HIV disease. There are numerous antiretroviral agents, and they are usually used in combinations called "cocktails." This combination treatment is called *highly active antiretroviral therapy* (HAART). About half of HIV-infected patients respond to

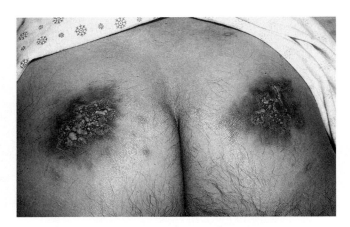

Fig. 19-59 Chronic herpes simplex.

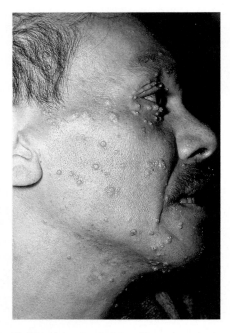

Fig. 19-60 Extensive facial molluscum contagiosum.

Primary HIV Infection (Acute Seroconversion Syndrome).
Several weeks after infection with HIV, an acute illness develops in a large proportion of individuals. The clinical syndrome is much like Epstein-Barr virus infection, with fever, sore throat, cervical adenopathy, a rash, and oral, genital, and rectal ulceration. The skin eruption can be polymorphous. Most characteristic is a papular eruption of discrete, slightly scaly, oval lesions of the upper trunk. The lesions have a superficial resemblance to pityriasis rosea, but the peripheral scale is not prominent, and there is focal hemorrhage in the lesions. A Gianotti-Crosti–like papular eruption may also occur. The mucosal erosions resemble aphthae but are larger and can affect all parts of the mouth, pharynx, esophagus, and anal mucosa. Dysphagia may be prominent. The helper T-cell count falls abruptly during seroconversion. The level of immune impairment may be adequate to allow oral candidiasis or even *Pneumocystis carinii* pneumonia to develop. The diagnosis should be suspected in any at-risk individual with the correct constellation of symptoms. A direct measurement of HIV viral load will confirm the diagnosis. Combination antiviral therapy is instituted immediately in these patients with the hope of improving the natural history of their disease.

HIV-Associated Pruritus. From early in the HIV epidemic, it was clear that pruritus was a marker of HIV infection throughout the world. Pruritus is not caused by HIV disease itself but is related to inflammatory dermatoses associated with the disease. "Papular pruritic eruption" is not a specific disease, but a wastebasket diagnosis used to encompass patients with many forms of HIV-associated pruritus. These pruritic eruptions are best subdivided as follicular and nonfollicular eruptions. The follicular eruptions are more common.

Eosinophilic folliculitis is the most common pruritic follicular eruption. It is seen in patients with a helper T-cell count of about 200. Clinically, it presents with urticarial follicular papules on the upper trunk, face, scalp, and neck. Pustular lesions are uncommon; pustules are usually smaller than in bacterial folliculitis and represent end-stage lesions. They are uncommonly seen, since the pruritus is so severe that they are excoriated before the lesion evolves to this degree. Ninety percent of lesions occur above the nipple line on the anterior trunk, and lesions typically extend down the midline of the back to the lumbar spine. The disease waxes and wanes in severity and may spontaneously clear, only to flare unpredictably. A peripheral eosinophilia may be present and the serum IgE level may be elevated, suggesting this is a disorder mediated by Th2 helper T cells. Histologically, an infiltrate of mononuclear cells and eosinophils is seen around the upper portion of the hair follicle at the level of the sebaceous gland. As lesions evolve, eosinophils and lymphocytes enter the follicular structure and the sebaceous glands. Pustules are formed late

this treatment and may have dramatic improvement of their HIV disease. HIV virus disappears from the blood and helper T-cell counts rise. As expected, in patients who respond to HAART, opportunistic infections no longer occur, and subsequently mortality decreases. This is also true of cutaneous infectious conditions but is not true of all the inflammatory disorders seen in patients with AIDS. HIV-associated psoriasis improves, especially if zidovudine is a part of the therapeutic cocktail. With the HAART combination treatment, however, eosinophilic folliculitis and drug eruptions may become more frequent or more severe.

and represent aggregates of eosinophils in the uppermost part of the follicle.

Initial treatment is with topical steroids and antihistamines. If the patient fails to respond, phototherapy (UVB or PUVA) or itraconazole 200 mg twice daily may be effective. In some patients repeated applications of permethrin (every other night for up to 6 weeks) may be of benefit. This latter therapy is directed at *Demodex* mites, which may be the antigenic trigger of this condition. Isotretinoin is also effective, often after a few months, in a dose of about 0.5 to 1 mg/kg/day. Staphylococcal folliculitis, which may be severely pruritic in patients with HIV disease, and pityrosporum folliculitis should be included in the differential diagnosis. These are excluded by bacterial culture and skin biopsy, respectively.

The other pruritic dermatoses that are not follicular can be divided into the primarily papular eruptions and the eczematous ones. The papular eruptions include scabies, insect bites, transient acantholytic dermatosis, granuloma annulare, and prurigo nodularis. The eczematous dermatoses include atopic-like dermatitis, seborrheic dermatitis, nummular eczema, xerotic eczema, photodermatitis, and drug eruptions. Patients may have multiple eruptions simultaneously, making differential diagnosis difficult. A skin biopsy from a representative lesion of every morphologic type on the patient may elucidate the true diagnoses. Treatment is determined by the diagnosis and is similar to treatment in persons without HIV infection with these same dermatoses. Special considerations in AIDS patients include the use of ivermectin for crusted scabies and thalidomide for prurigo nodularis and photodermatitis. Both these agents are very effective if used appropriately.

HIV-Associated Neoplasia.
Neoplasia is prominent in HIV infection and in some cases is highly suggestive of HIV infection. Kaposi's sarcoma (KS) is an example. Other common neoplasms seen in patients with HIV infection include superficial basal cell carcinomas of the trunk, squamous cell carcinomas in sun-exposed areas, genital HPV-induced squamous cell carcinoma, and extranodal B-cell and T-cell lymphoma.

Nonmelanoma skin cancers are very common in HIV-infected persons and usually occur as superficial multicentric basal cell carcinomas on the trunk in fair-skinned males in their twenties to fifties. The ratio of basal cell carcinoma to squamous cell carcinoma is not reversed in HIV disease, as it is in organ transplant recipients. Basal cell carcinomas behave in the same manner as they do in the immunocompetent host, and standard management is usually adequate.

Actinically induced squamous cell carcinomas are also quite common and present in the standard manner as nodules, keratotic papules, or ulcerations. In most cases their behavior is relatively benign and standard management is adequate. Removal of squamous cell carcinomas in sun-exposed areas by curettage and desiccation in patients with HIV infection is associated with an unacceptably high recurrence rate of about 15%; complete excision is therefore recommended. In a small subset of AIDS patients, the actinic squamous cell carcinomas can be very aggressive—they may double in size over weeks and may metastasize to regional lymph nodes or viscerally, leading to the death of the patient. Nonmelanoma skin cancers in the HIV-infected patient seem to have intermediate behavior between that of a normal host, and that of the organ transplant recipient. Basal cell carcinomas behave as expected, but squamous cell cancers arising in sun-exposed skin can be very aggressive.

Genital squamous cell carcinomas including cervical, vaginal, anal, penile, and nail bed squamous cell carcinoma all occur in patients with HIV infection. These neoplasms are increased in frequency, and the progression from HPV infection to neoplasia appears to be accelerated. This is analogous to the situation in organ transplant and other immunosuppressed patients. It appears that these cancers are associated with primarily "high-risk" human papillomavirus types.

For the dermatologist, there are three important manifestations of high-risk genital HPV infection in HIV. Most common is perianal dysplasia, seen most frequently in homosexual men with a history of receptive anal intercourse. Dysplasia in this area may present as velvety white or hyperpigmented plaques involving the whole anal area and extending into the anal canal. These lesions may erode or ulcerate. Histology will demonstrate squamous cell carcinoma in situ. The risk of progression of the lesions to anal squamous cell carcinoma is unknown but is estimated to be at least 10 times higher than the rate of cervical cancer in women in the general population. The management of such lesions is unclear, but regular follow-up is clearly indicated, and any masses in the anal canal should be immediately referred for biopsy.

The vulvar and penile skin may develop flat white or hyperpigmented macules from a few millimeters to several centimeters in diameter. These show squamous cell carcinoma in situ and are analogous to Bowenoid papulosis in the immunocompetent host. Rare cases of progression to squamous cell carcinoma have occurred. Such lesions are best managed conservatively as warts and are watched closely. Lesions of the penis and vulva, not at a transition zone or on mucosal surfaces, have a low risk of progressing to invasive squamous cell carcinoma. Lesions of the glans penis that are red and fixed should be undergo biopsy. If the changes of squamous cell carcinoma in situ are found, these should be managed aggressively as erythroplasia of Queyrat. Topical 5-FU and superficial radiation therapy are effective. Close clinical follow-up is indicated. Periungual squamous cell carcinoma has also been seen in patients with HIV infection and is felt to be associated with high-risk

HPV types. Any persistent keratotic or hyperpigmented lesion in the periungual area must be carefully evaluated. Management is surgical excision.

Extranodal B-cell and, less commonly, T-cell lymphomas are associated with the advanced immunosuppression of AIDS. The B-cell lymphomas and some of the T-cell lymphomas present as violaceous or plum-colored papules, nodules, or tumors. Once the diagnosis is established by biopsy, systemic chemotherapy is required. Epstein-Barr virus is found in some cases. Mycosis fungoides can also be seen in patients with HIV infection, often in patients who have not yet developed AIDS. It presents with pruritic patches or plaques and may progress to tumor stage. Epstein-Barr virus in not found in these cases.

Malignant melanoma is occasionally seen in persons with HIV infection. The patients demonstrate the same risk factors as do other melanoma patients, multiple nevi, fair skin type, and prior intermittent intense sun exposure. The prognosis of these patients is unknown, but the risk of metastasis has been suggested to be increased. Many fair-skinned patients infected with HIV complain of the new onset of atypical moles (analogous to organ transplant patients). Whether these confer an increased risk of melanoma is unknown.

AIDS and Kaposi's Sarcoma. Kaposi's sarcoma (KS) was, along with pneumocystis pneumonia, the harbinger of the AIDS epidemic. Many homosexual and bisexual men presented with this tumor in the early 1980s, with a prevalence of up to 25% in some cohorts. HHV-8, a gamma-herpesvirus, has been identified in these lesions and appears to be pathogenically related. The clinical features of KS in patients with AIDS are different than those seen in elderly men who do not have AIDS. Patients with AIDS present with symmetrical widespread lesions, often numerous. Lesions begin as macules that may progress to tumors of nodules (Figs. 19-61 and 19-62). Any mucocutaneous surface may be involved, but areas of predilection include the hard palate, trunk, penis, and lower legs and soles. Visceral disease may be present, and progressive. Edema may accompany lower leg lesions, and if it is significant, it is often associated with lymph node involvement in the inguinal area.

A diagnosis of KS is established by skin biopsy, which should be taken from the center of the most infiltrated plaque. Excessive bleeding is not usually a problem. Early macular lesions show atypical, angulated, ectatic vessels in the upper dermis associated with an inflammatory infiltrate containing plasma cells. Plaque lesions show aggregates of small vessels and endothelial cells in the upper dermis, and surrounding adnexal structures, especially the salivary glands. Nodules and tumors show the classic pattern of a spindle cell neoplasm with prominent extravasation of RBCs.

The treatment of AIDS-associated KS depends on the

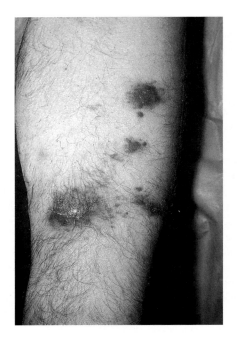

Fig. 19-61   Kaposi's sarcoma.

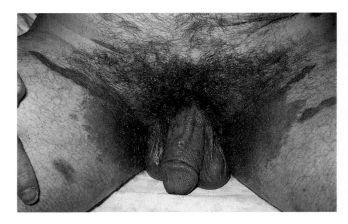

Fig. 19-62   Kaposi's sarcoma and seborrheic dermatitis.

extent and aggressiveness of the disease. Effective HAART after about 6 months is associated with involution of KS lesions. This should be the initial management in most patients with mild to moderate disease (fewer than 50 lesions, and fewer than 10 new lesions per month) who are not receiving anti-HIV treatment. Intralesional vinblastine 0.2 to 0.4 mg/ml can be infiltrated into lesions (as for a hypertrophic scar), and they will involve over several weeks. Hyperpigmentation usually remains. Cryotherapy is also effective but will leave postinflammatory hypopigmentation in pigmented persons. Persistent individual lesions and lesions of the soles and penis respond well to local irradiation therapy (one single treatment of 80 Gy or fractionated treatments to 150 Gy). For patients with symptomatic visceral disease, aggressive skin disease, marked edema, and pulmonary disease, systemic chemotherapy is indicated. Options include interferon alfa, vinca alkaloids, bleomycin, and liposomal doxorubicin as first-line therapies, and taxol for treatment failures.

Badger J, et al: HIV and psoriasis. *Clin Rev Allergy Immunol* 1997, 14:417.

Burdick AE, et al: Resolution of Kaposi's sarcoma associated with undetectable levels of human herpesvirus 8 DNA in a patient with AIDS after protease inhibitor therapy. *J Am Acad Dermatol* 1997, 37:648.

Kerschmann RL, et al: Cutaneous presentations of lymphoma in HIV disease. *Arch Dermatol* 1995, 131:1281.

Krown SE: Acquired immunodeficiency syndrome-associated Kaposi's sarcoma. *Med Clin North Am* 1997, 81:471.

Majors MJ, et al: HIV-related eosinophilic folliculitis. *Semin Cutan Med Surg* 1997, 6:219.

Maurer TA, et al: Cutaneous squamous cell carcinoma in human immunodeficiency virus infected patients. *Arch Dermatol* 1997, 133:577.

Pappert A, et al: Photosensitivity as the presenting illness in four patients with human immunodeficiency viral infection. *Arch Dermatol* 1994, 130:618.

Schacker TW, et al: Clinical and epidemiologic features of primary HIV infection. *Ann Intern Med* 1997, 126:174.

Stern RS: Epidemiology of skin disease in HIV infection. *J Invest Dermatol* 1994, 102(Suppl):34. _____ ▲

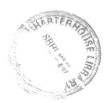

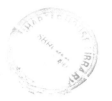

CHAPTER 20

Parasitic Infestations, Stings, and Bites

The major groups or phyla of animal parasites affecting humans are the Protozoa, Cnidaria (formerly Coelenterata), Nemathelminthes, Platyhelminthes, Annelida, Arthropoda, and Chordata.

Alexander J O'D: Arthropods and human skin. Berlin, 1984, Springer Verlag.

Fisher AA: Atlas of aquatic dermatology. New York, 1978, Grune & Stratton.

Mackey SL, et al: Dermatologic manifestations of parasitic diseases. *Infect Dis Clin North Am* 1994, 8:713.

Tornieporth NG, et al: Infectious considerations in the world traveler. *Dermatol Clin* 1997, 15:285.

Wong RC, et al: Spider bites. *Arch Dermatol* 1987, 123:98. ▲

Phylum Protozoa

The protozoa are one-celled organisms, divided into classes according to the nature of their locomotion. Class Sarcodina organisms move by temporary projections of cytoplasm (pseudopods); class Mastigophora by means of one or more flagella; class Ciliata by short, hairlike projections of cytoplasm (cilia); and class Sporozoa, with no special organs of locomotion.

CLASS SARCODINA

The ameba is the best known organism in this class. Of medical significance is *Entamoeba histolytica.*

Amebiasis Cutis

Most lesions begin as deep abscesses that rupture and form ulcerations with distinct, raised, cordlike edges and an erythematous halo approximately 2 cm wide. The base is covered with necrotic tissue and hemopurulent, glairy, pus-containing amebae. These lesions are from a few centimeters to 20 cm wide. They may occur on the trunk, abdomen, external genitalia, buttocks, or perineum. Those on the abdomen may result from hepatic abscesses. All ages are at risk.

Intestinal amebiasis, with bloody diarrhea and hepatic abscesses, may be present. Penile lesions are probably sexually acquired. The sole manifestation of early amebiasis may be chronic urticaria.

The causative organism, the trophozoite of *E. histolytica,* may be found in the base of the lesion by direct smear or shave biopsy.

Worldwide, an estimated 10% of the population is infected with *E. histolytica.* An estimated 10 million invasive cases occur annually, most of them in the tropics. In the United States, the disease occurs chiefly in institutionalized patients, world travelers, recent immigrants, migrant workers, and male homosexuals.

The histologic findings are those of a necrotic ulceration with many lymphocytes, neutrophils, plasma cells, and eosinophils. *E. histolytica* is found in the tissue, within blood and lymph vessels. The organism measures 50 to 60 μ in diameter, has basophilic cytoplasm, and a single eccentric nucleus with a central karyosome.

The organism is frequently demonstrable in fresh material from the base of the ulcer. Culture of the protozoa confirms the diagnosis. Indirect hemagglutination test results remain elevated for years after the initial invasive disease's onset, whereas the results of gel diffusion precipitation tests and counterimmunoelectrophoresis become negative at 6 months; this property can be used to test for recurrent or active disease in persons coming from endemic areas.

When the perianal or perineal areas are involved, granuloma inguinale, lymphogranuloma venereum, deep mycosis, and syphilis must be considered. In chronic urticaria, fresh stool examinations by a trained technician are necessary.

The treatment of choice is a combination of a specific drug with a luminal amebicide. Metronidazole (Flagyl), 750 mg orally three times a day for 10 days, followed by iodoquinol, 650 mg three times daily for 20 days, is recommended. Abscesses may require surgical drainage, but there is no need for resection of lesions.

Fujita WH, et al: Cutaneous amebiasis. *Arch Dermatol* 1981, 117:309.

Gullett J, et al: Disseminated granulomatous acanthamoeba infection presenting as an unusual skin lesion. *Am J Med* 1979, 67:891.

Martinez AJ: Acanthamoebiasis and immunosuppression. *J Neuropath Exp Neurol* 1982, 41:548.

Wortman PD: Acanthamoeba infection. *Int J Dermatol* 1996, 35:48. ▲

CLASS MASTIGOPHORA

The organisms belonging to this class are known as *flagellates*. Many have an undulating membrane with flagella along their crest.

Trichomoniasis

Trichomonas vulvovaginitis is a common cause of vaginal pruritus, with burning and a frothy leukorrhea. The vaginal mucosa appears bright red from inflammation and may be mottled with pseudomembranous patches. The male urethra may also harbor the organism; in the male it causes urethritis and prostatitis. Occasionally, men may develop balanoposthitis; Michalowski reported 16 cases of this, with erosive lesions on the glans and foreskin predominating. Pavithran reported it to be the cause of an abscess of the median raphae. Neonates may acquire the infection during passage through the birth canal, but they require treatment only if symptomatic or if colonization lasts more than 4 weeks. As this is otherwise nearly exclusively a sexually transmitted disorder, trichomonas vulvovaginitis in a child should make one suspect sexual abuse.

Trichomoniasis is caused by *Trichomonas vaginalis,* a colorless pyriform flagellate 5 to 15 μ long (Fig. 20-1). *T. vaginalis* is demonstrated in smears from affected areas. Testing by direct immunofluorescence is sensitive and specific.

Metronidazole, 2.0 g in a single oral dose, is the treatment of choice. Alternatively, 500 mg twice daily for 7 days may be given. Patients should be warned to not drink alcohol for 24 hours after the last dose because of the disulfiram type of effects of this medication. Male sex partners should also be treated. The use of metronidazole is contraindicated in pregnant women, and clotrimazole, applied intravaginally, at a dosage of 100 mg nightly for 2 weeks may be used in these cases.

Michalowski R: Trichomonal balanoposthitis. *Ann Dermatol Venereol* (Paris) 1981, 108:73.

Pavithran K: Trichomonal abscess of the median raphe of the penis. *Int J Dermatol* 1993, 32:820.

Sobel JD: Vulvovaginitis. *Dermatol Clin* 1992, 10:339.

STD treatment guidelines. *MMWR* 1998, 47:1. ▲

Leishmaniasis

Cutaneous leishmaniasis, American mucocutaneous leishmaniasis, and visceral leishmaniasis (kala-azar), which includes infantile leishmaniasis and post–kala-azar dermal

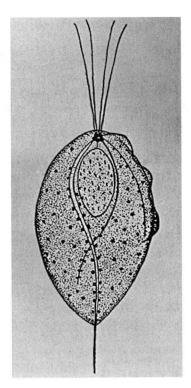

Fig. 20-1 *Trichomonas vaginalis.*

leishmaniasis, are all caused by morphologically and culturally indistinguishable protozoa of the family Trypanosomidae, called *Leishmania* (pronounced leesh-may´-nea). However, the clinical features of these diseases differ and they have, in general, different geographical distributions. The development of monoclonal antibodies that discriminate among organisms may lead to a clearer taxonomy, but this is in a state of flux.

Cutaneous Leishmaniasis. There are several types of lesions. All tend to occur on exposed parts as all are transmitted by the sandfly. Old World leishmaniasis is limited to the skin and has also been called *Baghdad boil* (Fig. 20-2), *Oriental sore, leishmaniasis tropica, Biskra button, Delhi boil, Aleppo boil, Kandahar sore,* and *Lahore sore.* Subtypes of New World infection with purely cutaneous involvement are *uta, pian bois,* and *bay sore* or *chiclero ulcer.*

CLINICAL FEATURES. In Old World leishmaniasis lesions may present in two ways. One distinct type is the moist or rural type, a slowly growing, indurated, livid, indolent papule, which enlarges in a few months to form a nodule that may ulcerate in a few weeks to form an ulcer as much as 5 cm in diameter (Fig. 20-3). Spontaneous healing usually takes place within 6 months, leaving a characteristic scar. This type is contracted from rodent reservoirs such as gerbils via the sandfly as the vector. The incubation period is relatively short—1 to 4 weeks. The dry or urban type has

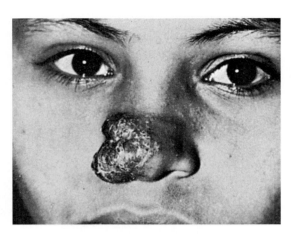

Fig. 20-2 Baghdad boil of 5 months' duration. (Courtesy Dr. G.F. Rahim, Baghdad.)

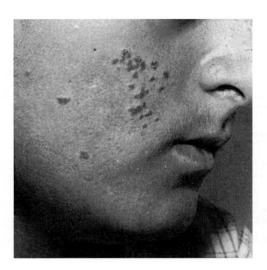

Fig. 20-4 Leishmaniasis recidivans. (Courtesy Dr. S. Ganos, Jerusalem.)

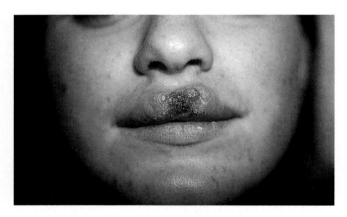

Fig. 20-3 Leishmaniasis in an American girl (condition was acquired while girl was in the Middle East).

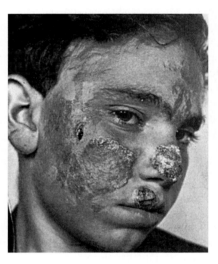

Fig. 20-5 Leishmaniasis recidivans.

a longer incubation period (2 to 8 months or longer), develops much more slowly, and heals more slowly than the rural type.

Rarely, after the initial or "mother" lesion is healed, there may appear at the borders of the healed area a few soft red papules covered with whitish scales and having the "apple jelly" characteristics of lupus vulgaris (Fig. 20-4). These spread peripherally on a common erythematous base and are the lupoid type (Fig. 20-5). This is also known as *leishmaniasis recidivans* and occurs most commonly with the urban type of disease, caused by *L. tropica*.

New World disease may also induce purely cutaneous lesions, of varied morphology. The primary papule may become nodular, verrucous, furuncular, or ulcerated, with an infiltrated red border (Figs. 20-6 to 20-8). Subcutaneous

peripheral nodules, which eventually ulcerate, may signal extension of the disease. A sporotrichoid pattern may occur with lymphadenopathy, and the nodes may rarely yield organisms (Fig. 20-9, *A* and *B*). Recidivans lesions are unusual in the New World form of disease.

In Yucatan and Guatemala, a subtype of New World disease exists: the chiclero ulcer. The most frequent site of infection is the ear (Fig. 20-10). The lesions ulcerate and occur most frequently in workers who harvest chicle for chewing gum in the forests, where there is high humidity. This form is a more chronic ulcer that may persist for years, destroying the ear cartilage and leading to deformity. The etiologic agent is *L. mexicana* and the vector, a sandfly, *Lutzomyia flaviscutellata*.

Uta is a term used by Peruvians for leishmaniasis

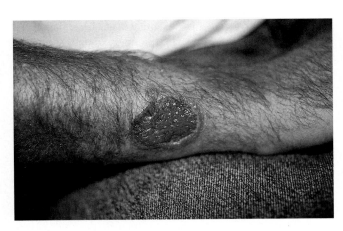

Fig. 20-6 Leishmania ulcer of the wrist, acquired in Panama by an American soldier.

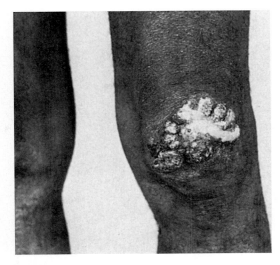

Fig. 20-8 Verrucous leishmaniasis on the knee. (Courtesy Dr. J. Convit.)

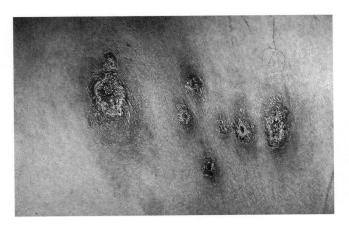

Fig. 20-7 New World leishmaniasis acquired in Costa Rica.

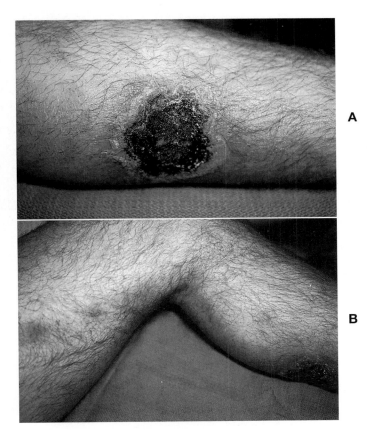

A

B

Fig. 20-9 **A,** Primary inoculation chancre with **B,** sporotrichoid extension up leg and thigh.

occurring in mountainous territory at elevations of 1200 to 1800 meters above sea level. The ulcerating lesions are found on exposed sites, and mucosal lesions do not occur.

Disseminated cutaneous leishmaniasis may be seen in both New and Old World disease. Multiple nonulcerated papules and plaques, chiefly on exposed surfaces, characterize this type (Fig. 20-11). It is caused by several subspecies of *L. mexicana; L. aethiopica* may cause this type of disease in Ethiopia and Kenya. The disease begins with a single ulcer, nodule, or plaque from which satellite lesions may develop and disseminate to cover the entire body (Fig. 20-12). The disease is progressive, and treatment is usually ineffective. It is characterized by anergy to the organism. The Montenegro reaction is negative. This type of leishmaniasis must be differentiated from lepromatous leprosy, xanthoma tuberosum, paracoccidioidal granuloma, Lobo's disease, and malignant lymphoma.

ETIOLOGIC FACTORS. Old World cutaneous leishmaniasis

may be caused by *L. tropica, L. major, L. aethiopia,* and *L. infantum,* the cause of Mediterranean visceral leishmaniasis. Purely cutaneous leishmaniasis is also caused by several species present in the New World. *L. mexicana* does not induce mucosal disease. *L. braziliensis guyanensis*

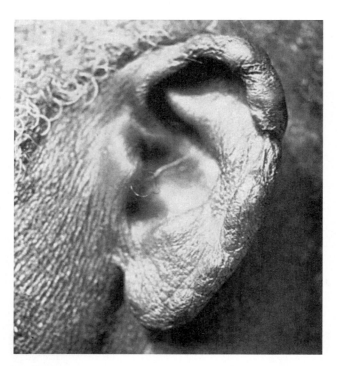

Fig. 20-10 Chiclero ulcer in leishmaniasis. (Courtesy Dr. Axel W. Hoke.)

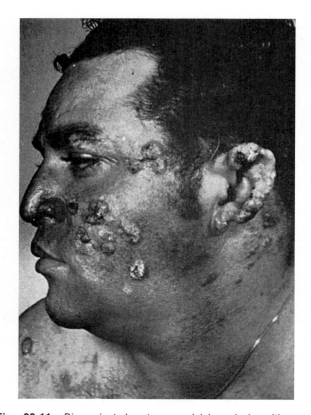

Fig. 20-11 Disseminated cutaneous leishmaniasis with nasal lesions, verrucous nodules, and mutilating ulcerations of the ear (chiclero ulcer). (Courtesy Dr. J. Convit, Venezuela.)

produces cutaneous disease, as does *L. braziliensis braziliensis and L. b. panamensis;* however, the latter two may also result in mucocutaneous disease.

EPIDEMIOLOGY. Cutaneous leishmaniasis is endemic in Asia Minor and to a lesser extent in many countries around the Mediterranean Sea. Iran and Saudi Arabia have a high occurrence rate. Purely cutaneous lesions are also found in Central and South America and nine patients who acquired their disease in Texas have been reported. Children are affected most often, since immunity is acquired from the initial infection. Deliberate inoculation on the thigh is sometimes practiced so that scarring on the face—a frequent site for Oriental sore—may be avoided.

PATHOGENESIS. The organism has an alternate life in a vertebrate and an insect host. Man and other mammals, such as dogs and rodents, are the natural reservoir hosts. The vector hosts are *Phlebotomus* sandflies in the Old World type and *Phlebotomus perniciosus* and *Lutzomyia* sandflies for the New World cutaneous leishmaniasis. After the insect has fed on blood, the flagellates (leptomonad, promastigote) develop in the gut in 8 to 20 days, after which migration occurs into the mouth parts; from here transmission into humans occurs by a bite. In humans, the flagella are lost and a leishmanial form (amastigote) is assumed.

HISTOPATHOLOGY. Cutaneous leishmaniasis shows the typical features of an ulcer, with a heavy infiltrate of histiocytes, lymphocytes, and polymorphonuclear leukocytes. Numerous organisms are present (mostly in histiocytes), which are nonencapsulated and contain a nucleus and a paranucleus. Wright's, Giemsa, and monoclonal antibody staining may be helpful in identifying the organisms. The parasitized histiocytes form tuberculoid granulomas in the dermis. Pseudoepitheliomatous hyperplasia may occur in the edges of the ulcer.

DIAGNOSIS. In endemic areas, the diagnosis is not too difficult. In other localities, cutaneous leishmaniasis may be confused with syphilis, yaws, lupus vulgaris, and pyogenic granulomas. The diagnosis is established by demonstration of the organism in smears. Parasites can be cultured from tissue fluid. A hypodermic needle is inserted into the normal skin and to the edge of the ulcer base. The needle is rotated to work loose some material and serum, which is then aspirated. A culture on Nicolle-Novy-MacNeal (NNN) medium at 22° to 35° C (71.6° to 95° F) is recommended to demonstrate the leptomonads. The leishmanin intradermal test (Leishman-Montenegro-Donovan) may be helpful in making the diagnosis in nonendemic populations. It becomes positive some 3 months after infection.

The sophisticated tests now being used to diagnose and classify subspecies involve detection of monoclonal antibodies with the use of immunoperoxidase, radiolabeling, or fluorescenation, DNA probes, DNA buoyancy, restriction–endonuclease fragment patterns of kinetoplast DNA, restriction–frequent length polymorphisms of nuclear DNA, and isoenzyme electrophoresis.

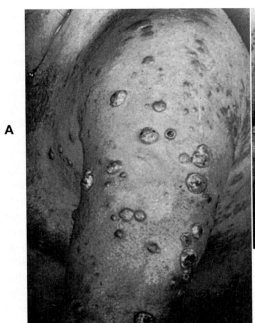
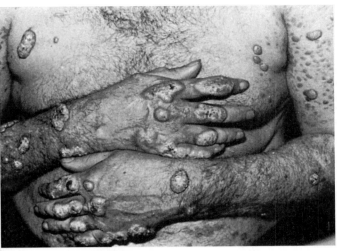

Fig. 20-12 **A,** Disseminated cutaneous leishmaniasis showing large nodules with one on deltoid area undergoing ulceration. **B,** Disseminated leishmaniasis. (**A,** Courtesy Dr. J. Convit, Venezuela; **B,** Courtesy Dr. F. Kerdel-Vegas.)

TREATMENT. Spontaneous healing occurs, usually within 12 to 18 months, shorter for Old World disease. The rationale of treating an ordinarily self-limited infection include avoiding disfiguring scars in exposed areas, notably the face; avoiding secondary infection; controlling disease in the population; and failure of spontaneous healing: in the diffuse cutaneous and recidivans types, the disease may persist for 20 to 40 years if not treated.

In areas in which localized cutaneous leishmaniasis is not complicated by recidive or sporotrichoid forms or mucocutaneous disease, treatment with such topical modalities as paromycin sulfate 15% plus methylbenzethonium chloride 12%, ketoconazole cream under occlusion, cryotherapy, local heat, and laser ablation, or with intralesional sodium stibogluconate antimony or emetine hydrochloride, may be effective and safe. Perilesional injections of interferon-gamma have also been reported to be effective but are expensive.

In patients who are immunosuppressed or who acquire disease in areas where mucocutaneous disease may occur, systemic therapy is recommended. As with topical treatment, many alternatives have been reported effective. Sodium antimony gluconate (sodium stibogluconate) solution is given intramuscularly or intravenously 20 mg/kg/day in two divided doses for 28 days. It can be obtained from the CDC Drug Service, Atlanta, GA 30333. Repeated courses may be given. Antimony *n*-methyl glutamine (Glucantime) is used more often in Central and South America because of its local availability.

Other systemic medications that are reported to be effective include ketoconazole (600 mg/day for 28 days), itraconazole, dapsone, rifampin, and allopurinol. Some of these have not been subjected to controlled clinical trials, as is true of most topical treatments. The recidive and disseminated cutaneous types may require prolonged courses or adjuvant interferon therapy. Amphotericin B may be used in antimony-resistant disease.

Control depends chiefly on the success of antifly measures taken by health authorities.

Mucocutaneous Leishmaniasis (Leishmaniasis Americana, Espundia)

CLINICAL FEATURES. The initial infection, which occurs at the site of the fly bite, is a destructive ulcer. Secondary lesions on the mucosa usually occur at some time during the next 5 years. The earliest mucosal lesion is usually hyperemia of the nasal septum with subsequent ulceration, which progresses to invade the septum and later the paranasal fossae. Perforation of the septum eventually takes place. For some time the nose remains unchanged externally, despite the internal destruction.

At first only a dry crust is observed, or a bright red infiltration or vegetation on the nasal septum, with symptoms of obstruction and small hemorrhages. Despite the mutilating and destructive character of leishmaniasis, it never involves the nasal bones. When the septum is destroyed, the nasal bridge and tip of the nose collapse, giving an appearance of a parrot beak, camel nose, or tapir nose.

It is important to recall that the four great chronic infections (syphilis, tuberculosis, leprosy, and leishmaniasis) have a predilection for the nose. The ulcer may extend to the lips (Fig. 20-13) and continue to advance to the pharynx, attacking the soft palate, uvula, tonsils, gingiva,

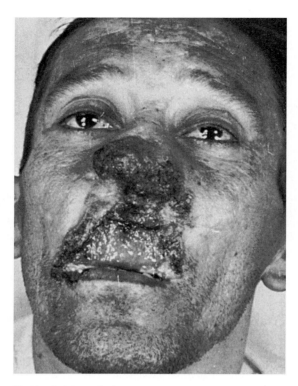

Fig. 20-13 Leishmaniasis americana (mucocutaneous). (Courtesy Dr. J. Convit.)

and tongue. The eventual mutilation is called *espundia*. Two perpendicular grooves at the union of the osseous palate and the soft tissues, in the midst of the vegetative infiltration of the entire pharynx is called the *palate cross of espundia*.

Only in exceptional cases does American leishmaniasis invade the genital or ocular mucous membranes. The frequency of mucous membrane involvement is variable. In Yucatan and Guatemala it is an exception; in other countries, such as Brazil, it may occur in 80% of the cases.

ETIOLOGIC FACTORS. Mucocutaneous leishmaniasis is caused by *L. braziliensis braziliensis* and *L. braziliensis panamensis*. Leishmania has two forms, the nonflagellated form or leishmania, which is found in the tissues of humans and in animals susceptible to the inoculation of the parasite, and the flagellated form or leptomonad, which is found in the digestive tract of the vector insect (*Lutzomyia* in mucocutaneous disease) and in cultures. The typical morphology of leishmania, as found in the vertebrates, is round or oval, usually with one extremity more rounded than the other, measuring 2 to 4 μ by 1.5 to 2.5 μ, with cytoplasm, nucleus, and blepharoplast or kinetoplast.

EPIDEMIOLOGY. Mucocutaneous leishmaniasis is predominantly a rural and jungle disease. It predominates in damp and forested regions. The disease can be contracted at any time of the year, but the risk is highest just after the rainy season. All ages and races and both sexes are equally affected.

HISTOPATHOLOGY. In cases of granulomatous infiltration, when intracellular parasites are found in histiocytes, leishmaniasis is one of several diseases to be considered, including rhinoscleroma, histoplasmosis, granuloma inguinale, and toxoplasmosis. The Leishman-Donovan body is nonencapsulated and shows a characteristic nucleus and parabasal body. Touch smears stained with Giemsa are helpful in many cases of cutaneous and mucocutaneous leishmaniasis.

In the ulcerous type, one can find marked irregular acanthosis and sometimes pseudoepitheliomatous hyperplasia. The dermis shows a dense infiltration of histiocytes, lymphocytes, and plasma cells. In new lesions some neutrophils are observed. Large Langhans' giant cells are occasionally seen. Typical tubercles are sometimes observed.

LABORATORY FINDINGS. Leishmania is demonstrated in the cutaneous and mucous membrane lesions by direct smears or cultures. In biopsy material stained with Wright's stain, one sees intracellular and extracellular organisms with typical morphology of two chromatic structures: nucleus and parabasal body. In later mucosal lesions the scarcity of parasites makes the identification difficult. The culture is done on Nicolle-Novy-MacNeal medium for leptomonads.

The intradermal Montenegro test is performed with a leptomonad suspension of 0.1 to 0.2 ml injected intradermally. The reading is made 48 to 72 hours later. A positive reaction is an area of induration greater than 5 mm in diameter 24 to 48 hours after injection (Fig. 20-14). This test is specific and sensitive, giving 95% positive results, but it can be negative in early cases of the disease, in which, however, it is always easy to find the parasites. Cross reactions occur with certain forms of cutaneous tuberculosis, but they are rare. Newer diagnostic techniques are under investigation as discussed above for cutaneous leishmaniasis, but most are only available at research centers.

PROPHYLAXIS. Although it is impractical to eliminate the insect vector, it is still the only valid measure for the control of this prevalent disease.

TREATMENT. Treatment is the same as described for cutaneous leishmaniasis except that antimony resistance is common in mucocutaneous disease. Combination therapy using antimonials with other drugs such as rifampin, or adding immunomodulators such as interferon gamma or interleukin-2 may result in cure. Amphotericin B treatment may be necessary.

Visceral Leishmaniasis (Kala-Azar, Dumdum Fever)

CLINICAL FEATURES. The earliest lesion is the cutaneous nodule or leishmanioma, which occurs at the site of the initial sandfly inoculation. *Kala-azar,* meaning "black fever," acquired its name because of the patchy macular darkening of the skin caused by deposits of melanin that develop in the later course of the disease. These patches are most marked over the forehead and temples, periorally, and on the midabdomen.

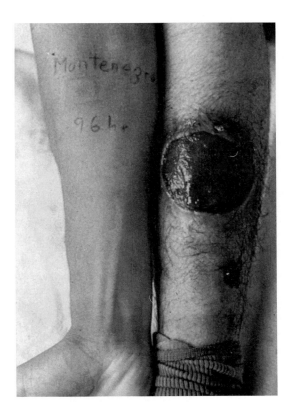

Fig. 20-14 Montenegro test in leishmaniasis. (Courtesy Dr. Axel W. Hoke.)

The primary target for the parasites is the reticuloendothelial system; the spleen, liver, bone marrow, and lymph nodes are attacked. The incubation period is 1 to 4 months. An intermittent fever, with temperatures ranging from 39° to 40° C (102° to 104° F). ushers in the disease. There are hepatosplenomegaly, agranulocytosis, anemia, and thrombocytopenia. Chills, fever, emaciation, weight loss, weakness, epistaxis, and purpura develop as the disease progresses. Susceptibility to secondary infection may produce pulmonary and gastrointestinal infection, ulcerations in the mouth (cancrum oris), and noma. Death occurs in about 2 years from onset in untreated individuals.

ETIOLOGIC FACTORS. *L. donovani* spp. *donovani, infantum,* and *chagasi,* cause visceral leishmaniasis and are parasites of rodents, canines, and humans. They are nonflagellate oval organisms some 3 μ in diameter, known as *Leishman-Donovan bodies.* In the sandfly it is a leptomonad form with flagella.

EPIDEMIOLOGY. *L.d. donovani* causes visceral leishmaniasis in India, with the major reservoir being humans and the vector being *Phlebotomus argentipes. L.d. infantum* occurs in China, Africa, the Near East and Middle East, and the Mediterranean littoral, where the major reservoirs are dogs, and *Phlebotomus perniciosus* and *P. ariasi* are the vectors of the Mediterranean type. American visceral leishmaniasis is caused by *L. donovani chagasi* and is transmitted by the sandfly *Lutzomyia longipalpis.* American visceral leishmaniasis principally affects domestic dogs, although explosive outbreaks of the human infection occur sporadically, when the number of *L. longipalpis* builds up to a high level in the presence of infected dogs. The principal foci of visceral leishmaniasis are in the drier, poorly forested areas of Latin America.

DIAGNOSIS. Leishman-Donovan bodies may be present in the blood in individuals with kala-azar of India. Specimens for examination, in descending order of utility, include spleen pulp, sternal marrow, liver tissue, and exudate from lymph nodes. Culturing on NNN medium may also reveal the organisms. The intradermal Montenegro test is also reliable.

TREATMENT. General supportive measures are essential. Pentavalent antimony has long been the drug of choice.

Post–Kala-Azar Dermal Leishmanoid.
In kala-azar, the leishmanoid (amastigote) forms may be widely distributed throughout apparently normal skin. During and after recovery from the disease, a special form of dermal leishmaniasis known as post–kala-azar dermal leishmanoid appears. This condition appears during or shortly after treatment in the African form, but its appearance may be delayed up to 10 years after treatment in the Indian form. It is common in India, occurring in up to 20% of patients, whereas in Africa only 2% develop it. There are two constituents of the eruption: a macular, depigmented eruption found mainly on the face, arms, and upper part of the trunk; and a warty, papular eruption in which amastigotes can be found. Because it may persist for up to 20 years, these patients may act as a chronic reservoir of infection. This condition closely resembles leprosy. There is evidence that patients who will develop this condition have as a marker interleukin-10 in their keratinocytes and sweat glands.

Viscerotropic Leishmaniasis.
Magill et al reported eight soldiers who developed systemic infection with *L. tropica* while fighting in Operation Desert Storm in Saudi Arabia. None had symptoms of kala-azar, but rather seven had fever, fatigue, malaise, cough, diarrhea, or abdominal pain. One patient was asymptomatic. None had cutaneous disease. In seven patients, diagnostic tests yielded positive results on bone marrow aspiration and one had lymph node involvement. Five of six treated with sodium stibogluconate improved.

Akufso H, et al: Administration of recombinant interleukin-2 reduces the local parasite load of patients with disseminated cutaneous leishmaniasis. *J Infect Dis* 1990, 161:775.

al Majali O, et al: A 2-year study of liquid nitrogen therapy in cutaneous leishmaniasis. *Int J Dermatol* 1997, 36:460.

Bahamdan KA, et al: Value of touch preparations (imprints) for diagnosis of cutaneous leishmaniasis. *Int J Dermatol* 1996, 35:558.

Ballou WR, et al: Safety and efficacy of high-dose sodium stibogluconate therapy of American cutaneous leishmaniasis. *Lancet* 1987, 2:13.

Berger TG, et al: Lymph node involvement in leishmaniasis. *J Am Acad Dermatol* 1985, 12:993.

Berman JD: Human leishmaniasis. *Clin Infect Dis* 1997, 24:684.

Bottasso O, et al: Successful treatment of antimony-resistant American mucocutaneous leishmaniasis. *Arch Dermatol* 1992, 128:996.

Cohen HA, et al: Treatment of leishmaniasis nodosa with intralesionally injected emetine hydrochloride. *J Am Acad Dermatol* 1987, 17:595.

Convit J, et al: Immunotherapy vs. chemotherapy in localized cutaneous leishmaniasis. *Lancet* 1987, 1:401.

Dauden E, et al: Leishmaniasis presenting as a dermatomyositis-like eruption in AIDS. *J Am Acad Dermatol* 1996, 35:316.

del Giudice, et al: Cutaneous leishmaniasis due to *Leishmania infantum. Arch Dermatol* 1998, 134:193.

Dogra J, et al: Dapsone in the treatment of cutaneous leishmaniasis. *Int J Dermatol* 1986, 25:398.

El Darouti MA, et al: Cutaneous leishmaniasis treatment with combined cryotherapy and intralesional stibogluconate injection. *Int J Dermatol* 1990, 29:56.

El On J, et al: Topical treatment of Old World leishmaniasis caused by *L. majore. J Am Acad Dermatol* 1992, 27:227.

Furner BB: Cutaneous leishmaniasis in Texas. *J Am Acad Dermatol* 1990, 27:368.

Gasim S, et al: High levels of plasma IL-10 and expression of IL-10 by keratinocytes during visceral leishmaniasis predict subsequent development of post-kala-azar dermal leishmaniasis. *Clin Exp Immunol* 1998, 111:64.

Goihanan Yahr M: American mucocutaneous leishmaniasis. *Dermatol Clin* 1994, 12:703.

Grevelink SA, et al: Leishmaniasis. *J Am Acad Dermatol* 1996, 34:257.

Herwaldt BL, et al: American cutaneous leishmaniasis in US travelers. *Ann Intern Med* 1993, 118:779.

Johhi RK, et al: Dermal leishmaniasis and rifampin. *Int J Dermatol* 1989, 28:612.

Kalter DC: Laboratory tests for the diagnosis and evaluation of leishmaniasis. *Dermatol Clin* 1994, 12:37.

Kenner JR, et al: The United States military and leishmaniasis. *Dermatol Clin* 1999, 17:77.

Kibbi AG, et al: Sporotrichoid leishmaniasis in patients from Saudi Arabia. *J Am Acad Dermatol* 1987, 17:759.

Kubba R, et al: Clinical diagnosis of cutaneous leishmaniasis (Oriental sore). *J Am Acad Dermatol* 1987, 16:1183.

Kubba R, et al: Dissemination in cutaneous leishmaniasis. *Int J Dermatol* 1988, 27:702.

Kurkuogla N, et al: Interferon gamma therapy for cutaneous leishmaniasis. *Arch Dermatol* 1990, 126:831.

Levine N: Cutaneous leishmaniasis treated with controlled localized heating. *Arch Dermatol* 1992, 128:759.

Magill AJ, et al: Visceral infection caused by *Leishmania tropica* in veterans of Operation Desert Storm. *N Engl J Med* 1993, 328:1387.

Martinez S, et al: Allopurinol in the treatment of American cutaneous leishmaniasis. *N Engl J Med* 1992, 326:741.

Mermel LA: Cutaneous leishmaniasis-chiclero ulcer in a Wisconsin native. *J Am Acad Dermatol* 1990, 230:1178.

Momeni AZ, et al: Treatment of cutaneous leishmaniasis with itraconazole. *Arch Dermatol* 1996, 132:784.

Mukherje CA, et al: Post-kala-azar dermal leishmaniasis. *J Cutan Pathol* 1993, 20:370.

Rames LV, et al: Efficacy of ketoconazole in post-kala-azar dermal leishmaniasis. *Arch Dermatol* 1992, 128:411.

Reed SG: Diagnosis of leishmaniasis. *Clin Dermatol* 1996, 14:471.

Rubio FA, et al: Leishmaniasis presenting as a psoriasiform eruption in AIDS. *Br J Dermatol* 1997, 136:792.

Samady JA, et al: Old World cutaneous leishmaniasis. *Int J Dermatol* 1997, 36:161.

Sangueza OP, et al: Mucocutaneous leishmaniasis. *J Am Acad Dermatol* 1993, 28:927.

Saurat JH: Cutaneous leishmaniasis treated with controlled localized heat. *Arch Dermatol* 1993, 129:510.

Sharguie KE, et al: Intralesional therapy of cutaneous leishmaniasis with sodium stibogluconate antimony. *Br J Dermatol* 1988, 1A:53.

Strick RA, et al: Recurrent cutaneous leishmaniasis. *J Am Acad Dermatol* 1983, 9:437.

Van Den Enden F, et al: Treatment of cutaneous leishmaniasis with itraconazole. *Int J Dermatol* 1994, 33:285.

Walsh DS, et al: Multiple lesions of sporotrichoid leishmaniasis in a Filipino expatriate. *J Am Acad Dermatol* 1997, 36:847.

Weinrauch L, et al: Topical treatment of New World cutaneous leishmaniasis in Belize. *J Am Acad Dermatol* 1993, 29:443. _____ ▲

Human Trypanosomiasis

Three species of trypanosomes are pathogenic to humans: *Trypanosoma gambiense* and *T. rhodesiense* in Africa, and *T. cruzi* in America. The skin manifestations are usually observed in the earlier stages of the disease as evanescent erythema, erythema multiforme, and edema, especially angioedema.

In the early stage of African trypanosomiasis, a trypanosome chancre may occur at the site of a tsetse fly bite. Then erythema with circumscribed swellings of angioedema, enlargement of the lymph glands, fever, malaise, headache, and joint pains ensue. In the West African (Gambian) form, the illness is chronic, lasting several years, with progressive deterioration, whereas the East African (Rhodesian) form is an acute illness, with a stormy, fatal course of weeks to months. The Rhodesian form is more often associated with cutaneous signs. Annular lesions and lesions resembling erythema nodosum are frequent manifestations. Lymphadenopathy is generalized, but frequently there is a pronounced enlargement of the posterior cervical group (Winterbottom's sign).

In American trypanosomiasis (Chagas' disease), similar changes take place in the skin. The reduviid bug *(kissing bug, assassin bug)* (Fig. 20-15) usually bites at night, frequently at mucocutaneous junctions, where the bug's infected feces are deposited when it feeds. The unsuspecting sleeping person rubs the feces into the bite and becomes infected. If the bite of the infected bug occurs near the eye, Romana's sign develops; this consists of unilateral conjunctivitis and edema of the eyelids, with an ulceration or chagoma in the area. The bite of a "kissing bug" becomes markedly swollen and red, whether trypanosomes are involved or not. Acute Chagas' disease is usually a mild illness consisting of fever, malaise, edema of the face and lower extremities and generalized lymphadenopathy. In chronic Chagas' disease, which occurs in 10% to 30% of infected persons years to decades later, the heart (myocarditis, arrhythmias, thromboembolism, and cardiac failure) and the gastrointestinal system (megaesophagus and megacolon) are the most commonly involved organs. The

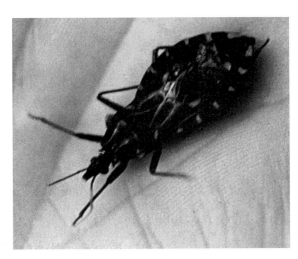

Fig. 20-15 Chagas' disease; the reduviid or "assassin" bug. (Courtesy Dr. Axel W. Hoke.)

remaining infected but asymptomatic indeterminate phase patients may pass the disease through transfusion.

Rhodesian trypanosomiasis is endemic among the cattle-raising tribes of East Africa, with the savannah habitat of the vectors determining its geographic distribution. Wild game and livestock are reservoir hosts, in addition to humans. The tsetse fly, *Glossina morsitans,* is the principal vector.

For Gambian trypanosomiasis, humans are the only vertebrate host and the palpalis group of tsetse flies is the invertebrate host. These flies are found close to the water, and their fastidious biologic requirements restrict their distribution, and thus that of the disease. Incidence is seasonal, with humidity and temperature being determining factors. The highest incidence is in males 20 to 40 years of age in the tropical areas of West and Central Africa.

Chagas' disease is prevalent in Central and South America from the United States to Argentina and Chile; the highest incidence is in Venezuela, Brazil, Uruguay, Paraguay, and Argentina. Approximately 29% of all male deaths in the 29- to 44-year-old age group in Brazil are ascribed to Chagas' disease.

Before central nervous system involvement has occurred, suramin, a complex, non–metal-containing, organic compound, is the treatment of choice. When the central nervous system is involved, melarsoprol is the drug of choice. For American trypanosomiasis, treatment is of limited efficacy. Nifurtimox and benzimidazole clear the parasitemia and reduce the severity of the acute illness. There is a high incidence of adverse effects, however. Conservative treatment is most appropriate for the patient with congestive heart failure from Chagas' myocarditis. Gastrointestinal complications may be treated surgically.

Cochran R, et al: African trypanosomiasis in the United States. *Arch Dermatol* 1983, 119:670.

Iborra C, et al: A traveler from Central Africa with fever and a skin lesion. *Clin Infect Dis* 1999, 28:679.
Kirchhoff LV: American trypanosomiasis. *N Engl J Med* 1993, 329:639.
McGovern TW, et al: Cutaneous manifestations of African trypanosomiasis. *Arch Dermatol* 1995, 131:1178. ▲

CLASS SPOROZOA
Toxoplasmosis

Toxoplasmosis is a zoonosis caused by a parasitic protozoan, *Toxoplasma gondii;* it is manifested by mild to severe forms of infection that may end in the host's death.

In humans, the infection may be either congenital or acquired. Congenital infection occurs from placental transmission. Abortion or stillbirth may result. However, a full-term child delivered to an infected mother may have a triad of hydrocephalus, chorioretinitis, and cerebral calcification. In addition, there may be hepatosplenomegaly and jaundice. Skin changes in toxoplasmosis are rare and clinically nonspecific.

In congenital toxoplasmosis, macular and hemorrhagic eruptions predominate. Blueberry muffin lesions, reflecting dermatoerythropoesis, may be seen. Occasionally, abnormal hair growth and exfoliative dermatitis have also been observed. Fine et al reviewed congenital toxoplasmosis and the differential diagnosis of the TORCH syndrome (toxoplasmosis, rubella, cytomegalovirus, and herpes simplex titer). In acquired toxoplasmosis, skin manifestations consist of cutaneous and subcutaneous nodules, macular, papular, and hemorrhagic eruptions, followed by scarlatiniform desquamation, roseola-like, erythema multiforme–like, and lichen planus–like eruptions as well as exfoliative dermatitis. As a rule, the exanthem is accompanied by high fever and general malaise. Pollock reported a case that clinically resembled dermatomyositis.

Diagnosis of acquired toxoplasmosis is of special importance to three groups of adults: healthy pregnant women concerned about recent exposure; adults with lymphadenopathy, fever, and myalgia, acute or chronic, who might have some other serious disease, such as lymphoma; and immunocompromised persons, such as patients with AIDS, in whom toxoplasmosis might be fatal. It is the most common cause of focal encephalitis in patients with AIDS. Hirschmann et al described an AIDS patient with a widespread papular eruption caused by toxoplasmosis.

As to pregnant women, 20% have already had the disease and are thus protected; they are identified by a positive test very early in pregnancy, or before they become pregnant. A high titer just before the twentieth week of gestation might make abortion advisable, or treatment indicated; or such a test before delivery would indicate treatment for the infant. Immunofluorescence or complement fixation tests are both informative. As to adults with lymphadenopathy, high or rising antibody titers at the time of onset or soon after are diagnostic. Characteristic histologic changes in lymph nodes may provide confirmation. In congenital cases (and, rarely, in acquired ones), chorioretinitis may occur a decade or more after infection. In congenitally acquired infection, chorioretinitis is usually bilateral, whereas in the acquired type it is usually unilateral.

Toxoplasma gondii is a crescent-shaped, oval, or round protozoan that can infect any mammalian or avian cell. The disease is often acquired through contact with animals, particularly cats. The two major routes of transmission of *T. gondii* in humans are oral and congenital. Meats used for human consumption may contain tissue cysts, thus serving as a source of infection when eaten raw or undercooked. There is no evidence of direct human-to-human transmission, other than from mother to fetus.

The diagnosis cannot be made on clinical grounds alone. The diagnosis of toxoplasmosis may be established by isolation of *T. gondii,* demonstration of the protozoa in tissue sections, smears, or body fluids by Wright's or Giemsa stain; characteristic lymph node histology; and serologic methods. Mouse inoculation with properly prepared tissue, such as a lymph node, spinal fluid, or peripheral blood, may isolate and identify the parasite if it is stained with Giemsa or Wright's stain. Antibodies are most commonly detected by the Sabin-Feldman dye test, which shows positivity 10 to 14 days after the initial infection. A maximum titer is attained in 4 to 5 weeks. The Jacobs-Lunde hemagglutination test, the complement fixation tests, the indirect fluorescent antibody test, and skin tests may also be used to establish the diagnosis.

Toxoplasmosis is worldwide in its distribution, with several areas having more than 90% seropositivity. It occurs in the eastern United States more frequently than in the western states. Reservoirs of infection have been reported in dogs, cats, cattle, sheep, pigs, rabbits, rats, pigeons, and chickens.

A combination of pyrimethamine (Daraprim), and sulfadiazine act synergistically and form an effective treatment. Dosages and total treatment time vary according to the age and immunologic competence of the infected patient. Pyrimethamine is a folic acid antagonist, so concomitant folinic acid therapy is recommended.

Fernandez DF: Acute cutaneous toxoplasmosis presenting as erythroderma. *Int J Dermatol* 1994, 33:129.

Fine JD, et al: The TORCH syndrome. *J Am Acad Dermatol* 1985, 12:697.

Hirschmann JV, et al: Skin lesions with disseminated toxoplasmosis in a patient with AIDS. *Arch Dermatol* 1988, 124:1446.

Leyva WH, et al: Cutaneous toxoplasmosis. *J Am Acad Dermatol* 1986, 14:600.

Pollack JL: Toxoplasmosis appearing to be dermatomyositis. *Arch Dermatol* 1979, 115:736. _____ ▲

Phylum Cnidaria

The cnidarians include the jellyfish, hydroids, corals, and sea anemones. These are all radial marine animals, living mostly in ocean water. When a swimmer's skin contacts these organisms, a toxin is released through small spicules.

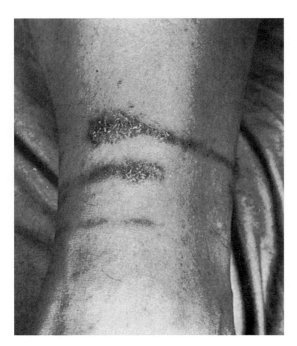

Fig. 20-16 A Portuguese man-of-war (*Physalia physalis*) sting on shin, resembling whiplash.

Portuguese Man-of-War Dermatitis

Stings by the Portuguese man-of-war (*Physalia physalis* in the Atlantic, or the much smaller *P. utriculus* or "bluebottle" in the Pacific) are characterized by linear lesions that are erythematous, urticarial, and even hemorrhagic (Fig. 20-16). The forearms, sides of the trunk, thighs, and feet are common sites of involvement. The usual local manifestations are sharp, stinging, and intense pain. Internally there may be severe dyspnea, prostration, nausea, abdominal cramps, lacrimation, and muscular pains. Death may occur if the areas stung are large in relation to the patient's size.

The fluid of the nematocysts contains toxin that is carried into the human victim through barbs along the tentacle. The venom is a neurotoxic poison that can produce marked cardiac changes.

Each Portuguese man-of-war is a colony of symbiotic organisms consisting of a blue to red float or pneumatophore with a gas gland, several gastrozooids measuring 1 to 20 mm, reproductive polyps, and the fishing tentacles bearing the nematocysts from which the barbs are ejected. The hydroid is found most frequently along the southeastern Florida coastline and in the Gulf of Mexico, and on windward coasts throughout the mid-Pacific and South Pacific.

Jellyfish Dermatitis

This produces lesions similar to those of the Portuguese man-of-war, except that the lesions are not so linear (Fig. 20-17). Delayed and persistent lesions were described by Reed et al from stings incurred in the Aegean and Caribbean

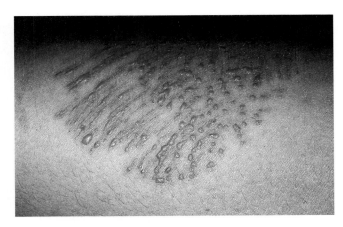

Fig. 20-17 Jellyfish sting. (Courtesy Dr. A. Slagel.)

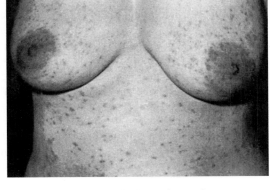

Fig. 20-18 Seabather's eruption.

areas. Burnett et al have reviewed the jellyfish envenomation syndromes and also have reported prolonged hypersensitivity reactions that were associated with specific antijellyfish immunoglobulins.

The Australian sea wasp, *Chironex fleckeri,* which is colorless and transparent, is the most dangerous of all, with a sting that is often fatal. Another sea wasp, *Carybdea marsupialis,* much less dangerous, occurs in the Caribbean.

Seabather's eruption is an acute dermatitis that begins a few hours after bathing in the ocean. Erythematous macules and papules appear that may develop into pustules or vesicles. Urticarial plaques are also present in a smaller number of patients. Crops of new lesions may occur for up to 72 hours, and the eruption persists for 10 to 14 days on average. It is quite pruritic.

Compared with cercarial dermatitis, seabather's eruption occurs along the coast of the Atlantic Ocean and affects covered areas of the body (Fig. 20-18). Cnidarian larvae become entrapped under the bathing suit and the nematocyst releases its toxin because of external pressure. Thus the buttocks and waist are affected primarily, with the breast also involved in women.

Wong et al and Tomchick et al described outbreaks that implicated larvae of the thimble jellyfish *Linuche unguiculata* as the "black dots" patients report being seen in the water or in their suits. Freudenthal et al reported small "pink seeds," the larvae of the sea anemone *Edwardstella lineata,* as the cause of seabather's eruption in Long Island, New York. This organism also has nematocysts, thus the mechanism of the eruption is the same as with the Florida jellyfish-induced eruption. It is likely that different cnidarian envenomations in different waters produce a similar clinical picture. Other reports focus on spring plants, dinoflagellates, protozoans, or crustaceans as potential causes. It appears that trapping of cnidarian larvae with their nematocysts or other toxic or irritant substances under the suit accounts for this eruption. It has been noted that seabathers who take off their suit and shower soon after leaving the water may limit the eruptions.

Hydroid, Sea Anemone, and Coral Dermatitis

Patients contacting the small marine hydroid *Halecium* may develop a dermatitis. The organism grows like a centimeter-thick coat of moss on the submerged portions of vessels or pilings. Sea anemones produce reactions similar to those produced by jellyfish and hydroids. Coral cuts are injuries caused by the exoskeleton of the corals, Milleporina. They have a largely undeserved reputation for becoming inflamed and infected and for delayed healing. The combination of implantation of fragments of coral skeleton and infection (since the cuts occur most commonly on the feet) probably accounts almost entirely for these symptoms. Detoxification as soon as possible after the injury is advisable for all of these types of stings or cuts.

TREATMENT OF STINGS AND CUTS. Therapy for these injuries, as well as those of the fire coral, hydroids, jellyfish, and sea anemone, is the same. The wound should be soaked in 5% acetic acid (vinegar). The leading alternative is isopropyl alcohol (40% to 70%). Meat tenderizer has been reported to be effective but is not as reliable as vinegar. The detoxicant should be applied continuously for at least 30 minutes.

Next, any large visible tentacles should be removed with forceps in a double-gloved hand. Finally, the remaining nematocysts should be removed by applying a layer of shaving cream and shaving the area gently. Fresh water and abrasion will worsen the envenomation. Topical anesthetics or steroids may be applied after decontamination. Systemic reactions may occur either through large amounts of venom or a previously sensitizing exposure from which anaphylaxis may result, and systemic treatment with epinephrine, antihistamines, or corticosteroids may be needed. Specific antivenin is available for the box-jellyfish, *Chironex flexeri.* This should be administered intravenously to limit myonecrosis.

Sponges and Bristleworms

Sponges have horny spicules of silicon dioxide and calcium carbonate. Some sponges produce dermal irritants such as halitoxin and okadaic acid, and others may be colonized by cnidaria. Allergic or irritant reactions may result. Bristleworms may also produce stinging. All of these may be treated by first using adhesive tape to remove the spicules, then applying vinegar soaks, as described earlier, and finally, applying topical corticosteroid agents.

Sea Urchin Injuries

Puncture wounds inflicted by the brittle, fragile spines of sea urchins, mainly of genus *Diadema* or *Echinothrix,* are stained blue-black by the black spines and may contain fragments of the spines. These are rarely large enough to require removal. Foreign-body or sarcoidlike granulomas may develop. Burke et al have reported a sea urchin sting that led to a vesicular hypersensitivity reaction 10 days later. Injuries by spines of the genus *Tripneustes* have been reported to cause fatal envenomation, but this genus is not found on U.S. coasts.

Starfish also have thorny spines that can sting and burn if they are stepped on or handled. Several different types of stinging fish also produce puncture wounds. Such envenomations may be caused by stingrays, scorpionfish, stonefish, catfish, and weaverfish.

These wounds should be immersed in nonscalding water (45° C [113° F]) for 30 to 90 minutes or until the pain subsides. Calcified fragments may be visible on x-ray evaluation, with fluoroscopy guiding extraction of spines, especially on the hands and feet. Debridement and possibly antibiotic therapy for deep puncture wounds of the hands and feet are recommended. There is a specific antivenin for stonefish stings.

Seaweed Dermatitis

Although this is caused by a marine alga and not by an animal, it deserves mention with other problems associated with swimming or wading. The dermatitis occurs 3 to 8 hours after the individual emerges from the ocean. The distribution is in parts covered by a bathing suit: scrotum, penis, perineum, and perianal area. The dermatitis is caused by a marine plant, *Lyngbya majuscula Gomont.* It has been observed only in bathers swimming off the windward shore of Oahu, Hawaii. Seabather's eruption, clamdigger's itch, and swimmer's itch must be differentiated from seaweed dermatitis caused by marine algae.

Prophylaxis is achieved by refraining from swimming in waters that are turbid with such algae. One should shower within 5 minutes after swimming. Active treatment in severe cases is the same as for acute burns.

Dogger Bank Itch

Dogger Bank itch is an eczematous dermatitis caused by the sea chervil, *Alcyondium hirsutum,* a seaweedlike animal colony. These sea mosses or sea mats are found on the Dogger Bank, an immense shelflike elevation under the North Sea between Scotland and Denmark.

Auerbach PS: Marine envenomations. *N Engl J Med* 1991, 325:486.

Burke WA, et al: Delayed hypersensitivity reaction following a sea urchin sting. *Int J Dermatol* 1986, 25:699.

Burnett JW: Seabather's eruption. *Cutis* 1992, 50:98.

Burnett JW, et al: Jellyfish envenomation syndromes. *J Am Acad Dermatol* 1986, 14:100.

Burnett JW, et al: Recurrent eruptions following unusual solitary coelenterate envenomations. *J Am Acad Dermatol* 1987, 17:86.

Burnett JW, et al: Studies on the serologic response to jellyfish envenomation. *J Am Acad Dermatol* 1983, 9:229.

Burnett JW, et al: Venomous coelenterates. *Cutis* 1987, 39:191.

Freudenthal AR, et al: Seabather's eruption. *N Engl J Med* 1993, 329:542.

Reed KM, et al: Delayed and persistent cutaneous reactions to coelenterates. *J Am Acad Dermatol* 1984, 10:462.

Tamanaha RH, et al: Persistent cutaneous hypersensitivity reaction after a Hawaiian box jellyfish sting *(Carybdea alata). J Am Acad Dermatol* 1996, 35:991.

Tomchick RS, et al: Clinical perspectives on seabather's eruption, also known as "sea lice." *JAMA* 1993, 269:1669.

Tong DW: Skin hazards of the marine aquarium industry. *Int J Dermatol* 1996, 35:153.

Wong DE, et al: Seabather's eruption. *J Am Acad Dermatol* 1994, 30:399.
▲

Phylum Platyhelminthes

Phylum Platyhelminthes includes the flatworms, of which two classes, trematodes and cestodes, are parasitic to humans. The trematodes, or blood flukes, parasitize human skin or internal organs. The cestodes are segmented, ribbon-shaped flatworms that inhabit the intestinal tract as adults and involve the subcutaneous tissue, heart, muscle, and eye in the larval form. This is encased in a sac that eventually becomes calcified.

CLASS TREMATODA
Schistosome Cercarial Dermatitis

Cercarial dermatitis is a severely pruritic, widespread, papular dermatitis caused by cercariae of schistosomes for which humans are not hosts (the usual animal hosts are waterfowl and rodents such as muskrats).

The eggs in the excreta of these animals, when deposited in water, hatch into swimming miracidia. These enter a snail, where further development occurs. From the snail, the free-swimming cercariae emerge to invade human skin on accidental contact. The swimming, colorless, multicellular organisms are a little less than a millimeter long. Exposure to cercariae occurs when a person swims, or more often, wades in water containing them. They attack by burrowing into the skin, where they die. The species that causes this eruption cannot enter the bloodstream or deeper tissues.

After coming out of the water, the bather begins to itch

and a transient erythematous eruption appears, but after a few hours, the eruption subsides, together with the itching. Then after a quiescent period of 10 to 15 hours, the symptoms recur, and erythematous macules and papules develop throughout the exposed parts that were in the water (Fig. 20-19). After several days the dermatitis heals spontaneously. There are two types: the freshwater swimmer's itch, and the saltwater marine dermatitis or clam digger's itch. It is not communicable.

Various genera and species of organisms have been reported from various locations worldwide. An outbreak of cercarial dermatitis was reported from Delaware in 1991 in which the avian schistosome *Microbilharzia variglandis* was implicated as the causative organism. *Schistosoma spindale* cercaria caused another recently reported epidemic in Southern Thailand.

The disease can be prevented by thoroughly washing, then drying with a towel after exposure. Rubbing with alcohol is an additional preventive measure advocated by some.

Visceral Schistosomiasis (Bilharziasis)

The cutaneous manifestation of bilharziasis may begin with mild itching and a papular dermatitis of the feet and other parts after swimming in polluted streams containing cercariae. The types of schistosomes causing this disease can penetrate into the bloodstream and eventually inhabit the venous system draining the urinary bladder (*Schistosoma haematobium*) or the intestines *(S. mansoni or S. japonicum)*. After an asymptomatic incubation period, there may be a sudden illness with fever and chills, pneumonitis, and eosinophilia. Petechial hemorrhages may occur.

Cutaneous schistosomal granulomas most frequently involve the genitalia, perineum, and buttocks (Figs. 20-20 and 20-21). These bilharziomas are usually caused by the eggs of *S. haematobium* or *S. mansoni*. Vegetating, soft, cauliflower-shaped masses occur. Fistulous tracts and extensive hard masses occur; these are riddled by sinuses that exude a seropurulent discharge with a characteristic odor. Phagedenic ulcerations and pseudoelephantiasis of the scrotum, penis, or labia are sometimes encountered. Histologically, the nodules contain bilharzial ova undergoing degeneration, with calcification and a surrounding cellular reaction of histiocytes, eosinophils, and occasional giant cells. In some cases, eventual malignant changes in these granulomas have been noted.

Infrequently, ectopic or extragenital lesions may occur, mainly on the trunk (Fig. 20-22). This is a papular eruption tending to group in plaques and become darkly pigmented and scaly.

A severe urticarial eruption known as *urticarial fever* or *Katayama fever* is frequently present along with a *S. japonicum* infection; it occurs with the beginning of oviposition, 4 to 8 weeks after infection. This condition occurs mainly in China, Japan, and the Philippines. In

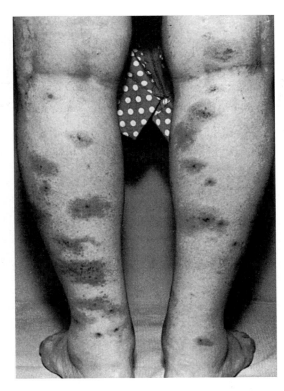

Fig. 20-19 Schistosome cercarial dermatitis.

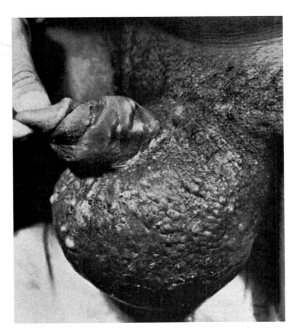

Fig. 20-20 Schistosomal granulomas of the scrotum. (Courtesy Dr. M. El-Zawahry, United Arab Republic.)

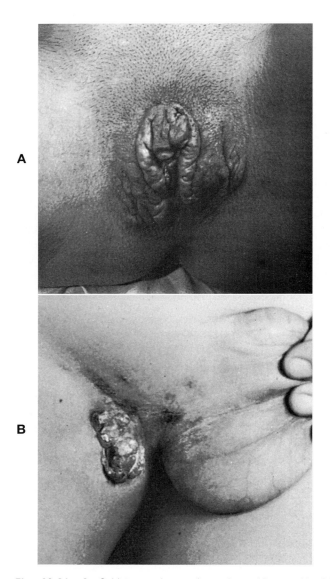

Fig. 20-21 **A,** Schistosomal granuloma in a 16-year-old girl. **B,** Intercrural granuloma of schistosomiasis. These granulomas are found most frequently in the genital and perineal areas. (**A,** Courtesy Dr. M. El-Zawahry; **B,** Courtesy Dr. A.M. El-Mofty, United Arab Republic.)

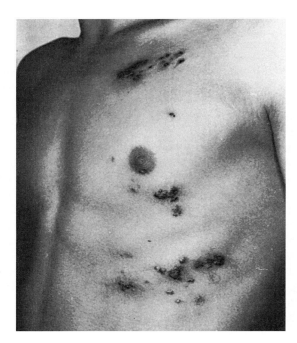

Fig. 20-22 Cutaneous schistosomiasis on the trunk, a typical site other than the genital and perineal areas. (Courtesy Dr. A.M. El-Mofty, United Arab Republic.)

(Biltricide) 20 mg/kg orally for each of two treatments in 1 day is the treatment of choice. *S. japonicum* treatment requires three doses in 1 day.

Schistosomicides exhibit toxicity for the host as well as for the parasite, and the risk of undesirable side effects may be enhanced by concomitant cardiac, renal, or hepatosplenic disease.

addition to the urticaria, fever, malaise, abdominal cramps, arthritis, and liver and spleen involvement are seen. This is felt to be a serum sickness–like reaction.

Preventive measures include reducing infection sources, preventing contamination by human excreta of snail-bearing waters, control of snail hosts, and avoiding exposure to cercaria-infested waters.

Prophylactic measures are constantly sought to control one of the world's worst parasitic diseases, but as yet none has been found to be practical.

For both *S. haematobium* and *S. mansoni,* praziquantel

Amer M: Cercaria dermatitis outbreak at a state park-Delaware, 1991. *Arch Dermatol* 1992, 128:945.

Amer M: Cutaneous schistosomiasis. *Dermatol Clin* 1994, 12:713.

Farrell AM, et al: Ectopic cutaneous schistosomiasis: extragenital involvement with progressive upward spread. *Br J Dermatol* 1996, 135:110.

Kullavanijaya P, et al: Outbreak of cercarial dermatitis in Thailand. *Int J Dermatol* 1993, 32:113.

Torres VM: Dermatologic manifestations of schistosomiasis mansoni. *Arch Dermatol* 1976, 112:1539.

Ulthman MAE, et al: Cutaneous schistosomal granuloma. *Int J Dermatol* 1990, 29:659.

Walther RR: Chronic papular dermatitis of the scrotum due to *Schistosoma mansoni. Arch Dermatol* 1979, 115:869. _____ ▲

Cysticercosis Cutis

The natural intermediate host of the pork tapeworm, *Taenia solium,* is the pig, but under some circumstances humans act in this role. The larval stage of *T. solium* is *Cysticercus cellulosae.* Infection takes place by the ingestion of food contaminated with the eggs, or by reverse peristalsis of eggs or proglottides from the intestine to the stomach. Here the eggs hatch, freeing the oncospheres. These enter the general circulation and form cysts in various parts of the body, such as striated muscles, brain, eye, heart, and lung.

In the subcutaneous tissues the lesions are usually painless nodules that contain cysticerci. They are more or less stationary, usually numerous, and often calcified, and are therefore demonstrable radiographically. Pain and ulceration may accompany the lesions. The disease is most prevalent in countries in which pigs feed on human feces. It may be confused with gumma, lipoma, and epithelioma. A positive diagnosis is established solely by incision and examination of the interior of the calcified tumor, where the parasite will be found.

Praziquantel given in doses as low as 10 mg/kg of body weight is the treatment of choice for intestinal tapeworms; five times this dose for 15 days is required if the central nervous system is involved. This regimen has no effect on calcified parasites, however, which need to be surgically removed.

Falanga V, et al: Cerebral cysticercosis. *J Am Acad Dermatol* 1985, 12:304.

Levin JA, et al: Praziquantel in the treatment of cysticercosis. *JAMA* 1986, 256:349.

O'Grady TC, et al: Subcutaneous cysticercosis simulating metastatic breast carcinoma. *Int J Dermatol* 1993, 32:62.

Puppin D Jr, et al: Subcutaneous cystercosis of the tongue mimicking a tumor. *Int J Dermatol* 1993, 32:818.

Schmidt DK, et al: Cerebral and subcutaneous cysticercosis treated with albendazole. *Int J Dermatol* 1995, 34:574.

Wortman PD: Subcutaneous cysticercosis. *J Am Acad Dermatol* 1991, 25:409. ▲

Sparganosis

Sparganosis is caused by the larva of the tapeworm of the species *Spirometra*. The adult tapeworm lives in the intestines of dogs and cats. This is a rare tissue infection occurring in two forms. *Application sparganosis* occurs when an ulcer or infected eye is poulticed with the flesh of an infected intermediate host (such poultices are frequently used in the Orient). The larvae become encased in small nodules in the infected tissue. *Ingestion sparganosis* occurs when humans ingest inadequately cooked meat, such as snake or frog, or when a person drinks water that is contaminated with *Cyclops,* which are infected with plerocercoid larvae. One or two slightly pruritic or painful nodules may form in the subcutaneous tissue or on the trunk and legs.

Humans are the accidental intermediate host of the Sparganum, which is the alternative name for the plerocercoid larva. Treatment is surgical removal or ethanol injection of the infected nodules. This may be difficult because of the swelling and extensive vascularity.

Griffin MP, et al: Cutaneous sparganosis. *Am J Dermatopathol* 1996, 18:70.

Sarma DP, et al: Human sparganosis. *J Am Acad Dermatol* 1986, 15:1145. ▲

Echinococcosis

Echinococcosis is also known as *hydatid disease.* In humans, infection is produced by the ova reaching the mouth by the hands, in food, or from containers soiled by ova-contaminated feces from an infected dog. This leads to *Echinococcus granulosus* infestation of the liver and the lungs. Soft, fluctuating, semitranslucent, cystic tumors may occur in the skin, sometimes in the supraumbilical area as fistulas from underlying liver involvement. These tumors become fibrotic or calcified after the death of the larva. Eosinophilia or intractable urticaria and pruritus may be present. The treatment is excision, with care being taken to avoid rupturing the cyst. Albendazole combined with percutaneous drainage may also be used.

Bresson-Hadni S, et al: Skin localization of alveolar echinococcosis of the liver. *J Am Acad Dermatol* 1996, 34:873. ▲

Phylum Annelida

LEECHES

Leeches, of the class Hirudinea, are of marine, freshwater, or terrestrial types. After attaching to the skin, they secrete an anticoagulant, *hirudin,* and then engorge themselves with blood. Local symptoms at the site of the bite may include bullae, hemorrhage, pruritus, whealing, necrosis, or ulceration. Allergic reactions, including anaphylaxis, may result. They may be removed by applying salt, alcohol, or vinegar, or by use of a match flame. Bleeding may then be stopped by direct pressure or by applying a styptic pencil to the site.

Leeches may be used medicinally to salvage tissue flaps that are threatened by venous congestion. However, aeromonas infection and anetoderma may be complications of their attachment.

Blackshear JL, et al: Leeching, hirudin, and coagulation tests. *Ann Intern Med* 1994, 121:151.

Haycox CL, et al: Indications and complications of medicinal leech therapy. *J Am Acad Dermatol* 1995, 33:1053.

Ross MS: The leech: of dermatologic interest. *Arch Dermatol* 1983, 119:276. ▲

Phylum Nemathelminthes

Phylum Nemathelminthes includes the roundworms, both the free-living and the parasitic forms. Multiplication is usually outside the host. Both the larval and adult stages may infect humans.

CLASS NEMATODA

Enterobiasis (Pinworm Infection, Seatworm Infection, Oxyuriasis)

The chief symptom of pinworm infestation, which occurs most frequently in children, is nocturnal pruritus ani. There is intense itching accompanied by excoriations of the anus, perineum, and pubic area. The vagina may become infested with the gravid pinworms. Restlessness, insomnia, enuresis, and irritability are but a few of the many symptoms ascribed to this exceedingly common infestation. Buslau et al described a papular pruritic dermatosis of the trunk and extremities in a child with enterobiasis presumed to be secondary to a systemic allergic mechanism.

Oxyuriasis is caused by the roundworm *Enterobius vermicularis* (Fig. 20-23), which may infest the small intestines, cecum, and large intestine of humans. The worms, especially gravid ones, migrate toward the rectum and at night emerge to the perianal and perineal regions to deposit thousands of ova, then the worm dries and dies outside the intestine. These ova are then carried back to the mouth of the host on the hands. The larvae hatch in the duodenum and migrate into the jejunum and ileum, where they reach maturity. Fertilization occurs in the cecum, thus completing the life cycle.

Humans are the only known host of the pinworm, which probably has the widest distribution of all the helminths. Infection occurs from hand-to-mouth transmission, often from handling soiled clothes, bedsheets, and other household articles. Ova under the fingernails are a common source of autoinfection. Ova may also be airborne and collect in dust that may be on furniture and the floor. Investigation may show that all members of the family of an affected person also harbor the infection. It is common in orphanages and mental institutions and among people living in communal groups.

Rarely is it feasible to identify a dead pinworm in the stool. Diagnosis is best made by demonstration of ova in smears taken from the anal region early in the morning before the patient bathes or defecates. With the patient in the knee-chest position, a smear is obtained from the anus with a small eye curette. This is placed on a glass slide with a drop of saline solution. It is also possible to use Scotch tape, looping the tape sticky-side out over a tongue depressor and then pressing it several times against the perianal region. The tape is then smoothed out on a glass slide. A drop of a solution containing iodine in xylol may be placed on the slide before the tape is applied to facilitate detection of any ova. These tests should be repeated on 3 consecutive days to rule out infection. Ova may be detected under the fingernails of the infected person.

Albendazole, 400 mg, or mebendazole, 100 mg repeated

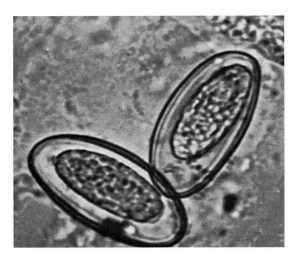

Fig. 20-23 Ova of *Enterobius vermicularis*. (Courtesy Dr. H.W. Brown.)

in 2 weeks, is effective. Personal hygiene and cleanliness at home are important. Fingernails should be cut short and scrubbed frequently; they should be thoroughly cleaned on arising, before each meal, and after using the toilet. Sheets, underwear, towels, pajamas, and other clothing of the affected person should be laundered thoroughly and separately.

Buslau M, et al: Papular eruption of helminth infection. *Acta Derm Venereol* (Stockh) 1990, 70:526.
Fiumara NJ, et al: Folliculitis of the buttocks and pinworms. *Sex Transm Dis* 1986, 13:45. ⎯⎯⎯⎯⎯⎯⎯⎯⎯⎯⎯⎯ ▲

Hookworm Disease (Ground Itch, Uncinariasis, Ancylostomiasis, Necatoriasis)

The earliest skin lesions (ground itch) are erythematous macules and papules, which in a few hours become vesicles. These itchy lesions usually occur on the soles, toe webs, and ankles; they may be scattered or in groups. The contents of the vesicles rapidly becomes purulent. These lesions are produced by the invasion of the skin by the *Ancylostoma* or *Necator* larvae and precede the generalized symptoms of the disease by 2 or 3 months. The cutaneous lesions last less than 2 weeks before the larvae continue their human life cycle. There may be as high as 40% eosinophilia around the fifth day of infection.

The onset of the constitutional disease is insidious and is accompanied by progressive iron deficiency anemia and debility. During the course of the disease urticaria often occurs. The skin ultimately becomes dry and pale or yellowish.

Hookworm is a specific communicable disease caused by *Ancylostoma duodenale* or *Necator americanus*. In the soil, under propitious circumstances, they attain the stage of infective larvae in 5 to 7 days. These tiny larvae (which can scarcely be seen with a small pocket lens), when they come into accidental contact with the bare feet, penetrate the skin and reach the capillaries. They are carried in the circulation to the lungs, where they pass through the capillary walls into the bronchi. They move up the trachea to the pharynx and, being swallowed, eventually reach their habitat in the small intestine. Here they bury their heads in the mucosa and begin their sexual life.

Hookworm is prevalent in most tropical and subtropical countries and is often endemic in swampy and sandy localities in the temperate zones. In these latter regions the larvae are killed off each winter, but the soil is again contaminated from human sources the following summer. *Necator americanus* prevails in the Western Hemisphere, Central and South Africa, South Asia, Australia, and the Pacific islands.

The defecation habits of infected individuals in the endemic areas are largely responsible for its widespread distribution, as is the use of human feces for fertilization in many parts of the world. In addition, the climate is usually such that people go barefoot because of the heat or because they cannot afford shoes. Infection is thereby facilitated, especially through the toes.

Finding the eggs in the feces of the suspected individual establishes the diagnosis. The ova appear in the feces about 5 weeks after the onset of infection. The eggs may be found in direct fecal films if the infection is heavy, but in light infections it may be necessary to resort to zinc sulfate centrifugal flotation or other concentration methods. Mixed infections frequently occur.

Treatment is by expulsion of the parasites from the body and by preventing reinfection through proper disposal of human feces. Albendazole, 100 mg once, or mebendazole, 100 mg twice daily for 3 days, is effective. Prophylaxis is largely a community problem and depends on preventing fecal contamination of the soil. This is best attained by proper sanitary disposal of feces, protecting individuals from exposure by educating them about sanitary procedures, and mass treatment through public health methods.

Nematode Dermatitis

Miller et al described a patient who developed a persistent widespread folliculitis caused by *Ancyclosforma caninum*. It was apparently acquired by his lying in grass contaminated by the droppings of his pet dogs and cats. A biopsy revealed hookworm larvae within the hair follicle. Oral thiabendazole was curative.

Creeping Eruption (Larva Migrans)

Creeping eruption is a term applied to twisting, winding linear skin lesions produced by the burrowing of larvae. People who go barefoot at the beaches, children playing in sandboxes, carpenters and plumbers working under homes, and gardeners are often victims. The most common areas involved are the feet, buttocks, genitals, and hands.

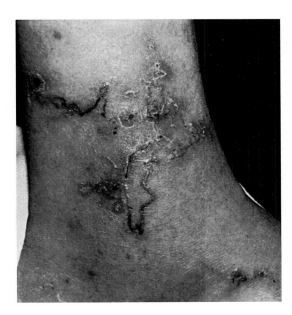

Fig. 20-24 Creeping eruption on ankle caused by *Ancylostoma braziliense.*

The onset is characterized by slight local itching and the appearance of papules at the sites of infection resulting from the migrations of the larvae. Intermittent stinging pain occurs, and thin, red, tortuous lines are formed in the skin (Figs. 20-24 and 20-25). The migrations begin 4 days after inoculation and progress at the rate of about 2 cm daily. However, the larvae may remain quiescent for several days or even months before beginning to migrate. The linear lesions are often interrupted by papules that mark the sites of resting larvae. As the eruption advances, the old parts tend to fade, but sometimes there are purulent manifestations caused by secondary infection; erosions and excoriations caused by scratching frequently occur. If the progress of the disease is not interrupted by treatment, the larvae usually die in 2 to 8 weeks, with resolution of the eruption, although rarely it has been reported to persist for up to 1 year. At times the larvae are removed from the skin by the fingernails in scratching. Eosinophilia may be present.

Loeffler's syndrome, consisting of a patchy infiltrate of the lungs and eosinophilia as high as 50% in the blood and 90% in the sputum, may complicate creeping eruption.

The majority of cases in this country are caused by penetration by the larvae of a cat and dog hookworm, *Ancylostoma braziliense*, acquired from body contact with damp sand or earth that has been contaminated by the excreta of dogs and cats. A similar dermatitis is rarely produced by the larvae of *A. caninum*, which also infests the dog and the cat. Creeping eruption caused by *A. braziliense* is common along the coast of the southeastern United States.

Ivermectin 150 µg/kg, generally given as a single 12-mg dose, or albendazole, 200 mg twice daily for 3 days, are

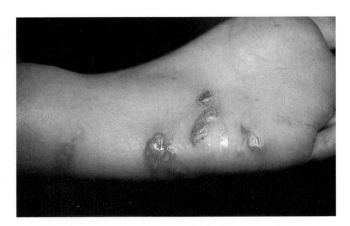

Fig. 20-25 Larva migrans on the elbow. Notice extreme eczematization from scratching. (Courtesy Dr. J. Penner.)

effective treatments. Criteria for successful therapy are relief of symptoms and cessation of tract extension, which usually occurs within a week.

Topical treatment with thiabendazole 10% oral suspension four times daily will result in marked relief from pruritus in 3 days, and the tracts become inactive in 1 week. Davies et al used 15% thiabenbendazole cream that they compounded and found it effective in 98% of their 53 patients who were treated.

Another condition, not to be confused with this helminthic disease, which also is called *creeping eruption* (or *sandworm,* as it is known in South Africa, particularly in Natal and Zululand), is caused by a small mite about 300 μ long that tunnels in the superficial layers of the epidermis.

Gnathostomiasis

Human gnathostomiasis is characterized by migratory, intermittent, erythematous, urticarial plaques. Each episode of painless swelling lasts from 7 to 10 days and recurs every 2 to 6 weeks. Movement of the underlying parasite may be as much as 1 cm/hr. The total duration of the illness may be 10 years. Histopathologic examination of the skin swelling will demonstrate eosinophilic panniculitis. The clinical manifestation has been called *larva migrans profundus.*

The nematode *Gnathostoma dolorosi* or *spinigerum* is the cause; most cases occur in Asia or South America. Eating raw flesh from the second intermediate host, most commonly freshwater fish, in such preparations as sashimi and ceviche allows humans to become the definitive host. Eating raw snake flesh was the cause of an infestation in six patients reported by Kurokawa et al. As the larval cyst in the flesh is digested, the larva becomes motile and penetrates the gastric mucosa, usually within 24 to 48 hours of ingestion. Symptoms then occur as migration of the parasite continues. Surgical removal is the treatment of choice, if the parasite can be located. This may be combined with albendazole 400 mg daily or twice daily for 21 days. Several

of Kurokawa et al's patients responded to treatment with only albendazole or mebendazole.

Several recent reports of creeping eruption in Japan have been found to be caused by a newly recognized causative parasite of the nematode superfamily Spiruroidea. Eating raw squid was associated with the onset of long, narrow lesions that were pruritic, linear, and migratory. Surgical removal is necessary; chemotherapy has been unsuccessful.

Larva Currens

Intestinal infections with *Strongyloides stercoralis* may be associated with a perianal larva migrans syndrome, called *larva currens,* because of the rapidity of larval migration (*currens* means "running" or "racing"). Larva currens is an autoinfection caused by penetration of the perianal skin by infectious larvae as they are excreted in the feces. An urticarial band is the prominent primary lesion of cutaneous strongyloidiasis (Fig. 20-26). Strongyloidiasis, and the creeping eruption secondary to it, is often a chronic disease. In 1985, Pelletier et al reported a case acquired in the Vietnam War, and other studies on prisoners of war from World War II have shown infections may persist for more than 40 years. Approximately one third of patients infected are asymptomatic.

Symptoms of systemic strongyloidiasis include abdominal pain, diarrhea, constipation, nausea, vomiting, pneumonitis, urticaria, and a peripheral eosinophilia. The skin lesions originate within 30 cm of the anus and characteristically extend as much as 10 cm/day.

Fatal cases of hyperinfection occur in immunocompromised patients. In such patients the parasite load increases dramatically and can produce a fulminant illness. Widespread petechiae and purpura are helpful diagnostic signs of disseminated infection and chronic urticaria is a possible presenting sign. Periumbilical ecchymoses may appear as if they were caused by a thumbprint.

Administration of ivermectin, 200 μg/kg/day for 2 days, or albendazole, 400 mg/day for 3 days, is the treatment of choice. Immunosuppressed hosts may be treated with thiabendazole 25 mg/kg twice daily for 7 to 10 days.

There are free-living strongyloides known as *Pelodera* that can produce a creeping eruption also. Jones et al reported a case of widespread follicular, erythematous, dome-shaped papules and pustules that began within 24 hours of working under a house. This eruption persisted for 1 month before presentation. Scraping the lesions revealed live and dead larvae of the free-living soil nematode *Pelodera strongyloides.* Treatment with oral thiabendazole led to resolution.

Amer M, et al: Larva currens and systemic disease. *J Invest Dermatol* 1981, 20:402.

Bank DE, et al: The thumb print sign. *J Am Acad Dermatol* 1990, 27:324.

Caumes E, et al: Efficacy of ivermectin in the therapy of cutaneous larva immigrant. *Arch Dermatol* 1992, 128:994.

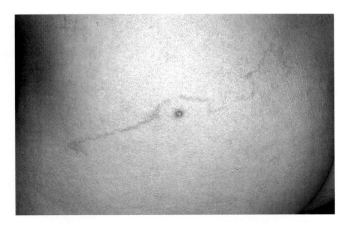

Fig. 20-26 Larva currens of the buttock. *Strongyloides stercoralis* was recovered from the patient's stool specimen.

Davies HD, et al: Creeping eruption. *Arch Dermatol* 1993, 129:588.

Elgart ML: Creeping eruption. *Arch Dermatol* 1998, 134:619.

Feinstein RJ, et al: Gnathostomiasis, or larva migrans profundus. *J Am Acad Dermatol* 1984, 11:738.

Gordon SM: Disseminated strongyloidiasis with cutaneous manifestations in an immunocompromised host. *J Am Acad Dermatol* 1994, 31:255.

Jacob CI, et al: *Strongyloides stercoralis* infection presenting as generalized prurigo nodularis and lichen simplex chronicus. *J Am Acad Dermatol* 1999, 41:357.

Jones CC, et al: Cutaneous larva migrans due to *Pelodere strongyloides.* *Cutis* 1991, 48:123.

Kagen CN, et al: Gnathostomiasis. *Arch Dermatol* 1984, 120:508.

Kalb RE, et al: Periumbilical purpura in disseminated strongyloidiasis. *JAMA* 1986, 256:1170.

Kao D, et al: Disseminated strongyloidiasis in a patient with acquired immunodeficiency syndrome *Arch Dermatol* 1996, 132:977.

Kurokawa M, et al: Cutaneous and visceral larva migrans due to Gnathostoma dolorosa infection via an unusual route. *Arch Dermatol* 1998, 134:638.

Miller AC, et al: Hookworm folliculitis. *Arch Dermatol* 1991, 127:547.

Okazak A, et al: Creeping disease due to larva of spiruroid nematode. *Int J Dermatol* 1993, 32:813.

Ollague W, et al: Human gnathostomiasis in Ecuador (nodular migratory eosinophilic panniculitis). *Int J Dermatol* 1984, 23:647.

Orihuela AR, et al: Single dose of albendazole in treatment of cutaneous larva migrans. *Arch Dermatol* 1990, 126:398.

Pelletier LL Jr, et al: Chronic strongyloidiasis in Vietnam veterans. *Am J Med* 1985, 78:139.

Ronan SG, et al: Disseminated strongyloidiasis presenting as purpura. *J Am Acad Dermatol* 1989, 21:1123.

Tanigachi Y, et al: Creeping eruption due to larvae of the suborder spirurina. *Int J Dermatol* 1994, 33:279.

Von Kuster LC, et al: Cutaneous manifestations of strongyloidiasis. *Arch Dermatol* 1988, 124:1826.

Williams HC, et al: Creeping eruption stopped in its tracks by albendazole. *Clin Exp Dermatol* 1989; 14:355. _____ ▲

Dracunculiasis (Guinea Worm Disease, Dracontiasis, Medina Worm)

Guinea worm disease is endemic in India, southwest Asia, northeast South America, the West Indies, and Africa. It is caused by *Dracunculus medinensis* and is contracted through drinking water that has been contaminated with

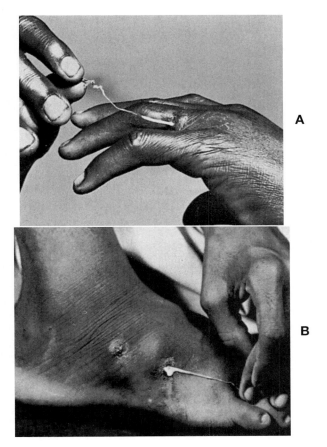

Fig. 20-27 **A,** Guinea worm disease, dracunculiasis. Guinea worm is protruding from bleb. **B,** The guinea worm is protruding from one bleb; proximally is another bleb still unbroken. (**A,** Courtesy Dr. G.H.V. Clarke, Wales; **B,** Courtesy Dr. M. El-Zawahry, United Arab Repulic.)

infected water fleas in which *Dracunculus* is parasitic. In the stomach, the larvae penetrate into the mesentery, where they mature sexually in 10 weeks. Then the female worm burrows to the cutaneous surface to deposit her larvae and thus causes the specific skin manifestations. As the worm approaches the surface, it may be felt as a cordlike thickening and forms an indurated cutaneous papule (Fig. 20-27). The papule may vesiculate and a painful ulcer develops, usually on the leg. The worm is often visible. When the parasite comes in contact with water, the worm rapidly discharges its larvae, which are ingested by water fleas (*Cyclops*), contaminating the water.

The cutaneous lesion is usually on the lower leg, but it may occur on the genitalia, buttocks, or arms. In addition to the ulcers on the skin there may be urticaria, gastrointestinal upsets, eosinophilia, and fever.

The disease may be prevented by boiling drinking water, providing safe drinking water through boreholes, or filtering the water through mesh fibers. Native treatment consists of gradually extracting the worm a little each day, with care not to rupture it; in the event of such an accident, the larvae escape into the tissues and produce fulminating inflammation. Surgical removal is the treatment of choice. Metronidazole 500 mg daily resolves the local inflammation and permits easier removal of the worm. Immersion in warm water promotes emergence of the worm.

Edungbola LD, et al: The impact of UNICEF-assisted rural water project on the prevalence of Guinea worm in Asia, Kwana State, Nigeria. *Am J Trop Med Hyg* 1988, 39:79.

Elgart ML: Onchocerciasis and dracunculosis. *Dermatol Clin* 1989, 7:323.

Watts, SJ: Dracunculiasis in Africa in 1986. *Am J Trop Med Hyg* 1987, 37:119. ▲

Filariasis

Elephantiasis Tropica (Elephantiasis Arabum). Filariasis is a widespread tropical disorder caused by infestation with filarial worms of *Wuchereria bancrofti, Brugia malayi,* or *B. timori.* It is characterized by lymphedema, with resulting hypertrophy of the skin and subcutaneous tissues, and by enlargement and deformity of the affected parts, usually the legs, scrotum, or labia majora. The disease occurs more frequently in young men than in women.

The onset of elephantiasis is characterized by recurrent attacks of acute lymphangitis in the affected part, associated with chills and fever (elephantoid fever) that lasts for several days to several weeks. These episodes recur over several months to years. After each attack the swelling subsides only partially, and as recrudescences supervene, thickening and hypertrophy become increasingly pronounced. The overlying epidermis becomes stretched, thin, and shiny, and in the course of years, leathery, insensitive, and verrucous or papillomatous from secondary pyogenic infection. There may be a dozen or more attacks in a year.

In addition to involvement of the legs and scrotum, the scalp, vulva, penis, female breasts, and arms are at times affected, either alone or in association with the other regions. The manifestations vary according to the part involved. When the legs are attacked, both are usually affected in a somewhat symmetrical manner, the principal changes occurring on the posterior aspects above the ankles and on the dorsa of the feet. At first, the thickening may be slight and associated with edema that pits on pressure. Later, the parts become massive and pachydermatous, the thickened integument hanging in apposing folds, between which there is a fetid exudate (Fig. 20-28).

When the scrotum is affected, it gradually reaches an enormous size and the penis becomes hidden in it (Fig. 20-29). The skin, which at first is glazed, later is coarse and verrucous, or, in far-advanced cases, ulcerated or gangrenous. Resistant urticaria may occur. Filarial orchitis and hydrocele are common. A testicle may enlarge rapidly to the size of an apple and be extremely painful. The swelling may subside within a few days, or the enlargement may be permanent. As a result of obstruction and dilation of the

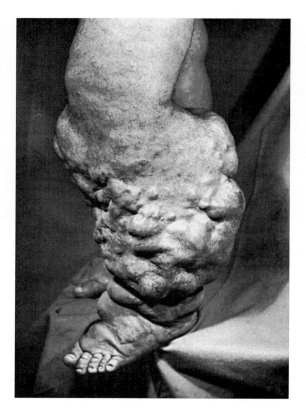

Fig. 20-28 Elephantiasis. An extremely advanced case. (Courtesy Dr. M. El-Zawahry, United Arab Republic.)

thoracic duct or some of its lower abdominal tributaries into the urinary tract, chyle appears in the urine, which assumes a milky appearance. Lobulated swellings of the inguinal and axillary glands, called *varicose glands,* are caused by obstructive varix and dilation of the lymphatic vessels.

Filaria are transmitted person-to-person by the bites of a variety of mosquitoes of the *Culex, Aedes,* and *Anopheles* species. The adult worms are threadlike, cylindrical, and creamy white. The females are 4 to 10 cm long. Microfilarial embryos may be seen coiled each in its own membrane near the posterior tip. Fully grown, sheathed microfilariae are 130 to 320 μ long. The adult worms live in the lymphatic system, where they produce microfilariae. These either remain in the lymphatic vessels or enter the peripheral bloodstream. An intermediate host is necessary for the further development of the parasite.

The disease is endemic in Africa, India, South China, Japan, Samoa, and Taiwan. It also occurs in the West Indies and Costa Rica. In Malaya, Ceylon, Indonesia, China, and Korea, there is Malayan filariasis caused by *B. malayi. B. timori* is restricted to the eastern Indonesian archipelago. *W. bancrofti* or *B. malayi* has been known in India since the sixth century BC. It is estimated that 250 million people are infected with these parasites.

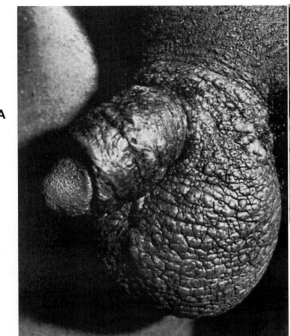

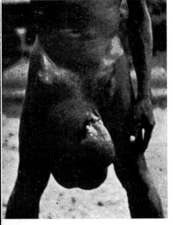

Fig. 20-29 A, Early elephantiasis. **B,** Elephantiasis of scrotum, with hyperplasia of inguinal glands. (**A,** Courtesy Dr. G.H.V. Clarke, Wales.)

It is important to realize that infestation by the filaria is often asymptomatic, and elephantiasis usually occurs only if hundreds of thousands of mosquito bites are suffered over a period of years, with episodes of intercurrent streptococcal lymphangitis. Filariasis was endemic in the considerable Samoan population of Hawaii for half a century, and only one case of elephantiasis has occurred among this group.

There is a striking periodicity to the time of the appearance and disappearance of the microfilariae in the skin and superficial vessels. *Culex fatigans* bites at night, and the microfilariae of *W. bancrofti* are found in the peripheral circulation at midnight (nocturnal periodicity) but rarely during the daytime. In the South Pacific, it is nonperiodic.

Search for the microfilariae should be made on fresh coverslip films of blood from the finger or ear and examined with a low-power objective lens. Specimens should be taken at midnight. Calcified adult worms may be demonstrated on x-ray examination, and sometimes adult filariae are found in abscesses or in material taken for pathologic examination. The filarial worm can be traced fluorescently, as the microfilariae and adult worms have an affinity for the tetracyclines, which fluoresce in ultraviolet radiation in a dark room. The filarial complement fixation test and skin tests, although only group specific, are useful in seeking the cause of lymphedema. The prognosis in regard to life is good, but living becomes burdensome unless the condition is alleviated.

Ivermectin, 100 to 440 μg/kg in one dose, is the treatment of choice. This regimen (as well as alternative treatment with diethylcarbamazine) will clear microfilariae but not adult worms. Surgical operations have been devised to remove the edematous subcutaneous tissue from the scrotum and breast. Prophylactic measures consist of appropriate mosquito control. Diethylcarbamazine has been effective in mass prophylaxis.

Ottensen EA, et al: A controlled trial of ivermectin and diethyl carbanazine in lymphatic filariasis. *N Engl J Med* 1990, 232:1113.
Routh HB, et al: Filariasis. *Dermatol Clin* 1994, 12:719. ▲

Loaiasis (*Loa loa,* Calabar Swelling, Tropical Swelling, Fugitive Swelling)

Infection with *Loa loa* is often asymptomatic. However, more or less painful localized subcutaneous nonpitting edema, or fugitive swellings called *calabar swellings,* occur. In infected persons, the parasite develops slowly and there may even be an interval of as much as 3 years between infection and the appearance of symptoms, although the usual interval is 1 year.

Calabar swellings are one or more slightly inflamed, edematous, transient swellings, usually about the size of a hen's egg. They usually last a few days and then subside, although recurrent swellings at the same site may eventually lead to a permanent cystlike protuberance. These swellings may result from hypersensitivity to the adult worm or to materials elaborated by it. Eosinophilia may be as high as 90% and often is between 60% and 80%.

The filariae may be noticed subcutaneously in the fingers, breasts, eyelids, or submucosally under the conjunctivae. The worm may be in the anterior chamber of the eye, the myocardium, or other sites. It has a predilection for loose tissues such as the eye region, the frenum of the tongue, and the genitalia. The wanderings of the adult parasite may be noticed by a tingling and creeping sensation. The death of the filaria in the skin may lead to the formation of fluctuant cystic lesions.

Loaiasis is a form of filariasis caused by *Loa loa*, widely distributed in west and central Africa. It is transmitted by the mango fly, *Chrysops dimidia* or *C. silacea*. This fly bites only in the daytime. Humans are the only important reservoir for the parasite.

The observation of the worm under the conjunctiva, calabar swellings, and eosinophilia establish the diagnosis. Demonstration of the characteristic microfilariae in the blood during the day is possible in only some 20% of patients. Complement fixation and intradermal tests may be helpful.

Removal of the adult parasite whenever it comes to the surface of the skin is mandatory. This must be done quickly by seizing the worm with forceps and placing a suture under it before cutting down to it. Worms that are not securely and rapidly grasped quickly escape into the deeper tissues.

Diethylcarbamazine kills both adults and microfilariae and is given for 21 days. On days 1 and 2, 50 mg is given three times daily; on day 3, 100 mg is given three times; and on days 4 through 21, 2 mg/kg is given three times daily.

In regions in which onchocerciasis and loiasis are both endemic and ivermectin is used in a community-based elimination strategy for onchocerciasis, simultaneously infected patients with a high *Loa loa* load have a high risk of serious side effects. If ivermectin treatment of these patients is undertaken, proper monitoring and appropriate supportive treatment should be available in anticipation of this risk. Diethylcarbamazine is an effective chemopreventive, using 300 mg weekly in temporary residents of regions of Africa where *Loa loa* is endemic. It occasionally causes nausea as a side effect.

Gardon J, et al: Serious reactions after mass treatment of onchocerciasis with ivermectin in an area endemic for *Loa loa* infection. *Lancet* 1997, 350:18.

Mackey SL, et al: Dermatologic manifestations of parasitic diseases. *Infect Dis Clin North Am* 1994, 8:713.

Marriott WRV: Loaiasis. *Int J Dermatol* 1985, 25:329.

Nutman TB, et al: Diethylcarbamazine prophylaxis for human loaiasis. *N Engl J Med* 1988, 319:752.

Rakita RM, et al: *Loa loa* infection as a cause of migratory angioedema. *Clin Infect Dis* 1993, 17:691. _____ ▲

Onchocerciasis

The skin lesions are characterized by pruritus, dermatitis, and onchocercomata. The dermatitis is variable in its appearance and probably relates to chronicity of infection, the age of the patients, the geographic area in which it was acquired, and the relative immune responsiveness. Early in the course of the infection an itchy papular dermatitis may

occur, and in visitors who acquire the infection, this may be localized to one extremity. In Central America, papules may appear only on the head and neck area. This unusual localization of insect bite–appearing papules with excoriations may lead to the diagnosis in travelers returning to their home countries. In Central America, another manifestation of the acute phase is acute swelling of the face with erythema and itching known as *erisipela de la costa*. In Zaire and Central America, an acute urticarial eruption is seen. The inflammation, which is accompanied by hyperpigmentation, is known as *mal morado.*

As time passes, the dermatitis becomes chronic and remains papular; however, thickening, lichenification, and dyspigmentation occur (Fig. 20-30). Later, atrophy may supervene. When the depigmentation is spotted, it is known as *leopard skin;* when the skin is thickened, it is called *elephant skin.* When local edema and thickened, wrinkled, dry dermatitic changes predominate, it is sometimes called *lizard skin.*

In Saudi Arabia, Yemen, and East Africa, a localized type of onchocerciasis exists called *sowda,* which is Arabic for "black." It is characterized by localized, pruritic, asymmetrical, usually darkly pigmented, chronic lichenified dermatitis of one leg or one body region. It is also known as the chronic hyperreactive type, and an association with antidefinsin antibodies suggests a reason for this enhanced reactivity against the parasite.

After a time, firm subcutaneous nodules, pea-sized or larger, develop on various sites of the body (Figs. 20-31 and 20-32). These nodules are onchocercomas containing myriad microfilariae. These occur in crops, are frequently painful, and their site varies. In parts of Africa, where natives are wholly or nearly unclothed, the lesions occur on the trunk, axillae, groin, and perineum. In Central and South America the head, especially the scalp, is the usual site of involvement.

Firm, nontender lymphadenopathy is a common finding in patients with chronically infected onchocerciasis. "Hanging groin" describes the loose, atrophic skin sack that contains these large inguinal nodes.

In about 5% of affected persons, serious eye lesions arise late in the disease, gradually leading to blindness.

Onchocerciasis is caused by *Onchocerca volvulus,* which is transmitted to humans by the bite of the black fly of the genus *Simulium,* which breeds in fast-flowing streams of water. When the black fly bites, it introduces larvae into the wound. The larvae reach adulthood in the subdermal connective tissue in about 1 year. Then millions of the progeny migrate back into the dermis and the aqueous humor of the eye.

Onchocerciasis occurs in Africa on the west coast, in the Sahara, Sudan, and the Victoria Nile division, where this disease is known as *river blindness.* In Central and South America, it is to be found in Guatemala, Brazil, Venezuela, and southern Mexico, where it is endemic in the provinces

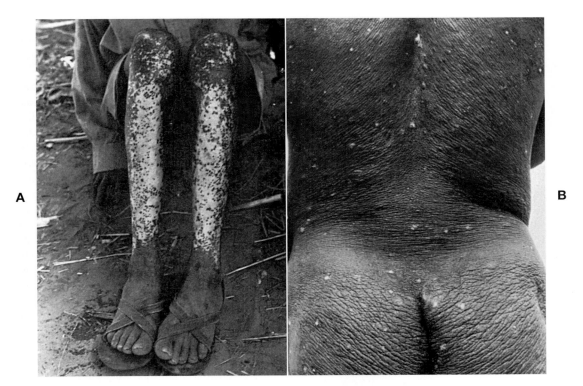

Fig. 20-30 **A,** Pretibial depigmentation in chronic onchocerciasis. **B,** Generalized onchocerciasis of long duration with thickening, edema, and atrophy of the skin with excoriation. (Courtesy Dr. Anthony Bryceson, London.)

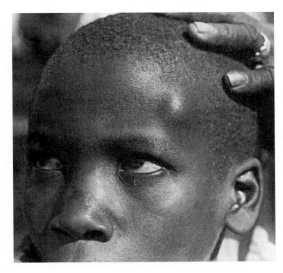

Fig. 20-31 Nodule of onchocerciasis on forehead. The skin is of normal appearance. The danger of blinding eye lesions is increased. (Courtesy Dr. Anthony Bryceson, London.)

of Oaxaca and Chiapas. In a survey in Chiapas, 50% of the population was found to be infected. Onchocerciasis constitutes one of Mexico's major public health problems: 20 million people are said to be infected.

The presence of eosinophilia, skin lesions, and onchocer-comas with ocular lesions is highly suggestive in endemic areas. Frequently the microfilariae may be found in skin shavings or dermal lymph, even when no nodules are detectable. The scapular area is the favorite site for procuring specimens for examination by means of a skin snip. This is performed in the field or office by lifting the skin with an inserted needle and then clipping off a small, superficial portion of the skin with a sharp knife or scissors. The specimen is laid in a drop of normal saline solution on a slide, covered with a coverslip, and examined under the microscope. The filariae wriggle out at the edges of the skin slice.

Specific serologic and polymerase chain reaction–based diagnostic tests from blood and skin biopsies are available on a research basis. Other filarial parasites can be detected in similar systems. A patient suspected of having onchocerciasis may be given a single oral dose of 50 mg of diethylcarbamazine. A reaction consisting of edema, itching, fever, arthralgias, and an exacerbation of pruritus is described as a positive Mazzotti test reaction, which supports the diagnosis of onchocerciasis.

Onchocercomas may be surgically excised whenever feasible. Ivermectin as a single oral dose of 150 µg/kg is the drug of choice. Skin microfilaria counts remain low at the end of 6 months' observation. It should be repeated every 6 months to suppress the dermal and ocular microfilarial counts, since no medicine kills the adult worms. If there is

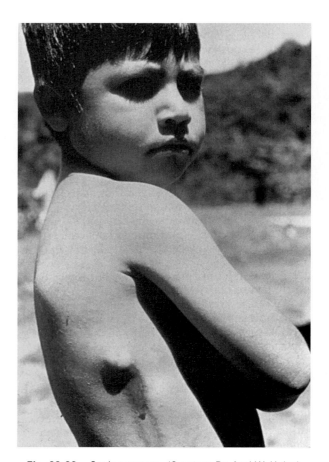

Fig. 20-32 Onchocercoma. (Courtesy Dr. Axel W. Hoke.)

eye involvement prednisone 1 mg/kg should be started several days before treatment with ivermectin.

There are community-based treatment protocols that have as the objective eliminating onchocerciasis from endemic areas. Severe reactions may occur in patients simultaneously infected with *Loa loa.*

Gallin MY, et al: Human autoantibody to defensin: disease association with hyperreactive onchocerciasis (sowda). *J Exp Med* 1995, 182:41.

Gardon J, et al: Serious reactions after mass treatment of onchocerciasis with ivermectin in an area endemic for *Loa loa* infection. *Lancet* 1997, 350:18.

Lazarov A, et al: Onchocerciasis. *Arch Dermatol* 1997, 133:382.

Siddiqui MA, et al: The black disease of Arabia, sowda-onchocerciasis. *Int J Dermatol* 1991, 30:130.

Stingl P: Onchocerciasis. *Int J Dermatol* 1997, 36:23.

Yarzabal L: The immunology of onchocerciasis. *Int J Dermatol* 1985, 25:349.

Zimmerman PA, et al: Polymerase chain reaction-based diagnosis of *Onchocera valvulus* infection. *J Infect Dis* 1994, 169:686. ———— ▲

Trichinosis

Ingestion of *Trichinella spiralis* larva–containing cysts in inadequately cooked pork, bear, or walrus meat may cause trichinosis. It usually causes a puffy edema of the eyelids, redness of the conjunctivae, and sometimes urticaria associated with hyperpyrexia, headache, erythema, gastrointestinal symptoms, muscle pains, and neurologic signs and symptoms. In 20% of cases a macular or petechial eruption occurs, and splinter hemorrhages are occasionally present. Eosinophilia is not constant, but may be as high as 80%. In the average patient, eosinophilia begins about 1 week after infection and attains its height by the fourth week.

Rapidly fatal cases of proven trichinosis have been reported without eosinophilia. Gay et al reported a patient, infected from uncooked sausage meat, who died 5 weeks after onset of brain involvement with right parietal hemorrhage, despite a regimen of 16 mg of dexamethasone daily. The intradermal skin test may give an immediate (15-minute) response, but it usually does not yield a positive result before the third week of infection, and it is not considered reliable enough for diagnosis.

The immunofluorescence antibody test has the greatest value in establishing a diagnosis. The bentonite flocculation test, an enzyme-linked immunosorbent assay (ELISA) test, and other serologic tests are limited by their inability to detect infection until the third or fourth week.

Diagnosis is confirmed by a muscle biopsy that demonstrates larvae of *Trichinella spiralis* in striated muscle. Unfortunately, trichinae cannot usually be demonstrated unless the infection is very heavy, of over a month's duration, and the biopsy specimen is very large. A 2 mm thick slice of the muscle biopsy may be compressed between two glass slides to demonstrate the cysts.

The condition is treated with albendazole 400 mg twice daily for 14 days. Corticosteroidal agents are effective as a means of controlling the often severe symptoms and should be given at doses of 40 to 60 mg per day.

Chaudhry AZ, et al: Cutaneous manifestations of intestinal helminthic infections. *Dermatol Clin* 1989, 7:275.

Gay T, et al: Fatal CNS trichinosis. *JAMA* 1982, 247:1024.

Hanada K, et al: Cutaneous changes in trichinellosis seen in Japan. *J Dermatol* 1987, 14:086.

Herrera R, et al: Dermatomyositis-like syndrome caused by trichinae. *J Rheumatol* 1985, 12:782. ———————————— ▲

Phylum Arthropoda

The following classes are of dermatologic significance: Myriapoda, Insecta, and Arachnida. This phylum contains more species than all the other phyla put together. Because of its complexity, the class and order of the organisms in this phylum will be given in many instances.

Injury from venoms of the arthropods (envenomization) is a common hazard in temperate and tropical regions. Arthropodal venoms may be mixtures of the following toxin types: vesicating toxin, producing vesicles and bullae;

neurotoxins, attacking the nervous system and producing respiratory paralysis and death; hemolytic toxin; and hemorrhagic toxin. Anaphylactic shock is the most serious type of reaction encountered from envenomization; however, this happens rarely. About 25,000 envenomizations occur each year that cause severe injury, with about 25 resulting deaths.

CLASS MYRIAPODA
Centipede Stings

Centipede stings are manifested by paired hemorrhagic puncta surrounded by an erythematous swelling that may progress into a brawny edema or lymphangitis and lymphadenopathy. Locally there may be intense itching and pain, sometimes associated with toxic constitutional symptoms.

The western United States species of *Scolopendra,* which will sting, attain a length of 15 to 20 cm; their size is frightening. In the eastern United States, the common house centipede, *Scutigera coleopterata,* does not sting humans. *Scolopendra subspinipes,* in Hawaii, inflicts a painful sting. Rubbing the area with raw garlic, using a cut clove, may rapidly relieve the pain, but injection of a topical anesthetic into the bite site is more effective.

Millipede Burns

Millipedes' bodies secrete a toxic liquid that when it comes in contact with human skin, causes a brownish pigmentation that progresses over the next 24 hours to intense erythema and finally vesiculation. Intense stinging and burning pain occurs. Washing off the toxin as soon as possible will curb the toxic effects. Topical corticosteroid agents should be helpful.

CLASS INSECTA
Order Lepidoptera

Order Lepidoptera includes the butterflies and moths and their larval forms, the caterpillars.

Caterpillar Dermatitis. Irritation is produced by the nettling hairs coming in contact with the skin, the toxin in the hairs producing local pruritic erythematous macules and wheals at the area of contact. Edwards et al documented a case in which both contact urticaria and delayed allergic contact dermatitis resulted from contact with a saddleback caterpillar. If the hairs get into the clothing, widespread dermatitis with conjunctivitis, nausea, and vomiting may result. Not only the caterpillars but their egg covers and cocoons may have the stinging hairs that produce irritation. Stinging caterpillars abound seasonally in the fall and are frequently seen on campers, children playing in trees, and lumberjacks in pine forests.

In the United States the most common caterpillars are the brown-tail moth caterpillar *(Nygmia phoeorrhoea),* puss caterpillar *(Megalopyge opercularis),* saddleback caterpillar *(Sibine stimulae),* crinkled flannel moth *(Megalopyge crispata),* slug caterpillar, and flannel moth *(Norape cretata).* The hairs of the processionary caterpillar *(Thaumetopoea processionea)* of Europe are especially dangerous to the eyes. The urticating apparatus remains in the forest environment all year long and remains a persistent risk for causing painful skin reactions. Most of the papular eruption will resolve in 48 hours after administration of antihistamines.

Moth Dermatitis. The malady is initiated by the hairs of the brown-tail moth *(Euproctis chrysorrhoea),* the goat moth *(Cossus cossus),* the puss moth *(Dicranura vinula),* the gypsy moth *(Lymantria dispar),* and the Douglas fir tussock moth *(Hemenocampa pseudotsugata).*

In Latin America, the moths of the genus *Hylesia* are most frequently the cause of moth dermatitis. Severe conjunctivitis and pruritus are the first signs; shortly afterward, erythematous papules and occasional ecthymatous lesions appear over the entire body, including the covered parts. Usually the lesions subside in about 1 week, but a miniepidemic of Caripito itch (named for Caripito, Venezuela) reported by Dinehart et al lasted for more than 3 weeks in the crew of a ship that was, however, overwhelmingly infested with dead moths and urticating setae (hairs). Berger detailed an outbreak of Korean yellow moth dermatitis caused by *Euproctis flava* Bremer.

Topical applications of various analgesics, antibiotics, and oral antihistaminics are of no help. Topical or oral corticosteroid medications were useful in the patients of Allen et al. Bathing and changing clothes may help prevent or limit the reaction if done soon after exposure.

Allen VT, et al: Gypsy moth caterpillar dermatitis revisited. *J Am Acad Dermatol* 1991, 24:979.

Berger TG: Korean yellow moth dermatitis. *J Assoc Milit Dermatol* 1986, 12:32.

Berman BA, et al: Gypsy moth caterpillar dermatitis. *Cutis* 1983, 31:251.

Dinehart SM: Caripito itch. *J Am Acad Dermatol* 1985, 13:743.

Edwards EK Jr, et al: Contact urticaria and allergic contact dermatitis to the saddleback caterpillar with histologic correlation. *Int J Dermatol* 1986, 25:467.

Gardner TL, et al: Painful papulovesicles produced by the puss caterpillar. *Cutis* 1997, 60:125.

Shenefelt PD: Moth cocoon dermatitis. *Arch Dermatol* 1991, 127:424. ▲

Order Hemiptera

The bugs represent order Hemiptera. They have two pairs of wings, usually modified, and a sucking mouth part. Among this order are bedbugs, water bugs, chinch bugs, stink bugs, squash bugs, and conenose bugs (kissing bugs, assassin bugs). The latter are vectors of South American trypanosomiasis.

Cimicosis (Bedbug Bites). The bedbug *(Cimex lectularius)* is a smelly parasite with nonfunctioning wings; it is found all over the world. It hides in crevices during the daytime and feeds on human blood at night. When the bedbug punctures the skin the bite is painless, but saliva is released, and resulting hypersensitivity to a protein in the saliva leads to an urticarial or purpuric reaction about the punctum several hours later.

One bedbug may produce several bites in the course of the night, chiefly on the exposed surfaces, these often being arranged in a line (Fig. 20-33). The bite is at first painless, and some persons react to it scarcely at all. They may not be aware of what has happened until they awake in the morning to find their nightclothes and bed stained with blood. Other persons react violently, with pronounced urticaria and pain. Papular urticaria and even extensive erythemas, urticaria, and even anaphylaxis have been reported, associated with the bites. Sansom et al reported the delayed onset of skin reaction to the bedbug bite in two women, one of whom did develop a papular eruption 9 days after exposure. Itching hives that are worse in the morning are suggestive.

The bedbug is an oval, flattened, brown bug, about 5 mm long, with three pairs of legs. The female must have a blood meal to lay eggs, which are deposited into the corners of wooden bedsteads and other crevices. The bedbug may survive starvation for many months and is readily transported in baggage and clothing.

The 1-mm operculated eggs are laid at the rate of two daily and hatch in 4 to 10 days. The bugs mature in about 6 weeks, after several moltings. The life span is up to a year. Hepatitis B surface antigen has been repeatedly demonstrated in the bugs, and it is thought that hepatitis may be transmitted in this way.

Treatment is by the use of soothing antipruritic lotions containing menthol or phenol. Topical steroid creams are effective, and in extensive reactions systemic antihistaminics are useful. Crevices in the furniture, floor, and walls should be sprayed with 0.1% trichlorfon spray or a pyrethrum spray. Malathion 0.5% spray is also effective. A 0.5% solution of lindane may be used. An infested house may also be treated by methyl bromide fumigation. Crissey urges obtaining the professional services of an exterminator; amateur efforts, he suggests, are likely to be unsuccessful.

Crissey JT: Bedbugs. *Intern Dermatol* 1981; 20:411.
Sansom JE, et al: Delayed reaction to bedbug bites. *Arch Dermatol* 1992, 128:272. ──────────────────────── ▲

Kissing Bug (Reduviid) Bites. Kissing bugs (assassin bugs, or conenoses) do not infest humans but descend on them individually, often when the person is asleep, and feed on an

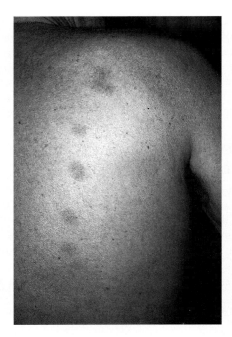

Fig. 20-33 Bedbug bites. Note linear arrangements. (Courtesy Dr. Axel W. Hoke).

exposed area of skin, often on the face; hence the name "kissing bug." The bite is painless but somewhat itchy. The bug immediately defecates, and if it is an intestinal carrier of *Trypanosoma cruzi,* the organism is rubbed into the bite—a regular manner of spread of this disease. In nonendemic areas, the bite is often followed by a red swelling suggestive of cellulitis, which soon subsides. Anaphylaxis has also occurred, and Rohr et al reported successful immunotherapy for immediate hypersensitivity to the bite of *T. protracta,* a variety commonly encountered in Southern California.

Burnett JW, et al: Triatoma. *Cutis* 1987, 39:399.
Rohr AS, et al: Successful immunotherapy for *Triatoma protraeta*-induced anaphylaxis. *J Allerg Clin Immunol* 1984, 73:369. ──────────── ▲

Order Anoplura

Pediculosis (Phthiriasis). Three varieties of these flattened, wingless insects commonly attack humans, although others infest the lower animals and may become temporarily deposited on human hosts. They are *Pediculus humanus* var. *capitis* (head louse), *P. humanus* var. *corporis* (body louse), and *Phthirus pubis* (pubic or crab louse).

Each variety of louse has a predilection for certain parts of the body and rarely migrates to other regions. Lice attach themselves to the skin and live on the blood they suck. In piercing the skin, the parasites exude an antigenic salivary secretion. This, together with the mechanical puncture, produces a pruritic dermatitis. In addition, the louse may be a carrier of disease and through its bite or excretions may

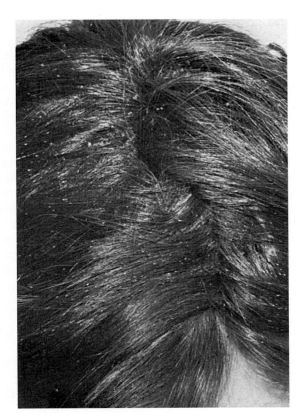

Fig. 20-34 Nits on scalp hair infected with *P. humanus* var. *capitis.*

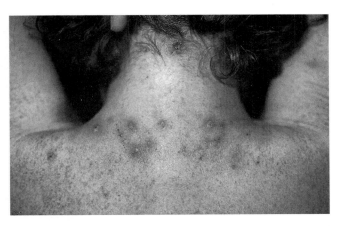

Fig. 20-35 Secondary pyoderma of scalp, posterior neck, and upper back seen in patients with pediculosis capitis.

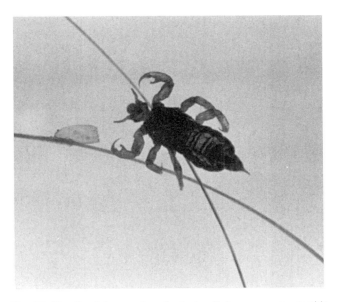

Fig. 20-36 Head louse of pediculosis, *P. humanus* var. *capitis.* (Courtesy Dr. Axel W. Hoke.)

transmit an infectious disease—epidemic typhus, relapsing fever, or trench fever.

Pediculosis Capitis. Pediculosis capitis is encountered principally in children, but occurs in adults also. Usually there is intense pruritus of the scalp, and the affected hairs become lusterless and dry (Fig. 20-34). Because of the itching, secondary complications with impetigo and furunculosis are common (Fig. 20-35). The pediculi may be seen on the scalp (Fig. 20-36), but more often only the nits are seen (Fig. 20-37). As a result of secondary infection, the cervical lymph nodes may become enlarged.

The diagnosis usually presents no difficulties, but occasionally pediculi and nits are so sparse that repeated examination is necessary to discover them. The disease should be suspected in cases of impetigo or furunculosis of the scalp or face in children. It is easy to mistake peripilar keratin (hair) casts encircling hair shafts, or the breaks of trichorrhexis nodosa, for nits. Scott et al have reviewed peripilar casts in detail.

Treatment of pediculosis capitis aims at destruction of the lice and ova. Permethrin 1% creme rinse (Nix) and a 5% prescription cream form (Elimite) are available. These contain a synthetic pyrethroid that is a relatively nontoxic and efficacious agent. The 1% cream rinse must be applied after shampooing and drying the hair completely. The medication is then applied for 10 minutes and rinsed off; shampooing should not take place for 24 hours afterward. Applying to dry hair lessens dilution of the medication; use of a conditioner or silicone shampoo coats the hair, so this also lessens the efficacy of the rinse.

Because of the increasing resistance of head lice to this standard treatment, some leave the rinse on for 30 to 60 minutes before rinsing. Others apply the 5% cream under a shower cap to increase efficacy.

Pyrethrins, combined with piperonyl butoxide (RID, A-200, R+C Shampoo), are sold over the counter. All are applied for 10 minutes after washing the hair. These are less and less useful, however, as the problem of resistance increases.

Retreatment in a week is necessary, since no treatment is oviducal. Combing with a nit comb, such as Licemeister on wet hair rinsed with a conditioner is an important adjunctive measure. Nit removal should be meticulous in the week between treatments. Use of an enzymatic egg remover, such as CLEAR or the plant-oil-derived Hair Clean 1-2-3, are other important aids to nit removal. Family members and contacts should be treated, since up to 6% of carriers are asymptomatic. Combs and brushes should be washed.

Pediculosis Corporis. Pediculosis corporis is also known as pediculosis vestimenti, or "vagabond's disease." The lice causing this condition live chiefly in the seams of clothing, especially wherever there is pressure (and therefore warmth), such as beneath a belt or collar or in bedding. The parasite is rarely discovered on the skin but obtains its nourishment from it by descending to the skin and piercing it with its teeth. The disease causes generalized itching, which may be accompanied by erythematous macules or urticarial wheals resulting from the punctures, or by excoriated papules, parallel linear scratch marks, and a pigmented thickening of the skin from continued rubbing (Fig. 20-38). Secondary furunculosis is common.

In the act of feeding, the louse bores with its stylets into the skin until a blood space is reached. Instantly the blood of the victim is pumped into the louse with such force that its abdomen is distended and its color changes, so that the young louse appears as a small pink spot. As fresh blood flows in one end, excreta are discharged from the other.

The diagnosis is, as a rule, readily established by the generalized itching, by parallel scratch marks, by hyperpigmentation, and by erythematous macules. It is differentiated from scabies by the freedom of the hands and feet from involvement and by its predilection for the upper back. Pruritus and urticaria may cause some confusion. The diagnosis is positively established by finding the lice or nits in the seams of clothing or in bedding.

Destruction of the lice is accomplished by laundering the clothing and bedding. Clothing placed in a dryer for 30 minutes at 65° C (149° F) should be disinfected. Dry cleaning destroys lice on wool garments. Pressing woolens with an iron, especially the seams, is also satisfactory. The patient should bathe thoroughly with soap and water. One percent malathion powder or 10% DDT may be dusted onto the inner surface of the underwear, with particular attention given to the seams. If discarding the clothing is feasible, this is best. Lice may live in clothing for 1 month without a blood meal. Examination of sex partners, their clothes, and the bedding will identify secondary cases.

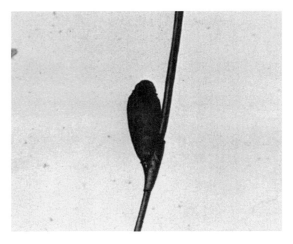

Fig. 20-37 Nit attached to hair shaft.

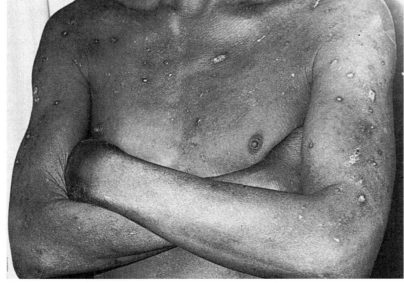

Fig. 20-38 Pediculosis corporis. (Courtesy Dr. J. Stricker.)

Pediculosis Pubis (Crabs). Pediculosis pubis is contracted chiefly by adults as the result of sexual intercourse, and not infrequently from bedding. *Phthirius pubis,* the crab louse (Fig. 20-39), usually limits its incursions to the genital region and hypogastrium or, rarely, the axillae or eyelashes (pediculosis palpebrarum) (Fig. 20-40). The lice are found on the skin, to which they cling tightly, appearing as yellowish brown or gray specks (Fig. 20-41). Because they are almost the color of the skin, they are difficult to identify, and for this reason the infestation may exist a long time before its recognition. The nits are attached to the hairs at an acute angle. The symptoms vary from slight discomfort to intolerable itching.

Pediculosis pubis frequently coexists with other sexually transmitted diseases, particularly gonorrhea and trichomoniasis, and to a lesser extent scabies, nongonococcal urethritis, genital warts, candidiasis, and syphilis. A diagnosis of pediculosis pubis should initiate a search for other sexually transmitted diseases, including HIV disease.

Occasionally, peculiar bluish or slate-colored macules that do not itch or that disappear on diascopic pressure occur in association with pediculosis pubis. These macules, about 0.5 cm in diameter, are located chiefly on the sides of the trunk and on the inner aspects of the thighs. They are most noticeable in blondes. The spots, called *maculae ceruleae,* are probably caused by altered blood pigments of an infested human, or to an excretion product from the louse's salivary gland. The spots may persist for several months.

Treatment of pediculosis pubis aims at destruction of the lice and the ova. Permethrin 1% creme rinse (Nix) and a 5% prescription cream form (Elimite) are available. They contain a synthetic pyrethroid that is relatively nontoxic and highly efficacious. Pyrethrins combined with piperonyl butoxide (RID, A-200, R+C Shampoo) are sold over the counter. All are applied for 10 minutes after washing the hair. An enzymatic egg remover such as CLEAR may also be used.

Retreatment in 1 week is recommended. The affected person's sexual contacts should be treated simultaneously. For eyelash involvement, a thick coating of petrolatum can be applied twice daily for 8 days, followed by mechanical removal of any remaining nits. Fluorescein drops are also effective. Clothing and fomites should be washed and dried by machine or laundered and ironed.

Altschuler DZ, et al: Pediculicide performance, profit, and the public health. *Arch Dermatol* 1986, 122:259.

Brown S: Treatment of ectoparasitic infections. *Clin Infect Dis* 1995, 20(Suppl):104.

Burkhart CG, et al: An assessment of topical and oral prescription and over-the-counter treatments for head lice. *J Am Acad Dermatol* 1998, 38:979.

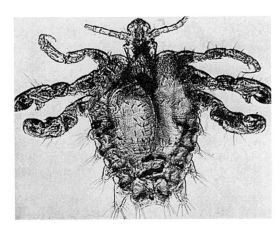

Fig. 20-39 Crab louse, female *(Pthirus pubis).* (×60.) (Courtesy Army Medical Museum.)

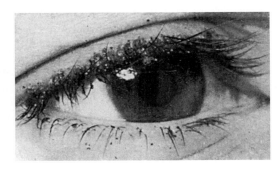

Fig. 20-40 Pediculosis palpebrarum in association with pediculosis pubis. (Courtesy Dr. C.S. Wright.)

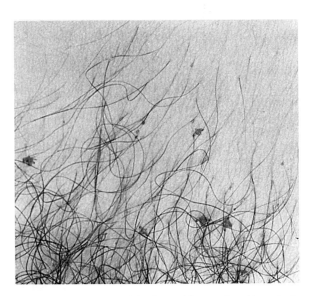

Fig. 20-41 Pediculosis pubis. Several lice on the skin and nits on the hair shafts are visible.

Gillis D, et al: Seasonality and long-term trends of pediculosis capitis and pubis on a young adult population. *Arch Dermatol* 1990, 126:638.

Kalter DC, et al: Treatment of pediculosis pubis. *Arch Dermatol* 1987, 123:1315.

Meinking TL, et al: Comparative efficacy of treatments for pediculosis capitis infestations. *Arch Dermatol* 1986, 122:267.

Meinking TL, et al: Update on scabies and pediculosis. *Adv Dermatol* 1999, 15:67.

Mumcuoglu KY, et al: Clinical observations related to head lice infestation. *J Am Acad Dermatol* 1991, 25:248.

Scott MJ Jr, et al: Hair casts. *J Am Acad Dermatol* 1983, 8:27.

Taplin D, et al: Pyrethrins and pyrethroids in dermatology. *Arch Dermatol* 1990, 126:213.

Urcuyo FG, et al: Malathion lotion as an insecticide and ovicide for head louse infestation. *Int J Dermatol* 1986, 25:60. ─────────── ▲

Order Diptera

Order Diptera includes the two-winged biting flies. Both the adults and the larvae parasitize humans in many ways. Because there is a tremendous number of species, only a few will be mentioned here, according to family.

Tabanidae include the horsefly, deerfly, gadfly, and others; these inflict extremely painful bites.

Muscidae include the housefly, stablefly, and the tsetse fly (which transmits trypanosomiasis). Tsetse fly bites usually cause no reaction the first time; however, repeated bites will cause severe reactions, so that desensitization may be necessary. Larvae of these flies may infest the skin (myiasis).

Simulidae are represented by the black fly, buffalo gnat, and coffee fly, some of which are vectors of onchocerciasis. These flies are usually dark colored and "hunchbacked." They may produce extremely painful bites that may be associated with fever, chills, and lymphadenitis. Black flies are seasonal annoyances in the northern United States and Canada.

Psychodidae are small, hairy flies (sandflies). *Phlebotomus* flies are of importance as vectors of cutaneous leishmaniasis, mucocutaneous leishmaniasis, and verruga peruana.

Culicidae, or mosquitoes, are vectors of many important diseases, such as filariasis, malaria, dengue, and yellow fever. Their bites may cause severe urticarial reactions.

Ceratopogonidae, the biting midges or gnats, fly in swarms and produce erythematous, edematous lesions at the site of their bite.

Steffen C: Clinical and histopathologic correlation of midge bites. *Arch Dermatol* 1981, 117:785. ─────────── ▲

Three specific problems created by members of the Diptera order will be discussed.

Mosquito Bites. The blood-sucking mosquitoes belong to the subfamily of *Culicinae*. Moisture, warmth, carbon dioxide, estrogens, and L-lactic acid in sweat attracts mosquitoes to hosts. The cutaneous reaction to a mosquito bite may be, in its simplest form, a pruritic local wheal that promptly subsides. A more severe reaction is an immediate allergic response, with a subsequent delayed reaction and even with a systemic response. Urticaria is not an unusual reaction, especially in visitors or new residents; this may be intermittent, continuing for approximately 1 week.

Treatment of mosquito bites usually offers no great problems. For the ordinary bite, application of one of the corticosteroid creams is satisfactory. The use of mosquito repellents on the skin and clothing is recommended for individuals who are sensitive to mosquito bites.

Diethyltoluamide (DEET) has been found to be the most effective repellent. Other good repellents are chlorodiethyl benzamide, ethyl hexanediol, and dimethyl phthalate. These are available in over-the-counter creams, liquids, sprays, and sticks.

Klenerman P: Mosquitoes. *Int J Dermatol* 1989, 28:370.

Peng Z, et al: Immunologic mechanisms in mosquito allergy. *Ann Allergy Asthma Immunol* 1996, 77:238.

Penneys NS, et al: Mosquito salivary gland antigens identified by circulating human antibodies. *Arch Dermatol* 1989, 125:219.

Tokura Y, et al: Severe hypersensitivity to mosquito bites associated with natural killer cell lymphocytosis. *Arch Dermatol* 1990, 126:362. ─── ▲

Ked Itch. The sheep ked *(Melophagus ovinus)* crawls into the sheep's wool and feeds by thrusting its sharp mouth parts into the skin and sucking blood. Occasionally it attacks woolsorters and sheepherders, causing pruritic, often hemorrhagic papules, nearly always with a central punctum. Deer keds attack people in a similar way. The papules are very persistent and may last for up to 12 months. Favorite locations are the hips and the abdomen.

Rantanen T, et al: Persistent pruritic papules from deer ked bites. *Acta Derm Venereol* 1982, 62:307. ─────────── ▲

Myiasis. The invasion of mammalian tissues by dipterous (fly) larvae is known as *myiasis*. The larvae of several varieties of flies produce cutaneous manifestations. The eggs, living larvae, or both are deposited on the skin or mucous membranes. The eggs hatch and produce larvae that then burrow into the skin and cause mild or severe inflammatory changes. Others migrate to folds of skin and burrow into the subcutaneous tissue, producing an inflammatory reaction that gives the appearance of a furuncle, at the center of which maggots may be seen.

Some varieties of flies puncture the skin and extrude the ova beneath the surface (furuncular myiasis), whereas others deposit their eggs on open wounds or ulcers (traumatic or wound myiasis). In this type of wound myiasis, larvae hatch out on the skin and maggots crawl about in the dirty, ulcerated area (Fig. 20-42).

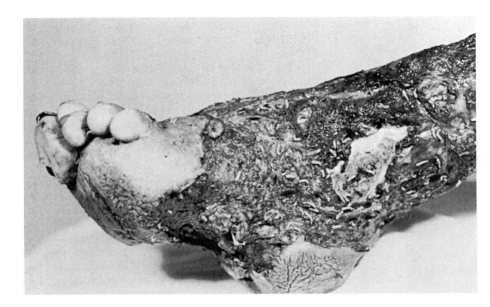

Fig. 20-42 Maggots in ulcer on leg. (Courtesy Dr. F. Kerdel-Vegas.)

A third type, known as *creeping eruption,* develops when the larvae of the *Gasterophilus* wander intradermally. The most common species are *G. nasalis* and *G. intestinalis.* An itching pink papule develops, followed by a tortuous line that extends by 1 to 30 cm daily. The larva may be picked out with a needle once localized.

The human botfly, *Dermatobia hominis,* is a common cause of furuncular myiasis in the neotropical region of the New World. It is a serious economic pest when it affects cattle. It has an interesting life cycle. The female glues its eggs to the body of a mosquito, stablefly, or tick. When the unwitting vector punctures the skin by biting, the larvae emerge from the egg and enter the skin through the puncture wound. Over a period of several days a painful furuncle develops in which the larva is present (Fig. 20-43).

In tropical Africa the Tumbu fly, or ver du cayor (*Cordylobia anthropophaga*), deposits her eggs on the ground, and the active young maggot attacks and penetrates the skin of its host. Dome-shaped furuncular-appearing lesions develop on the skin part exposed to the ground (Fig. 20-44). The fly usually attacks mammals other than humans. Ockenhouse et al provided an excellent reference in their report of a soldier infected on the Ivory Coast.

Another species of fly that causes furuncular myiasis in North America is the *Wohlfahrtia vigil.* This fly can penetrate infant skin, but not adult skin. Thus, nearly all reported cases have occurred in infants. Other larvae that frequently cause furuncular lesions in North America are the common cattle grub *(Hypoderma lineatum)* and the rabbit botfly *(Cuterebra cuniculi).*

The screw worm that most frequently infects animals and humans in the southern United States and American tropics is *Cochliomyia hominivorax.* The larvae of these flies, and those of *Callitroga americana* and *Callitroga macellaria,* account for the majority of cases of wound myiasis in

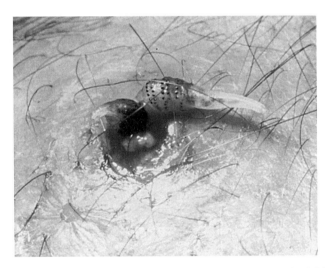

Fig. 20-43 Myiasis *(Dermatobia hominis).* (Courtesy Dr. Axel W. Hoke.)

the United States. The black blowfly *(Phormia regina),* which principally affects goats and sheep and occasionally humans, is also an important cause in this country. This fly is common around houses, privies, and packing establishments.

Treatment of furuncular myiasis is by injection of a local anesthetic into the skin, which anesthetizes both the skin and the larva. Then the larva is surgically removed by incising the lesion or by pushing the larva out with pressure from beneath. Inhabitants of endemic areas apply pork fat to the skin. This is occlusive, and the larva migrates out of the skin to avoid asphyxiation. Either bacon or petrolatum applications are similarly effective. Topical ivermectin was successfully used in a patient from Colombia.

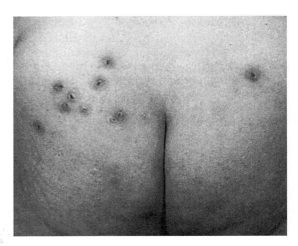

Fig. 20-44 Tumbu fly myiasis. Dome-shaped furuncular lesion with central craters through which maggots are evacuated. (Courtesy Dr. W.E. Schorr and *Arch Dermatol* 95:61, 1967.)

Treatment of wound myiasis is by surgical removal of the maggots and douching of the wound for 30 minutes with 15% chloroform dissolved in any light vegetable oil.

Arosemena R, et al: Cutaneous myiasis. *J Am Acad Dermatol* 1993, 28:254.

Jelinek T, et al: Cutaneous myiasis. *Int J Dermatol* 1995, 34:624.

Kron MA: Human infestation with *Cochliomyia hominivorax. J Am Acad Dermatol* 1992, 27:127.

Lodi A, et al: Myiasis due to *Cordylobia anthrophphaga. Int J Dermatol* 1994, 33:127.

Noutsis C, et al: Myiasis. *Dermatol Clin* 1994, 12:729.

Nunzio E, et al: Removal of *Dermatobia hominis* larvae. *Arch Dermatol* 1986, 122:140.

Ockenhouse CF, et al: Cutaneous myiasis caused by the African Tumbu-fly. *Arch Dermatol* 1990, 126:199.

Spigel GT: Opportunistic cutaneous myiasis. *Arch Dermatol* 1988, 124:1014.

Victoria J, et al: Myiasis: a successful treatment with topical ivermectin. *Int J Dermatol* 1999, 38:142. _____ ▲

Order Coleoptera

Blister Beetle Dermatitis. Blister beetle dermatitis occurs after contact with three major groups of beetles. The *Meloidae* and *Oedemeridae* families produce injury to the skin by releasing a vesicating agent, cantharidin, abundant in its reproductive organs. A third group of blister beetles belonging to the family *Staphylinidae* (species of the genus *Paederus*) contain a different vesicant, pederin. None of the beetles bite or sting; rather, they exude their blistering fluid if they are brushed against, pressed, or crushed on the skin.

Slight burning and tingling of the skin occur in a few minutes, and within a day single (Fig. 20-45) or multiple bullae develop, which are often arranged in a linear fashion. "Kissing lesions" are observed when the blister beetle's excretion is deposited in the flexures of the elbows or other folds. In South America, rove beetles (genus *Paederus*)

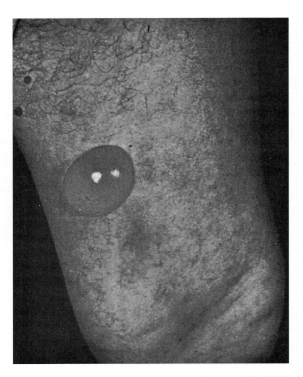

Fig. 20-45 Blister beetle bulla above knee. (Courtesy Dr. C. March.)

produce a patchy or linear erythematous vesicular eruption commonly known as *podo*. It occurs frequently during the rainy season and appears predominantly on the neck and exposed parts.

Several species are used medicinally. The best known among these is the "Spanish fly" *(Lytta vesicatoria),* which is prevalent in southern Europe. Blister beetles are common in all parts of the world.

Treatment consists of drainage of the bullae and application of cold wet compresses and topical corticosteroid preparations. Preliminary cleansing with acetone, ether, soap, or alcohol may be helpful.

Carpet Beetle Dermatitis. Papulovesicular and urticarial dermatitis is caused by the common carpet beetle *(Anthrenus scrophulariae).* The eruption involves the chest, neck, and forearms. The larvae inhabit warm houses throughout the winter months. They are reddish brown, fusiform, about 6 mm long, and covered by hairs.

A generalized pruritic eruption from larvae of a carpet beetle infesting two wool rugs was reported by Ahmed et al; the beetle was identified as *A. verbasci.* Fumigation of the house with sulfuryl fluoride (Vikane) abolished the larvae and solved the problem.

Ahmed AR, et al: Carpet beetle dermatitis. *J Am Acad Dermatol* 1981, 5:428.

Burnett JW, et al: Blister beetles: "Spanish fly." *Cutis* 1987, 39:22.

Nicholls DSH, et al: Oedemerid blister beetle dermatitis. *J Am Acad Dermatol* 1990, 22:815. _____ ▲

Order Hymenoptera

Hymenoptera includes the bees, wasps, hornets, and ants. Stings by any of these may manifest the characteristic clinical and histologic features of eosinophilic cellulitis (Wells' syndrome) complete with flame figures.

Bees and Wasps. Bees, or apids, are stinging insects that produce their sting by the ovipositor of the female abdomen. The venom contains many chemicals. Of importance in producing the clinical effects are histamine, mellitin, hyaluronidase, a high-molecular-weight substance with acid phosphatase activity, and phospholipase A. The barbed ovipositor of the honeybee is torn out of the bee and remains in the skin after stinging. The bumble bee, wasp, and hornet are able to withdraw their stinger.

There are many types of wasps, or vespids: hunting wasps, social wasps, digger wasps, yellowjackets, and hornets. Yellowjackets are the principal cause of allergic reaction to insect stings, because they nest in the ground or in walls and are disturbed by outdoor activity, such as gardening or lawn mowing. Bees are generally docile and sting only when provoked. The allergens in vespid venom are phospholipase, hyaluronidase, and a protein known as *antigen 5*.

The reaction to these stings may be mild local edema, pain and pruritus, large local reactions that may last for 2 to 7 days, serum sickness characterized by fever, urticaria, and joint pain that occur 7 to 10 days after the sting, or severe anaphylactic shock and death within minutes of the sting. Hypersensitivity reactions have been shown to be mediated by specific IgE antibodies to the venom of individual members of this order. Anaphylaxis has in some cases been the presenting symptom of mastocytosis. In some of these individuals there is no demonstrable specific IgE against wasp venom.

The imbedded ovipositor of the honeybee contains the poison sac, which should be scraped away with a sharp knife. Grasping the sac to pull out the stinger expresses more poison into the surrounding tissue. Removal is necessary, since the stinger is not absorbed and will act as an irritant source as long as it remains imbedded.

Treatment of local reactions consists of immediate application of ice packs and rubbing with a dilute solution of meat tenderizer. Oral antihistamines to allay pruritus and analgesics for the pain are also given. If meat tenderizer is not available, a pulverized aspirin tablet may be rubbed into the moistened site. Moistening it again will renew the relief. The site of any painful or inflamed sting may be injected with 1 or 2 ml of a mixture of equal parts of 1% triamcinolone diacetate (or acetonide) suspension and 2% lidocaine or procaine hydrochloride. Relief is instantaneous and usually permanent. Oral prednisone, 40 mg/day for 2 to 3 days, is another option for severe local reactions.

For severe systemic reactions, 0.3 ml epinephrine (1:1000 aqueous solution) is injected subcutaneously. This may need to be repeated for severe reactions. Corticoste-roids and epinephrine may be required for several days following severe reactions.

For persons who are frequently exposed to the hazard, hyposensitization procedures may be indicated. Reisman has reviewed the indications and guidelines for venom immunotherapy. It is effective in reducing the risk of anaphylaxis in people at risk. Susceptible persons should also carry a kit (Ana-Kit) containing syringe, epinephrine for injection, and antihistaminics.

Ewan PW: Allergy to insect stings. *J R Soc Med* 1985, 78:234.

Graft DF, et al: A prospective study of the natural history of large local reactions after hymenoptera stings in children. *J Pediatr* 1984, 104:664.

Janniger CK, et al: Childhood insect bite reactions to ants, wasps, and bees. *Cutis* 1994, 54:14.

Kors JW, et al: Anaphylactoid shock following *Hymenoptera* sting as a presenting symptom of systemic mastocytosis. *J Intern Med* 1993, 233:255.

Reisman RE: Insect stings. *N Engl J Med* 1994, 331:523.

Schorr WF: Eosinophilic cellulitis (Wells' syndrome) in arthropod bite reactions. *J Am Acad Dermatol* 1984, 11:1043.

VonWitt R: Topical aspirin for wasp stings. *Lancet* 1980, 2:1379. ▲

Ants. The sting of most ants is painful, but that of the fire ants *(Solenopsis saevissima, S. invicta, S. geminata, or S. xyloni)* is especially painful. *S. saevissima* is ferocious and vicious and will produce many burning, painful stings within seconds if its nest is molested. The sting causes intense pain, whealing develops, and a hemorrhagic punctum may appear that later develops into a vesicle, and finally umbilicated sterile pustules develop. Seizures and mononeuropathy have been reported. The sting of harvester ants and soldier ants may produce similar reactions. Little or nothing can alleviate the severe pain except perhaps intralesional injections of triamcinolone. In the case of multiple stings, epinephrine and systemic steroids are of decided benefit.

Cohen PR: Imported fire ant stings. *Pediatr Dermatol* 1992, 9:44.

deShazo RD, et al: Reactions to the stings of imported fire ants. *N Engl J Med* 1990, 323:462.

Ross EV, et al: Meat tenderizer in the acute treatment of imported fire ant stings. *J Am Acad Dermatol* 1987, 16:1189. ▲

Order Siphonaptera

Fleas are wingless, with highly developed legs for jumping. They are blood-sucking parasites, infesting most warm-blooded animals. The flea's body is armored with chitin, and the mouth is highly specialized for penetration and sucking.

Pulicosis (Flea Bites). Fleas exist universally among animals and human beings. The three species of fleas most commonly attacking humans in this country are the human flea *(Pulex irritans)* (Fig. 20-46), the cat flea *(Ctenocephalides felis)* (Fig. 20-47), and the dog flea *(Ctenocephalides canis)*. The mouse flea *(Leptopsylla*

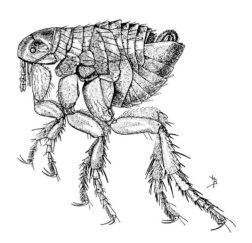

Fig. 20-46 Human flea, male *(Pulex irritans)*. (Courtesy U.S. Department of Agriculture.)

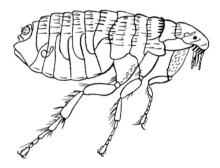

Fig. 20-47 Cat flea, female *(Ctenocephalides felis)*. (Courtesy C. J. Stojanovich, USPHS.)

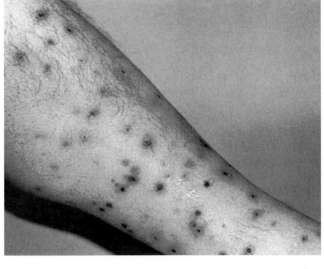

Fig. 20-48 Severe flea bites on the leg. (Courtesy Dr. Alex W. Hoke.)

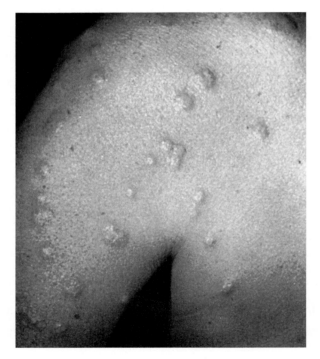

Fig. 20-49 Papular urticaria caused by flea bites.

segnis) and the chicken flea *(Ceratophyllus gallinae)* may occasionally be implicated.

Fleas are small, brown insects about 1/16 inch long, very flat from side to side, with long hind legs. They slip into clothing or jump actively when disturbed. They are known to be extraordinary jumpers, which facilitates travel from host to host. They bite especially about the legs and waist and may be troublesome in houses where there are dogs or cats. They extract their blood meal from the superficial capillaries, causing hemorrhagic puncta surrounded by an erythematous and urticarial patch (Fig. 20-48). The lesions are often grouped and may be arranged in zigzag lines. The irritation is produced by the injection into the skin of a fluid secreted by the salivary glands of the parasite. Some persons have hypersensitivity to this secretion and manifest immediate or delayed reactions at the site of the bite, which assumes the clinical appearance of papular urticaria (Fig. 20-49) or bullae (Fig. 20-50). Soothing lotions and corticosteroid creams, lotions, or sprays give prompt relief of symptoms at the bite sites. Extensive excoriations, eosinophilic cellulitis (Wells' syndrome), and furunculosis may also occur.

Vectors of Disease. Fleas are important because the rat flea, *Xenopsylla cheopis,* as well as *X. braziliensis* are vectors of plague and endemic typhus. When the infected rat dies, the flea seeks another host, which can be humans or

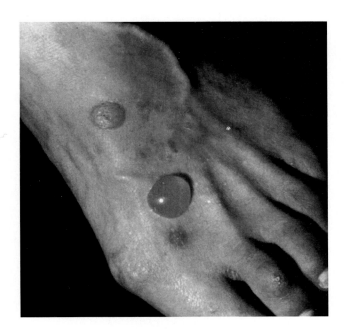

Fig. 20-50 Bullae from flea bites.

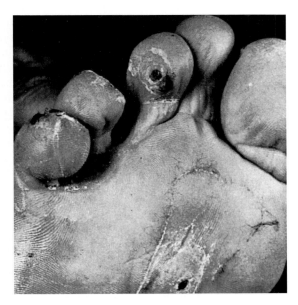

Fig. 20-51 Tungiasis. (Courtesy Dr. F. Reiss.)

other rats. Plague and tularemia are also transmitted by the squirrel flea, *Diamanus montanus*. Several species of fleas are intermediate hosts of the dog tapeworm and rat tapeworm, which may be an incidental parasite of humans.

Flea Control. Liquid and dust sprays are the most effective means of control. Rat nests and sleeping places of cats and dogs should be treated, since the larvae live on the excreta of animals, dried blood, and other debris. In extensive rat control measures, spraying should be done first so that the fleas do not seek other hosts, such as humans. Spraying should include carpets, floors, and stuffed furniture. Some of the effective sprays are 5% malathion powder or 1% lindane dust, 0.5% malathion, or chlordane in kerosene. Insect repellents should be used. Off! and other preparations containing DEET and pyrethrum are some of the effective repellents.

Tungiasis. Tunga penetrans is known as *nigua* in Latin America. In other localities it is also known as *chigoe, sand flea*, or *jigger*. It is a reddish brown flea about 1 mm long. It resides in equatorial Africa, Central and South America, India, and Pakistan. It was first reported in crewmen who sailed with Christopher Columbus. In the United States, it has been reported in travelers returning home from trips to endemic areas. Sanusi et al reviewed these cases.

The sand flea attacks the skin of humans, swine, and many lower animals. The impregnated female chigoe burrows into the skin. The eggs develop and drop to the ground. These eggs develop into larvae, which form cocoons from which the insects emerge in about 10 days.

The lesions are pruritic swellings the size of a small pea.

These usually occur on the ankles, feet, soles (Fig. 20-51), and toes, particularly about the toenails and, less often, about the anogenital areas. The lesions become extremely painful and secondarily infected, producing extensive painful ulcers, which can be crippling.

Curettage or excision of the burrows is recommended. Thiabendazole, 25 mg/kg/day, is a successful oral therapy in heavily infested patients. Antibiotics should be used for the secondary infection and tetanus prophylaxis given. These lesions can be prevented by the wearing of shoes. Infested ground and buildings may be disinfected by the use of insecticides.

Brown M, et al: Insect repellents. *J Am Acad Dermatol* 1997, 36:243.

Howard R, et al: Papular urticaria in children. *Pediatr Dermatol* 1996, 13:246.

Mashek H, et al: Tungiasis in New York. *Int J Dermatol* 1997, 36:276.

Milgraum SS, et al: A subungual nodule of recent onset. *Arch Dermatol* 1988, 124:429.

Sanusi JD, et al: Tungiasis. *J Am Acad Dermatol* 1989, 20:941.

Schorr WF, et al: Eosinophilic cellulitis (Wells' syndrome). *J Am Acad Dermatol* 1984, 11:1043. _____ ▲

CLASS ARACHNIDA

Arachnida includes the ticks, mites, spiders, and scorpions. Adult arachnids have four pairs of legs. Their bodies consist of cephalothorax and abdomen.

Order Acarina

Tick Bite. Several varieties of the family *Ixodidae* (hard ticks) and *Argasidae* (soft ticks) occasionally attack human skin. In the United States, the wood tick *(Dermacentor andersoni)* is the chief offender in the western United States; its habitat is in wooded districts, where it is found especially on pine trees and in the underbrush. Wood ticks are also found in the grass or bushes, from which they launch themselves and attach to human beings, dogs, and cattle. This and the lone star tick *(Amblyomma americanum)* from Texas are the carriers of Rocky Mountain spotted fever, tularemia, and tickborne encephalitis. *Ixodes ricinus* in Europe and *I. scapularis* and *I. pacificus* in the United States transmit *Borrelia burgdorferi,* the cause of Lyme disease. The kangaroo tick, *Amblyomma trigutatum,* and many other species of the hard ticks transmit Q fever to sheep. The dog ticks *Dermacentor variabilis* (Fig. 20-52) and *Rhipephalus sanguineus* are important because the former is a vector of tularemia and the latter carries *Rickettsia conorii,* the cause of Boutonneuse fever.

The female tick attaches itself to the skin by sticking its proboscis into the flesh to suck blood from the superficial vessels. The insertion of the hypostome is generally unnoticed by the subject. The attached tick may be mistaken by the patient as a new mole. In some patients a few hours after attachment an urticarial wheal appears at the puncture site (Fig. 20-53), which itches and is painful for several days. The parasite becomes engorged and then falls off. During this time, which may last for 7 to 12 days, the patient may suffer from fever, chills, headache, abdominal pain, and vomiting. This is called *tick bite pyrexia.* Removal of the engorged tick causes a subsidence of the general symptoms in 12 to 36 hours.

If an attempt is made to pull the tick off, the head is likely to be broken off and left in the skin. One method of removal involves tying a slipknot in a piece of thread, tightening it around the neck of the tick, and pulling gently on it for 3 or 4 minutes, until the tick withdraws its head voluntarily. Then it can safely be crushed under foot. Needham, an acarologist, has confirmed that gentle traction is superior to other methods, in a comparative study. If a portion of the tick is left in the skin, it should be removed by excision.

The bites may be followed by small, severely pruritic, fibrous nodules (tick bite granulomas) that persist for months or even a year or two, or by pruritic circinate and arciform localized erythemas that may continue for months.

Tick Paralysis. Tick paralysis occurs rarely, usually in children, and it may be fatal unless the tick, lodged in the patient's skin, is removed promptly. Paralysis occurs about 6 days after attachment of the tick, commonly on the neck and back of the head. Usually there is no fever, but there may be slight fever, with rapid pulse and respiration. The flaccid paralysis attacks the legs, then the arms, and finally the neck, resembling Landry-Guillain-Barré syndrome. Bulbar paralysis, dysarthria, dysphagia, and death from

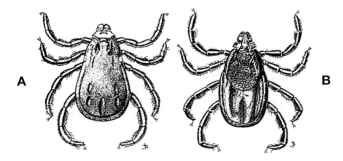

Fig. 20-52 American dog tick *(Dermacentor variabilis).* **A,** Female. **B,** Male. (Courtesy U.S. Department of Agriculture.)

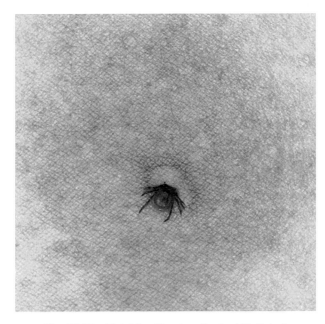

Fig. 20-53 Tick bite. (Courtesy Dr. Axel W. Hoke.)

respiratory failure may occur. Prompt recovery occurs if the tick is found and removed before the terminal stage.

It is thought that toxins elaborated by the tick causes a presynaptic neuromuscular blockade with involvement of the peripheral nerves.

Other Tick Bite Disorders. Several species of ticks of the genus *Ixodes* (notably *I. dammini, I. ricinus,* and *I. pacificus*) are of importance as vectors of *Borrelia burgdorferi,* the causative agent of Lyme disease. Erythema migrans, annular and concentric with the bite, and spreading centrifugally, occurs at the bite site.

Ronnen et al reported a case of ornithodoriasis that preceded a *Borrelia duttonii* infection, the agent of African endemic relapsing fever. The bite of the tick *Ornithodorus tholozani* produced a typical small inflammatory nodule, surrounded by a zone of normal skin, with a circumferential brownish ring. Other diseases besides Lyme disease and relapsing fever that are transmitted by ticks include the

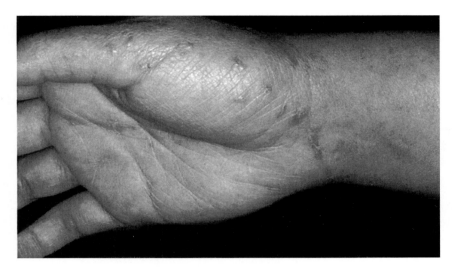

Fig. 20-54 Scabies on the wrist. (Courtesy Dr. Axel W. Hoke.)

rickettsioses (Rocky Mountain spotted fever, Q fever, boutonneuse fever, tick typhus), tularemia, babesiosis, ehrlichiosis, arbovirus and ungrouped viral encephalitides, and hemorrhagic fevers.

Subcutaneous hemorrhage, chronic ulcerations, localized swelling, erythema, blistering, pruritus, induration, gangrene, or necrosis, lymphoma-like tumors, or generalized erythema, urticaria, or psoriasiform dermatitis may occur. A patchy alopecia without erythema or scarring may present 1 to 2 weeks after tick bites on the scalp. Regrowth begins within 2 weeks and resolves completely over a 2-month period.

Protection from tick bites is best accomplished by the use of repellents in clothing, although these are only partially effective. The most effective of these have been found to be DEET, indalone, dimethyl carbamate, and dimethyl phthalate.

Brown M, et al: Insect repellents. *J Am Acad Dermatol* 1997, 36:243.

Jones BE: Human seed tick infestation. *Arch Dermatol* 1981, 117:812.

Leker RR, et al: Ornithordorus tholozani bites. *J Am Acad Dermatol* 1992, 27:1025.

Needham GR: Evaluation of five popular methods for tick removal. *Pediatrics* 1985, 75:997.

Ronnen M, et al: Ornithodoriasis preceding *Borrelia* infection. *Arch Dermatol* 1984, 120:1520. ▲

Mites. Mites may parasitize humans in several ways. Both the adult and larval form may invade the skin: some attack the skin only for feeding, others complete their life cycles in the skin.

SCABIES. Scabies is characterized by pruritic papular lesions and also burrows, which house the female mite and her young. Sites of predilection are chiefly the finger webs, wrists, antecubital fossae, axillae, areolae, and areas around the umbilicus, the lower abdomen, genitals, and buttocks (Figs. 20-54 and 20-55). An imaginary circle intersecting

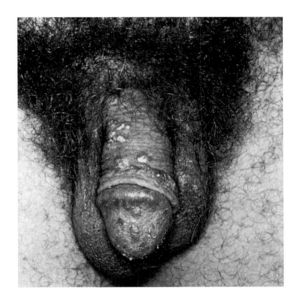

Fig. 20-55 Scabies. Note lesions on glans penis.

the main sites of election—axillae, elbow flexures, wrists and hands, and crotch—has long been called the *circle of Hebra*. In adults the scalp and face are usually spared, but in infants lesions are present over the entire cutaneous surface (Fig. 20-56). In immune-suppressed individuals, the face and scalp may be heavily infested.

The burrows form characteristic lesions barely discernible to the naked eye. These are slightly elevated, grayish, straight or tortuous lines in the skin. A vesicle or pustule may be produced at the end of the burrow, especially in infants and children.

The eruption varies considerably, depending on the manner of infection and previous treatment. It may also vary with climate and the host's immunologic status. In patients who are clean and bathe frequently, the eruption is seldom

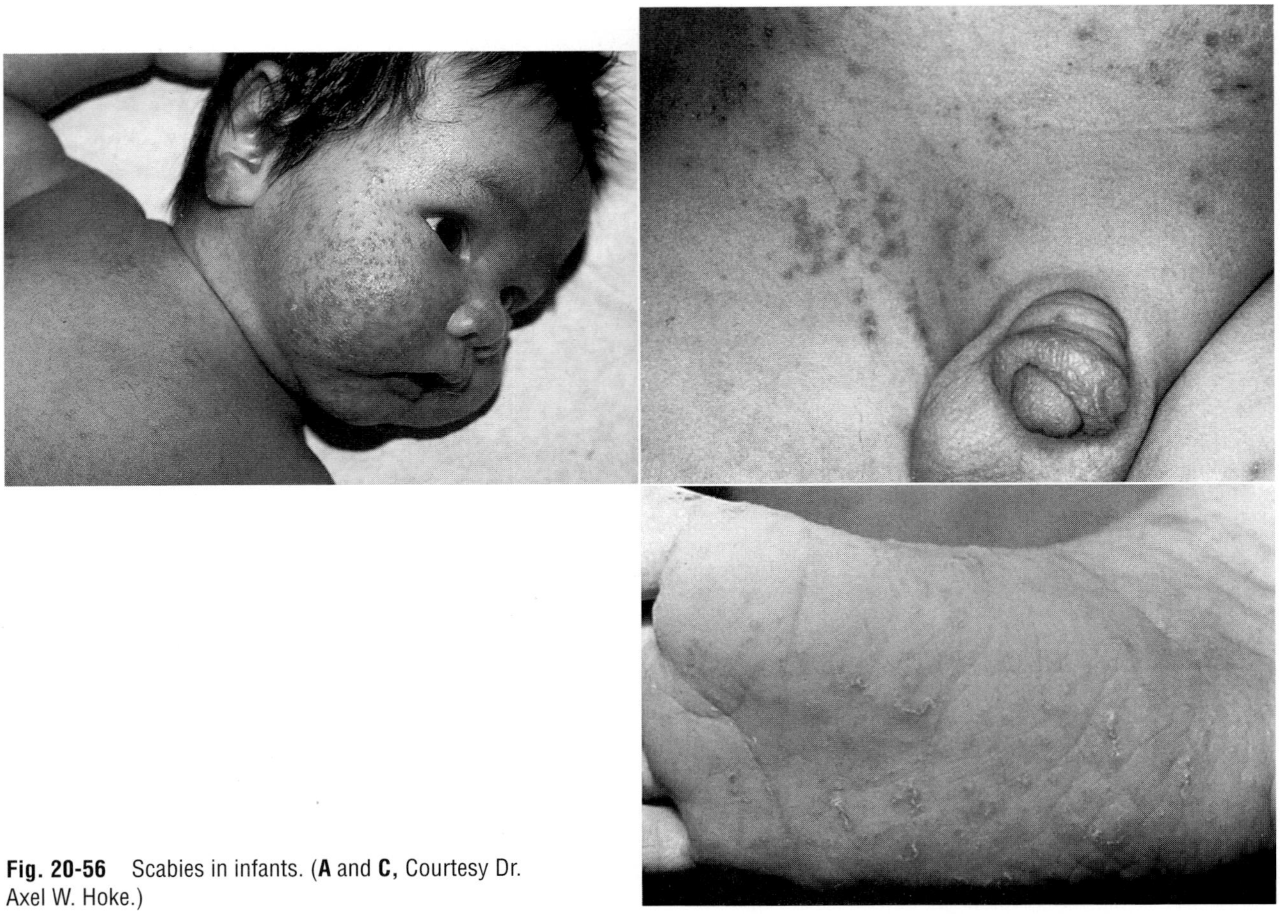

Fig. 20-56 Scabies in infants. (**A** and **C**, Courtesy Dr. Axel W. Hoke.)

pronounced, which usually makes the clinical diagnosis much more difficult. Nevertheless, in highly sensitized individuals, it may be profuse and extensive. Bullous lesions are seen in such patients at times, and also are frequent in infants and young children. The diagnosis must often be made, however, from the distribution of the itching and the lesions present. When the disease has been present a long time, eczematization, lichenification, impetigo, and furunculosis may be present.

Dull red nodules may appear during active scabies; these are 3 to 5 mm in diameter, may or may not itch, and persist on the scrotum, penis, or other areas for weeks or months after scabies has been cured (Fig. 20-57). Intralesional steroids, tar, or excision are methods of treatment of this troublesome condition, termed *nodular scabies*. Histologically, the lesions may suggest lymphoma.

Crusted scabies (Norwegian, or hyperkeratotic, scabies) is the form that is found in immunocompromised or institutionalized individuals, in whom it assumes a heavily scaling and crusted appearance. Crusts and scales teem with acari, and there is involvement of the face and especially the scalp. Itching may be slight. In full-blown cases there is psoriasis-like scaling, especially around and under the nails.

The tips of the fingers are swollen and crusted; the nails are distorted. There are subungual and palmar hyperkeratoses (Fig. 20-58) and severe fissuring and scaling of the genitalia and buttocks. Crusted purulent lesions are present on the face and scalp. The pressure-bearing areas are the sites of predilection for the heavy keratotic lesions, in which the mites may abound.

This curious form of infestation is seen most frequently in malnourished patients; those with neurologic disorders, especially Down syndrome; and in immunosuppressed patients. This type of infection may occur in patients with renal or other organ transplants, graft-versus-host disease, adult T-cell leukemia, leprosy, AIDS, or persons living in institutions under unsanitary conditions.

Funkhouser et al discussed both the typical hyperkeratotic form and a diffuse, uniform eruption of 3- to 5-mm papules that they observed in patients with late-stage AIDS. A patient with ordinary scabies may average a total of some 12 mites; those with keratotic scabies may have thousands of mites in the skin. This type of scabies infestation is believed to be caused by a reduced immunologic response.

Sarcoptes scabiei, the itch mite, is the causative organism. It is an oval, ventrally flattened mite. The female

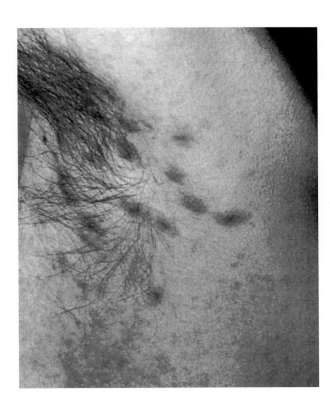

Fig. 20-57 Nodular scabies. (Courtesy Dr. Axel W. Hoke.)

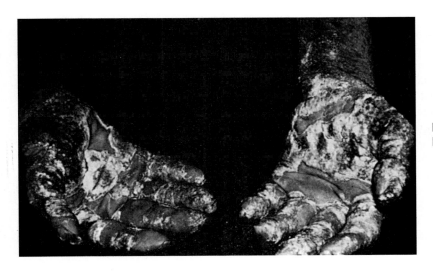

Fig. 20-58 Crusted (Norwegian) scabies. (Courtesy Dr. W.R. Hubler.)

mite is 0.3 to 0.5 mm long. The fertilized female burrows into the stratum corneum and there deposits her eggs (Fig. 20-59). A few hours after the start of the burrow, egg laying begins; two or three eggs are laid daily continuously for nearly 4 to 6 weeks. The male dies after copulation; the female dies after laying the eggs. The eggs hatch into larvae in 3 to 4 days. The larvae are transformed into nymphs, and these in turn into adults.

Scabies is usually contracted by close personal contact, such as nursing an infested patient; overcrowding and close living quarters, as occurs with institutionalized patients; or sleeping together; and infrequently, by the common use of contaminated towels, bed linen, and clothing. The female *S. scabiei* can survive only 2 or 3 days away from warm skin. Arlian et al reviewed the question of infestivity and survival of *S. scabiei* in detail, and also the question of cross-infestation; they concluded that all varieties of the organism prefer certain hosts but do not insist on them. In a related study they found the mites respond to both host odor and thermal stimuli as a means of host-seeking behavior.

Sensitization begins about 2 to 4 weeks after onset of infection. During this time the parasites may be on the skin

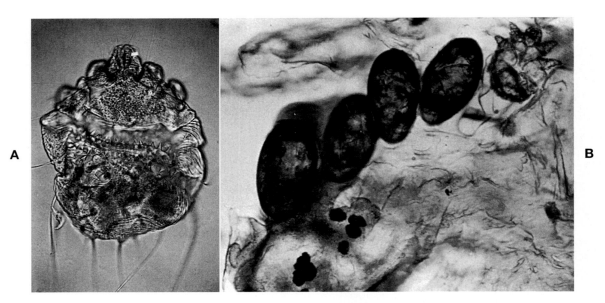

Fig. 20-59 **A,** Acarus. **B,** Photomicrograph of *Sarcoptes scabiei* burrow. (**B,** Courtesy Dr. Axel W. Hoke.)

and may burrow into it without causing pruritus or discomfort. Severe itching begins with sensitization of the host. In reinfections, itching begins immediately and the reaction may be clinically more intense.

The diagnosis is usually based on the presence of fierce itching at night, whereas during the daytime the pruritus is tolerable but persistent. The eruption does not involve the face or scalp in adults. In women, itching of the nipples associated with a generalized pruritic papular eruption is characteristic; in men, itchy papules on the scrotum and penis are equally typical. When more than one member of the family has pruritus, a suspicion of scabies should be aroused—and, because scabies cannot be excluded by examination, treatment on presumption of scabies is advisable.

Positive diagnosis is made only by the demonstration of the mite under the microscope with a low-power objective. A burrow is sought and the position of the mite is determined. A surgical blade or sterile needle is used to remove the parasite. A strong light and a magnifying glass are essential to detect the glistening speck with dark margins. The tunnel can be gently slit open by the blade. With the point touching the mite, transfer is made to a glass slide for microscopic examination. Another technique is to place a drop of mineral or immersion oil on a lesion and gently scrape away the epidermis beneath it. Black ink is applied to the burrow, and when the excess is wiped off, the outline of the burrow may be clearly seen, helping to identify scybala, ova, or mites. The majority of the mites are found on the hands and wrists, less frequently (in decreasing order) at the elbows, genitalia, buttocks, and finally, the axillae.

Patients with scabies in whom sexual transmission is suspected should be examined for other sexually transmitted diseases, including HIV infection.

In addition to scabies, other common diseases that usually affect the trunk but not the face are pityriasis rosea, tinea versicolor, pediculosis corporis, and lichen planus, all of which are readily distinguishable from scabies. In pediculosis corporis the interscapular area is the commonest site of lesions.

Permethrin 5% cream (Elimite) is the safest as well as the most effective medication for scabies. Permethrin is a synthetic pyrethroid that is lethal to mites and has extremely low toxicity for humans.

Permethrin cream or lindane (gamma-benzene hexachloride, Kwell) lotion, which for some years was the standard treatment, is thoroughly rubbed into the skin from the neck to the feet, with particular attention given to the creases, perianal areas, and the free nail edge and folds. It is washed off 8 to 10 hours later. It should be applied a second time in 1 week. Clothing and bed linens are changed and laundered thoroughly. Lindane is readily absorbed, and its neurotoxicity for infants and even to young children is a hazard. These drugs are not safe for use in pregnant women or nursing mothers. Davies et al and Friedman reviewed rare instances of poisoning by lindane.

In babies and pregnant women, 6% to 10% precipitated sulfur in petrolatum is perfectly safe and very effective. Sulfur should be applied nightly for 3 nights. Crotamiton (Eurax) cream or lotion cures only 50% to 60% of patients. It should be applied on 5 successive nights and washed off 24 hours after the last use.

Treatment for crusted scabies is difficult topically.

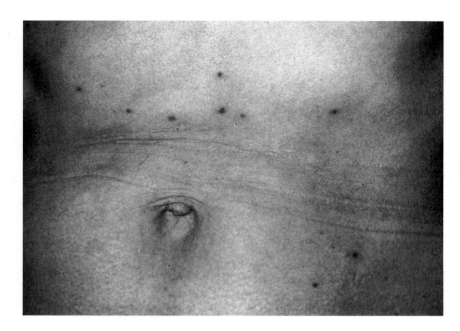

Fig. 20-60 Animal scabies. (Courtesy Dr. Axel W. Hoke.)

Ivermectin, an oral semisynthetic derivative of a family of macrocyclic lactones, has been used to control onchocerciasis since 1987. Numerous publications now attest to its efficacy and safety in treating scabies, particularly the crusted type. It is given at a dose of 200 mg/kg. It may be repeated two or three times at intervals separated by 1 to 2 weeks. Other circumstances in which it may be a better option than topical therapy include cases refractory to conventional topical treatment, epidemic or endemic scabies in institutions, or superinfected scabies. If topical treatment is utilized for crusted scabies, then the following is recommended: the hyperkeratotic lesions should be treated with keratolytics, 40% urea may aid in treating nail involvement, permethrin should be applied once each week for 6 weeks, on the other 6 days of each week either precipitated sulfur 6% or crotamiton is applied, and at the 3-week mark the environment should be meticulously treated. Special attention to treating the scalp, head and neck, and under the nails should be given.

Ideally, persons in close contact with the patient should be closely inspected and treated if they are affected; however, in practice, since examination cannot exclude the diagnosis, all contacts who itch, all sexual contacts, and all family members should be treated. Scabies in long-term health care institutions is an increasing problem. Large numbers of residents, staff, and visitors may be affected. Yonkosky et al found that an aggressive educational campaign combined with treating all residents, staff, and frequent visitors as well as their symptomatic family members helped eradicate the infestation.

ANIMAL SCABIES. Various acari affect animals with which humans come in close contact. Frequently, a reaction resembling scabies occurs in humans; it is contracted from infested dogs, cats, poultry, birds, camels, or horses. The parasites do not find the human skin a favorable habitat, however, so human cases acquired from such sources generally run a mild course. They are self-limited, have no burrows, and mites are not usually found. Bites are likely to be on surfaces in contact with the owner when the pet is held (Fig. 20-60).

CHEYLETIELLA **DERMATITIS.** *Cheyletiella yasguri, C. blakei,* and *C. parasitovorax* are three species of nonburrowing mites that are parasitic on dogs, domestic cats, and rabbits, respectively, and that may bite humans if there is close contact with the animals, producing an itchy dermatitis vaguely resembling scabies. The mites are a little smaller than *Sarcoptes scabiei* and are most easily found by brushing the animal's hair over a dark piece of paper. It may be better to leave its discovery to a veterinarian, to whom the only necessary treatment—treatment of the pet—had best be left anyway.

DEMODEX **MITES.** Demodices are usually found in adults over 30 years of age; children rarely have them. The reported percentage of adults in whom at least a few *Demodex* mites are demonstrated varies from investigator to investigator. Marples cites from 27% to 10%. The organisms are not significant unless they are numerous. *Demodicidosis* is an alternative name.

The larval form of *Demodex folliculorum* is a vermiform mite about 0.9 mm long that inhabits the sebaceous glands of the nose, especially the alae nasi, and, to a lesser extent, of the forehead, chin, and scalp. In mammals such as dogs, the lesions of demodectic mange contain numerous demodices. The larva has a flattened head; on the ventral aspect are four pairs of short, peglike legs, and behind these is an elongated abdomen (Fig. 20-61). The life cycle lasts 14

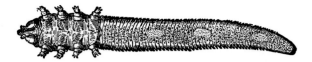

Fig. 20-61 *Demodex folliculorum,* ventral surface, as seen under the microscope. (×300.)

days, of which the egg stage totals 60 hours; larva, 36 hours; several nymph stages, about 132 hours; and the adult stage, about 120 hours. Fertilization occurs at the pilosebaceous orifice, after which the female burrows down the hair follicle to the sebaceous gland, where the eggs are deposited. After they have hatched, there are several stages of moult; during the final moult, the deutonymph emerges from the glandular opening and enters another follicle, where fertilization takes place to begin the next generation.

Demodex brevis is a little over half as long, tends to be solitary, and is found in sebaceous glands or ducts. It is rare at any age and its occurrence is especially rare in patients over age 70.

The pathogenicity of the *Demodex* has been conjectural for many years, because the demodices may be readily found in adults without any evidence of disease. On the other hand, some rosacea and rosacea-like lesions are thought by some to be caused by *Demodex* if the number of mites per follicle is large or if the mite comes in contact with the dermis after rupture of the follicle (Figs. 20-62 and 20-63). Published studies continue to be at odds; however, the importance of *Demodex* in rosacea is generally minimal. Occasional rosacea-like patients whose disease has been resistant to the usual treatments may respond to permethrin or lindane.

A papulonodular eruption caused by *Demodex* in two patients with AIDS was reported by Dominey et al. Lesions on the head and neck, revealing numerous mites on scraping, were cleared by permethrin creme rinse in one patient and by lindane in the other. Others have reported similar cases. Dominey et al also described six patients with pityriasis folliculorum, characterized by diffuse facial flushing and follicular plugging, which gave the skin a frosted appearance. They felt this was caused by *Demodex.* The condition responded to lindane lotion, permethrin cream rinse, and topical tretinoin. Demodicosis was first described in 1930 by Ayers and has been a controversial entity since.

Demodex may be readily demonstrated by expressing the contents of the sebaceous gland duct with a comedo expressor and placing the contents on a slide with a drop of glycerin. A coverslip flattens out the specimen to make the *Demodex* readily discernible under the microscope with a low-power objective.

Treatment of the eruptions in which *Demodex* has been implicated consists of applying benzyl benzoate emulsion

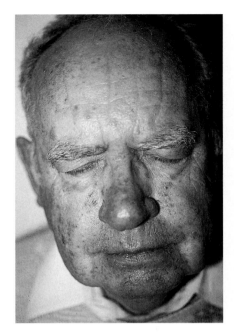

Fig. 20-62 Demodicidosis in rosacea.

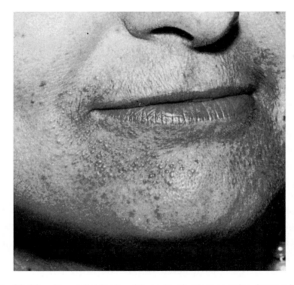

Fig. 20-63 Demodicidosis with perioral micropapules from which demodices were demonstrated in groups of four to ten from one lesion.

twice daily, permethrin cream, or lindane (Kwell). Applying a 5% benzoyl peroxide lotion to which 5% precipitated sulfur has been added is also successful. Usually after 3 days of therapy, *Demodex* can no longer be seen in the treated area.

OTHER MITE DISEASES

Chigger bite. The trombiculid mites are known as *chiggers, mower's mites,* or *red bugs.* They are common parasites, red, and measure 0.3 to 0.5 mm in length. In North America *Eutrombicula alfreddugesi* attacks humans and animals. In Europe it is the harvest mite, *Neotrombicula autumnalis.*

Attacks occur chiefly during the summer and fall, because individuals have more frequent contact with mite-infested grass and bushes. The lesions occur chiefly on the legs and at the belt line and other sites at which clothing causes constriction. They consist of severely pruritic hemorrhagic puncta surrounded by red swellings (Fig. 20-64). At times there are scratch marks, urticarial lesions, and widespread erythema. Tense bullae may be present.

Trombidiasis caused by *Parascoschoengastia nunezi* attacks the scalp, neck, back, axillae, and retroaural folds. It causes petechiae, pustules, crusts, scratch marks, scars, and at times high fever, leukocytosis with eosinophilia, and malaise. Several varieties of trombiculid mites exist in endemic areas of the Far East and South Pacific. They may be vectors of scrub typhus, (tsutsugamushi fever, "dangerous bug" fever).

A good chigger repellent is dimethylphthalate (DMP) solution. The bite site itself should be washed to get rid of larvae on the skin and treated with a topical steroid cream to relieve the pruritus.

Gamasoidosis. Persons who handle canaries, pigeons, and poultry are especially liable to gamasoidosis. This occurs chiefly on the hands and arms. The bite produces an inflammatory, itchy papule. Any area on the body may be attacked but the more common sites are the groin, areolae, umbilicus, face, and scalp.

A diagnosis of urticaria is usually made, but on questioning the patient it may be discovered that other persons similarly exposed are also affected. The mites may wander from birds' nests as soon as the young birds begin to fly, and they may infest terrace cushions and furniture. In large metropolitan areas, especially where pigeons tend to gather, it is not unusual to see pigeons roosting on window ledges. Through the open windows or even through air conditioners the pigeon mites attack humans and cause urticarial and papular eruptions. The starling mite *(Ornithonyssus bursa),* widely prevalent in wild birds in both continental United States and Hawaii, may do this. Lesions persist and itch for about a week longer than those caused by most biting arthropods.

Two genera of mites, *Ornithonyssus* and *Dermanyssus,* commonly infest birds. *O. bursa* and *O. sylvarium* are the two common species of feather mites. These and others of the genus characteristically live their life span in the feathers. *Dermanyssus gallinae,* the red or chicken mite, is also a common parasite of birds. Mites of both genera derive their sustenance from the blood of the host. *Dermanyssus,* however, is found on the bird only at night. It comes out of the cracks and recesses of the poultry house or the bird nest during darkness, feeds on the host, and withdraws again

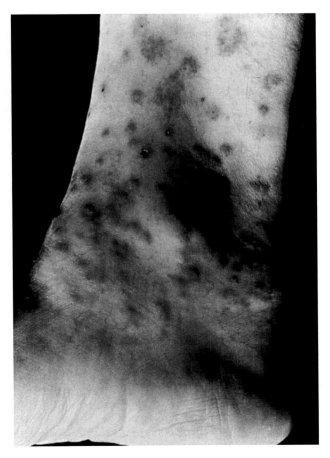

Fig. 20-64 Chigger bites.

during the daylight hours. It readily attacks humans. Apartments may become infested.

Dermanyssus gallinae is killed without direct treatment of the bird. Thorough spraying of the surroundings with malathion is effective. Mites of the Ornithonyssus group require, in addition, treatment of the birds themselves.

Grocer's itch. This is a pruritic dermatitis of the forearms, with occasional inflammatory and urticarial papules on the trunk. It results from the handling of figs, dates, and prunes when it is caused by *Carpoglyphus passularum,* or from the handling of cheese, in which case the infection is caused by *Acarus siro* and *Tyrophagus longior.* This must be distinguished from grocer's eczema caused by sensitization to flour, sugar, cinnamon, chocolate, and similar items.

Grain itch. Grain itch is also known as straw itch, barley itch, mattress itch, and prairie itch. The small causative mite, *Pyemotes tritici,* lives in grain and may temporarily attack the human skin. Those chiefly affected are harvesters of wheat, hay, barley, oats, and other cereals, or farm hands and packers who have contact with straw. Grain itch has a typical lesion consisting of an urticarial papule on which is a small vesicle. There is intense pruritus, with lesions occurring predominantly on the trunk. Frequently there is a central hemorrhagic punctum in the beginning that rapidly turns into an ecchymosis with hemosiderin pigmentation. One report traced a series of straw itch mite dermatoses to a host, the furniture beetle *(Anobium punctatum),* which was harboring the straw itch mite *(Pyemotes tritici).* This unusual source may help to explain those cases in which there has been no exposure to a straw mattress or to grain and in which the mite may not be demonstrable, mainly because it resides on the patient only briefly.

There have been outbreaks of *P. boylei* bites in homes fumigated for termites. Although mites do not appear capable of survival when forced to share an environment with termites, they thrive in locations in which there are termite carcasses.

House floors should be sprayed with a 2% deodorized malathion emulsion. Beetle infestation of wood should be counterattacked with a spray solution of 10-dichlorobenzene.

Other mite-related dermatitis. Vanillism is a dermatitis caused by *A. siro* and occurs in workers handling vanilla pods. Copra itch occurs on persons handling copra who are subject to *Tyrophagus longior* mite bites. Coolie itch is found in tea plantations in India and is caused by *Rhizoglyphus parasiticus.* It causes sore feet. Rat mite itch caused by *Ornithonyssus bacoti,* the tropical rat mite, may result in an intensely pruritic dermatitis. It may transmit endemic typhus and relapsing fever. This papulovesicular urticarial eruption is seen in workers in stores, factories, warehouse, and stockyards. Feather pillow dermatitis is a pruritic papular dermatitis traced to the Psoroptid carpet mite, *Dermatophagoides scheremetewskyi,* which may infest feather pillows. Finally, the house mouse mite, *Liponyssoides sanguineus,* is the vector of *Rickettsia akari,* the causative organism of rickettsialpox. Otherwise, it does not attack humans.

Arlian LG, et al: Cross infestivity of *Sarcoptes scabiei. J Am Acad Dermatol* 1984, 10:979.

Arlian LG, et al: Host-seeking behavior of *Sarcoptes scabiei. J Am Acad Dermatol* 1984, 11:594.

Arlian LG, et al: Prevalence of *Sarcoptes scabiei* in the homes and nursing homes of scabietic patients. *J Am Acad Dermatol* 1988, 19:806.

Arlian LG, et al: Survival and infestivity of *Sarcoptes* scabies var. *canis* and var. *hominis. J Am Acad Dermatol* 1984, 11:210.

Ashack RJ, et al: Feather pillow dermatitis caused by an unusual mite, *Dermatophagoides scheremetewskyi. J Am Acad Dermatol* 1985, 13:680.

Ashack RJ, et al: Papular pruritic eruption of *Demodex* folliculitis in patients with AIDS. *J Am Acad Dermatol* 1989, 21:306.

Baselga E, et al: Avian mite dermatitis. *Pediatrics* 1996, 97:743.

Bonnar E, et al: The *Demodex* mite population in rosacea. *J Am Acad Dermatol* 1993, 28:443.

Buntin DM, et al: Sexually transmitted diseases. *J Am Acad Dermatol* 1991, 25:527.

Chakrabarti A: Human notoedric scabies from contact with cats infested with *Notoedres cati. Int J Dermatol* 1986, 25:646.

Chouela EN, et al: Equivalent therapeutic efficacy and safety of invermectin and lindane in the treatment of human scabies. *Arch Dermatol* 1999, 135:651.

Cvancara JL, et al: Bullous eruption in a patient with systemic lupus erythematosus: mite dermatitis caused by *Cheyletiella blakei. J Am Acad Dermatol* 1997, 37:265.

Davies JE, et al: Lindane poisonings. *Arch Dermatol* 1983, 119:142.

del Giudice P, et al: Ivermectin. *Arch Dermatol* 1999, 135:705.

DePaoli RT, et al: Crusted (Norwegian) scabies. *J Am Acad Dermatol* 1987, 17:136.

Dominey A, et al: Papulonodular demodicidosis associated with AIDS. *J Am Acad Dermatol* 1989, 20:197.

Fox JG: Outbreak of tropical rat mite dermatitis in laboratory personnel. *Arch Dermatol* 1982, 118:676.

Friedman SJ: Lindane neurotoxic reaction in nonbullous congenital ichthyosiform erythroderma. *Arch Dermatol* 1987, 123:1056.

Frost M, et al: Acral hyperkeratosis with erythroderma. *Arch Dermatol* 1988, 124:121.

Funkhouser ME, et al: Management of scabies in patients with HIV disease. *Arch Dermatol* 1993, 129:911.

Gupta AK, et al: Chronic pruritus: an uncommon cause (avian mite dermatitis). *Arch Dermatol* 1988, 124:1101.

Holness DL, et al: Scabies in chronic health care institutions. *Arch Dermatol* 1992, 128:1257.

Jaramillo-Ayerbe F, et al: Ivermectin for crusted Norwegian scabies induced by use of topical steroids. *Arch Dermatol* 1998, 134:143.

Jucowics P, et al: Norwegian scabies in an infant with AIDS. *Arch Dermatol* 1987; 125:1670.

Lee BW: Cheyletiella dermatitis. *Cutis* 1991, 49:111.

Magee KL, et al: Crushed scabies in a patient with chronic graft-versus-host disease. *J Am Acad Dermatol* 1991, 25:889.

Orkin M: Scabies, other mite diseases, and papular urticaria. *Semin Dermatol* 1993, 12:1.

Parish LC, et al: Zoonoses of dermatological interest. *Semin Dermatol* 1993, 12:57.

Ramelet AA, et al: Rosacea. *Ann Dermatol Venereol* 1985, 115:801.

Rivers JK, et al: Walking dandruff and *Cheyletiella* dermatitis. *J Am Acad Dermatol* 1986, 15:1130.

Sarro RA, et al: An unusual demodicidosis manifestation in a patient with AIDS. *J Am Acad Dermatol* 1998, 38:120.

Schultz MW, et al: Comparative study of 5% permethrin cream and 1% lotion for the treatment of scabies. *Arch Dermatol* 1990, 126:167.

Schulze KE, et al: Dove-associated gamasoidosis. *J Am Acad Dermatol* 1994, 30:278.

Siberge S, et al: Rosacea. *J Am Acad Dermatol* 1992, 26:590.

Taplin D, et al: Community control of scabies. *Lancet* 1991, 337:1016.

Taplin D, et al: Pyrethrias and pyrethroids in dermatology. *Arch Dermatol* 1990, 126:213.

Wolf R, et al: Atypical crusted scabies. *J Am Acad Dermatol* 1987, 17:434.

Yonkosky D, et al: Scabies in nursing homes. *J Am Acad Dermatol* 1990, 23:1133. ▲

Order Scorpionidae

Scorpion Sting. Scorpions are different from other arachnids in that they have an elongated abdomen ending in a stinger. They also have a cephalothorax, four pairs of legs, pincers, and mouth pincers. Two poison glands in the back of the abdomen empty into the stinger. Scorpions are found all over the world, especially in the tropics. They are nocturnal and hide during the daytime in closets, shoes, and folded blankets. Ground scorpions may burrow into gravel and children's sandboxes.

Scorpions sting only by accident or in self-defense, but

any sting by a large scorpion should be considered dangerous, since scorpions produce both hemolytic and neurotoxic venom. The hemolytic venom causes mostly a painful swelling at the site of the sting, with little or no other effect. The neurotoxic venom may produce numbness at the sting site, laryngeal edema, profuse sweating and salivation, cyanosis, nausea, and paresthesia of the tongue. There is little or no visible change at the site of the sting. Death may occur from cardiac or respiratory failure, especially in children. The sting of the Egyptian scorpion *(Leiurus quinquestriatus)* has a mortality rate of 50% in children. Centruroides sculpturatus is the most common cause of scorpion stings in the continental United States. The sting of the now rare small Hawaiian scorpion, *Isometrus maculatus,* is no worse than that of a hornet.

Treatment for systemic reactions involves immediate first aid measures: application of a tourniquet if the sting is on an extremity and refrigeration of the site with ice or ethyl chloride spray. Specific antivenin, if available, should also be given. Phentolamine may be used to block the acute sympathetic and parasympathetic stimulation caused by the Old World species venom; and atropine will block the cholinergic effect. Barbiturates best counteract the central nervous system excitability and convulsions that are most prominent with *Centruroides* stings.

Debris such as loose rocks, mattresses, and boards should be removed from sites of human habitation or sprayed with 2% chlordane and 0.5% dieldrin.

Order Arachnidae

Arachnidism. Spiders are prevalent throughout the world; most of them are beneficial to humans in that they trap many insects, including mosquitoes, for food. However, a few among the species may be dangerous to humans.

Campbell et al described the bites of the wolf spider, and Wong et al reviewed the cutaneous effects of all types of spider stings, including those caused by tarantulas, the orb weaver, the green lynx spider, the broad-faced sack spider, the black jumping spider, the parson spider, and others. This article and an accompanying editorial by King are excellent general references for this subject. Schorr et al have reported that spider bites may cause eosinophilic cellulitis (Wells' syndrome). Latrodectism and loxoscelism are the two most important types of clinical manifestations of spider stings.

Latrodectism. The various species of *Latrodectus* have similar toxins and cause similar reactions in humans. Of these the black widow spider, *Latrodectus mactans,* is of chief concern in the continental United States.

It is 13-mm long, coal black, with an orange-red hourglass-shaped marking on its abdomen (Fig. 20-65). The legs are long, with a spread of some 4 cm. The black widow spider inhabits dry, dark places under rocks, in cellars, under privy seats, and in wood piles. It avoids strong sunlight and usually bites only when disturbed.

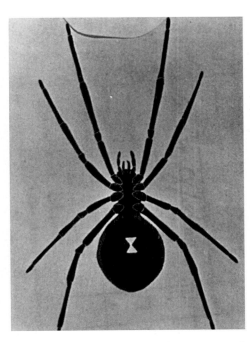

Fig. 20-65 Black widow spider *(Latrodectus mactans)* with red hourglass-shaped patch on abdomen. (×4.) (Courtesy Drs. H.C. Scott and C.J. Stojanovich.)

The sting itself is inconspicuous. Severe pains usually develop within a few minutes and spread throughout the extremities and trunk. Within a few hours there may be chills, vomiting, violent cramps, delirium or partial paralysis, spasms, and abdominal rigidity. The abdominal pains are frequently most severe. These symptoms may be mistaken for appendicitis, colic, or food poisoning. Symptoms begin to subside in about 2 days; however, such bites may bring death to young children. Toxic morbilliform erythema may occur. The venom of *Latrodectus* is neurotoxic.

Clark et al reviewed their experience in treating 163 patients with black widow spider envenomation. A combination of parenteral opioid and benzodiazepine was effective in relieving pain in most cases. Specific antivenin should be used only in patients with severe envenomation who have no allergic contraindications and in whom parenteral analgesics have failed. They found calcium gluconate not useful.

Loxoscelism. Not until 1957 did the toxic effects of the small brown recluse spider *(Loxosceles reclusa)* become known in North America. The house spider *(L. laeta)* has been known for many years in South America for its similar toxic effects.

Two types of reactions occur from the bite of the brown spider. In the localized type, known as *necrotic cutaneous loxoscelism,* a lesion with extensive gangrene develops. A

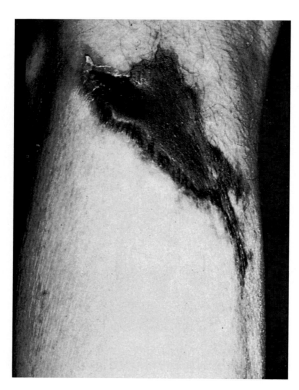

Fig. 20-66 Necrotic reaction to bite of the brown recluse spider in the left popliteal space. (Courtesy Dr. G.T. Jansen.)

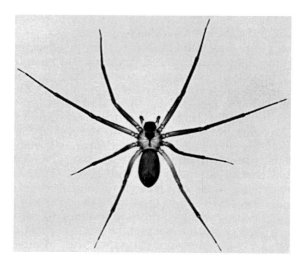

Fig. 20-67 Brown recluse spider. Note the inverted violin configuration on the cephalothorax. (×4.) (Courtesy Dr. G.T. Jansen.)

painful severe edematous reaction occurs within the first 8 hours, with development of a bulla with surrounding zones of erythema and ischemia. In about a week the central portion becomes dark, demarcated, and gangrenous (Fig. 20-66). This may produce a large necrotic ulceration, becoming many centimeters wide and lasting months before healing.

Viscerocutaneous loxoscelism fortunately is rare. There is the same local reaction, but there are fever of 39° to 40° C (102.2° to 104° F), chills, vomiting, joint pain, and hematologic pathology. Hematuria almost invariably occurs on the first day, with hemolytic anemia, thrombocytopenia, and other blood dyscrasias. The skin may show a petechial or morbilliform eruption. Shock and death may ensue.

The venom contains a phospholipase enzyme, sphingomyelinase D, which is responsible for both the dermonecrosis and hemolysis. It damages cell membranes.

This reclusive spider may be identified by a dark, violin-shaped band over the cephalothorax and three pairs of "eyes" on the anterior portion of the cephalothorax (Fig. 20-67). It is light to dark brown, about 1 cm long, and is found in the house in storage closets among clothing. Outdoors it has been found in grass, on rocky bluffs, and in barns. It stings only in self-defense. Most cases of loxoscelism have been found in the southern central United States.

TREATMENT. The advised treatment is (1) ice bags, compression, and elevation; (2) rest; (3) no hot packs or surgery; and (4) antibiotics and aspirin. Dapsone is effective in a dose of 100 mg twice daily and should be instituted early. Surgical intervention, however, should be delayed 4 to 6 weeks. Early surgical procedures increase the potential for complications. Tetanus toxoid should be given if the patient is not up to date with this, and antibiotics should be used if necrosis is incipient. Aspirin is used to prevent deep vein thrombosis. There is no benefit to be obtained from giving intralesional injections or from excision of the bite site.

Anderson PC: Spider bites in the United States. *Dermatol Clin* 1997, 15:307.

Burnett JW, et al: Brown recluse spider. *Cutis* 1985, 37:197.

Burnett JW, et al: Latrodectism: black widow spider bites. *Cutis* 1983, 37:121.

Campbell DS, et al: Wolf spider bites. *Cutis* 1987, 39:113.

Carbonaro PA, et al: Scorpion sting reactions. *Cutis* 1996, 57:139.

Clark RF, et al: Clinical presentation and treatment of black widow spider envenomation. *Ann Emerg Med* 1992, 21:782.

King LE Jr: Spider bites. *Arch Dermatol* 1987, 123:41.

King LE Jr, et al: Treatment of brown recluse spider bites. *J Am Acad Dermatol* 1986, 14:691.

Knutson CA, et al: Spider bite with lymphangistic streaking. *Arch Dermatol* 1992, 128:255.

Pennell TC, et al: The management of snake and spider bites in the Southeastern United States. *Am Surg* 1987, 53:193.

Rees RS, et al: Brown recluse spider bites. *Ann Surg* 1985, 202:659.

Schorr WF, et al: Eosinophilic cellulitis (Wells' syndrome). *J Am Acad Dermatol* 1984, 11:1043.

Wong RC, et al: Spider bites. *Arch Dermatol* 1987, 123:78. ▲

Phylum Chordata

Stingray Injury

The two stingray families (*Dasyatidae* and *Myliobatidae*) are among the most venomous fish known to man. Attacks generally occur as a result of an unwary victim stepping on a partially buried stingray. A puncture-type wound that later ulcerates occurs about the ankles or feet. Sharp, shooting pain develops immediately, with edema and cyanosis. Symptoms of shock may occur.

Persons wading in shallow, muddy waters where stingrays may be found should shuffle their feet through the mud to frighten the fish away. Successful treatment is usually attained by immersing the injured part in hot water for 30 to 60 minutes. The water should be as hot as can be tolerated, since the venom is detoxified by heat. Meperidine hydrochloride administered intravenously or intramuscularly may be necessary. If the ulcer remains unhealed after 8 weeks, excision is indicated.

Snake Bite

Venomous snake bites are a serious problem in some parts of the world. In the United States the rattlesnake, cottonmouth moccasin, and copperhead are the venomous snakes most frequently encountered. There are nearly 30 enzymes found in snake venom, most of which are hydrolases. Snake venom has an anticoagulant action and causes hemolysis and an increase in capillary permeability. These effects may be combated with fresh whole blood transfusions. Neurotoxins are the most toxic of venom constituents. Other toxins include myotoxins and cardiotoxins. Antivenin is of great value.

In all bites on the extremities, if the victim cannot be transported at rest within 1 hour to a definitive care facility, a tourniquet should be applied so as to obstruct venous and lymph flow but not arterial flow. Incision and suction should be instituted as quickly as possible, since they are effective only during the first 15 to 30 minutes following the bite. The incision is made around the fang marks and the edge of the swelling. Suction should be vigorous; if available, a small piece of thin rubber sheeting may be placed between the mouth and the wound for added protection against ingestion of the venom. It is necessary to use copious amounts of antivenin intramuscularly after a routine skin sensitivity test. In addition, antibiotics should be given and appropriate antitetanus measures begun. Indications for surgical intervention, and a review of snakebite therapy, have been published by Sprenger et al and Burnett et al.

Lizard Bite

Heloderma suspectum (the Gila monster) is found chiefly in Arizona and New Mexico. Another venomous lizard is the beaded lizard of southwestern Mexico *(H. horridum)*. Bites from these poisonous lizards may cause paralysis, dyspnea, and convulsions. Death rarely ensues. Local treatment is the same as for snake bite.

Burnett JW, et al: Venomous snakebites. *Cutis* 1986, 38:299.

Russell FE: Stingray injury. *JAMA* 1966, 195:708.

Sprenger TR, et al: Snakebite treatment in the United States. *Int J Dermatol* 1986, 25:479.

Streiffer RH: Bite of the venomous lizard, the Gila monster. *Postgrad Med* 1986, 79:297. ▲

CHAPTER 21

Chronic Blistering Dermatoses

In the principal chronic blistering (vesicular or bullous) dermatoses, the cause of blistering is an autoimmune reaction, and the pattern of immunofluorescence (IF), direct or indirect, is generally more authoritative than the clinical findings in establishing the diagnosis. Usually antibodies are bound at the site of the earliest lesions. Salt-split skin preparations are useful in determining the site of deposition of the autoantibodies. Immunoprecipitation and immunoblotting have helped to define the molecular targets of the autoantibodies.

Transient acantholytic dermatosis (Grover's disease) is a vesiculobullous disease that may be chronic, but a workup of the patient shows no findings on direct IF. Specific dermatoses of pregnancy are discussed under the differential diagnosis of herpes gestationis.

Beutner EH, et al: Immunofluorescence tests. *Int J Dermatol* 1985, 24:405.

Domloge-Hultsch N, et al: Direct IF microscopy of 1 mol/L sodium chloride–treated patient skin. *J Am Acad Dermatol* 1991, 24:846.

Gammon WR, et al: Immunofluorescence on split skin for the detection and differentiation of basement membrane zone autoantibodies. *J Am Acad Dermatol* 1992, 27:79.

Ghohestani RF, et al: Diagnostic value of indirect immunofluorescence of sodium chloride-split skin in differential diagnosis of subepidermal bullous dermatoses. *Arch Dermatol* 1997, 133:1102.

Helm KF, et al: The immunologically mediated vesiculobullous diseases. *Mayo Clin Prac* 1991, 66:187.

Mutasim DF: The accuracy of indirect immunofluorescence on sodium chloride-split skin in differentiating subepidermal bullous diseases. *Arch Dermatol* 1997, 133:1158.

Yancey KB: The diagnosis and biology of bullous diseases. *Arch Dermatol* 1994, 130:983.

Yancey KB, et al: Advances in the diagnosis of subepidermal bullous diseases. *Arch Dermatol* 1996, 132:220. ▲

PEMPHIGUS VULGARIS

CLINICAL FEATURES. Pemphigus vulgaris is characterized by thin-walled, relatively flaccid, easily ruptured bullae that appear on either apparently normal skin and mucous membranes or on erythematous bases (Fig. 21-1). The fluid in the bulla is clear at first but may become hemorrhagic or even seropurulent. The bullae soon rupture to form erosions, that is, raw surfaces that ooze and bleed easily (Fig. 21-2). The denuded areas soon become partially covered with crusts that have little or no tendency to heal; these enlarge by confluence (Fig. 21-3). The healed lesions often leave hyperpigmented patches with no scarring.

Pemphigus vulgaris may begin in many ways, but usually the lesions appear first in the mouth and next most commonly in the groin, scalp, face, neck, axillae, or genitals. Usually, at the beginning, bullae are sparse and seem inconsequential, but extensive, generalized lesions may develop in a few weeks, or they may be limited to one or more sites for several months.

The Nikolsky sign is present; that is, there is an absence of cohesion in the epidermis, so the upper layers are easily made to slip laterally by slight pressure or rubbing. This sign is variously elicited: The upper layers of the epidermis may easily be removed by a twisting pressure with the fingertip, leaving a moist surface. The lack of cohesion of the skin layers may also be demonstrated with the "bulla-spread phenomenon" by pressure on an intact bulla, gently forcing the fluid to wander under the skin away from the pressure site (the Asboe-Hansen sign).

The mouth lesions appear first in 60% of cases (Fig. 21-4). The short-lived bullae quickly rupture to involve most of the mucosa with painful erosions (Fig. 21-5). The lesions extend out onto the lips and form heavy, fissured crusts on the vermilion (Fig. 21-6). Involvement of the throat produces hoarseness and difficulty in swallowing. The mouth odor is offensive and penetratingly unpleasant. The esophagus may be involved, and sloughing of its entire lining in the form of a cast (esophagitis dissecans superficialis) has been reported. The conjunctiva, nasal mucosa, vagina, penis, and anus may also be involved. Cytologic results of testing on vaginal cells may be mistaken for a malignancy when vaginal lesions are present.

EPIDEMIOLOGY. Pemphigus vulgaris occurs with equal frequency in men and women, usually in their fifth and sixth decades. It is rare in young persons. The condition occurs more often in Jews and in people of Mediterranean descent.

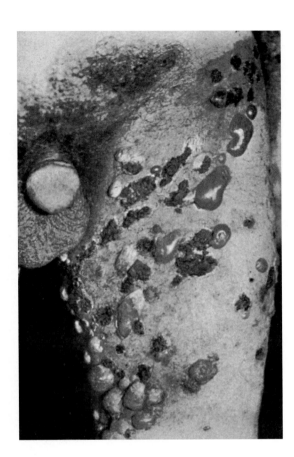

Fig. 21-1 Pemphigus vulgaris. Bullous lesions arising from apparently normal skin surface, with crusts.

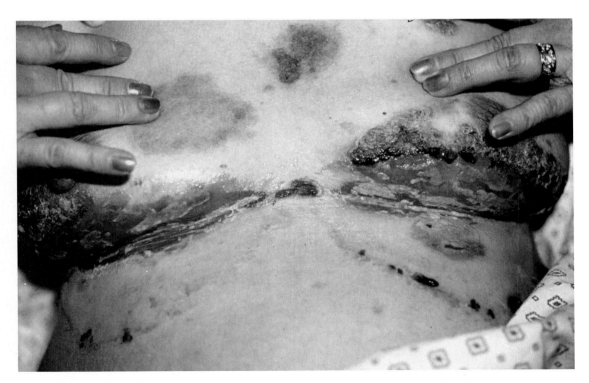

Fig. 21-2 Pemphigus vulgaris of inframammary areas with erosions.

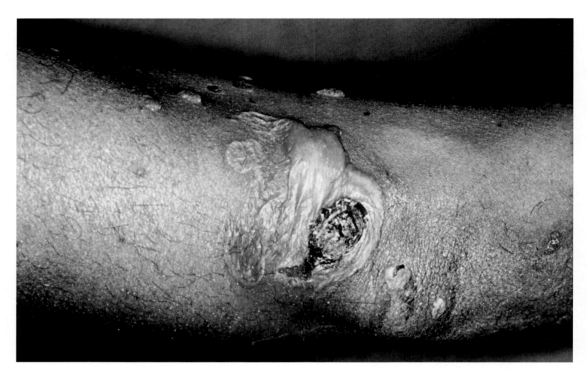

Fig. 21-3 Pemphigus vulgaris. Flaccid bullae with crusts.

Fig. 21-4 Desquamative gingivitis of pemphigus vulgaris.

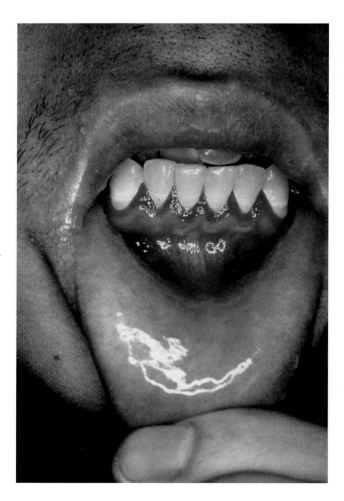

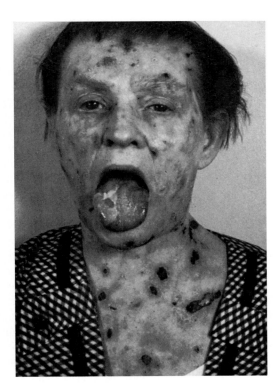

Fig. 21-5 Pemphigus vulgaris. Note the membranous sheet on the tongue.

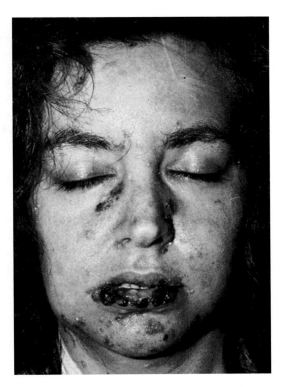

Fig. 21-6 Pemphigus vulgaris. (Courtesy Dr. S. Hochman.)

ETIOLOGIC FACTORS. Pemphigus vulgaris is an autoimmune blistering disease mediated by intercellular antibodies (IC). They are demonstrable throughout the epidermis and the oral epithelium, and circulating intercellular antibodies are present in the patient's serum. Direct IF is of great value in the early diagnosis of pemphigus vulgaris. The direct IF test shows intercellular IgG throughout the epidermis or the oral epithelium. IgG is found in both involved and clinically normal skin in nearly all patients with pemphigus. In acantholytic areas, C3 deposition is also reliably found. The direct IF test is a very reliable diagnostic tool, more so than the indirect IF test. Test results for direct IF become positive very early in the disease, often before the indirect IF test has become positive. Direct IF results remain positive for a long time and may still be positive many years after clinical remission.

With the indirect IF technique, circulating IC antibodies can be demonstrated in 80% to 90% of patients with pemphigus vulgaris. Indirect IF testing may yield a negative result in patients with early localized disease at a time when a positive test result would be of particular diagnostic value. Using indirect testing as a means of evaluating disease severity has been shown to be unreliable. However, circulating IC antibody titers often parallel disease activity. Antibodies to desmogleon-3 may be detected by a specific and sensitive enzyme-linked immunosorbent assay (ELISA). It is objective and automated.

Circulating IC antibodies have occasionally been reported in patients with various other autoimmune diseases and with burns, bullous drug eruptions, and maculopapular eruptions resulting from penicillin therapy. These IC antibodies differ from true pemphigus IC antibodies in that they do not fix to the epidermis in vivo and may be removed from serum samples by absorption with ABO blood-group antigens. On indirect testing it appears coarse, granular, and nonuniform. In pemphigus there is smooth, uniform staining.

Stanley showed that the serum of a patient with pemphigus vulgaris immunoprecipitates a disulfide-bonded 210-KD complex of 130 KD (desmoglein 3) and 85 KD (plakoglobin). If autoantibodies are only directed against desmoglein 3, mucosal lesions predominate. The autoantibodies of some patients with pemphigus vulgaris target desmoglein 1 in addition to desmoglein 3, and these patients express mucocutaneous disease. It is clear that the target antigen is a specific cell-surface glycoprotein that is synthesized by keratinocytes and mediates cell-cell adhesion. The pemphigus vulgaris antigen (130-KD transmembrane desmosomal glycoprotein) shows homology with the cadherin family of calcium-dependent cell adhesion molecules.

These IF test results aid in the differential diagnosis of such bullous dermatoses as bullous pemphigoid, cicatricial pemphigoid, dermatitis herpetiformis, chronic bullous dermatosis of childhood, herpes gestationis, epidermolysis bullosa, erythema multiforme, bullous drug eruptions, toxic epidermal necrolysis, and familial benign pemphigus of Hailey-Hailey.

Penicillamine treatment of rheumatoid arthritis has induced pemphigus, most often of the foliaceous type. Of the cases reported, nearly all have had a positive direct IF and more than half have had positive indirect IF. Yokel et al showed penicillamine and captopril may induce acantholysis in organ explant culture in the absence of autoantibody. The doses responsible for induction of disease have ranged from 250 to 1500 mg a day, and were taken for an average of 13 months before the onset of pemphigus. Only 10% to 15% have had oral lesions. Most such reactions have resolved when the medication is discontinued; some have persisted for many months, however, and a few have been fatal.

Captopril, penicillin, thiopronine, interleukin-2, and rifampin, among many other drugs, have also been reported to induce pemphigus. Many drugs implicated in inducing pemphigus contain sulfa groups. Korman et al showed that a patient with drug-induced pemphigus vulgaris had circulating autoantibodies against the pemphigus vulgaris antigen. Ultraviolet light may exacerbate the disease, and PUVA given for psoriasis was reported to have initiated disease onset. Low et al reviewed eight patients in whom ionizing radiation induced the disease.

Other autoimmune diseases have infrequently been reported to occur in association with pemphigus; however, the association of myasthenia gravis and thymoma has been reported by several authors.

Many studies have indicated a genetic predisposition to pemphigus exists. Statistical analysis shows a skewed distribution of various HLA antigens among patients with pemphigus. Most patients are of HLA phenotype DR4 or DR6. In addition, a specific HLA-DQ beta restriction fragment has been identified in many patients with pemphigus. Thus, there may be a genetically inherited susceptibility to the disease. Additionally, a predisposition to develop other autoimmune diseases may occur in relatives of pemphigus patients.

PATHOGENESIS. The pathologic changes in pemphigus vulgaris are acantholysis, clefts, and blister formation in the intraepidermal areas just above the basal cell layer. Acantholysis is the separation of keratinocytes from one another. The loss of cohesion or contact between cells begins with the detachment of tonofilaments from the desmosomes. Evidence indicates that it is the IgG autoantibody that induces these changes.

Anhalt induced pemphigus in newborn mice by passive transfer of IgG from patients with pemphigus. Normal IgG caused no pemphigus, but 39 of 55 mice injected with pemphigus antibody reacted with histologically, ultrastructurally, and immunologically typical pemphigus blisters, and the effect was dose dependent.

Others have shown that pemphigus antibody, when incubated with either normal skin or cultured keratinocytes, binds to the cell surfaces and induces acantholysis. Complement is not required. Hashimoto et al showed that plasminogen activator is released during this process. Thus,

it seems that the probable mechanism of blister formation in pemphigus is the binding of circulating antibody to a cell-surface glycoprotein, with resulting activation of plasmin, which causes enzymatic destruction of intercellular cement and desmosomes.

Tope et al reported a child born with pemphigus vulgaris to a mother who was in complete remission throughout pregnancy. They reviewed 10 reported cases and found there were three stillbirths. All seven neonates healed within 2 to 3 weeks with either no treatment or the use of topical antibiotics. Goldberg et al documented a mother with active disease and an antibody titer of 1:640 whose newborn child was free of lesions. They reviewed the risk factors of neonatal disease and made recommendations for the treatment of pemphigus vulgaris during pregnancy.

HISTOPATHOLOGY. The characteristic findings consist of acantholysis, intraepidermal cleft and blister formation, and the presence of acantholytic cells lining the bulla as well as lying free in the bulla cavity. These cells show no intercellular bridges; the large nuclei are surrounded by a lightly staining halo in the cytoplasm and then a darkly staining cytoplasm at the periphery of the cell. Smears from the base of a bulla stained by the Tzanck method using Giemsa stain will show the typical acantholytic or Tzanck cells.

Eosinophils may collect in the spongiotic epidermis of patients with pemphigus, a phenomenon called *eosinophilic spongiosis*. It is a harbinger of acantholysis when seen in pemphigus; however, it far more commonly presages pemphigoid, and, exceptionally, occurs in a great many other dermatoses. Occasionally, neutrophilic spongiosis may be seen in pemphigus.

BIOPSY MATERIAL. Because the bullae of pemphigus become large and flaccid in a short time, it is important that a small, early, intact blister be secured. Asboe-Hansen's modification of the Nikolsky test may be used to extend the bulla beyond its original margin to where secondary degenerative changes have not taken place. The site of the biopsy is frozen with an aerosol refrigerant spray so that the punch may include firm tissue. Normal-appearing perilesional skin should be used to obtain tissue for direct IF.

TREATMENT. Before the advent of corticosteroids, treatment was mainly supportive and was usually inadequate to combat this severe disease, which was often fatal. Both topical and systemic therapies are used.

Topical treatment. The skin lesions are extremely painful in advanced cases. When there are extensive raw surfaces, prolonged daily baths are helpful in removing the thickened crusts and reducing the foul odor. Silver sulfadiazine (Silvadene) 1%, widely used for local therapy of burns, is an effective topical antimicrobial agent. Painful ulcerations of the lips and mouth may benefit from topical application of a mixture of equal parts of Maalox and elixir of diphenhydramine hydrochloride (Benadryl) or viscous xylocaine, especially before meals. The various commercial antiseptic mouthwashes are helpful in alleviating discomfort and malodor.

Systemic therapy. The sooner the diagnosis is established and the sooner treatment is given, the more favorable the prognosis. Corticosteroid therapy is the standard treatment. Prednisone, given orally 60 to 100 mg/day, alone or (better) in combination with one or several immunosuppressants (azathioprine, cyclophosphamide, or methotrexate), is used to suppress the blistering disease. The therapeutic effects are estimated by the number of new vesicles per day and the rate of healing of the new lesions. In addition, pemphigus antibody titers are performed every 4 weeks, watching for a fall in titer. If after 4 to 8 weeks of treatment new blister formation is not suppressed, prednisone dosage may be increased to 150 mg/day, or one of several other options discussed next may be employed. The dosage adjustments are, of course, made more frequently and aggressively in severe, progressive disease. Dividing the daily dose will usually result in greater efficacy. Additionally, intravenous pulse therapy with megadose corticosteroids (Solu-medrol) at a dose of 1 g/day over a period of 2 to 3 hours, repeated daily for 5 days, may be employed for cases that are unresponsive to oral doses.

Medication is continued until clinical disease is suppressed and pemphigus antibody disappears from the serum. Once the antibody is no longer present, a direct IF test is repeated. After both direct and indirect IF yield negative results, the treatment is gradually but completely withdrawn.

The addition of an immunosuppressant (azathioprine is one of the best) is helpful in diminishing the need for corticosteroids. The clinician should remember that today the risk of death in pemphigus from the side effects of oral prednisone is greater than the risk of death from the disease itself. Death from sepsis and other complications of therapy occurs in 5% to 10% of treated cases. Ahmed et al found the primary cause of death to be infection, with *Staphylococcus aureus* most commonly isolated; the usual sites of infection are blood, the lungs, and skin. Untreated disease is usually fatal.

Immunosuppressive therapy. Immunosuppressant therapy alone has been reported as a successful treatment of early stable pemphigus vulgaris. If a contraindication to the use of corticosteroids exists or only limited disease is present, these may be used as single agents. In general, however, combined treatment with corticosteroids is superior in gaining early control of the disease. These drugs are less commonly used in dermatology and have significant side effect profiles, so thorough knowledge of their pharmacology, dosage guidelines, monitoring guidelines, and adverse effects is needed. Wolverton and Wilkin's book, *Systemic Drugs for Skin Diseases,* is an excellent resource in this regard.

Gendler reviewed the use of azathioprine in dermatologic disorders, and Snow et al have reported on the role of thiopurine methyltransferase activity in the observed efficacy and side effects of this medicine in dermatologic patients. Aberer et al reviewed their own prospective study of 29 patients and found the combination of prednisone and azathioprine effective. Cyclophosphamide has been reviewed by Ahmed et al, who thought it to be a good alternative when azathioprine therapy fails. Fleishli et al reported the use of pulse intravenous cyclophosphamide in nine patients in an effort to reduce dosage and possibly side effects. Kaur et al used dexamethasone and cyclophosphamide pulse therapy for pemphigus. Both authors continued oral cyclophosphamide 50 mg/day additionally. Less experience exists with methotrexate than with azathioprine or cyclophosphamide, but methotrexate has been recommended as adjunctive therapy. Adding cyclosporin to corticosteroids may improve the patient's condition without further increasing the steroid dose.

Mycophenolate mofetil has been studied as monotherapy and as a steroid-sparring agent in pemphigus and pemphigoid. Although the number of patients studied is low, the reports detail impressive results, including several whose antibody titer became undetectable and who did not relapse on discontinuation of therapy. It inhibits proliferation of T and B lymphocytes through inhibition of inosine monophosphate. It is usually given at a dose of 1 g twice daily, with adverse reactions mainly being gastrointestinal and myelosuppression and immunosuppression. It has few side effects on the liver and thus may be used in some patients unable to tolerate azathioprine.

Gold therapy. Gold sodium thiomalate (Myochrysine) has been reported to be effective in the treatment of pemphigus. The oral formulation, auranofin, has been tried in a few patients; the results are difficult to evaluate. It is infrequently used today. Pruritic macular and papular eruptions may be produced, although resumption of therapy does not regularly result in reproducing them. Bone marrow suppression and nephrotoxicity may occur.

Other therapeutic options. In severe cases plasmapheresis may be useful if combined with therapies that prevent new synthesis of pemphigus antibody. Tan-Lin et al reported their experience with 11 patients. Chaffins et al used nicotinamide and tetracycline in six patients and reported that two were controlled on this combination alone. Alpsoy et al treated 10 patients with this combination, however ,and had only one satisfactory result. The role of intravenous immunoglobulin, if any, remains to be investigated. Extracorporeal photochemotherapy has been useful as adjunctive therapy in five patients with drug-resistant pemphigus vulgaris. Dapsone may be of value as a steroid-sparing agent or maintenance drug. Intralesional steroid injections may control limited recalcitrant lesions, such as may be present in the mouth or on the scalp.

PEMPHIGUS VEGETANS

Pemphigus vegetans is a variant of pemphigus vulgaris and is believed to be connected with the amount of resistance these patients have to their disease. Some authorities recognize two types of pemphigus vegetans: the Neumann type and the Hallopeau type (pyodermite vegetante). Despite the benign course of the latter type and the fact that the lesions are not bullae but pustules, immunofluorescent studies indicate that both forms are simply mild variants of pemphigus vulgaris, the clinical spectrum of which has to be extended to include them. The Neumann type often begins and ends as typical pemphigus vulgaris, with vegetations developing during the course of disease.

Pemphigus vegetans is characterized by flaccid bullae that become erosions and form fungoid vegetations or papillomatous proliferations, especially in body folds (Fig. 21-7). Although the onset may be manifested solely by broken bullae in the mouth or about the genitals or umbilicus, the bullae rupture and their moist bases become exuberant with verrucous vegetations, capped by crusts and surrounded by a zone of inflammation. The tongue often shows cerebriform morphologic features early in the course. At times there is a tendency for the lesions to coalesce to form large patches or to arrange themselves into groups or configurate patterns.

Pemphigus vegetans begins insidiously, usually on the nose or in the mouth, as does pemphigus vulgaris. Other areas frequently affected are the scalp, axillae, groin (Fig. 21-8), genitalia, perineum, and flexural extremities. The subjective symptoms are slight, and there are often long remissions in the course of the disease. At times, however, high fever and other constitutional symptoms develop as a result of sepsis.

The laboratory findings, etiologic factors, epidemiology, pathogenesis, and treatment of pemphigus vegetans are the same as those of pemphigus vulgaris. Storer's report of a child with congenital pemphigus vulgaris born to a mother who had had pemphigus vegetans 16 months earlier and Pinto et al's report of captopril-induced pemphigus vegetans are other factors that on a clinical basis strongly suggest that pemphigus vegetans is simply modified pemphigus vulgaris.

Histologic findings are identical with those of pemphigus vulgaris, but there is an increased papillary proliferation and marked epidermal hyperplasia. Frequently, intraepidermal abscesses filled with eosinophils are present; they are characteristic of this variant of pemphigus.

Pemphigus vegetans must be differentiated from the fungating iodide eruption, which occurs without regard to sites of predilection and is not accompanied by autoantibodies that characterize pemphigus. Syphilitic condylomata, granuloma inguinale, condyloma acuminatum, and mycotic and amebic granulomas may resemble the disease, especially when it occurs in the anogenital region.

Pyodermite vegetante (Hallopeau type) has also been called *dermatitis vegetans* and benign *pemphigus vegetans*. It has no bullae but rather begins with pustules. IF findings in cases of this so-called Hallopeau type are typical of pemphigus vulgaris, so it should be regarded as a variant of pemphigus vulgaris.

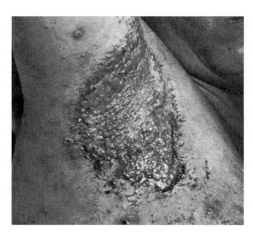

Fig. 21-7 Pemphigus vegetans of axilla. (Courtesy Dr. M. Costello.)

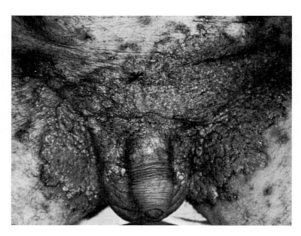

Fig. 21-8 Pemphigus vegetans with sharply delineated exudative vegetating lesions.

Ahmed AR, et al: Linkage of pemphigus vulgaris antibody to the major histocompatibility complex in healthy relations of a patient. *J Exp Med* 1993, 177:419.

Ahmed AR, et al: Use of cyclophosphamide in azathioprine failures in pemphigus. *J Am Acad Dermatol* 1987, 17:437.

Alpsoy E, et al: Is the combination of tetracycline and nicotinamide effective in pemphigus? *Arch Dermatol* 1995, 133:1339.

Amagai MJ, et al: Pemphigus. *Adv Dermatol* 1996, 11:319.

Amagai MJ, et al: Pemphigus vulgaris antigen (desmoglein 3) is localized in the lower epidermis, the site of blister formation in patients. *J Invest Dermatol* 1996, 106:351.

Amagai MJ, et al: The clinical phenotype of pemphigus is defined by the anti-desmoglein autoantibody profile. *J Am Acad Dermatol* 1999, 40:163.

Anhalt GJ: Making sense of antigens and antibodies in pemphigus. *J Am Acad Dermatol* 1999, 40:763.

Barthelemy H, et al: Plasmapheresis therapy of pemphigus. *Arch Dermatol* 1988, 124:1702.

Barthelemy H, et al: Treatment of nine cases of pemphigus vulgaris with cyclosporine. *J Am Acad Dermatol* 1988, 18:1262.

Brandsen R, et al: Circulating pemphigus IgG in families of patients with pemphigus. *J Am Acad Dermatol* 1997, 36:44.

Brenner S, et al: Recognition of pemphigus antigens in drug-induced pemphigus vulgaris and pemphigus foliaceus. *J Am Acad Dermatol* 1997, 36:919.

Bystryn JC, et al: The adjuvant therapy of pemphigus. *Arch Dermatol* 1996, 132:203.

Castle WN, et al: Chronic balanitis owing to pemphigus vegetans. *J Urol* 1987, 137:289.

Chaffins ML, et al: Treatment of pemphigus and linear IgA dermatosis with nicotinamide and tetracycline. *J Am Acad Dermatol* 1993, 28:998.

Chan E, et al: Pemphigus vulgaris of the cervix and upper vaginal vault. *Arch Dermatol* 1998, 134:1485.

Enk AH, et al: Mycophenolate is effective in the treatment of pemphigus vulgaris. *Arch Dermatol* 1999, 135:54.

Firooz A, et al: Prevalence of autoimmune diseases in family members of patients with pemphigus vulgaris. *J Am Acad Dermatol* 1994, 31:434.

Fitzpatrick RE, et al: Correlation of disease activity and antibody titers in pemphigus. *Arch Dermatol* 1980, 116:285.

Fleishli ME, et al: Pulse intravenous cyclophosphamide therapy in pemphigus. *Arch Dermatol* 1999, 135:57.

Fryer EJ, et al: Pemphigus vulgaris after initiation of psoralens and UVA therapy for psoriasis. *J Am Acad Dermatol* 1994, 30:651.

Gendler E: Azathioprine for use in dermatology. *J Am Acad Dermatol* 1984, 10:462.

Goldberg NS, et al: Pemphigus vulgaris and pregnancy. *J Am Acad Dermatol* 1993, 28:877.

Ho VC, et al: Cyclosporine in nonpsoriatic dermatoses. *J Am Acad Dermatol* 1990, 23:1249.

Ho VC, et al: Penicillamine-induced pemphigus. *J Rheumatol* 1985, 12:583.

Hoss DM, et al: Neutrophilic spongiosis in pemphigus. *Arch Dermatol* 1996, 132:315.

Jiao D, et al: Sensitivity of indirect immunofluorescence, substrate specificity, and immunoblotting in the diagnosis of pemphigus. *J Am Acad Dermatol* 1997, 37:211.

Jolles S, et al: Dermatological uses of high-dose intravenous immunoglobulin. *Arch Dermatol* 1998, 134:80.

Kaplan RP, et al: Drug-induced pemphigus related to angiotensin-converting enzyme inhibitors. *J Am Acad Dermatol* 1992, 26:364.

Korman N: Pemphigus. *J Am Acad Dermatol* 1988, 18:1219.

Korman N, et al: Drug-induced pemphigus. *J Invest Dermatol* 1991, 96:273.

Lenz P, et al: Desmoglein 3-ELISA. *Arch Dermatol* 1999, 135:195.

Low GL, et al: Ionizing radiation-induced pemphigus. *Arch Dermatol* 1990, 126:1319.

Nishikawa T, et al: Desmoglein ELISAs. *Arch Dermatol* 1999, 135:195.

Nousari HC, et al: Mycophenolate mofetil in autoimmune and inflammatory skin disorders. *J Am Acad Dermatol* 1999, 40:265.

Pandya AG, et al: Treatment of pemphigus vulgaris with pulse IV cyclophosphamide. *Arch Dermatol* 1992, 128:1626.

Prussick R, et al: Recurrence of pemphigus vulgaris associated with interleukin 2 therapy. *Arch Dermatol* 1994, 130:890.

Rodan KP, et al: Malodorous intertriginous pustules and plaques. *Arch Dermatol* 1987, 123:393.

Rook AH, et al: Extracorporeal photochemotherapy for drug resistant pemphigus vulgaris. *Ann Intern Med* 1990, 112:303.

Roujeau JC: Pulse glucocorticoid therapy. *Arch Dermatol* 1996, 132:1499.

Ruiz E, et al: Eosinophilic spongiosis. *J Am Acad Dermatol* 1994, 30:973.

Snow JL, et al: The role of genetic variation in thiopurine methyltransferase activity and the efficacy and/or side effects of azathioprine therapy in dermatologic patients. *Arch Dermatol* 1995, 131:193.

Stanley JR: Therapy of pemphigus vulgaris. *Arch Dermatol* 1999, 135:76.

Stanley JR: Update: structure and function of pemphigus vulgaris antigen. *J Dermatol* 1997, 24:741.

Storer JS, et al: Neonatal pemphigus vulgaris. *J Am Acad Dermatol* 1982, 6:929.

Tan-Lin R, et al: Effect of plasmapheresis therapy on circulating levels of pemphigus vulgaris antibodies. *J Am Acad Dermatol* 1990, 22:35.

Tope WD, et al: Neonatal pemphigus vulgaris in a child born to a woman in remission. *J Am Acad Dermatol* 1993, 29:480.

Trattner A, et al: Esophageal involvement in pemphigus vulgaris. *J Am Acad Dermatol* 1991, 24:223.

Virgili A, et al: Sudden vegetation of the mouth. *Arch Dermatol* 1992, 128:397.

Weissman-Kutzenelson DM, et al: The usefulness of IF tests in pemphigus patients in clinical remission. *Br J Dermatol* 1989, 120:391.

Werth VP: Treatment of pemphigus vulgaris with brief, high-dose intravenous glucocorticoids. *Arch Dermatol* 1996, 132:1435.

Wolverton SE, Wilkin JK, editors: Systemic drugs for skin diseases. Philadelphia, 1991, WB Saunders.

Yokel BY, et al: Induction of acantholysis in organ explant culture by penicillamine and captopril. *Arch Dermatol* 1991, 125:1367. ▲

PEMPHIGUS FOLIACEUS

Pemphigus foliaceus (PF) is a relatively mild, chronic variety of pemphigus characterized by flaccid bullae and localized or generalized exfoliation. Pemphigus foliaceus begins with small, flaccid bullae that rupture almost as they evolve to form crusting, below which is a moist surface with a tendency to bleed (Fig. 21-9). After a time, the exfoliative characteristics predominate, with few bullae. The bullae are scattered over the scalp, face (Fig. 21-10), and trunk, or the lesions may spread symmetrically until the entire integument is involved with a moist, red, edematous, exfoliative, and malodorous condition (Fig. 21-11). A variant of pemphigus that has clinical features suggestive of dermatitis herpetiformis but has immunologic features of pemphigus has been called *herpetiform pemphigus.* Ishii et al found the serum of 16 of 20 patients had antibodies to desmoglein 1 and four against desmoglein 3, with no overlap. Thus most of these patients express a clinical variant of pemphigus foliaceus, with the remainder being pemphigus vulgaris patients.

Nikolsky's sign is present in PF. Oral lesions are rarely seen, and then only as superficial erosive stomatitis. This may be because desmoglein 1, which is inhibited by PF antibodies, is present in the superficial portion of the oral mucosa; however, the function of desmoglein 3, present throughout the epithelium, is unaltered in PF and compensates by providing enough adherence to maintain clinical integrity.

Generally, patients with PF are not severely ill. They complain of burning and pain and at times of severe pruritus. The lesions may persist for many years without affecting the general health. PF occurs mostly in adults between 40 and 50 years of age; however, it has been reported to occur in children as young as 3. Walker et al reported a newborn who developed transient pemphigus foliaceus after passive transfer of IgG across the placental membrane. This rarely occurs, however, because distribution of desmoglein 1 and 3 in newborn skin is similar to that found in the oral mucosa, and the unaltered desmoglein 3 probably compensates for the functionally impaired desmoglein 1. The sexes are affected equally. Prevalence of PF in people of Jewish heritage is much less than with pemphigus vulgaris. There is an unusually high incidence of pemphigus

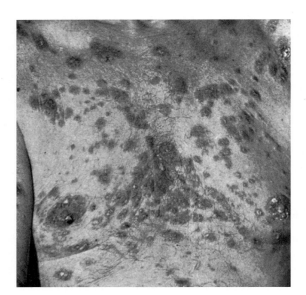

Fig. 21-9 Pemphigus foliaceus.

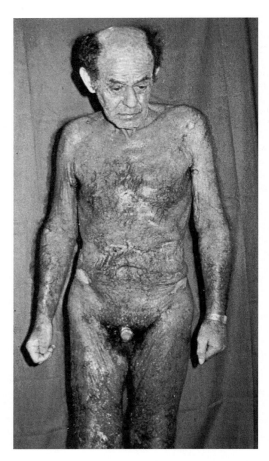

Fig. 21-11 Pemphigus foliaceus. Generalized exfoliative erythroderma.

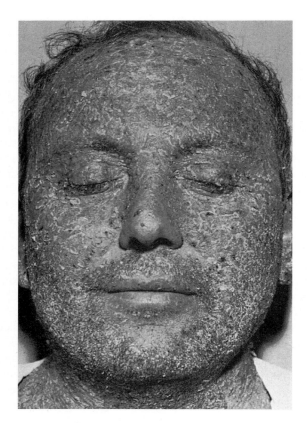

Fig. 21-10 Pemphigus foliaceus.

foliaceus in young Tunisian women. Drugs such as penicillamine and others listed under pemphigus vulgaris more commonly induce pemphigus foliaceus. The drugs induce an antibody response that is identical on a molecular level to the naturally occurring disease.

The principal histologic finding consists of acantholysis in the upper epidermis, usually in the granular layer, leading to the formation of a cleft that may develop into a bulla in a superficial (often subcorneal) position, with acantholysis present at the floor as well as at the roof of the bulla.

Direct IF demonstrates intercellular IgG throughout the epidermis; indirect IF, in most patients, gives a positive result, demonstrating a circulating antibody directed against the cell surface of keratinocytes. Stanley et al characterized a pemphigus foliaceus complex by immunoprecipitation consisting of polypeptides of 260-, 160-, and 85-KD molecular weight. The 260-KD molecule is a complex of the 160 and 85-KD polypeptides. The pemphigus foliaceous antibody binds to a 160-KD glycoprotein extracted from normal epidermis. This glycoprotein is identical to desmoglein 1, a desmosomal glycoprotein. The 85-KD glycoprotein is *plakoglobulin,* a desmosomal and adherens junction–associated molecule. A sensitive and specific ELISA for detecting antibodies to desmoglein 1 has been described. It is automated and objective. If it is positive and the anti-desmoglein 3 ELISA is negative, then the patient has pemphigus foliaceus. Occasional cases are being reported in which the patient manifests pemphigus vulgaris clinically and immunopathologically and over time develops PF, complete with altered antibody specificity.

TREATMENT. Treatment is similar to that for pemphigus vulgaris; however, less vigorous treatment is often required, which circumvents the side effects common to prolonged oral corticosteroid therapy. Judicious use of topical corticosteroids may avoid the necessity of oral doses of prednisone in some cases. Dapsone may be useful, either alone in mild cases or to reduce the steroid dose level.

Chaffins et al reported that nicotinamide, 1.5 g/day, and tetracycline, 2 g/day, obtained a response in four of five patients treated. Alopsy et al, however, reported failure in their two patients. Hymes et al reported three patients who responded to hydroxychloroquine 200 mg twice daily as an adjunctive therapy. In severe cases immunosuppressants such as azathioprine, mycophenolate mofetil, or cyclophosphamide may be needed.

BRAZILIAN PEMPHIGUS (FOGO SELVAGEM)

Brazilian pemphigus is an endemic form of pemphigus foliaceous found in the tropical regions, mostly in certain interior areas of Brazil. Fifteen percent of cases are familial. It is also known that fogo selvagem is common in children, adolescents, and young adults, with about one third of cases occurring before age 20 and two thirds by age 40. The initial lesions may be flaccid bullae, but later lesions are eczematoid, psoriasiform, impetiginous, or seborrheic in appearance. The midfacial areas may be involved. Melanoderma and verrucous vegetative lesions are not unusual, and exfoliative dermatitis may occur. The mucous membranes are not often involved. Nikolsky's sign is present. Diaz et al have published major clinical and epidemiologic studies of this disease. They feel that the immunologic alterations may be initiated by an infectious agent, possibly carried by mosquitoes or black flies. Their two major reviews are recommended.

Histologically and immunohistologically, fogo selvagem is identical to pemphigus foliaceus. Stanley et al demonstrated that patients with fogo selvagem have serum antibodies that specifically bound to desmoglein I, a 160-KD desmosomal glycoprotein.

The course of this disease is like that of pemphigus foliaceus, of which it is a forme fruste. It may run a chronic course from 5 to 20 years. Death is usually from some intercurrent disease.

Beneficial effects have been described from administration of quinine and quinacrine, but the corticosteroids are the treatment of choice, as for pemphigus. Movement from the rural environment to the city and potent topical steroids are other adjuvant therapeutic measures. Immunosuppressants may be necessary in severe cases.

PEMPHIGUS ERYTHEMATOSUS (SENEAR-USHER SYNDROME)

In Senear-Usher syndrome, the early lesions are circumscribed patches of erythema and crusting that clinically resemble lupus erythematosus and are immunopathologi-

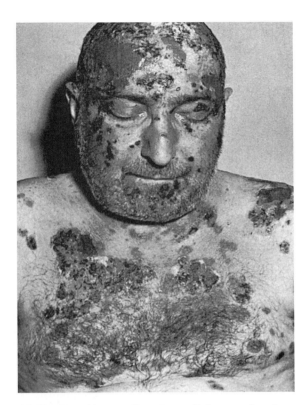

Fig. 21-12 Pemphigus erythematosus. Note moon face from oral prednisone therapy. Note also the predilection for the scalp and sternal area.

cally positive for the lupus band in 80% of patients. The lesions are erythematous and thickly crusted, bullous, or even hyperkeratotic. These are usually localized on the nose, cheeks, and ears—the sites frequently affected by lupus erythematosus. In addition, crusting and impetiginous lesions appear amid bullae on the scalp, chest, and extremities (Fig. 21-12). Bullae occur on the trunk from time to time (Fig. 21-13). This is a comparatively benign and usually localized type of chronic pemphigus in which the general health remains unimpaired.

The histopathology is that of PF. Immunofluorescent stains show IgG and complement localized in both intercellular and basement membrane sites, adding to the link between this and lupus erythematosus. The antinuclear antibody is present in low titer in 30% of patients.

The dosage of prednisone that has to be administered is usually much smaller than in pemphigus foliaceus. A favorable response to localized pemphigus erythematosus may occur with the use of topical steroids and sunscreens. Immunosuppressants may be needed in severe cases.

Alopsy E, et al: Is the combination of tetracycline and nicotinamide therapy alone effective in pemphigus? *Arch Dermatol* 1995, 133:1339.
American ML, et al: Pemphigus erythematosus. *J Am Acad Dermatol* 1984, 10:215.

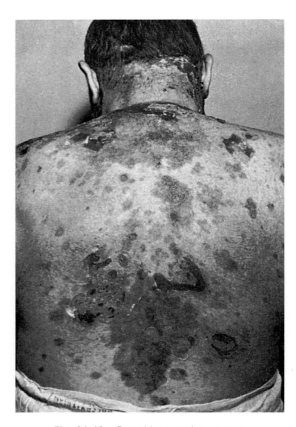

Fig. 21-13 Pemphigus erythematosus.

Azana JM, et al: Severe pemphigus foliaceus treated with extracorporeal photochemotherapy. *Arch Dermatol* 1997, 133:287.

Basset N, et al: Dapsone in initial treatment of superficial pemphigus. *Arch Dermatol* 1987, 123:783.

Bastuji-Garon S, et al: Comparative epidemiology of pemphigus in Tunisia and France. *J Invest Dermatol* 1995, 104:302.

Brenner S, et al: Recognition of pemphigus antigens in drug-induced pemphigus vulgaris and pemphigus foliaceus. *J Am Acad Dermatol* 1997, 36:919.

Chaffins ML, et al: Treatment of pemphigus and linear IgA dermatosis with nicotinamide and tetracycline. *J Am Acad Dermatol* 1993, 28:998.

Cruz PD Jr, et al: Concurrent features of cutaneous lupus erythematosus and pemphigus erythematosus following myasthenia gravis and thymoma. *J Am Acad Dermatol* 1987, 16:472.

Delvadi-Banta LJ, et al: Superficial erosions with oozing and marked coughing. *Arch Dermatol* 1993, 129:633.

Diaz LA, et al: Endemic pemphigus foliaceus (fogo selvagem). *J Invest Dermatol* 1989, 92:4.

Diaz LA, et al: Endemic pemphigus foliaceus (fogo selvagem). *J Am Acad Dermatol* 1989, 20:657.

Eyre RW, et al: Maternal pemphigus foliaceus with cell surface antibody bound to neonatal epidermis. *Arch Dermatol* 1988, 124:25.

Hymes SR, et al: Pemphigus foliaceus. *Arch Dermatol* 1992, 128:1462.

Ishii K, et al: Characterization of autoantibodies in pemphigus using antigen-specific ELISAs with baculovirus-expressed recombinant desmogleins. *J Immunol* 1997, 159:2010.

Ishii K, et al: Desmoglein 1 and desmoglein 3 are the target antigens in herpetiform pemphigus. *Arch Dermatol* 1999, 135:943.

Kawana S, et al: Changes in clinical features, histologic findings, and antigen profiles with development of pemphigus foliaceus from pemphigus vulgaris. *Arch Dermatol* 1994, 130:1535.

Korman NJ: Pemphigus. *J Am Acad Dermatol* 1988, 18:1219.

Korman NJ, et al: Drug-induced pemphigus. *J Invest Dermatol* 1991, 96:273.

Korman NJ, et al: The pemphigus foliaceus and pemphigus vulgaris antigen complexes contain plakoglobulin. *J Invest Dermatol* 1989, 92:463.

Morini JP, et al: Pemphigus foliaceus in young women. *Arch Dermatol* 1993, 129:69.

Rivitti EA, et al: Pemphigus foliaceus autoantibodies bind both epidermis and squamous mucosal epithelium, but tissue injury is detected only in the epidermis. *J Am Acad Dermatol* 1994, 31:954.

Shelton RM: Pemphigus foliaceus associated with enalapril. *J Am Acad Dermatol* 1991, 24:503.

Shirakata Y, et al: Lack of mucosal involvement in pemphigus foliaceus may be due to low expression of desmoglein 1. *J Invest Dermatol* 1998, 110:76.

Stanley JR: The enigma of fogo selvagem. *J Am Acad Dermatol* 1989, 20:675.

Stanley JR, et al: Antigenic specificity of fogo selvagem autoantibodies is similar to North American pemphigus foliaceus and distinct from pemphigus vulgaris autoantibodies. *J Invest Dermatol* 1986, 87:197.

Walker DC, et al: Neonatal pemphigus foliaceus. *Arch Dermatol* 1995, 133:1308. ▲

PARANEOPLASTIC PEMPHIGUS

In 1990, Anhalt et al described five patients with underlying neoplasms who presented with painful mucosal ulcerations and polymorphous skin lesions, which progressed to blistering eruptions on their trunk and extremities. Many subsequent reports of more than 150 patients and a characteristic antibody profile has affirmed this is a newly recognized unique disease.

The mucosal lesions may appear lichenoid or more commonly Stevens-Johnson–like with crusting of the lips. The skin lesions may appear as erythematous macules, lichenoid lesions, erythema multiforme–like lesions, flaccid bullae and erosions typical of pemphigus, or tense, more deep-set bullae. Horn et al and Anhalt et al have reviewed the histology and report epidermal acantholysis, suprabasal cleft formation, dyskeratotic keratinocytes, vacuolar change of the basalar epidermis, and epidermal exocytosis of inflammatory cells are major features. The combination of suprabasalar acantholysis and dyskeratotic keratinocytes is particularly suggestive.

Immunopathologic evaluation reveals IgG and C3 deposition in the intercellular spaces of the epithelium. There is also observed a linear or granular IgG and/or C3 at the basement membrane zone in some cases. Indirect immunofluorescence reveals intercellular IgG in the epithelium. Lin et al reported the use of rat bladder as a specific screen for these autoantibodies. Helou et al agree it is a useful screen. About 25% of cases will be negative and some erythema multiforme major cases may be falsely positive. Immunoprecipitation is the definitive test. It reveals a complex immune response with autoantibodies directed against four high–molecular-weight keratinocyte proteins. Antibody targets include desmoplakin 1 (250 KD), envoplakin

(210 KD), the major plaque protein of hemidesmosomes BPAg1 (230 KD), and periplakin (190 KD). Many cases also recognize an additional antigen at 170 KD. Finally, by ELISA testing antibodies to desmoglein 3 and 1 are frequently present.

A wide variety of both benign and malignant tumors are seen in these patients. Ostezan et al reported a patient with no known neoplasm. Most commonly non-Hodgkin's lymphoma, chronic lymphocytic leukemia, Castleman's tumor, sarcoma, and thymoma are associated. Therapy for the underlying disease should be initiated. Unfortunately, most reported patients have died from their tumor. Even when associated with a benign tumor such as Castleman tumor, the disease may be fatal, as Chorzelski et al's patient who died from bronchiolitis obliterans. Therapy for the bullous dermatoses with prednisone and/or immunosuppressive agents should be balanced with treatment of the tumor. To the many agents used for severe autoimmune blistering diseases Nousari et al have added immunoablative high-dose cyclophosphamide without stem cell rescue.

Individual cases of other unique bullous eruptions occurring with neoplasia have been reported and await further investigation to characterize them.

Anhalt GJ, et al: Paraneoplastic pemphigus. *Adv Dermatol* 1997, 12:77.

Anhalt GJ, et al: Paraneoplastic pemphigus. *N Engl J Med* 1990, 323:1729.

Camisa C, et al: Paraneoplastic pemphigus is a distinct neoplasia-induced autoimmune disease. *Arch Dermatol* 1993, 129:883.

Chorzelski TP, et al: Paraneoplastic pemphigus associated with Castleman tumor, myasthenia gravis, and bronchiolitis obliterans. *J Am Acad Dermatol* 1999, 41:393.

Chorzelski TP, et al: Unusual acantholytic bullous dermatosis associated with neoplasia and IgG and IgA antibodies against bovine desmocollins I and II. *J Am Acad Dermatol* 1994, 31:351.

Fullerton SH, et al: Paraneoplastic pemphigus with autoantibody deposition in bronchial epithelium after autologous bone marrow transportation. *JAMA* 1992, 267:1500.

Helou J, et al: Accuracy of indirect IF testing in the diagnosis of paraneoplastic pemphigus. *J Am Acad Dermatol* 1995, 32:441.

Horn TD, et al: Histologic features of paraneoplastic pemphigus. *Arch Dermatol* 1992, 128:1091.

Lee IJ, et al: Paraneoplastic pemphigus associated with follicular dendritic cell sarcoma arising from Castleman's tumor. *J Am Acad Dermatol* 1999, 40:294.

Lin AY, et al: Indirect Immunofluorescence on rat bladder transitional epithelium. *J Am Acad Dermatol* 1993, 28:696.

Nousari HC, et al: Immunoablative high-dose cyclophosphamide without stem cell rescue in paraneoplastic pemphigus. *J Am Acad Dermatol* 1999, 40:750.

Ostezan LB, et al: Paraneoplastic pemphigus in the absence of a known neoplasm. *J Am Acad Dermatol* 1995, 33:312.

Robinson ND, et al: The new pemphigus variants. *J Am Acad Dermatol* 1999, 40:649.

Stevens SR, et al: Paraneoplastic pemphigus presenting as a lichen planus pemphigiodes-like eruption. *Arch Dermatol* 1993, 129:866.

Su WPD, et al: Paraneoplastic pemphigus. *J Am Acad Dermatol* 1994, 30:841.

Watsky KL, et al: Figurate and bullous eruptions in association with breast carcinoma. *Arch Dermatol* 1990, 126:649. ⎯⎯⎯⎯⎯⎯⎯⎯ ▲

INTRAEPIDERMAL NEUTROPHILIC IgA DERMATOSIS

In 1985, Huff et al reported the case of an elderly man with a chronic bullous dermatosis with unique histologic and immunopathologic findings. Clinically, there were generalized flaccid bullae, which rapidly ruptured and crusted. There was no scarring when the dermatosis healed. No mucosal lesions were present, and the distal extremities, face, and neck were spared. Neither grouping nor symmetry were present.

Histologic findings consisted of neutrophilic exocytosis and in some areas neutrophils arranged in a linear fashion at the dermal-epidermal junction. Later, intraepidermal abscesses were formed; no acantholysis was present. Direct IF repeatedly showed an intercellular deposition of IgA within the epidermis, with minimal staining of the basal layer. No circulating antibodies were found.

Since this report, many additional patients with intraepidermal IgA deposition have been described. They have been classified as belonging in two subsets, one more closely mimicking pemphigus and the second simulating subcorneal pustular dermatosis. The former starts with vesicles that become pustular within a few days, enlarge peripherally, and rupture in the center; then a crust forms. Continued peripheral vesiculation may lead to a flowerlike appearance. The head, neck, and trunk are frequent sites of involvement. Histologically, intraepidermal bullae with neutrophils, some eosinophils, and acantholysis is seen. Direct IF shows intraepidermal IgA deposition, usually throughout the epidermis and IIF may reveal circulating autoantibody that binds to the same location. There is evidence that the IgA specificity in individual cases may be directed at either the pemphigus vulgaris or pemphigus foliaceus antigens. One patient had concurrent IgG intercellular antibodies and a monoclonal IgA gammopathy.

A second subset of patients develop disease that more closely simulates subcorneal pustular dermatosis. They present much like Sneddon-Wilkinson patients, with serpiginous and annular pustules. There is a positive direct IF with IgA present in a linear or superficial intraepidermal fashion in the subcorneal zone. These IgA autoantibodies are directed against desmocollin 1. There is at times a circulating IgA monoclonal gammopathy. Granulocyte–macrophage colony stimulating factor has been reported to induce this condition. Whether the IF positive and IF negative cases are separate diseases or are a disease spectrum remains to be determined. Some cases of IF-negative Sneddon-Wilkinson also have an IgA gammopathy.

Therapy with dapsone is often effective, and may be so even at doses as low as 25 mg/day. Oral corticosteroids may be necessary, however, and in some resistant cases, immunosuppressive agents and plasmapheresis have been required. In the subcorneal pustular dermatosis subtype colchicine cleared one patient.

Beutner EH, et al: IgA pemphigus foliaceus. *J Am Acad Dermatol* 1989, 20:89.

Caputo R, et al: IgA pemphigus in a child. *J Am Acad Dermatol* 1991, 25:383.

Chorzelski TP, et al: IgA pemphigus foliaceus with a clinical presentation of pemphigus herpetiformis. *J Am Acad Dermatol* 1991, 21:839.

Hodak E, et al: Effect of colchicine in the subcorneal pustular dermatosis type of IgA pemphigus. *J Am Acad Dermatol* 1999, 40:91.

Huff JC, et al: Intraepidermal neutrophilic IgA dermatosis. *N Engl J Med* 1985, 313:1643.

Kuan YZ, et al: Intraepidermal neutrophilic IgA dermatosis. *J Am Acad Dermatol* 1995, 22:917.

Miyagawa S, et al: Atypical pemphigus associated with monoclonal IgA gammopathy. *J Am Acad Dermatol* 1995, 32:352.

Myers SA, et al: Intraepidermal neutrophilic IgA dermatosis in an HIV-infected patient. *J Am Acad Dermatol* 1994, 31:502.

Prost C, et al: IgA autoantibodies bind to pemphigus vulgaris antigen in a case of intraepidermal neutrophilic IgA dermatitis. *J Am Acad Dermatol* 1991, 25:846.

Robinson ND, et al: The new pemphigus variants. *J Am Acad Dermatol* 1999, 40:649.

Teraki Y, et al: Intercellular IgA dermatosis of childhood. *Arch Dermatol* 1991, 127:221.

Wallach D: Intraepidermal IgA pustulosis. *J Am Acad Dermatol* 1992, 27:993. ▲

BULLOUS PEMPHIGOID

CLINICAL FEATURES. Bullous pemphigoid (BP) was identified and named by Lever in 1953. Bullous pemphigoid is characterized by large, tense, subepidermal bullae (Fig. 21-14) that may be localized to some part of the body, with a predilection for the groin, axillae, and flexor surfaces of the forearms. The reported proportion of oral involvement varies from 8% to 39%, with 20% frequently quoted. Involvement of the pharynx, larynx, nasal mucosa, vulva, urethra, and eye is rare. Kornstadt et al reported a case in which epiglottal lesions led to acute airway obstruction.

After the bullae rupture, large denuded areas are seen (Fig. 21-15), but these do not materially increase in size as they do in pemphigus vulgaris. Instead, the denuded areas show a tendency to heal spontaneously. In addition to the bullae, there often are erythematous patches and urticarial plaques, with a tendency to central clearing. These patches and plaques may be present without bullae early in the course of the disease. Sometimes, targetoid lesions may be seen (Fig. 21-16).

Bullous pemphigoid may begin at a localized site, frequently on the shins. It may remain localized throughout the course of the disease or eventuate in generalized pemphigoid. Cases of the localized disease in which a vesicular eruption was limited to the soles (dyshidrosiform pemphigoid) are occasionally observed. Young girls may be initially seen with localized vulvar erosions and ulcers that resemble the signs of child abuse. These localized varieties have been shown to have circulating IgG antibody, which immunoprecipitates the 230-KD bullous pemphigoid antigen. The disease may be limited to areas of radiation therapy or burns.

Many other variants of bullous pemphigoid have been described. A vesicular variant manifested by tense, small,

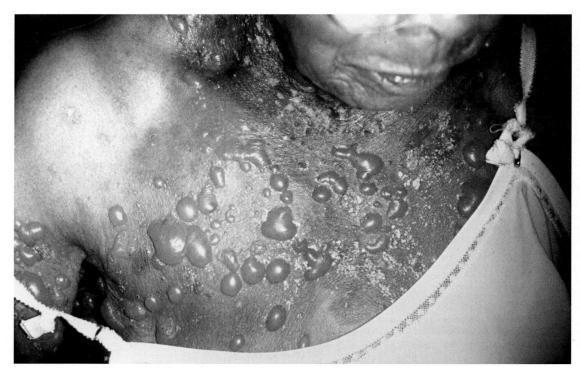

Fig. 21-14 Bullous pemphigoid. Note tense blisters.

occasionally grouped blisters is termed vesicular pemphigoid. Other patients, mostly women, have papules and nodules of the scalp and extremities, with sparing of the mucous membranes, in a pattern resembling prurigo nodularis (pemphigoid nodularis). Cases resembling pemphigus vegetans, but with IgG and C3 at the basement membrane zone, are occasionally observed (pemphigoid vegetans). Erythroderma may be present (erythrodermic pemphigoid) or there may be no bullae at all (nonbullous variant). The latter type may be observed in pruritic eczema or urticarial eruptions with peripheral eosinophilia.

Bullous pemphigoid occurs most frequently in the elderly. The age of onset averages 65 to 75 years. It also occurs, however, in young children (Fig. 21-17). Nemeth et al reviewed childhood bullous pemphigoid in a study of the 33 reported cases. Although most findings are similar to that in adult disease, they found that many cases begin with hand and foot bullae, and facial involvement is common in children. Also, the course of disease is usually less than 1 year, with most cases of the disease having a duration of 5 months or less.

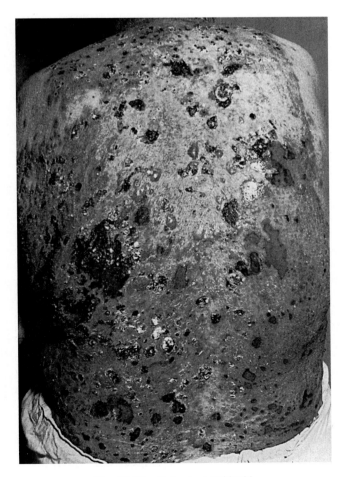

Fig. 21-15 Bullous pemphigoid.

In patients with lichen planus, a bullous eruption similar to bullous pemphigoid may develop. This so-called lichen planus pemphigoides is still the subject of debate regarding whether the circulating autoantibody targets the bullous pemphigoid antigen. Reports vary; the 230-KD antigen, the 180-KD antigen, and a unique 200-KD antigen all have been suggested target antigens in different reports.

Bullous pemphigoid is not a marker for, or a manifestation of, underlying malignancy.

Chan et al described a patient with a nonscarring eruption of acute onset with widespread erosions and severe mucous membrane involvement. The clinical pattern resembled toxic epidermal necrolysis or pemphigus vulgaris, but these investigators named the condition anti-p105 pemphigoid. The patient had linear IgG and C3 deposited in the basement membrane zone on direct and indirect IF, and Western blot testing showed that his autoantibodies reacted with a 105-KD antigen found in the lower portion of the lamina lucida.

ETIOLOGIC FACTORS. Circulating basement membrane zone (BMZ) antibodies of the IgG class are present in approximately 70% of patients with bullous pemphigoid. In most instances the antibodies fix complement in vitro, in contrast to pemphigus antibodies, which fail to do so. Complement is activated by both the classic and alternate pathways. No close correlation exists between the titer of antibodies and clinical disease activity.

The direct IF test in bullous pemphigoid is, just as in pemphigus, a much more reliable test than the indirect IF test is. In a positive test result, linear IF is seen along the BMZ. IgG or C3 or both are regularly found in biopsies from involved as well as uninvolved skin. A positive direct IF test result is found in nearly 100% of patients, with C3 most commonly present (approximately 100% of cases), and IgG present in about 80% of cases. The best area to biopsy is perilesional skin. IgA and IgM are each occasionally present.

The site of IgG binding has been localized to the lamina lucida, with accentuation near hemidesmosomes. Bullous pemphigoid antigen 1 (BPAg1) is synthesized by the keratinocyte and is an intracytoplasmic hemidesmosomal plaque protein of 230 KD molecular weight with disulfide-linked chains. A second BP antigen (BPAg2) is a transmembranous hemidesmosomal protein with an extracellular collagen domain and a molecular weight of 180 KD. The antibody to BPAg2 is likely the pathogenic factor. Approximately 90% of patients identify BPAg1 and BPAg2.

BP has occasionally been reported to be associated with other diseases, such as diabetes mellitus, rheumatoid arthritis, pemphigus foliaceus, dermatomyositis, ulcerative colitis, multiple autoimmune diseases, and myasthenia gravis and thymoma in one case. Drugs have been reported to induce bullous pemphigoid; these include penicillamine, furosemide, captopril, penicillin, sulfasalazine, nalidixic acid, and enalapril. Smith et al have shown that a patient

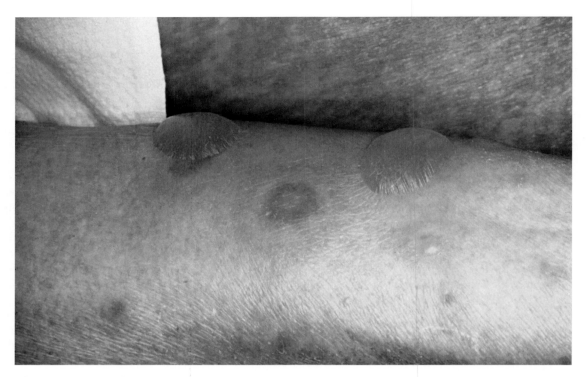

Fig. 21-16 Bullous pemphigoid. Note targetoid lesion between tense bullae.

taking the latter drug had circulating antibody targeting the 230-KD BP antigen.

As discussed under epidermolysis bullosa acquisita (EBA) (p. 597), it is recommended that indirect IF testing be performed on salt-split skin to differentiate EBA from BP. The autoantibody will react with primarily the epidermal side in BP and the dermal side in EBA.

Additionally, type IV collagen may be mapped on skin biopsy blisters; it will be on the base of the blister in BP, and on the roof in EBA. Tissue taken for direct IF may be salt-split and reactants found primarily on the epidermal side in BP and the dermal side in EBA. Finally, C3 deposition is nearly always present in BP, whereas it may be absent in EBA.

PATHOGENESIS. The initial event is apparently the binding of the IgG autoantibody to the BP antigen in the lamina lucida. Complement is activated, which produces factors with anaphylatoxic and chemotactic activity. Mast cells are activated and degranulated, which releases eosinophil chemotactic factors. Eosinophils accumulate in the dermis and eventually adhere to the basement membrane zone, where they release tissue-destructive enzymes and reactive oxygen intermediates. Resultant injury to this zone causes dermoepidermal separation and blister formation.

HISTOPATHOLOGY. The histologic changes are characterized by subepidermal bullae, by the absence of acantholysis, and by a superficial dermal infiltrate containing many eosino-phils. The amount of inflammatory infiltrate varies, and consequently, the subepidermal bullae and the underlying skin may be "infiltrate poor" or "infiltrate rich." Often the infiltrate is pronounced and contains many eosinophils. Eosinophilic spongiosis occurs; Crotty et al and Ruiz et al found BP to be the most frequently associated disease. In fact, peripheral blood eosinophilia is present in 50% of pemphigoid patients.

TREATMENT. Treatment should be the same as for pemphigus, with the expectation that the disease will respond more readily to relatively lower doses of corticosteroids. Localized variants may respond to topical steroids alone. In exceptionally severe cases, an effective measure is pulse therapy with methylprednisolone, giving 15 mg/kg in 16 ml of bacteriostatic water over a period of 30 to 60 minutes daily for three doses. Sodium succinate salt (Solu-Medrol) is used. It is followed with oral prednisone if necessary, 0.4 mg/kg daily, for at least 1 week. Blistering often stops completely after the third dose is given.

Immunosuppressive therapy may be necessary in resistant cases; azathioprine is most commonly used. Paul et al reported methotrexate to be useful in elderly patients when given in low doses in connection with low-dose corticosteroidal agents. Heilborn et al used methotrexate as monotherapy in 11 consecutive patients and found it effective in doses of 5 to 12.5 mg per week. Finally, mycophenolate mofetil, as discussed under pemphigus vulgaris, has also

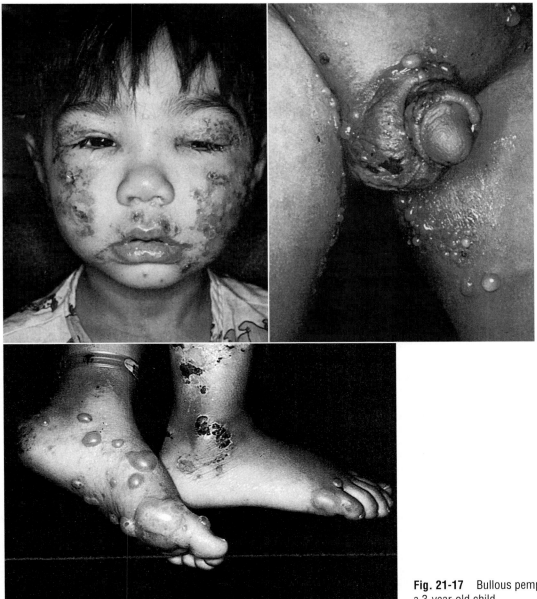

Fig. 21-17 Bullous pemphigoid in a 3-year-old child.

been reported to be effective in indivudual patients with bullous pemphigus.

Fivenson et al found 500 mg of nicotinamide three times daily combined with 500 mg of tetracycline four times daily to be an effective combination in inducing complete or partial responses in 10 of the 14 patients so treated. The use of tetracycline alone has been reported to be successful, as has tetracycline and nicotinamide given orally, combined with topical application of clobetasol.

Person et al reported that 10% of patients with bullous pemphigoid responded to sulfapyridine or dapsone. The patients who responded tended to be younger (mean age, 54) and tended to have more neutrophils than eosinophils in the infiltrate. Fox et al reported that two patients treated with erythromycin demonstrated improvement.

COURSE AND PROGNOSIS. Bullous pemphigoid is usually self-limited over a 5- to 6-year period. Some patients die within 6 months to 1 year of diagnosis. Many are elderly and have concomitant cardiovascular or other systemic disease. Bernard et al report that the presence of circulating anti-BP 180 antibodies, but not anti-BP230, was associated with a statistically increased chance of death in the first year after diagnosis. The childhood form generally clears in less than 1 year. With adequate therapy, response is usually complete: most patients have a lasting remission. In 10% to 15% of patients, relapse occurs once therapy is stopped.

Alcalay J, et al: Bullous pemphigoid mimicking bullous erythema multiforme. *J Am Acad Dermatol* 1988, 18:345.

Amato DA, et al: Bullous pemphigoid. *Int J Dermatol* 1988, 27:560.

Anhalt GJ, et al: Mechanisms of immunologic injury: pemphigus and bullous pemphigoid (editorial). *Arch Dermatol* 1983, 119:711.

Bassett N, et al: Dapsone as initial treatment in superficial pemphigoid. *Arch Dermatol* 1987, 123:783.

Berk MA, et al: The treatment of bullous pemphigoid with tetracycline and niacinamide. *Arch Dermatol* 1986, 122:670.

Bernard P, et al: Anti-BP180 autoantibodies as a marker of poor prognosis in bullous pemphigoid: a cohort analysis of 94 elderly patients. *Br J Dermatol* 1997, 136:694.

Borradori L, et al: Localized pretibial pemphigoid and pemphigus nodularis. *J Am Acad Dermatol* 1992, 27:863.

Bushkill LL, et al: Bullous pemphigoid: a cause of peripheral blood eosinophilia. *J Am Acad Dermatol* 1983, 8:648.

Chan LS, et al: A novel immune-mediated subepidermal dermatosis characterized by IgG autoantibodies to a lower lamina lucida component. *Arch Dermatol* 1994, 130:343.

Chan LS, et al: Pemphigoid vegetans represents bullous pemphigoid variant. *J Am Acad Dermatol* 1993, 28:331.

Chuang T, et al: Increased frequency of diabetes mellitus in patients with bullous pemphigoid. *J Am Acad Dermatol* 1984, 11:1099.

Cliff S, et al: Pemphigoid nodularis. *Br J Dermatol* 1997, 136:398.

Crotty C, et al: Eosinophilic spongiosis: a clinicopathologic review of 71 cases. *J Am Acad Dermatol* 1983, 8:337.

Descamps U, et al: Dyshidrosiform pemphigoid. *J Am Acad Dermatol* 1992, 26:651.

Domloge-Hultsch N, et al: A bullous skin disease patient with antibodies against separate epitopes in 1 mol/L sodium chloride split skin. *Arch Dermatol* 1992, 128:1096.

Domloge-Hultsch N, et al: Autoantibodies from patients with localized and generalized bullous pemphigoid immunoprecipitates the same 230-KD keratinocyte antigen. *Arch Dermatol* 1990, 126:1337.

Domloge-Hultsch N, et al: Direct IF microscopy of 1 mol/L sodium chloride-treated patient skin. *J Am Acad Dermatol* 1991, 24:946.

Duschet P, et al: Bullous pemphigoid after radiation therapy. *J Am Acad Dermatol* 1988, 18:441.

Fivenson DP, et al: Nicotinamide and tetracycline therapy of bullous pemphigoid. *Arch Dermatol* 1994, 130:753.

Fox BJ, et al: Erythromycin therapy of bullous pemphigoid. *J Am Acad Dermatol* 1982, 7:504.

Ghohestani RF, et al: Diagnostic value of indirect immunofluorescence on sodium chloride–split skin in differential diagnosis of subepidermal autoimmune bullous dermatoses. *Arch Dermatol* 1997, 133:1102.

Glover M, et al: Dermatomyositis pemphigoides. *J Am Acad Dermatol* 1992, 27:849.

Gruber GG, et al: Vesicular pemphigoid. *J Am Acad Dermatol* 1980, 3:619.

Grundemann-Kollmann M, et al: Mycophenolate mofetil. *J Am Acad Dermatol* 1999, 40:957.

Guenther LC, et al: Localized childhood vulvar pemphigoid. *J Am Acad Dermatol* 1990, 22:762.

Guillaume JC, et al: Controlled trial of azathioprine and plasma exchange in addition to prednisolone in the treatment of bullous pemphigoid. *Arch Dermatol* 1993, 12:49.

Haase C, et al: Detection of IgG autoantibodies in the serum of patients with bullous and gestasional pemphigoid. *J Invest Dermatol* 1997, 110:282.

Heilborn JD, et al: Low-dose oral pulse methotrexate as monotherapy in elderly patients with bullous pemphigoid. *J Am Acad Dermatol* 1999, 40:741.

Hernando LB, et al: Lichen planus pemphigoides. *J Am Acad Dermatol* 1992, 26:124.

Hornschuh B, et al: Treatment of 16 patients with bullous pemphigoid with oral tetracycline and niacinamide and topical clobetasol. *J Am Acad Dermatol* 1997, 36:101.

Ishiko A, et al: Combined features of pemphigus foliaceus and bullous pemphigoid. *Arch Dermatol* 1995, 131:732.

Jiao D, et al: Relation between antibodies to BP180 and gender in bullous pemphigoid. *J Am Acad Dermatol* 1999, 41:269.

Jung M, et al: Increased risk of bullous pemphigoid in male and very old patients. *J Am Acad Dermatol* 1999, 41:266.

Korman N: Bullous pemphigoid. *J Am Acad Dermatol* 1987, 16:907.

Kornstadt JW, et al: Refractory bullous pemphigoid leading to respiratory arrest and successfully treated with plasmapheresis. *Arch Dermatol* 1990, 126:1241.

Lynfield YL, et al: Bullous pemphigoid and multiple autoimmune diseases. *J Am Acad Dermatol* 1983, 9:257.

Maceyko RF, et al: Oral and cutaneous lichen planus pemphigoides. *J Am Acad Dermatol* 1992, 27:889.

Milligan A, et al: The use of chlorambucil in the treatment of bullous pemphigoid. *J Am Acad Dermatol* 1995, 22:796.

Mueller S, et al: A230 KD basic protein is the major bullous pemphigoid antigen. *J Invest Dermatol* 1989, 92:33.

Nagaro T, et al: Childhood bullous pemphigoid. *J Am Acad Dermatol* 1994, 30:884.

Nemeth AJ, et al: Childhood bullous pemphigoid. *Arch Dermatol* 1991, 127:378.

Ogasawara M, et al: Pemphigoid vegetans. *J Am Acad Dermatol* 1994, 30:649.

Paul MA, et al: Low dose methotrexate treatment in elderly patients with bullous pemphigoid. *J Am Acad Dermatol* 1994, 31:620.

Pereyo NG, et al: Generalized bullous pemphigoid controlled by tetracycline therapy alone. *J Am Acad Dermatol* 1995, 32:138.

Person JR, et al: Bullous pemphigoid responding to sulfapyridine and sulfones. *Arch Dermatol* 1977, 113:610.

Ross JS, et al: Unusual variants of pemphigoid. *J Cutan Pathol* 1993, 19:212.

Roujeau JC, et al: High risk of death in elderly patients with extensive bullous pemphigoid. *Arch Dermatol* 1998, 134:465.

Ruiz E, et al: Eosinophilic spongiosis. *J Am Acad Dermatol* 1994, 30:973.

Saad RW, et al: Childhood localized vulvar pemphigoid is a true variant of bullous pemphigoid. *Arch Dermatol* 1992, 128:807.

Saitoh A, et al: Erythrodermic bullous pemphigoid. *J Am Acad Dermatol* 1993, 28:124.

Scola F, et al: Dyshidrosiform pemphigus. *J Am Acad Dermatol* 1995, 32:516.

Siegel J, et al: High-dose methylprednisolone in treatment of bullous pemphigoid. *Arch Dermatol* 1984, 120:1157.

Smith EP, et al: Antigen identification in drug-induced bullous pemphigoid. *J Am Acad Dermatol* 1993, 29:879.

Smoller BR, et al: Differences in direct IF staining patterns in EBA and bullous pemphigoid. *J Am Acad Dermatol* 1992, 27:674.

Stanley JR, et al: Characterization of BP antigen. *Cell* 1981, 24:897.

Strohal R, et al: Nonbullous pemphigoid. *J Am Acad Dermatol* 1993, 29:293.

Tamada Y, et al: Lichen planus pemphigoides. *J Am Acad Dermatol* 1995, 32:883.

Taylor G, et al: Bullous pemphigoid and autoimmunity. *J Am Acad Dermatol* 1993, 29:181.

Thomas I, et al: Treatment of generalized bullous pemphigoid with oral tetracycline. *J Am Acad Dermatol* 1993, 28:74.

Vassileva S, et al: Burn-induced bullous pemphigoid. *J Am Acad Dermatol* 1994, 30:1027.

Weigand DA: Effect of anatomic region on IF diagnosis of bullous pemphigoid. *J Am Acad Dermatol* 1985, 12:274.

Westerhof W: Treatment of bullous pemphigoid with topical clobetasol propionate. *J Am Acad Dermatol* 1989, 20:458.

Zhu XJ, et al: Molecular identification of major and minor BP antigens. *J Am Acad Dermatol* 1990, 23:876. ▲

HERPES GESTATIONIS (PEMPHIGOID GESTATIONIS)

CLINICAL FEATURES. Herpes gestationis (HG) has many clinical, histologic, and immunopathologic similarities to bullous pemphigoid; thus the suggested name of pemphigoid gestationis. It is a rare (approximate incidence, 1 in 50,000 pregnancies), pruritic, inflammatory, bullous disease with onset either during pregnancy or during the postpartum period.

The onset of the disease is most often during the second trimester of pregnancy (average onset, 21 weeks' gestation). Urticarial plaques and papules develop around the woman's umbilicus and extremities, with subsequent spread over the abdomen, back, chest, and extremities, including the palms and soles. The face, scalp, and oral mucosa are usually spared. Within the infiltrated erythematous plaques, tense vesicles and bullae erupt, often in an annular or polycyclic configuration (Figs. 21-18 and 21-19). Pruritus is severe and may be paroxysmal.

The disease will often flare within a few days after delivery and then remit spontaneously, usually within 3 months. There may be recurrences with the taking of oral contraceptives, with subsequent menstrual periods, and nearly always with subsequent pregnancies. There is no scarring, except that caused by excoriations or secondary infections.

Maternal health is not affected. Lawley et al found a significant adverse effect on fetal survival; however, studies by Holmes et al, Shornick et al, and Mascaro et al failed to confirm this. Infants whose mothers have HG are more commonly premature and small for gestational age. In fewer than 5% of cases, infants may manifest the disease in the form of urticarial lesions or bullae. These cases are of limited extent and severity and clear spontaneously without the need for therapy.

ETIOLOGIC FACTORS. HG is an autoimmune, antibody-mediated disease. A complement-fixing IgG anti-basement-zone antibody is present in the serum. This is deposited in the lamina lucida, and fixes complement at the site of dermal-epidermal separation. The 180-KD bullous pemphigoid antigen (BPAg2) is the antigen targeted by the HG factor.

Studies have documented an increased frequency of HLA-DR3, DR 4, and C4 null alleles in patients with HG. Women may have antibodies directed against their husbands' HLA antigens. Black women rarely manifest HG; it is theorized this may be related to the low incidence of HLA-DR4 in American blacks. There is an increased frequency of Graves' disease in HG patients.

PATHOGENESIS. Pathogenesis is similar to that of bullous pemphigoid. However, hormonal factors influence the disease manifestation. In addition to being seen in pregnant patients, menstruating women, and those taking oral contraceptives, the disease may occur in association with hydatidiform mole and choriocarcinoma.

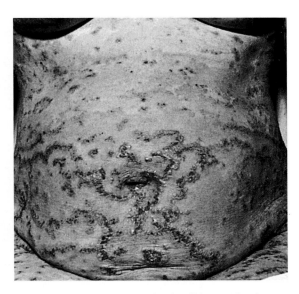

Fig. 21-18 Herpes gestationis in the fifth month of a seventh pregnancy. During only two pregnancies, the patient was free of lesions. (Courtesy Dr. B.M. Kesten.)

HISTOPATHOLOGY. A subepidermal, teardrop-shaped vesicle with a granulocyte-rich infiltration of the upper dermis with eosinophils and neutrophils is present. On direct IF, all patients have C3 deposited in a linear pattern at the dermoepidermal junction. Approximately 25% to 40% have IgG there as well. By conventional indirect IF testing, approximately 25% of patients have a circulating IgG anti-basement-zone antibody, but in nearly 75% the *HG factor,* a complement-fixing IgG antibody, can be demonstrated by complement-enhanced IF. Immunoelectron microscopy has demonstrated that the blister occurs at the level of the lamina lucida, with deposition of C3 and IgG at this site, exactly as in BP.

DIFFERENTIAL DIAGNOSIS. The main diagnosis to be considered is pruritic urticarial papules and plaques of pregnancy (PUPPP). There are, however, several diseases that are associated with or uniquely occur in pregnancy. Some, like PUPPP, are well-accepted, well-defined clinical entities. Others, such as papular dermatitis of pregnancy, are more controversial in that their very existence is questioned. All of these pregnancy-related dermatoses will be discussed together.

The differential diagnosis of herpes gestationis also includes diseases or conditions that are not specific for pregnancy but that may occur coincidentally. These include erythema multiforme, bullous pemphigoid, pemphigus, and drug reactions. Acrodermatitis enteropathica has also been reported to flare as a bullous eruption with each pregnancy.

TREATMENT. The use of topical steroid medications may be adequate in some milder cases of herpes gestationis. Prednisone in an oral dose of 40 mg/day will be effective in

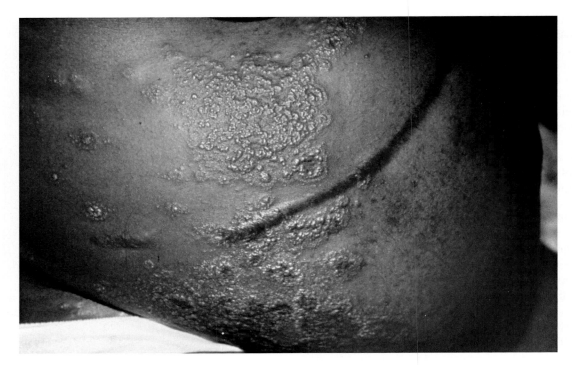

Fig. 21-19 Herpes gestationis.

most of the remainder of cases, and is ideally tapered to the lowest effective dose given on alternate days. Pyridoxine has been reported to have helped.

Borradori L, et al: Specific dermatoses of pregnancy. *Arch Dermatol* 1994, 130:778.

Castle SP, et al: Chronic herpes gestationis and antiphospholipid antibody syndrome successfully treated with cyclophosphamide. *J Am Acad Dermatol* 1996, 34:333.

Holmes RC, et al: HG persisting for 12 years post partum (letter). *Arch Dermatol* 1986, 122:375.

Holmes RC, et al: The fetal prognosis in pemphigoid gestationis (HG). *Br J Dermatol* 1984, 110:67.

Holmes RC, et al: The specific dermatoses of pregnancy. *J Am Acad Dermatol* 1983, 8:405.

Kelly SE, et al: Pemphigoid gestations. *J Cutan Pathol* 1988, 15:319.

Lawley TJ, et al: Fetal and maternal risk factors in HG. *Arch Dermatol* 1978, 114:552.

Mascaro JM Jr, et al: Fetal morbidity in HG. *Arch Dermatol* 1995, 131:1209.

Morrison LH, et al: Herpes gestationis autoantibodies recognize a 180 KD human epidermal antigen. *J Clin Invest* 1988, 81:2023.

Roger D, et al: Specific dermatoses of pregnancy. *Arch Dermatol* 1994, 130:734.

Shornick JK: Herpes gestationis. *J Am Acad Dermatol* 1987, 17:539.

Shornick JK: Herpes gestationis in blacks. *Arch Dermatol* 1984, 12:511.

Shornick JK: Secondary autoimmune diseases in herpes gestationis. *J Am Acad Dermatol* 1992, 26:563.

Shornick JK, et al: Complement polymorphism in herpes gestationis. *J Am Acad Dermatol* 1993, 29:545.

Shornick JK, et al: Fetal risks in herpes gestationis. *J Am Acad Dermatol* 1992, 26:63.

Shornick JK, et al: Herpes gestationis: clinical and histologic features of twenty-eight cases. *J Am Acad Dermatol* 1983, 8:214. _____ ▲

PREGNANCY-RELATED DERMATOSES

A working classification of specific dermatoses of pregnancy includes herpes (pemphigoid) gestationis, intrahepatic cholestasis of pregnancy or prurigo gravidarum, and the pruritic inflammatory dermatoses of pregnancy.

Intrahepatic Cholestasis of Pregnancy (Prurigo Gravidarum)

This pregnancy-related disease has no primary skin lesions, and is usually manifested only by generalized pruritus and jaundice. Secondary excoriations may be present. It is caused by cholestasis, occurs late in pregnancy, resolves after delivery, and recurs with subsequent pregnancies. There is an increased incidence of fetal complications. Roger et al found it to occur in 0.5% of 3192 pregnancies. Dexamethasone, 12 mg daily for 7 days, followed by discontinuation over 3 days, led to disappearance or relief of itching in all 10 patients treated by Hirvioja et al. Use of epomediol has also been reported to be effective.

Polymorphic Eruption of Pregnancy

Some investigators propose to include all of the pruritic inflammatory dermatoses of pregnancy into the designation *polymorphic eruption of pregnancy*. Certainly, by using this classification, the multitude of nonspecific pruritic dermatoses and their respective names would be simplified. These include toxemic rash of pregnancy, prurigo annularis, erythema multiforme gestationis, late-onset prurigo of pregnancy, pruritic urticarial papules and plaques of pregnancy, prurigo gestationis of Besnier, early onset prurigo of pregnancy, papular dermatitis of pregnancy, and pruritic folliculitis of pregnancy.

This subset of pruritic inflammatory dermatoses of pregnancy occur more frequently than any others, if they are placed under one heading. In approximately 1 of every 120 to 240 pregnancies, such an eruption will be manifested. Some of these will be discussed separately, but we like the proposed grouping of these disorders, because no consistent defining hormonal or immunopathogenetic factors reliably separate them. Also, treatment is similar and prognosis identical.

Pruritic Urticarial Papules and Plaques of Pregnancy.

Lawley et al first reported seven patients under the name *pruritic urticarial papules and plaques of pregnancy* (PUPPP) in 1979. This eruption is characterized by erythematous papules and plaques that begin as 1- or 2-mm lesions within the abdominal striae. They then spread over the course of a few days to involve the abdomen, buttocks, thighs, and in some cases the arms and legs (Fig. 21-20). The upper chest, face, and mucous membranes are generally spared. The lesions coalesce to form urticarial plaques, sometimes in configurate patterns, and occasionally spongiotic vesicles are present. Intense pruritus is characteristic, but only rarely are there excoriations.

This eruption occurs in primigravidas 75% of the time, and usually does not recur with subsequent pregnancies. It begins late in the third trimester and resolves with delivery. Many studies have investigated the relationship of maternal weight gain to the development of this dermatosis. Although results vary, the evidence seems to support the fact that patients with PUPPP, on average, gain more weight than those who remain free of disease. In contrast to herpes gestationis, postpartum onset or exacerbation is rare. Fetal and maternal outcomes are not affected by this eruption, and only rarely do newborns manifest transient lesions of PUPPP.

Histologic findings consist of a perivascular lymphohistiocytic infiltrate in the upper dermis and often mid-dermis, with a variable number of eosinophils and with dermal edema. The epidermis is usually normal, although focal spongiosis, parakeratosis, or scales or crust may be present. The results of a direct IF test are invariably negative.

Frequently, treatment with topical steroidal medications suffices, and if not, systemic steroidal agents may be used to bring the eruption under control. Beltrani et al reported on a patient who underwent cesarean section and early delivery for symptom relief.

Papular Dermatitis of Pregnancy.

Papular dermatitis of pregnancy is quite controversial, with very few cases reported. It is defined as a pruritic, generalized eruption of 3- to 5-mm erythematous papules surmounted by a small, firm, central crust. The lesions may erupt at any time during

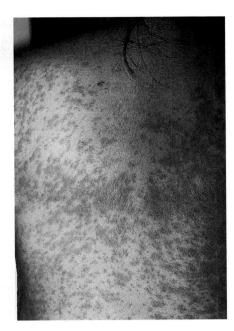

Fig. 21-20 Pruritic urticarial papules and plaques of pregnancy (PUPPP).

pregnancy and usually resolve with delivery, although a case reported by Michand et al continued to develop papules premenstrually for 11 months following delivery. A laboratory finding necessary to support the diagnosis of papular dermatitis of pregnancy is a marked elevation of the 24-hour urinary chorionic gonadotropin.

Administration of systemic corticosteroids is reportedly effective in controlling the eruption. The high incidence of fetal deaths reported by Spangler is now felt to have been overstated. Treatment may prevent any adverse effects. The condition may recur in subsequent pregnancies.

Prurigo Gestationis (Besnier).

This eruption consists of pruritic, excoriated papules of the proximal limbs and upper trunk; these occur most often between the twentieth and thirty-fourth week of gestation. It clears in the postpartum period and usually does not recur.

Therapy with potent topical steroidal agents is recommended. No adverse effects on maternal or fetal health are seen. This eruption may simply be an expression of atopic dermatitis in pregnancy.

Pruritic Folliculitis of Pregnancy.

Several authors have reported on pruritic folliculitis in gravid women with small follicular pustules scattered widely over the trunk that appear during the second or third trimester, resolving by 2 or 3 weeks after delivery. Acute folliculitis and focal spongiosis with exocytosis of polymorphonuclear leukocytes are present on biopsy, and direct IF results are negative. This condition may be a type of hormonally induced acne.

Linear IgM Dermatosis of Pregnancy. In 1988, Alcalay et al described a woman who developed small, red, follicular papules and pustules that on IF testing showed linear deposits of IgM. This is not, however, a specific finding, and should not be considered a "new" dermatosis of pregnancy.

Impetigo Herpetiformis. Impetigo herpetiformis (IH) is a form of severe pustular psoriasis occurring in pregnancy. It consists of an acute, usually febrile onset of grouped pustules on an erythematous base, which begins in the groin, axillae, and neck (Fig. 21-21). Extension of these lesions occurs until large areas of skin are involved. There is a high peripheral white blood cell count, and hypocalcemia may be present. The histopathology is that of pustular psoriasis.

The condition resolves with delivery, but recurrences with subsequent pregnancies may be expected. Fetal death is not uncommon; it results from placental insufficiency. Treatment is with systemic corticosteroids, 40 to 60 mg of oral prednisone a day.

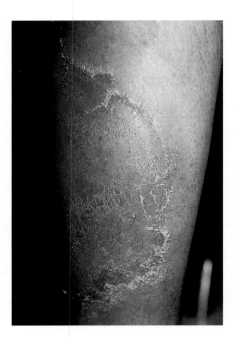

Fig. 21-21 Impetigo herpetiformis. Note pustules at the edge of scale. (Courtesy Dr. Axel W. Hoke).

Alcalay J, et al: Linear IgM dermatosis of pregnancy. *J Am Acad Dermatol* 1988, 18:412.

Beckett MA, et al: Pruritic urticarial papules and plaques of pregnancy and skin distention. *Arch Dermatol* 1991, 127:125.

Beltrani VP, et al: Pruritic urticarial papules and plaques of pregnancy. *J Am Acad Dermatol* 1992, 26:266.

Borradori L, et al: IgM autoantibodies to 180- and 230- to 240-kd human epidermal proteins in pregnancy. *Arch Dermatol* 1995, 131:43.

Borradori L, et al: Specific dermatoses of pregnancy. *Arch Dermatol* 1994, 130:778.

Gonzalez MC, et al: Epomediol ameliorates pruritus in patients with intrahepatic cholestasis of pregnancy. *J Hepatol* 1992, 16:241.

Helm TN, et al: Continuous dermoepidermal junction IgM detected by direct immunofluorescence: a report of nine cases. *J Am Acad Dermatol* 1992, 26:203.

Hirvioja ML, et al: The treatment of intrahepatic cholestasis of pregnancy by dexamethasone. *Br J Obstet Gynaecol* 1992, 99:109.

Holm AL, et al: Impetigo herpetiformis associated with hypocalcemia of congenital rickets. *Arch Dermatol* 1991, 127:91.

Holmes RC, et al: The specific dermatoses of pregnancy. *J Am Acad Dermatol* 1983, 8:405.

Jones SAV, et al: Pregnancy dermatoses. *J Am Acad Dermatol* 1999, 40:233.

Lawley TJ, et al: Pruritic urticarial papules and plaques of pregnancy. *JAMA* 1979, 241:1696.

Lotem M, et al: Impetigo herpetiformis. *J Am Acad Dermatol* 1989, 20:338.

Morrison LH, et al: Herpes gestationis autoantibodies recognize a 180 KD human epidermal antigen. *J Clin Invest* 1988, 81:2023.

Nguyen LO, et al: Papular dermatitis of pregnancy. *J Am Acad Dermatol* 1990, 22:690.

Oumeish OY, et al: Some aspects of impetigo herpetiformis. *Arch Dermatol* 1982, 118:103.

Pauwels C, et al: Pruritic urticarial papules and plaques of pregnancy. *Arch Dermatol* 1994, 130:806.

Reid R, et al: Fetal complications of obstetric jaundice. *Br Med J* 1976, 1:182.

Roger D, et al: Specific dermatoses of pregnancy. *Arch Dermatol* 1994, 130:734.

Thio HB, et al: Hypocalcemia in impetigo herpetiformis. *Arch Dermatol* 127:1587.

Winton GB, et al: Dermatoses of pregnancy. *J Am Acad Dermatol* 1982, 6:977. ———————————————————— ▲

CICATRICIAL PEMPHIGOID (BENIGN MUCOSAL PEMPHIGOID)

In 1953, Lever suggested the designation *benign mucosal pemphigoid* for what had previously been called *ocular pemphigus, cicatricial pemphigoid,* or *essential shrinkage of the conjunctiva.* Because of its scarring nature, the designation cicatricial pemphigoid has gained acceptance. The discussion that follows is a compilation of literature that characterizes all patients with such scarring lesions. It is clear that these conditions actually may be subdivided into many different diseases with varying clinical, laboratory, therapeutic response patterns and prognoses. Some of them are presently more clearly defined than others, but as antibody specificity is determined precisely, the disease states will come into better focus.

Cicatricial pemphigoid is characterized by the predilection for evanescent vesicles, which quickly rupture, leaving behind erosions and ulcers. They primarily occur on the mucous membranes, especially the conjunctiva and oral mucosa. Oral lesions occur in approximately 90% of cases and conjunctival lesions in 66%.

The oral mucosa is almost always involved, and may be the only affected site for years. Desquamative gingivitis, a diffuse erythema of the marginal and attached mucosa associated with areas of ulceration, vesiculation, and

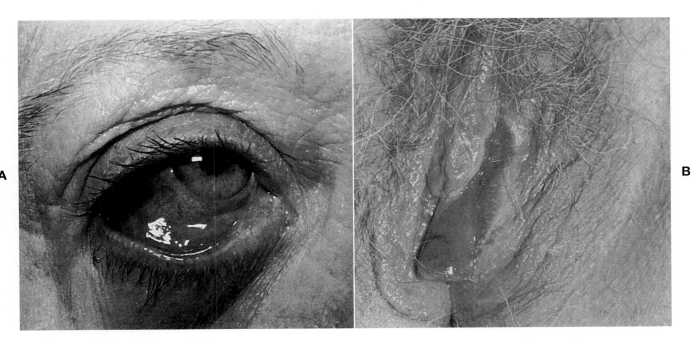

Fig. 21-22 Cicatricial pemphigoid with **A,** ocular and **B,** vaginal involvement. (Courtesy Dr. Axel W. Hoke.)

desquamation, is often the presenting sign. The buccal gingivae are almost always involved, the lingual surfaces less regularly. Like cicatricial pemphigoid as a whole, desquamative gingivitis tends to affect middle-aged to elderly women. The female to male ratio is approximately two to one. Of 41 patients with desquamative gingivitis, Rogers et al classified 18 as localized oral pemphigoid (gingival involvement only, without progression over 3-year average follow-up), 18 as cicatricial pemphigoid, and only two as pemphigus, one as lichen planus, one as epidermolysis bullosa, and one as contact stomatitis. By contrast, the dental literature and our experience indicate that at least half of all patients presenting with desquamative gingivitis have lichen planus by biopsy and immunofluorescent criteria. Other portions of the oral mucosa that may be involved by cicatricial pemphigoid are the palate, tongue, and tonsillar pillars.

The disorder is a chronic disease that may lead to a slowly progressive shrinkage of the ocular mucous membranes and connective tissues secondary to scarring and eventually (untreated) to blindness. It is usually bilateral and associated with redness and flaccid vesicles on the conjunctiva, xerosis, fibrous adhesions (symblepharon), and scarring of the conjunctivae (Fig. 21-22, *A*). Entropion, trichiasis, and corneal opacities develop and ultimately, the adhesions attach both lids to the eyeball and narrow the palpebral fissure. Associated scarring may develop following attacks of inflammation, vesicles, and denudation in the pharynx, esophagus, larynx and nose, and on the glans penis and vagina (Fig. 21-22, *B*) and anal mucosa. Stricture of the esophagus may occur. Deafness, suspected of being the

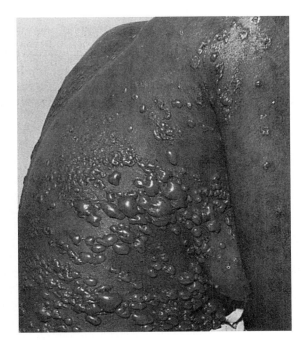

Fig. 21-23 Skin bullae in benign mucosal pemphigoid.

result of middle ear involvement, was reported by Thomson et al in one case.

Cutaneous lesions are seen in approximately 25% of patients. These lesions are tense bullae, similar to those seen in bullous pemphigoid (Fig. 21-23). The bullae, which heal with or without scarring, occur on the face, scalp, neck, and the inguinal region and extremities. Generalized lesions may also occur. Some of these patients will have circulating antibodies targeted against the classic bullous pemphigoid antigens, and should be classified as mucosal predominate bullous pemphigoid. Some of these patients may have secondary IgG antibodies against other antigens, or IgA antibodies, which may explain the scarring tendency of the mucosal lesions.

The patient's general health is usually not jeopardized; a chronic course is usually experienced. In contrast to bullous pemphigoid, cicatricial pemphigoid shows little tendency for remission. Cicatricial pemphigoid may be induced by penicillamine or by clonidine.

In Brunsting-Perry pemphigoid there are no mucosal lesions, but one or several circumscribed erythematous patches develop on which recurrent crops of blisters appear. Ultimately, atrophic scarring results. Generally, the areas of involvement are confined to the head and neck. The average age at onset is 58 with a 2:1 male-to-female ratio. Some of these patients have been discovered to have epidermolysis bullosa acquisita when the IgG autoantibody was found to target type VII collagen.

In a large study by Chan et al they found one subset of patients who clearly showed only eye involvement and who were frequently positive on both direct and indirect IF. Of patients with only mucous membrane lesions, one of 14 had antibodies that targeted the minor bullous pemphigoid antigen, suggesting some of these patients may have mucosal predominant bullous pemphigoid. The possibility exists that some of these will prove to have epidermolysis bullosa acquisita.

Domloge-Hultsch et al identified a subset of patients with a mucosal-predominant blistering disorder in which their circulating IgG autoantibodies target a glycoprotein complex, laminin 5. Although most patients exhibit antibodies to the α subunit of laminin 5, antibodies to the β3 and γ2 chains may also occur. These patients, who were initially reported under the designation *antiepiligrin cicatricial pemphigoid,* represent yet another subset of the phenotypic presentation of cicatricial pemphigoid. Other patients have been found to have autoantibodies that react with both laminin 6 as well as laminin 5, prompting the proposed designation of this subset as *antilaminin cicatricial pemphigoid.* Using similar approaches it is likely other subsets of patients targeting unique basement membrane zone antigens will be identified.

The histologic findings are identical to those of bullous pemphigoid, with the exception that fibrosis and scarring may be present in the upper dermis. Basement membrane separation occurs in the lamina lucida, as is the case in bullous pemphigoid.

Direct IF testing of lesional or perilesional skin or mucosa in cicatricial pemphigoid reveals C3 and IgG at the lamina lucida in 80% to 95% of the patients. The basement membrane zone of mucosal glands stains as well. IgA may be found occasionally. A circulating antibody to the BMZ is found by IIF in about 20% of cases. Immunoelectron microscopy shows the antibodies bind to the lamina lucida,

and, with suction-blistered or salt-split skin, binding is seen to occur at a deeper level than with bullous pemphigoid. Most IIF-positive cases, however, show IgG binding to the epidermal side of salt-split skin, although combined staining and dermal staining alone may be present in different subtypes. The epidermal side binding autoantibodies usually target BPAg2. It is the dermal side binding autoantibodies that have specificity for laminin.

In mild cases, topical steroids, either Decadron elixir, 0.5 mg/5 ml, or Temovate ointment mixed with equal parts of Orabase, applied several times a day, may be effective. Intralesional triamcinolone acetonide at a dilution of 5.0 to 7.5 mg/ml may be useful if given every 2 to 4 weeks. Vinyl inserts may be crafted by the dentist to serve as trays that occlude topical steroids on the gingiva. They are most useful in desquamative gingivitis and may be used for the gingival lesions in more widespread disease.

A similar appliance may be made for vaginal occlusive treatment of lesions of this site. Iontophoresis of steroids may also help localized areas. Topical sucralfate suspension may decrease the pain and healing time of the oral and genital ulcers. Cyclosporine washes have some efficacy but are too expensive for general use. More aggressive cases, especially when ocular scarring threatens, may require treatment with dapsone, alone or combined with prednisone. Azathioprine or cyclophosphamide is required in severe, unresponsive disease.

Ahmed AR, et al: Cicatricial pemphigoid. *J Am Acad Dermatol* 1991, 24:987.

Alpsoy E, et al: The use of sucralfate suspension in the treatment of oral and genital ulceration in Behçet disease. *Arch Dermatol* 1999, 135:529.

Azana JM, et al: Topical cyclosporins for cicatricial pemphigoid. *J Am Acad Dermatol* 1993, 28:124.

Bauco-van der Wal V, et al: Topical tetracycline in cicatricial pemphigoid. *J Am Acad Dermatol* 1997, 36:492.

Bernard P, et al: Cicatricial pemphigoid. *J Invest Dermatol* 1989, 92:402.

Chan LS, et al: Cicatricial pemphigoid. *Arch Dermatol* 1990, 126:1466.

Chan LS, et al: Immune-mediated subepithelial blistering diseases of the mucous membranes. *Arch Dermatol* 1993, 129:448.

Chan LS, et al: Laminin-6 and laminin-5 are recognized by autoantibodies in a subset of cicatricial pemphigoid. *J Invest Dermatol* 1997, 108:848.

Domloge-Hultsch H, et al: Anti epiligrin cicatricial pemphigoid. *Arch Dermatol* 1994, 130:1521.

Fleming MG, et al: Mucous gland basement membrane IF in cicatricial pemphigoid. *Arch Dermatol* 1988, 124:1407.

Fujimoto W, et al: Anti-epiligrin cicatricial pemphigoid with IgG autoantibodies to the β and γ subunits of laminin 5. *J Am Acad Dermatol* 1999, 40:637.

Ghohestani RF, et al: Diagnostic value of indirect immunofluorescence on sodium chloride-split skin in differential diagnosis of subepidermal autoimmune bullous dermatoses. *Arch Dermatol* 1997, 133:1102.

Gibson GE, et al: Anti-epiligrin (laminin 5) cicatricial pemphigoid and lung carcinoma. *Br J Dermatol* 1997, 137:780.

Joly P, et al: Brunsting-Perry cicatricial bulbous pemphigoid. *J Am Acad Dermatol* 1993, 28:89.

Kurzhals G, et al: Acquired EBA with the clinical features of Brunsting-Perry cicatricial bullous pemphigoid. *Arch Dermatol* 1991, 127:391.

Kurzhals G, et al: Localized cicatricial pemphigoid of the Brunsting-Perry type with transition into disseminated CP. *Arch Dermatol* 1995, 131:580.

Lazarova Z, et al: Reactivity of autoantibodies from patients with defined subepidermal bullous diseases against 1 mol/L salt-split skin: specificity, sensitivity, and practical considerations. *J Am Acad Dermatol* 1996, 35:398.

Lee MS, et al: Oral insertable prosthetic device as an aid in treating oral ulcers. *Arch Dermatol* 1991, 127:479.

Leverkus M, et al: Antiepiligrin cicatricial pemphigoid. *Arch Dermatol* 1999, 135:1091.

Lish KM, et al: Anti-epiligrin cicatricial pemphigoid in a patient with HIV. *J Am Acad Dermatol* 1997, 36:486.

Marren P, et al: Vulval cicatricial pemphigoid may mimic lichen sclerosus. *Br J Dermatol* 1996, 134:522.

Nayar M, et al: Association of autoimmunity and cicatricial pemphigoid. *J Am Acad Dermatol* 1991, 25:1011.

Nousari HC, et al: Anti-epiligrin cicatricial pemphigoid with antibodies against the γ2 subunit of laminin 5. *Arch Dermatol* 1999, 135:173.

Pandya AG, et al: Cicatricial pemphigoid successfully treated with pulse intravenous cyclophosphamide. *Arch Dermatol* 1997, 133:245.

Rogers RS III, et al: Desquamative gingivitis: clinical, histopathologic, immunopathologic, and therapeutic observations. *J Am Acad Dermatol* 1982, 7:729.

Rogers RS III, et al: Treatment of cicatricial pemphigoid with dapsone. *J Am Acad Dermatol* 1982, 6:215.

Silverman S Jr, et al: Oral mucous membrane pemphigoid. *Oral Surg* 1986, 61:233.

Vincent SC, et al: Clinical, historic, and therapeutic features of cicatricial pemphigoid. *Oral Surg Oral Med Oral Path* 1992, 76:453.

Walsh D, et al: A vaginal prosthetic device as an aid in treating ulcerative lichen planus of the mucous membrane. *Arch Dermatol* 1995, 131:265.

▲

EPIDERMOLYSIS BULLOSA ACQUISITA

For many years this nonhereditary bullous dermatosis was considered to be a noninflammatory scarring mechanobullous eruption that occurred in the elderly population. Exclusionary criteria for making the diagnosis of epidermolysis bullosa acquisita (EBA) were proposed in 1971 by Roenigk et al to be (1) clinical lesions of dystrophic EB, including increased skin fragility, trauma-induced blistering with erosions, atrophic scarring, milia over extensor surfaces, and nail dystrophy (Fig. 21-24); (2) adult onset; (3) lack of a family history of EB; and (4) exclusion of all other bullous diseases such as porphyria cutanea tarda, pemphigoid, pemphigus, dermatitis herpetiformis, and bullous drug eruption. In 1981, Roenigk et al extended these criteria to include (5) IgG at the basement membrane zone by direct immunofluorescence; (6) the demonstration of blister formation beneath the basal lamina; and (7) deposition of IgG beneath the basal lamina.

Although all of the above except adult onset hold true, extension of the clinical spectrum to an inflammatory type and knowledge of antibody specificity now allow definitive diagnostic criteria.

IIF studies reveal circulating antibasement membrane zone antibodies in approximately half of cases. Woodley et al showed that these antibodies are directed against the globular C-terminal domain of type VII collagen, the major structural component of anchoring fibrils. Patients with bullous systemic lupus erythematosus (SLE) have circulating antibodies with the same specificity.

The noninflammatory clinical presentation of EBA is the most commonly recognized type. It may manifest, in addition to the clinical criteria mentioned earlier, severe oral and esophageal mucosal scarring. The association of EBA with many systemic diseases, such as myeloma, granulomatous colitis, diabetes, lymphoma, leukemia, amyloidosis, and carcinoma is well established. In rare instances, cases of this noninflammatory subset may mimic either bullous or cicatricial pemphigoid. Lang et al reported a case in which severe eye involvement so dominated the clinical picture that it led to an initial diagnosis of cicatricial

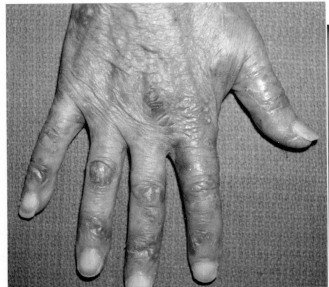

A

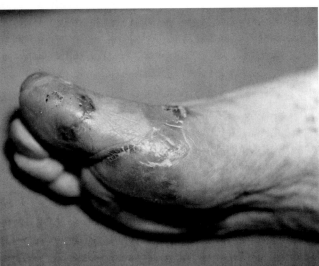

B

Fig. 21-24   Epidermolysis bullosa acquisita of **A,** dorsal hand and fingers and **B,** great toe area.

pemphigoid. Additionally, two cases that were thought to be Brunsting-Perry cicatricial pemphigoid based on clinical signs appeared by immunoelectron microscopy to be EBA. Zambruno et al described a patient with a papulovesicular eruption, scarring, and severe mucosal lesions with blindness. Direct IF revealed linear IgA deposits, indirect IF showed dermal side staining, immunoelectron microscopy showed the IgA deposits to be associated with anchoring fibrils, and the IgA reacted with the 290-KD antigen on Western blot analysis. This was a form of IgA-mediated EBA. Finally, when the onset is in childhood hereditary dystrophic EB may be considered. Arpey et al reviewed the six cases reported as of 1991, and other reports, such as that of Roger et al, have followed.

In 1982, Gammon et al described a patient with generalized inflammatory bullous disease that resembled bullous pemphigoid clinically, but with immunologic and ultrastructural features of EBA. Since that time many cases of this inflammatory subset of disease have been reported. Many have associated diabetes mellitus, are HLA-DR2 positive, and progress to the trauma-induced scarring type of EBA in the course of long-term follow-up. Data collected by Gammon et al suggest that this type of onset of EBA may occur in as many as 50% of all EBA patients. By analyzing sera of 85 patients diagnosed as having bullous pemphigoid, they were able to imply that possibly 10% of patients referred to medical centers as having BP may actually have EBA. Zhu et al found 5 of their 100 patients with circulating antibasement membrane zone antibodies to have EBA.

Differentiation may be suggested by the fact that histologically, EBA patients usually have a predominance of neutrophils over eosinophils. IIF-tested EBA patients are more likely to have linear IgG staining without concomitant C3 deposition than are patients with BP. Incubation of skin with sodium chloride causes a split to occur at the lamina lucida. This allows differentiation of the majority of cases without needing to resort to immunoblot techniques or immunoelectron microscopy. By direct IF testing of the patient's salt-split skin biopsy EBA will manifest IgG deposition only on the dermal side of the split, whereas the majority of BP patients will have IgG bound only to the epidermal side or to both sides. As demonstrated by indirect IF, the same results apply in the majority of cases. Additionally, this method may detect antibasement membrane zone antibodies in patients who had negative IIF results when tested by routine methods. Absolute differentiation of these diseases is obtained by immunoelectron microscopy or immunoblot findings. In BP the antibody is deposited in the lamina lucida and identifies hemidesmosomal proteins of 230-KD and 180-KD molecular weight to be the target antigens. In EBA the antibody is deposited in the upper dermis on the anchoring fibrils and identifies 290-KD and 145-KD proteins on immunoblotting. It has been shown that the antibody is targeting type VII collagen.

Because bullous SLE and EBA share antibasement membrane zone antibodies of identical specificity and there is clinical and histologic overlap as well, this differential diagnosis may be difficult.

The following features help to identify EBA: skin fragility, predilection for traumatized areas, and healing with scars and milia. In SLE, sun-exposed skin is involved by preference, the patient has a diagnosis of SLE established by American Rheumatism Association criteria, and in bullous SLE there is usually a dramatic response to dapsone. In addition to the cases of bullous SLE that show linear IgG staining below the lamina densa with circulating IgG autoantibodies to the 290-KD and 145-KD antigens, some patients will show granular staining of IgG at the basement membrane zone without circulating IgG.

In general, the results of treatment of EBA are unsatisfactory. A few patients with an inflammatory condition respond to steroids with or without azathioprine or dapsone, and these are worthy of a trial. Other immunosuppressives, colchicine, plasmapheresis, and intravenous immunoglobulin have all had reported successes in individual cases but are not effective in the majority of patients. Cyclosporine has been reported to be effective in a number of cases and deserves further study. The noninflammatory types of bullous conditions are often best managed by supportive therapy, including control of infection, careful wound management, and maintenance of good nutrition.

Arpey CS, et al: Childhood epidermolysis bullosa acquisita. *J Am Acad Dermatol* 1991, 24:706.

Boh E, et al: Epidermolysis bullosa acquisita preceding the development of SLE. *J Am Acad Dermatol* 1990, 22:587.

Borradori L, et al: Positive transfer of autoantibody from a patient with mutilating epidermolysis bullosa acquisita induces specific alterations in the skin of mice. *Arch Dermatol* 1995, 131:590.

Briggaman RA, et al: Epidermolysis bullosa acquisita and other acquired blistering diseases manifesting autoimmunity to type VII collagen. *Curr Prob Dermatol* 1991, 3:47.

Callot-Mellot C, et al: Epidermolysis bullosa acquisita in childhood. *Arch Dermatol* 1997, 133:1122.

Connolly SM, et al: Treatment of epidermolysis bullosa acquisita with cyclosporine. *J Am Acad Dermatol* 1987, 16:890.

Crow LL, et al: Clearing of epidermolysis bullosa acquisita with cyclosporine. *J Am Acad Dermatol* 1988, 19:937.

Cunningham BB, et al: Colchicine for epidermolysis bullosa acquisita. *J Am Acad Dermatol* 1996, 34:781.

Domloge-Hultsch N, et al: Direct IF microscopy of 1 mol/L sodium chloride-treated patient skins. *J Am Acad Dermatol* 1991, 24:946.

Gammon WR, et al: Epidermolysis bullosa acquisita presenting as an inflammatory bullous disease. *J Am Acad Dermatol* 1982, 7:382.

Gammon WR, et al: Increased frequency of HLA-DR2 in patients with autoantibodies to epidermolysis bullosa acquisita antigen. *J Invest Dermatol* 1988, 91:228.

Ghohestani RF, et al: Diagnostic value of indirect immunofluorescence on sodium chloride-split skin in differential diagnosis of subepidermal autoimmune bullous dermatoses. *Arch Dermatol* 1997, 133:1102.

Gordon KB, et al: Treatment of refractory epidermolysis bullosa acquisita with extracorporeal photochemotherapy. *Br J Dermatol* 1997, 136:415.

Jolles S, et al: Dermatological uses of high-dose intravenous immunoglobulin. *Arch Dermatol* 1998, 134:80.

Joly P, et al: Brunsting-Perry cicatricial BP. *J Am Acad Dermatol* 1993, 28:89.

Kofler H, et al: Intravenous immunoglobulin treatment in therapy-resistant epidermolysis bullosa acquisita. *J Am Acad Dermatol* 1997, 36:331.

Kubo A, et al: Epidermolysis bullosa acquisita exacerbated by systemic estrogen and progesterone treatment and pregnancy. *J Am Acad Dermatol* 1997, 36:792.

Kurzhals G, et al: Acquired EB with the clinical features of Brunsting-Perry cicatricial BP. *Arch Dermatol* 1991, 127:391.

Lang PG, et al: Severe ocular involvement in a patient with epidermolysis bullosa acquisita. *J Am Acad Dermatol* 1987, 16:439.

Luke MC, et al: Mucosal morbidity in patients with epidermolysis bullosa acquisita. *Arch Dermatol* 1999, 135:954.

McCuaig CC, et al: Epidermolysis bullosa acquisita in childhood. *Arch Dermatol* 1989, 125:944.

Meier F, et al: Epidermolysis bullosa acquisita. *J Am Acad Dermatol* 1992, 29:334.

Richter BJ, et al: The spectrum of epidermolysis bullosa acquisita. *Arch Dermatol* 1979, 115:1325.

Roenigk HH, et al: Epidermolysis bullosa acquisita. *Arch Dermatol* 1981, 117:383.

Roger H, et al: Epidermolysis bullosa acquisita in a 3½ year old child. *J Am Acad Dermatol* 1992, 27:858.

Smoller BR, et al: Differences in direct IF staining patterns in epidermolysis bullosa acquisita and bullous pemphigoid. *J Am Acad Dermatol* 1992, 27:674.

Stewart MI, et al: Epidermolysis bullosa acquisita and associated symptomatic esophageal webs. *Arch Dermatol* 1991, 127:373.

Woodley DT: IF on salt-split skin for the diagnosis of epidermolysis bullosa acquisita. *Arch Dermatol* 1990, 126:229.

Woodley DT, et al: Identification of the skin basement-membrane autoantigen in epidermolysis bullosa acquisita. *N Engl J Med* 1984, 310:1007.

Wuepper KD: Repeat direct IF to discriminate pemphigoid from epidermolysis bullosa acquisita. *Arch Dermatol* 1990, 126:1365.

Zachariae H: Cyclosporine A in epidermolysis bullosa acquisita. *J Am Acad Dermatol* 1987, 17:1058.

Zambruno G, et al: Linear IgA bullous dermatosis with autoantibodies to a 290-KD antigen of anchoring fibrils. *J Am Acad Dermatol* 1994, 31:884.

Zhu XS, et al: Epidermolysis bullosa acquisita. *Arch Dermatol* 1990, 126:171. ─────────────────────────── ▲

DERMATITIS HERPETIFORMIS (DUHRING'S DISEASE)

CLINICAL FEATURES. Dermatitis herpetiformis (DH) is a chronic, relapsing, severely pruritic disease with grouped, symmetrical, polymorphous, erythematous-based lesions (Fig. 21-25). The eruption may be papular, papulovesicular, vesiculobullous, bullous, or urticarial in nature (Fig. 21-26). On involution there may rarely be hyperpigmentation. Itching and burning are usually intense, and their paroxysmal quality provokes scratching to the point of bleeding and, at times, scarring. Spontaneous remissions lasting as long as a week and terminating abruptly with a new crop of lesions are a highly characteristic feature of the disease. Perimenstrual flares may occur.

The eruption is usually strikingly symmetrical. Sites of predilection are the scalp, nuchal area, posterior axillary folds, sacral region, buttocks, knees, and forearms, especially the extensor surfaces near the elbows. The lesions are acutely inflammatory, and the eruption is characteristically

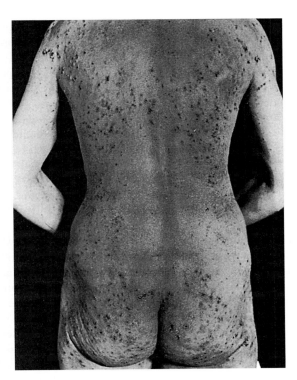

Fig. 21-25   Dermatitis herpetiformis. Note the symmetry and the large clear areas separating groups of lesions.

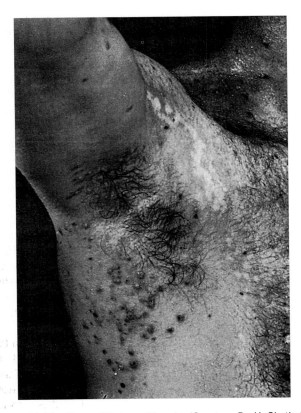

Fig. 21-26   Dermatitis herpetiformis. (Courtesy Dr. H. Shatin.)

polymorphous. The manifestations differ widely according to the type of lesions and the distribution. Pruriginous papules are a common feature of most eruptions, and the edema in some of these is sufficient to produce vesicopapules. Mild eruptions may resemble prurigo or urticaria. Vesicular and bullous lesions, if present, are thick-walled and usually tense, and at first have clear contents, but after a time these become somewhat purulent if scratching has not unroofed them. Vesicles are more common than bullae; however, all types of these lesions may be present in one patient. Pigmented spots alone over the lumbosacral region should arouse suspicion of DH. The mucous membranes are involved in rare cases, mostly when bullae are numerous. Laryngeal lesions may manifest as hoarseness.

The course of the disease is generally lifelong, with prolonged remissions being a rare event. The general health is not directly affected in Duhring's disease. It is remarkable, in view of the frequently associated gluten-sensitive enteropathy (GSE), how very few patients with DH ever have diarrhea.

Several large series have now been published documenting the occurrence of DH in childhood. These studies document that children present with disease clinically similar to the adult type, have identical histologic and immunofluorescent findings, and have a high incidence of HLA-B8 and -DR3 and abnormal jejunal biopsies. Karpati et al reported finding unusual palmer blisters or brown, hemorrhagic, purpuric macules in 30 of 47 children with DH, in every one of whom the diagnosis had been confirmed by finding granular IgA deposits in the skin. They were not present in patients who were asymptomatic or who had responded to treatment with a gluten-free diet or dapsone or sulfapyridine. They were seldom found on the feet. These palmar lesions may also be seen in many adult patients. Treatment with sulfones results in prompt response, as in adults.

Seventy-seven percent to 87% of patients with DH and IgA deposits in the skin are HLA-B8 positive; the frequency of this specificity equals that observed in ordinary GSE. Two other HLA antigens, DR3 and DQw2, have been shown to occur in ordinary GSE at a higher frequency than the HLA-B8 itself; similarly, they are more frequent as HLA-B8 in DH. Black and Asian patients are infrequent and some studies indicate this may be because of HLA differences. These HLA markers are associated with other autoimmune diseases and are a marker of patients who appear to have an overactive immune response to common antigens. DH is unexpectedly frequent in family members, undoubtedly owing to genetic predisposition.

One common antigen that patients with DH appear to be antigenically stimulated by is gluten, a protein found in cereals except for rice, oats, and corn. Villous atrophy of the jejunum and inflammation of the small bowel occurs. IgA antibodies are apparently formed. Whether these form IgA-immune complexes that are then carried to and de-

posited in the skin, or whether the IgA antibodies bind to antigenically similar skin proteins, is not known. IgA is bound to the skin, and this apparently activates complement, primarily via the alternate pathway. Once it is activated, the resulting inflammation of the skin with the development of lesions follows.

Patch tests with 50% potassium iodide in petrolatum produce a bulla in uncontrolled DH, but only exceptionally in patients controlled by a gluten-free diet or by sulfone therapy. There is no difference in the presence or amount of IgA or C3 between the induced bullae and the normal skin.

ASSOCIATED DISEASE. Thyroid disorders are increased in incidence in patients with DH. Cunningham et al found thyroid disease in 26 of 50 patients they examined. Leonard et al found an increased incidence of malignancy in their patients (relative risk, 2.38). The incidence of small bowel lymphoma is higher than expected, as is non-Hodgkin's lymphoma (relative risk, 5.4).

ENTEROPATHY. It has been found that about 70% of the patients with DH have abnormalities in the jejunal mucosa. If given a high-gluten diet, nearly all of these patients will develop abnormal findings that are indistinguishable from celiac disease. The enteropathy seldom reaches the clinical horizon.

The dapsone requirement in DH is not significantly decreased, according to most reports, until a gluten-free diet has been followed for 3 to 6 months, and improvement in the skin lesions on the diet alone takes an equally long time to become manifest. Fry et al showed that nearly all patients who adhere to a strict gluten-free diet, if followed long enough, are able to either stop their medication or significantly reduce the dosage. The diet is a difficult one, and in patients who are successful, expressions such as "highly motivated" and "dedicated" occur frequently.

DIAGNOSIS. The clinical distinction between pemphigoid, erythema multiforme, and bullous DH may sometimes be difficult. The distinction from linear IgA bullous dermatosis is often clinically impossible. Other conditions considered in the differential diagnosis at times are scabies, contact dermatitis, atopic dermatitis, nummular eczema, neurotic excoriations, insect bites, and chronic bullous disease of childhood. The finding of IgA in a granular pattern in the dermal papillae in normal skin is specific and pathognomonic for DH.

Autoantibodies. Circulating IgA antibodies against the smooth muscle cell endomysium are present in 70% of DH patients, in nearly all active celiac disease patients, and almost never in other conditions. Direct IF of noninvolved skin reveals deposits of IgA alone or together with deposits of C3 arranged in a granular pattern in the dermal papillae. IgM and IgG deposits are occasionally observed in association with IgA. Deposits may be focal, so that multiple biopsies may be needed, and the deposits of antibody are more often seen in previously involved skin or normal-appearing skin adjacent to involved skin. By immunoelectron microscopy one observes IgA either alone or in conjunction with C3, IgG, or IgM as clumps in the upper dermis. A fibrillar staining pattern exists when the immune deposits are along dermal microfibrils.

INCIDENCE AND PREVALENCE. This disease has equal male-to-female incidence; the average age of onset is between 20 and 40 years. It does occur with some frequency in children. Blacks and Asians are rarely affected.

HISTOPATHOLOGY. The initial changes are first noted at the tips of the dermal papillae, where edema and an eosinophilic and neutrophilic exudate occur to produce a subepidermal separation. This eventually leads to bulla formation. The papillae tips degenerate, the epidermis separates, and the confluence of several dermal tips produces the vesicles. The cellular infiltrate contains many neutrophils and few eosinophils. The biopsy should always include a good piece of the surrounding erythematous portion of the lesion where there is no apparent vesicle.

Histologic differentiation of linear IgA bullous dermatosis from DH is extremely difficult. Smith et al have devised an elaborate quantitative scheme in which the number of rete tips with neutrophils in basal vacuoles and the length of the basement membrane zone associated with them (greater in IgA bullous dermatosis), and the number of microabscesses in the dermal papillae (greater in DH) are counted or measured.

TREATMENT. The drugs chiefly used are dapsone and sulfapyridine. The most effective sulfone is diaminodiphenylsulfone (dapsone). The dose varies between 50 and 300 mg daily, usually starting with 100 mg daily and increasing gradually to an effective level or until side effects occur. Once a favorable response is attained, the dosage is decreased to the minimum that does not permit recurrence of signs and symptoms. Hemolytic anemia, leukopenia, methemoglobinemia, and rarely, agranulocytosis or peripheral neuropathy may occur. Acute hemolytic anemia (which may be severe) occurs in patients with glucose-6-phosphate dehydrogenase deficiency, therefore a G6PD level should be done before therapy. So rare is this deficiency, however, that many prefer simply to use a low starting dose (50 mg/day) and warn and watch the patient closely for dark urine. The patient should be warned to report by telephone any incident of red or brown urine or blue nail beds or lips. Hematocrit determination should be done weekly for 4 weeks, bimonthly for the 2 months, and every 2 to 6 months thereafter. A white blood cell count should be obtained weekly for 8 weeks, and patients should be advised to seek medical advice if fever develops. Liver function tests should be monitored bimonthly for the first 4 months, then checked with the hematologic studies every 4 to 6 months.

Sulfapyridine also has long been used for the treatment of Duhring's disease. Sulfapyridine and dapsone response was regarded, before the availability of immunofluorescence, as a specific test for the diagnosis; if the patient did not respond to one of them, Duhring's disease was not diagnosed. After a test dose of 0.5 g of sulfapyridine, one tablet (0.5 g) four times daily is given. The dose is then increased if necessary, or reduced if possible. Usually 1 to 4 g is required for good control. Sulfasalazine, 2 to 4 g/day, may also be used, since sulfapyridine is a metabolic product. In rare patients in whom it is necessary to find alternatives to the sulfa drugs, tetracycline and nicotinamide and colchicine have controlled individual patients.

GLUTEN-FREE DIET. If a gluten-free diet is followed strictly, the patient will almost certainly be able to take less medication or stop it altogether. Also some evidence suggests this may decrease the incidence of associated malignancy. It is a very difficult diet to follow; however, the Celiac Society or the American Celiac Society may be able to help in planning it. Addresses for the two organizations follow:

Celiac Society
P.O. Box 31700
Omaha, NE 68131-0700

American Celiac Society
58 Musano Court
West Orange, NJ 07052

Cunningham MJ, et al: Thyroid abnormalities in dermatitis herpetiformis. *Ann Intern Med* 1985, 102:194.

Emmacora E, et al: Long-term follow-up of dermatitis herpetiformis in children. *J Am Acad Dermatol* 1986, 15:24.

Fry L, et al: Long-term follow-up of dermatitis herpetiformis with and without dietary gluten withdrawal. *Br J Dermatol* 1982, 107:631.

Garioch JJ, et al: 25 years experience of gluten-free diet in the treatment of dermatitis herpetiformis. *Br J Dermatol* 1994, 131:541.

Giblin WJ, et al: Bizarre widespread vesicular eruption. *Arch Dermatol* 1990, 126:527.

Goldstein BG, et al: Sulfasalizine in dermatitis herpetiformis. *J Am Acad Dermatol* 1990, 22:697.

Haffenden GP, et al: The potassium iodide patch test in dermatitis herpetiformis in relation to treatment with gluten-free diet and dapsone. *Br J Dermatol* 1980, 103:313.

Hall RP, et al: Dermatitis herpetiformis in two American blacks. *J Am Acad Dermatol* 1990, 22:469.

Hall RP, et al: Dietary management of dermatitis herpetiformis. *Arch Dermatol* 1987, 123:1378.

Hardman CM, et al: Absence of toxicity of oats in patients with dermatitis herpetiformis. *N Engl J Med* 1997, 337:1884.

Hornsten P, et al: The incidence of agranulocytosis during treatment of dermatitis herpetiformis with dapsone as reported in Sweden. *Arch Dermatol* 1990, 126:919.

Jenkins D, et al: Histiocytic lymphoma occurring in a patient with dermatitis herpetiformis. *J Am Acad Dermatol* 1983, 9:252.

Karpati S, et al: Palmar and planter lesions in children with dermatitis herpetiformis Duhring. *Cutis* 1986, 37:184.

Katz SI, et al: Dermatitis herpetiformis: the skin and the gut. *Ann Intern Med* 1980, 93:857.

Kawana S, et al: Confocal laser scanning in microscopic and immuno-electron microscopic studies of the anatomical distribution of fibrillar IgA deposits in dermatitis herpetiformis. *Arch Dermatol* 1993, 129:456.

Kumar V, et al: Serologic markers of gluten-sensitive enteropathy in bullous diseases. *Arch Dermatol* 1992, 128:1474.

Leitao EA, et al: Perimenstrual nonvesicular dermatitis herpetiformis. *J Am Acad Dermatol* 1990, 22:331.

Leonard J, et al: Gluten challenge in dermatitis herpetiformis. *N Engl J Med* 1983, 308:816.

Leonard JN, et al: Increased incidence of malignancy in dermatitis herpetiformis. *Br Med J Clin Res Ed* 1983, 286:16.

Lewis HM, et al: Protective effect of gluten-free diet against development of lymphoma in dermatitis herpetiformis. *Br J Dermatol* 1996, 135:363.

McFadden JP, et al: Laryngeal involvement in dermatitis herpetiformis. *J Am Acad Dermatol* 1990, 22:325.

McGovern TW, et al: Palmar purpura. *Pediatr Dermatol* 1994, 11:319.

Meyer LJ, et al: Familial incidence of dermatitis herpetiformis. *J Am Acad Dermatol* 1987, 17:643.

Peters MS, et al: IgA antiendomysial antibodies in dermatitis herpetiformis. *J Am Acad Dermatol* 1989, 21:1225.

Pierce DK, et al: Purpuric papules and vesicles of the palms in dermatitis herpetiformis. *J Am Acad Dermatol* 1987, 16:1274.

Reunala T, et al: Diseases associated with dermatitis herpetiformis. *Br J Dermatol* 1997, 136:315.

Sigurgeirsson B, et al: Risk of lymphoma in patients with dermatitis herpetiformis. *Br Med J* 1994, 308:13.

Silvers DN, et al: Treatment of dermatitis herpetiformis with colchicine. *Arch Dermatol* 1980, 116:1373.

Smith SB, et al: Linear IgA bullous dermatosis vs dermatitis herpetiformis. *Arch Dermatol* 1984, 120:324.

Stenveld HJ, et al: Efficacy of cyclosporine in two patients with dermatitis herpetiformis resistant to conventional therapy. *J Am Acad Dermatol* 1993, 28:1014.

van der Meer JB: Gluten-free diet and elemental diet in dermatitis herpetiformis. *Int J Dermatol* 1990, 29:679.

Zemstov A, et al: Successful treatment of dermatitis herpetiformis with tetracycline and nicotinamide in a patient unable to tolerate dapsone. *J Am Acad Dermatol* 1992, 28:505.

Zone JJ, et al: Deposition of granular IgA relative to clinical lesions in dermatitis herpetiformis. *Arch Dermatol* 1996, 132:912.

Zone JJ, et al: Granular IgA is decreased or absent in never involved skin in dermatitis herpetiformis. *J Invest Dermatol* 1985, 84:332.

▲

LINEAR IgA BULLOUS DERMATOSIS

Linear IgA bullous dermatosis is characterized by subepidermal blisters, a neutrophilic infiltrate, a circulating IgA antibasement membrane zone antibody, and deposition of this IgA antibody at the dermoepidermal junction by direct IF. Zone et al defined a 97-KD antigen in the lamina lucida that the IgA is directed against. In reports in which the antibody specificities are meticulously defined, individual patients with bullous disease and linear IgA deposits are best grouped into epidermolysis bullosa acquisita, bullous pemphigoid, cicatricial pemphigoid, or various subtypes of linear IgA dermatosis. Most of the clinical characteristics presented below represent data obtained when lumping all patients with linear IgA deposition together, as the recognition that these patients have multiple definable diseases has been only recently appreciated. Although there is considerable overlap of the adult and childhood cases, these will be discussed separately.

Adult Form

This acquired, autoimmune blistering disease may present with a clinical pattern of vesicles indistinguishable from

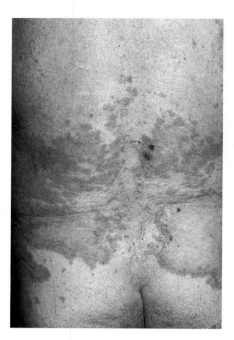

Fig. 21-27 Linear IgA in an adult. (Courtesy Dr. J. Fitzpatrick.)

dermatitis herpetiformis, or more commonly with vesicles and bullae in a bullous pemphigoid–like appearance (Fig. 21-27). There may be urticarial lesions, and in as many as half the cases mucous membrane involvement may occur. Oral and conjunctival lesions may dominate the presentation, and eye lesions may be scarring in nature. There is no association with enteropathy or with HLA-B8. The disease tends to remit over several years in approximately 60% of patients.

Linear IgA dermatosis may occur as a drug-induced disease. Kuechle et al have reviewed the literature. In these cases the eruption is self-limited, has less mucosal involvement, and usually does not have circulating autoantibody. Further, the IgA is usually deposited in the subbasal lamina area. Drugs implicated have included vancomycin (Fig. 21-28), lithium, amiodarone, captopril, penicillin, PUVA, furosemide, oxaprozin, interleukin-2, interferon-gamma immunotherapy, phenytoin, diclofenac, and glibenclamide. The antigen identified may be the 97-KD antigen, the 230-KD BP antigen, or the 180-KD bullous pemphigoid antigen. Sporadic reports have linked single cases with dermatomyositis, rheumatoid arthritis, and multiple sclerosis, although these are probably fortuitous associations.

McEvoy et al reviewed 12 patients who had a variety of associated malignancies. Smith et al discuss other anecdotal reports of immunologic stressors such as immunizations and infection that may exacerbate linear IgA dermatosis.

On histologic examination there may be papillary dermal microabscess with neutrophils and, at times, eosinophils, or a subepidermal bullae may be seen, again commonly with a

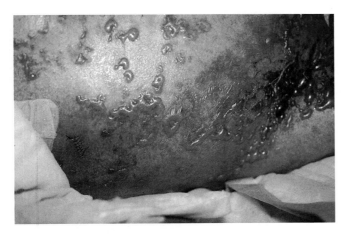

Fig. 21-28 Linear IgA drug eruption secondary to the use of vancomycin.

mixture of neutrophils and eosinophils. By direct IF evaluation, a homogeneous linear deposition of IgA is present at the BMZ. Some authors emphasize a frequent lack of C3 deposition. Some cases will have both linear IgA and IgG in combination at the BMZ. The lack of C3 may be a clue that both immunoglobulins recognize the 97-KD antigen, as Chan et al reported.

By indirect IF evaluation, only a minority will have circulating IgA autoantibody with anti-BMZ specificity, and this is usually present in low titer. On salt-split skin, deposition may occur on the roof, base, or a combination of the two. This correlates with the fact that on immunoelectron microscopy deposition of the autoantibody is present in the lamina lucida in some cases, in the sublamina densa in some cases, and in both in others. As stated above, this is because only recently has the heterogeneous nature of these patients been realized. True linear IgA disease has lamina lucida deposits, and the IgA is directed against the 97-KD peptide that Zone et al identified. Zambruno et al found as has Rusenko et al that some patients with this presentation will have IgA specificity against type VII collagen. These patients with sublamina densa deposits with immunoglobulins directed against the 290-KD antigen then have epidermolysis bullosa acquisita. Several patients with linear IgA disease whose IgA antibody identified the 230-KD or the 180-KD BP antigens have been described. Further definition of subsets of patients will undoubtedly be separated in the future.

Dapsone should be initially used in doses similar to that described for dermatitis herpetiformis as it may control the disease as a sole agent. Other cases require topical or systemic steroids in addition, or as sole treatment. A combination of tetracycline, 2 g/day, and nicotinamide, 1.5 g/day; intravenous immunoglobulin, or colchicine, 0.6 mg two to three times daily, may be effective.

Aboobaker J, et al: The localization of the binding site of circulating IgA antibodies in linea IgA disease of adults, chronic bullous disease of childhood, and childhood cicatricial pemphigoid. *Br J Dermatol* 1987, 116:293.

Acostamadiedo JM, et al: Phenytoin-induced linear IgA bullous disease. *J Am Acad Dermatol* 1998, 38:352.

Adachi A, et al: Immunoelectron microscopic differentiation of linear IgA bullous dermatosis of adults with coexistence of IgA and IgG deposition from bullous pemphigoid. *J Am Acad Dermatol* 1992, 27:394.

Aram H: Linear IgA bullous disease: successful treatment with colchicine. *Arch Dermatol* 1984, 120:960.

Bhogal B, et al: Linear IgA bullous dermatosis of adults and children. *Br J Dermatol* 1987, 117:289.

Carpenter S, et al: Vancomycin-associated linear IgA dermatosis. *J Am Acad Dermatol* 1992, 26:45.

Chaffins MC, et al: Treatment of pemphigus and linear IgA dermatosis with nicotinamide and tetracycline. *J Am Acad Dermatol* 1992, 28:998.

Chan LS, et al: Linear IgA bullous dermatosis. *Arch Dermatol* 1995, 31:1432.

Chan LS, et al: Oral manifestations of linear IgA disease. *J Am Acad Dermatol* 1990, 22:362.

Collier PM, et al: Linear IgA disease and pregnancy. *J Am Acad Dermatol* 1994, 30:407.

Ghohestani RF, et al: Linear IgA bullous dermatosis with IgA antibodies exclusively directed against the 180- or 230-KDa epidermal antigens. *J Invest Dermatol* 1997, 108:854.

Khan IU, et al: Linear IgA bullous dermatosis in a patient with chronic renal failure. *J Am Acad Dermatol* 1999, 40:485.

Kuechle MK, et al: Drug-induced linear IgA bullous dermatosis. *J Am Acad Dermatol* 1994, 30:187.

McEvoy MT, et al: Linear IgA dermatosis. *J Am Acad Dermatol* 1990, 22:59.

Miller JB, et al: Factors that exacerbate linear IgA disease. *J Am Acad Dermatol* 1995, 33:320.

Paul C, et al: Drug-induced linear IgA disease: target antigens are heterogeneous. *Br J Dermatol* 1997, 136:406.

Peoples D, et al: Linear IgA bullous dermatosis. *J Am Acad Dermatol* 1992, 26:498.

Peters MS, et al: IgA deposition at the cutaneous basement membrane zone. *J Am Acad Dermatol* 1989, 20:761.

Peterson MJ, et al: A case of linear IgA disease presenting initially with IgG immune deposits. *J Am Acad Dermatol* 1986, 14:1014.

Primka EJ III, et al: Amiodarone-induced linear IgA diseases. *J Am Acad Dermatol* 1994, 31:809.

Rusenko KW, et al: Type VII collagen is the antigen recognized by IgA anti–sub lamina densa autoantibodies. *J Invest Dermatol* 1989, 92:510.

Smith JB, et al: Factors that exacerbate linear IgA disease. *J Am Acad Dermatol* 1995, 33:321.

Webster G, et al: Cicatrizing conjunctivitis as a predominant manifestation of linear IgA bullous dermatosis. *J Am Acad Dermatol* 1994, 30:355.

Wojnarowska F, et al: Linear IgA disease: a heterogeneous disease. *Dermatology* 1994, 189(Suppl):52.

Zambruno G, et al: Linear IgA bullous dermatosis with autoantibodies to a 290-KD antigen of anchoring fibrils. *J Am Acad Dermatol* 1994, 31:884.

Zone JJ, et al: Identification of the cutaneous basement membrane zone antigen and isolation of antibody in linear IgA bullous dermatosis. *J Clin Invest* 1990, 85:812. ▲

Childhood Form (Chronic Bullous Disease of Childhood)

Chronic bullous disease of childhood (CBDC) is an acquired, self-limited bullous disease that may begin by the time the patient is age 2 or 3 and usually remits by age 13. The average age at onset is 5 years. Bullae develop on either erythematous or normal-appearing skin, preferentially involving the lower trunk, buttocks, genitalia, and thighs. Perioral and scalp lesions are common, and oral mucous membrane lesions are not uncommon. Indeed, Wojnarowska et al reported seeing them in 74% of their 29 patients. Bullae are often arranged in a rosette or annular array, the so-called cluster of jewels configuration (Fig. 21-29, *A*). Tense individual bullae similar to those present in bullous pemphigoid are also seen (Fig. 21-29, *B*). Pruritus is often severe.

The prime histologic finding is the presence of a subepidermal bulla filled with a preponderance of neutrophils. In some cases eosinophils predominate, as in BP. Direct IF reveals a linear deposition of IgA at the basement membrane zone. Indirect immunofluorescence is positive for circulating IgA anti-BMZ antibodies, usually in low titer, in approximately 50% of cases. Immunoelectron microscopy and immunomapping studies have been conflicting; in some cases the IgA has been within the lamina lucida, some have had it below the lamina densa and some patients a combination of both sites. Additionally, some children with both IgG and IgA deposits and circulating antibodies have been reported.

Zone et al showed that many patients who have an autoantibody in the lamina lucida are targeting a 97-KD peptide, as in linear IgA bullous dermatosis. Similar to adults with linear IgA bullous dermatosis, some children with subbasal lamina deposits may target type VII collagen and have epidermolysis bullosa acquisita. Patients with only IgA or with both IgG and IgA circulating autoantibodies may have specificity for the 230-KD and at times the 180-KD BP antigen. Darling et al reported a child who had a combination of IgA against the 97-KD peptide, and IgG against BPAg 1 and 2. The clinical and histologic features of this case were those of chronic bullous disease of childhood. Definition of other subsets of patients will undoubtedly occur in the future.

The untreated disease runs a variably chronic and remitting course, with eventual spontaneous resolution by adolescence being common. Treatment is most often successful with either sulfapyridine or dapsone. Occasional cases respond to topical steroids alone. Systemic steroidal medications are necessary in some cases, although a conservative approach is to be followed, since this is usually a benign, self-remitting disorder. Zeharia et al reported that colchicine was useful in their patient, in whom dapsone was contraindicated.

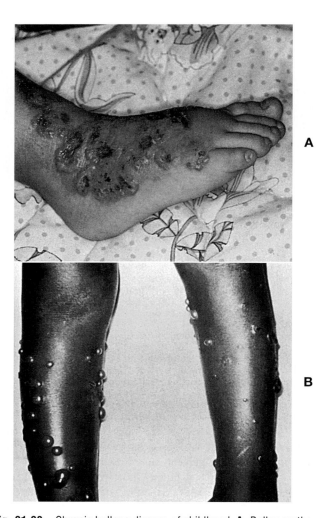

Fig. 21-29 *Chronic bullous disease of childhood.* **A,** Bullae on the feet in rosette configuration at the periphery. **B,** Large, tense bullae on the legs. (**A,** Courtesy Dr. J. Schiffner. **B,** Courtesy Dr. S. Prystowsky.)

Aboobaker J, et al: The localization of the binding site of circulating IgA antibodies in linea IgA disease of adults, chronic bullous disease of childhood, and childhood cicatricial pemphigoid. *Br J Dermatol* 1987, 116:293.

Darling TN, et al: A child with antibodies targeting both linear IgA bullous dermatosis and BP antigens. *Arch Dermatol* 1995, 131:1438.

Horiguchi Y, et al: Immunoelectron microscopic observations in a case of linear IgA bullous dermatitis of childhood. *J Am Acad Dermatol* 1986, 14:593.

Kanitakis J, et al: Linear IgA bullous dermatosis of childhood with autoantibodies to a 230 KD epidermal antigen. *Pediatric Dermatol* 1994, 11:139.

Marsden RA, et al: A study of benign chronic bullous dermatosis of childhood and comparison with dermatitis herpetiformis and bullous pemphigoid in childhood. *Clin Exp Dermatol* 1980, 5:159.

Rogers M, et al: Chronic bullous disease of childhood: aspects of management. *Australas J Dermatol* 1982, 23:62.

Sweren RJ, et al: Benign chronic bullous dermatosis of childhood: a review. *Cutis* 1982, 29:350.

Wojnarowska F, et al: A comparative study of benign chronic bullous disease of childhood and linear IgA disease of adults. *Br J Dermatol* 1985, 113(Suppl):16.

Wojnarowska F, et al: Chronic bullous disease of childhood, childhood cicatricial pemphigoid, and linear IgA disease of adults. *J Am Acad Dermatol* 1988, 19:792.

Yeager JK, et al: Vesicles, pustules, and erosions in a child. *Arch Dermatol* 1993, 129:897.

Zeharia A, et al: Successful treatment of chronic bullous disease of childhood with colchicine. *J Am Acad Dermatol* 1994, 30:660.

Zone JJ, et al: IgA antibodies in chronic bullous disease of childhood react with 97-KDa basement membrane zone protein. *J Invest Dermatol* 1996, 106:1277. ▲

TRANSIENT ACANTHOLYTIC DERMATOSIS

In 1970, Grover described a new dermatosis that occurred predominantly in persons over 50 years of age consisting of a sparse eruption, often of limited extent, and nearly always of limited duration. The lesions were fragile vesicles that rapidly turned to crusted and keratotic erosions, usually under 1 cm in diameter. In 1976, Simon et al reported a case persisting for 3 years; they called it *persistent acantholytic dermatosis*. In our experience, it is not uncommon for this eruption to follow a prolonged course. The distribution is predominantly limited to the chest or shoulder girdle area and upper abdomen, although more diffusely present, widespread lesions may rarely be observed.

There are four histologic types resembling, respectively, Darier's disease, pemphigus vulgaris, benign familial pemphigus, and simple spongiosis. Often two or more types can be found in a single biopsy specimen. Direct IF studies yield negative results.

Grover reviewed his 375 patients with the disease in 1984. Many of them were asymptomatic and were discovered in the course of examining the sun-exposed skin of patients with skin cancer. He had only five cases in patients under age 40; most were 60 to 69. Asteatotic eczema occurred five times as often among them as in controls. Skin cancer was almost twice as common, but of course there was a selection bias. The male-female ratio was 3:1.

In immunocompromised patients with cancer, four patients treated with recombinant human interleukin-4 and one patient with ionizing radiation have been reported to develop transient acantholytic dermatosis (TAD). Excessive heat, sweating, and/or fever are hypothesized to be causally associated.

The treatment of choice is potent topical steroids. In the few patients who do not respond and who are symptomatic, isotretinoin is an alternative treatment that is usually effective. Treatment with approximately 0.5 mg/kg for 2 to 6 months may be required. Relapse after discontinuation is variable, but permanent remission may result. Paul et al reported a case with extensive skin lesions, only partly controlled with oral prednisone and not at all by 300,000 units/day of vitamin A, in whom 50 mg of methoxsalen and 2 J/cm^2 of UVA twice a week, increased by 0.5 J/cm^2 each time, first flared the eruption and then improved it slowly. A shielded control patch 10 cm in diameter did not improve, but it improved when shielding was removed. Finally, dapsone may be given for unresponsive symptomatic disease, with reasonable hope for relief.

Grover RW: Transient acantholytic dermatosis. *Arch Dermatol* 1970, 101:426.

Grover RW, et al: The association of transient acantholytic dermatosis with other skin diseases. *J Am Acad Dermatol* 1984, 11:253.

Held JL, et al: Grover's disease provoked by ionizing radiation. *J Am Acad Dermatol* 1988, 19:137.

Helfman RJ: Grover's disease treated with isotretinoin. *J Am Acad Dermatol* 1985, 12:1981.

Liss WA, et al: Zosteriform transient acantholytic dermatosis. *J Am Acad Dermatol* 1993, 29:797.

Mahler SJ, et al: Transient acantholytic dermatosis induced by recombinant human interleukin 4. *J Am Acad Dermatol* 1993, 29:206.

Parsons JM: Transient acantholytic dermatosis (Grover's disease). *J Am Acad Dermatol* 1996, 35:653.

Paul BS, et al: The response of transient acantholytic dermatosis to photochemotherapy. *Arch Dermatol* 1984, 120:121.

Simon RS, et al: Persistent acantholytic dermatosis. *Arch Dermatol* 1976, 112:1429. ▲

CHAPTER 22

Nutritional Diseases

A nutritional disease is caused either by insufficiency or, less often, by excess of one or more dietary essentials. Nutritional diseases are particularly common in underdeveloped tropical countries. Infants and children are particularly at risk for deficiency states, especially malnutrition. Frequently, patients have features of several of these disorders if their diets have been generally restricted. In addition, many of the nutritional disorders have overlapping features. For example, the periorificial dermatitis of zinc deficiency also may be seen in essential fatty acid deficiency, and kwashiorkor. This occurs because these nutrients are essential to overlapping metabolic pathways with a final common expression: abnormal differentiation of the skin. For the same reason, the histologic findings in many types of nutritional dermatoses are similar.

In developed countries, alcoholism is the main cause of nutritional diseases. Nutritional diseases should also be suspected in postoperative patients; psychiatric patients, including those with anorexia nervosa and bulimia; patients on unusual diets; and patients with surgical or inflammatory bowel dysfunction, especially Crohn's disease. Cystic fibrosis may be initially accompanied by nutritional deficiency dermatitis. Deficiency states caused by inborn errors of metabolism are discussed in Chapter 26.

Brooke P: Diseases of nutrition and metabolism. *Adv Dermatol* 1993, 8:155.

Miller SJ: Nutritional deficiency and the skin. *J Am Acad Dermatol* 1989, 21:1.

Olumide YM: Nutritional dermatoses in Nigeria. *Int J Dermatol* 1995, 34:11.

Prendiville JS: Skin signs of nutritional disorders. *Semin Dermatol* 1992, 11:88. _____ ▲

VITAMIN A
Hypovitaminosis A (Phrynoderma)

Vitamin A is a fat-soluble vitamin found as retinyl esters in milk, fish oil, liver, and eggs, and as carotenoids in plants. Vitamin A deficiency is common in children in the developing world. It is rare in developed countries, where it is most commonly associated with diseases of fat malabsorption, such as Crohn's disease, celiac disease, cystic fibrosis, and cholestatic liver disease. Vitamin A is required for the normal keratinization of many mucosal surfaces. When deficient, the resultant abnormal keratinization leads to increased mortality from inflammatory disease of the gut and lung—diarrhea and pneumonia (especially in rubeola). Vitamin A supplementation of 200,000 IU/day for 2 days is recommended for children with rubeola.

The skin eruption, termed *phrynoderma*, or "toadskin," resembles keratosis pilaris. It consists of keratotic papules of various sizes, distributed over the extremities and shoulders, surrounding and arising from the pilosebaceous follicles. Individual lesions are firm, pigmented papules containing a central intrafollicular keratotic plug, which projects from the follicle as a horny spine and leaves a pit when expressed. The eruption usually begins on the anterolateral aspect of the thighs or the posterolateral aspect of the upper arms (Fig. 22-1). It then spreads to the extensor surfaces of both the upper and lower extremities, shoulders, abdomen, back, and buttocks, and finally reaches the face and posterior aspect of the neck. The hands and feet are not involved, and only occasionally are there lesions on the midline of the trunk or in the axillary and anogenital areas. On the face, the eruption resembles acne because of the presence of many large comedones, but it differs from acne in respect to dryness of the skin. The whole skin displays dryness and fine scaling.

In vitamin A deficiency, eye findings are prominent and often pathognomonic. These include night blindness, an inability to see bright light, xerophthalmia, xerosis corneae, and keratomalacia. The earliest finding is delayed adaptation to the dark (nyctalopia). Sometimes there are circumscribed areas of xerosis of the conjunctiva lateral to the cornea, occasionally forming well-defined white spots (Bitot's spots). These are triangular, with the apex toward the canthus. Vitamin A deficiency is a major cause of blindness in children in the developing world. The histologic findings of vitamin A deficiency are hyperkeratosis, horny plugs in the upper portion of the hair follicle, coiled hairs in the upper part of the follicle, severe atrophy of the

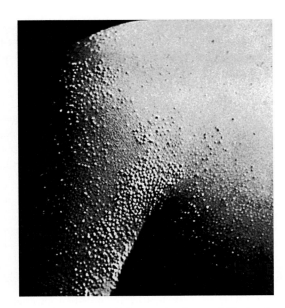

Fig. 22-1 Vitamin A deficiency showing a follicular keratotic eruption. (Courtesy Drs. C.N. Frazier and Ch'uan-K'uei Hu, China.)

sebaceous glands, and squamous metaplasia of the secretory cells of the eccrine sweat glands. If the follicles rupture, perifollicular granulomatous inflammation is found.

The diagnosis of vitamin A deficiency is usually based on the typical eye findings. The diagnosis may be aided by determination of the serum vitamin A level. The treatment is 100,000 IU/day for 2 days and an additional dose of 200,000 IU at the time of discharge, followed by the recommended dietary requirement.

Hypervitaminosis A

Because the skin findings of hypervitaminosis A are similar to the side effects of synthetic retinoid therapy, they are well recognized by most dermatologists. Children are at greater risk for toxicity than adults. Excess megavitamin ingestion may be the cause. In adults, as little as 25,000 IU daily may lead to toxicity, especially in persons with hepatic compromise from alcoholic, viral, or medication-induced hepatitis. Dialysis patients also are at increased risk. If the patient is taking a synthetic retinoid, all vitamin A supplementation should be stopped.

Most of the cases of chronic hypervitaminosis A have been reported in children. There is loss of hair and coarseness of the remaining hair, loss of the eyebrows, exfoliative cheilitis, generalized exfoliation and pigmentation of the skin, and clubbing of the fingers. Moderate widespread itching may occur. Hepatomegaly, splenomegaly, hypochromic anemia, depressed serum proteins, and elevated liver function tests may be found. Bone growth may be retarded by premature closure of the epiphyses in children. Pseudotumor cerebri with papilledema may occur very early, before any other signs appear. In infants this may present as a bulging fontanelle.

In adults, the early signs are dryness of the lips and anorexia. These may be followed by joint and bone pains, follicular hyperkeratosis, branny desquamation of the skin, fissuring of the corners of the mouth and nostrils, dryness and loss of scalp hair and eyebrows, and dystrophy of the nails. Fatigue, myalgia, depression, anorexia, headache (from pseudotumor cerebri), strabismus, and weight loss commonly occur. Liver disease may be progressive and may lead to cirrhosis with chronic toxicity. Hypercalcemia commonly occurs in dialysis patients. Retinoids are teratogens, and birth defects may occur with excess vitamin A supplementation during pregnancy.

Barr DJ, et al: Bypass phrynoderma. *Arch Dermatol* 1984, 120:919.
Fishbane S, et al: Hypervitaminosis A in two hemodialysis patients. *Am J Kidney Dis* 1995, 25:346.
Roe DA: Assessment of risk factors for carotenodermia and cutaneous findings of hypervitaminosis A in college-aged populations. *Semin Dermatol* 1991, 10:303.
Sharieff GX, et al: Pseudotumor cerebri and hypercalcemia resulting from vitamin A toxicity. *Ann Emerg Med* 1996, 27:518.
Silverman AK, et al: Hypervitaminosis A syndrome: a paradigm of retinoid side effects. *J Am Acad Dermatol* 1987, 16:1027. ▲

VITAMIN D

Although active vitamin D is produced in the skin, deficiency of vitamin D has no skin manifestations, except for alopecia. The elderly have decreased vitamin D cutaneous photosynthesis by reason of decreased sun exposure and poor intake of vitamin D, both of which predispose them to osteomalacia. Other patients at risk include those who are debilitated with limited sun exposure, those taking anticonvulsants, and those with fat malabsorption. Supplementation for these patients should be considered. Extensive sun protection and sunscreen use does not appear to lead to vitamin D deficiency.

Sollitto RB, et al: Normal vitamin D levels can be maintained despite rigorous photoprotection. *J Am Acad Dermatol* 1997, 37:942. ▲

Vitamin D Excess

Vitamin D overdose causes hypercalcemia and generalized calcinosis. Metastatic calcification may occur in the skin.

Hochberg Z, et al: Calcitriol-resistant rickets with alopecia. *Arch Dermatol* 1985, 121:646.
Holick MF: Vitamin D resistance and alopecia. *Arch Dermatol* 1985, 121:601. ▲

VITAMIN E DEFICIENCY

Most common in infants with low birth weight, vitamin E deficiency presents with peripheral edema, progressive neuromyopathy, and ophthalmoplegia.

Granot E, et al: Vitamin E deficiency and peripheral edema. *Ann Intern Med* 1989, 111:859. _____ ▲

VITAMIN K DEFICIENCY

Dietary deficiency of vitamin K, a fat-soluble vitamin, does not occur in adults because it is synthesized by bacteria in the large intestine. However, deficiency may occur in adults because of malabsorption caused by biliary disease, malabsorption syndromes, cystic fibrosis, or anorexia nervosa. Liver disease of all causes produces deficiency. Drugs such as coumarin, salicylates, cholestyramine, and perhaps the cephalosporins may induce a deficiency state. Newborns of mothers taking coumarin or phenytoin or premature infants with an uncolonized intestine can be vitamin K-deficient. The result is a decrease in the vitamin K-dependent clotting factors II, VII, IX, and X. The cutaneous manifestations that result are purpura, hemorrhage, and ecchymosis. Treatment is 5 mg to 10 mg/day of intramuscular vitamin K for several days. In acute crises, fresh frozen plasma is used.

VITAMIN B$_1$ DEFICIENCY

Vitamin B$_1$ (thiamine) deficiency results in beriberi. The skin manifestations are limited to edema. Peripheral neuropathy is common.

Comabella M, et al: Iatrogenic fulminant beriberi. *Lancet* 1995, 346:182. _____ ▲

VITAMIN B$_2$ DEFICIENCY

Vitamin B$_2$ (riboflavin) deficiency is seen most often in alcoholic patients; however, phototherapy for neonatal icterus, acute boric acid ingestion, hypothyroidism, and chlorpromazine use have been reported to cause it also. The classic findings are the oral-ocular-genital syndrome. The lips are prominently affected with angular cheilitis (perlèche) and cheilosis. The tongue is atrophic and magenta. A seborrheic-like dermatitis with follicular keratosis around the nares, primarily affects the face. Genital dermatitis is worse in men than it is in women who have riboflavin deficiency. There is a confluent dermatitis of the scrotum, sparing the midline, with extension onto the thighs. Photophobia and blepharitis angularis occur. The response to 5 mg of riboflavin daily is dramatic.

Roe DA: Riboflavin deficiency. *Semin Dermatol* 1991, 10:293. _____ ▲

VITAMIN B$_6$
Pyridoxine Deficiency

Pyridoxine deficiency may occur in cases of uremia and cirrhosis, as well as with the use of certain pharmacologic agents. Skin changes include a seborrheic dermatitis–like eruption, atrophic glossitis with ulceration, angular cheilitis, conjunctivitis, and intertrigo. Occasionally, a pellagra-like eruption may occur. Neurologic symptoms include somnolence, confusion, and neuropathy.

Pyridoxine Excess

Friedman et al reported a case of a patient who ingested large doses of pyridoxine (vitamin B$_6$) and developed a subepidermal vesicular dermatosis and sensory peripheral neuropathy. The bullous dermatosis resembled epidermolysis bullosa acquisita.

Friedman MA, et al: Subepidermal vesicular dermatosis and sensory peripheral neuropathy caused by pyridoxine abuse. *J Am Acad Dermatol* 1986, 14:915. _____ ▲

VITAMIN B$_{12}$ DEFICIENCY

Vitamin B$_{12}$ (cyanocobalamin) is absorbed through the distal ileum after binding to gastric intrinsic factor in an acid pH. Deficiency is caused mainly by gastrointestinal abnormalities such as a deficiency of intrinsic factor, achlorhydria, ileal diseases, and malabsorption syndromes resulting from pancreatic disease or sprue. Congenital lack of transcobalamin II can also produce B$_{12}$ deficiency. Because of the large body stores in adults, deficiency occurs 3 to 6 years after gastrointestinal abnormalities.

Glossitis, hyperpigmentation, and canities are the main dermatologic manifestations. The tongue is bright red, sore, and atrophic. The hyperpigmentation is generalized, but it is more commonly accentuated in exposed areas such as the face and hands and in the palmar creases and flexures, resembling Addison's disease. The nails may be pigmented. Premature gray hair may occur paradoxically. Megaloblastic anemia is present. Weakness, paresthesias, numbness, ataxia, and other neurologic findings occur.

Parenteral replacement with intramuscular injections, 1 mg/week for 1 month, then 1 mg/month, leads to a reversal of the pigmentary changes in the skin, nails, mucous membranes, and hair. Neurologic defects may or may not improve.

Marks VJ, et al: Hyperpigmentation in megaloblastic anemia. *J Am Acad Dermatol* 1985, 12:914.
Noppakun N, et al: Reversible hyperpigmentation of skin and nails with white hair due to vitamin B$_{12}$ deficiency. *Arch Dermatol* 1986, 122:896. ▲

FOLIC ACID DEFICIENCY

Diffuse hyperpigmentation, glossitis, cheilitis, and megaloblastic anemia, identical to vitamin B$_{12}$ deficiency, occur in folic acid deficiency.

Downham TF, et al: Hyperpigmentation and folate deficiency. *Arch Dermatol* 1976, 112:562. _____ ▲

SCURVY

Scurvy, or vitamin C deficiency, is the deficiency disease most commonly diagnosed by dermatologists, since cutaneous manifestations are early and prominent features. Elderly male alcoholics and psychiatric patients on restrictive diets are most commonly affected.

The four *H*s are characteristic of scurvy: *h*emorrhagic signs, *h*yperkeratosis of the hair follicles, *h*ypochondriasis, and *h*ematologic abnormalities. Perifollicular petechiae are the characteristic finding. In addition, ecchymoses of various sizes, especially on the lower extremities, are common (Fig. 22-2, *A*). These may be associated with tender nodules (subcutaneous and intramuscular hemorrhage) and subperiosteal hemorrhage, leading to pseudoparalysis in children. Woody edema may be present. Subungual, subconjunctival, intramuscular, and intraarticular hemorrhage may also occur. The consulting diagnosis is often vasculitis.

Another characteristic finding is keratotic plugging of the hair follicles, chiefly on the anterior forearms, abdomen, and posterior thighs (Fig. 22-2, *B*). The hair shafts are curled in follicles capped by keratotic plugs (Fig. 22-2, *C*). This distinctive finding has been named "corkscrew hairs."

Hemorrhagic gingivitis (Fig. 22-2, *D*) occurs adjacent to teeth and presents as swelling and bleeding of the gums. The teeth are loose, and the breath is foul. Gingival disease may be absent, especially in the edentulous and in those with good oral hygiene. Epistaxis, delayed wound healing, and depression also may occur. Frequently, anemia is present and may be the result of blood loss or associated deficiencies of other nutrients such as folate.

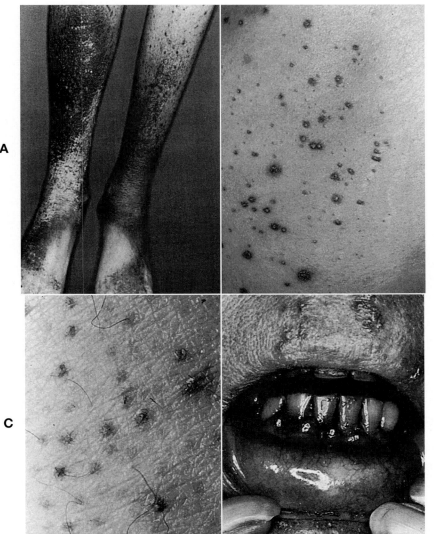

Fig. 22-2 Scurvy. **A,** Extensive ecchymoses of the lower extremities. **B,** Keratotic plugging and perifollicular hemorrhage of the skin. **C,** Corkscrew hairs and perifollicular hemorrhage. **D,** Swollen, hemorrhagic gingiva. (**C,** Courtesy Dr. Axel W. Hoke.)

The diagnosis of scurvy is usually made on clinical grounds and confirmed by a positive response to vitamin C. A biopsy will exclude vasculitis and demonstrate follicular hyperkeratosis, coiled hairs, and perifollicular hemorrhage in the absence of inflammation. Serum ascorbic acid levels may be confirmatory in unusual cases. Treatment is with ascorbic acid, 800 to 1000 mg daily for 1 week.

Adelman HM: Scurvy resembling cutaneous vasculitis. *Cutis* 1994, 54:111.
Ghorbani AJ, et al: Scurvy. *J Am Acad Dermatol* 1994, 30:881.
Ural AB, et al: Scurvy presenting with cutaneous and articular signs and decrease in red and white blood cells. *Int J Dermatol* 1996, 35:879.

NIACIN DEFICIENCY (PELLAGRA)

Pellagra usually results from a deficiency of nicotinic acid (niacin, vitamin B_3) or its precursor amino acid, tryptophan. It is associated classically with a diet almost entirely composed of corn, millet, or sorghum. Other vitamin deficiencies (especially pyridoxine) or malnutrition, which interfere with the conversion of tryptophan to niacin, often coexist and are required for the signs and symptoms of pellagra to occur. In the developed countries, most cases of pellagra occur in alcoholics. Other possible causes of pellagra are as follows:
- Carcinoid tumors, which divert tryptophan to serotonin
- Hartnup disease (impaired absorption of tryptophan)
- Intestinal parasites, especially hookworm
- Gastrointestinal disorders, for example, Crohn's and gastrointestinal surgery
- Prolonged intravenous supplementation
- Psychiatric disease, including anorexia nervosa

Pellagra also has been induced by certain medications, most commonly isoniazid, azathioprine (and its metabolite 6-mercaptopurine), and 5-fluorouracil, and less commonly the hydantoins, phenobarbital, ethionamide, protionamide, and pyrazinamide.

Clinical Features

Pellagra is a chronic disease affecting the gastrointestinal tract, the nervous system, and the skin; hence, the mnemonic of the 3 *D*s: *d*iarrhea, *d*ementia, and *d*ermatitis (Figs. 22-3 to 22-5).

Four types of dermatitis are seen in cases of pellagra: (1) a photosensitive eruption, (2) perineal lesions, (3) thickening and pigmentation over bony prominences, and (4) seborrheic dermatitis–like eruption on the face. The most characteristic is the photosensitive eruption, which worsens in the spring and summer. It occurs symmetrically on the face, neck, and upper chest (Casal's necklace); extensor arms; and backs of the hands. Initially, there is erythema and swelling after sun exposure, accompanied by itching and burning or pain. In severe cases, the eruption may be vesicular or bullous (wet pellagra). When compared with normal sunburn, the pellagrous skin takes about four

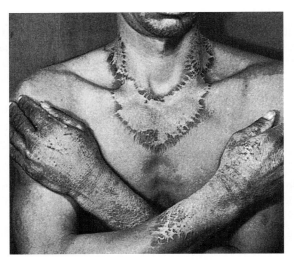

Fig. 22-3 Pellagra with typical "Casal's necklace" and lesions on the hands and forearms. (Courtesy Dr. M. el-Zawahry, Egypt.)

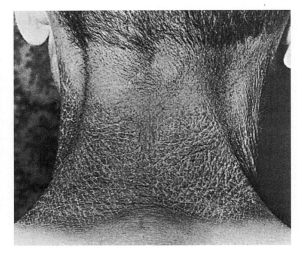

Fig. 22-4 Pellagra on the neck. (Courtesy Dr. M. el-Zawahry, Egypt.)

times longer to recover from the acute phototoxic injury. After several phototoxic events, thickening, scaling, and hyperpigmentation of the affected skin occurs. The skin has a copper or mahogany hue. In protracted cases, the skin ultimately becomes dry, smooth, paper-thin, and glassy with a parchment-like consistency. Scarring rarely occurs.

The nose is fairly characteristic. There is dull erythema of the bridge of the nose, with fine, yellow, powdery scales over the follicular orifices (sulfur flakes). The eruption resembles seborrheic dermatitis, except for its location. Plugs of inspissated sebum may project from dilated orifices on the nose, giving it a rough appearance.

Scrotal and perineal erythema and erosions are common. The mucous membranes of the mouth and vagina are

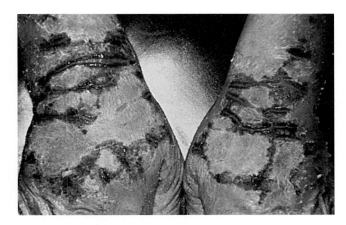

Fig. 22-5 Pellagra in an alcoholic patient. (Courtesy Dr. Axel W. Hoke.)

affected by painful fissures, ulcerations, and atrophy. Angular cheilitis occurs.

At the onset, there is weakness, loss of appetite, abdominal pain, diarrhea, mental depression, and photosensitivity. Skin lesions may be the earliest sign, with phototoxicity being the presenting symptom in some cases. Neurologic and gastrointestinal symptoms can occur without skin changes. In the later stages of the disease, the neurologic symptoms may predominate. Apathy, depression, muscle weakness, paresthesias, headaches, and attacks of dizziness or falling are typical findings. Hallucinations, psychosis, seizures, dementia, neurologic degeneration, and coma may develop. The disease is progressive, and the majority of patients die within 4 or 5 years if it goes untreated.

Pathology

Histologically, the findings in the skin vary according to the stage of the disease. There may be orthokeratosis or slight confluent parakeratosis; basilar pigmentation is increased. Papillary dermal vessels are dilated with papillary dermal edema. The most characteristic finding is pallor and vacuolar changes of the keratinocytes in a band in the upper layers of the stratum malpighii, just below the granular cell layer, which may be attenuated. If marked, a cleft may form in the upper epidermis, correlating with the blistering seen in wet pellagra.

Diagnosis and Treatment

If the characteristic skin findings are present, the diagnosis is not difficult clinically. Dietary treatment to correct the malnutrition is essential. Animal proteins, eggs, milk, and vegetables are beneficial and should be supplemented with 100 mg nicotinamide four times daily. Fluid and electrolyte loss from diarrhea should be replaced, and in patients with gastrointestinal symptoms, possibly interfering with absorption, initial intravenous supplementation should be considered. Within 24 hours after niacin therapy is begun, the skin lesions begin to resolve, confirming the diagnosis. Alcoholism must be treated if present, and the factors that may have led to pellagra must be corrected. If these are not addressed, complications of pellagra, which are sometimes fatal, may occur without reappearance of the skin eruption.

Hendricks WM: Pellagra and pellagra-like dermatoses. *Semin Dermatol* 1991, 10:282.
Jarrett P, et al: Pellagra, azathioprine, and inflammatory bowel disease. *Clin Exp Dermatol* 1997, 22:44.
Judd LE, et al: Pellagra in a patient with an eating disorder. *Br J Dermatol* 1991, 125:71.
Oakley A, et al: Hartnup disease presenting in an adult. *Clin Exp Dermatol* 1994, 19:407.
Rapaport MJ: Pellagra in a patient with anorexia nervosa. *Arch Dermatol* 1985, 121:125.
Stevens HP, et al: Pellagra secondary to 5-fluorouracil. *Br J Dermatol* 1993, 128:578. ▲

BIOTIN DEFICIENCY

Biotin is universally available and is produced by intestinal bacteria. Therefore, deficiency is rare but can occur in patients with short gut or malabsorption. Sometimes it occurs in individuals taking antibiotics or receiving parenteral nutrition. Ingestion of avidin, found in raw egg white, may bind biotin, leading to deficiency. The two inherited syndromes of multiple carboxylase deficiency—holocarboxylase synthetase deficiency (neonatal type) and biotinidase deficiency (juvenile type)—have similar features. The presentations are variable, with some patients having only some of the characteristic features.

A dermatitis similar to that found in cases of zinc deficiency and essential fatty acid deficiency is seen. It is periorificial and characterized by patchy, red, eroded lesions on the face and groin. *Candida* is regularly present on the lesions. Alopecia, sometimes total, including loss of the eyebrows and eyelashes can occur. Conjunctivitis may be present. Neurologic findings are prominent. In adults, these include depression, lethargy, hallucinations, and limb paresthesias. In infants, neurologic findings include hypotonia, lethargy, a withdrawn behavior, seizures, and developmental delay. Death may occur. The diagnosis of the inherited forms is made by detecting organic aminoaciduria with 3-hydroxyisovaleric acid. Treatment consists of 10 mg of biotin daily. Skin lesions resolve rapidly, but the neurologic damage may be permanent.

Mock DM: Skin manifestations of biotin deficiency. *Semin Dermatol* 1991, 10:296. ▲

ZINC DEFICIENCY

Zinc deficiency may be an inherited abnormality, acrodermatitis enteropathica, or it may be acquired. Presentation in infancy is the most common type. Premature infants are at particular risk because of inadequate body zinc stores, suboptimal absorption, and high zinc requirements. Normally, human breast milk has adequate zinc, and weaning classically precipitates clinical zinc deficiency in premature infants and in infants with acrodermatitis enteropathica. However, clinical zinc deficiency may occur in full-term and premature infants still breast-feeding. This is due to either low maternal breast milk zinc levels or a higher zinc requirement by the infant than the breast milk can provide (even though the zinc level in the breast milk is normal).

Parenteral nutrition without adequate zinc content may lead to zinc deficiency. Acquired zinc deficiency also occurs in alcoholics as a result of poor nutritional intake and increased urinary excretion; as a complication of malabsorption, inflammatory bowel disease, or jejunoileal bypass; and, occasionally, in cases of anorexia nervosa and AIDS. Zinc requirements increase during metabolic stress; so symptomatic deficiency may present during infections, after trauma or surgery, with malignancy, during pregnancy, and with renal disease. Diets containing mainly cereal grains are high in phytate, which binds zinc and causes endemic zinc deficiency in certain areas of the Middle East and North Africa.

The dermatitis found in all forms of zinc deficiency is pustular and bullous, with an acral and periorificial distribution. On the face, in the groin, and in other flexors there is a patchy, red, dry scaling with exudation and crusting (Figs. 22-6 and 22-7). Angular cheilitis and stomatitis are present. The periungual areas are erythematous, scaling, and sometimes have superficial, flaccid pustules. Nail dystrophy may result. Chronic lesions may be more psoriasiform. Generalized alopecia is characteristic.

Diarrhea is present in most cases. Growth retardation, ophthalmic findings, impaired wound healing, and central nervous system manifestations occur. Patients are particularly irritable and emotionally labile. Many abnormalities of the immune response occur in zinc deficiency.

The histologies of acquired and hereditary zinc deficiency are identical. There is vacuolation of the keratinocytes of the upper stratum malpighii. These areas of vacuolation may become confluent, forming a subcorneal bulla. In larger lesions, there may be total epidermal necrosis with subepidermal blister formation. Neutrophils are typically present.

The diagnosis of zinc deficiency should be suspected in at-risk individuals with acral or periorificial dermatitis. Particularly, chronic diaper rash with diarrhea in an infant should lead to evaluation for zinc deficiency. The diagnosis can be confirmed by low serum zinc levels. A low serum alkaline phosphatase, a zinc-dependent enzyme, may be a valuable adjunctive test where the serum zinc level is normal or near normal. In some patients, even if the zinc level is in the normal range, if the skin lesions are characteristic, a trial of zinc supplementation should be considered. Replacement is with zinc sulfate 1 to

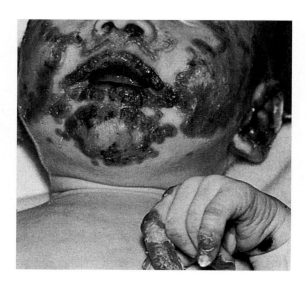

Fig. 22-6 Typical perioral and facial lesions of acrodermatitis enteropathica.

2 mg/kg/day (50 mg of elemental zinc per 220 mg zinc sulfate tablet). In acquired cases, transient treatment and addressing the underlying condition are adequate. In cases of acrodermatitis enteropathica, supplementation is 3 mg/kg/day and should be lifelong.

Bailly A, et al: Acrodermatitis enteropathica and Crohn's disease. *J Am Acad Dermatol* 1984, 11:525.

Borroni G, et al: Bullous lesions in acrodermatitis enteropathica. *Am J Dermatopathol* 1992, 14:304.

Fraker PJ, et al: Zinc deficiency and immune function. *Arch Dermatol* 1987, 123:1699.

Gaveau D, et al: Cutaneous manifestations of zinc deficiency in alcoholics. *Acta Derm Venereol* 1987, 114:39.

Kanekura T, et al: Zinc deficiency. *Cutis* 1991, 48:161.

Krasovec M, et al: Acrodermatitis enteropathica secondary to Crohn's disease. *Dermatology* 1996, 193:361.

Kuramoto Y, et al: Acquired zinc deficiency in breast-fed infants. *Semin Dermatol* 1991, 10:309.

Lee MG, et al: Transient symptomatic zinc deficiency in a full-term breast-fed infant. *J Am Acad Dermatol* 1990, 23:375.

Reichel M, et al: Acrodermatitis enteropathica in a patient with AIDS. *Arch Dermatol* 1992, 128:415.

Van Voorhees AS, et al: Acquired zinc deficiency in association with anorexia nervosa. *Pediatr Dermatol* 1992, 9:268.

West BL, et al: Alcohol and acquired acrodermatitis enteropathica. *J Am Acad Dermatol* 1986, 15:1305. ──────────────── ▲

ESSENTIAL FATTY ACID DEFICIENCY

Essential fatty acid (EFA) deficiency can occur in infants with low birth weight, gastrointestinal anomalies, inflammatory bowel disease, intestinal surgery, and prolonged parenteral nutrition without EFA supplementation. The resulting dermatitis is similar to that seen in zinc and biotin deficiency. There is a generalized xerosis, since EFAs

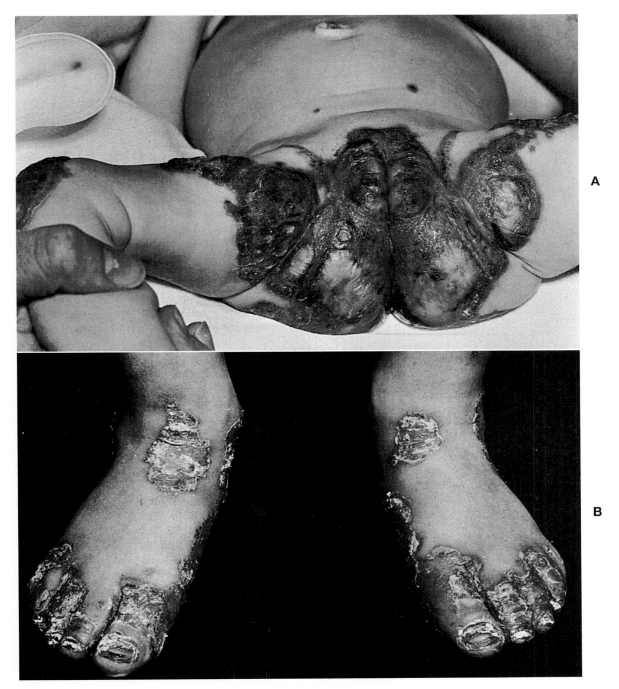

Fig. 22-7 A and **B** Acrodermatitis enteropathica. (**A,** From Wells BT, Winkelman RK: *Arch Dermatol* 1961, 84:40. **B,** Courtesy Dr. D. Bloom.)

constitute up to one quarter of the fatty acids of the stratum corneum and are required for normal epidermal barrier function. Widespread erythema and an intertriginous weeping eruption are seen. The hair becomes lighter in color, and diffuse alopecia is present. Poor wound healing, growth failure, and increased risk of infection may occur. There is a decrease in linoleic acid and an increase in palmitoleic and oleic acids. A ratio of eicosatrienoic acid to arachidonic acid of more than 0.4 is diagnostic of EFA deficiency. Intravenous lipid therapy with Intralipid 10% reverses the process. Topical safflower oil emulsion or sunflower seed oil applications may not be able to prevent or treat EFA deficiency and may predispose patients to α-linolenic acid deficiency.

Sacks GS, et al: Failure of topical vegetable oils to prevent essential fatty acid deficiency in a critically ill patient receiving long-term parenteral nutrition. *J Parenter Enteral Nutr* 1994, 18:274. _____ ▲

IRON DEFICIENCY

Iron deficiency is common, especially among actively menstruating women, particularly if they have little red meat in their diets, and have not made an effort to replace their losses with other foods. Mucocutaneous findings include koilonychia, glossitis, angular cheilitis, pruritus, and telogen effluvium diffuse hair loss. Plummer-Vinson syndrome is the combination of microcytic anemia, dysphagia, and glossitis, seen almost entirely in middle-aged women. The lips are thin and the opening of the mouth is small and inelastic, so that there is a rather characteristic appearance. Smooth atrophy of the tongue is pronounced. Koilonychia is present in 40% to 50% of patients, and alopecia may be present.

An esophageal web in the postcricoid area may occur, presenting as difficulty swallowing, or the feeling that food is stuck in the throat. The diagnosis is confirmed by measuring the serum iron level. Treatment consists of iron sulfate supplementation, 325 mg three times daily.

Sato S: Iron deficiency. *Semin Dermatol* 1991, 10:313. _____ ▲

SELENIUM DEFICIENCY

Selenium deficiency occurs in patients on parenteral nutrition, in areas where soil selenium content is poor, and in low–birth-weight infants. Manifestations in children include hypopigmentation of the skin and hair (pseudoalbinism). Leukonychia and Terry's-like nails have been reported. Cardiomyopathy, muscle pain, and weakness with elevated muscle enzymes are the major features. Treatment consists of 3 μg/kg/day of selenium.

PROTEIN-ENERGY MALNUTRITION

Protein-energy malnutrition is a spectrum of related diseases including marasmus, kwashiorkor, and marasmic kwashiorkor. These conditions are endemic in the developing world. Marasmus represents prolonged deficiency of protein and calories and is diagnosed in children who are below 60% of their ideal body weight without edema or hypoproteinemia. Kwashiorkor occurs with protein deficiency but a relatively adequate caloric intake. It is diagnosed in children between 60% and 80% of their ideal body weight with edema or hypoproteinemia. Marasmic kwashiorkor shows features of both conditions and is diagnosed in children who are less than 60% of

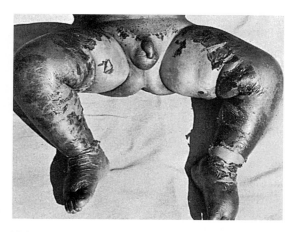

Fig. 22-8 Kwashiorkor with distinctive skin changes. (Courtesy Dr. E.B. Adams, Durban, Natal.)

their ideal body weight with features of edema or hypoproteinemia.

These conditions are rare in developed countries, but occasionally, kwashiorkor may occur as a result of cystic fibrosis or severe dietary restrictions instituted to improve infantile atopic dermatitis. Of infants with cystic fibrosis, 3% to 13% develop protein-calorie malnutrition, and in some a skin eruption is an early finding. The exact cause of this eruption is unknown, but deficiencies of zinc, essential fatty acids, protein, or some combination of these have been proposed. Untreated, this may be associated with severe morbidity and mortality.

Darmstadt GL, et al: Dermatitis as a presenting sign of cystic fibrosis. *Arch Dermatol* 1992, 128:1358.

McLaren DS: Skin changes in protein energy malnutrition. *Arch Dermatol* 1987, 123:1674.

Phillips RJ, et al: Cystic fibrosis presenting as kwashiorkor with florid skin rash. *Arch Dis Child* 1993, 69:446. _____ ▲

Marasmus

In cases of marasmus, the skin is dry, wrinkled, and loose because of marked loss of subcutaneous fat. The "monkey facies," caused by loss of the buccal fat pad, is characteristic. In contrast to kwashiorkor, there is no edema or dermatosis.

Kwashiorkor

Kwashiorkor produces hair and skin changes (Fig. 22-8), edema, impaired growth, and the characteristic potbelly (Fig. 22-9). The hair and skin changes are usually striking. Africans call the victims of kwashiorkor "red children." The hair is hypopigmented, varying in color from a reddish yellow to gray or even white. The hair is dry and lusterless; curly hair becomes soft and straight; and marked scaling

The skin lesions are hypopigmented on dark skin and erythematous or purple on fair skin. Lesions first appear in areas of friction or pressure: the flexures, groin, buttocks, and elbows. Hyperpigmented patches occur with slightly raised edges. As they progress, they resemble old, dark, deteriorating enamel paint with peeling or desquamation. This has been described variously as "crazy pavement," "crackled skin," "mosaic skin," "enamel paint," and "flaky paint." In severe cases, the peeling leaves pale, ulcerated hypopigmented areas with hyperpigmented borders.

Buno IJ, et al: The enamel paint sign in the dermatologic diagnosis of early-onset kwashiorkor. *Arch Dermatol* 1998, 134:107.

Latham MC: The dermatosis of kwashiorkor in young children. *Semin Dermatol* 1991, 10:270. ————————————— ▲

CAROTENEMIA AND LYCOPENEMIA

Excessive ingestion of carrots, oranges, squash, spinach, yellow corn and beans, butter, eggs, rutabagas, pumpkins, yellow turnips, sweet potatoes, or papaya may lead to a yellowish discoloration of the skin, which is especially prominent on the palms, soles, and central face. Carotenemia occurs most commonly in vegetarians and food faddists. The sclerae are spared. In lycopenemia, excess ingestion of red foods such as tomatoes, beets, chili beans, and various fruits and berries leads to a reddish discoloration of the skin.

Svensson A, Vahlquist A: Metabolic carotenemia and carotenoderma in a child. *Acta Derm Venereol* 1995, 75(1):70. ————————— ▲

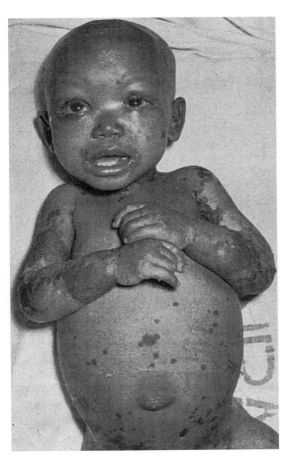

Fig. 22-9 Typical potbelly of kwashiorkor. (Courtesy Dr. E.B. Adams, Durban, Natal.)

(crackled hair) is seen. Especially striking is the flag sign, affecting long, normally dark hair. The hair grown during periods of poor nutrition is pale, so that alternating bands of pale and dark hair can be seen along a single strand, indicating alternating periods of good and poor nutrition. The nails are soft and thin.

CHAPTER 23

Diseases of Subcutaneous Fat

An inflammatory disorder that is primarily localized in the subcutaneous fat is termed a *panniculitis*. This group of disorders may be very difficult both for the clinician and the dermatopathologist. Clinically, lesions present as subcutaneous nodules, and because of their depth many disorders appear similar. Histopathologically, the subcutaneous fat is a rather homogenous tissue, and inflammatory processes may show considerable overlap. One way of looking at panniculitis is to separate erythema nodosum, as the prototypical septal panniculitis, from those processes that primarily involve the fat lobules—the lobular panniculitides. Some lobular panniculitides are due to diseases, such as a vasculitis, which are discussed in other chapters. The remaining lobular panniculitides are categorized by their pathogenesis.

Sanz Vico MD, et al: Erythema nodosum versus nodular vasculitis. *Int J Dermatol* 1993, 32:108.

White WL, et al: Panniculitis. *Semin Cutan Med Surg* 1996, 15:278. ▲

SEPTAL PANNICULITIS (ACUTE AND CHRONIC ERYTHEMA NODOSUM)

Erythema nodosum (EN) is a common inflammatory panniculitis. It occurs in two forms: acute, which is common, and chronic, which is rarer. Acute EN may occur at any age and in both sexes, but most cases occur in young adult women. The eruption consists of bilateral, symmetrical, deep, tender nodules 1 to 10 cm in diameter (Fig. 23-1). Usually there are up to 10 lesions, but in severe cases many more may be found. Initially, the skin over the nodules is red, smooth, slightly elevated, and shiny. The most common location is the pretibial area. In general, the lesions should be primarily on the anterior rather than posterior calf. Lesions may also be seen on the upper legs, extensor arms, neck, and rarely the face. The onset is acute, frequently associated with malaise, leg edema, and arthritis or arthralgias (usually of the ankles, knees, or wrists). Fever, headache, conjunctivitis, and various gastrointestinal complaints may also be present. Over a few days, the lesions flatten, leaving a purple or blue-green color resembling a deep bruise (erythema contusiforme). Ulceration does not occur, and the lesions resolve without atrophy or scarring. The natural history is for the nodules to last a few days or weeks, appearing in crops, and then slowly involute.

Acute EN is a reactive process. It is commonly associated with a streptococcal infection. Tuberculosis was at one time an important causative factor, especially in children. Intestinal infection with *Yersinia, Salmonella,* or *Shigella* may precipitate EN. Other infectious causes include systemic fungal infections (coccidioidomycosis, histoplasmosis, sporotrichosis, and blastomycosis) and toxoplasmosis. Erythema nodosum–like lesions have been described in other infectious diseases such as *Campylobacter* septicemia, brucellosis, psittacosis, cat-scratch disease, and many others. These cases have been inadequately evaluated to exclude the possibility that they represent localized infections in the fat caused by these organisms.

Sarcoidosis may present with fever, cough, joint pains, hilar adenopathy, and EN. This symptom complex, known as *Lofgren's syndrome,* is especially common in Scandinavia. Erythema nodosum is frequently seen in patients with inflammatory bowel disease, more commonly regional enteritis than ulcerative colitis.

Erythema nodosum has been rarely reported in association with various hematologic malignancies, but this is less common than Sweet's syndrome or pyoderma gangrenosum. In fact, when carefully evaluated, these cases of "EN and lymphoma" often represent subcutaneous lymphoma rather than EN.

Drugs may also induce erythema nodosum. The bromides, iodides, and sulfonamides were once the most frequent causative agents. Currently, oral contraceptives are the most common drug inducing EN. This association, the predominance in young women, and the occurrence of EN in pregnancy suggest that estrogens may predispose to the development of EN.

Erythema nodosum–like lesions have been described in Behçet's syndrome and Sweet's syndrome, and probably represent these inflammatory processes occurring in the fat, rather than the coexistence of two disorders.

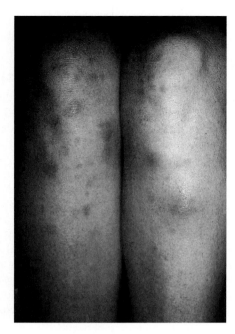

Fig. 23-1 Erythema nodosum.

Chronic Erythema Nodosum (Erythema Nodosum Migrans, Subacute Migratory Panniculitis)

This form of septal panniculitis is much less common than acute EN. It is distinguished from acute EN by the following features:

1. The lesions tend to occur in older women.
2. Lesions are unilateral or asymmetrical if bilateral.
3. They are not associated with systemic symptoms except arthralgias.
4. Lesions are painless or less tender than acute EN lesions.
5. They are not associated with underlying diseases.
6. They begin as a single lesion that tends to resolve but migrates centrifugally, forming annular plaques of subcutaneous nodules with central clearing.
7. They have a prolonged course of months to years.

In the differential diagnosis of EN one must consider other forms of panniculitis. Erythema induratum usually affects primarily the posterior calves alone and runs a slower course, with the possibility of ulceration and scarring. Syphilitic gummas, as well as the nodules of sporotrichosis, are, as a rule, unilateral. Subcutaneous fat necrosis associated with pancreatitis and nodular vasculitis may also occur on the shins, but associated clinical features and/or histologic features will allow the differentiation to be made. In most cases, the classic picture of the acute onset of symmetrical, red, tender nodules on the anterior shins of a young woman will allow the diagnosis of EN to be easily made without a biopsy.

Erythema nodosum is a septal panniculitis; the inflammatory infiltrate principally involves the connective-tissue septa between fat lobules throughout the evolution of the lesion. The infiltrate may be composed of either neutrophils (early) or lymphocytes and other mononuclear cells (later), or a mixture, depending on what stage the lesion is biopsied. In older lesions histiocytes and multinucleate giant cells may predominate. Fat lobules are only secondarily affected by the inflammation, but some foamy histiocytes may be seen in the evolution of the lesions. Meischer's radial granulomas, aggregates of histiocytes around stellate clefts, are characteristic but not diagnostic of EN. Leukocytoclastic vasculitis is not a histologic feature of erythema nodosum. In chronic EN septal fibrosis and septal granulomas of epithelioid macrophages are seen.

Treatment of Erythema Nodosum

Any underlying abnormality should be treated. Bed rest is of great value and may be all that is required in mild cases. Gentle support hose are also helpful. Curtailing vigorous exercise during the acute attacks will shorten the course. Aspirin, nonsteroidal antiinflammatory drugs (NSAIDs), and indomethacin are often helpful. Potassium iodide is safe and effective treatment. As a supersaturated solution, 5 drops three times a day, increased by 1 drop per dose per day up to 15 drops three times a day, is one easy-to-remember dose schedule. As a tablet, the dose is one 300-mg tablet three times a day. Induction of hypothyroidism by prolonged iodide therapy should be watched for. Once controlled the therapy is gradually reduced over 2 to 3 weeks. Intralesional corticosteroid injections will control persistent lesions. Systemic steroids will result in rapid resolution of lesions, if not contraindicated by the underlying precipitating cause.

For chronic erythema nodosum, SSKI is also effective. In refractory cases, antimalarials or colchicine may be tried.

The prognosis usually is good, the attack running its course in 3 to 6 weeks. Recurrences do occur, especially if the underlying condition or infection is still present. Chronic lesions should suggest an alternative diagnosis, such as nodular vasculitis.

Arsura EL, et al: Erythema nodosum in pregnant patients with coccidioidomycosis. *Clin Infect Dis* 1998, 27:1201.

Bartralot R, et al: Liquefactive panniculitis in the inguinal area as the first sign of chronic renal brucellosis. *J Am Acad Dermatol* 1996, 35:339.

Cribier B, et al: Erythema nodosum and associated diseases. *Int J Dermatol* 1998, 37:667.

Horio T, et al: Potassium iodide in erythema nodosum and other erythematous dermatoses. *J Am Acad Dermatol* 1983, 9:77.

Jarrett P, et al: Hydroxychloroquine and chronic erythema nodosum. *Br J Dermatol* 1996, 134:372.

Matsuoka LY: Neoplastic erythema nodosum. *J Am Acad Dermatol* 1995, 32:361.

Tami LF: Erythema nodosum associated with *Shigella* colitis. *Arch Dermatol* 1985, 121:590.

Veloso FT, et al: Immune-related systemic manifestations of inflammatory bowel disease. *J Clin Gastroenterol* 1996, 23:29. _____ ▲

Lobular panniculitis

VESSEL-BASED LOBULAR PANNICULITIS

Thrombosis of blood vessels may lead to fat necrosis caused by ischemia. This can occur in the primary vasculopathies such as polyarteritis nodosa and Churg-Strauss, in metabolic disorders such as oxalosis and calciphylaxis, with atheromatous emboli, and with heparin and Coumadin necrosis and various coagulopathies. These entities are discussed in other chapters. The two disorders that present as a lobular panniculitis and are due to other vascular abnormalities are nodular vasculitis and sclerosing panniculitis.

Nodular Vasculitis

Clinically and histologically, nodular vasculitis is identical to erythema induratum. Nodular vasculitis presents as tender, subcutaneous nodules of the calves of middle-aged, thick-legged women. Lesions are bilateral, less red and tender than erythema nodosum, often ulcerate, and recur over years (Fig. 23-2).

The early lesions show a suppurative vasculopathy, proposed by various authors to be an arteritis, a venulitis, or both. As opposed to other vasculopathies of the septal vessels, nodular vasculitis results in substantial lobular necrosis of adipocytes with suppuration. As lesions evolve, the fat becomes increasingly necrotic, forming microcysts, and suppuration progresses to the point where it may perforate through the epidermis, forming ulceration. Granulomatous inflammation appears adjacent to areas of fat necrosis, and eventually lesions resolve with fibrosis.

Nodular vasculitis must be distinguished from erythema induratum. Because clinical and pathologic features are identical, the differentiation is made by searching for tuberculous infection in the patient. If this is negative, polymerase chain reaction of the affected tissue may reveal the DNA of *Mycobacterium tuberculosis,* confirming the diagnosis of erythema induratum.

Treatment of nodular vasculitis is usually SSKI as outlined for erythema nodosum. This is effective in about half of cases. In the others trials of colchicine, antimalarials, NSAIDs, and systemic steroids may be attempted.

Sclerosing Panniculitis (Hypodermitis Sclerodermiformis, Lipodermatosclerosis)

Sclerosing panniculitis occurs primarily on the medial lower third of the lower legs of women older than age 40, usually bilaterally, but more commonly or more severely on the left leg. Typically, there is marked woody induration in a stocking distribution resulting in calves that resemble inverted champagne bottles. This induration results from fibrosis in the subcutaneous fat without the primary inflammatory panniculitis ever being clinically observed. It occurs multifocally and microscopically throughout the affected area. This pattern was called hypodermitis sclerodermiformis. When the areas of fat necrosis are larger, they present as erythematous, tender, subcutaneous nodules or plaques (Fig. 23-3). This was designated sclerosing panniculitis.

It is now recognized that these are two aspects of the same disease with a common pathogenesis—venous insufficiency. These patients may have venous varicosities, superficial thrombophlebitis, deep venous thrombosis, or several of these conditions. Even when venous disease is not clinically evident, evaluation of the venous system of the lower leg will reveal insufficiency. Venous insufficiency results in hypoxia in the center of the fat lobule, necrosis of fat, inflammation, and eventual fibrosis. If hypoxemia is present from other causes such as pulmonary disease, sclerosing panniculitis may be more severe.

The histologic features of sclerosing panniculitis are characteristic, but not all features may be seen on every biopsy, since the histologic features change over time within the lesion. The overlying dermis frequently shows changes of stasis with vascular proliferation of thick-walled vessels, hemosiderin deposition, fibrosis, and atrophy. In early lesions there is ischemic necrosis in the center of the fat

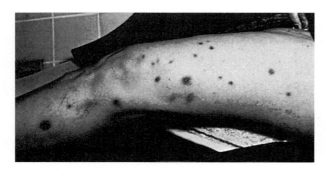

Fig. 23-2   Nodular vasculitis.

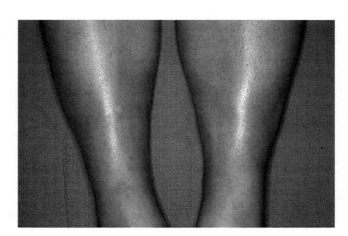

Fig. 23-3   Sclerosing panniculitis.

lobules manifested as "ghost cells"—pale cell walls with no nuclei. There is a sparse lymphocytic infiltrate in the fat septa. As the lesions evolve, the septa are thickened and fibrosed, and there is a mixed inflammatory infiltrate of lymphocytes, plasma cells, and macrophages. Foamy histiocytes are present around the areas of fat necrosis. Fat microcysts are characteristic and appear as small cysts with feathery remnants of adipocytes lining the cyst cavity, so-called lipomembranous fat necrosis. In later lesions, these microcysts collapse and are replaced by fibrosis. Despite these characteristic features, biopsy should be avoided in these patients. Biopsies heal poorly and may lead to chronic leg ulcers. If a biopsy must be performed, it should be from the most proximal edge of involvement.

This diagnosis can be clinically confirmed if a careful vascular evaluation is performed. The location on the lower medial calf is unusual for erythema nodosum. Most other panniculitides favor the posterior mid-calf. The gradual progression from the ankles proximally is characteristic of sclerosing panniculitis and not other forms of lobular panniculitis.

The treatment of sclerosing panniculitis is very difficult. Fibrotic areas may be irreversible. Graded-compression stockings and elevation, standard treatments for venous insufficiency, are most effective in this condition. Unfortunately, some patients cannot tolerate compression because of the pain of the lesions. Stanozolol, 2 to 5 mg twice daily, increases intravascular fibrinolytic activity and decreases pericapillary fibrin. This results in decreased pain within 3 weeks and decreased induration within 8 to 10 weeks. Compression stockings can then be added to the treatment, and the stanozolol dose reduced and eventually discontinued. Blood pressure and liver function tests should be monitored during stanozolol treatment.

Jorizzo JL, et al: Sclerosing panniculitis. *Arch Dermatol* 1991, 127:554.
Kirsner RS, et al: The clinical spectrum of lipodermatosclerosis. *J Am Acad Dermatol* 1993, 28:623.
Snow JL, et al: Lipomembranous (membranocystic) fat necrosis. *Am J Dermatopathol* 1996, 18:151. ▲

PHYSICAL PANNICULITIS

This category includes processes in the fat that occur from physical factors. Some are characterized by the presence of needlelike clefts—sclerema neonatorum, subcutaneous fat necrosis, and poststeroid panniculitis. Infants and children are most frequently affected, and in all these disorders metabolic differences in fat are apparently pathogenically important. Hypothermia or cold is frequently associated in some forms (cold panniculitis, sclerema, and subcutaneous fat necrosis). Traumatic fat necrosis occurs from damage to the subcutaneous fat resulting from trauma. All the conditions just mentioned are treated supportively, and in all

except sclerema neonatorum, spontaneous and complete recovery is expected.

Sclerema Neonatorum

Sclerema neonatorum is the most severe and rarest disorder in this group. It affects premature neonates who are gravely ill for other reasons. Affected neonates usually die, unless the underlying diseases can be reversed. In the first few days of life, the skin begins to harden, usually initially on the buttocks or lower extremities, and rapidly spreads to involve the whole body. The skin on the palms, soles, and genitalia is spared. The skin becomes dry, livid, cold, rigid, and boardlike, so that the mobility of the parts is limited. The skin in the involved areas cannot be picked up. The skin of the entire body may appear half frozen and is yellowish white. Visceral fat may also be involved.

Histologically, adipocytes are enlarged and filled with needlelike clefts in a radial array. Affected fat cells undergo necrosis. There is sparse inflammation, and histiocytes containing needlelike clefts are rare.

Jardine D, et al: Sclerema neonatorum and subcutaneous fat necrosis of the newborn in the same infant. *Eur J Pediatr* 1990, 150:125. ▲

Subcutaneous Fat Necrosis of the Newborn

Subcutaneous fat necrosis of the newborn occurs during the first 4 weeks of life in otherwise healthy, term or postterm infants. A history of perinatal hypothermia, asphyxia, or difficult labor is common. Maternal cocaine use and hypothermic cardiac surgery have also been associated, suggesting subcutaneous fat necrosis is pathogenically related to cold panniculitis. Asymptomatic, firm to rubbery, erythematous nodules appear, usually on the upper back, buttocks, cheeks, or proximal extremities. Lesions may fuse to form plaques and resolve spontaneously over a few months with no scarring. In general, the infants remain well; however, rarely hypercalcemia may occur. The hypercalcemia is associated with elevated 1,25 hydroxyvitamin D levels and increased gut absorption of calcium. Hypercalcemia may result in failure to thrive, seizures, and renal failure.

Histologically, subcutaneous fat necrosis is a lobular panniculitis, with granular necrosis of adipocytes. Needle-shaped clefts are arranged radially within histiocytes, and multinucleate foamy histiocytes are present. Lesions may resolve with calcification and fibrosis. Fine-needle aspiration has confirmed this diagnosis.

Carraccio C, et al: Subcutaneous fat necrosis of the newborn: link to maternal use of cocaine during pregnancy. *Clin Pediatr* 1994, 33(5):317.
Chuang SD, et al: Subcutaneous fat necrosis of the newborn complicating hypothermic cardiac surgery. *Br J Dermatol* 1995, 132:805.

Craig JE, et al: Fat necrosis after ice application for supraventricular tachycardia termination. *J Pediatr* 1998, 133:727.

Gu LL, et al: Nephrocalcinosis and nephrolithiasis due to subcutaneous fat necrosis with hypercalcemia in two full-term asphyxiated neonates. *Pediatr Radiol* 1995, 25:142.

Gupta RK, et al: Fine needle aspiration cytodiagnosis of subcutaneous fat necrosis of the newborn. *Acta Cytol* 1995, 39:759.

Lum CK, et al: Asymptomatic hypercalcemia in subcutaneous fat necrosis. *Clin Pediatr* 1999, 38:547.

Mather MK, et al: Subcutaneous fat necrosis of the newborn. *Int J Dermatol* 1997, 36:435.

Sharata H, et al: Subcutaneous fat necrosis, hypercalcemia, and prostaglandin E. *Pediatr Dermatol* 1995, 12:43.

Urban J, et al: Subcutaneous fat necrosis of the newborn. *Cutis* 1994, 54:383. ▲

Cold Panniculitis

Infants and young children are particularly predisposed to cold panniculitis. It has been described in children who suck on ice or Popsicles *(Popsicle panniculitis)*, in the upper outer thighs of women riding horses in the cold *(equestrian panniculitis)*, in the scrotum of prepubertal males, and in infants treated for supraventricular tachycardia with the application of cold packs to the face. Most affected infants reported have been black. Lesions occur within a few days of the application of the cold, and appear as slightly erythematous, nontender, firm subcutaneous nodules. The typical patient with fat necrosis of the scrotum is a prepubertal (9- to 14-year-old) boy, heavy-set or even obese, with scrotal swelling, usually bilateral, associated with mild to moderate pain (Fig. 23-4). The gait is often guarded and broad-based. There is a lack of systemic complaints and no symptoms related to voiding. The scrotal masses are bilateral and symmetrical in most cases. However, the lesions may be unilateral and there may be more than two. The masses are firm, tender, and do not transmit light. The overlying scrotal skin will be normal or red. Cryptorchidism is not unusual. The most common location of the lesions is near the perineum, consistent with the area of greatest concentration of scrotal fat in children. The adult scrotum lacks this fatty tissue. Without treatment lesions resolve over several days to weeks.

Histologically, there is necrosis of adipocytes within lobules of the upper subcutaneous fat adjacent to the lower dermis. A mixed inflammatory infiltrate of lymphocytes, neutrophils, and foam cells is present, and microcysts sometimes occur. This histology is not specific, and the diagnosis relies largely on obtaining a history of cold exposure.

Ter Poorten JC, et al: Cold panniculitis in a neonate. *J Am Acad Dermatol* 1995, 33:383. ▲

Poststeroid Panniculitis

This rare form of panniculitis occurs predominately in children treated acutely with high doses of systemic

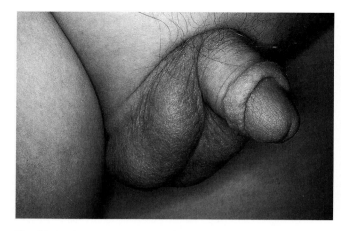

Fig. 23-4 Cold panniculitis of the scrotum secondary to prolonged cold water exposure.

corticosteroids during rapid corticosteroid withdrawal. Substantial weight gain usually occurred during the corticosteroid therapy. Firm subcutaneous nodules begin to appear within a month of tapering the corticosteroids. Areas of abundant subcutaneous fat are favored—the cheeks, trunk, and proximal extremities. Most cases resolve spontaneously, but if severe, the steroids must be reinstituted and tapered more slowly.

Histologically, the changes are identical to those seen in subcutaneous fat necrosis of the newborn. There is a lobular panniculitis with necrosis of adipocytes and needle-shaped clefts in both adipocytes and histiocytes. Foamy histiocytes are also present.

Silverman RA, et al: Poststeroid panniculitis. *Pediatr Dermatol* 1992, 5:92. ▲

Traumatic Panniculitis

Accidental trauma to the skin may induce necrosis of the fat. This is most common on the trunk and on the breasts of women. The prior history of trauma is frequently not recalled. Lesions present like a lipoma, as a firm, mobile, subcutaneous mass of variable tenderness.

Histologically, there is a granulomatous lobular panniculitis with foamy histiocytes, membranous fat necrosis, and microcysts. Lesions heal with fibrosis of the septa.

Winkelmann RK, et al: Factitial traumatic panniculitis. *J Am Acad Dermatol* 1985, 13:988. ▲

Factitial Panniculitis

Self-induced panniculitis is rarely reported but not uncommon. It may be induced by the injection of organic materials, povidone, and oils. In many cases, ulceration will occur. Factitial trauma may also induce a panniculitis.

Medical personnel are at risk because they have ready access to syringes and needles. Pointed, detailed questioning of the patient may identify inconsistencies in the history, or the underlying cause for the behavior (e.g., attention seeking, revenge, malingering).

The clinician must have a high index of suspicion in cases in which the clinical pattern is not characteristic of a known form of panniculitis. Inspection of early lesions for tell-tale healing injection sites may help confirm the diagnosis. A biopsy is often required. Careful evaluation of the biopsy material with polarization may identify foreign material. When the suspicion is high and no foreign material can be seen in the tissue, special evaluation by incineration and mass spectroscopy may identify the injected substance.

Kossard S, et al: Povidone panniculitis. *Arch Dermatol* 1980, 116:704. ▲

Sclerosing Lipogranuloma

Sclerosing lipogranuloma describes the granulomatous and fibrotic reaction that occurs in the panniculus from the injection of silicone or mineral oils. In Mexico the substance injected frequently is guayacol. In most cases the injections are intentional and cosmetic. The time from injection to onset of symptoms may be months to more than 10 years.

Lesions are usually localized to the penis, scrotum, breasts, and buttocks. The overlying skin is hyperpigmented and erythematous. Lesions are frequently initially diagnosed as cellulitis. On palpation, the skin is indurated and cannot be picked up between the fingers. The subcutaneous tissue is indurated, thickened, and lumpy. In some cases, there will be focal ulceration. The injected material will frequently migrate locally, extending beyond the sites of implantation. In some cases it is carried to other tissues, specifically the lymphoreticular system and lungs. Hepatosplenomegaly and pulmonary fibrosis may occur.

Up to two thirds of patients in some series develop autoimmune findings such as a positive antinuclear antibody, arthralgias, Raynaud's phenomenon, Sjögren's syndrome, and sclerodactyly. Up to 10% will meet criteria for the diagnosis of a connective tissue disease, usually scleroderma.

Histologically, the panniculus is replaced by the injected material, which is in various sized vacuoles, giving the affected tissue a "Swiss cheese" appearance. Because the material is usually washed out during the tissue processing, the material itself is not seen, only the spaces it occupied in the tissue in vivo. The vacuoles are surrounded by histiocytes, many of which have ingested the material giving their cytoplasm a vacuolated appearance. Fibrosis may be prominent.

Behar TA, et al: Sclerosing lipogranulomatosis. *Plast Reconstruct Surg* 1993, 91:352.

Cabral AR, et al: Clinical, histopathological, immunological and fibroblast studies in 30 patients with subcutaneous injections of modelants including silicone and mineral oils. *Rev Invest Clin* 1994, 46:257.

Newcomer VD, et al: Sclerosing lipogranuloma resulting from exogenous lipids. *Arch Dermatol* 1986, 73:361. _____ ▲

Enzyme-related panniculitis

This category includes panniculitis induced by enzymes that damage fat (pancreatic panniculitis) and panniculitis caused by the absence of an enzyme critical in preventing tissue inflammation after injury (alpha$_1$-antitrypsin).

PANCREATIC PANNICULITIS (SUBCUTANEOUS FAT NECROSIS)

Subcutaneous fat necrosis may result from pancreatitis or pancreatic carcinoma. Men outnumber women. Alcoholic pancreatitis is the most common cause, but it can also occur from cholelithiasis, stricture of the pancreatic or common bile ducts, medication-induced pancreatitis, and from traumatic pancreatitis and a pancreatic pseudocyst. In cases associated with pancreatic carcinoma, acinar cell carcinoma is most common. Even metastatic pancreatic carcinoma with no residual tumor in the pancreas may induce the syndrome. In 40% of cases, the skin lesions are the first symptom of the underlying pancreatic pathology, and therefore represent an important clue to the diagnosis.

Skin lesions frequently precede other findings and appear as tender or painless erythematous subcutaneous nodules from 1 to 5 cm in diameter (Fig. 23-5). The lower leg is the most common location, being affected in more than 90% of cases. Subcutaneous fat elsewhere may also be affected, except rarely on the head and neck. The number of lesions is usually less than 10 but may number in the hundreds. In most cases the lesions involute, leaving an atrophic scar. If the fat necrosis is severe, however, the lesion develops into a sterile abscess that may break down, draining a thick, brown, oily material.

Subcutaneous fat necrosis is frequently accompanied by a constellation of findings related to fat necrosis in other organs. Importantly, abdominal symptoms may be completely absent. Arthritis is found in 54% to 88% of cases, and may be monoarticular, oligoarticular, and rarely polyarticular. The arthritis may be intermittent, migratory, or persistent. Examination of the joint fluid reveals the presence of free fatty acids, suggesting it is due to fat necrosis adjacent to the joint space. Other findings are medullary fat necrosis of bone, polyserositis, and pulmonary infiltrates or embolism.

Laboratory evaluation is useful in establishing the diagnosis. In most patients the amylase or lipase, or both, are elevated. In many cases, however, one of the tests may be normal and the other markedly abnormal, so both tests must be performed. Sixty percent of patients with pancreatic

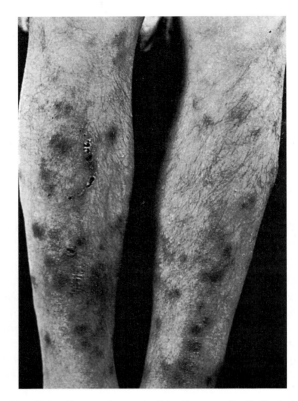

Fig. 23-5 Pancreatic panniculitis. (Courtesy Dr. H. Shatin.)

carcinoma and subcutaneous fat necrosis will have a peripheral eosinophilia.

The histologic features of pancreatic panniculitis are diagnostic. They include focal areas of fat necrosis with anucleate "ghost cells"; finely stippled basophilic material, representing calcium, within the residual rim of the necrotic cells and at the periphery of the affected foci; and a dense inflammatory polymorphous infiltrate at the periphery of the affected fat. The affected necrotic areas are relatively acellular. Several reports have suggested that the early features are those of a septal panniculitis, resembling erythema nodosum. This may have represented sampling error but does indicate that if the initial sample is not diagnostic, another, perhaps more adequate sample of a more advanced lesion should be considered.

The necrosis of fat at all affected sites is due to the release of fat-digesting enzymes, lipases, from the affected pancreatic tissue. These lipases spread hematogenously to the affected sites.

Erythema nodosum represents the primary differential consideration, since pancreatic panniculitis may not have abdominal symptoms, also favors the lower legs, and may be accompanied by joint symptoms. The distinction can be made by skin biopsy, serum amylase and lipase determinations, and especially if eosinophilia is present, a search for a pancreatic neoplasm.

Treatment revolves mainly around treating the cause of the pancreatitis. Obstruction or stenosis of ducts should be repaired, pseudocysts drained, and in the case of pancreatic carcinoma, octreotide administered, if necessary.

Ball NJ, et al: Possible origin of pancreatic fat necrosis as a septal panniculitis. *J Am Acad Dermatol* 1996, 34:362.

Cheng KS, et al: Recurrent panniculitis as the first clinical manifestation of recurrent acute pancreatitis secondary to cholelithiasis. *J Royal Soc Med* 1996, 89:105.

Dahl PR, et al: Pancreatic panniculitis. *J Am Acad Dermatol* 1995, 33:413.

Detlefs RL: Drug-induced pancreatitis presenting as subcutaneous fat necrosis. *J Am Acad Dermatol* 1985, 13:305.

Durden FM, et al: Fat necrosis with features of erythema nodosum in a patient with metastatic pancreatic carcinoma. *Int J Dermatol* 1996, 35:39.

Francombe J, et al: Panniculitis, arthritis and pancreatitis. *Br J Rheumatol* 1995, 34:680.

Lambiase P, et al: Resolution of panniculitis after placement of pancreatic duct stent in chronic pancreatitis. *Am J Gastroenterol* 1996, 91:1835.

Lee MS, et al: Subcutaneous fat necrosis following traumatic pancreatitis. *Austral J Dermatol* 1995, 36:196.

Shbeeb MI, et al: Subcutaneous fat necrosis and polyarthritis associated with pancreatic disease. *Arthritis Rheum* 1996, 39:1922. ▲

ALPHA₁-ANTITRYPSIN DEFICIENCY PANNICULITIS

Alpha$_1$-antitrypsin is the most abundant anti-protease in the circulation, and a potent and irreversible inactivator of neutrophil elastase. Heterozygous deficiency of this enzyme occurs in 1 of 50 persons and homozygous deficiency in 1 in 2500 persons of European descent. Emphysema and liver disease are the most common manifestations of deficiency. A small percentage of patients with homozygous deficiency and the PiZZ phenotype, and rarely heterozygotes with the PiMZ phenotype, will develop a panniculitis.

The panniculitis usually appears between ages 20 and 40 but can occur in childhood. Both sexes are equally affected. Lesions appear after relatively minor trauma and present as painful nodules on the extremities or trunk. They may spontaneously drain. Multiple draining sinus tracts can occur, with lesions coalescing into large, draining plaques.

The histologic findings in this form of panniculitis are dependent on the stage of the lesion. Early lesions show neutrophils splaying the collagen of the reticular dermis and subcutaneous septae. More fully evolved lesions show dissolution of the septae, with islands of normal fat floating in the spaces that represented the destroyed septae. This later finding is considered diagnostic by some. Elastic tissue stains may reveal decreased elastic tissue in the affected areas.

The clinical and histologic differential diagnosis is factitial panniculitis. This is not surprising since trauma produces both lesions, and in the case of the enzyme deficiency, the inflammation-produced enzymes are simply not inactivated, leading to more pronounced lesions than that degree of trauma would be expected to produce.

Replacement of the deficient enzyme will lead to resolution of the skin lesions. Dapsone (and perhaps doxycycline) can also be therapeutic apparently by their ability to reduce neutrophil chemotaxis. Colchicine can be attempted if dapsone is not tolerated. These agents can reduce the requirement for enzyme replacement and should be considered as maintenance treatment in previously affected patients. Systemic steroids may exacerbate the panniculitis. Liver transplantation leads to normal levels of the enzyme and resolution of the panniculitis.

Gaillard MC, et al: A case of systemic nodular panniculitis associated with M1 (Val213) Z phenotype of alpha 1-protease inhibitor. *Int J Dermatol* 1997, 36:276.

Geller JD, et al: A subtle clue to the histopathologic diagnosis of early alpha 1-antitrypsin deficiency panniculitis. *J Am Acad Dermatol* 1994, 31:241.

O'Riordan K, et al: Alpha 1-antitrypsin deficiency-associated panniculitis. *Transplantation* 1997, 63:480. ▲

CYTOPHAGIC HISTIOCYTIC PANNICULITIS

Cytophagic histiocytic panniculitis (CHP) is a multisystem disease characterized by widespread erythematous, painful subcutaneous nodules, which may occasionally become ecchymotic or break down and form crusted ulcerations. There is a progressive febrile illness, with hepatosplenomegaly, pancytopenia, hypertriglyceridemia, and liver dysfunction. These result from the proliferation of benign-appearing histiocytes, which have a marked phagocytic capacity and extensively involve the reticuloendothelial system. Some patients progress to a terminal phase characterized by profound cytopenia, liver failure, and a terminal hemorrhagic diathesis.

Cytophagic histiocytic panniculitis represents a spectrum of disease that occurs in children and adults. Some cases are triggered by viral infections (Epstein-Barr virus [EBV] and human immunodeficiency virus [HIV]), and others represent subcutaneous B- or T-cell lymphomas. The benign cases are reportedly EBV negative and the lymphoma-associated cases are EBV positive.

Histologically, there is infiltration of the lobules of subcutaneous fat by histiocytes and inflammatory cells (primarily helper T cells), with fat necrosis and hemorrhage. The characteristic cell is a "bean bag" cell: a histiocyte stuffed with phagocytized red blood cells, lymphocytes, neutrophils, platelets, or fragments of these cells. These "bean bag" cells are not diagnostic of CHP and can be seen uncommonly in other panniculitides, especially lupus profundus. The presence of atypical lymphocytes or the detection of a clonal B- or T-cell proliferation supports the diagnosis of subcutaneous lymphoma in cases of CHP.

The treatment of CHP is difficult. If malignancy cannot be detected, cyclosporine has been very effective in all reported cases treated with this agent, inducing a permanent remission. If malignancy is detected, aggressive chemotherapy and perhaps bone marrow transplantation may be considered.

Craig AJ, et al: Cytophagic histiocytic panniculitis. *J Am Acad Dermatol* 1998, 39:721.

Harada H, et al: Detection of Epstein-Barr virus genes in malignant lymphoma with clinical and histologic features of cytophagic histiocytic panniculitis. *J Am Acad Dermatol* 1994, 31:379.

Iwatsuki K, et al: Latent Epstein-Barr virus infection is frequently detected in subcutaneous lymphoma associated with hemophagocytosis but not in nonfatal cytophagic histiocytic panniculitis. *Arch Dermatol* 1997, 133:787.

Koizumi K, et al: Effective high-dose chemotherapy followed by autologous peripheral blood stem cell transplantation in a patient with the aggressive form of cytophagic histiocytic panniculitis. *Bone Marrow Transplant* 1997, 20:171.

Matsue K, et al: Successful treatment of cytophagic histiocytic panniculitis with modified CHOP-E. *Am J Clin Oncol* 1994, 17:470.

Ostrov BE, et al: Successful treatment of severe cytophagic histiocytic panniculitis with cyclosporine A. *Semin Arthritis Rheum* 1996, 25:404.

Perniciaro C, et al: Fatal cytophagic panniculitis. *J Am Acad Dermatol* 1995, 32:1062.

Schuval SJ, et al: Panniculitis and fever in children. *J Pediatr* 1993, 122:372. ▲

Miscellaneous forms of panniculitis

EOSINOPHILIC PANNICULITIS

Eosinophilic panniculitis is defined by the prominent infiltration of the subcutaneous fat with eosinophils. It is not a specific disease but is due to a variety of clinical conditions, including arthropod bites, parasitic infections, vasculitis, atopic dermatitis, contact dermatitis, Well's syndrome, bacterial infections, and injection reactions.

Adame J, et al: Eosinophilic panniculitis. *J Am Acad Dermatol* 1996, 34:229.

Samlaska CP, et al: Eosinophilic panniculitis. *Pediatr Dermatol* 1995, 12:35. ▲

GOUTY PANNICULITIS

Uric acid crystals may deposit initially in the subcutaneous fat, leading to lesions resembling other forms of panniculitis. Histologically, there is a lobular panniculitis with necrosis of adipocytes and infiltration of polymorphonuclear leukocytes.

LeBoit PE, et al: Gout presenting as lobular panniculitis. *Am J Dermatopathol* 1987, 9:334. ▲

LIPODYSTROPHY (LIPOATROPHY)

The lipodystrophies are rare conditions in which there is markedly reduced subcutaneous fat. The lipodystrophies can be generalized (total), partial, or localized, and may be present at birth (congenital), or appear after birth (acquired). These syndromes are rare, and their genetic basis and pathogenesis are not completely clarified. Therefore, the classification schemes rely largely on family history and phenotypic characteristics. In addition, localized fat loss can be a consequence of therapeutic injections into the fat.

Total Lipodystrophy

There are two forms of total lipodystrophy: the congenital form *(Beradinelli-Seip syndrome)* and the acquired form *(Seip-Lawrence syndrome)*. These two forms have many similar features. In both types females are more frequently reported, but this may simply reflect the increased severity of the syndromes in females, rather than a true female gender predominance (Fig. 23-6). Diabetes mellitus occurs, hence the term *lipoatrophic diabetes.*

Beradinelli-Seip syndrome has an autosomal recessive inheritance, and parental consanguinity is common. The variability of cases from different regions of the world suggests that the syndrome may be genetically heterogenous. From birth there is an extreme paucity of fat in the subcutaneous tissue and other adipose tissues. The children have a voracious appetite and are hypermetabolic. They have increased height and height velocity, advanced bone age, muscular hypertrophy, and a masculine habitus. This habitus plus enlargement of the genitalia in infancy can lead to the misdiagnosis of precocious puberty. Scalp hair is abundant and curly, and there is generalized hypertrichosis and hyperhidrosis. The abdomen is protuberant as the result of an enlarged liver and spleen. Acanthosis nigricans is invariably present and often generalized. Affected persons have mild mental retardation. Hyperinsulinemia, insulin resistance, and diabetes appear often around puberty. The diabetes mellitus resists insulin and oral hypoglycemic therapy, but ketoacidosis does not occur. Hypertriglyceridemia occurs and can produce eruptive xanthomas. Hypertrophic cardiomyopathy and peripheral pulmonary stenoses occur. Life span is shortened, with patients frequently dying in their young adult life as a result of complications of diabetes or liver or heart disease. Treatment is difficult, but fenfluramine, 2 mg/kg/day, will reduce the hypermetabolic state and decrease appetite, and can lead to resolution of some of the cutaneous features. Multiple smaller meals are required to compensate for the absence of a caloric reservoir in the adipose tissue.

Seip-Lawrence syndrome, acquired generalized lipodystrophy (AGL), shares many features with Berardinelli-Seip syndrome, except it begins after birth. Most cases begin before age 15, and often before age 5. A well-defined illness frequently precedes the onset of AGL in about one third of cases, including infections and autoimmune or connective tissue diseases. The anabolic features are less striking,

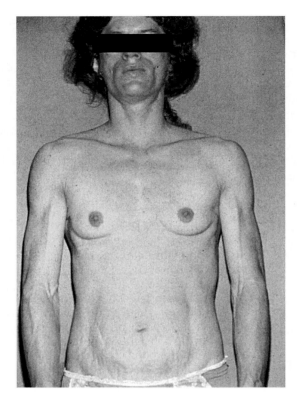

Fig. 23-6 Total lipodystrophy in a patient with insulin-resistant diabetes and hyperlipidemia. (Courtesy Dr. Axel W. Hoke.)

acanthosis nigricans also occurs, frank diabetes mellitus occurs earlier, and liver involvement may be more severe, with death from liver failure being common. Loss of fat may begin locally and generalize, or begin generalized. Etretinate treatment has improved the acanthosis nigricans in one patient.

Leprechaunism must be distinguished from generalized lipodystrophy. These patients have decreased or absent subcutaneous fat in a generalized distribution, wrinkled loose skin, acanthosis nigricans, hypertrichosis, rugae at the orifices, hyperkeratosis, dysplastic nails, thick lips, and gingival hypertrophy. They also have insulin resistance but apparently no organomegaly or liver disease. Also separating them from congenital total lipodystrophy is the presence of muscular wasting, retarded bone age, retarded growth, and early death.

Seip M, et al: Generalized lipodystrophy, congenital and acquired (lipoatrophy). *Acta Paediatr Suppl* 1996, 4413:2. _____ ▲

Partial Lipodystrophy

The syndromes of partial lipodystrophy are a mixed group. Several well-defined forms have been described: two familial forms inherited in an autosomal dominant manner (Kobberling-Dunnigan syndrome and the insulinopenic form with the Rieger anomaly), and an acquired form

(Barraquer-Simons' syndrome). Patients with familial partial lipodystrophy (Kobberling-Dunnigan syndrome) have normal fat distribution at birth and early childhood. At the time of puberty subcutaneous adipose tissue is lost from the extremities, gluteal, and truncal areas. Simultaneously, fat accumulates on the face and neck (giving a cushingoid appearance), intraabdominally, in the axillae, on the back, and in the labia majora. Other features include acanthosis nigricans, hirsutism, menstrual abnormalities, and polycystic ovaries. Diabetes mellitus (insulin resistant but without ketoacidosis), hypertriglyceridemia, and low HDL cholesterol appear after age 20. Because the syndrome is readily diagnosed in females, most reported cases are of the female gender. The genetic defect has been localized to the long arm of chromosome 1.

The other inherited form of partial lipodystrophy affects males and females equally. The onset is in early infancy, with loss of fat limited to the face and the buttocks. Acanthosis nigricans is not present, and growth, bone age, and dentition are retarded. Diabetes mellitus occurs but much later in life, and it is not associated with high levels of insulin as in congenital generalized lipodystrophy and familial partial lipodystrophy. The Rieger anomaly (eye and tooth abnormalities) occurs in this syndrome.

The most common form of lipodystrophy is acquired partial lipodystrophy, also called *progressive lipodystrophy* or *Barraquer-Simons' syndrome*. Girls outnumber boys. It presents in the first and second decades, often after a febrile viral illness. This progressive fat disorder is characterized by a diffuse and progressive loss of the subcutaneous fat that usually begins in the face and scalp (Figs. 23-7 and 23-8) and progresses downward as far as the iliac crests, sparing the lower extremities. The upper half of the body seems emaciated, and the cheeks sink in. There is an apparent, and sometimes a real, adiposity of the buttocks, thighs, and legs. The onset is insidious, with no discomfort or inflammation in the areas of fat loss. Histologically, the skin is normal except for the absence of fat. Most patients with this form of lipodystrophy have reduced levels of C3 resulting from the presence of a serum C3 nephritic factor. Proteinuria caused by mesangioproliferative glomerulonephritis occurs in about 50% of patients with low C3 and lipodystrophy. Diabetes mellitus, insulin resistance, and hyperlipidemia may also occur. Third-trimester intrauterine death may occur.

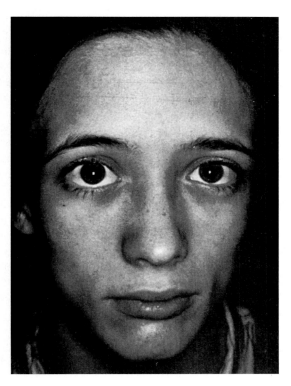

Fig. 23-7 Partial lipodystrophy in a young woman with chronic hypocomplementemic glomerulonephritis.

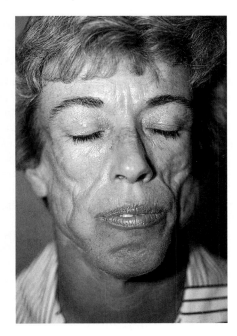

Fig. 23-8 Partial lipodystrophy.

Aarskog D, et al: Autosomal dominant partial lipodystrophy associated with Rieger anomaly, short stature and insulinopenic diabetes. *Am J Med Genet* 1983, 15:29.

Fitch N, et al: Progressive partial lipodystrophy and third-trimester intrauterine fetal death. *Obstet Gynecol* 1987, 156:1195.

Gurbuz O, et al: Partial lipodystrophy. *Int J Dermatol* 1995, 34:36.

Peters JM, et al: Localization of the gene for familial partial lipodystrophy (Dunnigan variety) to chromosome 1q21-22. *Nat Genet* 1998, 18:292.

Spranger S, et al: Barraquer-Simons syndrome. *Am J Med Genet* 1997, 71:397. _____ ▲

Centrifugal and Semicircular Lipoatrophy

"Lipodystrophia centrifugalis abdominalis infantilis" was the unwieldy name given to this entity by Imamura et al, who first reported it in 1971. Most cases have been reported from a single region of Japan. It is almost invariably a disease of childhood; 90% of cases begin by age 5. It is characterized by depression of the skin caused by loss of fat in the abdominal, and much less commonly, the axillary area. The atrophic area enlarges slowly centrifugally for 3 to 8 years in most cases. Histologically, most or all of the fat is lost, with minimal inflammatory infiltrate. Regional lymph node swelling occurred in about two thirds of cases. By the age of 8 to 13 years, the progression stops, and within a year or two, normal contours are restored in almost all cases.

Semicircular lipoatrophy affects primarily adult women and appears as single or multiple, asymptomatic, symmetrical depressions over the anterolateral upper thighs. The process is noninflammatory, and trauma precedes the lipoatrophy. Most cases resolve in a few years.

Annular atrophic connective tissue panniculitis of the ankles is a rare disorder affecting the ankles bilaterally in children and young adults. There is a band of lipoatrophy about 10 cm across that is asymptomatic. In its initial phase, this process shows little inflammation clinically, but a lipophagic panniculitis histologically.

Franks A, et al: Unilateral localized idiopathic lipoatrophy. *Clin Exp Dermatol* 1993, 18:468.

Nagore E, et al: Lipoatrophia semiciruclaris. *J Am Acad Dermatol* 1998, 39:879.

Roth DE, et al: Annular atrophic connective tissue panniculitis of the ankles. *J Am Acad Dermatol* 1989, 21:1152.

Zachary CB, et al: Centrifugal lipodystrophy. *Br J Dermatol* 1984, 110:107. ————————————————— ▲

Lipoatrophia Annularis (Ferreira-Marques)

Lipoatrophia annularis affects primarily women and usually affects the upper extremity. The lipoatrophy may be preceded by erythema, a bracelet-shaped swelling, and tenderness of the entire extremity. This is followed by loss of subcutaneous fat so that the arm is divided into two parts by a depressed, atrophic, braceletlike constriction. The depressed band is usually about 1 cm wide and up to 2 cm in depth. Arthralgias and pain of the affected extremity precede and accompany the process. The band persists for up to 20 years. The histology shows atrophy of the subcutaneous fat. The cause is unknown.

Rongioletti F, et al: Annular and semicircular lipoatrophies. *J Am Acad Dermatol* 1989, 20:433. ————————————————— ▲

Connective Tissue Panniculitis

Connective tissue panniculitis is a rare form of panniculitis occurring in both adults and children. Inflammatory nodules affect the trunk and extremities. Histologically, the lesions show a lymphocytic lobular panniculitis initially and the fat replaced by foamy macrophages in later lesions. Marked atrophy on healing is characteristic. Patients have evidence of autoimmunity including positive antinuclear antibodies,

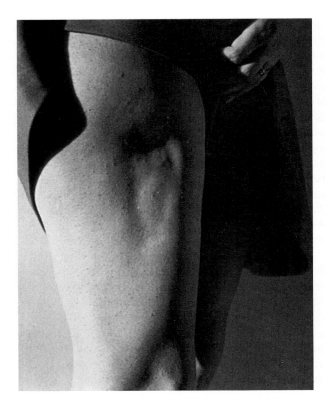

Fig. 23-9 Lipodystrophy secondary to insulin injections. (Courtesy Dr. Axel W. Hoke.)

Hashimoto's thyroiditis, and juvenile rheumatoid arthritis. Connective tissue panniculitis is distinguished from lupus profundus by its more extensive distribution and the lack of the typical histologic features of lupus profundus. Lipophagic panniculitis has been used to describe a series of similar patients in childhood.

Handfield-Jones SE, et al: The clinical spectrum of lipoatrophic panniculitis encompasses connective tissue panniculitis. *Br J Dermatol* 1993, 129:619.

Winkelmann RK, et al: Lipophagic panniculitis of childhood. *J Am Acad Dermatol* 1989, 21:971. ————————————————— ▲

Localized Lipodystrophy

Six months to 2 years after the initiation of insulin injections, localized atrophy of fat may develop at the sites, more frequently in children or women than in men (Fig. 23-9). This dystrophic change may resolve if patients are switched to human insulin. Much less often, insulin injections may result in lipohypertrophy. Rarely, injections of other medications may result in lipoatrophy.

Field LM: Successful treatment of lipohypertrophic insulin lipodystrophy with liposuction surgery. *J Am Acad Dermatol* 1988, 19:520.

Kayikcioglu A, et al: Semicircular lipoatrophy after intragluteal injection of benzathine penicillin. *J Pediatr* 1996, 129:166.

Samadaei A, et al: Insulin lipodystrophy, lipohypertrophic type. *J Am Acad Dermatol* 1987, 17:506.

Valenta LJ, et al: Insulin-induced lipodystrophy in diabetic patients resolved by treatment with human insulin. *Ann Intern Med* 1985, 102:790. _____ ▲

HIV-Associated Lipodystrophy

In a substantial portion of HIV-infected patients, most of whom are being treated with combination anti-HIV therapy, an unusual form of fat redistribution occurs. The fat of the face, especially the buccal fat pads, buttocks, and the limbs is lost (Fig. 23-10). There is increased fat deposition in other areas, especially the neck, upper back (buffalo hump), and intraabdominally ("Crix belly"). The cause of this fat redistribution is unknown, but it is unrelated to cortisol or other hormone levels. It is associated with effective combination anti-HIV antiretroviral therapy, especially with nucleoside reverse transcriptase inhibitors and protease inhibitors. Hypertriglyceridemia, hypercholesterolemia, and insulin resistance may occur.

Carr A, et al: Diagnosis, prediction, and natural course of HIV-1 protease inhibitor-associated lipodystrophy, hyperlipidemia, and diabetes mellitus. *Lancet* 1999, 353:2093.

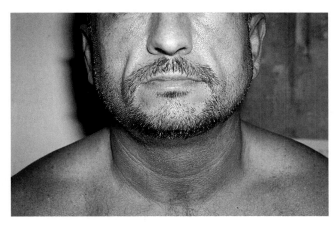

Fig. 23-10 Sunken cheeks and broad neck of HIV-associated lipodystrophy.

Lo JC, et al: "Buffalo hump" in men with HIV infection. *Lancet* 1998, 351:867.

Madge S, et al: Lipodystrophy in patients naïve to HIV protease inhibitors. *AIDS* 1999, 13:735.

Miller, KD, et al: Visceral abdominal-fat accumulation associated with use of indinavir. *Lancet* 1998, 351:871. _____ ▲

CHAPTER 24

Endocrine Diseases

The skin interacts with the endocrine system in many ways. Some of them are discussed in this chapter.

Feingold KR, et al: Endocrine-skin interactions. *J Am Acad Dermatol* 1987, 17:921.

Feingold KR, et al: Endocrine-skin interactions. *J Am Acad Dermatol* 1988, 19:1.

Grando SA: Physiology of endocrine skin interrelations. *J Am Acad Dermatol* 1993, 28:981.

Thiboutot DM: Dermatological manifestations of endocrine disorders. *J Clin Endocrinol Metab* 1995, 80:3082. _____ ▲

ACROMEGALY

In acromegaly, changes in the soft tissues and in the bones form a characteristic syndrome. In association with the well-known changes in the facial features caused by gigantic hypertrophy of the chin, nose, and supraorbital ridges, there is thickening, reddening, and wrinkling of the forehead, and exaggeration of the nasolabial grooves. The lips and tongue are thick. Cutis verticis gyrata is present in approximately 30% of patients. The hands and feet enlarge, and there is gradual growth of the fingertips until they resemble drumsticks. There is diffuse hypertrophy of the skin. This is at least partly due to deposition of colloidal-iron–positive material in the papillae and reticular dermis. Ferguson et al showed that increased skin thickness could be demonstrated in lateral radiographs of the heel, with reversal toward normal after treatment. Skin thickness did not correlate well with growth hormone levels at the time of diagnosis. Hypertrichosis, hyperpigmentation, and hyperhidrosis occur in many patients. The clinical changes may suggest the leonine facies of leprosy, as well as Paget's disease, myxedema, and pachydermoperiostosis.

The cause of acromegaly is hypersecretion of growth hormone by the pituitary, usually because of a mixed chromophobe and eosinophilic adenoma of the gland. It may occur as one of the manifestations of Carney's complex.

The currently preferred treatment is a combination of irradiation and transphenoidal microsurgical excision of the tumor. For patients who do not benefit from surgery, for those awaiting the effects of radiotherapy, or for those whom radiotherapy and/or surgery is contraindicated, octreotide is a superior medical therapy to the dopamine agonist bromocriptine. Octreotide is a potent and long-acting inhibitor of growth hormone (a somatostatin analogue). Fatigue, hyperhidrosis, paresthesias, and headaches improve rapidly with moderate doses of octreotide acetate (200 to 300 mg/day). With continuous treatment soft-tissue swelling and facial coarsening improve as growth hormone levels decline in almost all patients. After 18 to 24 months of therapy 50% of patients will completely normalize.

Camisa C: Somatostatin and a long-acting analogue, octreotide acetate. *Arch Dermatol* 1989, 125:407.

Chalmers RJ, et al: Acne vulgaris and hidradenitis suppurativa as presenting features of acromegaly. *Br Med J* 1983, 287:1346.

Ferguson JK, et al: Skin thickness in acromegaly and Cushing's syndrome and response to treatment. *Clin Endocrinol* (Oxf) 1983, 18:347.

Klein I, et al: Colonic polyps in patients with acromegaly. *Ann Intern Med* 1982, 97:27.

Kolawole TM, et al: Cutis verticis gyrata. *Eur J Radiol* 1998, 27:145. ▲

CUSHING'S SYNDROME

In 1932, when Cushing first described pituitary basophilism, relatively little was known about the delicately balanced hypothalamic-pituitary-adrenal (HPA) axis. He noted, however, the frequent association of pituitary basophilic tumors with adrenal cortical hyperplasia. Hyperfunction of the adrenocortical tissue is directly responsible for this syndrome when it has not been iatrogenically induced by overdosage with corticosteroid hormones either topically or, more often, systemically.

Among the most prominent features of this syndrome is the obesity, affecting the face, neck, trunk, and markedly the abdomen, but sparing the limbs. There may be deposition of fat over the upper back, or a buffalo hump. This may be treated with liposuction. The face becomes moon-shaped, being wide and round. In noniatrogenic cases, women are affected four times more frequently than men, and the peak ages of onset are the twenties and thirties.

The striking and distressing skin changes include hypertrichosis, dryness, and fragility of the skin, with facial acne and susceptibility to superficial dermatophyte and pityrosporon infections; a dusky flushing that may be associated with an actual polycythemia; and the characteristic purplish, atrophic striae on the abdomen and thighs. Women develop facial and body hypertrichosis, with thinning of the scalp hair. Ferguson et al have shown that the thinning of the skin can be demonstrated and measured in lateral radiographs of the heels. There is reversal with treatment. Occasionally there may be livedo reticularis, purpura, ecchymosis, or brownish pigmentation. Poikiloderma-like changes have been observed.

There is usually hypertension and marked generalized arteriosclerosis, with progressive weakness, prostration, and pains in the back, limbs, and abdomen; also kyphosis of the dorsal spine occurs, accentuating the buffalo appearance. There is a reduction in bone density, with osteoporosis. There is generally a loss of libido. In 20% of patients a disturbance in carbohydrate metabolism develops with hyperglycemia, glycosuria, and diabetes mellitus.

These varied symptoms indicate a marked and widespread disturbance caused by the hyperactive adrenal cortex. When microadenomas of the pituitary produce these clinical findings, it is referred to as Cushing's disease. This accounts for only 10% of patients, and contrary to Cushing's original description, most adenomas are chromophobic. Forty percent to 60% of additional cases are due to increased adrenocorticotropic hormone (ACTH) production by the pituitary, but no adenoma is identified. Adrenal adenomas and carcinomas, and ectopic production of ACTH by other tumors, account for the remainder of cases of noniatrogenic Cushing's syndrome. Primary pigmented nodular adrenocortical disease leading to Cushing's syndrome occurs in 30% of patients with Carney's complex. A rapid screening test for Cushing's syndrome consists of oral administration of 1 mg dexamethasone at 11 PM followed at 8 AM by a fluorometric determination of plasma cortisol. A cortisol level below 10 μg/100 ml essentially rules out Cushing's syndrome, except for the iatrogenic variety, in which there is adrenocortical hypoplasia, and the serum cortisol level is very low even without dexamethasone suppression. Kim et al has observed an unusual erysipelas-type presentation of sporotrichosis in a patient with Cushing's disease. When treated with 400 mg/day of itraconazole, the heightened cortisol level was suppressed to normal values. This lowering of cortisol is a well-known side effect of high-dose itraconazole, but such suppression may occur in doses of 400 mg/day even when cortisol secretion is driven by a pituitary tumor.

Ferguson JK, et al: Skin thickness in acromegaly and Cushing's syndrome and response to treatment. *Clin Endocrinol* (Oxf) 1983, 18:347.

Freda PU, et al: Differential diagnosis in Cushing syndrome. *Medicine* (Baltimore) 1995, 74:74.

Kim S, et al: Erysipeloid sporotrichosis in a woman with Cushing's disease. *J Am Acad Dermatol* 1999, 40:272.

Narins RS: Liposuction surgery for a buffalo hump caused by Cushing's disease. *J Am Acad Dermatol* 1989, 21:307.

Sawin CT: Measurement of plasma cortisol in the diagnosis of Cushing's syndrome. *Ann Intern Med* 1968, 68:624.

Stratakis CA, et al: Carney's complex. *J Clin Invest* 1996, 97:699. ▲

ADDISON'S DISEASE

Adrenal insufficiency is manifested in the skin primarily by hyperpigmentation. It is diffuse but most prominently observed in sun-exposed areas and sites exposed to recurrent trauma or pressure. The axillae, perineum, and nipples are also affected. Palmar crease darkening in whites, scar hyperpigmentation, and darkening of nevi, mucous membranes, hair, and nails may all be seen. Ibsen et al reported the eruptive onset of multiple new nevi as an early sign of Addison's disease. Fibrosis and calcification of the pinnae of the ears are rare complications. Addison's disease may be seen alone or as part of a polyglandular autoimmune disease. In the latter case hypoparathyroidism, chronic candidiasis, and vitiligo may also occur.

Baker JR Jr: Autoimmune endocrine disease. *JAMA* 1997, 278:1931.

Betterle C, et al: Complement-fixing activity to melanin-producing cells preceding the onset of vitiligo in a patient with type 1 polyglandular failure. *Arch Dermatol* 1992, 128:123.

Ibsen HH, et al: Eruptive nevi in Addison's disease. *Arch Dermatol* 1990 126:1239. ▲

PANHYPOPITUITARISM

Pituitary failure results in many changes in the skin, hair, and nails as a result of the absence of pituitary hormone action on these sites. Pale, thin, dry skin is seen. Diffuse loss of body hair, with axillary, pubic, and head hair being especially thin, is present. The nails are thin, fragile, and opaque and grow slowly. Yamaguchi et al documented a patient who manifested palmoplantar pustulosis, lymphocytic hypophysitis, and eosinophilia. The hypophysitis led to panhypopituitarism, diabetes insipidus, and hyperprolactinemia.

Yamaguchi T, et al: Lymphocytic hypophysitis, pustulosis palmaris et plantaris, and eosinophilia. *Intern Med* 1994, 33:150. ▲

ANDROGEN-DEPENDENT SYNDROMES

The androgen-dependent syndromes are caused by the excessive production of adrenal androgens by adrenal adenomas, carcinoma, or hyperplasia. The differential diagnosis includes Leydig's cell tumors in men, and arrhenoblastomas and Stein-Leventhal syndrome in women.

The cutaneous signs of excessive androgen include acne, hirsutism, temporal baldness, seborrhea, enlargement of the clitoris, and decreased breast size. Hyperpigmentation of the skin, areolae, genitalia, palmar creases, and buccal mucosa develops in some patients.

In the congenital adrenogenital syndrome, excess androgen is produced by an inherited defect in any of the five enzymatic steps required to convert cholesterol to cortisol. The formation of inadequate amounts of cortisol stimulates the pituitary to secrete excessive ACTH, which stimulates excess androgen production. In boys, precocious puberty results. In girls, masculinization occurs, with the prominent cutaneous signs of excess androgen production. Among these may be childhood acne. DeRave et al reported this in two girls whose acne began before age 9. It manifested as primarily comedonal lesions in the central face and was associated with advanced bone age. Many other children with this presentation, however, revealed no abnormality.

Treatment of the cutaneous signs of androgen excess is successful with the androgen-blocking agents cyproterone acetate, flutamide, and finasteride. Spironolactone, which competes for the androgen cytosol receptors, has proved useful as a systemic antiandrogen in the treatment of hirsutism, acne, adrenal-androgenic female pattern alopecia, and polycystic ovary syndrome. Chorionic villous biopsy may identify homozygous adrenogenital female fetuses, which will allow for dexamethasone therapy to prevent intrauterine virilization of the external genitalia.

Braithwaite SS, et al: Hirsutism. *Arch Dermatol* 1983, 119:279.

DeRave L, et al: Prepubertal acne. *J Am Acad Dermatol* 1995, 32:181.

Falsetti L, et al: Treatment of hirsutism by finasteride and flutamide in women with polycystic ovary syndrome. *Gynecol Endocrinol* 1997, 11:251.

Lucky AW: Androgens and the skin. *Arch Dermatol* 1987, 123:193.

McKenna TJ: Pathogenesis and treatment of polycystic ovary syndrome. *N Engl J Med* 1988, 318:558.

Reingold SB, et al: The relationship of mild hirsutism or acne in women to androgens. *Arch Dermatol* 1987, 123:209.

Shaw JC: Antiandrogen and hormonal treatment of acne. *Dermatol Clin* 1996, 14:803.

Sperling LC, et al: Androgen biology as a basis for the diagnosis and treatment of androgenic disorders in women. *J Am Acad Dermatol* 1993, 28:669, 901.

Traupe H, et al: Acne of the fulminans type following testosterone therapy in three excessively tall boys. *Arch Dermatol* 1988, 124:414.

Watson RE, et al: Hirsutism: evaluation and management. *J Gen Intern Med* 1995, 10:283.

Zemtsov A, et al: Successful treatment of hirsutism in HAIR-AN syndrome using flutamide, spironolactone, and birth control therapy. *Arch Dermatol* 1997, 133:431. _____ ▲

HYPOTHYROIDISM

Hypothyroidism is a deficiency of circulating thyroid hormone, or rarely peripheral resistance to hormonal action.

The condition produces various clinical manifestations, depending on when in life it occurs and on its severity. Middle-aged women are the most commonly affected adults. An autosomal recessive variant of ectodermal dysplasia reported as *ANOTHER* (*a*lopecia, *n*ail dystrophy, *o*phthalmic complications, *t*hyroid dysfunction, *h*ypohidrosis, *e*phelides and *e*nteropathy, and *r*espiratory tract infections) *syndrome* has been reported by Pike et al.

Cretinism

Thyroid deficiency in fetal life produces the characteristic picture of cretinism at birth and in the next few months of life. Depending on the degree of thyroid deficiency, a wide variety of signs and symptoms may be evident.

The person with cretinism has cool, dry, pasty white to yellowish skin. Disturbances in the amount, texture, and distribution of the hair with patchy alopecia are common. Pigmentation is less than normal after exposure to sunlight. Sweating is greatly diminished. The lips are pale, thick, and protuberant. The tongue is usually enlarged, and there is delayed dentition. The face is characterized by wide-set eyes; a broad, flat nose; periorbital puffiness; and a large, protruding tongue (Fig. 24-1). A protuberant abdomen with umbilical hernia; acral swelling; coarse, dry, brittle nails; a clavicular fat pad, and hypothermia with cutis marmorata are also seen.

Myxedema

When lack of secretion of thyroid hormone is severe, the systemic mucinosis called *myxedema* is produced. The skin

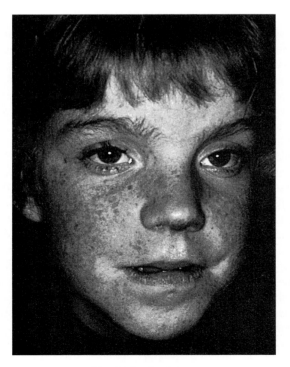

Fig. 24-1 Cretinism.

becomes rough and dry, and in severe cases of primary myxedema, ichthyosis vulgaris may be simulated. The facial skin is puffy; the expression is often dull and flat; macroglossia, swollen lips, and a broad nose are present; and chronic periorbital infiltration secondary to deposits of mucopolysaccharides frequently develops (Fig. 24-2). Forgie et al described a patient with erythema and thickening of the forehead skin, which on biopsy proved secondary to mucin. Carotenemia may cause a yellow tint in the skin that is especially prominent on the palms and soles. Diffuse hair loss is common, and the outer third of the eyebrows is shed. The hair becomes coarse and brittle. The free edges of the nails break easily, and onycholysis may occur.

Mild Hypothyroidism

Lesser degrees of deficiency are common and far less easily diagnosed. Coldness of hands and feet in the absence of vascular disease, sensitivity to cool weather, lack of sweating, tendency to put on weight, need for extra sleep, drowsiness in the daytime, or constipation all suggest possible hypothyroidism and the need for appropriate tests. Palmoplantar keratoderma may be a sign of hypothyroidism and will resolve after thyroid replacement is given. T3, T4, and thyroid-stimulating hormone (TSH) tests are recommended for screening.

Bijlmer-Iest JC, et al: Thyroid and the skin. *Curr Prob Dermatol* 1991, 20:34.

Forgie JC, et al: Myxedematous infiltrate of the forehead in treated hypothyroidism. *Clin Exp Dermatol* 1994, 19:168.

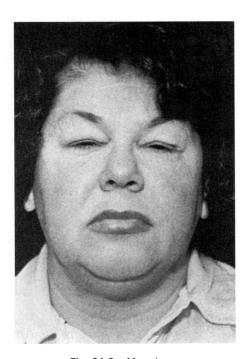

Fig. 24-2 Myxedema.

Good JM, et al: Keratoderma of myxedema. *Clin Exp Dermatol* 1988, 13:339.

Heymann WR: Cutaneous manifestations of thyroid disease. *J Am Acad Dermatol* 1992, 26:885.

Miller JJ, et al: Palmoplantar keratoderma associated with hypothyroidism. *Br J Dermatol* 1998, 139:741.

Nakatsui T, et al: Onycholysis and thyroid disease. *J Cutan Med Surg* 1998, 3:40.

Pike MG, et al: A distinctive type of hypohidrotic ectodermal dysplasia featuring hypothyroidism. *J Pediatr* 1986, 108:109.

Signore RJ, et al: Alopecia of myxedema. *J Am Acad Dermatol* 1991, 25:902. _____ ▲

HYPERTHYROIDISM

Excessive quantities of circulating thyroid hormone, produced in a variety of ways, affect various organs. The skin changes are distinctive in hyperthyroidism. The cutaneous surface is warm, moist, and smooth textured. Palmar erythema or facial flushing may be seen. The hair is thin and has a downy texture, and nonscarring alopecia may be observed. The skin may be diffusely pigmented to produce a bronzed appearance or melanoderma; sometimes even melasma of the cheeks is seen. Nail changes are present in approximately 5% of patient with Plummer's nails, a concave contour and distal onycholysis being characteristic. Hyperhidrosis may be noted.

Graves' disease has a female-to-male ratio of 7:1, and the peak age at onset is 20 to 30 years. Thyroid acropachy, seen in approximately 1% of Graves' patients, is characterized by digital clubbing and diaphyseal proliferation of the periosteum in acral and distal long bones (tibia, fibula, ulna, and radius). It usually occurs in association with past hyperthyroidism, untreated and treated, and frequently accompanies exophthalmos and pretibial myxedema. Thyroid acropachy has been recognized in euthyroid and hypothyroid patients. It can be confused clinically with acromegaly, pachydermoperiostosis, pulmonary osteoarthropathy, or osteoperiostitis, but the radiologic findings are pathognomonic.

Pretibial myxedema (Fig. 24-3) consisting of bilateral, localized, cutaneous accumulations of glycosaminoglycans, occurs in 4% of patients who have or have had Graves' disease. It may uncommonly also occur during the course of Hashimoto's thyroiditis and primary hypothyroidism. Patients with pretibial myxedema regularly have associated ophthalmopathy and occasionally have thyroid acropachy. Elevated serum levels of thyroid-stimulating antibodies usually accompany the presence of pretibial myxedema. Worstman et al reported that five of nine consecutively evaluated patients with Graves' disease had mucopolysaccharide deposition in the preradial area of the extensor aspects of the forearms. Lesions of the shoulder and thigh have been reported. Improvement in the plaques of pretibial myxedema has resulted from intralesional injections of triamcinolone acetonide and with clobetasol solution under Duoderm occlusion, applied once weekly for 4 to 6 weeks. Systemic steroids are of no benefit. Antonelli et al reported

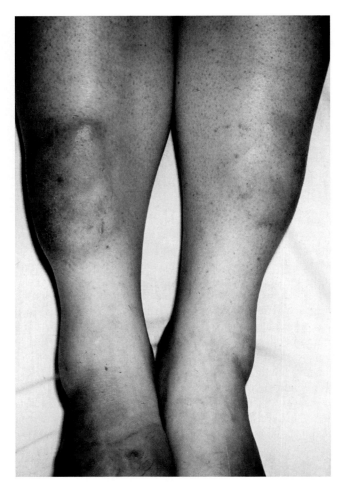

Fig. 24-3 Pretibial myxedema.

seven patients who improved with intravenous immunoglobulin. Skin, eye, and immunologic parameters were all affected positively.

Vitiligo is associated with hyperthyroidism in 7% of patients with Graves' disease and is seen with an increased frequency in Hashimoto's thyroiditis.

Antonelli A, et al: Pretibial myxedema and high dose IVIG treatment. *Thyroid* 1994, 4:399.
Goette DK: Thyroid acropachy. *Arch Dermatol* 1980, 116:205.
Heymann WR: Advances in the cutaneous manifestations of thyroid disease. *Int J Dermatol* 1997, 36:641.
Heymann WR: Cutaneous manifestations of thyroid disease. *J Am Acad Dermatol* 1992, 26:885.
Stevens CJ, et al: The dermal mucinoses. *Adv Dermatol* 1993, 8:201.
Truhan AP, et al: The cutaneous mucinoses. *J Am Acad Dermatol* 1986, 14:1.
Worstman J, et al: Preradial myxedema in thyroid disease. *Arch Dermatol* 1981, 117:635. _____ ▲

HYPOPARATHYROIDISM

Varied changes in the skin and its appendages may be evident. Most pronounced is faulty dentition when hypoparathyroidism is present during development of the permanent teeth. The skin is dry and scaly. A diffuse scantiness of the hair and complete absence of axillary and pubic hair may be found. The nails are brittle and malformed. Onycholysis with fungal infection may be present. Of patients with idiopathic hypoparathyroidism 15% develop mucocutaneous candidiasis. Hypoparathyroidism is the most frequent endocrine abnormality present in patients with the APECED (autoimmune polyendocrinopathy, candidiasis, ectodermal dystrophy) syndrome. Hypoparathyroidism with resultant hypocalcemia has been reported to trigger bouts of impetigo herpetiformis or pustular psoriasis, as in a case reported by Moynihan et al.

Pseudohypoparathyroidism (PH) is an autosomal-dominant or X-linked inherited disorder characterized by end-organ unresponsiveness to parathyroid hormone. The parathyroid hormone and phosphorus levels are high, whereas the serum calcium is low. The typical clinical findings include short stature; obesity; round face; prominent forehead; low nasal bridge; attached earlobes; short neck; short, wide nails; delayed dentition; mental deficiency; amenorrhea; blue sclera; and cataracts. Brachycephaly, microcephaly, and shortened metacarpals or metatarsals, especially of the fourth and fifth digits, occur because of premature epiphyseal closure. The latter results in short, stubby fingers and toes, with dimpling over the metacarpophalangeal joints (Albright's sign). Subcutaneous calcification and ossification occur commonly in this disorder as it may in pseudopseudohypoparathyroidism (PPH), which has the same phenotype but patients have normal serum and calcium levels. PH and PPH are the two types of Albright's hereditary osteodystrophy. In PH type 1a there is a defect in a G protein that couples receptors for several hormones to adenylate cyclase. This causes a generalized resistance to agents acting through the cAMP pathway and explains the frequent association of hypothyroidism and hypogonadism.

Ahonen P, et al: Clinical variation in APECED in a series of 68 patients. *N Engl J Med* 1990, 322:1829.
Kaplan FS: Skin and bones. *Arch Dermatol* 1996, 132:815.
Kinard RE, et al: Pseudohypoparathyroidism. *Arch Intern Med* 1979, 139:204.
Lang PG Jr: The clinical spectrum of parathyroid disease. *J Am Acad Dermatol* 1981, 5:733.
Miller ES, et al: Progressive osseous heteroplasia. *Arch Dermatol* 1996, 132:787.
Moynihan GD, et al: Impetigo herpetiformis and hypoparathyroidism. *Arch Dermatol* 1985, 121:1330.
Raimer SS, et al: Metastatic calcinosis cutis. *Cutis* 1983, 32:543. _____ ▲

HYPERPARATHYROIDISM

Multiple endocrine neoplasia (MEN) type I is characterized by tumors of the parathyroids, endocrine pancreas, anterior pituitary, thyroid, and adrenal glands. The most commonly observed abnormality is hypercalcemia from hypersecreting tumors of the parathyroid glands. This autosomal dominantly inherited disease usually presents in the fourth decade of life with clinical symptoms related to hypersecretion of hormone. Darling et al reported that patients with this syndrome were found to have multiple angiofibromas and collagenomas. Others had café au lait macules, lipomas, confetti-like hypopigmentation, and gingival macules. The angiofibromas were smaller and less numerous than those present in tuberous sclerosis. The tumors in both MEN I and tuberous sclerosis apparently arise because of abnormalities within a tumor suppressor gene. The MEN I gene, which is present on chromosome 11, has a protein product termed *menin* whose function is yet to be delineated.

Darling TN, et al: Multiple facial angiofibromas and collagenomas in patients with multiple endocrine neoplasia type 1. *Arch Dermatol* 1997, 133:853. _____ ▲

ACANTHOSIS NIGRICANS

Acanthosis nigricans (AN) is characterized by hyperpigmentation and papillary hypertrophy, which are symmetrically distributed. The regions affected may be the face, neck, axillae, external genitals, groin, inner aspects of the thighs, flexor surface of the elbows and knees, umbilicus, and anus (Fig. 24-4, *A*). With extensive involvement, lesions can be found on the areolae, around the umbilicus, on the eyelids, the conjunctiva, and on the lips and buccal mucosa (Fig. 24-4, *B*). Rarely the involvement may be almost universal. The color of the patches is grayish, brownish, or black. The palms or soles may show hyperkeratoses. Small, papillomatous, nonpigmented lesions and pigmented macules may occasionally be found in the mucous membranes of the mouth, pharynx, and vagina.

Type I: Acanthosis Nigricans Associated with Malignancy

The "malignant" type of AN may either precede (18%), accompany (60%), or follow (22%) the onset of the internal cancer. This rare type generally is the most striking clinically, both from the standpoint of extent of involvement and the pronounced nature of the lesions. Most cases are associated with adenocarcinoma, especially of the gastrointestinal tract (60% stomach), lung, and breast; less often the gallbladder, pancreas, esophagus, liver, prostate, kidney, colon, rectum, uterus, and ovaries. Other types of cancer and lymphomas may be seen also. A few cases of this type of AN have been observed in childhood, but most begin after puberty or in adulthood. This type should be highly suspected if widespread lesions develop in a nonobese male over age 40.

Tripe palms (acanthosis palmaris) are characterized by thickened, velvety palms with pronounced demoglyphics. In 77 patients reviewed by Cohen et al, 95% occurred in patients with cancer, and 77% were seen in conjunction with

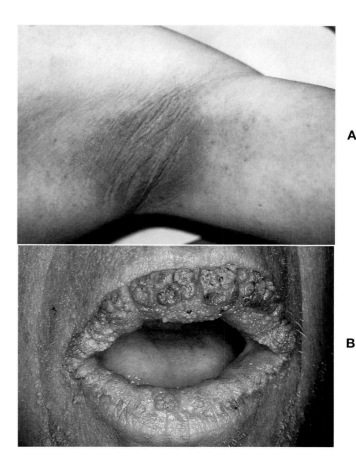

Fig. 24-4   Acanthosis nigricans **(A)** of the axilla and **(B)** of the lips in a man with adenocarcinoma of the stomach.

acanthosis nigricans. In 40% of these cases they were the presenting sign of an undiagnosed malignancy. If only the palms were involved, lung cancer was most common, whereas in tripe palms associated with AN gastric cancer was most frequent.

Type II: Familial Acanthosis Nigricans

This exceedingly rare type is present at birth or may develop during childhood (Fig. 24-5). It is commonly accentuated at puberty. It resembles ichthyosis hystrix clinically, but histologic differences are seen. It is not associated with an internal cancer, and it is inherited in an autosomal dominant manner.

Type III: Acanthosis Nigricans Associated with Obesity, Insulin-Resistant States, and Endocrinopathy

Type III is the most common variety of AN. It presents as a grayish, velvety thickening of the skin of the sides of the neck, axillae, and groins (Fig. 24-6). It occurs in obesity, with or without endocrine disorders. It also occurs in acromegaly and gigantism, Stein-Leventhal syndrome, Cushing's syndrome, diabetes mellitus, hypothyroidism, Addison's disease, hyperandrogenic states, hypogonadal syndromes, and the various well-recognized inulin-resistant states, including lipoatrophic diabetes; leprechaunism; pine-aloma (Rabson-Mendenhall syndrome); acral hypertrophy syndrome; type A syndrome, where there is a defect in insulin-receptor or postreceptor pathways; and type B syndrome, where autoantibodies to the insulin receptor are present. Whereas both types A and B occur most commonly in black females, type A predominates in young children with hyperandrogenic manifestations. Type B is seen in middle-aged patients with autoimmune disease. Flier, among others, suggests that most, if not all, of patients with AN may have either clinical or subclinical insulin resistance, and recommends investigation of this possibility in

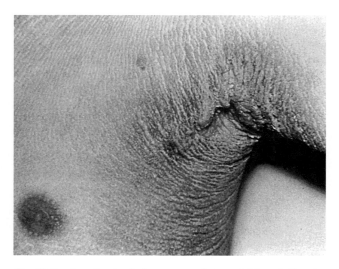

Fig. 24-5 Acanthosis nigricans present since childhood. (Courtesy Dr. Axel W. Hoke.)

these patients. Many of the conditions associated with insulin resistance and AN manifest as hyperandrogenism and have been dubbed the *HAIR-AN syndrome*. In one group of women with hirsutism, obesity, and hyperandrogenism, vulvar AN was present in all patients, with other sites less frequently involved.

AN may occur in various syndromes such as Bloom's syndrome, Alström syndrome, ataxia-telangiectasia, Costello syndrome, MORFAN syndrome (mental retardation, overgrowth, remarkable face, and AN), Capozucca syndrome, Prader-Willi syndrome, Beare-Stevenson cutis gyrata syndrome, Crouzon's syndrome, Rud's syndrome, and Wilson's disease. Drugs known to induce AN are nicotinic acid, niacinamide, diethylstilbestrol, triazineate, oral contraceptives, and glucocorticoids. Approximately 10% of renal transplant patients have AN.

The histopathology shows papillomatosis without thickening of the Malpighian layer. The term *acanthosis* was applied here to indicate the clinical, not the histologic, bristly thickening of the skin. Hyperkeratosis and slight hyperpigmentation of the basal layer is present in most cases; it appears, however, that the clinically observed hyperpigmentation is due to hyperkeratosis and clinical thickening rather than to melanin.

The differential diagnosis includes ichthyosis hystrix and several disorders of reticulated hyperpigmentation, including confluent and reticulated papillomatosis (Gougerot-Carteaud syndrome), Dowling-Degos' disease, Haber's syndrome, and acropigmentatio reticularis of Kitamura. Dowling-Degos' disease is a familial nevoid anomaly with delayed onset in adult life. There is progressive, brown-to-black hyperpigmentation of flexures with associated soft fibromas and follicular hyperkeratoses. Pitted acneform scars occur periorally.

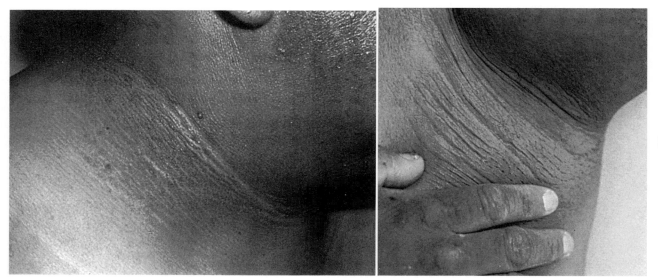

Fig. 24-6 **A** and **B**, Acanthosis nigricans associated with obesity. (Courtesy Dr. Axel W. Hoke.)

Treatment of the type associated with malignancy consists of finding and removing the causal tumor. Early recognition and treatment may be lifesaving. The type occurring with obesity usually improves with weight loss. If there is associated endocrinopathy, it must be treated as well. One patient with lipodystrophic diabetes improved markedly during dietary supplementation with fish oil, and etretinate and tretinoin have been reported as successful treatments.

Akoudyan VA, et al: Successful treatments of AN with etretinate. *J Am Acad Dermatol* 1994, 31:118.

Barbieri RL: Hyperandrogenism, insulin resistance and acanthosis nigricans. *J Reprod Med* 1994, 39:327.

Brown WG: Reticulate pigmentation anomaly of the flexures. *Arch Dermatol* 1982, 118:490.

Cohen PR, et al: Tripe palms and cancer. *J Clin Oncol* 1989, 7:669.

Cruz PD, et al: Excessive insulin binding to insulin-like growth receptors. *J Invest Dermatol* 1992, 98:825.

Darmstadt GL, et al: Treatment of acanthosis nigricans with tretinoin. *Arch Dermatol* 1991, 127:1139.

Esperanza LE, et al: HAIR-AN syndrome: spontaneous remission in a 15 year old girl. *J Am Acad Dermatol* 1996, 34:892.

Flier JS: Metabolic importance of acanthosis nigricans. *Arch Dermatol* 1985, 121:193.

Grasinger CC, et al: Vulvar acanthosis nigricans. *Fertil Steril* 1993, 59:583.

Holdiness MR: Acanthosis nigricans. *Arch Dermatol* 1985, 121:588.

Kalter DC: Acquired intertriginous pigmentation. *Arch Dermatol* 1985, 121:399.

Ober KP: Acanthosis nigricans and insulin resistance associated with hypothyroidism. *Arch Dermatol* 1985, 121:229.

Przylepa KA, et al: Fibroblast growth factor receptor 2 mutations in Beare-Stevenson cutis gyrata syndrome. *Nat Genet* 1996, 13:492.

Rendon MI, et al: Acanthosis nigricans. *J Am Acad Dermatol* 1989, 21:461.

Richards GE, et al: Obesity acanthosis nigricans, insulin resistance, hyperandrogenemia. *J Pediatr* 1985, 107:893.

Schwartz RA: Acanthosis nigricans. *J Am Acad Dermatol* 1994, 31:1.

Seemanova E, et al: Morfan: a new syndrome characterized by mental retardation, pre- and postnatal overgrowth, remarkable face and acanthosis nigricans in 5-year-old boy. *Am J Med Genet* 1993, 45:525.

Sherertz EF: Improved acanthosis nigricans with lipodystrophic diabetes during dietary fish oil supplementation. *Arch Dermatol* 1988, 124:1094.

Tasjian D, et al: Familial acanthosis nigricans. *Arch Dermatol* 1984, 120:1351.

Teebi AS, et al: Further delineation of Costello syndrome. *Am J Med Genet* 1993, 47:166. ▲

CHAPTER 25

Abnormalities of Dermal Connective Tissue

Disorders included in this chapter are characterized by abnormalities of the dermal connective tissue fibers. Alterations of mucopolysaccharide ground substance are discussed in Chapter 9 or Chapter 26. The changes may primarily involve either the elastic fibers or the collagen fibers, and they may be either inherited or acquired. Perforating disorders result in the transepidermal elimination of collagen, elastin, and related cellular matrix components through the epidermis and include elastosis perforans serpiginosa, perforating folliculitis, reactive perforating collagenosis, and Kyrle's disease/perforating disorder of uremia. The perforating disorders may have a common mechanism. Elevated serum and tissue concentrations of fibronectin may be responsible for inciting increased epithelial migration and proliferation culminating in perforation.

Morgan MB, et al: Fibronectin and the extracellular matrix in the perforating disorders of the skin. *Am J Dermatopathol* 1998, 20:147. ▲

COLLAGEN

More than 19 different kinds of collagens have been identified in tissues of vertebrates (Table 25-1). There are four families of collagens. *Fibrillar collagens* (types I, II, III, V, and XI) form fibrils that are among the most abundant proteins in the body. Type I collagen accounts for 60% to 90% of the dry weight of skin, ligaments, and demineralized bone. *Basement membrane-associated collagen* is made up of types IV and VII. *Fiber-associated collagens* (types VIII, IX, and XIV) are found on the surface of type I and II collagens and are believed to serve as flexible spacers among fibrils. *Fibril-associated collagens with interrupted triple helices* (FACITs) do not form fibrils themselves but are found attached to the surfaces of preexisting fibrils of the fibril-forming collagens. FACITs are composed of types IX, XII, XIV, XVI, and XIX. *Network-forming collagens* are produced from types VIII and X forming sheets. Studies on types XV, XVII, and XIX demonstrate widespread presence in basement membranes, particularly vascular endothelium, which may be a new subgroup of collagens associated with angiogenic and pathologic processes.

Berthod F, et al: Differential expression of collagens XII and XIV in human skin and in reconstructed skin. *J Invest Dermatol* 1997, 108:737.

Myers JC, et al: Biochemical and immunohistochemical characterization of human type XIX defines a novel class of basement membrane zone collagens. *Am J Pathol* 1997, 151:1729.

Prockop DJ, et al: Collagen: molecular biology, diseases and potentials for therapy. *Annu Rev Biochem* 1995, 64:403.

van der Rest M, et al: Collagen family of proteins. *FASEB J* 1991, 5:2814. ▲

Elastosis Perforans Serpiginosa

In 1953, Lutz described a chronic keratopapular eruption in an arciform shape located on the sides of the nape of the neck. In elastosis perforans serpiginosa (EPS), the skin-colored keratotic papules, 2 to 5 mm in diameter, are confluently grouped in a serpiginous or horseshoe-shaped arrangement with the area inside of the arc normal or slightly atrophic (Fig. 25-1). Although these lesions typically occur on the neck, other sites may be involved, such as the upper arms, face, lower extremities, and rarely the trunk. Disseminated lesions occur in Down syndrome. EPS is most common in young adults. Men outnumber women four to one. The disease runs a variable course with spontaneous resolution often occurring from 6 months to 5 years after onset. Often, atrophic scarring remains. It has been reported from all over the world. The etiology is unknown.

Approximately one third of cases occur in patients with associated diseases, the most frequent concomitant disorder being Down syndrome. Of persons with Down syndrome 1% have EPS. In this situation the lesions are likely to be extensive and persistent. In addition to Down syndrome, Ehlers-Danlos syndrome (Fig. 25-2), osteogenesis imperfecta, Marfan syndrome, Rothmund-Thomson syndrome, acrogeria, systemic sclerosis, morphea, XYY syndrome, and renal disease have been associated.

TABLE 25-1

Genetic Heterogeneity of Collagen

Collagen Type	Gene*	Chromosome	Tissue Distribution
I	COL1A1-2	17q21.3-q22	Skin, bone, tendon
I-trimer			Tumors, cell cultures, skin, liver
II	COL2A1	7q21.3-q22	Cartilage, vitreous
III	COL3A1	12q13-q14	Fetal skin, blood vessels, intestines
IV	COL4A1-6	13q34, 2q35-q37, Xq22	Basement membranes
V	COL5A1-3	9q34.2-q34.3	Ubiquitous
VI	COL6A1-3	21q22.3, 2q37	Aortic intima, placenta
VII	COL7A1	3p21	Amnion, anchoring fibrils
VIII	COL8A1-2	3q12-q13.1, 1p32.3-p34.3	Endothelial cell cultures
IX	COL9A1-3	6q12-q14, 1p32	Cartilage, type II collagen tissue
X	COL10A1	6q12-q22	Cartilage
XI	COL11A1-2, COL2A1	1p21	Cartilage, skin
XII	COL12A1	6	Skin, cartilage, cornea, limbal
XIII	COL13A1	10q22	Ubiquitous
XIV	COL14A1	8q23	Ubiquitous, fetal hair follicles, basement membranes
XV	COL15A1	9q21-22	Skin hemidesmosomes, kidney, liver, spleen
XVI	COL16A1	1p34-35	Ubiquitous
XVII	COL17A1	10q24.3	Skin hemidesmosomes
XVIII	COL18A1	21q22.3	Ubiquitous, basement membranes
XIX	COL19A1	6q12-q14	Ubiquitous, basement membranes

*Hyphenation denotes a series of genes (i.e., COL1A1-2 means COL1A1 and COL1A2).

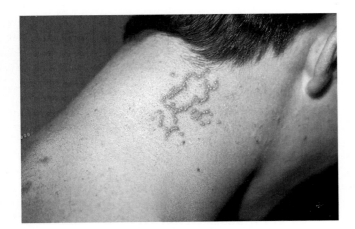

Fig. 25-1   Elastosis perforans serpiginosa on neck.

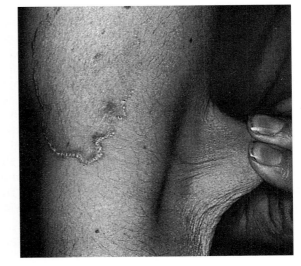

Fig. 25-2   Elastosis perforans serpiginosa in a patient with Ehlers-Danlos syndrome.

Reports of EPS associated with pseudoxanthoma elasticum are probably examples of perforating pseudoxanthoma elasticum. Several publications have detailed patients with Wilson's disease under prolonged treatment with penicillamine who developed EPS.

The distinctive histopathologic changes consist of elongated, tortuous channels in the epidermis into which red-staining elastic tissue perforates and is extruded from the dermis. There is degeneration and alteration of the elastic tissue, with an inflammatory response.

Treatment is difficult, but individual lesions may resolve following liquid nitrogen cryotherapy.

Armstrong DK, et al: Elastosis perforans serpiginosa associated with unilateral atrophoderma of Pasini and Pierini in an individual with 47,XYY karyotype. *Br J Dermatol* 1997, 137:158.

Iozumi K, et al: Penicillamine-induced degenerative dermatoses: report of a case and brief review of such dermatoses. *J Dermatol* 1997, 24:458.

Kuhn CA, et al: Acneiform papules on the neck: elastosis perforans serpiginosa (EPS). *Arch Dermatol* 1995, 131:341.

Scherbenske JM, et al: Cutaneous and ocular manifestations of Down syndrome. *J Am Acad Dermatol* 1990, 22:933.

Sehgal VN, et al: Perforating dermatoses: a review and report of four cases. *J Dermatol* 1993, 20:329.

Tuyp EJ, et al: Elastosis perforans serpiginosa: treatment with liquid nitrogen. *Int J Dermatol* 1990, 29:655. ▲

Reactive Perforating Collagenosis

In 1967, Mehregan et al reported a rare, familial, nonpruritic skin disorder characterized by papules on the extremities, face, or buttocks (Fig. 25-3). Lesions begin to appear in the first or second decade. Although the individual lesions involute after 6 to 8 weeks as a rule, there may be recurrent crops for many years. The linear configuration of the lesions and the observation that lesions appear in areas of skin injury and can be experimentally induced strongly suggests this is an aberrant reaction to connective tissue injury. Histologically similar lesions can occur sporadically, supporting this view.

An acquired form of reactive perforating collagenosis (RPC) has been reported in association with diabetes mellitus, renal disease, liver disease, lymphoma, hyperparathyroidism, hypothyroidism, neurodermatitis, and acquired immunodeficiency syndrome (AIDS). Pruritus is present in all cases and is usually severe. Superficial trauma induced by scratching induces the lesions. Acquired RPC is best viewed as a nonspecific reaction to skin injury. Some authors have used the terminology "acquired perforating dermatosis" for this phenomenon. This condition in the setting of renal failure represents a part of the spectrum of perforating disorder of renal failure (see Chapter 33). The treatment for these acquired cases is to treat the underlying disease and its associated pruritus.

Bang SW, et al: Acquired reactive perforating collagenosis: unilateral umbilicated papules along the lesions of herpes zoster. *J Am Acad Dermatol* 1997, 36:778.

Briggs PL, et al: Reactive perforating collagenosis of diabetes mellitus. *J Am Acad Dermatol* 1995, 32:521.

Faver IR, et al: Acquired reactive perforating collagenosis. *J Am Acad Dermatol* 1994, 30:575.

Herzinger T, et al: Reactive perforating collagenosis: transepidermal elimination of type IV collagen. *Clin Exp Dermatol* 1996, 21:279. ▲

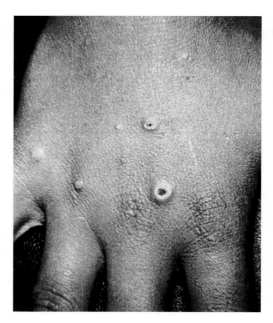

Fig. 25-3 Reactive perforating collagenosis. (Courtesy Dr. A.H. Mehregan.)

Pseudoxanthoma Elasticum

Pseudoxanthoma elasticum (PXE) is an inherited disorder involving the connective tissue of the skin, eye, and cardiovascular system. Many cases appear to be sporadic. In familial cases, both a recessive and a dominant inheritance pattern have been reported, with the recessive form apparently more common. The skin changes are small, circumscribed, yellowish to cream-colored, crepelike, lax, redundant folds, flecked with yellow papules, the so called "plucked chicken skin" appearance (Fig. 25-4). Nuchal comedones and milia en plaque may also be seen. The characteristic exaggerated nasolabial folds may remind one of the face of a hound dog. In addition, the inguinal, periumbilical, and periauricular skin, as well as the mucosa of the soft palate, inner lip, stomach, rectum, and vagina may be involved (Fig. 25-5).

The characteristic retinal change is the angioid streak (Fig. 25-6), which is the result of breaks in the elastic membrane of Bruch. PXE can be demonstrated in more than half of patients with angioid streaks, and 85% of PXE patients will have clinical evidence of retinal findings. The angioid streaks appear earlier than the skin changes, so that most cases are discovered by ophthalmologists. Angioid streaks may be the only sign of the disease for years. In such patients biopsies of the midportions of old scars may be diagnostic of PXE. The association of the skin lesions with angioid streaks is called *Grönblad-Strandberg syndrome*. Angioid streaks may also be seen in Ehlers-Danlos syndrome, Paget's disease of bone, diabetes, hemochromatosis, hemolytic anemia, hypercalcinosis, solar elastosis,

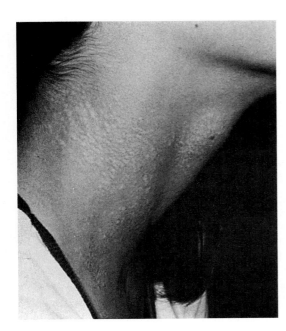

Fig. 25-4   Pseudoxanthoma elasticum in a young woman.

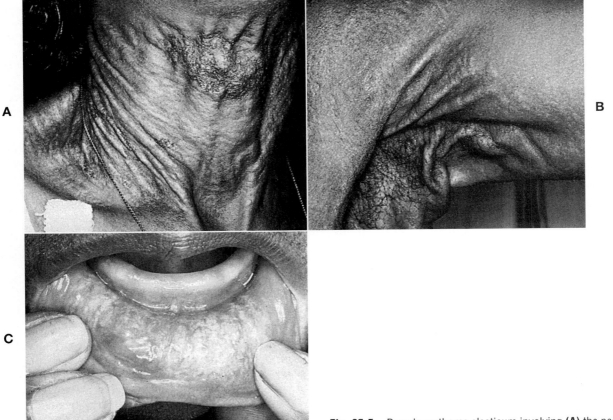

Fig. 25-5   Pseudoxanthoma elasticum involving **(A)** the neck, **(B)** the axillae, and **(C)** the labial mucosa of a 52-year-old woman.

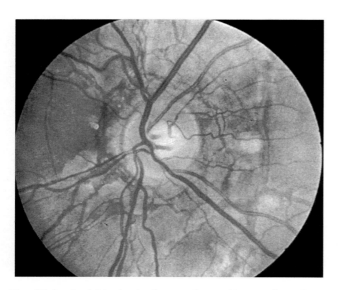

Fig. 25-6 Angioid streaks in a patient with pseudoxanthoma elasticum. (Courtesy Dr. Axel W. Hoke.)

neurofibromatosis, Sturge-Weber syndrome, tuberous sclerosis, myopia, sickle cell anemia, trauma, lead poisoning, hyperphosphatemia, pituitary disorders, and intracranial disorders. PXE, Paget's disease of the bone, and sickle cell disease account for the vast majority of cases with angioid streaks.

On funduscopic examination a reddish brown band is evident around the optic disk, from which glistening streaks extend along the vessels. With fluorescent photography early fluorescence of the angioid streaks and macular lesions are noted. In addition, there may be hemorrhages and exudates. Progressive loss of vision often starts after minor trauma to the eye.

Involvement of the cardiovascular system occurs with a propensity to hemorrhage. These vascular events are caused by the degeneration of the elastic fibers in the vascular media. Gastric hemorrhage occurs in 10% of patients, and viewed by gastroscopy diffuse rather than focal bleeding is found. Epistaxis occurs frequently, hematuria rarely. PXE affects the elastic tissue of the cardiac valves, myocardium, and pericardium. In one study mitral valve prolapse was found in 71% of 14 patients examined. Hypertension occurs in many patients older than age 30 as a result of involvement of the peripheral vessels. Any patient with hypertension at a young age should be examined for stigmata of pseudoxanthoma elasticum. Leg cramps and intermittent claudication occur in young persons. The peripheral pulses are diminished or absent. Calcification of peripheral arteries is seen in many patients over age 30 and may be detected by radiograph. Accelerated coronary artery disease can occur, especially in association with hypertension.

Histologically, throughout the mid-dermis the elastic fibers are swollen and fragmented or granular. They are more gray-blue than normal, and are twisted, curled, and broken, suggesting "raveled wool." Characteristic of PXE is the calcification of these abnormal elastic tissue fibers. Blind biopsies of scars or axillary skin in patients with a family history of PXE or with angioid streaks may sometimes show early changes of PXE. Screening such biopsies with calcium stains is recommended. The actual defect in PXE is unknown. The genetic locus is on the short arm of chromosome 16, and is not the gene for elastin, which is on chromosome 7.

The differential diagnosis includes PXE-like papillary dermal elastolysis, perforating calcific elastosis, and cutis laxa. Patients with PXE-like papillary dermal elastolysis may have cobblestoned, yellow papules on the neck, similar to PXE, but lack any retinal or vascular alterations and lack the typical fragmentation of elastic fibers with calcium deposition on histology. Penicillamine may induce similar clinical and histologic features in patients with Wilson's disease or homocystinuria.

No definitive therapy is available. Usually the skin presents only cosmetic problems; however, there is a progressive loss of vision. Limiting dietary calcium and phosphorus to minimal daily requirement levels has been recommended by some authors. Plastic surgery is helpful for loose folds.

Bolognia JL, et al: Pseudoxanthoma-elasticum-like skin changes induced by penicillamine. *Dermatology* 1992, 184:12.

Cho SH, et al: Milia en plaque associated with pseudoxanthoma elasticum. *J Cutan Pathol* 1997, 24:61.

Contri MB, et al: Matrix proteins with high affinity for calcium ions are associated with mineralization within the elastic fibers of pseudoxanthoma elasticum dermis. *Am J Pathol* 1996, 148:569.

Lebwohl M, et al: Pseudoxanthoma elasticum and mitral valve prolapse. *N Engl J Med* 1982, 307:228.

Orlandi A, et al: Familial occurrence of pseudoxanthoma-elasticum-like papillary dermal elastolysis. *J Eur Acad Dermatol Venereol* 1998, 10:175.

Rongioletti F, et al: Pseudoxanthoma elasticum–like papillary dermal elastolysis. *J Am Acad Dermatol* 1992, 26:648.

Sapadin AN, et al: Periumbilical pseudoxanthoma elasticum associated with chronic renal failure and angioid streaks: apparent regression with hemodialysis. *J Am Acad Dermatol* 1998, 39:338.

Schultz PN, et al: Angioid streaks and pseudoxanthoma elasticum. *JAMA* 1991, 265:45.

Uitto J, et al: International centennial meeting on pseudoxanthoma elasticum: progress in PXE research. *J Invest Dermatol* 1998, 110:840. ▲

Perforating Calcific Elastosis

Also known as *periumbilical perforating PXE* and *localized acquired cutaneous PXE,* perforating calcific elastosis is an acquired, localized cutaneous disorder, most frequently found in obese, multiparous, middle-aged women. Yellowish, lax, well-circumscribed, reticulated or cobblestoned plaques occur in the periumbilical region with keratotic surface papules. It is a distinct disorder that shares some features of PXE. Like PXE there may be calcific elastosis in

TABLE 25-2

Features of Ehlers-Danlos Syndromes

Ehlers-Danlos Type	Gene	Inheritance*	Molecular Abnormality	Clinical Features
I	COL5A1-2†	AD	Type V collagen	Gravis type: Joint laxity, skin hyperextensibility
II	COL5A1-A2	AD	Type V collagen	Mitis type: Same as EDS I but less severe
III		AD	Unknown	Hypermobility
IV	COL3A1	AD AR	Type III procollagen	Thin skin, brusing, ruptured blood vessels and viscera
V		X-linked	Unknown	Skin hyperextensibility, easy brusing
VI		AR	Lysyl hydroxylase deficiency	Severe eye defects and scoliosis
VIIA, VIIB	COL1A1-A2	AD	Type I procollagen	Arthrochalasis, subluxations, moderate skin stretchability
VIIC		AR	Procollagen peptidase deficiency	Dermatosparaxis, severe stretchability, redundant skin
VIII		AD	Unknown	Same as EDS I and II, periodontitis
X		AR	Fibronectin	Brusing

*AR, autosomal recessive; AD, autosomal dominant; X-linked.
†COL5A1-A2 means COL5A1 and COL5A2 genes.

the mid-dermis; however, hereditary PXE rarely causes perforating channels. None of the systemic features of PXE occur in perforating calcific elastosis.

It is suggested that repeated trauma of pregnancy, obesity, and/or abdominal surgery promotes elastic fiber degeneration, resulting in localized disease. PXE can cause periumbilical lesions, and in the absence of documented perforation, evaluations to exclude PXE should be performed. There is no effective therapy.

Karp DL, et al: A yellow plaque with keratotic papules on the abdomen: perforating calcific elastosis (periumbilical perforating pseudoxanthoma elasticum [PXE], localized acquired cutaneous PXE). *Arch Dermatol* 1996, 132:224. _____ ▲

Ehlers-Danlos Syndromes

Synonyms: Cutis hyperelastica, India rubber skin, and elastic skin

Cutis hyperelastica is a group of genetically distinct connective tissue disorders characterized by excessive stretchability and fragility of the skin with a tendency toward easy scar formation, calcification of the skin to produce pseudotumors, and hyperextensibility of the joints, especially the fingers, toes, and knees. Currently, there are nine remaining numeric types of Ehlers-Danlos syndromes (EDS), the salient features of which are listed in Table 25-2. Type IX EDS, allelic to Menkes' disease,

is now known as *occipital horn syndrome* and is identical to X-linked cutis laxa.

A new classification scheme has been proposed, grouping the disorders into six major categories as follows:

1. Classic type (Gravis–EDS type I and Mitis II)
2. Hypermobility type (hypermobile–EDS III)
3. Vascular type (arterial-ecchymotic–EDS type IV)
4. Kyphoscoliosis type (ocular-scoliotic–EDS type VI)
5. Arthrochalasia type (arthrochalasis multiplex congenita–EDS type VIIA and VIIB)
6. Dermatosparaxis type (human dermatosparaxis–EDS type VIIC)

A seventh category comprises other forms (X-linked EDS–EDS type V, periodontitis–EDS type VIII, fibronectin-deficient EDS–EDS type X, familial hypermobility syndrome—formerly EDS type XI, progeroid EDS, and unspecified forms). Major and minor criteria for each category have been established and reviewed by Beighton et al. Beighton believes that the original Gravis and Mitis types (type I and II) are actually one entity based on mutations in COL5A1 or COL5A2 genes.

In those types with hyperextensible skin (types I, II, III, V, VII, and VIII) the integument may be stretched out like a rubber band and snaps back with equal resiliency. This rubbery skin is most pronounced on the elbows, neck, and sides of the abdomen (Fig. 25-7). The skin is velvety in appearance and feels like wet chamois. Minor trauma may produce a gaping "fish-mouth" wound with large hemato-

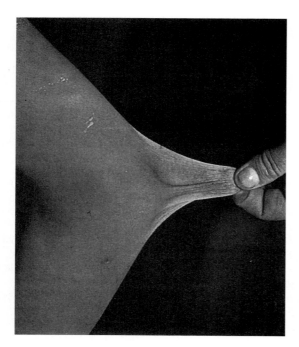

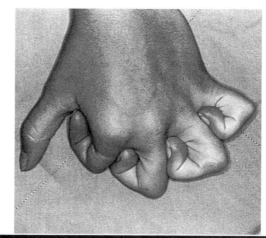

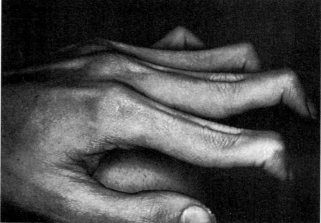

Fig. 25-7 Cutis hyperelastica with stretched skin at elbow. (Courtesy Dr. F. Ronchese.)

mas underneath. The subcutaneous calcifications are 2- to 8-mm oval nodules, mostly on the legs. Trauma over the shins, knees, and elbows produces cigarette-paper–thin scars. Approximately 50% of these patients can touch the tip of the nose with their tongue (Gorlin's sign), compared with 10% of persons without the disorder.

Two types of growths may occur in patients with Ehlers-Danlos syndromes. The molluscum pseudotumor is a soft, fleshy nodule seen in easily traumatized areas such as the ulnar forearms and shins. Spheroids are hard subcutaneous nodules that become calcified and are probably the result of fat necrosis.

Specific features are associated with the various subtypes. Atlantoaxial subluxation may occur in patients with type IV EDS. Patients with type IV EDS have thin, translucent skin; a predisposition for vascular fragility or rupture (arterial, intestinal, or uterine); extensive bruising; and characteristic facial features. Type V patients have clinical features that are similar to the Gravis/Mitis form. Microcornea, retinal detachment, and glaucoma, as well as scoliosis, may be found in type VI EDS. In type VIIA and VIIB EDS there is marked joint hypermobility (Fig. 25-8) and moderate cutaneous elasticity. Joint dislocations of the large joints, such as the hips, are common. Type VIIC, the autosomal recessive form, is referred to as *dermatosparaxis*. Patients with this type have severe skin fragility and sagging, redundant skin. Type VIII EDS manifests easy bruising, which is followed on the shins by scarring, and generalized periodontitis. Type IX EDS has been redefined as an X-linked recessive condition allelic to Menkes'

Fig. 25-8 Ehlers-Danlos syndrome.

syndrome. The original type X EDS patient had hypermobile joints, easy bruising, fish-mouth scars, mitral valve prolapse, and platelets resistant to aggregation with collagen and adenosine diphosphate (ADP) reagents. A qualitative deficiency of fibronectin was the suggested cause, although never confirmed. The familial joint hypermobility syndrome, EDS type XI, was removed from the classification scheme in 1988. Its relationship to EDS is not yet defined.

Hydroxylysylpyridinoline (HP) and lysylpyridinoline (LP) are two nonreducible collagen cross-links derived from hydroxylysyl and lysyl residues of collagen generated by the hydroxylysine pathway. In persons without the disorder the ratio of HP/LP in urine is stable, ranging from 9:1 to 10:1. Acil et al showed reverse ratios in patients with type VI EDS (1:3 to 1:7), a finding that could be used as a diagnostic marker.

It has been demonstrated that types I, II, III, and one subtype each of types IV, VII, and possibly VIII of EDS are transmitted by the autosomal dominant mode; one subtype of type IV, VI, VII, and type X, by the autosomal recessive mode; and type V by an X-linked inheritance pattern (Fig. 25-9). Ehlers-Danlos syndrome must be differentiated from

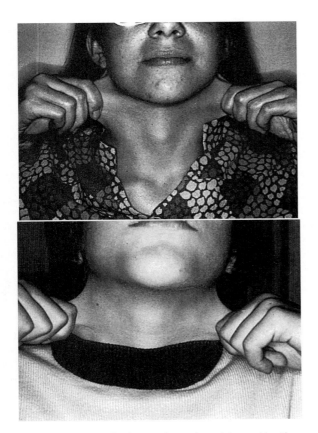

Fig. 25-9 Ehlers-Danlos syndrome in a sister and brother.

Marfan syndrome, pseudoxanthoma elasticum, osteogenesis imperfecta, and cutis laxa. Treatment is supportive, with avoidance of trauma to skin and joints.

Acil Y, et al: Ehlers-Danlos syndrome type VI: cross-link pattern in tissue and urine sample as a diagnostic marker. *J Am Acad Dermatol* 1995, 33:522.

Beighton P, et al: Ehlers-Danlos syndromes: revised nosology, Villefranche, 1997. *Am J Med Genet* 1998, 77:31.

Burrows NP, et al: The gene encoding collagen alpha1(V)(COL5A1) is linked to mixed Ehlers-Danlos syndrome type I/II. *J Invest Dermatol* 1996, 106:1273.

Byers PH, et al: Ehlers-Danlos syndrome: recent advances and current understanding of the clinical and genetic-heterogeneity. *J Invest Dermatol* 1994, 103:47.

Byers PH, et al: Ehlers-Danlos syndrome type VIIA and VIIB result from splice-junction mutations or genomic deletions that involve exon 6 in the COL1A1 and COL1A2 genes of type I collagen. *Am J Med Genet* 1997, 72:94.

Halko GJ, et al: Patients with type IV Ehlers-Danlos syndrome may be predisposed to atlantoaxial subluxation. *J Rheumatol* 1995, 22:2152.

Sasaki T, et al: Ehlers-Danlos syndrome. *Arch Dermatol* 1987, 123:76.

Smith LT, et al: Mutations in the COL3A1 gene result in the Ehlers-Danlos syndrome type IV and alterations in the size and distribution of the major collagen fibrils of the dermis. *J Invest Dermatol* 1997, 108:241.

Yeowell HN, et al: The Ehlers-Danlos syndromes. *Semin Dermatol* 1993, 12:229. _____ ▲

Marfan Syndrome

Marfan syndrome is a disorder of connective tissue transmitted as an autosomal dominant trait with skeletal, cardiovascular, and ocular involvement. It is one of the more common inherited diseases, with estimated incidence rates of 1/10,000 in the United States. Among the important abnormalities are tallness, loose-jointedness, a dolichocephalic skull, high-arched palate, arachnodactyly, pigeon breast, pes planus, poor muscle tone, and large, deformed ears. The aorta, chordae tendineae, and aortic and mitral valves are often involved. Ascending aortic aneurysm and mitral valve prolapse are commonly seen. Ectopia lentis, extensive striae over the hips and shoulders, dental anomalies, and, rarely, elastosis perforans serpiginosa has been reported. Several cases document the occasional occurrence of spontaneous pneumothorax and congenital lung abnormalities. Striae are common in patients with Marfan syndrome.

Marfan syndrome is caused by a gene defect localized to chromosome 15 producing abnormal elastic tissue in fibrillin 1 (aorta adventitia, the suspending ligaments of the lens, skin) and fibrillin 2 (elastin orientation in cartilage, aortic media, bronchi, and all tissues rich in elastin).

Boileau C, et al: Contribution of genetics to pathogenicity and diagnosis of Marfan syndrome. *Arch Mal Coeur Vaiss* 1997, 90(Suppl):1707.

Cohen PR, et al: Clinical manifestations of the Marfan syndrome. *Int J Dermatol* 1989, 28:291.

Pyeritz RE, et al: The Marfan syndrome: diagnosis and management. *N Engl J Med* 1979, 300:772.

Sidhu-Malik NK, et al: The Ehlers-Danlos syndromes and Marfan syndrome: inherited diseases of connective tissue with overlapping clinical features. *Semin Dermatol* 1995, 14:40. _____ ▲

Cutis Laxa (Generalized Elastolysis)

Synonyms: Dermatomegaly, dermatolysis, chalazoderma, and pachydermatocele

Cutis laxa is characterized by loose, redundant skin, hanging in folds. Around the eyelids, cheeks, and neck the drooping skin produces a bloodhound-like facies. Usually the entire integument is involved. The shoulder girdle skin may look like that of a St. Bernard dog. The abdomen is frequently the site of large, pendulous folds.

There are two well-described genetic forms of cutis laxa, the autosomal dominant and recessive types. The dominant form is primarily a cutaneous, cosmetic form, with a good prognosis. The recessive form is associated with significant internal involvement, including hernias, diverticula, pulmonary emphysema, cor pulmonale, aortic aneurysm, dental caries, and osteoporosis. Affected individuals die young. X-linked recessive cutis laxa is now known as *occipital horn syndrome* (formerly type IX Ehlers-Danlos syndrome). It is caused by a mutation in the copper-binding ion transporting ATPase, ATP7A, and is allelic to another X-linked disorder, Menkes' disease.

Nonfamilial cases of cutis laxa have been regularly

reported, with onset from childhood to the late fifties. Lesions may be localized to prior inflammatory lesions, or generalized. Some cases have been associated with an underlying disease or a preceding inflammatory skin process. These include urticaria, eczema, lupus erythematosus, glomerulonephritis, plasma cell dyscrasias, and systemic amyloidosis. Some cases associated with preceding urticarial lesions (Marshall's syndrome) have been shown to be associated with alpha$_1$-antitrypsin deficiency. This protective tissue enzyme has potent antielastase activity, and these cases probably represent enhanced connective tissue damage by elastases produced in the skin by inflammatory cells caused by the absence of normal protective factors. Generalized acquired cutis laxa may affect the pulmonary, vascular, and gastrointestinal connective tissues. Emphysema, pulmonary fibrosis, tracheobronchomegaly, cardiomegaly, cor pulmonale, aortic dilation, pulmonary artery stenosis, esophageal diverticula, esophageal dilation, gastric ulcers, hernias, cystocele, rectocele, prolapsed uterus, and ruptured patellar tendon can all occur. These complications can lead to premature death. Finally, an acrolocated variant may be seen as an isolated finding or associated with myeloma. The skin of the distal digits is loose and inelastic.

Histologically, inherited and acquired cutis laxa are similar. In the acquired form there may be a preceding inflammatory phase that contains large numbers of interstitial neutrophils or eosinophils. Even if no preceding inflammatory phase is noted, in some cases of acquired cutis laxa, macrophages engulfing elastic fibers may be found. There is eventually a diminution of the elastic fibers in the affected area, best detected by elastic tissue stains. The number of fibrocytes is decreased, and the collagen bundles are thinned in the reticular dermis.

The differential diagnosis of cutis laxa includes Ehlers-Danlos syndrome, Marfan syndrome, mid dermal elastolysis, postinflammatory elastolysis and cutis laxa, pseudoxanthoma elasticum, and granulomatous slack skin (a variant of cutaneous T-cell lymphoma).

Mid-dermal elastolysis is an acquired, nonfamilial condition affecting primarily young women. The whole skin surface is affected with widespread atrophic wrinkling. Histologically, elastic tissue is absent from the mid-dermis (as opposed to the whole reticular dermis as in cutis laxa). The cause is unknown, and its relationship to other forms of acquired connective tissue loss is unknown. Postinflammatory elastolysis and cutis laxa is a similar syndrome described originally in Africa and South America. There is a preceding inflammatory phase consisting of indurated plaques. Insect bites may be the trigger of these inflammatory lesions. Once the inflammatory lesions resolve, marked cutaneous atrophy resembling cutis laxa results.

Treatment has been generally disappointing. Multiple surgical procedures to remove the sagging tissue have been largely unsuccessful, since new folds develop in time at the sites of removal.

Chun SI, et al: Acquired cutis laxa associated with chronic urticaria. *J Am Acad Dermatol* 1996, 33:896.

Gardner LI, et al: Congenital cutis laxa syndrome. *Arch Dermatol* 1986, 122:1241.

Jung K, et al: Autosomal recessive cutis laxa syndrome: a case report. *Acta Derm Venereol* 1996, 76:298.

Kochs E, et al: Acquired cutis laxa. *Pediatr Dermatol* 1985, 2:282.

Martin MJ, et al: Acrolocalized acquired cutis laxa. *Br J Dermatol* 1996, 134:973.

McCarty MJ, et al: Cutis laxa acquisita associated with multiple myeloma: a case report and review of the literature. *Cutis* 1996, 57:267.

Mouly F, et al: Cutaneous T-cell lymphoma associated with granulomatous slack skin. *Dermatology* 1996, 192:288.

Nikko A, et al: Acquired cutis laxa associated with a plasma cell dyscrasia. *Am J Dermatopathol* 1996, 18:533.

Randle HW, et al: Generalized elastolysis with systemic lupus erythematosus. *J Am Acad Dermatol* 1983, 8:869. ▲

Blepharochalasis

In blepharochalasis the eyelid skin becomes so lax that it falls in redundant folds over the lid margins. It is an uncommon condition, occurring in young people at about the time of puberty. Recurrent transitory swellings of the lids, lasting 2 or 3 days, are first noted; each is accompanied by a little more stretching, thinning, and wrinkling of the lids, with slowly progressive hyperpigmentation. The condition gives the appearance of fatigue. Most cases are bilateral, but unilateral involvement may occur. Rarely, elastolysis of the earlobes may accompany blepharochalasis. It is generally sporadic, but a dominantly inherited form has been described. Biopsy shows lack of elastic fibers, and abundant IgA deposits have been demonstrated. In elderly patients a similar appearance occurs. Sequelae include excess thin skin, fat herniation, lacrimal gland prolapse, ptosis, blepharophimosis, pseudoepicanthic fold, proptosis, conjunctival injection and cysts, entropion, and ectropion.

Ascher syndrome consists of progressive enlargement of the upper lip and blepharochalasis. The minor salivary glands of the affected areas are hypotrophic and inflamed, resulting in superfluous folds of mucosa, giving the appearance of a double lip. There is a superficial resemblance to angioedema. Treatment is by surgical correction.

Collin JR: Blepharochalasis: a review of 30 cases. *Ophthal Plast Reconstr Surg* 1991, 7:153.

Grassegger A, et al: Immunoglobulin A (IgA) deposits in lesional skin of a patient with blepharochalasis. *Br J Dermatol* 1996, 135:791.

Sanchez MR, et al: Ascher syndrome: a mimicker of acquired angioedema. *J Am Acad Dermatol* 1993, 29:650. ▲

Anetoderma (Macular Atrophy)

The anetodermas, a group of disorders characterized by looseness of the skin, are due to loss of elastic tissue (and perhaps other connective tissue components) without other apparent changes in the skin. Although all disorders that result in tissue atrophy could be included in this group, dermatologists have tended to include in this category those skin diseases characterized by small (usually 1 cm or less) lesions. The category is divided into the primary anetodermas, where no preceding skin inflammatory process has occurred, and the secondary anetodermas, where another skin condition has resulted in anetoderma-like lesions. Because the primary anetodermas largely occur in adulthood and are nonfamilial, they may in reality be secondary to conditions that have not yet been identified. Histologically, as in cutis laxa, there is loss of elastic tissue in the dermis. The old term, *macular atrophy,* is confusing and best discarded.

The clinical findings in both primary and secondary anetoderma, 5- to 10-mm, atrophic plaques, are well defined. The lesions protrude from the skin, and on palpation have less resistance than the surrounding skin, producing the "button hole" sign identical to a neurofibroma (Fig. 25-10). The surface skin may be slightly shiny, white, and crinkly. The usual locations are the trunk, especially on the shoulders, upper arms, and thighs. Intervening skin is normal.

The etiology of primary anetoderma is unknown, but up to half of cases have an accompanying condition. These include Graves' disease, lupus anticoagulant, scleroderma, hypocomplementemia, hypergammaglobulinemia, autoimmune hemolysis, and infection with the human immunodeficiency virus (HIV).

Secondary anetoderma is known to occur after macular and papular secondary syphilis, measles, lupus erythematosus, leprosy, sarcoidosis, tuberous xanthoma, acne, and varicella, and after involution of infiltrative lesions of lymphoreticular malignancy.

Prizant et al described nine cases of anetoderma occurring in premature infants, which they believe to be a distinct subtype termed *anetoderma of prematurity.* Considerations as to cause include pressure, chemical (adhesive), changes in flow of ions or water under monitor leads, or metabolic abnormalities (hypoxemia, hypothermia, or immature metabolic pathways) in susceptible prenatal skin. Intrauterine borreliosis has been implicated in one case. This condition has also been referred to as *congenital anetoderma.*

Abere E, et al: Congenital anetoderma induced by intrauterine infection. *Arch Dermatol* 1997, 133:526.

Hodak E, et al: Immunologic abnormalities associated with primary anetoderma. *Arch Dermatol* 1992, 128:799.

Karrer S, et al: Primary anetoderma in children. *J Am Acad Dermatol* 1996, 13:382.

Olivo MP, et al: Anetoderma: anetoderma, the primary type. *Arch Dermatol* 1993, 129:106.

Prizant TL, et al: Spontaneous atrophic patches in extremely premature infants. *Arch Dermatol* 1996, 132:671.

Stephansson EA, et al: Antiphospholipid antibodies and anetoderma: are they associated? *Dermatology* (Switzerland) 1995, 191:204.

Zellman GL, et al: Congenital anetoderma in twins. *J Am Acad Dermatol* 1997, 36:483. _____ ▲

Striae Distensae

Also known as *striae atrophicae,* striae (pronounced "strye-ee") distensae are depressed lines or bands of thin, reddened skin, which later become white, smooth, shiny, and depressed. These occur on the abdomen during and after pregnancy (striae gravidarum) (Fig. 25-11), on the breasts after lactation, or in those who have suddenly gained weight or muscle mass (weight lifters). Similar striae occur on the

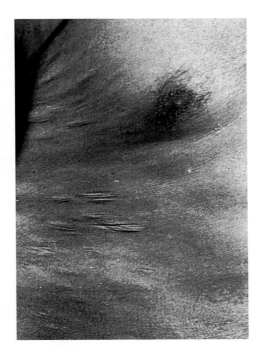

Fig. 25-10 Macular atrophy.

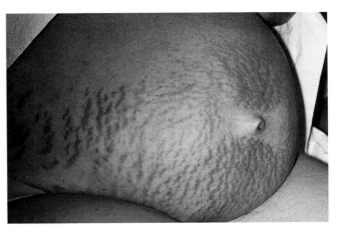

Fig. 25-11 Striae gravidarum.

buttocks and upper, outer, or inner thighs; in the inguinal areas; and over the knees and elbows in children during the growth spurt of puberty. Cushing's syndrome, either endogenous or induced by systemic steroid treatment, is a frequent cause of striae. Striae are common in patients with Marfan syndrome. Prolonged application of topical corticosteroid preparations, especially under occlusion or in folds, will regularly produce striae. In early striae the color may be pink or purple and an initial inflammatory component may be present.

The histologic findings in early striae are of a superficial and deep perivascular and interstitial infiltration of lymphocytes and sometimes eosinophils. In older lesions the infiltrate is much less prominent and the primary changes are in the connective tissue. The collagen of the upper dermis is decreased; the bundles are thinned, and they lie parallel to the overlying epidermis (as in a scar). Elastic tissue appears increased and closer together, probably caused by loss of collagen in excess of elastic tissue. Dilated upper dermal vessels running parallel to the skin surface are present.

Over time striae become less noticeable. Suggested treatments include topical tretinoin and vascular lasers. Low-dose tretinoin provided no benefit after 7 months of treatment in a well-controlled study by Pribanich et al.

Alster TS: Laser treatment of hypertrophic scars, keloids, and striae. *Dermatol Clin* 1997, 15:419.

Barkey WF: Striae and persistent tinea corporis related to prolonged use of betamethasone dipropionate 0.05% cream/clotrimazole 1% cream. *J Am Acad Dermatol* 1987, 17:518.

Elson ML: Treatment of striae distensae with topical tretinoin. *J Dermatol Surg Oncol* 1990, 16:267.

Pribanich S, et al: Low-dose tretinoin does not improve striae distensae. *Cutis* 1994, 54:121.

Tsuji T, et al: Elastic fibers in striae distensae. *J Cutan Pathol* 1988, 15:215. ▲

Linear Focal Elastosis (Elastotic Striae)

Burket et al originally described linear focal elastosis in three elderly men. They presented with asymptomatic, palpable, striaelike yellow lines of the middle and lower back. Subsequent reports have confirmed this not uncommon clinical picture, which can also be seen in young men and women. Histologically, there is increased elastic fibers characterized by thin, wavy, elongated, as well as fragmented, elastic fiber bundles. Electron microscopy reveals elongated thin, irregular shaped, swollen elastic fibers with degenerative changes.

This condition is distinguished from striae in that the linear bands are elevated, not depressed, and yellow, not pink or white. Some cases are also described to have striae distensae.

Burket JM, et al: Linear focal elastosis (elastotic striae). *J Am Acad Dermatol* 1989, 20:633.

Tamada Y, et al: Linear focal elastosis: a review of three cases in young Japanese men. *J Am Acad Dermatol* 1997, 36:301.

Vogel PS, et al: Linear focal elastosis. *Arch Dermatol* 1995, 131:855. ▲

Acrodermatitis Chronica Atrophicans

This acquired diffuse thinning of the skin begins with an early reddish appearance of the extensor surfaces of the extremities, and progresses to smooth, soft, atrophic skin. It is reviewed in Chapter 14 since it results from infection with *Borrelia*.

Osteogenesis Imperfecta

Osteogenesis imperfecta (OI), also known as *Lobstein's syndrome*, affects the bones, joints, eyes, ears, and skin. It is estimated to affect approximately 10,000 persons in the United States (4 to 5 per 100,000). There are four recognized forms, types I through IV. Types I and IV have only an autosomal dominant inheritance, whereas types II and III have both autosomal dominant and autosomal recessive forms. Fifty percent of OI patients have the type I form. The type II form is lethal, and deaths usually occur within the first week of life.

Brittle bones is a dramatic feature resulting from a defect in the collagenous matrix of bone. Fractures occur early in life, sometimes in utero. Loose-jointedness may be striking, and dislocation of joints can be a problem. Blue sclerae, when present, are a valuable clue to diagnosis. The ocular features are of minimal functional importance. Deafness develops in many by the second decade of life and is audiologically indistinguishable from otosclerosis. The skin is thin and rather translucent, and healing wounds result in spreading atrophic scars. Elastosis perforans serpiginosa has been described in patients with osteogenesis imperfecta. Some patients experience unusual bruisability but no consistent defects of the coagulation mechanism have been demonstrated. This is probably due to a structural defect in either the blood vessel wall or the supporting dermal connective tissue.

The basic defect is abnormal collagen synthesis, resulting in type I collagen of abnormal structure. In several patients the precise defect has been identified. In type I (blue scleral dominant) there is diminished type I collagen with a mutation of COL1A1 gene; in type II (perinatal lethal) there is diminished type I collagen synthesis and decreased integrity of the helical domain of α_1 (I) gene; in type III (progressive deforming) there is delayed secretion of type I collagen with altered mannosylation; and in type IV (white sclerae dominant) there is a defective pro α_1 (I) gene.

The major causes of death in osteogenesis imperfecta, attributed to the disease, are respiratory failure secondary to severe kyphoscoliosis and head trauma, mostly observed in type III disease. Patients with type I and type IV disease have a normal life span.

Pamidronate (biphosphonate) is a potent inhibitor of bone resorption, and preliminary studies in treating patients with osteogenesis imperfecta are encouraging. Devogelaer et al in an open trial noted significant increased bone density in patients treated with oral or intravenous pamidronate. Astrom et al reported similar results with intravenous pamidronate in children treated over a 2- to 5-year period with no significant side effects. The patients reported major improvement in well-being, pain, and the performance of activities of daily living.

Astrom E, et al: Beneficial effect of bisphosphonate during five years of treatment of severe osteogenesis imperfecta. *Acta Paediatr* 1998, 87:64.

Devogelaer JP, et al: Use of pamidronate in chronic and acute bone loss conditions. *Medicina* (B Aires) 1997, 1(Suppl):101.

Korkko J, et al: Analysis of the COL1A1 and COL1A2 genes by PCR amplification and scanning by conformation-sensitive gel electrophoresis identifies only COL1A1 mutations in 15 patients with osteogenesis imperfecta type I. *Am J Hum Genet* 1998, 62:98.

McAllion SJ, et al: Causes of death in osteogenesis imperfecta. *J Clin Pathol* 1996, 49:627. _____ ▲

Homocystinuria

Homocystinuria, an inborn error in the metabolism of methionine, is characterized by the presence of homocystine in the urine and systemic abnormalities of the connective tissue. Activity of the enzyme cystathionine synthetase is deficient and as a result cystine is required in the diet of these patients. Among the signs of homocystinuria are genu valgum, kyphoscoliosis, pigeon breast deformity, and frequent fractures. Generalized osteoporosis, arterial and venous thrombosis, and mental retardation are features of homocystinuria not found in Marfan syndrome.

The facial skin has a characteristic flush, especially on the malar areas; the color becomes violaceous when the patient is reclining. Elsewhere the skin is blotchy red, suggestive of livedo reticularis. The hair is fine, sparse, and blond. The teeth are irregularly aligned. Downward dislocation of the lens, as opposed to the upward displacement seen in Marfan syndrome, is a prominent feature. Treatment with hydroxocobalamin and cyanocobalamin produces variable results.

Andersson HC, et al: Biochemical and clinical response to hydroxocobalamin versus cyanocobalamin treatment in patients with methylmalonic acidemia and homocystinuria (cblC). *J Pediatr* 1998, 132:121.

CHAPTER 26

Errors in Metabolism

Amyloidosis

Amyloid is a material deposited in the skin and other organs that is eosinophilic, homogeneous, and hyaline in appearance. It represents beta-pleated sheet forms of various host-synthesized molecules processed into this configuration by host cells.

Amyloidosis can be classified as primary (which often has skin manifestations), secondary (which has very rare skin manifestations), primary localized amyloidosis (also called *primary cutaneous amyloidosis* when the skin is affected), and secondary cutaneous or tumor-associated amyloidosis. Rare familial syndromes may be complicated by secondary amyloidosis or have genetic defects that lead to amyloid deposition (heredofamilial amyloidosis). Classification of cutaneous amyloidoses is shown below.

   I. Systemic amyloidosis
      A. Primary (myeloma-associated) systemic amyloidosis
      B. Secondary systemic amyloidosis
  II. Cutaneous amyloidosis
      A. Macular amyloidosis
      B. Lichen amyloidosis
      C. Nodular amyloidosis
      D. Secondary (tumor-associated) cutaneous amyloidosis
 III. Heredofamilial amyloidosis

All forms of amyloid have relatively identical histologic and electron microscopic findings. The amyloid in all forms is made up of three distinct components: protein-derived amyloid fibers, amyloid P component (about 15% of amyloid), and ground substance. It is the protein-derived amyloid fibers that differ among the various forms of amyloid.

Amyloid is weakly periodic acid-Schiff (PAS) positive and diastase resistant, Congo-red positive, purple with crystal violet, and positive with thioflavin T. Amyloid stained with Congo red exhibits apple-green birefringence under polarized light. Secondary systemic amyloid (AA amyloid) loses its birefringence after treatment with po-

tassium permanganate, whereas primary and localized cutaneous forms do not.

Amyloid stains an intense, bright orange with cotton dyes such as Pagoda red, RIT Scarlet No. 5, or RIT Cardinal red No. 9. Ultrastructurally, amyloid has a characteristic fibrillar structure that consists of straight, nonbranching, nonanastomosing, often irregularly arranged filaments 60 to 100 nm in diameter. If the type of amyloid is known, specific antibodies against the protein component can be used. Only 50% of cases of primary systemic amyloidosis stain with antisera to kappa or lambda chains, because the amyloid protein frequently contains only the variable portion of the immunoglobulin light chain. Because amyloid substance P is present in all forms of amyloid, immunoperoxidase staining against this component will stain all forms of amyloid. In addition, since serum amyloid P (SAP) is avidly bound to amyloid, radiolabeled highly purified SAP can be used to localize amyloidosis, determine the extent of organ infiltration, study progression of disease, and see if therapy reduces the amount of amyloid in various organs.

SYSTEMIC AMYLOIDOSES
Primary Systemic Amyloidosis

Primary systemic amyloidosis involves mesenchymal tissue, the tongue, heart, gastrointestinal tract, and skin. Cutaneous manifestations occur in approximately 40% of cases of primary systemic amyloidosis. Myeloma-associated amyloidosis is included in this category. The amyloid fibril proteins in primary systemic (so-called immunocytic or plasma cell dyscrasia–associated) amyloidosis are composed of protein AL. This is derived from the immunoglobulin light chains, usually of the lambda subtype, and is often only a fragment of the light chain, particularly from the amino terminal end or variable region. Ninety percent of patients will also have this immunoglobulin fragment in the serum or urine. This same type of amyloid, AL, is also found in nodular or tumefactive cutaneous amyloidosis, which is best considered a localized plasmacytoma-producing amyloid.

In primary systemic amyloidosis, the cutaneous eruption usually begins as shiny, smooth, firm, flat-topped, or spherical papules of waxy color, which, because of their tenseness, have the appearance of translucent vesicles. These lesions coalesce to form nodules and plaques of various sizes and, in some cases, bandlike lesions. The regions about the eyes, nose, mouth, and mucocutaneous junctions are commonly involved. Vulvar lesions may resemble giant condylomata.

Purpuric lesions and ecchymoses occur in about 15% of patients and are the most common cutaneous manifestation of primary systemic amyloidosis. They result from amyloid infiltration of blood vessels. Purpura chiefly affects the eyelids, limbs, and oral cavity (Fig. 26-1). Purpura typically occurs after trauma (pinch purpura). Purpuric lesions also classically appear after actions or procedures that result in increased pressure in the vessels of the face, such as after vomiting, coughing, proctoscopic examination, or pulmonary function testing.

Glossitis, with macroglossia, occurs in at least 20% of cases, may be an early symptom, and can lead to dysphagia (Fig. 26-2). The tongue becomes greatly enlarged, and furrows develop. The lateral aspects show indentations from the teeth. Papules or nodules, sometimes with hemorrhage, occur on the tongue.

Bullous amyloidosis is a rare but important clinical manifestation of amyloidosis. Skin fragility and tense, hemorrhagic bullae appear at areas of trauma, usually the hands, forearms, and feet. Lesions heal with scarring and milia. Histologically, the lesions are subepidermal and pauciinflammatory. Epidermolysis bullosa acquisita and porphyria cutanea tarda are the differential diagnoses. Amyloid staining may yield negative results, and direct immunofluorescence may be falsely positive (because of AL protein deposition at the dermoepidermal junction). The diagnosis is confirmed by evaluation of the patient's serum and urine for immunoglobulin fragments and by electron microscopy of the skin biopsies, which will demonstrate the amyloid.

A diffuse or patchy alopecia, cutis verticis gyrata, a scleroderma-like, scleromyxedema-like, or a cutis laxa–like appearance have also rarely been described. The nail matrix may be infiltrated resulting in atrophy of the nail plate, presenting as longitudinal striae, partial anonychia, splitting, and crumbling of the nail plate. Cordlike thickening along blood vessels can also occur.

Patients may present with or develop a plethora of systemic findings. Most characteristically they develop carpal tunnel syndrome, other peripheral neuropathies, a rheumatoid arthritis–like arthropathy of the small joints, orthostatic hypotension, gastrointestinal bleeding, nephrotic syndrome, and cardiac disease. These patients may appear to have prominent deltoid muscles as a result of deposition of amyloid in the muscles (shoulder pad sign). Cardiac arrhythmias and congestive heart failure are common causes of death.

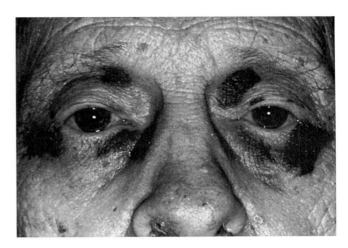

Fig. 26-1 Primary systemic amyloidosis.

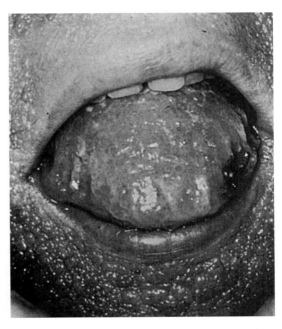

Fig. 26-2 Primary systemic amyloidosis. Progressive enlargement of the tongue with translucent papules and purpura of the tongue and skin.

The prognosis for patients with primary systemic amyloidosis is poor. The median survival averages 13 months for patients without myeloma, and 5 months for myeloma-associated cases. Patients presenting with neurologic findings survive longer than patients presenting with cardiac disease.

Treatment is very difficult. Systemic chemotherapy (usually melphalan) and prednisone or dexamethasone have been reported to be beneficial, but in general the prognosis is poor. Secondary malignancies may complicated alkylating therapy. Hematopoetic stem cell transplantation has led to remission in some patients.

Secondary Systemic Amyloidosis

Secondary systemic amyloidosis is amyloid involvement of the adrenals, liver, spleen, and kidney as a result of some chronic disease, such as tuberculosis, lepromatous leprosy, Hodgkin's disease, Behçet's disease, rheumatoid arthritis, ulcerative colitis, schistosomiasis, or syphilis. The parenchymatous organs are involved, but the skin is not. Certain dermatoses, such as hidradenitis suppurativa, stasis ulcers, psoriatic arthritis, and dystrophic epidermolysis bullosa may be complicated by systemic amyloidosis.

The amyloid fibrils in secondary systemic amyloidosis, and in the type associated with Muckle-Wells syndrome and with familial Mediterranean fever, are designated *AA*. The protein component is unrelated to immunoglobulin. Its precursor is serum amyloid A protein *(SAA)*, which is an acute-phase reactant that is increased in various inflammatory states. Biopsy of normal skin in secondary systemic amyloidosis may be positive for perivascular amyloid in slightly more than half the cases. The treatment of secondary systemic amyloidosis is to treat the underlying condition optimally.

In patients undergoing hemodialysis, carpal tunnel syndrome is frequent; its prevalence is related to the duration of dialysis. This finding is now known to be associated with amyloid deposition in synovium, causing not only carpal tunnel syndrome but also trigger finger, bone cysts, and spondyloarthropathy. The protein component of dialysis-related amyloidosis is beta 2-microglobulin, altered by uremia to have advanced glycation end products.

CUTANEOUS AMYLOIDOSIS
Primary Cutaneous Amyloidosis

The primary cutaneous amyloidoses have been divided into two forms—macular and lichen amyloid. Most patients have only one form, but rarely, patients may be seen with both patterns. Chronic rubbing of the skin resulting from pruritus or the use of nylon brushes during bathing (frictional amyloidosis) appears contributory. Individuals of Asian, Hispanic, or Middle Eastern ancestry seem to be predisposed. The deposited amyloid material contains keratin as its protein component, strongly suggesting that traumatic damage to basal keratinocytes results in the deposits. Why only certain individuals are affected is unknown. A rare form localized to the conchae has been described.

The histologic picture of both forms of primary cutaneous amyloidosis is similar, the only difference being the size of the amyloid deposits and the extent of the overlying epidermal changes. The overlying epidermis is frequently hyperkeratotic. Focal necrotic keratinocytes may be observed in the basal cell layer. Dermal papillae are expanded by the amorphous deposits of amyloid that may abut immediately below the epidermis. Melanin deposits are classically present in the amyloid. In all cases of postin-

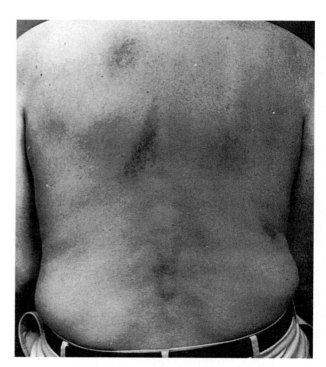

Fig. 26-3 Macular amyloidosis of the back.

flammatory hyperpigmentation with incontinence of pigment, one should carefully examine the texture of the areas of dermal melanosis to exclude amyloidosis. Systemic amyloidosis is excluded by the absence of amyloid deposits around blood vessels. Special stains may be used to confirm the diagnosis, but this is rarely required if the classic histology is found. In difficult cases, immunoperoxidase stains for keratin will stain the amyloid deposits and confirm the diagnosis of primary cutaneous amyloidosis. Direct immunofluorescence may demonstrate immunoglobulin (usually IgM) in a globular pattern in the keratin-derived cutaneous amyloidoses, but this is caused by passive absorption rather than by specific deposition. This phenomenon is seen in all disorders with prominent apoptosis of keratinocytes.

Macular Amyloidosis. Typical cases exhibit moderately pruritic, brown, rippled macules characteristically located in the interscapular region of the back (Fig. 26-3). Pigmentation is typically not uniform, giving the lesions a "salt and pepper" appearance. Notalgia paresthetica is localized to the same sites, and most cases of macular amyloid between the scapulae probably result from rubbing dysesthetic areas of notalgia paresthetica. Occasionally the thighs, shins, arms, breasts, and buttocks may be involved, and these more diffuse cases are usually associated with diffuse pruritus (Fig. 26-4). Macular amyloidosis is a chronic condition.

Lichen Amyloidosis. Lichen amyloidosis is characterized by the appearance of paroxysmally itchy lichenoid papules,

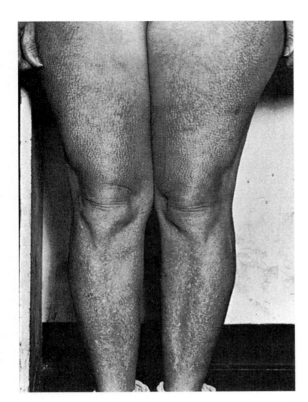

Fig. 26-4 Macular amyloidosis cutis of both shins and thighs. Note parallel ripples. (Courtesy Drs. R. Montgomery and W.B. Hurlburt.)

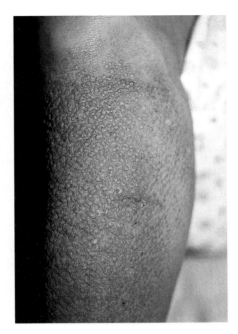

Fig. 26-5 Lichen amyloidosis.

typically appearing bilaterally on the shins (Fig. 26-5). The primary lesions are small, brown, discrete, slightly scaly papules that group to form infiltrated large moniliform plaques. It may, less commonly, occur on the thighs, the forearms, and even on the upper back, in addition to the shins.

Treatment of the primary cutaneous amyloidoses is frequently unsatisfactory. Reducing the friction to the skin is critical. Identifying the cause of the rubbing, whether it is habit, pruritus, or neuropathy (as in notalgia paresthetica), directs treatment. Occlusion plays a major role, because it both enhances topical treatments and provides a physical block to prevent trauma to the skin. Administration of topical high-potency corticosteroid agents can be beneficial, as can intralesional corticosteroid therapy when small areas are involved. Oral retinoids, cyclophosphamide, and dermabrasion have also been reported to be beneficial.

Nodular Amyloidosis. Nodular amyloidosis is a rare form of primary localized cutaneous amyloidosis in which single, or rarely, multiple nodules or tumefactions may be found on the extremities, trunk, genitals, or face. The overlying epidermis may appear atrophic, and lesions may resemble large bullae. The dermis and subcutis may be seen microscopically to be diffusely infiltrated with amyloid. The lesions may contain numerous plasma cells, and are

best considered isolated plasmacytomas. The amyloid in these patients is immunoglobulin-derived AL, as is seen in primary systemic amyloidosis, and is unrelated to keratinocyte-related amyloid or to AA amyloid. Treatment is physical removal or destruction of the lesion with shave removal and desiccation or CO_2 laser.

Secondary Cutaneous Amyloidosis

Following PUVA therapy and in benign and malignant cutaneous neoplasms, deposits of amyloid may be found. Most frequently the associated neoplasms are nonmelanoma skin cancers or seborrheic keratoses. In all cases, this is keratin-derived amyloid.

FAMILIAL SYNDROMES ASSOCIATED WITH AMYLOIDOSIS (HEREDOFAMILIAL AMYLOIDOSIS)

Familial syndromes have been reported that have either systemic or localized amyloidosis. In familial Mediterranean fever and Muckle-Wells syndrome, the amyloid protein is AA; these are hereditary inflammatory diseases commonly complicated by secondary systemic amyloidosis. Multiple endocrine neoplasia IIA can be complicated by keratin-derived amyloid. Poikiloderma-like cutaneous amyloidosis and other very rare hereditary variants of cutaneous amyloidosis exist.

Most forms of familial amyloidosis, however, present with neurologic disease and are now designated *familial amyloidotic polyneuropathy.* Peripheral neuropathy, and, less commonly, autonomic neuropathy and cardiomyopathy occur. Four types have been identified: FAP I through IV. FAP I (Portuguese/Japanese/Swedish) and FAP II (Maryland-German/Indiana-Swiss) are caused by genetic defects in transthyretin. These are autosomal dominant syndromes, and most affected patients are heterozygotes. FAP III is caused by a genetic defect in apolipoprotein A-1 and FAP IV by a defect in gelsolin.

Beber T, et al: Hemorrhagic bullous amyloidosis. *Arch Dermatol* 1988, 124:1683.

Benson MD: Familial amyloidosis. *J Intern Med* 1992, 232:525.

Breathnach SM: Amyloid and amyloidosis. *J Am Acad Dermatol* 1988, 18:1.

De Pietro WP: Primary familial cutaneous amyloidosis. *Arch Dermatol* 1981, 117:639.

Falk RH, et al: The systemic amyloidoses. *N Engl J Med* 1997, 337:898.

Fritz DA, et al: Unusual longevity in primary systemic amyloidosis. *Am J Med* 1989, 86:245.

Gejyo F, et al: Beta 2-microgobulin-associated amyloidoses. *J Intern Med* 1992, 232, 531.

Gertz MA, et al: Amyloidosis. *Mayo Clin Proc* 1999, 74:490.

Gertz MA, et al: Familial amyloidosis. *Mayo Clin Proc* 1992, 67:428.

Hashimoto K, et al: Nylon brush macular amyloidosis. *Arch Dermatol* 1987, 123:633.

Hicks BC, et al: Primary cutaneous amyloidosis of the auricular concha. *J Am Acad Dermatol* 1988, 18:19.

Husby G: Nomenclature and classification of amyloid and amyloidoses. *J Intern Med* 1992, 232:511

Kitajima Y, et al: Nodular primary cutaneous amyloidosis. *Arch Dermatol* 1986, 122:1425.

Kyle, RA: Primary systemic amyloidosis. *J Intern Med* 1992, 232:523.

Marschalko M, et al: Etretinate for the treatment of lichen amyloidosis. *Arch Dermatol* 1988, 124:657.

Miyata T, et al: Diagnosis, pathogenesis, and treatment of dialysis-related amyloidosis. *Miner Electrolyte Metab* 1999, 25:114.

Northcutt AD, et al: Nodular cutaneous amyloidosis involving the vulva. *Arch Dermatol* 1985, 121:518.

Olsen KE, et al: The use of subcutaneous fat tissue for amyloid typing by ELISA. *Am J Clin Pathol* 1999, 111:355.

Robert, C, et al: Bullous amyloidosis. *Medicine* 1993, 72:38.

Scheinberg MA, et al: DMSO and colchicine therapy in amyloid disease. *Ann Rheum Dis* 1989, 93:421.

Sezer O, et al: Rapid reversal of nephrotic syndrome due to primary systemic AL amyloidosis after VAD and subsequent high dose chemotherapy with autologous stem cell support. *Bone Marrow Transplant* 1999, 23:967.

Touart, DM, et al: Cutaneous deposition diseases. *J Am Acad Dermatol* 1998, 39:149.

Truhan AP, et al: Nodular primary localized cutaneous amyloidosis. *J Am Acad Dermatol* 1986, 14:1058.

Tuneau A, et al: A waxy plaque on the leg (nodular amyloidosis). *Arch Dermatol* 1988, 124:769.

Vasily DB, et al: Familial primary cutaneous amyloidosis. *Arch Dermatol* 1978, 114:1173.

Wang WJ, et al: Response of systemic amyloidosis to dimethyl sulfoxide. *J Am Acad Dermatol* 1986, 15:402.

Weyers W, et al: Lichen amyloidosis. *J Am Acad Dermatol* 1997, 37:923.

Wheeler GE, et al: Alopecia universalis. *Arch Dermatol* 1981, 117:815.

Wong C-K, et al: Dermabrasion for lichen amyloidosis. *Arch Dermatol* 1982, 118:302.

Yanagihara M, et al: Staining of amyloid with cotton dyes. *Arch Dermatol* 1984, 120:1184 _____ ▲

Porphyrias

Porphyrinogens are the building blocks of all the hemoproteins, including hemoglobin and the cytochrome enzymes. They are produced primarily in the liver and bone marrow or erythrocytes. In certain inherited and acquired disease states, called the *porphyrias,* these intermediate metabolites of hemoglobin synthesis are increased.

Each form of porphyria has now been associated with a deficiency in an enzyme in the metabolic pathway of heme synthesis. Cutaneous disease, characterized by photosensitivity, is observed in some forms of porphyria. The photosensitivity in porphyria is caused by the absorption of ultraviolet radiation in the Soret band (400 to 410 nm) by increased porphyrins. These activated porphyrins are unstable, and as they return to a ground state, they transfer energy to oxygen, creating reactive oxygen species. These unstable oxygen species interact with biologic systems, primarily plasma and lysosomal membranes, causing tissue damage. Mediators released from mast cells and polymorphonuclear leukocytes, acting through complement, eicosanoids, or factor XII pathways may augment tissue effects.

Understanding the biosynthetic pathway of heme has clarified the biochemical basis of the porphyrias. Delta-aminolevulinic acid (dALA) is synthesized in the mitochondria via dALA synthetase. From it are formed, successively, porphobilinogen, uroporphyrin III, coproporphyrin III, and protoporphyrin IX. This reenters the mitochondrion, to be acted on by ferrochelatase to produce heme. Each step in this process is catalyzed by a specific enzyme. Heme, by negative feedback, represses the production, or activity, of dALA synthetase. If heme is inadequate, dALA synthetase activity may be increased, leading to the production of more porphyrins. Because this enzyme system is "inducible," medications that increase the cytochrome drug metabolizing system in the liver can lead to exacerbation of the porphyrias by increasing the production of the porphyrin intermediates.

The current grouping of the porphyrias is based on the primary site of increased porphyrin production, either liver or bone marrow—the hepatic or erythropoietic porphyrias, respectively. Some include a hepatoerythropoietic category. Congenital erythropoietic porphyria (CEP), erythropoietic protoporphyria (EPP), and erythropoietic coproporphyria (ECP) are the erythropoietic forms. Acute intermittent porphyria (AIP), ALA dehydratase deficiency, hereditary coproporphyria (HCP), variegate porphyria (VP), and porphyria cutanea tarda (PCT) are the hepatic forms. Hepato-erythrocytic porphyria (HEP) has been classified as either a hepatic or hepatoerythropoietic type.

The porphyrias are diagnosed by identifying characteristic clinical and biochemical abnormalities, typically elevated levels of porphyrins in the urine, serum, or stool. Because there is some clinical overlap, biochemical testing should be performed to confirm any diagnosis of porphyria. The clinical syndromes may be chronic or have intermittent exacerbations with relative quiescent periods. The latter are called the *acute porphyrias*.

PORPHYRIA CUTANEA TARDA

Porphyria cutanea tarda (PCT) is the most common type of porphyria. It is characterized by photosensitivity resulting in bullae, especially on sun-exposed parts. The dorsal hands and forearms, ears, and face are primarily affected (Fig. 26-6). The bullae are not surrounded by erythema, and rupture easily to form erosions or shallow ulcers. These heal with scarring, milia, and dyspigmentation. Lesions on the legs, especially the shins and dorsal feet, occur primarily in women. In addition, patients frequently complain of skin fragility in affected areas. There is hyperpigmentation of the skin, especially of the face, neck, and hands. Hypertrichosis of the face, especially over the cheeks and temples, is seen (Fig. 26-7). The face and neck, especially in the periorbital area, may show a pink to violaceous tint. Sclerodermatous thickenings may develop on the back of the neck, in the preauricular areas, or on the thorax, fingers, and scalp (Fig. 26-8). In the latter instance, there is associated alopecia (Fig. 26-9). Friedman et al reported a direct relationship between the levels of uroporphyrins in the urine and sclerodermatous changes.

Liver disease is frequently present in patients with PCT. A history of alcoholism is common. Hepatitis C virus infection has been found in 17% (Northern Europe), 20% (Australia/New Zealand), 65% (Southern Europe), and 94% (United States) of patients with PCT. All PCT patients should be screened for hepatitis C infection. Iron overload in the liver is frequently found in patients with PCT. This may be as a consequence of chemical or viral liver damage, or because some patients with PCT are heterozygous for the gene for hemochromatosis and tend to deposit iron in their livers. Hepatocellular carcinoma may rarely produce PCT.

PCT has been frequently associated with other diseases. It is estimated that diabetes mellitus occurs in 15% to 20% of patients with PCT. Numerous cases of lupus erythematosus concomitant with PCT have been reported. Patients may have both systemic and/or purely cutaneous lupus, and either disease may present initially. The pathogenesis of this association is unclear.

PCT occurs not infrequently in patients infected with the human immunodeficiency virus (HIV). This is not solely related to coexistent hepatitis C virus infection, which is increased in some risk groups of HIV-infected persons. Subtle porphyrin abnormalities are found in HIV disease, but the porphyrin levels are well below those capable of

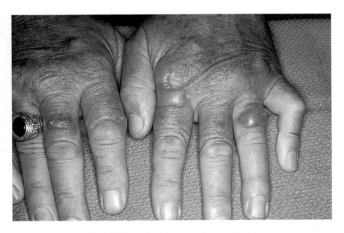

Fig. 26-6 Porphyria cutanea tarda.

inducing clinical disease. Other risk factors, such as alcoholism, are frequently present. HIV-infected patients with PCT should be evaluated for other causes of PCT, and the existence of PCT should not be attributed to the HIV disease alone. However, effective anti-HIV therapy has led to improvement of PCT in one HIV/hepatitis C-infected patient.

Estrogen treatment is associated with the appearance of PCT by an unknown mechanism. Before oral contraceptives were introduced, PCT cases occurred predominantly among men, but in most recent series, 60% of cases occurred in men and 40% in women. Men treated with estrogens for prostate cancer may also develop PCT.

Porphyria cutanea tarda is related to a deficiency in the enzyme uroporphyrinogen decarboxylase. Several types have been described. The most common is the sporadic, nonfamilial form, which represents about 80% or more of cases. Enzymatic activity of uroporphyrinogen decarboxylase is abnormal in the liver but normal in other tissues, and there are no mutations of the enzyme detected. With remission, the enzyme activity in the liver may return to normal. Patients present in midlife, averaging about age 45.

The second, or familial type, is an autosomal dominantly inherited deficiency of uroporphyrinogen decarboxylase in the liver and red blood cells of patients and also of clinically unaffected family members. There is an approximate 50% decrease in both the activity and concentration of the enzyme. Multiple genetic defects have been reported producing the same phenotype. Familial PCT tends to present at an earlier age, and development of PCT before age 20 strongly suggests familial PCT. A third nonfamilial form (acquired toxic PCT) is associated with acute or chronic exposure to hepatotoxins, specifically polyhalogenated hydrocarbons, such as hexachlorobenzene and dioxin. These patients have biochemical and clinical features identical to those of patients with sporadic and familial CT.

A diagnosis of PCT can be strongly suspected on clinical grounds. A useful confirmatory test that can be performed in

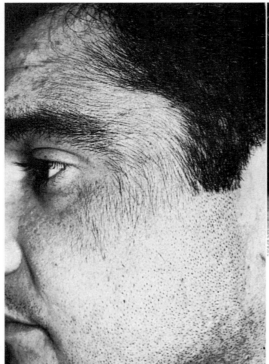

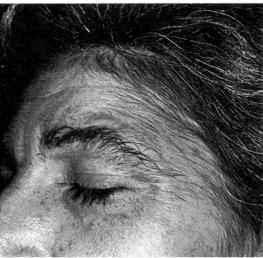

Fig. 26-7 Hypertrichosis over the forehead, temples, and malar eminences in a man and in a woman, both with porphyria cutanea tarda. (Courtesy Dr. C.P. DeFeo.)

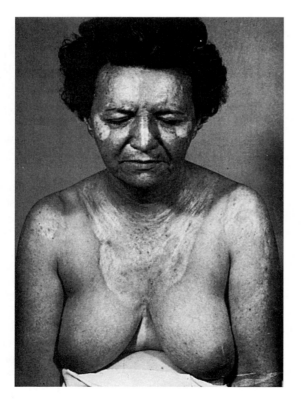

Fig. 26-8 Porphyria cutanea tarda with sclerodermoid patches on the sun-exposed areas.

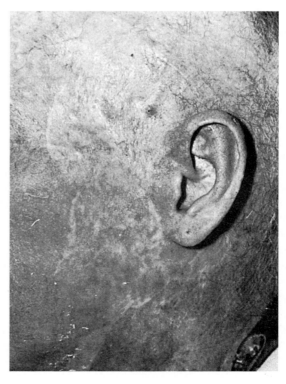

Fig. 26-9 Sclerodermid plaques and alopecia in a 65-year-old woman with porphyria cutanea tarda.

the office is the characteristic pink or coral-red fluorescence of a random urine specimen under a Wood's light. A 24-hour collected urine specimen usually contains less than 100 µg porphyrins in a normal individual; in PCT it may range from 300 µg to several thousand micrograms. The ratio of uroporphyrins to coproporphyrins in PCT is typically 3:1 to 5:1, distinguishing PCT from variegate porphyria.

Biopsy of a blister reveals a noninflammatory subepidermal bulla with an undulating, festooned base. PAS-positive thickening of blood vessel walls in the upper and mid-dermis is present. A useful and highly characteristic—but not diagnostic—feature is the presence of the so-called caterpillar bodies. These eosinophilic, elongated, wavy structures are present in the lower and midepidermis and lie parallel to the basement membrane zone. They stain positively with PAS and are positive for type IV collagen and laminin, suggesting they represent basement membrane material present in the epidermis. Direct immunofluorescence of involved skin shows IgG and C3 at the dermoepidermal junction and in the vessel walls in a linear pattern.

Initial treatment of PCT involves removal of all precipitating environmental agents such as alcohol and medications. This may lead to sufficient improvement that further therapy is not required. Physical barrier protection of affected areas by wearing gloves and a hat is also encouraged. Chemical sunscreens are of little value since they do not typically absorb radiation in the near-visible UVA range. Barrier sunscreens such as titanium dioxide and zinc oxide may be more beneficial.

Phlebotomy is an effective form of treatment. Uroporphyrinogen decarboxylase is inhibited by iron, and removal of hepatic iron may therefore lead to recovery of enzyme activity. Typically, phlebotomy of 500 ml at 2-week intervals is performed until the hemoglobin reaches 10 g/dL or the serum iron 50 to 60 µg/dL. Urinary porphyrin excretion initially increases, but gradually, 24-hour uroporphyrin levels are markedly reduced, with most patients able to achieve normal levels. This process takes several months, usually requiring a total of six to ten phlebotomies. As the porphyrins fall, the skin lesions also involute. Initially, blistering improves, then skin fragility decreases, and even the cutaneous sclerosis and hypertrichosis can eventually reverse. A common error in management is coadministration of oral iron supplementation during the phlebotomies to treat the anemia.

Antimalarials are an alternative to phlebotomy and may be combined with phlebotomy in difficult cases. Full doses of antimalarials may produce a severe hepatotoxic reaction. The initial dose is 200 mg of hydroxychloroquine or 125 mg of chloroquine twice weekly. Improvement is gradual, but can be more rapid than phlebotomy.

After both phlebotomy and antimalarial therapy, a remission is induced that may last many years. If the patient relapses, these treatments can be repeated. Alternative treatments, which are rarely required, include desferrioxamine (iron chelation) and erythropoietin treatment. Erythropoietin may be combined with phlebotomy. PCT in renal failure may respond to renal transplantation. If hepatitis C virus infection coexists, interferon alpha treatment of the hepatitis C infection may lead to improvement of the PCT.

PSEUDOPORPHYRIA

In certain settings patients develop blistering and skin fragility identical to PCT with the histologic features of PCT but with normal urine and serum porphyrins. Hypertrichosis, dyspigmentation, and cutaneous sclerosis do not occur. This condition is called *pseudoporphyria*. Most commonly this is caused by medications, typically an NSAID, usually naproxen (Fig. 26-10). Other NSAIDs and tetracycline can cause a similar picture. Sunbed use can also cause pseudo-PCT. Some patients on hemodialysis develop a similar PCT-like picture. Less commonly, dialysis patients develop true PCT (Fig. 26-11). In the anuric dialysis patient

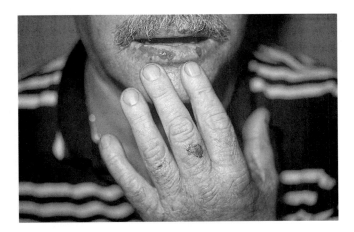

Fig. 26-10 Pseudoporphyria involving lips and dorsal hand secondary to NSAID therapy.

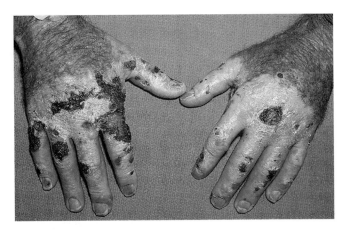

Fig. 26-11 Porphyria cutanea tarda in renal failure.

true PCT and pseudo-PCT are distinguished by analysis of serum porphyrins in a laboratory knowledgeable in the normal porphyrin levels in patients undergoing hemodialysis. The treatment of pseudoporphyria is physical sun protection and discontinuance of any inciting medication. Those cases induced by medications usually resolve over several months; the management of those associated with hemodialysis is much more difficult.

HEPATOERYTHROPOIETIC PORPHYRIA

Hepatoerythropoietic porphyria (HEP) is a very rare form of porphyria that is inherited as an autosomal recessive trait. HEP is the homozygous form of PCT. It is caused by a homozygous or compound heterozygous deficiency of uroporphyrinogen decarboxylase, which is about 10% of normal in both the liver and erythrocytes. The biochemical abnormalities are similar, but more marked, than those in PCT, but the clinical features are similar to congenital erythropoietic porphyria. Dark urine is usually present from birth, but may be noted later. In infancy vesicles occur in sun-exposed skin, followed by sclerodermoid scarring, hypertrichosis, pigmentation, red fluorescence of the teeth under Wood's light examination, and nail damage. Neurologic disease has been reported in one patient. The diagnosis is confirmed by abnormal urinary uroporphyrins, as seen in PCT, elevated erythrocyte protoporphyrins, and increased coproporphyrins in the feces. In congenital erythropoietic porphyria (CEP) uroporphyrins are elevated in the erythrocytes, allowing differentiation from HEP.

ACUTE INTERMITTENT PORPHYRIA

Acute intermittent porphyria (AIP), the second most common form of porphyria, is characterized by periodic attacks of abdominal colic, gastrointestinal disturbances, paralyses, and psychiatric disorders. Skin lesions do not occur, since the elevated porphyrin precursors are not photosensitizers. It is inherited as an autosomal dominant trait and is caused by a deficiency in porphobilinogen deaminase, which has 50% activity in affected persons. Only 10% of those with the genetic defect develop disease, but all may be at risk for primary liver cancer. AIP is particularly common in Scandinavia, especially Lapland. AIP usually presents after puberty in young adulthood, and women outnumber men by 1.5 to 2:1.

Severe abdominal colic is most often the initial symptom of AIP. Usually there is no abdominal wall rigidity, although tenderness and distension are present. Nausea, vomiting, and diarrhea or constipation accompany the abdominal pain. Peripheral neuropathy, mostly motor, is present. Severe pain in the legs occurs. Optic atrophy, diaphragmatic weakness, respiratory paralysis, flaccid quadriplegia, facial palsy, and dysphagia are but a few of the many neurologic signs.

Psychiatric disturbances are varied and frequently apparent. Attacks may be induced by numerous medications.

A diagnosis of AIP is established by finding elevated levels of urinary porphobilinogen (PBG) and increased delta-aminolevulinic acid (dALA) in the plasma and urine. Erythrocyte and fecal porphyrin levels are normal.

No specific treatment is available for AIP. It is important for the patient to avoid such precipitating factors as certain medications, sex steroid hormones, and starvation. Glucose loading has been used extensively and appears to be beneficial in many cases. Hematin infusions, or heme arginate, results in clinical improvement and a marked decrease in ALA and PBG excretion. Early treatment may ameliorate attacks. The phenothiazines (chlorpromazine) may be helpful for pain; opiates and propoxyphene are also useful for analgesia. Oral contraceptives may prevent attacks in women with premenstrual symptoms.

HEREDITARY COPROPORPHYRIA

Hereditary coproporphyria (HCP) is a rare, autosomal dominant porphyria resulting from a deficiency of coproporphyrinogen oxidase (CPO). About one third of these patients are photosensitive, with blistering similar to but less severe than in VP. Affected persons are prone to attacks with gastrointestinal and neurologic symptoms similar to those seen in AIP and VP. Fecal coproporphyrin is always increased; urinary coproporphyrin, ALA, and PBG are increased only during attacks.

Harderoporphyria is caused by a homozygous defect of coproporphyrinogen oxidase with patients having 10% of normal activity. Children present with photosensitivity, hypertrichosis, and hemolytic anemia. Harderoporphyrin is the natural intermediate between coproporphyrinogen and protoporphyrinogen.

VARIEGATE PORPHYRIA

Variegate porphyria (VP) is also known as *mixed porphyria, South African genetic porphyria,* and *mixed hepatic porphyria.* Variegate porphyria has an autosomal dominant inheritance, with a high penetrance. It results from a decrease in activity of protoporphyrinogen oxidase. The majority of affected relatives have silent VP, in which there is reduced enzyme activity but no clinical lesions. Such persons should be identified and counseled to avoid known precipitating medications.

VP is characterized by the combination of the skin lesions of PCT and the gastrointestinal and neurologic disease of AIP. Seventy percent of patients develop skin lesions; in 50%, this is the presenting finding. Vesicles and bullae with erosions, especially on the sun-exposed areas, are the chief manifestations. In addition, hypertrichosis is seen in the temporal area, especially in women. Hyperpigmentation of sun-exposed areas is also a feature. Facial scarring and thickening of the skin may give the patient a prematurely aged appearance.

The presence of VP should be suspected in a patient when findings indicate both PCT and AIP, especially if there is a history of South African ancestry. Fecal coproporphyrins and protoporphyrins are always elevated, and during attacks urine porphobilinogen and ALA are elevated. Urinary coproporphyrins are increased over uroporphyrins, distinguishing VP from PCT. A finding in the plasma of the "X porphyrin" with unique fluorescence at 626 nm is characteristic of VP and distinguishes it form all other forms of porphyria. Treatment is symptomatic and as outlined for PCT and AIP.

ERYTHROPOIETIC PROTOPORPHYRIA

Erythropoietic protoporphyria (EPP) is an inherited disorder with both autosomal dominant and autosomal recessive forms. The ferrochelatase activity is 10% to 25% of normal in affected persons. EPP typically presents early in childhood (2 to 5 years of age), but presentation late in adulthood can occur.

Unique among the more common forms of porphyria is an immediate burning of the skin on sun exposure. Because the elevated protoporphyrin IX absorbs both in the Soret band and also at 500 to 600 nm, visible light through window glass or in the operating room may precipitate symptoms. Infants simply cry when exposed to sunlight. Erythema, plaquelike edema, and wheals such as those seen in hydroa aestivale or solar urticaria can be seen. These lesions appear solely on sun-exposed areas. In severe cases, purpura is seen in the sun-exposed areas.

With repeated exposure, the skin develops a weather-beaten appearance. Shallow linear or elliptical scars, waxy thickening and pebbling of the skin on the nose, cheeks, and the over the metacarpophalangeal joints, and atrophy of the rims of the ears have been described (Fig. 26-12).

Many EPP patients have mildly elevated liver function tests. Severe liver disease develops in 10% of patients, and 1% of EPP patients die of liver failure. Excessive porphyrins are deposited in the liver, porphyrin gallstones are frequently found, and affected livers are cirrhotic. Autosomal recessive inheritance of EPP may be a risk factor for the development of liver failure. Liver failure requires liver transplantation. A mild microcytic anemia is present in 25% of patients with EPP, but therapy with iron should be used only if iron deficiency is detected, since it may exacerbate symptoms.

Histologically, there is prominent ground glass, PAS-positive material in the upper dermis mostly perivascularly. This material is type IV collagen. On direct immunofluorescence IgG and C3 may be found perivascularly.

A diagnosis of EPP can usually be suspected on clinical grounds, especially if both the acute symptoms and chronic skin changes are found. Because protoporphyrin IX is not water soluble, urine porphyrin levels are normal. Erythrocyte protoporphyrin is elevated, and can be detected by RBC fluorescence. Erythrocyte, plasma, and fecal protoporphyrin can also be assayed to confirm the diagnosis. Erythrocyte protoporphyrin levels in affected persons may range from several hundred to several thousand micrograms per 100 ml of packed RBC (normal values, less than 35 μg/100 ml of packed RBCs).

The differential diagnosis of EPP includes hydroa vacciniforme, xeroderma pigmentosa, and solar urticaria. In infancy, before the appearance of the chronic skin changes, erythrocyte porphyrins may need to be screened to confirm

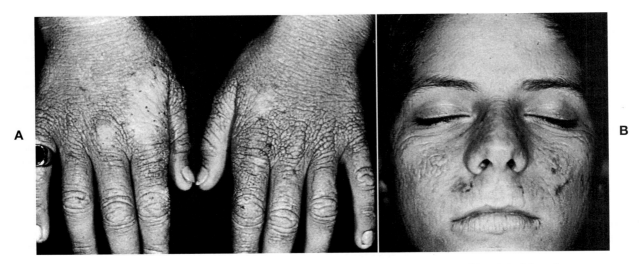

Fig. 26-12 Erythropoietic protoporphyria. Note **A,** weather-beaten appearance of hands in this male adolescent and **B,** shallow scars on the face.

the diagnosis. Once chronic changes are present, a skin biopsy will confirm the diagnosis.

The treatment consists of protection from exposure to sunlight with clothing and barrier sunscreens with titanium dioxide or zinc oxide. Beta carotene, 60 to 180 mg daily, to maintain a serum level of from 400 to 600 μg/100 ml, provides some protection for most cases. As the child grows, the dose must be increased to maintain adequate tissue levels. Phototherapy (PUVA or narrow-band UVB) to increase skin thickness and epidermal melanin may be of benefit. Cysteine at a dose of 500 mg twice daily can reduce symptoms. Transfusions of washed packed red blood cells may be used to treat anemia, if the patient is symptomatic.

Cholestyramine, oral bile acids, hematin, and a high-carbohydrate diet have all been proposed to prevent or slow the progression of liver disease, but no definitive therapy has been developed.

CONGENITAL ERYTHROPOIETIC PORPHYRIA

Congenital erythropoietic porphyria (CEP) is a rare form of porphyria, also known as *erythropoietic porphyria* or *Gunther's disease*. It is inherited as an autosomal recessive trait and is caused by a homozygous defect of the enzyme uroporphyrinogen III synthase.

CEP presents soon after birth with the appearance of red urine (noticeable on the diapers). Severe photosensitivity occurs, and may result in immediate pain and burning so that the affected child screams when exposed to the sun. Redness, swelling, and blistering occur and result in scarring of the face, dorsal hands and scalp (with subsequent alopecia). Ectropion can occur with subsequent corneal damage and loss of vision. Erythrodontia of both deciduous and permanent teeth is also characteristic (Fig. 26-13). This phenomenon is demonstrated by the coral-red fluorescence of the teeth when exposed to a Wood's light. Mutilating scars, especially on the face, and the always-present hypertrichosis, with hair on the cheeks, profuse eyebrows, and long eyelashes, has prompted the terms "monkey face" or "werewolf" for these unfortunate individuals. Other features seen in CEP include growth retardation, hemolytic anemia, thrombocytopenia, porphyrin gallstones, osteopenia, and increased fracturing of bones.

A diagnosis of CEP can be easily suspected when an infant has dark urine and is severely photosensitive. Milder forms of the disease resemble adult PCT. Abnormally high amounts of uroporphyrin I and coproporphyrin I are found in urine, stool, and red cells. There is stable red fluorescence of erythrocytes. On biopsy there is a subepidermal bulla identical to that seen in PCT.

Treatment is strict avoidance of sunlight, and sometimes splenectomy for the hemolytic anemia. Oral activated charcoal is efficacious; presumably it retards the absorption of endogenous porphyrins. Repeated transfusions of packed red cells, enough to maintain the hematocrit level at 33%,

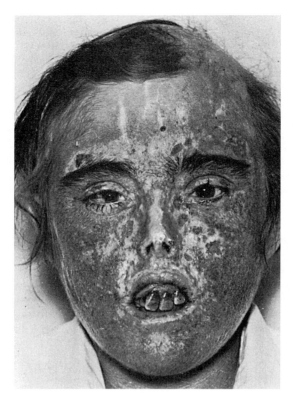

Fig. 26-13 Congenital erythropoietic porphyria (Gunther's disease) in a 17-year-old girl with lesions since she was 7 months old. (Courtesy Dr. H.R. Vickers, England.)

turns off the demand for heme and reduces porphyrin production. Bone marrow transplantation can be an effective treatment.

TRANSIENT ERYTHROPORPHYRIA OF INFANCY (PURPURIC PHOTOTHERAPY-INDUCED ERUPTION)

Paller et al reported seven infants exposed to 380 to 700 nm blue lights for the treatment of indirect hyperbilirubinemia who developed marked purpura in the skin exposed to ultraviolet light. Extensive blistering and erosions occurred in one case. Biopsies of the skin show hemorrhage without epidermal changes in the cases associated with purpura, and a pauciinflammatory, subepidermal bulla in the case with blistering. The infants had all received transfusions. Elevated plasma coproporphyrins and protoporphyrins were found in the four infants examined. The pathogenesis is unknown.

Anderson KE, et al: Erythropoietin for the treatment of porphyria cutanea tarda in a patient on long-term hemodialysis. *N Engl J Med* 1990, 322:315.
Bonkovsky HL, et al: Porphyria cutanea tarda, hepatitis C, and HFE gene mutations in North America. *Hepatology* 1998, 27:1661.

Bruch-Gerharz D, et al: Erythropoietic protoporphyria and terminal hepatic failure. *Acta Derm Venereol* 1996, 76:453.

Bulaj ZJ, et al: Clinical and biochemical abnormalities in people heterozygous for hemochromatosis. *N Engl J Med* 1996, 335:1799.

Camagna A, et al: Erythrocyte uroporphyrinogen decarboxylase activity. *Am J Med Sci* 1998, 315:59.

Checketts SR, et al: Nonsteroidal anti-inflammatory–induced pseudoporphyria. *Cutis* 1999, 63:223.

Chuang TY, et al: Porphyria cutanea tarda and hepatitis C virus. *J Am Acad Dermatol* 1999, 41:31.

Cox TM: Erythropoietic protoporphyria. *J Inherit Metab Dis* 1997, 20:258.

Crawford RI, et al: Transient erythroporphyria of infancy. *J Am Acad Dermatol* 1996, 35:833.

Cribier B, et al: Abnormal urinary coproporphyrin levels in patients infected by hepatitis C virus with or without HIV. *Arch Dermatol* 1996, 132:1448.

Egbert BM, et al: Caterpillar bodies. *Am J Dermatopathol* 1993, 15:199.

Ewing S, et al: Renal transplantation for PCT. *N Engl J Med* 1997, 336:811.

Farr, PR, et al: Inhibition of photosensitivity in erythropoietic protoporphyria with terfenadine. *Br J Dermatol* 1990, 122:809.

Felsher BF, et al: Decreased hepatic uroporphyrinogen decarboxylase activity in porphyria cutanea tarda. *N Engl J Med* 1982, 306:766.

Frank J, et al: Homozygous variegate porphyria. *J Invest Dermatol* 1998, 110:452.

Friedman SJ, et al: Sclerodermoid changes of porphyria cutanea tarda: possible relationship to urinary uroporphyrin levels. *J Am Acad Dermatol* 1985, 13:70.

Fritsch C, et al: Congenital erythropoietic porphyria. *J Am Acad Dermatol* 1997, 36:594.

Gibson GE, et al: Coexistence of lupus erythematosus and porphyria cutanea tarda in 15 patients. *J Am Acad Dermatol* 1998, 38:569.

Gibson GE, et al: Cutaneous abnormalities and metabolic disturbance of porphyrins in patients on maintenance hemodialysis. *Clin Exp Dermatol* 1997, 22:124.

Glynn P, et al: Bullous dermatoses in end-stage renal failure. *Am J Kidney Dis* 1999, 34:155.

Gross U, et al: Hormonal oral contraceptives, urinary porphyrin excretion, and porphyrias. *Horm Metab Res* 1995, 27:379.

Harvey E, et al: Pseudoporphyria cutanea tarda. *J Pediatr* 1992, 121:749.

Henderson CA, et al: Erythropoietic protoporphyria presenting in an adult. *J Roy Soc Med* 1995, 88:476.

Huang J, et al: Congenital erythropoietic porphyria. *J Am Acad Dermatol* 1996, 34:924.

Ingrish G, et al: Oxaprozin-induced pseudoporphyria. *Arch Dermatol* 1996, 132:1519.

Krischer J, et al: Pseudoporphyria induced by nabumetone. *J Am Acad Dermatol* 1999, 40:492.

Lim HW, et al: Hepatoerythropoietic porphyria: a variant of childhood onset porphyria cutanea tarda. *J Am Acad Dermatol* 1984, 11:1103.

Lim HW, et al: The porphyrias. *Clin Dermatol* 1996, 14:375.

Mansourati FF, et al: PCT and HIV/AIDS. *Int J STD AIDS* 1999, 10:51.

Mathews-Roth MM, et al: A double-blind study of cysteine photo protection in erythropoietic protoporphyria. *Photodermatol Photoimmunol Photomed* 1994, 10:244.

Milligan A, et al: Erythropoietic protoporphyria exacerbated by oral iron therapy. *Br J Dermatol* 1988, 119:63.

Moder KG: A coproporphyria-like syndrome induced by glipizide. *Mayo Clin Proc* 1991, 66:312.

Moran MJ, et al: Hepatic uroporphyrinogen decarboxylase activity in PCT patients. *Hepatology* 1998, 27:584.

Murphy GM, et al: Late-onset erythropoietic protoporphyria with unusual cutaneous features. *Arch Dermatol* 1985, 121:1309.

Nomura N, et al: Abnormal serum porphyrin levels in patients with AIDS with or without hepatitic C virus infection. *Arch Dermatol* 1996, 132:906.

Nordmann Y, et al: Harderoporphyria: a variant hereditary coproporphyria. *J Clin Invest* 1983, 72:1139.

O'Conner WJ, et al: PCT and HIV virus. *Mayo Clin Proc* 1998, 73:895.

Okano J, et al: Interferon treatment of PCT associated with chronic hepatitis type C. *Hepatogastroenterology* 1997, 44:525.

O'Reilly FM, et al: Screening of patients with iron overload to identify hemochromatosis and PCT. *Arch Dermatol* 1997, 133:1098.

Paller AS, et al: Purpuric phototherapy-induced eruption in transfused neonates. *Pediatrics* 1997, 100:360.

Parsons JL, et al: Neurologic disease in a child with hepatoerythropoietic porphyria. *Pediatr Dermatol* 1994, 11:216.

Pimstone NR, et al: Therapeutic efficacy or oral charcoal in congenital erythropoietic porphyria. *N Engl J Med* 1987, 316:390.

Piomelli S, et al: Complete suppression of the symptoms of congenital erythropoietic porphyria by long-term treatment with high level transfusions. *N Engl J Med* 1986, 314:1029.

Poh-Fitzpatrick MB: Human protoporphyria. *J Am Acad Dermatol* 1997, 36:40.

Poux JM, et al: Porphyria cutanea tarda in a dialyzed patient with hepatitis C infection. *Am J Med* 1997, 103:163

Rocchi E, et al: High weekly doses of desferrioxamine in PCT. *Br J Dermatol* 1987, 117:393.

Rocchi E, et al: Iron removal therapy in porphyria cutanea tarda: phlebotomy versus slow subcutaneous desferrioxamine infusion. *Br J Dermatol* 1986, 114:621.

Roelandts R, et al: Photo(chemo)therapy and general management of erythropoietic protoporphyria. *Dermatology* 1995, 190:330.

Romseo I, et al: Erythropoietic protoporphyria terminating in liver failure. *Arch Dermatol* 1982, 118:668.

Sampietro M, et al: Iron overload in PCT. *Haematologica* 1999, 84:248.

Sarkany RPE, et al: Autosomal recessive EPP. *Q J Med* 1995, 88:541.

Seubert S, et al: A PCT-like distribution pattern of porphyrins in plasma, hemodialysate, hemofiltrate, and urine of patients on chronic hemodialysis. *J Invest Dermatol* 1985, 85:107.

Thomas C, et al: Correction of congenital erythropoietic porphyria by bone marrow transplantation. *J Pediatr* 1996, 129:453.

Toback AG, et al: Hepatoerythropoietic porphyria. *N Engl J Med* 1987, 316:645.

Topi GC, et al: Recovery from porphyria cutanea tarda with no specific therapy other than avoidance of hepatic toxins. *Br J Dermatol* 1984, 111:75.

Tsukazaki N, et al: Porphyria cutanea tarda and hepatitis C virus infection. *Br J Dermatol* 1998, 138:1015. _____ ▲

Calcinosis cutis

Cutaneous calcification results from deposits of calcium and phosphorous in the skin. Calcinosis cutis is divided into four forms. *Dystrophic calcinosis* includes those conditions in which calcification occurs in damaged tissue (usually collagen or elastic tissue). Serum calcium and phosphorus levels are normal. Dermatomyositis is a classic example. *Metastatic calcification* refers to deposition of calcium resulting from elevated serum levels of calcium or phosphorus. Hyperparathyroidism is an example of this form of calcification. *Iatrogenic* and *traumatic calcinosis* is associated with medical procedures or occupational exposures that may involve both tissue damage and local elevated calcium concentrations. *Idiopathic calcinosis* cutis refers to those forms of cutaneous calcification of unknown cause with normal serum calcium. In osteoma cutis, true bone is formed in the skin.

DYSTROPHIC CALCINOSIS CUTIS

Damage to connective tissue may lead to deposition of calcium in the skin. Systemic calcium metabolism is normal, and lesions affect the skin only. This may be divided into localized (calcinosis circumscripta) and widespread (calcinosis universalis) types. Localized calcinosis cutis occurs most commonly as small deposits of chalky granular material around the fingers and on the elbows. This may spontaneously extrude from the skin. It occurs most commonly in limited scleroderma (the CREST syndrome: calinosis cutis, Raynaud's phenomenon, esophageal disorders, sclerodactyly, and telangiectasia) but may also be seen in progressive systemic sclerosis and systemic lupus erythematosus. Pancreatic and lupus panniculitis typically demonstrate dystrophic calcification, but the process tends to remain microscopic. Calcinosis universalis is usually seen in children with dermatomyositis. It affects the skin, muscles, and tendons as well as more diffusely. This calcification can persist for many years after the dermatomyositis is inactive. Dystrophic calcification is treated with limited surgical removal as needed to control discomfort. Long-term diltiazem treatment has been reported to lead to dramatic improvement of dystrophic calcification in patients with CREST and dermatomyositis.

METASTATIC CALCINOSIS CUTIS

This rare entity is characterized by calcifications in the skin, elevated serum calcium, and sometimes hyperphosphatemia. Metastatic calcinosis is often associated with bone loss or destruction, the bone providing the source of the elevated serum calcium. Conditions associated with metastatic calcinosis include parathyroid neoplasms, primary hyperparathyroidism, hypervitaminosis D, sarcoidosis, and excessive intake of milk and alkali. Destruction of bone by osteomyelitis, leukemia, Paget's disease of the bone, and metastatic carcinoma may lead to elevated serum calcium and metastatic calcification. In calcinosis cutis with hyperparathyroidism, the skin manifestations are numerous, small, firm, white papules, about 1 to 4 mm in diameter, occurring symmetrically in the popliteal fossae, over the iliac crests, and in the posterior axillary lines.

The most common metabolic condition associated with metastatic calcification is renal failure. Usually there is an elevated phosphorus level and secondary hyperparathyroidism, resulting in high calcium-phosphorous production and deposition of calcium phosphate in tissues. Less commonly, cutaneous calcification in renal disease can occur with normal serum calcium and phosphorus levels. Three forms of cutaneous calcification in renal disease have been described: tumoral calcinosis, calcifying panniculitis, and calciphylaxis. Often the latter two conditions occur in the same patient at the same time, suggesting that they may be of a common pathogenesis. Isolated, firm, indurated nodules, usually on the legs or thighs, in the subcutaneous fat have been called *calcifying panniculitis*. Most frequently they are seen with livedo reticularis and calciphylaxis.

The most severe complication of the abnormal calcium and phosphorus metabolism of renal disease is calciphylaxis. Patients at risk tend to have high calcium-phosphorus products and secondary hyperparathyroidism. The high calcium-phosphorus product is the most important variable, but some patients do develop calciphylaxis in the face of normal calcium and phosphorous levels. Affected patients usually show extensive medial calcification of blood vessels on x-ray evaluation. The exact pathogenesis is unknown, but in the susceptible patient, certain trigger factors, such as trauma, albumin, sepsis, iron supplementation, oral calcium carbonate and corticosteroid therapy, can precipitate the syndrome. In some patients a reduced functional factor C level is found, but this may reflect consumption of this antithrombotic product by the widespread intravascular thrombosis.

Clinically, patients with calciphylaxis present with livedo reticularis and ischemic tissue necrosis. Painful red-to-purple livedoid plaques develop that may involve the full thickness of the skin, including the subcutaneous tissue. Over a few days these areas become necrotic, eventually leading to extensive ulcerations. Lesions most commonly occur below the knees, and if restricted to below midcalf and the fingers (distal type), the prognosis is good, with a 70% survival rate. Extensive lesions (proximal type) usually affect the buttocks, thighs, shoulders, and trunk. This portends a very bad prognosis, with a mortality rate of more than 85% in some series. Death is usually from sepsis. Histologically, there is necrosis of affected areas. The media of blood vessels in the involved tissue is usually calcified. The affected vessels may show intravascular thrombosis, without inflammation. There is no vasculitis.

Although calciphylaxis most commonly occurs in the setting of chronic renal failure, it can rarely occur in other conditions. Breast carcinoma with widespread bony metastases, primary hyperparathyroidism, and end-stage liver disease have all been associated.

Treatment of calciphylaxis is difficult. It is best prevented, if possible, by management of the elevated phosphorus levels with binding agents. Once lesions begin to appear, parathyroidectomy may be considered. The parathyroids are removed and some transplanted. If the process continues, the transplanted parathyroids are also removed. Hyperbaric oxygen therapy and administration of prednisone, cimetidine, and systemic corticosteroids have been suggested as therapeutic. In general, the extent of disease at the onset predicts the outcome.

Tumoral calcinosis is a very rare complication of renal disease. It occurs in patients with the same metabolic abnormalities as calciphylaxis. Managing these metabolic abnormalities may led to resolution of the tumoral calcinosis.

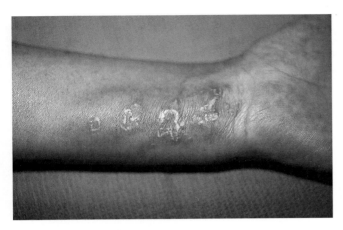

Fig. 26-14 Iatrogenic calcinosis cutis secondary to extravasation of calcium chloride infusion.

IATROGENIC AND TRAUMATIC CALCINOSIS CUTIS

Medical procedures that may inadvertently introduce calcium into tissue in association with tissue trauma may lead to cutaneous calcification. This has been reported after extravasation of calcium chloride infusion (Fig. 26-14) and after electroencephalography or electromyography. The electrode paste is high in calcium, and the skin is traumatized during the procedure, leading to calcifications at the sites of electrode insertion. The most common setting is on the scalps of children. Lesions spontaneously resolve over months. Performing frequent heel sticks in neonates has led to similar lesions.

Traumatic calcinosis may occur as a result of occupational exposure to calcium-containing materials, as in the cases reported in oil field workers and coal miners. Exposure of the skin to cloth sacks of calcium chloride, limewater compresses, and refrigerant calcium chloride can all cause calcinosis cutis.

IDIOPATHIC CALCINOSIS CUTIS
Idiopathic Scrotal Calcinosis

Idiopathic scrotal calcinosis is the most common form of idiopathic calcinosis cutis. Lesions present in young to middle-aged adult men as multiple, bilaterally symmetrical, asymptomatic, firm, round, yellow papules from several millimeters up to 1 cm in diameter. The papules resemble infundibular follicular cysts. Similar lesions may be seen less commonly in women on the labia majora. Histologically, there are localized deposits of calcium surrounded by foreign body reaction. Although dermatopathologists debate the point, at least some portion of these cases are calcifications of scrotal infundibular cysts. Why they have such a high proclivity to calcification at this anatomic location is unclear. Treatment is not required, but surgical removal cures individual lesions.

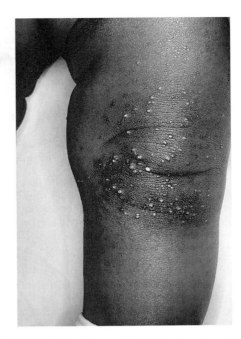

Fig. 26-15 Subepidermal calcified lesions in an infant.

Subepidermal Calcified Nodule

Subepidermal calcified nodule is an uncommon but distinct type of idiopathic calcinosis; it occurs most frequently as one or a few lesions on the scalps or faces of children. Males outnumber females in a ratio of nearly 2:1, and the average age at onset is 7 years. Lesions present as fixed, uninflamed papules that look very much like those of molluscum contagiosum with a central umbilication (Fig. 26-15). Histologically, there is an upper dermal deposit of calcium surrounded by multinucleated giant cells. On level sections the calcium is found to be transepidermally eliminated, producing the umbilication on the lesion. Treatment is not required, but surgical removal will cure any individual lesion.

Tumoral Calcinosis

Tumoral calcinosis is a rare disease of unknown cause that can be divided into two forms. The idiopathic, primary, or nomophosphatemic form is seen in young adults, primarily in African natives. It is not familial, lesions are usually solitary, and antecedent trauma is frequently present. Primary hyperphosphatemic tumoral calcinosis is a familial disease, primarily of black males. Most cases present before the second decade of life. Three quarters of these individuals have affected siblings, but the exact mode of inheritance is unknown. Multiple lesions predominate, and there is no preceding history of trauma. The serum calcium level is normal, but serum phosphorus and calcitriol levels are elevated.

Lesions in both types present as large subcutaneous masses of calcium overlying pressure areas and large joints, usually the hips, elbows, shoulders, or knees. Skin involvement, apart from the tumoral masses, is extremely rare but may occur as localized calcinosis cutis. The internal organs are not involved, and serum calcium levels are generally normal. Surgical excision has been the mainstay of therapy; however, recurrences are frequent after incomplete removal. Various dietary restrictions to lower calcium and phosphorus intake have shown some success.

OSTEOMA CUTIS

Bone formation within the skin may be primary in cases where there was no preceding lesion; metastatic (associated with abnormalities of parathyroid metabolism); or dystrophic, where ossification occurs in a preexisting lesion or inflammatory process.

Other types of primary osteoma cutis include either widespread or single, plaquelike osteomas present at birth or in early life, single osteomas occurring in later life, or miliary osteomas of the face usually in women. Some feel the latter are dystrophic because they occur in patients with acne and are associated with scars. If tetracycline is ingested for treatment of the acne, the cutaneous osteomas may be pigmented and will fluoresce with ultraviolet light.

Progressive osseous heteroplasia is a rare form of cutaneous ossification initially seen between birth and 6 months of age, often in the first month of life. Females are preferentially affected. Lesions begin as small papules that can coalesce to large plaques. Lesions are randomly distributed and may be unilateral or only involve one anatomic area. There is no preceding trauma or inflammatory phase. Serum calcium, phosphorus, PTH and calcitriol are normal, but alkaline phosphatase, LDH, and creatinine phosphokinase (CPK) may be elevated indicating increased bone formation (alkaline phosphatase) or muscle destruction (CPK and LDH). The cause of the condition is unknown. Histologically, the lesions represent heterotopic bone and can affect the soft tissues as well as skin. Only calcification without ossification may not be found in superficial dermal biopsies, so a deep biopsy including subcutaneous fat may be required to confirm the diagnosis. The condition is progressive and can lead to serious sequelae, including ulceration, infection, and severe pain. Familial cases have been described. The relationship of this condition to plate-like osteoma cutis is unclear, but the latter is usually not progressive.

Metastatic osteoma cutis occurs most frequently in pilomatricomas; however, other lesions in which bone formation may occur are basal cell epithelioma, intradermal nevi, mixed tumor of the skin, scars, scleroderma, and dermatomyositis.

Chan YL, et al: The vascular lesions associated with skin necrosis in renal disease. *Br J Dermatol* 1983, 109:85.

Coskey RJ, et al: Calcinosis cutis in a burn scar. *J Am Acad Dermatol* 1984, 11:666.

Elamin EM, et al: Calcifying panniculitis with renal failure. *Dermatology* 1996, 192:156.

Gibney MD, et al: Firm plaque of the forearm in a patient with Hodgkin lymphoma. *Arch Dermatol* 1999, 134:101.

Gilson RT, et al: Calciphylaxis. *Cutis* 1999, 63:149.

Goldsminz D, et al: Calcinosis cutis following extravasation of calcium chloride. *Arch Dermatol* 1988, 124:922.

Hironaga M, et al: Cutaneous calcinosis in a neonate following extravasation of calcium gluconate. *J Am Acad Dermatol* 1982, 6:392.

Janigan DT, et al: Acute skin and fat necrosis during sepsis in a patient with chronic renal failure and subcutaneous arterial calcification. *Am J Kidney Dis* 1992, 20:643.

Leung A: Calcification following heel sticks. *J Pediatr* 1985, 106:168.

Levin A, et al: Mathematical formulation to help identify the patient at risk of ischemic tissue necrosis. *Am J Nephrol* 1993, 13:448.

Mallory SB, et al: Solitary congenital nodule of the ear. *Arch Dermatol* 1988, 124:769.

Mastruserio DN, et al: Calciphylaxis associated with metastatic breast carcinoma. *J Am Acad Dermatol* 1999, 41:295.

Mehta RL, et al: Skin necrosis associated with acquired protein C deficiency in patients with renal failure and calciphylaxis. *Am J Med* 1990, 88:252.

Michl UHG, et al: Idiopathic calcinosis of the scrotum. *Scand J Urol Nephrol* 1994, 28:213.

Miller ES, et al: Progressive osseous heteroplasia. *Arch Dermatol* 1996, 132:787.

Oh DH, et al: Five cases of calciphylaxis and a review of the literature. *J Am Acad Dermatol* 1999, 40:979.

Oliveri MD, et al: Regression of calcinosis during diltiazem treatment in juvenile dermatomyositis. *J Rheumatol* 1996, 23:2152.

Pecovnik-Balon B, et al: Tumoral calcinosis in patients on hemodialysis. *Am J Nephrol* 1997, 17:93.

Poch E, et al: Calciphylaxis in a hemodialysis patient. *Am J Kidney Dis* 1992, 19:285.

Pursley TV, et al: Cutaneous manifestations of tumoral calcinosis. *Arch Dermatol* 1979, 115:1100.

Redmond WJ, et al: Keloidal calcification. *Arch Dermatol* 1983, 119:270.

Song DH, et al: Idiopathic calcinosis of the scrotum. *J Am Acad Dermatol* 1988, 19:1095.

Smack DP, et al: Proposal for a pathogenesis-based classification of tumoral calcinosis. *Int J Dermatol* 1996, 35:265.

Speer ME, et al: Calcification of superficial scalp veins secondary to intravenous infusion of sodium bicarbonate and calcium chloride. *Cutis* 1983, 32:65.

Touart DM, et al: Cutaneous deposition diseases. *J Am Acad Dermatol* 1998, 39:527.

Vassa N, et al: Hyperbaric oxygen therapy in calciphylaxis-induced skin necrosis in a peritoneal dialysis patient. *Am J Kidney Dis* 1994, 23:878.

Wang W-J, et al: Calcinosis cutis in juvenile dermatomyositis: remarkable response to aluminum hydroxide therapy. *Arch Dermatol* 1988, 124:1721.

Wheeland RG, et al: Calcinosis cutis resulting from percutaneous penetration and deposition of calcium. *J Am Acad Dermatol* 1985, 12:172.

Young PC, et al: Widespread livedo reticularis with painful ulcerations. *Arch Dermatol* 1995, 131:786.

Zacharias JM, et al: Calcium use increases risk of calciphylaxis. *Perit Dial Int* 1999, 19:248. ▲

ALBRIGHT'S HEREDITARY OSTEODYSTROPHY

Albright's syndrome, or Albright's hereditary osteodystrophy, is characterized by short, stocky stature; short metacarpals and phalanges (brachymetaphalangism or Albright dimpling sign); round facies; developmental delay; and cutaneous ossification. The thumbs are short and the fourth metacarpal and proximal phalanges are short, causing the skin to dimple over the fourth knuckle when a fist is made.

Other features of Albright's include large pigmented macules of the skin (café au lait spots), fibrous dysplasia of the long bones, and precocious puberty in girls. Various associated endocrinopathies have been reported. The café au lait spots of Albright's syndrome are present soon after birth, are usually unilateral, stop abruptly at the midline, and involve the forehead, nuchal area, and buttocks most commonly. Albright described them as darker and more jagged in outline than those seen in neurofibromatosis, but this is not always the case. The pigmentation may follow the lines of Blaschko. Spotty pigmentation may also occur periorally.

The cutaneous ossifications may be noted soon after birth and are usually multiple, small, superficial plaques. They favor the scalp, hands, and feet, periarticular regions, abdomen, and chest wall. Small lesions are of little consequence, but large subcutaneous masses may disrupt underlying structures. There are five forms of pseudohypoparathyroidism, three of which can be associated with Albright's. Albright's hereditary osteodystrophy (AHO) may be seen in both pseudohypoparathyroidism and pseudopseudohypoparathyroidism (PHP and PPHP). In PHP, there is hypocalcemia and no response to parathyroid hormone; in PPHP, serum calcium is normal. The disease is believed to be the result of a lethal gene surviving by mosaicism. Mutations in the Gs alpha gene that inactivate its activity and at chromosome 2q37 have been described in Albright's osteodystrophy. Some patients, however, have no mutations in these regions, suggesting other genetic mutations can produce a similar phenotype.

Kaplan FS: Skin and bones. *Arch Dermatol* 1996, 132:815.

Ringel MD, et al: Clinical implications of genetic defects in G proteins: the molecular basis of McCune-Albright syndrome and Albright's hereditary osteodystrophy. *Medicine* 1996, 75:171.

Ringel MD, et al: Melanotic macules following Blaschko's lines in McCune-Albright syndrome. *Br J Dermatol* 1994, 130:215.

Sakaguchi H, et al: A case of Albright's hereditary osteodystrophy–like syndrome complicated by several endocrinopathies: normal Gs alpha gene and chromosome 2q37. *J Clin Endocrin Metabol* 1998, 83:1563.

Shenker A, et al: Severe endocrine and nonendocrine manifestations of the McCune-Albright syndrome associated with activating mutations of stimulatory G protein GS. *J Pediatr* 1993, 123:509.

Wilson LC, et al: Albright's hereditary osteodystrophy. *J Med Genet* 1994, 31:779. ▲

Lipid disturbances

XANTHOMATOSIS

Xanthomatosis is a cutaneous manifestation of lipidosis in which the plasma lipoproteins and free fatty acids are changed quantitatively. There is accumulation of lipids in large foam cells in the tissues. Cholesterol or triglycerides are usually found, but when cholesterol levels are normal,

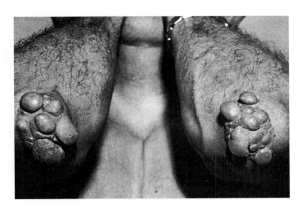

Fig. 26-16 Xanthoma tuberosum on elbows.

beta-sitosterol, campesterol, or stigmasterol (plant sterols), or cholestanol may rarely be at fault.

The cutaneous manifestations of xanthomatosis are named based on clinical morphology. Several different genetic diseases may present with similar cutaneous xanthoma patterns. The morphologies are relatively specific for the associated elevated lipid, however, with eruptive xanthomas seen with hypertriglyceridemia and other forms of xanthomas seen with elevations in cholesterol.

Xanthoma Tuberosum

Beginning at any age, tuberous xanthomata are variously found as flat or elevated and rounded, grouped, yellowish or orange nodules located over the joints, particularly on the elbows and knees (Fig. 26-16). The lesions are indurated and tend to coalesce. They may also occur over the face, knuckles, toe joints, axillary and inguinal folds, and buttocks. Solitary lesions may occur. Early lesions are usually bright yellow or erythematous; older lesions tend to become fibrotic and lose their color. Pedunculated, fissured, and suppurative nodules may also be seen.

Xanthoma tuberosum is associated with primary hyperlipoproteinemias with elevated cholesterol levels, such as familial hypercholesterolemia and familial dysbetalipoproteinemia. It also occurs in biliary cirrhosis, myxedema, phytosterolemia, and normocholesterolemic dysbetalipoproteinemia.

XANTHOMA TENDINOSUM

Papules or nodules 5 to 25 mm in diameter are found in the tendons, more especially in extensor tendons on the backs of the hands and dorsa of the feet and in the Achilles tendons (Fig. 26-17). These predominate in conditions with elevated cholesterol, such as the primary hyperlipoproteinemias of familial hypercholesterolemia and familial hyperbetalipoproteinemia. They are seen in association with tuberous xanthomas and xanthelasma. They also occur in obstructive liver disease, diabetes, myxedema, cerebrotendinous xanthomatosis, and phytosterolemia.

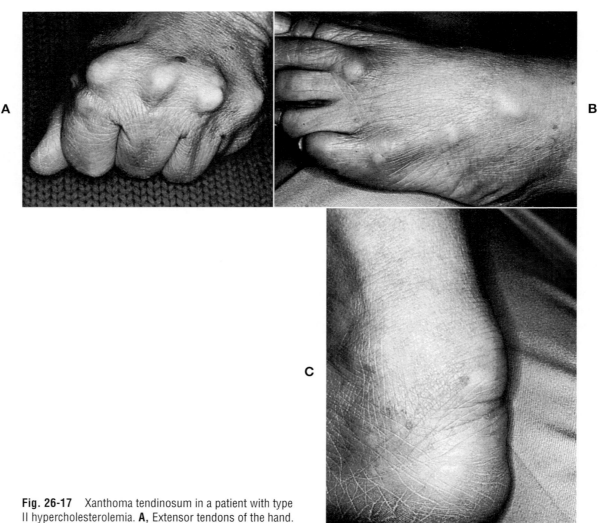

Fig. 26-17 Xanthoma tendinosum in a patient with type II hypercholesterolemia. **A,** Extensor tendons of the hand. **B,** Extensor tendons of the feet and **C,** Achilles tendon.

Eruptive Xanthoma

Xanthoma eruptivum consists of small yellowish orange to reddish brown papules that appear in crops over the entire body (Fig. 26-18). These occur in association with markedly elevated triglycerides. Causes for such elevations are genetic deficiency of lipoprotein lipase, familial deficiency of apoprotein CII, and endogenous familial hypertriglyceridemia. Certain diseases or drugs raise the triglyceride level either by increased production, decreased catabolism, or decreased excretion. These include diabetes mellitus, obesity, pancreatitis, chronic renal failure, hypothyroidism, and treatment with estrogens, corticosteroids, isotretinoin, or acitretin.

The papules may be surrounded by an erythematous halo and may be grouped in various favored locations such as the buttocks, flexor surfaces of the arms and thighs, knees, inguinal and axillary folds, and oral mucosa. Koebnerization may occur. Pruritus is variable.

Xanthoma Planum (Plane Xanthoma)

These xanthomas appear as flat macules or slightly elevated plaques with a yellowish tan or orange coloration of the skin that is spread diffusely over large areas. They are frequently associated with biliary cirrhosis and myeloma but have been described in patients with high-density lipoprotein (HDL) deficiency, monoclonal gammopathy, lymphoma, leukemia, serum lipoprotein deficiency, and in xanthomas following erythroderma (Fig. 26-19). Characteristically, plane xanthomas may occur about the eyelids, neck, trunk, shoulders, or axillae (Fig. 26-20). These well-defined macular patches may be situated on the inner surface of the thighs and antecubital and popliteal spaces. Xanthelasma palpebrarum may be associated with xanthoma planum elsewhere.

Palmar Xanthomas

These consist of nodules and irregular yellowish plaques involving the palms and flexural surfaces of the fingers.

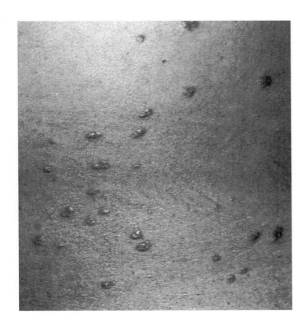

Fig. 26-18 Eruptive xanthoma on the torso in a patient with adult-onset diabetes mellitus.

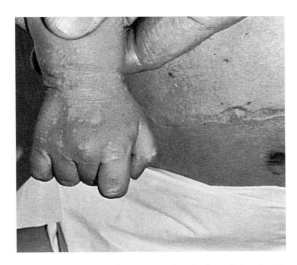
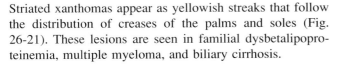

Fig. 26-19 Xanthoma planum on the backs of the hands and elsewhere in a 9-month-old child with biliary atresia.

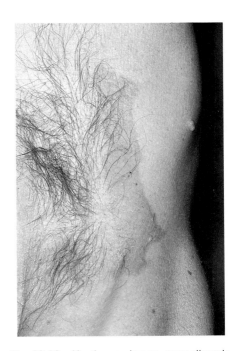

Fig. 26-20 Xanthoma planum, normolipemic.

Striated xanthomas appear as yellowish streaks that follow the distribution of creases of the palms and soles (Fig. 26-21). These lesions are seen in familial dysbetalipoproteinemia, multiple myeloma, and biliary cirrhosis.

Xanthelasma Palpebrarum (Xanthelasma)

Xanthelasma is the most common type of xanthoma. It occurs on the eyelids and is characterized by soft, chamois-colored or yellowish orange oblong plaques, usually near the inner canthi (Fig. 26-22). The xanthelasmata vary from 2

to 30 mm in length. Frequent symmetry, with a tendency to be permanent, progressive, multiple, and coalescent, is also characteristic. Frequently xanthelasmata are associated with other types of xanthomas, but they are usually present without any other disease.

The disorder is encountered chiefly in patients of middle age. It is common among women who have hepatic or biliary disorders. Xanthelasma may be seen in the various familial hyperlipoproteinemias, especially in familial hypercholesterolemia; however, half or more of the patients are

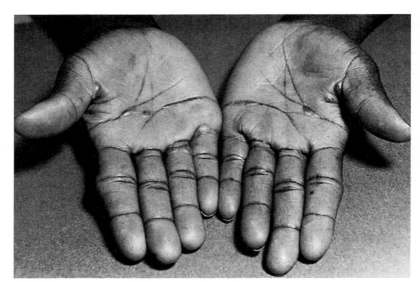

Fig. 26-21 Xanthoma striatum palmare.

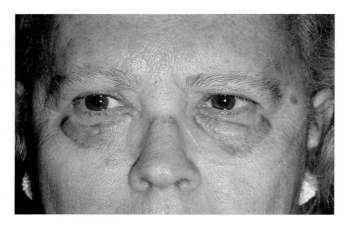

Fig. 26-22 Xanthelasma palpebrarum.

normolipemic. It is a common finding in generalized xanthoma planum, in obstructive liver disease, myxedema, diabetes, and phytosterolemia.

Several studies have found abnormalities in apolipoprotein E phenotypes or other lipoprotiens more frequently than in controls. We consider it prudent to evaluate new patients with a full lipoprotein profile as well as a careful history and physical examination.

Treatment of xanthelasma is discussed here because of its uniqueness among the xanthomas, in that surgical therapy is often successful. The best method is surgical excision. The anesthetized lesion is grasped with mouse-tooth forceps and clipped off with scissors, and the skin edges undermined and sutured with fine silk. Excellent cosmetic results are obtained, even if the wound is not closed. Fulguration, trichloracetic acid cauterization, and CO_2 laser vaporization are other methods. Complete removal of the lesions does not preclude the possibility that other new lesions will develop.

Tuberoeruptive Xanthomas

These xanthomas are red papules and nodules that appear inflamed and tend to coalesce. They are associated with familial dysbetalipoproteinemia.

Nodular Xanthomas

These are multiple, yellowish, dome-shaped lesions, 4 to 5 mm or larger in diameter; they may be discrete or confluent and may occur on the earlobes, neck, elbows, and knees. They are usually associated with biliary cirrhosis and atresia of the bile ducts.

The histologic features in all varieties of xanthoma are similar, characterized by the presence of numerous large xanthoma or foam cells, which are phagocytes (fat-laden histiocytes). They may be multinucleated. In addition to the foam cells, giant cells of the Touton type occur. Clefts representing cholesterol and fatty acids dissolved by embedding agents may be noted. There is generally a connective tissue reaction about the nests of foam cells, and in old lesions most of the foam cells are replaced with fibrosis. To demonstrate lipids in the histologic sections, frozen sections should be stained with lipid stains (scarlet red).

PRIMARY HYPERLIPOPROTEINEMIAS

Cutaneous xanthomas are usually manifestations of some disorder of lipid metabolism. The blood lipids, with the exception of free fatty acids, are bound to circulating plasma proteins and are mainly cholesterol, phospholipid, and triglyceride. The total serum lipids have a range of 400 to 1000 mg%. Of this, serum cholesterol values vary according to age. Generally a serum cholesterol below 200 mg/dl is normal, while a level of more than 240 mg requires further evaluation. A triglyceride level of more than 250 mg/dl is considered abnormal.

Lipoprotein fractions may be demonstrated by paper electrophoresis. Four lipoprotein bands may be evident: the alpha lipoprotein band (high-density lipoprotein), beta lipoprotein (low-density lipoprotein, LDL), prebeta lipoprotein (very low-density lipoprotein, VLDL), and the chylomicron band. When the lipoproteins are subjected to ultracentrifugation it is found that the high-density alpha lipoproteins (HDL) are composed mostly of phospholipid and esterified cholesterol. The beta lipoproteins (low density, LDL) are composed mostly of cholesterols. The prebeta lipoproteins (very low density, VLDL) are fractions of still lower density that are the main carriers of endogenous triglycerides. The lowest density chylomicrons are the exogenous triglycerides.

Frederickson classified hyperlipoproteinemias into six types on the basis of electrophoretic patterns, as follows:

Type I: Excess chylomicrons
Type IIa: Excess beta lipoprotein
Type IIb: Excess beta lipoprotein with slightly elevated VLDLs
Type III: Increased intermediate-density (remnant) lipoprotein
Type IV: Increased prebeta lipoprotein
Type V: Increased prebeta lipoproteins and chylomicrons

Although this phenotypic classification has been useful for many years, advances in the understanding of lipoprotein metabolism and transport, coupled with new knowledge of molecular defects which result in these phenotypes, has led to the use of a genetic classification of lipoproteinemias.

Lipoprotein metabolism may be viewed based on the lipid source: an exogenous and an endogenous category. Exogenous lipids in the diet are absorbed and incorporated into triglyceride-rich chylomicrons. These are hydrolyzed by the action of lipoprotein lipase and certain cofactors, among them apoprotein CII. The resulting remnants are taken up by the liver. Endogenously produced VLDLs are synthesized in the liver and (again through the action of lipoprotein lipase) are connected to cholesterol-rich intermediate-density lipoproteins (IDLs) and eventually into LDLs.

These are then available for uptake by peripheral tissues, as well as by the liver. The uptake of LDL, IDL, and chylomicron remnants is dependent on specific receptors. Abnormalities of lipoprotein lipase, the apolipoproteins, cofactors, receptors, or stimulators or retarders of endogenous production or catabolism, whether on a genetic or sporadic basis, may accelerate or block the pathway in different areas. If blockade occurs early and results in elevation of triglyceride-rich particles, eruptive xanthoma may result. If a defect occurs later in the pathway, and cholesterol-rich particles accumulate, xan-

thelasma, tuberous xanthomas, and tendinous xanthomas are to be expected, along with premature atherosclerotic cardiovascular disease.

Lipoprotein Lipase Deficiency. Lipoprotein lipase deficiency causes type I disease (chylomicronemia) early in life. As patients grow older, their VLDLs (type V) become elevated.

Familial Apoprotein CII Deficiency. Patients with familial apoprotein CII deficiency lack lipoprotein lipase activator; very high triglyceride levels, up to 10,000 mg/dl, result. The condition is very rare.

Familial Hypertriglyceridemia. In familial hypertriglyceridemia, increased hepatic production of VLDLs occurs first (type IV), but overloaded removal mechanisms result in accumulation of dietary lipids, and chylomicrons accumulate, so a type V pattern results. Eruptive xanthomas are common, and atherosclerotic heart disease may occur. Cholelithiasis is common. Polyarthritis and arthralgia frequently occur.

Familial Dysbetalipoproteinemia (Broad Beta Disease). In this disorder, remnant lipoproteins increase, LDLs and HDLs are reduced, and triglyceride and cholesterol levels are increased. The cholesterol-rich IDLs form a broad band on electrophoresis, extending from prebeta lipoproteins to beta lipoproteins: hence *broad beta* disease. Xanthomas (tuberous, eruptive, palmar, or tendinous) are common; xanthelasmas are infrequent. Atherosclerosis is common, as are diabetes, gout, and obesity.

Familial Hypercholesterolemia. Familial hypercholesterolemia is Frederickson's type II disease: LDLs (beta lipoproteins) are found in high levels in the plasma; there may be a moderate increase in VLDLs and in the triglycerides that they carry. There is overproduction of LDL cholesterol (caused by loss of normal feedback inhibition) and impaired removal of it (because of impaired formation of LDL receptors). There is elevated plasma beta lipoprotein from birth in heterozygotes, and symptoms begin in the third to sixth decade, when tendinous or tuberous xanthomas, xanthelasmas, and atherosclerotic disease appear. Homozygotes generally get coronary atherosclerosis before age 20, and more than 40% get xanthelasmas, tendinous xanthomas, or tuberous xanthomas in childhood. Cultured amniotic fluid cells permit prenatal diagnosis in homozygotes.

Familial Combined Hyperlipidemia or Multiple-Type Hyperlipoproteinemia. This, the commonest of the genetic lipoproteinemias, has a high risk of myocardial infarction and diabetes, and a low incidence of tuberous or tendinous xanthomas.

SECONDARY HYPERLIPOPROTEINEMIA
Obstructive Liver Disease (Xanthomatous Biliary Cirrhosis)

This type of hyperlipoproteinemia shows increase of the serum phospholipid and cholesterol, giving a type II lipoprotein pattern. This is caused by the presence of lipoprotein X, which is secreted by the liver in cholestasis. It has the ability to carry large quantities of free cholesterol and phospholipids. The triglycerides are not elevated and the plasma is clear, showing no chylomicrons.

The xanthomatous lesions are plane xanthomas, with lesions on the face, the flexor surfaces of the extremities, and the trunk. Striate palmar and plantar lesions and xanthelasmas are also seen. Tuberous xanthomas may also occur. Pruritus is extremely severe. Hepatomegaly and jaundice are present.

Cholestyramine is of help in allaying pruritus. Alagille's syndrome is a congenital disorder characterized by intrahepatic bile ductular atresia, patent extrahepatic bile ducts, a characteristic facies (prominent forehead; deeply set eyes; straight nose; small, pointed chin), cardiac murmur, vertebral and ocular abnormalities, low intelligence, and hypogonadism. It is an autosomal dominantly inherited condition. There is persistent cholestasis early in life with pruritus and hyperbilirubinemia. Lipid levels elevate by age 2 and planar or papular xanthomas may occur. This is a treatable condition with cholestyramine and fat-soluble vitamins leading to prolonged improvement.

Hematopoietic Diseases

Xanthomas may occur secondarily in myelomas; Waldenström's macroglobulinemia; cryoglobulinemia and occasionally, lymphoma; and hemochromatosis. These xanthomas are usually generalized plane xanthomas of the eyelids, periorbital areas, sides of the neck, shoulders, and upper back. The lipoproteinemia may be of type I, V, or IIa pattern. In some patients no lipoprotein abnormality is present. These patients may have paraproteins that bind to the lipoproteins, preventing their metabolism.

Xanthoma Diabeticorum

Eruptive xanthomas may occur secondarily, especially in young persons unresponsive to insulin. Cardiovascular disease and hepatomegaly are common. Insulin is necessary for the normal plasma triglyceride clearing action of lipoprotein lipase. Therefore, in insulin deficiency, an acquired lipoprotein lipase deficiency exists, which leads to impaired clearance of chylomicrons or VLDLs, or both. This results in a type I, IV, or V lipoprotein pattern and hypertriglyceridemia. When the diabetes is brought under control, the triglyceride levels are lowered and prompt involution of the lesions is seen. Weight reduction and carbohydrate intake restriction are also helpful. Identical phenomena may occur in von Gierke's disease, a form of glycogen storage disease in which there is a lack of hepatic glucose-6-phosphatase.

Chronic Renal Failure

If plasma protein levels are reduced by urinary loss in the nephrotic syndrome (or by plasmapheresis or repeated bleeding), a compensatory increase of lipoproteins may occur, with hyperlipidemia and various kinds of xanthoma.

Renal failure with or without dialysis may cause hypertriglyceridemia. In long-term dialysis there is increased cardiovascular disease because of increased levels of VLDL as well as lowered HDLs. Type IV and V profiles are most commonly seen.

Myxedema

Lipoprotein lipase needs thyroid hormone to work, and its failure may lead to type I, IV or V disease; or thyroid hormone deficiency may lead to hypercholesterolemia, because thyroid hormone is needed in the oxidation of hepatic cholesterol to bile salts. Xanthelasma and xanthomas are common in myxedema.

Pancreatitis

Hyperlipidemia in the hyperchylomicronemic syndromes (types I and V) may cause pancreatitis; in type V it may be recurrent, and pancreatic necrosis and death may occur. Alternatively, pancreatitis (perhaps initiated by ethanol) may cause type I or V hyperlipoproteinemia by inducing insulin deficiency and a relative lack of lipoprotein lipase activity.

Medication-Induced Hyperlipoproteinemia

Estrogens, by decreasing lipoprotein lipase activity and increasing VLDL synthesis, may cause type I or type IV patterns. Eruptive xanthomas may occur. Oral prednisone may induce insulin deficiency and cause type IV or V patterns to develop. Isotretinoin and acitretin sometimes increase triglycerides carried in VLDL, and eruptive xanthomas may occur.

Normolipoproteinemic Xanthomatoses

The normolipoproteinemic xanthomatoses are conditions in which serum cholesterol and lipoproteins are normal, yet secondary lipid deposition in the skin occurs.

Cerebrotendinous Xanthomatosis. Cerebrotendinous xanthomatosis is an autosomal recessive disease caused by an accumulation of cholestanol in plasma lipoproteins and xanthomatous tissue. It appears that the underlying abnormality is a deficiency of the hepatic enzyme 26-hydrolase, necessary for the complete oxidation of cholesterol to bile acids. Cholestanol, an intermediate, accumulates as a result. It accumulates in tendons, brain, heart, lungs, and the ocular lenses. There may be tendinous xanthomas, especially of the Achilles tendons; progressive neurologic dysfunction; cerebellar ataxia; dementia; spinal cord paresis; cataracts; atherosclerotic coronary disease; and endocrine abnormalities. Urinary gas chromatography is a specific test for this disease. The condition is treated with chenodeoxycholic acid and cholic acid.

Phytosterolemia. In phytosterolemia, a rare disorder, plant sterols such as beta-sitosterol, stigmasterol, and campesterol are absorbed from the gastrointestinal tract in excessive amounts. They accumulate in the body as xanthelasmas, tendinous xanthomas, and cutaneous xanthomas. In most patients there is also type IIa hyperlipoproteinemia. There is a risk of hemolysis, arthritis, and premature atherosclerosis.

Verruciform Xanthoma. Verruciform xanthoma (VX) is an uncommon lesion that occurs as a reddish orange or paler hyperkeratotic plaque or papillomatous growth with a pebbly or verrucous surface. The most common site is the oral mucosa. It has also been reported on other mucosal surfaces, the genitalia, the lower extremities, and elsewhere. The type of epidermal nevus that is present in CHILD syndrome may have characteristics of VX. Additionally, VX has been reported in psoriatic lesions undergoing PUVA therapy and in psoriasiform skin lesions in an HIV+ patient. Histologically, there is acanthosis without atypia, parakeratosis, and xanthoma cells in the papillary dermis. The etiology is unknown.

Familial Alphalipoprotein Deficiency (Tangier Disease). Generally, xanthomas do not occur in Tangier disease; the characteristic finding is yellow, enlarged tonsils from accumulation of lipid in this localized area. One patient was reported to have a generalized papular eruption in which clinically uninvolved skin showed extracellular deposits of cholesterol esters outside the dermal cells.

Bergman R: The pathogenesis and clinical significance of xanthelasma palpebrarum. *J Am Acad Dermatol* 1994, 30:236.

Bickley LK: Yellow papules in a middle-aged woman. *Arch Dermatol* 1989, 125:287.

Bouwres Bavinc JN, et al: Capillary gas chromatography of urine samples in diagnosing cerebrotendinous xanthomatosis. *Arch Dermatol* 1986, 122:1269.

Caputo R, et al: Normolipemic eruptive cutaneous xanthomatosis. *Arch Dermatol* 1986, 122:1294.

Chyu J, et al: Verruciform xanthoma of the lower extremity. *J Am Acad Dermatol* 1987, 17:695.

Cruz PO, et al: Dermal, subcutaneous, and tendon xanthomas. *J Am Acad Dermatol* 1988, 19:95.

Cuozzo D, et al: Verruciform xanthoma of the penis. *J Urol* 1995, 153:1625.

Eckel RH: Lipoprotein lipase. *N Engl J Med* 1989, 320:1060.

Friedman SJ, et al: Xanthoma striatum palmare associated with multiple myeloma. *J Am Acad Dermatol* 1987, 16:1272.

Gerber LE, et al: Changes in lipid metabolism during retinoid administration. *J Am Acad Dermatol* 1982, 6:664.

Goldstein GD: The Koebner response with eruptive xanthomas. *J Am Acad Dermatol* 1984, 10:1064.

Gomez JA, et al: Apolipoprotein E phenotypes, lipoprotein composition, and xanthelasma. *Arch Dermatol* 1988, 124:1230.

Happle R: Epidermal nevus syndromes. *Semin Dermatol* 1995, 14:111.

Hobbs HH, et al: Deletion in the gene for the low-density lipoprotein receptor in a majority of French Canadians with familial hypercholesterolemia. *N Engl J Med* 1987, 317:737.

Huang JS, et al: Verruciform xanthoma: case report and literature review. *J Periodontol* 1996, 67:162.

Hwang SY, et al: Cerebrotendinous xanthomatosis. *J Dermatol* 1990, 17:115.

Low LC, et al: Phytosterolemia and pseudohomozygous type II hypercholesterolemia in two Chinese patients. *J Pediatr* 1991, 118:746.

Matsuo I, et al: Phytosterolemia and type IIa hyperlipoproteinemia with tuberous xanthoma. *J Am Acad Dermatol* 1981, 4:47.

McCadden ME, et al: Mycosis fungoides associated with dystrophic xanthomatosis. *Arch Dermatol* 1987, 123:91.

Mountcastle EA, et al: Verruciform xanthoma of the digits. *J Am Acad Dermatol* 1989, 20:313.

Parker F: Normocholesterolemic xanthomatosis. *Arch Dermatol* 1986, 122:1253.

Parker F, et al: Xanthomas and hyperlipidemias. *J Am Acad Dermatol* 1985, 13:1.

Pasternak RC, et al: Effect of combination therapy with lipid-reducing drugs in patients with coronary heart disease and "normal" cholesterol levels. *Ann Intern Med* 1996, 125:529.

Ribera M, et al: Lipid metabolism and apolipoprotein E phenotypes in patients with xanthelasma. *Am J Med* 1995, 99:485.

Russo GG: Hyperlipidemias. *Clin Dermatol* 1996, 14:367.

Shulman RS, et al: Beta-sitosterolemia and xanthomatosis. *N Engl J Med* 1977, 14:651.

Smith KJ, et al: Changes of verruciform xanthoma in an HIV-1+ patient with diffuse psoriasiform skin disease. *Am J Dermatopathol* 1995, 17:185.

Watts GF, et al: Cerebrotendinous xanthomatosis. *QJM* 1996, 89:55.

Williford PM, et al: The spectrum of normolipemic plane xanthoma. *Am J Dermatopathol* 1993, 15:572.

Yamamoto T, et al: Verruciform xanthoma in a psoriatic patient under PUVA therapy. *Dermatology* 1995, 191:254. ━━━━━━━━ ▲

NIEMANN-PICK DISEASE

This rare disease most frequently occurs in Jewish infants during their first year of life. It is characterized by hepatosplenomegaly, lymphadenopathy, and the accumulation of foam cells in the bone marrow. Cherry-red spots in the maculae retinae, pulmonary infiltration, and mental retardation are also seen. Still rarer are the adult, juvenile, and Nova Scotia forms.

Cutaneous changes consist of distinctive yellowish coloration of the skin and occasionally of lesions resembling eruptive xanthomas. Black macular patches may occur on the mucous membranes. The disease is associated with the accumulation of sphingomyelin and cholesterol in large foam cells throughout the body. Only rarely is the skin affected. Kimura reported characteristic inclusions in sweat gland epithelium. The enzyme sphingomyelinase is deficient. The course of the disease is progressive, and the

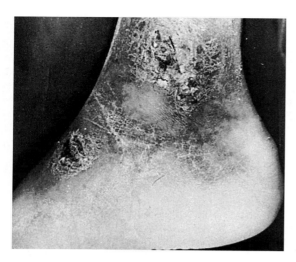

Fig. 26-23 Gaucher's disease. (Courtesy Dr. F. Daniels, Jr.)

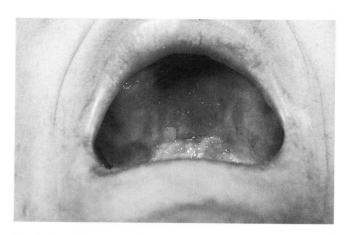

Fig. 26-24 Lipoid proteinosis. Note infiltrative lesions on the soft palate.

patient usually dies within the first 3 years of life. There is no treatment.

Kimura S: Sweat gland pathology in neurodegenerative diseases. *No To Hattatsu* 1991, 23:20.

Toussaint M, et al: Specific skin lesions in a patient with Niemann-Pick disease. *Br J Dermatol* 1994, 131:895. _____ ▲

GAUCHER'S DISEASE

Gaucher's disease is a rare autosomal recessive disorder of the reticuloendothelial system. Betaglucocerebrosidase is lacking, with a resulting accumulation of glucocerebrosides in the brain and in the reticuloendothelial cells of the liver, spleen, and marrow. The disease occurs at any age, but three forms are recognized: type 1 (adult type), without neurologic involvement; type 2 disease, the infantile form, with acute early neurologic manifestations; and type 3, the juvenile chronic neuropathic type.

Some type 2 patients have congenital ichthyosis that preceded neurologic manifestations, and some have been born with a collodian membrane. Epidermal ultrastructural and biochemical abnormalities occur in all type 2 patients. The adult type is characterized by hepatosplenomegaly, rarefaction of the long bones, pingueculae of the sclera, and a distinctive bronze coloration of the skin from melanin. A deeper pigmentation may extend from the knees to the feet (Fig. 26-23). This is often caused by hemosiderin and may be accompanied by thrombocytopenia and splenomegaly.

The disease occurs most frequently among Ashkenazi Jews. Approximately 1 in 20 carry the defective gene, the lack of which leads to the accumulation of glucocerebroside in histiocytes in the bone marrow and spleen, and Kupffer cells in the liver, forming Gaucher cells. These are large, 20 to 100 μ in diameter, with one nucleus or a few small nuclei and pale cytoplasm that stains faintly for fat but is PAS

positive. Elevated plasma acid phosphatase occurs and is a useful clue to the diagnosis. There is thinning of the cortex of the long bones.

Bone marrow transplantation performed before neurologic deficits occur has a high mortality rate (20% to 50%) but when successful has halted neurologic progression. Enzyme therapy is successful in treating some of the manifestations of the adult form, but it is limited by cost. Symptomatic treatment includes radiation therapy to the long bones to relieve bone pain and splenectomy for hypersplenism (anemia and thrombocytopenia, with petechiae and bruising). With the identification of the gene defect, carrier screening and prenatal diagnosis are possible.

Beaudet AL: Gaucher's disease. *N Engl J Med* 1987, 316:619.

Charrow J, et al: Gaucher's disease. *Arch Int Med* 1998, 158:1754.

Fujimoto A, et al: Congenital ichthyosis preceding neurologic symptoms in two sibs with type 2 Gaucher disease. *Am J Med Genet* 1995, 59:356.

Isuji S: A mutation in the human glucocerebrosidase gene in neuropathic Gaucher's disease. *N Engl J Med* 1987, 316:570.

Rappeport JM, et al: Bone-marrow transplantation in severe Gaucher's disease. *N Engl J Med* 1984, 311:84.

Sidransky E, et al: Epidermal abnormalities may distinguish type 2 from type 1 and type 3 of Gaucher's disease. *Pediatr Res* 1996, 39:134.

Spada M, et al: Cardiac response to enzyme-replacement therapy in Gaucher's disease. *N Engl J Med* 1998, 339:1165. _____ ▲

LIPOID PROTEINOSIS

Also known as *Urbach-Wiethe disease* and *hyalinosis cutis et mucosae,* this rare autosomal recessive disturbance is characterized by yellowish white infiltrative deposits on the inner surfaces of the lips, the undersurface of the tongue, the fauces, and the uvula. Other parts of the upper respiratory tract are also affected (Fig. 26-24). In the early stage, crops of bullae and pustules occur; these heal, leaving acnelike

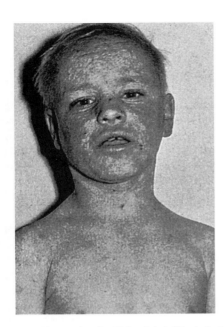

Fig. 26-25 Lipoid proteinosis. Yellowish infiltrated plaques over the entire face, lips, and buccal mucosa. Notice the enlargement of the tongue. (Courtesy Dr. J.C.M. Grosfeld et al, The Netherlands.)

scars (Fig. 26-25). Changes in the larynx lead to a marked degree of hoarseness, which usually appears within the first few weeks of life. Failure to cry and a hoarse, gravelly voice are suggestive signs.

The patient's tongue is "like wood" and moves only with difficulty. The patient is unable to protrude the tongue. Marked changes occur in the epiglottis. The vocal cords are thickened by an infiltration of grayish yellow material, giving rise to the hoarseness observed so early. In some patients, similar yellowish and cream-colored deposits are sometimes observed on the labia majora, urethral orifice, scrotum, gluteal folds, and the axillae. Severe xerostomia and poor salivation may result from infiltration of the salivary glands. Patchy alopecia is common.

Hyperkeratotic wartlike or nodular lesions are found on the dorsal aspects of the hands, fingers, elbows, and knees. The eyelid margins contain small, yellowish, transparent, pearly papules in about two thirds of patients. Drusen of Bruch's membrane are seen in the fundi in half of the patients. Sickle-shaped calcifications found dorsal and lateral to the sella turcica in skull x-ray films are pathognomonic.

Distinctive histologic features include extreme dilation of the blood vessels, thickening of their walls, progressive hyalinization of sweat glands, and infiltration of the dermis and subcutaneous tissue with extracellular hyaline deposits, which are also demonstrable in the vessel walls. Normal skin and mucous membranes also show changes of endothelial proliferation of the subpapillary vessels and a homogeneous thickening of the walls of the deeper vessels.

Types IV and V collagen are increased around vessels, and types I and III collagen are reduced in quantity and abnormally hydrolyzed in the dermis. Elevated alpha-1 (IV) collagen mRNA levels occur. Thus, it is hypothesized that the defect affects endothelial cells, with a resultant increase in the production of basement membrane zone collagen, and it also affects fibroblasts by a decreased synthesis of altered fibrous collagen. Differentiation from erythropoietic protoporphyria may be difficult, especially histologically. Gruber et al reported that use of etretinate improved some skin conditions; however, the follow-up was limited.

Cannata G, et al: An edentulous woman with warty lesions. *Arch Dermatol* 1996, 132:1240.

Disdier P, et al: Specific xerostomia during Urbach-Wiethe disease. *Dermatology* 1994, 188:50.

Gruber F, et al: Treatment of lipoid proteinosis with etretinate. *Acta Derm Venereol* 1996, 76:154.

Konstantinov D, et al: Lipoid proteinosis. *J Am Acad Dermatol* 1992, 27:293.

Olsen DR, et al: Expression of basement membrane zone genes coding for type IV procollagen and laminin by human skin fibroblasts in vitro. *J Invest Dermatol* 1988, 90:734.

Rizzo R, et al: Lipoid proteinosis. *Pediatr Dermatol* 1997, 14:22.

Touart DM, et al: Cutaneous deposition diseases. *J Am Acad Dermatol* 1998, 39:149. ▲

ANGIOKERATOMA CORPORIS DIFFUSUM (FABRY'S DISEASE)

Also known as *glycolipid lipidosis* and *Fabry's* or *Anderson-Fabry's disease,* in angiokeratoma corporis diffusum (ACD), a storage disease, ceramide trihexoside (galactosyl galactosyl glucosyl ceramide) accumulates in the skin and viscera. The skin lesions are widespread punctate telangiectatic vascular papules that on first inspection suggest purpura. Some show hyperkeratotic tops, but this is less prominent than in other forms of angiokeratoma. Myriad tiny telangiectatic papules are seen, especially on the lower extremities, scrotum and penis, lower trunk, axillae, ears, and the lips, where the small, sometimes linear, angiokeratomas are most numerous on the midline of the lower lip (Fig. 26-26). Hair growth is scanty.

The deposits of glycolipids (ceramide trihexoside) occur in the endothelial cells, fibroblasts, and pericytes of the dermis, in the heart, kidneys, and autonomic nervous system. Cardiac disease (cardiomyopathy) and renal insufficiency bring death, usually in the fifth decade. Edema of the ankles, paralyses, paresthesias manifested by a burning sensation of the hands and feet, and hypohidrosis are often present. Abnormal vascular structures are noted in the conjunctiva and eye-grounds. Distinctive whorl-like opacities of the cornea occur in 90%, and 50% develop characteristic spokelike cataracts in the posterior capsular location. The urine, in addition to albuminuria, may show "Maltese cross" material on polaroscopy, and glycolipids

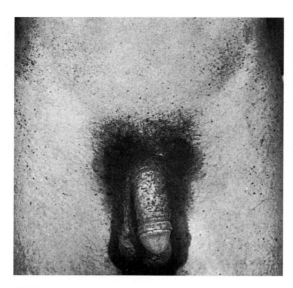

Fig. 26-26 Angiokeratoma corporis diffusum. (Courtesy Dr. H.B. Curry.)

may be seen in the form of "mulberry cells" in the sediment.

The cause of the disease is a deficiency of alpha-galactosidase A. Inheritance is by an X-linked recessive route. Female heterozygotes may show evidence of the disease in varying degrees. The diagnosis can be confirmed by finding diminished levels of alpha-galactosidase A in leukocytes, serum, tears, skin fibroblasts, or amniotic fluid cells.

Histologically, there is dilation of capillaries in the papillary dermis, resulting in endothelium-lined lacunae filled with blood and surrounded by acanthotic and hyperkeratotic epidermis. Electron microscopy reveals characteristic electron-dense bodies in endothelial cells, pericytes, and fibroblasts. They have also been found in normal skin in affected adults and in a young boy without telangiectases.

Laser treatment of the angiokeratomas is cosmetically helpful. Phenytoin has been reported to afford significant relief of pain. Infusions of normal plasma, hemodialysis, and renal transplantation have been tried; the latter, however, has not afforded symptomatic relief or consistent improvement of overall prognosis.

FUCOSIDOSIS

Angiokeratomas identical with those of Fabry's disease occur in this rare disorder. It can be distinguished clinically by the frequent presence of coarse thickening of the skin of the face, severe mental retardation, weakness, spasticity, and seizures.

Histologically, there are granule-filled vacuoles in endothelial and other cells. The defect, a lack of alpha-L-fucosidase, is transmitted as an autosomal recessive trait.

Progressive mental and motor deterioration begins in infancy and progresses, with death by age 18 to 20 as a rule.

SIALIDOSIS

Another disease presenting with Fabry's-like angiokeratomas is caused by type II neuraminidase deficiency, which causes intracellular accumulation of sialilated oligosaccharides. Mental retardation, myoclonus, cerebellar ataxia, skeletal abnormalities, and coarse facies have been reported.

BETA-MANNOSIDASE DEFICIENCY

Rodriguez-Serna et al reported the twelfth case of this autosomal recessive disorder of glycoprotein metabolism. The patient's sole manifestation was Fabry's-like amgiokeratomas. Mental retardation was a constant finding in ten of the other patients and many other abnormalities such as hearing loss, aggressive behavior, peripheral neuropathy, recurrent infections, epilepsy, coarse facies, and skeletal abnormalities were also often present.

Several patients with rare lysosomal enzyme disorders, such as galactosialidosis, aspartylglycosaminuria, adult-onset GM_1 gangliosidosis, and alpha-N-acetylgalactosaminidase deficiency (Kanzaki's disease) have been reported to have Fabry's-like angiokeratomas. Finally, several patients without any detectable enzyme deficiency have been reported. Among them was a family with autosomal dominantly inherited Fabry's-like angiokeratomas associated with arteriovenous malformations. It should be emphasized that there are many normal patients who have widespread small petechia-like lesions that erupt in adulthood. This is a variant of cherry angiomas.

Calzavara-Pinton PG, et al: Angiokeratoma corporis diffusum and arteriovenous fistulas with dominant transmission in the absence of metabolic disorders. *Arch Dermatol* 1995, 131:57.

Chesser RS, et al: Perioral telangiectases: a new cutaneous finding in Fabry's disease. *Arch Dermatol* 1990, 126:1655.

Crovato F, et al: Angiokeratoma corporis diffusum and normal enzyme activities. *J Am Acad Dermatol* 1985, 12:885.

Fleming C, et al: Cutaneous manifestations of fucosidosis. *Br J Dermatol* 1997, 136:594.

Kang WH, et al: Generalized anhidrosis associated with Fabry's disease. *J Am Acad Dermatol* 1987, 17:883.

Kanzaki T, et al: Angiokeratoma corporis diffusum with glycopeptiduria due to deficient lysosomal alpha-N-acetylgalactosaminidase activity. *Arch Dermatol* 1993, 129:460.

Lapins J, et al: Angiokeratomas in Fabry's disease and Fordyce's disease: successful treatment with copper vapor laser. *Acta Derm Venereol* 1993, 73:133.

Marsden J, et al: Widespread angiokeratomas without evidence of metabolic disease. *Arch Dermatol* 1987, 123:1125.

Rodriguez-Serna M, et al: Angiokeratoma corporis diffusum associated with beta-mannosidase deficiency. *Arch Dermatol* 1996, 132:1219.

Shelley ED, et al: Painful fingers, heat intolerance, and telangiectases of the ear. *Pediatr Dermatol* 1995, 12:215.

Tabata H, et al: Hair abnormality of Fabry disease. *Int J Dermatol* 1996, 35:576. ▲

NECROBIOSIS LIPOIDICA (NECROBIOSIS LIPOIDICA DIABETICORUM)

Necrobiosis lipoidica is characterized by well-circumscribed, hard, depressed, waxy, yellow-brown, atrophic plaques on the skin of persons (women three times more commonly than men) who may also have diabetes mellitus (Fig. 26-27).

The earliest clinical lesions are sharply bordered, elevated, red papules 2 mm in diameter; these may be capped by a slight scale and do not disappear under diascopic pressure. Later the lesions develop into irregularly round or oval scleroderma-like lesions with well-defined borders and a smooth, glistening (glazed) surface. The center becomes depressed and sulfur-yellow, so that a firm yellowish lesion forms, surrounded by a broad violet-red or pink border. In the yellow portion numerous telangiectases are evident. Ulceration is not unusual. Rarely, squamous cell carcinoma may occur in chronic ulcers.

The most common location of the lesions is on the shins. About 85% of the lesions occur on the legs. A much less common site is on the forearms, and lesions have been reported on the trunk, face, scalp, palms, and soles. Only rarely are they present exclusively in sites other than the legs.

Sixty percent of patients with necrobiosis lipoidica have diabetes mellitus; another 20% will have glucose intolerance or a family history of diabetes. In 15%, necrobiosis lipoidica precedes the onset of frank diabetes by an average of 2 years. Control of the diabetes does not influence the course of the disease. Its incidence is 3 to 7 per 1000 diabetic patients. The average age of onset is 34 years—22 years, on average, in insulin-dependent patients and 49 years in non–insulin-dependent patients.

Histologically, well-developed lesions of necrobiosis lipoidica demonstrate a superficial, deep, and interstitial inflammatory process that involves the whole reticular dermis and often the panniculus. The inflammatory cells include lymphocytes, histiocytes, multinucleate giant cells, and plasma cells. At low magnification there are palisaded granulomas that contain degenerated collagen centrally, surrounding which the inflammatory infiltrate is arrayed. In contradistinction to granuloma annulare, mucin is not increased in the centers of the granulomas. The overlying epidermis tends to be thinned, with loss of the normal rete ridge pattern.

Treatment, after control of the diabetes is achieved, is not completely satisfactory. The best results have occurred after intralesional injections of triamcinolone suspension into the inflammatory papules and active advancing edges. Goette reported a complete response to topical clobetasol propionate under occlusion. Some cases have benefited by excision and skin grafts, but others have had recurrences in the grafts or at the edges of the grafts.

A combination of dipyridamole (Persantine) 225 mg and aspirin 1 g daily has been reported to be effective. These

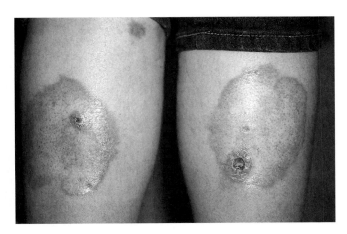

Fig. 26-27 Necrobiosis lipoidica.

may have to be continued for 3 or 4 months before results are obtained. Trental (pentoxifylline) may also be helpful in doses of 400 mg three times daily. This may be especially helpful in healing ulcers. Hyperbaric oxygen, topically applied bovine collagen, and cyclosporine are other reported options for chronic ulcers.

Petzelbauer et al reported that systemic corticosteroids given over a 5-week period was effective in all six patients treated and did not recur after a mean follow-up period of 7 months. Control of the diabetes was achieved by oral hypoglycemics or insulin. The atrophy did not improve. Heymann has reported topical tretinoin to be helpful in diminishing the atrophy in one case. Spontaneous resolution may occur in 13% to 19% of patients after 6 to 12 years.

Boulton AJM, et al: Necrobiosis lipoidica. *J Am Acad Dermatol* 1988, 18:530.

Clement M, et al: Squamous cell carcinoma arising in long-standing necrobiosis lipoidica. *Arch Dermatol* 1985, 121:24.

Goette DK: Resolution of necrobiosis lipoidica with exclusive clobetasol propionate treatment. *J Am Acad Dermatol* 1990, 22:855.

Heymann WR: Necrobiosis lipoidica treated with topical tretinoin. *Cutis* 1996, 58:53.

Littler CM, et al: Pentoxifylline for necrobiosis lipoidica. *J Am Acad Dermatol* 1987, 17:314.

Lowitt MH, et al: Necrobiosis lipoidica. *J Am Acad Dermatol* 1991, 25:735.

Noz KC, et al: Ulcerating necrobiosis lipoidica effectively treated with pentoxifylline. *Clin Exp Dermatol* 1993, 18:78.

Petzelbauer P, et al: Necrobiosis lipoidica: treatment with systemic corticosteroids. *Br J Dermatol* 1992, 126:542.

Quimby SR, et al: The cutaneous immunopathology of necrobiosis lipoidica diabeticorum. *Arch Dermatol* 1988, 124:1364.

Smith K: Ulcerating necrobiosis lipoidica resolving in response to cyclosporine A. *Dermatol Online J* 1997, 3:2.

Spenceri EA, et al: Topically applied bovine collagen in the treatment of ulcerative necrobiosis lipoidica diabeticorum. *Arch Dermatol* 1997, 133:817.

Stratham B, et al: A randomized double blind comparison of an aspirin dipyridamole combination in the treatment of necrobiosis lipoidica. *Acta Dermatol* 1981, 61:220.

Weisz G, et al: Treatment of necrobiosis lipoidica by hyperbaric oxygen. *Acta Derm Venereol* 1993, 73:447. ▲

OTHER DIABETIC DERMADROMES

In addition to NL there are many cutaneous signs in this common endocrinopathy.

Diabetic Dermopathy (Shin Spots)

Dull-red papules that progress to well-circumscribed, small, round, atrophic, hyperpigmented lesions on the shins are the most common cutaneous sign of diabetes (Fig. 26-28). Although they occur individually in people who do not have diabetes, if four or more are present the specificity is high for microvascular disease in other tissues. They are present in 50% of people with diabetes, most commonly in men.

Diabetic Bullosis

Noninflammatory, spontaneous, painless blistering, most often in acral locations, is characteristic (Fig. 26-29). Lesions heal spontaneously in 4 to 5 weeks, usually without scarring.

Toonstra reported a case of diabetes with spontaneous bullae on the hands alone, and reviewed 44 published cases, in 21 of which a biopsy was done. Six were subepidermal and 13 intraepidermal—but might have been subepidermal initially. Electron microscopic studies show separation at the lamina lucida level. Direct immunofluorescence is negative. Ultraviolet light, trauma, neuropathy, and cation imbalance have all been hypothesized to be inciting factors to the blistering. Bernstein et al reported a reduced threshold to suction-induced blistering in insulin-dependent diabetics.

Carotenosis

Carotenosis is a yellowish discoloration of the skin, especially of the palms and soles, that is sometimes seen in diabetic patients who have carotenemia. Of the 50% of diabetic persons who have carotenemia, about 10% have carotenosis. The sclerae remain white. There may be night blindness (delayed dark adaptation) as a result of reduced conversion of carotene to vitamin A in the liver.

Limited Joint Mobility and Waxy Skin

Limited joint mobility and waxy skin are important not only because of the 30% to 50% prevalence of these conditions in diabetic patients with long-standing disease, but also because these are associated with microvascular complications, such as nephropathy and retinopathy. Joint symptoms begin with limitation of joint mobility in the fifth finger at the metacarpophalangeal and proximal joints and progress radially to the other fingers. It is bilateral, symmetrical, and painless. Involvement of the feet also occurs and is thought

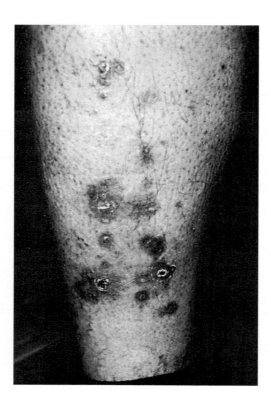

Fig. 26-28   Diabetic dermopathy.

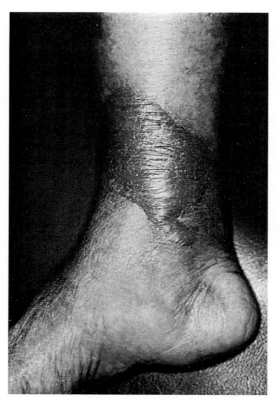

Fig. 26-29   Bullous eruption of diabetes mellitus.

to contribute to the development of chronic ulcerations. Such open sores on the neuropathic, microvascularly compromised, infection-prone diabetic foot pose a constant threat to life and limb.

Other Associated Conditions in Patients with Diabetes

Erysipelas-like erythema of the legs or feet; sweating disturbances; paresthesias of the legs; mal perforans ulcerations; a predisposition to certain infections such as mucormycosis, group B streptococcal infections, nonclostridial gas gangrene, and malignant external otitis resulting from *Pseudomonas;* disseminated granuloma annulare; eruptive xanthomas; rubeosis of the face; acanthosis nigricans, Dupuytren's contracture; and finger-pebbling are various abnormalities often seen in patients with diabetes.

Arkkila PE, et al: Dupuytren's disease in type 1 diabetic patients. *Clin Exp Rheumatol* 1996, 14:59.

Benson PM, et al: Group B streptococcal blistering distal dactylitis in an adult diabetic. *J Am Acad Dermatol* 1987, 17:310.

Bernstein JE, et al: Reduced threshold to suction-induced blister formation in insulin-dependent diabetics. *J Am Acad Dermatol* 1983, 8:790.

Flier JS: Metabolic importance of acanthosis nigricans. *Arch Dermatol* 1985, 121:193.

Hanna W, et al: Pathologic features of diabetic thick skin. *J Am Acad Dermatol* 1987, 16:546.

Huntley AC: The cutaneous manifestations of diabetes mellitus. *J Am Acad Dermatol* 1982, 7:427.

Huntley AC: Eruptive lipofibromata. *Arch Dermatol* 1983, 119:612.

Huntley AC: Finger pebbles: a common finding in diabetes mellitus. *J Am Acad Dermatol* 1986, 14:612.

Huntley AC: Threshold to suction-induced blister formation in insulin-dependent diabetics. *J Am Acad Dermatol* 1984, 10:305.

Kahana M, et al: Skin tags: a cutaneous marker for diabetes mellitus. *Acta Derm Venereol* (Stockh) 1987, 67:175.

Kakourou T, et al: Limited joint mobility and lipodystrophy in children and adolescents with insulin-dependent diabetes mellitus. *Pediatr Dermatol* 1994, 11:310.

Sibbald RG, et al: Skin and diabetes. *Endocrinol Metab Clin North Am* 1996, 25:463.

Toonstra J: Bullosis diabeticorum. *J Am Acad Dermatol* 1985, 13:799. ▲

Other metabolic disorders

NEONATAL CITRULLINEMIA

Citrullinemia is an autosomal dominantly inherited deficiency of the enzyme argininosuccinic acid synthetase. This enzyme converts citrulline and aspartic acid to argininosuccinic acid, as a part of the urea cycle. Low plasma arginine levels result, and the hypothesis is that since keratin is 16% arginine, dermatitis may occur. Goldblum et al reported a patient with erosive, erythematous, scaling patches and plaques that were prominent in the perioral, lower abdominal, diaper, and buttock regions. This eruption cleared with arginine supplementation. Two patients with this disease have had short, sparse hair.

In carbamoyl phosphate synthetase deficiency, low plasma arginine levels may also occur, and similar cutaneous findings have been reported in this second metabolic defect of the urea cycle.

Diets high in arginine will heal the skin lesions.

Goldblum OM, et al: Neonatal citrullinemia associated with cutaneous manifestations and arginine deficiency. *J Am Acad Dermatol* 1986, 14:321.

Kline J, et al: Arginine deficiency syndrome. *Am J Dis Child* 1981, 135:437. ▲

HARTNUP DISEASE

Hartnup disease is an inborn error of tryptophan excretion; it was named after the Hartnup family, in which it was first noted. The outstanding findings are a pellagra-like dermatitis following exposure to sunlight, intermittent cerebellar ataxia, psychiatric manifestations, and constant aminoaciduria.

The dermatitis occurs on exposed parts of the skin, chiefly the face, neck, hands, and legs. The erythematous scaly patches flare up into a hot, red, exudative state after exposure to sunlight, followed after subsidence by hyperpigmentation. Stomatitis and vulvitis also occur. The disease becomes milder with increasing age. Hartnup disease is an autosomal recessive trait. Large amounts of indole-3-acetic acid and indican are secreted in the urine. The skin lesions respond to niacinamide, 200 mg a day.

Galadari E, et al: Hartnup disease. *Int J Dermatol* 1993, 32:904.

Oakley A, et al: Hartnup disease presenting in an adult. *Clin Exp Dermatol* 1994, 19:407. ▲

PROLIDASE DEFICIENCY

Prolidase deficiency is an autosomal recessive inherited inborn error of metabolism. Prolidase cleaves dipeptides containing C-terminal proline or hydroxyproline. When this enzyme is deficient, the normal recycling of proline residues obtained from collagen degradation is impaired. A buildup of iminodipeptides results, with disturbances in connective tissue metabolism and excretion of large amounts of iminodipeptides in the urine.

Clinically, 85% of patients have some dermatologic manifestations. The most important cutaneous signs, which almost always appear before the affected person is 12 years old, are skin fragility, ulceration, and scarring of the lower extremities; photosensitivity and telangiectasia; poliosis; scaly, erythematous, maculopapular, and purpuric lesions; and thickening of the skin with lymphedema. Systemic signs and symptoms include mental deficiency, splenomegaly, and recurrent infections. An unusual facial appearance is noted at times, with low hairline, frontal bossing, and saddle nose. Prolidase measurement may be determined in erythrocytes, leukocytes, or fibroblasts. Leoni et al reported structural abnormalities of collagen and elastin after electron microscopic study. Many therapeutic options have been described, such as oral supplements of manganese and ascorbic acid, both modulators of prolidase activity; however, results of treatment are highly variable.

Berardesca E, et al: Blood transfusions in the therapy of a case of prolidase deficiency. *Br J Dermatol* 1992, 126:193.

Bissonnette R, et al: Prolidase deficiency. *J Am Acad Dermatol* 1993, 29:818.

Cantatore FP, et al: Chronic leg ulcers resembling vasculitis in two siblings with prolidase deficiency. *Clin Rheumatol* 1993, 12:410.

Leoni A, et al: Prolidase deficiency in two siblings with chronic leg ulcers. *Arch Dermatol* 1987, 123:493.

Milligan A, et al: Prolidase deficiency. *Br J Dermatol* 1989, 121: 405. ▲

PHENYLKETONURIA

Also known as *phenylpyruvic oligophrenia*, phenylketonuria (PKU), an autosomal recessive disorder of phenylalanine metabolism, is characterized by mental deficiency; epileptic seizures; the presence of phenylpyruvic acid in the urine; pigmentary dilution of skin, hair, and eyes; psuedoscleroderma; and dermatitis. It is most common in whites. Phenylalanine hydroxylase is lacking in the liver and also in peripheral lymphocytes. Phenylalanine is therefore not oxidized to tyrosine.

Affected children are blue eyed, with blond hair and fair skin. They are usually extremely sensitive to light, and about 50% have an eczematous dermatitis that is clinically similar to atopic dermatitis, with a predilection for the flexures. It is worst in the youngest patients, may improve with dietary treatment, and has been exacerbated by phenylalanine challenge in a carrier of the recessive gene. Skin lesions may be sclerodermatous in nature. Indurations of the thighs and buttocks are present early in infancy and increase with time.

Blood levels of phenylalanine are high. The presence of phenylpyruvic acid in the urine is demonstrated by a characteristic deep-green color when a few drops of ferric chloride solution are added to it. Green diapers occur in histidinemia as well as in phenylketonuria.

Young infants should be treated by a diet low in phenylalanine; this may bring about normal development if it is begun shortly after birth.

Fisch RO, et al: Studies of phenylketonurics with dermatitis. *J Am Acad Dermatol* 1981, 4:284.

Guillet GY, et al: Pseudoscleroderma and phenylketonuria. *Int J Dermatol* 1983, 22:422.

Nova MP, et al: Scleroderma-like skin indurations in a child with phenylketonuria. *J Am Acad Dermatol* 1992, 26:329. ▲

ALKAPTONURIA AND OCHRONOSIS

Alkaptonuria, inherited as an autosomal recessive trait, is caused by the lack of renal and hepatic homogentisic acid oxidase, the enzyme necessary for the catabolism of homogentisic acid to acetoacetic and fumaric acids. It is characterized by the excretion of homogentisic acid in the urine to produce a black-staining urine, the deposition of a grossly brown-black pigment in the connective tissue, and ochronotic arthropathy.

In patients with alkaptonuria the voided urine is dark and turns black on standing from the homogentisic acid. For many years, the dark urine may be the only indication of the presence of alkaptonuria. In the meantime, large amounts of homogentisic acid are accumulated in the body tissues. By the third decade of life the deposition of pigment becomes apparent. Cartilage is preferentially affected. The early sign is the pigmentation of the sclera (Osler's sign) and the cartilage of the ears (Figs. 26-30 and 26-31). Later the cartilage of the nose and the tendons, especially those on the hands, become discolored.

Blue or mottled brown macules appear on the skin. The bluish macules have a predilection for the fingers, ears, nose, genital regions, apices of the axillae, and the buccal mucosa. Palmoplantar pigmentation may occur. The sweat glands are rich in ochronotic pigment granules, and intradermal injection of epinephrine into the skin of the axillary vault will yield brown-black sweat droplets in the follicular orifices (Fig. 26-32). The cerumen is often black. Internally, the larynx, great vessels and valves of the heart, kidneys, esophagus, tonsils, and the dura mater may be involved.

Histologically, there are large, irregular collagen bundles within the reticular dermis. They are yellow-brown with routine hematoxylin and eosin, and stain black with crystal violet or methylene blue.

Ochronotic arthropathy involves the spinal joints first, resembling osteoarthritis. Next affected are the knees, shoulders, and hips. Radiographic films show a characteristic appearance of early calcification of the intervertebral

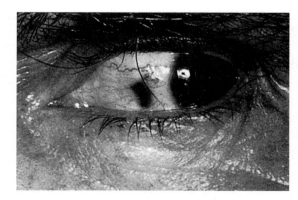

Fig. 26-30 Pigmented macule on sclera—Osler's sign. An early sign of ochronosis. (Courtesy Dr. J.M. Hitch.)

disk and later narrowing of the intervertebral spaces with eventual disk collapse.

There is no effective treatment.

Exogenous Ochronosis

Topically applied phenolic intermediates such as hydroquinone, carbolic acid (phenol), picric acid, and resorcinol may produce exogenous ochronosis. Hydroquinone specifically inhibits the enzyme homogentisic acid oxidase locally, resulting in accumulation of this substance on the collagen fibers in tissues where it is applied. Histologically, exogenous ochronosis and alkaptonuria have identical changes on skin biopsy. Treatment with dermabrasion and the CO_2 laser has been effective. Annular granulomatous inflammation present within the areas of exogenous ochronosis may represent sarcoidosis.

Albers SE, et al: Alkaptonuria and ochronosis. *J Am Acad Dermatol* 1992, 27:609.

Bruce S, et al: Exogenous ochronosis resulting from quinine injections. *J Am Acad Dermatol* 1986, 15:357.

Cherian S: Palmoplantar pigmentation. *J Am Acad Dermatol* 1994, 30:264.

Diven DG, et al: Hydroquinone-induced localized exogenous ochronosis treated with dermabrasion and CO_2 laser. *J Dermatol Surg Oncol* 1990, 16:1018.

Gutzmer R, et al: Alkaptonuric ochronosis. *J Am Acad Dermatol* 1997, 37:305.

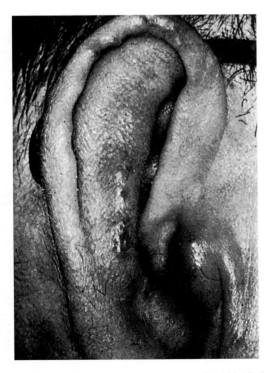

Fig. 26-31   Ochronosis on ear. (Courtesy Dr. J.M. Hitch.)

Jacyk WK: Annular granulomatous lesions in exogenous ochronosis are manifestations of sarcoidosis. *Am J Dermatopathol* 1995, 17:18.

Lawrence N, et al: Exogenous ochronosis in the United States. *J Am Acad Dermatol* 1988, 18:1207.

Micali G, et al: Endogenous ochronosis (alkaptonuria). *Arch Dermatol* 1998, 134:98.

Snider RL, et al: Exogenous ochronosis. *J Am Acad Dermatol* 1993, 28:662.

Touart DM, et al: Cutaneous deposition diseases (II). *J Am Acad Dermatol* 1998, 39:527.   ▲

WILSON'S DISEASE (HEPATOLENTICULAR DEGENERATION)

Wilson's disease is an autosomal recessive derangement of copper metabolism. Affected persons develop hepatomegaly, splenomegaly, and neuropsychiatric changes. Slurred speech, a squeaky voice, salivation, dysphagia, tremors, incoordination, and spasticity may all occur. There is progressive, fatal hepatic and central nervous system degeneration. The body retains an excessive amount of copper, leading to damage in the liver and brain. As a result, azure lunulae (sky-blue moons) of the nails occur in 10% of patients, and the smoky, greenish brown Kayser-Fleischer rings develop at the edges of the corneas. Hyperpigmentation develops on the lower extremities in most patients. A vague greenish discoloration of the skin on the face, neck, and genitalia may also be present. Feldman et al reported a patient who developed an idiopathic blistering eruption that ceased with treatment of Wilson's disease. The changes of cirrhosis (vascular spiders and palmar erythema) may occur. Low ceruloplasmin level in the serum is diagnostic.

The disease is caused by the inability of the body to synthesize a normal amount of ceruloplasmin. The treatment is D-penicillamine, which removes copper by chelating it. The dose is 1 or 2 g/day orally. Potential side effects include pemphigus, cutis laxa, and elastosis perforans

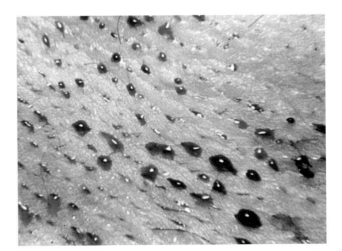

Fig. 26-32   Black sweat after intradermal injection of epinephrine in a patient with ochronosis. (Courtesy Dr. Axel W. Hoke.)

serpiginosa, which has been reported repeatedly in Wilson's patients on penicillamine. Treatment must be continued for life.

Baban NK, et al: Wilson's disease. *South Med J* 1997, 90:535.
Feldman SR, et al: A blistering eruption associated with Wilson's disease *J Am Acad Dermatol* 1989, 21:1030. _____ ▲

TYROSINEMIA II (RICHNER-HANHART SYNDROME)

Tyrosinemia is an autosomal recessive syndrome resulting from a deficiency of hepatic tyrosine aminotransferase. Serum tyrosine ranges from 200 to 300 µmol/100 ml (normal, 10 or less). Clinical features are mild to severe keratitis, and hyperkeratotic and erosive lesions of palms and soles, often with mental retardation. Photophobia and tearing commonly occur as the keratitis begins, and ultimately neovascularization is seen. Painful palmar and plantar erosions and hyperkeratoses usually appear within the first year of life, weeks to months after the eye lesions. Thigh skin, grafted to the heel, is spared. A low-tyrosine, low-phenylalanine diet (Mead Johnson 3200 AB) may improve or prevent the eye and skin lesions but may or may not benefit the mental retardation.

Crovato F, et al: Richner-Hanhart syndrome spares plantar autograft. *Arch Dermatol* 1985, 121:539.
Goldsmith L: Tyrosinemia II. *Int J Dermatol* 1985, 24:293.
Jimenez-Acosta F: Painful plantar calluses and mental retardation. *Arch Dermatol* 1994, 130:507.
Rabinowitz LG, et al: Painful keratoderma and photophobia. *J Pediatr* 1995, 126:266.
Tallab TM: Richner-Hanhart syndrome. *J Am Acad Dermatol* 1996, 35:857. _____ ▲

WAARDENBURG SYNDROME

Waardenburg syndrome (WS), is an autosomal dominant pigmentary disorder. Four variants are described. Abnormalities of transcription factors PAX3 (WS types 1 and 3) and MITF (WS type 2) have been identified in these patients. MITF transactivates the gene for tyrosinase, critical to melanocyte differentiation, and PAX3 transactivates the MITF promoter, explaining the relationship between these mutations and the clinical features of the syndrome. Clinical findings consist of white forelock, depigmented macules, unilateral or bilateral deafness (as a result of the absence of melanocytes in the organ of Corti), lateral displacement of the inner canthi, a broad nasal root, heterochromia of the iris, and confluent eyebrows (Fig. 26-33). There are at least two distinct types. Type 1 has associated dystopia canthorum, whereas type 2 does not. The incidence of deafness is lower (25%) in type 1 than in

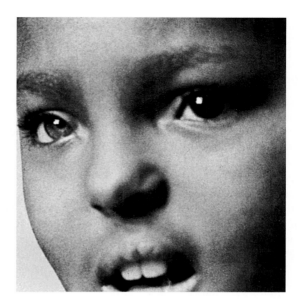

Fig. 26-33 Waardenburg syndrome in an 8-year-old girl whose two siblings are similarly affected with deafness, heterochromia of the eyes (*right,* blue; *left,* brown), broad nasal root, lateral displacement of inner canthi, and partial albinism. (Courtesy Dr. Y. Rapp.)

type 2 (50%). Patients with the musculoskeletal abnormalities of the upper extremities are said to have Klein-Waardenburg syndrome (type 3). Chang et al reported two patients who demonstrated spontaneous repigmentation of congenital leukodermic patches. Type 4 Waardenburg syndrome, also called *Waardenburg-Shah syndrome,* has deafness and pigmentary abnormalities plus Hirschsprung's disease. It is due to a genetic defect in the SOX10 gene.

Cambiaghi S, et al: What syndrome is this? *Pediatr Dermatol* 1998, 15:235.
Chang T, et al: Spontaneous contraction of leukodermic patches in Waardenburg syndrome. *J Dermatol* 1993, 20:707.
Dourmishev AL, et al: Waardenburg syndrome with facial palsy and lingua plicata. *Cutis* 1999, 63:139.
Liu-X, et al: Hearing loss and pigmentary disturbances in Waardenburg syndrome with reference to WS type II. *J Laryngol Otol* 1995, 109:96.
Pingault V, et al: JOX10 mutations in patients with Waardenburg-Hirschsprung disease. *Nat Genet* 1998, 18:171.
Watanabe A, et al: Epistatic relationship between Waardenburg syndrome genes MITF and PAX3. *Nat Genet* 1998, 18:283. _____ ▲

HURLER'S SYNDROME (MUCOPOLYSACCHARIDOSIS I)

Hurler's syndrome, or gargoylism, is an autosomal recessive disorder of mucopolysaccharide metabolism. A deficiency of alpha-L-iduronidase is the causative defect. It is characterized by mental retardation, hepatosplenomegaly, umbilical and inguinal hernia, genital infantilism, corneal opacities, and skin abnormalities. Patients with Hurler's syndrome have gargoylelike features, with broad saddle nose, thick lips, and a large tongue. The skin is thickened, with ridges and grooves, especially on the upper half of the body. Fine lanugo hair is profusely distributed all over the body. Large, coarse hair is prominent, especially on the extremities. The skeletal system is deformed, with hydrocephalus and kyphosis and gibbus (cat-back shape). The hands are broad and have clawlike fingers. The joints are distorted.

The two acid mucopolysaccharides, dermatan sulfate and heparan sulfate, are produced excessively in gargoylism, so that in many tissues there is an accumulation, and they are excreted in the urine in large amounts. Dried urine on filter paper will show a purple color when acetic acid followed by toluidine blue reagent is added.

Prenatal diagnosis is possible. Bone marrow transplantation is the most effective treatment of Hurler's syndrome. It can prevent dementia if performed early enough.

Field RE, et al: Bone marrow transplantation in Hurler's syndrome. *J Bone Joint Surg Br* 1994, 76:975.

Hambrick GW Jr, et al: Studies of the skin in Hurler's syndrome. *Arch Dermatol* 1962, 89:455.

Muenzer J: Mucopolysaccharidoses. *Adv Pediatr* 1986, 33:269. ▲

HUNTER'S SYNDROME

Hunter's syndrome is X-linked mucopolysaccharidosis (MPS) II. The clinical features are similar to those of Hurler's syndrome and are characterized by an excessive storage and excretion of mucopolysaccharides. The relative mildness and the mode of inheritance distinguish it from Hurler's syndrome. The pebbly lesions of MPS II in the skin over the inferior angles of the scapulas represent the only distinctive skin changes of the mucopolysaccharidoses. These are firm, flesh-colored to white papules and nodules, which coalesce. They are most common on the back, but may be seen on the pectoral areas, the nape of the neck, and the lateral aspects of the arms and thighs. They generally occur at about age 10.

The deficient enzyme is iduronate sulfatase. Dermatan sulfate and heparin sulfate are excreted in the urine in large amounts. Bone marrow transplantation does not benefit.

Downs AT, et al: Hunter's syndrome and oral manifestations. *Pediatr Dent* 1995, 17:98.

Zivony DI, et al: Ivory-colored papules in a young boy. *Arch Dermatol* 1995, 131:81. ▲

MORQUIO'S DISEASE

This autosomal recessive disorder is characterized by dwarfism, prognathism, corneal opacities, deafness, progressive kyphoscoliosis, flat feet, and knock-knees. The standing position is a crouch. There is increased excretion of keratan sulfate. The enzyme deficiencies are galactosamine-6-sulfate sulfatase in Morquio A and beta-galactosidase in Morquio B.

Groebe H, et al: Morquio's syndrome associated with beta-galactosidase deficiency. *Am J Hum Genet* 1980, 32:258.

Muenzer J: Mucopolysaccharidoses. *Adv Pediatr* 1986, 33:269. ▲

HYALUONIDASE DEFICIENCY

Natowicz et al reported a 14-year-old girl with complete absence of the enzyme hyaluronidase. The patient had short stature, erosions of the acetabula, and multiple periauricular soft-tissue masses.

Natowicz MR, et al: Clinical and biochemical manifestations of hyaluronidase deficiency. *N Engl J Med* 1996, 335:1029. ▲

LAFORA'S DISEASE

Lafora's disease is an autosomal recessive form of progressive epilepsy beginning at puberty. It is characterized by myoclonic jerks followed by progressive ataxia, dysphagia, dysarthria, dementia, and death in early adulthood. Diagnosis is established in the proper clinical setting by demonstration of characteristic PAS-positive cytoplasmic inclusion bodies in the eccrine ducts, axillary apocrine myoepithelial cells, and peripheral nerves. The best site to biopsy is the axilla. Other conditions in which similar polyglucosan inclusions can be seen include normal aging (amyloid bodies), double athetosis syndrome, amyotrophic lateral sclerosis, and glycogen storage disease, type IV.

Cutaneous manifestations are rare. Papulonodular lesions on the ears and indurated, thickened plaques on the arms have been reported. Large amounts of acid mucopolysaccharides were demonstrated histologically in these lesions. The disease is felt to be caused by an enzyme defect in the mucopolysaccharide metabolic pathway.

Samlaska CP, et al: Lafora's disease. *J Am Acad Dermatol* 1989, 21:791. ▲

FARBER'S DISEASE

First described by Sidney Farber in 1952, and also known as *fibrocytic dysmucopolysaccharidosis* and *lipogranulomatosis,* Farber's disease is characterized by periarticular swellings; a weak, hoarse cry; pulmonary failure; painful joint deformities; and motor and mental retardation. The onset is during the first months of life; death can be expected before the patient reaches age 2.

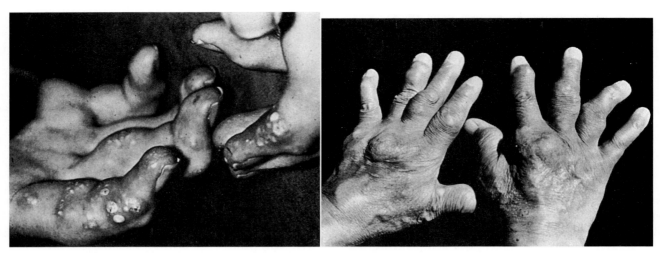

Fig. 26-34 Gout.

The rubbery subcutaneous nodules have a distinct yellowish hue and are 1 to 2 cm in diameter. They are usually located over the joints, lumbar spine, scalp, and weight-bearing areas. Histologically, they are granulomas. Diagnosis can be aided by finding Farber bodies (curvilinear bodies) within the cytoplasm or phagosomes of fibroblasts, histiocytes, or endothelial cells, banana-shaped bodies within Schwann cells, and zebra bodies within endothelial cells and neurons.

In Farber's disease, an accumulation of ceramide and its degradation products in foam cells and a specific deficiency of acid ceramidase in cultured fibroblasts and white blood cells have been demonstrated.

Rauch HJ, et al: Banana bodies in disseminated lipogranulomatosis (Farber's disease). *Am J Dermatopathol* 1983, 5:263. _____ ▲

ADRENOLEUKODYSTROPHY (SCHILDER'S DISEASE)

Adrenoleukodystrophy (ALD) is an X-linked disorder in which cerebral white matter becomes progressively demyelinated and serious adrenocortical insufficiency usually occurs. Skin hyperpigmentation often calls attention to the adrenal disease, and mental deterioration indicates the even graver diagnosis of ALD. Computed tomography may help indicate the site for a diagnostic brain biopsy. A mild ichthyotic appearance to the skin of the trunk and legs and sparse hair with trichorrhexis nodosa–like features may occur. Skin biopsies may show characteristic vacuolization of eccrine secretory coils (duct cells being spared), and biopsies of the skin and conjunctiva may show diagnostic clefts in Schwann cells surrounding myelinated axons. The abnormal gene encodes for a protein ALDP, known to be important in peroxisomal beta-oxidation. Bone marrow transplantation may prevent dementia and result in a better quality of life.

Crum BA, et al: 26-year-old man with hyperpigmentation of skin and lower extremity spasticity. *Mayo Clin Proc* 1997, 72:479.
Krivit W, et al: The future for treatment by bone marrow transplantation for adrenoleukodystrophy, metachromatic leukodystrophy, globoid cell leukodystrophy and Hurler syndrome. *J Inherit Metab Dis* 1995, 18:398.
Papini M, et al: Adrenoleukodystrophy: dermatological findings and skin surface lipid study. *Dermatology* 1994, 188:25. _____ ▲

GOUT

In chronic cases of gout (podagra), monosodium urate monohydrate may be deposited in the subcutaneous tissues, forming nodules called tophi. These vary from pinhead-sized to pea-sized or, rarely, even baseball-sized. They are commonly found on the rims of the ears and over the distal interphalangeal articulations (Fig. 26-34). Tophi are of a yellow or cream color. In the course of time they tend to break down and discharge sodium urate crystals, afterward healing and perhaps breaking down again. The diagnosis is verified histologically by finding the characteristic long, needle-shaped crystals of monosodium urate. Because these deposits are dissolved by routine processing, fixation in absolute ethanol or freezing is optimal for their demonstration. Ninety-five percent of patients are men.

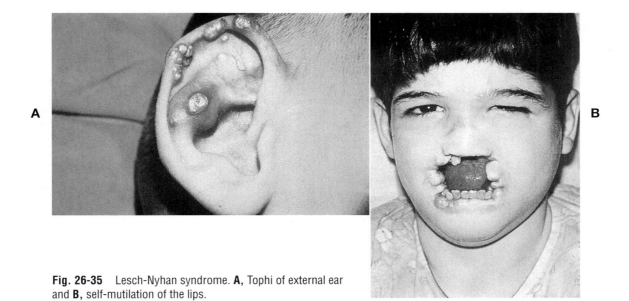

Fig. 26-35 Lesch-Nyhan syndrome. **A,** Tophi of external ear and **B,** self-mutilation of the lips.

LESCH-NYHAN SYNDROME

Also known as *juvenile gout,* Lesch-Nyhan syndrome is a rare, X-linked, recessively inherited disorder characterized by childhood hyperuricemia (Fig. 26-35, *A*), choreoathetosis, progressive mental retardation, and self-mutilation.

The cutaneous lesions are distinctive. Massive self-mutilation of lips with the teeth occurs (Fig. 26-35, *B*). The fingers are also badly chewed. The ears and nose are occasionally mutilated. An early diagnostic clue is orange crystals in the diaper. The blood uric acid is increased and allopurinol, 200 to 400 mg daily, is given. There is a marked deficiency in an enzyme of purine metabolism, hypoxanthine guanine phosphoribosyltransferase (HGPRT).

Conejo Mir J, et al: Panniculitis and ulcers in a young man. *Arch Dermatol* 1998, 134:501.

Eng AM, et al: Finger pad deposits. *Arch Dermatol* 1994, 130:1435.

Fam AG, et al: Intradermal urate tophi. *J Rheumatol* 1997, 24:1126.

Schepis C, et al: What syndrome is this? Lesch-Nyhan syndrome. *Pediatr Dermatol* 1996, 13:169.

Watts DJ, et al: Gouty tophi. *Dermatol Surg* 1996, 22:118. ▲

CHAPTER 27

Some Genodermatoses and Acquired Syndromes

Genetic disorders are often grouped into three categories: chromosomal, single gene, and multifactorial. Chromosomal disorders can be either numerical, such as trisomy and monosomy, or structural, resulting from translocations, deletions, and duplications. *Mosaicism* is the presence of two or more genetically distinct cell lines in a single individual, producing diverse phenotypes. A good example of mosaicism is linear and whorled nevoid hypermelanosis, which produces pigmentary anomalies along the lines of Blaschko. Most genodermatoses show single-gene or mendelian inheritance (autosomal dominant, autosomal recessive, or X-linked recessive genes).

Autosomal (non–sex chromosomal) dominant conditions require only a single gene to produce the phenotype. Usually the patient has one affected parent, and the disease is transmitted from generation to generation. Autosomal recessive traits, on the other hand, require a homozygous state to produce the abnormality. The pedigree here will often reveal parental consanguinity; parents will be clinically unaffected but often have affected siblings.

X-linked conditions occur when the mutant gene is carried on the X chromosome. If a disease is X-linked recessive, it occurs almost exclusively in males, who cannot transmit the disease to their sons, but all of their daughters will be carriers. Carrier females who are heterozygous (having one normal and one abnormal X chromosome) occasionally may show some subtle evidence of the disease. X-linked dominant disease states, if lethal in males (as incontinentia pigmenti is theorized to be), explain pedigrees in which more than one female is affected but no males express the disease. If such conditions are not lethal in males, the pedigree may resemble an autosomal dominant pattern of inheritance; however, an affected male will transmit the disorder to all of his daughters, but none of his sons. Genetic counseling is a mainstay for patients and their families in most of the conditions that will be discussed next.

Kumar S, et al: Common genodermatoses. *Int J Dermatol* 1996, 35:685.
Nehal KS, et al: Analysis of 54 cases of hypopigmentation and hyperpigmentation along the lines of Blaschko. *Arch Dermatol* 1996, 132:1167.
Paller AS: Pigmentary patterning as a clinical clue of genetic mosaicism. *Arch Dermatol* 1996, 132:1234. _____ ▲

X-LINKED, MOSAIC, AND RELATED DISORDERS
Incontinentia Pigmenti

Also known as *Bloch-Sulzberger's disease,* incontinentia pigmenti is characterized by spattered pigmentation on the trunk preceded by urticarial, vesicular, or verrucous inflammatory changes. It appears in girls during the first weeks of life. Most lesions are evident by time the infant is 4 to 6 weeks old. The highly distinctive findings are initially vesicular in 87% of cases. This first stage begins in most individuals before 6 weeks of age and is replaced by verrucous lesions after several weeks to months. The second (verrucous) stage follows the blistering in two thirds of patients, occurring in a similar distribution. Although these usually resolve by 1 year of age, lesions may persist for many years.

Following the inflammatory and verrucous stages, the third, or pigmentary phase occurs: pigmented macules scattered over the trunk, upper arms, and upper legs. The pigmentation is capriciously patterned, dendritic, and bizarre, with irregularly shaped splashes, lines, streaks, whorls, polyangular flecks, and spidery and fountain-spray splatters (Figs. 27-1 to 27-3). The eruption follows the lines of Blaschko. Although cases have been reported in which the inflammatory stages do not necessarily precede the typical pigmentation (there is frequent overlap of the three stages, and the blistering and verrucous stages may not occur at all in some patients), these individuals may actually have linear and whorled nevoid hypermelanosis. The pigmentary stage may last for many years and then fade away, leaving no sequelae. A fourth stage may be seen

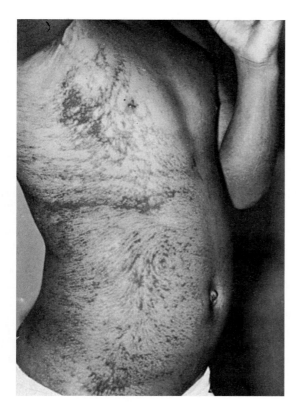

Fig. 27-1 Incontinentia pigmenti with whorls and fountain-spray splatters. (Courtesy Dr. J.P. Ruppe.)

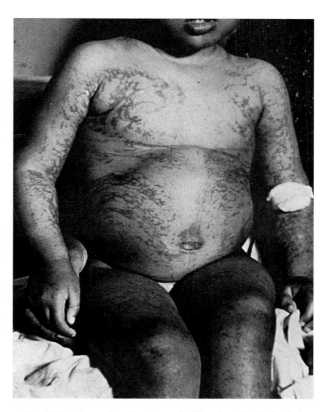

Fig. 27-2 Incontinentia pigmenti. (Courtesy Dr. H. Curth.)

in some adult women, manifesting subtle, faint, hypochromic or atrophic linear lesions, most commonly on the extremities.

Other cutaneous changes include patchy alopecia at the vertex of the scalp, atrophic changes simulating acrodermatitis chronica atrophicans on the hands, onychodystrophy, subungual tumors with underlying lytic bone lesions, and palmoplantar hyperhidrosis. Extracutaneous manifestations occur in 70% to 80% of patients. Most commonly involved are the teeth (65%), central nervous system (33%), eyes (25% to 35%), and the bones. Immune dysfunction with defective neutrophil chemotaxis and elevated IgE has been reported. Eosinophilia is common.

Dental abnormalities usually manifest by the time the individual is 2 years old. Partial anodontia occurs in 43% and pegged teeth in 30%. The most common central nervous system findings are seizures (13%), mental retardation (12%), spastic paralysis (11%), microcephaly, destructive encephalopathy, and motor retardation. The eye changes, half of them serious, include strabismus (most common), cataracts, retinal detachments, optic atrophy, blue sclerae, and exudative chorioretinitis. Skeletal abnormalities include syndactyly, skull deformities, dwarfism, spina bifida, clubfoot, supernumerary ribs, hemiatrophy, and shortening of the legs and arms.

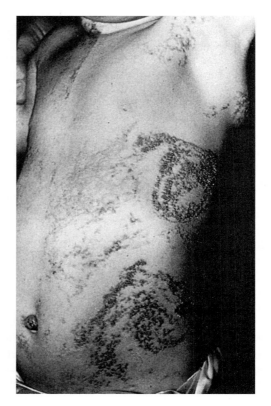

Fig. 27-3 Incontinentia pigmenti with whorled verrucous lesions.

Incontinentia pigmenti is caused by a mutation on the X chromosome, localized to Xq28. Of the 48 male patients reported most were identified before 1961, when chromosome analysis became available. More recent male cases (five boys) were shown to have Klinefelter's syndrome (47,XXY). Boys with one abnormal X chromosome are believed to die in utero with severe disease, and there is an increased incidence of spontaneous abortion in affected women. An additional explanation for surviving males is a spontaneous mutation during replication in the gamete, resulting in mosaicism.

Histologically, in the blistering stage, vesicles are intraepidermal and associated with marked spongiosis and eosinophils (eosinophilic spongiosis). Individual necrotic keratinocytes are present. Acanthosis, hyperkeratosis, and papillomatosis occur in the second stage, with persistent presence of necrotic keratinocytes. The end-stage of pigmentation is due to melanin in melanophages in the upper dermis.

In the differential diagnosis, epidermolysis bullosa and childhood bullous pemphigoid are easily distinguished. Incontinentia pigmenti differs from the Franceschetti-Jadassohn syndrome in that the latter has a reticular pigmentation rather than sprays or spatters; also, no abnormal dentition and no eye lesions are present. Incontinentia pigmenti achromians differs in that it is a negative image, with hypopigmentation; it is autosomal dominant in inheritance; it has no vesicular or verrucous stages; and it has a higher incidence of central nervous system abnormalities. Patients with linear and whorled nevoid hypermelanosis lack the vesicular and verrucous phases. Happle syndrome (X-linked dominant chondrodysplasia punctata) has ichthyosiform erythroderma along lines of Blaschko, cataracts, asymmetrical limb shortening, and calcified stippling of the epiphyses of long bones. Follicular atrophoderma replaces the erythroderma after the first year.

There is no treatment for incontinentia pigmenti. Use of ruby lasers to treat pigmented lesion in infants and young children is not necessary and may worsen the condition. Usually the end-stage of streaks of incontinentia pigmenti start to fade out at age 2, and by adulthood there may be little residuum.

Naegeli-Franceschetti-Jadassohn Syndrome

Also known as the *chromatophore nevus of Naegeli,* Naegeli-Franceschetti-Jadassohn syndrome differs from incontinentia pigmenti in that the pigmentation is reticular and there are no preceding inflammatory changes, vesiculation, or verrucous lesions. Vasomotor changes and hypohidrosis are present. There is reticulate pigmentation involving the neck, flexural skin, and perioral and periorbital areas. Diffuse keratoderma and punctiform accentuation of the palms and soles may occur. Dermatoglyphics are abnormal, producing atrophic or absent ridges on fingerprints.

Congenital malalignment of the great toenails may be found in some individuals. Dental abnormalities are common, and many patients are edentulous. Both sexes are equally affected. This has been reported in three families in which the disease occurred as an autosomal dominant trait.

Dutheil P, et al: Incontinentia pigmenti late sequelae and genotypic diagnosis: a three-generation study of four patients. *Pediatr Dermatol* 1995, 12:107.

Itin PH, et al: Natural history of the Naegeli-Franceschetti-Jadassohn syndrome and further delineation of its clinical manifestations. *J Am Acad Dermatol* 1993, 28:942.

Nagase T, et al: Extensive vesiculobullous eruption following limited ruby laser treatment for incontinentia pigmenti. *Australas J Dermatol* 1997, 38:155.

Sahn EE, et al: Incontinentia pigmenti. *J Am Acad Dermatol* 1994, 31:852.

Scheuerle AE: Male cases of incontinentia pigmenti. *Am J Med Genet* 1998, 77:201.

Yang JH, et al: Destructive encephalopathy in incontinentia pigmenti. *J Dermatol* 1995, 22:340. ▲

Incontinentia Pigmenti Achromians (Hypomelanosis of Ito)

Incontinentia pigmenti achromians is characterized by various patterns of bilateral or unilateral hypopigmentation (instead of hyperpigmentation, as is seen in the Bloch-Sulzberger incontinentia pigmenti). The lesions suggest the "negative image" of incontinentia pigmenti and usually develop by the first year of life. The female-to-male ratio is about 2.5:1. Three fourths of affected individuals have associated anomalies of the central nervous system, eyes, hair, teeth, skin, nails, musculoskeletal system, or internal organs.

More than half of these patients are found to have chromosomal abnormalities, with most demonstrating mosaicism for aneuploidy or unbalanced translocations. No inflammatory changes or vesiculation are found before the development of the hypopigmentation, and there is no liquefaction of the basal layer or incontinence of pigment. There is no treatment, but eventual repigmentation is the rule.

Failla P, et al: Hypomelanosis of Ito: a syndrome requiring a multisystem approach. *Australas J Dermatol* 1997, 38:65.

Ruiz-Maldonado R, et al: Hypomelanosis of Ito: diagnostic criteria and report of 41 cases. *Pediatr Dermatol* 1992, 9:1.

Sybert VP: Hypomelanosis of Ito: a description, not a diagnosis. *J Invest Dermatol* 1994, 103(Suppl):141. ▲

Linear and Whorled Nevoid Hypermelanosis

This disorder of pigmentation develops within a few weeks of life and progresses for 1 to 2 years before stabilizing. There is linear and whorled hyperpigmentation following the lines of Blaschko without preceding bullae or verrucous lesions. Sparing of mucous membranes, eyes, palms, and soles is also a major feature. The number of cases with congenital anomalies, such as mental retardation, cerebral palsy, atrial septal defects, dextrocardia, auricular atresia, and patent ductus arteriosus, is increasing. There is no sexual predilection. Biopsy of pigmented areas demonstrates increased pigmentation of the basal layer and prominence of melanocytes without incontinence of pigment.

Most cases appear to be sporadic although familial cases have been reported. Sporadic forms have been attributed to mosaicism. Because of confusion with other pigmented disorders, such as incontinentia pigmenti, early linear epidermal nevi, hypomelanosis of Ito, and nevus depigmentosus, it is likely that linear and whorled nevoid hypermelanosis may be more common than previously appreciated.

Akiyama M, et al: Familial linear and whorled nevoid hypermelanosis. *J Am Acad Dermatol* 1994, 30:831.
Alvarez J, et al: Linear and whorled nevoid hypermelanosis. *Pediatr Dermatol* 1993, 10:156.
Harre J, et al: Linear and whorled pigmentation. *Int J Dermatol* 1994, 33:529.
Kubota Y, et al: Linear and whorled nevoid hypermelanosis in a child with chromosomal mosaicism. *Int J Dermatol* 1992, 31:345.
Schepis C, et al: Linear and whorled nevoid hypermelanosis in a boy with mental retardation and congenital defects. *Int J Dermatol* 1996, 35:654. ▲

Chondrodysplasia Punctata

A variant of the original Conradi-Hünermann syndrome or chondrodystrophia calcificans congenita, chondrodysplasia punctata is characterized by ichthyosis of the skin similar to that of the collodion baby, followed by hyperkeratotic "whirl and swirl" patterns on erythematous skin. In addition to the reddening, the waxy, shiny skin has hyperkeratotic scales of a peculiar crushed-eggshell configuration. As the child grows, follicular atrophoderma and pseudopelade develop. Usually the ichthyosis clears within the first year of life but may leave behind hyperpigmentation similar to that seen in incontinentia pigmenti. Additional features include minor nail defects, such as platonychia and onychoschizia.

There are four forms of chondrodysplasia punctata, which are classified by their inheritance patterns. The Conradi-Hünermann type is associated with autosomal dominant inheritance, facial dysmorphia with a low nasal bridge, short stature, mild disease, cataracts, and few skin lesions. The rhizomelic form has autosomal recessive inheritance, marked shortening of the extremities, cataracts, ichthyosis, and nasal hypoplasia; the patient dies in infancy. The X-linked recessive type has been described as part of contiguous gene deletion syndromes, with short stature, telebrachydactyly, and nasal hypoplasia. The X-linked dominant form (Happle syndrome) is lethal in males. The skeletal defects revealed on radiographic evaluation show irregular calcified stippling of the cartilaginous epiphyses in the long bones, costal cartilages, and vertebral diaphysis. The stippling occurs in the fetus and persists until age 3 or 4. The humeri and femurs may be shortened, and there may be joint dysplasia. Histologic evaluation of the ichthyotic

lesions reveals a thinned, granular cell layer, calcification of keratotic follicular plugs, and focal hyperpigmentation of basal keratinocytes. The keratotic follicular plugs and calcium deposits are characteristic of this disease and very helpful in establishing the diagnosis in newborns.

Bruch D, et al: Ichthyotic and psoriasiform skin lesions along Blaschko's lines in a woman with X-linked chondrodysplasia punctata. *J Am Acad Dermatol* 1995, 33:356.
Yanagihara M, et al: Usefulness of histopathologic examination of thick scales in the diagnosis of X-linked dominant chondrodysplasia punctata (Happle). *Pediatr Dermatol* 1996, 13:1. ▲

Klinefelter's Syndrome

Klinefelter's syndrome consists of hypogonadism, gynecomastia, eunuchoidism, small or absent testicles, and elevated gonadotropins. There may be a low frontal hairline, sparse body hair with only a few hairs in the axillary and pubic areas, scanty or absent facial hair in men, and shortening of the fifth digit of both hands.

Thrombophlebitis and recurrent or chronic leg ulcerations may be a presenting manifestation; these may be more common than previously reported. The cause of the hypercoagulable state is believed to be an increase in plasminogen activator inhibitor-1 levels. Patients are at an increased risk of a variety of cancers, especially male breast cancer and germ tumors, hematologic malignancies, and sarcomas (retinoblastoma and rhabdomyosarcoma).

Many of these patients are tall; some are obese. Dull mentality or misbehavior is frequent, and psychiatric disorders occur in about one third of these patients. Klinefelter's syndrome is most frequently associated with an XXY sex chromosome pattern, although other variations occur as the number of X chromosomes increases. Marked improvement in appearance has been achieved by injection of testosterone.

XXYY Genotype

The XXYY genotype is considered to be a variant of Klinefelter's syndrome. In addition to the changes seen in Klinefelter's, there are vascular changes, such as cutaneous angiomas, acrocyanosis, and peripheral vascular disease leading to stasis dermatitis.

Humphreys M, et al: Klinefelter syndrome and non-Hodgkin lymphoma. *Cancer Genet Cytogenet* 1997, 97:111.
Spier C, et al: Recurrent leg ulcerations as the initial clinical manifestation of Klinefelter's syndrome. *Arch Dermatol* 1995, 131:230.
Veraart JC, et al: Leg ulcers and Klinefelter's syndrome. *Arch Dermatol* 1995, 131:959.
Zollner TM, et al: Leg ulcers in Klinefelter's syndrome: further evidence for an involvement of plasminogen activator inhibitor-1. *Br J Dermatol* 1997, 136:341. ▲

Turner's Syndrome

Turner's syndrome, also known as *gonadal dysgenesis,* is characterized by a webbed neck, low posterior hairline margin, increased carrying angle at the elbow (cubitus valgus), a triangular mouth, alopecia of the frontal area on the scalp, sometimes koilonychia, cutis laxa, cutis hyperelastica, and patchy alopecia on the scalp (Fig. 27-4). Patients tend to have numerous melanocytic nevi and an increased risk of melanoma has been suggested. There may be mental retardation, short stature, infantilism, and retarded sexual development with primary amenorrhea.

It has been shown that these patients have only 45 chromosomes rather than the normal 46 chromosomes. An X chromosome is missing, resulting in an XO genotype. Mosaicism, structural abnormalities of the X chromosome, or a partial deficiency of one sex chromosome may account for a number of the variations in gonadal dysgenesis. No specific treatment is available. Growth hormone has been shown to be effective in treating the short stature, but its use is controversial.

Becker B, et al: Melanocytic nevi in Turner syndrome. *Pediatr Dermatol* 1994, 11:120.

Gare M, et al: Malignant melanoma in Turner's syndrome. *Int J Dermatol* 1995, 34:823.

Leichtman DA, et al: Familial Turner's syndrome. *Ann Intern Med* 1978, 89:473.

Rosenfeld RG, et al: Six-year results of a randomized, prospective trial of human growth hormone and oxandrolone in Turner syndrome. *J Pediatr* 1992, 121:49. ▲

Noonan's Syndrome

Noonan's syndrome is an autosomal dominant disease that in many respects mimics Turner's syndrome. Males and females are equally affected, and the chromosome number is normal in Noonan's syndrome. The major features are a characteristic facies with hypertelorism, prominent ears, webbed neck, short stature, undescended testicles, low posterior neck hairline, cardiovascular abnormalities (pulmonary stenosis and hypertrophic cardiomyopathy),

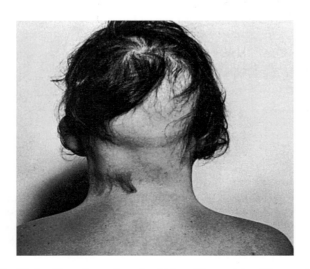

Fig. 27-4 Alopecia areata and webbing of the neck in a 14-year-old girl with Turner's syndrome.

and cubitus valgus. Some 25% to 40% of patients have dermatologic findings: lymphedema; short, curly hair; dystrophic nails; a tendency toward keloid formation; soft, elastic skin; keratosis pilaris atrophicans; and abnormal dermatoglyphics.

Daoud MS, et al: Noonan syndrome. *Semin Dermatol* 1995, 14:140.

Sharland M, et al: A clinical study of Noonan syndrome. *Arch Dis Child* 1992, 67:178. ▲

Cardio-Facio-Cutaneous Syndrome

Cardio-facio-cutaneous syndrome is a congenital condition manifested by numerous anomalies. It may resemble Noonan's syndrome, and some authors believe it to be a variant of Noonan's syndrome. Typical features include a characteristic craniofacial appearance, psychomotor and growth retardation, congenital cardiac defects, and skin and hair abnormalities. The most frequent dermatologic finding is hair that is sparse, curly, fine or thick, woolly or brittle. In more than half of the reported cases, the patient has dry, scaly, or "hyperkeratotic," ichthyotic skin.

Other cutaneous findings include sparse or absent eyebrows and eyelashes, low posterior hairline, patchy alopecia, scant body hair, follicular hyperkeratosis, keratosis pilaris, keratosis pilaris atrophicans faciei, palmoplantar keratoderma, seborrheic dermatitis, eczema, lymphedema, hemangiomas, café au lait spots, pigmented nevi, hyperpigmented macules or stripes, cutis marmorata, and sacral dimples. Nail dystrophy, koilonychia, and dysplastic teeth have also been reported.

The differential diagnosis includes Noonan's syndrome, Ullrich-Turner syndrome, C syndrome, Pallister mosaic aneuploid syndrome, and Crowe-Dickermann syndrome. The difficulty often arises in assessing the facial features, which are similar in all of these syndromes. The tremendous variation in clinical findings further adds to the difficulty in diagnosis, without more specific criteria or genetic mapping.

Borradori L, et al: Skin manifestations of cardio-facio-cutaneous syndrome. *J Am Acad Dermatol* 1993, 28:815.

Krajewska-Walasek M, et al: The cardio-facio-cutaneous (CFC) syndrome: two possible new cases and review of the literature. *Clin Dysmorphol* 1996, 5:65.

Ward KA, et al: The cardio-facio-cutaneous syndrome: a manifestation of the Noonan syndrome? *Br J Dermatol* 1994, 131:270.

Wieczorek D, et al: Cardio-facio-cutaneous (CFC) syndrome: a distinct entity? Report of three patients demonstrating the diagnostic difficulties in delineation of CFC syndrome. *Clin Genet* 1997, 52:37. ▲

Phakomatoses

The phakomatoses are the various inherited disorders of the central nervous system that have congenital retinal tumors and cutaneous involvement. They include tuberous sclerosis, von Recklinghausen's disease (neurofibromatosis), von

Hippel-Lindau's disease (angiomatosis retinae), ataxia-telangiectasia, basal cell nevus syndrome, nevus sebaceus, and Sturge-Weber syndrome.

TUBEROUS SCLEROSIS (EPILOIA, BOURNEVILLE'S DISEASE)

Tuberous sclerosis is also called *epiloia* (*epi* = epilepsy, *loi* = low intelligence, *a* = adenoma sebaceum).

This classic triad of adenoma sebaceum, mental deficiency, and epilepsy, however, is present in only a minority of patients. Other associated features may include periungual fibromas, shagreen plaques, oral papillomatosis, ash-leaf hypomelanotic macules, skin fibromas, and café au lait spots.

Adenoma sebaceum are 1- to 3-mm, yellowish red, translucent, discrete, waxy papules that are distributed symmetrically, principally over the cheeks, nose, and forehead (Figs. 27-5 and 27-6). They have also been reported in patients with multiple endocrine neoplasia (MEN). These lesions are present in 90% of patients over 4 years of age, persist indefinitely, and may increase in number. Histologically, the facial lesions are angiofibromas.

Shagreen patch is named after a type of leather tanned in a particular way to produce granulated-texture greenish knobs on the surface, resembling shark skin (Fig. 27-7). Patches of this type of "knobby" skin, varying from 1 to 8 cm in diameter, are found on the trunk, most commonly on the lumbosacral area. They are connective tissue nevi. They occur in 40% of patients and develop in the first decade of life.

Koenen's tumors are distinctive when present; they occur in 50% of patients. The tumors are small, digitate, protruding, asymptomatic periungual and/or subungual (Fig. 27-8). Histologically, they are angiofibromas. They have their onset at puberty. Similar lesions may occur on the gingiva.

Congenital white leaf-shaped macules, called *hypomelanotic macules*, are found in 85% of patients with tuberous sclerosis, the number ranging from 1 to 100. These may be detected at birth in most patients, although occasional patients may not develop them until they are 6 to 8 years of age. They may be shaped like an ash leaf (Fig. 27-9), but linear and confetti-type white macules may also be present. Wood's light examination should be performed when evaluating a patient for tuberous sclerosis. Focal poliosis (localized tufts of white hair) may be present at birth. Solitary ash-leaf macules are not uncommon in the general

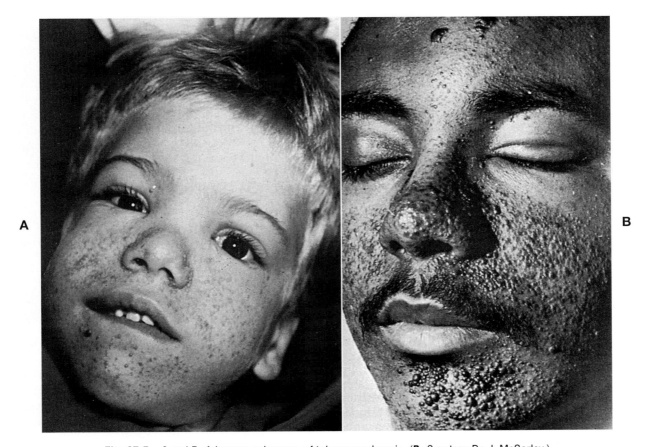

Fig. 27-5 **A** and **B**, Adenoma sebaceum of tuberous sclerosis. (**B**, Courtesy Dr. J. McSorley.)

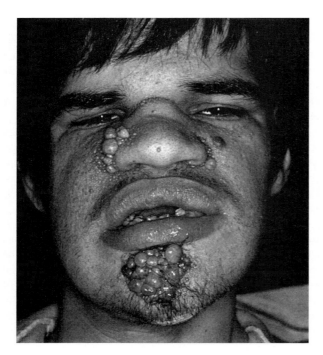

Fig. 27-6 Patient with tuberous sclerosis, mental retardation, and a convulsive disorder. (Courtesy Dr. Axel W. Hoke.)

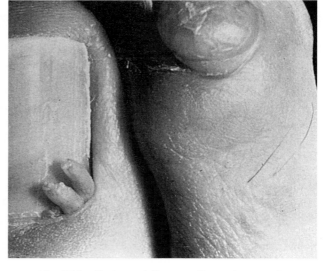

Fig. 27-8 Periungual fibromas (Koenen's tumors).

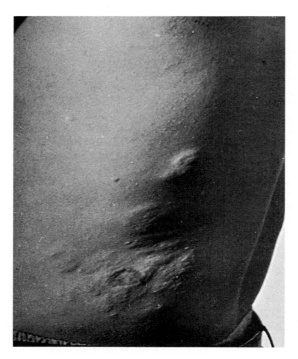

Fig. 27-7 Shagreen skin in tuberous sclerosis on the flank.

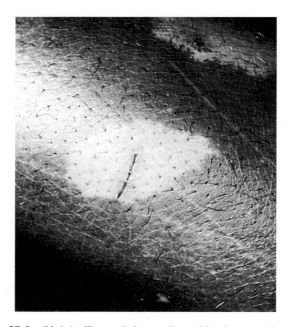

Fig. 27-9 "Ash-leaf" macule in a patient with tuberous sclerosis.

population and may be confused for other hypopigmented macules, such as nevus depigmentosus.

Mental deficiency, usually seen early in life, is present in 40% to 60% of patients, varying widely in its manifestations. Epilepsy also occurs, is variable in its severity, and usually also presents early in life. Eighty percent to 90% of patients have seizures or nonspecific electroencephalographic abnormalities. Hamartomatous proliferations of glial and neuronal tissue produce potato-like nodules or brain stones in the cortex. X-ray evaluation will reveal these once they are calcified, but CT scans, cranial ultrasonography, and MRIs may define these lesions as early as 6 weeks of age and thus are useful in making an early diagnosis. These brain tumors may progress to gliomas. Subependymal nodules (candle drippings) are similar lesions in the ventricular walls. Astrocytomas may also occur.

Retinal tumors (phakomas) occur, which are optic nerve or retinal nerve hamartomas. Various ophthalmologic findings, such as pigmentary changes, nystagmus, and angioid streaks, occur in 50% of patients.

Renal hamartomas (angiomyolipomas [45%], cystic disease [18%], fibroadenomas, or mixed tumors) and cardiac tumors (rhabdomyomas [43%]) may also occur. In the familial variety of tuberous sclerosis, 80% of patients have angiomyolipomas, which are often bilateral and frequently cause severe problems, including renal failure.

A few patients—almost all women of childbearing age—have pulmonary lymphangioleiomyomas, and the suggestion has been made that pulmonary lymphangioleiomyomatosis may be a forme fruste of tuberous sclerosis.

Nearly half of patients with epiloia have bony abnormalities such as bone cysts and sclerosis, which can be seen on x-ray evaluation. Five or more pits in the enamel of permanent teeth are a marker for this disease.

Tuberous sclerosis is a common inherited autosomal dominant disease with highly variable penetrance. Prevalence estimates range from 1 per 5800 to 1 per 15,000. Up to 50% of cases may occur as a result of spontaneous mutations.

There are two genes, the mutations of which produce indistinguishable phenotypes—9q34 (TSC1) and 16p13.3 (TSC2). TSC1 and TSC2 are tumor suppressor genes. TSC2 encodes for tuberin, a putative GTPase-activating protein for rap1 and rab5. TSC1 encodes for hamartin, a novel protein with no significant homology to tuberin or any other vertebrate protein. Hamartin and tuberin associate physically in vivo, suggesting that they function in the same complex rather than in separate pathways. This interaction of tuberin and hamartin explains the indistinguishable phenotypes caused by mutations in either gene.

Diagnosis

The ash-leaf macules—most easily seen with a Wood's light—may be present at birth and are an indication for skull x-ray evaluation. If this fails to show calcified intracranial nodules, ultrasonography, a CT scan or MRI, which are more sensitive, should be performed. Funduscopic examination, hand and foot x-ray evaluation, and renal ultrasonography are often rewarding in a patient with few clinical findings, since up to 31% of asymptomatic parents have been identified using these tests.

Solitary periungual fibromas are not an uncommon finding in patients without risk for systemic involvement, and caution should be exercised in making the diagnosis

of tuberous sclerosis in these individuals. Likewise, the prevalence of hypopigmented macules in the general population has been underestimated, and detection of a few macules without further evidence suggesting tuberous sclerosis need not prompt an extensive evaluation. Molecular analysis for TSC1 and TSC2 may be the only way to ultimately identify "mildly affected" individuals.

HISTOPATHOLOGY AND TREATMENT. Adenoma sebaceum is a vascular and connective tissue tumor (angiofibromatous hamartoma). Similar histologic features are seen with subungual and gingival tumors.

Adenoma sebaceum can be treated by shaving, dermabrasion, or laser therapy. Lesions are likely to recur, requiring repeat treatment. Cranial irradiation of astrocytomas should be avoided because this may result in the subsequent development of glioblastomas.

Castro M, et al: Pulmonary tuberous sclerosis. *Chest* 1995, 107:189.

Gil-Mateo MP, et al: Widespread angiokeratomas and tuberous sclerosis. *Br J Dermatol* 1996, 135:280.

Griffiths PD, et al: Tuberous sclerosis complex: the role of neuroradiology. *Neuropediatrics* 1997, 28:244.

Kwiatkowski DJ, et al: Tuberous sclerosis. *Arch Dermatol* 1994, 130:348.

Matsumura H, et al: Glioblastoma following radiotherapy in a patient with tuberous sclerosis. *Neurol Med Chir* 1998, 38:287.

McGrae JD Jr, et al: Unilateral facial angiofibromas. *Br J Dermatol* 1996, 134:727.

Roach ES, et al: Tuberous sclerosis. *Dermatol Clin* 1995, 13:151.

Schnur RE: Tuberous sclerosis: the persistent challenge of clinical diagnosis. *Arch Dermatol* 1995, 131:1460.

Torres OA, et al: Early diagnosis of subependymal giant cell astrocytoma in patients with tuberous sclerosis. *J Child Neurol* 1998, 13:173.

Vanderhooft SL, et al: Prevalence of hypopigmented macules in a healthy population. *J Pediatr* 1996, 129:355.

van Slegtenhorst M, et al: Identification of the tuberous sclerosis gene TSC1 on chromosome 9q34. *Science* 1997, 277:805.

van Slegtenhorst M, et al: Interaction between hamartin and tuberin, the TSC1 and TSC2 gene products. *Hum Mol Genet* 1998, 7:1053.

Verheyden CN: Treatment of the facial angiofibromas of tuberous sclerosis. *Plast Reconstr Surg* 1996, 98:777.

Webb DW, et al: The cutaneous features of tuberous sclerosis: a population study. *Br J Dermatol* 1996, 135:1.

Zeller J, et al: The significance of a single periungual fibroma: report of seven cases. *Arch Dermatol* 1995, 131:1465. _____ ▲

NEUROFIBROMATOSIS (VON RECKLINGHAUSEN'S DISEASE, NF)

von Recklinghausen's disease is an autosomal dominantly inherited syndrome manifested by developmental changes in the nervous system, bones, and skin. Several types have been described. Type 1 NF, which includes more than 85% of cases, is classic neurofibromatosis. Patients have many neurofibromas that measure a few millimeters to a few centimeters in diameter, many café au lait spots, widely distributed, and few or no central nervous system lesions (Figs. 27-10 and 27-11). Lisch nodules can be found in the irises of about one fourth of patients under 6 years of age and in 94% of older patients. Type 2, central or acoustic neurofibromatosis, is distinguished by bilateral acoustic neuromas. Type 3 (mixed) and 4 (variant) forms resemble type 2 but may have more numerous cutaneous neurofibromas. Patients with these types are at greater risk for developing optic gliomas, neurilemomas, and meningiomas.

These forms are inherited as autosomal dominant traits. Type 5, segmental (dermatomal) neurofibromatosis, is considered to arise from a postzygotic somatic mutation and is not generally heritable. It may be bilateral. Type 6 NF has

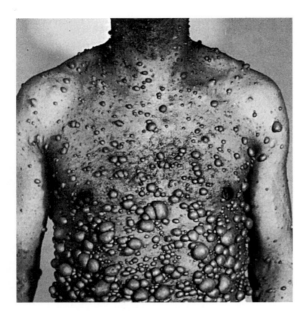

Fig. 27-10 Multiple neurofibromas in type 1 NF.

no neurofibromas, only café au lait spots, and must occur in two generations to be diagnosed. Type 7 NF, late-onset neurofibromatosis, does not begin to manifest neurofibromas before patients are in their twenties. It is not yet known whether it is inherited.

The characteristic skin lesions occur in several forms of NF, chiefly neurofibromas, but also café au lait macules, axillary freckles, bronzing, giant pigmented hairy nevi ("neuronevi"), sacral hypertrichosis, cutis verticis gyrata, and macroglossia.

The cutaneous neurofibromas are dermal tumors that vary from pinhead sized to large, pendulous, flabby masses weighing several kilograms that may cause great disfigurement. Many of the small, soft tumors can be pushed down into the panniculus by light pressure with the finger ("buttonholing") and spring back when released, which distinguishes them from lipomas. Neurofibromas of the areolae occur in more than 90% of women with this disease.

Subcutaneous plexiform neurofibromas occur as discrete, slowly growing nodules along peripheral nerves. On palpation they are described as feeling like a "bag of worms." Later, the single subcutaneous tumor may be associated with other growths, frequently along the same nerve trunk.

The café au lait macule is a hallmark of this disease (see Fig. 27-11). Usually it is a uniformly pigmented light brown macule, unevenly round or oval, from 1.5 to 15 cm in diameter, most often present at birth and almost always present by the time the patient is 1 year of age. The finding of six or more of these lesions at least 1.5 cm in diameter is diagnostic, usually indicating type 1 neurofibromatosis. In children, the minimum diameter for a significant lesion is 0.5 cm. Histologically, giant melanosomes may be seen.

Fig. 27-11 von Recklinghausen's disease. Numerous neurofibromas on the upper back and several café au lait patches are apparent.

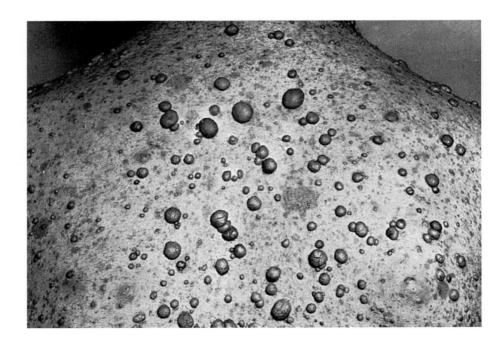

Axillary freckling (Crowe's sign) may occur, extending to the neck and involving the inguinal regions extending to the perineal areas (Fig. 27-12). Bronzing or hyperpigmentation of the skin may be present. Xanthogranulomas may occur. A plexiform neurofibroma and bony dysplasia may be signaled by a giant café au lait macule overlying this defect.

Many organ systems may be involved. Such endocrine disorders as acromegaly, cretinism, hyperparathyroidism, myxedema, pheochromocytoma (less than 1%), or precocious puberty may be present. Lisch nodules occur in 94% of postpubertal patients. Bone changes (usually erosive) may produce lordosis, kyphosis, and pseudoarthrosis, as well as spina bifida, dislocations, and atraumatic fractures (Fig. 27-13). Neuromas of spinal nerves may cause various paralyses. Patients with neurofibromatosis type 1 are four times more likely to develop malignancies than the general population are. Cutaneous neurofibromas may rarely develop into neurofibrosarcomas and malignant schwannomas. Wilms' tumor, rhabdomyosarcomas, gastrointestinal malignancies, and chronic myelogenous leukemia have also been reported. Children with neurofibromatosis type 1 are 200 to 500 times more likely to develop malignant myeloid disorders.

Mental retardation, dementia, epilepsy, and a variety of intracranial malignancies may occur. Hypertelorism heralds a severe expression of neurofibromatosis with brain involvement. Diffuse interstitial lung disease occurs in 7% of patients. There have been reports of other skin disorders in NF-1, such as juvenile xanthogranuloma (increased association with juvenile chronic myelogenous leukemia), and giant cell tumors. Melanoma does not appear to be a true association.

Neurofibromatosis is autosomal dominantly inherited, except for type 5, which is believed to be caused by a postzygotic somatic mutation. Approximately 50% of cases represent new mutations. The gene for NF-1 is in the pericentric region of chromosome 17q11.2 and codes for neurofibromin, a protein that negatively regulates signals transduced by Ras proteins. The gene for NF-2 is on the long arm of chromosome 22q11-q13 and encodes for merlin (schwannomin), a protein that links the actin cytoskeleton to cell surface glycoproteins and functions as a negative growth regulator.

Histologically, neurofibromas consist of faintly eosinophilic, thin, wavy spindle cells with spindle-shaped nuclei. The background contains excess mucin, and mast cells are increased.

Diagnosis

The diagnosis of type 1 neurofibromatosis requires two or more of the following criteria: (1) six or more café au lait macules of more than 5 mm in greatest diameter in prepubertal individuals and more than 15 mm in greatest diameter in postpubertal individuals; (2) two or more neurofibromas of any type or one plexiform neurofibroma;

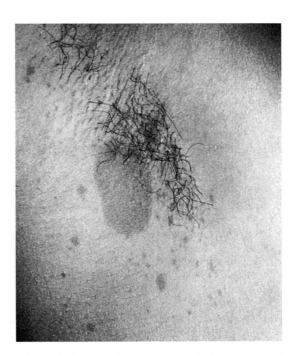

Fig. 27-12 Axillary freckles (Crowe's sign) in a patient with neurofibromatosis. (Courtesy Dr. Axel W. Hoke.)

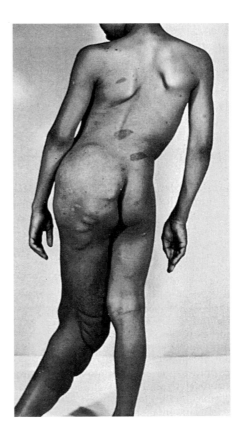

Fig. 27-13 Kyphoscoliosis, café au lait macules, and enormous plexiform neurofibromas (elephantiasis neurofibromatosus).

(3) freckling in the axillary or inguinal regions; (4) optic glioma; (5) two or more Lisch nodules; (6) a distinctive osseous lesion, such as a sphenoid dysplasia or thinning of the long bone cortex with or without pseudarthrosis; and (7) a first-degree relative (parent, sibling, or offspring) with the disease.

A diagnosis of type 2 neurofibromatosis requires either of the following: (1) bilateral eighth nerve masses as demonstrated on CT or MRI or (2) having a first-degree relative with neurofibromatosis 2 and either unilateral eighth nerve mass or two of the following: a neurofibroma, meningioma, glioma, schwannoma, or juvenile posterior subcapsular lenticular opacity.

Screening and Monitoring for Complications

Wolkenstein et al followed 152 patients with type 1 neurofibromatosis in the hope of defining which screening measures might prove useful. X-ray evaluation, cerebral imaging, abdominal ultrasonography, and urinary catecholamines detected 21 abnormalities. There were only two cases in which the evaluation altered treatment, in contrast to 22 complications from these investigations that required intervention. Of interest in 93 asymptomatic patients who underwent cerebral imaging, 12 optic gliomas were detected, suggesting that screening MRIs or CT scans may be justified. The authors concluded that screening tests are unwarranted and that annual clinical examinations and a problem-focused approach with testing performed based on clinical evaluation is the more prudent approach. Multidisciplinary management, as outlined by Gutmann et al, is recommended.

TREATMENT. There is no treatment for the neurofibromas except excision. Deaths have been reported from intracranial meningiomas and gliomas, peripheral nerve sarcomas, and other associated malignancies. The disease tends to be exacerbated during pregnancy, and treatment-resistant hypertension may occur.

Cnossen MH, et al: A prospective 10-year follow-up study of patients with neurofibromatosis type 1. *Arch Dis Child* 1998, 78:408.

Duve S, et al: Cutaneous melanoma in a patient with neurofibromatosis. *Br J Dermatol* 1994, 131:290.

Goldberg NS: Neurofibromatosis. *Adv Dermatol* 1996, 11:179.

Gutmann DH, et al: The diagnostic evaluation and multidisciplinary management of neurofibromatosis 1 and neurofibromatosis 2. *JAMA* 1997, 278:51.

Gutmann DH, et al: Juvenile xanthogranuloma, neurofibromatosis 1, and juvenile chronic myeloid leukemia. *Arch Dermatol* 1995, 131:904.

Ingorado V, et al: Segmental neurofibromatosis: is it uncommon or underdiagnosed? *Arch Dermatol* 1995, 131:959.

Paik SC, et al: Bilateral segmental neurofibromatosis with speckled lentiginous nevus. *Int J Dermatol* 1996, 35:360.

Sahn EE, et al: Multiple cutaneous granular cell tumors in a child with possible neurofibromatosis. *J Am Acad Dermatol* 1997, 36:327.

Shaw RJ, et al: Localization and functional domains of the neurofibromatosis type II tumor suppressor, merlin. *Cell Growth Differ* 1998, 9:287.

Side L, et al: Homozygous inactivation of the NF1 gene in bone marrow cells from children with neurofibromatosis type 1 and malignant myeloid disorders. *N Engl J Med* 1997, 336:1713.

Wolkenstein P, et al: Usefulness of screening investigations in neurofibromatosis type 1: a study of 152 patients. *Arch Dermatol* 1996, 132:1333.

Wong SS: Bilateral segmental neurofibromatosis with partial unilateral lentiginosis. *Br J Dermatol* 1997, 136:380.

Xu HM, et al: Merlin differentially associates with the microtubule and actin cytoskeleton. *J Neurosci Res* 1998, 51:403.

Zoller ME, et al: Malignant and benign tumors in patients with neurofibromatosis type 1 in a defined Swedish population. *Cancer* 1997, 79:2125. _____ ▲

PROTEUS SYNDROME

Although not a phakomatosis, Proteus syndrome may be confused with neurofibromatosis. This rare disease, named for the Greek god Proteus (the polymorphous) has protean manifestations that include partial gigantism of the hands and feet, plantar hyperplasia, hemangiomas, lipomas, linear verrucous epidermal nevi, patchy dermal hypoplasia, macrocephaly, hyperostosis, and hypertrophy of the long bones. Many investigators believe that Joseph Merrick, who was known as "the Elephant Man," had Proteus syndrome rather than neurofibromatosis. It is believed to be caused by a somatic mutation, lethal in the nonmosaic state.

Biesecker LG, et al: Proteus syndrome: diagnostic criteria, differential diagnosis and patient evaluation. *Am J Med Genet* 1999, 84:389.

del Rosario Barona-Mazuera M, et al: Proteus syndrome: new findings in seven patients. *Pediatr Dermatol* 1997, 14:1.

Happle R, et al: Patchy dermal hypoplasia as a characteristic feature of Proteus syndrome. *Arch Dermatol* 1997, 133:77.

Samlaska C, et al: Proteus syndrome. *Arch Dermatol* 1989, 125:1109.

Tattelbaum AG, et al: Proteus syndrome: a newly recognized hamartomatous syndrome with significant craniofacial dysmorphology. *J Craniofac Surg* 1995, 6:151. _____ ▲

VON HIPPEL-LINDAU SYNDROME

von Hippel-Lindau syndrome is an autosomal dominant disorder consisting of retinal angiomas, cerebellar medullary angioblastic tumors, pancreatic cysts, and renal tumors and cysts. Usually the skin is not involved, although occasionally angiomas may occur in the occipitocervical region.

Ten percent to 20% of cerebellar hemangioblastomas produce erythropoietin and are accompanied by a secondary polycythemia. Ocular lesions may lead to retinal detachment. Ten percent of hypernephromas and less than 8% of renal cysts also produce erythropoietin. Pheochromocytoma has been associated in several kindreds with von Hippel-Lindau disease.

Karsdorp N, et al: Von Hippel-Lindau disease: new strategies in early detection and treatment. *Am J Med* 1994, 97:158.

Neumann HP, et al: Pheochromocytomas, multiple endocrine neoplasia type 2, and von Hippel-Lindau disease. *N Engl J Med* 1994, 329:1531. ▲

ATAXIA-TELANGIECTASIA

Also known as *Louis-Bar syndrome,* ataxia-telangiectasia consists of cerebellar ataxia, oculocutaneous telangiectasia, and sinopulmonary infection. It is familial and is usually first noted when the child begins to walk. There is awkwardness and a swaying gait, which by about 10 years of age results in the child's being confined to a wheelchair. Choreic and athetoid movements and pseudopalsy of the eyes are other features. Fine telangiectases of venous origin appear on the exposed surfaces of the conjunctiva at about age 3. Nystagmus is present. Telangiectases also appear later on the butterfly area of the face, inside the helix and over the backs of the ears, in the roof of the mouth, the necklace area, the bends of the elbows and knees, and over the dorsa of the hands and feet. Other stigmata are café au lait patches, hypopigmented macules, seborrheic dermatitis, premature graying and sparsity of the hair, and progeroid features. The skin tends to be dry and coarse, and in time becomes tight and inelastic, as in scleroderma. Atrophic, granulomatous, scarring plaques may occur. Early death from bronchiectasis occurs in more than half of these patients, most of whom suffer from recurrent sinus and lung infections that begin when the patient is between 3 and 8 years of age.

Patients may have a marked IgA deficiency, with decreased lymphocytes and a small to absent thymus. The most common types of malignancies are lymphomas, usually of the B cell type, and leukemias. It has been shown that homozygous patients also have a higher risk of breast cancer—100 times higher when compared with age-matched control subjects. An increased risk may also occur in heterozygous family members.

Ataxia-telangiectasia is transmitted as an autosomal recessive trait, and heterozygotes, although they lack clinical findings, are believed to be cancer prone. The gene mutated has been designated *ATM* and is a member of a family of phosphatidylinositol-3-kinase–like enzymes that are involved in cell-cycle control, meiotic recombination, telomere length monitoring, and DNA-damage response. Affected cells are hypersensitive to ionizing radiation and are defective at the G1/S checkpoint after radiation damage. The ATM gene is located on chromosome 11q22.3. Translocations are common in these patients, particularly for chromosomes 7 and 14.

Two specific abonormal findings are cerebellar alterations in CT scan results and elevated serum alpha-fetoprotein levels. Serum carcinoembryonic antigen levels are also high. Early diagnosis can be difficult and the most frequent misdiagnosis is cerebral palsy. In the series by Cabana et al, telangiectasia occurred before the diagnosis was established in 34 of 48 patients. Evaluation of alpha-fetoprotein levels is the best screening test for children with persistent ataxia.

Cabana MD, et al: Consequences of the delayed diagnosis of ataxia-telangiectasia. *Pediatrics* 1998, 102:98.

Drolet BA, et al: Cutaneous granulomas as a presenting sign in ataxia-telangiectasia. *Dermatology* 1997, 194:273.

Gatti RA: Ataxia-telangiectasia. *Dermatol Clin* 1995, 13:1.

Gatti RA, et al: Ataxia-telangiectasia: an interdisciplinary approach to pathogenesis. *Medicine* 1991, 70:99.

Joshi RK, et al: Cutaneous granuloma with ataxia-telangiectasia: a case report and review of the literature. *Clin Exp Dermatol* 1993, 18:458.

Shafman T, et al: Interaction between ATM protein and c-Abl in response to DNA damage. *Nature* 1997, 387:520.

Swift M, et al: Incidence of cancer in 161 families affected by ataxia-telangiectasia. *N Engl J Med* 1991, 325:1831. _____ ▲

EPIDERMOLYSIS BULLOSA

Epidermolysis bullosa (EB) is a group of rare genetic disorders that have in common the formation of blisters on minor physical injury. A comprehensive classification is as follows:

Intraepidermal
    EB simplex, generalized (Koebner)
    EB simplex, localized (Weber-Cockayne)
    EB herpetiformis (Dowling-Meara)
    EB simplex (Ogna)
    EB simplex with mottled pigmentation
    EB with muscular dystrophy

Junctional (intralamina lucida)
    JEB atrophicans generalisata gravis (Herlitz; EB letalis)
    JEB atrophicans generalisata mitis
    JEB atrophicans localisata
    JEB atrophicans inversa
    JEB progressiva
    JEB with pyloric atresia
    Generalized atrophic benign EB (GABEB)
    Cicatricial junctional EB

Dermolytic or dystrophic (sublamina densa)
Dominant forms
    Dystrophic EB, hyperplastic variant (Cockayne-Touraine)
    Dystrophic EB, albopapuloid variant (Pasini)
    Bart's syndrome
    Transient bullous dermolysis of the newborn
    Acrokeratotic poikiloderma (Weary-Kindler)
Recessive forms
    Generalized (gravis or mitis)
    Localized
    Inverse

Epidermolysis bullosa acquisita is an autoimmune disease. It is discussed in Chapter 21.

Internal involvement may occur in several of these subtypes of EB. Esophageal and laryngeal complications are seen primarily in recessive dystrophic EB, but may be present in junctional EB (Herlitz). Pyloric atresia is reported to occur in junctional EB. Ocular lesions may be severe in dystrophic EB, and mild lesions have been reported in simplex and junctional disease.

Clinical findings should not be relied on for diagnosis. Additionally, routine histologic evidence is misleading. Definition of disease types must rely on electron microscopic studies or immunofluorescent mapping. These can identify the level of the epidermal separation, and in addition may define other defects, such as absence of anchoring fibrils or hypoplasia of hemidesmosomes. In RDEB, electron microscopy reveals the cleavage is below the basal lamina and that anchoring fibrils are diminished or absent.

Immunofluorescent mapping may define the level of the split without resorting to electron microscopy. By staining biopsy specimens for normal components of the basement membrane zone, such as bullous pemphigoid antigen, laminin, type IV collagen, or LDA-1 antigen, one may determine the level of the split by whether the antigen localizes at the roof or base of the blister. In simplex types, all will be at the base; in dystrophic types, all will be at the roof; and in junctional types bullous pemphigoid antigen will be on the roof, while type IV collagen and LDA-1 will be at the base. KF-1 has been found to be absent or diminished in dystrophic EB. The specific keratin abnormalities along with the abnormal genes have been identified for many of these disorders, and commercial applications will provide the ultimate diagnostic test. In general, EB simplex is caused by defects in genes encoding for keratins 5 and 14. In junctional EB there are defective genes encoding for kallidin/laminin 5. Dystrophic forms result from mutations in type VII collagen gene COL7A1.

Intraepidermal Forms

Epidermolysis Bullosa Simplex (Koebner)

The generalized type of epidermolysis bullosa simplex (EBS), dominantly inherited, with complete penetrance, occurs in 1 in 500,000 births. It is characterized by the development of vesicles, bullae, and milia over the joints of the hands, elbows, knees, and feet, and other sites subject to repeated trauma (Fig. 27-14). The child is affected at birth or shortly thereafter, with improvement within the first few months, only to recur when the child begins crawling or later in childhood, but in some patients (with homozygous keratin 14), the blistering may be more protracted and generalized. The blistering is worse during the summer and improves during the winter. The lesions are sparse and do not lead to severe atrophy. The Nikolsky sign is negative. Usually the mucous membranes and nails are not involved. EBS is usually milder than other forms of EB.

Inherited as an autosomal dominant trait, EBS is a disease in which keratin gene mutations cause the production of defective intermediate filaments, which lead to epidermal basal cell fragility and subsequent blistering. Gene mutations producing abnormalities in keratin 5 and keratin 14, keratins expressed in the basal cell layer, have

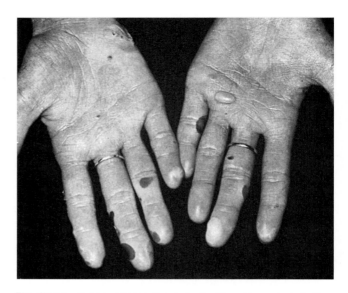

Fig. 27-14   Palmar lesions in a patient with epidermolysis bullosa simplex.

been reported. Patients heterozygous for abnormal keratin 14 have blistering limited to the hands and feet, but homozygotes have more severe and widespread blistering of the skin and mucous membranes.

Separation occurs through the basal cell layer. Rubbing skin with an eraser may lead to a subclinical lesion that may be diagnostic histologically.

TREATMENT AND PROGNOSIS. In general, with all forms of EB this consists of prevention of trauma, decompression of large blisters, and treatment of infection. EBS tends to have periods of exacerbation, but with passage of time blistering decreases considerably.

Localized Epidermolysis Bullosa Simplex

Recurrent bullous eruption of the hands and feet (Weber-Cockayne) is autosomal dominantly determined and appears in a chronic form in infancy or at times later in life (Fig. 27-15). The lesions exacerbate during hot weather and when the patient is subjected to prolonged walking or marching, as is experienced in military service. Hyperhidrosis may be an associated finding. In localized EBS, the bullae are intraepidermal and suprabasal, and healing occurs without scarring.

TREATMENT. Application of aluminum chloride hexahydrate in anhydrous ethanol (Drysol) on the normal skin of hands and feet twice a day has been shown to be effective. After 2 weeks of daily therapy the patient can be switched to once or twice weekly applications.

EB Herpetiformis (Dowling-Meara)

An autosomal dominant variant of EBS, active blisters with circinate configuration occur in infancy. Milia may develop, but there is no scarring. The oral mucosa is involved. Nails are shed but may regrow, sometimes with dystrophy. Blistering lessens with age. Hyperkeratosis of the palms and

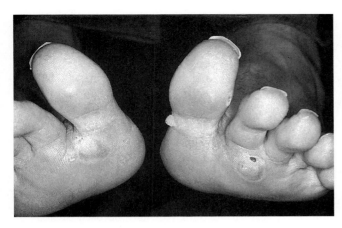

Fig. 27-15   EB simplex, Weber-Cockayne.

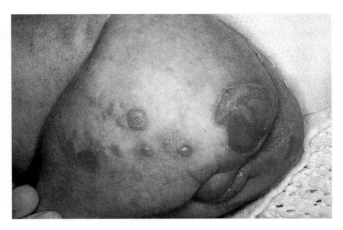

Fig. 27-16   Junctional epidermolysis bullosa.

soles may occur. Histologically, the split is through the basal layer, and tonofilaments are clumped on electron microscopy. Point mutations have been shown in keratin 5 and keratin 14 genes.

EB Simplex (Ogna)

In this condition affecting a single Norwegian kindred, generalized bruising and hemorrhagic blisters occur. It is transmitted as an autosomal dominant trait. At birth there are small, acral traumatic sanguinous blisters. The basal keratinocytes in this syndrome do not stain with anti-plectin antibodies.

EB Simplex with Mottled Pigmentation

One Swedish family with autosomal dominant inheritance pattern has been reported with EB simplex, whose members were born with scattered hyper- and hypopigmented macules, which faded slowly. The remaining features are similar to those of generalized EB simplex. Ultrastructural studies show vacuolization of the basal cell layer.

EB Simplex with Muscular Dystrophy

There is a form of EB simplex associated with late-onset neuromuscular disease. It is inherited as an autosomal recessive trait. There is widespread blistering at birth associated with scarring, milia, atrophy, nail dystrophy, dental anomalies, laryngeal webs, and urethral strictures. Progressive muscular dystrophy with weakness and wasting begins in childhood or later. This disease is caused by a mutation in the plectin gene, with affected patients having absent plectin in their skin and muscles.

Junctional Forms

Junctional Epidermolysis Bullosa (Epidermolysis Bullosa Letalis, Herlitz)

In junctional epidermolysis bullosa, a rare type, which has autosomal recessive transmission, severe generalized blistering may be present at birth, and extensive denudation may prove fatal within a few months. There is generalized blistering with relative sparing of the hands and characteristic perioral and perinasal hypertrophic granulation tissue (Fig. 27-16). Eventually the lesions heal without scarring or milia formation. Erosions may persist for years, however. Dysplastic teeth are common. Laryngeal and bronchial lesions may cause respiratory distress and even death. Additional systemic complications include gastrointestinal tract, gallbladder, corneal, and vaginal disease. In patients who survive infancy, there is growth retardation, and moderate to severe refractory anemia is frequent. Separation occurs in the lamina lucida, as shown by electron microscopy.

Herlitz junctional epidermolysis bullosa is caused by mutations in three genes: LAMA3, LAMB3, or LAMC2, which code for polypeptide subunits of laminin 5. The LAMB3 gene has been localized to chromosome 1q32.

Supportive therapy and intensive systemic corticosteroid therapy are recommended during life-threatening periods. Epidermal autographs of cultured keratinocytes, isolated from clinically uninvolved skin and grown on collagen sponges, for chronic facial erosions may be useful. Complete reepithelialization is achieved over 7 to 10 months.

Junctional EB with Pyloric Atresia

This rare autosomal recessively inherited form of junctional EB presents at birth with severe mucocutaneous fragility and gastric outlet obstruction. Even if the pyloric atresia is repaired, the neonates may die because of the severity of their skin disease. If they survive the neonatal period, the blistering diminishes. Persistent scarring of the urinary tract may occur, however, with stenosis of the ureteral-vesicular junction, requiring numerous urologic procedures. This syndrome is caused by a genetic mutation in either the alpha 6 or beta 4 integrin genes (ITGA6 and ITGB4). This alpha 6–beta 4 integrin complex is uniquely expressed on epithelial surfaces.

Generalized Atrophic Benign Epidermolysis Bullosa

Most cases of generalized atrophic benign EB are characterized by onset at birth, generalized blisters and atrophy, mucosal involvement, and thickened, dystrophic, or absent nails. Enamel defects in deciduous and permanent teeth and atrophic alopecia are prominent features. Multiple cutaneous squamous cell carcinomas have been reported. Cleavage is within the lamina lucida; hemidesmosomes are reduced or absent; the basal lamina and anchoring fibrils, collagen fibers, and dermal microfibril bundles are unaltered. Inheritance is autosomal recessive. In contrast to EB Herlitz, patients often survive to adulthood. Studies have shown mutations in the COL17A1 gene encoding for type XVII collagen (BPAg2), a transmembrane component of hemidesmosomes.

Cicatricial Junctional Epidermolysis Bullosa

In 1985, Haber et al described another type of junctional EB, which they named *cicatricial junctional epidermolysis bullosa*, because the blisters heal with scarring, which may produce syndactyly and contractures, and there is stenosis of the anterior nares. Electron microscopy reveals junctional bullae with rudimentary hemidesmosomes. The bases of the bullae are covered by an intact basal lamina with normal anchoring fibrils.

Dermolytic or Dystrophic Forms

The cause of dystrophic EB in both autosomal dominantly and recessively inherited forms is mutations in the COL7A1 gene encoding for type VII collagen. The anchoring fibrils in these patients are defective or deficient.

Dominant Dystrophic Epidermolysis Bullosa (DDEB)

On the extensor surfaces of the extremities vesicles and bullae appear; these are most pronounced over the joints, especially over the toes, fingers, knuckles, ankles, and elbows. Spontaneous, flesh-colored, scarlike (albopapuloid) lesions may appear on the trunk, often in adolescence, with no previous trauma. The nails may be thickened. Usually the Nikolsky sign is present, and frequently the accumulated fluid in a bulla can be moved under the skin several centimeters away from the original site. Healing usually occurs with scarring and atrophy. Epidermal cysts (milia) are often present on the rims of the ears, on the dorsal surfaces of the hands, and on the extensor surfaces of the arms and legs.

The mucous membranes are frequently involved. Bullae, vesicles, and erosions are encountered on the buccal mucosa, tongue, palate, esophagus, pharynx, and larynx. The latter involvement is manifested by persistent hoarseness in some of these patients. There may be angular contractures at the gingivolabial sulcus and dysphagia from faucial and pharyngeal scarring. Scarring on the tip of the tongue is typical. The teeth are normal. Usually the conjunctiva is not involved.

Other changes include nail dystrophy, partial alopecia of the scalp, absence of body hair, dwarfism, and the formation of contractures and clawlike hands, with atrophy of the phalangeal bones and pseudosyndactylism. The albopapuloid type (Pasini) is the more severe expression of DDEB. The Cockayne-Touraine type is more limited in extent and severity, and no albopapuloid lesions are seen.

Histologically, a noninflammatory subepidermal bulla is present. On electron microscopy, cleavage occurs beneath the basal lamina, and anchoring fibrils are rudimentary and reduced in number. In blistered areas they are not demonstrable. Type VII collagen staining is normal.

Autologous meshed split-thickness skin grafts and allogeneic cultured keratinocytes may be used in treating nonhealing skin defects. In many patients with DDEB, blistering reduces with time and only nail dystrophy may be present in adulthood.

Bart's Syndrome

Bart et al reported congenital localized defects of the skin, mechanoblisters, and nail deformities with autosomal dominant inheritance. Although the clinical and histologic picture of this syndrome is one of a mildly scarring mechanobullous dermatosis with a favorable prognosis, associations with mandibulofacial dysostosis, renal aplasia, and congenital abnormalities of the lower extremities have been reported. Bart's syndrome is a clinical variant of DDEB, based on identification of a defect in the COL7A1 gene (chromosome 3p) encoding for type VII collagen.

Transient Bullous Dermolysis of the Newborn

In 1985, Hashimoto et al reported a newborn who developed blisters from every minor trauma. Separation was below the basal lamina, with degeneration of collagen and anchoring fibrils. There was rapid healing by 4 months of age. Nails were not damaged, and there was no scarring.

They considered as criteria for this entity (1) vesiculobullous lesions present at birth or induced by friction; (2) spontaneous recovery at a few months of age; (3) no dystrophic scars; (4) subepidermal blisters beginning in the dermal papillae; (5) ultrastructurally observed collagenolysis and damaged anchoring fibrils; and (6) enormous dilation of rough endoplasmic reticulum, with stellate bodies of keratinocytes in their vacuoles.

The cause has been shown in one family to be a transversion mutation in COL7A1 gene encoding for type VII collagen, and it is therefore allelic with other variants of DDEB. The mechanism for the transient nature of reduced amounts of type VII collagen along the dermoepidermal junction remains to be defined.

Acrokeratotic Poikiloderma (Weary-Kindler)

In 1954, Kindler reported a combination of poikiloderma congenitale and traumatic blistering of the feet from minor trauma. Fewer than 100 cases have been described. It is believed to be a variant of DDEB. Characteristic features include acral bullae, generalized poikiloderma with prominent atrophy, photosensitivity, and acral keratoses. Pseudo-ainhum and sclerotic bands were reported in one case. Erythematous and erosive gingiva and rapidly progressive periodontal disease may also occur. The principal histologic change is absence of elastic fibers in the papillary dermis and fragmented ones in the mid-dermis.

Recessive Dystrophic Epidermolysis Bullosa (Hallopeau-Siemens)

There are three variants of recessive dystrophic epidermolysis bullosa (RDEB)—generalized, localized, and inverse. The generalized type has two variants, a mild or mitis form and the severe (Hallopeau-Siemens) variety. Generalized RDEB in its mild (mitis) form has blisters limited primarily to the hands, feet, elbows, and knees and limited complications. The more severe variety characteristically begins at birth with generalized cutaneous and mucosal blistering.

Digital fusion with encasement of the fingers and toes in scar tissues, forming a "mittenlike" deformity, is characteristic of the severe form of RDEB, occurring in up to 90% of patients by age 25 (Figs. 27-17 to 27-20). Dental complications may be severe, such as rampant dental caries and microstomia. Esophageal stricture may be present. Anemia and growth retardation are frequently seen in the most severe cases, and progressive nutritional deficiency can result in fatal cardiomyopathy. Fatal systemic amyloidosis (AA type) has also been reported. There is a high risk of developing cutaneous squamous cell carcinomas (SCCs) (Fig. 27-21), with up to 50% of patients affected by age 35. These SCCs may be multiple and can metastasize and cause death.

TREATMENT. Treatment remains primarily palliative. Debilitating oral lesions produce pain, scarring, and microstomia. Aggressive dental intervention is recommended. Nutritional support is of critical importance. Autologous meshed split-thickness skin grafts and allogeneic cultured

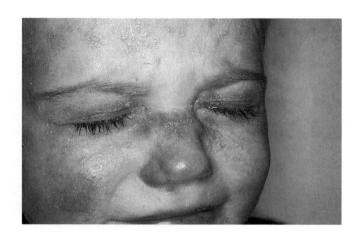

Fig. 27-17 Generalized RDEB in a child. Note numerous milia.

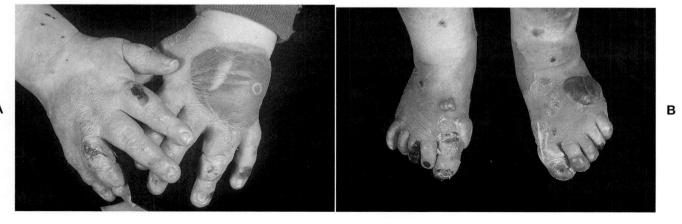

Fig. 27-18 Generalized RDEB in a child. **A,** Dorsal hands and fingers. **B,** Dorsal feet and toes. (Courtesy Dr. James Cook.)

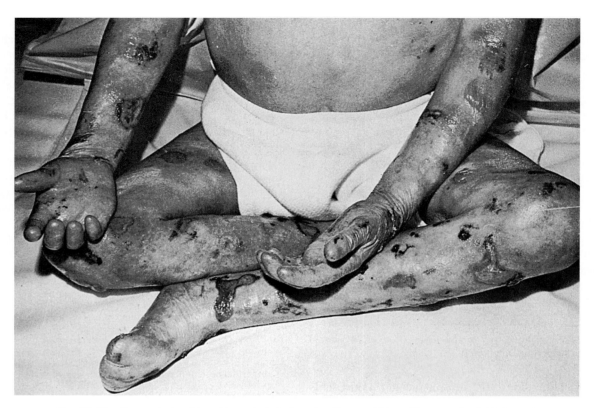

Fig. 27-19 Severe dystrophic epidermolysis bullosa in a 7-year-old boy. (Courtesy Dr. J. McSorley.)

Fig. 27-20 RDEB in an 8-year-old boy. (Courtesy Dr. J. McSorley.)

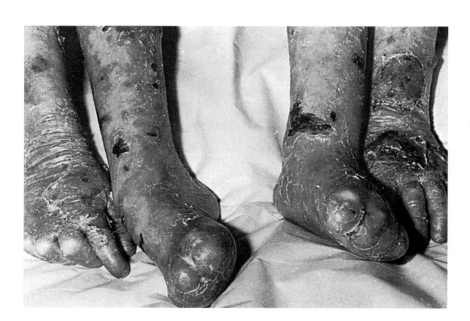

keratinocytes have been shown to be useful in treating nonhealing cutaneous defects, or they may be used for closure after removal of large cutaneous malignancies. Family education and referral to DEBRA (Dystrophic Epidermolysis Bullosa Research Association of America, 141 Fifth Ave., New York, New York, 10010) is strongly recommended.

Allman S, et al: Nutrition in dystrophic epidermolysis bullosa. *Pediatr Dermatol* 1992, 9:231.

Banwell BL, et al: Myopathy, myesthemic syndrome, and epidermolysis bullosa simplex due to plectin deficiency. *J Neuropathol Exp Neurol* 1999, 58:832.

Bourke JF, et al: Fatal systemic amyloidosis (AA type) in two sisters with dystrophic epidermolysis bullosa. *J Am Acad Dermatol* 1995, 33:370.

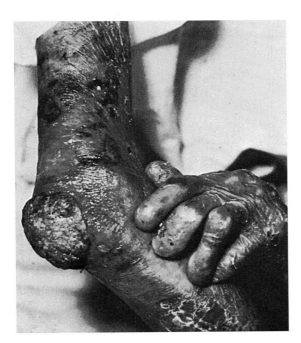

Fig. 27-21 Squamous cell carcinoma on elbow of 34-year-old male with RDEB.

Caldwell-Brown D, et al: Lack of efficacy of phenytoin in recessive dystrophic epidermolysis bullosa. Epidermolysis Bullosa Study Group. *N Engl J Med* 1992, 327:163.

Chan YM, et al: Genetic analysis of a severe case of Dowling-Meara epidermolysis bullosa simplex. *J Invest Dermatol* 1996, 106:327.

Christiano AM, et al: Genetic basis of Bart's syndrome: a glycine substitution mutation in the type VII collagen gene. *J Invest Dermatol* 1996, 106:1340.

Christiano AM, et al: Genetic basis of dominantly inherited transient bullous dermolysis of the newborn: a splice site mutation in the type VII collagen gene. *J Invest Dermatol* 1997, 109:811.

Combemale P, et al: Epidermolysis bullosa simplex with mottled pigmentation. *Dermatology* 1994, 189:173.

Darling TN, et al: A deletion mutation in COL17A1 in five Austrian families with generalized atrophic benign epidermolysis bullosa represents propagation of an ancestral allele. *J Invest Dermatol* 1998, 110:170.

Darling TN, et al: Generalized atrophic benign epidermolysis bullosa. *Adv Dermatol* 1997, 13:87.

Furumura M, et al: Three neonatal cases of epidermolysis bullosa herpetiformis (Dowling-Meara type) with severe erosive skin lesions. *J Am Acad Dermatol* 1993, 28:859.

Goldstein AM, et al: Junctional epidermolysis bullosa: diagnosis and management of a patient with the Herlitz variant. *J Pediatr Surg* 1998, 33:756.

Haynes L, et al: Gastrostomy and growth in dystrophic epidermolysis bullosa. *Br J Dermatol* 1996, 134:872.

Hovnanian A, et al: Characterization of 18 new mutations in COL7A1 in recessive dystrophic epidermolysis bullosa provides evidence for distinct molecular mechanisms underlying defective anchoring fibril formation. *Am J Hum Genet* 1997, 61:599.

Hu ZL, et al: Partial dominance of a keratin 14 mutation in epidermolysis bullosa simplex: increased severity of disease in a homozygote. *J Invest Dermatol* 1997, 109:360.

Kirtschig G, et al: Acquired junctional epidermolysis bullosa associated with IgG autoantibodies to the beta subunit of laminin-5. *Br J Dermatol* 1998, 138:125.

Krunic AL, et al: Hereditary bullous acrokeratotic poikiloderma of Weary-Kindler associated with pseudo-ainhum and sclerotic bands. *Int J Dermatol* 1997, 36:529.

Martin RW III, et al: Congenital absence of skin and blistering in a neonate: Bart's syndrome and mandibulofacial dysostosis. *Arch Dermatol* 1995, 131:1197.

Mazzanti C, et al: 180-kDa bullous pemphigoid antigen defective generalized atrophic benign epidermolysis bullosa: report of four cases with an unusually mild phenotype. *Br J Dermatol* 1998, 138:859.

Mellerio JE, et al: Prognostic implications of determining 180 kDa bullous pemphigoid antigen (BPAG2) gene/protein pathology in neonatal junctional epidermolysis bullosa. *Br J Dermatol* 1998, 138:661.

Mellerio JE, et al: Pyloric atresia-junctional epidermolysis bullosa syndrome. *Br J Dermatol* 1998, 139:862.

Melville C, et al: Fatal cardiomyopathy in dystrophic epidermolysis bullosa. *Br J Dermatol* 1996, 135:603.

Pulkkinen L, et al: Hemidesmosomal variants of epidermolysis bullosa. *Exp Dermatol* 1998, 7:46.

Puvabanditsin S, et al: Epidermolysis bullosa associated with congenital localized absence of skin, fetal abdominal mass, and pyloric atresia. *Pediatr Dermatol* 1997, 14:359.

Ricketts DN, et al: Kindler syndrome: a rare cause of desquamative lesions of the gingiva. *Oral Surg Oral Med Oral Pathol Oral Radiol Endod* 1997, 84:488.

Shimizu H, et al: Epidermolysis bullosa simplex associated with muscular dystrophy. *J Am Acad Dermatol* 1999, 41:950.

Swensson O, et al: Generalized atrophic benign epidermolysis bullosa in two siblings complicated by multiple squamous cell carcinomas. *Arch Dermatol* 1998, 134:199.

Takizawa Y, et al: Maternal uniparental meroisodisomy in the LAMB3 region of chromosome 1 results in lethal junctional epidermolysis bullosa. *J Invest Dermatol* 1998, 110:828.

Terril PJ, et al: The surgical management of dystrophic epidermolysis bullosa (excluding the hand). *Br J Plast Surg* 1992, 45:426.

Uitto J, et al: Molecular basis of the dystrophic and junctional forms of epidermolysis bullosa: mutations in the type VII collagen and kallidin (laminin 5) genes. *J Invest Dermatol* 1994, 103(Suppl):39.

Verplancke P, et al: Treatment of dystrophic epidermolysis bullosa with autologous meshed split-thickness skin grafts and allogeneic cultured keratinocytes. *Dermatology* 1997, 194:380.

Wright JT, et al: Hereditary epidermolysis bullosa. *Semin Dermatol* 1994, 13:102.

Zelickson B, et al: Bart's syndrome: ultrastructure and genetic linkage. *Arch Dermatol* 1995, 131:663. _____ ▲

FAMILIAL BENIGN CHRONIC PEMPHIGUS (HAILEY-HAILEY DISEASE)

In 1939, Hailey and Hailey described a familial disease characterized by persistently recurrent bullous and vesicular dermatitis of the sides of the neck, axillae, flexures, and apposing surfaces (Figs. 27-22 to 27-25). The eruption may remain localized or may become widespread. The onset is usually in the late teens or early twenties. The primary lesion is a vesicle or bulla arising on seemingly normal skin. After rupture of the bulla, an erosion is seen; this soon becomes thickly crusted and may resemble impetigo. Sometimes the center becomes dry and crusted and there is an actively inflammatory border that spreads peripherally, producing circinate and configurate patterns.

The lesions appear in crops and run their course in several weeks; however, lesions are often more protracted during the summer. Lesions recur at the original sites. A

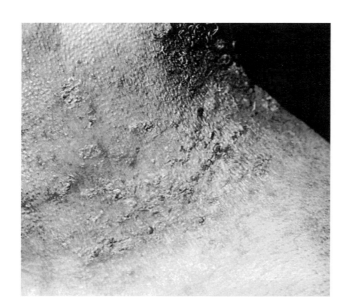

Fig. 27-22   Hailey-Hailey of the neck. (Courtesy Dr. Axel W. Hoke.)

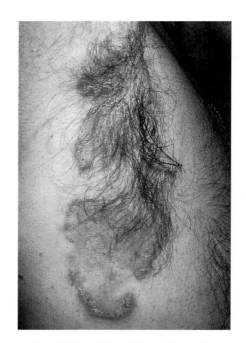

Fig. 27-23   Hailey-Hailey of the axilla.

Fig. 27-24   Hailey-Hailey of the inner thigh.

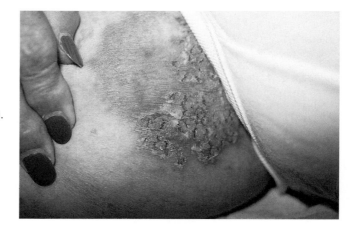

Fig. 27-25   Hailey-Hailey.

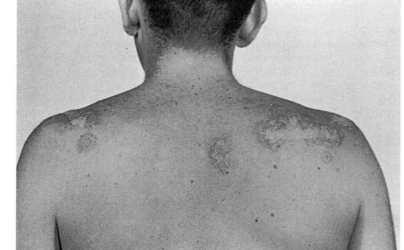

papular variant in the genital area has been described, simulating condylomata. There may be tenderness and enlargement of the regional lymph glands caused by secondary bacterial infection. Involvement of the esophagus, mouth, and labia majora is rare. Hailey-Hailey disease is inherited in an autosomal dominant manner. Thirty percent of patients are new mutations. The disease is due to a genetic defect in a calcium ATPase.

In predisposed persons with Hailey-Hailey disease, skin trauma, bacterial or fungal infection, and dermatoses may trigger lesions. Drug eruptions may produce devastating results requiring intensive management. Sunburn may also exacerbate the disease.

The histopathologic picture is unique. There are prominent intraepidermal vesicles and bullae. There is acantholysis and the formation of clefts above the basal cell layer into which the acantholytic cells "tumble," or disassociate like a "dilapidated brick wall." The basal cell layer remains attached to the dermis.

The treatment of Hailey-Hailey is difficult. Many cases improve with the use of systemic antibiotics effective against *Staphylococcus aureus,* topical clindamycin, antifungal agents, or mupirocin. Corticosteroids, administered topically, systemically, or both, have shown response. Cyclosporine, oral retinoids, and dapsone have been used in severe cases. Dermabrasion and CO_2 laser vaporization have been shown to be effective. Grafting has also been helpful in the most severe forms of the disease.

Berth-Jones J, et al: Benign familial chronic pemphigus (Hailey-Hailey disease) responds to cyclosporin. *Clin Exp Dermatol* 1995, 20:70.

Burge SM: Hailey-Hailey disease: the clinical features, response to treatment and prognosis. *Br J Dermatol* 1992, 126:275.

Cooley JE, et al: Hailey-Hailey disease keratinocytes: normal assembly of cell-cell junctions in vitro. *J Invest Dermatol* 1996, 107:877.

Hamm H, et al: Hailey-Hailey disease: eradication by dermabrasion. *Arch Dermatol* 1994, 130:1143.

Hunt MJ, et al: Vesiculobullous Hailey-Hailey disease: successful management with oral retinoids. *Australas J Dermatol* 1996, 37:196.

Ikeda S, et al: Localization of the gene whose mutations underlie Hailey-Hailey disease to chromosome 3q. *Hum Mol Genet* 1994, 3:1147.

Ikeda S, et al: Successful management of Hailey-Hailey disease with potent topical steroid ointment. *J Dermatol Sci* 1993, 5:205.

Kartamaa M, et al: Familial benign chronic pemphigus (Hailey-Hailey disease): treatment with carbon dioxide laser vaporization. *Arch Dermatol* 1992, 128:646.

Meffert JJ, et al: Bullous drug eruption to griseofulvin in a man with Hailey-Hailey disease. *Cutis* 1995, 56:279. ——————————— ▲

DISORDERS OF CORNIFICATION (ICHTHYOSES AND ICHTHYOSIFORM SYNDROMES)

The term *ichthyosis* is derived from the Greek word *ichthys,* meaning "fish." Ichthyosis is not one disease but a group of diseases in which the homeostatic mechanism of epidermal cell kinetics or differentiation is altered, resulting in the clinical appearance of scale. It has become apparent in recent years that although phenotypic similarities exist, there are multiple genotypically distinct entities. Because these disorders manifest as abnormal differentiation of the epidermis, the term *disorders of cornification* is preferred to ichthyosis.

TREATMENT. Many forms respond well to the same therapeutic interventions. Symptomatic treatment with alphahydroxy acids, such as lactic acid or 12% ammonium lactate lotion (Lac-Hydrin), is helpful (except in ichthyosis vulgaris associated with atopic dermatitis). Other compounds with hydrating and keratolytic properties are also beneficial. Simple lubricating creams, 10% urea cream, and 3% to 6% salicylic acid preparations may also be useful. However, widespread use of topical salicylic acid in children may lead to salicylism, and these keratolytic preparations are best reserved for localized thicker areas. Salt water baths may help by hydrating the horny layer. Application of a 40% to 60% solution of propylene glycol in water, then having the patient don an occlusive suit for several nights, removes the scales and may give the patient a normal appearance for 1 to 2 weeks. This can be repeated as frequently as needed.

Ichthyosis Vulgaris

Ichthyosis vulgaris is autosomal dominantly inherited and is characterized by onset in early childhood, usually between 3 and 12 months of age, with fine scales that appear "pasted-on" over the entire body (Fig. 27-26). Varying degrees of dryness of the skin may be evident. The scales are coarser on the lower extremities than they are on the trunk. The extensor surfaces of the extremities are most prominently involved (Fig. 27-27). The axillary and the gluteal folds are usually not involved. Although the antecubital and popliteal fossae are usually spared by ichthyosis vulgaris, atopic changes may be present. Accentuated skin markings and hyperkeratosis of the palms are common features. Keratosis pilaris is frequently associated. The scalp is involved, with only slight scaling. Keratotic lesions may be found on the palmar creases (keratosis punctata). Atopy manifested as hay fever, eczema, asthma, or urticaria is frequently present. The course is favorable, with limited findings by the time the patient is an adult.

Histologically, there is a moderate degree of hyperkeratosis. The granular layer is reduced or absent, and keratohyalin granules are spongy or fragmented on electron microscopy. The spinous layer is of normal thickness. Filaggrin is not detectable in involved epidermis, and profilaggrin mRNA is unstable in keratinocytes. This is a retention hyperkeratosis, with a normal rate of epidermal turnover.

The differential diagnosis includes severe xerosis, X-linked ichthyosis, acquired ichthyosis, and other more benign forms of ichthyosis. X-linked ichthyosis may be the most difficult to distinguish clinically, and specific tests may be required.

X-Linked Ichthyosis

X-linked ichthyosis is transmitted only to males by heterozygous mothers as an X-linked recessive trait. Scales

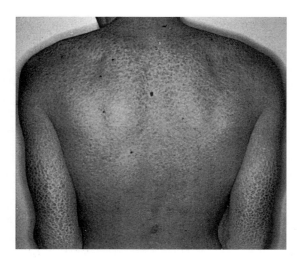

Fig. 27-26 Ichthyosis vulgaris.

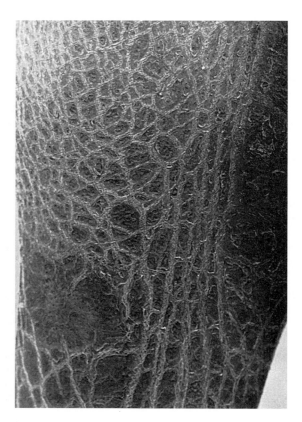

Fig. 27-27 Ichthyosis vulgaris on the thigh of a 23-year-old man. (Courtesy Dr. H. Shatin.)

are large and prominent on the anterior neck, extensor surfaces of the extremities, and the trunk. The sides of the neck are invariably involved, giving the child an unwashed look. Parents and patients alike often scrub these regions vigorously. The elbow and knee flexures are relatively

spared, as are the face and scalp; the palms and soles are nearly always spared.

A diagnosis of X-linked ichthyosis is also more likely if the abdomen is more involved than the back and if the ichthyosis extends down the entire dorsum of the leg. This condition occurs once in every 2000 to 5000 male births, and onset is usually before 3 months of age. Spontaneous parturition has often failed to occur when these patients were born, owing to a placental sulfatase deficiency.

Keratosis pilaris is not present. The incidence of atopy is not abnormally high. Corneal opacities (which do not affect vision) are seen by slit-lamp examination on the posterior capsule or Descemet's membrane in about 50% of affected males and female carriers. Another extracutaneous feature is a 12% to 15% incidence of cryptorchidism and an independently increased risk of testicular cancer. Warm weather ameliorates the scale.

There is usually a deletion at Xp22.3. Steroid sulfatase (aryl sulfatase C) is lacking in these patients' fibroblasts, leukocytes, and keratinocytes, and cholesterol sulfate accumulates as a result, causing the abnormal cornification.

Clinical differentiation from ichthyosis vulgaris at times may be difficult. The diagnosis can be made (or confirmed) by lipoprotein electrophoresis, because the increase in cholesterol sulfate makes the low-density lipoproteins migrate much more rapidly, and cholesterol sulfate is elevated in serum, erythrocyte membranes, and keratin. The reduced enzyme activity can be assessed in fibroblasts, keratinocytes, leukocytes, and prenatally in amniocytes.

Unlike ichthyosis vulgaris, X-linked ichthyosis does not improve with age, but gradually worsens in both extent and severity. Ten percent cholesterol cream and topical calcipotriol ointment have been shown to be effective. In severe cases acitretin is useful.

Multiple Sulfatase Deficiency

Patients with multiple sulfatase deficiency display an overlap of steroid sulfatase deficiency, mucopolysaccharidosis, and metachromatic leukodystrophy. The scaling is sometimes milder than X-linked recessive ichthyosis. There may be developmental delay, spastic quadriparesis, and coarse facial features. Histologic examination shows hyperkeratosis with a normal granular cell layer. This autosomal recessive disorder is caused by a lack of or deficiency in all known sulfatases.

Autosomal Recessive Ichthyosis

Biochemical and genetic studies have helped to define the specific subtypes. Clinical features often overlap, and in the past, the severity of the disease determined the classification. Identification of specific defects, such as transglutaminase 1, and profilaggrin/filaggrin are important to define each disorder and are the basis for classification of ichthyotic disorders.

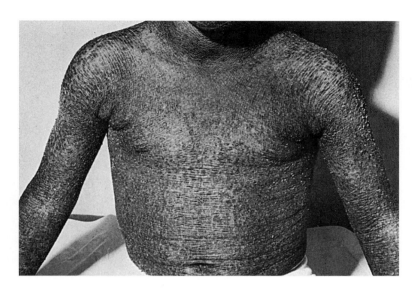

Fig. 27-28 Lamellar ichthyosis in a 6-year-old girl.

Lamellar Ichthyosis

Lamellar ichthyosis is present at birth or becomes apparent soon after and almost always involves the entire cutaneous surface (Figs. 27-28 and 27-29). Usually a collodion-like membrane encases babies with lamellar ichthyosis at birth, but this desquamates over the first 2 to 3 weeks of life.

It is characterized by large (5 to 15 mm), grayish brown scales, which are strikingly quadrilateral, free at the edges and adherent in the center. In severe cases, the scales may be so thick that they are like armor plate. Moderate hyperkeratosis of the palms and soles is frequently present. The follicles in most instances have a crateriform appearance. Ectropion is almost always present and is a helpful diagnostic sign.

Lamellar ichthyosis is inherited as an autosomal recessive trait. About half of patients will be found to have decreased or absent transglutaminase 1 (TGM1) activity. The specific TGM1 genes are heterogeneous (chromosomes 14q11 and 2q33-35).

Lamellar ichthyosis responds partially to alpha-hydroxy acids and other creams recommended for the treatment of ichthyosis vulgaris. Topical calcipotriol, tazarotene (Tazorac), and a variety of emollients have been shown to be effective. Systemic treatment with orally administered 13-cis retinoic acid (Accutane) or acitretin can greatly improve symptoms in patients with lamellar ichthyosis, although the adverse effects associated with prolonged use of these products make their use for long-term maintenance therapy difficult.

Nonbullous Congenital Ichthyosiform Erythroderma

Most infants with nonbullous congenital ichthyosiform erythroderma (CIE) are born enclosed in a constricting parchmentlike or collodion-like membrane that limits motion; they also have ectropion of the eyelids. Within 24

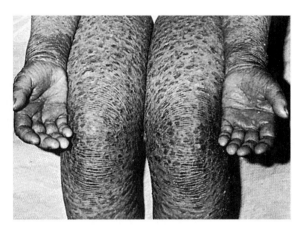

Fig. 27-29 Lamellar ichthyosis in a 6-year-old girl. Her sister has a similar skin problem. Note the glazed and thickened palms.

hours, fissuring and peeling begin, and large keratinous lamellae are cast off in 10 to 14 days, coincident with rapid improvement. As the membrane is shed, underlying redness and scaling are apparent. Generalized involvement is the rule, including face, palms, soles, and flexures. Cicatricial alopecia, nail dystrophy, and some ectropion are common. Scales may be large and platelike on the legs but are likely to be fine on the trunk, face, and scalp. The condition has been found in association with neutral lipid storage disease.

"Collodion babies" are most often seen with CIE (Fig. 27-30). The process may also occur, however, with patients who eventually have normal skin (lamellar exfoliation of the newborn) and with lamellar ichthyosis, as well as with isolated cases of other ichthyoses.

Maintaining a humid environment in the isolette, attention to possible infection in fissured areas, and avoiding use

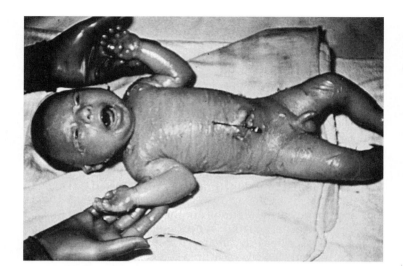

Fig. 27-30 Lamellar exfoliation of the neonate (collodion fetus).

of keratolytics are recommended. Simple emollients are safest during the exfoliative stage.

Harlequin Fetus

Harlequin fetus is a severe, recessively inherited disorder that affects the skin in utero, causing thick, horny, armorlike plates covering the entire surface. The ears are rudimentary or absent, and eclabium and ectropion are severe. The child is often stillborn or dies soon after delivery; however, with aggressive management there have been long-term survivors; some have lived more than 9 years. These survivors develop features of congenital ichthyosiform erythroderma. Three biochemical phenotypes have been identified— failure to convert profilaggrin to fillagrin, and K6 and K16 expression in the epidermis—suggesting that it is a distinct disorder. Aggressive skin care and systemic retinoid therapy have significantly extended survival.

Akiyama M, et al: Cornified cell envelope proteins and keratins are normally distributed in harlequin ichthyosis. *J Cutan Pathol* 1996, 23:571.

Bernhardt M, et al: Report of a family with an unusual expression of recessive ichthyosis: review of 42 cases. *Arch Dermatol* 1986, 122(4):428.

Bichakjian CK, et al: Prenatal exclusion of lamellar ichthyosis based on identification of two new mutations in the transglutaminase 1 gene. *J Invest Dermatol* 1998, 110:179.

Castano SE, et al: Ichthyosis: the skin manifestation of multiple sulfatase deficiency. *Pediatr Dermatol* 1997, 14:369.

Crowe MA, et al: X-linked ichthyosis. *JAMA* 1993, 270:2265.

Cuevas-Covarrubias SA, et al: Accuracy of the clinical diagnosis of recessive X-linked vs ichthyosis vulgaris. *J Dermatol* 1996, 23:594.

Del-Rio E, et al: Keratosis punctata of the palmar creases: a report on three generations, demonstrating an association with ichthyosis vulgaris and evidence of involvement of the acrosyringium. *Clin Exp Dermatol* 1994, 19:165.

Fleckman P, et al: Harlequin ichthyosis keratinocytes in lifted culture differentiate poorly by morphologic and biochemical criteria. *J Invest Dermatol* 1997, 109:36.

Ghadially R, et al: Ichthyoses and hyperkeratotic disorders. *Dermatol Clin* 1992, 10:597.

Gnemo A, et al: Lamellar ichthyosis is markedly improved by a novel combination of emollients. *Br J Dermatol* 1997, 137:1017.

Haftek M, et al: A longitudinal study of a harlequin infant presenting clinically as non-bullous congenital icthyosiform erythroderma. *Br J Dermatol* 1996, 135:448.

Hennies HC, et al: Kinetic and immunohistochemical detection of mutations inactivating the keratinocyte transglutaminase in patients with lamellar ichthyosis. *Hum Genet* 1998, 102:314.

Keren DF, et al: Low maternal serum unconjugated estriol during prenatal screening as an indication of placental steroid sulfatase deficiency and X-linked ichthyosis. *Am J Clin Pathol* 1995, 103:400.

Kragballe K, et al: Efficacy, tolerability, and safety of calcipotriol ointment in disorders of keratinization: results of a randomized, double-blind, vehicle-controlled, right/left comparative study. *Arch Dermatol* 1995, 131:556.

Lavrijsen AP, et al: Reduced skin barrier function parallels abnormal stratum corneum lipid organization in patients with lamellar ichthyosis. *J Invest Dermatol* 1995, 105:619.

Lucker GP, et al: Effect of topical calcipotriol on congenital ichthyosis. *Br J Dermatol* 1994, 131:546.

Mevorah B, et al: Genodermatoses in women. *Clin Dermatol* 1997, 15:17.

Nirunsuksiri, W, et al: Reduced stability and bi-allelic, coequal expression of profilaggrin m-RNA in keratinocytes cultured from subjects with ichthyosis vulgaris. *J Invest Dermatol* 1998, 110:854.

Paller AS: Laboratory tests for ichthyosis. *Dermatol Clin* 1994, 12:99.

Parmentier L, et al: Mapping of a second locus for lamellar ichthyosis to chromosome 2q33-35. *Hum Mol Genet* 1996, 5:862.

Prasad RS, et al: Management and follow-up of harlequin siblings. *Br J Dermatol* 1994, 130:650.

Roberts LJ: Long-term survival of a harlequin fetus. *J Am Acad Dermatol* 1989, 21:335.

Santolaya-Forgas J, et al: Prenatal diagnosis of X-linked ichthyosis using molecular cytogenetics. *Fetal Diagn Ther* 1997, 12:36.

Sato J, et al: Cholesterol sulfate inhibits proteases that are involved in desquamation of stratum corneum. *J Invest Dermatol* 1998, 111:189.

Shwayder T, et al: All about ichthyosis. *Pediatr Clin North Am* 1991, 38:835.

Stege H, et al: Topical application of tazarotene in the treatment of nonerythrodermic lamellar ichthyosis. *Arch Dermatol* 1998, 134:640.

Steijlen PM, et al: Acitretin in the treatment of lamellar ichthyosis. *Br J Dermatol* 1994, 130:211.

Williams ML: Ichthyosis: mechanisms of disease. *Pediatr Dermatol* 1992, 9:365. _____ ▲

Epidermolytic Hyperkeratosis (Bullous Ichthyosiform Erythroderma)

An autosomal dominantly inherited disorder, epidermolytic hyperkeratosis, or bullous congenital ichthyosiform erythroderma, is usually manifested by blisters at or shortly after birth (Figs. 27-31 and 27-32). Later, thickened, horny, warty, ridged scales may cover the entire body. Soon after birth, the scales are shed to leave a raw surface that forms scales anew. These thick, grayish brown, sometimes verruciform scales prominently involve the flexures and the intertriginous areas. Other parts of the skin may be involved, but to a lesser extent. There is remarkable heterogeneity, particularly in regard to extent of body surface involvement, presence or absence of erythroderma, and palm and sole involvement. Epidermal nevi of the epidermolytic type are mosaic expressions of epidermolytic hyperkeratosis.

Although great variability exists, one subtype has been described in enough detail to merit its own name, *ichthyosis*

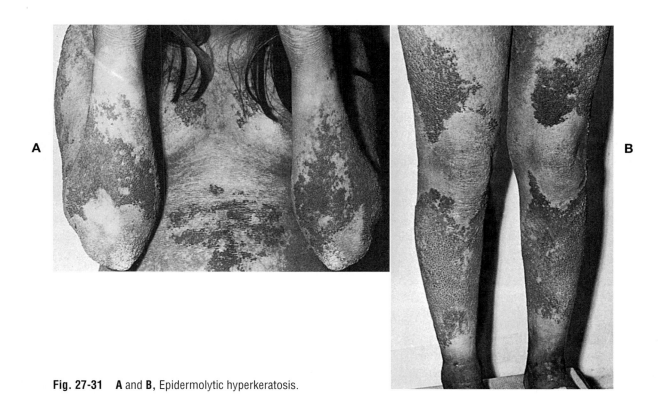

A   B

Fig. 27-31   **A** and **B,** Epidermolytic hyperkeratosis.

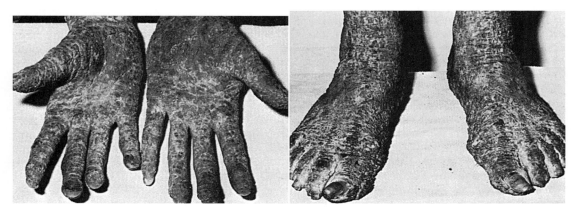

Fig. 27-32   Epidermolytic hyperkeratosis on hands and feet.

bullosa of Siemens. This condition is characterized by a lack of erythema, the "masering phenomenon" (a superficial molting or peeling of the skin), and by confinement of the epidermolytic change to the superficial layers of the epidermis.

There are defects in keratins K1 and K10. Keratin distribution patterns in keratinocytes are abnormal, suggesting that there is an altered assembly process of cornified cell envelopes in epidermolytic hyperkeratosis.

The histologic picture is distinctive, but not pathognomonic. Hyperkeratosis is marked. The granular layer is markedly thickened and contains coarse keratohyaline granules. Epidermal cells detach in the granular cell layer. Electron microscopy reveals the formation of perinuclear haloes. These findings allow prenatal diagnosis by fetal skin biopsy. Epidermolytic hyperkeratosis has been described in normal skin, skin adjacent to benign and malignant epidermal tumors, and normal oral mucosa.

Short intensive therapy with high-dose vitamin A (750,000 units of Aquasol A daily) for 2 weeks produced modest clinical improvement. Others have tried administering systemic retinoids, with similar results; however, the patients' blistering may worsen, despite clinical improvement of the scales. The application of 0.1% retinoic acid (Retin-A cream) has also been used successfully. Pyogenic infection is a common problem, and appropriate antibiotics should be administered. A water solution of 10% glycerin and 3% lactic acid has been effective when applied to wet skin. The disease tends to become less severe with age.

Bale SJ, et al: Epidermolytic hyperkeratosis. *Semin Dermatol* 1993, 12:202.

DiGiovanna JJ, et al: Clinical heterogeneity in epidermolytic hyperkeratosis. *Arch Dermatol* 1994, 130:1026.

Ishida-Yamamoto A, et al: Altered distribution of keratinization markers in epidermolytic hyperkeratosis. *Arch Dermatol Res* 1995, 287:705.

Leigh IM, et al: Mutations in the genes for epidermal keratins in epidermolysis bullosa and epidermolytic hyperkeratosis. *Arch Dermatol* 1993, 129:1571.

Otley CC, et al: Epidermolytic hyperkeratosis. *Int J Dermatol* 1996, 35:579.

Paller AS, et al: Genetic and clinical mosaicism in a type of epidermal nevus. *N Engl J Med* 1994, 331:1408.

Reddy BS, et al: Generalized epidermolytic hyperkeratosis in a child born to a parent with systematized epidermolytic linear epidermal nevus. *Int J Dermatol* 1997, 36:198.

Smack DP, et al: Keratin and keratinization. *J Am Acad Dermatol* 1994, 30:85. ▲

Restrictive Dermopathy

More than 24 cases of this rare, lethal, autosomal recessively inherited disease have been reported. Virtually all cases are afflicted with prematurity, fixed facial expression, micrognathia, mouth in the "O" position, rigid and tense skin with erosions and denudations, and multiple joint contractures. At least eight patients also had wide cranial sutures, small pinched nose, low-set ears, microstomia, rocker-bottom feet, scaly skin, and respiratory insufficiency. Natal teeth were found in two of these patients, and ectropion or chemosis was noted in three.

Sillevis Smitt JH, et al: Restrictive dermopathy: report of 12 cases. *Arch Dermatol* 1998, 134:577. ▲

Ichthyosis Linearis Circumflexa

Ichthyosis linearis circumflexa is a term applied to a disorder of cornification in which bizarre migratory annular and polycyclic patches occur (Fig. 27-33). It is an inherited autosomal recessive disease. On the trunk and extremities is a widespread polycyclic serpiginous eruption characterized by constantly changing patterns; this clears from day to day in previously involved areas and develops new circinate lesions. In about a week the lesions attain their maximum diameter and involute, leaving no atrophy, scarring, or pigmentation. Most are found to have bamboo hair (trichorrhexis invaginata). The association of ichthyosiform dermatitis, hair abnormality, and atopic diathesis is called *Netherton's syndrome* (see Chapter 33). Because of coexistent atopic dermatitis, the scalp, face, and eyebrow regions are erythematous and scaly. The lesions may clear almost completely during the summertime, but this is a lifelong condition.

It may start as newborn erythroderma and demonstrate clinical and histologic findings that are most consistent with an atopic diathesis. These patients are often severely ill; fatal complications occur in up to one third. Ichthyosis linearis circumflexa and Netherton's syndrome should be considered in the differential diagnosis of neonatal erythroderma.

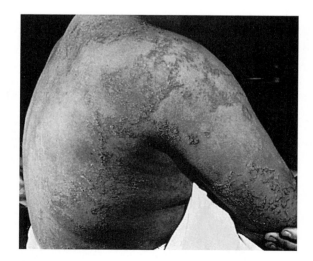

Fig. 27-33 Ichthyosis linearis circumflexa. Widespread polycyclic serpiginous circinate lesions in a 12-year-old girl whose brother has same eruption. (Courtesy Dr. F.J. McCauley.)

Histologic examination shows a remarkable thickening of the horny layer, with parakeratosis and acanthosis. The granular layer is thickened, and dyskeratosis is present.

PUVA and acitretin are the recommended treatments; however, the use of retinoids should be avoided in erythrodermic neonates. Otherwise, palliative topicals can be helpful.

Hausser I, et al: Severe congenital generalized exfoliative erythroderma in newborns and infants: a possible sign of Netherton syndrome. *Pediatr Dermatol* 1996, 13:183.

Judge MR, et al: A clinical and immunological study of Netherton's syndrome. *Br J Dermatol* 1995, 133:153. _____ ▲

Neutral Lipid Storage Disease

Chanarin-Dorfman syndrome is a rare autosomal recessive disorder characterized by an ichthyosiform eruption, myopathy, and vacuolated leukocytes. Lipid vacuoles are present in all circulating granulocytes and monocytes, as well as dermal cells, keratinocytes, and acrosyringia. Other organ systems, such as the CNS, liver, muscles, ears, and eyes, may also have deposits. Associated cutaneous disorders include poikiloderma atrophicans vasculare and bullous congenital ichthyosiform erythroderma. The disorder is caused by a regulatory defect that alters the rates of synthesis and degradation of the major cellular phospholipids, particularly triacylglycerol-derived diacylglycerol. Electron microscopic findings show electron-lucent globular inclusions in lamellar structures. Dietary intervention, with modulation of dietary fats, has been shown to aid in controlling the disease.

Igal RA, et al: Neutral lipid storage disease: a genetic disorder with abnormalities in the regulation of phospholipid metabolism. *J Lipid Res* 1998, 39:31.

Judge MR, et al: Neutral lipid storage disease. *Br J Dermatol* 1994, 130:507.

Kakourou T, et al: Neutral lipid storage disease–response to dietary intervention. *Arch Dis Child* 1997, 77:184.

Wollenberg A, et al: Dorfman-Chanarin syndrome: a neutral lipid storage disease. *Hautarzt* 1997, 48:753. _____ ▲

Ichthyosis Follicularis

Ichthyosis follicularis is characterized by striking alopecia, severe photophobia, and generalized cutaneous follicular projections that are flesh-colored and spiny. There is xerosis of nonspiny skin. It has also been called *ichthyosis follicularis, alopecia, and photophobia* (IFAP) *syndrome*. Males outnumber females in a ratio of 5:1. The main considerations in differential diagnosis are the keratitis, ichthyosis, and deafness (KID) syndrome and keratosis follicularis spinulosa decalvans (KFSD). The disorder may be transmitted by an X-linked recessive gene, although an autosomal dominant form has also been reported.

Eramo LR, et al: Ichthyosis follicularis with alopecia and photophobia. *Arch Dermatol* 1985, 121:1167.

Hazell M, et al: Follicular ichthyosis. *Br J Dermatol* 1984, 111:101.

Keyvani K, et al: Ichthyosis follicularis, alopecia, and photophobia (IFAP) syndrome: clinical and neuropathological observations in a 33-year-old man. *Am J Med Genet* 1998, 78:371.

Rothe MJ, et al: Ichthyosis follicularis in two girls: an autosomal dominant disorder. *Pediatr Dermatol* 1990, 7:287. _____ ▲

Syndromes with Ichthyosis

Ichthyosis is a feature of several genetic disorders. These are rare disorders, and the associated ichthyosis may be mild.

Sjögren-Larsson Syndrome

Sjögren-Larsson syndrome is characterized by ichthyosis, spastic paralysis, oligophrenia, mental retardation, and a degenerative retinitis. The ichthyosis is usually generalized, with little or no involvement of the scalp, hair, or nails (Fig. 27-34). There is a flexural and lower abdominal accentuation. The central face is spared, ectropion is unusual, and palms and soles are involved. Beginning by age 2 or 3, there is spastic paralysis consisting of a stiff, awkward movement of the extremities, typical of Little's disease. Electron microscopy reveals prominent Golgi apparatus and increased numbers of mitochondria in keratinocytes. Usually, a severe mental deficiency is present; no mentally normal patients have been reported. The epilepsy is of the grand mal type. This syndrome is of autosomal recessive inheritance, localized to chromosome 17p11.2. These patients have a fibroblast and leukocyte deficiency in fatty aldehyde dehydrogenase (FALDH).

De Laurenzi V, et al: Sjögren-Larsson syndrome is caused by a common mutation in northern European and Swedish patients. *J Invest Dermatol* 1997, 109:79.

Sillen A, et al: Detailed genetic and physical mapping in the Sjögren-Larsson syndrome gene region in 17p11.2. *Hereditas* 1998, 128:245. _____ ▲

Refsum's Syndrome

Refsum's syndrome is ichthyosis with atypical retinitis pigmentosa, hypertrophic peripheral neuropathy, cerebellar ataxia, nerve deafness, and various electrocardiographic changes. The ichthyosis resembles ichthyosis vulgaris. It may be generalized or localized to the palms and soles; it is of delayed onset and shows lipid vacuoles in the basal layer, and the epidermal cell turnover rate is increased. This is an autosomal recessively inherited disorder. Biochemically the disease is characterized by excessive accumulation of phytanic acid in tissues and body fluids resulting from a deficiency of phytanoyl-CoA hydroxylase, localized on chromosome 10. Reduction of phytanic acid–containing vegetables in the diet affords clinical improvement.

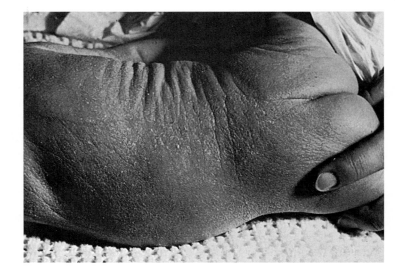

Fig. 27-34 Sjögren-Larsson syndrome. Diffuse erythroderma with scaling of the trunk. (Courtesy Drs. W.B. Reed and A. Heijer.)

Alli N, et al: Keratitis, ichthyosis and deafness (KID) syndrome. *Int J Dermatol* 1997, 36:37.

Caceres-Rios H, et al: Keratitis, ichthyosis, and deafness (KID syndrome). *Pediatr Dermatol* 1996, 13:154.

Chahal A, et al: Restoration of phytanic acid oxidation in Refsum disease fibroblasts from patients with mutations in the phytanoyl-CoA hydroxylase gene. *FEBS Lett* 1998, 429:119.

Ostergaard JR, et al: The central nervous system in Tay syndrome. *Neuropediatrics* 1996, 27:326.

Powers JM, et al: Peroxisomal disorders: genotype, phenotype, major neuropathologic lesions, and pathogenesis. *Brain Pathol* 1998, 8:101. ▲

Rud's Syndrome

Rud's syndrome is characterized by ichthyosis, hypogonadism, small stature, mental retardation, epilepsy, macrocytic anemia, and, rarely, retinitis pigmentosa. It is believed to be of autosomal recessive inheritance, although some patients with this disease have been found to have steroid sulfatase deficiencies of the X-linked variety. Although there are at least 55 cases reported in the literature, most geneticists have dismissed Rud's syndrome as a distinct entity as a result of new understanding of the ichthyoses. Cases of Rud's disease are believed to be either atypical variants of the well-described disorders Sjögren-Larsson syndrome or Refsum syndrome.

Kaufman LM: A syndrome of retinitis pigmentosa, congenital ichthyosis, hypergonadotropic hypogonadism, small stature, mental retardation, cranial dysmorphism, and abnormal electroencephalogram. *Ophthalmic Genet* 1998, 19:69. ▲

Congenital Ichthyosiform Syndrome with Deafness and Keratitis (KID Syndrome)

Several reports detail children with a syndrome characterized by an extensive congenital ichthyosiform eruption, neurosensory deafness, hypotrichosis, partial anhidrosis,

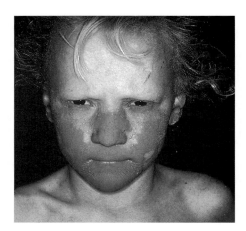

Fig. 27-35 KID syndrome.

vascularization of the cornea, nail dystrophy, and tight heel cords (Fig. 27-35). Distinctive leathery, verrucoid plaques involve the central portion of the face and the ears. These changes, with absent eyebrows and eyelashes, and furrows about the mouth and chin, give the children a unique facies. Isotretinoin treatment may exacerbate and promote corneal vascularization. The most frequent findings are: neurosensory deafness (90%), erythrokeratoderma (89%), vascularizing keratitis (79%), alopecia (79%), and reticulated hyperkeratosis of the palms and soles (41%). This condition is either of autosomal recessive inheritance or sporadic mutation.

Alli N, et al: Keratitis, ichthyosis and deafness (KID) syndrome. *Int J Dermatol* 1997, 36:37.

Caceres-Rios H, et al: Keratitis, ichthyosis, and deafness (KID syndrome). *Pediatr Dermatol* 1996, 13:105.

Kone-Paut I, et al: Keratitis, ichthyosis, and deafness (KID) syndrome in half sibs. *Pediatr Dermatol* 1998, 15:219. ▲

Congenital Hemidysplasia with Ichthyosiform Erythroderma and Limb Defects (CHILD) Syndrome

Present at birth, *c*ongenital *h*emidysplasia with *i*chthyosiform erythroderma and *l*imb *d*efects (CHILD) syndrome is characterized by unilateral inflammatory epidermal nevi and ipsilateral limb hypoplasia or limb defect. Features may vary widely, from complete absence of an extremity to defects of internal organs involving the musculoskeletal, cardiovascular, or central nervous systems. It is believed to be X-linked dominant and lethal in hemizygous males. It has also been suggested that lyonization may occur, producing cutaneous patterns following the lines of Blaschko, similar to incontinentia pigmenti or X-linked dominant chondrodysplasia. The pathogenesis is related to altered prostaglandin metabolism resulting from a diminished activity of two peroxisomal enzymes, catalase and dihydroxyacetone phosphate acyltransferase.

Emami S, et al: Peroxisomal abnormality in fibroblasts from involved skin of CHILD syndrome. *Arch Dermatol* 1992, 128:1213.

Fink-Puches R, et al: Systematized inflammatory epidermal nevus with symmetrical involvement: an unusual case of CHILD syndrome? *J Am Acad Dermatol* 1997, 36:823.

Happle R, et al: How many epidermal nevus syndromes exist? *J Am Acad Dermatol* 1992, 26:1027.

Happle R, et al: The CHILD nevus. *Dermatology* 1995, 191:210. ▲

Erythrokeratodermia Variabilis

Erythrokeratodermia variabilis (EKV), also called *erythrokeratodermia figurata variabilis, erythrokeratodermia variabilis,* and *Mendes da Costa type erythrokeratodermia,* is a rare genetic disorder characterized by erythematous patches and hyperkeratotic plaques of sparse but generalized distribution. The erythematous patches may assume bizarre geographic configurations that are sharply demarcated; in a short time (hours or days), these change their shape or size or involute completely. The keratotic plaques are reddish brown, often polycyclic, and fixed in location. The extensor surfaces of the limbs, buttocks, axillae, groins, and face are most often involved. Keratoderma of the palms and soles sometimes occurs. Hair, nails, and mucous membranes are spared.

The onset of the condition is shortly after birth or, rarely, at birth or in early adult life, after which there is usually some improvement with age, particularly after menopause. Exacerbations have been seen during pregnancy. The configurate erythematous component may be accentuated from exposure to heat, cold, or wind; emotional upsets may also be a factor.

The inheritance is autosomal dominant. The gene has been mapped to 1p34-p35 coding for a gap junction protein alpha-4 (connexin 31). Histologically, there is hyperkeratosis and parakeratosis and a diminished granular layer. Acanthosis may occur. Ultrastructurally, epidermal keratinosomes are diminished.

Isotretinoin restores the deficient keratinosomes and clears the hyperkeratotic plaques and (partially) the migratory erythematous patches in some patients. The disease often relapses when therapy is discontinued.

Hendrix JD Jr, et al: Erythrokeratodermia variabilis present at birth: case report and review of the literature. *Pediatr Dermatol* 1995, 12:351.

Itin P, et al: Family study of erythrokeratodermia figurata variabilis. *Hautarzt* 1992, 43:500.

Knipe RC, et al: Erythrokeratoderma variabilis: case report and review of the literature. *Pediatr Dermatol* 1995, 12:21.

Richard G, et al: Mutations in the human connexin gene GJB3 cause erythrokeratodermia variabilis. *Nat Genet* 1998, 20:366. ▲

Progressive Symmetric Erythrokeratodermia

Progressive symmetric erythrokeratodermia is a rare, autosomal dominantly inherited disorder that manifests soon after birth with erythematous, hyperkeratotic plaques that are symmetrically distributed on the extremities, buttocks, and face, sparing the trunk (Fig. 27-36). Palmoplantar keratoderma may be present. The lesions may regress at puberty. The cause in one kindred was related to an insertion mutation in the loricrin gene. Topical treatments, including keratolytics, corticosteroids, and retinoids have had variable success. Acitretin is another consideration.

Gray LC, et al: Progressive symmetric erythrokeratodermia. *J Am Acad Dermatol* 1996, 34:858.

Ishida-Yamamoto A, et al: The molecular pathology of progressive symmetric erythrokeratoderma. *Am J Hum Genet* 1997, 61:581.

Kiesewetter F, et al: Progressive partially symmetric erythrokeratodermia with deafness. *Dermatology* 1993, 186:222. ▲

Acquired Ichthyosis

Ichthyosis that is clinically similar to ichthyosis vulgaris may develop in patients of any age with several systemic diseases. Acquired ichthyosis has been reported to develop in patients with Hodgkin's disease weeks or months after other manifestations of the disease, but it may be a presenting symptom. It has also occurred in association with non-Hodgkin's lymphomas, mycosis fungoides, multiple myeloma, and carcinomatosis. In hypothyroidism, patients may develop fine scaling of the trunk and extremities as well as carotenemia and diffuse alopecia. Characteristic ichthyosiform lesions may develop in patients with sarcoidosis, particularly over the lower extremities, which on biopsy show granulomas (Fig. 27-37). Ichthyosiform changes have also been reported in patients with leprosy, in gross nutritional deficiency, AIDS, lupus erythematosus, and dermatomyositis, and secondary to multiple drugs including nicotinic acid, triparanol, and butyrophenones.

PITYRIASIS ROTUNDA

This remarkable dermatosis is manifested as perfectly circular, hyperkeratotic, hypopigmented macules, character-

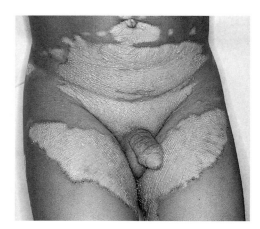

Fig. 27-36 Progressive symmetric erythrokeratodermia.

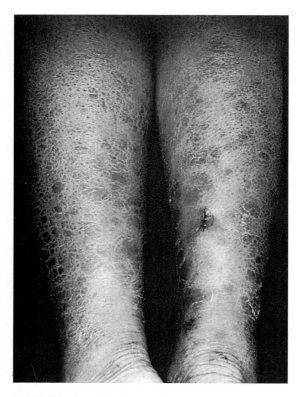

Fig. 27-37 Sarcoidosis presenting as acquired ichthyosis.

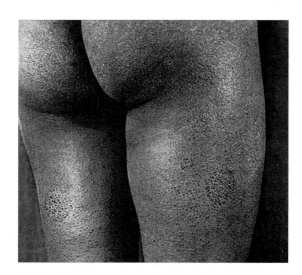

Fig. 27-38 Pityriasis rotunda. Three patches are present on the posterior thighs. (Courtesy Dr. H. El-Hefnaw, U.A.R.)

Two forms of the disease occur: type I is found in blacks or Asians; has hyperpigmented lesions, less than 30 in number; is nonfamilial; and may be associated with systemic disease or malignancies; type II disease occurs in white patients; has hypopigmented lesions, more than 30 in number; is often familial; and usually is not associated with internal disease.

There is a strong ethnic predisposition: cases have been reported in Japanese, Koreans, and Italians; in Tanzanian, South African, West Indian, and American blacks; and in an Egyptian woman. The disease persists for many years, except in those few patients with an accompanying malignancy, in whom it has cleared rapidly when the malignancy was treated. Malnutrition has been implicated in some cases.

The differential diagnosis includes tinea versicolor, tinea corporis, erythrasma, leprosy, fixed drug eruptions, and pityriasis alba. Unfortunately, treatment is of little benefit unless there is an accompanying malignancy that responds to oncologic therapy.

Aste N, et al: Pityriasis rotunda: a survey of 42 cases observed in Sardinia, Italy. *Dermatology* 1997, 194:32.

Gibbs S: Pityriasis rotunda in Tanzania. *Br J Dermatol* 1996, 135:491.

Griffin LJ, et al: Acquired ichthyosis and pityriasis rotunda. *Clin Dermatol* 1993, 11:27.

Grimalt R, et al: Pityriasis rotunda: report of a familial occurrence and review of the literature. *J Am Acad Dermatol* 1994, 31:866.

Kurzrock R, et al: Cutaneous paraneoplastic syndromes in solid tumors. *Am J Med* 1995, 99:662.

Pinto GM, et al: Pityriasis rotunda. *Cutis* 1996, 58:406.

ized by hyperorthokeratosis, on the trunk and extremities (Fig. 27-38). They appear in childhood and extend over most of the skin surface within a few years, slowly enlarging to as much as 20 cm in diameter. About a third of those greater than 5 or 6 cm in diameter are slightly oval. Pruritus may occur. There may be summer remissions and winter exacerbations.

KERATOSIS PILARIS

Keratosis pilaris is an autosomal dominantly inherited condition that may be limited in mild cases to the posterior upper arms, and results from a horny plug in each hair follicle. The thighs are the next most common site. In severe cases the plugs may occur on the face, forearms, and legs, and may become widespread (Fig. 27-39). Facial involvement may be mistaken for acne vulgaris.

The individual lesions are small, acuminate, follicular papules. These may or may not be erythematous; more often they appear grayish because of the superimposed keratotic cone. The latter is composed of cornified keratinocytes collected about a hair shaft, which at times is found coiled within it. Sometimes these corneous plugs are the most prominent feature of the eruption, whereas at other times they are present only in small numbers, and most of the lesions are punctate erythematous papules. Occasionally, inflammatory acneiform pustules and papules may appear.

Forcible removal of one of the plugs leaves a minute cup-shaped depression at the apex of the papule, which is soon filled by new keratotic material. The lesions tend to be arranged in poorly defined groups, dotting the otherwise normal skin in a fairly regular pattern. They are prone to appear in xerotic or atopic subjects. This common dermatosis usually appears between the ages of 2 and 3 and then flourishes until age 20, subsiding in adulthood.

Other conditions associated with keratosis pilaris are ichthyosis follicularis, atrichia with papular lesions, cardio-facio-cutaneous syndrome, ectodermal dysplasia with corkscrew hairs, and KID syndrome.

Treatment is very difficult in all but mild cases. Twelve percent lactic acid (Lac-Hydrin lotion) is the most effective agent, used once or twice daily to the affected area. Treatment with topical tretinoin is usually beneficial; it is most often used for facial lesions. Topical vitamin D creams and ointments have also been shown to be effective.

Abramovits-Ackerman W, et al: Cutaneous findings in a new syndrome of autosomal recessive ectodermal dysplasia with corkscrew hairs. *J Am Acad Dermatol* 1992, 27:917.

Borradori L, et al: Skin manifestations of cardio-facio-cutaneous syndrome. *J Am Acad Dermatol* 1993, 28:815.

Gassia V, et al: Management of keratosis pilaris. *Ann Dermatol Venereol* (France) 1991, 118:69.

Poskitt L, et al: Natural history of keratosis pilaris. *Br J Dermatol* 1994, 130:711. ———————————————————————— ▲

FOLLICULAR ATROPHODERMA

Follicular atrophoderma consists of follicular indentations, approximately 1 mm wide, without hairs, notably occurring on extensor surfaces of the hands, legs, and arms (Fig. 27-40). Scrotal (fissured) tongue may also be found. It has been described repeatedly in association with other genetically determined abnormalities; X-linked dominant chondrodysplasia punctata (see p. 685), Bazex's syndrome (follicular atrophoderma type), and keratosis palmoplantaris disseminata.

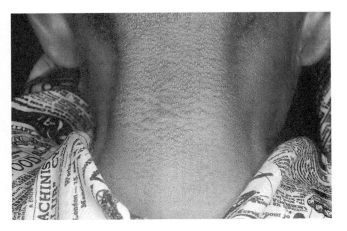

Fig. 27-39   Keratosis pilaris in a patient with atopic dermatitis.

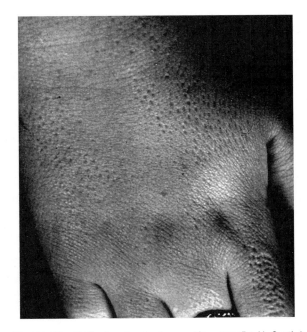

Fig. 27-40   Follicular atrophoderma. (Courtesy Dr. H. Curth.)

KERATOSIS PILARIS ATROPHICANS

Keratosis pilaris atrophicans is seen in three syndromes: (1) keratosis pilaris atrophicans faciei, (2) atrophodermia vermiculata, and (3) keratosis pilaris follicularis spinulosa decalvans. Keratosis pilaris atrophicans has been reported associated with woolly hair and Noonan's syndrome. Overlap between the three entities may occur.

Keratosis Pilaris Atrophicans Faciei and Ulerythema Ophryogenes

Keratosis pilaris atrophicans faciei is characterized by persistent erythema and small horny follicular papules with onset during childhood. On involution these leave pitted scars and atrophy with resulting alopecia. It involves the

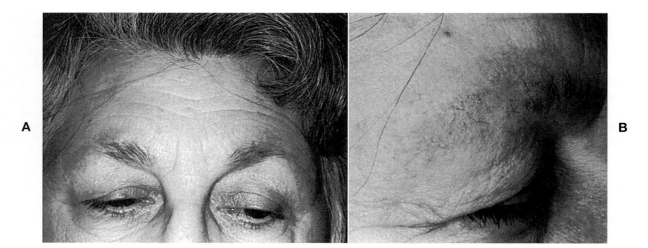

Fig. 27-41 **A** and **B,** Ulerythema ophryogenes.

eyebrows, from which it may rarely spread to the neighboring skin and even to the scalp (Fig. 27-41). Classically, the term *ulerythema ophryogenes* is used to describe cases with involvement limited to the lateral third of the eyebrows.

Lesions may also begin on the cheeks or temples, rather than the eyebrows. The follicles become reddened, then develop papules, later pigmentation, and finally, follicular atrophy. In keratosis pilaris atrophicans faciei the follicular involvement extends to the cheeks and forehead.

These rare dermatoses are characterized by a follicular hyperkeratosis of the upper third of the hair follicle. A small depressed scar forms when the lesion heals. It may occur with atopy, and some authors consider it a marker for Noonan's syndrome, which is often associated with it. It may also be found in patients with cardio-facio-cutaneous syndrome. Transmission is autosomal dominant. Keratolytic ointments or mild tar ointments have been therapeutic. Lac-Hydrin lotion (used cautiously on the face) and Retin-A may be helpful.

Atrophodermia Vermiculata

Atrophodermia vermiculata is also known as *atrophodermia ulerythematosa, folliculitis ulerythematosa reticulata,* and *honeycomb atrophy.* Atrophodermia reticulata is characterized by symmetrical involvement of the face by numerous closely crowded small areas of atrophy separated by narrow ridges, producing a cribriform or honeycomb surface (Fig. 27-42). This almost worm-eaten ("vermiculata") appearance results from atrophy of not only the follicles but also the epidermis and dermis. Each atrophic area is an abrupt, pitlike depression 1 to 3 mm in diameter. Among the ridges a few milia may be seen.

The skin covering the ridges is even with the normal skin and is contrasted with it by being somewhat waxy, firmer, and apparently stretched. On close inspection through a

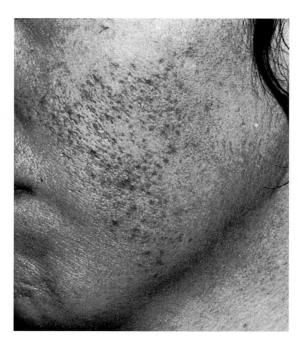

Fig. 27-42 Atrophodermia vermiculata.

magnifying glass redness is apparent, which is usually caused by a ramification of fine capillaries.

The cause of the disease is undetermined but familial occurrence has been noted, and it may be associated with other diseases such as congenital heart block, other cardiac anomalies, neurofibromatosis, oligophrenia, or Down syndrome.

Histologically, the epidermis is slightly atrophic with diminution in size of the interpapillary projections. In the dermis the capillaries are dilated and the vessels have a moderate lymphocytic perivascular infiltration. Some of the follicles are enlarged, tortuous, dilated, and hyperkeratotic.

In addition, there are cystlike cavities lined with epithelium and containing keratin (horn cysts). The sebaceous glands are sparse. Isotretinoin was effective in treating one case.

Rombo Syndrome

Two patients have been reported with features of "grainy skin," multiple basal cell carcinomas, trichoepitheliomas, hypotrichosis, and a peculiar cyanosis of the hands and feet. The associated vermicular atrophoderma produces a coarse, grainy skin texture. The syndrome is inherited in an autosomal dominant fashion. It must be distinguished from Bazex's syndrome, Rasmussen's syndrome (milia, trichoepithelioma, and cylindroma), and multiple trichoepitheliomas.

Keratosis Follicularis Spinulosa Decalvans

In keratosis follicularis spinulosa decalvans (KFSD), keratosis pilaris begins on the face and, at any age up to adolescence, progresses to involve the limbs and trunk. There is hyperkeratosis of the palms and soles. This is followed by loss of hair and scarring. Cicatricial alopecia of the scalp and eyebrows is a hallmark of the disease. Atopy, photophobia, and corneal abnormalities are commonly associated. Deafness, physical and mental retardation, recurrent infections, nail abnormalities, and aminoaciduria have also been purported associations. The inheritance may be X-linked recessive, X-linked dominant, or autosomal dominant. In one X-linked form the defective genetic site is in Xp22.13-p22.2. Topical treatment is most effective, although systemic retinoids may be warranted in some individuals.

Arrieta E, et al: Honeycomb atrophy on the right cheek (atrophoderma vermiculatum). *Arch Dermatol* 1988, 124:1101.

Ashinoff R, et al: Rombo syndrome. *J Am Acad Dermatol* 1993, 28:1011.

Baden HP, et al: Clinical findings, cutaneous pathology, and response to therapy in 21 patients with keratosis pilaris atrophicans. *Arch Dermatol* 1994, 130:500.

Burnett JW, et al: Ulerythema ophryogenes with multiple congenital anomalies. *J Am Acad Dermatol* 1988, 18:437.

Maroon M, et al: Keratosis pilaris and scarring alopecia. *Arch Dermatol* 1992, 128:397.

McHenry PM, et al: The association of keratosis pilaris atrophicans with hereditary woolly hair. *Pediatr Dermatol* 1990, 7:202.

Neild VS, et al: The association of keratosis pilaris atrophicans and woolly hair, with and without Noonan's syndrome. *Br J Dermatol* 1984, 110:357.

Oranje AP, et al: Keratosis pilaris atrophicans: one heterogeneous disease or a symptom in different clinical entities? *Arch Dermatol* 1994, 130:500.

Porteous ME, et al: Keratosis follicularis spinulosa decalvans. *J Med Genet* 1998, 35:336.

Romine KA, et al: Cicatricial alopecia and keratosis pilaris. *Arch Dermatol* 1997, 133:381.

Tuzun Y, et al: Follicular atrophoderma with scrotal tongue. *Pediatr Dermatol* 1987, 4:328.

Weightman W: A case of atrophoderma vermiculatum responding to isotretinoin. *Clin Exp Dermatol* 1998, 23:89. _____ ▲

POROKERATOSIS

Porokeratosis is a heterogeneous group of disorders that are inherited in an autosomal dominant fashion. Except for the punctate type, they are characterized by distinct clinical findings of a keratotic ridge that corresponds to the cornoid lamella on histology. Immunosuppression; immunosuppressive diseases, such as AIDS; ultraviolet exposure; and radiation therapy may exacerbate porokeratosis and promote the development of skin cancers. There is a 7.5% risk of developing cutaneous malignancies, and patients with the linear type are at greatest risk.

Plaque-Type Porokeratosis (Mibelli)

Plaque-type porokeratosis is a chronic, progressive disease characterized by the formation of slightly atrophic patches surrounded by an elevated, warty border (Figs. 27-43 to 27-46). The lesions begin as a small keratotic papule, which spreads peripherally and atrophies in the center, so that eventually there is formed a circinate or serpiginous well-defined plaque surrounded by a keratotic wall or collar, giving rise to a festooned appearance. This wall is grayish or brownish and frequently is surmounted by a tiny groove or linear ridge running along its summit. The enclosed central portion of the plaque consists of dry, smooth, atrophic skin, the lanugo hairs generally being absent when the patches occur in hairy areas.

Sometimes, minute horny projections are visible, representing follicular orifices. In areas subject to friction and rubbing where the skin is thick, the ridges about the patches are particularly pronounced. In other regions the atrophy is more prominent, chiefly on the hands and ankles, but both the keratosis and the atrophy are less distinct in areas, such as the axillae, where the skin is thinner and moist. Linear or zosteriform distribution of the lesions may also occur. If the nail matrix is involved, nail dystrophy may develop.

Sites of predilection are the surfaces of the hands and fingers, and the feet and ankles. The disease also occurs on the face and scalp (where it produces bald patches), on the buccal mucosa (where the ridge becomes macerated by moisture and appears as a milky white, raised cord), and on the glans penis (where it causes erosive balanitis).

The onset of the disease is early in life; it persists indefinitely, with a tendency to slow, irregular progress. The disease is twice as common in males as in females.

Histologically, the principal changes are in the epidermis, where there is marked hyperkeratosis, parakeratosis, and acanthosis. The epidermis is atrophic in the central area. The cornoid lamella is a thickened column of keratin containing parakeratotic nuclei extending outward from a notch in the malpighian layer. The granular cell layer is absent beneath the cornoid lamella. Changes in the dermis consist of mild, perivascular inflammatory infiltrate. There is a tendency for malignant transforma-

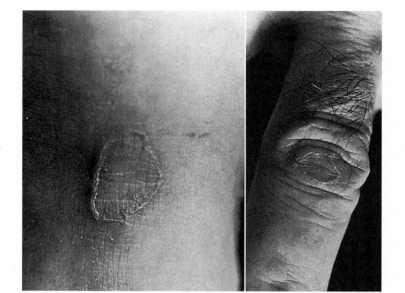

Fig. 27-43 Porokeratosis of Mibelli on the antecubital fossa and midfinger. (Courtesy Dr. H. Shatin.)

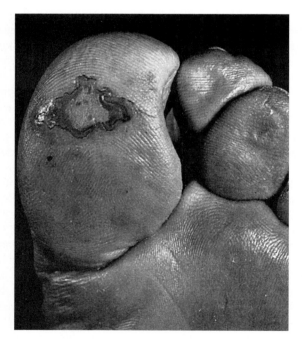

Fig. 27-44 Porokeratosis of Mibelli. (Courtesy Dr. H. Shatin.)

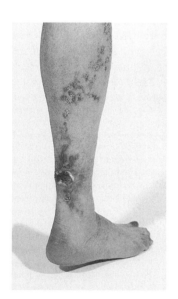

Fig. 27-45 Linear porokeratosis of Mibelli with squamous cell carcinoma.

tion, but subsequent squamous cell carcinomas are rarely aggressive.

It has been suggested that porokeratosis develops because of a localized point of faulty keratinization caused by an abnormal clone of keratinocytes with disordered metabolism or increased growth rate. Appearance or exacerbation of lesions has occurred during chemotherapy for malignancy, after renal transplantation, while on PUVA treatment, and in areas of chronic sun damage, or chemical exposure, such as benzylhydrochlorothiazide.

Treatment with topical undiluted 5-FU solution under occlusion, or in the disseminated superficial type by 5% 5-FU cream, has been reported to be effective. Several reports of acitretin and isotretinoin therapy document improvement while on the medication. There is a tendency to recurrence on discontinuing the retinoid. Carbon dioxide

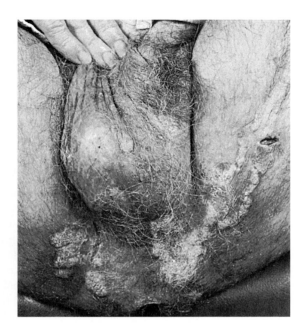

Fig. 27-46 Extensive porokeratosis of Mibelli in the perineal area. Ulceration on posterior thigh is biopsy site. (Courtesy Dr. H. Shatin.)

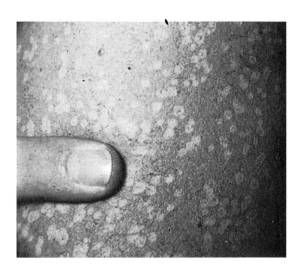

Fig. 27-47 Disseminated superficial actinic porokeratosis on upper arm.

laser ablation and excision are other methods available for localized lesions.

Disseminated Superficial Actinic Porokeratosis

Disseminated superficial actinic porokeratosis (DSAP) is characterized by numerous superficial, annular, keratotic, brownish red macules found on the sun-exposed areas (Fig. 27-47). It is more common in women. The individual lesions enlarge over the years and may be as much as 5 cm in diameter. The centers become depressed and the edge becomes a sharp ridge. On careful observation one often finds lesions with a distinct furrow along the edge. The histopathology is identical to the common form of porokeratosis.

The distribution of the lesions on the sun-exposed areas indicates that actinic radiation is an important factor in its pathogenesis, and new lesions have been induced by exposure to commercial tanning salons. Exacerbations have occurred in about two thirds of cases during the height of the summer season. Not all cases can be described as being related to actinic damage; however, since there are patients with lesions in non–sun-exposed areas. Immunosuppression is well-documented to exacerbate the disease. It has been seen in patients with AIDS, cirrhosis, and Crohn's disease. Organ transplant patients may develop DSAP. Improvement of the immunosuppression may lead to resolution of the lesions.

Cryotherapy is effective in treating individual lesions; however, it is impractical in generalized disease. Topical 5-fluorouracil (Efudex) is well-established therapy.

Linear Porokeratosis

Linear porokeratosis may be segmental or generalized. It may be identified during the newborn period, and when found in the segmental pattern, may follow the lines of Blaschko. Ulcerations and erosions involving the face or extremities may delay the correct diagnosis, and linear porokeratosis should be included in the differential diagnosis of ulcerative lesions occurring in the neonatal period. This form of porokeratosis has the highest risk of developing cutaneous malignancies. James et al reviewed 29 patients in whom squamous cell carcinoma (21 patients), Bowen's disease (eight cases), or basal cell carcinoma (three occurrences) was found within lesions of porokeratosis. Most occurred in the linear type, and most were on the legs. Happle believed that increased risk for malignant degeneration in this form of porokeratosis is related to allelic loss. Oral retinoids have been effective in some patients.

Porokeratosis Palmaris, Plantaris, et Disseminata

In this distinctive form of porokeratosis, lesions first appear on the palms or soles, or more often both, of patients in their twenties, and slowly extend over the entire body. In porokeratotic eccrine ostial and dermal duct nevus, the presentation clinically appears as a nevus comedonicus of the palm or sole. However, histologic analysis reveals multiple comedoid lamella-like parakeratotic columns. In porokeratosis punctata palmaris et plantaris or punctate porokeratosis, lesions are limited to the hands and feet. Treatment with isotretinoin may be effective; however, the condition often recurs when medication is discontinued.

Bencini PL, et al: Porokeratosis and immunosuppression. *Br J Dermatol* 1995, 132:74.

Breneman DL, et al: Cutaneous T-cell lymphoma mimicking porokeratosis of Mibelli. *J Am Acad Dermatol* 1993, 29:1046.

Fisher CA, et al: Linear porokeratosis presenting as erosions in the newborn period. *Pediatr Dermatol* 1995, 12:318.

Goldman GD, et al: Generalized linear porokeratosis treated with etretinate. *Arch Dermatol* 1995, 131:496.

Fleischer AB Jr, et al: Tanning salon porokeratosis. *J Am Acad Dermatol* 1993, 29:787.

Happle R: Cancer proneness of linear porokeratosis may be explained by allelic loss. *Dermatology* 1997, 195:20.

Herranz P, et al: High incidence of porokeratosis in renal transplant recipients. *Br J Dermatol* 1997, 136:176.

James WD, et al: Squamous cell carcinoma arising in porokeratosis of Mibelli. *Int J Dermatol* 1986, 25:389.

Kanitakis J, et al: Disseminated superficial porokeratosis in a patient with AIDS. *Br J Dermatol* 1994, 131:284.

Matsushita S, et al: A case of disseminated superficial actinic porokeratosis subsequent to renal transplantation. *J Dermatol* 1997, 24:110.

Morton CA, et al: Porokeratosis and Crohn's disease. *J Am Acad Dermatol* 1995, 32:894.

Parks BS, et al: Disseminated superficial porokeratosis in a patient with chronic liver disease. *J Dermatol* 1997, 24:485.

Rabbin PE, et al: Treatment of porokeratosis of Mibelli with CO$_2$ laser vaporization versus surgical excision with split-thickness skin graft: a comparison. *J Dermatol Surg Oncol* 1993, 19:199.

Rahbari H, et al: Destructive facial porokeratosis. *J Am Acad Dermatol* 1995, 33:1049.

Rodriguez EA, et al: Porokeratosis of Mibelli and HIV infection. *Int J Dermatol* 1996, 35:402.

Romani J, et al: Disseminated superficial porokeratosis developing after electron-beam total skin irradiation for mycosis fungoides. *Clin Exp Dermatol* 1996, 21:310.

Sasson M, et al: Porokeratosis and cutaneous malignancy: a review. *Dermatol Surg* 1996, 22:339.

Sawai T, et al: Squamous cell carcinoma arising from giant porokeratosis: a case with extensive metastasis and hypercalcemia. *J Am Acad Dermatol* 1996, 34:507.

Schamroth JM, et al: Porokeratosis of Mibelli: overview and review of the literature. *Acta Derm Venereol* 1997, 77:207.

Tangoren IA, et al: Penile porokeratosis of Mibelli. *J Am Acad Dermatol* 1997, 36:479.

Tsambaos D, et al: Disseminated superficial porokeratosis: complete remission subsequent to discontinuation of immunosuppression. *J Am Acad Dermatol* 1993, 28:651. ▲

DARIER'S DISEASE (KERATOSIS FOLLICULARIS)

Darier's disease is characterized by dirty, warty, papular excrescences that tend to coalesce into patches on symmetrical areas of the face, trunk, and flexures of the extremities (Figs. 27-48 and 27-49). The early lesions are small, firm papules, almost the color of normal skin. Each of these soon becomes covered with a greasy, gray, brown or black crust that fits into a small concavity in the summit of the papule. As the lesions grow older, their color becomes darker. In the course of years the papules grow and may fuse to form malodorous papillomatous and vegetating growths. These are fissured and eroded and may be covered with an offensive purulent exudate.

The neck and shoulders, the face, the extremities, the front of the chest, and the midline of the back are sites of predilection for the disease, but as the eruption spreads, the entire trunk, buttocks, genitals, and other parts of the skin may be involved. A frequent site for the earliest lesions is behind the ears.

Vegetations appear chiefly in the axillae, gluteal crease,

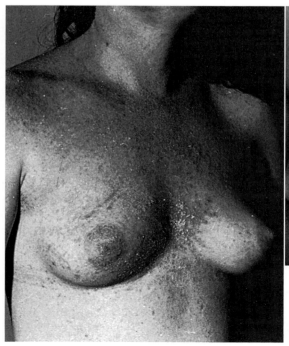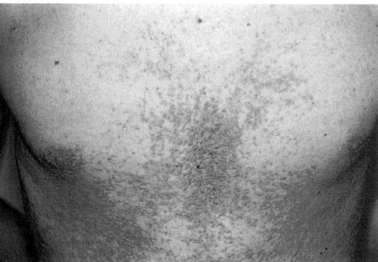

Fig. 27-48 Darier's disease.

groin, and behind the ears. The scalp is generally covered with greasy crusts. Lesions on the face are particularly severe about the nose. The lips may be crusted, fissured, swollen, and superficially ulcerated, and there may be a patchy keratosis with superficial erosions on the dorsum of the tongue. Usually, small white papules are present on the gingiva and palate, or there may be pebbly areas with verrucous white plaques. Punctate keratoses, either raised or with a central pit, are frequently noted on the palms and soles. A general horny thickening of the palms and soles may be present because of innumerable closely set small papules. On the dorsa of the hands and on the shins the flat verrucous papules may resemble verrucae planae. The nails show subungual hyperkeratosis, fragility, and splintering, with longitudinal alternating white and red streaks, and triangular nicking of the free edges (Fig. 27-50). Involvement with Darier's disease of the oropharynx, esophagus, hypopharynx, larynx, and anorectal mucosa has been reported. Disseminated cutaneous herpes simplex may be a complication of the disease.

Usually the eruption is symmetrical and widespread, but striking unilateral or zosteriform (Blaschkoian) involvement may also occur. Localized Darier's disease almost always occurs in this linear fashion. The trunk is a favorite site. A biopsy usually establishes the diagnosis. These cases of limited or nevoid distribution probably represent

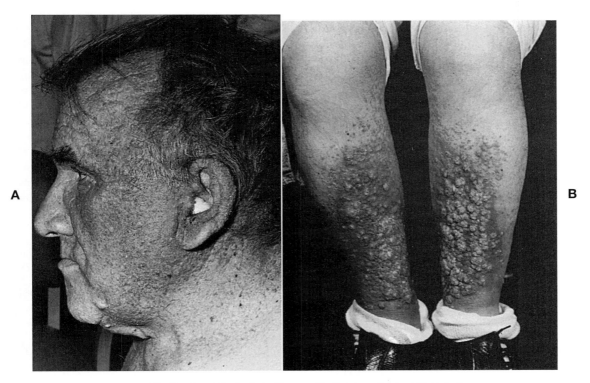

Fig. 27-49 **A** and **B**, Darier's disease. (**B**, Courtesy Dr. Axel W. Hoke.)

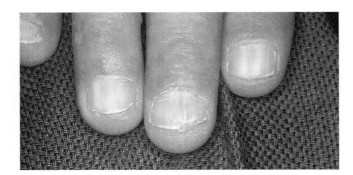

Fig. 27-50 Typical nail changes of Darier's disease.

postzygotic mutations. The possibility of genetic transmission cannot be absolutely excluded, however, since the germ cells (sperm or ova) may also contain the mutation.

Darier's disease is usually worse in the summer, patients being heat sensitive. It may begin after severe sunburn (photo-Koebner). In some patients the lesions may be reproduced with suberythema doses of UVB. Most cases tend to improve or clear in winter. The patient usually has severe itching and discomfort from the skin erosions; these also cause pain, bleed readily, and have an offensive odor. Lithium carbonate has been shown to induce Darier's disease in some individuals.

Darier's disease is a genodermatosis of autosomal dominant inheritance producing abnormalities in keratinization. There is abnormal dissolution of desmosomal plaque proteins, specifically, desmoplakin I and II, plakoglobin, and desmoglein. Vesicle formation occurs as a result of deficiency in the tonofilament/desmosome attachment. Calcium (2+)-dependent cell-cell adhesion molecules (epithelial cadherins) are markedly reduced on the acantholytic cells of patients with Darier's disease. The Darier gene has been localized to 12q23-24.1 and codes for a calcium ATPase (SERCA2).

EPIDEMIOLOGY. Darier's disease occurs in all races, with males and females affected equally. Prevalence estimates range from 1 in 50,000 to 1 in 100,000. It usually has its onset during childhood.

HISTOLOGY. Darier's disease shows hyperkeratosis, parakeratosis, acanthosis, formation of a suprabasal cleft lacuna via acantholysis, with villi in the lacunae. In the lacunae, acantholytic dyskeratotic keratinocytes, termed *corps ronds,* and grains are present. Corps ronds are keratinocytes with a basophilic nucleus surrounded by a halo. Grains are small, dark cells with a pyknotic nucleus, seen most frequently in the stratum corneum.

TREATMENT. For localized disease, topical retinoids may be effective. Tazarotene (Tazarac) and adalpene may also be effective. Isotretinoin and acitretin are the drugs of choice for most severe cases. Cyclosporine may control severe flares. For hypertrophic lesions, dermabrasion, laser excision, or excision and grafting can be considered. Secondary infection with *Staphylococcus aureus* is responsible for some flares and should be sought and managed aggressively.

Burge SM, et al: Darier-White disease: a review of the clinical features in 163 patients. *J Am Acad Dermatol* 1992, 27:40.

Burge SM, et al: Topical isotretinoin in Darier's disease. *Br J Dermatol* 1995, 133:924.

Burkhart CG, Brukhart CN: Tazarotene gel for Darier's disease. *J Am Acad Dermatol* 1998, 38:1001.

Furukawa F, et al: Roles of E- and P-cadherin in the human skin. *Microsc Res Tech* 1997, 38:343.

Gautam RK, et al: Localized Darier's disease and its nosologic status. *Int J Dermatol* 1996, 35:355.

Hur W, et al: Acral Darier's disease: report of a case complicated by Kaposi's varicelliform eruption. *J Am Acad Dermatol* 1994, 30:860.

O'Malley MP, et al: Localized Darier disease: implications for genetic studies. *Arch Dermatol* 1997, 133:1134.

Rubin MB, et al: Lithium-induced Darier's disease. *J Am Acad Dermatol* 1995, 32:674.

Sakuntabhai A, et al: Mutations in ATP2A2, encoding a Ca2+ pump, cause Darier's disease. *Nat Genet* 1999, 21:271.

Salopek TG, et al: Case report of Darier disease localized to the vulva in a 5-year-old girl. *Pediatr Dermatol* 1993, 10:146.

Shadidullah H, et al: Darier's disease: severe eczematization successfully treated with cyclosporin. *Br J Dermatol* 1995, 133:492.

Speight EL: Vesiculobullous Darier's disease responsive to oral prednisolone steroids (letter). *Br J Dermatol* 1998, 139:934.

Steijlen PM, et al: Topical treatment of ichthyoses and Darier's disease with 13-cis-retinoic acid: a clinical and immunohistochemical study. *Arch Dermatol Res* 1993, 285:221. ▲

ACROKERATOSIS VERRUCIFORMIS (HOPF)

This rare genodermatosis is characterized by numerous flat verrucous papules occurring on the backs of the hands, insteps, knees, and elbows (Fig. 27-51). The papules are closely grouped and resemble warts except that they are flatter and more localized. It is inherited as an autosomal dominant trait. Verrucous lesions similar to these occur not infrequently in Darier's disease, and in at least one instance, the two diseases were seen in different members of the same family.

Histologically, hyperkeratosis, thickening of the granular layer, and acanthosis characterize the disease. Papillomatosis with a resemblance of the epidermal elevations to church spires is present. Available treatment methods are liquid nitrogen therapy, shave excision, and CO_2 laser ablation. Recurrence is common.

Chapman-Rolle L, et al: Persistent flat-topped papules on the extremities: acrokeratosis verruciformis (AKV) of Hopf. *Arch Dermatol* 1994, 130:508.

Hafner O, et al: Acrokeratosis verruciformis-like changes in Darier disease. *Hautarzt* 1997, 48:572. ▲

PACHYONYCHIA CONGENITA

In 1906, Jadassohn and Lewandowsky described a rare, often familial, anomaly of the nails to which they gave the name *pachyonychia congenita*. It is characterized by distinctively and excessively thickened nails of all fingers and toes; palmar and plantar hyperkeratoses; follicular keratosis of the skin, especially on the knees and elbows; blister formation, especially under and around callosities; palmar and plantar hyperhidrosis; and leukokeratosis of the mucous membranes (Figs. 27-52 to 27-54). The nail changes consist of great thickening, which increases toward the free borders. The nail plates are extremely hard and are firmly attached to the nail beds. The nail bed is filled with yellow, horny, keratotic debris, which may cause the nail to project upward at the free edge. Paronychial infection is frequently present. Paller et al reported a series of patients with delayed onset pachyonychia in their twenties and thirties, predominantly manifesting nail disease.

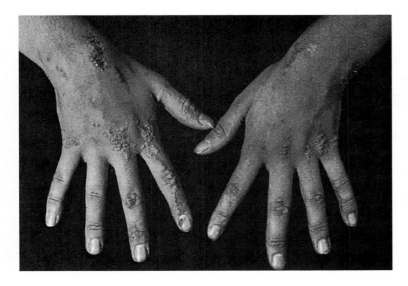

Fig. 27-51 Acrokeratosis verruciformis of Hopf.

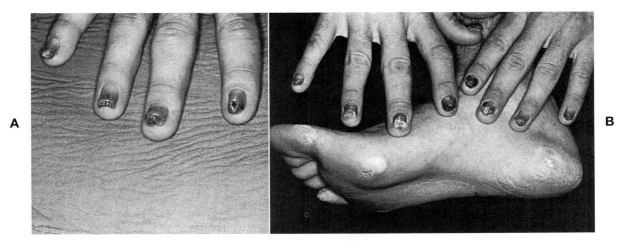

A

B

Fig. 27-52 **A** and **B,** Nail involvement and plantar keratoderma in pachyonychia congenita.

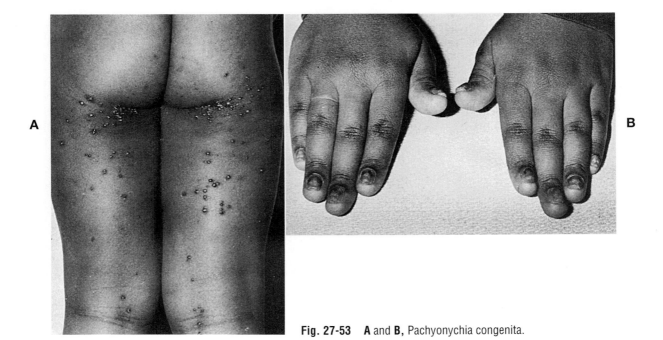

A

B

Fig. 27-53 **A** and **B,** Pachyonychia congenita.

On the extensor surfaces of the extremities, buttocks, and lumbar regions are follicular, keratotic, grayish black papules, having in their centers horny cones that fit into craterlike depressions. The removal of these central cones is fairly easy and leaves a slightly bleeding cavity. The eruption on the outer aspects of the upper and lower extremities is also follicular, resembling keratosis pilaris. This latter condition is not constant and disappears at times.

Painful friction blisters may develop on the plantar aspects of the toes or heels or along the edges of the feet. Cases have been misdiagnosed as epidermolysis bullosa. Leukokeratosis of the tongue and oral mucosa, as well as occasional laryngeal involvement with hoarseness, may occur. This oral leukokeratosis is not predisposed to the development of malignancy.

Pachyonychia congenita is divided into four types, the above-described type being most common, and designated type I *(Jadassohn-Lewandowsky syndrome)*. Type II *(Jackson-Sertoli syndrome)* has the same features as type I, with the additional features of natal teeth and steatocystoma multiplex. Type III *(Schafer-Branauer syndrome)* is like type I with the addition of leukokeratosis of the corneas. *Pachyonychia congenita tarda* was suggested as the name for late-onset disease (type IV). Type IV disease has been described with hyperpigmentation around the neck, waist, axillae, thighs, flexures of the knees, buttocks, and abdomen. Pigmentary incontinence and amyloid deposition are seen in biopsy specimens.

Pachyonychia congenita is usually inherited as an autosomal dominant trait although recessive forms have also been reported. There is a genetic mutation of keratin 6 or 16 in type I and keratin 17 in type II disease.

Numerous measures to relieve the pachyonychia have proved marginally effective. Avulsion of the nails brings about only temporary relief. Removal of the nail matrix fails to provide relief. Vigorous curettage of the matrix and nail bed is the simplest and most effective therapy.

The keratoderma may also produce physical disability, and topical keratolytics are to date the best treatment for this: lactic acid or Lac-Hydrin (ammonium lactate 12%) lotion, salicylic acid, and urea preparations may all be helpful. Isotretinoin clears the keratotic papules and the oral leukokeratosis but does not improve the palms or soles. Acitretin has been shown to be effective in treating the late-onset form.

Chang A, et al: Pachyonychia congenita in the absence of other syndrome abnormalities. *J Am Acad Dermatol* 1994, 30:1017.

Dahl PR, et al: Jadassohn-Lewandowski syndrome (pachyonychia congenita). *Semin Dermatol* 1995, 14:129.

Fujimoto W, et al: Pachyonychia congenita type 2: keratin 17 mutation in a Japanese case. *J Am Acad Dermatol* 1998, 38:1007.

Lucker GP, et al: Pachyonychia congenita tarda. *Clin Exp Dermatol* 1995, 20:226.

Paller AS, et al: Pachyonychia congenita tarda: a late-onset form of pachyonychia congenita. *Arch Dermatol* 1991, 127:701.

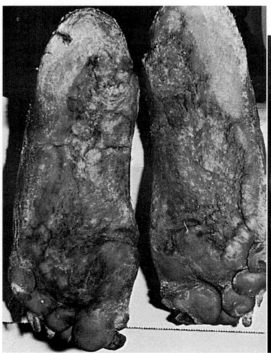
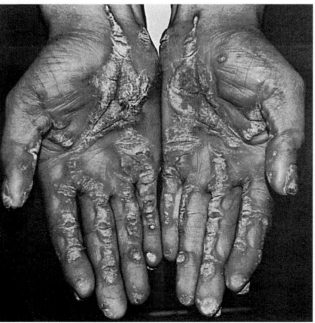

Fig. 27-54 Pachyonychia congenita on the palms, soles, and nails of a 21-year-old-man.

Pryce DW, et al: A family of pachyonychia congenita affecting the nails only. *Clin Exp Dermatol* 1994, 19:521.

Rohold AE, et al: Pachyonychia congenita: therapeutic and immunologic aspects. *Pediatr Dermatol* 1990, 7:307.

Smith FJ, et al: Missense mutations in keratin 17 cause either pachyonychia congenita type 2 or a phenotype resembling steatocystoma multiplex. *J Invest Dermatol* 1997, 108:220. _____ ▲

DYSKERATOSIS CONGENITA

Dyskeratosis congenita is a rare congenital syndrome characterized by atrophy and a reticular pigmentation of the skin, dystrophy of the nails, and leukoplakia (Fig. 27-55), together with multisystem ectodermal and some mesodermal changes. The striking feature of the skin is the tan-gray mottled hyperpigmented or hypopigmented macules or reticulated patches that on some areas appear like a fine network. Atrophy and telangiectasia are also present. These lesions are located typically on the upper torso, neck, and face, although the extremities may also be involved.

The nails may be dystrophic, with thinning, tapering, and distortion resulting from atrophy. Ridging and longitudinal fissuring are seen in mild cases. This is the first component of the syndrome to appear, becoming apparent between the ages of 5 and 15. The other cutaneous lesions follow within 3 to 5 years, as a rule. Leukoplakia may occur, mostly on the buccal mucosa, where extensive involvement with verru-

cous thickening may be present. The anus, vagina, conjunctiva, and the urethral meatus can be involved. Malignant neoplasms of the skin, mouth, nasopharynx, esophagus, rectum, and cervix have been seen in these patients more frequently than in the unaffected similar age group, often occurring in sites of leukoplakia.

Other manifestations of dyskeratosis congenita may be hyperhidrosis of the palms and soles, bullous conjunctivitis, gingival disorders, dysphagia resulting from esophageal strictures and diverticula, skeletal abnormalities, aplastic anemia, mental deficiency, and hypersplenism. In many cases, a Fanconi type of anemia develops, beginning with leukopenia and thrombocytopenia, and then severe pancytopenia occurs. Pulmonary complications may also occur including interstitial and *Pneumocystis carinii* pneumonia.

The disease usually begins in childhood, affecting significantly more males than females. The most common mode of inheritance is as an X-linked recessive trait. The genetic defect is located on Xq28, associated with Zinsser-Cole-Engman syndrome. The defective gene is called *dyskerin,* a nucleolar protein with a role in the biogenesis of ribosomes and rRNA precursors. Autosomal dominant inheritance has also been reported; some of these cases have anemia and reticulated pigmentation following the lines of Blaschko. Graft-versus-host disease may show similar nail changes. In patients with aplastic anemia treated with bone

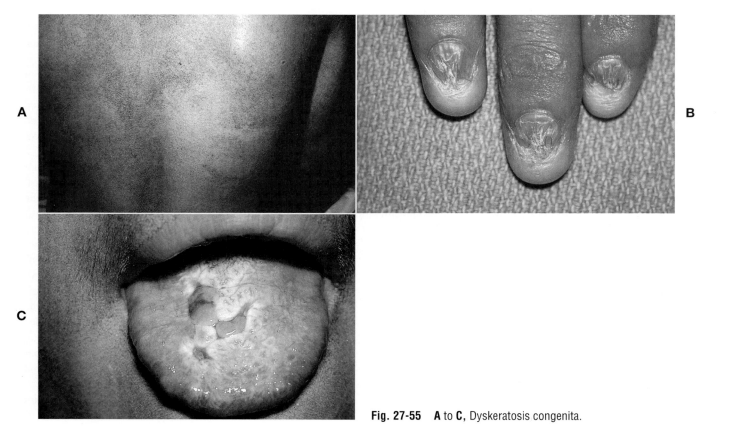

A   **B**   **C**

Fig. 27-55 **A** to **C**, Dyskeratosis congenita.

marrow transplantation, the development of graft-versus-host disease can become a diagnostic dilemma. Granulocyte colony–stimulating factor and erythropoietin may provide short-term benefits in treating bone marrow failure. Bone marrow transplantation is the only potential long-term treatment option for this disease.

Alter BP, et al: Treatment of dyskeratosis congenita with granulocyte colony–stimulating factor and erythropoietin. *Br J Haematol* 1997, 97:309.

Baselga E, et al: Dyskeratosis congenita with linear areas of severe cutaneous involvement. *Am J Med Genet* 1998, 75:492.

Dokal I: Severe aplastic anemia including Fanconi's anemia and dyskeratosis congenita. *Curr Opin Hematol* 1996, 3:453.

Drachtman RA, et al: Dyskeratosis congenita. *Dermatol Clin* 1995, 13:33.

Heiss NS, et al: X-linked dyskeratosis congenita is caused by mutations in a highly conserved gene with putative nucleolar functions. *Nat Genet* 1998, 19:32.

Ho CL, et al: Dyskeratosis congenita in an ethnic Chinese girl. *Int J Dermatol* 1996, 35:659.

Ivker RA, et al: Dyskeratosis congenita or chronic graft-versus-host disease? A diagnostic dilemma in a child eight years after bone marrow transplantation for aplastic anemia. *Pediatr Dermatol* 1993, 10:362.

Joshi RK, et al: Dyskeratosis congenita in a female. *Br J Dermatol* 1994, 130:520.

Imokawa S, et al: Dyskeratosis congenita showing usual interstitial pneumonia. *Intern Med* 1994, 33:226.

Limmer RL, et al: Abnormal nails in a patient with severe anemia: dyskeratosis congenita. *Arch Dermatol* 1997, 133:97.

Phillips RJ, et al: Dyskeratosis congenita: delay in diagnosis and successful treatment of pancytopenia by bone marrow transplantation. *Br J Dermatol* 1992, 127:278.

Rose C, et al: Another case of *Pneumocystis carinii* pneumonia in a patient with dyskeratosis congenita (Zinsser-Cole-Engman syndrome). *Clin Infect Dis* 1992, 15:1056. ▲

FANCONI'S SYNDROME

Also known as *familial pancytopenia* or *familial panmyelophthisis,* Fanconi's syndrome may be associated with diffuse pigmentation of the skin (hypopigmentation, hyperpigmentation, and café au lait macules), absence of the thumbs, aplasia of the radius, severe hypoplastic anemia, thrombocytopenia, retinal hemorrhage, strabismus, generalized hyperreflexia, and testicular hypoplasia. The syndrome is associated with increased risk of myelomonocytic leukemia, squamous cell carcinoma, and hepatic tumors. No hypersensitivity to UV light, x-rays, or chemical agents is present.

Chromosome patterns are frequently abnormal. Heterogeneity has been shown; however, some patients manifest short stature, failure to thrive, absent thumbs, short palpebral fissures, and typical skin abnormalities, which are suggestive of Fanconi's, without hematologic abnormalities. In the series reported by Giampietro et al of an autosomal recessive variant chromosomal breakage was demonstrated in fibroblasts but not in lymphocytes. A case with similar clinical features was reported by Papadopoulos et al and Milner et al. It remains to be determined whether these clinically phenotypic forms of Fanconi's (absent the anemia) are variants of Fanconi's syndrome or a separate entity.

Complementation analysis has shown five complementation groups (FA-A, -B, -C, -D, and -E) and therefore five associated genes. The genes play an important role in hematopoiesis, and abnormal gene expression has been shown to increase apoptosis. FA-A has been localized to 16q24.3, and FA-D to 3p22.26.

Auerbach AD: Fanconi anemia. *Dermatol Clin* 1995, 13:41.

Giampietro PF, et al: New recessive syndrome characterized by increased chromosomal breakage and several findings which overlap with Fanconi anemia. *Am J Med Genet* 1998, 78:70.

Milner RD, et al: A new autosomal recessive anomaly mimicking Fanconi's anaemia phenotype. *Arch Dis Child* 1993, 68:101.

Papadopoulos NG, et al: A case of non-Fanconi bone marrow dysfunction with familial involvement. *Pediatr Hematol Oncol* 1998, 15:277. ▲

CONGENITAL ECTODERMAL DEFECTS

The ectodermal dysplasias are a clinically and genetically heterogenous group of genodermatoses in which the cardinal features are the abnormal, absent, incomplete, or delayed development during embryogenesis of one or more of the epidermal appendages or oral mucosa (hair, sebaceous glands, nails, teeth, or mucosal glands).

Hypohidrotic Ectodermal Dysplasia (Anhidrotic Ectodermal Dysplasia)

The classic triad of this disorder consists of hypotrichosis, anodontia, and hypohidrosis to anhidrosis. This disease is often called *Christ-Siemens-Touraine syndrome.* Absent or reduced sweating is a prominent feature. Despite appropriate heat stress, either environmental or fever-induced sweating is absent or slight, and febrile seizures may occur. Biopsy confirms that eccrine glands are absent or rudimentary, and prenatal diagnosis may be based on this.

The appearance of these patients is typical and conspicuous, since they have a facies suggestive of congenital syphilis. The cheekbones are high and wide, whereas the lower half of the face is narrow (Fig. 27-56). The supraorbital ridges are prominent; the nasal bridge is depressed, forming a saddleback nose (Fig. 27-57). The tip of the nose is small and upturned, and the nostrils are large and conspicuous. The eyebrows are scanty. The eyes slant upward, simulating a Mongolian facies. At the buccal commissures there are radiating furrows (pseudorhagades), and on the cheeks there are telangiectases and small yellow papules (sebaceous gland hyperplasia), simulating milium and adenoma sebaceum. The lips are thickened, with the upper lip particularly protrusive. Absent mammary glands and nipples have been reported.

Hypotrichosis is generalized. Complete alopecia is not present; rather the hair is scraggly, thin, sparse, and dry. In addition to the scalp, other areas are affected, such as the

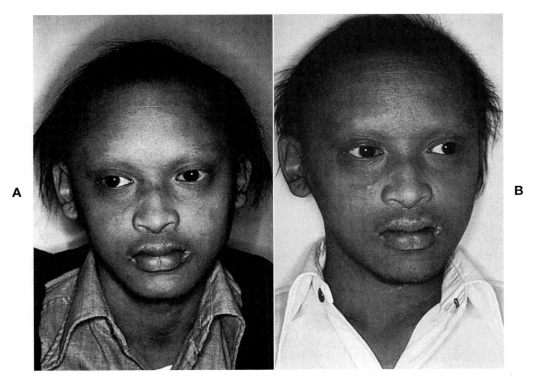

Fig. 27-56 **A** and **B,** Hypohidrotic ectodermal defect and atopic dermatitis in brothers.

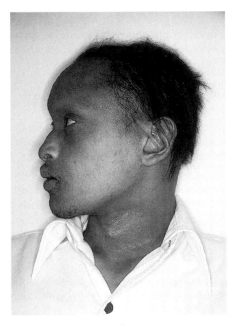

Fig. 27-57 Hypohidrotic ectodermal dysplasia. Note hypotrichosis, saddle nose, and protrusive upper lip.

beard area, axillae, pubic area, and trunk. There is partial or total anodontia. Nails may be thinned, brittle, and ridged; the skin is soft, thin, dry, and smooth. Mental retardation is present in some cases, possibly as a consequence of hyperthermic episodes in childhood.

The inheritance pattern is almost always expressed through an X-linked recessive gene (Xq11-12). Ten percent of female carriers may have partial expression of this disorder. Both autosomal recessive and dominant modes of inheritance have been described. The gene for autosomal dominant hypohidrotic ectodermal dysplasia has been mapped to 2q11-q13.

Hidrotic Ectodermal Dysplasia

The hidrotic type of congenital ectodermal dysplasia is often referred to as *Clouston's syndrome*. The eccrine sweat glands are active and the facial features are normal, without the typical saddle nose. An autosomal dominant gene is responsible in these cases. Alopecia, nail dystrophy, palmoplantar hyperkeratosis, and eye changes such as cataracts and strabismus are the features of hidrotic ectodermal dysplasia. The defective gene has been identified on 13q11-q12.1.

AEC Syndrome (Hay-Wells Syndrome)

*A*nkyloblepharon, *e*ctodermal defects, and *c*left lip and/or palate constitute the AEC syndrome. It has an autosomal dominant pattern of inheritance. There may or may not be fusion or partial fusion of the lids (ankyloblepharon) at birth. Sparse hair, dental defects, cleft palate and lip, dystrophic nails, hypospadias, syndactyly, short stature, absent lacrimal puncta, and stenotic auditory canals and short stature are a few of the possible anomalies. An erosive scalp dermatitis is more likely to be observed in AEC than in other ectodermal disorders and is a helpful distinguishing feature. The scalp dermatitis is often extensive, difficult to treat, and persists or recurs.

EEC Syndrome

*E*ctodermal dysplasia, *e*ctrodactyly, and *c*left lip/palate are defining features of EEC syndrome. It must be distinguished from AEC and Rapp-Hodgkin ectodermal dysplasia. EEC lacks scalp dermatitis, has mild hypohidrosis, and ectrodactyly (congenital absence of all or part of a digit) is a prominent feature.

Rapp-Hodgkin Ectodermal Dysplasia Syndrome

Characteristic features of Rapp-Hodgkin ectodermal dysplasia syndrome include anomalies of hair (pili torti, pili canaliculi, alopecia, thinning of eyebrows/lashes), cleft lip/palate, onychodysplasia, dental caries, adontia, craniofacial abnormality, hypohidrosis, otitis media (hearing deficits), and hypospadias. It is usually inherited in an autosomal dominant manner. Some authors believe this disorder to be a variant of AEC.

Ectodermal Dysplasia with Corkscrew Hairs

Abramovits-Ackerman et al described this new disorder in 27 patients from seven families who live on Margarita Island, northeast of Venezuela. Salient features include corkscrew hairs (exaggerated pili torti), scalp keloids, follicular plugging, keratosis pilaris, xerosis, eczema, palmoplantar keratodermia, syndactyly, onchodysplasia, and conjunctival neovascularization. Typical facies, anteverted pinnae, malar hypoplasia, cleft lip and palate, and dental abnormalities may also be found. Inheritance is autosomal recessive. Anhidrosis or hypohidrosis are not features.

Odonto-Tricho-Ungual-Digital-Palmar Syndrome

First described by Mendoza et al in two brothers, their mother, and 18 other relatives from five generations, the salient clinical features are natal teeth, trichodystrophy, prominent interdigital folds, simian-like hands with transverse palmar creases, and ungual digital dystrophy, inherited as an autosomal dominant trait. Hypoplasia of the first metacarpal and metatarsal bones and distal phalanges of the toes may also occur.

Costello Syndrome

Costello syndrome is characterized by growth retardation, coarse facies, redundant skin on the neck, palms, soles, and fingers, dark skin, acanthosis nigricans, and nasal papillomata. It is divided into two phases: phase 1 begins with severe failure to thrive within the first few months, which, with vigorous support, evolves into phase 2, normal weight gain. Cardiomyopathy is frequently found, but other visceral organs are usually spared. Hydrocephalus may occur. Mild to moderate mental deficiency is frequently discovered, and most patients exhibit a characteristic so-

ciable and friendly personality. Papillomata, which may arise later in life, loose skin, hyperpigmentation, and typical facies allow for an early diagnosis.

Lenz-Majewski Syndrome

Lenz-Majewski syndrome has some overlapping features with Costello syndrome. Considered one of the craniotubular dysplasias, the main features include craniodiaphyseal dysplasia, failure to thrive, mental retardation, proximal symphalangism, enamel hypoplasia, and loose skin. Cases have been sporadic.

Naegeli-Franceschetti-Jadassohn Syndrome

The syndrome consists of reticulate pigmentation, hypohidrosis, absent dermatoglyphics, abnormal teeth leading to early or total loss, and palmoplantar keratoderma. The reticulate pigmentation often fades after puberty and may disappear completely in older adults. Some patients may develop congenital malalignment of the great toenails. The syndrome is inherited as an autosomal dominant trait (see p. 684).

CHIME Syndrome

The CHIME syndrome, a rare neuroectodermal disorder, comprises *c*olobomas of the eye, *h*eart defects, *i*chthyosiform dermatosis, *m*ental retardation, and *e*ar defects. Other features may include facial anomalies, epidermal nevi, developmental delay, infantile macrostomia, recurrent infections, acute lymphoblastic leukemia, and duplicated renal collecting system. The inheritance is believed to be autosomal recessive.

Pachydermoperiostosis

Pachydermoperiostosis, also known as *Touraine-Solente-Gole syndrome,* is characterized by thickening of the skin in folds and accentuation of creases on the face and scalp, clubbing of the fingers, and periostosis of the long bones (Fig. 27-58). The changes are especially prominent on the forehead, where the horizontal lines are deepened and the skin becomes shiny. The eyelids, particularly the upper ones, are thickened. Likewise there is thickening of the ears and of the lips. The tongue is enlarged. The scalp may be thickened and show cutis verticis gyrata (pachydermie vorticelle). The extremities, especially the elbows, knees, and hands, are enlarged and spade shaped. The fingers become club shaped (Fig. 27-59). The palms are rough, and the thenar and hypothenar eminences are enlarged. Hyperhidrosis is common. Hyperkeratotic linear lesions of the palms and soles may be present. These lines are rippled, resembling sand of the "wind-blown desert." Movements of the muscles may be painful. There are inherited and acquired forms.

There are a number of causes of the acquired form. Clubbing of the fingers and toes and osteoarthropathy have long been known to occur in chronic pulmonary, mediasti-

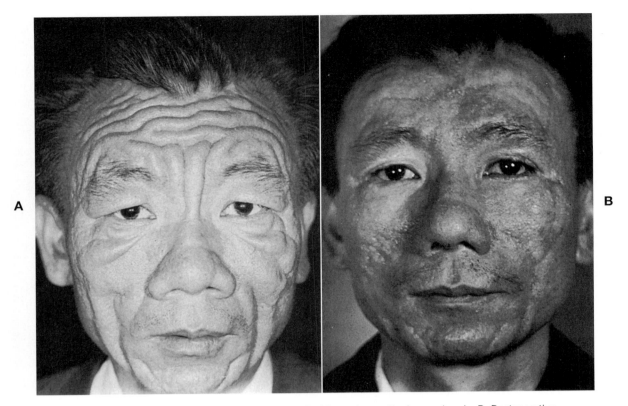

Fig. 27-58 **A,** Pachydermoperiostosis with marked furrowing on the face and scalp. **B,** Postoperative results. (Courtesy Drs. F. Reiss and M.M. Shuster.)

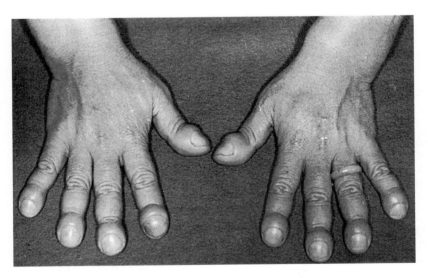

Fig. 27-59 Clubbing of the fingertips in patient shown in Fig. 27-58. (Courtesy Dr. F. Reiss.)

nal, and cardiac diseases that are associated with chronic low-grade anoxemia in peripheral tissues. Some cases of pachydermoperiostosis have been associated with bronchogenic carcinoma. When such an association occurs, the enlargement of the forehead, hands, and fingers may antedate the recognition of the tumor or may develop after the tumor is known to be present. Bronchogenic carcinoma–

associated pachydermoperiostosis occurs almost exclusively in men over age 40, whereas Touraine-Solente-Gole syndrome usually occurs as a familial autosomal dominant disorder not associated with malignant disease. More prominent signs are seen in males, and onset occurs in late adolescence and in the twenties. Sinha et al described a family with pachydermoperiostosis inherited in an autosomal recessive fashion. Cleft palate and congenital heart defects were manifested in recessive homozygous individuals.

The condition may be confused with acromegaly based on clinical features, and lung cancer should be considered in older patients. Treatment is centered mostly on improvement of the cosmetic appearance via plastic surgical repair.

Abramovits-Ackerman W, et al: Cutaneous findings in a new syndrome of autosomal recessive ectodermal dysplasia with corkscrew hairs. *J Am Acad Dermatol* 1992, 27:917.

Aswegan AL, et al: Autosomal dominant hypohidrotic ectodermal dysplasia in a large family. *Am J Med Genet* 1997, 72:462.

Camacho F, et al: Rapp-Hodgkin syndrome with pili canaliculi. *Pediatr Dermatol* 1993, 10:54.

Cambiaghi S, et al: Rapp-Hodgkin syndrome and AEC syndrome: are they the same entity? *Br J Dermatol* 1994, 130:97.

Fosko SW, et al: Ectodermal dysplasias associated with clefting: significance of scalp dermatitis. *J Am Acad Dermatol* 1993, 29:505.

Hizli S, et al: Anhidrotic ectodermal dysplasia (Christ-Siemens-Touraine syndrome) presenting as a fever of unknown origin in an infant. *Int J Dermatol* 1998, 37:132.

Ho L, et al: A gene for autosomal dominant hypohidrotic ectodermal dysplasia (EDA3) maps to chromosome 2q11-q13. *Am J Hum Genet* 1998, 62:1102.

Itin PH, et al: Natural history of the Naegeli-Franceschetti-Jadassohn syndrome and further delineation of its clinical manifestations. *J Am Acad Dermatol* 1993, 28:942.

Jansen T, et al: Pachydermoperiostosis. *Hautarzt* 1995, 46:429.

Matucci-Cerinic M, et al: The clinical spectrum of pachydermoperiostosis (primary hypertrophic osteoarthropathy). *Medicine* 1991, 70:208.

Mendoza HR, et al: A newly recognized autosomal dominant ectodermal dysplasia syndrome: the odonto-tricho-ungual-digital-palmar syndrome. *Am J Med Genet* 1997, 71:144.

Micali G, et al: Structural hair abnormalities in ectodermal dysplasia. *Pediatr Dermatol* 1990, 7:27.

Nishimura G, et al: Craniotubular dysplasia with severe postnatal growth retardation, mental retardation, ectodermal dysplasia, and loose skin: Lenz-Majewski-like syndrome. *Am J Med Genet* 1997, 71:87.

Nordgarden H, et al: Salivary gland involvement in hypohidrotic ectodermal dysplasia. *Oral Dis* 1998, 4:152.

O'Donnell BP, et al: Rapp-Hodgkin ectodermal dysplasia. *J Am Acad Dermatol* 1992, 27:323.

Philip N, et al: Costello syndrome. *J Med Genet* 1998, 35:238.

Pratesi R, et al: Costello syndrome in two Brazilian children. *J Med Genet* 1998, 35:54.

Rowan DM: Scalp dermatitis, ectodermal dysplasia and cleft lip and palate: Rapp-Hodgkin or AEC syndrome? *Austral J Dermatol* 1996, 37:102.

Schnur RE, et al: Acute lymphoblastic leukemia in a child with the CHIME neuroectodermal dysplasia syndrome. *Am J Med Genet* 1997, 72:24.

Sinha GP, et al: Pachydermoperiostosis in childhood. *Br J Rheumatol* 1997, 36:1224.

Taylor TD, et al: Confirmation of linkage of Clouston syndrome (hidrotic ectodermal dysplasia) to 13q11-q12.1 with evidence for multiple independent mutations. *J Invest Dermatol* 1998, 111:83. ▲

Cutis Verticis Gyrata

Cutis verticis gyrata is characterized by folds and furrows on the scalp (Fig. 27-60). Most frequently the vertex is involved, but other areas may have the distinctive furrowing. There may be 2 to 20 folds. The hair itself is usually black and of normal growth.

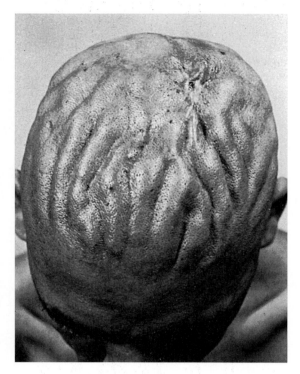

Fig. 27-60 Cutis verticis gyrata. (Courtesy Dr. H. Shatin.)

Cutis verticis gyrata has been reported to occur primarily in males, with a male-to-female ratio of 6:1. Onset is usually in puberty, with more than 90% of patients developing it before age 30. The condition may be familial when it occurs as a component of pachydermoperiostosis. It has been reported to be the result of developmental anomalies, inflammation, trauma, tumors, nevi, or proliferative diseases.

Cutis verticis gyrata is frequently found in patients with mental retardation or chronic schizophrenia. Rarely, a cerebriform intradermal nevus may be mistaken for this disorder. In severely involved cases, excision with grafting or scalp reduction may be indicated.

Jeanfils S, et al: Cerebriform intradermal nevus: a clinical pattern resembling cutis verticis gyrata. *Dermatology* 1993, 186:294.

Passarini B, et al: Cutis verticis gyrata secondary to acute monoblastic leukemia. *Acta Derm Venereol* 1993, 73:148.

Schepis C, et al: Primary cutis verticis gyrata or pachydermia verticis gyrata: a peculiar scalp disorder of mentally retarded adult males. *Dermatology* 1995, 191:292. ▲

Aplasia Cutis Congenita

Aplasia cutis congenita, a congenital defect of the skin, is a rare anomaly of the newborn, with a predilection for the midline of the vertex of the scalp. A small bleb in fetal life may develop into a coin-sized or larger absence of skin and subcutaneous tissue, very rarely penetrating into the cranium. Also rare, multiple symmetrical defects may occur on the skin, generally on the lower extremities, which are believed to be a variant of aplasia cutis congenita. At times nevocellular nevi with associated alopecia are confused with this disorder. An association with thyroid disease and thyroid medications (methimazole) has been implicated as a cause. There is a tendency for these aplasias to heal spontaneously; however, some case are quite severe requiring surgical intervention.

Drolet et al described a series of six patients with aplastic cutis congenita who demonstrated a ring of dark, long hair encircling the congenital scalp lesion, called "the hair collar sign." The authors proposed that this is a subtype of aplasia cutis congenita, referred to as *membranous aplasia cutis.* They believe it represents the form fruste of a neural tube defect.

Classen DA: Aplasia cutis congenita associated with fetus papyraceous. *Cutis* 1999, 64:104.

Drolet B, et al: "Membranous aplasia cutis" with hair collars: congenital absence of skin or neuroectodermal defect? *Arch Dermatol* 1995, 131:1427.

Kalb RE, et al: The association of aplasia cutis congenita with therapy of maternal thyroid disease. *Pediatr Dermatol* 1986, 3:327.

Kruk-Jeromin J, et al: Aplasia cutis congenita of the scalp: report of 16 cases. *Dermatol Surg* 1998, 24:549.

Martinez-Frias ML, et al: Methimazole in animal feed and congenital aplasia cutis. *Lancet* 1992, 339:742.

Mastruseria DN, et al: Nevocellular nevus associated with alopecia presenting as aplasia cutis congenita. *Int J Dermatol* 1998, 37:37.

Tekinalp G, et al: Bilateral abdominal aplasia cutis congenita associated with atrial septal defect: a case report. *Pediatr Dermatol* 1997, 14:117.

Theile RJ, et al: Reconstruction of aplasia cutis congenita of the scalp by split rib cranioplasty and a free latissimus dorsi muscle flap in a nine month old infant. *Br J Plast Surg* 1995, 48:507.

Vogt T, et al: Aplasia cutis congenita after exposure to methimazole: a causal relationship? *Br J Dermatol* 1995, 133:994. _____ ▲

Adams-Oliver Syndrome

Features of Adams-Oliver syndrome include severe aplasia cutis congenita of the scalp, which may involve both skin and cranium, extensive cutis marmorata telangiectatica congenita, and limb defects. Other associations include hemangiomas, retro- and micrognathia, strabismus, and atrial septal defect. It is a rare autosomal dominantly inherited neuroectodermal syndrome.

Bork K, et al: Multifocal aplasia cutis congenita, distal limb hemimelia, and cutis marmorata telangiectatica in a patient with Adams-Oliver syndrome. *Br J Dermatol* 1992, 127:160.

Dyall-Smith D, et al: Adams-Oliver syndrome: aplasia cutis congenita, terminal transverse limb defects and cutis marmorata telangiectatica congenita. *Australas J Dermatol* 1994, 35:19.

Frank RA, et al: Adams-Oliver syndrome: cutis marmorata telangiectatica congenita with multiple anomalies. *Dermatology* 1993, 187:205.

Swartz EN, et al: Vascular abnormalities in Adams-Oliver syndrome: cause or effect? *Am J Med Genet* 1999, 82:49. _____ ▲

Focal Dermal Hypoplasia (Goltz's Syndrome)

Goltz's syndrome is characterized by multiple abnormalities of mesodermal and ectodermal tissues. Reddish tan, atrophic, often linear or cribriform patches in conjunction with herniations of yellowish brown (fat) nodules may be present prominently on the buttocks, axillae, and thighs. The lesions are strikingly linear and often serpiginous, following lines of Blaschko. Brown, atrophic, sharply circumscribed patches appear. Telangiectases are commonly present. Papillomas, small and reddish tan, have occurred around the orifices of the mouth, anus, and vagina. They may be misdiagnosed as condyloma acuminata.

The bone changes involve mostly the extremities, where there may be syndactyly, oligodactyly, and adactyly (Fig. 27-61). Scoliosis, spina bifida, and hypoplasia of the clavicle have also been reported. Eighty percent of patients have skeletal defects. Variable ocular, dental, hair, and nail abnormalities have been described. Forty percent to 50% of patients have ocular and dental abnormalities. Coloboma is the most common ocular defect. The large majority of reported patients have been female. An X-linked dominant trait is believed to be the hereditary pattern, with lethality in males, and females protected by X chromosome mosaicism, identical to the situation in incontinentia pigmenti. Treatment of atrophic erythematous patches have been successful using a flashlamp-pumped pulsed dye laser.

Alster TS, et al: Focal dermal hypoplasia (Goltz's syndrome): treatment of cutaneous lesions with the 585-nm flashlamp-pumped pulsed dye laser. *Arch Dermatol* 1995, 131:143.

Arnold WP, et al: Focal dermal hypoplasia (Goltz-Gorlin syndrome). *Br J Dermatol* 1993, 129:214.

Kore-Eda S, et al: Focal dermal hypoplasia (Goltz syndrome) associated with multiple giant papillomas. *Br J Dermatol* 1995, 133:997.

Pereyo NG, et al: Atrophic macules in an infant: Goltz syndrome (focal dermal hypoplasia [FDH] syndrome). *Arch Dermatol* 1993, 129:897. ▲

Cockayne's Syndrome

One of the syndromes of premature aging, Cockayne described a condition he named *dwarfism with retinal atrophy and deafness.* The various dermatologic features are photodermatitis related to sensitivity to sunlight, which results in telangiectasia, atrophy, hyperpigmentation, and scarring. The hands, legs, and feet are cyanotic, cold, and disproportionately large (Fig. 27-62). Other changes are microcephaly, sunken eyes, a characteristic facial appearance, severe flexion contractures, dorsal kyphosis, cryptorchidism, cataracts, retardation of growth, severe mental retardation, hypothalamic and cerebellar dysfunction, and retinitis pigmentosa with optic atrophy. Dermal fibroblasts and lymphoblastoid cell lines, as well as cultured amniotic fluid cells from an affected fetus, demonstrate impaired colony-forming ability, and decreased DNA and RNA synthesis after ultraviolet light exposure (254 nm). There

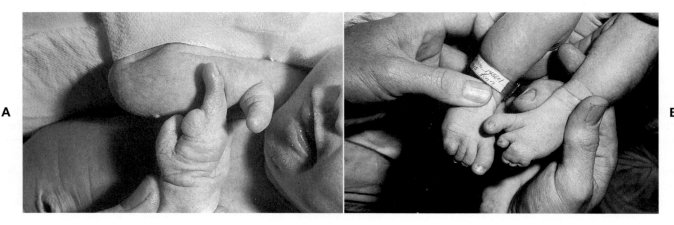

Fig. 27-61 Focal dermal hypoplasia. Note **A,** oligodactyly and **B,** syndactyly.

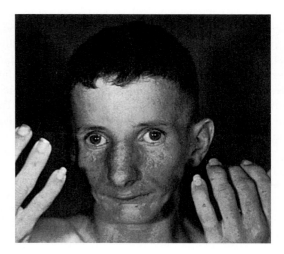

Fig. 27-62 Cockayne's syndrome. (Courtesy Dr. V.J. Derbes.)

is progressive neurologic disturbance with a shortened life-span. There is no increased carcinogenesis. Inheritance is autosomal recessive with complete penetrance. The genetic defect is in the XPB DNA helicase.

Cooper PK, et al: Defective transcription-coupled repair of oxidative base damage in Cockayne syndrome patients from XP group G. *Science* 1997, 275:990.

Francis MA, et al: UV-induced reactivation of a UV-damaged reporter gene suggests transcription-coupled repair is UV-inducible in human cells. *Carcinogenesis* 1999, 20:19.

Inoue T, et al: An adult case of Cockayne syndrome without sclerotic angiopathy. *Intern Med* 1997, 36:565.

Moriwaki S, et al: DNA repair and ultraviolet mutagenesis in cells from a new patient with xeroderma pigmentosum group G and Cockayne syndrome resemble xeroderma pigmentosum cells. *J Invest Dermatol* 1996, 107:647.

Van Gool AJ, et al: The Cockayne syndrome B protein, involved in transcription-coupled DNA repair, resides in an RNA polymerase II-containing complex. *EMBO J* 1997, 16:5955. _____ ▲

Werner's Syndrome (Adult Progeria)

Werner's syndrome is a premature-aging syndrome characterized by many metabolic and structural abnormalities involving the skin, hair, eyes, muscles, fatty tissues, bones, blood vessels, and carbohydrate metabolism (Fig. 27-63).

The most characteristic findings are premature aging and arrest of growth at puberty, senile cataracts developing in the late twenties and thirties, premature balding and graying, and scleroderma-like lesions of the skin. A characteristic change is the loss of subcutaneous tissue and wasting of muscles, especially the extremities, so that the legs become spindly and the trunk becomes stocky.

Additional changes may be painful callosities with ulcerations around the malleoli, Achilles tendons, heels, and toes. Hair thins on the eyebrows, axillae, and pubis. The skin over the cheek bones becomes taut to produce proptosis and beaking of the nose. Cataracts develop early. The vocal cords become thickened so that a weak, high-pitched voice ensues. Premature arteriosclerosis and sexual impotence are frequently observed. Diabetes is frequent, and areas of calcinosis circumscripta occur.

A high rate of malignancy is associated with Werner's syndrome. Uterine sarcoma, hepatoma, carcinoma of the breast, fibrosarcoma, and thyroid adenocarcinoma have occurred. Histologic changes in the skin may include atrophy of the epidermis and fibrosis of the dermis.

Consanguinity and familial incidence are encountered, to suggest a mendelian recessive mode of transmission. Five markers for the Werner gene (WS) have been found on chromosome 8. WS-3 has been localized to 8p11-p12, which encodes for a protein that confers adhesive properties to macromolecular proteins like fibronectin.

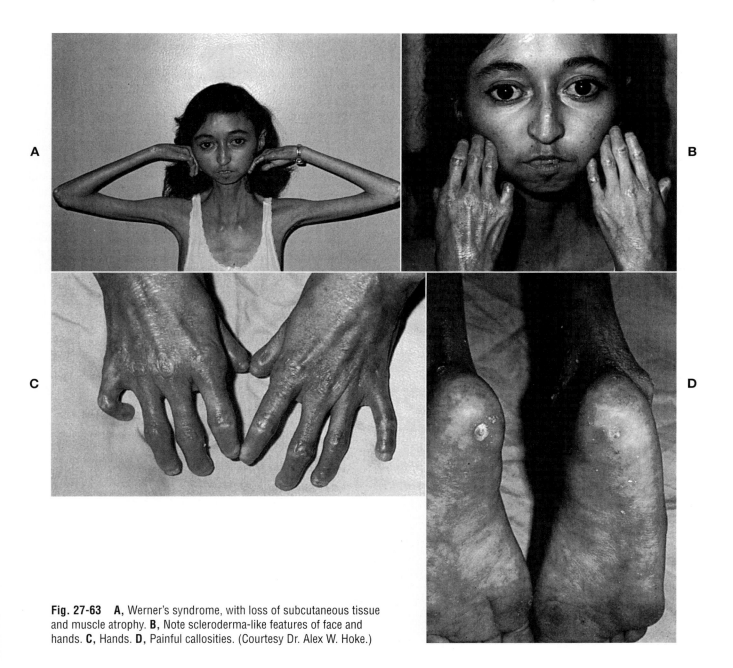

Fig. 27-63 **A,** Werner's syndrome, with loss of subcutaneous tissue and muscle atrophy. **B,** Note scleroderma-like features of face and hands. **C,** Hands. **D,** Painful callosities. (Courtesy Dr. Alex W. Hoke.)

Werner's syndrome should be differentiated from scleroderma, atopic dermatitis (cataracta dermatogenes), ectodermal dysplasia, dystrophia myotonica, lipoatrophic diabetes, Rothmund's syndrome, progeria with nanism, and Turner's syndrome.

Progeria (Hutchinson-Gilford Syndrome)

Progeria, or Hutchinson-Gilford syndrome, is characterized by dwarfism, alopecia, generalized atrophy of the skin and muscles, enlarged head with prominent scalp veins, and a high incidence of generalized atherosclerosis, usually fatal

by the second decade. There are usually sclerodermatous plaques on the extremities. Treatment is symptomatic: chiefly, control of diabetes mellitus and treatment of leg ulcerations.

Cottoni F, et al: Werner's syndrome associated with myelofibrosis. *J Am Acad Dermatol* 1994, 30:1034.

Duvic M, et al: Werner's syndrome. *Dermatol Clin* 1995, 13:163.

Ichikawa K, et al: Cloning and characterization of a novel gene, WS-3, in human chromosome 8p11-p12. *Gene* (Netherlands) 1997, 189:277.

Ishikawa Y, et al: Unusual features of thyroid carcinoma in Japanese patients with Werner syndrome and possible genotype-phenotype relations to cell type and race. *Cancer* 1999, 85:1345.

Morita K, et al: Werner's syndrome associated with basal cell epithelioma. *J Dermatol* 1995, 22:693.

Pesce K, et al: The premature aging syndromes. *Clin Dermatol* 1996, 14:161.

OTHER CONGENITAL ANOMALIES
Congenital Fistulas of the Lower Lip

Variously known as *labial fistulae, lip pits,* or *congenital pits of the lower lip,* these are characterized as paired circular or slitlike depressions on either side of the center of the lower lip at the edge of the vermilion border. The fistulous tract in the center of the depression may extend 5 to 25 mm into the lip. Frequently, these are associated with cleft lip and cleft palate, and/or preauricular sinuses. Originally described by Van der Woude in 1954, these occur in about 1 in 200,000 births.

An autosomal dominant inheritance is frequently found. Other reported associations include hypodontia, absence of second premolars, natal teeth, ankyloglossia, syndactyly, equinovarus foot deformity, and congenital heart disease. Lower lip pits may be found in other congenital disorders, such as popliteal pterygium syndrome (cleft palate, popliteal web, toenail dysplasia, syndactyly of the toes, and genital anomalies), and occasionally in orofaciodigital syndrome type I (oral frenula and clefts, hypoplasia of alae nasi, and digital asymmetry). Surgical excision is the treatment of choice.

Franceschetti-Klein Syndrome

First associated with Treacher Collins in 1900, Franceschetti and Klein wrote extensively about the disease in the 1940s and coined the term *mandibulofacial dysostosis,* which consists, when complete, of palpebral antimongoloid fissures, hypoplasia of the facial bones, macrostomia, vaulted palate, malformations of both the external and internal ear, buccal-auricular fistula, abnormal development of the neck with stretching of the cheeks, accessory facial fissures, and skeletal deformities. Patients who have the complete syndrome usually die in infancy, but patients with the abortive type may live to an old age. The abortive type is called *Treacher Collins syndrome* (Fig. 27-64). The syndrome is inherited as an autosomal dominant trait. The identified gene mutations have been localized to chromosome 5q31.3-32.

Congenital Auricular Fistula

This anomaly occurs in the preauricular region, often in several members and generations of a family. On each side

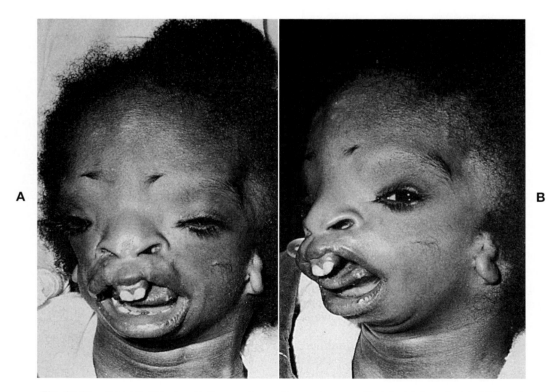

Fig. 27-64 **A** and **B,** Treacher Collins syndrome (incomplete mandibulofacial dysostosis). Wide-set eyes, deformed nose and ears, enlarged mouth, small lower jaw. (Courtesy Dr. G. Salinger.)

just anterior to the external ear there is a small dimple, pore, or fistulous opening that may extend even into the middle ear (Fig. 27-65). Occasionally, cysts or granulomatous nodules that simulate scrofuloderma or epidermal inclusion cysts may develop at these sites.

Branchial Cleft Cyst

Developmental anomalies of the branchial clefts may occur as cysts, sinus tracts, or cartilage remnants in the skin (Fig. 27-66). They may be bluish in color. These anomalies appear in a line extending from a point anterior to the ears downward on the neck to the insertion of the sternomastoid muscle into the sternum. Most frequently, cysts or sinus

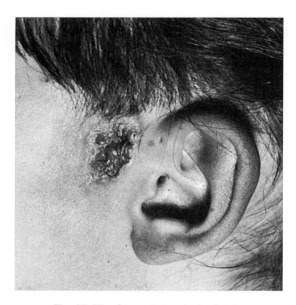

Fig. 27-65 Congenital auricular fistula.

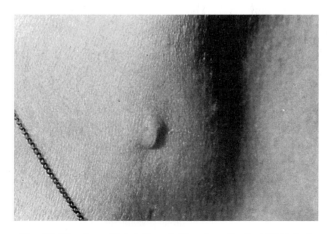

Fig. 27-66 Branchial cleft cyst. (Courtesy Dr. Axel W. Hoke.)

tracts are seen. They are soft, tender lesions from which rancid, sebumlike material may exude. Frequently, secondary infection calls attention to the disorder. Inheritance pattern is autosomal dominant with incomplete penetrance.

The differential diagnosis should include tuberculous lymphadenitis, epidermoid cyst, and primary as well as metastatic carcinoma must be considered. If the subcutaneous mass is blue, one should suspect lymphadenopathy, epidermal inclusion cyst, blue nevus, pilomatricoma, other adnexal tumors, vascular lesions, carotid and thyroid tumors, metastatic carcinoma, and other cysts (thyroglossal, bronchogenic, and thymic). Treatment is excision by a well-qualified head-and-neck surgeon since the lesions, especially in sinus tracts, may extend deeply into areas encompassing vital structures.

Popliteal Pterygium Syndrome

Pterygia or skinfolds may extend from the thigh down to the heel and thus prevent extension or rotation of the legs (Fig. 27-67). In addition, crural pterygia may be present. Cryptorchism, bifid scrotum, agenesis of the labia majora, cleft lip and palate, adhesions between the eyelids, syndactyly, and talipes equinovarus are all commonly seen in this syndrome. An autosomal dominant inheritance trait is presumed.

Apert's Syndrome (Acrocephalosyndactyly)

Apert's syndrome, a disorder that is autosomal dominantly inherited, is characterized by synostosis of the feet, hands, carpi, tarsi, cervical vertebrae, and skull. The facial features are distorted and the second, third, and fourth fingers are fused into a bony mass with a single nail. Oculocutaneous albinism and severe acne vulgaris have been reported with Apert's syndrome. The molecular basis is specific: two adjacent amino acid substitutions (S252W or P253R) occurring in the linking region between the second and third immunoglobulin domains of the fibroblast growth factor receptor (FGFR) 2 gene. Isotretinoin is useful in treating the severe acne.

Whistling Face Syndrome

Also known as *cranio-carpo-tarsal syndrome, Freeman-Sheldon syndrome, Windmill-Vane-Hand syndrome,* and *distal arthrogryposis type 2,* in this rare disorder the child appears to be whistling all the time. This configuration is the result of microstomia, deep-set eyes, flattened midface, coloboma, and alterations of the nostrils. Ulnar deviation of the fingers, kyphoscoliosis, and talipes equinovarus may be present. Brain anomalies have also been reported. An autosomal dominant trait is responsible for this syndrome, although a nonlethal recessive variant has also been reported. The prenatal diagnosis can be made on ultrasound. Surgical intervention may be required for some patients.

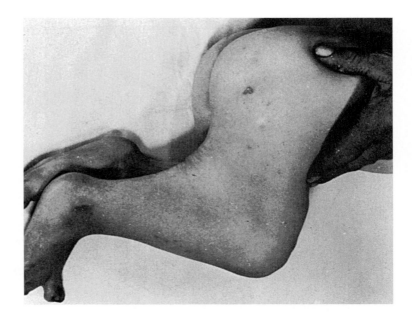

Fig. 27-67 Popliteal pterygium syndrome. (Courtesy Dr. R.J. Gorlin.)

Cardoso ER, et al: A recessively inherited non-lethal form of popliteal pterygium syndrome. *Br J Oral Maxillofac Surg* 1998, 36:138.

Cohen MM Jr, et al: An updated pediatric perspective on the Apert syndrome. *Am J Dis Child* 1993, 147:989.

Cruickshanks GF, Brown S, Chitayat D: Anesthesia for Freeman-Sheldon syndrome using a laryngeal mask airway. *Can J Anaesth* 1999, 46:783.

Dizon MJ: Treacher Collins syndrome. *Hum Mol Genet* 1996, 5:1391.

Lajeunie E, et al: Clinical variability in patients with Apert's syndrome. *J Neurosurg* 1999, 90:443.

Limova M, et al: A nodule on the side of the neck in a child: branchial cleft cyst. *Arch Dermatol* 1992, 128:1397.

Marasovich WA, et al: Otolaryngologic findings in whistling face syndrome. *Arch Otolaryngol Head Neck Surg* 1989, 115:1373.

Marres HA, et al: The Treacher Collins syndrome: a clinical, radiological, and genetic linkage study on two pedigrees. *Arch Otolaryngol Head Neck Surg* 1995, 121:509.

Robbins-Furman P, et al: Prenatal diagnosis of Freeman-Sheldon syndrome (whistling face). *Prenat Diagn* 1995, 15:179.

Soekarman D, et al: Variable expression of the popliteal pterygium syndrome in two three-generation families. *Clin Genet* 1995, 47:169.

Velez A, et al: Congenital lower lip pits (Van der Woude syndrome). *J Am Acad Dermatol* 1995, 32:520.

Zampino G, et al: Severe form of Freeman-Sheldon syndrome associated with brain anomalies and hearing loss. *Am J Med Genet* 1996, 29:293. _____ ▲

CHAPTER 28

Dermal and Subcutaneous Tumors

The dermis and subcutaneous tissue contain many cellular elements, all capable of both reactive and neoplastic proliferation. In this chapter, such processes, which are derived from vascular endothelial cells, fibroblasts, myofibroblasts, smooth muscle cells, Schwann cells, and lipocytes, will be reviewed. We will also discuss several neoplasms of cells invading or aberrantly present in the dermis, such as metastatic cancer, endometriosis, and meningioma.

CUTANEOUS VASCULAR ANOMALIES

It is difficult to classify cutaneous vascular anomalies: some lesions fulfill criteria for both hyperplasia and neoplasms but eventually undergo complete regression; some have similar clinical appearances but vary in histologic findings and prognosis. We will follow the classification scheme that divides these anomalies into hamartomas, malformations, dilation of preexisting vessels, hyperplasias, benign neoplasms, and malignant neoplasms.

Mulliken JB: Classification of vascular birthmarks. In Mulliken JB, Young AE, editors: Vascular birthmarks: hemangiomas and malformations. Philadelphia, 1988, WB Saunders.
Requena L, et al: Cutaneous vascular anomalies. Part I. *J Am Acad Dermatol* 1997, 37:523.
Requena L, et al: Cutaneous vascular neoplasms. Part II. *J Am Acad Dermatol* 1997, 37:887.
Requena L, et al: Cutaneous vascular neoplasms. Part III. *J Am Acad Dermatol* 1998, 38:143. _____ ▲

Hamartomas

Hamartomas are characterized by an abnormal arrangement of tissues normally present.

Phakomatosis Pigmentovascularis.
Patients with a combination of vascular malformations and melanocytic or epidermal nevi are grouped into four subtypes of this disorder. All have nevus flammeus. Those with a coexisting epidermal nevus have type I; if aberrant mongolian spots are present, it is classified as type II; if a nevus spilus is seen, it is classified as type III; and when both ectopic mongolian spots and nevus spilus are present, it is classified as type IV. The last three categories may or may not have associated nevus anemicus. If cutaneous disease only is present, the patient's condition is designated subgroup a; if there is associated systemic disease, subtype b is appended. Associated systemic findings may include intracranial and visceral vascular anomalies, ocular abnormalities, and hemihypertrophy of the limbs. Type II is the most common (85%); type III has been associated with multiple granular cell tumors. Nearly all patients reported have been Asian.

Gilliam AC, et al: Phakomatosis pigmentovascularis type IIb with iris mammillations. *Arch Dermatol* 1993, 129:340.
Guiglia MC, et al: Multiple granular cell tumors associated with giant speckled lentiginous nevus and nevus flammeus in a child. *J Am Acad Dermatol* 1991, 24:359.
Libow LF: Phakomatosis pigmentovascularis type IIIb. *J Am Acad Dermatol* 1993, 29:305.
Mahroughan M, et al: Phakomatosis pigmentovascularis. *Pediatr Dermatol* 1996, 13:36.
Van Gysel D, et al: Phakomatosis pigmentovascularis. *Pediatr Dermatol* 1996, 13:33. _____ ▲

Eccrine Angiomatous Hamartoma (Sudoriparous Angioma).
Eccrine angiomatous hamartoma usually appears as a solitary nodular lesion on the acral areas of the extremities, particularly the palms and soles. This lesion appears at birth or in early childhood and is often associated with pain and hyperhidrosis. The lesion is a dome-shaped, tender, bluish hemangioma that will vary from 12 to 20 mm in diameter. When stroked or pinched, the dark-red, dusky, moderately soft lesion forms characteristic drops or beaded rings of perspiration (Fig. 28-1).

Histologically, there is a combination of lobules of mature eccrine glands and ducts with thin-walled blood vessels. The condition is benign and slow growing; however, excision may be necessary because of pain.

Calderone DC, et al: Eccrine angiomatous hamartoma. *J Dermatol Surg Oncol* 1994, 20:837.

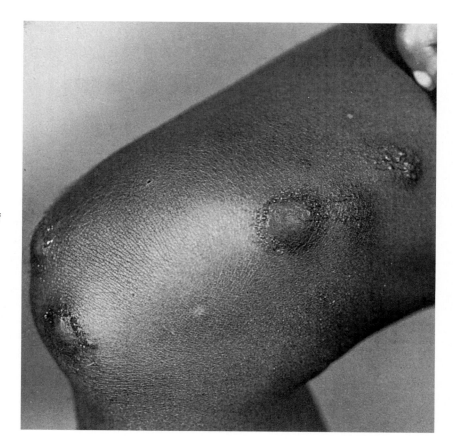

Fig. 28-1 Eccrine angiomatous hamartoma on the thigh of a 3-year-old child. Notice the beads of perspiration on the periphery, induced by stroking. (Courtesy Dr. Louis Shapiro.)

Diaz-Landaeta L, et al: Hyperhidrotic, painful lesion. *Arch Dermatol* 1993, 129:107.
Smith C, et al: Eccrine angiomatous hamartoma. *Pediatr Dermatol* 1996, 13:139. ▲

Malformations

These are abnormal structures that result from an aberration in embryonic development. The abnormality may result from a functional alteration as in nevus anemicus, or from an anatomic malformation. The latter are then subdivided according to the type of vessel involved: capillary, venous, arterial, lymphatic, or combined.

Nevus Anemicus.

Nevus anemicus is a congenital disorder characterized by macules of varying size and shape that are paler than the surrounding skin and cannot be made red by trauma, cold, or heat. The nevus resembles vitiligo, but there is a normal amount of melanin. Wood's light does not accentuate it, and diascopy causes it to merge into the surrounding blanched skin. The patches are usually round and well defined with irregular edges. Sometimes the condition occurs as a linear lesion that may appear in any location. Rarely, it may occur in neurofibromatosis, tubercular sclerosis, or as one component of phakomatosis pigmentovascularis. In nevus anemicus the triple response of Lewis lacks a flare, but outside the nevus a flare does develop after rubbing the skin. Histologic, pharmacologic, and exchange transplant studies have demonstrated donor dominance and suggested that the defect is attributable to increased sensitivity of the blood vessels to catecholamines.

Mizutani H, et al: Loss of cutaneous delayed hypersensitivity reactions in nevus anemicus. *Arch Dermatol* 1997, 133:617.
Mountcastle EA, et al: Nevus anemicus. *J Am Acad Dermatol* 1986, 14:628. ▲

Nevus Oligemicus.

In 1981, Davies et al reported from St. John's Hospital a 46-year-old man with a large patch of erythema on the flank that had persisted for 14 years. It did not look like an angioma clinically or histologically. It was cooler than normal skin and had decreased blood flow. Davies and his colleagues thought that this was because of vasoconstriction in deep vessels; the vasodilation remained unexplained. They named it *nevus oligemicus,* considering it a variant of nevus anemicus. Two other cases have since been reported; the clinical lesions were of a livid color.

Davies MG, et al: Nevus oligemicus. *Arch Dermatol* 1981, 117:111.
Plantin P, et al: Nevus oligemicus. *J Am Acad Dermatol* 1992, 26:268. ▲

Cutis Marmorata Telangiectatica Congenita (Congenital Phlebectasia, Van Lohuizen's Syndrome).

Cutis marmorata telangiectatica congenita is characterized by the presence of a purplish, reticulated vascular network with a generalized or segmental distribution (Fig. 28-2), phlebectasia, telangiectasia, and at times ulcerations, usually involving the extremities. The mottling is pronounced and is made more distinct by crying, vigorous activity, and cold. There is a female preponderance.

Other common anomalies associated with this disorder include varicosities, nevus flammeus, and hypoplasia and hypertrophy of soft tissue and bone. These and other more unusual associated anomalies, such as generalized congenital fibromatosis and rectal and genital anomalies, occur in about 50% of cases.

The differential diagnosis includes residual vascular lesions from neonatal lupus and Bockenheimer's syndrome. Bockenheimer's syndrome appears in childhood and shows progressive development of large venous ectasias involving one limb. No treatment is required. Many will become less noticeable with time.

Carrascosa JM, et al: Cutis marmorata telangiectatica congenita or neonatal lupus? *Pediatr Dermatol* 1996, 13:230.

Del Giudice SM, et al: Cutis marmorata telangiectatica with multiple congenital anomalies. *Arch Dermatol* 1986, 122:1060.

Pehr K, et al: Cutis marmorata telangiectatica congenita. *Pediatr Dermatol* 1993, 10:6.

Weilepp AE, et al: Association of glaucoma with cutis marmorata telangiectatica congenita. *J Am Acad Dermatol* 1996, 35:276. ▲

Nevus Flammeus.

Nevus flammeus nuchae, or "stork bite," is a common congenital capillary malformation of the skin, present in from 25% of newborns. It may persist in at least 5% of the population. It usually is a pink-red macule situated on the posterior midline between the occipital protuberance and the tip of the spine of the fifth cervical vertebra. The long axis is usually up and down. A similar appearing midline nevus flammeus or "salmon patch" on the glabellar region or on one upper eyelid is common in infants. They are present in approximately 15% of newborns. They tend to fade or even disappear during childhood.

The port-wine stain variant (Fig. 28-3) occurs in an estimated 3 in 1000 children, is present at birth, and ranges from small red macules to large red patches that are partially or completely blanched by diascopic pressure. They vary in color from pink to dark or bluish red. The lesions are usually unilateral and located on the face and neck, although they may be widespread and involve as much as half the body. The most common site is a unilateral distribution on the face (Fig. 28-4). The mucous membrane of the mouth may be involved. Although the surface of a nevus flammeus is usually smooth, small vascular nodular outgrowths or warty excrescences may be present or develop in the course of life

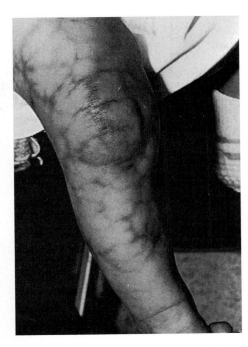

Fig. 28-2 Congenital phlebectasia in a 14-month-old child. (Courtesy V.M. Torres-Rodriguez.)

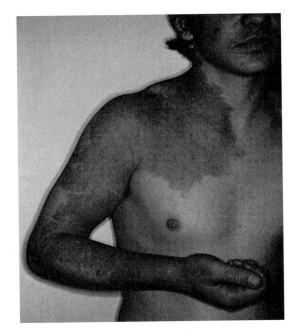

Fig. 28-3 Nevus flammeus in a young man.

(Fig. 28-5). These lesions often become more bluish or purple with age; however, they sometimes become fainter but rarely disappear. Several reports document multiple basal cell carcinomas occurring in adult life over sites of long-standing nevus flammeus. Rarely, nevus flammeus

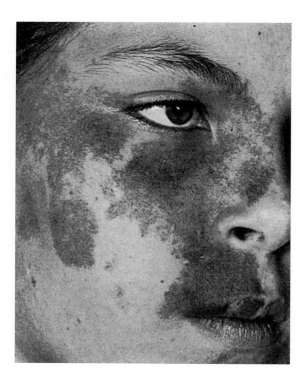

Fig. 28-4 Nevus flammeus (port-wine stain).

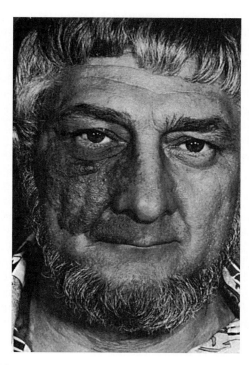

Fig. 28-5 Nevus flammeus in an adult. (Courtesy Dr. J. Cook.)

may appear as an acquired condition, usually with onset after trauma.

Nevus flammeus in the area supplied by the ophthalmic division of the trigeminal cranial nerve is a component of the Sturge-Weber syndrome (encephalotrigeminal angiomatosis). In Enjoiras et al's review of port-wine stains, they found that 90 of 106 patients had only the cutaneous vascular abnormality, without any leptomeningeal component. Thus, Sturge-Weber syndrome is present in only 10% of patients with all or most of the V1 branch of the trigeminal nerve involved. Bilateral port-wine stains occur in 40% of these patients (Fig. 28-6). Homolateral leptomeningeal angiomatosis, when present, may clinically manifest as epilepsy, mental retardation, hemiplegia, hemisensory defects, and homonymous hemianopsia. Characteristic calcifications are present in the outer layers of the cerebral cortex; these consist of double-contoured "tram lines" that follow the brain convolutions. Ocular abnormalities such as glaucoma, buphthalmos, retinal detachment, and blindness affect approximately 50% of patients. These may be present without leptomeningeal involvement.

Overgrowth of soft tissue and underlying bone may occur in an affected extremity, giving rise to the Klippel-Trenaunay syndrome. The Klippel-Trenaunay syndrome is characterized by port-wine malformations in association with deep venous system malformations, superficial varicosities, and bony and soft tissue hypertrophy. Management is commonly affected by deeper vessel involvement, which will be discussed later in this chapter.

Port-wine stains are components of many rare congenital disorders. Occasionally, nevus flammeus may be associated with nevus anemicus, pigmented nevi such as nevus spilus or atypical Mongolian spots, or epidermal nevi. Such patients have a condition called *phakomatosis pigmentovascularis*. The Beckwith-Wiedemann syndrome may comprise facial port-wine stain, macroglossia, omphalocele, visceral hyperplasia, occasionally hemihypertrophy, and hypoglycemia. Cobb syndrome (cutaneous meningospinal angiomatosis) is a nonfamilial disorder characterized by a port-wine hemangioma or other vascular malformation, found in or very close to the dermatome, supplied by a segment of the spinal cord, and containing a venous or arteriovenous malformation. Kyphoscoliosis is common and multiple neurologic, gastrointestinal, urologic, and skeletal abnormalities may also be present. Proteus syndrome is characterized by vascular malformations including nevus flammeus, hemihypertrophy, macrodactyly, verrucous epidermal nevus, soft-tissue subcutaneous masses, and cerebriform overgrowth of the plantar surface. Roberts' syndrome consists of a facial port-wine stain and hypomelia, hypotrichosis, growth retardation, and cleft lip. The Wyburn-Mason syndrome consists of unilateral retinal arteriovenous malformation associated with ipsilateral port-wine stain near the affected eye. This may be present in association with Sturge-Weber syndrome. The TAR syndrome is defined by congenital thrombocytopenia, bilateral absence or hypoplasia of the radius, and port-wine stain. Coats' disease manifests retinal telangiectasia and ipsilateral facial port-

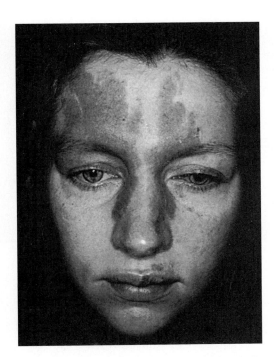

Fig. 28-6 Sturge-Weber syndrome, with bilateral nevus flammeus, retinal detachment, and cerebral calcification.

wine stain. Histologic changes are not conspicuous: there is only moderate dilation of capillaries in the subpapillary network.

Laser therapy has been used with satisfactory results. The laser of choice is the flashlamp pumped pulsed dye laser. This laser localizes heat within ectatic vessels through its 450-microsecond pulse and is operated at 577 or 585 nm. It has been hypothesized that the best results occur with thinner lesions in younger patients; however, similar clinical results have been achieved in adults and children. Treatment in patients before school age is often desirable. Lightening the lesion without scarring is generally possible after multiple treatments.

Ashinoff R, et al: Flashlamp pumped pulsed-dye laser for port-wine stains in infancy. *J Am Acad Dermatol* 1991, 24:467.

Duhra P, et al: Basal-cell carcinoma complicating a port-wine stain. *Clin Exp Dermatol* 1991, 16:63.

Enjoiras O, et al: Facial port-wine stains and Sturge-Weber syndrome. *Pediatrics* 1985, 76:48.

Fitzpatrick RE, et al: Flashlamp-pumped pulsed-dye laser treatment of port-wine stains. *J Dermatol Surg Oncol* 1994, 20:743.

Flint ID, et al: Acquired persistent erythematous patch on the neck. *Arch Dermatol* 1994, 130:509.

Garden JM, et al: Laser treatment of port-wine stains and hemangiomas. *Dermatol Clin* 1997, 15:373.

Goldberg NS, et al: Sacral hemangiomas and multiple congenital anomalies. *Arch Dermatol* 1986, 122:684.

Haedersdal M, et al: Changes in skin redness, pigmentation, echostructure, thickness, and surface contour after 1 pulsed-dye laser treatment of port-wine stains in children. *Arch Dermatol* 1998, 134:175.

Jacob AG, et al: Klippel-Trenaunay syndrome. *Mayo Clin Proc* 1998, 73:28.

Mahroughan M, et al: Phakomatosis pigmentovascularis. *Pediatr Dermatol* 1996, 13:36.

Osburn K, et al: Congenital pigmented and vascular lesions in newborn infants. *J Am Acad Dermatol* 1987, 16:788.

Paller AS: The Sturge-Weber syndrome. *Pediatr Dermatol* 1987, 4:300.

Requena L, et al: Cutaneous vascular anomalies. *J Am Acad Dermatol* 1997, 37:523.

Rosen S, et al: Port-wine stain. *J Am Acad Dermatol* 1987, 17:164.

Smoller BR, et al: Port-wine stains. *Arch Dermatol* 1986, 122:177.

Truhan AP, et al: Magnetic resonance imaging: its role in the neuroradiologic evaluation of neurofibromatosis, tuberous sclerosis, and Sturge-Weber syndrome. *Arch Dermatol* 1993, 129:219.

van der Horst CC, et al: Effect of the timing of treatment of port-wine stains with the flash-lamp-pumped pulsed-dye laser. *N Engl J Med* 1998, 338:1028. ▲

Verrucous Vascular Malformation. This is a vascular malformation with typical features, clinically and histologically, of a malformation of dermal and subcutaneous capillaries and veins. The difference is that this congenital vascular lesion develops a later secondary characteristic: a verrucous component. These are bluish red, well-defined lesions occurring on the lower extremities mostly, but also on the chest or forearm (Fig. 28-7). Angiokeratoma circumscriptum is a designation that is less favorable, as angiokeratomas occur secondary to dilation of existing blood vessels whereas this lesion is a vascular malformation with a hyperkeratotic surface.

Wong DS, et al: Unilateral keratotic vascular lesion on the leg: verrucous hemangioma. *Arch Dermatol* 1996, 132:705. ▲

Venous Malformation. The old term for this lesion was *cavernous hemangioma;* however, it is not a neoplasm but rather a congenital malformation of veins. They present as rounded, bright red or deep purple, spongy nodules. The consistency may be varied by the admixture of fibrous connective tissue; however, it is usually readily compressible. The lesions occur chiefly on the head and neck (Fig. 28-8) but may be found in any region, including the mucous membranes (Fig. 28-9). They may occur as a localized venous malformation; however, there is usually a deep component where there is connection by capillaries or veins to the venous circulation. This leads to venous ectasias that may be complicated by recurrent thrombophlebitis. Calcified phleboliths, localized hyperhidrosis, and pressure on surrounding structures such as nerves are signs and symptoms that may be seen in this otherwise generally asymptomatic lesion. There may be a chronic consumptive coagulopathy in these slow flow malformations. These malformations persist and because of the deep components are not amenable to laser therapy or even surgical resection. Compression may be helpful. Customized, snug-fitting garments are preferable to elastic bandages.

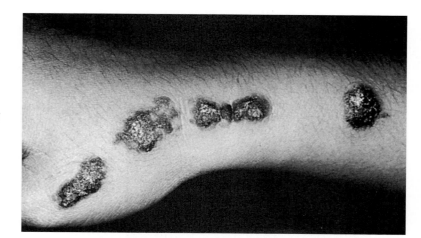

Fig. 28-7 Verrucous vascular malformation. (Courtesy Dr. T. Mathias.)

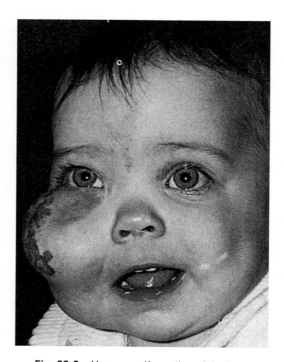

Fig. 28-8 Venous malformation of the face.

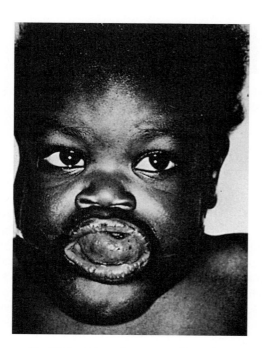

Fig. 28-9 Intraoral venous malformation.

Several syndromes are associated with venous malformations. The *Bannayan-Riley-Ruvalcaba syndrome* may include multiple cutaneous and visceral venous, capillary, and lymphatic malformations, macrocephaly, pseudopapilledema, systemic lipoangiomatosis, spotted pigmentation of the penis, hamartomatous intestinal polyps, and rarely trichilemmomas. The presence of the latter raises the possibility that this syndrome is caused by a genetic defect closely related to Cowden's disease. Inheritance is by autosomal dominance.

Maffucci's syndrome, also known as *dyschondroplasia with hemangiomata,* is characterized by multiple vascular

malformations with dyschondroplasia. The dyschondroplasia is manifested by uneven bone growth as a result of the defects of ossification, with enchondromatous changes that result in multiple and frequent fractures in the period of bone growth. During the prepubertal years, 1- to 2-cm nodules appear on the small bones of the hand or foot (Fig. 28-10). Later, larger nodules, the enchondromas, appear on the long bones (Fig. 28-11). Much later, similar lesions appear on the trunk. Sarcomatous degeneration occurs in 50% of patients. The distribution of the lesions is mostly unilateral. Multiple venous malformations of the skin and mucous membranes are present in this nonhered-

eroded flexural skin. In penicillamine-induced dermopathy there is a hemorrhagic macular stain that is often surmounted by milia.

The method of treatment depends on the cause. If lymphangiectasis results from cancer infiltration and pressure, treatment of the primary process may reopen the lymphatic drainage and lead to resolution. If the condition results from penicillamine or topical steroid application, decreasing the dose or discontinuance may result in improvement. If the underlying process is fibrosis and scarring and the involved part is amenable to pressure dressings or a pump, the chylous discharge may be improved. If recurrent erysipelas is a recurrent complication long-term oral antibiotic prophylaxis may prevent this.

Ambrojo P, et al: Cutaneous lymphangiectases after therapy for carcinoma of the cervix: a case with unusual clinical and histological features. *Clin Exp Dermatol* 1990, 15:57.

Buckley DA, et al: Vulvar lymphangiectasia due to recurrent cellulitis. *Clin Exp Dermatol* 1996, 21:215.

DiLeonardo M, et al: Acquired cutaneous lymphangiectasias secondary to scarring from scrofuloderma. *J Am Acad Dermatol* 1986, 14:688.

Goldstein JB, et al: Penicillamine dermopathy with lymphangiectases. *Arch Dermatol* 1989, 125:92.

Leshin B, et al: Lymphangioma circumscriptum following mastectomy and radiation therapy. *J Am Acad Dermatol* 1986, 115:1117.

Moon SE, et al: Acquired cutaneous lymphangiectasia. *Br J Dermatol* 1993, 129:193.

Pena JM, et al: Cutaneous lymphangiectases associated with severe photoaging and topical corticosteroid application. *J Cutan Pathol* 1996, 23:175.

Stone MS: Central-facial papular lymphangiectases. *J Am Acad Dermatol* 1997, 36:493. _____ ▲

Hyperplasias

Angiolymphoid Hyperplasia with Eosinophilia. Patients with angiolymphoid hyperplasia with eosinophilia (AHLE) usually present with pink to red-brown, dome-shaped, dermal papules or nodules of the head or neck, especially about the ears and on the scalp (Fig. 28-22). AHLE may also occur in the mouth, trunk and extremities, penis, and vulva. Grouped lesions merge to form plaques or grapelike clusters. There is a female preponderance, and the average age of onset is 32 years. Symptoms can be pain or pruritus; these may occur after trauma. An underlying arteriovenous shunt may occur as a result of damage to and repair of an artery or vein.

Histologically, anomalous vascular hyperplasia with varying degrees of mixed cellular infiltrate that is dominated by lymphocytes and eosinophils are present in well-circumscribed dermal nodules.

Lesions do not spontaneously regress. Treatment with surgical excision is successful in 65% of cases. Recurrence after excision will be the case if an underlying arteriovenous shunt is present and not excised. Intralesional corticosteroids and pulsed dye laser therapy are also excellent treatments. Cryotherapy, pentoxifylline, indomethacin, and

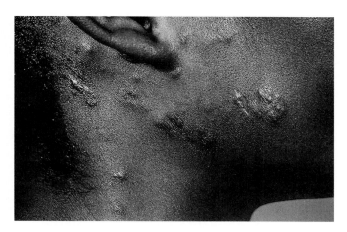

Fig. 28-22 Angiolymphoid hyperplasia with eosinophilia.

electrodesiccation have also been successful in isolated cases. Difficult cases have been controlled with vinblastine, and partial responses to intralesional cytotoxic agents have been reported.

Much confusion in the literature has centered on distinguishing AHLE from Kimura's disease. The latter is an inflammatory disorder that presents as massive subcutaneous swelling in the periauricular and submandibular region in young Asian men. Histologically, prominent germinal centers with eosinophils are present in the subcutaneous tissue. Although blood vessels are abundant, changes are less prominent than in AHLE. Additionally Kimura's is frequently accompanied by lymphadenopathy, peripheral blood eosinophilia, and an elevated IgE level. Thus, Kimura's is an inflammatory disorder, whereas AHLE is a hyperplasia of the vessels of the dermis.

Bartralot R, et al: Angiolymphoid hyperplasia with eosinophilia affecting the oral mucosa. *Br J Dermatol* 1996, 134:744.

Chun SI, et al: Kimura's disease and angiolymphoid hyperplasia with eosinophilia. *J Am Acad Dermatol* 1992, 27:954.

Lertzman BH, et al: Pulsed dye laser treatment of angiolymphoid hyperplasia with eosinophilia lesions. *Arch Dermatol* 1997, 133:920.

Olsen TG, et al: Angiolymphoid hyperplasia with eosinophilia. *J Am Acad Dermatol* 1985, 12:781.

Requena L, et al: Cutaneous vascular proliferation. *J Am Acad Dermatol* 1997, 37:887. _____ ▲

Pyogenic Granuloma. A pyogenic granuloma is a small, almost always solitary, sessile or pedunculated, raspberry-like vegetation of exuberant granulation tissue ("proud flesh") (Fig. 28-23). The lesion occurs chiefly in children and is a dull red color. It occurs most often on an exposed surface: on the hands, forearms, or face, or at sites of trauma (Fig. 28-24). The lesion also occurs in the mouth, especially on the gingiva, most often in pregnant women (granuloma gravidarum) (Fig. 28-25). The sole of the foot or the nail fold of a toe or finger (Fig. 28-26) may also be the site of

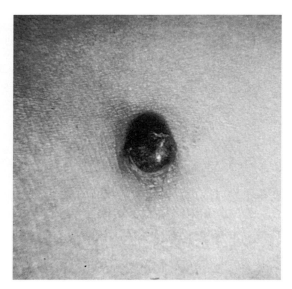

Fig. 28-23 Pyogenic granuloma.

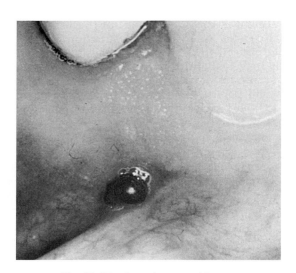

Fig. 28-25 Granuloma gravidarum.

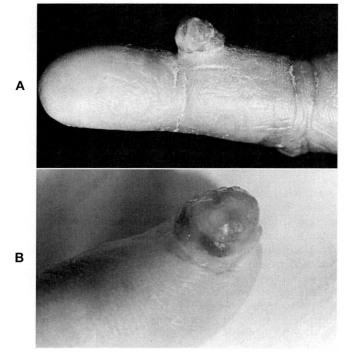

Fig. 28-24 A, Pyogenic granuloma. Note collarette at base. **B,** Pyogenic granuloma occurring in pregnancy. (Courtesy Dr. Axel W. Hoke.)

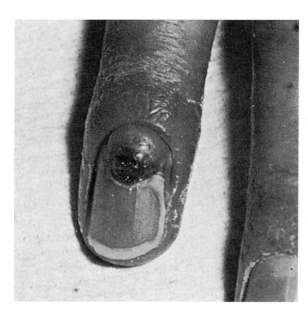

Fig. 28-26 Pyogenic granuloma resembling malignant melanoma of the nail bed.

such a lesion, where it may be mistaken for a melanoma. Such nail fold lesions may be seen in patients treated with isotretinoin or indinavir. Isotretinoin treatment of acne vulgaris can be complicated by numerous exuberant pyogenic granuloma–like proliferations on truncal lesions. Pyogenic granulomas bleed easily on the slightest trauma

and, if cut off superficially, promptly recur. Recurring lesions may have one or many satellite lesions (Fig. 28-27).

Histologically, the epidermis is thinned. Growth is composed of numerous newly formed capillaries suggestive of a capillary hemangioma. The capillaries are lined with endothelial cells in a single layer. There is also an

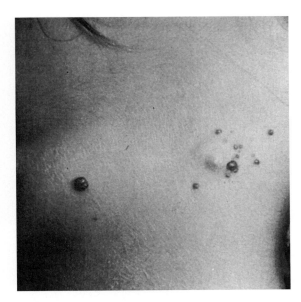

Fig. 28-27 Pyogenic granuloma with multiple satellites.

edematous fibroblastic proliferation in the stroma that surrounds the vascular tumor. Intraluminal papillary endothelial proliferation occurs in cases with satellite lesions.

Pyogenic granuloma is usually diagnosed easily; however, it can be mistaken for Kaposi's sarcoma (especially histologically), melanoma, melanotic whitlow, senile angioma, atypical fibroxanthoma, bacillary angiomatosis, and metastatic carcinoma.

Treatment is the shelling out of the lesion with a dermal curette or the performance of a deep shave excision, followed by destruction of the base by fulguration, under local anesthesia. At other times a recalcitrant lesion will persist after the above therapy has been followed, and excision or laser ablation may become necessary. The drug-induced variety will regress after lowering of the dose or discontinuation of the medication.

Bouscarat F, et al: Paronychia and pyogenic granuloma of the great toes in patients treated with indinavir. *N Engl J Med* 1998, 338:1776.

Ceyhan M, et al: Pyogenic granuloma with multiple dissemination in a burn lesion. *Pediatr Dermatol* 1997, 14:213.

Patrice SJ, et al: Pyogenic granuloma. *Pediatr Dermatol* 1991, 8:267.

Shah M, et al: Eruptive pyogenic granulomas. *Br J Dermatol* 1995, 133:795.

Tay YK, et al: Treatment of pyogenic granuloma in children with the flashlamp-pumped pulsed-dye laser. *Pediatrics* 1997, 99:368. ▲

Intravascular Papillary Endothelial Hyperplasia.
Masson described in 1923, in infected hemorrhoids, intravascular papillary proliferation mimicking angiosarcoma. This reactive hyperplasia of endothelial cells may occur in the dermis, or subcutis, or intramuscularly. In the skin they appear as red or purplish 5-mm to 5-cm papules or nodules on the head, neck, or upper extremities. The condition may be present in a wide variety of underlying vascular lesions and is seen as a response to intravascular thrombosis and attendant organization.

Histologic examination reveals hyaline papillary projections lined by endothelial cells within a dilated, thin-walled vessel. Thrombi may still be present. Excision is curative as a rule.

Gordon ML, et al: Flesh-colored nodules on the forearm. *Arch Dermatol* 1988, 124:263.

Hashimoto H, et al: Intravascular papillary endothelial hyperplasia. *Am J Dermatopathol* 1983, 5:539.

Stewart M, et al: Multiple lesions of intravascular papillary endothelial hyperplasia (Masson's lesions). *Arch Pathol Lab Med* 1994, 118:315.

Wong RC, et al: Intravascular papillary endothelial hyperplasia. *J Am Acad Dermatol* 1984, 10:110. ▲

Benign Neoplasms

Angioma Serpiginosum.
Angioma serpiginosum, first described by Hutchinson in 1889, is characterized by minute, copper-colored to bright red angiomatous puncta that have a tendency to become papular. These puncta occur in groups, which enlarge through the constant formulation of new points at the periphery, whereas those at the center fade. In this manner small rings or serpiginous patterns are formed. No purpura is present, but a netlike or diffuse erythema forms the background. In the areas undergoing involution, a delicate tracery of rings and lines, a fine desquamation, and, at times, a semblance of atrophy are seen. Slight lichenification and scaling may be evident in the papular lesions. The eruption predominates on the lower extremities but may affect any region of the body (Fig. 28-28) except the palms, soles, and mucocutaneous junctions. Although it affects both sexes at all ages, 90% of cases occur in girls under 16. It is usually slowly progressive and chronic, and although involution may occur it is probably never complete. Treatment with a pulsed dye laser will improve or eliminate such lesions.

Angioma serpiginosum must be differentiated from the progressive pigmentary disease of Schamberg. In the latter, the so-called cayenne pepper spots are macules that tend to coalesce and form diffusely pigmented patches. Purpura annularis telangiectodes (Majocchi) is bilateral and is characterized by acute outbreaks of telangiectatic points that spread peripherally and form small rings. In lichenoid purpuric and pigmentary dermatosis of Gougerot and Blum, the primary lesion is a minute, lichenoid, reddish brown papule that is sometimes hemorrhagic. It has a tendency toward central involution and residual pigmentation.

In angioma serpiginosum, the most important histologic finding is dilated and tortuous capillaries in the dermal papillae and the upper dermis. No inflammatory infiltrate or extravasation of red cells is observed. The dilated capillaries show no alkaline phosphatase activity, in contrast to normal capillaries.

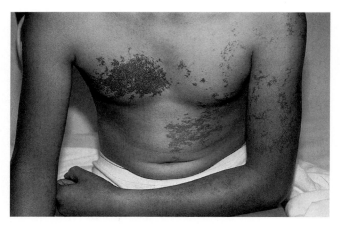

Fig. 28-28 Angioma serpiginosum.

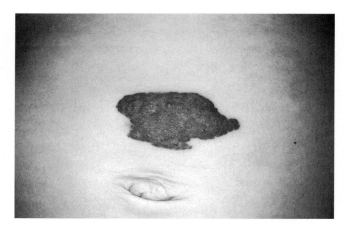

Fig. 28-29 Infantile hemangioma.

Kumakiri M, et al: Angioma serpiginosum. *J Cutan Pathol* 1980, 7:410.
Long CC, et al: Treatment of angioma serpiginosum using a pulsed tunable
dye laser. *Br J Dermatol* 1997, 136:631. _____ ▲

Infantile Hemangioma (Strawberry Hemangioma).

Strawberry (capillary) hemangiomas, the most common
benign tumor of childhood, may be present at birth in one
third of cases. The remainder appear very rapidly, in a
hitherto inconspicuous pale macule, when the child is 2
weeks to 2 months of age. The usual size is 1 to 60 mm in
diameter, although rarely, as much as an entire extremity
may be involved. Sixty percent are on the head and neck,
but they may occur anywhere (Fig. 28-29). The dome-
shaped lesion is usually a dull red, and when involution
begins, streaks or islands of white appear in the lesion as it
flattens (Fig. 28-30). The lesions have sharp borders; they
are soft and easily compressed.

Generally, they tend to grow over the first year or so,
remain stable for a while, and then in the course of months
or years, involute spontaneously. Approximately 30%
resolve by the third year, 50% by age 5, and 70% by the
time the patient is 7 years of age. The skin may appear
normal after involution, but more commonly, atrophy,
telangiectasia, or anetoderma-type redundancy is present.

The majority of these lesions occur sporadically, yet Blie
et al reported six kindreds in which infantile hemangiomas
and/or vascular malformations occurred among various
affected family members in an autosomal dominant fashion.
Approximately 7% of hemangiomas may occur in association with structural malformations.

One grouping of associated abnormalities is the PHACE
syndrome. This acronym, proposed by Frieden et al in 1996,
denotes the association of *p*osterior fossa brain malformations (primarily the Dandy-Walker malformation), *h*eman-
giomas, *a*rterial anomalies, *c*oarctation of the aorta and
cardiac defects, and *e*ye abnormalities. In three reported
cases, sternal clefting and abdominal raphae were present,
and designation in those cases could have been PHACES.

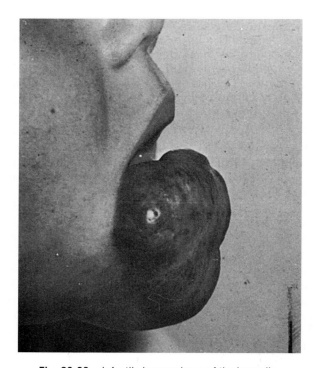

Fig. 28-30 Infantile hemangioma of the lower lip.

The hemangiomas present in the 43 cases reviewed by
Frieden et al tended to be large, plaquelike, and facial in
location, frequently involving more than one dermatome.
They recommended that brain imaging studies be performed
in all infants with such hemangiomas.

Multiple hemangiomas, usually 1 to 10 mm in size, may
appear in the first few weeks to months of life and can be
large in number. If they are purely cutaneous, generally they
involute without sequelae, and the term *benign neonatal
hemangiomatosis* is applied. However, visceral lesions may
be present in the central nervous system (CNS), the lungs,
the liver, or other organs. When internal lesions are present,
complications may occur, such as GI or CNS bleeding,

high-output cardiac failure, obstructive jaundice, or respiratory failure; this results in a high mortality rate among untreated patients. This more ominous variant is called *diffuse neonatal hemangiomatosis.*

Histologically, strawberry marks are composed of primitive endothelial cells similar to those that are found before the embryonic development of true venous channels. Ultrastructurally, they lack typical Weibel-Palade bodies but do have crystalloid inclusions typical of embryonic endothelium. They proliferate intraluminally. Later the endothelium flattens and the lumina are more apparent because of increased blood flow. In time, fibrosis becomes pronounced as involution progresses.

In most cases intervention detracts from the quality of the ultimate cosmetic result. Proponents of early treatment point out that many of these hemangiomas remain significant body image factors to children when they enter school. Cryotherapy or laser ablation of early lesions has generally not been successful. The pulsed dye laser can help the residual involuted lesions with residual telangiectasias; however, the depth of the hemangiomas does not allow the lasers to be effective in growing or stable childhood hemangiomas. The so-called Cyrano defect, a hemangioma that causes the end of the nose to become bulbous, may be successfully approached surgically in many cases before beginning school. Additionally, surgical intervention in small pedunculated hemangiomas and eyelid tumors may also be excellent options. Finally, compressive wraps may improve extremity hemangiomas.

Specific circumstances necessitate treatment. These are considered indications for intervention: severe hemorrhage, thrombocytopenia, threatened cardiovascular compromise from high-output cardiac failure, nasal or auditory canal obstruction, hepatic hemangiomatosis, skin ulceration, or threatened interference with vital functions such as feeding, respiration, passage of urine or stool, limb function, tissue destruction, or vision. There is a risk of occlusion amblyopia, astigmatism, and myopia from periorbital hemangiomas. Additionally, strong consideration should be given to treatment of those hemangiomas that may lead to permanent disfigurement or long-term psychologic consequences such as large hemangiomas of the ear, nose, glabellar area, or lips.

Intralesional steroids or oral prednisone may be employed. Oral treatment requires use of prednisone at a dose of 2 or 3 mg/kg/day. In the 30% of patients who respond well to treatment, the enlarging hemangioma stops growing in 3 to 21 days. Ulcerations will heal within 2 weeks. The lesion will usually shrink if treatment is continued for 30 to 90 days. Laryngeal involvement and stridor, if present, are usually dramatically relieved by treatment. Repeated courses of treatment may be undertaken if rebound of growth occurs on discontinuation of the steroidal agent. Some experts recommend prolonged low-dose oral steroids over a 12-month period to prevent this rebound phenome-

non. In another 40%, the clinical situation will stabilize with this treatment; however, the remaining 30% do not respond to treatment with prednisone. Treatment with recombinant interferon alfa-2a or -2b may result in a good response in 80% of patients. The dose is usually 1 to 3 million units/m^2/day. Many patients require prolonged therapy for 6 to 10 months or more. Thyroid dysfunction and neurotoxicity in the form of spastic diplegia may occur.

Achauer BM, et al: Management of hemangioma of infancy. *Plast Reconstr Surg* 1997, 99:1301.

Barlow CF, et al: Spastic diplegia as a complication of interferon alfa-2a treatment of hemangiomas of infancy. *J Pediatr* 1998, 132:527.

Blie F, et al: Familial segregation of hemangiomas and vascular malformations as an autosomal dominant trait. *Arch Dermatol* 1998, 134:718.

Chowdri NA, et al: Intralesional corticosteroid therapy for childhood cutaneous hemangiomas. *Ann Plast Surg* 1994, 33:46.

Drolet BA, et al: Hemangiomas in children. *N Engl J Med* 1999, 341:173.

Eichenfield LF: Evolving knowledge of hemangiomas and vascular malformations. *Arch Dermatol* 1998, 134:740.

Enjolras O, et al: Superficial hemangiomas: associations and management. *Pediatr Dermatol* 1997, 14:173.

Enjolras O, et al: Vascular tumors and vascular malformations. *Adv Dermatol* 1998, 13:375.

Esterly NB: Cutaneous hemangiomas, vascular stains and malformations, and associated syndromes. *Curr Probl Pediatr* 1996, 26:3.

Frieden IJ: Which hemangiomas to treat—and how? *Arch Dermatol* 1997, 133:1593.

Frieden IJ, et al: Guidelines of care for hemangiomas of infancy. American Academy of Dermatology Guidelines/Outcomes Committee. *J Am Acad Dermatol* 1997, 37:631.

Frieden IJ, et al: PHACE syndrome. *Arch Dermatol* 1996, 132:307.

Garden JM, et al: Laser treatment of port-wine stains and hemangiomas. *Dermatol Clin* 1997, 15:373.

Kaplan M, et al: Clinical pearl: use of self-adhesive, compressive wraps in the treatment of limb hemangiomas. *J Am Acad Dermatol* 1995, 32:117.

Management of hemangiomas. *Pediatr Dermatol* 1997, 14:57.

Stratte EG, et al: Multimodal management of diffuse neonatal hemangiomatosis. *J Am Acad Dermatol* 1996, 34:337.

Tamayo L, et al: Therapeutic efficacy of interferon alfa-2b in infants with life-threatening giant hemangiomas. *Arch Dermatol* 1997, 133:1567. ▲

Cherry Angiomas (Senile Angiomas, De Morgan Spots).

Oval or circular, slightly elevated, 0.5 to 6 mm in diameter, ruby-red papules are the commonest of vascular anomalies (Fig. 28-31). It is a rare 30-year-old person who does not have a few, and the number increases with age; probably every 70-year-old person has some. Most are on the trunk; they are rarely seen on the hands, feet, or face. Early lesions may mimic petechiae. When lesions are surrounded by a purpuric halo, amyloidosis should be suspected.

They are easily obliterated without scarring by light electrodesiccation or laser ablation, but most patients accept reassurance and do not request their removal.

Ross BS, et al: Laser treatment of acquired vascular lesions. *Dermatol Clin* 1997, 15:385.

Schmidt CP: Purpuric halos around hemangiomas in systemic amyloidosis. *Cutis* 1991, 48:141. ▲

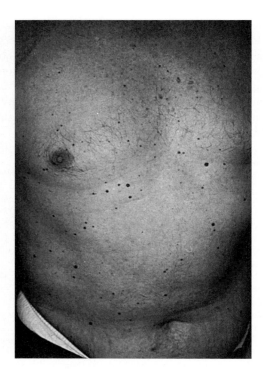

Fig. 28-31 Cherry angiomas.

Targetoid Hemosiderotic Hemangioma. In 1988, Santa Cruz and Aronberg described a lesion characterized by a central brown or violaceous papule that is surrounded by an ecchymotic halo. These acquired hemangiomas occur in the young to middle aged and are present on the trunk or extremities. They likely represent trauma to a preexisting hemangioma with thrombosis and subsequent recanalization. Carlson et al studied 33 cases and concluded that targetoid hemosiderotic hamangiomas (THH) are variants of solitary angiokeratomas. They found three patients had episodic changes of swelling, darkening, and/or involution.

Carlson JA, et al: Targetoid hemosiderotic hemangioma. *J Am Acad Dermatol* 1999, 41:215.
Morganroth GS, et al: Targetoid hemangioma associated with pregnancy and the menstrual cycle. *J Am Acad Dermatol* 1995, 32:282.
Santa Cruz DJ, Aronberg J, et al: Targetoid hemosiderotic hemangioma. *J Am Acad Dermatol* 1988, 19:550. _____ ▲

Microvenular Hemangioma. This recently described acquired benign vascular neoplasm presents as an asymptomatic, slowly growing, 0.5- to 2.0-cm reddish lesion on the forearms or other sites of young to middle-aged adults. Monomorphous, elongated blood vessels with small lumina involve the entire reticular dermis. The main differential diagnosis is that of Kaposi's sarcoma.

Black RJ, et al: Microvascular haemangioma. *Clin Exp Dermatol* 1995, 20:260.
Hunt SJ, et al: Microvenular hemangioma. *J Cutan Pathol* 1991, 18:235. ▲

Tufted Angioma (Angioblastoma). This lesion usually develops in infancy or early childhood on the neck and upper trunk. These angiomas are ill-defined, dull red macules with a mottled appearance; they vary from 2 to 5 cm. Some show clusters of smaller angiomatous papules superimposed on the main macular area. Histologic examination reveals small, circumscribed angiomatous tufts and lobules scattered in the dermis in a so-called cannonball pattern. Most lesions slowly extend with time, being progressive but benign in nature. Occasional spontaneous regression is documented; however, treatment with pulsed dye laser, excision, high-dose steroids, and interferon alfa has been successful in individual cases.

Bernstein EF, et al: Tufted angioma of the thigh. *J Am Acad Dermatol* 1994, 31:307.
Suarez SM, et al: Response of deep tufted angioma to interferon alfa. *J Am Acad Dermatol* 1995, 33:124.
Wilson Jones E, et al: Tufted angioma (angioblastoma). *J Am Acad Dermatol* 1989, 20:214. _____ ▲

Glomeruloid Hemangioma. This distinctive benign vascular neoplasm was described in 1990 and has only been reported in patients with POEMS syndrome (Crow-Fukase syndrome).

POEMS syndrome consists of *p*olyneuropathy (severe sensorimotor), *o*rganomegaly (heart, spleen, kidneys), *e*ndocrinopathy, *M* protein, and *s*kin changes (hyperpigmentation, hypertrichosis, thickening, sweating, clubbed nails, leukonychia, and angiomas). Small, firm, red to violaceous papules appear on the trunk and proximal extremities in approximately one third of patients. Histologically, they may be microvenular hemangiomas, cherry angiomas, multinucleated cell angiohistiocytomas or glomeruloid hemangiomas. The latter consists of ectatic vascular structures containing aggregates of capillary loops within a dilated lumina, simulating the appearance of a renal glomerulus.

Bardwick PA, et al: Plasma cell neoplasia with polyneuropathy, organomegaly, endocrinopathy, M protein and skin changes. *Medicine* 1980, 59:311.
Kanitakis J, et al: Cutaneous angiomas in POEMS syndrome. *Arch Dermatol* 1988, 124:695.
Perniciaro C: POEMS syndrome. *Semin Dermatol* 1995, 14:162.
Puig L, et al: Cutaneous angiomas in POEMS syndrome. *J Am Acad Dermatol* 1985, 12:961.
Rongioletti F, et al: Glomeruloid hemangioma: a cutaneous marker of POEMS syndrome. *Am J Dermatopathol* 1994, 16:175.
Shelley WB, et al: The skin changes in the Crow-Fukase (POEMS) syndrome. *Arch Dermatol* 1987, 123:85. _____ ▲

Kaposiform Hemangioendothelioma. Kaposiform hemangioendothelioma (KHE) is an uncommon vascular tumor that affects infants and young children. It was first designated KHE in 1993. Although it frequently occurs in the retroperitoneum, they may present as multinodular soft tissue masses, purpuric macules, plaques, and multiple telangiectatic papules. The lesions extend locally and usually involve the skin, soft tissues and even bone. The cutaneous variant may be associated with lymphangiomatosis. KHE is locally aggressive, may be complicated by platelet trapping and consumptive coagulopathy (Kasabach-Merritt syndrome), but distant metastases have not yet been reported.

Histologically, there are combined features of cellular infantile hemangioma and Kaposi's sarcoma. Additionally, in some tumors lymphangiomatosis is seen sharply separated from the vascular lesion. There is a multilobular appearance that closely resembles that of tufted angioma, but in KHE they are larger, less circumscribed, and involve the deep soft tissue and even bone.

The prognosis depends on the depth and location of the lesion. If localized to the skin they may be successfully excised. However, because of their tendency for deep and infiltrative growth this is usually not possible. Prednisone may shrink the tumor or limit tumor expansion. If Kasabach-Merritt phenomenon occurs prognosis will be more linked to this complication.

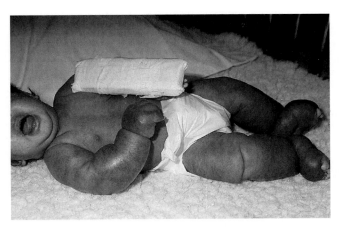

Fig. 28-32 Kasabach-Merritt syndrome.

Beaubien IR, et al: Kaposiform hemangioendothelioma. *J Am Acad Dermatol* 1998, 38:799.

Enjorlas O, et al: Vascular tumors and vascular malformations. *Adv Dermatol* 1998, 13:375.

Requena L, et al: Cutaneous vascular proliferations. Part II. *J Am Acad Dermatol* 1997, 37:887.

Vin Christian K, et al: Kaposiform hemangioendothelioma. *Arch Dermatol* 1997, 133:1573. _____ ▲

Kasabach-Merritt Syndrome (Hemangioma with Thrombocytopenia). This syndrome is seen in infants at an average age of 7 weeks. Before the onset of the acute event the infant will often have a reddish or bluish plaque or tumor on the limb or trunk, or in rare instances no lesion at all. None of these preexisting lesions are typical infantile "strawberry" hemangiomas. The lesions usually have an associated lymphatic component and are best classified as kaposiform hemangioendotheliomas. It should also be stated that some patients with venous malformations will have a chronic consumptive coagulopathy that occurs throughout life, and this is not to be confused with Kasabach-Merritt syndrome.

The infant suddenly develops a painful violaceous mass in association with purpura and thrombocytopenia (Fig. 28-32). The most striking sign is the bleeding tendency, especially in the hemangioma itself or into the chest or abdominal cavities. The spleen may be enlarged. Hemoglobin, platelets, fibrinogen, and factors II, V, and VIII are all reduced. Prothrombin time and partial thromboplastin time are prolonged, and fibrin split products are elevated. Cases of microangiopathic hemolytic anemia have also been described. Repeated episodes of bleeding may occur, and although these may be spontaneous, it is not uncommon for bleeding to be precipitated by surgery, directed either at the hemangioma or elsewhere. The mortality may be as high as 30%, with most deaths being secondary to bleeding complications.

Some authors emphasize that it is usually a self-limited disorder and recommend expectant observation as the best approach initially. If steroids, heparin, antiplatelet drugs, or interferon alfa-2a are considered, it is well to consult with a hematologist.

Carrington PR, et al: Kasabach-Merritt syndrome with bone involvement. *J Am Acad Dermatol* 1993, 29:117.

Enjorlas O, et al: Vascular tumors and vascular malformations. *Adv Dermatol* 1998, 13:375.

Esterly NB: Kasabach-Merritt syndrome. *J Am Acad Dermatol* 1983, 8:504. _____ ▲

Acquired Progressive Lymphangioma (Benign Lymphangioendothelioma). The term *acquired progressive lymphangioma* was introduced by Wilson-Jones in 1976 to designate a group of lymphangiomas that occur anywhere in young individuals, grow slowly, and present as bruiselike lesions or erythematous macules. The histologic appearance is that of delicate endothelium-lined spaces dissecting between collagen bundles. A similarity to the plaque stage of Kaposi's sarcoma may be striking. Simple excision is curative. Prednisolone has caused extensive lesions to regress.

Herron GS, et al: Benign lymphangioendothelioma. *J Am Acad Dermatol* 1994, 31:362.

Tudaki T, et al: Acquired progressive lymphangioma as a flat erythematous patch on the abdominal wall of a child. *Arch Dermatol* 1988, 124:699.

Watanabe M, et al: Acquired progressive lymphangioma. *J Am Acad Dermatol* 1983, 8:663. ⎯⎯⎯⎯⎯⎯⎯⎯⎯⎯⎯⎯⎯ ▲

Glomus Tumor (Glomangioma).

The solitary glomus or neuromyoarterial tumor, arising from a normal glomus, is most frequently a skin-colored or slightly dusky blue firm nodule 1 to 20 mm in diameter. The subungual tumor shows a bluish tinge through the translucent nail plate (Fig. 28-33). The tumor is usually extremely tender and paroxysmal pain occurs frequently. Sensitivity is likely to be present constantly, and when touched the tumor responds with severe radiating pain. However, nontender glomus tumors are encountered. The characteristic location is subungual, but it may occur on the fingers and arms, or elsewhere. Tsuneyoshi et al, in a review of 63 cases, found that 34 of 37 digital lesions were from women, and 19 of 26 lesions in other, widely scattered, sites were from men. High-resolution MRI will reliably detect the limits of the tumor before surgery is undertaken. Progressive growth may lead to ulceration.

Multiple glomangiomas also occur (Fig. 28-34). These usually nontender lesions are generally widely distributed over the body. These may be inherited as an autosomal dominant trait and can be congenital (Fig. 28-35). Clinically, they may resemble lesions of blue rubber bleb nevus. When grouped in one area they may appear as a confluent mass.

Histologically, the glomus tumor contains numerous vascular lumina lined by a single layer of flattened endothelial cells. Peripheral to the endothelial cells are a few to many layers of glomus cells, seen in the multiple and solitary types, respectively. Both solitary and multiple glomus tumors are related to the arterial segment of the cutaneous glomus, the Sucquet-Hoyer canal. The glomus cells are smooth-muscle cells and stain with vimentin.

Treatment of glomus tumors is best carried out by complete excision, which immediately produces relief from pain. The subungual tumors are most difficult to locate and eradicate since they are usually small, seldom more than a few millimeters in diameter.

Rare reports of glomangiosarcomas describe large, deeply located extremity lesions that consist of sarcomatous areas intermingled with areas of benign glomus tumor.

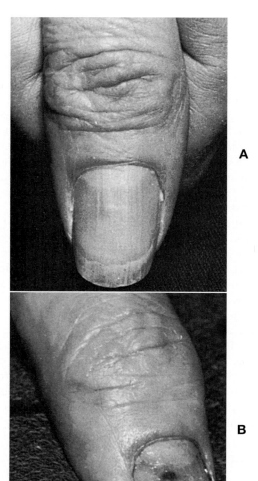

Fig. 28-33 Glomus tumor. **A,** A small area of discoloration under the right side of midline of the nail. **B,** The lesion showing more prominently after complete avulsion of the nail.

Baselga E, et al: Multiple acquired vascular nodules. *Pediatr Dermatol* 1997, 14:327.

Drape JL, et al: Standard and high resolution magnetic resonance imaging of glomus tumors of toes and fingertips. *J Am Acad Dermatol* 1996, 35:550.

Lopez-Rios F, et al: Glomangiosarcoma of the lower limb. *J Cutan Pathol* 1997, 24:571.

Naversen DN, et al: Giant glomangioma. *J Am Acad Dermatol* 1986, 14:1083.

Tsuneyoshi M, et al: Glomus tumor. *Cancer* 1982, 50:1601.

Yen A, et al: Multiple painful blue nodules. *Arch Dermatol* 1996, 132:704.

Yoon T-Y, et al: Giant congenital multiple patch-like glomus tumors. *J Am Acad Dermatol* 1999, 40:826. ⎯⎯⎯⎯⎯⎯⎯⎯⎯⎯⎯⎯ ▲

Hemangiopericytoma.

A hemangiopericytoma is a nontender, bluish red tumor that occurs on the skin or in the subcutaneous tissues on any part of the body. The firm, usually solitary nodule may be up to 10 cm in diameter.

Histologically, the tumor is composed of endothelium-lined tubes and sprouts that are filled with blood and surrounded by cells with oval or spindle-shaped nuclei (pericytes). Wide local excision is the treatment of choice, but radiation therapy may produce excellent palliation.

It is difficult to distinguish between benign and malignant forms of hemangiopericytoma. Nearly half of the

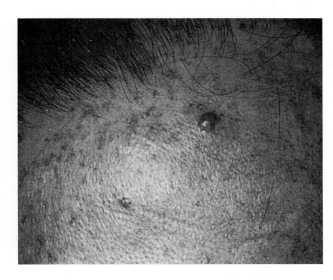

Fig. 28-34 Glomus tumors on the forehead of a 64-year-old man.

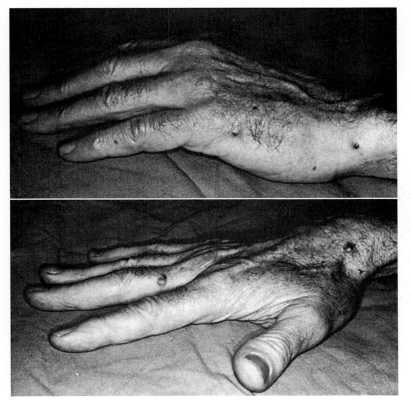

A

B

Fig. 28-35 **A** and **B,** Familial multiple glomangiomas.

malignant hemangiopericytomas of soft tissues metastasize (Fig. 28-36). The rate of metastases from lesions of the skin is closer to 20%. The most common cause of death is pulmonary metastasis.

An exception is found in tumors that arise at birth, or up to 7 months of age. These infantile tumors are almost always cutaneous or subcutaneous, and do not metastasize.

Ferreira CM, et al: Congenital hemangiopericytoma of the skin. *Int J Dermatol* 1997, 36:521.
Nunnery EW, et al: Hemangiopericytoma. *Cancer* 1981, 47:906. ▲

Proliferating Angioendotheliomatosis. The conditions that have historically fallen under the classification of

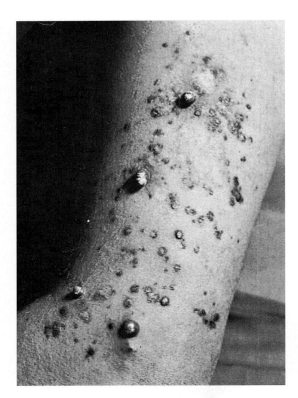

Fig. 28-36 Multiple hemangiopericytomata with malignant changes. (Courtesy Dr. W. Raab, Vienna, and Grosse-Edition, Berlin.)

proliferating angioendotheliomatosis are included here briefly, not because they are hemangiomas, but because histologically they may fall into the differential diagnosis of vascular proliferative lesions.

Diseases designated *angioendotheliomatosis* have historically been divided into two groups: a reactive, involuting type and a malignant, rapidly fatal type. They were reported to have similar clinical lesions and histologic findings but different basic mechanisms, the reactive type being an endothelial proliferation, and the malignant type a manifestation of lymphoma.

The reactive type of angioendotheliomatosis is uncommon. It occurs in patients who have subacute bacterial endocarditis, Chagas' disease, pulmonary tuberculosis, cryoproteinemia, severe atherosclerotic disease and in patients with no identifiable underlying process. They present with red to purple patches, plaques, nodules, petechiae, and ecchymoses, usually of the lower extremities. A variant of this is diffuse dermal angiomatosis, in which the lesions are associated with atherosclerosis. The lesion occurs in areas of vascular insufficiency and clears with revascularization.

Histologically, the capillaries in the dermis and subcutaneous tissue are dilated and are filled with proliferating endothelial cells, usually without atypia. The course in this type is characterized by involution over 1 to 2 years. Therapy for the underlying condition has been felt to hasten involution.

The malignant type of angioendotheliomatosis is actually a lymphoma and now is called *intravascular lymphoma*. It is a rapidly progressive disease: usually death ensues within 10 months of diagnosis. The mean age at onset is 55 years. Reddish purple plaques, nodules, or patches developing in the skin. Multisystem involvement is characteristic, with the CNS often involved. There may be progressive dementia or focal signs that reflect ischemic infarcts. Kidney, heart, lung, and gastrointestinal tract lesions may occur. Biopsy will show a proliferation of atypical cells that fill the lumen of cutaneous vessels. Immunochemical stains for leukocyte/common antigen have confirmed the lymphomatous nature of these cells. Angioendotheliomatosis is usually B cell in phenotype, but cases of T-cell lineage have been reported.

Doxorubicin alone, as well as in combination with vincristine, prednisone, and cyclophosphamide, has been effective in isolated cases.

Berger TG, et al: Angioendotheliomatosis. *J Am Acad Dermatol* 1988, 18:407.
Gupta AK, et al: Proliferating angioendotheliomatosis. *Arch Dermatol* 1986, 122:314.
Kimyai-Asadi A, et al: Diffuse dermal angiomatosis. *J Am Acad Dermatol* 1999, 40:257.
Lazova R, et al: Reactive angioendotheliomatosis. *Am J Dermatopathol* 1996, 18:63.
Perniciaro C, et al: Malignant angioendotheliomatosis is an angiotropic intravascular lymphoma. *Am J Dermatopathol* 1995, 17:242.
Wilson BB: Indurated telangiectatic plaques. *Arch Dermatol* 1992, 128:255. ▲

Malignant Neoplasms

Kaposi's Sarcoma. Moritz Kaposi (*cop-O-see*) described this vascular neoplasm in 1872 and called it multiple benign pigmented idiopathic hemorrhagic sarcoma. Since his description, the disease has been reported in five separate clinical settings, with different presentations, epidemiology, and prognoses.

The five subtypes of Kaposi's sarcoma (KS) are (1) classic KS, an indolent disease seen chiefly in middle-aged men of Southern and Eastern European origin; (2) African cutaneous KS, a locally aggressive process affecting middle-aged Africans in tropical Africa; (3) African lymphadenopathic KS, an aggressive disease of young patients, chiefly children under age 10; (4) KS in patients immunosuppressed by AIDS; or by (5) lymphoma or immunosuppressive therapy.

CLINICAL FEATURES

Classic Kaposi's sarcoma. The early lesions appear most commonly on the toes or soles as reddish, violaceous, or bluish black macules and patches that spread and coalesce to form nodules or plaques (Figs. 28-37 and 28-38). These have a rubbery consistency. There may be brawny edema of the affected leg. Macules or nodules may appear, usually much later, on the arms and hands, and rarely may extend to the face, ears (Fig. 28-39), trunk, genitalia (Fig. 28-40), or

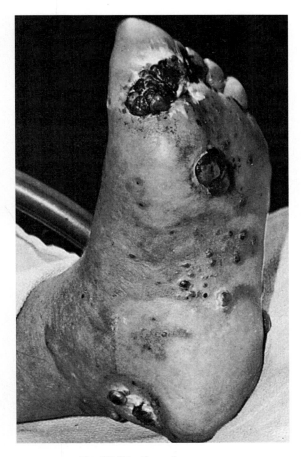

Fig. 28-37 Kaposi's sarcoma.

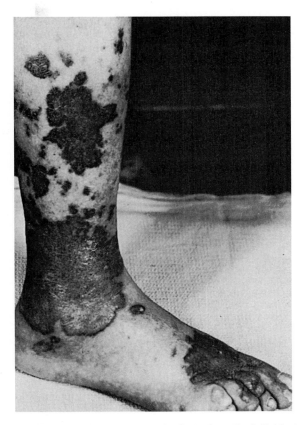

Fig. 28-38 Kaposi's sarcoma on the foot where the initial lesions are first seen. Large violaceous plaques, infiltrations, and angiomatous tumors may be present.

buccal cavity, especially the soft palate. The course is slowly progressive and may lead to great enlargement of the lower extremities as a result of lymphedema.

However, there may be periods of remission, particularly in the early stages of the disease, when nodules may undergo spontaneous involution. After involution there may be an atrophic and hyperpigmented scar.

African cutaneous Kaposi's sarcoma. Nodular, infiltrating, vascular masses occur on the extremities, mostly of men between ages 20 and 50. This form of KS is endemic in tropical Africa, and has a locally aggressive but systemically indolent course.

African lymphadenopathic Kaposi's sarcoma. Lymph node involvement, with or without skin lesions, may occur in children under 10 years of age. The course is aggressive, often terminating fatally within 2 years of the onset.

AIDS-associated Kaposi's sarcoma. Cutaneous lesions begin as one or several red to purple-red macules, rapidly progressing to papules, nodules, and plaques. There is a predilection for the head, neck, trunk, and mucous membranes (Figs. 28-41 and 28-42). A fulminant, progressive course with nodal and systemic involvement is ex-

pected. This may be the presenting manifestation of HIV infection.

Immunosuppression-associated Kaposi's sarcoma. The lesion's morphology resembles that of classic KS; however, the site of presentation is more variable.

INTERNAL INVOLVEMENT. The gastrointestinal tract is the site of the most frequent internal involvement in classic KS. The small intestine is probably the most commonly involved viscus. In addition, the lungs, heart, liver, conjunctiva, adrenal glands, and lymph nodes of the abdomen may be involved. Skeletal changes are characteristic and diagnostic. Bone involvement is always an indication of widespread disease. Changes noted are rarefaction, cysts, and cortical erosion.

African cutaneous KS is frequently accompanied by massive edema of the legs, caused by arborizing infiltrates along cutaneous lymphatics, and frequent bone involvement.

African lymphadenopathic KS has been reported among Bantu children, who develop massive involvement of the lymph nodes, especially the cervical nodes, preceding the appearance of skin lesions. The children also develop

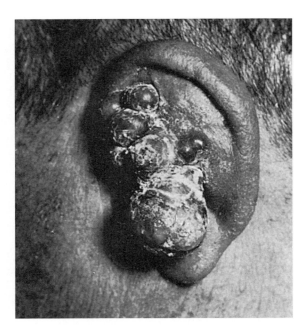

Fig. 28-39 Kaposi's sarcoma of the ear.

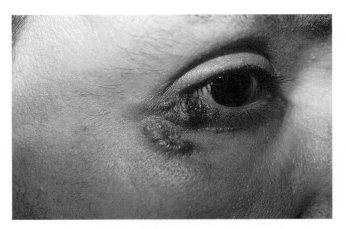

Fig. 28-41 AIDS-related Kaposi's sarcoma.

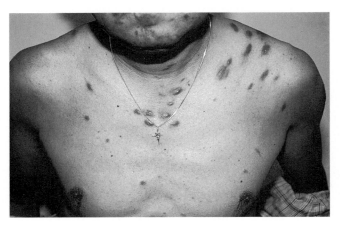

Fig. 28-42 AIDS-related Kaposi's sarcoma.

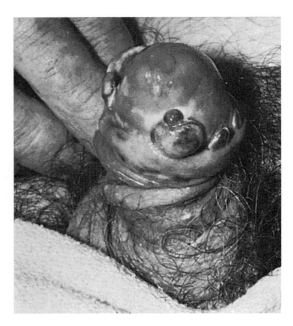

Fig. 28-40 Kaposi's sarcoma on glans penis. (Courtesy Dr. J. Teisch.)

lesions on the eyelids and conjunctiva from which masses of hemorrhagic tissue hang down. Eye involvement is often associated with swelling of the lacrimal, parotid, and submandibular glands with a picture similar to Mikulicz's syndrome.

In AIDS-associated KS, 25% of patients have cutaneous involvement alone, whereas 29% have visceral lesions only. The most frequent sites of visceral involvement are the lungs (37%), gastrointestinal tract (50%), and lymph nodes (50%). Visceral involvement ultimately occurs in more than 70% of patients with AIDS-associated KS.

Other immunosuppressed patients with KS may have visceral involvement in a variable percentage of cases.

EPIDEMIOLOGY. Kaposi's sarcoma is worldwide in distribution. In Europe there appear to be foci of classic KS in Galicia, near the Polish-Russian border, and extending southward to Austria and Italy. In New York City, KS has occurred mostly in elderly male Galician Jews and southern Italians. In Africa, KS occurs largely south of the Sahara. Northeast Congo and Rwanda-Burundi areas have the highest prevalence, and to a lesser extent, West and South Africa.

The highest prevalence of AIDS-related KS is among male homosexuals, with an average age of 35. Very few reports have documented the exceptional occurrence of KS in patients with AIDS who acquired their infection from intravenous drug use, or in Haitians, children, or people with hemophilia. As the HIV epidemic progresses, many fewer cases of KS occur than were occurring in the 1980s.

Patients at risk for developing KS associated with other causes of immunosuppression include those with iatrogenic suppression from oral prednisone or other chronic immunosuppressive therapies, as may be given to transplant patients.

Kaposi's sarcoma is associated with an increased risk of developing second malignancies, such as malignant lymphomas (Hodgkin's disease, T-cell lymphoma, non-Hodgkin's lymphoma), leukemia, and myeloma. The risk of lymphoreticular malignancy is about 20 times greater in KS patients than in the normal population.

ETIOPATHOGENESIS. Kaposi believed this disease to be of multicentric origin, and it is still so viewed. Kaposi's sarcoma is formed by proliferation of abnormal vascular endothelial cells. Human herpesvirus 8 (HHV-8) was first found in tissue of a patient with KS and was reported in 1994. Now it has been found in KS lesional tissue irrespective of clinical type. Detection of HHV-8 in HIV-infected individuals who do not have KS is predictive of the development of KS, usually within 2 to 4 years. It is considered at this time that sexual or fecal-oral transmission is the most likely means of acquiring this infection. The HHV-8 genome has many open reading frames that encode products that produce growth dysregulation or evasion of immune surveillance. How these orchestrate the formation and proliferation of spindle cells is under active investigation. Primary effusion lymphoma and Castleman's disease are other confirmed associations with HHV-8 infection.

HISTOLOGY. There is considerable variation in the histopathology according to the stage of the disease. Early lesions are of a chronic inflammatory or granulomatous nature, with new and dilated blood vessels, edema, hemorrhage, blood pigment, and dense perivascular infiltrations of lymphocytes and plasma and mast cells. The endothelial cells of the capillaries are large and protrude into the lumen, like buds. In the early patch stage, dilated, thin-walled vascular spaces with a jagged outline are present in the upper dermis. Other individual lesions are made up of capillaries and a fibrosarcoma-like tissue in greatly varying proportions, and often the capillaries show a marked tendency to anastomose. Extravasation of erythrocytes and deposits of hemosiderin are present. At this stage the lesions look like hemangiomas or angiosarcoma. In the later phases there is a spindle-cell proliferation that may be difficult to distinguish from sarcoma.

TREATMENT. Most tumor cells are latently, as opposed to lytically, infected with HHV-8, and treatment with antiherpetic medications has not been successful. All types of KS are radiosensitive. Radiation therapy has been used with considerable success, either by small fractionated doses, larger single doses to limited or extended fields, and by electron beam radiation. Local excision, cryotherapy, alitretinoin gel (Panretin), locally injected chemotherapy or interferon, or laser ablation has been used for troublesome, localized lesions. Alitretinoin gel is applied two to four times daily according to tolerance. Irritation is often the limiting factor. In responders improvement will be seen in 2 to 14 weeks.

Vincristine solution 0.1 mg/ml injected intralesionally, not more than 3 ml at one time and at intervals of 2 weeks, produces involution of tumors, some for as long as 8 months. These studies indicate that adequate control of the lesions may be had, at least for periods of 6 to 12 months. The development of resistance to medication seems to be inevitable.

Many other agents have been found to be effective; among the best are interferon, vinblastine, and actinomycin D. The response rate initially is high, but recurrent lesions, which are common, are generally less responsive. A combined approach using radiation therapy, chemotherapy, and immunotherapy may offer the most hope for the future. Systemic therapy is usually needed if more than 10 new KS lesions develop in 1 month, if there is symptomatic lymphedema, symptomatic pulmonary disease, or symptomatic visceral involvement.

COURSE. Classic KS progresses slowly, with rare lymph node or visceral involvement. Death usually occurs years later from unrelated causes. African cutaneous KS is aggressive, with early nodal involvement, and death from KS is expected within 1 to 2 years. AIDS-related KS, although widespread, is almost never fatal; nearly all patients die of intercurrent infection. The course of the disease is variable in patients who develop immunosuppression-related KS from causes other than AIDS. Removal of the immunosuppression may result in resolution of the KS without therapy.

Blauvelt A: The role of human herpesvirus 8 in the pathogenesis of Kaposi's sarcoma. *Adv Dermatol* 1999, 14:167.

Burdick AE, et al: Resolution of Kaposi's sarcoma associated with undetectable level of human herpesvirus 8 DNA in a patient with AIDS after protease inhibitor therapy. *J Am Acad Dermatol* 1997, 37:648.

Cooper JS, et al: Radiotherapy for epidemic Kaposi's sarcoma. *JAMA* 1984, 252:934.

Cooper JS, et al: The duration of local control of classic (non-AIDS-associated) Kaposi's sarcoma by radiotherapy. *J Am Acad Dermatol* 1988, 19:59.

El Akkad S, et al: Kaposi's sarcoma and its management by radiotherapy. *Arch Dermatol* 1986, 122:1396.

Ensoli B, et al: AIDS-Kaposi's sarcoma–derived cells express cytokines with autocrine and paracrine growth effects. *Science* 1989, 243:223.

Krischer J, et al: Regression of Kaposi's sarcoma during therapy with HIV-1 protease inhibitors. *J Am Acad Dermatol* 1998, 38:594.

Krown SE: Acquired immunodeficiency syndrome-associated Kaposi's sarcoma. *Med Clin North Am* 1997, 81:471.

Lebbe C: Human herpesvirus 8 as the infectious cause of Kaposi's sarcoma. *Arch Dermatol* 1998, 134:136.

Lemlich G, et al: Kaposi's sarcoma and acquired immunodeficiency syndrome. *J Am Acad Dermatol* 1987, 16:319.

Marchell N, et al: Successful treatment of cutaneous Kaposi's sarcoma by the 585-nm pulsed-dye laser. *Dermatol Surg* 1997, 23:973.

Myskowski PL, et al: AIDS-associated Kaposi's sarcoma. *J Am Acad Dermatol* 1988, 18:1299.

Piette WW: The incidence of second malignancies in subsets of Kaposi's sarcoma. *J Am Acad Dermatol* 1987, 16:855.

Rieber E, et al: Vincristine and Kaposi's sarcoma. *Ann Intern Med* 1984, 101:876.

Tappero JW, et al: Kaposi's sarcoma. *J Am Acad Dermatol* 1993, 28:371.

Tur E, et al: Treatment of Kaposi's sarcoma. *Arch Dermatol* 1996, 132:327. ▲

Epithelioid Hemangioendothelioma.

In 1982, Weiss et al described this rare tumor that both clinically and histologically is intermediate between angiosarcoma and hemangioma. It is usually a solitary, slowly growing papule or nodule on a distal area of an extremity. There is a male preponderance, and onset is frequently before the individual is 25 years of age. Histologically, there are two components: dilated vascular channels and spindle cell elements. Some may have cellular pleomorphism and mitotic activity. Wide excision is recommended with evaluation of regional lymph nodes. This is the usual site of metastases, and if they occur here, further surgery may be curative. In the minority of cases in which distant metastatic lesions develop, chemotherapy, radiation, or both may be employed. Of the 31 patients from the original series who had follow-up at an average of 18 months, 20 were alive and well.

Kanik AB, et al: Disseminated cutaneous epithelioid hemangioma. *J Am Acad Dermatol* 1996, 35:851.

Malane SL, et al: Epithelioid hemangioendothelioma associated with reflex sympathetic dystrophy. *J Am Acad Dermatol* 1992, 26:325.

Mentzel T, et al: Epithelioid hemangioendothelioma of skin and soft tissues. *Am J Surg Pathol* 1997, 21:363.

Polk P, et al: Isolated cutaneous epithelioid hemangioendothelioma. *J Am Acad Dermatol* 1997, 36:1026.

Weiss SW, et al: Epithelioid hemangioendothelioma. *Cancer* 1982, 50:970. ▲

Spindle-Cell Hemangioendothelioma.

Spindle-cell hemangioendothelioma is a vascular tumor that was first described in 1986; approximately 100 cases have now been reported. The condition commonly presents in a child or young adult who develops blue nodules of firm consistency on a distal extremity. Usually, multifocal lesions occur within an anatomic region. Histologically, a well-circumscribed dermal nodule will contain dilated vascular spaces with fascicles of spindle cells between them. They may repeatedly recur focally after excision.

Eltorky M, et al: Spindle cell hemangioendothelioma. *JDSO* 1994, 20:196.

Pellegrini AE, et al: Spindle cell hemangioendothelioma. *J Cutan Pathol* 1995, 22:173.

Weiss SW, et al: Spindle cell hemangioendothelioma. *Am J Surg Pathol* 1986, 10:521. ▲

Retiform Hemangioendothelioma.

Retiform hemangioendothelioma is another low-grade angiosarcoma, first described in 1994. It presents as a slow-growing exophytic mass, dermal plaque, or subcutaneous nodule. It most commonly occurs on the upper or lower extremities of young adults. Histologically, there are arborizing blood vessels reminiscent of normal rete testis architecture. Wide excision is recommended, although local recurrences are common. To date, no widespread metastases have occurred, although regional lymph nodes may develop tumor infiltrates.

Calonje E, et al: Retiform hemangioendothelioma. *Am J Surg Pathol* 1994, 18:115.

Duke D, et al: Multiple retiform hemangioendotheliomas. *Am J Dermatopathol* 1996, 18:606.

Sanz-Trelles A, et al: Retiform hemangioendothelioma. *J Cutan Pathol* 1997, 24:440. ▲

Endovascular Papillary Angioendothelioma (Dabska's Tumor).

Endovascular papillary angioendothelioma, a low-grade angiosarcoma, presents as a slow-growing tumor on the head, neck, or extremity of infants or young children. It shows multiple vascular channels with papillary plugs of endothelial cells surrounding central hyalinized cores that project into the lumina.

Wide excision and, in cases where they are involved, regional lymph node excision is usually curative.

Magnin PH, et al: Endovascular papillary angioendothelioma in children. *Pediatr Dermatol* 1987, 4:332.

Morgan J, et al: Malignant endovascular papillary angioendothelioma (Dabska tumor). *Am J Dermatopathol* 1989, 11:64.

Quecedo E, et al: Dabska tumor developing within a preexisting vascular malformation. *Am J Dermatopathol* 1996, 18:302. ▲

Angiosarcoma.

Angiosarcomas of the skin occur in four clinical settings. First and most common are those that occur in the head and neck of elderly people (Fig. 28-43). The male-to-female ratio is 2:1. The lesion often begins as an ill-defined bluish macule that may be mistaken for a bruise. Distinguishing features are the frequent occurrence of a peripheral erythematous ring, satellite nodules, the presence of intratumoral hemorrhage, and the tendency for the lesion to bleed spontaneously, or after minimal trauma. The tumor progressively enlarges asymmetrically, often becomes multicentric, and develops indurated bluish nodules and plaques. The sudden development of thrombocytopenia may herald metastatic disease or an enlarging primary tumor.

Histologically, anaplastic pleomorphic endothelial cells are present, with new vascular channels among them. Immunoperoxidase staining for factor VIII or other endothelial vascular markers aids in the diagnosis.

Early diagnosis and complete surgical excision followed by moderate dose very wide field radiotherapy offer the best prognosis for limited disease. Chemotherapy and

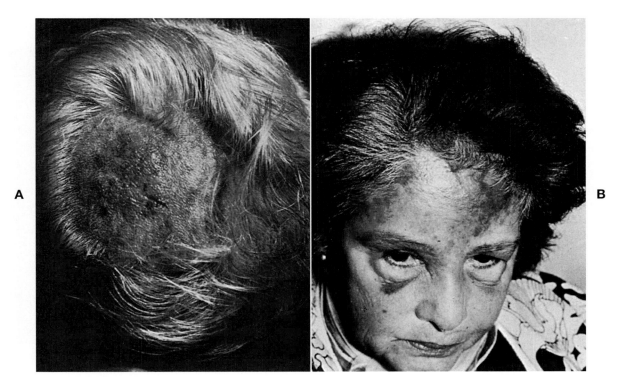

Fig. 28-43 **A,** Angiosarcoma on top of the scalp of a 73-year-old man. The dusky red infiltrated lesion, containing five small nodules. **B,** Angiosarcoma of the forehead and scalp.

radiation therapy for extensive disease are only palliative. Because of the multicentricity of lesions, the frequent occurrence on the face or scalp, and the rapid growth with early metastasis, death occurs in most patients within 2 years. Spieth et al reported a dramatic response in a 77-year-old man with recurrent angiosarcoma of the face and scalp after combination treatment with interferon alfa-2a and 13-cis-retinoic acid.

The second classic clinical situation in which angiosarcoma develops is in chronic lymphedematous areas, such as that which occurs in the upper arm after mastectomy, the so-called Stewart-Treves syndrome. This tumor appears approximately 11 to 12 years after surgery in an estimated 0.45% of patients. The prognosis is poor for these patients, with a mean survival of 19 to 31 months, and a 5-year survival rate of 6% to 14%. Metastases to the lungs is the most frequent cause of death. Early amputation offers the best hope.

A third setting includes tumors that develop in previously irradiated sites. If the condition for which radiation therapy was given was a benign one, the average interval between radiation and development of angiosarcoma is 23 years. If the preceding illness was a malignant condition, the interval is shortened to 12 years. Again, the prognosis is poor, with survival time generally between 6 months and 2 years after diagnosis.

Angiosarcomas develop in settings other than those previously described, and this small miscellaneous subset comprises the fourth category (Fig. 28-44).

Caldwell JB, et al: Cutaneous angiosarcoma arising in the radiation site of a congenital hemangioma. *J Am Acad Dermatol* 1995, 33:865.

Goette DK, et al: Post-irradiation angiosarcoma. *J Am Acad Dermatol* 1985, 12:922.

Hallel-Halevy D, et al: Stewart-Treves syndrome in a patient with elephantiasis. *J Am Acad Dermatol* 1999, 41:349.

Karuse KI, et al: Anterior abdominal wall angiosarcoma in a morbidly obese woman. *J Am Acad Dermatol* 1986, 15:327.

Kettler A, et al: A draining arm lesion in a female adult. *Arch Dermatol* 1985, 121:1455.

Kirchmann TT, et al: Cutaneous angiosarcoma as a second malignancy in a lymphedematous leg in a Hodgkin's disease survivor. *J Am Acad Dermatol* 1994, 31:861.

Kofler H, et al: Hemangiosarcoma in chronic leg ulcer. *Arch Dermatol* 1988, 124:1080.

Lapidus CS, et al: Angiosarcoma of the eyelid. *J Am Acad Dermatol* 1996, 34:308.

Mentzel T, et al: Cutaneous angiosarcoma of the face. *J Am Acad Dermatol* 1998, 38:837.

Morrison WH, et al: Cutaneous angiosarcoma of the head and neck. *Cancer* 1995, 76:319.

Satoh T, et al: Cutaneous angiosarcoma with thrombocytopenia. *J Am Acad Dermatol* 1999, 40:872.

Scheman AJ, et al: Purple nodules in the lower extremity following above-knee amputation. *Arch Dermatol* 1988, 124:263.

Spieth K, et al: Therapeutic efficacy of interferon alfa-2a and 13-cis-retinoic acid in recurrent angiosarcoma of the head. *Arch Dermatol* 1999, 135:1035. ▲

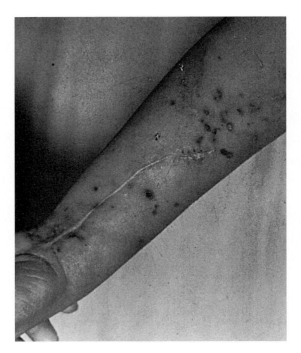

Fig. 28-44   Angiosarcoma in a 54-year-old man.

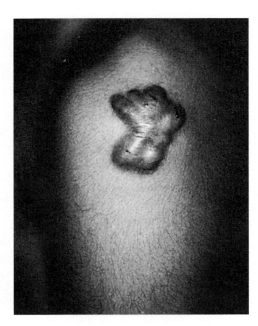

Fig. 28-45   Keloid in a vaccination site.

FIBROUS TISSUE ABNORMALITIES
Keloid

A keloid is a firm, irregularly shaped, thickened, hypertrophic, fibrous, pink or red excrescence. The growth usually arises as the result of a cut, laceration, or burn—or, less often, an acne pustule on the chest or upper back—and spreads beyond the limits of the original injury (Fig. 28-45), often sending out clawlike (cheloid) prolongations. The overlying epidermis is smooth, glossy, and thinned from pressure (Fig. 28-46). The early, growing lesion is red and tender and has the consistency of rubber. It is often surrounded by an erythematous halo, and the keloid may be telangiectatic. In the course of time the keloid generally becomes brown, is sometimes hypesthetic but often is extremely tender, painful, pruritic, hard, and stationary.

Keloids are often multiple, varying in size and number. Keloids may be as tiny as pinheads or as large as an orange. Those that follow burns and scalds are large. Lesions are often linear, and the surface may be larger than the base, so that the edges are overhanging. The most common location is the sternal region (Fig. 28-47), but keloids also occur frequently on the neck, ears, extremities, or trunk, and rarely on the face, palms, or soles. The earlobes are frequently involved as a result of ear piercing (Fig. 28-48). They are much more common, and grow to larger dimensions, in blacks than in other races.

Why certain persons develop keloids still remains unsolved. Trauma is usually the immediate causative factor, but this induces keloids only in those with a predisposition for its development. There is also a regional predisposition.

A keloid is a dense and sharply defined new growth of myofibroblasts and collagen in the dermis with a whorl-like arrangement of hyalinized bundles of collagenous fibers. The superficial collagen bundles lie parallel to the epidermis, but those lower down interlace in all directions. The ribbonlike bundles are more compact and prominent in older lesions. There is a paucity of elastic tissue. By pressure, the tumor causes thinning of the normal papillary dermis and atrophy of adjacent appendages, which it pushes aside. Mucopolysaccharides are increased, and often there are numerous mast cells.

Keloids are distinctive enough to cause little difficulty in distinguishing them from other dermatoses, except perhaps from a hypertrophic scar. The most pronounced distinction is the clawlike projections of the keloid that are absent in the hypertrophic scar. Moreover, the hypertrophic scar does not extend beyond the original wound as the keloid usually does (Fig. 28-49). Frequently there is a spontaneous improvement of the hypertrophic scar during the first 6 months, whereas in the keloid such does not occur.

The most gratifying type of treatment has been the intralesional injection of triamcinolone suspension. Using a 30-gauge needle on a 1-ml tuberculin Luer syringe, 0.02- to 0.04-ml aliquots of triamcinolone suspension (40 mg/ml) are injected into various parts of the lesion. This treatment is repeated at intervals of 6 to 8 weeks, as required. Flattening and cessation of itching are reliably achieved by this approach. The lesions are never made narrower, however. Another approach is the flashlamp pumped pulsed dye laser. Carbon dioxide laser vaporization of scars that are actively proliferating is not advised

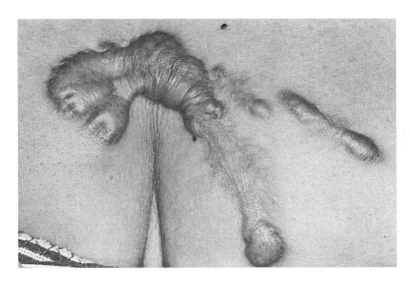

Fig. 28-46 Keloids in a white patient secondary to acne.

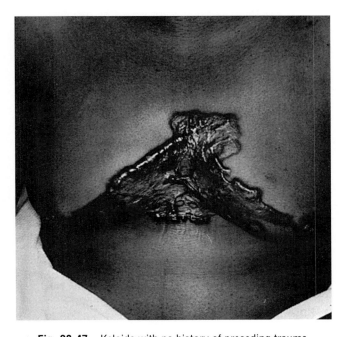

Fig. 28-47 Keloids with no history of preceding trauma.

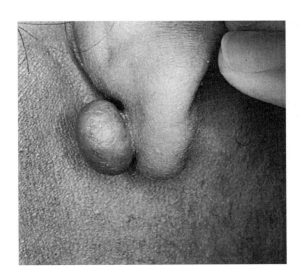

Fig. 28-48 Keloid resulting from ear piercing.

because of the high rate of recurrence or the potential for worsening of the condition.

If surgical removal by excision is feasible, and if narrowing of the keloid is a vitally important goal, the keloid may be excised. After the excision, intralesional injection of triamcinolone or interferon alfa-2b may be combined with postoperative x-ray irradiation. Silicone sheeting and pressure are other adjunctive methods used to try to limit recurrences. Unfortunately, superior results are not obtained with any of these tactics. Wittenberg et al could not demonstrate improvements in hypertrophic scars over controls with the flashlamp pumped pulsed dye laser and silicone gel sheeting.

Pierced-ear keloids occur with considerable frequency.

When the keloid is young, intralesional injection of triamcinolone is frequently sufficient to control the problem. In old keloids, excision of the lesion using lidocaine with triamcinolone, followed by injections at 2-week intervals, produces good results. CO_2 laser excision has also been successful in old mature keloids in this site.

Alster TS: Laser treatment of hypertrophic scars, keloids, and striae. *Dermatol Clin* 1997, 15:419.

Alster TS, et al: Treatment of scars. *Ann Plast Surg* 1997, 39:418.

Berman B, et al: Adjunct therapies to surgical management of keloids. *Dermatol Surg* 1996, 22:126.

Berman B, et al: Keloids. *J Am Acad Dermatol* 1995, 33:117.

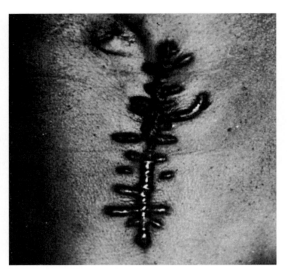

Fig. 28-49 Hypertrophic scar on the lower abdomen following laparotomy. Extension into suture marks is conspicuous.

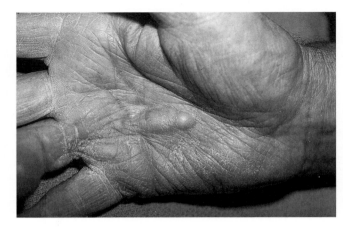

Fig. 28-50 Dupuytren's contracture.

Berman B, et al: Recurrence rates of excised keloids treated with postoperative triamcinolone acetonide injections or interferon alfa-2b injections. *J Am Acad Dermatol* 1997, 37:755.

Enhamre A, et al: Treatment of keloids with excision and postoperative x-ray irradiation. *Dermatologica* 1983, 167:90.

Fulton JE Jr: Silicone gel sheeting for the prevention and management of evolving hypertrophic and keloid scars. *Dermatol Surg* 1995, 21:947.

Janssen de Limpens AMP: A comparison of the treatment of keloids and hypertrophic scars. *Eur J Plast Surg* 1986, 9:18.

Janssen de Limpens AMP: The local treatment of hypertrophic scars and keloids with retinoic acid. *Br J Dermatol* 1980, 103:319.

Kantor GR, et al: Treatment of earlobe keloids with carbon dioxide laser excision. *J Dermatol Surg Oncol* 1985, 11:1063.

Klumpar DI, et al: Keloids treated with excision followed by radiation therapy. *J Am Acad Dermatol* 1994, 31:225.

Murray JC, et al: Keloids and hypertrophic scars. *Clin Dermatol* 1994, 12:27.

Novick NL, et al: Suppurative keloidosis in a black woman. *J Am Acad Dermatol* 1986, 16:1090.

Rubenstein R, et al: Atypical keloids after dermabrasion of patients taking isotretinoin. *J Am Acad Dermatol* 1988, 15:280.

Scholz TA, et al: Laser treatment of hypertrophic scars and keloids. *Dermatol Surg* 1998, 24:298.

Sclafani AP, et al: Prevention of earlobe keloid recurrence with postoperative corticosteroid injections versus radiation therapy. *Dermatol Surg* 1996, 22:569.

Wittenberg GP, et al: Prospective, single-blinded, randomized, controlled study to assess the efficacy of the 585-nm flashlamp-pumped pulsed-dye laser and silicone gel sheeting in hypertrophic scar treatment. *Arch Dermatol* 1999, 135:1049. ▲

Dupuytren's Contracture

Dupuytren's contracture is a fibromatosis of the palmar aponeurosis. The lesion arises most commonly in men between the ages of 30 and 50 as multiple firm nodules in the palm (Fig. 28-50). Usually three to five nodules about 1 cm in diameter develop, proximal to the fourth finger. Later the fibromatosis produces contractures, which may be disabling. It occurs at times with alcoholic cirrhosis, diabetes mellitus, and chronic epilepsy. It is also associated with Peyronie's disease, plantar fibromatosis, and knuckle pads. In some cases there is a familial predisposition. The fibrous nodules are composed of myofibroblasts.

Early intralesional triamcinolone may help, but surgical excision of the involved palmar fascia may be the only way to liberate severely contracted fingers.

Frey M: Risks and prevention of Dupuytren's contracture. *Lancet* 1997, 350:1568.

James WD, et al: The role of the myofibroblast in Dupuytren's contracture. *Arch Dermatol* 1980, 116:807.

McFarlane R: Dupuytren's disease. *J Hand Ther* 1997, 10:8. ▲

Plantar Fibromatosis

The plantar analog of Dupuytren's contracture, plantar fibromatosis occurs as slowly enlarging nodules on the soles that ultimately cause difficulty in walking or even weight-bearing. This is sometimes called *Ledderhose's syndrome*. The usual treatment, as for Dupuytren's, is wide excision of the plantar fascia, but improvement by the intralesional injection of triamcinolone acetonide, 30 mg/ml, monthly for 5 months has been reported. The triamcinolone can be diluted with lidocaine solution.

Classen DA, et al: Plantar fibromatosis and bilateral flexion contracture. *Ann Plast Surg* 1992, 28:475.

Pentland AP, et al: Plantar fibromatosis responds to intralesional steroids. *J Am Acad Dermatol* 1985, 12:212.

White S: Plantar fibromatosis. *Arch Dermatol* 1986, 117:376. ▲

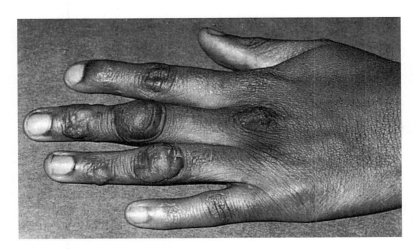

Fig. 28-51   Knuckle pads.

Knuckle Pads

Knuckle pads (heloderma) are well-defined, round, plaque-like, fibrous thickenings that develop on the extensor aspects of the proximal interphalangeal joints of the toes and fingers, including the thumbs (Fig. 28-51). They develop at any age and grow to be some 10 to 15 mm in diameter in the course of a few weeks or months, then persist permanently. They are flesh-colored or somewhat brown, with normal or slightly hyperkeratotic epidermis overlying them and adherent to them. They are a part of the skin and are freely movable over underlying structures.

Knuckle pads are sometimes associated with Dupuytren's contracture and camptodactylia (irreducible flexion contracture of one or more fingers). Some cases are familial. Families with knuckle pads, mixed hearing loss (sensorineural and conductive), and total leukonychia noted through many generations have been reported. The condition is inherited as an autosomal dominant trait.

Histologically, the lesions are fibromas. They are to be differentiated clinically from the nodular type of neurodermatitis and from the small hemispherical pitted papules that may develop over the knuckles after frostbite or in acrocyanosis, and from rheumatic nodules. Treatment with intralesional injection of corticosteroids may be beneficial.

Kodama BF, et al: Papules and plaques over the joint spaces. *Arch Dermatol* 1993, 129:1044.

Kose O, et al: Knuckle pads, leukonychia and deafness. *Int J Dermatol* 1996, 35:728. _____ ▲

Peyronie's Disease

Plastic induration of the penis is a fibrous infiltration of the intercavernous septum of the penis. This fibrosis results in the formation of nodules or plaques. As a result of these plaques, a fibrous chordee is produced, and curvature of the penis occurs on erection, sometimes so severe as to make intromission difficult or impossible. Sometimes pain may be severe. The association of this disease with Dupuytren's contracture has been recognized. Intralesional triamcinolone suspension injected or iontophoresed into the plaques and nodules may be curative.

Surgical correction tailored to the degree of deformity is often successful.

Connelly TS: Development of Peyronie's and Dupuytren's disease in an individual after single episodes of trauma. *J Am Acad Dermatol* 1999, 41:106.

Levine LA, et al: A surgical algorithm for the treatment of Peyronie's disease. *J Urol* 1997, 158:2149.

Muralidhar S, et al: Etiologic factors in Peyronie's disease. *Int J Dermatol* 1997, 36:579. _____ ▲

Desmoid Tumor

A large, deep-seated, well-circumscribed mass arising from the muscular aponeurosis characterizes this lesion. It most commonly occurs on the abdominal wall, especially in women during or soon after pregnancy. Desmoid tumors have been divided into five types: abdominal wall, extraabdominal, intraabdominal, multiple, and those occurring in Gardner's syndrome. They recur locally and can kill if they invade, surround, or compress vital structures. The most dangerous, then, are those at the root of the neck and the intraabdominal type. MRI will aid in the evaluation of soft tissue extension and recurrence following treatment.

Treatment may be with wide local excision, radiotherapy, or hormonal manipulation.

Pereyo NG, et al: Extraabdominal desmoid tumor. *J Am Acad Dermatol* 1996, 34:352. _____ ▲

Collagenous Fibroma

This slow-growing, deep-set, benign fibrous tumor is characterized by hypocellularity and dense bands of hyalinized collagen that may infiltrate into skeletal muscle.

Despite this, no tumors have been reported to metastasize or recur after excision.

Weisberg NK, et al: Collagenous fibroma. *J Am Acad Dermatol* 1999, 41:292. ———————————————————————— ▲

Aponeurotic Fibroma

Aponeurotic fibroma has also been called *juvenile aponeurotic fibroma* (calcifying fibroma). It is a tumorlike proliferation characterized by the appearance of slow-growing, cystlike masses that occur on the limbs.

Histologically, the distinctive lesions are sharply demarcated and composed of collagenous stroma showing acid mucopolysaccharides infiltrated by plump mesenchymal cells with oval nuclei. Hyalinized areas are also present, suggesting chondroid or osteoid metaplasia.

An aid to the diagnosis is stippled calcification, readily seen on roentgenograms. Surgical excision is the treatment.

Murphy BA, et al: Extra-acral calcifying aponeurotic fibroma. *J Cutan Pathol* 1996, 23:369. —————————————————— ▲

Congenital Generalized Fibromatosis (Infantile Myofibromatosis)

Congenital generalized fibromatosis is an uncommon condition that presents at birth or soon after. It is characterized by multiple firm dermal and subcutaneous nodules; skeletal lesions, primarily of the metaphyseal regions of the long bones, occur in 50% of patients. If only the skin and bones develop fibromas, the prognosis is excellent, with spontaneous resolution of the lesions without complications expected within the first 1 to 2 years of life. Some refer to this limited disease as *congenital multiple fibromatosis*.

The fibromas may involve the viscera, including the gastrointestinal tract, breast, lungs, liver, pancreas, tongue, serosal surfaces, lymph nodes, or kidney. Mortality in this more widespread subset is high; 80% of affected individuals die from obstruction or compression of vital organs. Those who survive past 4 months have spontaneous regression of their disease.

Histologically, fascicles of spindle cells occur in a whorled pattern. These nodules are composed of myofibroblasts. There is a suggestion in the literature of a familial pattern of the disease. Females more commonly get the generalized disease.

Barnes L, et al: Solitary nodule on the arm of an infant. *Arch Dermatol* 1986, 122:89.
Bellman B, et al: Infantile myofibromatosis. *Pediatr Dermatol* 1991, 8:306.
Parker RK, et al: Infantile myofibromatosis. *Pediatr Dermatol* 1991, 8:129.
Sonoda T, et al: Infantile myofibromatosis. *J Dermatol* 1994, 21:508.
Spraker MK, et al: Congenital generalized fibromatosis. *J Am Acad Dermatol* 1984, 10:365. ——————————— ▲

Juvenile Hyaline Fibromatosis

This syndrome begins in early childhood with soft nodular tumors of the scalp, face, and extremities, which may or may not be associated with flexion contractures, hypertrophic gums, osteolytic bone lesions, and stunted growth. Aberrant synthesis of glycosaminoglycans by fibroblasts appears to be present in the nodules. The disease has occurred in siblings and in a child from a consanguineous marriage.

In two cases reported with long-term follow-up, continued nodule formation, especially in the hands, with disabling contractures, osteolysis of phalanges, and surgical scarring were the prominent late findings.

Histologically, there are fibroblasts with fine intracytoplasmic eosinophilic granules, embedded in a homogeneous eosinophilic dermal ground substance.

Breier F, et al: Juvenile hyaline fibromatosis. *Arch Dis Child* 1997, 77:436.
Camarasa JG, et al: Juvenile hyaline fibromatosis. *J Am Acad Dermatol* 1987, 16:881.
Miyake I, et al: Juvenile hyaline fibromatosis. *Am J Dermatopathol* 1995, 17:584. —————————————————————— ▲

Infantile Digital Fibromatosis (Infantile Digital Myofibroblastoma)

Infantile digital fibromatosis is a rare neoplasm of infancy and childhood characterized by fibroblastic proliferations. Usually the lesions occur singly or severally on the dorsal or lateral aspects of the distal phalanges of the toes and fingers (Fig. 28-52). The thumb and great toe are usually spared. These asymptomatic, firm, red, smooth nodules, approximately 1 cm in diameter, occur during the first year of life; 47% occur in the first month of life. The lesions do not metastasize.

Histologically, the epidermis is normal, but the dermis is infiltrated with proliferating fibroblasts and collagen bundles. In addition, eosinophilic cytoplasmic inclusions in many of the fibroblasts are characteristic. The elongated cells are myofibroblasts ultrastructurally.

Treatment by surgical excision has a high risk of recurrence. It is preferable to procrastinate in the hope of spontaneous resolution.

Miyamoto T, et al: Posttraumatic occurrence of infantile digital fibromatosis. *Arch Dermatol* 1986, 122:915.
Ramsdell WM: Recurring digital fibroma of childhood. *Arch Dermatol* 1983, 119:702. ——————————————————— ▲

FIBROUS HAMARTOMA OF INFANCY

Fibrous hamartoma of infancy is a single dermal or subcutaneous firm nodule of the upper trunk that is present at birth. Biopsy shows a cell-poor fibrous lesion, with immature spindle cells present in a mucoid matrix. There is no recurrence after excision.

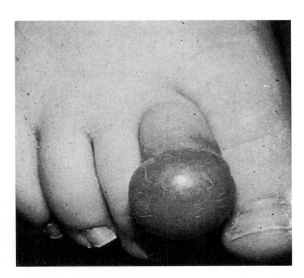

Fig. 28-52 Infantile digital fibromatosis. (Courtesy Dr. L. Shapiro.)

Paller AS, et al: Fibrous hamartoma of infancy. *Arch Dermatol* 1989, 125:88. _____ ▲

Fibromatosis Colli

In fibromatosis colli there is a fibrous tissue proliferation infiltrating the lower third of the sternocleidomastoid muscle at birth. Spontaneous remission occurs within a few months. Occasionally, some patients are left with a wryneck deformity; however, this complication is amenable to surgery.

Mehregan AH: Superficial fibrous tumors in childhood. *J Cutan Pathol* 1981, 8:321. _____ ▲

Diffuse Infantile Fibromatosis

This process occurs within the first 3 years of life and is usually confined to the muscles of the arms, neck, and shoulder area. There is a multicentric infiltration of muscle fibers with fibroblasts resembling those seen in aponeurotic fibromas. Calcification does not occur. Recurrence after excision occurs in about a third of cases.

Allen PW: The fibromatoses. *Am J Surg Pathol* 1977, 1:255, 305. _____ ▲

Aggressive Infantile Fibromatosis

The clinical presentation of this locally recurring, nonmetastasizing lesion involves single or multiple fast-growing masses that are present at birth or occur within the first year of life. Infantile fibromatosis may be seen in any location, although the arms, legs, and trunk are the usual sites. Histologically, it mimics malignancy.

Amoric JC, et al: Infantile aggressive fibromatosis. *Ann Dermatol Venereol* 1993, 120:762. _____ ▲

Giant Cell Tumor of the Tendon Sheath

This tumor, which is most commonly attached to the tendons of the fingers, hands, and wrists, has a predilection for the flexor surfaces. It is firm, measures from 1 to 3 cm in diameter, and does not spontaneously involute. It recurs after excision in approximately 25% of cases. Another tumor of the tendon sheath, fibroma of the tendon sheath, may represent a variant of the giant cell tumor. It also affects the flexural tendons of the fingers and hands, and morphologically, it and the giant cell tumor are identical. The condition tends to occur in younger men (the average age at onset is 30) than the giant cell variety, but the recurrence rate after surgery is identical.

Histologically, the giant cell tumor consists of lobules of densely hyalinized collagen. The characteristic giant cells have deeply eosinophilic cytoplasm and a variable number of nuclei. Lipophages and siderophages may be numerous. The fibroma of the tendon sheath generally lacks the lipophages, siderophages, and giant cells, with the lobules being composed of dense fibrocollagenous tissue.

Ciattaglia G, et al: Giant cell tumor of tendon sheath. *J Am Acad Dermatol* 1991, 25:728.
Cooper PH, et al: Fibroma of tendon sheath. *J Am Acad Dermatol* 1984, 11:625.
Richert B, et al: Laterosubungual giant cell tumor of the tendon sheath. *J Am Acad Dermatol* 1999, 41:347.
Schleicher SM: Giant cell tumor of tendon sheath. *Cutis* 1997, 59:133.
Watanabe T, et al: Sclerotic fibroma of tendon sheath. *Dermatology* 1997, 195:563. _____ ▲

Ainhum

Ainhum is also known as *dactylolysis spontanea, bankokerend,* and *sukhapakla.* Ainhum is a disease affecting the toes, especially the fifth toe, characterized by a linear constriction around the affected digit, which leads ultimately to the spontaneous amputation of the distal part (Fig. 28-53). It occurs chiefly among black men in Africa. Usually it is unilateral, but it may be bilateral.

The disease begins with a transverse groove in the skin on the flexor surface of the toe, usually beneath the first interphalangeal articulation. The furrow is produced by a ringlike fibrosis and an induration of the dermis. It deepens and extends laterally around the toe until the two ends meet, so that the digit becomes constricted as if in a ligature. The constricted part becomes swollen and soft and after a time greatly distended. Ulceration may result in a malodorous discharge, with pain and gangrene. The course of the disease is slow, but in 5 to 10 years spontaneous amputation occurs, generally at a joint.

The cause is unknown. The condition may result from chronic trauma and exposure to the elements by walking

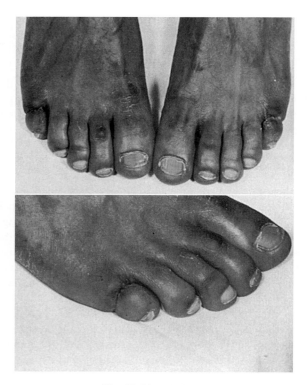

Fig. 28-53 Ainhum.

barefoot in the tropics. Fissuring followed by chronic inflammation and fibrosis may then result.

Treatment in the early cases by cutting the constricting band is unsuccessful; in advanced cases amputation of the affected member is advisable. Surgical correction by Z-plasty has produced good results. Intralesional injection of betamethasone (total, 15 injections) has also been successful.

Pseudo-Ainhum

Pseudo-ainhum has been a term used in connection with certain hereditary and nonhereditary diseases in which annular constriction of digits occurs. Hereditary disorders include hereditary palmoplantar keratodermas, especially Vohwinkel's syndrome and mal de Meleda, pachyonychia congenita, Ehlers-Danlos syndrome, erythropoietic protoporphyria, and congenital ectodermal defect. Nonhereditary disorders associated with constriction of digits are ainhum, leprosy, cholera, ancyclostomiasis, scleroderma, Raynaud's syndrome, pityriasis rubra pilaris, psoriasis, Olmstead syndrome, syringomyelia, ergot poisoning, and tumors of the spinal cord. Factitial pseudo-ainhum may be produced by self-application of a rubber band, string, or other ligature.

Congenital cases have been reported that may affect digits or limbs. It may occur as a familial condition or may result secondary to amniotic bands.

Treatment may be with surgery or intralesional injection of corticosteroids, as in ainhum, or retinoids may be used in diseases responsive to them.

McLaurin CI: Psoriasis presenting with pseudo-ainhum. *J Am Acad Dermatol* 1982, 7:130.
Park BS, et al: Pseudo-ainhum associated with linear scleroderma. *Arch Dermatol* 1996, 132:1520. _____ ▲

Connective Tissue Nevi

These uncommon lesions, although often very inconspicuous, may present as acquired isolated plaques, as multiple lesions either acquired or congenital, or as one finding in a more generalized disease. Biopsy findings in many cases do not appear very different from normal skin, although in some cases increased amounts of collagen or elastin may be identified.

These lesions characteristically occur on the trunk (Fig. 28-54), most often in the lumbosacral area. They may be solitary, but are often multiple, in which case they may show a zosteriform arrangement. Individual lesions are slightly elevated plaques 1 to 15 cm in diameter (Fig. 28-55), varying in color from light yellow to orange, with a surface texture resembling shagreen leather. In Proteus syndrome the connective tissue nevi are present as plantar, or occasionally, palmar masses with a cerebriform surface.

Connective tissue nevi of the acquired type have been classified as eruptive collagenomas, isolated collagenomas, or isolated elastomas, depending on the number of lesions and the predominant dermal fibers present. They cannot be differentiated clinically.

The hereditary types of connective tissue nevi discussed here include dermatofibrosis lenticularis disseminata in the Buschke-Ollendorff syndrome, familial cutaneous collagenoma, and the so-called shagreen patches seen in tuberous sclerosis.

Buschke-Ollendorff syndrome is an autosomal dominantly inherited disorder in which widespread dermal papules and plaques develop asymmetrically over the trunk and limbs. Elastic fiber thickening, highly variable fiber diameter, and desmosine increases threefold to sevenfold above normal have been described in some cases. The associated feature of osteopoikilosis is asymptomatic, but it is diagnostic in x-ray evaluation. Focal sclerotic densities are seen, primarily in long bones, the pelvis, and the hands.

Patients with familial cutaneous collagenomas may present with numerous symmetric asymptomatic dermal nodules on the back (Fig. 28-56). The age of onset is usually in the mid to late teens. In patients with the inherited disease multiple endocrine neoplasia type I multiple collagenomas were reported to be present in 23 of 32 patients by Darling et al. These were less than 3 millimeters in diameter and were on the upper torso, neck, and shoulders. They occurred in association with numerous other cutaneous findings such as angiofibromas, café au lait macules, and lipomas.

Connective tissue nevi are also associated with tuberous sclerosis. The inconspicuous, thickened "shagreen plaques" are present with the classic skin findings of adenoma sebaceum, periungual fibromas, and ash-leaf macules. Because at least half the cases of tuberous sclerosis result

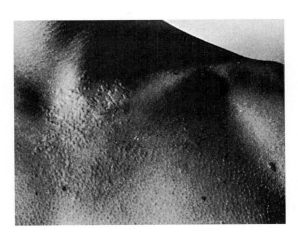

Fig. 28-54 Connective tissue nevus over the sternoclavicular junction. (Courtesy Dr. L. Fragola.)

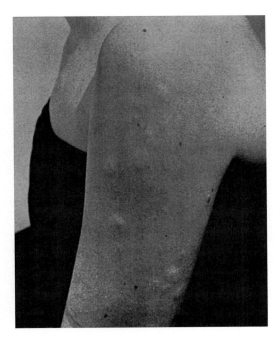

Fig. 28-55 Connective tissue nevus on the upper arm of a 12-year-old girl. (Courtesy Dr. J. Stephens.)

from new mutations, all patients with connective tissue nevi should be carefully studied for evidence of tuberous sclerosis, even in the absence of a family history of the disease.

Berberian BB, et al: Asymptomatic nodules on the back and abdomen. *Arch Dermatol* 1987, 123:811.

Darling TN, et al: Multiple facial angiofibromas and collagenomas in patients with multiple endocrine neoplasia type 1. *Arch Dermatol* 1997, 133:853.

Gautam RK, et al: Isolated collagenoma. *J Dermatol* 1996, 23:476.

Huilgol SC, et al: Familial juvenile elastoma. *Australas J Dermatol* 1994, 35:87.

Kwiatkowski DJ, et al: Tuberous sclerosis. *Arch Dermatol* 1994, 130:348.

Phillips JC, et al: Familial cutaneous collagenoma. *J Am Acad Dermatol* 1999, 40:255.

Samlaska CP, et al: Proteus syndrome. *Arch Dermatol* 1989, 125:1109.

Smith JB, et al: Multiple collagenomas in a patient with Down syndrome. *J Am Acad Dermatol* 1995, 33:835.

Trattner A, et al: Buschke-Ollendorff syndrome of the scalp. *J Am Acad Dermatol* 1991, 24:822.

Uitto J, et al: Connective tissue nevi of the skin. *J Am Acad Dermatol* 1980, 3:441. ▲

Elastofibroma Dorsi

Elastofibroma dorsi is a rare benign tumor usually located in the deep soft tissues in the subscapular region but sometimes at other sites. The tumor is firm, unencapsulated, and measures up to several centimeters in diameter. It is believed to represent an unusual response to repeated trauma. Histologically, the tumor consists of abundant compact sclerotic collagen mixed with large, swollen, irregular elastic fibers, often appearing as globules of elastic tissue. Excision is curative.

Bieger AK, et al: Elastofibroma dorsi. *Ann Plast Surg* 1994, 32:548.

Said S, et al: Subcapsular subcutaneous tumor. *Arch Dermatol* 1999, 135:341.

Schwarz T, et al: Ulcerating elastofibroma dorsi. *J Am Acad Dermatol* 1989, 21:1142. ▲

Angiofibromas

These skin-colored to reddish papules, which show fibroplasia and varying degrees of vascular proliferation in the upper dermis, may occur as a solitary nonhereditary form, the fibrous papule of the nose, as multiple nonhereditary lesions, pearly penile papules, or as multiple hereditary forms as in tuberous sclerosis (adenoma sebaceum. forehead plaques, Koenen's tumors and gingival lesions) and in multiple endocrine neoplasia type I. There have been isolated reports of agminated or segmental angiofibromas that have been hypothesized to be a segmental form of tuberous sclerosis. The multiple hereditary types are discussed in other chapters.

Anliker MD, et al: Unilateral agminated angiofibromas: a segmental expression of tuberous sclerosis? *Dermatology* 1997, 195:176.

Darling TN, et al: Multiple facial angiofibromas and collagenomas in patients with multiple endocrine neoplasia type 1. *Arch Dermatol* 1997, 133:853.

McGrae JD Jr, et al: Unilateral facial angiofibromas: a segmental form of tuberous sclerosis. *Br J Dermatol* 1996, 134:727. ▲

Fibrous Papule of the Nose. A dome-shaped, sessile, skin-colored, white, or reddish papule 3 to 6 mm in diameter, usually solitary, on or near the nose, in an adult (Fig. 28-57), is very likely to be a harmless lesion first described by Graham et al in 1965. It may be confused with a nevocytic nevus, neurofibroma, granuloma pyogenicum, or a basal cell carcinoma. Conservative excision is curative; recurrence is rare.

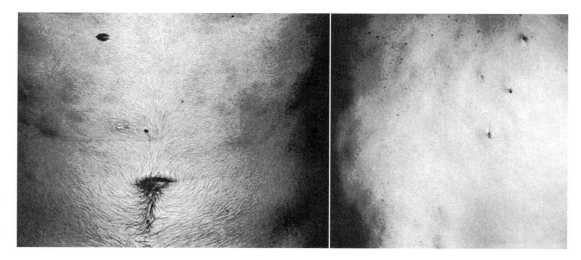

Fig. 28-56   Familial cutaneous collagenoma.

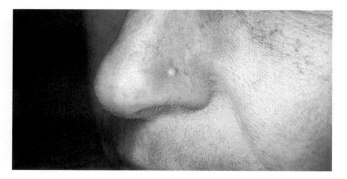

Fig. 28-57   Fibrous papule of the nose.

Cerio R: An immunohistochemical study of fibrous papule of the nose. *J Cutan Pathol* 1989, 16:194.
Nemeth AJ, et al: Fibrous papule. *J Am Acad Dermatol* 1988, 19:1102.
Rosen LB, et al: Fibrous papules. *Am J Dermatopathol* 1988, 10:109. ▲

Pearly Penile Papules. *Pearly penile papules* is the term given to pearly white, dome-shaped papules occurring circumferentially on the coronal margin and sulcus of the glans penis (Fig. 28-58). Occasionally, lesions are also present on the penile shaft. Pearly penile papules are not uncommon. Patients usually present around the age of 20 to 30 years concerned these are condylomata or are referred as treatment-resistant venereal warts.

These lesions should be distinguished from papillomas, hypertrophic sebaceous glands, and condyloma acuminatum.

No treatment is necessary, only reassurance. If treatment is desired laser ablation is best.

Magid M: Pearly penile papules. *J Dermatol Surg Oncol* 1989, 15:552.
Ocampo-Candiani J, et al: Cryosurgical treatment of pearly penile papules. *J Am Acad Dermatol* 1996, 35:486.

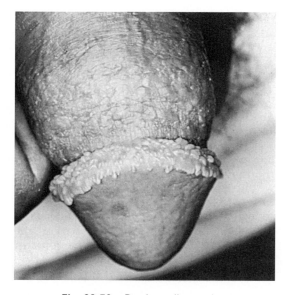

Fig. 28-58   Pearly penile papules.

O'Neil CA, et al: Pearly penile papules on the shaft. *Arch Dermatol* 1995, 131:491. ▲

Perifollicular Fibromas

Zackheim and Pinkus described a rare type of fibroma with a perifollicular pattern. Clinically, there are multiple, small, firm papules, either flesh-colored or pink, located on the face and neck. The appearance is not distinctive and may suggest a nevus or trichoepithelioma. They may also appear as solitary lesions. Reports have linked it to a colonic villous adenoma or colonic polyposis.

The pathologic changes are those of a benign fibroma of the connective tissue sheath of the hair follicle. The fibroma stems from the mesodermal portion of the pilary complex. Reports of this entity before the elucidation of fibrofolliculoma are difficult to evaluate because many reports of perifollicular fibromas show epithelial proliferation in association with perifollicular fibrosis, a finding characteristic of fibrofolliculomas. This problem was discussed by Ubogy-Rainey et al.

Junkins-Hopkins JM, et al: Multiple perifollicular fibromas. *J Cutan Pathol* 1994, 21:467.
Sasai S, et al: Coexistence of multiple perifollicular fibromas and colonic polyp and cancer. *Dermatology* 1996, 192:262.
Ubogy-Rainey Z, et al: Fibrofolliculomas, trichodiscomas, and acrochordons. *J Am Acad Dermatol* 1987, 16:452. _____ ▲

Acral Fibrokeratoma

Acral fibrokeratoma, often called *acquired digital fibrokeratoma,* is characterized by a pinkish, hyperkeratotic, hornlike projection occurring on a finger, toe, or palm (Fig. 28-59); the projection usually emerges from a collarette of elevated skin. Kint et al reviewed 50 new cases and found the average age of the patients was 40 years old; 39 lesions were on the fingers, six on the toes; the rest were on the palm, wrist, and calf. The lesion resembles a rudimentary supernumerary digit, cutaneous horn, and a neuroma.

The histologic features show a central core of thick collagen bundles interwoven closely in a vertical position. This is surrounded by capillaries and a fine network of reticulum fibers.

Simple surgical excision or laser ablation at the level of the skin surface is effective.

Berger RS, et al: Dermal papule on a distal digit. *Arch Dermatol* 1988, 124:1559.
Kint A, et al: Acquired (digital) fibrokeratoma. *J Am Acad Dermatol* 1985, 12:816. _____ ▲

Familial Myxovascular Fibromas

Multiple verrucous papules on the palms and fingers, which on biopsy show focal neovascularization and mucinlike changes in the papillary dermis, have been described. Clinically, these lesions closely resemble warts. They have been reported from several family members, with a probable autosomal dominant inheritance.

Coskey RJ, et al: Multiple vascular fibromas and myxoid fibromas of the fingers. *J Am Acad Dermatol* 1980, 2:425.
Moulin G, et al: Familial multiple acral mucinous fibrokeratomas. *J Am Acad Dermatol* 1998, 38:1998.
Peterson JL, et al: Familial myxovascular fibromas. *J Am Acad Dermatol* 1982, 6:470. _____ ▲

SUBUNGUAL EXOSTOSIS

Subungual exostosis is a solitary fibrous and bony nodule protruding from beneath the distal edge of the nail (Fig. 28-60), most commonly of the great toe. Rarely, the terminal phalanges of other toes, particularly the little toe or

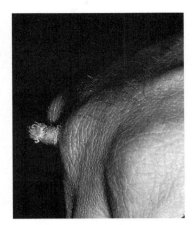

Fig. 28-59   Acral fibrokeratoma.

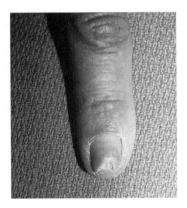

Fig. 28-60   Subungual exostosis.

even the fingers, may be involved. The exostosis is seen chiefly in women between the ages of 12 and 30. The first appearance is a small pinkish growth projecting slightly beyond the inner free edge of the nail. The overlying nail becomes brittle and either breaks or is removed, after which the tumor, being released, mushrooms upward and distally above the level of the nail. It grows slowly to a maximum diameter of about 8 mm. Pressure of the shoe on the lesion causes great pain.

Subungual exostosis must be differentiated from pyogenic granuloma, verruca vulgaris, pterygium inverum unguis, ingrowing nail, glomus tumor, and melanotic whitlow. If subungual exostosis is suspected, the diagnosis can be confirmed by radiographic examination. Complete excision or curettage is the proper method of treatment.

Davis DA, et al: Subungual exostosis. *Pediatr Dermatol* 1996, 13:212.
James MP: Digital exostosis causing enlargement of the fingertip. *J Am Acad Dermatol* 1988, 19:132.
Jetmalani SN, et al: Painful solitary subungual nodule. *Arch Dermatol* 1992, 128:849.
Warren KJ, et al: Subungual exostosis. *Dermatol Surg* 1998, 24:287. ▲

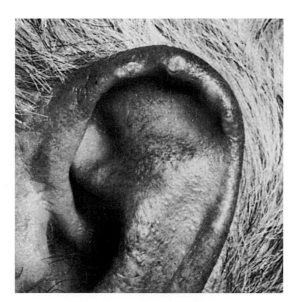

Fig. 28-61 Chondrodermatitis nodularis chronica helicis. Painful nodules on the edge of the upper helix. (Courtesy Dr. I. Abrahams.)

Chondrodermatitis Nodularis Chronica Helicis

This is a small, nodular, tender, chronic inflammatory lesion occurring on the outer helix of the ear (Fig. 28-61). Most patients are men. The lesions are not uncommon and sometimes as many as 12 nodules may arrange themselves along the edge of the upper helix. The lesions evolve slowly and are ovoid, well defined, slightly reddish, extremely tender masses, 2 to 4 mm in diameter. They are firmly attached to the underlying cartilage. At times the surface is covered by an adherent scale or a shallow ulcer. After the masses have reached a certain size, growth ceases, but the lesions persist unchanged for years. There is no tendency to malignant change. Similar lesions may occur on the anthelix, predominantly in women.

Often there is a history of frostbite, chronic trauma, or chronic actinic exposure with concomitant actinically in-duced lesions of the face and dorsal hands.

Histologically, degenerative changes of the collagen are the chief features. In addition, acanthosis and hyperkeratosis with plugging and thinning of the epidermis are noted. On excision one finds a projecting spur of altered cartilage about which the lesion is formed, apparently a chronic inflammatory response. This is a process of transepidermal elimination.

The lesions may be excised, together with the underlying spicule of cartilage.

Lawrence CM: The treatment of chondrodermatitis nodularis with cartilage removal alone. *Arch Dermatol* 1991, 127:530.
Long D, et al: Surgical planing in the treatment of chondrodermatitis nodularis chronica helicis of the antihelix. *J Am Acad Dermatol* 1996, 35:761.

Munnoch DA: Chondrodermatitis nodularis chronica helicis et antihelicis. *Br J Plast Surg* 1996, 49:473.
Taylor MB: Chondrodermatitis nodularis chronica helicis. *J Dermatol Surg Oncol* 1991, 17:862. _____ ▲

Submucous Fibrosis of the Palate

A distinctive fibrosis of the palate occurs in the western Pacific basin and south Asia among persons whose diet is heavily seasoned with chili or who chew betel, a compound of the nut of the areca palm, the leaf of the betel pepper, and lime. The irritation produced causes first a thickening of the palate, tonsillar pillars, and fauces secondary to dermal and muscular fibrosis. As the disease progresses opening of the mouth and protrusion of the tongue develops such that eating, swallowing, and speech are impaired. Later ulceration and leukoplakic areas occur and finally, in approximately 7% of patients, malignant transformation to squamous cell carcinoma develops. Treatment consists of the intralesional injection of dexamethasone and hyaluronidase, and in advanced cases surgical excision and grafting. Discontinuance of the offending substance and physical therapy are also needed.

Lai DR, et al: Clinical evaluation of different treatment methods for oral submucous fibrosis. *J Oral Pathol Med* 1995, 24:402.
Norton SA: Betel. *J Am Acad Dermatol* 1998, 38:81. _____ ▲

Fascial Hernia

Evanescent herniations in the form of nodules appear in the skin where the deep and superficial veins meet going through the fascia. These herniated nodules, seen most frequently on the lower extremities, become prominent when the underlying muscles contract. Treatment is not indicated.

Harrington AC, et al: Hernias of the anterior tibialis muscle. *J Am Acad Dermatol* 1990, 22:123. _____ ▲

Acrochordon (Cutaneous Tag, Papilloma Colli, Fibroma Pendulum, Cutaneous Papilloma, Fibroma Molluscum, Templeton's Skin Tags, Skin Tags)

Small, flesh-colored to dark brown, pinhead-sized and larger, sessile and pedunculated papillomas commonly occur on the neck (Fig. 28-62) often in association with small seborrheic keratoses. These tags are also seen frequently in the axillae and on the eyelids, less often on the trunk and groins, where the soft, pedunculated growths often hang on thin stalks (Fig. 28-63). These flesh-colored, teardrop-shaped tags when palpated feel like small bags. Occasionally, as a result of twisting of the pedicle, one will become inflamed, tender, and even gangrenous. The onset is between ages 10 and 50. Both sexes have the same

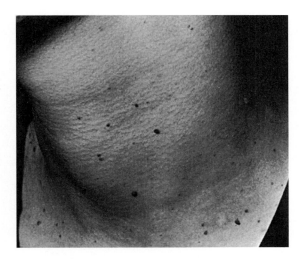

Fig. 28-62 "Cutaneous tags" of the neck: pedunculated seborrheic keratoses.

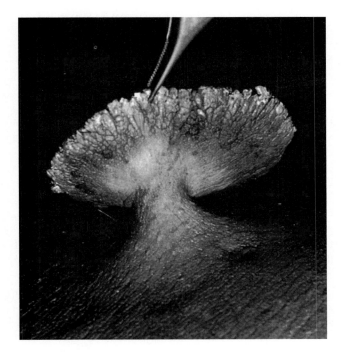

Fig. 28-63 Giant acrochordon on buttocks. (Courtesy Dr. Axel W. Hoke.)

incidence, with nearly 60% getting them by age 69. They often increase in number when the patient is gaining weight or during pregnancy. In patients preselected for gastrointestinal complaints, skin tags appear to be more prevalent in those with colonic polyps. This association has not been proved for the general population.

Histologically, acrochordons are characterized by a hyperplastic epidermis enclosing a dermal connective tissue stalk composed of loose collagen fibers. The baglike papillomas generally show a flattened epidermis. In a study of 1335 clinical specimens submitted as fibroepithelial polyps, Eads et al concluded that cutaneous lesions diagnosed by a dermatologist as typical skin tags need not be submitted for microscopic examination.

Most can be clipped off at the base with no anesthesia and aluminum chloride applied for hemostasis if needed. In larger lesions anesthesia and light electrodesiccation may be necessary.

An entity that is frequently reported as perianal acrochordons or skinfolds has now been named *infantile perianal pyramidal protrusions*. This occurs in young children, usually girls, in the midline anterior to the anus. This reduces with time and no treatment is necessary. Child abuse, genital warts, granulomatous lesions of inflammatory bowel disease, or rectal prolapse are in the differential diagnosis of these lesions.

Beitler M, et al: Association between acrochordons and colonic polyposis. *J Am Acad Dermatol* 1986, 14:1042.

Chobanian SJ: Skin tags and colonic polyps. *J Am Acad Dermatol* 1987, 16:407.

Eads TJ, et al: The utility of submitting fibroepithelial polyps for histological examination. *Arch Dermatol* 1996, 132:1459.

Gould BE, et al: Lack of association between skin tags and colon polyps in a primary care setting. *Arch Intern Med* 1988, 148:1799.

Kayashima K, et al: Infantile perianal pyramidal protrusion. *Arch Dermatol* 1996, 132:1481.

Lubach D, et al: Skin tags and colonic polyps. *J Am Acad Dermatol* 1987, 16:402.

Luk GD, et al: Colonic polyps and acrochordons do not correlate in familial colonic polyposis kindreds. *Ann Intern Med* 1986, 104:209. ▲

Dermatofibroma

This common nodular skin lesion has many names including histiocytoma cutis, fibroma durum, nodulus cutaneus, subepidermal nodular fibrosis, dermatofibroma lenticulare, and sclerosing hemangioma. The appearance is usually sufficiently characteristic to permit clinical diagnosis. It is generally a single round or ovoid papule or nodule about 1 cm in diameter (Fig. 28-64) that is reddish brown, sometimes with a yellowish hue. The sharply circumscribed nodule is more evident on palpation than is expected from inspection. The larger lesions may present an abrupt elevation at the border to form an exteriorized tumor resting on a sessile base.

The lesions may be elevated or slightly depressed. The hard nodule is adherent to the overlying epidermis, which may be thinner from pressure or even indented, so that there is a dell-like depression over the nodule. In such cases one sees only the depression but on palpation finds the true nature of the lesion. Fitzpatrick proposed the term *dimple sign* for the depression created over a dermatofibroma when it is grasped gently between thumb and forefinger.

Dermatofibromas seldom occur in children; they are encountered mostly in middle-aged adults. The size generally varies from 4 to 20 mm, although giant lesions greater

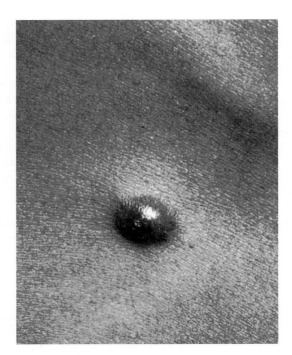

Fig. 28-64 Dermatofibroma (8 mm in diameter) on the infraclavicular area of a 12-year-old boy.

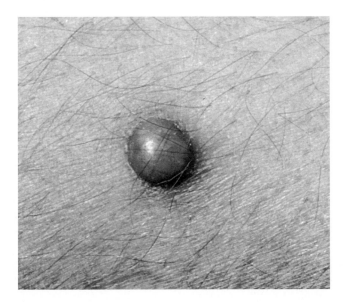

Fig. 28-65 Dermatofibroma on the leg. (Courtesy Dr. Axel W. Hoke.)

than 5 cm occur. After reaching this size, growth ceases and the harmless lump remains stationary. The principal locations are on the lower extremities (Fig. 28-65), above the elbows, or on the sides of the trunk. Some patients may develop multiple dermatofibromas. Systemic lupus erythematosus, treatment with prednisone or immunosuppressive drugs, and HIV infection have been associated with multiple dermatofibromas.

It is suspected that many of these are initiated by various injuries to the skin, such as insect bites or blunt trauma.

On histologic examination there is a dermal mass composed of close whorls of fibrous tissue in which are numerous cells with large nuclei rich in chromatin, epithelioid cells, or elongated spindle cells. At times the cells may be strikingly atypical and are referred to as monster cells. Alternatively a granular or even a translucent cytoplasm may predominate. The cells have features of fibroblasts and myofibroblasts, but are probably of primitive mesenchymal origin. Immunohistochemical studies show most cells are factor XIIIa positive, MAC387 negative, S-100 negative and CD34 negative.

Small or large amounts of pigment, hemosiderin, may be present, or alternatively foam cells and lipid deposits may be seen. There is a great variation in the vascular components. Rarely, the vascularization is pronounced and suggests a kind of hemangioma. The tumor is not well circumscribed and may extend into adjacent structures and surround individual collagen bundles at the periphery.

The changes in the epidermis are secondary and may be those of pressure atrophy or of acanthosis and hyperkeratosis. Basal cell carcinomas and basal cell carcinoma–like changes may overlie dermatofibromas but much more frequently, reactive changes such as acanthosis and pseudo-epitheliomatous hyperplasia are seen.

The clinical appearance of the lesion and its location, chiefly on the lower extremities, are distinctive. Clinically, granular cell tumor, dermatofibrosis lenticularis disseminata, clear cell acanthoma, and melanoma are some of the lesions to be considered. At times only a biopsy can differentiate these.

Progressive enlargement beyond 2 or 3 cm in diameter suggests a malignant fibrous histiocytoma or dermatofibrosarcoma protuberans, and excisional biopsy is indicated.

These lesions usually are asymptomatic and do not require treatment. Involution may occur within a few years if the lesion is left alone. Simple reassurance is suggested.

Goldblum JR, et al: CD34 and factor XIIIa immunoreactivity in dermatofibrosarcoma protuberans and dermatofibroma. *Am J Dermatopathol* 1997, 19:147.

Green C: Multiple nodules on the back. *Arch Dermatol* 1999, 135:341.

Lannigan SW, et al: Cryotherapy for dermatofibromas. *Clin Exp Dermatol* 1987, 12:121.

Lu I, et al: Multiple dermatofibromas in a woman with HIV infection and systemic lupus erythematosus. *J Am Acad Dermatol* 1995, 32:901.

Manente L, et al: Cutaneous epithelioid cell histiocytoma. *Am J Dermatopathol* 1997, 19:519.

Murphy SC, et al: Multiple eruptive dermatofibromas in an HIV-positive man. *Dermatology* 1995, 190:309.

Page EH, et al: Atrophic dermatofibroma and dermatofibrosarcoma protuberans. *J Am Acad Dermatol* 1987, 17:947.

Requena L, et al: The atrophic dermatofibroma. *J Dermatol* 1995, 22:334.

Requena L, et al: Giant dermatofibroma. *J Am Acad Dermatol* 1994, 30:714.

Setoyama M, et al: Case of dermatofibroma with monster cells. *Am J Dermatopathol* 1997, 19:312.

Sharata H, et al: Multiple hyperpigmented nodules. *Arch Dermatol* 1994, 130:650.

Soyer HP, et al: Granular cell dermatofibroma. *Am J Dermatopathol* 1997, 19:168.

Zelger BW, et al: Clear cell dermatofibroma. *Am J Surg Pathol* 1996, 20:483. _____ ▲

Dermatofibrosarcoma Protuberans

Dermatofibrosarcoma protuberans (DFSP) is characterized by bulky, protuberant, neoplastic masses (Fig. 28-66). Fifty percent to 60% occur on the trunk, with less common involvement of the proximal extremities and the head and neck. The disease begins with one or multiple elevated, erythematous, firm, nodules or plaques associated often with a purulent exudate or with ulceration (Fig. 28-67). Patients, usually middle-aged, complain of a firm, painless lump in the skin that has been slowly increasing in size for several years.

The course is slowly progressive, with pain becoming prominent as the lesion grows, and frequent recurrence after initial conservative surgical intervention. Severe pain, contractures, and invalidism gradually deplete the general health in untreated patients. There is little tendency to metastasize, although wide dissemination has been reported.

Histologically, the tumor shows a subepidermal fibrotic plaque with uniform spindle cells and variable vascular spaces. In many instances there is a cartwheel pattern of spindle cell arrangement surrounding a central area of collagen. Giant cells and histiocytes are also present but only in small numbers. Pigment-laden cells may occur and these lesions, which predominantly affect persons of color, are called *Bednar tumors.* Electron microscopic studies favor a fibroblastic origin, and several lesions have stained positively for vimentin, an intermediate filament protein of mesenchymal cells. CD34 positivity is characteristic and serves as a suitable marker to discern DFSP from dermatofibroma. S-100 is negative and may be used to separate melanoma from a Bednar tumor.

The differential diagnosis, especially in the early stage, is that of keloid and a large dermatofibroma.

Surgical excision by Mohs' technique is the treatment of choice. In a series of 50 patients the recurrence rate was 2%, whereas in other series of patients treated with wide local excision, recurrence was 11% to 50%.

Allan AE, et al: Clonal origin of DFSP. *J Invest Dermatol* 1993, 100:99.

Bouyssou-Gauthier ML, et al: DFSP in childhood. *Pediatr Dermatol* 1997, 14:463.

Elgart GW, et al: Bednar tumor occurring in a site of prior immunization. *J Am Acad Dermatol* 1999, 40:315.

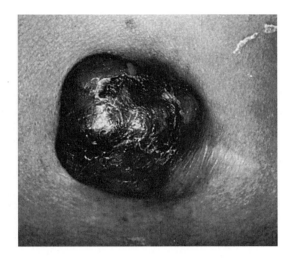

Fig. 28-66 Dermatofibrosarcoma protuberans.

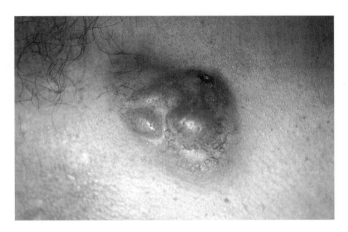

Fig. 28-67 Dermatofibrosarcoma protuberans.

Gloster HM Jr: DFSP. *J Am Acad Dermatol* 1996, 35:355.

Gutierrez G, et al: DFSP. *Int J Dermatol* 1984, 23:396.

Haycox CL, et al: Immunohistochemical characterization of DFSP with practical applications for diagnosis and treatment. *J Am Acad Dermatol* 1997, 37:438.

Kobayashi T, et al: A case of Bednar tumor. *Dermatology* 1997, 195:57.

Miettinen M, et al: Antibodies to intermediate filament proteins. *Arch Dermatol* 1985, 121:736.

Ratner D, et al: Mohs micrographic surgery for the treatment of DFSP. *J Am Acad Dermatol* 1997, 37:600.

Robinson J: DFSP resected by Mohs surgery. *J Am Acad Dermatol* 1985, 12:1093. _____ ▲

Nodular Fasciitis (Nodular Pseudosarcomatous Fasciitis)

Also known as *subcutaneous pseudosarcomatous fibromatosis* or *proliferative fasciitis,* this benign mesenchymal neoplasm occurs most often on the arms. Clinically, a firm, solitary, sometimes tender nodule develops in the deep fascia, and often extends into the subcutaneous tissue. It measures usually 1 to 4 cm in diameter. The lesion appears suddenly over a period of a few weeks, without apparent cause, in normal, healthy persons. Sex distribution is equal, and the average age at onset is 40.

Microscopic findings consist of myxoid, fibroblastic, and capillary proliferations. Lymphocytic-histiocytic infiltration is present, with many normal-looking mitotic figures. On electron microscopic examination, the component cells in the neoplasm have proved to be myofibroblasts.

Dermal, intravascular, and proliferating variants have been described. These are designated when the nodular masses arise in the dermis, in intimate association with blood vessels, or show giant cells within the infiltrative tumor respectively.

The proper treatment is complete excision. Recurrence is rare, and the prognosis is excellent. Graham et al described a patient with a rapid response to intralesional corticosteroids.

Cranial fasciitis of childhood is an uncommon variant of nodular fasciitis, manifesting as a rapidly enlarging mass in the subcutaneous tissue of the scalp, which may invade the cranium. It occurs in infants and children, resembles nodular fasciitis histologically, and usually does not recur after surgical excision.

Cartwright LE, et al: Rapidly growing asymptomatic subcutaneous nodules. *Arch Dermatol* 1988, 124:1559.

Chartier S, et al: Nodular fasciitis of the upper lip mimicking a sarcoma. *Int J Dermatol* 1994, 33:503.

Goodlad JR, et al: Intradermal variant of nodular "fasciitis." *Histopathology* 1990, 17:569.

Graham BS, et al: Nodular fasciitis. *J Am Acad Dermatol* 1999, 40:490.

Kiryu H, et al: Proliferative fasciitis. *Am J Dermatopathol* 1997, 19:396.

Lai FM M, et al: Nodular fasciitis of the dermis. *J Cutan Pathol* 1993, 20:66.

Meffert JJ, et al: Intradermal nodular fasciitis presenting as an eyelid mass. *Int J Dermatol* 1996, 35:548.

Montgomery EA, et al: Nodular fasciitis. *Am J Surg Pathol* 1991, 15:942.

Patterson JW, et al: Cranial fasciitis. *Arch Dermatol* 1989, 125:674.

Price SK, et al: Dermal and intravascular fasciitis. *Am J Dermatopathol* 1993, 15:539.

Shimizu S, et al: Nodular fasciitis. *Pathology* 1984, 16:161. ▲

Atypical Fibroxanthoma

Atypical fibroxanthoma (AFX) of the skin is a low-grade malignancy related to malignant fibrous histiocytoma, which it resembles histologically. Its smaller size and more superficial location account largely for its more favorable prognosis. The lesion occurs chiefly on the sun-exposed parts of the head or neck in white persons over age 50 (Fig. 28-68). The tumor is a small, firm nodule often with an eroded or crusted surface without characteristic morphologic features. A clinical variant, found in 25% of cases, occurs in a subset with an average age of 39; it presents as a slowly enlarging tumor on a covered area.

The lesion develops in the dermis and is separated from the epidermis by a thin band of collagen. The tumor consists

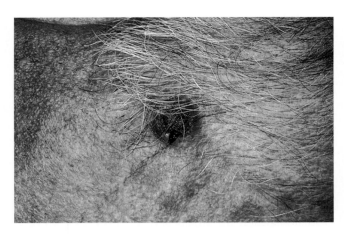

Fig. 28-68 Atypical fibroxanthoma.

of bizarre spindle cells mingled with atypical histiocytes. Some spindle cells have a vesicular nucleus. The cytoplasm may be vacuolated and resemble the xanthoma cell. Mitotic figures, prominent eosinophilic nucleoli, and the presence of biphasic tumor cell population are characteristic findings. S-100 staining is sparse when compared with melanoma, and prekeratin staining is negative: this helps to distinguish AFX from squamous cell carcinoma. Variants with clear cells and osteoclast-type cells have been described.

The treatment of choice is complete surgical excision. Mohs' microsurgery results in fewer recurrences than in wide excision. Although the prognosis is excellent, local recurrence after inadequate excision is usual, and cases of metastasizing AFX have been reported.

Davis JL, et al: A comparison of Mohs micrographic surgery and wide excision for the treatment of atypical fibroxanthoma. *Dermatol Surg* 1997, 23:105.

Holmes S, et al: Bleeding nodule on the forehead. *Arch Dermatol* 1999, 135:1113.

Kanitakis J, et al: Atypical fibroxanthoma in a renal graft recipient. *J Am Acad Dermatol* 1996, 35:262.

Kuwano H, et al: Atypical fibroxanthoma distinguishable from spindle cell carcinoma in sarcoma-like skin lesions. *Cancer* 1985, 55:172.

Limmer BL, et al: Cutaneous micrographic surgery for atypical fibroxanthoma. *Dermatol Surg* 1997, 23:553.

Patterson JW, et al: Atypical fibroxanthoma in a patient with xeroderma pigmentosum. *Arch Dermatol* 1987, 123:1066.

Wesson SK: Solitary nodule on the foot of a 37-year-old man. *Arch Dermatol* 1986, 122:1325.

Winkelmann RK, et al: Atypical fibroxanthoma. *Arch Dermatol* 1985, 121:753. ▲

Malignant Fibrous Histiocytoma (Malignant Histiocytoma)

Malignant fibrous histiocytoma (MFH) is the most common soft-tissue sarcoma of middle and late adulthood. It resembles dermatofibrosarcoma protuberans; both may present as a protruding rounded tumor from 1 cm to several centimeters in diameter, often reddish or dusky, and progressively enlarging. MFH arises deeply and is more likely to appear in the subcutaneous tissue. One third occur on the thigh or buttock. Peak incidence is in the seventh decade. They sometimes arise in an area of radiodermatitis or in a chronic ulceration.

Pleomorphic cellular elements and bizarre mitotic figures are characteristic. Atypical fibroxanthomas are smaller and more superficial tumors of the dermis, compared with the deeper muscular, subcutaneous or, uncommonly, deep dermal location of MFH. Epithelioid sarcoma, while it shares with MFH the presence of both polygonal and spindle cell types, lacks the latter's large, bizarre, multinucleated cell types. Several histologic variants of MFH have been described, including myxoid, inflammatory, and giant cell types. Cell staining is positive for vimentin.

The prognosis in MFH is related to the site; deeper and more proximally located tumors have a poorer prognosis. The myxoid variant is less likely to metastasize. An especially poor prognosis attends tumors arising in sites of radiodermatitis. Local recurrence after excision occurs in 25%, 35% metastasize, and the overall survival rate is 50%. Mohs' surgical removal may result in less recurrences.

A tumor that presents on the extremities of children as a slowly growing dermal or subcutaneous mass may be the angiomatoid type. It has been separated from the term malignant as it has a relatively good prognosis.

Alconchel MD, et al: Squamous cell carcinoma, malignant melanoma and malignant fibrous histiocytoma arising in burn scars. *Br J Dermatol* 1997, 137:793.
Biederman TM, et al: Subcutaneous nodule of the lower extremity. *Arch Dermatol* 1999, 135:1113.
Brown MD, et al: Treatment of malignant fibrous histiocytoma and atypical fibrous xanthomas with micrographic surgery. *J Dermatol Surg Oncol* 1989, 15:1287.
Chang P, et al: Malignant fibrous histiocytoma of the skin. *Int J Dermatol* 1994, 33:50.
Enzinger FM: Angiomatoid malignant fibrous histiocytoma. *Cancer* 1979, 44:2147.
Farber JN, et al: Malignant fibrous histioctyoma arising from discoid lupus erythematosus. *Arch Dermatol* 1988, 124:114.
Fletcher CDM, et al: Pleomorphic malignant fibrous histiocytoma. *Am J Surg Pathol* 1992, 16:213.
Goette DK, et al: Post-irradiation malignant fibrous histiocytoma. *Arch Dermatol* 1985, 122:535.
Pezzi CM, et al: Prognostic factors in 227 patients with malignant fibrous histiocytoma. *Cancer* 1992, 69:2098.
Routh A, et al: Malignant fibrous histiocytoma arising from chronic ulcer. *Arch Dermatol* 1985, 122:529. ▲

Epithelioid Sarcoma

Epithelioid sarcoma occurs chiefly in young adults, with onset usually being from 20 to 40 years of age. Two thirds of cases are in men. Nearly all lesions are on the extremities, half of them on the hands or wrists. It has, however, been reported from a wide variety of locations, including the genital region.

The tumor grows slowly among fascial structures and tendons, often with central necrosis of the tumor nodules and ulceration of the overlying skin. Recurrence after attempted excision occurs in three out of four cases, and late metastasis occurs in 45% of patients. Initial clinical diagnoses may include granuloma annulare, rheumatoid nodule, ganglion, fibroma, and inclusion dermoid cyst. It has also been mistaken for palisading granuloma, chronic inflammation, and squamous cell carcinoma.

Histologically, irregular nodular masses of large, deeply acidophilic polygonal cells merge with spindle cells and are frequently associated with large amounts of hyalinized collagen.

A cure may be achieved by wide local excision in the early stage of the disease. Women have a markedly more favorable prognosis. The smaller the tumor at diagnosis, the more likely the cure.

Bos GD, et al: Epithelioid sarcoma. *J Bone Joint Surg* (Am) 1988, 70:862.
Chase DR, et al: Epithelioid sarcoma. *Am J Surg Pathol* 1985, 9:241.
Evans HL, et al: Epithelioid sarcoma. *Semin Diag Pathol* 1993, 10:286.
Kodet R, et al: Epithelioid sarcoma in childhood. *Pediatr Pathol* 1994, 14:443.
Padilla RS, et al: Epithelioid sarcoma. *Arch Dermatol* 1985, 121:389.
Puissegur Lupo ML, et al: Epithelioid sarcoma. *Arch Dermatol* 1985, 121:394.
Shmookler BM, et al: Superficial epithelioid sarcoma. *J Am Acad Dermatol* 1986, 14:93.
Weissmann D, et al: Vulvar epithelioid sarcoma metastatic to the scalp. *Am J Dermatopathol* 1990, 12:462.
Zanolli MD, et al: Epithelioid sarcoma. *J Am Acad Dermatol* 1992, 26:302. ▲

Myxomas

Myxomas may be considered as two types of lesions: the digital mucous cyst and cutaneous myxomas. The latter may or may not be associated with cardiac myxomas and cutaneous spotty pigmentation.

Digital mucous cysts are taut, shiny, translucent, white to pink, dome-shaped lesions characteristically located on the dorsal aspect of the distal interphalangeal articulation. There may be an associated grooving or dystrophy of the nail. Either fingers or toes may be affected.

Digital mucous cysts, which are discussed in more detail in Chapter 9, should be differentiated from ganglions, which occur most frequently over the wrists, are herniations of joint linings, are deeper in location, and are often associated with exostoses. These have a lining to the cavity and require excision and grafting with removal of the cyst, the lining, and the pedicle to the joint.

Singh et al reported on cutaneous metaplastic synovial cysts, a tender subcutaneous or dermal nodule at the site of trauma or surgery. The cystic lining resembles hyperplastic synovium.

Cutaneous myxomas may be solitary, and appear as flesh-colored nodules on the face, trunk, or extremities.

They may also occur as part of a syndrome championed by Carney et al. They reported 41 patients with a disorder they refer to as myxomas, spotty pigmentation, and endocrine overactivity. This has also been reported under the eponyms NAME (*n*evi, *a*trial myxoma, *m*yxoid neurofibromas, and *e*phelides) and LAMB (*l*entigines, *a*trial myxoma, *m*ucocutaneous myxomas, *b*lue nevi) and simply as cutaneous lentiginosis with atrial myxoma.

The Carney complex consists of patients who have two or more of the following: (1) cardiac myxomas (79%), (2) cutaneous myxomas (not myxoid neurofibromas) (45%), (3) mammary myxoid fibromas (30%), (4) spotty mucocutaneous pigmentation, including lentiginoses (not ephelides) and blue nevi often of a distinctive epithelioid variety (65%), (5) primary pigmented nodular adrenocortical disease (45%), (6) testicular tumors (56% of male patients), and (7) pituitary growth hormone–secreting tumors (10%). A peculiar type of schwannoma featuring melanin and psammoma bodies may also be present.

The cutaneous myxomas occur as small (less than 1 cm), multiple, skin-colored papules having a predilection for development by a mean age of 18 years, and a tendency to occur on the ears, eyelids, and nipples. The lentigines are prominent on the face, lips, and genital mucosa. This condition is autosomal dominantly inherited and the defect maps to the short arm of chromosome 2. Recognition of this syndrome, with diagnosis and removal of the atrial myxomas, can be lifesaving.

A malignant counterpart, the myxosarcoma, is a tumor that arises in the subcutaneous fat and underlying soft tissues (Fig. 28-69). There is a tendency for local recurrence after wide and deep excision. Metastases are rare.

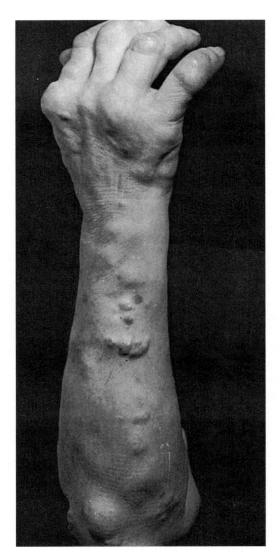

Fig. 28-69 Myxosarcoma. (Courtesy Dr. F. Daniels, Jr.)

Arnijo M: Mucoid cysts of the finger. *J Dermatol Surg Oncol* 1981, 7:317.

Carney JA: Carney complex: the complex of myxomas, spotty pigmentation, endocrine overactivity, and schwannomas. *Semin Dermatol* 1995, 14:90.

Carney JA: Cutaneous myxomas. *Arch Dermatol* 1986, 122:790.

Carney JA: The complex of myxomas, spotty pigmentation, and endocrine overactivity. *Medicine* 1985, 64:270.

Carney JA: The epithelioid blue nevus. *Am J Surg Pathol* 1996, 20:259.

Epstein E: A simple technique for managing digital mucous cysts. *Arch Dermatol* 1979, 115:1315.

Huerter CJ, et al: Treatment of digital mucous cysts with carbon dioxide laser vaporization. *J Dermatol Surg Oncol* 1987, 13:723.

Gourdin FW, et al: Cylindrical deformity of the nail plate secondary to subungual myxoma. *J Am Acad Dermatol* 1996, 35:846.

Macpherson M, et al: Ganglia of the ankle. *J Am Acad Dermatol* 1985, 13:873.

Reed OM, et al: Cutaneous lentiginosis with atrial myxoma. *J Am Acad Dermatol* 1986, 15:398.

Singh SR, et al: Multiple cutaneous metaplastic synovial cysts. *J Am Acad Dermatol* 1999, 41:330.

Stratakis CA, et al: Carney complex, a familial multiple neoplasia and lentiginosis syndrome. *J Clin Invest* 1996, 97:699.

Utiger CA, et al: Psammomatous melanotic schwannoma. *Arch Dermatol* 1993, 129:202.
_____ ▲

MASTOCYTOSIS (URTICARIA PIGMENTOSA)

Mastocytosis is a general term applied to local and systemic accumulations of mast cells. Urticaria pigmentosa is a manifestation of mastocytosis characterized by persistent pigmented, itchy skin lesions of various size that tend to urticate on mechanical or chemical irritation. Studies have revealed activating mutations in the c-KIT protooncogene. Its protein product is the transmembrane tyrosine kinase KIT receptor whose ligand is stem cell factor (also known as *mast cell growth factor*). Both clonality studies and mutational analysis indicate that at least some adult cases of mastocytosis result from a neoplastic proliferation of mast cells, while childhood mastocytosis reveals cytokine-driven hyperplasia.

CLINICAL FEATURES. Nettleship first described the disease in 1869. Urticaria pigmentosa may occur from birth to middle age. However, about half the cases have their onset before 6 months of age, and an additional fourth occur before puberty.

The cutaneous lesions may consist of macules, papules, nodules, plaques, vesicles, or bullae. Rarely, telangiectases, petechiae, or ecchymoses may occur. There may be no visible skin lesions at all, even though biopsy will prove the presence of high numbers of mast cells.

At their onset the lesions are similar to urticaria except that they are not evanescent. The lesions of urticaria pigmentosa persist and gradually become chamois- or slate-colored. When they are firmly stroked or vigorously rubbed, urticaria with a surrounding erythematous flare (Darier's sign) usually develops.

Frequently, the lesions are slightly elevated; the nodules may be firm and discrete or confluent and are usually of a brownish waxy appearance. Dermographism of clinically uninvolved skin is present in a third to half of patients. Flushing of a generalized type sometimes accompanied by syncope, may be present at the onset and may gradually decrease during the course of the disease.

Severe symptoms as a result of the massive liberation of histamine from mast cells may occur after ingestion of known mast cell degranulators such as alcohol, morphine, or codeine, or after extended rubbing. *Hymenoptera* stings may induce anaphylaxis.

Pruritus, the most frequent symptom, varies from a mild state to an intensity that may interfere with sleep and may be accompanied by fatigue, anorexia, diarrhea, and joint pains. Rarely, diarrhea may be the chief symptom. Cromolyn sodium generally controls explosive attacks, though patients may continue to have three or four bowel movements a day.

In the course of time, old lesions tend to disappear without sequelae. Spontaneous involution is especially likely in those patients whose cutaneous disease began in childhood.

Several types of lesions occur with the solitary mastocytoma, with bullous, pseudoxanthomatous, and diffuse cutaneous types being mostly seen in children and erythrodermas, telangiectasia macularis eruptiva perstans, and leukemia-associated types more common in adults.

Solitary mastocytoma. The solitary nodule may be present at birth or may develop during the first weeks of life. The tumor stems from a brown macule that urticates on stroking (Fig. 28-70). This macule develops into a papule or a raised round or oval plaque up to 20 mm in diameter. It may have a smooth or a slightly warty surface (peau d'orange). Although it may occur anywhere on the body, its favorite location is on the dorsum of the hand near the wrist. Edema, urtication, vesiculation, and even bulla formation may be observed in the lesion. Uncommonly, several of these mastocytomas may be present.

Although the generalized form may begin with a single lesion, dissemination usually occurs within 3 months of its appearance. Most solitary mastocytomas involute spontane-

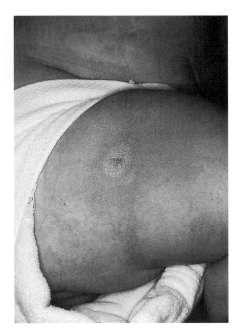

Fig. 28-70 Solitary mastocytoma on the leg.

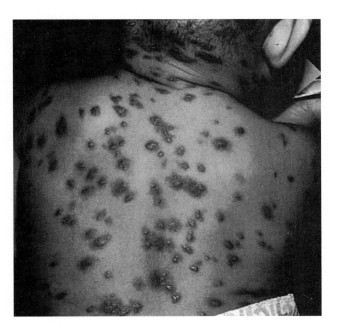

Fig. 28-71 Urticaria pigmentosa. (Courtesy Dr. Axel W. Hoke.)

ously by age 10 or earlier. They also respond favorably to excision. Progression to malignant disease does not occur.

Generalized eruption, childhood type. In the generalized form the eruption usually begins during the first weeks of life, presenting with rose-colored, pruritic, urticarial, slightly pigmented macules, papules, or nodules (Fig. 28-71). The lesions are oval or round, and vary in diameter between 5 and 15 mm and may coalesce (Fig. 28-72). The color varies from yellowish brown to yellowish red.

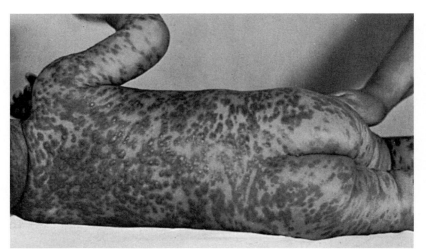

Fig. 28-72 Urticaria pigmentosa.

Vesicle and bulla formation is a frequent prominent feature early in the disease (Fig. 28-73). Indeed, vesicles and bullae may be the initial presenting signs however they usually persist no longer than 3 years. In the older age groups vesiculation rarely occurs.

Pigmentation and all evidence of the disease commonly disappears within a few years, generally before puberty. The eruption, however, may persist into adult life. Although systemic involvement is possible, malignant systemic disease is extremely rare.

Pseudoxanthomatous mastocytosis (xanthelasmoidea). An uncommon variant of urticaria pigmentosa is xanthelasmoidea, described as such by Tilbury Fox in 1875. Pale yellow nodules 1 mm to 2 cm in diameter usually are present in profusion at birth. The spleen may be enlarged. Erythema, but no urtication, is elicited by rubbing. A dense mast cell infiltrate is found histologically.

Diffuse cutaneous mastocytosis. In this form, with diffuse involvement, the entire integument may be thickened and infiltrated with mast cells to produce a peculiar orange color, giving rise to the term *homme orange*. There is an infiltrated doughy or boggy consistency to the skin, and lichenification may be present.

Generalized eruption, adult type. Most frequent are the pruritic brownish papular or nodular forms, with typical urtication of the lesion disseminated over most of the body but especially on the upper arms, legs, and trunk. These may be reddish-purple, rust colored, or brown. In the latter case they may closely resemble common nevi.

Erythrodermic mastocytosis. There is generalized erythroderma and the skin has a leather-grain appearance. Urtication can be produced over the entire surface.

Telangiectasia macularis eruptiva perstans. This is a persistent, pigmented, asymptomatic macular eruption, with a slightly reddish tinge (Fig. 28-74). Often little or no telangiectasia is evident. This form is a benign disorder, of cosmetic import only, in the great majority of cases,

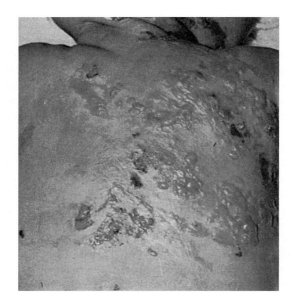

Fig. 28-73 Bullous mastocytosis. (Courtesy Dr. M. Orkin.)

although bone lesions and peptic ulcer disease may occur. Darier's sign may not be demonstrable.

Systemic mastocytosis. Mast cell proliferation not only may occur in the skin but may involve such organs as the lymph nodes, gastrointestinal system, bones, heart, blood, liver, and spleen. In fact, any organ system except the CNS may be affected. The process may be progressive or may remain stationary. Skin lesions are mostly of the nodular type, and the bone lesions are usually asymptomatic, with x-ray evaluation showing areas of radiolucency and radiodensity. Although usually bone lesions are silent and nonprogressive mast cell leukemia may rarely develop. Non–mast-cell leukemias and lymphomas may also complicate this disease.

The gastrointestinal tract may show mucosal changes,

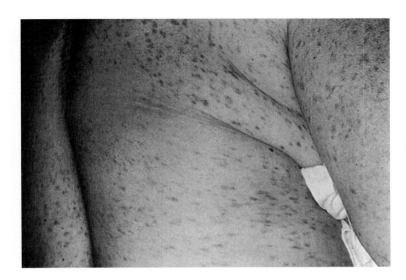

Fig. 28-74 Telangiectasia macularis eruptiva perstans.

which are distinctive. Abdominal pain, nausea, and vomiting are frequently present. Systemic mast cell disease occurs most frequently in the adult; however, about 10% of the patients with the juvenile disseminated type will have systemic involvement. Organ dysfunction may also result from secondary hypereosinophilic syndrome.

Excessive histamine release from the mast cells is believed to cause the systemic reactions, including flushing. A tendency to bleed may be manifested by hematemesis, epistaxis, melena, and ecchymoses. It is believed that elevated plasma heparin levels may be responsible for these signs. Anemia, leukopenia, and thrombocytopenia, with increased prothrombin time, are known to occur.

Malignant mast cell disease occurs when overwhelming infiltration of mast cells in the various organs disturbs their normal functions. Rarely, the cutaneous-visceral type may be fatal. This is more likely to occur in adults; however, extensive systemic infiltration may produce death in infants also. If mast cell leukemia develops, the prognosis is quite poor.

Familial urticaria pigmentosa. Mastocytosis of any kind is rarely familial. Fowler et al reviewed 47 reported cases of familial mastocytosis and concluded that it was usually transmitted by autosomal dominant inheritance with reduced expressivity, although other patterns may occur.

BIOCHEMICAL STUDIES. Human mast cells have been shown to contain histamine. Excess histamine is released from the mast cells into the bloodstream. At this time flushing, tachycardia, hypotension, headache, and gastrointestinal symptoms may occur. The increased amounts of histamine produce histaminuria. Although 60% of patients with systemic mastocytosis have an elevated 24-hour urine histamine level, the histamine metabolites methylhistamine and methylimidazole acetic acid are more sensitive and specific indicators. The demonstration of elevated tryptase

levels is also a useful marker as hypereosinophilic states can cause increases in histamine levels.

HISTOPATHOLOGY. The typical lesion shows a dense dermal aggregate of large mononuclear cells with abundant basophilic cytoplasm. When these large mononuclear cells are stained with Giemsa, azure A, or polychrome toluidine blue, the metachromatic granules are observed. Kasper et al described a method of counting tissue mast cells using morphometric point counting and a conjugated avidin stain; this method can useful in establishing the diagnosis. When blisters are present, the roof of the vesicle or bulla is subepidermal. The mast cells collect in a band below the vesicle. Infiltration of local anesthetic adjacent to the lesion rather than directly into it and the use of anesthetic without epinephrine may help to avoid mast cell degranulation.

DIAGNOSIS. The typical case of cutaneous mastocytosis is easily diagnosed by the presence of solitary or multiple pigmented papules or nodules that urticate when irritated by stroking or scratching. The diagnosis is confirmed by biopsy of the lesion with the demonstration of numerous mast cells. The bullous and vesicular lesions may be more difficult to diagnose; however, scrapings from the base of the bulla when stained with Giemsa or Wright stain will show mast cells in profusion.

Persistently elevated levels of histamine and two of its major metabolites, *N*-methylhistamine and *N*-methylimidazole acetic acid are present in the urine in many mastocytosis patients. Elevated levels also occur in chronic myelocytic leukemia and polycythemia vera.

DIFFERENTIAL DIAGNOSIS. Clinically, the solitary mastocytoma may most frequently resemble the pigmented nevus or juvenile xanthogranuloma. Urtication establishes the diagnosis. The disseminated lesions are also distinctive enough to give little or no difficulty in the diagnosis. The nodular form may resemble xanthomas; however, the presence of urtication is distinctive. The vesicular and bullous lesions are to be distinguished from various hereditary and nonhereditary bullous diseases and bullous impetigo. The main histologic similarity is to Langerhans' cell histiocytosis.

PROGNOSIS. In all forms of cutaneous mastocytosis without systemic involvement. the prognosis is good. In children with limited disease, most cases clear completely. The others improve, or the condition persists indefinitely. The solitary mastocytoma involutes spontaneously, usually within 3 years of onset.

TREATMENT. Symptomatic relief may be achieved in many cases by the use of antihistamines. Both H_1 and H_2 blockers and the antiserotonin drugs such as cyproheptadine (Periactin) may alleviate urtication, pruritus, and flushing. Oral methoxsalen and UVA (PUVA) therapy produces excellent clearing in most cases; unfortunately, however, recurrence on discontinuation is common. Godt et al reported that 14 of 20 patients improved and that in 25% the improvement lasted longer than 5 years. Intralesional triamcinolone or potent topical steroids under occlusion may also clear cutaneous lesions; however, the lesions recur after discontinuance. Also, concern about local atrophy, striae, and systemic absorption limit the utility of this treatment. Fairley et al have reported a response to nifedipine, an oral calcium channel blocker, in a dose of 10 mg three times a day. All symptoms ceased within 24 hours. It presumably acts by raising the mast cells' threshold for degranulation.

Control of diarrhea in systemic mastocytosis may be achieved by orally administered disodium cromoglycate. Cromolyn is more effective against gastrointestinal manifestations, and the antihistamines better against the cutaneous ones. A single dose of mithramycin resulted in the disappearance of bone pain in one patient, but had little effect on histamine release symptomatology.

It cannot be overemphasized that avoidance of physical stimuli, such as extremes of temperature and pressure and chemical degranulators of mast cells, is important. These include opiates, aspirin, alcohol, quinine, scopolamine, gallamine decamethonium, reserpine, amphotericin B, polymyxin B antibiotics, and D-tubocurarine. *Hymenoptera* stings may induce anaphylaxis; the patient (and the parents, if the affected individual is a child) should be taught to recognize the signs of anaphylactic shock and to provide treatment as appropriate.

Azana JM, et al: Urticaria pigmentosa. *Pediatr Dermatol* 1994, 11:102.

Barton J, et al: Treatment of urticaria pigmentosa with corticosteroids. *Arch Dermatol* 1985, 121:1516.

Ellis DL: Treatment of telangiectasia macularis eruptiva perstans with the 585-nm flashlamp pumped-dye laser. *Dermatol Surg* 1996, 22:33.

Fairley JA, et al: Urticaria pigmentosa responsive to nifedipine. *J Am Acad Dermatol* 1984, 11:740.

Fowler JF, et al: Familial urticaria pigmentosa. *Arch Dermatol* 1986, 122:80.

Godt O, et al: Short- and long-term effectiveness of oral and bath PUVA therapy in urticaria pigmentosa and systemic mastocytosis. *Dermatology* 1997, 195:35.

Henz BM: SCF and c-kit in mastocytosis: a Pandora's box holding more theories than proven facts. *J Invest Dermatol* 1998, 110:186.

James MP, et al: Familial urticaria with giant mast-cell granules. *Arch Dermatol* 1981, 117:713.

Kanwar AJ, et al: Diffuse cutaneous mastocytosis. *Pediatr Dermatol* 1993, 10:301.

Kasper CS, et al: Quantification of cutaneous mast cells using morphometric point counting and a conjugated avidin stain. *J Am Acad Dermatol* 1987, 16:326.

Kendall ME, et al: Cutaneous mastocytosis without clinically obvious skin lesions. *J Am Acad Dermatol* 1984, 10:903.

Kettelhut BV, et al: Pediatric mastocytosis. *Ann Allergy* 1994, 73:197.

Kors JW, et al: Long-term follow-up of indolent mastocytosis in adults. *J Intern Med* 1996, 239:157.

Krober SM, et al: Mastocytosis: reactive or neoplastic? *J Clin Pathol* 1997, 50:525.

Kunisada T, et al: Murine cutaneous mastocytosis and epidermal melanocytosis induced by keratinocyte expression of transgenic stem cell factor. *J Exp Med* 1998, 187:1565.

Longley BJ, et al: Chronically KIT-stimulated clonally derived human mast cells show heterogeneity in different tissue microenvironments. *J Invest Dermatol* 1997, 108:792.

Longley BJ, et al: Somatic c-KIT activating mutation in urticaria pigmentosa and aggressive mastocytosis: establishment of clonality in a human mast cell neoplasm. *Nat Genet* 1996, 12:312.

Longley J, et al: The mast cell and mast cell disease. *J Am Acad Dermatol* 1995, 32:545.

Mackey S, et al: Diffuse cutaneous mastocytosis. *Arch Dermatol* 1996, 132:1429.

McElroy EA Jr, et al: Systemic mast cell disease associated with the hypereosinophilic syndrome. *Mayo Clin Proc* 1998, 73:47.

Musette P, et al: Inguinal pigmented papules. *Arch Dermatol* 1999, 135:203.

O'Connell BM, et al: Pigmented papules in the axilla. *Arch Dermatol* 1988, 124:1421.

Oude-Elberink JN, et al: Fatal anaphylaxis after a yellow jacket sting, despite venom immunotherapy, in two patients with mastocytosis. *J Allergy Clin Immunol* 1997, 99:153.

Parks A, et al: Reddish-brown macules with telangiectasia and pruritus. *Arch Dermatol* 1988, 124:429.

Tharp MD: Mast cell disease and its diagnosis. *J Invest Dermatol* 1995, 104:885.

Tharp MD: Understanding mast cells and mastocytosis. *J Invest Dermatol* 1997, 108:698.

Topar G, et al: Urticaria pigmentosa. *Am J Clin Pathol* 1998, 109:279.

Van Gysel D, et al: Value of urinary N-methylhistamine measurements in childhood mastocytosis. *J Am Acad Dermatol* 1996, 35:556. ▲

ABNORMALITIES OF NEURAL TISSUE
Solitary Neurofibroma

The ordinary solitary cutaneous neurofibroma may be 2 to 20 mm in diameter. It is soft, flaccid, and pinkish white. Frequently the soft small tumor can be invaginated, as if through a ring in the skin by pressure with the finger (this is called "buttonholing").

Neurofibroma is either solitary or multiple (Fig. 28-75). When solitary (one or two lesions), they are spontaneous tumors without any internal manifestations. When three or more are present, the diagnosis of neurofibromatosis is made. Uncommonly, large pendulous masses occur in which numerous tortuous, thickened nerves can be felt; this has been likened to a "bag of worms." These plexiform

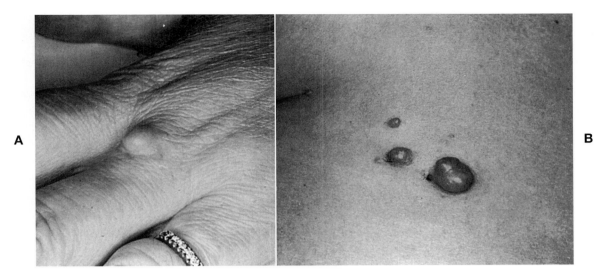

Fig. 28-75 **A,** Solitary neurofibroma. **B,** Localized neurofibromas.

neurofibromas, which often have overlying pigmentation, occur in neurofibromatosis. Neurofibromatosis is discussed in Chapter 27.

The distinctive histopathologic findings are characterized by three basic features: fibrils, cellular proliferation, and degenerative changes (fatty and myxomatous). The wavy fibrillar tissues with small cells containing ovoid nuclei are densley arranged. Cellular proliferation is in sheets or stellate clumps. Glycosaminoglycans may be greatly increased, and numerous mast cells may be present. Cholinesterase activity is markedly positive in the neurofibromas. Immunochemical staining shows positivity for S-100, vimentin, and myelin basic protein, markers for schwannian tissue.

Treatment of those lesions that are particularly objectionable is by surgical excision.

Oshman RG, et al: A solitary neurofibroma on the finger. *Arch Dermatol* 1988, 124:1185.

Requena L, et al: Benign neoplasms with neural differentiation. *Am J Dermatopathol* 1995, 17:75. ——————————————— ▲

Granular Cell Tumor

Granular cell tumor was described by Abrikossoff in 1926. It has been called *granular cell myoblastoma* or *schwannoma* for years, but many other synonyms have been used. About one third of the reported cases have occurred on the tongue, one third involved the skin, and one third occurred in the internal organs. The tumor is usually a well-circumscribed, solitary, firm nodule ranging from 5 to 30 mm with a brownish red or flesh tint, depending on nearness to the surface (Fig. 28-76).

Its surface is usually smooth and glistens, but infrequently it may ulcerate. Although usually solitary, it may be multiple in 10% to 15% of cases (Fig. 28-77).

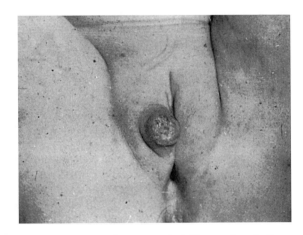

Fig. 28-76 Granular cell tumor on the labium majus of a 5-year-old child.

The solitary lesion may be located anywhere on the body, but nearly half of all tumors appear on the head or neck (Fig. 28-78). Usually the patients are in the third to fifth decades. About two thirds of patients are black, and two thirds are women. In most cases it grows very slowly, and when completely removed does not usually recur. However, local or multicentric recurrence may at times cause confusion in determining if a granular cell tumor is malignant.

The cells stain positively with vimentin, neuron-specific enolase, S-100, and myelin protein. These stains show that the granules are composed of myelin or myelin metabolic products.

The histologic picture is distinctive. The cells are large, pale, and irregularly polygonal, with a poorly defined cellular membrane, and contain coarsely granular cytoplasm. Some of the cells are multinucleated or contain vacuoles or small pyknotic or eosinophilic inclusions. At

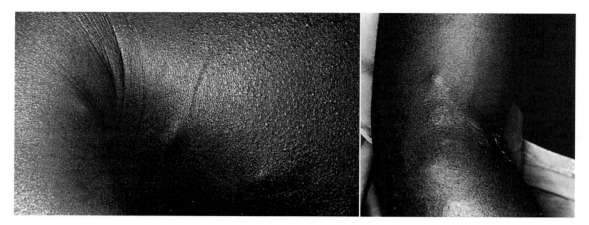

Fig. 28-77 Multiple granular cell tumors.

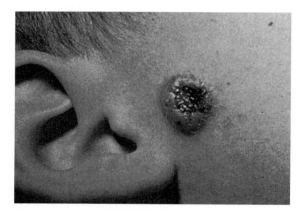

Fig. 28-78 Granular cell tumor on cheek of 12-year-old boy.

times the arrangement is in cords or sheets, in irregular alveolar masses, or even organoid. The similarity to xanthoma cells has been pointed out. However, with special stains no lipids are demonstrable. Pseudo-epitheliomatous hyperplasia is a regular feature, and has often led to a mistaken diagnosis of squamous cell carcinoma associated with xanthoma.

Malignant granular cell tumor is rare. Malignant lesions are much larger, with an average diameter of 9 cm; benign lesions average less than 2 cm. Rapidity of growth and invasion of adjacent tissue are other criteria to be weighed, because the histologic findings are not always reliable.

Aggressive surgery is the treatment of choice.

Alidina R, et al: A solitary tumor on the earlobe. *Arch Dermatol* 1994, 130:913.

Apisarnthanarax P: Granular cell tumor. *J Am Acad Dermatol* 1981, 5:171.

Lee J, et al: Plexiform granular cell tumor. *Am J Dermatopathol* 1994, 16:537.

Seo IS, et al: Multiple visceral and cutaneous granular cell tumors. *Cancer* 1984, 53:2104.

Toback AC: Arm tumor resembling a supernumerary nipple. *Arch Dermatol* 1985, 121:927.

Truhan AP: Firm linear plaque on the lip of a child. *Arch Dermatol* 1985, 121:1197. _____ ▲

Neuroma Cutis

Cutaneous neuromas are uncommon. Three true neuromas exist in the skin and mucous membranes: traumatic neuromas, multiple mucosal neuromas, and solitary palisaded encapsulated neuromas.

Traumatic neuromas result from the overgrowth of nerve fibers in the severed ends of peripheral nerves. The lesion may be tender or painful, and when scarring has occurred or the distal stump has been removed, a phantom limb syndrome may result. These often occur on the fingers, at sites of amputation of supernumerary digits, or on the sole, usually at the third metatarsal space.

Multiple mucosal neuromas occur as part of multiple mucosal neuroma syndrome (multiple endocrine neoplasia, type 2b). These patients have a marfanoid habitus, thickened protruding lips, and multiple neuromas of the oral mucosa (lips, tongue, and gingiva), the conjunctiva, and sometimes the sclera. A few have multiple cutaneous neuromas, usually limited to the face. There is a strong association with medullary carcinoma of the thyroid, bilateral pheochromocytomas, and diffuse alimentary tract ganglioneuromatosis.

The palisaded, encapsulated neuroma of the skin is a solitary, large, encapsulated tumor, usually of the face. It is a slow-growing, flesh-colored, dome-shaped, firm lesion usually appearing around the mouth or nose. It closely resembles a basal cell carcinoma or an intradermal nevus.

Argenyi ZB, et al: Plexiform and other unusual variants of palisaded encapsulated neuroma. *J Cutan Pathol* 1993, 20:34.

De Roos KP et al: Traumatic neuroma. *J Dermatol Surg Oncol* 1994, 20:681.

Dover JS, et al: Palisaded encapsulated neuromas. *Arch Dermatol* 1989, 125:386.

Fairchild P, et al: Palisaded encapsulated neuroma (PEN). *Arch Dermatol* 1994, 130:369.

Holloway KB, et al: Multiple endocrine neoplasia 2B (MEN 2B)/MEN 3. *Dermatol Clin* 1995, 13:99.

Kirk JF, et al: Multiple endocrine neoplasia type III. *Pediatr Dermatol* 1991, 8:124.

Lashgari AR, et al: The importance of early diagnosis in multiple endocrine neoplasia. *J Am Acad Dermatol* 1997, 36:296.

Megahed M: Palisaded encapsulated neuroma (solitary circumscribed neuroma). *Am J Dermatopathol* 1994, 16:120.

Rubin Z: Cutaneous neuroma. *Arch Dermatol* 1982, 118:960. _____ ▲

Neurothekeoma (Nerve Sheath Myxoma)

Gallager and Helwig described a benign cutaneous tumor they called a neurothekeoma, meaning a tumor of nerve sheath, composed of cords and nests of large cells packed among collagen bundles in close proximity to small nerves. Mitotic figures and nuclear atypia are sometimes seen, but the tumor is benign. This is probably the same lesion described by Harkin and Reed in 1969 as an axon sheath myxoma. These benign intradermal or subcutaneous tumors histologically are divided into two subtypes: myxoid and a more common cellular variant. The former occurs in middle-aged adults on the head, neck, and upper extremities primarily. It is twice as common in women. The cellular type occurs in childhood, with a high female preponderance, and a predilection for the head, neck, or shoulders. The cellular type does not stain with S-100 or HMB-45, useful facts in differentiating it from melanoma.

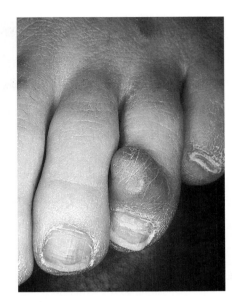

Fig. 28-79   Neurilemmoma.

Argenyi ZB, et al: Nerve sheath myxoma (neurothekeoma) of the skin. *J Cutan Pathol* 1993, 20:294.

Argenyi ZB, et al: Ultrastructural spectrum of cutaneous nerve sheath myxoma/cellular neurothekeoma. *J Cutan Pathol* 1995, 22:137.

Barnhill RL, et al: Studies on the cellular origin of neurothekeoma. *J Am Acad Dermatol* 1991, 25:80.

del Rio E, et al: Neurothekeoma. *Arch Dermatol* 1993, 129:1506.

Husain S, et al: Histologic spectrum of neurothekeoma and the value of immunoperoxidase staining for S-100 protein in distinguishing it from melanoma. *Am J Dermatopathol* 1994, 16:496. _____ ▲

Schwannoma (Neurilemmoma)

Peripheral schwannomas are usually a solitary nerve sheath tumor, most often seen in women. They occur almost exclusively along the main nerve trunks of the extremities (Fig. 28-79), especially the flexor surface of the arms, wrists, and knees, but they are also seen on the scalp, sides of the neck, and tongue. The solitary tumor is a nodule from 3 to 30 mm in diameter. It is soft or firm, pale pink or yellowish; it may or may not be painful.

Sometimes the tumors are multiple. When this occurs they may be seen with neurofibromatosis type 1 or as an entity independent of neurofibromatosis. Most commonly, however, they are associated with neurofibromatosis type 2 (NF-2). The independent type may be congenital or have a delayed onset. It may be sporadic or familial. Three clinical patterns are described: elevated dome-shaped nodules, pale brown indurated macules, and multiple papules coalescing into plaques from 2 to 100 mm broad, with a predilection for the trunk. Cases have occurred that appeared to be

unassociated with NF-2 that on further investigation of the individual or the family revealed them to have other signs of NF-2 and to carry the gene abnormality on chromosome 22.

Plexiform schwannomas may occur as single or multiple lesions, localized to a single anatomic site or more generalized, and arise in the dermis or subcutaneous tissue. They may occur as a solitary lesion, or associated with NF-1, NF-2, or multiple schwannomas. Another subtype of schwannoma is the melanotic psammomatous type that is seen in association with Carney's syndrome of spotty pigmentation, myxomas, and endocrine overactivity. A malignant variety occurs either as a solitary lesion, associated with NF-1, or in some cases associated with xeroderma pigmentosa.

Schwannomas occur in many other organs, and brain tumors such as meningiomas, gliomas, and astrocytomas may occur.

Histologically, the classic types are well encapsulated and composed of two types of tissue, referred to as *Antoni types A* and *B*. The diagnosis is affirmed by the finding of Verocay bodies. Bodian stain reveals very few or no nerve fibers. Numerous mast cells may be seen within the tumor. S-100, vimentin, and myelin basic protein stains are positive. Many histologic subtypes exist, and some distinctive ones are associated with syndromes as cited above.

Excision is almost invariably curative, except in the malignant variety.

Berger TG, et al: Agminated neurilemmomas. *J Am Acad Dermatol* 1987, 17:891.

Buscher CA, et al: A painful subcutaneous neurilemmoma attached to a peripheral nerve. *J Am Acad Dermatol* 1998, 38:122.

Demitsu T, et al: Malignant schwannoma arising in patients with von Recklinghausen's disease. *J Dermatol* 1995, 22:747.

Elston DM, et al: Schwannoma with sweat duct differentiation. *J Cutan Pathol* 1993, 20:254.

Evans DG, et al: Spinal and cutaneous schwannomatosis is a variant form of type 2 neurofibromatosis. *J Neurol Neurosurg Psychiatry* 1997, 62:361.

Honda M, et al: Neurofibromatosis 2 and neurilemmomatosis gene are identical. *J Invest Dermatol* 1995, 104:74.

Kikuchi A, et al: Solitary cutaneous malignant schwannoma. *Am J Dermatopathol* 1993, 15:15.

Prevoo R, et al: Multiple cutaneous neurilemmomas with abnormalities of the eyes and congenital rib deformities. *J Am Acad Dermatol* 1987, 17:1054.

Purcell SM, et al: Schwannomatosis. *Arch Dermatol* 1989, 125:390.

Reith JD, et al: Multiple cutaneous plexiform schwannomas. *Arch Pathol Lab Med* 1996, 120:399.

Sasaki T, et al: Congenital neurilemmomatosis. *J Am Acad Dermatol* 1992, 26:786.

Shishiba T, et al: Multiple cutaneous neurilemmomas as a skin manifestation of neurilemmomatosis. *J Am Acad Dermatol* 1984, 10:744.

Utiger CA, et al: Psammomatous melanotic schwannoma. *Arch Dermatol* 1993, 129:202.

Val Bernal JF, et al: Cutaneous plexiform schwannoma associated with neurofibromatosis type 2. *Cancer* 1995, 76:1181.

Wolkenstein P, et al: Schwannomatosis. *Dermatology* 1997, 195:228.

Yamashiro S, et al: Malignant trigeminal schwannoma associated with xeroderma pigmentosum. *Neurol Med Chir* 1994, 34:817. ▲

Infantile Neuroblastoma

Neuroblastoma is the most common malignant tumor of early childhood. Cutaneous nodules are most often seen in younger patients, being present in 32% of infants with the disease (Fig. 28-80). These occur as multiple 2- to 20-mm, firm, blue nodules that, when rubbed, blanch and form a halo of erythema. The blanching persists for 1 to 2 hours and is followed by a refractory period of several hours. Biopsy shows clusters of basophilic cells with large nuclear-to-cytoplasmic ratio, surrounded by eosinophilic fine fibrillar material. Two other findings that may be present are periorbital ecchymoses (the so-called raccoon eyes) and heterochromia of the irises.

For patients with skin involvement the prognosis is good, with either spontaneous remission or spontaneous transformation into benign ganglioneuromas expected.

Lucky AW, et al: Infantile neuroblastoma presenting with cutaneous blanching nodules. *J Am Acad Dermatol* 1982, 6:389. ▲

Ganglioneuroma

Ganglioneuroma has only rarely been described in the skin as an isolated entity. These tumors are composed of mature ganglion cells commingled with fascicles of spindle cells. They arise most often in von Recklinghausen's neurofibromatosis or with neuroblastomas, and usually occur in childhood. The tissue stains positively for both argyrophilic and argentaffin granules.

Gambini C, et al: Primary congenital cutaneous ganglioneuroma. *J Am Acad Dermatol* 1996, 35:353.

Geffner RE, et al: Ganglioneuroma of the skin. *Arch Dermatol* 1986, 122:377.

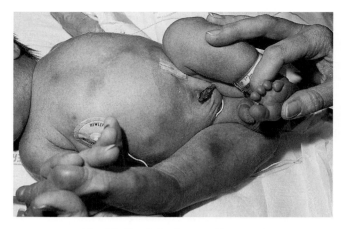

Fig. 28-80　Infantile neuroblastoma.

Hammond RR, et al: Cutaneous ganglioneuromas. *Hum Pathol* 1996, 27:735. ▲

Nasal Glioma (Cephalic Brainlike Heterotopias)

Nasal gliomas are rare, benign, congenital tumors. When they occur extranasally, they are easily confused with hemangiomas. They are ectopic neural tissue, with the histology of astrocytomas. The tumor is usually a firm, incompressible (unlike a hemangioma and encephalocele), reddish blue to purple lesion occurring on the nasal bridge or midline near the root (Fig. 28-81). It does not transilluminate or enlarge with crying, unlike some encephaloceles. They may also occur intranasally.

Nasal gliomas differ from encephaloceles in that the latter are connected to the subarachnoid space by a sinus tract, while the former lose this connection before birth. Clinically, these cannot be differentiated, so a biopsy should not be performed.

Radiography should be performed to detect possible skull involvement. Neurosurgical consultation is advisable.

Histologically, the nodule consists of glial tissue associated with glial giant cells, fibrous tissue, and numerous blood vessels. It is unencapsulated. The lesion does not involute spontaneously.

Fletcher CD, et al: Nasal glioma. *Am J Dermatopathol* 1986, 8:341.

Gebhart W, et al: Nasal glioma. *Int J Dermatol* 1982, 21:212.

Kennard CD, et al: Congenital midline nasal masses. *J Dermatol Surg Oncol* 1990, 16:1025.

Paller AS, et al: Nasal midline masses in infants and children. *Arch Dermatol* 1991, 127:362. ▲

Cutaneous Meningioma

Cutaneous meningioma is also known as *psammoma*. Primary cutaneous meningioma, also known as *rudimentary meningocele,* is a developmental defect. It results from the presence of meningocytes outside the calvarium. If actual brain remnants are present, the lesion is called a *rudimentary cephalocele*. Small, hard, fibrous, calcified nodules

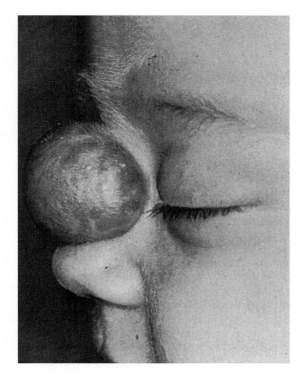

Fig. 28-81   Nasal glioma. (Courtesy Dr. H.C. Christianson.)

occur along the spine, in the scalp, on the forehead, or rarely in the external ear canal. Most occur over scalp, some have an underlying connection to the central nervous system or an underlying bony abnormality, and usually come to medical attention in the first year of life. On the scalp they may present with a dark tuft of hair or an alopecic area surrounded by a dark collar of hair (hair collar sign).

Cutaneous meningiomas may develop in the scalp secondary to an intracranial meningioma, either by means of erosion of the skull, or by extension through an operative defect of the skull. Finally, they may also arise from cranial or spinal nerves. Clinically, these lesions have no distinctive appearance. They are firm subcutaneous nodules adherent to the skin.

Diagnosis is made by histologic examination. The tumors consist of strands of cells with large oval vesicular nuclei and granular cytoplasm; these are hyaline bodies (psammoma bodies), which are calcified to some extent. Psammoma bodies have also been found in intradermal nevi, juvenile xanthogranuloma, the pituitary of the fetus and newborn, schwannomas associated with Carney's syndrome, meninges, choroid plexus, pineal gland, papillary carcinoma of the thyroid, ovarian neoplasms, and mammary intraductal papilloma.

Commens C, et al: Heterotropic brain tissue presenting as bald cysts with a collar of hypertrophic hair. *Arch Dermatol* 1989, 125:1253.
Fung MA, et al: Intracranial malignant meningioma mimicking frontalis-associated lipoma of the forehead. *J Am Acad Dermatol* 1996, 34:306.

Hu B, et al: Association of primary intracranial meningioma and cutaneous meningioma of external auditory canal. *Arch Pathol Lab Med* 1998, 122:97.
Iglesias ME, et al: Intracranial osteolytic meningioma affecting the scalp. *J Am Acad Dermatol* 1996, 35:641.
Penas PF, et al: Cutaneous meningioma underlying congenital localized hypertrichosis. *J Am Acad Dermatol* 1994, 30:363.
Stone MS, et al: Rudimentary meningocele presenting with a scalp hair tuft. *Arch Dermatol* 1994, 130:775. _____ ▲

ENCEPHALOCELE AND MENINGOCELE

Primary defects in the neural tube may lead to encephaloceles, meningoceles, or meningomyeloceles. They present in infancy along the midline of the face, scalp, neck, or back as soft, compressible masses that may transilluminate or enlarge with crying. Tufts of long, dark hair, or alopecia with a surrounding collar of dark hair may occur overlying them.

Many cutaneous lesions of the back may infer other malformations of the spinal cord and associated structures are present. Cutaneous manifestations of spinal dysraphism include depressed lesions, dermal lesions, dyschromic lesions, hairy lesions, polypoid lesions, neoplasms, and subcutaneous and vascular lesions. Midline masses require intensive radiologic and neurosurgical evaluation before biopsy because of the possible connection to the CNS.

Berry AD III, et al: Meningoceles, meningomyeloceles, and encephaloceles. *J Cutan Pathol* 1991, 18:164.
Davis DA, et al: Cutaneous stigmata of occult spinal dysraphism. *J Am Acad Dermatol* 1994, 31:892.
Enjolras O, et al: Cervical occult spinal dysraphism. *Pediatr Dermatol* 1995, 12:256.
Howard R: Cutaneous markers of congenital malformations. *Adv Dermatol* 2000, 15:1.
Wiss K: Midline developmental defects in children. *Adv Dermatol* 2000, 15:109. _____ ▲

Chordomas

These slow-growing, locally invasive neoplasms present as firm, smooth nodules in the sacrococcygeal region or at the base of the skull in middle-aged patients. They arise from notochord remnants. The pathologic appearance is that of incompletely encapsulated sheets, nests, and cords of large epithelioid cells with fibrous trabeculae present. They may metastasize late in their course.

Wide excision with postoperative radiation therapy is the treatment of choice.

Miller SD, et al: Multiple smooth skin nodules. *Arch Dermatol* 1997, 133:1579. _____ ▲

ABNORMALITIES OF FAT TISSUE
Lipomas

Lipomas are subcutaneous tumors composed of fat tissue, most commonly found on the trunk. They also occur frequently on the neck, forearms, and axillae. They are soft,

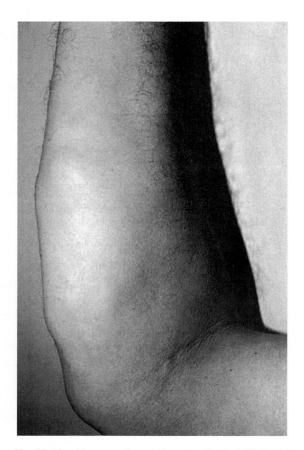

Fig. 28-82 Lipomas of arm. (Courtesy Dr. Axel W. Hoke.)

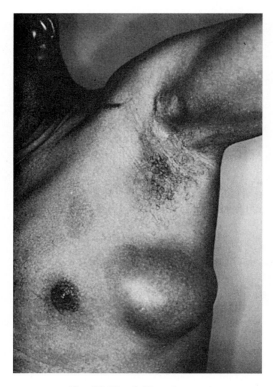

Fig. 28-83 Solitary lipoma.

single or multiple (Fig. 28-82), small or large (Fig. 28-83), lobulated, compressible growths, over which the skin on traction often becomes dimpled, although otherwise unchanged. They usually stop growing after attaining a certain size, then remain stationary indefinitely. Frontalis-associated lipomas of the forehead are relatively large lesions arising either within or deep to the frontalis muscle.

A lipoma located in the midline of the sacral region may be a marker for spinal dysraphism or other embryologic malformation. Other midline lesions, such as tufts of hair ("fawn's tail"), hemangiomas (Cobb's syndrome), skin tags, sinuses, or pigmented lesions should also raise one's suspicion for occult embryologic malformations. At least a radiographic evaluation of the lumbosacral region should be obtained. If spinal dysraphism is diagnosed, early treatment may be possible before irreversible damage has occurred. Do not attempt to biopsy a sacrococcygeal lipoma; call a neurosurgeon into consultation. It may be a lipomeningocele, with communicating sinuses to the dura.

Histologically, the lipoma is an encapsulated, lobulated tumor containing normal fat cells held together by strands of connective tissue. Occasionally, eccrine sweat glands may be associated and then they are called *adenolipomas*.

In the differential diagnosis, the epidermoid cyst should always be considered. At times it is difficult to distinguish the two. Others to be kept in mind are angiolipoma and hibernoma.

Lipomas may be left untreated unless they are large enough to be objectionable. If they are objectionable, they may be excised. Alternatively a cutting curette may be introduced through a 3-mm incision over the center of the lipoma and the globular tumor freed from the surrounding tissue, after which it is compressed laterally and extruded through the incision with gentle traction. Liposuction is another method of removal. More advanced surgical technique is necessary to remove the deep lesions on the forehead. Removal of these was discussed in detail by Zitelli et al and Salasche et al.

Solitary lipomas should be investigated for malignancy if they become 10 cm in diameter, especially when they occur on the upper thigh.

Multiple lipomas may occur in groups of two to hundreds of confluent painless tumors of various sizes over any part of the body. These lesions are sometimes painful when growing rapidly. When present in certain patterns, special designations are applied.

Madelung's disease (benign symmetric lipomatosis or multiple symmetric lipomatosis) occurs most commonly in

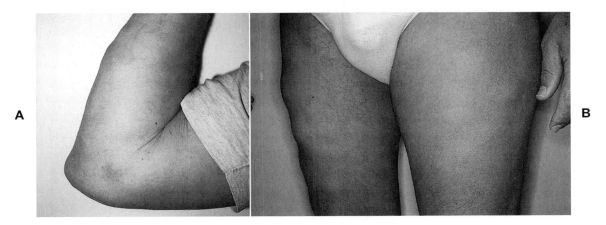

Fig. 28-84 **A** and **B,** Familial multiple lipomatosis.

middle-aged men, who may develop multiple, large, painless, coalescent lipomas around the neck, shoulders, and upper arms.

Dercum's disease (adiposis dolorosa) is characterized by obese or corpulent menopausal women who develop symmetrical, tender, circumscribed fatty deposits, often accompanied by weakness and psychiatric disturbances. Juhlin obtained relief of pain lasting for weeks in a 60-year-old woman by intravenous infusions of lidocaine, 1.3 g daily for 4 days.

Familial multiple lipomatosis is a dominantly inherited syndrome in which multiple asymptomatic lipomas of the forearms and thighs appear in the third decade of life (Fig. 28-84). The shoulders and neck are spared, and the lipomas are encapsulated and movable.

Several other conditions are characterized by multiple abnormalities including lipomas. Encephalocraniocutaneous lipomatosis is a rare neurocutaneous syndrome characterized by unilateral facial and scalp lesions, ipsilateral ocular abnormalities, and neurologic complications. Approximately 20 cases have been reported since its description by Haberland and Perou in 1970. The skin changes consist of unilateral lipomatous scalp tumors with overlying alopecia and connective tissue nevi. Ipsilateral lipodermoids, choristomas, and calcifications are the eye findings. Central nervous system abnormalities are unilateral cerebral atrophy, dilated ventricles, porencephaly, cerebral calcifications and lipomas of the leptomeninges. Seizures and mental retardation may occur. Some cases may have overlapping features of Proteus syndrome, which features multiple lipomas, epidermal nevi, cerebriform lesions of the plantar surfaces, vascular malformations, macrodactyly, hemihypertrophy, exostoses, and scoliosis.

Bannayan-Riley-Ruvalcaba syndrome is characterized by multiple subcutaneous lipomas and vascular malformations, lentigines of the penis and vulva, verrucae, and acanthosis nigricans. There is overlap in some of these cases with Cowden's syndrome. Both have been found to have abnormalities of the PTEN protein and thus share genetically similar if not identical abnormalities.

Multiple endocrine neoplasia type 1 (MEN1) has been found to have skin lesions consisting of multiple facial angiofibromas, collagenomas, café au lait spots, lipomas, confetti-like hypopigmented macules, and multiple gingival papules in addition to the tumors of the parathyroid glands, endocrine pancreas, and anterior pituitary.

Fröhlich's syndrome consists of multiple lipomas, obesity, and sexual infantilism.

Gardner's syndrome consists of multiple osteomas, fibromas, desmoid tumors, lipomas, fibrosarcomas, epidermal inclusion cysts, and leiomyomas, associated with intestinal polyposis exclusively in the colon and rectum. The coexistence of cutaneous cysts, leiomyomas, and osteomas (mostly on the skull) with intestinal polyposis is frequently not recognized until malignant degeneration of one of the polyps occurs and operative removal brings the syndrome to notice. Half of such patients develop carcinoma of the colon before age 30, and practically all these patients die before age 50 unless they have surgical treatment. In general, total colectomy is advised. Bony exostoses occur in 50% of patients and usually involve the membranous bones of the face and head. Cysts occur in 63% of patients, and again occur most commonly on the face and in the scalp. These are epidermal inclusion cysts; two thirds have within them foci of pilomatricoma. Traboulis et al described pigmented lesions of the ocular fundus in 90% of 41 patients with Gardner's syndrome and 46% of 43 first-degree relatives. They are usually multiple and bilateral, and, having been seen in a 3-month-old infant, are probably congenital. Gardner's syndrome is transmitted as an autosomal dominant disease. The defect is a mutation in the APC gene. In some families polyposis and carcinoma may occur without the skin and bone tumors.

Carlin MC, et al: Multiple symmetric lipomatosis. *J Am Acad Dermatol* 1988, 18:359.

Ciatti S, et al: Encephalocraniocutaneous lipomatosis. *J Am Acad Dermatol* 1998, 38:102.

Cooper PH, et al: Pilomatricoma-like changes in the epidermal cysts of Gardner's syndrome. *J Am Acad Dermatol* 1983, 8:639.

Darling TN, et al: Multiple facial angiofibromas and collagenomas in patients with multiple endocrine neoplasia type I. *Arch Dermatol* 1997, 133:853.

Economides NG, et al: Benign symmetric lipomatosis (Madelung's disease). *South Med J* 1986, 79:1023.

Fargnoli MC, et al: Clinicopathologic findings in the Bannayan-Riley-Rubvalcaba syndrome. *Arch Dermatol* 1996, 132:1214.

Field LM: Liposuction surgery for symmetric lipomatosis. *J Am Acad Dermatol* 1988, 18:1370.

Hardin FF: A simple technique for removing lipomas. *J Dermatol Surg Oncol* 1982, 8:316.

Herbert AA, et al: Sacral lipomas. *Arch Dermatol* 1987, 123:711.

Hitchcock MG, et al: Adenolipoma of the skin. *J Am Acad Dermatol* 1993, 29:82.

Juhlin L: Long-standing pain relief of adiposis dolorosa after intravenous infusion of lidocaine. *J Am Acad Dermatol* 1986, 15:383.

Leffell DJ, et al: Familial multiple lipomatosis. *J Am Acad Dermatol* 1986, 15:275.

McAtee-Smith J, et al: Skin lesions of the spinal axis and spinal dysraphism. *Arch Pediatr Adolesc Med* 1994, 148:740.

Nishisho I, et al: Mutations of chromosome 5q21 genes in FAP and colorectal cancer patients. *Science* 1991, 253:665.

Perniciaro C: Gardner's syndrome. *Dermatol Clin* 1995, 13:51.

Pinski KS, et al: Liposuction of lipomas. *Dermatol Clin* 1990, 8:483.

Ruzicka T, et al: Benign symmetric lipomatosis Launois-Bensaude: report of ten cases and review of the literature. *J Am Acad Dermatol* 1987, 17:663.

Salasche SJ, et al: Frontalis-associated lipoma of the forehead. *J Am Acad Dermatol* 1989, 20:462.

Samlaska CP, et al: Proteus syndrome. *Arch Dermatol* 1989, 125:1109.

Traboulis EI, et al: Prevalence and importance of pigmented ocular fundus lesions in Gardner's syndrome. *N Engl J Med* 1987, 316:661.

Zitelli JA: Subgaleal lipomas. *Arch Dermatol* 1989, 125:384. ▲

Angiolipoma

The angiolipoma is a painful subcutaneous nodule just slightly above the level of the skin, having all the other features of a typical lipoma. It is seen in young adults who have multiple painful lumps in the skin. Multiple subcutaneous angiolipomas have no invasive or metastatic potential.

Haustein UF, et al: Multiple bluish subcutaneous nodules. *Arch Dermatol* 1990, 126:666.

Kaneko T, et al: The treatment of multiple angiolipomas by liposuction surgery. *J Dermatol Surg Oncol* 1994, 20:690. ▲

Neural Fibrolipoma

Neural fibrolipoma is an overgrowth of fibro-fatty tissue along a nerve trunk that often leads to nerve compression. Patients are usually age 30 or younger and note a slowly enlarging subcutaneous mass with associated tenderness, decreased sensation, or parasthesia. The median nerve is most commonly involved. At times macrodactyly appears, with elongation and splaying of the phalanges. MRI will provide the diagnosis, but unfortunately there is no effective treatment.

Ricci RM, et al: Congenital painful pedal mass. *Arch Dermatol* 1999, 135:707. ▲

Spindle-Cell Lipoma

The spindle-cell lipoma is an asymptomatic, slow-growing subcutaneous tumor that has a predilection for the posterior back, neck and shoulders of older men. It is usually solitary, although multiple lesions may occur. Some patients who have a familial background of these have been described. The neoplasm consists of lobulated masses of mature adipose tissue with areas of spindle cell proliferation.

Duve S, et al: Spindle-cell lipoma of the skin. *Am J Dermatopathol* 1995, 17:529.

Fanburg-Smith JC, et al: Multiple spindle cell lipomas. *Am J Surg Pathol* 1998, 22:40. ▲

Painful Piezogenic Pedal Papules

Shelley and Rawnsley in 1968 described transitory, soft, sometimes painful papules on the sides of the heels (Fig. 28-85), elicited by weight-bearing (hence "piezogenic," produced by pressure) and disappearing when this is stopped. These occur in at least 75% of normal individuals, but are painful, presumably because of ischemia, in the few persons who complain of the condition. The painful papules are typically large, nearly 1 cm in diameter, and occur mostly in women over age 40. They consist of fat lobules forced out of the panniculus by the pressure of weight-bearing.

Suitable supportive shoes may alleviate the discomfort. There is no definitive therapy. Laing et al point out that with pressure piezogenic papules occur in the wrist area in 86 percent of patients.

Laing VB, et al: Piezogenic wrist papules. *J Am Acad Dermatol* 1991, 24:415.

van Straaten EA, et al: Piezogenic papules of the feet in healthy children and their possible relation with connective tissue disorders. *Pediatr Dermatol* 1991, 8:277. ▲

Nevus Lipomatosus Superficialis

Soft, yellowish papules or cerebriform plaques, usually of the buttock or thigh, less often of the ear or scalp, with a wrinkled rather than warty surface, characterize this tumor (Fig. 28-86). The distribution may be either zonal (as in the multiple lesions reported by Hoffmann and Zurhelle) or solitary. Solitary ones look rather like a fatty acrochordon. Onset before age 20 is the rule.

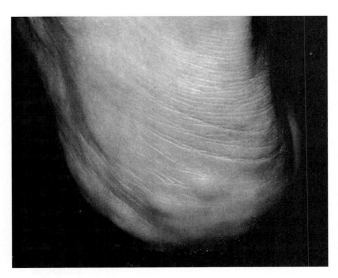

Fig. 28-85 Painful piezogenic pedal papules, when bearing weight. (Courtesy Dr. Axel W. Hoke.)

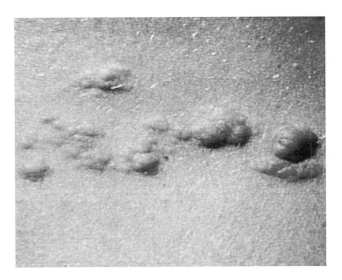

Fig. 28-86 Nevus lipomatosus cutaneus superficialis.

Chanoki M, et al: Nevus lipomatosus cutaneus superficialis of the scalp. *Cutis* 1989, 43:143.
Park HJ, et al: Nevus lipomatosus superficialis on the face. *Int J Dermatol* 1997, 36:435. _____ ▲

Folded Skin with Scarring (Michelin Tire Baby Syndrome)

In this rare syndrome, there are numerous deep, conspicuous, symmetrical, ringed creases around the extremities. The underlying skin may manifest a smooth muscle hamartoma, a nevus lipomatosis, or elastic tissue abnormalities. It may occur as an autosomal dominant trait, as a sporadic condition, as an isolated finding, associated with congenital facial and limb abnormalities, or with severe neurologic defects.

Glover MT, et al: Michelin tire baby syndrome resulting from diffuse smooth muscle hamartoma. *Pediatr Dermatol* 1989, 6:329.
Sato M, et al: Michelin tire syndrome. *Br J Dermatol* 1997, 136:583.
Schnur RE, et al: Variability in the Michelin tire syndrome. *J Am Acad Dermatol* 1993, 28:364. _____ ▲

Diffuse Lipomatosis

Diffuse lipomatosis is characterized by an early age of onset, usually before age 2; diffuse infiltration of muscle by an unencapsulated mass of histologically mature lipocytes; and progressive enlargement and extension of the tumor mass. It usually involves a large portion of the trunk or an extremity. Some cases are associated with distant lipomas or hemangiomas or with hypertrophy of underlying bone.

Klein JA, et al: Diffuse lipomatosis and tuberous sclerosis. *Arch Dermatol* 1986, 122:1298. _____ ▲

Hibernoma

Hibernoma (lipoma of brown fat) is a form of lipoma composed of finely vacuolated fat cells of embryonic type. Hibernomas have a distinctive brownish color and a firm consistency, and usually occur singly. These tumors are benign. They occur chiefly in the mediastinum and the interscapular region of the back but they also occur on the scalp, sternal region, and legs. They are usually about 3 to 12 cm in breadth and the onset is usually in adult life. Epidural lipomatosis, collections of fat in the epidural space, may cause acute chord compression in the course of systemic corticosteroid treatment. A case of this distinctive, uncommon side effect proved to be the result of deposits of brown fat.

Muszynski CA, et al: Scalp hibernoma. *Surg Neurol* 1994, 42:343.
Perling LH, et al: Epidural hibernoma as a complication of corticosteroid treatment. *J Neurosurg* 1988, 69:613. _____ ▲

Pleomorphic Lipoma

These lesions, like spindle-cell lipomas, occur for the most part on the backs or necks of elderly men. There are occasional lipoblast-like cells and atypical mitotic figures that requires differentiation from a liposarcoma. Fat cells of variable size interspersed with characteristic "floret" multinucleated giant cells are seen microscopically. Despite this alarming appearance, the lesions behave in a perfectly benign manner.

Digregorio F, et al: Pleomorphic lipoma. *J Dermatol Surg Oncol* 1992, 18:197.
Griffin TD, et al: Pleomorphic lipoma. *J Cutan Pathol* 1992, 19:330. _____ ▲

Benign Lipoblastomatosis

This tumor, frequently confused with a liposarcoma, affects exclusively infants and young children, with approximately 90% occurring before 3 years of age. It involves most commonly the soft tissues of the upper and lower extremities. A circumscribed and a diffuse form can be distinguished. The circumscribed form is superficially located and clinically comparable to a lipoma. The diffuse form is more deeply situated and is analogous to diffuse lipomatosis. Microscopically, both forms consist of lobulated immature adipose tissue composed of lipoblasts, a plexiform capillary pattern, and a richly myxoid stroma. Complete local excision is the treatment of choice.

Coffin CM, et al: Congenital lipoblastoma of the hand. *Pediatr Pathol* 1992, 12:857. _____ ▲

Liposarcoma

Liposarcoma is one of the less common mesenchymal neoplasms of the soft tissue. They usually arise from the intermuscular fascia, and only rarely from the subcutaneous fat. They do not arise from preexisting lipomas. The usual course is an inconspicuous swelling of the soft tissue that undergoes an imperceptibly gradual enlargement. When a fatty tumor becomes more than 10 cm in diameter liposarcoma should be seriously considered. The upper thigh is the most common site. Other frequent sites are the buttocks, groin, and upper extremities. Adult males are affected mostly.

Liposarcomas may be well or poorly differentiated, myxoid or pleomorphic, or dominated by round cells. Treatment is adequate radical excision of the lesion. In well-differentiated superficial lesions the prognosis is good; for deeper, high-grade lesions extension between fascial planes and small satellite nodules requires carefully planned surgery, which may be assisted by MRI guidance. For metastatic liposarcomas, radiation therapy may be effective.

Kessler A, et al: Liposarcoma of the scalp. *Otolaryngol Head Neck Surg* 1997, 117:412.

Yoshikawa H, et al: Dedifferentiated liposarcoma of the subcutis. *Am J Surg Pathol* 1996, 20:1525. _____ ▲

ABNORMALITIES OF SMOOTH MUSCLE
Leiomyoma

Cutaneous leiomyomas are smooth muscle tumors characterized by painful nodules that occur singly or multiply. They may be separated conveniently into solitary and multiple cutaneous leiomyomas arising from arrectores pilorum muscles (piloleiomyomas); solitary genital leiomyomas arising from the dartoic, vulvar, or mammillary muscle; and solitary angioleiomyomas arising from the muscles of veins.

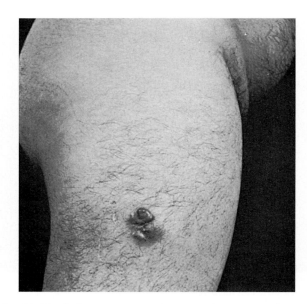

Fig. 28-87 Solitary cutaneous leiomyoma on thigh. (Courtesy Dr. H. Shatin.)

Leiomyomas are benign, and treatment is directed toward the removal of the pain source. Simple excision is the best method of removal of these small lesions.

Solitary Cutaneous Leiomyoma. The typical lesion is a deeply circumscribed, rounded nodule ranging from 2 to 15 mm in diameter (Fig. 28-87). It is freely movable. The overlying skin may have a reddish or violaceous tint. Although the lesion is insensitive at first, painful paroxysms may occur. Once pain commences, the tendency is for it to intensify.

Multiple Cutaneous Leiomyomas. These brownish, grouped, papular lesions vary from 2 to 23 mm in diameter and are the most common variety of leiomyomas (Fig. 28-88). Two or more sites of the skin surface may be involved. The firm, smooth, superficial, sometimes translucent, and freely movable nodules are located most frequently on the trunk and extremities. They often form linear or dermatomal patterns. These leiomyomas may occur on the tongue or, less often, elsewhere in the mouth as well.

Patients with these lesions often experience pain, especially in cool weather. Relief of pain may result by giving phenoxybenzamine, an alpha-adrenergic blocker or nifedipine, 10 mg three times a day. Calcium channel blockers may act by relaxing smooth muscle. An ice cube applied over the lesions often induces pain, and the effectiveness of therapy may be assessed by the length of time it takes the ice cube to cause pain.

Multiple leiomyomas are sometimes inherited by autosomal dominance. Women with this inherited type often have uterine leiomyomas as well.

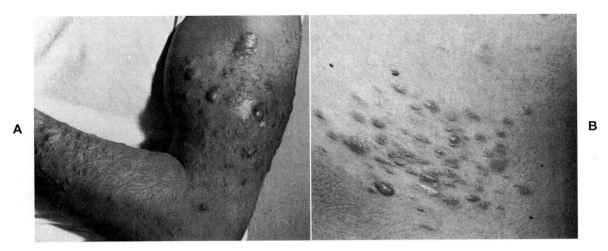

Fig. 28-88 Multiple cutaneous leiomyomas of **A**, the arm and **B**, the trunk.

Solitary Genital Leiomyoma. These lesions are located on the scrotum, on the labia majora, or rarely, on the nipples. They may be intracutaneous or subcutaneous in location. Most genital leiomyomas are painless.

Angioleiomyoma (Vascular Leiomyoma). This variety of leiomyoma arises from the muscle of veins. Pain, either spontaneous or provoked by pressure or cold, occurs in roughly half the cases. It is found mostly on the lower leg in middle-aged women. Solid tumors occur three times more frequently in women, and cavernous tumors occur four times more frequently in men. Solid lesions on the extremities are commonly painful; tumors of the head are rarely painful.

Histologically, the leiomyoma is made up of bundles and masses of smooth muscle fibers. Varying amounts of collagen are intermingled. The smooth muscle cells are finely fibrillated and are mostly vacuolated. The nuclei are typically long, thin, and rod shaped. The muscle bundles are irregularly separated by strands of collagen fibers.

Fitzpatrick et al reported eight patients with acquired, solitary, asymptomatic acral nodules. Seven were men and all were adults. Histologically, they were well-circumscribed subcutaneous tumors composed of smooth muscle cells, blood vessels, connective tissue and fat, thus earning the designation *angiolipoleiomyoma.*

Archer CB, et al: Assessment of treatment for painful cutaneous leiomyomas. *J Am Acad Dermatol* 1987, 17:141.

Fitzpatrick JE, et al: Cutaneous angiolipoleiomyoma. *J Am Acad Dermatol* 1990, 23:1093.

Hachisuga T, et al: Angioleiomyoma. *Cancer* 1984, 54:126.

Henderson CA, et al: Multiple leiomyomata presenting in a child. *Pediatr Dermatol* 1997, 14:287.

Ohtake N, et al: Leiomyoma of the scrotum. *Dermatology* 1997, 194:299.

Pujol RM, et al: A solitary papule on the nipple. *Arch Dermatol* 1991, 127:573.

Raj S, et al: Cutaneous pilar leiomyoma. *Am J Dermatopathol* 1997, 19:2.

Spencer JM, et al: Tumors with smooth muscle differentiation. *Dermatol Surg* 1996, 22:761.

Straka BF, et al: Multiple papules on the leg. *Arch Dermatol* 1991, 127:1717.

Yaghoobi R, et al: Multiple papular and nodular lesions in the extremities and trunk. *Arch Dermatol* 1999, 135:341. _____ ▲

Congenital Smooth Muscle Hamartoma

Congenital smooth muscle hamartoma is typically a skin-colored or lightly pigmented patch or plaque with hypertrichosis. It is often present at birth, usually on the trunk, with the lumbosacral area involved in two thirds of patients. Older patients may have perifollicular papules. They vary in size from 2 × 3 cm to 10 × 10 cm. The Michelin tire baby syndrome may result from a diffuse smooth muscle hamartoma. One case has presented with a linear reddish-purple plaque. Zvulunov et al report an incidence of 1 in 2600 newborns at their institution. Clinically, a mastocytoma may be mimicked, because transient elevation on rubbing may be seen (pseudo-Darier's sign) in 80%. A nevocellular nevus is also in the differential diagnosis.

Histologically, numerous thick, long, well-defined bundles of smooth muscle are seen in the dermis at various angles of orientation. There may be an increase in hair follicles.

Slifman et al believed this to be part of the spectrum of Becker's nevus. Classically, Becker's nevus is a unilateral (rarely bilateral) acquired hyperpigmentation, usually beginning as a tan macule on the shoulder or pectoral area of a teenage male. Over time hypertrichosis develops within it. Biopsy of such lesions shows acanthosis, papillomatosis, and increased basal cell pigmentation. Occasional congenital lesions manifesting hyperpigmentation and hypertrichosis have shown biopsy findings consistent with those of a Becker's nevus (no smooth muscle proliferation) and lesions with a typical late-onset history compatible with

Becker's nevus have occasionally shown smooth muscle–hamartoma-like changes in the dermis. Other cases of late-onset smooth muscle hamartomas are occasionally reported that are not hyperpigmented or hypertrichotic.

No treatment is necessary for either lesion. Mechanical epilation may be given to the occasional woman with a Becker's nevus.

Darling TN, et al: Acquired cutaneous smooth muscle hamartoma. *J Am Acad Dermatol* 1993, 28:844.

Gagne EJ, et al: Congenital smooth muscle hamartoma of the skin. *Pediatr Dermatol* 1993, 10:142.

Grau-Massanes M, et al: Congenital smooth muscle hamartoma presenting as a linear atrophic plaque. *Pediatr Dermatol* 1996, 13:222.

Hsiao GH, et al: Acquired genital smooth muscle hamartoma. *Am J Dermatopathol* 1995, 17:67.

Oku T, et al: Folded skin with an underlying cutaneous smooth muscle hamartoma. *Br J Dermatol* 1993, 129:606.

Person JR, et al: Becker's nevus. *J Am Acad Dermatol* 1984, 10:235.

Sahn EE, et al: A pigmented paraspinal plaque in an infant. *Arch Dermatol* 1995, 131:611.

Schnur RE, et al: Variability in the Michelin tire syndrome. *J Am Acad Dermatol* 1993, 28:364.

Slifman NR, et al: Congenital arrector pili hamartoma. *Arch Dermatol* 1985, 121:1034.

Zvulunov A, et al: Congenital smooth muscle hamartoma. *Am J Dis Child* 1990, 144:782. ▲

Leiomyosarcoma

Leiomyosarcomas of soft-tissue origin are extremely rare; occasionally, however, they may occur as a metastasis from an internal source. A cutaneous leiomyosarcoma appears in the dermis as a solitary nodule. This has a good prognosis, since metastasis to lymph nodes is rare, and rarely fatal. Subcutaneous leiomyosarcomas, on the contrary, have a guarded prognosis, since hematogenous metastases, especially pulmonary, prove fatal in about one third of the cases.

The clinical appearance of these lesions is not distinctive, so that the diagnosis is established by the histopathologic findings. These differ from the leiomyoma only by the nuclear pleomorphism, the numerous mitotic figures, and the disarray of the smooth muscle bundles. Collagen is found only in the septa.

The preferred method of treatment is wide local excision. The Mohs' surgical approach may be useful.

Bernstein SC, et al: Leiomyosarcoma of the skin. *Dermatol Surg* 1996, 22:631.

Grech C, et al: An erythematous noduloplaque on the trunk. *Arch Dermatol* 1999, 135:341.

Jensen ML, et al: Intradermal and subcutaneous leiomyosarcoma. *J Cutan Pathol* 1996, 23:458.

Kaddu S, et al: Cutaneous leiomyosarcoma. *Am J Surg Pathol* 1997, 21:979.

Landry MM, et al: Leiomyosarcoma of the buttock. *J Am Acad Dermatol* 1991, 24:618.

Moon TD, et al: Leiomyosarcoma of the scrotum. *J Am Acad Dermatol* 1989, 20:290.

Oliver GF, et al: Cutaneous and subcutaneous leiomyosarcoma. *Br J Dermatol* 1991, 124:252.

Wascher RA, et al: Recurrent cutaneous leiomyosarcoma. *Cancer* 1992, 70:490.

Yanguas I, et al: Cutaneous leiomyosarcoma in a child. *Pediatr Dermatol* 1997, 14:281. ▲

MISCELLANEOUS TUMORS AND TUMOR-ASSOCIATED CONDITIONS
Cutaneous Endometriosis

Endometriosis of the skin, described by von Recklinghausen in 1885, is characterized by the appearance of brownish papules at the umbilicus or in lower abdominal scars after gynecologic surgery in middle-aged women. The tumor, usually solitary, ranges from a few millimeters to 60 mm, averaging 5 mm, in diameter. The tender or painful lesion is bluish black from the bleeding that occurs cyclically in many of the patients.

Histopathologic findings are glandular structures with two cell types (glands and decidualized stroma), an infiltrating margin, and no mitotic figures. It is easily misdiagnosed as a malignant metastasis.

Treatment of choice is surgical excision. Preoperative treatment with danazol or leuprolide may reduce its size.

Albrecht LE, et al: Cutaneous endometriosis. *Int J Dermatol* 1995, 34:261.

Choi SW, et al: A case of cutaneous endometriosis developed in postmenopausal women receiving hormonal replacement. *J Am Acad Dermatol* 1999, 41:327.

Munoz H, et al: An ulcerated umbilical nodule. *Arch Dermatol* 1999, 135:1113.

Purvis RS, et al: Cutaneous and subcutaneous endometriosis. *J Dermatol Surg Oncol* 1994, 20:693.

Shwayder TA: Umbilical nodule and abdominal pain. *Arch Dermatol* 1987, 123:105.

Tidman MJ, et al: Cutaneous endometriosis. *J Am Acad Dermatol* 1988, 18:373. ▲

Teratoma

Teratomas may develop in the skin but are most common in the ovaries or testes. They have no characteristic clinical features, but on microscopic examination many types of tissue, representative of all three germ layers, are present. Hair, teeth, and functioning thyroid tissue are examples of fully differentiated tissues that may develop. Occasionally, malignancy may occur.

Boughton RS, et al: Malignant melanoma arising in an ovarian cystic teratoma in pregnancy. *J Am Acad Dermatol* 1987, 17:871.

Tsai TF, et al: A cystic teratoma of the skin. *Histopathology* 1996, 29:384. ▲

Metastatic Carcinoma

Malignant tumors are able to grow at sites distant from the primary site of origin; thus, dissemination to the skin may occur with any malignant neoplasm. These infiltrates may result from direct invasion of the skin from underlying tumors, may extend by lymphatic or hematogenous spread, or may be introduced by therapeutic procedures.

Five percent to 10% of patients with cancer develop skin metastases. The reported incidence figures vary widely according to the type of study undertaken and the site of primary tumor studied. The frequency of involvement of the skin is low when one considers other sites such as the lung, liver, lymph nodes, and brain. Usually, metastases occur as numerous firm, hard, or rubbery masses, with predilection for the chest, abdomen, or scalp, in an adult over age 40 who has had a previously diagnosed carcinoma. Many variations in morphology, number of lesions, site of growth, age at onset, and timing of metastases exist, however.

Clinically, the lesions are most commonly intradermal papules, nodules, or tumors that are firm, skin-colored to reddish, purplish, black or brown (Fig. 28-89); may be fixed to underlying tissues; and rarely ulcerate.

Several unusual morphologic patterns occur. Carcinoma en cuirasse is a diffuse infiltration of the skin that imparts an indurated and hidebound leathery quality to it. This sclerodermoid change, also referred to as scirrhous carcinoma, is produced by fibrosis and single rows of tumor cells. This type primarily occurs with breast carcinoma. Carcinoma telangiectaticum is another unusual type of cutaneous metastasis from breast carcinoma that presents as small pink to purplish papules, pseudovesicles, and telangiectases.

Inflammatory carcinoma (carcinoma erysipelatoides) is characterized by erythema, edema to the point of vesiculation at times, warmth, and tenderness, with a well-defined leading edge, similar to erysipelas in appearance (Fig. 28-90). This is usually caused by breast carcinoma, but has been reported with many other primary tumors. Alopecia neoplastica may present as a cicatricial localized area of hair loss, which on biopsy is usually caused by breast metastases in women and lung or kidney carcinoma in men.

The so-called Sister Mary Joseph nodule is formed by localization of metastatic tumors to the umbilicus. Powell et al reviewed 85 cases and found the most common primary sites to be the stomach, large bowel, ovary, and pancreas. Zosteriform, linear, or chancroidal ulcerations of the genitalia, and verrucous nodules of the legs, are other rarely reported clinical presentations.

The primary tumor is usually diagnosed before the appearance of metastases, and dissemination to the skin is often a late finding associated with metastatic disease to other more commonly involved organs such as the lung and the liver. A poor prognosis is thus the rule. Skin infiltrates may, however, be the first harbinger of a malignant visceral neoplasm and is quite often the first clinically apparent metastatic site.

The principal anatomic sites to which metastases localize are the chest, abdomen, and scalp, with the back and

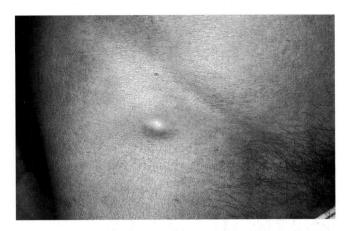

Fig. 28-89 Cutaneous metastasis from lung carcinoma.

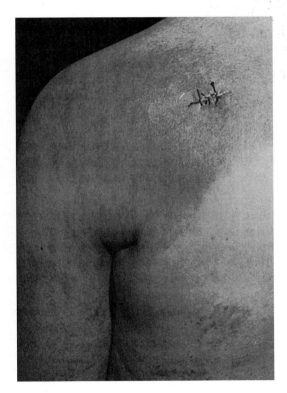

Fig. 28-90 Metastatic carcinoma of the breast with lesions on the chest, back, and arm. Erysipelas-like, diffuse infiltration of the skin occurred 4 months after breast amputation.

extremities being relatively uncommon areas. Involvement of the skin is likely to be near the area of the primary tumor. Thus, chest lesions are usually caused by breast carcinoma in women (Fig. 28-91) and lung carcinoma in men, abdominal or perineal lesions to colonic carcinoma, and the face to squamous cell carcinoma of the oral cavity. Extremity lesions, when they do occur, are most commonly caused by melanoma.

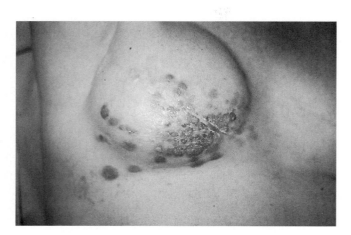

Fig. 28-91 Cutaneous metastases from breast carcinoma.

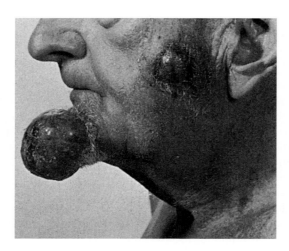

Fig. 28-93 Metastatic carcinoma on chin and left preauricular area with primary carcinoma of the lung. (Courtesy Dr. H. Shatin.)

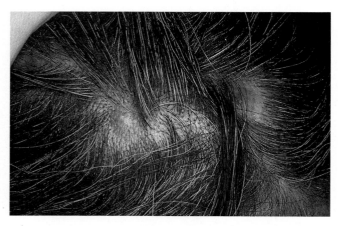

Fig. 28-92 Cutaneous metastases to scalp from breast carcinoma.

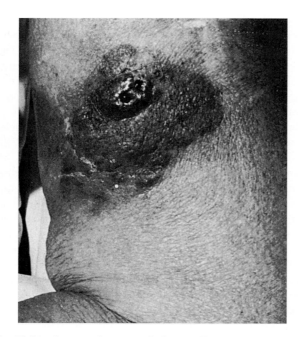

Fig. 28-94 Lympangiosarcoma in Stewart-Treves syndrome on the biceps area of an 84-year-old woman who had had a radical mastectomy followed by ionizing radiation therapy 12 years before.

Because of its overall high prevalence, breast cancer is the type most commonly metastatic to the skin in women (Fig. 28-92), and melanoma, followed by lung cancer, are the types seen in men (Fig. 28-93). Colon carcinoma is also common because of its high incidence in both sexes. Hypernephroma, or renal cell carcinoma, while less common, has a predilection for scalp metastases. Metastatic lesions are uncommon in children, but when they do occur neuroblastoma and leukemia are the most frequent causes.

Lymphangiosarcoma (Stewart-Treves syndrome) develops in a site of chronic lymphedema such as in breast cancer patients who have had lymph node resection (Fig. 28-94). Antikeratin and antidesmosomal antibodies are useful in identifying metastatic breast carcinoma, while antifactor VIII antibodies are positive in Stewart-Treves angiosarcoma.

Baum EM, et al: Alopecia neoplastica. *J Am Acad Dermatol* 1981, 4:688.

Dahl PR, et al: Thyroid carcinoma metastatic to the skin. *J Am Acad Dermatol* 1997, 36:531.

Lookingbill DP, et al: Cutaneous metastases in patients with metastatic carcinoma. *J Am Acad Dermatol* 1993, 29:228.

Meadows KP, et al: Vesicular carcinoma crysipelatodes. *J Am Acad Dermatol* 1999, 40:805.

Myhand RC, et al: Osteogenic sarcoma with skin metastases. *J Am Acad Dermatol* 1995, 32:803.

Powell FC, et al: Sister Mary Joseph's nodule. *J Am Acad Dermatol* 1984, 10:610.

Tschen EH, et al: Inflammatory metastatic carcinoma of the breast. *Arch Dermatol* 1981, 117:120. _____ ▲

Paraneoplastic Syndromes

Some cancers produce findings in the skin that indicate to the clinician that an underlying internal malignancy may be present. These may range from a specific eruption characteristic of a particular type of cancer, such as necrolytic migratory erythema, to a nonspecific cutaneous reaction pattern, among the causes of which may be an internal malignancy. Although many of these syndromes are discussed in other sections of the book a few will be mentioned here as illustrative examples of this phenomenon.

Bazex's syndrome, or acrokeratosis paraneoplastica, is characterized by violaceous erythema and scaling of the fingers, toes, nose, and aural helices. Nail dystrophy and palmoplantar keratoderma may be seen. These cases are secondary to primary malignant neoplasms of the upper aerodigestive tract or metastatic cancer to the lymph nodes.

Necrolytic migratory erythema, or the glucagonoma syndrome, is characterized by weight loss, glucose intolerance, anemia, glossitis, erythematous patches with bullae, and light brown papules with scales involving the face, groin, and abdomen. This is seen with glucagon-secreting tumors of the pancreas.

Erythema gyratum repens is a gyrate serpiginous erythema with characteristic wood-grain-pattern scales (Fig. 28-95); it is nearly always associated with an underlying malignancy. Hypertrichosis lanuginosa acquisita, or malignant down, is the sudden growth of profuse, soft, nonmedullated, nonpigmented, downy hair in an adult (Fig. 28-96). Jemic's review of 28 cases concluded that the most common sites of associated carcinoma were lung and colon.

The sign of Leser-Trelat is the sudden appearance of multiple pruritic seborrheic keratoses, associated with an internal malignancy. Trousseau's sign, or migratory thrombophlebitis, is usually associated with pancreatic carcinoma; it may, however, occur with other tumors, as reviewed by James. A form of pemphigus, paraneoplastic pemphigus is associated with lymphoma, chronic lymphocytic leukemia, and Castleman's disease most commonly.

Several cutaneous diseases that are not associated with internal malignancy with the frequency of the above paraneoplastic syndromes but that may be a sign of internal malignancy in some cases, are exfoliative erythroderma (lymphoproliferative disease), acanthosis nigricans (adenocarcinoma), multicentric reticulohistiocytosis, Sweet's syndrome (leukemia), nodular fat necrosis (pancreatic carcinoma), Paget's disease (underlying adnexal or breast carcinoma, or adenocarcinoma of the genitourinary tract or colon), dermatomyositis in patients over age 40, and acquired ichthyosis (lymphoproliferative).

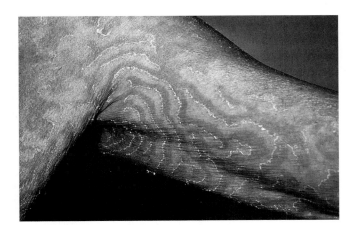

Fig. 28-95 Erythema gyratum repens.

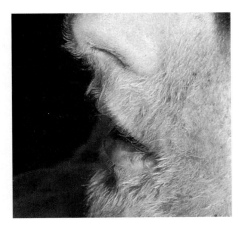

Fig. 28-96 Hypertrichosis lanuginosa acquisita (malignant down).

A variant of acquired ichthyosis, pityriasis rotunda, manifests circular, brown, scaly patches from 1 to 28 cm in diameter and varying in number from 1 to 20. They may occur on the trunk or extremities. These symptomless patches have been described in the Japanese, and in African and West Indian blacks. Berkowitz et al have shown it to be a pointer to the diagnosis of hepatocellular carcinoma in South African black patients. Tripe palms, considered by some to be acanthosis nigricans of the palms, is associated with carcinoma more than 90% of the time. Filiform hyperkeratosis of the palms may present in patients who develop cancer.

Anhalt GJ: Paraneoplastic pemphigus. *Adv Dermatol* 1997, 12:77.

Berkowitz I, et al: Pityriasis rotunda as a cutaneous marker of hepatocellular carcinoma. *Br J Dermatol* 1989, 120:545.

Bolognia JL: Bazex syndrome. *Semin Dermatol* 1995, 14:84.

Cohen PR, et al: Mucocutaneous paraneoplastic syndromes. *Semin Oncol* 1997, 24:334.

Cohen PR, et al: Sweet syndrome in patients with solid tumors. *Cancer* 1993, 72:2723.

Etoh T, et al: Pityriasis rotunda associated with multiple myeloma. *J Am Acad Dermatol* 1991, 24:303.

Grimwood RE, et al: Acrokeratosis paraneoplastica with esophageal squamous cell carcinoma. *J Am Acad Dermatol* 1987, 17:685.

Hovenden AL: Hypertrichosis lanuginosa acquisita associated with malignancy. *Clin Dermatol* 1993, 11:99.

Huang W, et al: A persistent periorificial eruption. *Arch Dermatol* 1997, 133:909.

James WD: Trousseau's sign. *Int J Dermatol* 1984, 23:205.

Jemic GBE: Hypertrichosis lanuginosa acquisita associated with multiple malignancies. *J Am Acad Dermatol* 1985, 12:1106.

Kaddu S, et al: Palmar filiform hyperkeratosis. *J Am Acad Dermatol* 1995, 33:337.

Kurzrock R, et al: Cutaneous paraneoplastic syndromes in solid tumors. *Am J Med* 1995, 99:662.

Kurzrock R, et al: Erythema gyratum repens. *JAMA* 1995, 273:594.

McLean DI: Cutaneous paraneoplastic syndromes. *Arch Dermatol* 1986, 122:765.

McLean DI: Toward a definition of cutaneous paraneoplastic syndrome. *Clin Dermatol* 1993, 11:11.

Mullans EA, et al: Tripe palms. *South Med J* 1996, 89:626.

Mustasim DF, et al: Bazex syndrome mimicking a primary autoimmune blistering disorder. *J Am Acad Dermatol* 1999, 40:822.

Schwartz RA: Sign of Leser-Trelat. *J Am Acad Dermatol* 1996, 35:88.

Wishner AJ, et al: Psoriasiform dermatitis in a cachectic man. *Arch Dermatol* 1988, 124:1851. ▲

Carcinoid

Carcinoid is characterized by distinctive involvement of the lungs, heart, gastrointestinal tract, and skin. The outstanding feature of the skin is the cutaneous flushing, usually of 5 to 10 minutes' duration. It involves chiefly the head and neck, producing a diffuse, scarlet color, with mottled red patches on the thorax and abdomen. Striking color changes may be occur, with salmon red, bluish white, and other colors appearing simultaneously on various portions of the skin. Cyanosis may also be present. As the episodic flushing continues over months to years, telangiectases and plethora appear, as though the patient had polycythemia vera. Gyrate and serpiginous patches of erythema and cyanosis flare up and subside, not only on the face but on all parts of the body and extremities.

Pellagroid changes may appear as a result of shunting of dietary tryptophan away from the kynurenine-niacin pathway and into the 5-hydroxyindole pathway. Periorbital swelling, edema of the face, neck, and feet, and scleroder-matous changes may occur. Disseminated deep dermal and subcutaneous metastatic nodules from a primary bronchial carcinoid tumor have been documented.

The clinical features of the carcinoid syndrome become evident only after hepatic metastases have occurred, or when the primary tumor is a bronchial carcinoid, or if the carcinoid arises in an ovarian teratoma, where the venous drainage bypasses the hepatic circulation.

The release of excessive amounts of serotonin and bradykinin into the circulation produces attacks of flushing of the skin, weakness, abdominal pain, nausea, vomiting, sweating, palpitation, diarrhea, and collapse. These attacks may last a few hours. Such symptoms may be induced in these patients by the injection of epinephrine, at which time kinin peptide is released.

ETIOLOGIC FACTORS. Carcinoid, also called *argentaffinoma*, is a tumor that arises from the argentaffin Kulchitsky chromaffin cells in the appendix or terminal ileum but also in other parts of the gastrointestinal tract, from the lungs as bronchial adenomas and rarely from ovarian or testicular teratomas. Some of these produce large amounts of serotonin (5-hydroxytryptamine), a derivative of tryptophan, and others do not. The primary lesion is more active in the production of serotonin than are the metastases. The tumor frequently metastasizes to the draining lymph glands or to neighboring organs, especially the liver, rarely to more distal sites.

LABORATORY FINDINGS. The diagnosis may be established by finding a high level of 5-hydroxyindolacetic acid (5-HIAA) in the urine. The normal urinary excretion of 5-HIAA is 3 to 8 mg daily, but in the presence of carcinoid it may reach 300 mg. Urinary values greater than 25 mg/day are diagnostic of carcinoid. Any value above the normal output is considered suspicious. The ingestion of bananas may cause significant elevations of 5-HIAA in the urine within a few hours, because banana pulp contains serotonin (4 mg per banana) and catecholamines. Tomatoes, red plums, pineapples, avocados, and eggplants also contain serotonin, but in much smaller amounts.

A screening test for 5-HIAA is the addition of ni-trosonaphthol to the urine. A purple color is produced when there is 40 mg of 5-HIAA excreted daily. Other serotonin metabolites besides 5-HIAA are found in the urine. The blood also contains serotonin in amounts of 0.2 to 0.4 mg%. In the presence of carcinoid the amount may be 10 times normal.

TREATMENT. The primary tumor, usually in the small intestine and occasionally in the lung, should be removed. Excision of metastatic lesions in the liver may also be considered. If this is impossible, chemotherapy for meta-static carcinoid usually includes 5-fluorouracil and strepto-zocin. It induces remission in approximately one third of patients and helps control symptoms in a higher percentage. Serotonin production should be reduced by drugs to inhibit cutaneous flushes, intestinal cramping, hypotension, and bronchospasm. Restriction of tryptophan-containing foods for short periods may limit serotonin production. Simultaneous use of H_1 and H_2 antihistamines, cimetidine and diphenhydramine, has been shown to block the flushes, as have in some instances clonidine, cyproheptadine, phenothi-azines, propranolol, and corticosteroids. A somatostatin analog, octreotide, 150 μg given subcutaneously two or three times daily, blocks the flushing and diarrhea. Methy-sergide maleate and parachlorophenylalanine may control the diarrhea. Vitamin supplementation with niacin is recommended.

Altman AR, et al: Treatment of malignant carcinoid. *Arch Dermatol* 1989, 125:394.

Bart RS, et al: Carcinoid tumor of skin. *J Am Acad Dermatol* 1990, 22:366.

Camisa C: Somatostatin and a long-acting analogue, octreotide acetate. *Arch Dermatol* 1989, 125:407.

Kvols LK, et al: Metastatic carcinoid tumors and the malignant carcinoid syndrome. *Ann N Y Acad Sci* 1994, 733:464.

Maton PN, et al: The carcinoid syndrome. *JAMA* 1988, 260:1602.

McCracken GA, et al: Metastatic cutaneous carcinoid. *J Am Acad Dermatol* 1996, 35:997.

Moertel CG, et al: A study of cyproheptadine in the treatment of metastatic carcinoid tumor and the malignant carcinoid syndrome. *Cancer* 1991, 67:33.

Pavlovic M, et al: Regression of sclerodermatous skin lesions in a patient with carcinoid syndrome treated by octreotide. *Arch Dermatol* 1995, 131:1207.

Rodriguez G, et al: Carcinoid tumor with skin metastasis. *Am J Dermatopathol* 1992, 14:263.

Schmidt KT, et al: Acanthosis nigricans and a rectal carcinoid. *J Am Acad Dermatol* 1991, 25:361. ⎯⎯⎯⎯⎯⎯⎯⎯⎯⎯⎯⎯ ▲

CHAPTER 29

Epidermal Nevi, Neoplasms, and Cysts

KERATINIZING EPIDERMAL NEVI

Keratinizing epidermal nevi are described by a great variety of terms; some of these are hard nevus of Unna, soft epidermal nevus, nevus verrucosus (verrucous nevus), nevus unius lateris, linear epidermal nevus, systematized nevi, and ichthyosis hystrix. Some of these terms, which denote some distinctive manifestation of the nevus, are described in this chapter. Hyperkeratosis without cellular atypia characterizes them all: nevus cells do not occur. Other types of epidermal nevi that include harmatomatous hyperplasia of adnexal structures, such as nevus sebaceus, are discussed later in this chapter.

Linear Verrucous Epidermal Nevus

The individual lesions are verrucous pink papules that may also be dirty gray or brown (Figs. 29-1 and 29-2). Interspersed in the localized patch may be horny excrescences (Fig. 29-3) and, rarely, comedones. The age of onset of epidermal nevi is generally at birth or within the first 10 years of life. On the extremities their course is longitudinal (Figs. 29-4 and 29-5) and on the trunk it is transverse or curved, as if along the distribution of the intercostal nerves, and virtually never extends past the mid-sagittal line, following the lines of Blaschko. The term *ichthyosis hystrix* is used to describe those cases with extensive bilateral involvement. The *systematized type* has linear hyperkeratotic papules and plaques (often showing a parallel arrangement), which may be unilateral or bilateral (often symmetrical). Happle believes the use of terminology such as *nevus unicius lateris,* originally used to describe localized forms, should be abandoned.

The histologic changes in the epidermis are hyperplastic and affect chiefly the stratum corneum and stratum malpighii. There is variable hyperkeratosis, acanthosis, and papillomatosis. Up to 62% of the histology of epidermal nevi have this pattern. About 16% show epidermolytic hyperkeratosis. At times other histologic patterns may be found, including a psoriatic type, an acrokeratosis verruciformis–like type, and a Darier's disease–like type. Mosaic mutations have been implicated, and epidermal nevi have shown chromosomal mosaicism within lesional skin.

Rare malignancies have been reported associated with epidermal nevi. Trichoepithelioma, keratoacanthoma, and verruciform xanthoma have also been purported. Topical management includes phenol, 5-fluorouracil, and tretinoin preparations. Shave excisions, cryotherapy, and CO_2 lasers have also been shown effective, but recurrence is common.

Bazex J, et al: Shave excision and phenol peeling of generalized verrucous epidermal nevus. *Dermatol Surg* 1995, 21:719.

Hamanaka S, et al: Multiple malignant eccrine poroma and a linear epidermal nevus. *J Dermatol* 1996, 23:469.

Hohenleutner U, et al: Carbon dioxide laser therapy of a widespread epidermal nevus. *Lasers Surg Med* 1995, 16:288.

Ichikawa T, et al: Squamous cell carcinoma arising in a verrucous epidermal nevus. *Dermatology* (Switzerland) 1996, 193:135.

Moss C, et al: Precocious puberty in a boy with a widespread linear epidermal naevus. *Br J Dermatol* 1991, 125:178.

Nelson BR, et al: Management of linear verrucous epidermal nevus with topical 5-flurouracil and tretinoin. *J Am Acad Dermatol* 1994, 30:287.

Paller AS, et al: Genetic and clinical mosaicism in a type of epidermal nevus. *N Engl J Med* 1994, 331:1447.

Reddy BS, et al: Generalized epidermolytic hyperkeratosis in a child born to a parent with systematized epidermolytic linear epidermal nevus. *Int J Dermatol* 1997, 36:198.

Stosiek N, et al: Chromosomal mosaicism in two patients with epidermal verrucous nevus. *J Am Acad Dermatol* 1994, 30:622. _____ ▲

Inflammatory Linear Verrucous Epidermal Nevus

Inflammatory linear verrucous epidermal nevus (ILVEN) is usually present at birth or appears during the first few years of life, though it may have its onset as late as the forties or fifties. It occurs mainly on an extremity in girls, is characteristically pruritic, pursues a chronic course, and is generally resistant to topical and intralesional treatments. It most commonly involves the lower extremity. It may occur in widely separated areas, usually on only one side of the body, but it may be bilateral.

Because of its psoriasiform histologic appearance, differentiation from linear psoriasis has created some controversy. Many believe it to be a type of epidermal nevus.

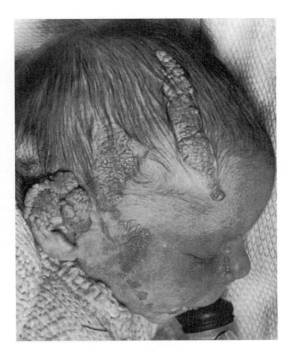

Fig. 29-1 Verrucous epidermal nevi.

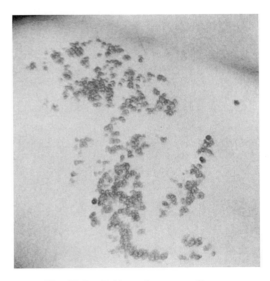

Fig. 29-2 Epidermal nevus on thorax.

Familial patterns have been reported, and sporadic mosaic forms most likely exist. It may be associated with CHILD syndrome (*c*ongenital *h*emidysplasia with *i*chthyosiform erythroderma and *l*imb *d*efects).

ILVEN must be differentiated from other forms of epidermal nevi and their associated disorders (see epidermal nevus syndrome in the following discussion). ILVEN is differentiated from linear epidermal nevus (LEN) by the presence of erythema and pruritus clinically and by the

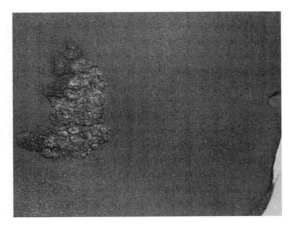

Fig. 29-3 Epidermal nevus on abdomen of a 7-year-old boy.

presence of inflammation and parakeratosis on biopsy. Treatment options include modalities already suggested for epidermal nevi. The flashlamp pumped pulsed dye laser is also therapeutic.

Alsaleh QA, et al: Familial inflammatory linear verrucous epidermal nevus (ILVEN). *Int J Dermatol* 1994, 33:52.

Alster TS: Inflammatory linear verrucous epidermal nevus: successful treatment with the 585 nm flashlamp-pumped pulsed dye laser. *J Am Acad Dermatol* 1994, 30:622.

Gatti S, et al: Treatment of inflammatory linear verrucous epidermal naevus with calcipotriol. *Br J Dermatol* 1995, 132:837.

Goldman K, et al: Adult onset of inflammatory linear verrucous epidermal nevus in a mother and her daughter. *Dermatology* (Switzerland) 1994, 189:170.

Mitsuhashi Y, et al: Treatment of inflammatory linear verrucous epidermal naevus with topical vitamin D₃. *Br J Dermatol* 1997, 136:134.

Oram Y, et al: Bilateral inflammatory linear verrucous epidermal nevus associated with psoriasis. *Cutis* 1996, 57:275. _____ ▲

Epidermal Nevus Syndrome

In 1968, Solomon et al described the epidermal nevus syndrome, consisting of extensive epidermal nevi with abnormalities of the central nervous system (CNS), skeleton, skin, cardiovascular system, and eyes. Cutaneous lesions other than epidermal nevi that may occur are café au lait spots, areas of pigmentary change, multiple nevus cell nevi, and cutaneous hemangiomas. The abnormalities seen are congenitally acquired.

Happle divides the epidermal nevus syndromes into five distinct types. These types are distinguished on clinical, histologic, and genetic criteria and are as follows:

1. *Schimmelpenning syndrome* (sebaceous nevus associated with cerebral anomalies, coloboma, and lipodermoid of the conjunctiva)
2. *Nevus comedonicus syndrome* (associated predominantly with cataracts)
3. *Pigmented hairy epidermal nevus syndrome* (Becker

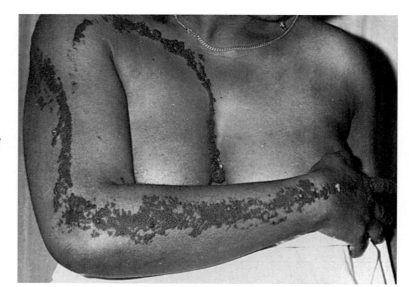

Fig. 29-4 Linear epidermal nevus. (Courtesy Dr. J. Stricks.)

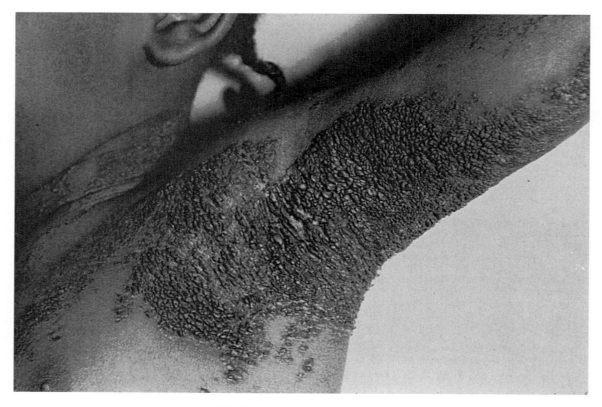

Fig. 29-5 Verrucous linear nevus.

nevus, ipsilateral hypoplasia of the breast, and skeletal defects such as scoliosis)
4. *Proteus syndrome* (the epidermal nevus is flat and velvety)
5. *CHILD syndrome*

Happle does not believe that keratinizing epidermal nevi are associated with systemic abnormalities. We disagree.

Several patients with ILVEN and wooly hair nevus have also been reported with associated internal findings.

Happle R: Epidermal nevus syndrome. *Semin Dermatol* 1995, 14:111.
Hodge JA, et al: The epidermal nevus syndrome. *Int J Dermatol* 1991, 30:91.
Rogers M, et al: Epidermal nevi and the epidermal nevus syndrome: a review of 131 cases. *J Am Acad Dermatol* 1989, 20:476.

Rogers M, et al: Epidermal nevi and the epidermal nevus syndromes: a review of 233 cases. *Pediatr Dermatol* 1992, 9:233. _____ ▲

Nevoid Hyperkeratosis of the Nipple

Nevoid hyperkeratosis of the nipple, a rare condition, is most common in women. There is verrucous thickening and brownish discoloration of the nipple or nipples and areola. It must be distinguished from epidermal nevi, ichthyosis, acanthosis nigricans, Darier's disease, cutaneous T-cell lymphoma, and other chronic skin disorders such as lichen simplex chronicus. Topical agents such as lactic acid lotions and other keratolytics should be tried first. Cryotherapy is alternative therapy. Oral retinoids are ineffective.

Alpsoy E, et al: Hyperkeratosis of the nipple: report of two cases. *J Dermatol* 1997, 24:43.

English JC III, et al: A man with nevoid hyperkeratosis of the areola. *Cutis* 1996, 57:354.

Ortonne JP, et al: Nevoid hyperkeratosis of the nipple and areola mammae: ineffectiveness of etretinate therapy. *Acta Derm Venereol* (Sweden) 1986, 66:175.

Revert A, et al: Nevoid hyperkeratosis of the areola. *Int J Dermatol* 1993, 32:745. _____ ▲

NEVUS COMEDONICUS

Nevus comedonicus is characterized by closely arranged, grouped, often linear, slightly elevated papules that have at their center keratinous plugs resembling comedones (Fig. 29-6). Cysts, abscesses, fistulas, and scars may develop. It may be localized to a small area or have an extensive nevoid type of distribution. Lesions occur mostly on the trunk, in a linear fashion. The lesions may develop any time from birth to middle age but are usually present by age 10. They are mostly unilateral; however, bilateral cases are also seen. Associated abnormalities of bone, CNS, skin, and eyes that may accompany epidermal nevi may also be seen in extensive nevus comedonicus, but these are very rare. Nevus comedonicus may be seen with other cutaneous disorders, including epidermal nevi. It has also been found in one patient with Alagille syndrome (arteriohepatic dysplasia).

The pilosebaceous follicles are dilated and filled with keratinous plugs. On the palms, pseudocomedones arise in sweat glands and resemble the changes found in poroma. Histologic examination may also reveal at times well-differentiated cutaneous lesions of follicular origin and occasionally, epidermolytic hyperkeratosis may be present.

Treatment consists of incision and expression of the comedones. Retinoic acid cream, gel, or swabs may be tried. One of the authors (WDJ) treated one patient with isotretinoin, and has knowledge of a second patient so treated. Both patients suffered from recurrent inflammatory cysts before therapy. Although the comedo-like lesions remained unchanged, the inflammatory lesions improved, becoming less troublesome and less frequent.

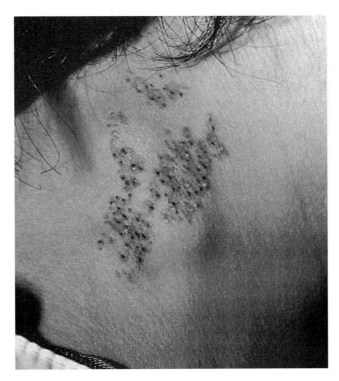

Fig. 29-6 Nevus comedonicus with underlying epidermoid cysts. (Courtesy Dr. Axel W. Hoke.)

Gonzalez-Martinez R, et al: Nevus comedonicus: report of a case with genital involvement. *Cutis* 1996, 58:418.

Happle R: How many epidermal nevus syndromes exist? *J Am Acad Dermatol* 1991, 25:550.

Woods KA, et al: Extensive naevus comedonicus in a child with Alagille syndrome. *Clin Exp Dermatol* 1994, 19:163. _____ ▲

CLEAR CELL ACANTHOMA (PALE CELL ACANTHOMA)

Clear cell acanthoma is also known as *Degos acanthoma* and *acanthome cellules claires of Degos and Civatte*. The typical lesion is a circumscribed, reddish, moist nodule with some crusting and peripheral scales; it is usually about 1 to 2 cm in diameter (Fig. 29-7). A collarette is commonly observed, and there may be pigmented variants. The favorite site is on the shin, calf, or occasionally the thigh, although others have reported other sites, such as the abdomen and scrotum. The lesion is asymptomatic and slow-growing, and can occur in either sex, usually after age 40. Solitary lesions are most common, but multiple ones have been described. Rarely, an eruptive form of the disease occurs, producing up to 400 lesions. Squamous cell carcinoma arising from clear cell acanthoma has also been reported.

The acanthotic epidermis consists of pale, edematous cells and is sharply demarcated. The basal cell layer is normal. In the dermis, underneath the acanthoma, dilated blood vessels produce increased vascularity. The clear

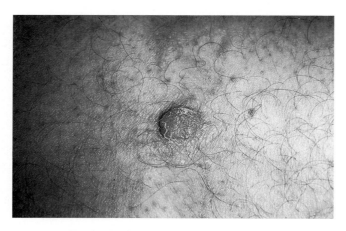

Fig. 29-7 Clear cell acanthoma on the leg.

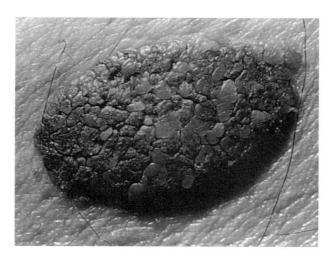

Fig. 29-8 Seborrheic keratosis. (Courtesy Dr. Axel W. Hoke.)

keratinocytes abound in glycogen, lack phosphorylase, and have reduced amounts of cytoplasmic cytochrome oxidase and succinic dehydrogenase. The histologic appearance is categorized into three architectural forms, with most being acanthotic types, followed by exophytic and psoriasiform variants.

Clear cell acanthoma must be differentiated from eccrine poroma, which appears most frequently on the hair-free part of the foot, and from clear cell hidradenoma, which occurs most frequently on the head, especially on the face and eyelids. Treatment is removal by fulguration and curettage after a shave biopsy or excision has been performed. Cryotherapy has also been used successfully.

Betti R, et al: Successful cryotherapy treatment and overview of multiple clear cell acanthomas. *Dermatol Surg* 1995, 21:342.

Breer WA: Asymptomatic papule on the lower leg: clear-cell acanthoma. *Arch Dermatol* 1993, 129:1506.

Burg G, et al: Eruptive hamartomatous clear-cell acanthomas. *Dermatology* (Switzerland) 1994, 189:437.

Innocenzi D, et al: Disseminated eruptive clear cell acanthoma: a case report with review of the literature. *Clin Exp Dermatol* 1994, 19:249.

Kavanagh GM, et al: Multiple clear cell acanthomas treated by cryotherapy. *Australas J Dermatol* 1995, 36:33.

Langer K, et al: Pigmented clear cell acanthoma. *Am J Dermatol* 1994, 16:134.

Parsons ME, et al: Squamous cell carcinoma in situ arising within clear cell acanthoma. *Dermatol Surg* 1997, 23:487. _____ ▲

SEBORRHEIC KERATOSIS

Seborrheic keratoses are multiple, oval, slightly raised, light brown to black, sharply demarcated papules or plaques (Fig. 29-8), rarely more than 3 cm in diameter, located mostly on the chest and back (Fig. 29-9) but also commonly involving the scalp (Fig. 29-10), face, neck, and extremities. Occasionally, genital lesions are seen (Fig. 29-11). The

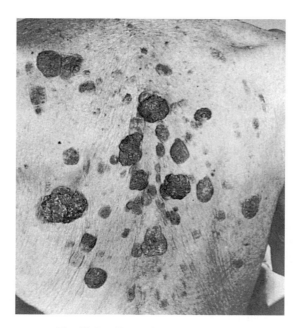

Fig. 29-9 Giant seborrheic keratoses.

palms and soles are spared; "seborrheic keratoses" in these areas are usually eccrine poromas. The individual nummular warty lesions often become crumbly, like a crust that is loosely attached. When this is removed a raw, moist base is revealed. Seborrheic keratoses may be associated with itching. Some patients have hundreds of these lesions on the trunk (Fig. 29-12). The age of onset is generally in the fourth to fifth decade.

Some believe the pathogenesis of seborrheic keratoses is a development resulting from a local arrest of maturation of keratinocytes that are normal in other respects. They usually originate de novo but may also evolve from lentigines. They may increase in number when the patient is gaining weight,

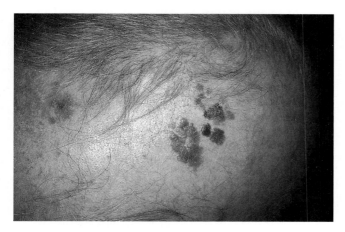

Fig. 29-10 Seborrheic keratoses on the scalp.

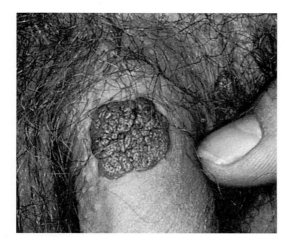

Fig. 29-11 Seborrheic keratosis on penis.

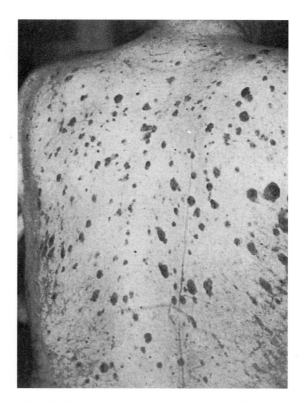

Fig. 29-12 Multiple seborrheic keratoses on the back.

and a sudden eruption of many seborrheic keratoses has been associated with inflammatory cutaneous disorders such as the case of a patient with exfoliative erythroderma.

The seborrheic keratosis is a combined hyperplasia of epidermis and supporting papillary connective tissue. In addition, small horn pseudocysts result from invagination of the stratum corneum. Usually there is some inflammatory reaction in the dermis. Six histologic types—hyperkeratotic, acanthotic, adenoid or reticulated, clonal, irritated, and melanoacanthoma—are distinguished. The histologic characteristics of these six types may be observed in any standard biopsy from lesions that otherwise demonstrate the typical clinical features of a seborrheic keratosis, unlike inverted follicular keratosis, dermatosis papulosa nigra, and stucco keratosis, which often have distinguishing clinical features. Melanoacanthoma differs from regular seborrheic keratosis by the presence of numerous dendritic melanocytes. Oral melanoacanthoma, which has also been called

melanoacanthosis, is clinically a reactive pigmented lesion seen primarily in young black patients. It is detailed further on p. 1002. Melanoacanthosis is perhaps a better term for this type of mucosal lesion, recognizing the different clinical features from melanoacanthoma found on the skin.

The differential diagnosis usually poses no problems in most cases, but clinically atypical lesions can be a challenge. The most difficult, especially for the nondermatologist, is to differentiate the solitary black seborrheic keratosis from melanoma (Fig. 29-13). The regularly shaped verrucous lesion is often different from the smooth-surfaced and slightly infiltrating pattern of melanoma. The actinic keratosis is usually erythematous, more sharply rough, and slightly scaly. The edges are not sharply demarcated, and they occur most often on sun-exposed surfaces, especially the face and backs of the hands, in light-skinned persons. Nevi may be closely simulated (Fig. 29-14). Rarely, intraepidermal nests suggestive of intraepidermal epithelioma of Jadassohn may be seen in the seborrheic keratosis; however, these are regarded as normal parts of the seborrheic keratosis. Rarely, squamous cell carcinomas and basal cell carcinomas arising within typical-appearing seborrheic keratoses may occur. It is prudent to biopsy any lesion that appears atypical, since even the most seasoned dermatologist has been humbled by the occasional diagnosis of melanoma in low-suspect histologic specimens.

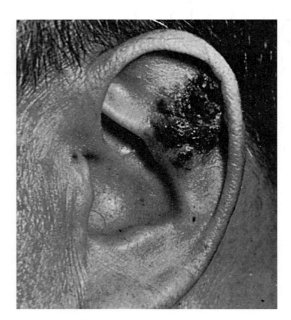

Fig. 29-13 Pigmented seborrheic keratosis resembling melanoma.

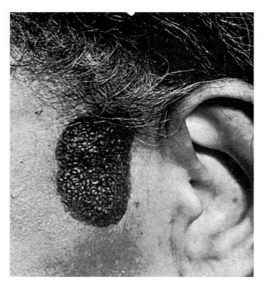

Fig. 29-14 Pigmented seborrheic keratosis resembling pigmented intradermal nevus.

Seborrheic keratoses are easily removed with liquid nitrogen and curettage. The spray freezes the lesion to make it brittle enough for easy removal with the curette. Scarring is not produced by this method. Light freezing with liquid nitrogen alone is also effective. So is simple curettage, either with or without local anesthesia. Light fulguration and CO_2 laser vaporization are other acceptable methods. Trichloracetic acid is usually not effective, and excision is not necessary.

Sign of Leser-Trelat

The sudden appearance of numerous itchy seborrheic keratoses in an adult constitutes this sign of internal malignancy, and the validity of the disorder continues to be debated. Sixty percent of the neoplasms have been adenocarcinomas, primarily of the stomach. The other most common malignancies found are lymphoma, breast cancer, and squamous cell carcinoma of the lung. The list also includes melanoma, neurofibrosarcoma, leukemia, hepatoma, ovarian adenocarcinoma, other gastrointestinal malignancies, and osteogenic sarcoma. To be accepted as having this sign the keratoses should begin at approximately the same time as the development of the cancer and run a parallel course in regard to growth and remission.

Akasaka T, et al: Two cases of basal cell carcinoma arising in seborrheic keratosis. *J Dermatol* 1997, 24:322.

Anderson PJ, et al: Squamous cell carcinoma arising within seborrheic keratosis. *Plast Reconstr Surg* 1998, 102:453.

Barron LA, et al: The sign of Leser-Trelat in a young woman with osteogenic sarcoma. *J Am Acad Dermatol* 1992, 26:344.

Burgess JT, et al: Seborrheic keratosis with trichilemmomas masquerading as melanoma. *Cutis* 1994, 54:351.

Cascajo CD, et al: Malignant neoplasms associated with seborrheic keratoses: an analysis of 54 cases. *Am J Dermatopathol* 1996, 18:278.

Field LM: Clinical misdiagnosis of melanoma as well as squamous cell carcinoma masquerading as seborrheic keratosis. *J Dermatol Surg* 1994, 20:222.

Goode RK, et al: Oral melanoacanthoma: review of the literature and report of ten cases. *Oral Surg Oral Med Oral Pathol* 1983, 56:622.

Lindelof B, et al: Seborrheic keratoses and cancer. *J Am Acad Dermatol* 1992, 26:947.

Maize JC, et al: Nonmelanoma skin cancers in association with seborrheic keratoses: clinicopathologic correlations. *Dermatol Surg* 1995, 21:960.

Richert CA, et al: Malignant melanoma simulating a seborrheic keratosis: a case report. *Dermatol Online J* 1997, 3:5.

Tomich CE, et al: Melanoacanthosis (melanoacanthoma) of the oral mucosa. *J Dermatol Surg Oncol* 1990, 16:231.

Yamamoto T, et al: Hereditary onset of multiple seborrheic keratoses: a variant of Leser Trelat sign? *J Dermatol* 1996, 23:191. _____ ▲

Inverted Follicular Keratosis (Basosquamous-Cell Acanthoma)

These benign epithelial tumors occur most frequently on the face or scalp of older persons as firm, skin-colored papules from 2 to 10 mm in diameter. Central scaling with a sharply marginated edge characterizes the lesion. Histologically, there are numerous squamous eddies composed of eosinophilic, flattened squamous cells arranged in an onion-peel configuration. There is endophytic proliferation of mature squamous cells.

This benign lesion responds readily to a shallow shave biopsy with subsequent hemostasis. We consider this lesion to be an irritated seborrheic keratosis. But others believe them to be warts. Hori was able to demonstrate positive results in one histologic specimen tested with papillomavirus common antibody.

Hori K: Inverted follicular keratosis and papillomavirus infection. *Am J Dermatopathol* 1991, 13:145.

Lever WF: Inverted follicular keratosis is an irritated seborrheic keratosis. *Am J Dermatopathol* 1983, 5:474.

Mehregan AH: Inverted follicular keratosis is a distinct follicular tumor. *Am J Dermatopathol* 1983, 5:467.

Sim-Davis D, et al: Inverted follicular keratosis: surprising variant of seborrheic wart. *Acta Derm Venereol* (Stockh) 1976, 56:337.

Spielvogel RL, et al: Inverted follicular keratosis is not a specific keratosis but a verruca vulgaris (or seborrheic keratosis) with squamous eddies. *Am J Dermatopathol* 5:427, 1983. _____ ▲

DERMATOSIS PAPULOSA NIGRA

Dermatosis papulosa nigra occurs in about 35% of blacks and is also relatively common in Asians. It usually begins in adolescence, showing first as minute, round, skin-colored or hyperpigmented papules that develop singly or in sparse numbers on the malar regions or on the cheeks below the eyes (Fig. 29-15). It has been described in a 3-year-old child. The lesions increase in number and in size, so that in the course of years the patient may have hundreds of lesions distributed over the periorbital regions initially, then onto the rest of the face, neck, and upper chest. These lesions closely simulate seborrheic keratoses and verrucae planae in both size and shape. They do not itch or produce other subjective symptoms. Scaling, crusting, and ulceration do not occur, and there is no tendency to disappear.

Microscopically, the chief alterations are in the epidermis and are characterized by an irregular acanthosis and deposits of uncommonly large amounts of pigment throughout the rete and particularly in the basal layer. Many believe it to be a form of seborrheic keratosis.

Treatment is made difficult by the tendency for the development of dyspigmentation. Light curettage with or without anesthesia; light, superficial liquid nitrogen application; and light electrodesiccation are effective therapeutic modalities in this entity. Aggressive techniques should be avoided to prevent pigmentary and scarring complications.

Babapour R, et al: Dermatosis papulosa nigra in a young child. *Pediatr Dermatol* 1993, 10:356.

Grimes PE, et al: Dermatosis papulosa nigra. *Cutis* 1983, 32:385.

Kauh YC, et al: A surgical approach for dermatosis papulosa nigra. *Int J Dermatol* 1983, 22:590. _____ ▲

STUCCO KERATOSIS

Keratoelastoidosis verrucosa of the extremities have been described as "stuck-on" keratoses occurring on the lower legs, especially in the vicinity of the Achilles tendon. They are also seen on the instep, dorsa of the feet, forearms, and backs of the hands. The palms, soles, trunk, and head are never affected. Varying in size from 1 to 5 mm in diameter, they are loosely attached, so that they can easily be scratched off. They vary in number from two to several

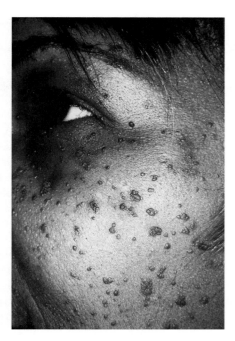

Fig. 29-15 Dermatosis papulosa nigra.

score. Stucco keratoses are common in the United States and Australia. They occur mostly in men aged 40 and over. Histologically, the picture is that of a hyperkeratotic type of seborrheic keratosis. The treatment, if any is required, consists of emollients, which soften the skin and cause the scaly lesions to fall off. Lac-Hydrin (12% ammonium lactate) lotion may be very effective.

Kocsard E, et al: Keratoelastoidosis verrucosa of the extremities (stucco keratosis of the extremities). *Dermatologica* 1966, 113:225.

Rees RB: For stucco keratoses, Lac-Hydrin. *Schoch Letter* 1985, 35:45.

Schnitzler L, et al: Stucco keratosis: histologic and ultrastructural study in 3 patients. *Ann Dermatol Venereol* 1977, 104:489. _____ ▲

MULTIPLE MINUTE DIGITATE HYPERKERATOSIS

There are three forms of multiple minute digitate hyperkeratosis: the inherited type (autosomal dominant), the sporadic type, and the postinflammatory form. All are characterized by multiple minute keratotic papules that are unassociated with follicular orifices. A spiked projection often occurs at the top of the papule. There are no associated abnormalities. Six families have been described. The postinflammatory variant is most often the result of irradiation therapy.

Balus L, et al: Multiple minute digitate hyperkeratoses. *J Am Acad Dermatol* 1988, 18:431.

Benoldi D, et al: Multiple minute digitate hyperkeratoses. *Clin Exp Dermatol* 1993, 18:261.

Mizuno K, et al: Postirradiation multiple minute digitate hyperkeratoses. *Clin Exp Dermatol* 1995, 20:425.

Ramselaar C, et al: Multiple minute digitate hyperkeratoses. *Eur J Dermatol* 1999, 9:460. _____ ▲

HYPERKERATOSIS LENTICULARIS PERSTANS (FLEGEL'S DISEASE)

Rough, yellow-brown keratotic plaques 2 to 5 mm in diameter and small psoriasiform discs, on the insteps, tops of the feet, and lower legs, characterize this distinctive dermatosis, described by Flegel in 1958 (Fig. 29-16). The palms, soles, and oral mucosa may rarely be involved.

Most of the known cases have begun in men in their thirties and forties. Bean suggests that this is a genodermatosis transmitted as an autosomal dominant trait. In one sibship basal cell carcinomas were an associated finding but were unrelated to the keratoses. Localized involvement may occur.

The histologic findings are distinctive, with hyperkeratosis and parakeratosis overlying a thinned epidermis, and irregular acanthosis at the periphery. A bandlike inflammatory infiltrate occurs in the papillary dermis. Topical corticosteroid creams, topical 5-fluorouracil, and acitretin (etretinate) have been useful. Lac-Hydrin may give relief, whereas tretinoin is ineffective. The lesions do not recur after shallow shave excision.

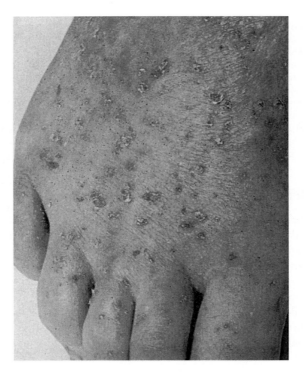

Fig. 29-16 Hyperkeratosis lenticularis perstans. (Courtesy Dr. E. Kocsard.)

Bean SF: Hyperkeratosis lenticularis perstans. *Arch Dermatol* 1969, 87:91.

Gutierrez MC, et al: Localized hyperkeratosis lenticularis perstans (Flegel's disease). *Cutis* 1991, 48:201.

Jang KA, et al: Hyperkeratosis lenticularis perstans (Flegel's disease): histologic, immunohistochemical, and ultrastructural features in a case. *Am J Dermatolpathol* 1999, 21:395.

Langer K, et al: Hyperkeratosis lenticularis perstans (Flegel's disease): ultrastructural study of lesional and perilesional skin and therapeutic trial of topical tretinoin versus 5-fluorouracil. *J Am Acad Dermatol* 1992, 27:812.

Miranda-Romero A, et al: Unilateral hyperkeratosis lenticularis perstans (Flegel's disease). *J Am Acad Dermatol* 1998, 39:655. _____ ▲

WARTY DYSKERATOMA

Warty dyskeratomas (Szymanski) are found on the face, neck, scalp, or axilla, and occasionally in the mouth. The lesion is a brownish red papule with a soft, yellowish, central keratotic plug. Histologically, the stratum corneum is hyperkeratotic and crusted. An invagination, filled with a keratotic plug, occurs to produce a cuplike depression. In the intraepidermal lacunae are acantholytic cells and pseudovilli. Corps ronds and grains may be seen in the lining of the crater. In the differential diagnosis keratoacanthoma, basal cell carcinoma, and syringocystadenoma papilliferum must be considered. Treatment consists of shave excision of the lesions.

Azuma Y, et al: Warty dyskeratoma with multiple lesions. *J Dermatol* 1993, 20:374.

Mesa ML, et al: Oral warty dyskeratoma. *Cutis* 1984, 33:293.

Rubenstein MH: Warty dyskeratoma. *Arch Dermatol* 1981, 117:746. ▲

BENIGN LICHENOID KERATOSES

Benign lichenoid keratoses are usually solitary dusky red to violaceous papular lesions (Fig. 29-17). They were first described in 1966 by Lumpkin and Helwig and by Shapiro and Ackerman. They occur most often on the distal forearms or hands, or chests, of middle-aged white women. Multiple lesions may simulate a photodermatitis. Some have found evidence of preexisting lentigo senilis histologically and by history and consider the benign lichenoid keratosis to be an involuting pigmented lesion. The role of sun exposure in the etiology is unsettled.

Histologically, there is parakeratosis, a lichenoid infiltrate with occasional plasma cells and eosinophils in addition to lymphocytes, and what may be remnants of lentigo senilis at the periphery. Direct immunofluorescence is positive, with clumped deposits of IgM in a lichenplanuslike pattern at the dermoepidermal junction. Cryotherapy with liquid nitrogen is effective.

Berger TG, et al: Lichenoid benign keratosis. *J Am Acad Dermatol* 1984, 11:635.

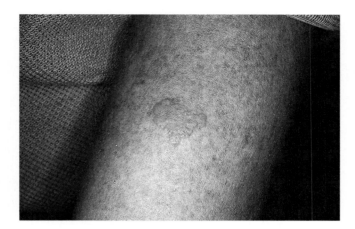

Fig. 29-17 Benign lichenoid keratosis.

Berman A, et al: The involuting lichenoid plaque. *Arch Dermatol* 1982, 118:93.

Bleicher PA, et al: Lichenoid dermatoses and related disorders. II. Lichen nitidus, lichen sclerosus et atrophicus, benign lichenoid keratoses, lichen aureus, pityriasis lichenoides, and keratosis lichenoides chronica. *J Am Acad Dermatol* 1990, 22:671.

Ramesh V, et al: Benign lichenoid keratosis due to constant pressure. *Australas J Dermatol* 1998, 39:177. _____ ▲

ARSENICAL KERATOSES

Arsenical keratoses are keratotic, pointed, 2- to 4-mm wartlike lesions on the palms (Fig. 29-18), soles (Fig. 29-19), and sometimes the ears of persons who have a history of drinking well water or "taking drops" (Fowler's solution) or pills (Asiatic pills), usually for asthma or atopic dermatitis, or psoriasis, often years previously. These lesions resemble verruca vulgaris on the palms and soles. When the lesion is picked off with the fingernails, a small dell-like depression is seen.

Arsenical keratoses may also occur on other areas of the skin, especially the trunk and extremities. These may or may not be associated with plantar and palmar keratoses and with arsenical hyperpigmentation. The latter is seen in about half of the patients and is discussed in Chapter 6. In addition to the keratoses and hyperpigmentation, Bowen's disease and invasive arsenical squamous carcinomata may be present, with the latent period being 10 years and 20 years, respectively. Superficial multicentric basal cell carcinomas may more rarely be seen. Internal carcinoma also occurs with increased frequency, after an average latent period of 30 years, with pulmonary and genitourinary carcinoma being most common. Arsenic has also been implicated in causing Merkel cell carcinoma.

Arsenic is an elemental metal that is ubiquitous, existing in nature as metalloids, alloys, and a variety of chemical compounds. These various forms of arsenic may be deposited into water, soil, and vegetation, producing serious

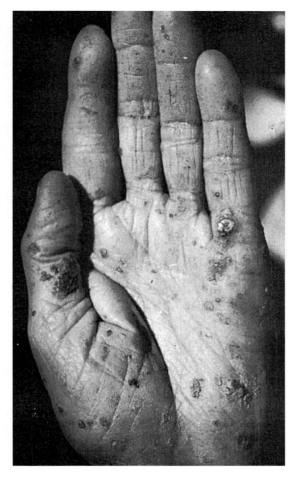

Fig. 29-18 Keratoses on the palm caused by inorganic arsenic in the drinking water. (Courtesy Dr. A Kaminsky, Buenos Aires.)

health risks. In West Bengal, India, an estimated 200,000 people have arsenic-induced skin disorders, and more than 1 million Indians are drinking arsenic-laced water from contaminated wells. Arsenic-contaminated water sources are a worldwide health concern also affecting countries such as Japan, Chile, Taiwan, and Mongolia. It is unknown what are safe levels of arsenic in drinking water. The World Health Organization (WHO) current permissible levels are under 0.01 mg/L.

Industries using arsenical compounds place their workers at risk of exposure. Use of arsenic pesticides and exposure to sodium arsenite, used as a veterinary pesticide exposing sheep-dip workers, has resulted in chronic arsenism. In the United States arsenic is used for pesticides, rodenticides, herbicides, insecticides, desiccants, feed additives, and wood preservatives. Pressure-treated lumber, particularly the marine-treated plywood, exposes carpenters and shipbuilders. The largest risk from wood products, however, occurs when pretreated wood is burned and the

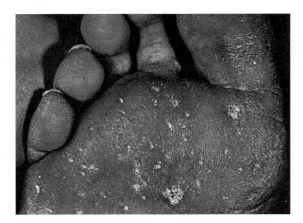

Fig. 29-19 Arsenical keratoses on the sole.

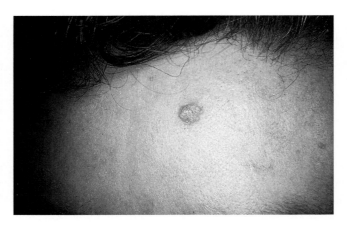

Fig. 29-20 Actinic keratosis on forehead.

arsenic fumes are inhaled. Electroplating silver may also require arsenic. Another potential source of exposure during the 1960s was American tobacco, resulting mostly from the use of arsenic-containing insecticides. Miners and individuals ingesting contaminated Chinese proprietary medicines are other major sources of exposure.

The histopathology shows hyperkeratosis, acanthosis, cellular atypia, and downward proliferation of the rete ridges. Histologic changes are the same as those of actinic keratosis, but without the basophilic degeneration of the dermis frequently associated with actinic damage. The palmar and plantar keratoses are easily diagnosed if there is hyperpigmentation of the skin, Bowenoid changes, or arsenical cancers. Multiple verruca and acrokeratosis verruciformis should also be considered. Treatment of arsenical keratoses is by cryotherapy, electrodesiccation and curettage, or topical application of 5-fluorouracil.

Bagla P, et al: India's spreading health crisis draws global arsenic experts. *Science* 1996, 274:174.

Col M, et al: Arsenic-related Bowen's disease, palmar keratosis, and skin cancer. *Environ Health Perspect* 1999, 107:687.

Maloney ME: Arsenic in dermatology. *Dermatol Surg* 1996, 22:301.

Person JR: Bowen's disease and arsenism from tobacco smoke: an association? *Cutis* 1996, 58:65.

Saha DP: Arsenic poisoning in West Bengal. *Science* 1996, 274:1287.

Schwartz RA: Arsenic and the skin. *Int J Dermatol* 1997, 36:241.

Wong SS, et al: Cutaneous manifestations of chronic arsenism: review of seventeen cases. *J Am Acad Dermatol* 1998, 38:179. _____ ▲

ACTINIC KERATOSIS (SOLAR KERATOSIS)

Although they are found chiefly on the chronically sun-exposed surfaces of the face (Fig. 29-20), ears, and backs of the hands and forearms, actinic keratoses may occur on any chronically or repeatedly sun-exposed part of the body. They are usually multiple, discrete, flat or elevated, verrucous or keratotic, red, pigmented, or skin colored.

Usually the surface is covered by an adherent scale, but sometimes it is smooth and shiny. The lesions are usually relatively small, measuring 3 mm to 1 cm. Rare variants do occur; in the spreading hypertrophic pigmented actinic keratosis, the lesion may be 1 to 2 cm in diameter. The hypertrophic type, which may lead to cutaneous horn formation, is most frequently present on the dorsal forearms and hands (Fig. 29-21). Squamous cell carcinoma may be present at the base.

Previously known as *senile keratosis* because it is usually seen in elderly persons, now it is known that excessive sun exposure induces the lesions, especially in fair-skinned, middle-aged and elderly persons. Development of actinic keratoses may occur in the twenties or thirties in patients who live in areas of high solar irradiation, are fair-skinned, and do not use sunscreens for protection. Clinical signs of solar damage, such as solar lentigines, facial telangiectasia, and poikiloderma of the neck, are strong risk factors for the development of skin cancer and solar keratoses.

Actinic keratoses are the most common epithelial precancerous lesions. The prevalence in other light-skinned whites is again related to the degree of sun exposure. In Japan the prevalence is much less, being 413.4 per 100,000. It is well accepted that these lesions have a propensity for the development of nonmelanoma cutaneous malignancies, with estimates ranging from 0.25% to 20%. Hyperkeratotic actinic plaques less than 1 cm in diameter on the dorsum of the hand, wrist, or forearms in white patients have been shown to have a malignancy rate of 50% in the series by Suchniak et al. Squamous cell carcinomas arising from the lip, temple (Fig. 29-22), and hand regions have a higher rate of metastasis than other skin sites. The risk of metastasis for cutaneous squamous cell carcinomas is also related to the tumor thickness and depth of invasion.

Histologically, the epidermal changes are characterized by acanthosis and dyskeratosis, and cellular atypia, the

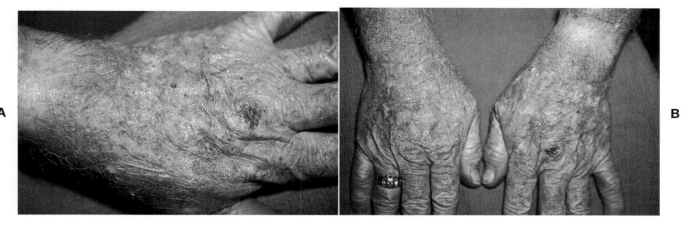

Fig. 29-21 A and **B,** Actinic keratoses on dorsum of hands.

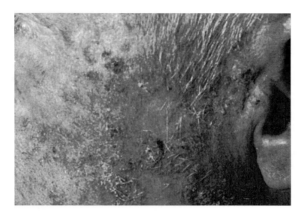

Fig. 29-22 Actinic keratoses. Patient subsequently died of squamous cell carcinoma metastases.

keratinocytes differing in size and shape and staining quality. Mitotic figures are common. The histologic picture may resemble Bowen's disease. There may be marked hyperkeratosis and areas of parakeratosis, with loss of the granular layer. Five types of actinic keratoses can be recognized histologically: hypertrophic, atrophic, bowenoid acantholytic, pigmented, and lichenoid. There is often a dense inflammatory infiltrate.

It has been demonstrated that the p53 chromosomal mutation, which is found in more than 90% of human cutaneous squamous cell carcinomas, is also frequently found in actinic keratoses. This is the consequence of long-term solar radiation; UV light exposure from artificial sources, such as tanning beds; x-irradiation; or exposure to polycylic aromatic hydrocarbons. Patients with arsenic exposure, thermal injuries, large scars, papilloma virus infections, and immunosuppressive states, such as organ transplants, are more susceptible to cutaneous malignancies and the malignant transformation of actinic keratosis.

The actinic keratosis is distinguished from discoid lupus erythematosus by the absence of dilated follicles and atrophy; from seborrheic keratosis by the absence of the greasy brown crust and sharply demarcated border; from Bowen's disease by the absence of infiltration and sharp outline; and from squamous cell carcinoma by the absence of infiltration and the extremely slow growth.

The treatment methods for actinic keratosis are varied. Cryotherapy with liquid nitrogen is most effective and practical when there are a limited number of sites. The individual lesion is frozen for a specific time (depending on many variables) using a bulky cotton applicator dipped into liquid nitrogen or a handheld nitrogen spray. We recommend using a C tip with continuous bursts of nitrogen spray in a circular motion, depending on the size of the lesion, attempting an even frosting. Only the lesion should be frosted. A long freeze that results in significant epidermal-dermal injury produces white scars. To avoid this try to freeze only the lesion and time the thawing rate. A complete thaw rate of from 15 seconds to a maximum of 30 seconds is recommended, depending on the thickness of the lesion. Repetitive superficial freezes (three cycles) is very effective and minimizes scarring. Healing usually occurs within a week on the face but may require up to 4 weeks on the arms and legs. Caution should be exercised when treating below the knee since wound healing in these regions is particularly poor.

For extensive, broad, or numerous lesions, 5-fluorouracil topically has been found to be extremely effective. Fluoroplex cream or solution, 1%, or Efudex, 2%, are recommended for the face; however, for the trunk, scalp, hands, arms, and neck we prefer 5% Efudex cream. It is rubbed in gently twice a day for 3 to 4 weeks on the head and neck, 4 to 6 weeks for other areas, or until there is a severe inflammatory reaction. The 1% solution is effective on the lips (Fig. 29-23). The medication should be applied with extreme care near the eyes and mouth. According to the individual's sensitivity, an erythematous burning reaction

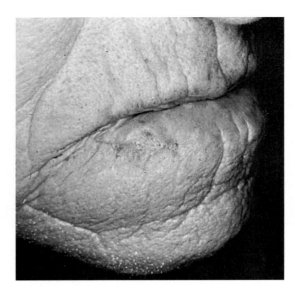

Fig. 29-23 Actinic keratosis on vermilion border of lip.

will occur within several days. Treatment is stopped when a peak response occurs characterized by a change in color from bright to dusky red, by reepithelialization, and by crust formation. Healing usually occurs within another 2 weeks after treatment has been stopped, depending on the treatment site. Another treatment cycle for 5-FU is four times daily application for 7 to 21 days. The shorter cycle may result in better compliance, and clinical results have been encouraging, as reported by Unis.

It has been observed that 5-fluorouracil "seeks out" the individual lesions of actinic keratosis even though the lesion is not clinically apparent. Excellent and lasting results are frequently observed. Clinically inapparent basal cell carcinomas may be detected during or on completion of the treatment. Topical tretinoin may be useful for long-term management of facial lesions but cannot compete with the effectiveness of the more rapid treatment modalities, such as Efudex and cryotherapy. A combination of 5-FU and isotretinoin has been shown effective for disseminated disease.

Many other treatments are possible. Topical application of a 20% solution of aminolevulinic acid to lesions followed by exposure to a red light source (580 to 740 nm) is referred to as *photodynamic therapy.* It has been reported to clear 66% of treated lesions; however, experience is limited. Its place in the treatment of actinic keratoses awaits more widespread use. Dermabrasion for severe actinic keratoses is most useful on the hairless scalp. A variety of chemical peels have been therapeutic. Carbon dioxide laser vaporization is also effective in the severest forms, and is the treatment of choice for severe actinic cheilitis. It has long been known in animal studies that dietary fats influence the incidence of sun-induced skin cancer. Black

et al showed that low-fat diets may decrease the number of actinic keratoses in humans; the mechanism of this response is unknown. Daily use of sunscreens is an effective, highly recommended method of preventing further chronic solar damage to the skin of patients with actinic keratoses.

Alirezai M, et al: Clinical evaluation of topical isotretinoin in the treatment of actinic keratoses. *J Am Acad Dermatol* 1994, 30:447.

Black HS, et al: Effect of a low-fat diet on the incidence of actinic keratosis. *N Engl J Med* 1994, 330:1272.

Callen JP, et al: Actinic keratoses. *J Am Acad Dermatol* 1997, 36:650.

Dinehart SM, et al: Metastases from squamous cell carcinoma of the skin and lip. *J Am Acad Dermatol* 1989, 21:241.

Dinehart SM, et al: Metastatic cutaneous squamous cell carcinoma derived from actinic keratosis. *Cancer* 1997, 79:920.

Dodson JM, et al: Malignant potential of actinic keratoses and the controversy over treatment: a patient-oriented perspective. *Arch Dermatol* 1991, 127:1029.

Goldberg LH, et al: Proliferative actinic keratosis. *Int J Dermatol* 1994, 33:341.

Kurwa HA, et al: A randomized paired comparison of photodynamic therapy and topical 5-fluorouracil in the treatment of actinic keratoses. *J Am Acad Dermatol* 1999, 41:414.

Naruse K, et al: Prevalence of actinic keratosis in Japan. *J Dermatol* 1997, 15:183.

Sander CA, et al: Chemotherapy for disseminated actinic keratoses with 5-fluorouracil and isotretinoin. *J Am Acad Dermatol* 1997, 36:236.

Schwartz RA: Premalignant keratinocytic neoplasms. *J Am Acad Dermatol* 1996, 35:223.

Schwartz RA: Therapeutic perspectives in actinic and other keratoses. *Int J Dermatol* 1996, 35:533.

Suchniak JM, et al: High rate of malignant transformation in hyperkeratotic actinic keratoses. *J Am Acad Dermatol* 1997, 37:392.

Unis ME: Short-term intensive 5-fluorouracil treatment of actinic keratoses. *Dermatol Surg* 1995, 21:121.

Weinstock MA, et al: Human papillomavirus and widespread cutaneous carcinoma after PUVA photochemotherapy. *Arch Dermatol* 1995, 131:701. ▲

CUTANEOUS HORN (CORNU CUTANEUM)

Cutaneous horns are encountered most frequently on the face and scalp (Fig. 29-24). Lesions may also occur on the hands, penis, and eyelids. They are skin-colored, horny excrescences, 2 to 60 mm long (Fig. 29-25), sometimes divided into several antlerlike projections. Their base is usually reddened and slightly thicker than their extremity.

These lesions are most often benign, with the hyperkeratosis being superimposed on an underlying seborrheic keratosis, verruca vulgaris, angioma, or trichilemmoma 50% to 60% of the time. However, 20% to 30% may overlie premalignant keratoses and 20% may overlie squamous cell carcinomas or basal cell carcinomas, and the prevalence is much higher in elderly fair-complected persons. In the series by Yu of 643 patients, 38.9% were due to malignant or premalignant epidermal lesions, and 61.1% from benign

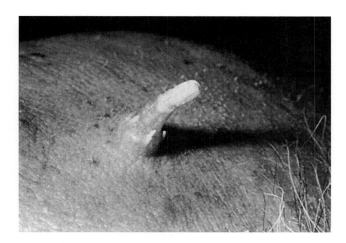

Fig. 29-24 Cutaneous horn. (Courtesy Dr. Axel W. Hoke.)

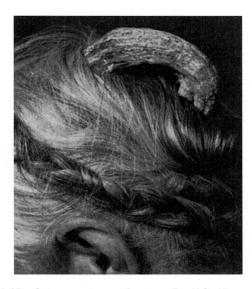

Fig. 29-25 Cutaneous horn. (Courtesy Dr. K.G. Higoumenakis, Athens.)

lesions. One third of penile horns are associated with underlying malignancies. Excisional biopsy with histologic examination of the base is necessary to determine the best therapy, which would be dictated by the diagnosis of the underlying lesion and by the apparent adequacy of removal.

Sehgal VN, et al: Palmoplantar keratoderma with cutaneous horns. *Int J Dermatol* 1992, 31:369.

Solivan GA, et al: Cutaneous horn of the penis: its association with squamous cell carcinoma and HPV-16 infection. *J Am Acad Dermatol* 1990, 23:269.

Yu RC, et al: A histopathological study of 643 cutaneous horns. *Br J Dermatol* 1991, 124:449. _____ ▲

LEUKOPLAKIA
Clinical Features

Leukoplakia presents as a whitish thickening of the epithelium of the mucous membranes, occurring as lactescent superficial patches of various shapes and sizes, that may coalesce to form diffuse sheets (Fig. 29-26). The surface is generally glistening and opalescent, often reticulated, and may even be somewhat pigmented. The white pellicle is adherent to the underlying mucosa and attempts to remove it forcibly cause bleeding. At times it is a thick, rough, elevated plaque (Fig. 29-27). The lips, gums, cheeks, and edges of the tongue are the most common sites, but the lesion may arise on the anus and genitalia. Leukoplakia is found chiefly in men over age 40.

Biopsy of these white lesions may reveal orthokeratosis or parakeratosis with minimal inflammation, or there may be evidence of varying degrees of dysplasia. There is a benign form that is usually a response to chronic irritation and that has very little chance of conversion into the precancerous dysplastic form. Premalignant leukoplakia, with atypical cells histologically, is present in only about 10% to 20% of leukoplakia. Unfortunately, clinically it is not possible to predict which lesions will be worrisome histologically, except that if ulceration or erosions are scattered throughout, the lesion is most likely precancerous. Therefore, biopsy is indicated.

The course of the disease is extremely chronic. In time an extensive, thick, white pellicle may cover the tongue or oral mucosa. In old lesions the epithelium may be desquamated and there may be fissures or ulcerations. Such changes are associated with more or less hyperemia and tenderness, and with a tendency to bleed after slight trauma. If transformation to carcinoma occurs, it generally follows a 1- to 20-year lag time.

When the lesion occurs on the lip, leukoplakia is closely related to chronic actinic cheilitis, which consists of a circumscribed or diffuse keratosis, almost invariably on the lower lip. It is preceded by an abnormal dryness of the lip and may be caused by biting the lips, by smoking (especially pipe smoking) (Fig. 29-28), or by chronic sun exposure. This type of leukoplakia is distinguished from squamous cell carcinoma of the lip by the absence of infiltration, from lichen planus and psoriasis of the lips and mouth by the absence of lesions elsewhere, and from lupus erythematosus by the absence of telangiectases. Biopsy is necessary, however, to fully differentiate these conditions.

Oral hairy leukoplakia is a term used to describe white, corrugated plaques that occur primarily on the sides of the tongue of patients with acquired immunodeficiency syndrome (AIDS). This is a virally induced lesion, discussed in Chapter 19, that has a characteristic histology.

Leukoplakia of the vulva usually occurs in obese women after menopause as grayish white, thickened, pruritic

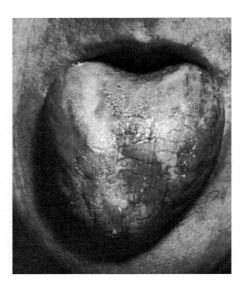

Fig. 29-26 Leukoplakia of the tongue. In 10 years this 75-year-old nonsmoking woman developed carcinomas in both tonsillar fossae and on the floor of the mouth. All were successfully treated with ionizing radiation.

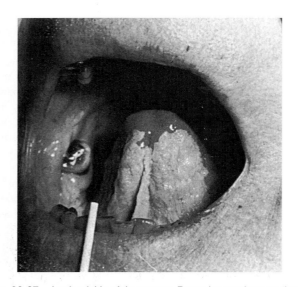

Fig. 29-27 Leukoplakia of the tongue. Extensive carcinomas developed in the mouth over 3 years.

patches that may become fissured and edematous from constant rubbing and scratching. Secondary infection with edema, tenderness, and pain may occur. It is differentiated from lichen planus by the absence of discrete, rectangular or annular flat papules of violaceous hue in the mucosa outside the thickened patches, or about the anus or on the buccal mucosa. Lichen planus may involve the skin as well as the mucocutaneous areas. Leukoplakia of the vulva is most frequently confused with lichen sclerosus et atrophicus and other vulval atrophies. On the penis, though leukoplakia

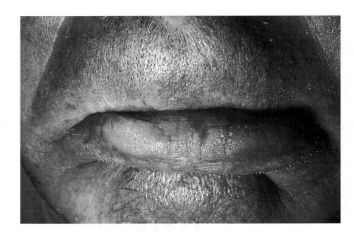

Fig. 29-28 Leukoplakia in a pipe smoker.

may occur, a similar precancerous process called *erythroplasia* (of Queyrat) is usually seen instead.

Etiology

Numerous factors are involved in the cause of leukoplakia. It may develop as a result of the excessive use of tobacco, poorly fitting dentures, sharp and chipped teeth, or improper oral hygiene. Extensive involvement of the lips and oral cavity with leukoplakia may exist for years without any indication of carcinoma. On the other hand, small inflamed patches may be the site of a rapidly growing tumor, which, with relatively insignificant local infiltration, may involve the cervical lymphatics. Carcinoma in leukoplakia usually begins as a localized induration, often about a fissure, or as a warty excrescence or a small ulcer. There is a 6% to 10% transformation rate of intraoral leukoplakia into squamous cell carcinoma. The red lesions of leukoplakia (erythroleukoplakia) have a much higher risk of malignant degeneration than uniform white lesions.

Warnakulasuriya et al have shown that the degree of epithelial atypia correlates with increased labeling with 3H thymidine and may be considered in staging the risk of developing malignancy. It has also been shown that there is an increased expression of p53 tumor-suppressor product in these lesions.

Treatment

It must be remembered that cancer develops so frequently on histologically dysplastic leukoplakia that its complete removal should be the goal in each case—first by conservative measures, then by surgery or destruction, if necessary. The use of tobacco should be stopped, and proper dental care obtained. Fulguration, simple excision, cryotherapy, and CO_2 laser ablation are effective methods of treat-

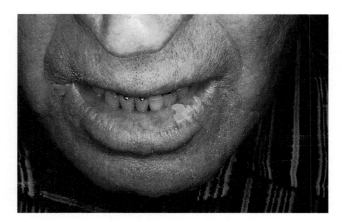

Fig. 29-29 Epidermization of the lower lip.

ment. In actinic cheilitis accompanying leukoplakia of the tongue, the mucous membrane of the exposed surface of the lip may be removed and replaced by sliding forward the mucosa from the inner aspect of the lip. Cryotherapy is effective. Isotretinoin, 1 to 2 mg/kg/day for 3 months, and 5-fluorouracil are good therapeutic considerations.

Leukoplakia with Tylosis and Esophageal Carcinoma

Leukoplakia associated with tylosis and esophageal carcinoma is extremely rare but may occur.

Epidermization of the Lip

Relatively smooth leukokeratosis of the lower vermilion, blending evenly into the skin surface distally and having a steep, sharp, irregular proximal margin, may easily be mistaken for precancerous leukoplakia clinically (Fig. 29-29). Histologically, it shows only hyperkeratosis, without parakeratosis or any cellular atypia at all. A shallow shave excision suffices to cure it and to rule out precancerous leukoplakia; no fulguration is required.

Axell T: Oral white lesions with special reference to precancerous and tobacco-related lesions. *J Oral Pathol Med* (Denmark) 1996, 25:49.

Warnakulasuriya KA, et al: Epithelial cell kinetics in oral leukoplakia. *J Oral Pathol Med* 1995, 24:165.

Wood MW, et al: Accumulation of the p53 tumor-suppressor gene product in oral leukoplakia. *Otolaryngol Head Neck Surg* 1994, 111:758. ————————————————— ▲

WHITE SPONGE NEVUS (FAMILIAL WHITE FOLDED MUCOSAL DYSPLASIA)

The mouth, vagina, or rectum may be the site of this spongy, white overgrowth of the mucous membrane, with acanthosis, vacuolated prickle cells, and acidophilic condensations in the cytoplasm of keratinocytes, which have been shown by electron microscopy to be aggregated

tonofilaments. The buccal mucosa is the most common site of involvement. There are no extramucosal lesions. There is no treatment. Progression of the disorder generally stops at puberty. The disease is inherited as an autosomal dominant disorder. A mutation in the mucosal keratin pair K4 and K13 have been identified as the inherited defect. HPV 16 DNA has been identified in some patients, the significance of which remains to be determined. Antibiotics, particularly tetracycline, provide significant improvement.

Alinovi A, et al: White sponge nevus: successful treatment with penicillin. *Acta Derm Venereol* (Sweden) 1983, 63:83.

Corden LD, et al: Human keratin disease: hereditary fragility of specific epithelial tissues. *Exp Dermatol* 1996, 5:297.

Cox MF, et al: Human papillomavirus 16 DNA in oral white sponge nevus. *Oral Surg Oral Med Oral Pathol* 1992, 73:476.

Hernandez-Martin A, et al: Diffuse whitening of the oral mucosa in a child. *Pediatr Dermatol* 1997, 14:316.

Lim J, et al: Oral tetracycline rinse improves symptoms of white sponge nevus. *J Am Acad Dermatol* 1992, 26:1003.

McDonagh AJ, et al: White sponge naevus successfully treated with topical tetracycline. *Clin Exp Dermatol* 1990, 15:152.

Nichols GE, et al: White sponge nevus. *Obstet Gynecol* 1990, 76:545.

Wright S, et al: White sponge naevus and ocular coloboma. *Arch Dis Child* 1991, 66:514. ————————————————— ▲

ORAL FLORID PAPILLOMATOSIS

Oral florid papillomatosis was originally described by Rock and Fisher in 1960 as a confluent papillomatosis covering the mucous membranes of the oral cavity. The distinctive picture is that of a white mass resembling cauliflower, covering the tongue and extending onto the other portions of the mucous membranes, including the oropharynx, larynx, and trachea. Usually there is no lymphadenopathy.

The course of the disease is progressive. Some lesions eventuate in squamous cell carcinoma, whereas others continue for many years, the patient dying of some intercurrent disease. Oral florid papillomatosis should be regarded as a verrucous carcinoma, which has been defined as a distinctive, slowly growing fungating tumor representing a well-differentiated squamous cell carcinoma in which metastases occur very late or not at all (Fig. 29-30). The histologic features are those of papillomatosis, acanthosis, and varying degrees of dysplasia of the epithelium, without disruption of the basement membrane. It is reasonable to expect the eventual development of epidermoid carcinoma in most patients. Ishii et al reported a case with esophageal involvement and keratotic papules of the extremities. In the differential diagnosis, leukoplakia, proliferative verrucous leukoplakia, candidiasis, acanthosis nigricans, and condyloma acuminatum should be considered. Treatment is recommended to be surgical excision; however, it is often followed by recurrence and spread. Recombinant-alpha 2a interferon in combination with a CO_2 laser has also been used.

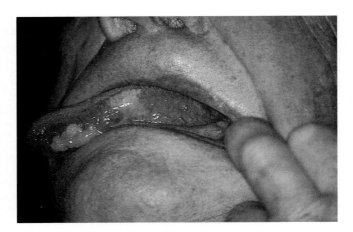

Fig. 29-30 Verrucous carcinoma.

Collangettes D, et al: Oral florid papillomatosis. *Eur J Cancer B Oral* 1993, 29B:81.

Ishii Y, et al: Oral florid papillomatosis and leukoplakia of the esophagus associated with keratoderma and showing transepidermal elimination. *J Dermatol* 1994, 21:974.

Schwartz RA: Verrucous carcinoma of the skin and mucosa. *J Am Acad Dermatol* 1995, 32:1. ⎯⎯⎯⎯⎯⎯⎯⎯⎯⎯⎯⎯ ▲

ELASTOTIC NODULES OF ANTHELIX

Elastotic nodules of the anthelix of the ear have been described by Carter et al. The bilateral, semitranslucent nodules appear exclusively on the upper part of the anthelix. The surface has an "orange peel" appearance. It is believed that sun damage causes these nodules.

Histologically, a marked hyperkeratosis with a normal granular and malpighian layer characterizes this lesion. Some show basal cell proliferation. In the dermis the collagen is replaced with elastotic fibers and amorphous elastic material is seen. Elastotic nodules are frequently mistaken for basal cell carcinoma. Other diagnoses frequently considered are rheumatoid nodules, gouty tophi, sarcoid, and calcinosis cutis. Treatment centers on removal of the lesions by shave excision and fulguration of the base. The removed specimen is used for biopsy.

Carter VH, et al: Elastotic nodules of anthelix. *Arch Dermatol* 1969, 100:282. ⎯⎯⎯⎯⎯⎯⎯⎯⎯⎯⎯⎯⎯⎯⎯ ▲

KERATOACANTHOMA

Clinical Features

There are four types of keratoacanthomas: solitary, multiple, eruptive, and keratoacanthoma centrifugum marginatum.

Sunlight appears to play an important role in the etiology, especially in the solitary types. Seasonal variations have been well documented, and the high index of sunlight exposure to the prevalence of keratoacanthomas is clearly correlated. In addition, light-skinned persons are more apt to develop keratoacanthoma than dark-skinned persons. Instances of keratoacanthomas arising from inoculation or as an isomorphic phenomenon may occur. In one series approximately 10% of lesions developed in areas of injury or previous skin disease.

Many reports have suggested an association of keratoacanthoma with internal malignancies. Many appear to be coincidental. An exception is Muir-Torre syndrome in which sebaceous tumors and keratoacanthomas occur in association with multiple low-grade malignancies.

Solitary Keratoacanthoma

This type of keratoacanthoma is a rapidly growing papule that enlarges from a 1-mm macule or papule to as much as 25 mm in 3 to 8 weeks. When fully developed it is a hemispheric, dome-shaped, skin-colored nodule in which there is a smooth crater filled with a central keratin plug (Fig. 29-31). The smooth shiny lesion is sharply demarcated from its surroundings (Fig. 29-32). Telangiectases may run through the lesion.

Atypical forms of keratoacanthoma occur frequently. Some resemble seborrheic keratoses or benign acanthomas; others may have a nodulovegetative appearance; some, craterlike depressions. An interesting type is the one in which there is progressive peripheral growth while the center heals at the same time (Fig. 29-33); *keratoacanthoma centrifugum* and *keratoacanthoma centrifugum marginatum* are terms applied to this form, whose features are distinctive enough to be considered as a separate type. Giant keratoacanthomas are defined as those larger than 2 cm in diameter and most commonly involve the nose and eyelids. They have been known to attain a diameter of 25 cm, and metastases have been reported. Many believe that those with metastatic disease were squamous cell carcinomas from the onset. This presumably reflects the untrustworthiness of diagnostic criteria rather than the ability of keratoacanthomas to metastasize. Another variety is the coral-reef keratoacanthoma, in which multiple lesions extend from the original central lesion. Coalescing plaques or nodules occurring on the forehead have also been described and named *keratoacanthoma dyskeratoticum et segregans*. Subungual keratoacanthomas are tender, have a destructive crateriform center, and often cause damage to the terminal phalanx. Subungual lesions often do not regress spontaneously and induce early underlying bony destruction, characterized on radiograph as a crescent-shaped lytic defect without accompanying sclerosis or periosteal reaction.

The solitary keratoacanthoma occurs mostly on sun-exposed skin, with the central portion of the face, the backs of the hands, and the arms being the most commonly

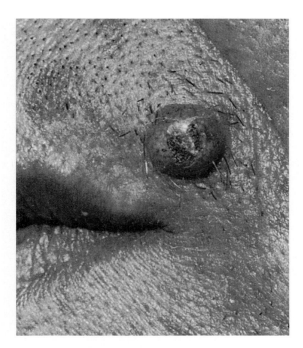

Fig. 29-31   Keratoacanthoma.

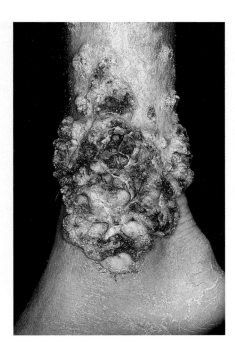

Fig. 29-33   Keratoacanthoma centrifugum marginatum.

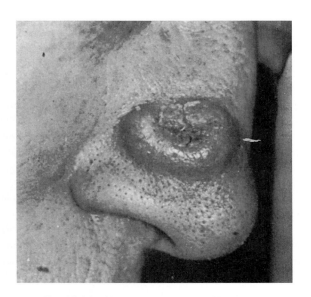

Fig. 29-32   Keratoacanthoma on side of nose.

involved sites. Less frequently, other sites are involved, such as the buttocks, thighs, penis, ears, and scalp. Women have fewer lesions on the dorsal hands, and keratoacanthomas on the calves and shins are common in women but unusual in men. Rarely, this tumor involves the mucous membranes of the oral cavity or the subungual region. Keratoacanthoma is seen mostly in middle-aged to elderly persons, with men being more frequently involved.

The most interesting feature of this disease is the rapid growth for some 2 to 6 weeks, followed by a stationary period for another 2 to 6 weeks, and finally a spontaneous involution for another 2 to 6 weeks to leave a slightly depressed scar. The stationary period and involuting phase are variable; some lesions may take 6 months to a year to completely resolve. It has been estimated that some 5% of treated lesions recur. Invasion along nerve trunks has been documented.

Multiple Keratoacanthomas

This type of keratoacanthoma is frequently referred to as the *Ferguson Smith type of multiple self-healing keratoacanthomas*. These lesions are identical clinically and histologically to the solitary type. They may occur in any number, but generally only some 3 to 10 lesions are noted, localized to one site. The most common sites are the face, trunk, and genitalia. Young men are most frequently affected.

A familial type of generalized keratoacanthoma has been reported, referred to as the *Ferguson Smith type of self-healing squamous epithelioma*. The unusual aspect is the severe pruritus over a number of years, leading to an erroneous diagnosis of prurigo nodularis.

Eruptive Keratoacanthomas

This type of keratoacanthoma is characterized by a generalized eruption of numerous dome-shaped, skin-colored papules from 2 to 7 mm in diameter (Fig. 29-34). The eruption is usually generalized but spares the palms and

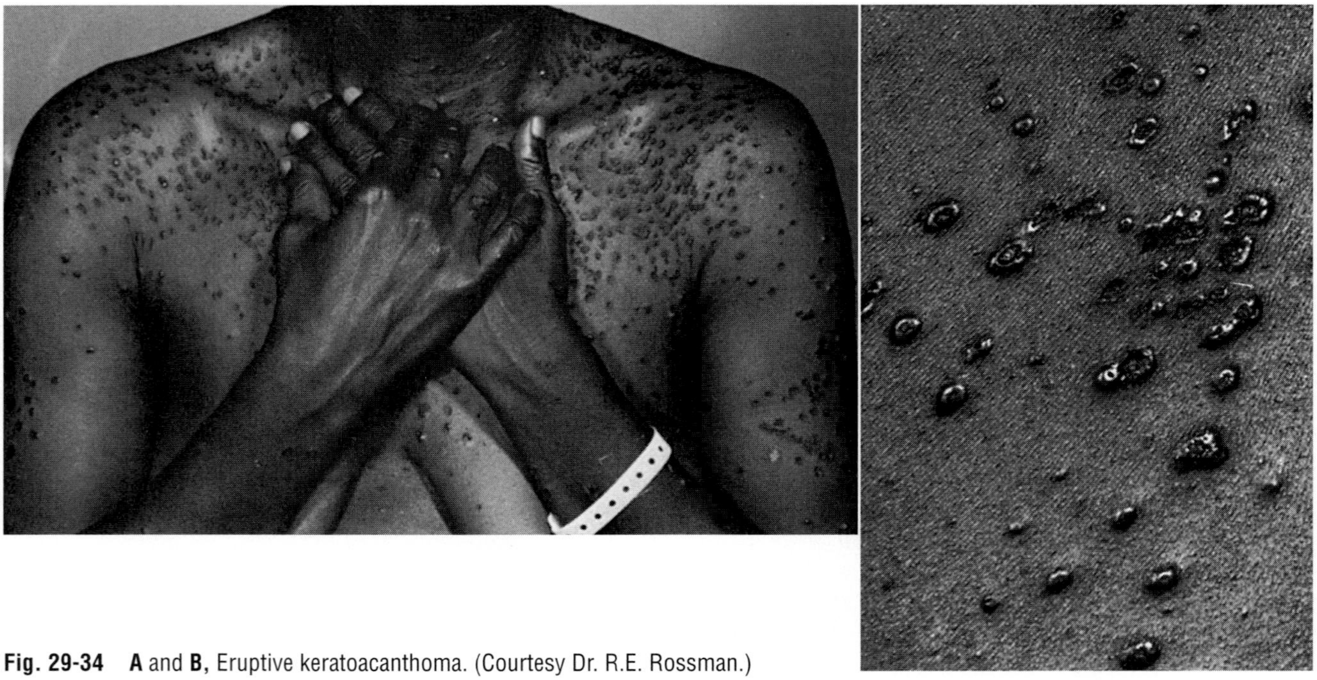

Fig. 29-34 **A** and **B,** Eruptive keratoacanthoma. (Courtesy Dr. R.E. Rossman.)

soles. The oral mucous membranes can be involved. Severe pruritus may be a feature in some, plus bilateral ectropion and narrowing of the oral aperture. Linear arrangement of some lesions, especially over the shoulders and arms, has also been noted. It appears to be associated with a higher incidence of immunosuppression than the other forms of keratoacanthomas. Lupus erythematosus, leukemia, leprosy, kidney transplantation, photochemotherapy, thermal burn, and radiation therapy have all been associated. Seasonal variations have also been documented, with worsening during the summer, once again implicating ultraviolet exposure.

Keratoacanthoma Centrifugum Marginatum

An uncommon variant (16 cases), keratoacanthoma centrifugum marginatum is characterized by progressive peripheral expansion and concomitant central healing leaving atrophy, and usually involves the dorsum of the hands and pretibial regions. Initially described by Miedzinski and Kozakewicz in 1962, the lesions can range from 5 to 30 cm in diameter. Unlike giant solitary keratoacanthomas there is no tendency for spontaneous involution. These unique features separate keratoacanthoma centrifugum marginatum from solitary keratoacanthoma.

Etiology

Many believe that keratoacanthomas are a variant of regressing squamous cell carcinoma, based on immunohistochemical studies, histologic features, and the detection of p53 oncoprotein expression that is equal to that documented in squamous cell carcinomas. Conditions known to promote progression of actinic keratosis and malignant degeneration of premalignant lesions, such as sun exposure, tar therapy, and immunosuppressed states, have been shown also to promote the expression and development of keratoacanthomas. Inflammatory cells in keratoacanthomas are mostly CD4+ T lymphocytes activated by interleukin 2 and adhesion molecules, not unlike inflammatory infiltrates observed in squamous cell carcinomas, again suggesting a common link.

Histopathology

The histologic findings of keratoacanthoma and a low-grade squamous cell carcinoma are so similar that it is frequently difficult to make a definite diagnosis on the histologic findings alone. When a properly sectioned specimen is examined under low magnification, the center of the lesion shows a crater filled with eosinophilic keratin. Over the sides of the crater, which seems to have been formed by invagination of the epidermis, a "lip" or "marginal buttress" of epithelium extends over the keratin-filled crater. At the base and sides of the crater, acanthosis in the form of pseudoepitheliomatous hyperplasia occurs. The epidermal cells are highly keratinized and have an eosinophilic, glassy cytoplasm. Outside of this keratinocyte proliferation a dense lymphocytic infiltrate is frequently seen.

In the eruptive keratoacanthoma the histologic findings are similar to the solitary type. Many of the lesions will show the typical picture of a keratin-filled crater with an overhanging epidermis that is acanthotic and actively proliferating. Other lesions may show dilated follicles with keratin-plugged orifices. Acanthosis is seen surrounding the follicle.

The keratoacanthoma is distinguished from squamous cell carcinoma by far faster growth (sometimes fully grown in 2 weeks), and by its typical central core of keratin, which is usually absent in squamous cell carcinoma. Immunohistochemical stain for involucrin, a soluble precursor of the envelope of stratified squamous epithelium, is a diagnostic aid in differentiating these tumors. Keratoacanthomas show a homogeneous staining pattern, whereas in squamous cell carcinomas it is usually highly irregular.

Keratoacanthoma is also to be distinguished from seborrheic keratosis, cutaneous horn, epidermoid cyst, pseudoepitheliomatous hyperplasia, iododerma and bromoderma, prurigo nodularis, verruca vulgaris, and hypertrophic lichen planus. Histologic examination of the lesion is frequently necessary. The eruptive keratoacanthomas are distinguished from pityriasis rubra pilaris, scleromyxedema, lichen amyloidosis, and Kyrle's disease. It may be necessary to examine several papular lesions before the distinctive features of keratoacanthoma are found.

Treatment

Although keratoacanthomas spontaneously involute it is impossible to predict how long it will take. The patient may be faced with an unsightly tumor for as long as a year. More importantly, grade I squamous cell carcinoma cannot be excluded even with a biopsy; therefore, biopsy excision or curettage and fulguration of an ordinary lesion less than 2 cm in diameter can and should be done in most cases. It is the safest course.

Intralesional injections of 5-fluorouracil solution, straight from the ampule, and intralesional (0.5 to 1 ml of 25 mg/ml methotrexate), as well as intramuscular (25 mg weekly) methotrexate, have been shown effective. Topical 5-FU cream may also work. Clearing with intralesional bleomycin (1 mg/ml diluted with an equal amount of lidocaine) has occurred within 20 days after start of treatment. For clinically typical lesions these modalities may be tried before resorting to surgical removal, especially if the latter presents any problem. We recommend excision if involution of the lesion is not complete after three consecutive injections 1 week apart or the failure within 3 weeks of topical therapy. Mohs' microsurgery is recommended for facial lesions that may be deforming.

Podophyllum in compound tincture of benzoin is useful in giant keratoacanthomas. Oral retinoids are therapeutic and may be particularly helpful in treating large or recalcitrant lesions, such as seen in the eruptive, giant multiple, or centrifugum marginatum forms. Eruptive forms tend to be very resistant to therapy; however, good results have been achieved with oral and topical retinoids and cyclophosphamide.

Radiation therapy may also be used on giant keratoacanthomas when surgical excision or electrosurgical methods are not feasible. We treat these lesions in the same way as squamous cell carcinomas when radiation therapy is indicated. Good results can be achieved using 5000 rads over 15 to 20 days. Radiation therapy is a good choice for patients with subungual keratoacanthomas.

Andreassi A, et al: Guess what! Keratoacanthoma treated with intralesional bleomycin. *Eur J Dermatol* 1999, 9:403.

Benest L, et al: Keratoacanthoma centrifugum marginatum of the lower extremity treated with Mohs micrographic surgery. *J Am Acad Dermatol* 1994, 31:501.

Cuesta-Romero C, et al: Intralesional methotrexate in solitary keratoacanthoma. *Arch Dermatol* 1998, 134:513.

de la Torre C, et al: Keratoacanthoma centrifugum marginatum: treatment with intralesional bleomycin. *J Am Acad Dermatol* 1997, 37:1010.

Dessoukey MW, et al: Eruptive keratoacanthomas associated with immunosuppressive therapy in a patient with systemic lupus erythematosus. *J Am Acad Dermatol* 1997, 37:478.

Dufresne RG, et al: Seasonal presentation of keratoacanthomas in Rhode Island. *Br J Dermatol* 1997, 136:227.

El-Hakim IE, et al: Squamous cell carcinoma and keratoacanthoma of the lower lip associated with "Goza" and "Shisha" smoking. *Int J Dermatol* 1999, 38:108.

Grine RC, et al: Generalized eruptive keratoacanthoma of Grzybowski: response to cyclophosphamide. *J Am Acad Dermatol* 1997, 36:786.

Janette A, et al: Solitary intraoral keratoacanthoma: report of a case. *J Oral Maxillofac Surg* 1996, 54:1026.

Kavanagh GM, et al: A case of Grzybowski's generalized eruptive keratoacanthomas. *Australas J Dermatol* 1995, 36:83.

Keeney GL, et al: Subungual keratoacanthoma. *Arch Dermatol* 1988, 124:1074.

Kerschmann RL, et al: p53 oncoprotein expression and proliferation index in keratoacanthoma and squamous cell carcinoma. *Arch Dermatol* 1994, 130:181.

Lee YS, et al: p53 expression in pseudoepitheliomatous hyperplasia, keratoacanthoma, and squamous cell carcinoma of skin. *Cancer* 1994, 73:2317.

Patel A, et al: Evidence that regression in keratoacanthoma is immunologically mediated: a comparison with squamous cell carcinoma. *Br J Dermatol* 1994, 131:789.

Reizner GT, et al: Keratoacanthoma in Japanese Hawaiians in Kauai, Hawaii. *Int J Dermatol* 1995, 34:851.

Santoso-Pham JC, et al: Aggressive giant keratoacanthoma of the face treated with intramuscular methotrexate and triamcinolone acetonide. *Cutis* 1997, 59:329.

Schaller M, et al: Multiple keratoacanthomas, giant keratoacanthoma and keratoacanthoma centrifugum marginatum: development in a single patient and treatment with oral isotretinoin. *Acta Derm Venereol* (Norway) 1996, 76:40.

Singal A, et al: Unusual multiple keratoacanthoma in a child successfully treated with 5-fluorouracil. *J Dermatol* 1997, 24:546.

Tamir G, et al: Synchronous appearance of keratoacanthomas in burn scar and skin graft donor site shortly after injury. *J Am Acad Dermatol* 1999, 40:870.

Warner DM, et al: Solitary keratoacanthoma (squamous cell carcinoma): surgical management. *Int J Dermatol* 1995, 34:17.

Watanabe D, et al: Keratoacanthoma centrifugum marginatum arising from a scar after skin injury. *J Dermatol* 1999, 26:541.

Wong WY, et al: Treatment of a recurrent keratoacanthoma with oral isotretinoin. *Int J Dermatol* 1994, 33:579. _____ ▲

BASAL CELL CARCINOMA

Synonyms: Basal cell epithelioma, basalioma, rodent ulcer, Jacobi's ulcer, rodent carcinoma

Clinical Features

Basal cell carcinoma is a tumor composed of one or a few small, waxy, semitranslucent nodules forming around a central depression that may or may not be ulcerated, crusted, and bleeding (Figs. 29-35 and 29-36). The edge of larger lesions has a characteristic rolled border (Fig. 29-37). Telangiectases course through the lesion. Bleeding on slight injury is a common sign.

As growth progresses, crusting appears over a central erosion or ulcer (Fig. 29-38), and when the crust is knocked or picked off, bleeding occurs and the ulcer becomes apparent. This ulcer is characterized by chronicity and gradual enlargement as time goes by. The lesions are asymptomatic, and bleeding is the only difficulty encountered. They rarely metastasize, because they are highly dependent on the connective-tissue stroma in which they lie. Metastasizing cases have almost always been subjected to repeated incomplete excisions or were so neglected that the lesion reached extremely large size without treatment.

The lesions are most frequently found on the face (85%

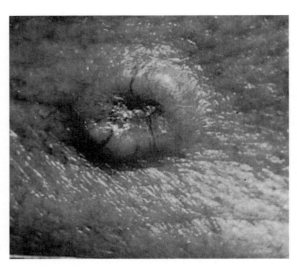

Fig. 29-35   Basal cell carcinoma, approximately 1 cm in diameter, showing rolled waxy edge, telangiectasia, and central ulceration.

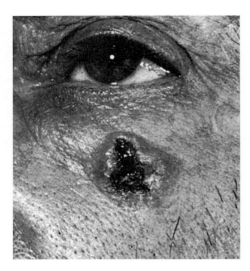

Fig. 29-37   Basal cell carcinoma on the cheek. (Courtesy Dr. H. Shatin.)

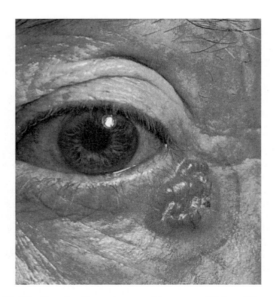

Fig. 29-36   Basal cell carcinoma of lower eyelid in a 65-year-old man. (Courtesy Dr. H. Shatin.)

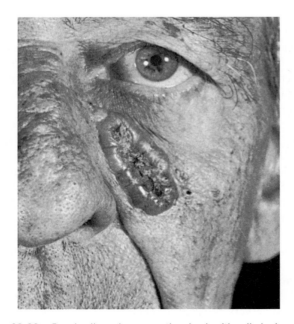

Fig. 29-38   Basal cell carcinoma on the cheek with rolled edge and central ulceration.

are found in the head and neck regions) and especially on the nose (Fig. 29-39) (25% to 30%). The forehead, ears (Figs. 29-40 and 29-41), the periocular areas (Figs. 29-42 and 29-43) and cheeks are also often involved. Any part of the body may be involved; however, the only other site of major frequency besides the head and neck (Fig. 29-44) is the upper trunk, where multiple lesions may occur simultaneously. An interesting observation is that basal cell carcinomas relatively rarely occur on the dorsal hand, where sun exposure and actinic keratoses and squamous cell

carcinomas abound. Squamous cell carcinoma is three times more common than basal cell carcinoma on the dorsum of the hand. In addition to the typical lesion just described, several clinical varieties are recognized. Awareness of these varieties is helpful not only in the diagnosis but also in the management of the tumor. The classic, or nodular type just

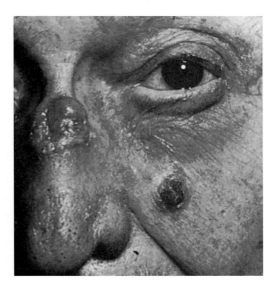

Fig. 29-39 Basal cell carcinomas on the bridge of the nose and left cheek of an 80-year-old woman.

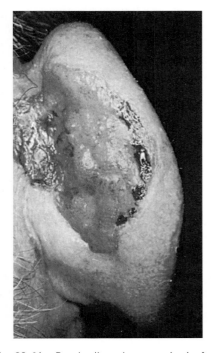

Fig. 29-41 Basal cell carcinoma on back of ear.

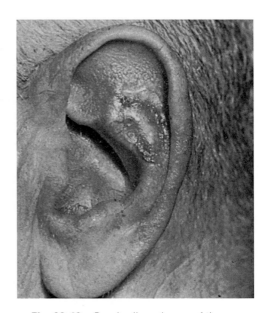

Fig. 29-40 Basal cell carcinoma of the ear.

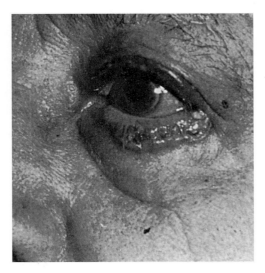

Fig. 29-42 Extensive basal cell carcinoma of lower eyelid. The lesion responded well to radiation therapy.

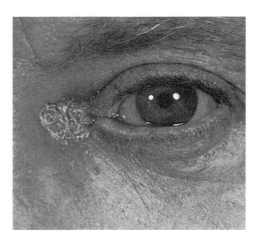

Fig. 29-43 Basal cell carcinoma of the inner canthus—a common site when eyelids are involved. (Courtesy Dr. H. Shatin.)

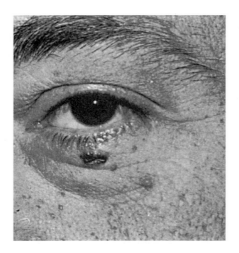

Fig. 29-45 Pigmented basal cell carcinoma on lower eyelid. Simple excision yielded excellent results.

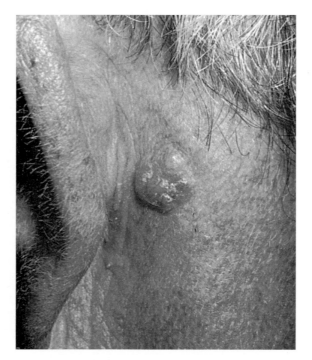

Fig. 29-44 Basal cell carcinoma, postauricular area. (Courtesy Dr. Axel W. Hoke.)

described, comprises 50% to 54% of all basal cell carcinomas.

Pigmented Basal Cell Carcinoma

This variety has all the features of the basal type and, in addition, brown or black pigmentation is present (Fig. 29-45). These are usually extremely slow in evolving. This type is seen more frequently in dark-complected persons such as Latin Americans or Japanese (not blacks). Carcinomas caused by arsenic ingestion are often of the pigmented basal cell variety or the superficial type and occur frequently on the trunk, but do not contain more arsenic than the surrounding normal skin. Pigmented basal cell carcinomas comprise 6% of all basal cell carcinomas. In the management of these lesions it should be known that, if ionizing radiation therapy is chosen as the therapeutic modality, the pigmentation remains at the site of the lesion.

Cystic Basal Cell Epithelioma

These dome-shaped, blue-gray cystic nodules are clinically similar to eccrine and apocrine hidrocystomas. They comprise 4% to 8% of all basal cell carcinoma.

Morphea-Like Epithelioma

This type of basal cell carcinoma demonstrates waxy white sclerotic plaques occurring in the head and neck region, with a conspicuous absence of a rolled edge. Ulceration and crusting are also absent, whereas telangiectasia is prominent. The unique histologic feature is the strands of basal cells interspersed amid densely packed connective tissue, and is a particularly aggressive form. Often the degree of infiltration far exceeds what is clinically apparent. Morphea-like epitheliomas comprise 2% of all basal cell carcinomas. This type is resistant to radiation and electrocautery forms of therapy.

Cicatricial Basal Cell Carcinoma

Called "field fire" epithelioma, cicatricial basal cell carcinoma resembles localized scleroderma that presents a cicatricial surface with nests of active lesions that are usually ulcerated. A fine waxy border or a threadlike raised edge, as well as telangiectases, are present. In our experience the cicatricial basal cell carcinoma occurs almost exclusively on the cheeks. The only other area noted to be involved has been the forehead. These lesions respond to excision, Mohs' microsurgery, or ionizing radiation therapy.

Rodent Ulcer

Also known as *Jacobi's ulcer,* rodent ulcer is a penetrating serpiginous ulcer that slowly progresses for many years to become a large, gnawed-out, mutilating lesion. It is a neglected basal cell carcinoma.

Superficial Basal Cell Carcinoma

Superficial basal cell carcinoma has been described under various names such as intraepidermal carcinoma, intraepidermal basal cell epithelioma of Borst-Jadassohn, and "multicentric" basal cell carcinoma. The multicentricity is merely an illusion created by the passing of the plane of histologic section through the branches of a single, multiply branching lesion. Pinkus has shown that in such lesions the characteristic stroma forms a solid, continuous plate.

This type frequently occurs as several dry, psoriasiform, scaly lesions on the trunk or limbs (Figs. 29-46 to 29-48). They are usually superficial flat growths that exhibit little tendency to invade or ulcerate, and enlarge only very slowly. These lesions may grow to be some 10 to 15 cm in diameter without ulceration. Close examination of the edges of the lesion will show a threadlike raised border. These erythematous plaques with telangiectasia may show atrophy or scarring occasionally, and infiltration is conspicuously absent. Sometimes the lesion will heal at one place with a white atrophic scar and then spread actively to the neighboring skin. There may be several dozen lesions, some of which may coalesce to form extensive plaques. There may be a history of medicinal arsenic ingestion over a long period. An association between frequent radiographs and radiation therapy has been suggested, but not proved. This type is often found in younger patients, with a mean age of 56.8 years, and comprise 9% to 11% of all basal cell carcinomas.

These lesions are not only frequently mistaken for plaques of psoriasis but also for Bowen's disease and extramammary Paget's disease.

Fibroepithelioma of Pinkus

First described by Pinkus as premalignant fibroepithelial tumor, the tumor is usually an elevated, skin-colored, sessile lesion on the lower trunk, the lumbosacral area, groin, or thigh (Fig. 29-49) and may be as large as 7 cm. The lesion is superficial and resembles a fibroma or papilloma and may be found occurring together with superficial basal cell carcinomas. It has also been reported overlying breast carcinomas.

Histologically, there are interlacing basocellular sheets that extend downward from the surface to form an epithelial meshwork enclosing a hyperplastic mesodermal stroma. A slight inflammatory infiltrate may also be present. Pinkus

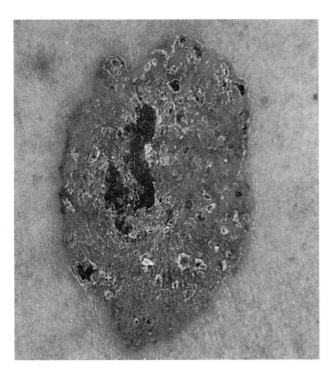

Fig. 29-46 Superficial basal cell carcinoma on scapular area.

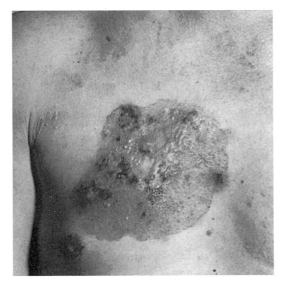

Fig. 29-47 Superficial basal cell carcinoma on right pectoral area.

regarded it as a neoplasm of the stromal element of a basal cell carcinoma. Simple removal by excision or electrosurgery is the treatment of choice.

Keloidal Basal Cell Carcinoma

Requena et al described this unusual variant, which presents as a nodular lesion on the face, clinically suggestive of

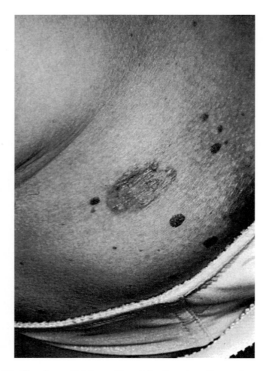

Fig. 29-48 Superficial multicentric basal cell carcinoma and smaller seborrheic keratoses on the breast of a black female.

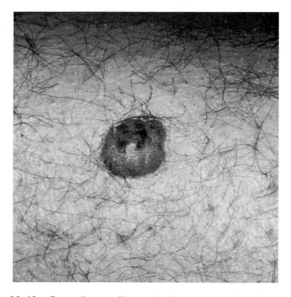

Fig. 29-49 Premalignant fibroepithelioma eventuating in a basal cell carcinoma. (Courtesy Drs. L. Shapiro and J. Penner.)

keloids. On biopsy there are characteristic basaloid nests intermingled with thick, sclerotic, keloidal collagen bundles in the stroma.

Aberrant Basal Cell Carcinoma

Even in the absence of any apparent carcinogenic factor such as arsenic, radiation, or chronic ulceration, basal cell carcinoma may occur in odd sites such as the scrotum, vulva, perineum, nipple, and axilla.

Solitary Basal Cell Carcinoma in Young Persons

These curious lesions are typically located in the region of embryonal clefts in the face and are often deeply invasive. Deep surgical excision is much safer than curettage for their removal. Cases in children and teenagers, unassociated with the basal cell nevus syndrome or nevus sebaceus, are well documented. Individuals with sun exposure risk, such as golfers, have been found to develop lesions at an early age.

Course

Basal cell carcinomas run a chronic course, during which new nodules develop, crusts form and fall off, and the ulceration enlarges. As a rule, there is a tendency for the lesions to bleed without pain or other symptoms. Some of the lesions tend to heal spontaneously and to form scar tissue as they extend. Peripheral spreading may produce configurate, somewhat serpiginous patches. The ulceration may burrow deep into the subcutaneous tissues, or even into cartilage and bone, causing extensive destruction and mutilation (Figs. 29-50 and 29-51). The floor of the ulcer is covered by viscid necrotic material, crusts, and some serosanguineous discharge. This type is termed *rodent ulcer,* but despite the well-documented tendency to invade locally, it does not usually metastasize.

METASTASIS. Although metastasis is extremely rare, more are being reported, and the relative rate is 0.0028% to 0.55%. Supporting stromal tissue is necessary for survival, which explains the infrequency of metastasis. More than 260 cases have been reported. The following criteria are now widely accepted for the diagnosis of these rare metastases:

1. The primary tumor must arise in the skin.
2. Metastases must be demonstrated at a site distant from the primary tumor and must not be related to simple extension.
3. Histologic similarity between the primary tumor and the metastases must exist.
4. The metastases must not be mixed with squamous cell carcinoma.

Males are involved twice as often as females. The head and neck region is the site of the primary tumor in the large majority of cases, with the regional lymph nodes the most frequent site of metastasis, followed by the lung, bone, skin, liver, and pleura. Spread is equally distributed between hematogenous and lymphatic. An average of 9 years elapses between the diagnosis of the primary tumor and metastatic disease, but the interval for metastasis ranges from under 1 year to 45 years. Fewer than 20% survive 1 year, and less than 10% will live past 5 years after metastasis. The appearance of metastatic deposits indicates a poor prognosis, with a median survival of 8 months. Morphea-like and adenocystic types are more aggressive than other histologic forms.

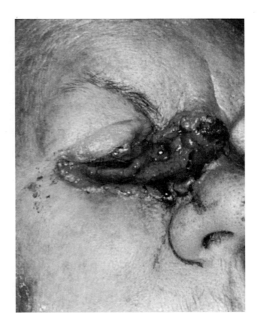

Fig. 29-50 Ulcerating basal cell carcinoma of the orbit and nose.

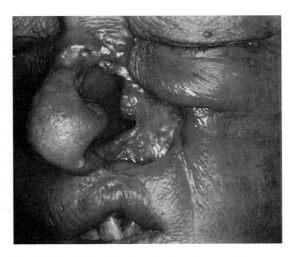

Fig. 29-51 Destructive basal cell carcinoma of the nose.

Management requires the skills of an oncologist, and combinations of chemotherapy, irradiation, and surgery are often required.

ASSOCIATION WITH INTERNAL MALIGNANCIES. Frisch et al reported a series of 37,674 patients with basal cell carcinomas followed over 14 years. Comparison of cancer rates for the general population was remarkable for 3663 new cancers compared with 3245 in the control population. Malignant melanoma and lip cancers were the most frequently found; however, internal malignancies were also noted to be excessive, involving the salivary glands, larynx, lung, breast, kidney, and lymphatics (non-Hodgkin's lymphoma). The rate of non-Hodgkin's lymphoma was particularly high.

Patients receiving the diagnosis of basal cell carcinoma before age 60 were found to have a higher rate of breast cancer, testicular cancer, and non-Hodgkin's lymphoma. The mechanism is believed to be related to the immunosuppressive effects of chronic sunlight exposure. Reports from the Cancer Prevention Study II, reported by Kahn et al, have confirmed these findings.

Epidemiology

There is a worldwide epidemic of skin cancer, particularly basal cell carcinoma. Nonmelanoma skin cancers constitute one third of all cancers diagnosed in the United States and of these basal cell carcinomas account for more than 75%. In 1995, 1.2 million estimated basal cell carcinomas were identified and treated within the United States. More than 99% of individuals with this malignancy are white, and 95% are between the ages of 40 and 79. Just over half of all patients are men. Approximately 30% to 40% of patients with a basal cell carcinoma will develop one or more similar lesions within 10 years.

Excessive sunlight exposure, chemical cocarcinogens, and genetic determinants are implicated as causes of basal cell carcinoma. For this reason it is seen mostly in middle-aged and elderly persons, since they have had years of cumulative chronic exposure to sunlight. In addition to age, the type of skin and its ability to pigment are important factors. Light-complected persons in regions of the world where they are exposed to large amounts of sunlight (such as in Australia) often demonstrate the effects of that excessive exposure. Dark-skinned persons are much less susceptible to skin cancers but not totally immune. The carcinogenic rays of the solar spectrum are between 290 and 400 nm. It has been shown that the highest incidence of skin cancer occurs among Anglo-Saxons who are fair-skinned and have blue eyes. Sailors, farmers, inveterate sunbathers, and outdoor sportspersons are especially prone to skin cancers.

Excessive chronic exposure to ionizing radiation, especially x-rays, radium, and artificially and naturally occurring radioactive substances, may also cause cancer. Physicians, dentists, technicians, and workers with radioactive substances are at risk, and careful handling, shielding and dosage exposure records should be maintained to minimize danger. Radiation therapy for acne has been responsible for skin cancers 20 or 30 years later.

Ionizing and ultraviolet radiation are carcinogenic; however, some individuals are genetically more at risk than others because of defective DNA repair mechanisms. Xeroderma pigmentosum, an autosomal recessive disorder, is such a disorder, in which cutaneous neoplasms, including basal cell carcinomas, occur with increased frequency.

Certain dermatoses of long-standing duration, such as nevus sebaceus, may degenerate into basal cell carcinoma. The epidermis overlying dermatofibromas also seems to be predisposed. Sites of long-standing scars may develop basal cell carcinomas (Fig. 29-52).

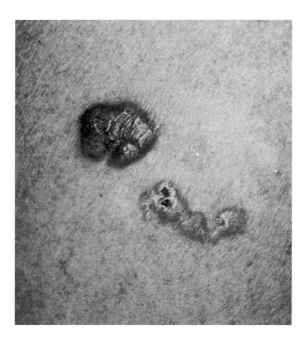

Fig. 29-52 Basal cell carcinoma developing in a vaccination site.

Immunosuppression

Suppression of defensive immune surveillance by immunosuppressive medications, as in renal transplantation or cancer treatment, increases the risk of skin cancers as well as their aggressiveness. Although squamous cell carcinoma is most common, basal cell carcinomas do occur. Local immunosuppression also occurs in areas of the skin exposed to UVB through the damaging action of ultraviolet light on the Langerhans cells. It is theorized that this may lead to a susceptibility to skin cancer formation, not only because immune responses are diminished, but also because Langerhans cells become tolerant to antigens to which they are exposed after UVB damage. Thus, if tumor antigens are present in skin exposed to chronic UVB, they may not respond to these altered antigens, and thus allow the cancer to grow.

Etiology and Pathogenesis

It appears that basal cell carcinomas arise from immature pluripotential cells. Mutations that activate the hedgehog pathway, which controls cell growth, may be a necessary, if not sufficient, step in basal cell carcinoma development. This most commonly occurs through inactivation mutations in the *patched* gene, a tumor suppressor gene. Activating mutations in associated genes *smoothened* and *hedgehog* are also seen. RAS and p53 mutations no doubt also contribute to the malignant characteristics of the tumors. There is little question that stromal factors are also important in the growth and propagation of basal cell carcinoma, but the exact mechanism is yet to be defined.

Histopathology

The early lesion shows small, darkly staining, polyhedral cells resembling those of the stratum germinativum, with swollen nuclei and small nucleoli. These occur within the epidermis as thickenings or immediately beneath the epidermis as downgrowths connected with it. After the growth has progressed, regular compact columns of these cells fill the tissue spaces of the dermis, and a connection with the epidermis may be difficult to demonstrate. At the periphery of the masses of cells, the columnar cells may be characteristically arranged like fence paling (palisading). This may be absent when the tumor cells are in cord arrangement or in small nests. A few mitoses are usually present. Cysts may form. The interlacing strands of tumor cells may present a latticelike pattern.

Subtypes occur histologically in which the immature cells differentiate toward a type of more mature tumor. Pilar, eccrine, apocrine, sebaceous, and squamous types of differentiation may be seen.

Pinkus indicated that the dermal stroma is an integral and important part of the basal cell carcinoma. The tumor does not terminate at the bottom of the epithelial nests but actually extends into its own newly formed connective tissue matrix to constitute a fibroepithelial neoplasm.

Electron microscopic studies show that the cells of the basal cell carcinoma have a greater nuclear/cytoplasmic ratio, fewer filaments, and fewer desmosomes than normal basal cells. No half-desmosomes facing the basement membrane are found in the tumor. On the other hand, the tumor cells are quite similar to the undifferentiated matrix of the human hair follicle.

DIFFERENTIATION. Occasionally a basal cell carcinoma occurs that has differentiated into structures resembling sweat ducts, hair follicles, or sebaceous gland acini. These are reported under varying names such as *eccrine epithelioma* or *apocrine epithelioma.*

Differential Diagnosis

Distinguishing between small basal cell and small squamous cell carcinomas is largely an intellectual exercise. Both are caused chiefly by sunlight; neither is likely to metastasize; neither is likely to be amenable to ordinary topical therapy with 5-fluorouracil; and both will have to be removed, usually by simple surgical excision or curettage.

Generalizations about location are both helpful and misleading. Both types of lesions may occur anywhere on the skin. However, the basal cell lesions are found chiefly on the face, especially on the nose, forehead, eyelids, temples, and upper lip, whereas the squamous cell growths are found principally on the face, at the mucocutaneous junctions, and on the extremities. Primary carcinoma on the vermilion surface of the lower lip is of the squamous cell type. The lesions on the backs of the hands are usually actinic keratoses, keratoacanthomas, or squamous cell carcinomas. Basal cell carcinomas rarely occur at this site.

The duration of the lesion may serve to differentiate the basal and squamous cell types of carcinoma from keratoacanthoma. If a lesion attains a diameter of 1 cm in less than 3 months, a diagnosis of squamous cell carcinoma or keratoacanthoma is likely. Cornification is distinctly a property of the squamous cell type and of keratoacanthoma. Horny material is usually clinically undetectable in basal cell lesions.

A waxy, nodular, rolled edge is fairly characteristic of basal cell growths. The squamous cell carcinoma is a dome-shaped, elevated, hard, and infiltrated lesion. The early basal cell carcinoma may easily be confused with sebaceous hyperplasia, which has a depressed center with yellowish small nodules surrounding the lesion. These lesions never bleed and do not become crusted.

Bowen's disease, Paget's disease, and actinic and seborrheic keratosis may also simulate basal cell carcinoma. Ulcerated basal cell carcinoma on the shins is frequently considered to be a stasis ulcer, and a biopsy may be the only way to differentiate the two. Pigmented basal cell epithelioma is frequently misdiagnosed as melanoma or as a pigmented nevus. The superficial basal cell carcinoma is easily mistaken for psoriasis. The careful search for the rolled edge of the peripheral nodules is important in differentiating basal cell carcinoma from all other lesions.

Treatment

Each lesion of basal cell carcinoma must be thoroughly evaluated individually. Age, sex, and the size, site, and type of lesion are important factors to be considered when choosing the proper method of treatment for an advanced lesion. No single treatment method is ideal for all lesions, be that excision, Mohs' microsurgery, ionizing radiation, cryosurgery, curettage, or electrosurgery. The choice of treatment will also be influenced by the experience and ability of the treating physician in the various treatment modalities.

The aim in treatment is for a permanent cure with the best cosmetic results. This is important because the most frequent site of the basal cell carcinoma is the face. Recurrences result from inadequate treatment and are usually seen during the first 4 to 12 months after treatment. Cure rates are still calculated in 5-year periods; however, it is uncommon to see recurrences later than 1 year after treatment. Five-year follow-up is indicated, however, to continue a search for new lesions, since the development of a second basal cell carcinoma is common.

PROPHYLAXIS. All light-skinned individuals, especially those with blue eyes and light hair, should avoid unnecessary exposure to the sun from childhood to old age. Sunscreen lotions and creams that are helpful and effective are available. They should be applied every morning and reapplied after swimming or vigorous outdoor activity.

BIOPSY. A biopsy should be performed in all cases of suspected basal cell carcinoma. When the lesion is small enough to be amenable to surgical removal, a biopsy excision is preferable.

EXCISION. The ideal treatment method for carcinomas greater than 5 to 7 mm in diameter is simple elliptic excision with suturing for most sites. The scalp, ear rim, forehead, cheeks, chin, neck, and the remainder of the body are sites where simple elliptic excision may be indicated. Wedge excision is a method that is ideally performed on the lips but should be avoided on the nasal rim and ears where alternative methods, such as full-thickness grafts for the nose and tissue advancement for the ears, produce better cosmetic results.

When lesions are much too large for simple elliptic excision or where closure is not feasible, excision with secondary intention healing or skin grafting or the use of skin flaps may be necessary. The skin grafts are either split-thickness or full-thickness grafts. Whether the split-thickness graft is to be thin, intermediate, or thick depends on the area to be covered.

Specimens should be examined histologically to confirm that the margins are clear. If the margins of the excision are involved, reexcision is necessary. The minimal margin generally necessary to totally eradicate the tumor in more than 95% of cases with tumors less than 2 cm in size is 4 mm.

MOHS' MICROSURGERY. Mohs introduced a method for the removal of accessible forms of cancer under microscope control. His pioneering work began in the late 1930s. For 30 years he microscopically controlled the surgery by fixing the neoplastic tissue in situ with zinc chloride paste, excising a layer of tissue, carefully marking, mapping, and color-coding the margins, cutting horizontal sections, examining them microscopically, and repeating the process until all cancer was removed. This method is time consuming, but the cure rate is high, determined by Mohs to be 99.3% of 9351 lesions. In 1970, Tromovitch modified the technique by eliminating the fixative paste and doing the procedure on fresh tissue. Multiple sections can be taken each day and allows for immediate repair. This type of surgery has an extremely high cure rate, usually more than 99% for primary basal cell carcinomas and more than 96% for recurrent lesions. The indications for this type of surgery have been expanding, because of its proven cure rate and wider availability. It is referred to as *Mohs' microsurgery,* acknowledging the abandonment of the ''chemical'' form of fixing tissue.

Consideration for Mohs' microsurgery should be allowed for primary tumors occurring in the ''H zone'' of the face (the nasolabial fold, nasal alae, periorbital region, and periauricular area) and certain scalp tumors; the histologic variants of more aggressive types such as morphea-like or sclerosing types and basal-squamous types; for lesions larger than 2 cm; and for clinical situations such as those lesions occurring in immunosuppressed patients. Recurrent basal cell carcinomas, especially in difficult areas, are also candidates for Mohs' microsurgery.

ELECTROSURGERY. Many skin cancers are treated satisfactorily with a good cure rate and good cosmetic results by curettage and fulguration. The proper use of various-sized dermal curettes in connection with the fulguration permits the easy seeking out of the cancerous tumor. The large, multiple superficial carcinomas found on the trunk are effectively and easily treated by thorough curettage and fulguration. Small lesions, 5 to 20 mm, of the nodular or cystic type, may be treated satisfactorily by this method in most locations.

A pliable, often white scar is formed with this method, and a high cure rate is attained in up to 96% in select cases. Central facial basal cell carcinomas and those of an infiltrating, micronodular or morphea-like histologic type are prone to recurrence if treated with curettage and desiccation. These lesions are thus better treated by methods, such as excision or Mohs' microsurgery, that permit examination of the margins.

CURETTAGE. McDaniel treated 437 basal cell carcinomas with curettage alone and has followed 328 treatment sites for more than 5 years. Cosmetic results have been excellent. Twenty-eight treatment failures were noted. He avoided utilizing this technique on the eyelids and lips and with morphea-like or infiltrating lesions. Careful patient selection is stressed.

IONIZING RADIATION THERAPY. The indications for radiation therapy are continually being modified, as Mohs' microsurgery becomes more available and advanced. In general, skin cancer should be treated by a modality that ensures margin control, such as excision or microsurgery. For individuals unable to tolerate surgical procedures, such as those with multiple medical problems, or in some cases the extremely elderly, radiation therapy offers an excellent alternative. In cases in which surgery would be mutilating this modality may also be considered; however, the ultimate consideration should be the probability of cure, which often then favors surgical intervention.

The amount of x-ray exposure for the treatment of carcinoma depends on the size, depth, and thickness of the lesion and also the type of radiation used. As a rule, ionizing radiation therapy to the ears requires great caution because of possible postradiation necrosis of the cartilage.

Cancers of the scalp and forehead are near to the skull, and the proximity of the bone to the lesion, as well as the probability of permanent alopecia, modifies the choice of therapy. Heavy radiation exposure is contraindicated because of the danger of bone necrosis. Most carcinomas of the scalp and forehead can be readily treated by surgical measures if these hazards are recognized.

Treatment failures are probably the result of errors in estimating the size and depth of tumors. Recurrence at the periphery of the lesion indicates inadequate field size of irradiation; recurrence in the center of the field results from insufficient tumor depth dose. Radiation should not be used in areas where recurrences might be catastrophic, as in the inner canthus or in young patients where radiation sequelae in the treated area will compromise the cosmetic result.

PSEUDORECIDIVE. *Pseudorecidive* is a term used to describe the appearance of a pseudoepitheliomatous reaction at the site of a previously irradiated basal cell carcinoma. This reaction occurs some 2 to 4 weeks after ionizing radiation therapy has been performed; it may persist for as long as 2 months before spontaneous disappearance occurs. The lesion may resemble a seborrheic keratosis or a keratoacanthoma.

TOPICAL CYTOTOXIC THERAPY. The topical application of 5-fluorouracil in various concentrations has been reported to be effective in the treatment of basal cell carcinomas, especially the superficial, multicentric type. Some have applied 5-FU after thorough curettage of the lesion. Mohs et al warn that topical fluorouracil treatment of invasive basal cell carcinoma of the face can result in partial or complete healing of the skin overlying deeper extensions of the neoplasm. This method is not an accepted treatment.

CRYOSURGERY. Cryotherapy for basal cell carcinomas, as well as other benign and malignant neoplasms, has been used since solid carbon dioxide became available. The use of a variety of probes and monitoring of tissue temperatures with thermocouples has allowed for excellent cure rates in some hands. These authors also report good cosmetic results, with hypopigmentation being the most common side effect. The down-side to the use of this modality is the long healing times, often requiring 6 to 8 weeks, and the lack of margin control.

LASER THERAPY. Wheeland et al reported their results treating 52 patients with 370 basal cell carcinomas of the superficial type with curettage and CO_2 laser vaporization. They had excellent results with the advantages of rapid healing, diminished postoperative pain, and excellent field visualization.

OTHER MODALITIES. Retinoids, imiquimod, immunotherapy (IL-1, IL-2, interferon alfa-2a, interferon-gamma), and photodynamic therapy have all been used with variable success. Chemotherapy used in treating metastatic disease may have a part in treating patients with multiple lesions. Systemic therapy including cisplatin, doxorubicin, cyclophosphamide, and adriamycin have all been used in various degrees. Bleomycin has provided mixed results. Chemotherapy may be used as adjunctive therapy in patients with numerous lesions treated with radiation therapy or suspected incomplete surgical excision. Use of these modalities is experimental.

Prevention

Sunscreens should be used daily by all patients with basal cell cancer to prevent further solar damage. Sun-protective clothing may also prove beneficial.

Abreo F, et al: Basal cell carcinoma in North American blacks: clinical and histopathologic study of 26 patients. *J Am Acad Dermatol* 1991, 25:1005.

Alcalay J, et al: Pedal basal cell carcinoma. *Int J Dermatol* 1991, 24:715.

Berti JJ, et al: Metastatic basal cell carcinoma to the lung. *Cutis* 1999, 63:165.

Betti R, et al: Basal cell carcinoma of covered and unusual sites of the body. *Int J Dermatol* 1997, 36:503.

Betti R, et al: Giant basal cell carcinomas: report of four cases and considerations. *J Dermatol* 1997, 24:317.

Beutner KR, et al: Therapeutic response of basal cell carcinoma to the immune response modifier imiquimod 5% cream. *J Am Acad Dermatol* 1999, 41:1002.

Bigler C, et al: Pigmented basal cell carcinoma in Hispanics. *J Am Acad Dermatol* 1996, 34:751.

Caccialanza M, et al: Results and side effects of dermatologic radiotherapy. *J Am Acad Dermatol* 1999, 41:589.

Crowson AN, et al: Basal cell carcinoma arising in association with desmoplastic trichilemmoma. *Am J Dermatopathol* 1996, 18:43.

Esquivias Gomez JI, et al: Basal cell carcinoma of the scrotum. *Australas J Dermatol* 1999, 40:141.

Frisch M, et al: Risk for subsequent cancer after diagnosis of basal-cell carcinoma. *Ann Intern Med* 1996, 125:815.

Gailani MR, Bale AE: Acquired and inherited basal cell carcinomas and the *patched* gene. *Adv Dermatol* 1999, 14:261.

Goldberg LH: Basal cell carcinoma. *Lancet* 1996, 347:663.

Goldberg LH: Basal-cell carcinoma as a predictor of other cancers. *Lancet* 1997, 349:664.

Goncalves JC: Fractional cryosurgery: a new technique for basal cell carcinoma of the eyelids and periorbital area. *Dermatol Surg* 1997, 23:475.

Grabski WJ, et al: Positive surgical excision margins of a basal cell carcinoma. *Dermatol Surg* 1998, 24:921.

Halpern AC, et al: Genetic predisposition to skin cancer. *Curr Opin Oncol* 1999, 11:132.

Kahn HS, et al: Increased cancer mortality following a history of nonmelanoma skin cancer. *JAMA* 1998, 280:910.

Kikuchi A, et al: Clinical histopathological characteristics of basal cell carcinoma in Japanese patients. *Arch Dermatol* 1996, 132:320.

Kuflik EG, et al: Recurrent basal cell carcinoma treated with cryosurgery. *J Am Acad Dermatol* 1997, 37:82.

Lawrence CM: Mohs' micrographic surgery for basal cell carcinoma. *Clin Exp Dermatol* 1999, 24:130.

Lindgren G, et al: Long-term follow-up of cryosurgery of basal cell carcinoma of the eyelid. *J Am Acad Dermatol* 1997, 36:742.

Lo JS, et al: Metastatic basal cell carcinoma: report of twelve cases with a review of the literature. *J Am Acad Dermatol* 1991, 24:715.

Maloney ME: Histology of basal cell carcinoma. *Clin Dermatol* 1995, 13:545.

Mansur CP: The regulation and function of the p53 tumor suppressor. *Adv Dermatol* 1998, 13:121.

McCormack CJ, et al: Differences in age and body site distribution of the histological subtypes of basal cell carcinoma: a possible indicator of differing causes. *Arch Dermatol* 1997, 133:593.

McDaniel WE: Therapy for basal cell epitheliomas by curettage only. *Arch Dermatol* 1983, 119:901.

Miller ES, et al: Vulvar basal cell carcinoma. *Dermatol Surg* 1997, 23:207.

Miller SJ: Biology of basal cell carcinoma (Part I). *J Am Acad Dermatol* 1991, 24:1.

Miller SJ: Biology of basal cell carcinoma (Part II). *J Am Acad Dermatol* 1991, 24:161.

Nahass GT, et al: Basal cell carcinoma of the scrotum: report of three cases and review of the literature. *J Am Acad Dermatol* 1992, 26:574.

Orengo IF, et al: Correlation of histologic subtypes of primary basal cell carcinoma and number of Mohs' stages required to achieve a tumor-free plane. *J Am Acad Dermatol* 1997, 37:395.

Randle HW: Basal cell carcinoma: identification and treatment of the high-risk patient. *Dermatol Surg* 1996, 22:255.

Requena L, et al: Keloidal basal cell carcinoma: a new clinicopathological variant of basal cell carcinoma. *Br J Dermatol* 1996, 134:953.

Rosso S, et al: The multicentre south European study "Helios." II: different sun exposure patterns in the aetiology of basal cell and squamous cell carcinomas of the skin. *Br J Cancer* (Scotland) 1996, 73:1447.

Rowe DE: Comparison of treatment modalities for basal cell carcinoma. *Clin Dermatol* 1995, 13:617.

Sahl WJ Jr, et al: Giant basal cell carcinoma: report of two cases and review of the literature. *J Am Acad Dermatol* 1994, 30:856.

Walsh DS: Molecular genetics of cancer. *Adv Dermatol* 1998, 13:167.

Wheeland RG, et al: Carbon dioxide laser vaporization and curettage in the treatment of large or multiple superficial basal cell carcinomas. *J Dermatol Surg Oncol* 1987, 13:119.

Wrone DA, et al: Increased proportion of aggressive-growth basal cell carcinoma in the Veterans Affairs population of Palo Alto, California. *J Am Acad Dermatol* 1996, 35:907. _____ ▲

NEVOID BASAL CELL CARCINOMA SYNDROME (GORLIN'S SYNDROME)

Nevoid basal cell carcinoma syndrome has frequently been miscalled the basal cell nevus syndrome and nevoid basalioma syndrome.

Clinical Features

The nevoid basal cell carcinoma syndrome is a hereditary disorder characterized by basal cell carcinomas; odontogenic cysts of the jaws; pitted depressions on the hands and feet; osseous anomalies of the ribs, spine, and skull; and multiple other disorders. Keratin cysts are frequently seen, and calcium deposits in skin, especially in the scalp, may be present. A characteristic facies is present, with frontal bossing, a hypoplastic maxilla, a broad nasal root, and true ocular hypertelorism being features.

Of 105 patients, 80% were white and 38% were black in the series reported by Kimonis et al. The first tumor developed by the mean age of 23 and 21 years for white and black patients, respectively. Palmar pits were seen in 87%. Jaw cysts were found in 74%, with 80% manifested by age of 20. The total number of cysts ranged from 1 to 28. Medulloblastomas developed in four patients, and three had cleft lip or palate. Physical findings in this series included "coarse face" (54%), macrocephaly (50%), hypertelorism (42%), frontal bossing (27%), pectus deformity (13%), and Sprengel deformity (11%). Previously described features not found in this series include short fourth metacarpal, scoliosis, cervical ribs, or spina bifida occulta.

Skin Tumors

The basal cell carcinomas occur at an early age or any time thereafter as multiple lesions, usually numerous. The usual age of appearance is between 17 and 35 years. Although any area of the body may be affected, there is a marked tendency toward involvement of the central facial area (Fig. 29-53), especially the eyelids, periorbital area, nose, upper lip, and

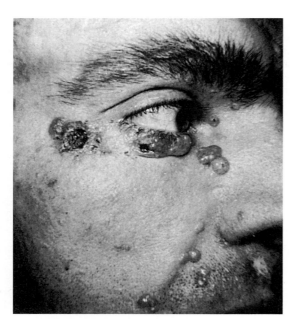

Fig. 29-53 Nevoid basal cell carcinoma syndrome in a 39-year-old man with ameloblastoma, multiple cysts of the jaw, calcification of falx cerebri, spina bifida, Marfan syndrome, and rheumatic heart disease. (Courtesy Dr. A.M. Lefkovitz.)

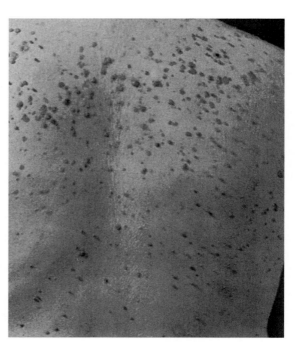

Fig. 29-54 Nevoid basal cell carcinoma in a 10-year-old girl. (Courtesy Dr. J.B. Howell.)

cheeks. Any variety of basal cell carcinoma may be present; among these may be nodular, pigmented, morphea-like, or ulcerated types. In children they may be pigmented papules resembling skin tags (Fig. 29-54).

Basal cell carcinomas in this syndrome may extend into the brain. Metastasis may also occur. It is for this reason that some authors prefer the designation of "nevoid basal cell carcinoma syndrome" as indicative of the possible mutilating and destructive characteristics of these tumors.

Jaw Cysts

Jaw cysts occur in 70% of patients. Both the mandible and the maxilla may show cystic defects by x-ray, with mandibular involvement occurring twice as often. The patient may complain of jaw pain and tenderness, fever, difficulty in closing the mouth, and swelling of the jaw. The cysts are uni- or multilocular and may occur anytime during life, with the first decade being the most common time of appearance. They may have a keratinized lining, and some are ameloblastomas.

Pits of Hands and Feet

An unusual pitting of palms and soles (Fig. 29-55) is a distinguishing feature of the disease. They usually become apparent in the second decade of life. Up to 87% of patients with nevoid basal cell carcinoma syndrome will have such findings. Some believe that they are minimal expressions of

a characteristic feature of basal cell carcinomas: inability to keratinize. Others regard them as intraepidermal basal cell carcinomas that may never become clinically or histologically manifest. If they do, they are usually unaggressive.

Skeletal Defects

Numerous skeletal defects are easily detected by roentgenograms; such defects may be spina bifida, deformed ribs, scoliosis, and kyphosis. An interesting finding is shortened fourth metacarpal and metatarsal bones. The shortened fourth metacarpal results clinically in a dimple over the fourth metacarpophalangeal joint (Albright's sign). Radiographic evidence of multiple lesions is highly suggestive of this syndrome, and since most are present congenitally, roentgenograms may be useful in diagnosing this syndrome in patients too young to manifest other abnormalities. Seventy percent to 75% of patients manifest skeletal abnormalities. In the series by Kimonis et al flame-shaped lucencies of the phalanges, metacarpal, and carpal bones of the hands were found in 30% of 105 patients. Other radiographic findings in this series include bifid ribs (26%), hemivertebra (15%), and fusion of the vertebral bodies (10%).

Disorders of the Central Nervous System

Roentgenograms of the skull may show early lamellar calcification of the falx cerebri, falx cerebelli, and dura or

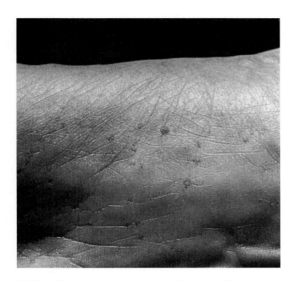

Fig. 29-55 Pits on the sole in nevoid basal cell carcinoma syndrome. (From Howell JB: *JAMA* 1964, 190:274.)

basal ganglia. In the series by Kimonis et al important radiographic signs included calcification of the falx cerebri (65%), calcification of the tentorium cerebelli (20%), and calcification of the bridged sella (68%). Varying mental problems may be encountered in patients.

Other Defects

Ophthalmologic abnormalities and mesenteric, ovarian, and mammary cysts, as well as uterine fibromas, lipomas, epithelial cysts, milia, and renal calculi, are known to occur at times in these patients. Calcified multinodular ovarian fibromas are characteristic.

Etiology

This is a genetic disorder with an autosomal dominant pattern. Penetrance may be as high as 95%. The mutation is located on chromosome 9q22.3. Mutations in the *patched* tumor suppressor gene and other activating mutations of the hedgehog pathway as described on p. 826 are responsible for this disease.

Histopathology

The histology of basal cell carcinomas arising in syndrome patients is identical to those arising in nonsyndrome patients, with the solid and superficial types being most common. The cutaneous keratocysts may show histologic findings similar to those seen in jaw keratocysts, and may be another cutaneous marker of this disease.

Differential Diagnosis

The skin tumors of the basal cell nevus syndrome have the following unique features that help to differentiate them from other tumors: Usually the lesions are multiple basal

cell carcinomas occurring over a span of years from early childhood to late in life. The tumors occur in other than sun-exposed areas, with a history of similar tumors in other family members through several generations.

Two other unique types of presentation of basal cell carcinomas should not be confused with this entity. One is the linear unilateral basal cell carcinoma syndrome, in which a linear arrangement of close-set papules, sometimes interspersed with comedones, is present at birth. Biopsy reveals basal cell epitheliomas; however, they do not increase in size with age of the patient. The second type, referred to as *Bazex's syndrome,* is an autosomal dominantly inherited disease comprising follicular atrophoderma of the extremities, localized or generalized hypohidrosis, hypotrichosis, and multiple basal cell carcinomas of the face, which often arise at an early age.

Treatment

The aggressiveness of the carcinomas varies, and owing to this and the multitude of lesions, Mohs' microsurgery provides the best cure rates and cosmetic appearance. Curettage and desiccation of the superficial lesions of the trunk and excision are other effective methods. Genetic counseling is essential.

Cohen MM Jr: Nevoid basal cell carcinoma syndrome: molecular biology and new hypothesis. *Int J Oral Maxillofac Surg* 1999, 28:216.

Gailani MR, Bale AE: Acquired and inherited basal cell carcinomas and the *patched* gene. *Adv Dermatol* 1999, 14:261.

Hall J, et al: Nevoid basal cell carcinoma syndrome in a black child. *J Am Acad Dermatol* 1998, 38:363.

Kimonis VE, et al: Clinical manifestations in 105 persons with nevoid basal cell carcinoma syndrome. *Am J Med Genet* 1997, 69:299.

Walter AW, et al: Complications of the nevoid basal cell carcinoma syndrome: a case report. *J Pediatr Hematol Oncol* 1997, 19:258.

INTRAEPIDERMAL EPITHELIOMA

This rare neoplasm has also been known as *Borst-Jadassohn epithelioma* and *intraepidermal epithelioma of Jadassohn.* Clinically, these single lesions present as a gray to tan-brown, keratotic, scaly, flat, sometimes verrucous, round to irregularly shaped plaque that clinically resembles Bowen's disease, multicentric basal cell carcinoma, epithelial nevus, seborrheic keratosis, nevus cell nevus, and melanotic freckle of Hutchinson. They appear on various parts of the body and may slowly grow to be several centimeters in diameter. Jadassohn's case had several superficial carcinomas at the same time.

Pinkus and Mehregan define intraepidermal epithelioma histologically as a neoplasm in which sharply defined nests of neoplastic cells are surrounded completely by normal keratinocytes. This is in contrast to carcinoma in situ, in which neoplastic cells range from the basement membrane to the epidermal surface. It has been suggested that these lesions may be only seborrheic keratoses, although intraepidermal nests may also occur in intraepidermal poromas and in Bowen's disease. Graham and Helwig believe that intraepidermal epithelioma represents a variety of carcinoma in situ arising from acrosyringium keratinocytes or pluripotential adnexal cells. When the dermoepidermal basement membrane is disrupted, it is considered to represent an adnexal eccrine carcinoma.

Simple local excision, and curettage and desiccation, are acceptable methods of treatment. Lesions showing carcinoma should be treated by wide local excision including subcutaneous fat.

Amichai B, et al: A seborrheic keratosislike lesion: intraepidermal epithelioma of Borst-Jadassohn. *Arch Dermatol* 1995, 131:1331.
Smith KJ, et al: Recent advances and controversies concerning adnexal neoplasms. *Dermatol Clin* 1992, 10:117. _____ ▲

SQUAMOUS CELL CARCINOMA
Synonyms: Prickle cell carcinoma, epidermoid carcinoma

Clinical Features
Squamous cell carcinoma occurs not only on the skin but also on the mucous membranes. Frequently, squamous cell carcinoma begins at the site of actinic keratosis on sun-exposed areas such as the face and backs of the hands. Basal cell carcinomas far outnumber squamous cell carcinomas on the facial skin, but squamous cell carcinomas on the hand occur three times more commonly than basal cell carcinomas. The lesion may be superficial, discrete, and hard, and arises from an indurated, rounded, elevated base (Fig. 29-56). It is dull red and contains telangiectases. In other instances, the tumors begin as small, erythematous, infiltrated, hard, scaly plaques, on skin that has been damaged by x-rays, scars, or chronic ulcers. In the course of a few months the lesion becomes larger, deeply nodular, and ulcerated. The ulcer is at first superficial and is hidden by a crust. When this is removed, a well-defined, papillary base is seen and on palpation a discrete hard disk is felt. In the early phases this tumor is localized, elevated, and freely movable on the underlying structures; later it gradually becomes diffuse, more or less depressed, and fixed. The growth eventually invades the underlying tissues (Fig. 29-57). The tumor above the level of the skin may be dome-shaped (Fig. 29-58), with a corelike center that later ulcerates. The surface in advanced lesions may be cauliflower-like, composed of densely packed, filamentous projections, between which are clefts filled with a viscid, purulent, malodorous exudate (Fig. 29-59).

In black patients squamous cell carcinomas are 20% more common than basal cell carcinomas. The most common sites are the face and lower extremities, with involvement of non–sun-exposed areas more common. Thus, as contrasted with white patients, the frequent predisposing

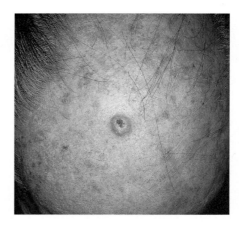

Fig. 29-56 Squamous cell carcinoma of the scalp.

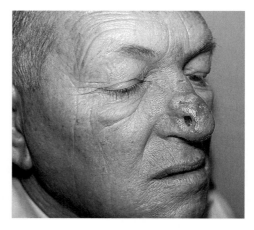

Fig. 29-57 Advanced squamous cell carcinoma of the nose.

conditions are scarring processes such as burns, leg ulcers, and hidradenitis suppurativa. Metastasis, with a mortality rate of 18%, is very low from sites of chronic sun damage, whereas it is relatively high (20% to 30%) in squamous cell carcinomas occurring in scarring processes.

On the lower lip, squamous cell carcinoma often develops on actinic cheilitis. From repeated sunburn the vermilion surface becomes dry, scaly, and fissured, and keratoses develop. Cancer usually arises on such a fissure or keratosis. At the beginning only a local thickening is noticeable. This then becomes a firm nodule. It may grow outward as a sizable tumor or grow inward with destructive ulceration (Fig. 29-60). A history of smoking is also frequent and a significant predisposing factor. Lower lip lesions far outnumber upper lip lesions, men far outnumber women (ratio 12:1), and the median age is the late sixties. Squamous cell carcinomas occurring on the lower lip metastasize approximately 10% to 15% of the time. Squamous cell carcinoma of the lip may also occur in areas of discoid lupus in black patients. Neoplastic transformation into squamous cell car-

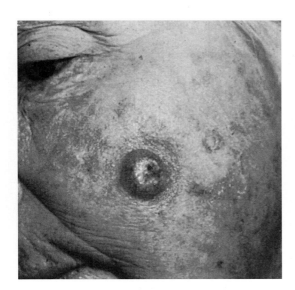

Fig. 29-58 Squamous cell carcinoma. Note dome shape of the tumor.

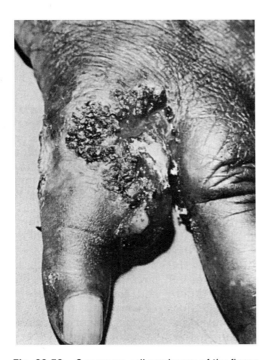

Fig. 29-59 Squamous cell carcinoma of the finger.

cinoma may develop in 0.3% to 3% of patients with the oral form of the disease (Fig. 29-61).

Subungual squamous cell carcinoma frequently presents with signs of swelling, erythema, and localized pain. It commonly arises in the nail folds of the hands (Fig. 29-62) (particularly the thumbs) of patients in the 50- to 69-year-old age range. Fifty percent of those x-rayed show changes in the terminal phalanx. There is a very low rate of

metastases, but local excision with Mohs' microsurgery is recommended to save as much normal tissue as possible. Radiation therapy is another consideration.

Biopsy of chronic, recalcitrant, indurated lesions in actinically damaged skin of the lip, or of such lesions in chronic scarred sites, should be done to make this diagnosis. Generally, incisional or excisional biopsies are recommended. Punch biopsies may not be diagnostic.

Etiology

Many causative factors have been identified in squamous cell carcinoma. Ultraviolet light certainly is a major factor in light-complected individuals and in individuals with significant childhood and adolescent exposure. Although UVB has long been known to be of prime importance, the role of UVA is also important. UVB may predispose to skin cancer not only through its DNA-damaging action but also via local injury to Langerhans cells.

Photochemotherapy, psoralens plus UVA light, as used in the United States, is associated with squamous cell carcinoma formation. Other situations that reveal the importance of ultraviolet light in squamous cell carcinoma formation include the relatively high incidence of this tumor in Africans; in hypopigmented black skin secondary to other dermatoses (albinism, postinflammatory disorders); and in patients with genetic inability to repair sun-induced DNA damage.

Thermal injury to the skin may produce thermal keratoses and squamous cell carcinoma. The constant exposure to hot tea as experienced by tea tasters may produce leukoplakia and oral cancer. The Kangri cancer (Fig. 29-63), occurring in Kashmir among natives who use the Kangri jar, a brazier of hot coals carried under the clothing for warmth, develops on the abdomen and upper thighs.

Chemical carcinogenesis is a classic cause of skin cancer. Best known are the effects of polycyclic aromatic hydrocarbons, which include 3,4-benzpyrene. This has been implicated as the cause of scrotal squamous cell carcinoma in mule spinners in the cotton textile industry. Other situations in which chemical carcinogenesis can play a role are scrotal cancers in chimney sweeps and patients with mycosis fungoides treated topically with nitrogen. Arsenic, paraffin, creosote, anthracene, tobacco smoke tars, and chromates are other important carcinogens.

Chronic radiation dermatitis from x-radiation or radium may produce squamous cell carcinomas, as in several patients who developed carcinoma of the fingers under rings contaminated with radioactive gold. Sarcomas, malignant fibrous histiocytomas, angiosarcomas, and basal cell carcinomas may also appear in these sites.

Human papillomavirus (HPV), especially of types 16, 18, 30, and 33, is associated with squamous cell carcinoma. It occurs in sun-exposed areas and with increased frequency in epidermodysplasia verruciformis (EV). In a study by

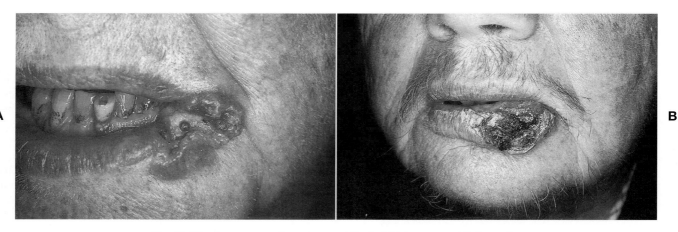

Fig. 29-60 Squamous cell carcinoma of the **A,** labial crease and **B,** lower lip.

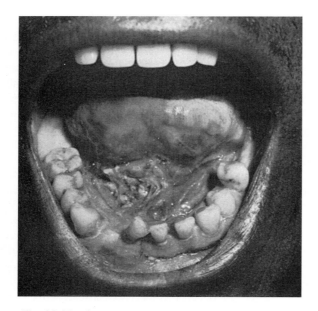

Fig. 29-61 Squamous cell carcinoma on floor of mouth.

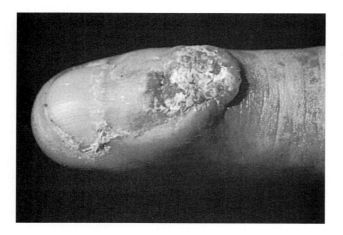

Fig. 29-62 Squamous cell carcinoma, subungual, mimicking a wart. (Courtesy Dr. Axel W. Hoke.)

Harwood et al of PUVA-associated nonmelanoma skin cancers, HPV DNA was detected in 15 of 20 (75%) of biopsies and the most common HPV types were HPV-5, -20, -21, -23, -24, and -38 (EV viral types). HPV is also associated with cervical cancer and may be related to the increase in skin cancer seen in renal transplant patients. Women sex partners of men with squamous cell carcinoma of the penis (Fig. 29-64) have been shown to be 1.65 times more likely to develop preinvasive and invasive cancer of the neck of the uterus.

The eponym *Marjolin's ulcer* is used when cancers, most of which are of the squamous cell type, arise in chronic ulcers, sinuses, and scars of various etiologies, although burns are the most common cause. Burns; fistulous tracts such as occur in hidradenitis suppurativa, acne conglobata, or pilonidal sinus; syphilis; lupus vulgaris; stasis ulcers; osteomyelitis sinuses; amputation stumps; smallpox vaccinations; decubitus ulcers; epidermolysis bullosa scars; granuloma inguinale; lymphogranuloma venereum; and discoid lupus scars have been implicated as processes that predispose to the development of squamous cell carcinoma. It may occur in chronic lymphedema and unhealed wounds of Crohn's disease.

Certain dermatoses, such as porokeratosis of Mibelli, nevus sebaceus (Fig. 29-65), and lichen sclerosus et atrophicus, have been associated with an increased incidence of squamous cell carcinoma developing in them.

Histopathology

Squamous cell carcinoma is characterized by irregular nests of epidermal cells invading the dermis to varying degrees. The degree of cell differentiation has been used to grade squamous cell carcinoma. Although interpretations vary, it is believed that the greater the differentiation, the less the invasive tendency, thereby the better the prognosis. The Broders classification has four grades of cell differentiation. In grade I most of the cells are well differentiated, whereas in grade IV most of the cells are undifferentiated or

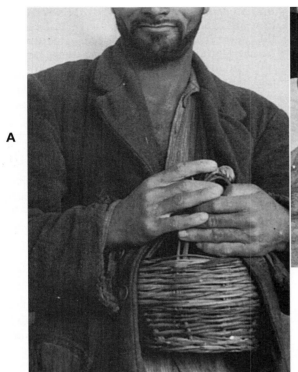

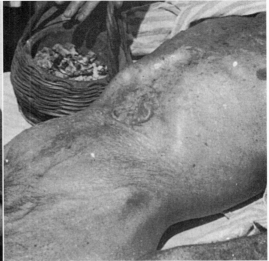

Fig. 29-63 **A,** Kangri (fire basket). **B,** Kangri cancer. The kangri is a small basket with an earthen pot inside in which glowing coals and Chinan leaves burn. The smoke and heat on the abdomen are said to induce cancers at that site. (Courtesy Dr. K.J. Ranadine, Bombay, India.)

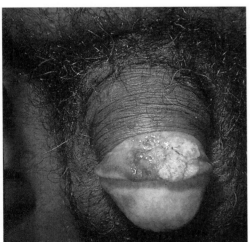

Fig. 29-64 Squamous cell carcinoma of the penis.

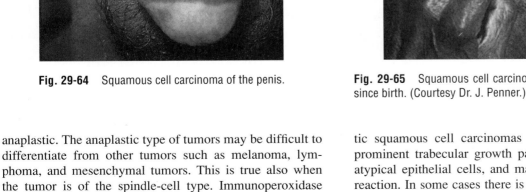

Fig. 29-65 Squamous cell carcinoma in nevus sebaceus present since birth. (Courtesy Dr. J. Penner.)

anaplastic. The anaplastic type of tumors may be difficult to differentiate from other tumors such as melanoma, lymphoma, and mesenchymal tumors. This is true also when the tumor is of the spindle-cell type. Immunoperoxidase staining for prekeratin or cytokeratin is useful. Desmoplas-

tic squamous cell carcinomas by light microscopy have prominent trabecular growth patterns, narrow columns of atypical epithelial cells, and marked desmoplastic stromal reaction. In some cases there is perineural and perivascular invasion.

Differential Diagnosis

Squamous cell carcinoma may be difficult to distinguish from keratoacanthoma. The rapid growth and the presence of a rolled border with a keratotic central plug are good indicators that one is dealing with a keratoacanthoma. The early squamous cell carcinoma may be confused with a hypertrophic actinic keratosis, and, indeed, the two may be indistinguishable clinically. Biopsy to include the base of the lesion is necessary to make the diagnosis. In the mouth it is to be distinguished from a chancre. The procedure in differentiating the two is to biopsy the lesion. Gummatous lesions of the skin are differentiated in the same manner.

Pseudoepitheliomatous hyperplasia is a histologic diagnosis to be considered. The clinical features are suggestive of a carcinoma occurring in some of the inflammatory diseases, especially in granulomatous reactions and ulcerations. Pseudoepitheliomatous hyperplasia may be seen in granular cell tumor, in bromoderma, blastomycosis, granuloma inguinale, and chronic pyodermas. It is frequently mistaken for squamous cell carcinoma in chronic stasis ulcers, ulcerations occurring in thermal burns, lupus vulgaris, leishmaniasis, and even in sporotrichosis. It may occur in a "dry" socket after dental extraction.

Architecturally, the epithelial hyperplasia is suggestive of squamous cell carcinoma; however, the atypical cells are absent and the nuclei show normal staining. Strands of epidermal cells may extend into the reticular dermis. In the dermis a pronounced inflammatory reaction is often present.

Metastases

The rate of squamous cell carcinoma metastasis from all skin sites ranges from 0.5% to 5.2%. Careful attention should be paid to regional lymph nodes draining the site of the squamous cell carcinoma.

Local recurrence and metastasis are related to: (1) treatment modality, (2) prior treatment, (3) location, (4) size, (5) depth, (6) histologic differentiation, (7) histologic evidence of perineural involvement, (8) histologic evidence of desmoplastic features, (9) precipitating factors other than ultraviolet light, and (10) host immunosuppression. In reference to metastatic disease, the highest rates occur from scars (37.9%), the lip (13.7%), and the external ear (8.8%). Risk of metastasis rises for lesions larger than 2 cm in diameter, skin lesions thicker than 4 mm, and lip lesions thicker than 8 mm. Patients with perineural spread have a local recurrence rate of 47.2% and a metastatic rate of 34.8%. Desmoplastic squamous cell carcinomas are six times more likely to metastasize than other histologic patterns, excluding neurotropic forms.

Patients with squamous cell carcinoma are at risk of developing other malignancies such as cancers of the respiratory organs, buccal cavity, pharynx, small intestines (in men), non-Hodgkin's lymphoma, and leukemia. Squamous cell lung cancer must not be confused with metastatic disease from skin.

Treatment

Because of the possibility of metastasis from squamous cell carcinoma, treatment should be thorough. Ideally an excisional surgical specimen with margin control should be obtained. Mohs' surgical technique, especially for recurrent disease, large lesions, those in the postauricular sulcus or ear, those in irradiated or scarred skin, neurotropic or desmoplastic forms, or those in areas requiring the salvage of as much normal skin as possible, as on the penis or the finger, is a preferred choice. Radiation therapy is also effective in select cases.

Retinoids, electrochemotherapy, photodynamic therapy, beta carotene, interferons, and intratumoral chemotherapy with fluorouracil/epinephrine injectable gel or bleomycin, are developing treatment alternatives. For metastatic or advanced disease cisplatin and doxorubicin or bleomycin are frequently used.

Prevention

It has been estimated that the regular use of a sunscreen with a sun protection factor of 15 or greater for the first 18 years of life would reduce the lifetime incidence of nonmelanoma skin cancers by 78%.

Akgunner M, et al: Marjolin's ulcer and chronic burn scarring. *J Wound Care* 1998, 7:121.

Breuninger H, et al: Desmoplastic squamous cell carcinoma of skin and vermilion surface: a highly malignant subtype of skin cancer. *Cancer* 1997, 79:915.

Dinehart SM, et al: Metastatic cutaneous squamous cell carcinoma derived from actinic keratosis. *Cancer* 1997, 79:920.

Dupree MT, et al: Marjolin's ulcer arising in a burn scar. *Cutis* 1998, 62:49.

English DR, et al: Case-control study of sun exposure and squamous cell carcinoma of the skin. *Int J Cancer* 1998, 77:347.

Fleming ID, et al: Principles of management of basal and squamous cell carcinoma of the skin. *Cancer* 1995, 75:699.

Fritsch C, et al: New primary cancers after squamous cell skin cancer. *Am J Epidemiol* 1995, 141:916.

Fritsch C, et al: Photodynamic therapy in dermatology. *Arch Dermatol* 1998, 134:207.

Fruland JE, et al: Skin necrosis with subsequent formation of squamous cell carcinoma after subcutaneous interferon beta injection. *J Am Acad Dermatol* 1997, 37:488.

Goldman GD: Squamous cell cancer: a practical approach. *Semin Cutan Med Surg* 1998, 17:80.

Gonzalez-Perez R, et al: Metastatic squamous cell carcinoma arising in Bowen's disease of the palm. *J Am Acad Dermatol* 1997, 36:635.

Harwood CA, et al: Detection of human papillomavirus DNA in PUVA-associated nonmelanoma skin cancers. *J Invest Dermatol* 1998, 111:123.

Harwood CA, et al: Human papillomavirus and the development of non-melanoma skin cancer. *J Clin Pathol* 1999, 52:249.

Haydon RC III: Cutaneous squamous carcinoma and related lesions. *Otolaryngol Clin North Am* 1993, 26:57.

Hayes AG, et al: Cutaneous metastasis from squamous cell carcinoma of the cervix. *J Am Acad Dermatol* 1992, 26:846.

Heller R, et al: Treatment of cutaneous and subcutaneous tumors with electrochemotherapy using intralesional bleomycin. *Cancer* 1998, 83:148.

Iversen T, et al: Squamous cell carcinoma of the penis and cervix, vulva and vagina in spouses: is there any relationship? An epidemiological study from Norway, 1960-92. *Br J Cancer* 1997, 76:658.

Johnson TM, et al: Squamous cell carcinoma of the skin (excluding lip and oral mucosa). *J Am Acad Dermatol* 1992, 26:467.

Kirsner RS, et al: Squamous cell carcinoma arising in osteomyelitis and chronic wounds: treatment with Mohs' micrographic surgery vs amputation. *Dermatol Surg* 1996, 22:1015.

Kraus S, et al: Intratumoral chemotherapy with fluorouracil/epinephrine injectable gel: a nonsurgical treatment of cutaneous squamous cell carcinoma. *J Am Acad Dermatol* 1998, 38:438.

Kwa RE, et al: Biology of cutaneous squamous cell carcinoma. *J Am Acad Dermatol* 1992, 26:1.

Levine N: Role of retinoids in skin cancer treatment and prevention. *J Am Acad Dermatol* 1998, 39:S62.

Lister RK, et al: Squamous cell carcinoma arising in chronic lymphoedema. *Br J Dermatol* 1997, 136:384.

Mendonca H, et al: Squamous cell carcinoma arising in hidradenitis suppurativa. *J Dermatol Surg Oncol* 1991, 17:830.

Mir LM, et al: Effective treatment of cutaneous and subcutaneous malignant tumours by electrochemotherapy. *Br J Cancer* 1998, 77:2336.

Petter G, et al: Squamous cell carcinoma of the skin: histopathological features and their significance for the clinical outcome. *J Eur Acad Dermatol Venereol* 1998, 11:37.

Rowe DE, et al: Prognostic factors for local recurrence, metastasis, and survival rates in squamous cell carcinoma of the skin, ear, and lip: implications for treatment modality selection. *J Am Acad Dermatol* 1993, 28:281.

Sarani B, et al: Squamous cell carcinoma arising in an unhealed wound in Crohn's disease. *South Med J* 1997, 90:940.

Suchniak JM, et al: High rate of malignant transformation in hyperkeratotic actinic keratoses. *J Am Acad Dermatol* 1997, 37:392.

Takeda H, et al: Multiple squamous cell carcinomas in situ in vitiligo lesions after long-term PUVA therapy. *J Am Acad Dermatol* 1998, 38:268.

Talmi YP, et al: Squamous cell and basal cell cancers directly invading major salivary glands. *Ann Plast Surg* 1991, 26:483. _____ ▲

ACANTHOLYTIC (ADENOID) SQUAMOUS CELL CARCINOMA

Pseudoglandular Squamous Cell Carcinoma

A fast-growing tumor, usually on sun-exposed areas of the face, ears, and backs of the hands, pseudoglandular squamous cell carcinoma may be found in various anatomic sites. The oral cavity and conjunctiva may also be involved. They arise from actinic keratoses and present the same clinical features as squamous cell carcinoma. Histologically, acantholysis is marked and there is often a distinctive adenoid proliferation. Metastasis occurs between 2% and 14% of the time. At times it may be mistaken for metastatic adenocarcinoma or angiosarcoma on histology. Surgical excision is the preferred treatment.

Bernstein SC, et al: The many faces of squamous cell carcinoma. *Dermatol Surg* 1996, 22:243.

Jones AC, et al: Oral adenoid squamous cell carcinoma: a report of three cases and review of the literature. *J Oral Maxillofac Surg* 1993, 51:676.

Mauriello JA Jr, et al: Adenoid squamous carcinoma of the conjunctiva: a clinicopathological study of 14 cases. *Br J Ophthalmol* 1997, 81:1001.

Nappi O, et al: Pseudovascular adenoid squamous cell carcinoma of the skin: a neoplasm that may be mistaken for angiosarcoma. *Am J Surg Pathol* 1992, 16:429.

Van der wal JE, et al: Adenoid cystic carcinoma of the palate with squamous metaplasia or basaloid-squamous carcinoma? *J Oral Patho Med* (Denmark) 1994, 23:461. _____ ▲

VERRUCOUS CARCINOMA (CARCINOMA CUNICULATUM)

First described by Ackerman, verrucous carcinoma is a distinct, well-differentiated variety of squamous cell carcinoma. The term is a collective one, which may include such entities as giant condyloma of Buschke and Lowenstein (Fig. 29-66), epithelioma cuniculatum, and oral florid papillomatosis. Verrucous carcinoma may also be found in the larynx, or on the glans penis, scrotum, vulva, scalp, face, back, nail bed, and sole (Fig. 29-67). The slow-growing and invading lesion may invade the bony structure around the tumor. Human papillomavirus may be involved in the induction of these tumors. Verrucous carcinoma developing from lichen planus has also been described.

Histologically, the lesion shows a characteristic picture of bulbous rete ridges that are topped by an undulating keratinized mass. The squamous epithelium is well differentiated. Pseudoepitheliomatous hyperplasia must also be considered.

Excision is the best treatment, and Mohs' microsurgery may be required in some cases. Radiotherapy may induce anaplastic transformation and should be avoided. Lymph node metastasis is rare, and the prognosis is favorable when complete excision is accomplished. In squamous cell carcinoma of the penis derived from verrucous forms the prognosis is much better than other causes of penile squamous cell carcinoma.

Carrozzo M, et al: An atypical verrucous carcinoma of the tongue arising in a patient with oral lichen planus associated with hepatitis C virus infection. *Oral Oncol* 1997, 33:220.

Castano E, et al: Verrucous carcinoma in association with hypertrophic lichen planus. *Clin Exp Dermatol* 1997, 22:23.

Kanik AB, et al: Penile verrucous carcinoma in a 37-year-old circumcised man. *J Am Acad Dermatol* 1997, 37:329.

Soria JC, et al: Squamous cell carcinoma of the penis: multivariate analysis of prognostic factors and natural history in monocentric study with a conservative policy. *Ann Oncol* 1997, 8:1089.

Van Geertruyden JP, et al: Verrucous carcinoma of the nail bed. *Foot Ankle Int* 1998, 19:327. _____ ▲

BOWEN'S DISEASE

Bowen's disease is an intraepidermal squamous cell carcinoma. It may ultimately become invasive.

Clinical Features

Bowen's disease may be found on any part of the body as an erythematous, slightly scaly and crusted, noninfiltrated

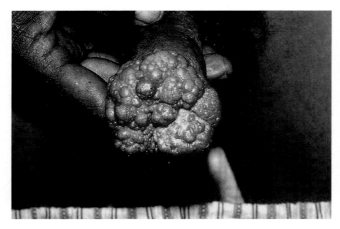

Fig. 29-66 Giant condyloma of Buschke-Lowenstein better termed *verrucous carcinoma of the penis.*

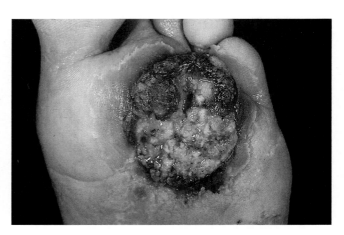

Fig. 29-67 Plantar verrucous carcinoma.

A

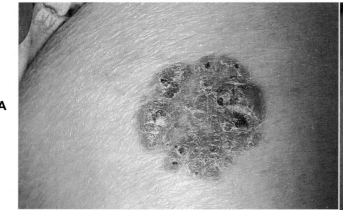

B

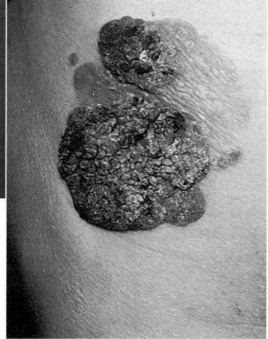

Fig. 29-68 A, Bowen's disease. **B,** Bowen's disease with marked hyperkeratosis. (**A,** Courtesy Dr. Axel W. Hoke. **B,** Courtesy Dr. Detlef K. Goette.)

patch from a few millimeters to many centimeters in diameter (Fig. 29-68). The lesion is sharply defined. The scale is often pronounced, and on its removal the exposed dull resurface may be papillary and moist.

As the lesion slowly enlarges, spontaneous cicatrization may develop in portions of the lesion. When the intra-epithelial growth becomes invasive, it does so by forming a nodular infiltration of the lesion, which becomes ulcerated and fungating. Squamous cell carcinoma is the type usually seen and may complicate Bowen's disease in up to 5% of cases. Sebaceous carcinoma occurring within Bowen's disease has also been reported.

The mucous membranes may be involved. The vulva, vagina, nasal mucosa, conjunctiva, and larynx are the sites of most frequent involvement. When squamous cell carcinoma in situ occurs on the glans penis it is referred to as *erythroplasia of Queyrat* (see p. 840).

Etiology

Bowen's disease affects mostly older white men, in whom the lesions occur primarily on sun-exposed surfaces (Fig. 29-69), and relates directly to the degree of chronic sun damage. Chronic arsenism produces Bowen's disease in non–sun-exposed sites as well as chemically exposed areas

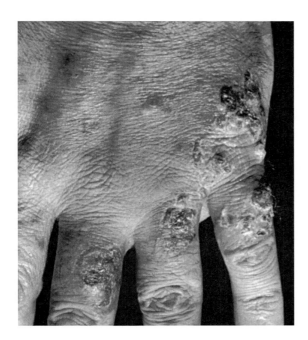

Fig. 29-69 Multiple lesions of Bowen's disease. (Courtesy Dr. Axel W. Hoke.)

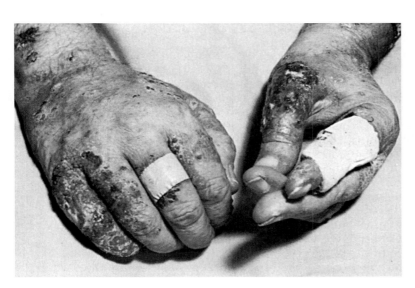

Fig. 29-70 Basal cell carcinomas and multiple Bowen's disease in a man with a history of arsenic ingestion for many years.

(Fig. 29-70). When this is the etiology, internal malignancies may later become manifest. Bowen's disease may develop in lesions of epidermodysplasia verruciformis caused by HPV-5. HPV-16 has been implicated in lesions involving the hands, fingers (Fig. 29-71), and genital regions (Fig. 29-72).

Histopathology

The epidermis shows hyperkeratosis, parakeratosis, acanthosis, and thickening of the rete ridges. The cellular architecture is disorganized, and individually keratinizing cells and atypical cells are seen at all levels of the epidermis. There is, however, a sharp delineation between dermis and epidermis, and the basement membrane is intact. The upper dermis usually shows a chronic inflammatory infiltrate.

Differential Diagnosis

Bowen's disease is frequently misdiagnosed as psoriasis, superficial multicentric basal cell carcinoma, nummular eczema, seborrheic keratosis, and actinic or arsenical dermatosis. Paget's disease, especially the extramammary type, not only clinically but also histologically may mimic Bowen's disease (Fig. 29-73). There is no dyskeratosis in Paget's disease, and the intervening nonvacuolated epidermal cells are not atypical in Paget's disease. Stains for mucin are positive in Paget's disease and negative in Bowen's disease. Bowen's disease may, at times, be heavily pigmented, especially when occurring in the anogenital region, and may resemble melanoma in these cases. Bowenoid papulosis (see Chapter 19) may histologically mimic Bowen's disease; however, its multicentricity and

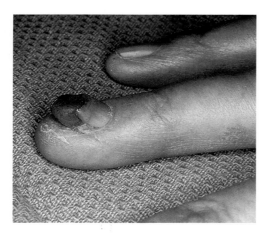

Fig. 29-71 Subungual Bowen's disease. Twenty-five-year history of a wart in the site. (Courtesy Dr. Detlef K. Goette.)

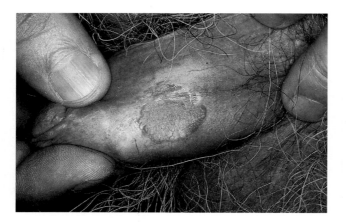

Fig. 29-72 Bowen's disease of the penis.

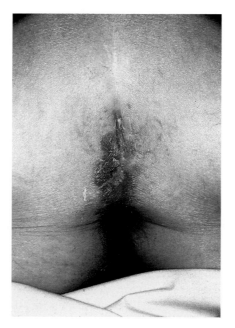

Fig. 29-73 Perianal Bowen's disease.

positive markers for HPV are usually helpful, although positive HPV detection has also been noted in Bowen's disease. When the lesion is in the scalp, it may be confused with seborrheic dermatitis. Tinea circinata must also be considered in diagnosing Bowen's disease.

Treatment

Simple elliptic excision of small lesions is the best treatment option. Fulguration and curettage, electrocautery, cryotherapy, laser ablation, 5-fluorouracil (used as iontophoretic therapy or as a topical ointment with or without occlusion), x-irradiation, photodynamic therapy, and shave excision have been used with variable success. Local recurrence may occur because of extension down the outer root sheaths of hair follicles. Large, ill-defined lesions, or lesions in which preservation of normal tissue is critical are indications for Mohs' microsurgery.

Ball SB, et al: Treatment of cutaneous Bowen's disease with particular emphasis on the problem of lower leg lesions. *Australas J Dermatol* 1998, 39:63.

Biediger TL, et al: Bilateral pigmented Bowen's disease of the lower lip. *Int J Dermatol* 1995, 34:116.

Cox NH, et al: Body site distribution of Bowen's disease. *Br J Dermatol* 1994, 130:714.

Cox NH, et al: Wound healing on the lower leg after radiotherapy or cryotherapy of Bowen's disease and other malignant skin lesions. *Br J Dermatol* 1995, 133:60.

Fitzgerald DA: Cancer precursors. *Semin Cutan Med Surg* 1998, 17:108.

Forslund O, et al: DNA analysis indicates patient-specific human papillomavirus type 16 strains in Bowen's disease on fingers and in archival samples from genital dysplasia. *Br J Dermatol* 1997, 136:678.

Gonzalez-Perez R, et al: Metastatic squamous cell carcinoma arising in Bowen's disease of the palm. *J Am Acad Dermatol* 1997, 36:635.

Holder JE, et al: Amelanotic superficial spreading malignant melanoma mimicking Bowen's disease. *Br J Dermatol* 1996, 134:519.

Jaeger AB, et al: Bowen disease and risk of subsequent malignant neoplasms. *Arch Dermatol* 1999, 135:790.

Murata Y, et al: Partial spontaneous regression of Bowen's disease. *Arch Dermatol* 1996, 132:429.

Reizner GT, et al: Bowen's disease (squamous cell carcinoma in situ) in Kauai, Hawaii: a population-based incidence report. *J Am Acad Dermatol* 1994, 31:596.

Sarveswari KN: Bowen's disease of the palm. *Int J Dermatol* 1998, 37:157.

Stables GI, et al: Large patches of Bowen's disease treated by topical aminolaevulinic acid photodynamic therapy. *Br J Dermatol* 1997, 136:957.

Uezato H, et al: Detection of human papilloma virus type 56 in extragenital Bowen's disease. *Acta Derm Venereol* 1999, 79:311.

Welch ML, et al: 5-fluorouracil iontophoretic therapy for Bowen's disease. *J Am Acad Dermatol* 1997, 36:956. ▲

ERYTHROPLASIA OF QUEYRAT

Queyrat's erythroplasia is histologically Bowen's disease of the glans penis. Clinically, it is characterized by single or multiple well-circumscribed, erythematous, moist, velvety or smooth, red-surfaced plaques on the glans penis of uncircumcised men, usually over age 40 (Fig. 29-74). It resembles Zoon's balanitis clinically.

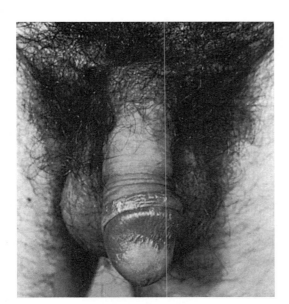

Fig. 29-74 Erythroplasia of Queyrat.

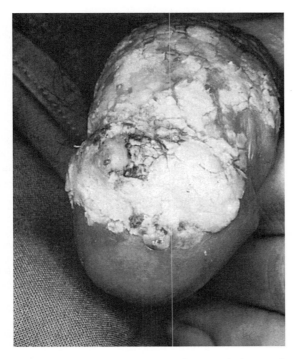

Fig. 29-75 Extensive erythroplasia of Queyrat of glans penis and prepuce with eventuation into squamous cell carcinoma.

Malignant transformation is more common than in Bowen's disease, and the resulting squamous cell carcinomas are more aggressive and tend to metastasize earlier than those that develop in Bowen's disease (Fig. 29-75). There is no evidence of an increase in internal malignancy in patients with erythroplasia. Conservative excision or, preferably topical 5-fluorouracil, is the recommended treatment. This is effective because of the absence of follicles on the glans. The CO_2 laser is another option.

Greenbaum SS, et al: Carbon dioxide laser treatment of erythroplasia of Queyrat. *J Dermatol Surg Oncol* 1989, 16:490.
Grossman HB: Premalignant and early carcinomas of the penis and scrotum. *Urol Clin North Am* 1992, 19:221. _____ ▲

BALANITIS PLASMACELLULARIS (ZOON)

Balanitis plasmacellularis is also known as *benign plasma cell erythroplasia* and *balanoposthitis chronica circumscripta plasmacellularis*. It is a benign inflammatory lesion with a plasma cell infiltrate. Clinically, it is characterized by a persistent inflammation, which is usually sharply demarcated and usually on the inner surface of the prepuce and the glans penis (Fig. 29-76). The lesion is erythematous, moist, and shiny. It occurs as a single lesion, but it may consist of several confluent macules. It is asymptomatic and does not produce inguinal adenopathy. Uncircumcised men from ages 24 to 85 are most often affected.

Vulvitis chronica plasmacellularis is the counterpart of balanitis in women. The vulva shows a striking lacquer-like luster. Erosions, punctate hemorrhage, synechiae, and a slate-to-ochre pigmentation may supervene.

Plasmacytosis circumorificialis is the same disease on the oral mucosa, lips, cheeks, and tongue, clinically suggestive of squamous cell carcinoma.

Histologically, the epidermis is atrophic with no other changes. In the papillary dermis a band of infiltrate consisting almost exclusively of plasma cells is present. Dilated vessels are also seen. This picture is strikingly different from that of the main clinical differential diagnosis, erythroplasia of Queyrat, in which the epidermis is principally involved, with individual cell keratinization in the thickened prickle cell layer. HPV has not been detected. Topical steroids are helpful and may even be curative. The CO_2 laser and circumcision have also provided treatment successes.

Baldwin HE, et al: The treatment of Zoon's balanitis with the carbon dioxide laser. *J Dermatol Surg Oncol* 1989, 15:491.
Ferrandiz C, et al: Zoon's balanitis treated with circumcision. *J Dermatol Surg Oncol* 1984, 10:622.
Gerbig AW: Griseofulvin ineffective in balanitis circumscripta plasmacellularis. *J Am Acad Dermatol* 1995, 33:319.
Kiene P, et al: No evidence of human papillomavirus infection in balanitis circumscripta plasmacellularis Zoon. *Acta Derm Venereol* 1995, 75:496.
McCreedy CA, et al: Vulvar erythema: vulvitis chronica plasmacellularis (Zoon's vulvitis). *Arch Dermatol* 1990, 126:1352.
Salopek TG, et al: Vulvitis circumscripta plasmacellularis (Zoon's vulvitis) associated with autoimmune polyglandular endocrine failure. *Br J Dermatol* 1996, 135:991.
Tamaki K, et al: Treatment of plasma cell cheilitis with griseofulvin. *J Am Acad Dermatol* 1994, 30:789. _____ ▲

PSEUDOEPITHELIOMATOUS KERATOTIC AND MICACEOUS BALANITIS

Pseudoepitheliomatous keratotic and micaceous balanitis was described by Lortat-Jacob and Civatte in 1966. The lesions occurring on the glans penis are verrucous excres-

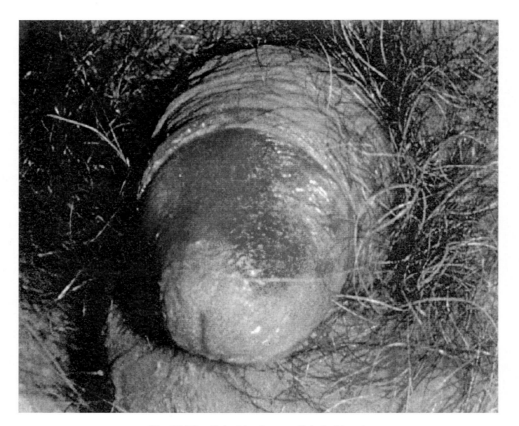

Fig. 29-76 Balanitis plasmacellularis (Zoon).

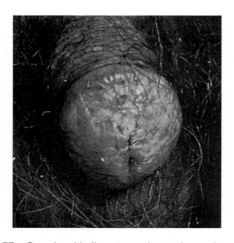

Fig. 29-77 Pseudoepitheliomatous keratotic and micaceous balanitis.

cences with scaling. Ulcerations, cracking, and fissuring on the surface of the glans frequently are present (Fig. 29-77). The keratotic scaling is usually micaceous and resembles psoriasis. Most patients are over age 50 and frequently have been circumcised for phimosis in adult life.

Histologically, there is marked hyperkeratosis and parakeratosis as well as pseudoepitheliomatous hyperplasia. Acanthotic masses give rise to a craterlike configuration.

Many believe it is a form of verrucous carcinoma. Treatment may require removal by Mohs' microsurgery, although treatment success has also been obtained with topical 5-fluorouracil. If topical chemotherapy is utilized, posttreatment biopsies are recommended.

Bargman H: Pseudoepitheliomatous, keratotic, and micaceous balanitis. *Cutis* 1985, 35:77.

Beljaards RC, et al: Is pseudoepitheliomatous, micaceous and keratotic balanitis synonymous with verrucous carcinoma? *Br J Dermatol* 1987, 117:641.

Ganem JP, et al: Pseudo-epitheliomatous keratotic and micaceous balanitis. *J Urol* 1999, 161:217.

Jenkins D Jr, et al: Pseudoepitheliomatous, keratotic, micaceous balanitis. *J Am Acad Dermatol* 1988, 18:419.

Krunic AL, et al: Pseudoepitheliomatous, keratotic and micaceous balanitis. *Urol Int* 1996, 56:125. ▲

PAGET'S DISEASE OF THE NIPPLE

Clinical Features

Paget's disease of the nipple is characterized by a unilateral sharply defined eczema caused by epidermal metastases from underlying ductal adenocarcinoma of the breast. The disease begins as an erythematous crusted or keratotic, circumscribed, pruritic patch (Fig. 29-78). It may simulate unilateral eczematous neurodermatitis. In the course of

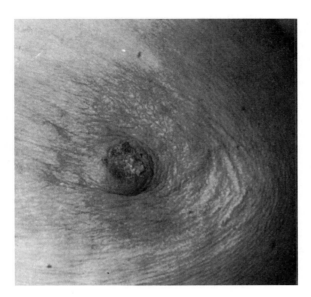

Fig. 29-78 Paget's disease still confined to the nipple.

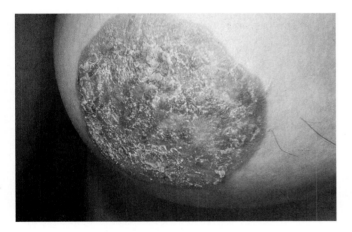

Fig. 29-79 Paget's disease of the breast of several years' duration.

months or years it may become infiltrated and ulcerated (Fig. 29-79). The nipple may or may not be retracted. The disease is less common, and carries a worse prognosis, in men than in women.

Histopathology

Paget's disease is characterized by the presence of Paget cells: large, round, clear-staining cells with large nuclei. Intercellular bridges are absent. The cells appear singly or in small nests between the squamous cells. Frequent mitoses are present. Acanthosis is usually present, the granular layer is preserved, and usually there is no parakeratosis. Frequently a layer of basal cells separates the Paget cells from the dermis; this is not seen in melanoma. In the dermis an inflammatory reaction is often present.

The Paget cell may take a periodic acid-Schiff stain even after diastase treatment, unlike the dyskeratotic cells in Bowen's disease. Immunoperoxidase stains may also be helpful. Carcinoembryonic antigen (CEA) and apocrine epithelial antigen are often positive.

Diagnosis

The presence of unilateral eczema of the nipple recalcitrant to simple treatment is indicative of Paget's disease, and the lesion should be biopsied. The presence of bilateral lesions suggests neurodermatitis, atopic dermatitis, or nummular eczema. The biopsy should be through the nipple with the removal of a liberal portion of the region involved. Unless an adequate specimen is obtained, small nests of Paget cells may be overlooked.

Papillary adenoma of the nipple clinically resembles Paget's disease, but on biopsy shows a papillary and adenomatous growth in the dermis with connection to the surface. There is a lining of apocrine type secretory epithelium. Hyperkeratosis of the nipple and areola may occasionally be unilateral, but histologically reveals only hyperkeratosis, acanthosis, and papillomatosis. Clear cell papulosis of the skin presents with scattered, white, flat-topped lesions distributed along the milk line in Taiwanese children (six cases reported). Histologic examination reveals benign pagetoid clear cells in the basal layer. The clear cells are antikeratin AE1 positive, which appears to be the best marker for this disorder.

Treatment

Surgical excision with margins and radiotherapy have been shown efficacious in treating Paget's disease of the nipple. Mastectomy may be required.

EXTRAMAMMARY PAGET'S DISEASE

The lesions of extramammary Paget's disease are similar to those of the nipple lesions, but may go undiagnosed longer and thus become more extensive. A nonhealing banal eczematous patch may persist in the anogenital or axillary region for several years before it causes concern (Fig. 29-80). Usually a single lesion occurs and is mistaken for a fungal infection, especially in the inguinal region. Intense pruritus is common, and sometimes pain may also be present. Bleeding is a late sign. Lesions may simulate lichen simplex chronicus or leukoplakia. If the primary lesions are associated with a reddish discoloration with edematous infiltration, then lymphatic infiltration by cancer cells is suggested. This underpants-pattern erythema begins in the inguinal area and extends centrifugally. All patients studied by Murata et al with this sign died of the disease within 13 months.

Extramammary Paget's disease is frequently associated with an underlying glandular adnexal carcinoma or a regional internal carcinoma with or without metastasis. The most common site is the vulva, followed by the perianal area, penis, scrotum, and groin in decreasing frequency.

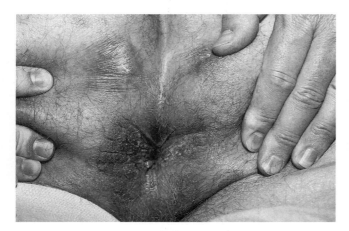

Fig. 29-80 Extramammary Paget's disease of the perianal area. (Courtesy Dr. Nicholas Lapins.)

Allan SJ, et al: Paget's disease of the scrotum: a case exhibiting positive prostate-specific antigen staining and associated prostatic adenocarcinoma. *Br J Dermatol* 1998, 138:689.

Becker-Wegerich PM, et al: Carbon dioxide laser treatment of extramammary Paget's disease guided by photodynamic diagnosis. *Br J Dermatol* 1998, 138:169.

Ho TC, et al: Pigmented Paget's disease of the male breast. *J Am Acad Dermatol* 1990, 23:338.

Koh KB, et al: Paget's disease of the scrotum: report of a case with underlying carcinoma of the prostate. *Br J Dermatol* 1995, 133:306.

Kollmorgen DR, et al: Paget's disease of the breast: a 33-year experience. *J Am Coll Surg* 1998, 187:171.

Kurzl RG: Paget's disease. *Semin Dermatol* 1996, 15:60.

Lee JY, et al: Clear cell papulosis of the skin. *Br J Dermatol* 1998, 138:678.

Miller L, et al: Erosive adenomatosis of the nipple: a benign imitator of malignant breast disease. *Cutis* 1997, 59:91.

Montemarano AD, et al: Superficial papillary adenomatosis of the nipple: a case report and review of the literature. *J Am Acad Dermatol* 1997, 36:871.

Murata Y, et al: Underpants-pattern erythema. *J Am Acad Dermatol* 1999, 40:949.

Ohno H, et al: Two cases of unilateral axillary Paget's disease. *J Dermatol* 1998, 25:260.

Pierce LJ, et al: The conservative management of Paget's disease of the breast with radiotherapy. *Cancer* 1997, 80:1065.

Takeuchi T, et al: Paget's disease arising near a male areola without an underlying carcinoma. *J Dermatol* 1999, 26:248.

Ward KA, et al: Dermatologic diseases of the breast in young women. *Clin Dermatol* 1997, 15:45.

Yugueros P, et al: Paget's disease of the groin: report of seven cases. *Plast Reconstr Surg* 1997, 100:336. ▲

About a quarter of patients will have an underlying cutaneous adnexal adenocarcinoma with a 46% mortality rate. A reported 12% to 50% will have an underlying internal malignancy within close proximity of the cutaneous Paget's. Prostate cancer and rectal, renal cell, cervical, and transitional cell carcinoma are just a few examples.

Histologically, the findings are similar to those found in the nipple: hyperkeratosis, parakeratosis, acanthosis, and the pale, vacuolated Paget's cells in rete ridges. Sialomucin, diastase-resistant, is observed on periodic acid-Schiff stains. In extramammary Paget's disease associated with prostate cancer, the intraepidermal tumor cells may express prostate-specific antigen.

In the anal, perianal, and perineal areas extramammary Paget's disease should be differentiated from other premalignancies and malignancies, such as squamous cell carcinoma, basal cell carcinoma, perianal Bowen's disease, cloacogenic carcinoma, and anorectal melanoma. It is also mistaken for chronic fungal infections, chronic irritant or contact dermatitis, lichen simplex chronicus, and inverse psoriasis. Histologically, it must be differentiated from Bowen's disease and superficial spreading or pagetoid malignant melanoma.

Surgical removal is the treatment of choice, which may require Mohs' microsurgery. The preoperative use of 5-fluorouracil topically may help delineate the tumor margins. Despite what appears to be adequate margins, recurrence rates are high because of the poor correlation between clinically evident disease compared with histologic findings, and the multifocal nature of extramammary Paget's disease. Serum CEA levels may be useful for monitoring the disease response and providing some determination of prognosis. In widespread disease that may preclude complete surgical removal, use of a CO_2 laser guided by photodynamic diagnosis has been used successfully in one elderly patient.

Trabecular Carcinoma (Merkel Cell Carcinoma)

This malignant tumor was first described by Toker in 1972. The cell of origin is thought to be a pluripotential cell that may differentiate in a neuroendocrine direction, as evidenced by the typical membrane-bound neurosecretory granules seen within the neoplastic cells by electron microscopy.

Clinically, it presents as a rapidly growing nodule on sun-exposed skin, most commonly in elderly patients. The mean age of onset is 68 years, women outnumber men, and the primary sites of involvement are the head and neck (44%), leg (28%), arm (16%), and buttock (9%). Unusual areas, such as the scrotum and vulva, may be involved. The rate of local recurrence is 26% to 44%, regional nodal metastases is 53%, distant metastases occur in 75%, and death resulting from tumor (5-year survival rates) ranges between 30% to 64%. The prognosis is worse than malignant melanoma.

Histologically, the tumor is composed of uniform round cells, with the cells being arranged in sheets. The main differential diagnosis is oat cell carcinoma metastatic to skin. Electron microscopy on properly fixed specimens reveals the granules typical of Merkel cells. These are not seen in formalin-fixed tissue; however, characteristic paranuclear whorls of intermediate filaments remain. Immunohistochemically, neuron-specific enolase may be positive, but the most discriminating marker is the antikeratin antibody, which stains the cells in a paranuclear inclusion-bodylike aggregate. The keratin has been shown to be of the simple epithelial type.

Complete surgical ablation is the treatment of choice, with Mohs' microsurgery as the preferred method because of the aggressiveness of this malignancy. Some recommend wide local excision with 3-cm margins. Both radiation therapy and chemotherapy are effective in palliating unresectable disease and may be curative in select cases. Intralesional tumor necrosis factor has also been shown effective. Of interest are the reports of spontaneous regression that have been documented in some patients, a feature that should not alter selection of treatment options.

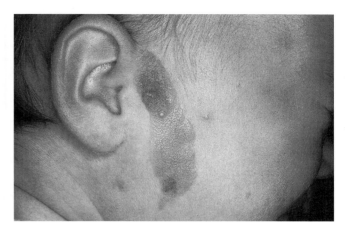

Fig. 29-81 Nevus sebaceus.

Al-Ghazal SK, et al: Merkel cell carcinoma of the skin. *Br J Plast Surg* 1996, 49:491.

Best TJ, et al: Merkel cell carcinoma of the scrotum. *Ann Plast Surg* 1994, 33:83.

Chen KT: Merkel's cell (neuroendocrine) carcinoma of the vulva. *Cancer* 1994, 73:2186.

Fenig E, et al: The role of radiation therapy and chemotherapy in the treatment of Merkel cell carcinoma. *Cancer* 1997, 80:881.

Ferrau F, et al: Merkel cell carcinoma of the scalp: dramatic resolution with primary chemotherapy. *J Am Acad Dermatol* 1994, 31:271.

Haag ML, et al: Merkel cell carcinoma: diagnosis and treatment. *Dermatol Surg* 1995, 21:669.

Hata Y, et al: Two cases of Merkel cell carcinoma cured by intratumor injection of natural human tumor necrosis factor. *Plast Reconstr Surg* 1997, 99:547.

House NS, et al: Malignant melanoma with clinical and histologic features of Merkel cell carcinoma. *J Am Acad Dermatol* 1994, 31:839.

O'Connor WJ, et al: Merkel cell carcinoma. *Dermatol Surg* 1996, 22:262.

Ohnishi Y, et al: Merkel cell carcinoma and multiple Bowen's disease: incidental association or possible relationship to inorganic arsenic exposure? *J Dermatol* 1997, 24:310.

Urbatsch A, et al: Merkel cell carcinoma occurring in renal transplant patients. *J Am Acad Dermatol* 1999, 41:289.

Yanguas I, et al: Spontaneous regression of Merkel cell carcinoma of the skin. *Br J Dermatol* 1997, 137:296. _____ ▲

SEBACEOUS NEVI AND TUMORS
Nevus Sebaceus (Organoid Nevus)

Nevus sebaceus of Jadassohn is a sharply circumscribed, yellow-orange, verrucous hamartoma varying from a few millimeters to several centimeters in diameter (Fig. 29-81). The solitary lesion is present at birth, most frequently near the vertex of the scalp but also commonly on the face or neck and may be linear. The lesions persist throughout life and are usually alopecic. In adulthood the nevus becomes more verrucous. Basal cell carcinoma may develop in approximately 5% to 10% of the lesions. A syringocystadenoma papilliferum has been found in approximately 10% of lesions also. Other tumors occurring more rarely are solid hidradenoma, sebaceous epithelioma, apocrine cystadenoma, apocrine carcinoma, eccrine porocarcinoma (metastatic), ductal sweat gland carcinoma, squamous cell carcinoma, spiradenoma, and keratoacanthoma. Deletions

of the *patched* gene have been identified in nevus sebaceus and may be responsible for the predisposition to the development of basal cell carcinomas and other tumors in this lesion.

Nevus sebaceus lesions, especially when large, may be associated with multiple internal abnormalities, similar to those reported in the linear epidermal nevus syndrome. Associated problems have included intracranial masses, seizures, mental retardation, skeletal abnormalities, pigmentary changes, ocular lesions, and hamartomas of the kidney. Mediastinal lipomatosis has also been reported.

Histologically, papillomatosis is present with hypergranulosis and hyperkeratosis. The hair follicles may range in their development from completely undifferentiated cells of the embryonic type, to just small hair shafts, to normal hair follicles. The sebaceous glands in the early lesions occur as immature lobules with incompletely formed hair follicles. In older lesions, well-developed sebaceous glands may be seen. Apocrine glands are common in the lesions of the adult. The dermis is thickened, with increased vascularity and fibrous connective tissue.

Because malignant changes may occur, the treatment of choice is to remove these nevi early by excision. Carbon dioxide lasers have been used to treat a patient with involvement of the nose; however, the long-term risk of developing malignant transformation remains high because of the deep involvement often observed with nevus sebaceus. Tissue expanders may be required for large lesions.

Ashinoff R: Linear nevus sebaceus of Jadassohn treated with the carbon dioxide laser. *Pediatr Dermatol* 1993, 10:189.

Chun K, et al: Nevus sebaceus: clinical outcome and considerations for prophylactic excision. *Int J Dermatol* 1995, 34:538.

Frodel JL Jr, et al: Primary reconstruction of congenital facial lesion defects with tissue expansion. *J Dermatol Surg Oncol* 1993, 19:1110.

Itin PH, et al: *Molluscum contagiosum* mimicking sebaceous nevus of Jadassohn, ecthyma and giant condylomata acuminata in HIV-infected patients. *Dermatology* (Switzerland) 1994, 189:396.

Jacyk WK, et al: Tubular apocrine carcinoma arising in a nevus sebaceus of Jadassohn. *Am J Dermatopathol* 1998, 20:389.

Kucukoduk S, et al: A new neurocutaneous syndrome: nevus sebaceus syndrome. *Cutis* 1993, 51:437.

Palazzi P, et al: Linear sebaceous nevus syndrome: report of a patient with unusual associated abnormalities. *Pediatr Dermatol* 1996, 13:22.

Shapiro M, et al: Spiradenoma arising in a nevus sebaceus of Jadassohn: case report and literature review. *Am J Dermatopathol* 1999, 21:462.

Snow JL, et al: Sudden nodular growth in a congenital facial lesion: squamous cell carcinoma arising in a nevus sebaceus Jadassohn (NSJ). *Arch Dermatol* 1995, 131:1069.

Taboada E, et al: Sebaceus naevus of Jadassohn and primary mediastinal lipomatosis. *Br J Plast Surg* (Scotland) 1993, 46:264.

Waltz KM, et al: The spectrum of epidermal nevi: a case of verrucous epidermal nevus contiguous with nevus sebaceus. *Pediatr Dermatol* 1999, 16:211.

Weng CJ, et al: Jadassohn's nevus sebaceus of the head and face. *Ann Plast Surg* 1990, 25:100.

Xin H, et al: The sebaceous nevus: a nevus with deletions of the PTCH gene. *Cancer Res* 1999, 59:1834. _____ ▲

Sebaceous Hyperplasia

Also known as *senile sebaceous hyperplasia* and *senile sebaceous adenoma,* these common lesions are scattered irregularly over the face, having a predilection for the forehead, infraorbital regions, and temples. The lesions are small, cream-colored or yellowish umbilicated papules 2 to 6 mm in diameter. The age at onset is usually past 40 although it has also been reported in children. Unusual sites may be affected, such as the areolas, nipples, neck, and penis. Histologically, the sebaceous glands are hypertrophied, with normal-appearing acini. The glands are multilobulated, each dividing into other lobules to produce a cluster resembling a bunch of grapes. Clinically, they may mimic an early basal cell carcinoma.

Premature sebaceous hyperplasia, also known as *familial presenile sebaceous hyperplasia*, presents with extensive sebaceous hyperplasia with onset at puberty and worsening with age. Familial patterns have been reported, inherited in an autosomal dominant fashion. It involves the face, neck, and upper thorax but spares the periorificial regions. It must be differentiated from rosacea, multiple sebaceous adenomas, trichoepitheliomas, and angiofibromas.

Treatment is mostly for cosmetic purposes. Electrodesiccation or an extremely fine fulgurating spark will remove these with good results, though curettage or a shallow shave biopsy may be desirable if there is the least doubt about the diagnosis. Isotretinoin (Accutane) has been used successfully; however, recurrence is common. Lasers are also effective.

Belinchon I, et al: Areolar sebaceous hyperplasia. *Cutis* 1996, 58:63.

Boonchai W, et al: Familial presenile sebaceous gland hyperplasia. *J Am Acad Dermatol* 1997, 36:120.

Grimalt R, et al: Premature familial sebaceous hyperplasia: successful response to oral isotretinoin in three patients. *J Am Acad Dermatol* 1997, 37:996.

Kumar A, et al: Band-like sebaceous hyperplasia over the penis. *Australas J Dermatol* 1999, 40:47.

Schonermark MP, et al: Treatment of sebaceous gland hyperplasia with the pulsed dye laser. *Lasers Surg Med* 1997, 21:313.

Sehgal VN, et al: Sebaceous hyperplasia in youngsters. *J Dermatol* 1999, 26:619. _____ ▲

Sebaceous Epithelioma

Clinically, sebaceous epitheliomas have the same morphologic characteristics as basal cell carcinomas. They appear as yellow or orange papules, nodules, or plaques, usually on the scalp, face, and neck. They may be associated with Muir-Torre syndrome, discussed on the facing page.

Histologically, the tumor consists of neat oval nests of irregularly shaped basaloid cells with differentiation toward sebaceous cells. Also there may be cystic spaces containing vacuolated amorphous hyaline-like material.

Dinneen AM, et al: Sebaceous epithelioma: a review of twenty-one cases. *J Am Acad Dermatol* 1996, 34:47.

Watanabe R, et al: Sebaceous epithelioma. *J Dermatol* 1994, 21:35. ▲

Sebaceous Gland Carcinoma

This rare carcinoma may arise on the eyelids from the meibomian or Zeis glands. It usually appears in the tarsal region of the upper eyelids (75%). The scalp, other areas of the face, and the trunk are the next most common areas involved. Sebaceous carcinoma can occur in any site that contains sebaceous glands. Rarely, it has been reported to involve the external genitalia, external auditory canal, sole, dorsum of the hands and feet, laryngeal/pharyngeal cavities, and the oral mucosa. Fatal metastatic disease occurs in 20% to 30% of eyelid cases, whereas this result is rare when the sebaceous carcinoma originates in other sites. It may also be seen in Muir-Torre syndrome (see facing page).

Histologically, the lobules contain sebaceous cells and many undifferentiated cells, with numerous mitotic figures. The cells vary greatly in size and shape. They are eosinophilic, and the nuclei are also lighter than those of the sebaceous epithelioma.

Treatment is by wedge resection of the tumor on the eyelid. Mohs' microsurgery is preferable and has been reported successful.

Damm DD, et al: Intraoral sebaceous carcinoma. *Oral Surg Oral Med Oral Pathol* 1991, 72:709.

Nelson BR, et al: Sebaceous carcinoma. *J Am Acad Dermatol* 1995, 33:1. ▲

Sebaceous Adenoma

Sebaceous adenoma is usually a solitary, skin-colored or yellowish papule or nodule of the head or neck, most often occurring in men over age 50 or 60. It may be seen in Muir-Torre syndrome. Microscopically, it is a sharply demarcated tumor in the upper dermis consisting of incompletely differentiated sebaceous lobules. Excision is curative.

Pehoushek JF, et al: Solitary facial lesion: sebaceous adenoma in association with Muir-Torre syndrome (MTS). *Arch Dermatol* 1997, 133:98. _____ ▲

Muir-Torre Syndrome

Sebaceous tumors of the skin of any sort at an early age or in large numbers were first reported by Muir in 1967 and Torre in 1968 to be associated with the development of low-grade internal malignancy, a combination that has been called the *Muir-Torre syndrome*. The internal tumors often occur a decade or two before the cutaneous lesions.

Most often colonic adenocarcinoma, but also neoplasms of the uterus, ovary, and kidney, may occur. The cutaneous lesions may be sebaceous adenomas, sebaceous carcinomas, sebaceous epitheliomas, keratoacanthomas, or basal cell carcinomas with sebaceous differentiation. The visceral tumors are usually not aggressive. At times the cutaneous lesions may precede or accompany the internal malignancies; therefore, screening of patients with the uncommon sebaceous neoplasms with a thorough history and physical, follow-up investigations of all abnormalities identified, and a colonoscopy and first morning urine for cytology are recommended. In some families genetic linkage to a locus on chromosome 2p has been identified. Although the molecular basis is likely heterogeneous, most patients have a germline mutation in the hMSH2 mismatch repair gene.

Exacerbation of the syndrome occurs with immunosuppression. Surgical excision of cutaneous lesions is recommended. Grossly involved lymph nodes should also be excised. Patients have responded well to 40 mg of isotretinoin a day, and may continue to experience good results with doses as low as 10 mg a day. Patients with this syndrome should have regular examinations for gastrointestinal and genitourinary cancer, including annual colonoscopy beginning at age 25 and first morning urine for cytology. Asymptomatic relatives should also be counseled and evaluated.

Akhtar S, et al: Muir-Torre syndrome: case report of a patient with concurrent jejunal and ureteral cancer and a review of the literature. *J Am Acad Dermatol* 1999, 41:681.

Cohen PR, et al: Muir-Torre syndrome. *Dermatol Clin* 1995, 13:79.

Davis DA, et al: Genitourinary tumors in men with the Muir-Torre syndrome. *J Am Acad Dermatol* 1995, 33:909.

Lynch HT, et al: Colorectal cancer and the Muir-Torre syndrome in a gypsy family: a review. *Am J Gastroenterol* 1999, 94:575.

Lynch HT, et al: The Muir-Torre syndrome in kindreds with hereditary nonpolyposis colorectal cancer (Lynch syndrome): a classic obligation in preventive medicine. *J Am Acad Dermatol* 1999, 41:797.

Rodenas JM, et al: Muir-Torre syndrome associated with a family history of hyperlipidemia. *J Am Acad Dermatol* 1993, 28:285.

Schwartz RA, et al: The Muir-Torre syndrome: a 25-year retrospect. *J Am Acad Dermatol* 1996, 35:493. _____ ▲

ECCRINE NEVI AND TUMORS
Syringoma

In syringoma small, translucent papules develop—yellowish, brownish, or pinkish; globoid; 1 to 3 mm in diameter; discrete and closely set—most frequently, and often exclusively, on the eyelids and upper cheeks (Figs. 29-82 and 29-83). They are disproportionately common, in these sites, in Japanese women. Other sites of involvement include the axilla, abdomen, forehead, penis, and vulva, and rarely they may be found in unilateral or linear groupings. Symmetrical distal extremity involvement has also been reported. Familial patterns may occur. They develop slowly and persist indefinitely without symptoms. Syringomas occur in 18% of adults with Down syndrome, particularly females. This is approximately 30 times the frequency seen in patients with other mental disabilities.

Microscopically, the syringoma is characterized by dilated cystic sweat ducts, some of which have small commalike tails to produce a distinctive picture, resembling tadpoles. Strands of epithelial cells may occur independently of the ducts. Usually, two rows of epithelial cells line

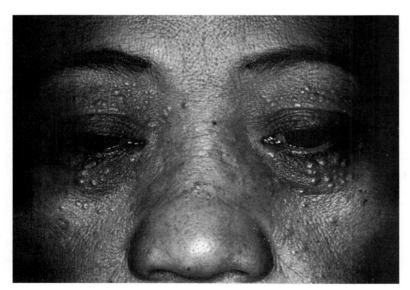

Fig. 29-82 Syringomas.

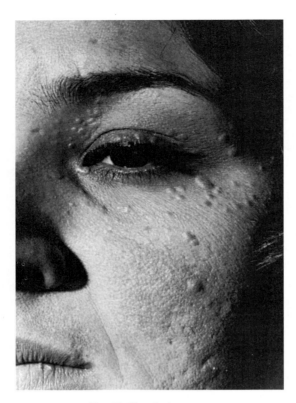

Fig. 29-83 Syringomas.

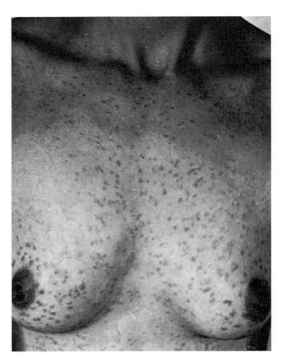

Fig. 29-84 Generalized syringomas. (Courtesy Dr. S.F. Rosen.)

the duct walls. Histochemical studies have shown that syringomas contain phosphorylase and hydrolytic enzymes typical of eccrine origin. They probably represent adenomas of intradermal eccrine ducts.

Treatment may be desirable because of the unsightly appearance. Electrodesiccation of each individual lesion, laser ablation, or cryotherapy with liquid nitrogen to each tumor are three methods that may help. However, destruction to the depth necessary to eliminate the tumor risks significant scarring.

Clear Cell Syringoma

This variant of syringoma is frequently associated with diabetes mellitus. Clinically, the lesions are identical to syringoma. There is no difference in age, sex, or distribution. The only difference between the two disorders, besides the histology, is the association of clear-cell syringomas with diabetes mellitus. Only a single case out of an estimated 60 cases in the literature did not have diabetes. Eruptive disease has been reported.

Nests of ordinary syringoma are commingled with nests of cells with clear ground-glass–like material surrounding a small, dark, oval nucleus. Immunohistochemical analysis of keratin expression has shown that it is a metabolic variant of conventional syringoma.

Eruptive Syringoma

First described by Darier, eruptive syringomas are histologically identical to syringoma of the eyelid but occur in an eruptive form of numerous lesions on the neck, chest, axillae, upper arms, and periumbilically, usually in young persons (Fig. 29-84). Generalized forms have been reported. The shiny, faintly rose-colored papules closely resemble lichen planus and secondary syphilid. This variant has been reported in Down syndrome, as a familial trait, and to have occurred in a diabetic woman with the clear-cell histology. Clinically, it may be confused with reticulated papillomatosis of Gougerot-Carteaud.

Other Variants

Many individual case reports exist of unusual clinical variants of syringomas. These include types limited to the scalp, causing alopecia; a unilateral linear or nevoid distribution; those limited to the vulva or penis; those limited to the distal extremities; and the lichen planus–like and milia-like morphologic types.

Akaraphanth R, et al: Eruptive syringoma in a Chinese boy. *Int J Dermatol* 1993, 32:202.

Azon-Masoliver A, et al: Multiple erythematous papules in both axillae: syringomas. *Arch Dermatol* 1993, 129:1609.

Biolcati G, et al: Eruptive syringoma. *J Am Acad Dermatol* 1993, 28:800.

Chi HI: A case of unusual syringoma: unilateral linear distribution and plaque formation. *J Dermatol* 1996, 23:505.

Di Lernia V, et al: Localized vulvar syringomas. *Pediatr Dermatol* 1996, 13:80.

Friedman S, et al: Syringoma presenting as milia. *J Am Acad Dermatol* 1987, 16:310.

Garcia C, et al: Multiple acral syringomata with uniform involvement of the hands and feet. *Cutis* 1997, 59:213.

Gomez MI, et al: Eruptive syringoma: treatment with topical tretinoin. *Dermatology* (Switzerland) 1994, 189:105.

Karam P, et al: Intralesional electrodesiccation of syringomas. *Dermatol Surg* 1998, 24:692.

Karam P, et al: Syringomas: new approach to an old technique. *Int J Dermatol* 1996, 35:219.

Kim SJ, et al: Unusual cases of syringoma of the forehead. *J Dermatol* 1996, 23:61.

Kudo H, et al: Generalized eruptive clear-cell syringoma. *Arch Dermatol* 1989, 125:1716.

Lee AY, et al: Generalized eruptive syringoma. *J Am Acad Dermatol* 1991, 25:570.

Lee MW, et al: Syringoma resembling confluent and reticulated papillomatosis of Gougerot-Carteaud. *Cutis* 1998, 61:227.

Ohnishi T, et al: Immunohistochemical analysis of keratin expression in clear cell syringoma: a comparative study with conventional syringoma. *J Cutan Pathol* 1997, 24:370.

Rongioletti F, et al: Unilateral multiple plaque-like syringomas. *Br J Dermatol* 1996, 135:623.

Saitoh A, et al: Clear cells of eccrine glands in a patient with clear cell syringoma associated with diabetes mellitus. *Am J Dermatopathol* 1993, 15:166.

Schepis C, et al: Palpebral syringomas and Down's syndrome. *Dermatology* (Switzerland) 1994, 189:248.

Sola Casas MA, et al: Syringomas localized to the penis (case report). *Clin Exp Dermatol* 1993, 18:384.

Trager JD, et al: Neck and vulvar papules in an 8-year-old girl. *Arch Dermatol* 1999, 135:203.

Weiss E, et al: Eruptive syringomas associated with milia. *Int J Dermatol* 1995, 34:193. _____ ▲

Eccrine Hidrocystomas

Eccrine hidrocystomas are 1- to 3-mm translucent papules that occasionally have a bluish tint (Fig. 29-85). They usually are solitary, occur on the face, and are more common in women. In some patients, multiple lesions may be present and they may be pigmented. They may become more prominent during hot weather. Microscopically, a single cystic cavity lined by two layers of small cuboidal epithelial cells is present. Treatment, if desired, is by excision for solitary lesions. Topical atropine ointment 1% or scopolamine, 0.01% (1.2 ml of 0.25% scopolamine eyedrops in 30 g of Eucerin) once daily, have been used with variable success. There may be systemic symptoms with the use of topical atropine.

Bourke JF, et al: Multiple pigmented eccrine hidrocystomas. *J Am Acad Dermatol* 1996, 35:480.

Clever HW, et al: Multiple eccrine hidrocystomas: a nonsurgical treatment. *Arch Dermatol* 1991, 127:422.

De Eusebio E, et al: Multiple hidrocystomas. *Dermatology* (Switzerland) 1996, 193:152.

Masri-Fridling GD, et al: Eccrine hidrocystomas. *J Am Acad Dermatol* 1992, 26:780. _____ ▲

Eccrine Poroma

Eccrine poroma is a benign, slow-growing, slightly protruding, sessile, soft, reddish tumor that may occur anywhere but most often on the sole or side of the foot (Figs. 29-86

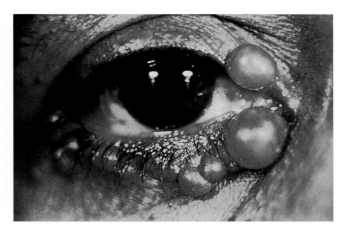

Fig. 29-85 Eccrine hidrocystomas. (Courtesy Dr. Michael Milligan.)

and 29-87). The 2- to 12-mm lesion will bleed on slight trauma. A striking finding is the frequent cup-shaped shallow depression from which the tumor grows and protrudes. It also may occur on the palms. Although the lesion tends to occur singly, multiple lesions may also occur. The lesions may recur. A rare variant is called *eccrine poromatosis*, in which more than 100 lesions may involve the palms and soles, and may be associated with hidrotic ectodermal dysplasia.

Histologically, solid masses of uniform, very small, basophilic epithelial cells are seen, with intercellular bridging. These cells tend to arrange themselves around cleftlike lumina with formation of a cuticle. Vascular dilation and hyperplasia of the capillaries may be present. Glycogen in the tumor cells may be demonstrable with periodic acid-Schiff stain.

The clinical differential diagnosis is from porocarcinoma, granuloma pyogenicum, melanoma (amelanotic and melanotic), Kaposi's hemorrhagic sarcoma, basal cell carcinoma, and seborrheic keratosis. The lesions are benign, and the treatment consists of simple excision.

Malignant Eccrine Poroma (Porocarcinoma)

Most porocarcinomas arise from long-standing eccrine poromas (50%), but the tumors may develop directly. Clinically, they are similar to poromas but may also manifest as a blue or black nodule, plaque, or ulcerated tumor. More than 120 cases have been reported, with a relatively equal male to female ratio and an average age of 70 years. The most frequent sites of involvement are the legs (30%), feet (20%), face (12%), thighs (8%), and arms (7%). Of interest is the rare involvement of the palms (one case) and soles (eight cases), despite having the greatest concentration of eccrine sweat glands. The average age from onset to treatment is 8 years, with 20% developing regional spread and about 10% developing distant metastasis. If metastasis occurs there is a 70% mortality rate.

Histologically, the tumor may be seen adjoining an eccrine poroma. Two neoplastic cell types may be found.

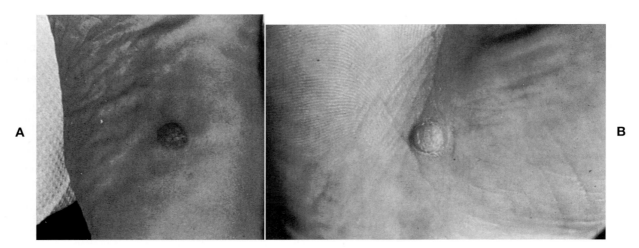

Fig. 29-86 **A,** Eccrine poroma on the sole of a 57-year-old man. **B,** Eccrine poroma on the palm.

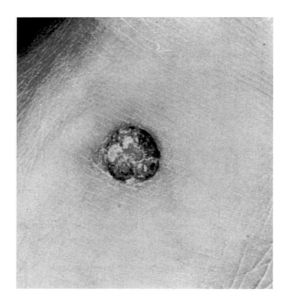

Fig. 29-87 Eccrine poroma on the dorsum of the foot.

The smaller, basophilic cells are monomorphous with small nuclei and scant, eosinophilic cytoplasm (periodic acid-Schiff positive, diastase labile) and tend to encircle numerous ducts. Other malignant cells have large hyperchromatic, irregularly shaped nuclei and may be multinucleated. The cells are rich in glycogen. Dendritic melanocytes containing melanin may be found. The tumor cells frequently demonstrate cytologic pleomorphism and frequent, abnormal mitotic figures.

Mohs' microsurgery is the treatment of choice for this aggressive malignancy, particularly on the face. If the lesion is small, wide simple excision may also be effective with aggressive margin checks. In histologically aggressive cases or large lesions, lymph node dissection may be indicated to evaluate for the possibility of regional metastasis. Clinical responses to isotretinoin and interferon alfa polychemotherapy have been somewhat successful in metastatic disease.

Barzi AS, et al: Malignant metastatic eccrine poroma: proposal for a new therapeutic protocol. *Dermatol Surg* 1997, 23:267.
Boynton JR, et al: Porocarcinoma of the eyelid. *Ophthalmology* 1997, 104:1626.
Johnson RC, et al: A painful step: eccrine poroma. *Arch Dermatol* 1992, 128:1530.
Kircik L, et al: Eccrine poroma in an unusual location. *Cutis* 1994, 54:183.
Lozano Orella JA, et al: Eccrine porocarcinoma: report of nine cases. *Dermatol Surg* 1997, 23:925.
Mousawi A, et al: Pigmented eccrine poroma: a simulant of nodular melanoma. *Int J Dermatol* 1995, 34:857.
Nakanishi Y, et al: Eccrine porocarcinoma with melanocyte colonization. *Br J Dermatol* 1998, 138:519.
Spencer DM, et al: Pedal papule: eccrine porocarcinoma (EPC) in association with poroma. *Arch Dermatol* 1995, 131:211.

Chondroid Syringoma

Chondroid syringoma was formerly called mixed tumor of the skin and pleomorphic sweat gland adenoma. Clinically, the tumor is usually a firm intradermal or subcutaneous nodule, most commonly located on the nose or cheeks (80% involve the head and neck regions) (Fig. 29-88). Intraosseous disease may occur. These tumors are usually asymptomatic and measure 5 to 30 mm in diameter.

Histologically, nests of cuboidal or polygonal epithelial cells in the corium give rise to tubuloalveolar and ductal structures and occasionally, keratinous cysts. These structures are embedded in a matrix varying from a faint bluish chondroid substance to an acidophilic hyaline material. This tumor is felt to be of eccrine origin.

Malignant Chondroid Syringoma

Synonyms for *malignant chondroid syringoma* include malignant mixed tumor of skin, aggressive chondroid

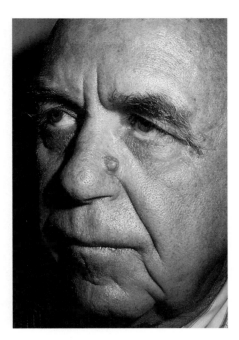

Fig. 29-88 Chondroid syringoma.

syringoma, and metastasizing chondroid syringoma. Most occur on the extremities but have also been reported to involve the face, scalp, back, and buttock. At presentation the masses range from 1 to 10 cm, with a median size of 4 cm, and often grow rapidly. The chance of metastasis is more than 50%, with a predilection for visceral spread. Metastases are usually as an adenocarcinoma, and the chondroid stroma found in primary lesions is often not found.

Histologic features that distinguish it from chondroid syringoma include cytologic atypia, pleomorphism, increased mitotic activity, and focal necrosis. Treatment is aggressive surgical excision. Adjuvant radiation therapy with or without chemotherapy has been recommended.

Barreto CA, et al: Intraosseous chondroid syringoma of the hallux. *J Am Acad Dermatol* 1994, 30:374.

Hong JJ, et al: Role of radiation therapy in the management of malignant chondroid syringoma. *Dermatol Surg* 1995, 21:781.

Onayemi O, et al: Chondroid syringoma: a neglected diagnosis. *Int J Dermatol* 1991, 30:441.

Steinmetz JC, et al: Malignant chondroid syringoma with widespread metastasis. *J Am Acad Dermatol* 1990, 22:845.

Watson JA, et al: Malignant chondroid syringoma: a rare cause of secondary bone tumor. *Clin Exp Dermatol* 1991, 16:306. ▲

Clear Cell Hidradenoma (Nodular Hidradenoma)

The wide array of names given to the *clear cell hidradenoma* attest to the confusion surrounding its histogenesis. Some of these names have been hidradenoma, cystic hidradenoma, porosyringoma, dermal sweat duct tumor, sweat gland epithelioma, clear cell myoepithelioma, nodular hidradenoma, eccrine acrospiroma, and eccrine sweat gland adenoma. It is classified as an eccrine sweat gland tumor.

The clear cell hidradenoma occurs as a single nodular, solid or cystic, occasionally protruding cutaneous mass, 5 to 30 mm in diameter. The flesh-colored or reddish lesion may be lobulated, with dome-shaped nodules. Ulceration is frequent. The lesions occur anywhere on the body, such as the axillae, arms, thighs, scalp, and pubic region, but the most common site is the head. Pain on pressure occurs in approximately 20% of patients. Multiple lesions on the eyelids have been reported. Its incidence is mostly between the ages of 20 and 50, and it occurs in women twice as commonly as in men.

Microscopically, the tumor is a circumscribed but unencapsulated mass of epithelial cells arranged into irregular or lobular masses extending deeply into the dermis. The distinctive cell is a large cuboidal or polyhedral cell with a clear cytoplasm suggestive of a single transparent vacuole surrounded by a clearly demarcated membrane. The round or oval nucleus is located at the edge of the cytoplasm. A second cell type present is fusiform or polyhedral, with basophilic cytoplasm. No mitoses are seen. The tumor is radioresistant, and extirpation is the treatment of choice.

Malignant Clear Cell Hidradenoma

Synonyms for malignant clear cell hidradenoma include *hidradenocarcinoma, malignant clear cell acrospiroma,* and *malignant nodular hidradenoma.* An extremely rare sweat gland neoplasm, it presents as a solitary nodule on the head, trunk, or distal extremity. More than 76 cases have been published, with a mean age of 57 years and an equal male-to-female ratio. Distribution in these cases was as follows: lower extremity (32.9%), upper extremities (27.6%), trunk (11.9%), head (26.3%), and neck (1.3%). Local recurrence is estimated at 50%, and metastasis occurs in 60%, with the regional lymph nodes and viscera being the most frequently involved sites. Distinguishing histologic features from clear cell hidradenoma are similar to other malignancies; namely, cellular atypia, tumor necrosis, and numerous mitoses. Treatment involves wide local excision, radiation, and chemotherapy.

Ashley I, et al: Sweat gland carcinoma: case report and review of the literature. *Dermatol Surg* 1997, 23:129.

Feldman AH, et al: Clear cell hidradenoma of the second digit: a review of the literature with case presentation. *J Foot Ankle Surg* 1997, 36:21.

Hamptom MT, et al: Recurrent draining cyst on the shoulder: clear cell hidradenoma (CCH) (nodular hidradenoma). *Arch Dermatol* 1992, 128:1531.

Kato N, et al: Clear cell hidradenoma: a tumor with basaliomatous changes in the overlying epidermis and follicular infundibula of surrounding skin. *J Dermatol* 1992, 19:436.

Schweitzer WJ, et al: Ulcerated tumor on the scalp: clear-cell hidradenoma. *Arch Dermatol* 1989, 125:985.

Touma D, et al: Malignant clear cell hidradenoma. *Dermatology* (Switzerland) 1993, 186:284.
Wong TY, et al: Clear cell eccrine carcinomas of the skin: a clinicopathologic study of nine patients. *Cancer* 1994, 73:1631. ▲

Eccrine Spiradenoma

Eccrine spiradenoma, first described by Kersting and Helwig, is clinically characterized by a solitary, 1-cm, deep-seated nodule occurring most frequently on the ventral surface of the body, especially over the upper half. Normal-appearing skin covers the nodule, which may be skin-colored, blue, or pink. Occasionally, multiple lesions may be present and may occur in a linear or zosteriform pattern. A striking symptom is pain appearing in paroxysms.

Eccrine spiradenoma has a generally benign clinical course and occurs most frequently between ages 15 and 35, although it has also been reported in infancy.

Microscopically, it is characterized as a multilobulated tumor surrounded by an adherent connective tissue capsule. The lobules are composed of basophilic cells arranged in characteristic small rosettes. Two cell types are those with large, pale, vesicular and ovoid nuclei and those with small, dark nuclei.

When painful, eccrine spiradenoma may be mistaken for leiomyoma, glomus tumor, neuroma, and angiolipoma. It also resembles fibroma, deep hemangioma, and neurofibroma. Treatment is simple excision.

Malignant Eccrine Spiradenoma

In long-standing eccrine spiradenoma, malignant degeneration may occur and may be lethal (Fig. 29-89). A breast tumor variant with features of eccrine spiradenoma has also been reported, showing typical local recurrence, but no metastasis. The deep location of the malignancy within the breast suggested origin within the breast parenchyma.

Berberian BJ, et al: Familial multiple eccrine spiradenomas with cylindromatous features associated with epithelioma adenoides cysticum of Brooke. *Cutis* 1990, 46:46.
Herzberg AJ, et al: Unusual case of early malignant transformation of spiradenoma. *Dermatol Surg Oncol* 1995, 21:1.
Kao GF, et al: Eccrine spiradenoma occurring in infancy mimicking mesenchymal tumor. *J Cutan Pathol* 1990, 17:214.
Lee MW, et al: Dermal cylindroma and eccrine spiradenoma. *Australas J Dermatol* 1996, 37:48.
Panico L, et al: An unusual, recurring breast tumor with features of eccrine spiradenoma: a case report. *Am J Clin Pathol* 1996, 106:665. ▲

Papillary Eccrine Adenoma

This uncommon benign sweat gland neoplasm was originally described in 1977 by Rulon and Helwig. Clinically, dermal nodules located primarily on the extremities of black patients are characteristic. Histologic findings consist of a well-circumscribed, dermal, unencapsulated growth composed of a bilayer of branching tubules. Immunohistochem-

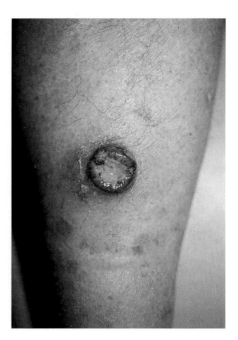

Fig. 29-89 Malignant eccrine spiradenoma.

ical analysis of the cells indicates differentiation toward the eccrine secretory coil. Because of its tendency to recur locally, complete surgical excision with clear margins is recommended.

Jerasutus S, et al: Papillary eccrine adenoma: an electron microscopic study. *J Am Acad Dermatol* 1989, 20:1111.
Sexton M, et al: Papillary eccrine adenoma. *J Am Acad Dermatol* 1988, 18:1114. ▲

Syringoacanthoma

Rahbari in 1984 reported 21 cases of this rare seborrheic keratosis–like neoplasm, 12 benign and 9 malignant. The cells contained fine glycogen particles and small accumulations of glycosaminoglycans. An extremely rare lesion, it has been reported to cause significant tissue destruction if left untreated. Its classification remains controversial, some believing it is a variant of eccrine poroma. It is derived from the acrosyringium. Just under half of all reported cases are believed to be malignant.

Cribier B, et al: Mutilating syringoacanthoma. *Dermatology* (Switzerland) 1994, 188:145.
Rahbari H: Syringoacanthoma. *Arch Dermatol* 1984, 120:751. ▲

Eccrine Syringofibroadenoma

First described by Mascaro in 1963, more than 44 cases have been reported, most presenting as a solitary, hyperker-

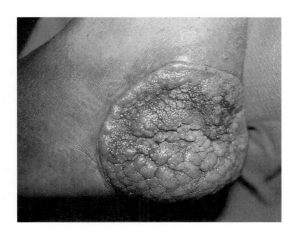

Fig. 29-90 Eccrine syringofibroadenoma.

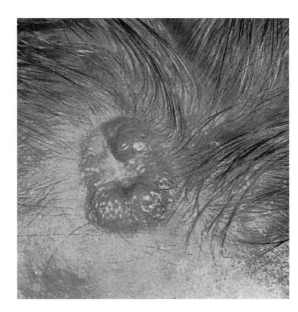

Fig. 29-91 Cylindroma on the forehead of a 60-year-old man. (Courtesy Dr. H. Shatin.)

atotic nodule or plaque involving the extremities (Fig. 29-90). At times they may have a linear quality. Four patients were associated with Schopf syndrome (hydrocystomas of the eyelids, hypotrichosis, hypodontia, and nail abnormalities), manifesting with multiple eccrine syringofibroadenomas in a mosaic pattern involving the palms and soles. Starink believes that multiple eccrine syringofibroadenomas are a characteristic marker of Schopf syndrome. Multiple lesions have also been reported without any other associated cutaneous findings. It is a neoplasm of eccrine acrosyringeal cells, resembling the premalignant fibroepithelial tumor of Pinkus, but with small, uniform, cuboidal cells instead of basaloid cells. There is one case of malignant eccrine syringofibroadenoma.

Hurt MA, et al: Eccrine syringofibroadenoma (mascaro). *Arch Dermatol* 1990, 126:945.

Ohnishi T, et al: Eccrine syringofibroadenoma. *Br J Dermatol* 1995, 133:449.

Starink TM: Eccrine syringofibroadenoma: multiple lesions representing a new cutaneous marker of the Schopf syndrome, and solitary nonhereditary tumors. *J Am Acad Dermatol* 1997, 36:569.

Trauner MA, et al: Eccrine syringofibroadenoma treated with a dual pulse width flashlamp pumped pulsed dye laser. *Dermatol Surg* 1999, 25:418.

Utani A, et al: Reactive eccrine syringofibroadenoma: an association with chronic foot ulcer in a patient with diabetes mellitus. *J Am Acad Dermatol* 1999, 41:650. _____ ▲

Cylindroma

Cutaneous cylindroma, also known as *dermal eccrine cylindroma, Spiegler's tumor, turban tumor,* and *tomato tumor,* occurs predominantly on the scalp and face as a solitary lesion with a firm but rubberlike nodule, pinkish

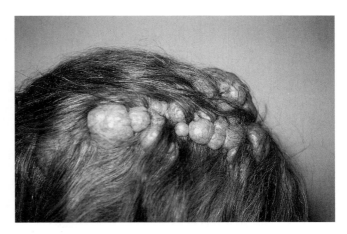

Fig. 29-92 Cylindromas or turban tumors.

to blue, and ranging from a few millimeters to several centimeters (Fig. 29-91). The solitary cylindroma is considered to be nonhereditary and may at times be found in areas other than the head and neck.

The dominantly inherited form manifests itself by the appearance soon after puberty of numerous rounded masses of various sizes on the scalp. The lesions resemble bunches of grapes or small tomatoes (Fig. 29-92). Sometimes they cover the entire scalp like a turban and are frequently associated with trichoepitheliomas and milia. In the familial form the cylindromas may be widespread.

Women are affected chiefly, beginning in early adult life. These lesions grow slowly and are benign. Cylindromas rarely undergo malignant degeneration, but aggressive behavior may be predicted by histologic findings such as lack of palisading and diminution or lack of hyalin sheaths. Occasionally, multiple lesions of cylindroma are associated with multiple trichoepitheliomas, eccrine spiradenomas, and other malignancies, such as basal cell carcinoma and other adnexal neoplasms. Malignant transformation occurs most often in the multiple-tumor form.

Differentiation is most often of apocrine origin; however, eccrine differentiation may occur in some. Histologically, these are cylindrical masses of epithelial cells surrounded and penetrated by a thick band of hyalin substance. Among the groups of epithelial cells are hyalin deposits and cystic cavities.

Cylindroma may be mistaken for epidermoid cyst, but the distinctive appearance and consistency makes diagnosis easy, especially in the multiple type. Treatment is by excision.

Antonescu CR, et al: Multiple malignant cylindromas of skin in association with basal cell adenocarcinoma with adenoid cystic features of minor salivary glands. *J Cutan Pathol* 1997, 24:449.

Cardenas AA, et al: Solitary violaceous nodule on the face: dermal cylindroma (also known as cylindroma, dermal eccrine cylindroma, Spiegler's tumor, turban tumor, and tomato tumor). *Arch Dermatol* 1993, 129:498.

Gerretsen AL, et al: Cutaneous cylindroma with malignant transformation. *Cancer* 1993, 72:1618.

Gerretsen AL, et al: Familial cutaneous cylindromas: investigations in five generations of a family. *J Am Acad Dermatol* 1995, 33:199.

Guzzo C, et al: Unusual abdominal location of a dermal cylindroma. *Cutis* 1995, 56:239.

Schirren CG, et al: A nevoid plaque with histological changes of trichoepithelioma and cylindroma in Brooke-Spiegler syndrome. *J Cutan Pathol* (Denmark) 1995, 22:563. _____ ▲

Sweat Gland Carcinoma

Malignant diseases of the sweat gland are rare, and those that have been described do not present a characteristic appearance clinically or histologically. They occur predominantly on the head and neck area and in patients aged 50 to 80. Although surgical excision is the treatment of choice, in metastatic disease, the role of chemotherapy and radiation therapy should be reevaluated since it may show good results in occasional patients. Several varieties have been reported. A listing of some of these follows.

Eccrine Carcinoma. Carcinoma of the eccrine glands does not have a characteristic clinical appearance but does have a high incidence of metastatic spread. It may arise anywhere in the skin. The microscopic pattern is that of an adenocarcinoma, which may create confusion with metastatic adenocarcinoma. In the "classic" type the histologic configuration varies from fairly well-differentiated tubular structures in some areas to anaplastic carcinoma in other areas.

Mucinous Eccrine Carcinoma. This tumor is commonly a round, elevated, reddish, and sometimes ulcerated mass,

usually located on the head and neck (75%). Forty percent occur on the eyelid. It grows slowly and is usually asymptomatic. Local recurrence is seen in 36%, but the incidence of metastasis is low (11%).

The lesions are often misdiagnosed as sebaceous cysts, hemangiomas, adenocystic basal cell carcinomas, lipomas, melanomas, or neuromas.

Histologically, tumors are characterized by the presence of large areas of mucin associated with tumor cells in ductlike structures. Histochemically, they have been shown to contain sialomucin, a nonsulfated mucoprotein. The recommended treatment is local surgical excision.

Snow SN, et al: Mucinous eccrine carcinoma of the eyelid. *Cancer* 1992, 70:2099.

Werner MS, et al: Mucinous eccrine carcinoma of the eyelid. *Ophthal Plast Reconstr Surg* 1996, 12:58. _____ ▲

Aggressive Digital Papillary Adenocarcinoma

This aggressive malignancy involves the digit between the nail bed and the distal interphalangeal joint spaces in most cases, presenting as a solitary nodule. Ulceration and bleeding can occur, and rarely the malignancy may be fixed to underlying tissues. Most patients are men in their fifties. More than 50% will experience recurrence, and just under 50% develop metastasis, particularly pulmonary. Immunohistochemical studies are remarkable for CEA positivity along luminal borders. A poor prognosis is expected when there is poor glandular differentiation, necrosis, prominent cellular atypia, and infiltration of underlying bone or vessels. All patients should have a chest roentgenogram. Complete excision is the treatment of choice. Wide local excision or even amputations may be required.

Ceballos PI, et al: Aggressive digital papillary adenocarcinoma. *J Am Acad Dermatol* 1990, 23:331.

Kao GF, et al: Aggressive digital papillary adenoma and adenocarcinoma. *J Cutan Pathol* 1987, 14:129.

Matysik TS, et al: Aggressive digital papillary adenoma. *Cutis* 1990, 46:125. _____ ▲

Primary Cutaneous Adenoid Cystic Carcinoma

This rare cutaneous tumor presents usually on the chest or scalp of middle- to older-aged persons. It is identical histologically to adenoid cystic carcinoma of the salivary gland. It may recur locally or, rarely, metastasize. Mohs' microsurgery is the treatment of choice.

Chesser RS, et al: Primary cutaneous adenoid cystic carcinoma treated with Mohs micrographic surgery. *J Dermatol Surg Oncol* 1992, 18:175.

Salzman MJ, et al: Primary cutaneous adenoid cystic carcinoma: a case report and review of the literature. *Plast Reconstr Surg* 1991, 88:140. _____ ▲

Microcystic Adnexal Carcinoma (Sclerosing Sweat Duct Carcinoma). Goldstein et al in 1982 described six cases of "microcystic adnexal carcinoma," closely resembling syringoma. Immunohistologic studies suggest both pilar and eccrine differentiation, an observation consonant with the many names that have been given this entity. It is also known as *sclerosing sweat duct carcinoma.*

The tumor is generally a very slow-growing plaque or nodule. It occurs most commonly on the upper lip in women, but occurs in other facial areas and in men. Histologically, it looks like a syringoma, with variable development of cords and ducts, embedded in a hyalinized stroma. Perineural infiltration is common and may be extensive. This explains the frequent recurrence after initial excision. Mohs' microsurgery is the treatment of choice. There have been no reports of metastases.

Burns MK, et al: Microcystic adnexal carcinoma. *J Dermatol Surg Oncol* 1994, 20:429.

Friedman PM, et al: Microcystic adnexal carcinoma: collaborative series and update. *J Am Acad Dermatol* 1999, 41:225.

Le Boit PE, et al: Microcystic adnexal carcinoma of the skin: a reappraisal of the differentiation and differential diagnosis of an underrecognized neoplasm. *J Am Acad Dermatol* 1993, 29:609.

Sebastien TS, et al: Microcystic adnexal carcinoma. *J Am Acad Dermatol* 1993, 29:840. _____ ▲

APOCRINE GLANDS
Ceruminoma

Ceruminous glands have features of both apocrine and eccrine differentiation and are classified as apoeccrine glands. Ceruminoma is a rare apoeccrine tumor that rarely becomes malignant. It is characterized by a firm nodular mass in the external auditory canal. Ulceration and crusting follow, with eventual growth that may obstruct the meatus.

Histologically, large masses of tumor cells with pale-staining nuclei are present. Miotic figures may be seen in some cases. There can also be associated adenoid tubular proliferation and cystic spaces. Mills et al reviewed 32 patients with tumors of the external auditory meatus over a 30-year period. Lesions diagnosed as ceruminoma were reclassified as adenoma, cylindroma, adenoid cystic carcinoma, or ceruminous adenocarcinoma. Whether ceruminoma is a true entity is being questioned.

Treatment is excision; however, recurrences are frequent in the malignant variants, ceruminous adenocarcinoma and adenoid cystic carcinoma, in which perineural and neural invasion predispose to recurrence.

Mansour P, et al: Ceruminous gland tumours: a reappraisal. *J Laryngol Otol* 1992, 106:727.

Mills RG, et al: "Ceruminoma": a defunct diagnosis. *J Laryngol Otol* 1995, 109:180.

Roland PS, et al: Disorders of the external auditory canal. *J Am Acad Audiol* 1997, 8:367. _____ ▲

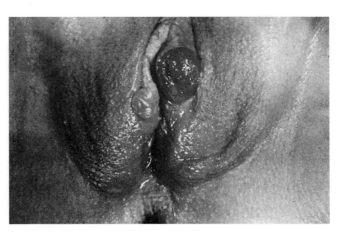

Fig. 29-93 Hidradenoma papilliferum.

Hidradenoma Papilliferum

Hidradenoma papilliferum is a benign solitary tumor that is located almost exclusively in the vulvar (Fig. 29-93) and anal areas, but also may involve the eyelid. The tumor is covered by normal skin. On palpation it is a firm nodule a few millimeters in diameter. Occasionally, bleeding, ulceration, discharge, itching, and pain are noted.

Microscopically, this is an adenoma of the apocrine glands. It is encapsulated and lies in the dermis and has no connection with the epidermis. There is a cystlike cavity lined with villi. The walls of the cavity and the villi are lined, occasionally with a single layer but usually a double layer of cells—luminal secretory cells and myoepithelial cells. Electron microscopy shows hidradenoma and myoepithelial cells, confirming the apocrine origin of hidradenoma papilliferum. This is a benign lesion, and the diagnosis and treatment are accomplished by excisional biopsy.

Goette DK: Hidradenoma papilliferum. *J Am Acad Dermatol* 1988, 19:133.

Netland PA, et al: Hidradenoma papilliferum of the upper eyelid arising from the apocrine gland of Moll. *Ophthalmology* 1990, 97:1593.

Vang R, et al: Ectopic hidradenoma papilliferum: a case report and review of the literature. *J Am Acad Dermatol* 1999, 41:115.

Veraldi S, et al: Hidradenoma papilliferum of the vulva: report of a case characterized by unusual clinical behavior. *J Dermatol Surg Oncol* 1990, 16:674. _____ ▲

Syringadenoma Papilliferum (Syringocystadenoma Papilliferum)

This lesion most commonly develops in a nevus sebaceus of Jadassohn on the scalp or face, around the time of puberty (Fig. 29-94). About half are present at birth, and approximately 25% arise on the trunk and the genital and inguinal regions during adolescence or adult life, without a preexisting lesion. The lesions are rose-red papules of firm consistency; they vary from 1 to 3 mm and occur in groups. Vesicle-like inclusions are seen, pinpoint to pinhead in size, filled with clear fluid. Some of the papules may be

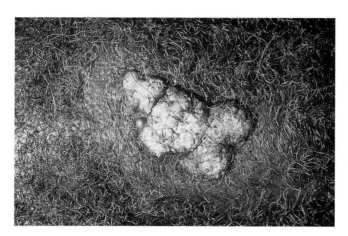

Fig. 29-94 Syringoadenoma papilliferum. (Courtesy Dr. Detlef K. Goette.)

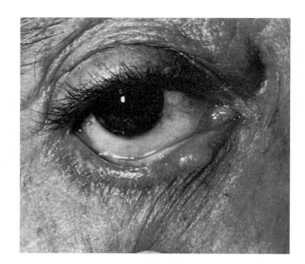

Fig. 29-95 Apocrine hidrocystoma of the lower eyelid margin.

umbilicated and simulate molluscum contagiosum. Extensive verrucous or papillary plaques may also be present.

It is differentiated from syringoma by the grouping of the lesions and by histologic studies, which show dilated and cystic changes in the sweat glands and ducts with numerous papillary projections extending into the lumina. The papillary projections are lined by glandular epithelium, often consisting of two rows of cells. The tumor stains positively for carcinoembryonic antigen by immunohistochemical methods.

Lesions around the eye may be mistaken for basal cell carcinoma. Although transition to carcinoma is rare, it has occurred, and excision is advisable. Radiation is ineffective.

Abanmi A, et al: Syringocystadenoma papilliferum mimicking basal cell carcinoma. *J Am Acad Dermatol* 1994, 30:127.

Nowak M, et al: Syringocystadenoma papilliferum of the male breast. *Am J Dermatopathol* 1998, 20:422.

Perlman JI, et al: Syringocystadenoma papilliferum of the eyelid. *Am J Ophthalmol* 1994, 117:647. ▲

Apocrine Hidrocystoma (Apocrine Retention Cyst)

Apocrine hidrocystoma or cystadenoma was described by Mehregan as a single benign tumor occurring chiefly on the face (Fig. 29-95). Other sites of involvement include the ears (Fig. 29-96), scalp, chest, and shoulders. Those reported on the penile shaft have been reclassified as median raphe cysts. The lesion is a dome-shaped, smooth-surfaced, translucent nodule, frequently bluish or brownish. A brownish fluid is noted in some incised lesions. They are usually solitary; however, multiple lesions may also be seen, particularly involving the eyelids.

Microscopically, these lesions are an adenomatous cystic proliferation of the apocrine glands. Large cystic spaces

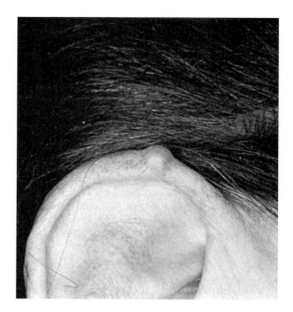

Fig. 29-96 Apocrine hidrocystoma.

lined by apocrine type secretory epithelium are present in the dermis. The cysts are surrounded by a fibrous stroma. From the cyst wall papillary projections extend into the cystic cavity.

Apocrine cystadenoma is to be differentiated from pigmented nevus, melanoma, blue nevus, or a cystic basal cell carcinoma. The lesion is benign, so that when feasible, simple excision is indicated for treatment.

De Eusebio E, et al: Multiple hidrocystomas. *Dermatology* (Switzerland) 1996, 193:152.

Milum EA: A solitary pigmented tumor of the face: apocrine hidrocystoma. *Arch Dermatol* 1991, 127:572.

Veraldi S, et al: Pigmented apocrine hidrocystoma: a report of two cases and review of the literature. *Clin Exp Dermatol* 1991, 16:18. ▲

Apocrine Gland Carcinoma

Apocrine gland carcinoma, unrelated to Paget's disease, is rare. The axilla is the most common site, but occasionally other areas with apocrine glands, such as the nipples and vulva, and also the eyelids and external auditory meatus, where Moll's glands and the ceruminous glands are found, may be involved. Some of these cases from the axillae and nipples may originate from aberrant mammary glands. Widespread metastases may occur.

Burket JM, et al: Tubular apocrine adenoma with perineural invasion. *J Am Acad Dermatol* 1984, 11:639.

Okun MR, et al: Apocrine adenoma versus apocrine carcinoma. *J Am Acad Dermatol* 1980, 2:322.

Paties C, et al: Apocrine carcinoma of the skin. *Cancer* 1993, 71:375.

Warkel RL, et al: Apocrine gland adenoma and adenocarcinoma of the axilla. *Arch Dermatol* 1971, 103:68. ▲

HAIR FOLLICLE NEVI AND TUMORS
Pilomatricoma (Calcifying Epithelioma of Malherbe)

Since 1880, when first described, this entity has had various names such as *Malherbe's calcifying epithelioma* and *pilomatrixoma*. Occurring usually as a single tumor, it is most commonly found on the face, neck, or arms, although it may also be located on the scalp, trunk, and lower extremities (Fig. 29-97). Pilomatricoma is an asymptomatic, deeply seated, 0.5- to 7.0-cm, firm nodule, covered by normal or pink skin, which on stretching may show the "tent sign," with multiple facets and angles. At times the lesions may have a bullous appearance. In the review of 209 patients by Julian et al the youngest patient reported was 18 months and the oldest 86 years. There was a bimodal age distribution. In the earlier years the peak age is between 5 to 15 years for females and up to 5 years for males. In adults it occurs mostly between 50 and 65 years.

The lesions may be seen in patients with myotonia atrophica (myotonic muscular dystrophy), together with frontoparietal baldness and Raynaud's phenomenon. Familial patterns may also occur. A few patients with multiple lesions have been reported. Multiple pilomatricomas have been reported in Rubinstein-Taybi and Gardner syndrome.

The histopathology shows an encapsulated mass. "Basophilic" and "shadow" cells are seen in solid masses, with a transition from the darkly staining basophilic cells to the shadow cells, which stain eosinophilic. Calcification takes place and in most instances appears as dusting of basophilic substances in the shadow cells or as solid purple amorphous masses. Ossification, melanin deposits, and foreign-body reaction with giant cells may all be present.

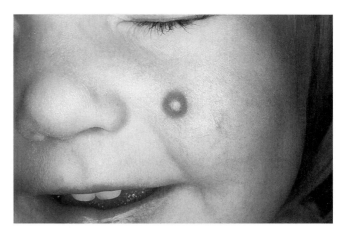

Fig. 29-97 Pilomatricoma on the cheek of a child.

Pilomatricoma is derived from hair matrix cells. Tumorigenesis results from activating mutations in beta-catenin.

Clinical differential diagnosis is usually impossible. The subcutaneous firm nodule with normal skin above should suggest the diagnosis, although the epidermoid cyst closely resembles pilomatricoma. Simple excision of the lesion for biopsy is the best procedure, though curettage of the cyst contents through a small incision or 2-mm punch biopsy hole has been used with success.

Malignant Pilomatricoma

Malignant pilomatricomas are rare, and in the series of 209 patients reported by Julian, only one malignant case was found. Fewer than 20 cases have been reported in the world literature and tend to occur in middle-aged patients. Histologic evidence typically shows proliferating basaloid cells with numerous abnormal mitoses with infiltration of underlying structures. They do not behave aggressively.

Alli N, et al: Perforating pilomatricoma. *J Am Acad Dermatol* 1996, 35:116.

Berberian BJ, et al: Multiple pilomatricomas in association with myotonic dystrophy and a family history of melanoma. *J Am Acad Dermatol* 1997, 37:268.

Cambiaghi S, et al: Multiple pilomatricomas in Rubinstein-Taybe syndrome: a case report. *Pediatr Dermatol* 1994, 11:21.

Chan EF, et al: A common skin tumor is caused by activating mutations in beta-catenin. *Nat Genet* 1999, 21:410.

Demircan M, et al: Pilomatricoma in children: a prospective study. *Pediatr Dermatol* 1997, 14:430.

Graells J, et al: Multiple familial pilomatricomas associated with myotonic dystrophy. *Int J Dermatol* 1996, 35:732.

Inui S, et al: Pilomatricoma with a bullous appearance. *J Dermatol* 1997, 24:57.

Julian CG, et al: A clinical review of 209 pilomatricomas. *J Am Acad Dermatol* 1998, 39:191.

Pujol RM, et al: Multiple familial pilomatricomas: a cutaneous marker for Gardner syndrome? *Pediatr Dermatol* 1995, 12:331.

Waxtein L, et al: Malignant pilomatricoma: a case report. *Int J Dermatol* 1998, 37:538. ▲

Trichofolliculoma

Originally described by Miescher, trichofolliculoma is a benign, highly structured adenoma of the pilosebaceous unit, characterized by a small, dome-shaped nodule some 5 mm in diameter on the face or scalp (Fig. 29-98). From the center of the flesh-colored nodule a small wisp of fine, immature hairs protrudes from a central pore. At times it may appear as a facial pore. It may occur at any age but mostly affects adults.

Histologically, the tumor consists of one or more large cystic follicles with smaller radiating follicular structures. The immature hair follicles range from an immature rudimentary matrix to formed hair papillae with fine hairs. Sebaceous glands and even a keratin cyst may be present in the tumor.

The benign nature of the tumor indicates only simple removal such as an excisional biopsy, or fulguration after a suitable shave biopsy has been obtained.

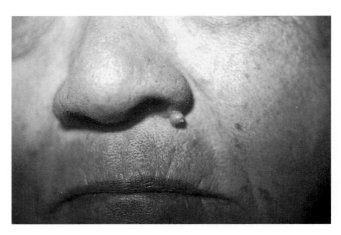

Fig. 29-98   Trichofolliculoma.

Ishii N, et al: A case of congenital trichofolliculoma. *J Dermatol* 1992, 19:195.

Kuttner BJ: A productive black facial pore: trichofolliculoma. *Arch Dermatol* 1989, 125:827.

Morton AD, et al: Recurrent trichofolliculoma of the upper eyelid margin. *Ophthal Plast Reconstr Surg* 1997, 13:287. _____ ▲

Trichoepithelioma (Epithelioma Adenoides Cysticum, Multiple Familial Trichoepitheliomas)

Clinical Features

Described by Brooke in 1892 as epithelioma adenoides cysticum and by Fordyce as multiple benign cystic epithelioma, multiple trichoepitheliomas are hereditary and occur as multiple cystic and solid nodules on the face, especially about the upper lip, nasolabial folds, and eyelids (Fig. 29-99). Other sites may be the scalp, neck, and trunk. At times they may be found in unusual configurations such as a large hemifacial plaque.

The lesions are characterized by multiple, small, rounded, smooth, shiny, slightly translucent, firm, circumscribed papules or nodules. The individual lesion is 2 to 4 mm in diameter and flesh-colored or slightly reddish. The center may be slightly depressed. Most frequently the lesions are grouped but discrete. On the face they are often symmetrical. The lesions begin during childhood or at the latest in early adulthood and tend to occur more commonly in females. Trichoepitheliomas are benign.

Although rare reports of degeneration into basal cell carcinomas have been reported, it is not believed to be a true association. The simultaneous presence of multiple trichoepithelioma and cylindroma has been observed repeatedly. It is due to a single autosomal dominant gene located on chromosome 9, which is capable of phenotypic dimorphism and variable penetrance.

Patients have been reported with generalized trichoepitheliomas, alopecia, and myasthenia gravis. Multiple linear and dermatomal trichoepitheliomas may rarely be seen.

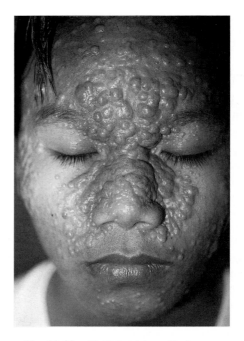

Fig. 29-99   Multiple trichoepitheliomas.

Solitary Trichoepithelioma

The singly occurring trichoepithelioma is nonhereditary and occurs mostly on the face (Fig. 29-100); however, it may also be found on the scalp, neck, trunk, upper arms, and thighs.

Giant Solitary Trichoepithelioma

Considered a distinct variant by some, the lesions may be several centimeters in diameter, occurring most commonly on the thigh or perianal regions. They are found in older adults.

Desmoplastic Trichoepithelioma

This lesion, which is difficult to differentiate from morphea-like basal cell carcinoma, occurs as solitary or multiple

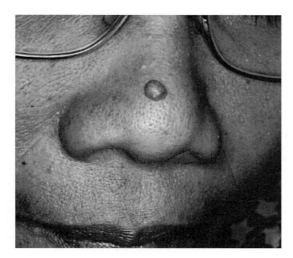

Fig. 29-100   Solitary trichoepithelioma.

lesions on the facies. They present on the face of young women most commonly and often have a raised annular border with a central nonnucleated center.

Among the most meaningful histologic criteria are this tumor's differentiation of pilar and sebaceous structures, its lack of any connection with the epidermis, and its non-invasion of cutaneous nerves or muscles. It behaves like an adenoma rather than an invasive malignancy.

Histology

Trichoepithelioma shows characteristic keratinous cysts and strands and masses of embryonal cells similar to those of the basal layer or those of the external root sheath of the hair follicle. In proliferating downward these strands form solid epithelial nests showing antlerlike branching. The cell nests contain granular horny or colloid material that forms cysts. The cells are small and mature. Adenoid structures may be present. Calcification of the cystic material and foreign-body giant cell reaction to it may also be seen. Trichoepitheliomas are best classified as an epithelioma of the hair germ. Histologically, trichoepithelioma must be differentiated from keratotic basal cell carcinoma, for which it is frequently confused. Complicating this are those cases in which basal cell carcinomas are found in association with trichoepitheliomas. In this regard a report linking overexpression of the *patched* gene to trichoepithelioma formation, similar to the findings in basal cell carcinomas, is provocative.

Differential Diagnosis

The multiple lesion type is distinguished from syringoma, which closely resembles it; in the solitary type it may be confused with basal cell carcinoma. Undoubtedly, some of the cases of basal cell carcinoma reported in children and adolescents have in fact represented solitary trichoepithelioma.

Treatment

Multiple lesions are difficult to treat satisfactorily since only the cosmetic results are important. Light fulguration or gentle electrodesiccation produces acceptable results. Cryotherapy with liquid nitrogen is at times satisfactory for small lesions. Dermabrasion is beneficial; however, the lesions tend to slowly recur. Solitary lesions are best removed by excisional surgery or laser such as the CO_2 laser.

Beck S, et al: Recurrent solitary giant trichoepithelioma located in the perianal area: a case report. *Br J Dermatol* 1988, 188:563.

Gerretsen AL, et al: Familial cutaneous cylindromas: investigations in five generations of a family. *J Am Acad Dermatol* 1995, 33:199.

Johnson SC, et al: Occurrence of basal cell carcinoma among multiple trichoepitheliomas. *J Am Acad Dermatol* 1993, 28:322.

Harada H, et al: Basal cell carcinoma occurring in multiple familial trichoepithelioma. *Arch Dermatol* 1997, 133:666.

Harada H, et al: The gene for multiple familial trichoepithelioma maps to chromosome 9p21. *J Invest Dermatol* 1996, 107:41.

Lorenzo MJ, et al: Cystic giant solitary trichoepithelioma. *Am J Dermatopathol* 1992, 14:155.

Oh DH, et al: A young boy with a large hemifacial plaque with histopathologic features of trichoepithelioma. *J Am Acad Dermatol* 1997, 37:881.

Rosenbach A, et al: Multiple trichoepitheliomas successfully treated with a high-energy, pulsed carbon dioxide laser. *Dermatol Surg* 1997, 23:708.

Sumithra S, et al: Desmoplastic trichoepithelioma and multiple epidermal cysts. *Int J Dermatol* 1993, 32:747.

Vorechovsky I, et al: Trichoepitheliomas contain somatic mutations in the overexpressed PTCH gene. *Cancer Res* 1997, 57:4677.

Votruba M, et al: The management of solitary trichoepithelioma versus basal cell carcinoma. *Eye* 1998, 12:43.

Wallace ML, et al: Trichoepithelioma with an adjacent basal cell carcinoma: transformation or collision? *J Am Acad Dermatol* 1997, 37:343.

West AJ, et al: Solitary facial plaque of long duration: desmoplastic trichoepithelioma. *Arch Dermatol* 1995, 131:213. _____ ▲

Trichoblastoma

These rare, benign neoplasms of follicular germinative cells present as asymptomatic 1- to 2-cm nodules of the scalp and face that tend to shell out during excision. They present in adulthood with an equal male-to-female ratio. Surgical excision is curative.

Albertini JG, et al: Asymptomatic scalp nodule present for 20 years. *Arch Dermatol* 1999, 135:707. _____ ▲

Trichilemmoma and Cowden's Disease (Multiple Hamartoma Syndrome)

Trichilemmoma is a benign neoplasm of the hair follicle that is derived from or differentiates toward cells of the outer sheath. It may occur as a small solitary papule on the face, particularly the nose and cheeks. Most lesions are clinically misinterpreted as basal cell carcinoma or verruca.

Trichilemmomas may also occur as multiple lesions (Fig. 29-101). These are a specific cutaneous marker for Cowden's syndrome, an autosomal dominantly inherited condition associated with multiple benign and malignant

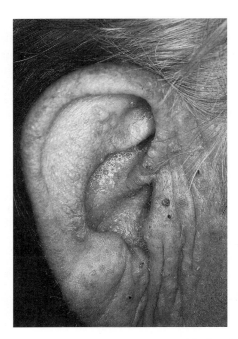

Fig. 29-101 Trichilemmomas in a man with Cowden's syndrome.

tumors. The trichilemmomas are generally limited to the head and neck area; however, unusual sites may be involved such as the sacral region. Eighty-seven percent of patients with Cowden's syndrome (the multiple hamartoma syndrome) have these facial papules. Other benign features include oral mucosal papules; acral keratotic papules; thyroid goiter, adenomatous or nodular; lipomas; gastrointestinal polyps; and fibrocystic breast disease. Thirty-eight percent develop malignancies, with breast cancer (25% to 36%) of women, thyroid carcinoma (7%), and colon adenocarcinoma being the most common. Tumors of the nervous system, including meningiomas, neurofibromas, and neuromas, have also been reported. A peculiar proliferation of abnormal neuronal elements of the cerebellum, known as *Lhermitte-Duclos disease,* may be closely associated with Cowden's disease, both having autosomal dominant inheritance. A number of mucocutaneous malignancies have been found in these patients to include melanoma, basal cell carcinoma, squamous cell carcinoma, Merkel cell carcinoma, and trichilemmomal carcinoma. A tumor suppressor gene (called *PTEN, MMACI,* or *TEPI*) believed responsible for Cowden's disease has been mapped to 10q22-23. Another disorder that may be linked to the disease is *Bannayan-Riley-Ruvalcaba syndrome* (autosomal dominantly inherited, macrocephaly, genital lentigines, motor and speech delay, mental retardation, hamartomatous polyps, myopathies, lipomas, and hemangiomas).

Microscopically, trichilemmomas show a verrucous epidermis and lobular acanthosis of glycogen-rich clear cells oriented about a follicle.

It is important that practitioners detect this disorder so as to monitor for the development of subsequent malignancies, especially of the breast. Isotretinoin has been used to treat the cutaneous lesions, and though they regress on medication, they tend to recur when it is discontinued. Some patients get satisfactory cosmetic results from dermabrasion or the CO_2 laser.

Albrecht S, et al: Cowden syndrome and Lhermitte-Duclos disease. *Cancer* 1992, 70:869.

Arch EM, et al: Deletion of PTEN in a patient with Bannayan-Riley-Ruvalcaba syndrome suggest allelism with Cowden's disease. *Am J Genet* 1997, 71:489.

De la Torre C, et al: Cowden's disease and Down syndrome: an exceptional association. *J Am Acad Dermatol* 1991, 25:909.

Hamby LS, et al: Parathyroid adenoma and gastric carcinoma as manifestations of Cowden's disease. *Surgery* 1995, 188:115.

Liaw D, et al: Germline mutations of the PTEN gene in Cowden's disease: an inherited disease, an inherited breast and thyroid cancer syndrome. *Nat Genet* 1997, 16:64.

Mallory SB: Cowden syndrome (multiple hamartoma syndrome). *Dermatol Clin* 1995, 13:27.

Marsh DJ, et al: PTEN mutation spectrum and genotype-phenotype correlations in Bannayan-Riley-Ruvalcaba syndrome suggest a single entity with Cowden syndrome. *Hum Mol Genet* 1999, 8:1461.

O'Hare AM, et al: Trichilemmomal carcinoma in a patient with Cowden's disease (multiple hamartoma syndrome). *J Am Acad Dermatol* 1997, 36:1021.

Sasake M, et al: Cowden's disease with pulmonary hamartoma. *Intern Med* (Japan) 1993, 32:39.

Steffen C, et al: A family with lesions on the face, hands, and buccal mucosa: Cowden's disease. *Arch Dermatol* 1993, 129:1505.

Yang JH, et al: Cowden's disease: report of the first case in a Chinese. *J Dermatol* 1994, 21:415. ▲

Trichilemmal Carcinoma

Trichilemmal carcinoma occurs in sun-exposed areas, most commonly involving the face and ears, presenting as a slow-growing epidermal papule, indurated plaque, or nodule with a tendency to ulcerate. Other locations include the trunk, arms, and legs. Mitoses and atypia are prominent, and metastasis may occur. Surgical removal is recommended.

Boscaino A, et al: Tricholemmal carcinoma: a study of seven cases. *J Cutan Pathol* 1992, 19:94.

Swanson PE, et al: Tricholemmal carcinoma: clinicopathologic study of 10 cases. *J Cutan Pathol* 1992, 19:100.

Wong TY, et al: Tricholemmal carcinoma: a clinicopathologic study of 13 cases. *Am J Dermatopathol* 1994, 16:463. ▲

Trichodiscoma, Fibrofolliculoma, and Birt-Hogg-Dubé Syndrome

Multiple small hamartomas of the mesodermal component of the hair discs (Haarscheibe) were identified as trichodiscomas in 1966 by Pinkus. Hundreds of flat or dome-shaped, skin-colored, asymptomatic papules, always in close proximity to a vellus hair, may develop at an early age over the face, trunk, and extremities. Such cases occur in families as an autosomal dominant trait. Histologically, there is a richly vascularized stroma, at the periphery of which is a hair follicle. When sectioned horizontally it appears that these actually are fibrofolliculomas because the epithelial proliferative component can be appreciated. Controversy exists whether trichodiscomas are a real entity.

Fibrofolliculomas are 2- to 4-mm skin-colored to white papules that may be solitary, or more commonly are multiple, scattered over the face, trunk, and extremities. Histologically, there is proliferation of the follicular epithelium as epithelial strands extending into a well-circumscribed mantle of connective tissue. Horizontal sectioning will facilitate its demonstration.

Patients with multiple fibrofolliculomas may also have acrochordons, collagenomas, lipomas, and/or oral fibromas. This dominantly inherited syndrome is known as *Birt-Hogg-Dubé syndrome* (BHD). A number of malignancies have been reported in patients with BHD, to include medullary carcinoma, colon cancer, and renal cell carcinoma. Toro et al screened 152 individuals with familial renal tumors and their asymptomatic at-risk relatives and found 3 kindreds in whom renal neoplasms and Birt-Hogg-Dubé segregated together. They recommend that BHD patients and their relatives undergo abdominal computed tomography and renal ultrasound screening for renal tumors. Treatment is dermabrasion or CO_2 laser.

Balus L, et al: Familial multiple trichodiscomas. *J Am Acad Dermatol* 1986, 15:603.

Birt AR, et al: Hereditary multiple fibrofolliculomas with trichodiscomas and acrochordons. *Arch Dermatol* 1977, 113:1674.

Junkins-Hopkins JM, et al: Multiple perifollicular fibromas. *J Cutan Pathol* 1994, 21:467.

Roth JS, et al: Bilateral renal cell carcinoma in the Birt-Hogg-Dubé syndrome. *J Am Acad Dermatol* 1993, 29:1055.

Toro JR, et al: Birt-Hogg-Dubé syndrome. *Arch Dermatol* 1999, 135:1195.

Ubogy-Rainey Z, et al: Fibrofolliculomas, trichodiscomas, and acrochordons. *J Am Acad Dermatol* 1987, 16:452.

Weinstein M, et al: Multiple hypopigmented papules: trichodiscoma. *Arch Dermatol* 1990, 126:1093. _____ ▲

Other Hair Follicle Tumors

Dilated Pore (Winer). First described by Winer, in dilated pore there is a central pore or giant comedo, usually occurring on the face as a solitary lesion (Fig. 29-102). It is most commonly found in adult males.

Pilar Sheath Acanthoma. Most often found on the face, particularly above the upper lip in adults, patients present with a solitary skin-colored nodule with a central pore. Histologically, pilar sheath acanthoma differs from a dilated pore by the presence of a large, irregular, branching cystic cavity.

Trichoadenoma. Presenting as a solitary growth ranging from 3 to 15 mm in diameter, clinically it has been mistaken as a seborrheic keratosis, having a vegetative or verrucous

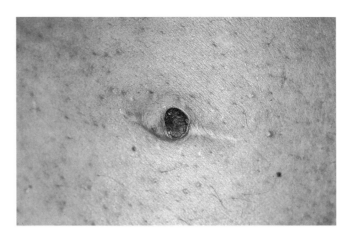

Fig. 29-102   Dilated pore.

appearance. Although most frequently found on the face, it may occur at other sites, such as the buttock, which is the second most common site. Histologically, it resembles a trichoepithelioma, having eosinophilic cells associated with islands of basophilic cells and numerous horn cysts.

Perifollicular Fibroma. Occurring as solitary or multiple papules, perifollicular fibromas are cutaneous hamartomatous proliferations of pilar connective tissue occurring on the face and trunk. Reports of autosomal dominant inheritance, association with colonic polyposis, fibrofolliculomas, trichodiscomas, and acrochordons are believed to represent cases of Birt-Hogg-Dubé syndrome. Histologically, perifollicular fibromas are characterized by a concentric arrangement of collagen fibers surrounding a generally unaltered hair follicle.

Generalized Follicular Hamartomas. Most often affecting the skin of the face and scalp, hamartomas are solitary or multiple skin-colored papules and infiltrating plaques associated with progressive hair loss in the affected areas. Congenital and adult cases have been found in association with alopecia, myasthenia gravis, and/or circulating autoantibodies (antinuclear and antiacetylcholine receptor antibodies). Cystic fibrosis and generalized follicular hamartomas have been reported in three siblings, suggesting a possible genetic linkage. Histologically, there are basaloid hamartomatous structures arising from the lower part of the pilosebaceous follicles in lesional and apparently normal skin.

Folliculosebaceous Cystic Hamartoma. First described by Kimura in 1991, folliculosebaceous cystic hamartoma presents as a flesh-colored sessile or pedunculated papule (0.5 to 1.4 cm) on the head, especially the central part of the face and nose. Onset ranges between 4 to 47 years. Diagnostic microscopic features include infundibular cystic structures with attached sebaceous glands, characteristic stroma, and stromal spindle cells positive for CD34.

Tumors of the Follicular Infundibulum. These flat, keratotic papules of the head and neck are usually solitary but may be multiple. There is a platelike proliferation of epidermal cells growing parallel to the epidermis and connecting to it at multiple sites. These are benign.

Alessi E, et al: Localized hair follicle hamartoma. *J Cutan Pathol* 1993, 20:364.

Headington JT: Tumors of the hair follicle. *Am J Pathol* 1976, 85:840.

Jaqueti G, et al: Verrucous trichoadenoma. *J Cutan Pathol* 1989, 16:145.

Junkins-Hopkins JM, et al: Multiple perifollicular fibromas. *J Cutan Pathol* (Denmark) 1994, 21:467.

Mascaro JM, et al: Congenital generalized follicular hamartoma associated with alopecia and cystic fibrosis in three siblings. *Arch Dermatol* 1995, 131:454.

Mehregan AH, et al: Pilar sheath acanthoma. *Arch Dermatol* 1978, 114:1495.

Mohri S: Pilar acanthoma. *J Dermatol* 1981, 8:479.

Sasai S, et al: Coexistence of multiple perifollicular fibromas and colonic polyp and cancer. *Dermatology* (Switzerland) 1996, 192:262.

Templeton SF: Folliculosebaceous cystic hamartoma. *J Am Acad Dermatol* 1996, 34:77.

Vin-Christian K, et al: Hypopigmented papules of the cheeks, neck, and shoulders. *Arch Dermatol* 1999, 135:463.

Winer L: The dilated pore. *J Invest Dermatol* 1954, 23:181.

Yamaguchi J, et al: A case of trichoadenoma arising in the buttock. *J Dermatol* 1992, 19:503. ▲

EPITHELIAL CYSTS AND SINUSES
Epidermal Cyst (Keratin Cyst, Sebaceous Cyst, Epidermoid Cyst)

The epidermal cyst is a commonly fluctuant, tense swelling varying from a half to several centimeters in diameter (Fig. 29-103). The surface of the overlying skin is usually smooth and shiny from the upward pressure. These nodules are freely movable over underlying tissue and are attached to the normal skin above them by the remains of the expanded gland duct, the opening of which frequently shows at a central point on the surface as a comedo. The pasty contents of the cysts are formed mostly of macerated keratin and cheesy, fatty material. Epidermoid cysts occur commonly on the face, neck, and trunk, but may be found almost anywhere. Their association with Gardner's syndrome is discussed elsewhere. Lesions of similar appearance found on the hairy scalp are usually pilar (trichilemmal) cysts. Penetrating injuries, such as with a sewing machine needle, may result in epidermoid cysts growing within bone, producing radiologic defects associated with a subcutaneous mass.

These cysts may rupture and induce a vigorous foreign body inflammatory response, after which they are most firmly adherent to surrounding structures and are more difficult to enucleate. Rarely, low-grade, nonmetastasizing

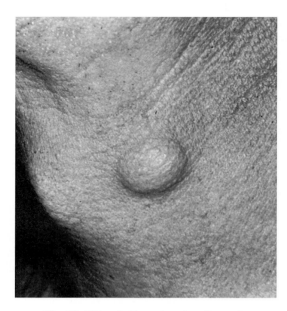

Fig. 29-103 Epidermal cyst on the neck.

squamous cell carcinoma may arise in the cyst wall. There is evidence that idiopathic scrotal calcinosis is due to end-stage dystrophic calcinosis associated with inflamed scrotal epidermoid cysts.

The epidermoid cyst is a keratinizing cyst, the wall of which is stratified squamous epithelium containing keratohyalin granules. It is differentiated from the pilar cyst by its location. Pilar cysts occur most frequently on the scalp. The lipoma closely resembles the epidermoid cyst, and at times it may be difficult to demonstrate the freely movable property of the cyst. Branchial cleft cysts and nodular fibromas should also be kept in mind.

The fastest and most definitive treatment is enucleation of the cyst through a small incision or even through a hole made with a 4- or even a 2-mm biopsy punch. Inflamed cysts do not lend themselves well to any of these procedures, and an incision and drainage is recommended. If any fragment of the cyst wall is left behind, recurrence usually occurs. In extremely large cysts the resulting surgical scar may be undesirable. In such cases a stabbing incision with an 11 blade followed by removal of most, if not all, of the cyst contents may be accomplished using a closed curette. At times the cyst wall may be "snagged" and withdrawn in smaller cysts but is unlikely with a larger one. Larger cysts treated this way will likely recur, but when they do they will be considerably smaller, allowing for a much smaller surgical procedure and a much more acceptable cosmetic result. The use of antibiotics for the treatment of ruptured epidermal inclusion cysts is controversial, since studies have shown no difference in the bacteria cultured from ruptured versus unruptured cysts. We generally do not place patients on antibiotics, unless they have other medical conditions that may make them predisposed to secondary infections. Drainage is the treatment of choice for ruptured cysts. Treatment with a copper ion and acid solution (Solcoderm) has been recommended by some.

Proliferating Epidermoid Cyst

Sau et al reported 96 cases of proliferating epithelial cysts, which comprise two types: proliferating epidermoid cysts and proliferating trichilemmal cysts (see the following discussion). Tumors derived from epidermoid cysts occur more commonly in men (64%), and the most frequent sites are the pelvic/anogenital areas (36%), scalp (21%), upper extremities (18%), and trunk (15%). Seventy-nine percent were located in areas other than the scalp. There may be carcinomatous changes on histology, with anaplasia, high mitotic rate, and deep invasion. They are locally aggressive, and distant metastasis is rare.

Akasaka T, et al: Pigmented epidermal cyst. *J Dermatol* (Japan) 1997, 24:475.

Bhawan J, et al: The so-called idiopathic scrotal calcinosis. *Arch Dermatol* 1983, 119:709.

Diven DG, et al: Bacteriology of inflamed and uninflamed epidermal inclusion cysts. *Arch Dermatol* 1998, 134:49.

Fisher BK, et al: Epidermoid cyst of the sole. *J Am Acad Dermatol* 1986, 15:1127.

Ronnen M, et al: Treatment of epidermal cysts with Solcoderm (a copper ion and acid solution). *Clin Exp Dermatol* 1993, 18:500.

Samlaska CP, et al: Intraosseous epidermoid cysts. *J Am Acad Dermatol* 1992, 27:454.

Sau P, et al: Proliferating epithelial cysts: clinicopathological analysis of 96 cases. *J Cutan Pathol* 1995, 22:394. ───────────────── ▲

Pilar Cyst (Trichilemmal Cyst)

The trichilemmal cyst, also known as a *wen,* is similar clinically to the epidermoid cyst except that about 90% of the pilar cysts occur on the scalp, and inheritance by the autosomal dominant mode is common (Fig. 29-104). It has been found rarely on the face, trunk, and extremities. The contents of this type of cyst are more keratinous and not so fatty as those of the epidermoid cyst. They are also odorless.

The trichilemmal cyst has a wall lined by keratinizing epithelium without a granular layer. Pinkus has shown that these trichilemmal cysts originate from the middle portion of the hair follicle epithelium.

Clinically, these lesions are indistinguishable from the epidermoid cyst. Differentiation from other lesions is fairly easily established, except for proliferating variants. Treatment is the same as that for the epidermoid cyst. They are much more easily enucleated, owing to their firm, coherent nature.

Proliferating Trichilemmal Cyst

These tumors were first named proliferating epidermoid cysts by Wilson Jones. These large (up to 25 cm) and exophytic neoplasms are confined almost exclusively to the scalp and back of the neck (Fig. 29-105). They are

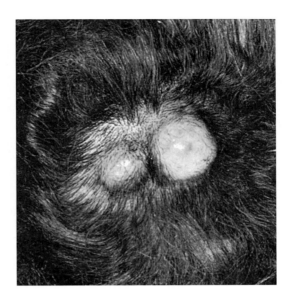

Fig. 29-104   Pilar cysts of the scalp.

approximately five times more common in women, and the mean age of patients is 65 years. They gradually enlarge and may undergo ulceration. These lesions have been misinterpreted both clinically and histologically as squamous cell carcinoma. They have been found in association with nevus sebaceus. They are believed to be derived from pilar cysts. Metastasis may occur, but most respond to surgical excision.

Histologic features include a sharply circumscribed pattern of convoluted lobules with definite margins, frequent continuity with the epidermis, extensive areas of tumor cell necrosis, and trichilemmal type keratinization with abrupt transition to dense keratin but without formation of a granular layer. Patterns of aggressive growth are occasionally present, and cytologic atypia may occur.

Arico M, et al: Proliferating tricholemmal tumour with lymph node metastases. *Br J Dermatol* 1989, 121:793.

Bulengo-Ransby SM, et al: Enlarging scalp nodule: proliferating trichilemmal cyst (PLC). *Arch Dermatol* 1995, 131:721.

Carlin MC, et al: Enlarging, painful scalp tumor. *Arch Dermatol* 1988, 124:935.

Hendricks DL, et al: A case of multiple pilar tumors and pilar cysts involving the scalp and back. *Plast Reconstr Surg* 1991, 87:763.

Rahbari H, et al: Development of proliferating trichilemmal cyst in organoid nevus. *J Am Acad Dermatol* 1986, 14:123.

Weiss J, et al: Malignant proliferating trichilemmal cyst. *J Am Acad Dermatol* 1995, 32:870. ───────────────── ▲

Dermoid Cyst

Dermoid cysts are congenital in origin and occur chiefly along the lines of cleavage (Fig. 29-106). They are the result of improper embryologic development, and there is a

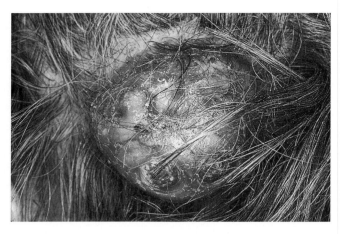

Fig. 29-105 Proliferating trichilemmal tumor.

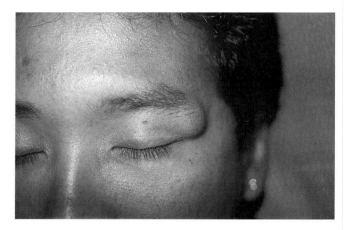

Fig. 29-106 Dermoid cyst.

potential for intracranial communication. In the sublingual region the soft, elastic, oval cysts may vary from a few millimeters to several centimeters in diameter. They may also occur about the eyes, root of the nose, and floor of the mouth. They are generally not attached to the skin but are freely movable. At times there may be a rim of bone surrounding the base of the cyst, particularly when there is intracranial extension. Dermoid cysts may produce visual impairment through extension into the orbit.

Histologically, the cyst wall is lined with stratified squamous epithelium containing skin appendages, including lanugo hair.

In a child attempts at surgical removal or biopsy of a cyst over cranial cleavage planes (including spinal, midline) should not be attempted without proper assessment to rule out a potential intracranial communication. A CT or MRI scan is required to rule this out. Any underlying bony changes detected by CT scan should be followed up with an MRI scan, since the cranial penetration by the cyst may at times be difficult to identify by CT scan. If an intracranial mass is detected the patient should be referred to a neurosurgeon. Dermoid cysts not found over cranial cleavage planes, such as the ear, can be safely removed surgically.

Bauer DJ, et al: Large asymptomatic mass on the ear: dermoid cyst of the auricle. *Arch Dermatol* 1994, 130:913.

Bonavolonta G, et al: Dermoid cysts: 16-year survey. *Ophthal Plast Reconstr Surg* 1995, 11:187.

Emerick GT, et al: Chewing-induced visual impairment from a dumbbell dermoid cyst. *Ophthal Plast Reconstr Surg* 1997, 13:57.

Nocini PF, et al: Dermoid cyst of the nose: a case report and review of the literature. *J Oral Maxillofac Surg* 1996, 54:357.

Paller AS, et al: Nasal midline masses in infants and children. *Arch Dermatol* 1991, 127:362.

Saito H, et al: Congenital dermal sinus with intracranial dermoid cyst. *Br J Dermatol* 1994, 130:235.

Sinclair RD, et al: Congenital inclusion dermoid cysts of the scalp. *Australas J Dermatol* 1992, 33:135. _____ ▲

Pilonidal Sinus

Pilonidal cyst or sinus is a midline hairy patch or pit in the sacral region with a sinus orifice in the bottom, or a cyst beneath it, in which hair is growing. It usually becomes symptomatic during adolescence and presents as a foreign body abscess, with hair as the offender. In theory, wide-open cystectomy and thorough debridement should suffice to cure it; but there are many failures. Hoehn has had great satisfaction for 30 years with a method proposed by Korb in 1951: opening the cyst widely, debriding it, and packing the cavity with silver nitrate crystals. By the third day, the sac has separated and can be lifted out and any remaining sinuses repacked with silver nitrate. The entire procedure is done without hospitalization. In recalcitrant disease more advanced surgical intervention may be required. Squamous cell carcinomas have been reported to arise from chronic inflammatory pilonidal disease.

Gur E, et al: Squamous cell carcinoma in perineal inflammatory disease. *Ann Plast Surg* 1997, 38:653.

Hoehn GH: A simple solution to the therapeutic dilemma of pilonidal cysts. *J Dermatol Surg Oncol* 1982, 8:56.

Jones DJ: ABC of colorectal diseases: silonidal sinus. *BMJ* 1992, 304:974. ▲

Steatocystoma Simplex

Brownstein reported a solitary steatocystoma in 16 women and 14 men. The site was on the face, limbs, or chest. It appears to be the nonheritable counterpart of the more familiar steatocystoma multiplex. It occurs as a rule between ages 15 and 70 (median age 39). The content of the cyst is an oily yellow fluid. The oral mucosa may also be involved. Simple excision is curative.

Brownstein MH: Steatocystoma simplex. *Arch Dermatol* 1982, 118:409.

Dailey T: Pathology of intraoral sebaceous glands. *J Oral Pathol Med* (Denmark) 1993, 22:241.

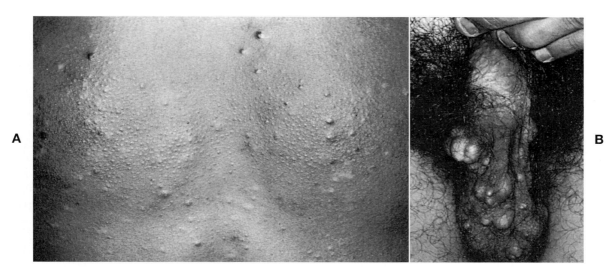

Fig. 29-107 Steatocystoma multiplex **A,** on the chest and **B,** on the scrotum.

Nakamura S, et al: A case of steatocystoma simplex on the head. *J Dermatol* 1988, 15:347. _____ ▲

Steatocystoma Multiplex

Steatocystoma multiplex consists of multiple, small, yellowish, cystic nodules 2 to 6 mm in diameter, located principally on the upper anterior portion of the trunk, upper arms, axillae, and thighs (Fig. 29-107). In severe cases, the lesions may be generalized, with sparing only of the palms and soles. At times the lesions may be limited to the face or scalp and is considered a specific variant by some. These cysts often contain a syruplike, yellowish, odorless, oily material.

Steatocystoma has a high familial tendency and probably has an autosomal dominant mode of transmission. However, numerous nonhereditary cases have been.

Histologically, there is a folded cyst wall consisting of several layers of epithelial cells, with flattened sebaceous lobules within or close to the wall. In some instances hair follicle type extensions occur in the wall, and lanugo-sized hairs may be present in the cavity. A relationship between eruptive vellus hair cysts has been suggested because of a similar clinical appearance, time of onset, and overlapping histologic features. It has been proposed that these clinical entities are a spectrum of the same disease process and should be classified as multiple pilosebaceous cysts.

In the differential diagnosis steatocystomata are easily differentiated from dermoid and epidermoid cysts by their multiplicity and sites and because of the characteristic oily contents.

The definitive treatment of individual lesions is excision. Elliptic excisions with one or at most two sutures produce excellent results. However, the sheer number of the cysts usually precludes this type of treatment. In such instances, incision and thorough expression of the cyst contents or aspiration using an 18-gauge needle is effective in temporarily reducing the lesions; however, recurrence is the rule.

Ahn SK, et al: Steatocystoma multiplex localized only in the face. *Int J Dermatol* 1997, 36:372.

Hansen KK, et al: Multiple papules of the scalp and forehead: steatocystoma multiplex (facial papular variant). *Arch Dermatol* 1995, 131:835.

Kiene P, et al: Eruptive vellus hair cysts and steatocystoma multiplex: variants of one entity? *Br J Dermatol* 1996, 134:365.

Moon SE, et al: Eruptive vellus hair cyst and steatocystoma multiplex in a patient with pachyonychia congenita. *J Am Acad Dermatol* 1994, 30:275.

Ohtake N, et al: Relationship between steatocystoma multiplex and eruptive vellus hair cysts. *J Am Acad Dermatol* 1992, 26:876.

Pamoukian VN, et al: Five generations with steatocystoma multiplex congenita: a treatment regimen. *Plast Reconstr Surg* 1997, 99:1142.

Requena L, et al: A facial variant of steatocystoma multiplex. *Cutis* 1993, 51:449.

Sato K, et al: Aspiration therapy in steatocystoma multiplex. *Arch Dermatol* 1993, 129:35. _____ ▲

Eruptive Vellus Hair Cysts

Esterly et al described this entity in 1977. Many ensuing publications have characterized it as an autosomal dominantly inherited disorder that appears as yellowish to reddish brown, small papules of the chest and proximal extremities. They may be congenital but usually have their onset between ages 17 and 24. Disseminated lesions have occurred as well as lesions limited to the face. Histologically, the cystic epithelium is of the stratified squamous type; the cyst contents are composed of laminated keratin and vellus hairs, and follicle-like invaginations may be present in the cyst wall. This is felt to be caused by an abnormality at the infundibular level of the vellus hair. Some authors believe this disorder and steatocystoma multiplex are within the spectrum of the same disease process (multiple pilosebaceous cysts). Treatment similar to that described for epidermal cysts may be effective.

Armstrong CR, et al: Multiple papulocystic lesions on the trunk: eruptive vellus hair cysts (EVHC). *Arch Dermatol* 1995, 131:343.

Grimalt R, et al: Eruptive vellus hair cysts: case report and review of the literature. *Pediatr Dermatol* 1992, 9:98.

Kiene P, et al: Eruptive vellus hair cysts and steatocystoma multiplex: variants of one disease? *Br J Dermatol* 1996, 134:365.

Nogita T, et al: Eruptive vellus hair cysts with sebaceous glands. *Br J Dermatol* 1991, 125:475.

Ohtake N, et al: Relationship between steatocystoma multiplex and eruptive vellus hair cysts. *J Am Acad Dermatol* 1992, 26:876. ▲

Pigmented Follicular Cysts

Single pigmented lesions occurring in men between ages 20 and 60, easily mistaken for moles, may be pigmented follicular cysts. These were first described by Mehregan and Medenica in 1982. The stratified squamous epithelial wall has rete ridges and papillae, and the cyst is full of thick, deeply pigmented hair shafts. Most occurred on the face or neck. It has been suggested to be a variant of multiple pilosebaceous cysts.

Mehregan AH, et al: Pigmented follicular cysts. *J Cutan Pathol* 1982, 2:423.

Salopek TG, et al: Multiple pigmented cysts: a subtype of multiple pilosebaceous cysts. *Br J Dermatol* 1996, 134:758.

Sandoval R, et al: Pigmented follicular cyst. *Br J Dermatol* 1994, 131:130. ▲

Milia

Milia are white keratinous cysts, 1 to 4 mm in diameter, appearing chiefly on the face, especially under the eyes (Fig. 29-108). Montgomery described them as "tiny pearly white globoid masses, often appearing like kernels of rice lying beneath a translucent layer of tissue." They may occur in great numbers, especially in middle-aged women. They occur in up to 50% of newborns.

Primary milia develop without a predisposing condition and are most commonly found in adults or during the newborn period. Secondary milia can develop in inflammatory conditions and skin diseases such as epidermolysis bullosa, pemphigus, bullous pemphigoid, porphyria cutanea tarda, herpes zoster, contact dermatitis, and after prolonged use of nonsteroidal antiinflammatory drugs. They also tend to occur after trauma, such as dermabrasion, or after a bullous or vesicular eruption has healed, or after long-term corticosteroid use, or after 5-FU therapy.

It has been associated with a number of genodermatoses, such as congenital ectodermal defect; reticular pigmented genodermatosis with milia (Naegeli-Franceschetti-Jadassohn syndrome); and congenital absence of dermal ridges, syndactyly, and facial milia.

Other variants have been reported. Multiple eruptive milia (MEM) occurs when crops of milia develop suddenly on the face and upper trunk. MEM may be associated with multiple trichoepitheliomas. MEM may also be familial, with autosomal dominant inheritance. Milia en plaque (MEP) presents with grouped milia forming plaques most commonly in the postauricular area; however, it may also involve the preauricular region and supraclavicular areas. MEP has been reported in one patient with pseudoxanthoma

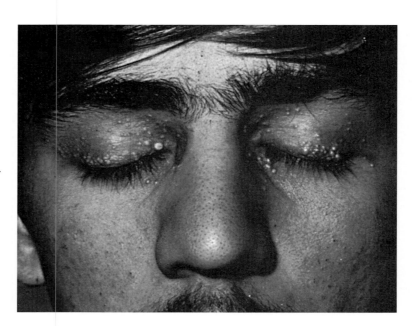

Fig. 29-108 Milia on the eyelids.

elasticum. The cause of MEP is unknown, but application of topical agents, such as perfumes, has been implicated.

Milia are viewed as retention cysts and are believed to be derived from vellus hairs at the most inferior point in primary disease. In secondary milia the cysts are derived from the eccrine sweat ducts or from aberrant epidermis or hair follicles.

Treatment is incision and expression of the contents with a comedo expressor. No anesthesia is needed for most patients. Topical tretinoin (Retin-A) has been effective in treating MEP and more generalized forms of milia involving the face. Minocycline has been used with some success to treat MEP.

Cho SH, et al: Milia en plaque associated with pseudoxanthoma elasticum. *J Cutan Pathol* 1997, 24:61.

Cirillo-Hyland VA, et al: Reevaluation of a kindred with congenital absence of dermal ridges, syndactyly, and facial milia. *J Am Acad Dermatol* 1995, 32:315.

Combemale P, et al: "Milia en plaque" in the supraclavicular area. *Dermatology* (Switzerland) 1995, 191:262.

Hisa T, et al: Post-bullous milia. *Australas J Dermatol* 1996, 37:153.

Keohane SG, et al: Milia en plaque: a new site and novel treatment. *Clin Exp Dermatol* 1996, 21:58.

Langley RGB, et al: Multiple eruptive milia: report of a case, review of the literature, and a classification. *J Am Acad Dermatol* 1997, 37:353.

Lee WS, et al: Milia arising in herpes zoster scars. *J Dermatol* 1996, 23:556.

Losada-Campa A, et al: Milia en plaque. *Br J Dermatol* 1996, 134:970.

Samlaska CP, et al: Milia en plaque. *J Am Acad Dermatol* 1989, 21:311.

Stork J: Retroauricular bilateral "milia en plaque." *Dermatology* (Switzerland) 1995, 191:260.

Tzermias C, et al: Reticular pigmented genodermatosis with milia: special form of Naegeli-Franceschetti-Jadassohn syndrome or a new entity? *Clin Exp Dermatol* 1995, 20:331. _____ ▲

Pseudocyst of the Auricle

Pseudocyst of the auricle clinically presents as a fluctuant, tense, noninflammatory swelling on the upper half of the ear (Fig. 29-109). It is believed to be associated with trauma. Localized degeneration of the cartilage leads to accumulation of fluid. Needle aspiration yields a yellow oily material. Treatment includes drainage of the cavity followed by application of a pressure dressing. Intralesional steroid injection has also been used successfully.

Christian MM, et al: Asymptomatic swelling of a man's ear: auricular pseudocyst. *Arch Dermatol* 1998, 134:1627.

Ichioka S, et al: Pseudocyst of the auricle: case reports and its biochemical characteristics. *Ann Plast Surg* 1993, 31:471.

Lee JA, et al: Endochondral pseudocyst of the auricle. *J Clin Pathol* 1994, 47:961.

Miyamoto H, et al: Steroid injection therapy for pseudocyst of the auricle. *Acta Derm Venereol* (Norway) 1994, 74:140.

Santos AD, et al: Bilateral pseudocyst of the auricle in an infant girl. *Pediatr Dermatol* 1995, 12:152.

Secor CP, et al: Auricular endochondral pseudocysts: diagnosis and management (review). *Plast Reconstr Surg* 1999, 103:1451. _____ ▲

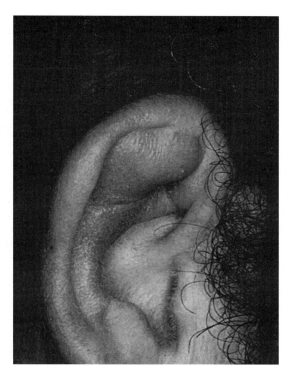

Fig. 29-109 Pseudocyst of the auricle.

Cutaneous Columnar Cysts

Four types of cysts that occur in the skin are lined by columnar epithelium. *Branchiogenic cysts* are small, solitary lesions just above the sternal notch. The cells may have cilia, and the wall contains smooth muscle and mucous glands. *Thyroglossal duct cysts* are similar clinically to branchiogenic cysts except they are usually located on the anterior aspect of the neck. Malignancies (papillary adenocarcinoma, follicular adenocarcinoma, mixed papillary/follicular adenocarcinoma, adenocarcinoma, and squamous cell carcinomas) arising from cysts have been reported in 1% of cases. Histologically, they simulate branchiogenic cysts also, except there is no smooth muscle in the wall, and frequently thyroid follicles are present. *Cutaneous ciliated cysts* are usually located on the legs in females. Men may also be affected. They have also been described in the perineum, vulva, and foot regions. The epithelium seen on biopsy resembles that seen in fallopian tubes. *Median raphe cysts* of the penis are developmental defects lying in the ventral midline of the penis, usually on the glans (Fig. 29-110). Ethanol injection sclerotherapy may be useful in treating thyroglossal duct cysts and branchial cleft cyst. Surgical intervention is standard therapy.

Ashton MA: Cutaneous ciliated cyst of the lower limb in a male. *Histopathology* 1995, 26:467.

Fraga S, et al: Branchiogenic cysts in the skin and subcutaneous tissue. *Am J Clin Pathol* 1971, 56:230.

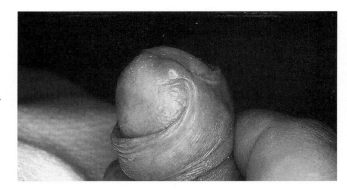

Fig. 29-110   Median raphe cyst.

Fukumoto K, et al: Ethanol injection sclerotherapy for Baker's cyst, thyroglossal duct cyst, and branchial cleft cyst. *Ann Plast Surg* 1994, 33:615.

Greinwald JH Jr, et al: Hereditary thyroglossal duct cysts. *Arch Otolaryngol Head Neck Surg* 1996, 122:1094.

Heymann WR: Cutaneous manifestations of thyroid disease. *J Am Acad Dermatol* 1992, 26:885.

Kang IK, et al: Ciliated cyst of the vulva. *J Am Acad Dermatol* 1995, 32:514.

Miller OF, et al: Cutaneous branchiogenic cysts with papilloma and sinus presentation. *J Am Acad Dermatol* 1984, 11:367.

Osada A, et al: Cutaneous ciliated cyst on the sole of the foot. *Br J Dermatol* 1995, 132:488.

Romani J, et al: Median raphe cyst of the penis with ciliated cells. *J Cutan Pathol* 1995, 22:378.

Sharkey MJ, et al: Postcoital appearance of a median raphe cyst. *J Am Acad Dermatol* 1992, 26:273.

Sidoni A, et al: Ciliated cyst of the perineal skin. *Am J Dermatopathol* 1997, 19:93. _____ ▲

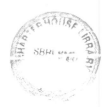

CHAPTER 30

Melanocytic Nevi and Neoplasms

Pigmented nevi and neoplasms may be composed of melanocytes or nevus cells. Melanocytes originate in the embryonal neural crest and migrate to the epidermis, the dermis, the leptomeninges, the retina, the mucous membrane epithelium, and the inner ear, cochlea, and vestibular system. Nevus cell precursors enter the epidermis, dermis, and panniculus, where they may aggregate to form clusters of cells, a feature that distinguishes them from melanocytes. They also do not have dendritic processes, whereas melanocytes do.

EPIDERMAL MELANOCYTIC LESIONS

The normal melanocyte occurring at the epidermal-dermal junction is a dendritic secretory cell that supplies all the normal melanin of the skin. These cells contain pigment granules (melanosomes). They stain with the dopa reaction and silver stains because they contain melanin. Melanocytes of the epidermis transfer the melanosomes through their thin dendritic processes into surrounding keratinocytes. The number and size of the melanosomes in the keratinocytes determine the pigmentation of the skin and hair.

Nevus Spilus

Nevus spilus is a pigmented, light brown or tan macule of varied diameter, speckled with smaller, darker-colored macules or papules (Fig. 30-1). It frequently occurs on the trunk and lower extremities. Two reports have indicated that approximately 2% of those studied had theses lesions.

The nevus spilus may be small, measuring less than 1 cm in diameter, or may be quite large. When large, these nevi may follow a dermatomal or nevoid type of distribution; frequently they do not cross the midline. When this pattern exists, the lesion may be referred to as a *zosteriform,* or sometimes a *speckled lentiginous nevus.* Multiple sites may be involved in the same individual; these sites may be widely separated by normal skin. Additionally, these nevi may be present in combination with a nevus flammeus, in which case the condition is called *phakomatosis pigmentovascularis.* A syndrome comprising an organoid nevus with sebaceous differentiation, hemiatrophy

with muscular weakness and other neurologic findings, and a speckled lentiginous nevus is called *phakomatosis pigmentokeratotica.*

Histologically, the flat tan background may show only basilar hyperpigmentation, such as is present in a café au lait spot, or may show lentiginous proliferation of the epidermis. The darker speckles usually contain nevus cells.

Because nevus cells are often present in the dark speckles, melanoma may arise in them with greater frequency than in normal skin. However, this possibility does not necessitate removal, in our opinion. Removal by Q-switched ruby laser has been reported to be effective.

Casanova D, et al: Management of nevus spilus. *Pediatr Dermatol* 1996, 13:233.

Grevelink JM, et al: Treatment of nevus spilus with the Q-switched ruby laser. *Dermatol Surg* 1997, 23:365.

Grinspan D, et al: Melanoma on dysplastic nevus spilus. *Int J Dermatol* 1997, 36:499.

Kopf AW, et al: Congenital nevus-like nevi, nevi spili, and cafe-au-lait spots in patients with malignant melanoma. *J Dermatol Surg Oncol* 1985, 11:275.

Kopf AW, et al: Prevalence of congenital nevus-like nevi, nevi spili, and cafe au lait spots. *Arch Dermatol* 1985, 121:766.

Libow LF: Phakomatosis pigmentovascularis type IIIb. *J Am Acad Dermatol* 1993, 29:305.

McLean DI, et al: "Sunburn" freckles, cafe-au-lait macules, and other pigmented lesions of schoolchildren. *J Am Acad Dermatol* 1995, 32:565.

Tadini G, et al: Phacomatosis pigmentokeratotica. *Arch Dermatol* 1998, 134:333.

Welch ML, et al: Widespread nevus spilus. *Int J Dermatol* 1993, 32:120.

▲

Lentigo

Lentigo Simplex. One, or far oftener, many of these sharply defined, rounded, brown or black macules may appear anywhere on the body surface or the mucosa. The lesions usually arise in childhood but may appear at any age. They are indistinguishable from junctional nevi. There is no predilection for areas of sun exposure.

Histologically, lentigo simplex shows elongation of the rete ridges, an increase in the number of melanocytes in the basal layer, an increase of melanin in both the melanocytes

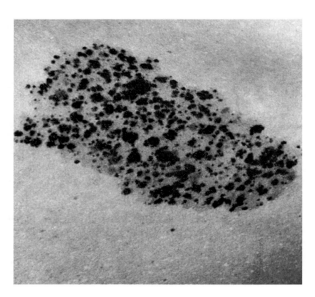

Fig. 30-1 Speckled lentiginous nevus.

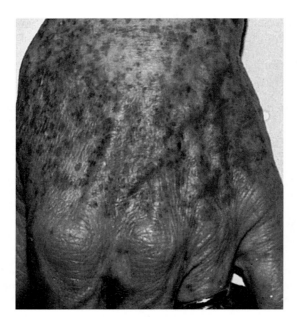

Fig. 30-2 Solar lentigines. Sparing of the knuckles is characteristic.

and basal keratinocytes, and melanophages in the upper dermis.

No therapy is indicated, because there is no predisposition to neoplastic change.

Solar Lentigines (Lentigo Senilis). Solar lentigines are commonly known as *liver spots*. They are persistent, benign, discrete, hyperpigmented macules of irregular shape, occurring on sun-exposed skin. The backs of the hands (Fig. 30-2) and the forehead are favorite sites in the typical middle-aged to older patient. Red-haired, light-skinned individuals, especially those with high solar exposure, may develop many of these on the shoulders and central upper chest, even at an early age. A markedly irregular, reticulated, dark black variant resembling a spot of ink on the skin may occur.

Histologically, the rete ridges appear club-shaped and show small, budlike extensions. There is a marked increase in the number of melanocytes, with increased pigmentation in the basal cell layer and adjacent keratinocytes. The upper dermis often contains melanophages.

Solar lentigines may be accompanied by depigmented macules, actinic purpura, and other chronic actinic degenerative changes in the skin. They may evolve into benign lichenoid keratoses and into seborrheic keratoses. Light application of liquid nitrogen with a cotton-tip applicator is an excellent treatment for these lesions of only cosmetic significance. The argon, Q-switched Nd:YAG, Er:YAG, Q-switched alexandrite, Q-switched ruby, and short pulsed dye lasers have been reported effective in the treatment of lentigines. They may recur, at times as a lentigo maligna or lentigo maligna melanoma. Patients should be told to return for reexamination if pigmentation reappears.

Protective measures, particularly sunscreens, should be taken to prevent excessive exposure to sunlight. Bleaching creams containing 4% or 5% hydroquinone may be used over a period of several months. This induces temporary lightening and may be reused as necessary. Chemical peels and topical tretinoin, either alone or in combination, and salicylic acid ointment are other treatment options.

Individuals receiving oral methoxsalen photochemotherapy (PUVA) or in those frequenting tanning salons may develop persistent lentigines in which there may be cellular atypia, on sites (such as the penis) that are normally protected from sunlight. Also, high-dose single exposures to radiation, such as occurred in accidents like Chernobyl, may result in lentigines in exposed skin.

Penile and Vulvar Melanosis. Penile and vulvar melanosis (Fig. 30-3) are localized pigmentary alterations that may show lentiginous changes on biopsy, but most often show only basilar hyperpigmentation. Occasionally, atypical melanocytes are also present. Mottling of pigmentation may appear in large patches or in smaller, well-demarcated lesions. Such changes may be present on the penis or female genitalia. In the latter location, the labia minora are most often affected.

Bannayan-Riley-Ruvalcaba Syndrome. Bannayan-Riley-Ruvalcaba syndrome is a rare autosomal dominant disorder that first manifests in childhood. Eighty percent of patients are male. The syndrome is characterized by genital

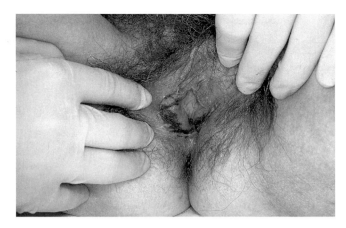

Fig. 30-3 Vulvar melanosis.

lentiginosis, macrocephaly, motor and speech delay, mental retardation, lipomas, hemangiomas, verruca vulgaris, and other types of facial papules, some of which may be syringomas or trichilemmomas, myopathies, and hamartomatous polyps. Additional features reported in some patients are café au lait spots, supernumerary nipples, angiokeratomas, lymphangiomas, acanthosis nigricans, enlarged testes and penis, diabetes, and thyroiditis. An interstitial deletion of 10q23.2-24.1 was reported in one patient. Of interest is the potential relationship to Cowden's disease, which has some minor overlap of clinical features, but its susceptibility gene has been mapped to chromosome 10q22-23. The PTEN gene, a tumor suppressor gene, is mutated in both of these syndromes. One family whose mother has Cowden's syndrome and the son has Bannayan-Riley-Ruvalcaba syndrome has been seen by Dr. Mark Lebwohl.

Multiple Lentigines Syndrome.
Multiple generalized lentigines may occur with a number of associated signs as a dominantly inherited syndrome. The lentigines are dark brown macules from 1 to 5 mm in diameter. There is a preponderance on the trunk, but other areas may also be involved, such as the palms and soles, buccal mucosa, genitalia, and scalp.

The lesions appear shortly after birth and develop a distinctive speckled appearance that has given rise to the designation *LEOPARD syndrome*. LEOPARD is Gorlin's mnemonic acronym for *l*entigines, *e*lectrocardiographic abnormalities, *o*cular hypertelorism, *p*ulmonary stenosis, *ab*normalities of genitalia, *r*etardation of growth, and *d*eafness.

Moynahan Syndrome.
Moynahan syndrome consists of multiple lentigines, congenital mitral stenosis, dwarfism, genital hypoplasia, and mental deficiency.

Generalized Lentiginosis.
An occasional patient will have generalized lentiginosis without associated abnormalities, as in the patient reported by Uhle et al.

Centrofacial Lentiginosis.
Centrofacial lentiginosis is characterized by lentigines on the nose and adjacent cheeks, variously associated with status dysraphicus, multiple skeletal anomalies, and central nervous system disorders. Mucous membranes are spared. Onset is in the first years of life.

Inherited Patterned Lentiginosis in Blacks.
O'Neill et al reported ten light-complexioned black patients who, through autosomal dominant familial inheritance, developed numerous lentigines in infancy or early childhood. The lentigines were distributed over the central face (Fig. 30-4), and lips, with variable involvement of the dorsal hands and feet, elbows, and buttocks. The mucous membranes were spared. No internal abnormalities are associated with this pigmentary pattern.

Partial Unilateral Lentiginosis.
Partial unilateral lentiginosis is a rare disorder of cutaneous pigmentation characterized by the presence of multiple lesions of simple lentigo, wholly or partially involving half of the body. Agminated lentiginosis appears to be a similar if not identical entity.

Carney's Syndrome.
Synonyms for Carney's syndrome are NAME syndrome and LAMB syndrome. This designation comprises cardiocutaneous myxomas, lentigines, blue nevi, and endocrine abnormalities. It is discussed in more detail with myxomas in Chapter 28.

Peutz-Jeghers Syndrome.
Peutz-Jeghers syndrome is an autosomal dominant syndrome consisting of pigmented macules on the lips, oral mucosa, and perioral and acral areas. Gastrointestinal polyps, especially prominent in the jejunum, are frequently associated. It is discussed further under disorders of pigmentation in Chapter 36.

Abel EA, et al: PUVA-induced melanocytic atypia. *J Am Acad Dermatol* 1985, 13:761.

Arch EM, et al: Deletion of PTEN in a patient with Bannayan-Riley-Ruvalcaba syndrome suggest allelism with Cowden's disease. *Am J Med Genet* 1997, 71:489.

Arnsmeier SL, et al: Pigmentary anomalies in the multiple lentigines syndrome. *Pediatr Dermatol* 1996, 13:100.

Berger TG, et al: Lichenoid benign keratoses. *J Am Acad Dermatol* 1984, 11:635.

Ber-Rahman S, et al: Lentigo. *Int J Dermatol* 1996, 35:229.

Bolognia JL: Reticulated black solar lentigo ("ink spot" lentigo). *Arch Dermatol* 1992, 128:934.

Coppin BD, et al: Multiple lentigines syndrome (LEOPARD syndrome or progressive cardiomyopathic lentiginosis). *J Med Genet* 1997, 34:582.

Fargnoli MC, et al: Clinicopathologic findings in the Bannayan-Riley-Ruvalcaba syndrome. *Arch Dermatol* 1996, 132:1214.

Giardello FM, et al: Increased risk of cancer in the Peutz-Jeghers syndrome. *N Engl J Med* 1987, 316:1511.

Humphreys TR, et al: Treatment of photodamaged skin with trichloroacetic acid and topical tretinoin. *J Am Acad Dermatol* 1996, 34:638.

Jackson R: Melanosis of the vulva. *J Dermatol Surg Oncol* 1984, 10:119.

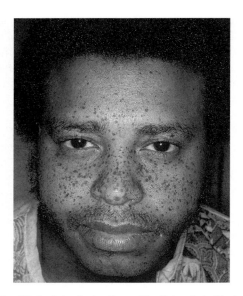

Fig. 30-4 Inherited patterned lentiginosis in blacks.

Jih DM, et al: A histopathologic evaluation of vulvar melanosis. *Arch Dermatol* 1999, 135:857.

Kanj LF, et al: Vulvar melanosis and lentiginosis. *J Am Acad Dermatol* 1992, 27:777.

Lee PK, et al: Failure of Q-switched ruby laser to eradicate atypical-appearing solar lentigo. *J Am Acad Dermatol* 1998, 38:314.

Leicht S, et al: Atypical pigmented penile macules. *Arch Dermatol* 1988, 124:1267.

Li J, et al: PTEN, a putative protein tyrosinase phosphatase gene mutated in human brain, breast, and prostate cancer. *Science* 1997, 75:1943.

Micali G, et al: Agminated lentiginosis. *Pediatr Dermatol* 1994, 11:241.

O'Neill JF, et al: Inherited patterned lentiginosis in blacks. *Arch Dermatol* 1989, 125:1231.

Peter RU, et al: Radiation lentigo. *Arch Dermatol* 1997, 133:209.

Pique E, et al: Partial unilateral lentiginosis. *Clin Exp Dermatol* 1995, 20:319.

Revuz J, et al: Penile melanosis. *J Am Acad Dermatol* 1989, 20:567.

Stratakis CA, et al: Carney complex, a familial multiple neoplasia and lentiginosis syndrome. *J Clin Invest* 1996, 97:699.

Swinehart JM: Salicylic acid ointment peeling of the hands and forearms. *J Dermatol Surg Oncol* 1992, 18:495.

Trattner A, et al: Partial unilateral lentiginosis. *J Am Acad Dermatol* 1993, 29:693.

Uhle P, et al: Generalized lentiginosis. *J Am Acad Dermatol* 1988, 18:444. ▲

MELANOACANTHOMA

Cutaneous melanoacanthoma is an uncommon lesion first described by Bloch. It is a benign epidermal melanocytic neoplasm, occurring on the head. Clinically, it resembles a pigmented seborrheic keratosis or pigmented basal cell carcinoma. Its onset is slow, and it occurs predominantly in white men older than 60 years of age.

Histologically, melanoacanthoma is a benign neoplasm composed of keratinocytes and large dendritic melanocytes, filled with pigment.

Oral melanoacanthoma is also a proliferation of two cell types, melanocytes and epithelial cells; however, it appears to be a reactive lesion. It occurs on the oral tissues, predominantly in young black women. A rapid onset and spontaneous resolution is typical.

Eisen D, et al: Oral melanoma and other pigmented lesions of the oral cavity. *J Am Acad Dermatol* 1991, 24:527.

Simon P, et al: How rare is melanoacanthoma? *Arch Dermatol* 1991, 127:583.

Zemtsov A, et al: Oral melanoacanthoma with prominent spongiotic intraepithelial vesicles. *J Cutan Pathol* 1989, 16:365. _____ ▲

CELLULAR NEVI

The common mole, also known as *nevus cell* or *nevocytic nevus* and *cellular nevus,* is not stable; it grows, going through changes of maturation, and even of senescence. They begin to appear in the first years of life and increase in prevalence and number of lesions over the following two to three decades, after which there is a steady decline. Females tend to have more nevi than males, and whites more than blacks. They are less common in doubly covered areas, such as the buttocks, except in the dysplastic nevus syndrome, or in other relatively sun-protected sites, such as the inner arms. They typically reach their maximum size within a few years and do not continue to enlarge.

The typical nevus cell is oval or cuboid and has a distinctly outlined homogeneous cytoplasm. The nucleus is large, round or oval, pale, and vesicular. Nevus cells show variations in appearance. In the upper dermis they appear epithelioid, while in the lower dermis, they may resemble fibroblasts or Schwannian cells. Nevus cells are apparently modified melanocytes without dendrites.

INCIDENCE AND PREVALENCE. The maximum number of nevi is present between ages 20 and 25, and the average number is 40. From then on the lesions flatten and fade, disappearing completely by age 90. Nevi begin as small, flat, pigmented macules called *junctional nevi.* Over time most develop into compound, and finally intradermal, nevi.

Sun exposure appears to increase the number of moles in the exposed skin. Australians have more moles than Europeans. Whites have more than blacks, and individuals with a light complexion have more nevi than those with a dark complexion. Women tend to have more nevi on the legs, and men more on the trunk; sun exposure presumably accounts for this. Blacks have more nevi than whites on the palms, soles, conjunctivae, and nail beds. Plantar nevi are slightly more common than palmar lesions, while conjunctival nevi occur in only about 1% of patients. Mucous membrane and nail bed nevi are unusual in all patients.

Eruptive nevi are rare but may occur after severe bullous disease such as toxic epidermal necrolysis, erythema multiforme, or severe sunburn, Addison's disease with HIV infection, or other types of immunosuppression including that seen in transplant patients or in individuals with leukemia. A halolike dermatitis may occur around nevi that, when it clears, leaves the nevus unchanged. The appearance of multiple so-called Myerson's nevi has been reported to occur during interferon alfa-2a given for Behçet's syndrome.

CLINICAL AND HISTOLOGIC FEATURES. The junctional nevus is a smooth, hairless, light to dark brown macule, varying in size from 1 to 6 mm in diameter. It may have the characteristic appearance of a target or a fried egg. It occurs at any site on the body surface. On the palms, soles (Fig. 30-5), or scrotum, pigmented nevi are usually of the junctional type. Junctional nevi may be present at birth (Figs. 30-6 and 30-7) but usually appear between 3 and 18 years of age. During adolescence and adulthood, some of these junctional nevi will become compound or intradermal. However, they may persist into or develop during adulthood.

The junctional nevus usually remains flat until the nevus cells extend into the dermis. The nevus is then said to become compound—that is, both junctional and intradermal (Figs. 30-8 and 30-9). Later, junctional proliferation ceases and the nevus cells become separated from the epidermis by a band of connective tissue to produce the intradermal nevus, which is the type usually found in middle-aged persons. The lesions may be dome-shaped, sessile, warty or smooth papules, flesh-colored or brown to black, and with or without hairs (Fig. 30-10).

The junctional nevus is characterized by the presence of single melanocytes, or theques of them, in the lower levels of the epidermis. The compound nevus is one that is still manifesting so-called junctional activity (accumulation of melanocytes in theques in the epidermis) but has the formed structure of a cellular nevus in the dermis as well. The intradermal nevus is simply a compound nevus in which junctional activity—that is, theques of melanocytes in the epidermis or at the dermoepidermal junction—has ceased, and all the nevus cells are in the dermis.

MALIGNANT DEGENERATION. The signs of malignant transformation in pigmented nevi are recent enlargement, an irregular or scalloped border, asymmetry, changes or variegation in color (especially red, white, or blue), surface changes (scaling, erosion, oozing, crusting, ulceration, or bleeding), development of a palpable thickening, development of pain or tenderness, signs of inflammation, or the appearance of satellite pigmentation. The "ugly duckling" sign refers to the fact that nevi in an individual generally share a common profile, so one that does not share the same characteristics as the majority of other lesions should be considered for biopsy. Likewise, clinically atypical nevi are less likely to be melanoma if other nevi in the patient share similar features, such as may be present in the dysplastic nevus syndrome. Nevi with small dark dots that do not lie entirely within the lesion, but produce a small extension

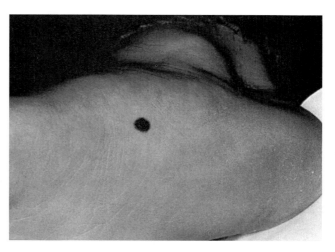

Fig. 30-5 Junctional nevus on the sole.

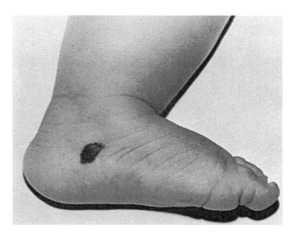

Fig. 30-6 Junctional nevus near the heel of an infant.

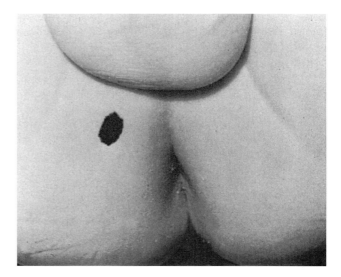

Fig. 30-7 Junctional nevus near the perineum of an infant.

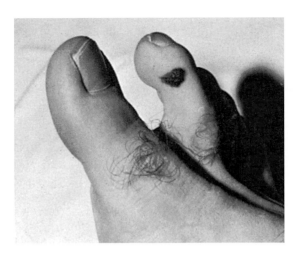

Fig. 30-8   Compound nevus. The lesion is slightly elevated.

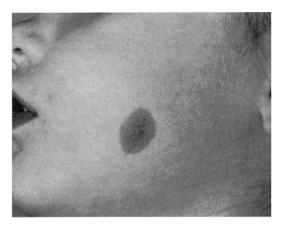

Fig. 30-9   Compound nevus. Note the fine dark hairs.

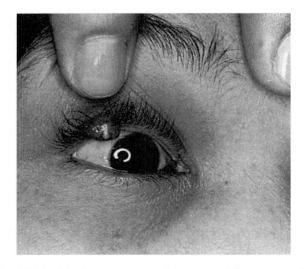

Fig. 30-10   Intradermal nevus on the margin of the upper eyelid.

beyond the border, may represent melanoma. The clinician should alert the pathologist about this dot and the pathologist should section through the appropriate area. Variegation in color may also be present when there is perifollicular hypopigmentation. This benign occurrence may be present at the edge of the nevus and give the lesion outline a notched appearance.

The development of what appears to be a new pigmented nevus in a patient over 35 years of age should alert the physician to possible melanoma, because approximately half of melanomas occur in preexisting nevi, but half develop in previously normal skin. Patients without the dysplastic nevus syndrome usually do not develop new nevi at this age.

Features that suggest benignancy are as follows: diameter of 3 mm or less; perfectly uniform pigmentation; flaccid epidermis; smooth, uniform border; and an unchanging size and color.

There may be clinical changes with pregnancy or with oral contraceptive use. Nevi from normal persons have no estrogen or progesterone receptors; there may be positive estrogen receptor binding in nevi from pregnant women, as is also found in malignant melanoma. Although some changes in nevi during pregnancy are not unexpected, if a lesion develops signs of malignant transformation biopsy is indicated. The pathologist should be alerted to the clinical situation as nevocellular nevi may have unusual histologic features during pregnancy and in children.

TREATMENT. The management of nevi is a perplexing problem. Clearly, if all moles were removed, thousands of melanomas would be prevented. Just as obviously, this would be impossibly impractical, and too costly. There are too many. Acquired (as opposed to congenital) nevi should be removed if they show signs of malignant transformation (see above), or if the patient desires removal for cosmetic reasons—and if they are so unsightly that a keloid or hypertrophic scar could look no worse. Nevi of the neckline, beltline, or other areas that are irritated may be removed to relieve the patient of the irritation.

Nevi within the hairy scalp are uncommon. They should be removed if atypical, because it is impractical to try to watch them. If a solitary pigmented lesion is present on the oral or vaginal mucous membrane, a biopsy should be performed, because nevi are uncommon in these locations. When melanomas are diagnosed, they are frequently deeply invasive, because these sites are less likely to be routinely observed. Nail matrix nevi produce a pigmented nail band. Most commonly these bands are produced by melanocytic activation and not by nevi or melanoma but it is impossible to distinguish them clinically. Hutchinson's sign of pigmentation over the nail fold as an indicator of melanoma is at times hard to distinguish from the pigmentation of the overlying transparent cuticle and proximal nail fold (pseudo-Hutchinson's sign). Biopsy of an acquired longitudinal pigmented band in an adult involving only one nail is necessary to ascertain the cause. Nail matrix melanoma in children is exceptional, and routine nail biopsy has not been recommended in these cases.

Conjunctival nevi occur, and most can be serially followed if the lesion has been present since childhood or has shown no evidence of growth. Suspicion of melanoma should arise if conjunctival nevi occur in the palpebral or forniceal conjunctiva, if they are not hinged at the limbus and are immovable, if they extend into the cornea, if there is canalicular obstruction that leads to tearing, or if a leash of vessels is noted in a nevus.

Biopsy should always be performed in tarsal pigmentation. Because there are several other pigmented lesions besides the nevocellular nevus, some of which are premalignant, such as the flat, golden to chocolate brown, unilateral, primary acquired melanosis, changing pigmented lesions and those acquired after childhood are best evaluated by an ophthalmologist.

Bolognia JL, et al: Perifollicular hypopigmentation. *Arch Dermatol* 1992, 128:514.

Bolognia JL, et al: The significance of eccentric foci of hyperpigmentation (small dark dots) within melanocytic nevi. *Arch Dermatol* 1994, 130:1013.

Buchner A, et al: Pigmented nevi of the oral mucosa. *Oral Surg* 1987, 63:676.

Christiansen WN, et al: Histologic characteristics of vulvar nevocellular nevi. *J Cutan Pathol* 1987, 14:87.

Coleman WP, et al: Nevi, lentigines, and melanomas in blacks. *Arch Dermatol* 1980, 116:548.

Eisen D, et al: Oral melanoma and other pigmented lesions of the oral cavity. *J Am Acad Dermatol* 1991, 24:527.

Ellis DL, et al: Increased nevus estrogen and progesterone ligand binding related to oral contraceptives or pregnancy. *J Am Acad Dermatol* 1986, 14:25.

Farber M, et al: Pigmented lesions of the conjunctiva. *J Am Acad Dermatol* 1998, 38:971.

Fitzsimons CP, et al: A study of the total number and distribution of melanocytic nevi in a British population. *Br J Dermatol* 1984, 111(Suppl):9.

Foucar E, et al: A histopathologic evaluation of nevocellular nevi in pregnancy. *Arch Dermatol* 1985, 121:350.

Grin JM, et al: Ocular melanomas and melanocytic lesions of the eye. *J Am Acad Dermatol* 1998, 38:716.

Grob JJ, et al: The "ugly duckling" sign. *Arch Dermatol* 1998, 134:103.

Harrison SL, et al: Body-site distribution of melanocytic nevi in young Australian children. *Arch Dermatol* 1999, 135:47.

Holly EA, et al: Number of melanocytic nevi as a major risk factor for malignant melanoma. *J Am Acad Dermatol* 1987, 17:459.

Kirscher J, et al: Interferon alfa-2a-induced Myerson's nevi in a patient with dysplastic nevus syndrome. *J Am Acad Dermatol* 1999, 40:105.

Luther H, et al: Increase of melanocytic nevus counts in children during 5 years of follow-up and analysis of associated factors. *Arch Dermatol* 1996, 132:1473.

Mackie RM, et al: The number and distribution of benign pigmented moles in a healthy British population. *Br J Dermatol* 1985, 113:167.

Pennoyer JW, et al: Changes in size of melanocytic nevi during pregnancy. *J Am Acad Dermatol* 1997, 36:378.

Pope DJ, et al: Benign pigmented nevi in children. *Arch Dermatol* 1992, 128:1201.

Rampen FHJ, et al: Frequency of moles as a key to melanoma incidence? *J Am Acad Dermatol* 1986, 15:1200.

Richert S, et al: Widespread eruptive dermal and atypical melanocytic nevi in association with chronic myelocytic leukemia. *J Am Acad Dermatol* 1996, 35:326.

Shoji T, et al: Eruptive melanocytic nevi after Stevens-Johnson syndrome. *J Am Acad Dermatol* 1997, 37:337.

Swerdlow AJ, et al: Benign melanocytic nevi as a risk factor for malignant melanoma. *Br Med J* 1986, 292:1555.

Tosti A, et al: Nail matrix nevi. *J Am Acad Dermatol* 1996, 34:765. ▲

Pseudomelanoma (Recurrent Nevus)

Melanotic lesions clinically resembling a superficial spreading melanoma may occur at the site of a recent removal (usually by shave excision) of a melanocytic nevus. Although some recurrent nevi may simulate melanoma histologically, there is fibrosis in the upper dermis, often remnants of the original nevus beneath this zone of fibrosis, and sharp lateral demarcation corresponding to the clinical confinement of the pigmentation to the scar.

Dwyer CM, et al: Pseudomelanoma after dermabrasion. *J Am Acad Dermatol* 1993, 28:263.

Goldenhersh MA, et al: Recurrent melanocytic nevi after Solcoderm therapy. *J Am Acad Dermatol* 1992, 27:1012.

Park HK, et al: Recurrent melanocytic nevi. *J Am Acad Dermatol* 1987, 17:285. ▲

Balloon Cell Nevus

The balloon cell nevus is a pigmented nevus, varying in size from 1 to 5 mm, usually occurring on the head, neck, trunk, and occasionally elsewhere, such as the arm and the foot. Clinically, the lesions are indistinguishable from the ordinary pigmented or nonpigmented nevus.

Histologically, the lesions are composed of peculiar vesicular cells that appear to be foamy and form large pale polyhedral balloon cells that may be multinucleated giant cells. In addition, nevus cells are also evident. The two types of cells form nests or theques throughout the epidermis and dermis. Occasionally, the lesions are composed entirely of balloon cells.

These nevi are not considered potentially malignant, and treatment is along the conventional lines of other nevi. Balloon cell melanoma does exist, but here the cells are pleomorphic, the nuclei are larger, the cytoplasm is scantier, and mitoses can be observed.

Cote J, et al: Halo balloon cell nevus. *J Cutan Pathol* 1986, 13:123.

Goette DK, et al: Balloon cell nevus. *Arch Dermatol* 1978, 114:109. ▲

Halo Nevus

Halo nevus is also known as *Sutton's nevus, perinevoid vitiligo,* and *leukoderma acquisitum centrifugum.* The halo nevus is characterized by a pigmented nevus, with a surrounding depigmented zone. The nevus is usually a compound or intradermal nevus with a concentric area of depigmentation that has a regular, sharply demarcated border (Fig. 30-11). It may be single or multiple and occurs most frequently on the trunk (Fig. 30-12). These lesions develop mostly in teenagers.

Immunologically induced rejection of melanin or of a melanoma beginning in the nevus has been suggested as the mode of pathogenesis. There may be associated vitiligo (Fig. 30-13). Of course, melanoma in a state of regression may have associated leukoderma; however, the pattern is usually more haphazard and wholly within the pigmented lesion. This suggests commonality of etiologic factors; indeed, patients with halo nevi possess antibodies to melanocytes and cell-mediated immunity to melanoma cells.

Although the nevocellular nevus is the tumor most frequently found surrounded by a halo, many other lesions may also have a surrounding zone of leukoderma. These are the blue nevus, the neurofibroma, the neural nevus, the spindle and epithelioid cell nevus, congenital nevus, and melanoma.

Histologically, amelanotic dopa-positive melanocytes may be found in the leukodermic halo. In the central lesion the nevus cells form a compound or intradermal nevus with an associated dermal infiltrate.

Treatment of the halo nevus is not indicated. The central nevus will usually disappear in time. The leukodermic area will remain depigmented for an unpredictable time, but eventually repigmentation may take place. Full mucocutaneous examination at the time of diagnosis is indicated to exclude a concurrent melanoma.

Baranda L, et al: Presence of activated lymphocytes in the peripheral blood of patients with halo nevi. *J Am Acad Dermatol* 1999, 41:567.

Berman B, et al: Halo giant congenital melanocytic nevus. *J Am Acad Dermatol* 1988, 19:954.

Mooney MA, et al: Halo nevus or halo phenomenon? *J Cutan Pathol* 1995, 22:342.

Zeff RA, et al: The immune response in halo nevi. *J Am Acad Dermatol* 1997, 37:620. _____ ▲

Congenital Nevocytic Nevus

Giant Pigmented Nevus (Giant Hairy Nevus, Bathing Trunk Nevus). The giant pigmented nevus is a distinctive pigmented nevus characterized by a large, darkly pigmented

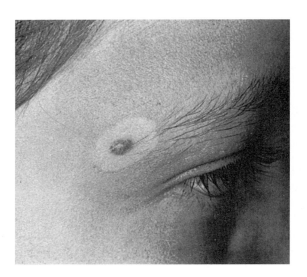

Fig. 30-11 Halo nevus on the lateral aspect of the forehead.

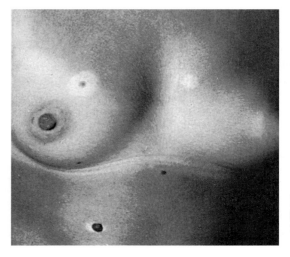

Fig. 30-12 Multiple halo nevi.

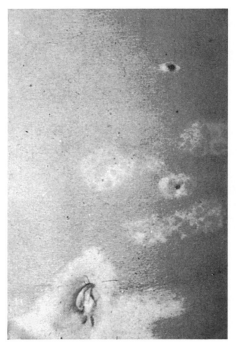

Fig. 30-13 Perinevoid vitiligo and vitiligo on upper abdomen.

hairy patch (Fig. 30-14) in which smaller, darker patches are interspersed or present as small satellite lesions. The skin may be thickened and verrucous. A tendency to follow a dermatome distribution results in a typical picture in most instances. The trunk is a favored site (Fig. 30-15), more especially the upper or lower parts of the back (Fig. 30-16). Giant hairy nevi are present at birth and grow proportionally to the site of the body on which they are located. By definition they measure more than 20 cm in diameter. When a large congenital nevus involves the axial skin, there may be an associated *neurocutaneous melanocytosis*. Some congenital melanocytic nevi may have associated placental infiltration by benign melanocytes.

The incidence of melanomas developing in giant congenital pigmented nevi is approximately 3% to 7%. About 40% of the malignant melanomas seen in children occur in large congenital nevi. The risk is apparently greatest for axial lesions: DeDavid et al did not observe any melanomas that developed in the associated small satellite lesions or solely

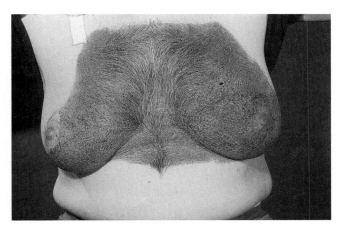

Fig. 30-14   Giant pigmented nevus.

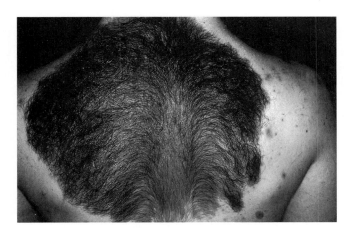

Fig. 30-15   Giant pigmented nevus.

in extremity giant congenital nevi (although the number of the latter patients was small in their study). Furthermore, if neurocutaneous melanosis is present, which can be detected by magnetic resonance imaging scans, the risk of dying at a young age is high secondary to hydrocephalus or the development of leptomeningeal melanoma.

Histologically, giant nevi classically include nevus cells in the lower two thirds of the dermis, occasionally extending into the subcutis. These cells are found between collagen bundles and in association with eccrine or pilosebaceous structures in the midreticular dermis or below. Immunohistochemical staining or serial sections may at times be necessary to delineate some of these findings. Also, estrogen and progesterone binding is present in giant, as well as smaller, congenital nevi. These receptors are commonly present in other precursor lesions of melanoma, such as dysplastic nevi but are generally absent from common acquired nevi.

Most authorities recommend total surgical excision of the entire giant pigmented nevus and resurfacing with autografts. This does not eliminate the risk of leptomeningeal melanoma in patients with leptomeningeal melanosis. Because these children have a poor prognosis, the decision may be made to spare them extensive surgical intervention. Conversely, excision would eliminate a large area of involved skin, and serial scans and close neurosurgical observation could result in the early detection of a melanoma of the brain at a time at which it could be resectable. Additionally, current data indicate satellite lesions and extremity lesions may have a lower incidence of neoplastic conversion. Finally, some lesions are not amenable to excision as they are so extensive or involve functionally critical areas.

Alternative approaches to treatment—dermabrasion, curettage, and laser ablation—are designed to eliminate some of the nevus cells, with theoretic lowering of the melanoma risk, and to improve the cosmetic appearance of these large lesions. Although approximately two thirds of melanomas occurring in congenital nevi arise from nonepidermal sites, which compromises early detection, lifelong periodic cutaneous examinations and general medical evaluations are indicated.

Small and Medium-Sized Congenital Nevocytic Nevus.
Small congenital nevocytic nevi are defined as less than 1.5 cm in greatest diameter, and medium-sized lesions measure more than 1.5 cm but less than 20 cm (Fig. 30-17). They are found in about 1% of newborns. About half eventually become hairy. Walton et al found pigmented lesions in 2.5% of newborns, but only about a third were nevocytic nevi.

Histologically, these are similar to acquired nevi, but they often have deeper involvement, consisting of spindle cells that may extend into the subcutaneous tissue and also may surround the adnexa, vessels, and nerves. Sometimes these features may also occur in acquired nevi.

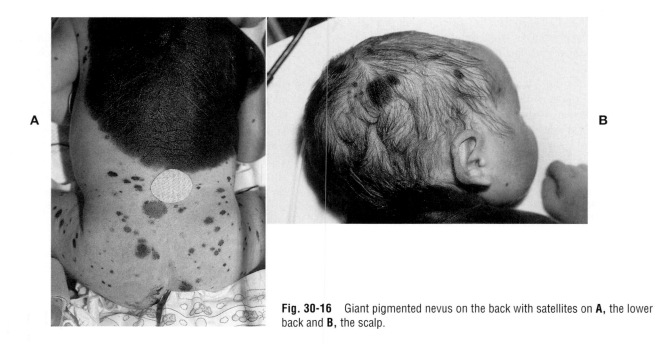

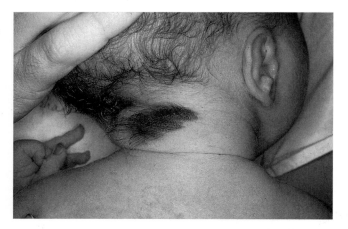

Fig. 30-16 Giant pigmented nevus on the back with satellites on **A,** the lower back and **B,** the scalp.

Fig. 30-17 Congenital nevocytic nevus, medium-sized.

Data are starting to accumulate regarding the frequency of melanoma occurring in these relatively common lesions. These are reassuring that such lesions, which involve unexcisable structures, or those without unusual features that are present in an area easily observed by the patient, can be observed as long as lifelong medical observation is followed. Excision is recommended for lesions of the hairy scalp, or those of great cosmetic concern or nevi that have unusual clinical features. Illig et al reviewed 52 cases in which melanoma had occurred in congenital nevi less than 10 cm in diameter. All occurred in patients over 18 and originated within the epidermis. If the physician and patient determine that excision is appropriate for this size congen-ital nevi, a reasonable course is to follow these lesions until they can be excised under local anesthesia.

Alper J: Congenital nevi. *Arch Dermatol* 1985, 121:734.

Alper J: The incidence and significance of birthmarks in a cohort of 4,641 newborns. *Pediatr Dermatol* 1983, 1:58.

Ball RA, et al : Congenital melanocytic nevi with placental infiltration by melanocytes. *Arch Dermatol* 1998, 134:711.

Barnhill RL, et al: Histologic features of congenital melanocytic nevi in infants 1 year of age or younger. *J Am Acad Dermatol* 1995, 33:780.

Carroll CB, et al: Severely atypical medium-sized congenital nevus with widespread satellitosis and placental deposits in a neonate. *J Am Acad Dermatol* 1994, 30:825.

Casanova D, et al: Early curettage of giant congenital naevi in children. *Br J Dermatol* 1998, 138:341.

Ceballos PI, et al: Melanoma in children. *N Engl J Med* 1995, 332:656.

Coskey RJ, et al: Congenital subungual nevus. *J Am Acad Dermatol* 1983, 9:747.

DeDavid M, et al: A study of large congenital melanocytic nevi and associated malignant melanomas. *J Am Acad Dermatol* 1997, 36:409.

DeDavid M, et al: Neurocutaneous melanosis. *J Am Acad Dermatol* 1996, 35:529.

DeRaeve LE, et al: Neonatal curettage of giant congenital melanocytic nevi. *Arch Dermatol* 1996, 132:20.

Egan CL, et al: Cutaneous melanoma risk and phenotypic changes in large congenital nevi. *J Am Acad Dermatol* 1998, 39:1998.

Ellis DL, et al: Estrogen and progesterone receptors in congenital nevocytic nevi. *J Am Acad Dermatol* 1985, 12:235.

Ellis DL, et al: Estrogen and progesterone receptors in melanocytic lesions. *Arch Dermatol* 1985, 121:1282.

Frieden IJ, et al: Neonatal curettage of giant congenital melanocytic nevi. *J Am Acad Dermatol* 1994, 31:423.

Grevelink JM, et al: Clinical and histological responses of congenital melanocytic nevi after single treatment with Q-switched lasers. *Arch Dermatol* 1997, 133:349.

Illig L, et al: Congenital nevi <10 cm as precursors to melanoma. *Arch Dermatol* 1985, 121:1274.

Imayama S, et al: Long- and short-term histological observations of congenital nevi treated with the normal-mode ruby laser. *Arch Dermatol* 1999, 135:1211.

Keipert JA, et al: Giant pigmented nevi. *Aust J Dermatol* 1985, 26:81.

Kopf AW, et al: Prevalence of congenital nevus-like nevi, nevi spili, and cafe-au-lait spots. *Arch Dermatol* 1985, 121:766.

Kroon S, et al: Incidence of congenital melanocytic nevi in newborn babies in Denmark. *J Am Acad Dermatol* 1987, 17:422.

Management of congenital melanocytic nevi. *Pediatr Dermatol* 1996, 13:321.

Marghoob AA, et al: Large congenital melanocytic nevi and the risk for the development of malignant melanoma. *Arch Dermatol* 1996, 132:170.

National Institutes of Health Consensus Development Conference. *J Am Acad Dermatol* 1984, 10:683.

Nickoloff BJ, et al: Immunohistologic patterns of congenital nevocellular nevi. *Arch Dermatol* 1986, 122:1263.

Rhodes AR, et al: A histologic comparison of congenital and acquired nevomelanocytic nevi. *Arch Dermatol* 1985, 121:1266.

Rhodes AR, et al: Congenital nevomelanocytic nevi. *J Am Acad Dermatol* 1996, 34:51.

Rompel R, et al: Dermabrasion of congenital nevocellular nevi. *Dermatology* 1997, 194:261.

Ruiz-Maldonado R, Orozco-Covarrubias ML: Malignant melanoma in children: a review. *Arch Dermatol* 1997, 133:363.

Sahin S, et al: Risk of melanoma in medium-sized congenital melanocytic nevi. *J Am Acad Dermatol* 1998, 39:428.

Shpall S, et al: Risk of malignant transformation of congenital melanocytic nevi in blacks. *Pediatr Dermatol* 1994, 11:204.

Swerdlow AJ, et al: The risk of melanoma in patients with congenital nevi. *J Am Acad Dermatol* 1995, 32:595.

Ueda S, et al: Normal-mode ruby laser for treating congenital nevi. *Arch Dermatol* 1997, 133:355.

Waldorf HA, et al: Treatment of small and medium congenital nevi with the Q-switched ruby laser. *Arch Dermatol* 1996, 132:301.

Walton RG, et al: Pigmented lesions in newborn infants. *Br J Dermatol* 1976, 95:389.

Williams ML, et al: Melanoma, melanocytic nevi, and other melanoma risk factors in children. *J Pediatr* 1994, 124:833.

Yosipovitch G, et al: Poliosis associated with a giant congenital nevus. *Arch Dermatol* 1999, 135:859. ─────────────── ▲

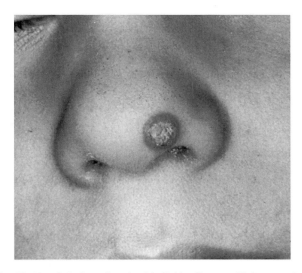

Fig. 30-18 Spindle-cell and epithelioid cell nevus (Spitz nevus) on the nose of child.

Epithelioid and Spindle-Cell Nevus (Benign Juvenile Melanoma, Spitz Nevus)

The Spitz nevus is a smooth-surfaced, raised, round, slightly scaly, firm papule with a distinctive pink, brownish red, or purplish red color (Fig. 30-18). Most frequently, Spitz nevi occur during the first two decades of life, although it occurs in adulthood in about a third of the cases. Typical is the firm, rosy papule on the face, especially on the cheek, some 3 to 10 mm in diameter; however, the legs are the most frequent site of the pigmented type. There is a female predominance. Spitz nevi are rarely diagnosed in persons of color.

Infrequently, multiple lesions are present and they may occasionally occur as agminate lesions (clustered papules) in children and adults. These frequently develop on a hyperpigmented base. Widespread eruptive Spitz nevi occur rarely.

The Spitz nevus is a variant of the compound nevus. Microscopic analysis reveals that the epidermal changes are mainly those of irregular acanthosis, striking pseudoepithe-liomatous hyperplasia, and thinning of the epidermis. In the upper dermis, edema and ectasia of the various vascular elements may be present. The nevus cells are pleomorphic. They are mostly spindle-shaped (fusiform) cells or, less frequently, polygonal (epithelioid) cells. Giant cells with eosinophilic cytoplasm and a large nucleus may be seen. Multinucleated giant cells are observed less frequently. Many of these giant cells are prominent, because they are surrounded by intense edema. In adults, increased fibrosis in the deep dermis may be seen, although no features distinguish the childhood lesion from that of the adult type. Eosinophilic globules with fibrillar microstructure (Kamino bodies) are found in 60% to 85% of Spitz nevi. They may also be present in melanomas (12%) and compound nevi (8%), but they are fewer and smaller than in Spitz nevi. Immunohistochemical staining for MIB-1 and bcl-2 will distinguish most Spitz nevi from melanoma; melanomas are immunoreactive, whereas Spitz nevi generally are not.

Most frequently, Spitz nevus is misdiagnosed clinically as a pyogenic granuloma, mastocytoma, juvenile xanthogranuloma, or melanoma.

The Spitz nevus should be completely excised and a specimen examined histologically. Full excision is recommended to prevent confusion with melanoma in the unlikely event of recurrence.

Arbuckle S, et al: Eosinophilic globules in the Spitz nevus. *J Am Acad Dermatol* 1982, 7:324.

Bullen R, et al: Multiple agminated Spitz nevi. *Pediatr Dermatol* 1995, 12:156.

Casso EM, et al: Spitz nevi. *J Am Acad Dermatol* 1992, 27:901.

Kanter-Lewensohn L, et al: Immunohistochemical markers for distinguishing Spitz nevi from malignant melanomas. *Mod Pathol* 1997, 10:917.

Kaye VN, et al: Spindle and epithelioid cell nevus (Spitz nevus). *Arch Dermatol* 1990, 126:1581.

Merot Y: Transepidermal elimination of nevus cells in spindle and epithelioid cell (Spitz) nevus. *Arch Dermatol* 1988, 124:1441.

Prose NS, et al: Multiple benign juvenile melanoma. *J Am Acad Dermatol* 1983, 9:236.

Sau P, et al: Pigmented spindle cell nevus. *J Am Acad Dermatol* 1993, 28:565.

Smith SA, et al: Eruptive widespread Spitz nevi. *JAMA* 1986, 15:1155.

Spatz A, et al: The Spitz tumor 50 years later. *J Am Acad Dermatol* 1999, 40:223. ▲

Dysplastic Nevus

In 1978, Clark et al described families with unusual nevi and multiple melanomas, a condition they referred to as the *B-K mole syndrome* (after Family B and Family K). About the same time, Lynch et al recognized similar findings in families they were studying, and they designated this the *familial atypical multiple mole–melanoma syndrome.* Since that time our understanding of this autosomal dominant syndrome has grown rapidly. The most widely accepted term for the marker lesions is *dysplastic nevus,* with the patients' condition called the *dysplastic nevus syndrome* (DNS). Patients with dysplastic nevi who have at least two blood relatives with dysplastic nevi and melanoma have the worst prognosis for development of melanoma; some investigators estimate there is a 100% lifetime risk. An associated increased risk of developing pancreatic carcinoma is present in some families. Some studies have indicated ocular melanomas may occur in these patients; however, other authors dispute these findings.

The genetic basis for familial melanoma is being elucidated. A quarter to a third of patients have germline mutations on chromosome 9p in the CDKN2A tumor-suppressor gene (also known as *p16, MTS1,* and *p16INK4A*). It encodes for an inhibitor of a cyclin-dependent kinase 4 (CDK4) that functions to suppress proliferation. In patients with mutations that impair the function of the p16 suppressor protein, referred to as the *p16M alleles,* there is a concomitant predisposition to pancreatic cancer. In other families where this is not present and who have 16W alleles, the predisposition to melanoma does not correlate with an elevated risk of pancreatic cancer.

Mutations in the CDK4 gene have also been found to be responsible for a lesser number of cases of familial melanomas. This was to be expected, because the products of this gene interact with the same cell growth cycle process as p16. Other hereditary gene mutations await discovery.

Dysplastic nevi may also occur commonly in patients without a personal or family history of melanoma, with 5% to 20% of patients having at least one clinically dysplastic nevus, depending on the criteria used in the study. In this situation, the importance appears to be threefold: (1) the nevi need to be histologically differentiated from melanoma in some cases; (2) they serve to initiate a careful history, and in some cases an inspection of other family members, for

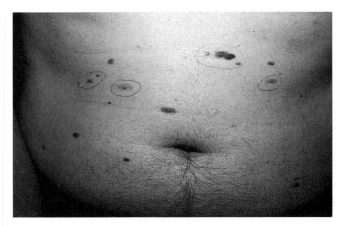

Fig. 30-19 Dysplastic nevi.

the presence of melanoma or dysplastic nevi; and (3) they provide another risk factor for melanoma predisposition, together with such other findings as total nevus count, skin type, freckle density, eye color, and history of blistering sunburns. The relative risk defined by the presence of these lesions is strong, in the order of threefold to forty-threefold, depending on the number of dysplastic nevi present.

Dysplastic nevi (Fig. 30-19) differ from common acquired nevi in several respects. The typical dysplastic nevus is clinically characterized by a variegated tan, brown, and pink coloration, with the pink hues seen mainly in the macular portion of the nevus. A macular component is always present and may comprise the entire lesion but frequently surrounds a papular center. The nevi are larger than are common nevi, usually 5 to 12 mm in diameter (common nevi usually measure 6 mm or less). The shape of dysplastic nevi is very irregular, with frequent angulated, indistinct borders. There is marked lesion-to-lesion variability. The unusual nevi are most commonly seen on the back. Exposure to sun promotes the development of these lesions in individuals with DNS. The number of lesions per individual varies; however, in patients with the familial variety 75 to more than 100 lesions are not unusual. In diametric contrast to typical nevi, patients with dysplastic nevi have a disproportionate predilection to have nevi on non–sun-exposed areas, such as the buttocks, scalp, and breasts. Finally, although the dysplastic nevi may not be evident until puberty in affected children, these nevi continue to develop over their lifetime, whereas the common nevocytic nevus usually develops in childhood or the early adult years only.

Most authorities feel there is a definite histologic correlation to the clinical lesions; however, criteria for its diagnosis vary among dermatopathologists. The National Institutes for Health (NIH) consensus conference published the following as typical histologic features: basilar melanocytic hyperplasia with elongation of the rete ridges; spindle-shaped or occasionally, epithelioid melanocytes arranged horizontally and aggregating in nests that fuse with adjacent rete ridges; lamellar and concentric superficial dermal infiltrate; and cytologic atypia, usually present but not essential for diagnosis.

When a patient with clinically dysplastic nevi is seen, initial examination should include a total body inspection, including the scalp. A family history should be obtained with special attention paid to items such as moles, skin cancer, and melanoma. Baseline dermatologic photography may aid surveillance examinations. Although excision of individually atypical nevi may be indicated to ensure melanoma is not present biopsy confirmation of the dysplastic nature of the nevi is not necessary as the clinical entity is the proven risk factor. It should be emphasized that while melanomas may arise within preexisting dysplastic nevi these lesions serve mostly as a marker for patients who are at increased risk of developing melanoma and that most melanomas that occur in these patients arise on normal appearing skin. In spite of this all lesions that are difficult to follow clinically (especially those of the scalp) may be excised, as well as those with very atypical morphology. There should be prudent sun avoidance and sunscreen use. Patients should be educated in self-examination techniques and encouraged to examine themselves monthly. Physician examination every year is also prudent.

In patients with dysplastic nevi and a positive family or personal history of melanoma, physician examination every 3 to 6 months is recommended, with excision of those nevi that change in clinical appearance. The use of photographs with measured scale is helpful in following lesions.

Abadir MC, et al: Case-control study of melanocytic nevi on the buttocks in atypical mole syndrome. *J Am Acad Dermatol* 1995, 33:31.

Arndt KA: Precursors to malignant melanoma. *JAMA* 1984, 251:1882.

Barnes LM, et al: The natural history of dysplastic nevi. *Arch Dermatol* 1987, 123:1059.

Bataille V, et al: Risk of cutaneous melanoma in relation to the numbers, types and sites of naevi. *Br J Cancer* 1996, 73:1605.

Bergman W, et al: Familial melanoma and pancreatic cancer. *N Engl J Med* 1996, 334:471.

Cannon-Albright LA, et al: A review of inherited predisposition to melanoma. *Semin Oncol* 1996, 23:667.

Clark WH Jr, et al: Origin of familial malignant melanoma from heritable melanocytic lesions. *Arch Dermatol* 1978, 114:732.

Clark WH Jr, et al: The dysplastic nevus syndrome. *Arch Dermatol* 1988, 124:1207.

Crutcher WA, et al: Prevalence of dysplastic naevi in a community practice. *Lancet* 1984, 1:729.

Goldstein AM, et al: Increased risk of pancreatic cancer in melanoma-prone kindreds with p16INK4 mutations. *N Engl J Med* 1995, 333:970.

Greene MH, et al: High risk malignant melanoma in melanoma-prone families with dysplastic nevi. *Ann Intern Med* 1985, 102:458.

Grin JM, et al: Ocular melanomas and melanocytic lesions of the eye. *J Am Acad Dermatol* 1998, 38:716.

Hille ET, et al: Excess cancer mortality in six Dutch pedigrees with the familial atypical multiple mole-melanoma syndrome from 1830 to 1994. *J Invest Dermatol* 1998, 110:788.

Kang S, et al: Melanoma risk in individuals with clinically atypical nevi. *Arch Dermatol* 1994, 130:999.

Kelly JW, et al: A high incidence of melanoma found in patients with multiple dysplastic naevi by photographic surveillance. *Med J Aust* 1997, 167:191.

Kopf AW, et al: Relationship of lumbosacral nevocytic nevi to sun exposure in dysplastic nevus syndrome. *Arch Dermatol* 1986, 122:1003.

Kopf AW, et al: Relationship of nevocytic nevi to sun exposure in dysplastic nevus syndrome. *J Am Acad Dermatol* 1985, 12:650.

Knoell KA, et al: Nonpigmented dysplastic melanocytic nevi. *Arch Dermatol* 1997, 133:992.

Kraemer KH, et al: Dysplastic nevi and cutaneous melanoma risk. *Lancet* 1984, 1:1076.

Lynch HT, et al: Familial atypical multiple mole-melanoma syndrome. *J Med Genet* 1978, 15:352.

Maize JC: Dysplastic melanocytic nevi in histologic association with primary cutaneous melanomas. *J Am Acad Dermatol* 1984, 10:831.

Marghoob AA, et al: Risk of cutaneous malignant melanoma in patients with "classic" atypical-mole syndrome. *Arch Dermatol* 1994, 130:993.

National Institutes of Health Consensus Development Conference. *J Am Acad Dermatol* 1984, 10:683.

Novakovic B, et al: Melanocytic nevi, dysplastic nevi, and malignant melanoma in children from melanoma-prone families. *J Am Acad Dermatol* 1995, 33:631.

Piepkorn MW: Genetic basis of susceptibility to melanoma. *J Am Acad Dermatol* 1994, 31:1022.

Rhodes AR, et al: Dysplastic melanocytic nevi in histologic association with 234 primary cutaneous melanomas. *J Am Acad Dermatol* 1983, 9:563.

Rhodes AR, et al: Intervention strategy to prevent lethal cutaneous melanoma. *J Am Acad Dermatol* 1998, 39:262.

Schneider JS, et al: Risk factors for melanoma incidence in prospective follow-up. *Arch Dermatol* 1994, 130:1002.

Seykora J, et al: Dysplastic nevi and other risk markers for melanoma. *Semin Oncol* 1996, 23:682.

Skender-Kalnenas TM, et al: Benign melanocytic lesions. *J Am Acad Dermatol* 1995, 33:1000.

Slade J, et al: Atypical mole syndrome. *J Am Acad Dermatol* 1995, 32:479.

Snels DG, et al: Risk of cutaneous malignant melanoma in patients with nonfamilial atypical nevi from a pigmented lesions clinic. *J Am Acad Dermatol* 1999, 40:686.

Sober AJ, et al: Precursors to skin cancer. *Cancer* 1995, 75:645.

Sterry W, et al: Quadrant distribution of dysplastic nevus syndrome. *Arch Dermatol* 1988, 124:926.

Tucker MA, et al: Clinically recognized dysplastic nevi. *JAMA* 1997, 277:1439.

Tucker MA, et al: Dysplastic nevi on the scalp of prepubertal children from melanoma-prone families. *J Pediatr* 1983, 103:65.

Weinstock MA, et al: Reliability of the histopathologic diagnosis of melanocytic dysplasia. *Arch Dermatol* 1997, 133:953.

Wolfel T, et al: A p16INK4a insensitive mutant targeted by cytolytic T lymphocytes in a human melanoma. *Science* 1995, 269:1281.

Zuo L, et al: Germline mutations in the p16INK4a binding domain of CDK4 in a familial melanoma. *Nat Genet* 1996, 12:97. ▲

MELANOMA (MALIGNANT MELANOMA)

Melanomas originate almost invariably from melanocytes at the epidermal-dermal junction. Approximately half will develop in preexisting nevi, but the rest will develop on previously normal appearing skin. Usually there is a prolonged, noninvasive, horizontally oriented growth phase in which the lesion enlarges asymmetrically. Eventually, a tumor nodule develops, reflecting a vertical growth phase. Invasion into deeper levels of skin occurs and the risk of metastatic disease increases markedly. It is during the early horizontal phase that the patient may be saved; if the melanoma is excised during this time, survival is nearly ensured, whereas once the tumor spreads from its site of origin treatment results are poor and the prognosis is dismal.

To help everyone, including the public, recognize and be suspicious of such curable lesions, the ABCD criteria have been developed. The letters stand for *a*symmetry, *b*order irregularity, *c*olor variegation, and a large *d*iameter (greater than 6 mm). Patients should be taught to do monthly self-examination for new and changing lesions. This can result in earlier diagnosis and less loss of life, as Berwick et al reported. This probably occurs because patients identify melanomas when they are smaller and thinner, as shown by Richert et al. Epiluminescence microscopy is a noninvasive technique for examining pigmented lesions that makes subsurface structures visible. Although a science surrounds this, complete with terminology and diagnostic criteria, its usefulness is restricted to experienced investigators. Digital videomicroscopy may prove to be a clinically valuable addition to our diagnostic armamentarium in the future.

One in 80 Americans will develop a melanoma. The incidence of melanomas has increased 1000% in the past 50 years, probably as a result of increased exposure to ultraviolet radiation. It occurs most often in light-skinned people. Melanoma is not commonly encountered in the darker races. The lowest incidence is found among Asians. The incidence of melanoma is low until after puberty. Children may manifest either congenital melanoma or acquired melanoma. The former may occur because of transplacental transmission from an affected mother, as a primary intrauterine lesion, as a melanoma that occurs on a congenital nevus in utero, or as prenatal metastatic lesions from neurocutaneous melanosis. All of these have a poor prognosis. In children, melanomas occur at least half of the time from preexisting normal skin, where the clues to diagnosis are the same as in adults, but there is often delayed recognition because of its overall low incidence in this population. Melanomas may also develop in preexisting nevi, most importantly the congenital giant type, as discussed earlier in this chapter.

During pregnancy, pigmented nevi often become uniformly darker, and may enlarge symmetrically. Estrogen and progesterone receptors develop on the melanocytes and these changes are likely hormonally induced. If, however, changes occur that would normally incite worry about melanoma, such as irregular pigmentation or asymmetrical growth, they should be heeded and a biopsy performed. Women who develop melanoma during pregnancy have a shorter disease-free interval following excision; however, there is no adverse survival effect.

ETIOLOGIC FACTORS. Light complexions, light eyes, blond or red hair, the occurrence of blistering sunburns in childhood, heavy freckling, and tendency to tan poorly and sunburn easily indicate increased risk for melanoma, given comparable sunlight exposure.

Rampen found blondness and ease of sunburning correlated with number of moles and that the distribution pattern of these corresponded with the sex and site distribution of melanomas. Nevus pattern is an important risk factor with large numbers of common nevi, the presence of large nevi, and especially the presence of clinically dysplastic lesions all increase the risk of melanoma. Twenty percent to 50% of melanomas develop in a preexisting nevus. The presence of a large congenital nevus or of mutations in the p16-CDK4 interactions in the cell growth cycle, as has been discussed earlier with dysplastic nevi, are other predisposing factors to melanoma. The risk of developing multiple primary melanomas is elevated if there is a family history of melanoma, if there are clinically or histologically atypical nevi, if there are greater than 50 benign nevi, and if the patient is a nonuser of sunscreen.

Kopf et al concluded that there is considerable circumstantial evidence that sunlight plays a role in the etiologic factors of melanoma, though a less essential and direct one than in the case of nonmelanoma skin cancer. Sunscreens applied daily to sun-exposed areas are recommended to decrease not only nonmelanoma skin cancers but, as Holly et al showed, also limit melanoma development. Other factors implicated in predisposing patients to melanoma include PUVA, tanning lamps, xeroderma pigmentosum, the occasional development of melanoma in large burn scars, and the presence of genetic immunodeficiency syndromes or acquired states of immunodeficiency including chemotherapy, HIV infection, or organ transplantation rejection prophylaxis. An association between administration of levodopa therapy for Parkinson's disease and the onset of melanoma has been implied in some 19 case reports gathered by Rampen, but it remains unproved.

Melanoma Types

There are four recognized clinicohistologic types of melanoma. They are as follows:

1. Lentigo maligna (melanoma in situ, noninvasive melanoma)
2. Superficially spreading melanoma
3. Acral-lentiginous melanoma
4. Nodular melanoma

In addition, pedunculated and polypoidal melanomas, inflammatory melanomas, amelanotic melanomas, and hyperkeratotic and verrucous melanomas are clinical findings that may be observed. Desmoplastic, neurotropic, myxoid, balloon cell, and signet cell patterns are variants seen at the microscopic level.

The subject of melanoma is now enormous and complex enough for a separate textbook. It will be dealt with only in summary here.

Lentigo Maligna (Melanoma in Situ, Noninvasive Melanoma). Lentigo maligna begins as a tan macule that extends peripherally, with gradual uneven darkening, over

the course of several years (Fig. 30-20). The spread and darkening are usually so slow that little attention is paid to this insidious lesion. Its edge becomes irregular with time, and its color variegated, due to areas of regression. After a radial growth period of 5 to 20 years, vertically growing melanoma usually develops within it. The lesion is then called *lentigo maligna melanoma* (Fig. 30-21). A palpable nodule within the original macular lesion is the best evidence that this has occurred, though there may be darkening or bleeding as well (Fig. 30-22).

This lesion occurs equally in men and women, usually in their sixties or seventies, in chronically sun-damaged skin, most often on the face. It accounts for about 5% of all melanomas.

Superficially Spreading Melanoma. Superficially spreading melanoma is the commonest type, constituting 70% of melanomas (Fig. 30-23). It affects adults of all ages, with the median age in the fifth decade. It has no preference for sun-damaged skin. The upper back of both sexes and the shins in women are the commonest sites. It may occur anywhere, however. There is a tendency to multicoloration, not just with different shades of tan, but variegated black, red, brown, blue, and white. Bolognia et al found that 5% of eccentric foci of hyperpigmentation, a roundish area of brown or black that measures 3 mm or less in diameter and located peripherally, are melanomas arising within the nevus. It is necessary to ensure that the pathologist sections through the black dot to make this early diagnosis. In all cases of melanoma the small dark dot did not lie entirely within the borders of the remainder of the lesion but produced a small extension beyond the border. The border is often notched by focal regression or asymmetrical growth (Fig. 30-24). As stated earlier, this reflects a prolonged, noninvasive, horizontally oriented growth phase in which the lesion enlarges in an asymmetrically. As vertical growth develops, skin markings disappear (Fig. 30-25). If regression occurs, these may reappear. These lesions grow as much in a year as lentigo maligna does in 3 to 5 years. Easy bleeding is a sign of malignancy, as is erosion or ulceration. Horizontal or lateral growth into the adjoining epidermis continues for 1 to 5 years, before invasion into the dermis takes place.

Acral-Lentiginous Melanoma. Acral-lentiginous melanoma lies midway between the lentigo maligna and the superficially spreading melanoma in respect to speed of horizontal growth into adjacent epidermis. Mucosal and

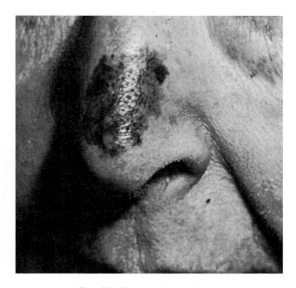

Fig. 30-20 Lentigo maligna.

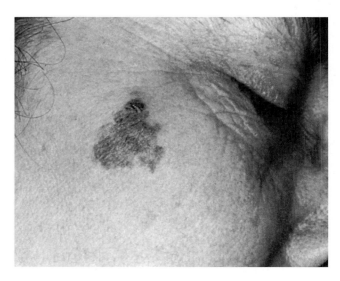

Fig. 30-21 Lentigo maligna melanoma.

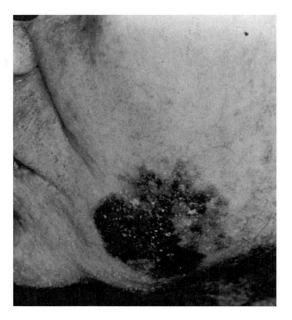

Fig. 30-22 Lentigo maligna melanoma of several years' duration.

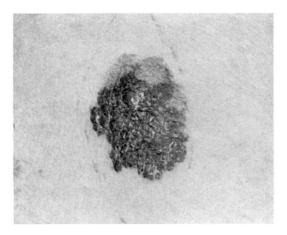

Fig. 30-23 Superficially spreading melanoma in a preexisting nevus of 30 years' duration.

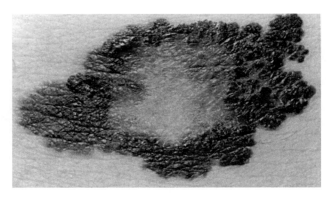

Fig. 30-24 Superficially spreading melanoma. (Courtesy Dr. Axel W. Hoke.)

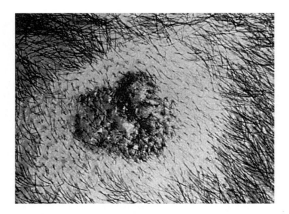

Fig. 30-25 Superficially spreading melanoma of the scalp.

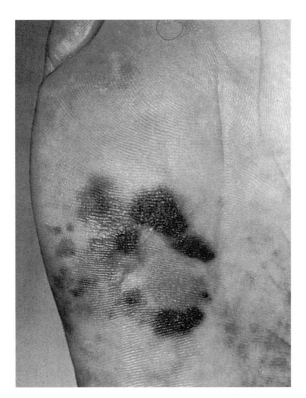

Fig. 30-26 Acral-lentiginous melanoma. (Courtesy Dr. Axel W. Hoke.)

subungual lesions are classified within this category. They account for 10% of lesions overall; however, they are the most common type among Japanese, blacks, Hispanics, and Native Americans. This is because the frequency of occurrence of the other types is low in these patients, not because the incidence of acral-lentiginous melanoma is any higher than in whites. The median age is 50 years, with equal sex distribution. The most common site of melanoma in blacks is the foot, with 60% of patients having subungual or plantar lesions.

Perhaps its most important feature is that it is so easily overlooked histologically that the first biopsy may give a false impression of a benign lesion. Nevertheless, it must be excised in toto or it will, like others, become a nodular melanoma. An irregular, enlarging black macule on palm, sole (Fig. 30-26), digit tip, or nail fold (Fig. 30-27) or bed is virtually diagnostic. Hutchinson's sign, a black discoloration of the proximal nail fold at the end of a pigmented streak (melanonychia striata) is ominous and may signal the site of melanoma in the matrix of the nail. However, there are several benign conditions, as well as Bowen's disease of the nail unit, that may have associated periungual hyperpigmentation.

The early changes may be simply a light brown, dark brown, or black discoloration. The thumb and hallux (Fig. 30-28) are more frequently involved than the other digits. In time, the lesion becomes nodular and later ulcerates. Metastases to the epitrochlear and axillary nodes develop in the late stage of the disease and are common, because there is often a delay in diagnosis.

Subungual melanoma may be misdiagnosed as onycho-

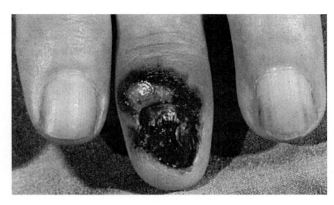

Fig. 30-27 Acral-lentiginous melanoma (melanotic whitlow). (Courtesy Dr. Axel W. Hoke.)

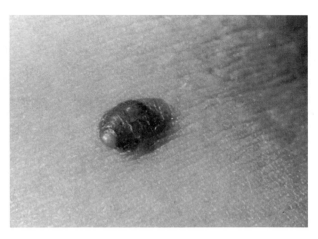

Fig. 30-29 Nodular melanoma. (Courtesy Dr. Axel W. Hoke.)

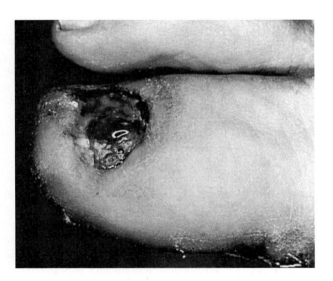

Fig. 30-28 Subungual acral-lentiginous melanoma.

mycosis, verruca vulgaris, chronic paronychia, subungual hyperkeratosis, pyogenic granuloma, Kaposi's sarcoma, glomus tumor, and subungual hematoma.

Primary melanoma of the mucous membranes is rare. It may occur in the nasal mucosa, chiefly as a polypoid tumor, with or without pigment. On the lip it is apt to be an indolent ulcer. In the mouth the lesion is usually pigmented and ulcerated. Rapini et al reviewed 177 cases in 1985 and found that the commonest site was the palate. The upper jaw was involved more often than the lower. Most patients are elderly, and the prognosis is poor. Melanoma of the vulva is manifested by a tumor, often ulcerated, with bleeding and pruritus; however, it is most often detected after metastasis to the groin has occurred.

Nodular Melanoma. Although a wide variety of clinical lesions of nodular melanoma exist, the typical lesion may be

described as a pigmented papule or nodule of varying size, present for a few months (Fig. 30-29). These lesions arise without a clinically apparent radial growth phase, but usually large atypical melanocytes can be found in the epidermis for several rete ridges beyond the region of vertical growth, at all margins of the excised lesion.

Nodular melanoma constitutes about 15% of all melanomas. It occurs twice as often in men as in women, primarily on sun-exposed areas of the head, neck, and trunk.

Although the tumors are at first 1 to 4 mm wide, they may grow much larger and become papillary, fungoid, or ulcerated. Bleeding is usually a late sign. The color is usually not uniform throughout the tumor but is likely to be scattered irregularly and is grayish brown, bluish black, or black.

Other Morphologic Features

Polypoid melanoma. This is a variant of nodular melanoma; it is a pedunculated tumor. At its base the polypoid melanoma does not appear to descend for any appreciable distance into the dermis. Nevertheless it behaves as a level IV or V tumor; the 5-year survival rate is only 42%, compared with 57% for nodular melanoma.

Verrucous melanoma. Steiner et al have reviewed this hyperkeratotic, relatively uniformly pigmented, sharply demarcated variant.

Desmoplastic melanoma. This deeply infiltrating type of melanoma usually has a spindle-cell pattern histologically in which collagen fibers extend between the tumor cells. It most often occurs on the head or neck of older men, many times within a lentigo maligna. One third of cases present with only a palpable dermal irregularity and when a tumor is present most are amelanotic. S100 and other stains are often necessary for diagnosis. The HMB-45 is negative. Neurotropic spread is often seen.

Inflammatory melanoma. The clinical phenomenon of inflammation in or near the site of a melanoma signifies a poor prognosis. Haupt et al reported two such cases, which metastasized widely in a short time.

Amelanotic melanoma. The nonpigmented melanoma differs from the other melanomas only in its lack of pigment. The lesion is pink, erythematous, or flesh colored, but otherwise the appearance of growth and ulceration is the same as that in the pigmented variety. The lesion is easily mistaken for granuloma pyogenicum, even by the experienced. Amelanotic melanoma is the typical variant seen in albinos.

DIFFERENTIAL DIAGNOSIS. Melanoma may clinically simulate a wide variety of lesions. In our experience melanoma may most frequently resemble the pigmented basal cell carcinoma, which is indurated, usually has a rolled edge, and occurs chiefly in deeply pigmented persons; a darkly pigmented seborrheic keratosis, which is usually verrucous and greasy, and seems to rest on the top of the skin; a pyogenic granuloma; and Kaposi's sarcoma. Other melanoma-simulating lesions are subungual traumatic hematoma, senile angioma, and junctional and compound nevi. Nevi are differentiated from melanomas by the latter's tendency for later onset, steady growth, slow change in color and its mottling. Breast carcinomas may be pigmented and mimic melanoma both clinically and histologically. Bowen's disease, as well as Paget's disease, may likewise be pigmented and simulate melanoma.

A lesion that resembles melanoma histologically is the clear cell sarcoma, or as it is also known, *melanoma of the soft parts.* These tumors often contain melanin, and in the majority of cases melanosomes are present. In addition, they stain positively for S-100 and HMB-45. It occurs most frequently on the lower extremities of young people. The average age at onset is 27. The history is of an enlarging often painful mass on an extremity, with the foot or ankle involved 43% of the time. The tumors arise in and are bound to the aponeuroses, tendons, or fascia and only uncommonly invades the overlying skin. Histologically, there are compact nests and fascicles of polygonal or fusiform cells with a clear cytoplasm present between dense fibrous tissue septa that connect with tendonous or aponeurotic tissue. Multinucleated cells are frequent. Metastases are often present at first diagnosis and the prognosis is poor. Local recurrence or distant metastases after the initial excision are frequent and result in death in more than 50% of reported cases. Treatment is with wide excision and lymph node dissection. Radiotherapy and chemotherapy are used as an adjunct in some cases. The lesion appears to arise from neural crest cells. Frequently translocations of chromosomes 12 and 22 are present.

BIOPSY. When the size of the lesion lends itself to simple surgical excision, this is the best method to establish the diagnosis. If the biopsy shows melanoma, then definitive surgery may be performed.

In lesions too large for simple excision, an incisional or punch biopsy, deep enough to permit measurement of thickness, has no effect on prognosis, and is considered good practice. When melanoma is suspected in the melanotic freckle or in a giant pigmented nevus, biopsy should be done through the thickest and most atypical area and multiply sectioned to find the deepest area of involvement.

HISTOPATHOLOGY. Pinkus and Mehregan set forth the following criteria for the diagnosis of malignancy in melanotic tumors: presence of mitoses, inflammatory reaction composed of lymphocytes and perhaps plasma cells, dermoepidermal junctional activity (which is the site of origin for all melanomas except those occurring in the giant pigmented nevus), and the absence of dermal stroma, which is destroyed in malignant melanoma.

Atypical melanocytes are scattered throughout the epidermis, singly and in irregular nests. There is asymmetry, poor circumscription, and failure of melanocytic maturation.

The findings depend considerably on the age of the lesion. At first atypical melanocytes are found at the dermoepidermal junction. As the melanocytes proliferate, the dermoepidermal border becomes irregular, while the melanocytic cells may form nests at the junction to give it a moth-eaten appearance. There is often extension of these atypical cells down the follicular orifices. As the atypical cells extend into the dermis ("vertical growth"), an invasive melanoma develops and metastasis is a possibility.

METASTASIS. In the beginning this is usually manifested by pigmented nodules appearing around the site of the excision (Fig. 30-30). Early remote metastases occur via the lymphatics, and regional lymphadenopathy may be the first sign. The lymph nodes are hard and discrete. Later, metastases occur via the blood stream, and may become widespread. The chief site for metastatic melanoma is the skin (Fig. 30-31), but all other organs are at risk. Central nervous system metastasis is the most common cause of death. Although most metastatic spread occurs in the first 5 years after diagnosis late onset metastases occurs. In Raderman et al's series of 18 patients who suffered metastases after 10 years, 16 were premenopausal women. Melanemia, melanuria, and cachexia are likely to occur in terminal disease. In extreme cases, the entire integument may become deeply pigmented (generalized melanosis), either by individual melanoma cells, or by melanophages alone. Occasionally, patients are seen with metastatic melanoma from an unknown source. Full-body skin examination may reveal a depigmented or telangiectatic or irregularly pigmented atrophic patch. Such patients are estimated to have a 40% chance of 5-year survival.

WORKUP AND FOLLOW-UP. The initial workup of a patient with melanoma concentrates on establishing a family history, doing a thorough review of systems, and examining for evidence of metastatic disease via a thorough physical examination. Whether additional studies such as chest

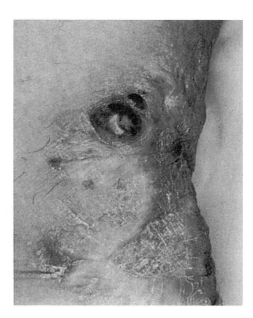

Fig. 30-30 Metastatic melanoma developing after excision of a melanoma on the heel of a woman.

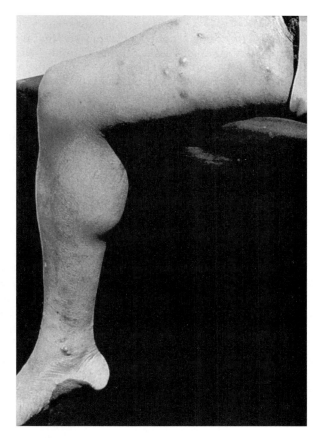

Fig. 30-31 Cutaneous metastasis from melanoma of the sole. (Courtesy Dr. Axel W. Hoke.)

radiographs and laboratory tests should be ordered for asymptomatic patients with localized disease is controversial. Some argue that the false-positive rate, in a population with few true positives, is relatively high and the value of treatment in those identified from these tests low. However, at times, limited metastatic disease can be resected and lead to long-term remission. A consensus conference in 1992 concluded that a staging workup was not indicated for melanomas below 1.0 mm thickness. Many experienced physicians, however, obtain chest radiographs and an LDH. Further information is needed to guide clinicians on the indications for these or other more extensive testing such as CT or MRI scans.

Many schedules are recommended for following patients with melanoma. The principles are an increased number of visits early in the disease course, when spread is most likely, and follow-up for life, since late recurrences, new primary melanomas, and metastases occur in some patients. Chest radiographic evaluation is useful in detecting early metastases to the lungs. It is worthwhile to detect these, since surgical removal of solitary pulmonary metastases may result in cure. As in the initial workup, more information and a consensus statement would help to establish indications for testing in these patients. Consultation with an oncologist regarding this workup is worthwhile, because protocols may be available to help answer some of these questions.

STAGING. In 1992, the American Joint Committee on Cancer developed a staging system for cutaneous melanoma. The system's categories depend on definitions for primary tumors, lymph node involvement, and distant metastases:

- pTis refers to melanoma in situ (Clark level I).
- pT1 are tumors 0.75 mm or less in thickness that invade the papillary dermis (Clark level II).
- pT2 are tumors more than 0.75 mm thick but not more than 1.5 mm thick and/or tumors that invade to the papillary reticular dermal interface (Clark level III).
- pT3 are tumors of more than 1.5 mm thick but less than 4 mm in thick and/or tumors that invade the reticular dermis (Clark level IV).
- pT4 are tumors of more than 4 mm thick and/or tumors that invade the subcutaneous tissue (Clark level V) and/or satellites within 2 cm of the primary tumor.

In cases in which there is a discrepancy between thickness and level, the pT category is based on the less favorable finding. Lymph node staging is based on size with less than or greater than 3 cm being the dividing point between N1 and N2 (N0 means no regional lymph node metastases). If no distant metastases are present, the designation is M0; if metastases are present, the designation is M1. Stages I and II occur in localized melanoma, with the dividing line at 1.50 mm of thickness. Stage III is for regional node metastases, and stage IV is for distant metastases.

PROGNOSIS. The prognosis for a patient with stage I melanoma is primarily related to tumor thickness:

- In situ lesions should have 100% survival.
- Lesions less than 0.76 mm have an excellent prognosis, with only 2% to 4% mortality over 5 years.
- Lesions 0.76 to 1.49 mm thick have an approximate 86% to 90% survival rate.
- Lesions 1.50 to 3.99 mm thick have a 66% to 70% survival rate.
- Lesions more than 4 mm have a 53% to 55% survival rate.

If grouped according to stage for localized primary melanoma, the overall survival rate is 80%. If regional lymph node disease is present, the survival rate drops to 30% to 35% and for distant metastases, the 5-year survival is only 10%. Spontaneous regression has been documented in cases of melanoma, even with metastases.

Many other variables have been reported to influence survival, and some of these are taken into account in various prognostic tables that have been published over the years. These other factors include the presence of tumor infiltrating lymphocytes (brisk response is best), mitotic rate (zero is best, and greater than $6/mm^2$ is worst), ulceration (if present, this has been reported to be adverse effect in some series), location (hair-bearing limbs yield a better prognosis than when lesions are present on the trunk, head, neck, palm, or sole), sex (women have a better prognosis than men), age (younger patients have a better prognosis), the presence of leukoderma at distal sites (improves the prognosis), and regression (associated with a poorer prognosis in some series). Multivariant analysis shows that many of these are not independently predictive and others are of variable significance in different series. Tumor thickness is presently the factor that is used to determine therapy.

TREATMENT. Early diagnosis and excision remain the hope for cure of melanoma. A margin of 0.5 to 1.0 cm is recommended for excision of a melanoma in situ, a 1.0 cm margin for melanomas less than 2.0 mm thick, and a 3-cm margin for those thicker than 2.0 mm. However, Zitelli et al warned that wider margins were needed to remove melanomas on the head, neck, hands, and feet than those on the trunk and extremities in their study of 535 patients treated by Mohs' microsurgery. They recommended a minimum surgical margin of 1.5 cm for lesions of the head, neck, hands, and feet, unless Mohs' microsurgery is used. In their series they were able to conserve tissue by using this method and still maintain 5-year survival rates and metastatic rates equivalent to or better than historical controls. This technically difficult method is not frequently employed to remove melanoma.

Nail apparatus melanoma may necessitate amputation of a digit or skin grafting. Banfield et al treated a patient with fixed-tissue Mohs' microsurgery who had in situ melanoma causing longitudinal melanonychia with excellent functional and cosmetic results.

Performing regional elective lymph node dissection (ELND) at the time of initial surgery is controversial. If palpable lymph nodes are present at the time of diagnosis, distant metastases are present in 70% to 85% of patients and the 5-year survival rate is only 30%. ELND may be recommended, however, for palliative purposes. Tumors less than 1.0 mm thick so rarely metastasize that ELND is not indicated. For tumors more than 4.0 mm thick, survival is uniformly poor and, although ELND may be useful for staging purposes, it is not indicated for therapeutic reasons. For patients with lesions 1 to 4 mm thick, ELND is controversial. A randomized clinical trial found a significantly higher survival rate for patients 60 years of age or younger, patients with a primary tumor of 1- to 2-mm thickness, and those whose primary tumor was not ulcerated.

Because of the controversy about the benefits of ELND and its attendant cost and morbidity, an alternative method of assessing lymph node involvement has been used over the past several years. It is called *intraoperative lymphatic mapping*. Because in most cases lymph node involvement occurs in the first node of the drainage channel closest to the site of tumor, this node is identified during removal of the primary tumor by injecting either a dye or a radioactive tracing agent. The sentinel node is then removed and examined. If no melanoma cells are found, no more surgery is done; if the node is involved, the remainder of the nodes are removed. Studies are now underway to see if this technique may be used to extend survival.

High-dose interferon alfa-2b therapy was reported to increase survival as adjuvant therapy in patients with melanoma of greater than 4 mm; however, subsequent data did not confirm this. Toxicity is marked. Adjuvant interferon alfa-2a treatment has been reported to diminish the occurrence of metastases and thus prolongs disease-free survival in patients with melanoma of greater than 1.5 mm thick. Long-term survival advantage has not been shown, however. Thus, the role for interferon in the treatment of melanoma still awaits further definition. Chemotherapy is not very effective in the treatment of melanoma; the most effective agent identified is dacarbazine (DTIC). Combination chemotherapy trials are ongoing; however, the response remains poor. High-dose chemotherapy and autologous bone marrow transplantation is a toxic, risky therapy for patients with widely disseminated melanoma. It may benefit selected patients.

Adoptive immunotherapy with lymphokine-activated killer cells plus interleukin-2, or high-dose interleukin-2 alone is another toxic treatment, with some response obtained in some patients. Many new trials testing various more specific genetic immunotherapy models are underway. Guidelines on current treatment and many other controversial areas continue to change rapidly.

Perfusion chemotherapy has been used for extremity melanoma. This technique establishes a temporary oxygenated and hyperthermic circuit through the vessels supplying the tumor and limits the distribution of the chemotherapeutic agent with the use of a tourniquet. It is effective for regionally confined advanced disease and has virtually eliminated the need for amputation.

Radiation therapy is not very successful; its use lies largely in symptomatic treatment of metastatic disease to bone or the central nervous system.

Arbiser JL: Melanoma. *Arch Dermatol* 1998, 134:1027.

Banfield CC, et al: Mohs micrographic surgery for the treatment of in situ nail apparatus melanoma: a case report. *J Am Acad Dermatol* 1999, 40:98.

Baran R, et al: Hutchinson's sign. *J Am Acad Dermatol* 1996, 34:87.

Barnhill RL, et al: Tumor vascularity, proliferation, and apoptosis in human melanoma micrometastases and macrometastases. *Arch Dermatol* 1998:134;991.

Berwick M: Why are people still dying of melanoma? *Arch Dermatol* 1999, 135:1534.

Berwick M, et al: Screening for cutaneous melanoma by self-examination. *J Natl Cancer Inst* 1996, 88:17.

Black WC, et al: Melanoma within a southwestern Hispanic population. *Arch Dermatol* 1987, 123:1331.

Bolognia JL, et al: The significance of eccentric foci of hyperpigmentation ("small dark dots") within melanocytic nevi. *Arch Dermatol* 1994, 130:1013.

Bondi EE, et al: Skin markings in malignant melanoma. *JAMA* 1983, 250:503.

Briggs JC, et al: Late recurrence of cutaneous melanoma. *J Am Acad Dermatol* 1988, 18:147.

Burden AD, et al: Genetic and environmental influences in the development of multiple primary melanoma. *Arch Dermatol* 1999, 135:261.

Bystryn JC, et al: Prognostic significance of hypopigmentation in malignant melanoma. *Arch Dermatol* 1987, 123:1053.

Carli P, et al: Cutaneous melanoma histologically associated with a nevus and melanoma de novo have a different profile of risk. *J Am Acad Dermatol* 1999, 40:549.

Chang P, et al: Metastatic melanoma of unknown primary. *Cancer* 1982, 49:1106.

Chung EB, et al: Malignant melanoma of soft parts: a reassessment of clear cell sarcoma. *Am J Surg Pathol* 1983, 7:405.

Cliff S, et al: Amelanotic lentigo maligna melanoma of the face. *Clin Exp Dermatol* 1997, 22:177.

Cohen LM: Lentigo maligna and lentigo maligna melanoma. *J Am Acad Dermatol* 1995, 33:923.

Cotton J, et al: Melanoma-in-transit presenting as panniculitis. *J Am Acad Dermatol* 1998, 39:876.

Day CL, et al: Predictors of late death among patients with clinical stage I melanoma who have not had bony or visceral metastases within the first 5 years after diagnosis. *J Am Acad Dermatol* 1983, 8:864.

Farber M, et al: Pigmented lesions of the conjunctiva. *J Am Acad Dermatol* 1998, 38:971.

Friedman RJ, et al: Favorable prognosis for malignant melanomas associated with acquired melanocytic nevi. *Arch Dermatol* 1983, 119:455.

Glass FL, et al: Lymphatic mapping and sentinel node biopsy in the management of high-risk melanoma. *J Am Acad Dermatol* 1998, 39:603.

Grin JM, et al: Ocular melanomas and melanocytic lesions of the eye. *J Am Acad Dermatol* 1998, 38:716.

Gross EA: Initial evaluation of melanoma. *Arch Dermatol* 1998, 134:623.

Gutman M, et al: Acral melanoma. *Br J Surg* 1985, 72:610.

Hall HI, et al: Update on the incidence and mortality from melanoma in the United States. *J Am Acad Dermatol* 1999, 40:35.

Haupt HM, et al: Inflammatory melanoma. *J Am Acad Dermatol* 1984, 10:52.

Holly EA. et al: Cutaneous melanoma in women. *Am J Epidemiol* 1995, 141:923.

Horton S, et al: Erythematous nodule of the nail bed. *Arch Dermatol* 1999, 135:1113.

Huang CL, et al: Laboratory tests and imaging studies in patients with cutaneous malignant melanoma. *J Am Acad Dermatol* 1998, 39:451.

Johanson CR, et al: Radiotherapy in nodular melanoma. *Cancer* 1983, 51:226.

Johnson TM, et al: Advances in melanoma therapy. *J Am Acad Dermatol* 1998, 38:731.

Johnson TM, et al: Multiple primary melanomas. *J Am Acad Dermatol* 1998, 39:422.

Kato T, et al: Malignant melanoma of mucous membranes. *Arch Dermatol* 1987, 123:216.

Kirckwood JM, et al: Interferon alfa-2b adjuvant therapy of high-risk resected cutaneous melanoma. *J Clin Oncol* 1996, 14:7.

Klaus MV, et al: Generalized melanosis caused by melanoma of the rectum. *J Am Acad Dermatol* 1996, 35:295.

Kopf AW, et al: Sun and malignant melanoma. *J Am Acad Dermatol* 1984, 11:694.

Kossard S, et al: Neurotropic melanoma. *Arch Dermatol* 1987, 123:907.

Kraemer KH, et al: Xeroderma pigmentosum. *Arch Dermatol* 1987, 123:241.

Lederman JS, et al: Skin markings in the diagnosis and prognosis of cutaneous melanoma. *Arch Dermatol* 1984, 120:1449.

Lederman JS, et al: Does biopsy type influence survival in clinical stage I melanoma? *J Am Acad Dermatol* 1985, 13:983.

Lienard D, et al: Isolated limb perfusion in primary and recurrent melanoma. *Semin Surg Oncol* 1998, 14:202.

Mackey SL, et al: Melanoma of the soft parts (clear cell sarcoma). *J Am Acad Dermatol* 1998, 38:815.

Manci EA, et al: Polypoid melanoma, a virulent variant of the nodular growth pattern. *Am J Clin Pathol* 1981, 75:810.

Milton FW, et al: Subungual malignant melanoma. *Australas J Dermatol* 1985, 26:61.

Mraz Germhard, et al: Prediction of sentinel lymph node micrometastasis by histological features in primary cutaneous malignant melanoma. *Arch Dermatol* 1998, 134:983.

Nordlund JJ: Hypopigmentation, vitiligo, and melanoma. *Arch Dermatol* 1987, 123:1005.

Oguchi S, et al: Characteristic epiluminescent microscopic features of early malignant melanoma on glabrous skin. *Arch Dermatol* 1998, 134:563.

Paladugu RR, et al: Acral lentiginous melanoma. *Cancer* 1983, 52:161.

Parker T, et al: Malignant melanoma. *Dermatol Surg* 1996, 22:234.

Pehamberger H, et al: Adjuvant interferon alfa-2a treatment in resected primary stage II cutaneous melanoma. *J Clin Oncol* 1998, 16:1425.

Peters MS, et al: Balloon cell malignant melanoma. *J Am Acad Dermatol* 1985, 13:351.

Raderman D, et al: Late metastases (beyond ten years) of cutaneous malignant melanoma. *J Am Acad Dermatol* 1986, 15:374.

Rapini RP, et al: Primary malignant melanoma of the oral cavity. *Cancer* 1985, 55:1543.

Reed KM, et al: Prognosis for polypoidal melanoma is determined by primary tumor thickness. *Cancer* 1986, 57:1201.

Reintgen DS, et al: Malignant melanoma and pregnancy. *Cancer* 1985, 55:1340.

Rhodes AR, et al: Risk factors for cutaneous melanomas. *JAMA* 1987, 258:3146.

Richert SM, et al: Cutaneous melanoma. *J Am Acad Dermatol* 1998, 39:571.

Rodriquez E, et al: t(12;22)(q13;13) and trisomy 8 are nonrandom aberration in clear cell sarcoma. *Cancer Genet Cytogenet* 1992, 64:1992.

Rosenberg SA, et al: A progress report in the treatment of 157 patients with advanced cancer using lymphokine-activated killer cells and interleukin-2, or high-dose interleukin-2 alone. *N Engl J Med* 1987, 316:889.

Rosenberg SA, et al: Use of tumor-infiltrating lymphocytes and interleukin-2 in immunotherapy of patients with metastatic melanoma. *N Engl J Med* 1988, 319:1676.

Ruiz-Maldonado, et al: Malignant melanoma in children. *Arch Dermatol* 1997, 133:363.

Sau P, et al: Bowen's disease of the nail bed and periungual area. *Arch Dermatol* 1994, 130:204.

Sau P, et al: Pigmented breast carcinoma. *Arch Dermatol* 1989, 125:536.

Seidenari S, et al: Digital videomicroscopy improves diagnostic accuracy for melanoma. *J Am Acad Dermatol* 1998, 39:175.

Skelton HG, et al: Desmoplastic malignant melanoma. *J Am Acad Dermatol* 1995, 32:717.

Steiner A, et al: Verrucous malignant melanoma. *Arch Dermatol* 1988, 124:1534.

Stern RS, et al: Malignant melanoma in patients treated for psoriasis with PUVA. *N Engl J Med* 1997, 336:1041.

Swerdlow AJ, et al: Benign melanocytic nevi as a risk factor for malignant melanoma. *Br Med J* 1986, 292:1555.

Swerdlow AJ, et al: Do tanning lamps cause melanoma? *J Am Acad Dermatol* 1998, 38:89.

Takematsu H, et al: Subungual melanoma. *Cancer* 1985, 55:2725.

Terhune MH, et al: Use of chest radiography in the initial evaluation of patients with localized melanoma. *Arch Dermatol* 1998, 134:569.

Vaszuez M, et al: Melanoma of volar and subungual skin in Puerto Ricans. *J Am Acad Dermatol* 1984, 10:39.

Wagner RF Jr, et al: Paraneoplastic syndromes, tumor markers, and other unusual features of malignant melanoma. *J Am Acad Dermatol* 1986, 14:249.

Whitacker DC, et al: Desmoplastic malignant melanoma. *J Am Acad Dermatol* 1992, 26:704.

Zacarian SA: Cryosurgical treatment of lentigo maligna. *Arch Dermatol* 1982, 118:89.

Zitelli JA, et al: Mohs micrographic surgery for the treatment of primary cutaneous melanoma. *J Am Acad Dermatol* 1997, 37:236.

Zitelli JA, et al: Surgical margins for excision of primary cutaneous melanoma. *J Am Acad Dermatol* 1997, 37:422. _____ ▲

DERMAL MELANOCYTIC LESIONS

At birth, melanocytes may be present in the dermal portion of the skin of the scalp, the backs of the hands, and the sacrum. These dermal melanocytes are large ameboid cells that normally disappear shortly after birth.

Mongolian Spot

The Mongolian spot is a bluish gray macule varying in size from 2 to 8 cm in diameter. It occurs typically in the sacral region of the newborn, in 80% to 90% of Asians, Southern Europeans, American blacks, and Native Americans. The Mayan Indians uniquely take great pride in it as an indicator of pure Mayan inheritance. The Mongolian spot may be situated in other locations. Multiple spots may occur in a

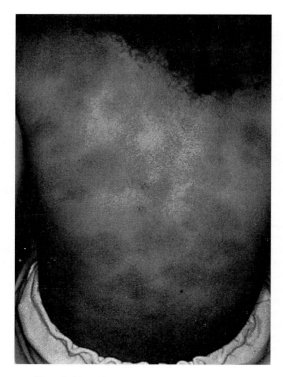

Fig. 30-32 Mongolian spots on a young girl.

widespread distribution (Fig. 30-32); these have been called *generalized dermal melanocytosis* or *dermal melanocytic hamartomas*. If associated with a nevus flammeus phakomatosis pigmentovascularis is the designation.

Histologically, the Mongolian spot shows elongated dermal melanocytes, widely scattered among the collagen bundles. It usually disappears during childhood, although rarely, it may persist into adulthood.

Bashiti HM, et al: Generalized dermal melanocytosis. *Arch Dermatol* 1981, 117:791.

Burkhart CG, et al: Dermal melanocytic hamartoma. *Arch Dermatol* 1981, 117:102.

Kikuchi I: Mongolian spots remaining in schoolchildren. *J Dermatol* 1980, 7:213.

Kikuchi I, et al: Natural history of the Mongolian spot. *J Dermatol* 1980, 7:449.

Park KD, et al: Extensive aberrant Mongolian spot. *J Dermatol* 1995, 22:330.

Van Gysel D, et al: Phakomatosis pigmentovascularis. *Pediatr Dermatol* 1996, 13:33. _____ ▲

Nevus of Ota (Oculodermal Melanocytosis)

This nevus, described by Ota, is also known as *nevus fuscoceruleus ophthalmomaxillaris* (Fig. 30-33). It is usually present at birth in the two of three affected patients who have ocular involvement. Other lesions may not begin until the teen years. The conjunctiva and the skin about the eye

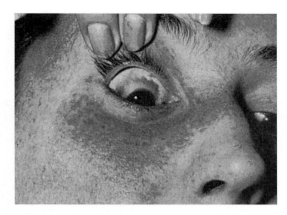

Fig. 30-33 Nevus of Ota. Nevus fuscoceruleus ophthalmomaxillaris. (Courtesy Dr. F. Kerdel-Vegas, Venezuela.)

supplied by the first and second branch of the trigeminal nerve, as well as the sclera, ocular muscles, retrobulbar fat, periosteum, and buccal mucosa, may be involved. On the skin, brown, slate gray, or blue-black macules grow slowly larger and deeper in color. It persists throughout life. Eighty percent occur in females; 5% are bilateral. Although the lesion is benign, malignant melanoma may rarely occur. Dutton et al reviewed 32 cases of melanoma occurring in nevus of Ota and found it to be proportionally more frequent in white patients, and reported the most common site of malignancy was the choroid. Glaucoma may also occasionally complicate nevus of Ota.

Histologically, elongated dendritic dermal melanocytes are seen scattered in the upper portion of the dermis.

Nevus of Ito

Also known as *nevus fuscoceruleus acromiodeltoideus,* the nevus of Ito has the same features as nevus of Ota except that it occurs in the distribution of the posterior supraclavicular and lateral cutaneous brachial nerves, to involve the shoulder, side of the neck, and supraclavicular areas (Fig. 30-34).

The results of treatment with the Q-switched ruby laser are dramatic.

Alster TS, et al: Treatment of nevus of Ota by the Q-switched alexandrite laser. *Dermatol Surg* 1995, 21:592.
Chang CJ, et al: Q-switched ruby laser treatment of oculodermal melanosis (nevus of Ota). *Plast Reconstr Surg* 1996, 98:784.
Dutton JJ, et al: Orbital malignant melanoma and oculodermal melanocytosis. *Opthalmology* 1984, 91:497.
Grin JM, et al: Ocular melanomas and melanocytic lesions of the eye. *J Am Acad Dermatol* 1998, 38:716.
Patel BC, et al: Cutaneous malignant melanoma and oculodermal melanocytosis (nevus of Ota). *J Am Acad Dermatol* 1998, 38:862.
Shimbashi T, et al: Treatment of nevus of Ota by Q-switched ruby laser. *Aesthetic Plast Surg* 1997, 21:118. _____ ▲

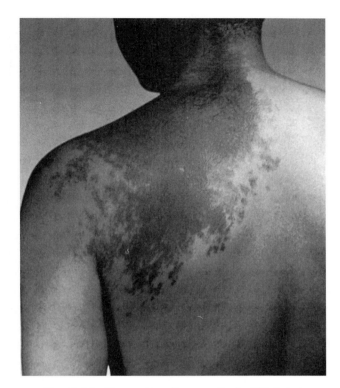

Fig. 30-34 Nevus of Ito. (Courtesy Dr. Axel W. Hoke.)

Blue Nevus

The blue nevus consists of two distinct types, the blue nevus of Jadassohn-Tiche (common blue nevus) and the cellular blue nevus. Rarely, they may occur as a congenital lesion, as eruptive or disseminated lesions, as familial multiple lesions, or histologically as a combined nevus where the blue nevus is seen in association with another type of nevus.

Blue Nevus of Jadassohn-Tiche. The typical common blue nevus, nevus ceruleus, is a steel-blue nodule that begins in early life. The slowly growing lesion is rarely more than 2 to 10 mm in diameter. The lesion occurs most frequently on the dorsal hands, feet (Figs. 30-35 and 30-36), forearms, shins, face, and the buttocks.

Histologically, dermal melanocytes, fibrocytes, and melanophages are found to be increased and situated deep in the dermis. The flattened melanocytes are more abundant than seen in the Mongolian spot.

Cellular Blue Nevus. Usually the cellular blue nevus is a large, firm, blue or blue-black nodule. It is most frequently seen on the buttock and sacrococcygeal region, and occasionally is present at birth. The nodular tumors are multilobulated and well circumscribed. Women have cellular blue nevus 2.5 times as frequently as men; the average age of the patient seen with this lesion is 40 years. Uncommonly, these

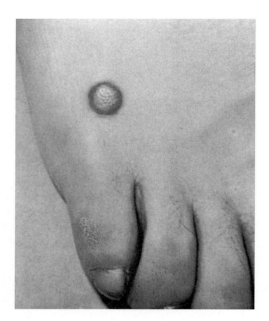

Fig. 30-35 Blue nevus on the dorsum of the foot. (Courtesy Dr. G. Sorensen.)

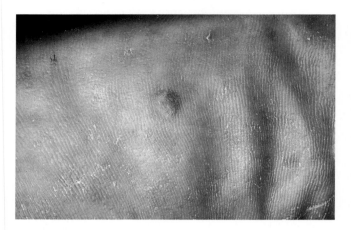

Fig. 30-36 Blue nevus resembling a melanoma on the sole of a 36-year-old man.

may invade underlying structures such as the skull in scalp lesions.

Histologically, in addition to deeply pigmented dendritic melanocytes, one observes cellular islands, composed of large spindle-shaped cells with ovoid nuclei and abundant pale cytoplasm, containing little or no pigment.

Epithelioid Blue Nevus. This newly described lesion is important because of its strong association with Carney's complex. This syndrome consists of myxomas, spotty skin pigmentation, endocrine overactivity, and schwannomas. The blue nevi occur on the extremities and trunk, less frequently on the head and neck, and are at times multiple. They are darkly pigmented, domed, and less than 1 cm. Microscopically, they are heavily pigmented, poorly circumscribed, dermal lesions that display two types of melanocytes: one intensely pigmented, globular, and fusiform; the other lightly pigmented, polygonal, and spindle. The melanocytes are situated among the dermal collagen bundles singly, in short rows and small groups, and occasionally in fascicles. Nuclei of the lightly pigmented, polygonal and spindle cells are vesicular with very pale chromatin and a single prominent nucleolus.

Malignant Blue Nevus. The cellular blue nevus may rarely undergo malignant transformation into a malignant melanoma. Clinically, there is a sudden increase in size, and ulceration. Pleomorphism of nuclei, mitotic figures, and invasion of clusters of malignant cells into the deep dermis and fatty tissue are seen; there is no junctional activity in the malignant blue nevus.

Excision has been the mainstay of treatment for blue nevi. Successful results have now been reported with the use of the Q-switched ruby laser. Treatment of the malignant variety is the same as for a malignant melanoma.

Balloy BC, et al: Disseminated blue nevus. *Arch Dermatol* 1998, 134:245.

Boni R, et al: Malignant blue naevus with distant subcutaneous metastasis. *Clin Exp Dermatol* 1996, 21:427.

Carney JA, et al: The epithelioid blue nevus. *Am J Surg Pathol* 1996, 20:259.

Goldenhersh MA, et al: Malignant blue nevus. *J Am Acad Dermatol* 1988, 19:712.

Kawasaki T, et al: Congenital giant common blue nevus. *J Am Acad Dermatol* 1993, 28:653.

Knoell KA, et al: Familial blue nevi. *J Am Acad Dermatol* 1998, 39:322.

Lambert WC, et al: Nodal and subcutaneous cellular blue nevi. *Arch Dermatol* 1984, 120:367.

Micali G, et al: Cellular blue nevus of the scalp infiltrating the underlying bone. *Pediatr Dermatol* 1997, 14:199.

Milgraum SS, et al: Treatment of blue nevi with the Q-switched ruby laser. *J Am Acad Dermatol* 1995, 32:307.

Ozgur F, et al: Metastatic malignant blue nevus. *Ann Plast Surg* 1997, 39:411.

Shenfield HT, et al: Multiple agminated blue nevi. *J Dermatol Surg Oncol* 1980, 6:725.

Suchniak JM, et al: Acquired multiple blue nevi on an extremity. *J Am Acad Dermatol* 1995, 33:1051. ▲

CHAPTER 31

Macrophage/Monocyte Disorders

PALISADED GRANULOMATOUS DERMATOSES
Granuloma Annulare

Granuloma annulare (GA) is a relatively common idiopathic disorder of the dermis and subcutaneous tissue. The disease occurs in all races and at all ages. Pathogenically, IgM and C3 in the blood vessels of the skin lesions are found in about half of patients. At the periphery of GA lesions, a leukocytoclastic vasculitis is sometimes seen. These findings suggest an immunoglobulin-mediated vasculitis in the pathogenesis of granuloma annulare. Epstein-Barr virus (EBV) has been found in some cases, and resolution with antiviral therapy suggests there may be a causal relationship. Granuloma annulare is common in patients infected with the human immunodeficiency virus (HIV), and lesions of GA occur in resolved lesions of herpes zoster.

Many clinical types of GA exist. Usually, patients exhibit primarily one clinical type during the course of their illness, except in the subcutaneous form, in which typical papular or localized GA may also occur.

Localized Granuloma Annulare. This form of GA tends to affect young adults. Localized GA usually appears on the lateral or dorsal surfaces of the fingers or hands, elbows, dorsal feet, and ankles (Fig. 31-1). Lesions are white or pink, flat-topped papules, which slowly spread peripherally, at the same time undergoing central involution, so that roughly annular lesions are formed (Fig. 31-2). The overlying skin remains completely normal. Lesions may coalesce and sometimes form scalloped patterns or firm plaques. The lesions never ulcerate and on resolving leave no residua. The lesions develop slowly and often involute spontaneously. Although up to three fourths of patients clear within 2 years, 25% have no resolution in 8 years.

Generalized Granuloma Annulare. This form of GA affects mostly women past middle age. Diabetes has been reported to occur in up to 20% of cases. Generalized GA presents as a diffuse papular eruption. Lesions favor the nape of the neck, upper trunk, and proximal upper extremities (Fig. 31-3). The face and genital area are usually spared. In some cases sun exposure seems to be a trigger (see actinc granuloma on p. 896). Some patients are completely asymptomatic, whereas others complain of severe pruritus. Spontaneous clearing usually occurs but at variable times. The average duration is 3 to 4 years but may be as short as 4 months or longer than a decade.

Macular Granuloma Annulare. Flat or only slightly palpable lesions occur, especially on the feet, ankles, and upper medial thighs. Individual lesions average 1 to 4 cm in diameter but may be much larger. On careful palpation, small papules can be felt in some cases, and on stretching the skin the papules or small annular lesions can be seen. Such papules are the most fruitful sites for biopsies.

Subcutaneous Granuloma Annulare (Deep GA, Pseudorheumatoid Nodule). Subcutaneous GA is most common in children, with boys affected twice as commonly as girls. Childhood cases appear at any age from 1 year to adolescence, with half of cases appearing in children ages 5 to 12. Lesions tend to occur on the lower legs but may also occur on the distal upper extremity or scalp. Multiple lesions are usually present. There is often a history of trauma to the affected area preceding the appearance of a lesion. Superficial papular lesions are present in about one fourth of patients with subcutaneous GA. Lesions in general are asymptomatic and resolve over a few years. The major clinical problem occurs when the initial pathologic interpretation is rheumatoid nodule, and an unnecessary extensive rheumatologic workup is performed.

Perforating Granuloma Annulare. Perforating granuloma annulare usually appears on the dorsal hands and presents as papules with a central keratotic core. This core represents transepidermal elimination of the degenerated material in the center of GA lesions.

Granuloma Annulare in HIV Disease. GA may occur in persons with HIV infection at all stages of disease. Lesions are typically papular, and generalized GA is more common (60%) than localized GA (40%). Photodistributed and perforating lesions may also occur. The histology is identical to GA in the normal host. The natural history of GA in HIV is unknown.

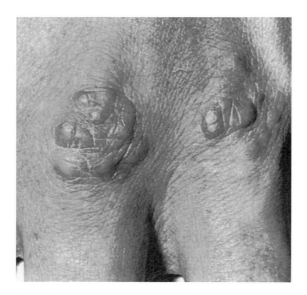

Fig. 31-1   Granuloma annulare in a typical location on the knuckles.

Granuloma Annulare and Lymphoma. The occurrence of GA and lymphoma in the same patient is rare. The lymphoma may be of any type, and it may occur before or after the GA. In those cases, however, where there is a close temporal relationship between the lymphoma and the GA, the GA is often atypical. The GA lesions can be painful and located in unusual sites such as the face or palms. Typical lesions of GA may represent one form of granulomatous inflammation seen in lymphoma.

Because there are many clinical patterns of GA, skin biopsies are often performed to confirm the diagnosis. In general, there are two histopathologic patterns that often coexist in the same patient. The classic pattern of GA is a palisading granuloma characterized by histiocytes and epithelioid cells surrounding a central zone of altered collagen. In well-developed lesions, there is mucin deposition within the foci of altered collagen. Fibrin and nuclear dust may also be present in the degenerated foci. Lesions are most typically located in the upper and mid-reticular dermis, but may involve the deep dermis or subcutaneous tissue. At the periphery of lesions a leukocytoclastic vasculitis may rarely be found.

The second pattern of GA is the interstitial pattern. It may represent early or macular lesions and is seen adjacent to well-formed palisaded lesions. A diffuse dermal infiltrate of histiocytes and other mononuclear cells with some neutrophils is interspersed between collagen bundles. Even in this interstitial pattern, however, at lowest power it can be

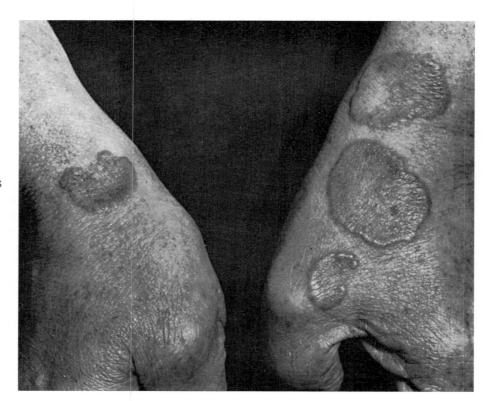

Fig. 31-2   Granuloma annulare on wrists of a 57-year-old woman; GA cleared with intralesional corticosteroid suspension injections. (Courtesy Dr. Axel W. Hoke.)

seen to be localized to certain foci within the dermis, with normal dermis between the affected foci. Interstitial mucin is often present in the affected areas. Although these features are sufficient to confirm the diagnosis of GA, further sectioning may reveal typical palisaded granulomas.

Necrobiosis lipoidica can be distinguished from GA by the tendency of the former to involve the deep dermis and subcutis, and to be diffuse, with no intervening normal collagen; and by the absence of mucin. Plasma cells are often present in the infiltrates of necrobiosis lipoidica Rheumatoid nodules are distinguished by the clinical history and by the histologic tendency for the lesions to have abundant fibrin at the center of larger palisaded granulomas.

Treatment

Patients regularly report that a biopsy of the lesion will cause its involution. Because the lesions are often asymptomatic and spontaneous involution occurs, no treatment is required in many mild cases. The intralesional injection of triamcinolone suspension is effective for individual lesions and is a reasonable initial treatment. Most cases relapse within 3 to 7 months. Topical vitamin E, cryotherapy, intralesional gamma interferon, and surgical excision have all been reported as effective, and are alternatives for individual lesions.

Generalized cases represent a major therapeutic challenge. Although systemic steroids may be very effective, the high doses required and the usual immediate relapse as the steroids are tapered make this approach untenable in most situations. In addition, because diabetes may be present, systemic steroids may complicate the management of the diabetes. A long list of systemic agents have been reported as effective, but few have been tested in large numbers of cases or in blinded or controlled fashion. These include dapsone, 100 mg once or twice daily; nicotinamide, 1.5 g daily; potassium iodide (SSKI), to 10 drops three times daily; cyclosporine to 5mg/kg/day; PUVA; UVA-1 phototherapy; and antimalarials. Systemic retinoids, both isotretinoin (Accutane) and etretinate, appear to be effective in some cases. As with all treatments, relapse may occur with discontinuation.

Barksdale SK, et al: Granuloma annulare in patients with malignant lymphoma. *J Am Acad Dermatol* 1994, 31:42.

Czarnecki DB, et al: The response of generalized granuloma annulare to dapsone. *Acta Derm Venereol* (Stockh) 1986, 66:82.

Dabski K, et al: Generalized granuloma annulare. *J Am Acad Dermatol* 1989, 20:28, 39.

Evans MJ, et al: Pseudorheumatoid nodule (deep GA) of childhood. *Pediatr Dermatol* 1994, 11:6.

Ho VC: Cyclosporine in the treatment of generalized granuloma annulare. *J Am Acad Dermatol* 1995, 32:298.

Ma A, et al: Response of generalized granuloma annulare to high-dose niacinamide. *Arch Dermatol* 1983, 119:836.

McFarland JP, et al: Periorbital granuloma annulare. *Arch Dermatol* 1982, 118:190.

Muchenberger S, et al: Phototherapy with UV-A-I for generalized granuloma annulare. *Arch Dermatol* 1997, 133:1605.

Shelley WB, et al: Surgical treatment of tumor-sized granuloma annulare of the fingers. *J Am Acad Dermatol* 1997, 37:473.

Simon M, et al: Antimalarials for control of disseminated granuloma annulare in children. *J Am Acad Dermatol* 1994, 31:1064.

Smith JB, et al: Potassium iodide in the treatment of disseminated granuloma annulare. *J Am Acad Dermatol* 1994, 30:791.

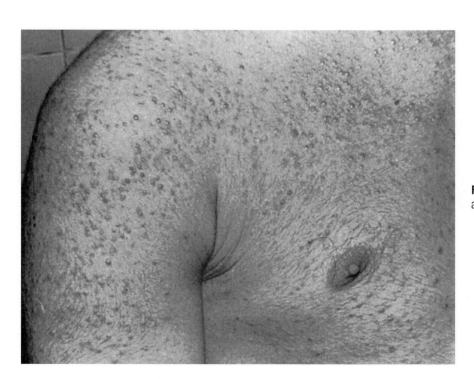

Fig. 31-3 Generalized papular granuloma annulare.

Steiner A, et al: Sulfone treatment of granuloma annulare. *J Am Acad Dermatol* 1985, 13:1004.

Toro JR, et al: Granuloma annulare and HIV infection. *Arch Dermatol* 1999, 135:1341.

Weiss JM, et al: Treatment of granuloma annulare by local injections with low-dose recombinant human interferon gamma. *J Am Acad Dermatol* 1998, 39:117. ⬛ ▲

Annular Elastolytic Giant Cell Granuloma (Meischer's) and Actinic Granuloma (O'Brien)

Annular elastolytic giant cell granuloma and actinic granuloma are unified by their histopathologic appearance. It is currently unclear whether they simply represent variants of GA occurring on sun-damaged skin or are distinct diseases.

Annular elastolytic giant cell granuloma typically presents as a single, asymptomatic, atrophic-appearing, yellow, thin plaque on the forehead. Clinically, this pattern resembles facial necrobiosis lipoidica more than GA. Multiple trunk lesions can occur with or without the facial lesions. The condition is chronic and refractory to treatment.

Actinic granuloma (O'Brien) presents as papules and plaques on sun-exposed skin. Lesions are frequently numerous and may coalesce to cover much of the exposed skin (Fig. 31-4). The diagnosis is suspected by a history of onset after significant sun exposure and the distribution on physical examination. A few lesions may occur on sun-protected sites or spill over from affected areas to more photoprotected sites. This condition affects older adults (usually over age 50), is more common in men, and can be intensely pruritic. It is not associated with diabetes mellitus, but there are numerous reports of it occurring in patients with temporal arteritis. It is speculated that the vasculitis is

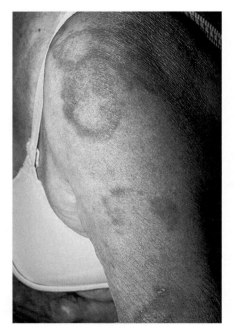

Fig. 31-4 Actinic granuloma.

also due to actinic injury to the connective tissue surrounding the temporal artery. Actinic granuloma is difficult to manage and refractory to treatment. Systemic retinoids may provide some benefit.

Histologically, both these conditions show a characteristic histology. The dermal infiltrate of macrophages is largely interstitial, and well-formed palisaded granulomas are rare. Multinucleated giant cells, often quite large, are numerous. Mucin is scant or lacking. The macrophages characteristically contain fragments of actinically damaged elastic tissue (elastophagocytosis). When this typical histology is seen in concert with the classic clinical features noted above, it may be reasonable to make these specific diagnoses. These conditions cannot, however, be diagnosed based on clinical or histologic grounds alone.

Davies MG, et al: Actinic granuloma in a young woman following prolonged sunbed usage. *Br J Dermatol* 1997, 136:797.

Lau H, et al: Actinic granuloma in association with giant cell arteritis. *Pathology* 1997, 29:260.

McGrae JD: Actinic granuloma. *Arch Dermatol* 1986, 122:43.

Ratnavel RC, et al: O'Brien's actinic granuloma. *J R Soc Med* 1995, 88:528P.

Revenga F, et al: Annular elastolytic giant cell granuloma: actinc granuloma. *Clin Exp Dermatol* 1996, 21:51.

Sina B, et al: Generalized elastophagocytic granuloma. *Cutis* 1992, 49:355. ▲

Granuloma Multiforme (Leiker)

Granuloma multiforme is seen only in central Africa, where it is a common disorder. It affects adults over age 40 and is more common in females. Lesions are most frequent on the upper trunk and arms. It begins as small papules that evolve into round or oval plaques up to 15 cm wide within a year's time. The active edge of lesions may be elevated to as much as 4 mm in height, and the center may be slightly depressed and hypopigmented. Pruritus can occur, and coalescing lesions may form unusual polycyclic shapes. The course is chronic. It is most importantly separated from tuberculoid leprosy. Histologically, it resembles GA, but multinucleated giant cells are prominent. Giant cells typically contain phagocytosed connective tissue, and elastic tissue is decreased in the areas affected by the granulomas. In these regards it shares features with annular elastolytic giant cell granuloma.

Meyers WM, et al: Histologic characteristics of granuloma multiforme (Mkar disease). *Int J Lepr Other Mycobact Dis* 1970, 38:241. ▲

SARCOIDOSIS

Sarcoidosis has also been known as *Besnier-Boeck-Schaumann disease, Boeck's sarcoid, Besnier's lupus pernio,* and *Schaumann's benign lymphogranulomatosis.* Sarcoidosis is a systemic granulomatous disease of undetermined etiology and pathogenesis that involves the skin and many of the internal organs with a persistent course interrupted by remissions and relapses. In addition to the skin, which is involved in between 9% and 37% of cases, other sites of involvement are lungs, mediastinal and peripheral lymph nodes, eyes, phalangeal bones, myocardium, central nervous system (CNS), kidneys, spleen, liver, and parotid glands.

Sarcoidosis occurs worldwide. In Europe it is most prevalent in the Scandinavian countries, especially in Sweden, where up to 140 cases per 100,000 occur in certain rural forested areas. In the United States the southeastern states and certain areas in New York City show the highest prevalence. The disease begins most frequently between ages 20 and 40. People of Irish, African, and Afro-Caribbean heritage are more frequently affected. In the United States, blacks are three times more likely to develop sarcoidosis than whites. In addition, blacks are affected more severely. Among blacks in England, the United States, and South Africa, two thirds to three quarters of patients are women, whereas in whites men and women are equally affected. Children may also develop sarcoidosis. The average age is 13 years, with a gender ratio of 1:1.

Cutaneous involvement in sarcoidosis may be classified as *specific*, which reveals granulomas on biopsy, or *nonspecific*, which is mainly reactive, such as erythema nodosum. In about 20% of cases the skin lesions appear before the systemic disease, in 50% there is simultaneous appearance of the skin and systemic lesions, and in 30% the skin lesions appear up to 10 years after the systemic disease has occurred. This is often coincident with the tapering of systemic steroids for pulmonary sarcoidosis. The cutaneous manifestations of sarcoidosis are quite varied, and numerous morphologic lesion types have been described. The morphology of the lesions in sarcoidosis might include papules, nodules, plaques, subcutaneous nodules, scar sarcoidosis, erythroderma, ulcerations, and verrucose, ich-

thyosiform, hypomelanotic, psoriasiform, and alopecia. Sarcoid, like syphilis, is a great mimic of other skin diseases and should be considered in the differential diagnosis of many different skin disorders. In sarcoidosis lesions are usually multiple and firm and elastic when palpated, and extend to involve the entire thickness of the dermis. The overlying epidermis may be slightly thinned, discolored, telangiectatic, or scaly. The color is faint, showing dull tints of red, purple, brown, or yellow according to the stage of development. Usually the lesions are asymptomatic, but approximately 10% to 15% of patients itch. There is a racial difference in the frequency of cutaneous lesions in sarcoidosis. Among white patients erythema nodosum is as frequent as the specific cutaneous manifestations, and both types of cutaneous involvement occur in about 10% of patients with sarcoidosis. In blacks, erythema nodosum is much less common; however, specific cutaneous manifestations occur in 50% or more of patients.

Papular Sarcoid. Papules are the most common form of cutaneous sarcoidosis. Lesions may be localized or generalized, in which case small papules predominate. This is also known as *miliary sarcoid*. The papules are especially numerous over the face, eyelids, neck, and shoulders (Figs. 31-5 to 31-8). In time the lesions involute to faint macules. Verrucous lesions are a rare variant (Fig. 31-9). The differential diagnosis includes syringoma, xanthelasma, lichen planus, or trichoepithelioma.

Annular Sarcoidosis. Papular lesions may coalesce or be arranged in annular patterns. Central clearing with hypopigmentation, atrophy, and scarring may occur (Figs. 31-10 and 31-11). Lesions favor the head and neck and are usually associated with chronic sarcoidosis.

Hypopigmented Sarcoidosis. Hypopigmentation may be the earliest sign of sarcoidosis and is usually diagnosed in

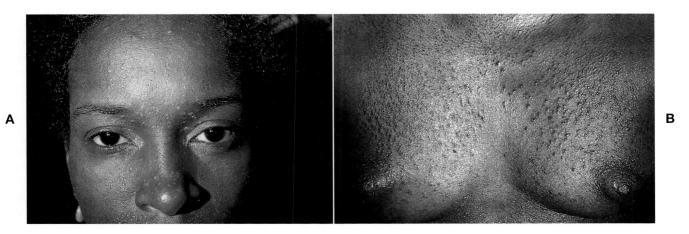

Fig. 31-5 **A** and **B**, Papular sarcoidosis.

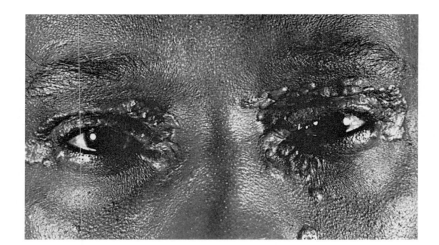

Fig. 31-6 Sarcoidosis. (Courtesy Dr. H. Shatin.)

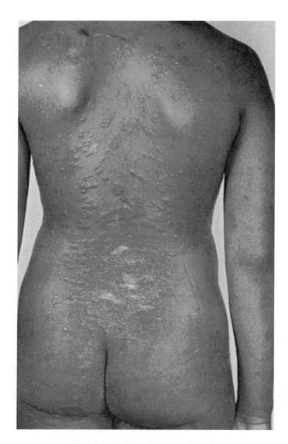

Fig. 31-7 Papular sarcoidosis.

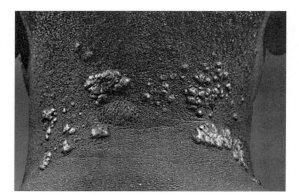

Fig. 31-8 Sarcoidosis resembling acne keloidalis nuchae. (Courtesy Dr. H. Shatin.)

Lupus Pernio. In three quarters of cases of lupus pernio, chronic fibrotic respiratory tract involvement is found. Lesions typically are violaceous, smooth, and shiny plaques on the head and neck, especially the nose, cheeks, lips, forehead, and ears. Lesions may be disfiguring. Involvement of the nasal mucosa and underlying bone may occur and lead to nasal perforation. In 43% of cases, lupus pernio is associated with granulomas in the bones (punched-out cysts), most commonly of the fingers. Chronic ocular lesions occur in 37% of cases. Lupus pernio is typically seen in women in their fourth or fifth decade of life. The skin lesions rarely involute spontaneously.

Ulcerative Sarcoidosis. Ulcerative sarcoidosis is very rare. It affects primarily black women in young adulthood. In half of cases it is the presenting finding of sarcoidosis (Fig. 31-13). The ulcerations may occur de novo or in sarcoidal plaques. Lesions favor the lower extremities. The clinical appearance may not be specific, but skin biopsies are diagnostic. Lupus pernio may also be present. Many patients

darkly pigmented races, especially blacks (Fig. 31-12). Lesions vary from a few millimeters to more than a centimeter in diameter and favor the extremities. Although they appear macular by visual inspection, on palpation a dermal or subcutaneous component is often palpable in the center of the lesion.

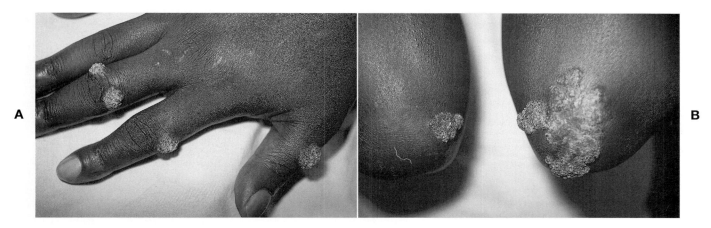

Fig. 31-9 A and B, Verrucose sarcoidosis.

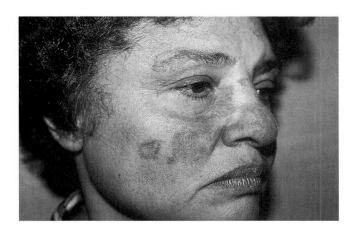

Fig. 31-10 Annular sarcoidosis.

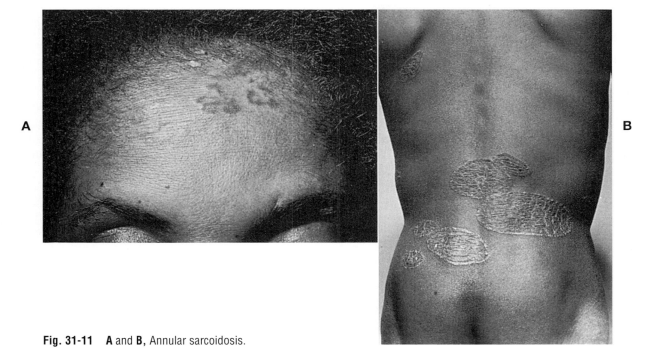

Fig. 31-11 A and B, Annular sarcoidosis.

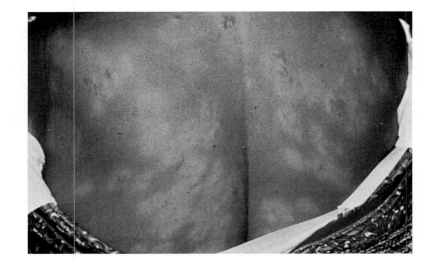

Fig. 31-12 Hypopigmented sarcoidosis. (Courtesy Dr. K. Stein.)

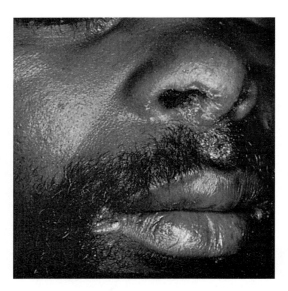

Fig. 31-13 Ulcerative sarcoidosis with mild destructive changes on the nose.

have multisystem sarcoidosis, although uncommonly no other evidence of sarcoidosis is found.

Subcutaneous Sarcoidosis. Subcutaneous sarcoidosis is also known as *Darier-Roussy sarcoid* and consists of a few 1- to 3-cm deep-seated nodules on the trunk and extremities; only rarely do they appear on the face. The overlying epidermis may be slightly violaceous. A biopsy is usually required to confirm the diagnosis. Five percent or fewer patients with sarcoidosis have subcutaneous nodules. This form of sarcoidosis may be associated with acute or chronic disease and is therefore not of predictive value.

Sarcoidosis in Scars (Scar Sarcoid). Sarcoid lesions may develop in old scars from various causes. Infiltration of tattoos and involvement of areas with foreign body material are two variants of scar sarcoid (Fig. 31-14). Previously

flat scars raise up and may become erythematous or violaceous. These lesions closely resemble keloids. Scar sarcoid may sometimes occur in patients with acute disease but most frequently is found in patients with chronic sarcoidosis.

Plaques. These distinctive lesions, first reported by Hutchinson, are flat-surfaced, slightly elevated plaques that appear with greatest frequency on the cheeks, limbs, and trunk symmetrically (Fig. 31-15). Superficial nodules may be superimposed, and coalescence of plaques may lead to serpiginous lesions. Involvement of the scalp may lead to permanent alopecia. Granuloma annulare, necrobiosis lipoidica, and cutaneous syphilis must be distinguished.

Erythrodermic Sarcoidosis. Erythrodermic sarcoidosis is an extremely rare form of sarcoidosis. A diffuse infiltrative erythroderma of the skin usually begins as erythematous, scaling patches that merge to involve large portions of the body.

Ichthyosiform Sarcoidosis. Ichthyosiform sarcoidosis resembles ichthyosis vulgaris, with fine scaling usually on the distal extremities (Fig. 31-16). Although the lesions have no palpable component, a biopsy will reveal dermal noncaseating granulomas.

Alopecia. Alopecia subsequent to sarcoidosis is seen in two settings. Plaques may extend into and involve the scalp leading to scarring hair loss. More rarely, macular lesions from one to several centimeters in diameter appear on the scalp and closely resemble alopecia areata. This form may be permanent or reversible. A biopsy of both forms of alopecic sarcoid will reveal dermal granulomas and sometimes loss of follicular structures.

Morpheaform Sarcoid. Very rarely, specific cutaneous lesions of sarcoidosis may be accompanied by substantial

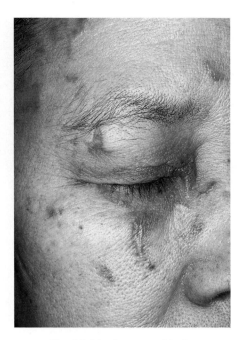

Fig. 31-14 Scar sarcoidosis.

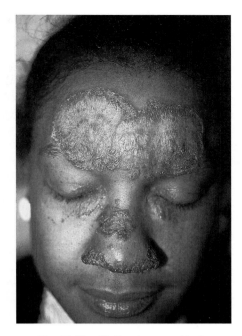

Fig. 31-15 Disfiguring sarcoidosis.

dermal fibrosis and simulate morphea. Lesions are more typically generalized plaques but may be localized and resemble linear morphea. Skin biopsy will demonstrate noncaseating granulomas. Some patients respond to antimalarial therapy.

Mucosal Sarcoid. The lesions in the mouth are characterized by pinhead-size papules that may be grouped and fused together to form a flat plaque. The hard palate, tongue, buccal mucosa, or posterior pharynx may be involved. In lupus pernio the nasal mucosa is frequently involved.

Erythema Nodosum in Sarcoidosis. Erythema nodosum is the most common nonspecific cutaneous finding in sarcoidosis. Sarcoidosis may first appear with fever, polyarthralgias, uveitis, bilateral hilar adenopathy, fatigue, and erythema nodosum. This combination, known as *Lofgren's syndrome,* occurs frequently in Scandinavian whites and is uncommon in American blacks. The typical red, warm, and tender subcutaneous nodules of the anterior shins are distinctive and are most frequently seen in young women. The face, upper back, and extensor surfaces of the upper extremities may less commonly be involved. There is a strikingly elevated erythrocyte sedimentation rate, frequently above 50. Erythema nodosum is associated with a good prognosis, with the sarcoidosis involuting within 6 months of onset in 80% of cases.

Systemic Sarcoidosis. Many instances of sarcoidosis are asymptomatic, and it is only when routine radiographs of the chest reveal some abnormality that sarcoidosis is suspected. Fever may be the only symptom of the disease.

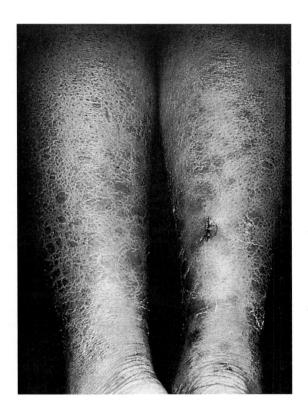

Fig. 31-16 Ichthyosiform sarcoidosis.

In other instances the disease begins insidiously, with fever, weight loss, fatigue, and malaise.

Intrathoracic lesions, including lung lesions and hilar adenopathy, are the most common manifestation of the disease. Pulmonary changes, usually bilateral, consist of large, dense shadows with extensions radiating outward and with reticulation of the lower lobes. The large, dense shadows may resemble metastatic tumor. Hilar adenopathy is usually present and if alone is often associated with a good prognosis; however, chronic pulmonary fibrosis rarely involutes. Lymphadenopathy, especially of the mediastinal and hilar nodes, and generalized adenopathy, or adenopathy confined to the cervical or axillary areas, may be an initial sign of sarcoidosis or occur during the course of the disease.

Polyarthralgias may be seen with acute sarcoidosis or as a component of chronic disease. Chronic arthritis may occur. Osseous involvement is often present in chronic disease. The most characteristic changes are found radiographically in the bones of the hands and feet, particularly in the phalanges (Fig. 31-17). They consist of round, punched-out, lytic, cystic lesions. These are seen frequently in patients with lupus pernio. The bone lesions represent epithelioid granulomas. Ocular involvement is present in some 25% to 30% of patients, with granulomatous uveitis the most frequent lesion. The lacrimal gland may be involved unilaterally or bilaterally by painless nodular swellings. With lacrimal gland changes there may be associated enlargement of the submaxillary, salivary, and cervical lymph glands, or the parotid glands may become involved (Mikulicz's syndrome). Lesions of the iris are nodular and painless. There may also be lesions of the retina, choroid, sclera, and optic nerve. Ophthalmic disease is highly correlated with systemic involvement.

Parotid gland and lacrimal gland enlargement with uveitis and fever may occur in sarcoidosis; this is known as *uveoparotid fever* or *Heerfordt's syndrome* and usually lasts 2 to 6 months if not treated. Facial nerve palsy and CNS disease frequently are seen in this syndrome.

Liver involvement occurs in about 20% of patients clinically; however, a blind liver biopsy will reveal granulomas in 60% of cases. Hepatomegaly with elevation of serum alkaline phosphatase, biliary cirrhosis with hypercholesterolemia, and portal hypertension with esophageal varices are some of the manifestations. Liver biopsy showing hepatic tubercles is an excellent means of confirming the diagnosis of sarcoidosis.

Renal disease may be due to direct involvement with granulomas or secondary to hypercalcemia. Nephrolithiasis may result. Virtually every other organ may be involved. Among these are the heart, with primary myocardial sarcoidosis; the spleen, with hypersplenism; the muscles, with sarcoidal granulomas; and the nervous system, with peripheral and CNS findings.

Most patients with sarcoidosis have an increased erythrocyte sedimentation rate. Leukopenia, lymphopenia, anemia, eosinophilia, and thrombocytopenia may be found. Elevated serum proteins occur because of polyclonal hyperglobulinemia. With liver or bone lesions, serum alkaline phosphatase may be elevated. If hypercalcemia is present, anorexia, vomiting, muscle weakness, and polyuria may

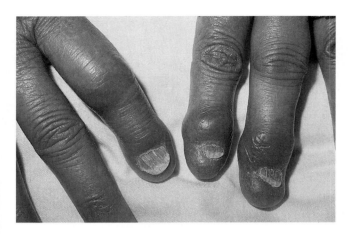

Fig. 31-17 Sarcoidosis affecting bones and nails of fingers.

occur. Hypercalcemia is found in about 11% of patients, but hypercalcuria in 40%. Renal stones and failure can occur.

Angiotensin-converting enzyme (ACE) levels may be elevated in all granulomatous diseases, including sarcoidosis. An elevated ACE level is suggestive, but not diagnostic, for granulomatous inflammation. A normal ACE level cannot be used to rule out sarcoidosis, and an elevated level does not necessarily indicate the presence of multisystem involvement. If elevated, ACE levels may be used to monitor the activity of the disease.

Cell-mediated immune responses in sarcoidosis are altered in the following respects:

- Skin-test responses are lost or at least diminished.
- The proliferative response of lymphocytes to antigens and mitogens is reduced.
- Circulating helper T cells are reduced more than suppressor cells are increased.
- Activated T cells are increased.
- Humoral (B cell) reactions are increased, with polyclonal elevation of serum immunoglobulin.
- The humoral response to certain antigens is exaggerated.
- Serum antibodies to *Mycoplasma* and several viruses are increased.
- Circulating immune complexes occur in the blood in about half the patients with acute disease.
- Autoantibodies to rheumatoid factor and antinuclear antibody can occur.

The Kveim-Siltzbach test is performed by the intradermal injection of 0.2 ml Kveim antigen in the forearm. The antigen is produced from affected sarcoidal tissue. After 6 weeks the site of injection is biopsied. The presence of typical "naked" epithelioid cell tubercles signifies a positive Kveim reaction. The Kveim reaction is expected to be positive in about 80% of active cases of sarcoidosis. The test becomes negative when the patient goes into remission. The test is quite specific for sarcoidosis, with only 2%

false-positives. It is not usually performed in the United States.

The cause of sarcoidosis remains elusive. Two theories predominate. One is that sarcoidosis represents a reaction to an as yet unidentified antigen or infectious agent. The "transmission" of sarcoidosis by cardiac and bone marrow transplantation supports the infectious theory. The second is that there is a genetic predisposition. Among black patients 19% have a family history of sarcoidosis. These theories are not mutually exclusive.

The histology of sarcoidosis in all affected tissues is identical. The characteristic finding is that of the "naked tubercle" composed of collections of large, pale-staining, epithelioid histiocytes. There may be small foci of necrosis in the center of the granulomas, and multinucleate giant cells, sometimes with inclusions (asteroid bodies and Schaumann bodies), may be present. Although classically there are few lymphocytes around the granulomas, they may be numerous. The granulomas may be nodular, diffuse, or tubular along neurovascular structures.

The histologic differential diagnosis is broad, and the diagnosis of sarcoidosis cannot be definitely made histologically. Allergic granulomas caused by zirconium or beryllium are histologically identical to sarcoidosis. Other foreign-body granulomas (especially as a result of silica), granulomatous rosacea, granulomatous secondary syphilis, tuberculoid leprosy, and leishmaniasis may closely simulate sarcoidosis.

The diagnosis of sarcoidosis is established by the demonstration of involvement consistent with sarcoidosis in two different organ systems. This is usually done histologically. A positive Kveim test may help to confirm the diagnosis.

If cutaneous sarcoidal granulomas are identified in a patient with no prior history of sarcoidosis, the first diagnostic test to be performed should be a chest radiograph. If this is abnormal, pulmonary function testing may be indicated. Ophthalmologic evaluation and conjunctival biopsy may be useful. Blind biopsy of the minor salivary glands may demonstrate sarcoidal granulomas. Otherwise, histologic evaluation of any involved tissue may be considered.

Sarcoidosis and Immunologic Abnormalities

Numerous reports exist of sarcoidosis occurring in patients with various forms of immunodeficiency, both congenital and acquired. This includes patients with various malignancies, especially Hodgkin's disease. It is unclear whether these represent true sarcoidosis or are sarcoidlike reactions caused by immune dysregulation. Interestingly, there are numerous reports documenting the appearance of cutaneous sarcoidal granulomas in association with interferon alfa therapy. In one report, cutaneous lesions, pulmonary findings, or both, as well as other features of sarcoidosis, occurred in 5% of patients treated with interferon for hepatitis C.

Treatment

Numerous therapies have been reported as beneficial in cutaneous sarcoidosis, usually after anecdotal observation. There is virtually no information regarding what types of therapy are best for which of the various cutaneous manifestations. The cutaneous disease may spontaneously remit without treatment. Because most skin lesions are asymptomatic, the major indication for treatment is cosmetic (except for disfiguring facial lesions).

Systemic corticosteroids are virtually always beneficial in cutaneous sarcoidosis. Unfortunately, the doses required to control cutaneous disease may be too high (usually in excess of 15 mg daily) to be ideal for long-term use. For limited skin disease intralesional injection of 2.5 mg/ml to 5.0 mg/ml of triamcinolone acetonide suspension is very effective. For thinner lesions, the superpotent steroids may even be effective.

Corticosteroid therapy is indicated when there is acute systemic involvement with fever and weight loss, in active eye disease, in sarcoidal involvement of the myocardium, in active pulmonary disease with functional disability, in hypersplenism, in hypercalcemia, and in symptomatic CNS involvement.

Antimalarials, both chloroquine and hydroxychloroquine, have been used to treat extensive cutaneous sarcoidosis in doses of 250 mg or 200 to 400 mg daily, respectively. About three quarters of patients appear to respond partially or completely. In some cases the associated pulmonary disease also improves. These agents may also be used to reduce the dose of systemic steroids required.

Methotrexate in doses of 15 to 25 mg weekly is also efficacious and seems to help patients with severe lupus pernio or ulcerative sarcoidosis who are otherwise very difficult to treat. Methotrexate-induced hepatitis occurs in 15% of patients with sarcoidosis treated with methotrexate. Allopurinol, 300 mg daily, has been reported to lead to clearing of refractory and widespread cutaneous lesions. With all the treatments just mentioned, response begins after a few weeks of treatment. The retinoids, principally isotretinoin, are also beneficial in some patients, usually at doses of 0.5 to 1.0 mg/kg. Response is usually seen after 6 or more weeks. Thalidomide, 50 to 100 mg daily, has led to improvement of the skin lesions after several months. *It should not be used to treat pregnant patients, however, because of possible teratogenic effects to the fetus.* Tranilast has been reported to be of benefit. Lupus pernio lesions may be complicated by a dusky purple color and telangiectasias. These may respond to pulsed dye laser therapy.

Albertini JG, et al: Ulcerative sarcoidosis. *Arch Dermatol* 1997, 133:215.

Banse-Kupin L, et al: Ichthyosiform sarcoidosis. *J Am Acad Dermatol* 1987, 17:616.

Bower JS: Pulmonary evaluation of patients presenting with cutaneous manifestations of sarcoidosis. *Int J Dermatol* 1981, 20:385.

Brechtel B, et al: Allopurinol: a therapeutic alternative for disseminated cutaneous sarcoidosis. *Br J Dermatol* 1996, 135:307.

Burov EA, et al: Morpheaform sarcoidosis. *J Am Acad Dermatol* 1998, 39:345.

Callen JP, et al: Serum angiotensin I-converting enzyme level in patients with cutaneous sarcoidal granuloma. *Arch Dermatol* 1982, 118:232.

Diestelmeier MR, et al: Sarcoidosis manifesting as eyelid swelling. *Arch Dermatol* 1982, 118:356.

Eggelmeuer F, et al: An unusual presentation of sarcoidosis. *J Rheumatol* 1991, 18:1936.

Goodman MM, et al: Treatment of lupus pernio with the flashlamp pulsed dye laser. *Laser Surg Med* 1992, 12:549.

Healsmith MF, et al: The development of scar sarcoidosis in the site of desensitization injections. *Clin Exp Dermatol* 1992, 17:369.

Hebel JL, et al: Lofgren's syndrome. *Cutis* 1993, 52:223.

Hess SP, et al: Ichthyosiform and morpheaform sarcoidosis. *Clin Exp Dermatol* 1990, 8:171.

Heyll A, et al: Possible transmission of sarcoidosis via bone marrow transplantation. *Bone Marrow Transplant* 1994, 14:161.

Hoffman RM, et al: Sarcoidosis associated with interferon-alpha therapy for hepatitis C. *J Hepatol* 1998, 28:1058.

Jones E, et al: Hydroxychloroquine is effective therapy for control of cutaneous sarcoidal granulomas. *J Am Acad Dermatol* 1990, 23:487.

Kalb RE, et al: Sarcoidosis with subcutaneous nodules. *Am J Med* 1988, 85:731.

Kerdel FA, et al: Sarcoidosis. *J Am Acad Dermatol* 1984, 11:1.

Mana J, et al: Cutaneous involvement in sarcoidosis. *Arch Dermatol* 1997, 133:882.

Matarasso SL, et al: Ichthyosiform sarcoidosis. *Cutis* 1991, 47:405.

Mitchell IC, et al: Ulcerative and hypopigmented sarcoidosis. *J Am Acad Dermatol* 1986, 15:1062.

Nessan VJ, et al: Biopsy of the minor salivary glands in the diagnosis of sarcoidosis. *N Engl J Med* 1979, 301:922.

Newman LS, et al: Sarcoidosis. *N Engl J Med* 1997, 336:1224.

Patel KB, et al: Nails in sarcoidosis. *Arch Dermatol* 1983, 119:272.

Rasmussen JE: Sarcoidosis in young children. *J Am Acad Dermatol* 1981, 5:566.

Robert C, et al: Malignant melanoma and granulomatosis. *Br J Dermatol* 1997, 137:787.

Rousseau L, et al: Cutaneous sarcoidosis successfully treated with low doses of thalidomide. *Arch Dermatol* 1998, 134:1045.

Scott TH, et al: Sarcoidosis with nodular lesions of the palm and sole. *Arch Dermatol* 1984, 120:1239.

Smith C, et al: Sarcoidosis in Johannesburg. *S Afr Med J* 1991, 80:423.

Sowden JM, et al: Sarcoidosis presenting with granulomatous reaction confined to tattoos. *Clin Exp Dermatol* 1992, 17:446.

Spiteri MA, et al: Lupus pernio. *Br J Dermatol* 1985, 112:315.

Vainsencher D, et al: Subcutaneous sarcoidosis. *Arch Dermatol* 1984, 120:1028.

Veien NK, et al: Cutaneous sarcoidosis in Caucasians. *J Am Acad Dermatol* 1987, 16:534.

Verdegem TD, et al: Cutaneous ulcers in sarcoidosis. *Arch Dermatol* 1987, 123:1531.

Waldinger TP, et al: Treatment of cutaneous sarcoidosis with isotretinoin. *Arch Dermatol* 1983, 119:1003.

Walsh NMG, et al: Cutaneous sarcoidosis and foreign bodies. *Am J Dermatopathol* 1993, 15:203.

Webster GF, et al: Methotrexate therapy in cutaneous sarcoidosis. *Ann Int Med* 1989, 111:538.

Yamada H, et al: Treatment of cutaneous sarcoidosis with tranilast. *J Dermatol* 1995, 22:149.

Yavorkovsky LL, et al: Cutaneous sarcoidosis in a patient with Philadelphia-positive chronic myelogenous leukemia treated with interferon alpha. *Am J Hematol* 1998, 58:80.

Zic JA, et al: Treatment of cutaneous sarcoidosis with chloroquine. *Arch Dermatol* 1991, 127:1034. _____ ▲

HISTIOCYTOSES

Certain syndromes that are well defined clinically and histologically include the term *histiocyte* in their name. They are characterized by infiltrates with prominent macrophages and have been grouped under the term *histiocytoses*. This classification is less than ideal, since the term *histiocyte* is poorly defined, but until a clear classification scheme is developed, these conditions will be grouped together. One point of agreement is that there are two separate groups within these disorders: the Langerhans' cell (or X-type) histiocytoses and the non-Langerhans' types (or non-X histiocytoses). The value of immunohistochemical markers and electron microscopic findings (other than Birbeck granules) in classifying these disorders is unclear.

Fowler JF, et al: Cutaneous non-X histiocytosis. *J Am Acad Dermatol* 1985, 13:645.

Gianotti F, et al: Histiocytic syndromes: a review. *J Am Acad Dermatol* 1985, 13:383.

Headington JT: The histiocyte. *Arch Dermatol* 1986, 122:533.

Ringel E, et al: Primary histiocytic dermatoses. *Arch Dermatol* 1985, 121:1531. _____ ▲

Non-X histiocytoses

Juvenile Xanthogranuloma

Juvenile xanthogranuloma (JXG) is the most common non-Langerhans' histiocytosis. Between 5% and 17% are present at birth, and 40% to 70% appear in the first year of life. In adults lesions tend to occur in the late twenties to early thirties. JXG is 10 times more common in whites than blacks but occurs in all races. In childhood JXG is 1.5 times more common in males than females, but the gender distribution in adults is equal.

Sixty percent to 80% of JXG are solitary. They begin as well-demarcated, firm, rubbery, round to oval papules or nodules from 5 to 20 mm in diameter (Fig. 31-18). Early lesions are pink to red with a yellow tinge and become tan/brown over time. Most lesions are asymptomatic. The head and neck are the most common location, followed by the upper trunk and upper extremities. Gianotti classified multiple childhood JXGs into two forms: small nodular and large nodular types (Figs. 31-19 to 31-21). The small type has lesions of 2 to 5 mm and are more numerous, whereas lesions in the large type are 10 to 20 mm and fewer in number. Often one patient will have both types of lesions. Skin lesions regress spontaneously within 3 to 6 years in children. In adults lesions are often more persistent. Hyperpigmentation, atrophy, or anetoderma may remain after lesions resolve.

Multiple atypical presentations have been described. These include hyperkeratotic nodules; macronodular tumors from 2 to 10 cm in diameter; clustered forms; flat, plaquelike lesions; and pedunculated lesions. Atypical sites

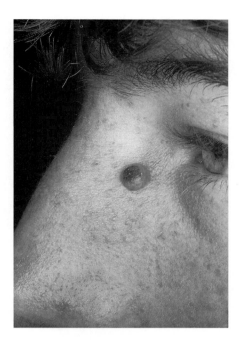

Fig. 31-18   Solitary juvenile xanthogranuloma in an adult.

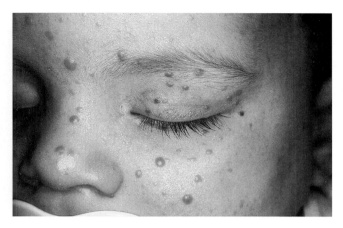

Fig. 31-19   Juvenile xanthogranuloma.

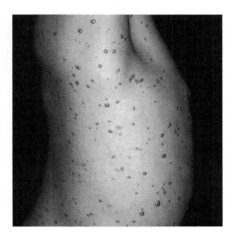

Fig. 31-20   Juvenile xanthogranuloma on the trunk.

of involvement include the genitalia, lips, palms, soles, earlobes, and fingers (Fig. 31-22). Subcutaneous masses can occur on the head and neck, or trunk or upper extremity. Oral JXG usually develops after age 3 and is most frequently a solitary lesion of the lateral tongue or midline of the hard palate.

Extracutaneous JXG is uncommon. It may appear with or without cutaneous lesions, but if cutaneous lesions are present, they are always multiple. Ocular involvement occurs in about 0.4% of children with multiple JXGs, and 41% of children with ocular JXGs have skin lesions. Skin lesions appear after eye lesions in 45% of cases. Eye lesions usually occur during the first 2 years of life. The most common location is the iris, where JXG can present as a tumor, as unilateral glaucoma, as a unilateral uveitis, with spontaneous hyphema, or as heterochromia iridis. The eyelid or posterior eye may also be involved. Other extracutaneous sites and their presentations, in order of frequency, include the lung (respiratory distress and nodular opacities on chest radiograph), liver (hepatomegaly), testis (mass), and rarely, the CNS, kidney, spleen, and retroperitoneum. Ocular screening is reserved for children with multiple cutaneous lesions before the age of 2 years. Other evaluations for extracutaneous JXGs are not indicated unless there are symptoms or findings suggesting their presence. Extracutaneous lesions also spontaneously regress.

JXGs have been reported in association with both neurofibromatosis (NF-1) and juvenile chronic myelogenous leukemia (JCML). JCML and NF-1 are known to be linked, but since JCML occurs in infancy or early child-hood, often café au lait macules are the only findings of NF-1 at that time. Sometimes all three conditions affect the same patient, with males having a 3:1 predominance, and commonly a maternal history of NF-1. Children with JXG should be examined for stigmata of NF-1. If these stigmata are found, especially in a boy with a maternal history of NF-1, the pediatrician should be alerted of the possible, although uncommon, occurrence of JCML.

Lesions appear histologically as nonencapsulated, but circumscribed, proliferations in the upper and mid reticular dermis and may extend more deeply into the subcutaneous tissue, or abut directly on the epidermis with no grenz zone. Epidermotropism does not occur. The histopathology varies in accordance with the stage of the lesion. Very early lesions are composed of mononuclear cells with abundant amphophilic cytoplasm that is poorly lipidized or vacuolated. Later the cells become more vacuolated, and multinucleated forms appear. In mature lesions, foam cells, multinucleated foam cells (Touton giant cells) and foreign-body giant cells are present. Touton giant cells are characteristic of

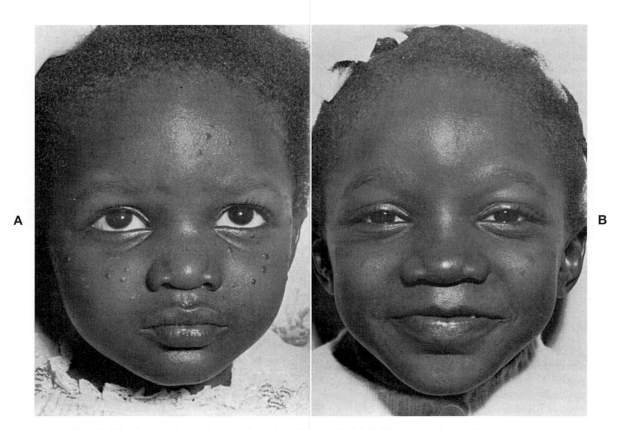

Fig. 31-21 **A,** Juvenile xanthogranuloma in a 3-year-old girl. **B,** Three years later with no treatment.

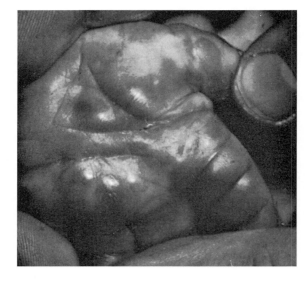

Fig. 31-22 Juvenile xanthogranuloma on the palm of a 6-month-old child.

JXG but not specific for it. The inflammatory infiltrate consists of lymphocytes, eosinophils, and neutrophils, and lacks plasma cells. Fibrosis occurs in the older lesions. The macrophages in JXG stain with Factor XIIIa, sometimes with peanut agglutinin, rarely with CD1, and not with S-100 or Mac 387.

JXG must be distinguished from Langerhans' cell his-tiocytosis. The features favoring JXG include lack of crusting or scale and the distribution and uniformity of size of lesions. Histologic evaluation is definitive in difficult cases, since JXGs are negative for markers that stain Langerhans' cells (S-100, CD1). Benign cephalic histiocy-tosis (BCH) may be difficult to distinguish both clinically and histologically, but in BCH lesions tend to be flatter and are mainly on the head and neck. Papular xanthoma can be distinguished histologically. Mastocytosis clinically will urticate when scratched (Darier's sign) and can be distinguished histologically. Solitary JXG appearing in a child must be distinguished from a Spitz nevus, usually requiring a biopsy.

Chang MW, et al: The risk of intraocular juvenile xanthogranuloma. *J Am Acad Dermatol* 1996, 34:445.

Gutmann DH, et al: Juvenile xanthogranuloma, neurofibromatosis 1, and juvenile chronic myeloid leukemia. *Arch Dermatol* 1996, 132:1390.

Hernandez-Martin A, et al: Juvenile xanthogranuloma. *J Am Acad Dermatol* 1997, 36:355.

Mann RE, et al: Urticaria pigmentosa and juvenile xanthogranuloma. *Pediatr Dermatol* 1996, 13:122.

Neuman CC, et al: Nonlipidized juvenile xanthogranuloma. *Pediatr Dermatol* 1997, 14:98.

Zelger B, et al: Juvenile and adult xanthogranuloma. *Am J Surg Pathol* 1994, 18:126.

Zvulunov A: Juvenile xanthogranuloma, neurofibromatosis, and juvenille chronic myelogenous leukemia. *Arch Dermatol* 1996, 132:712. _____ ▲

Benign Cephalic Histiocytosis

Benign cephalic histiocytosis (BCH) is a rare condition affecting boys twice as commonly as girls. The onset is between 2 and 34 months of age, most occurring in the second half of the first year of life. The disease begins initially on the head, often the cheeks, then involves the neck and upper trunk. The lesions are slightly raised, multiple, reddish yellow papules 2 to 3 mm in diameter. Lesions may coalesce to give a reticulate appearance. The mucosa and viscera are not involved. Lesions spontaneously involute over 2 to 8 years, leaving behind atrophic pigmented lesions. Some view it as a localized childhood variant of generalized eruptive histiocytoma. Histologically, there is a diffuse dermal infiltration of nonlipidized histiocytic cells. S-100 stains are negative.

Gianotti R, et al: Benign cephalic histiocytosis. *Am J Dermatopathol* 1993, 15:315.

Pena-Penabad C, et al: Benign cephalic histiocytosis. *Pediatr Dermatol* 1994, 11:164. _____ ▲

Reticulohistiocytosis

Two distinct forms of reticulohistiocytosis occur: reticulohistiocytic granuloma (solitary and multiple reticulohistiocytoma) and multicentric reticulohistiocytosis. The two forms have identical histology; however, clinically their manifestations are quite distinct.

Reticulohistiocytic Granuloma.

Reticulohistiocytic granuloma usually occurs as a solitary, firm, dermal lesion of less than 1 cm in diameter. Multiple lesions may rarely occur and can be quite extensive and diffuse. Solitary lesions and multiple lesions without systemic involvement, in contrast to multicentric reticulohistiocytosis, have been described mainly in adult men and rarely in children.

These solitary lesions are to be distinguished from xanthogranuloma, granular cell tumor and dermatofibroma, and multiple lesions from granuloma annulare, Langerhans cell histiocytosis, and granular cell tumor.

Multicentric Reticulohistiocytosis.

Multicentric reticulohistiocytosis is a multisystem disease beginning usually in the fifth decade. It is two to three times more common in women than in men and affects all races. About 30% of reported cases have had an associated malignancy, but no specific type of malignancy is more prevalent. Solid tumors, lymphomas, melanoma, and sarcomas have all coexisted. The skin lesions usually appear before the diagnosis of the malignancy, but synchronous behavior of the skin lesions and the underlying malignancy is uncommonly reported. It is unclear whether multicentric reticulohistiocytosis should be considered a true paraneoplastic syndrome, like acanthosis nigricans, for example. Given the high frequency of underlying malignancy, however, an evaluation for underlying cancer should be undertaken in a patient with multicentric reticulohistiocytosis.

Clinically, there may be a few to a few hundred firm, skin-colored to red-brown papules and nodules mostly 2 to 10 mm in diameter, but some reaching several centimeters in size. These occur most frequently on the fingers and hands, with a tendency to cause paronychial lesions (Fig. 31-23). In about half the cases lesions will be arranged about nail folds, giving a so-called "coral bead" appearance, which may be associated with nail dystrophy. The upper half of the body, including the arms, scalp, face, ears, and neck are also common sites (Fig. 31-24). Ninety percent of patients have lesions on the face and hands. Characteristic are nodular and papular involvement of the pinnae and a symmetrical distribution of the lesions, especially over joints. The nodules on the arms, elbows, and knees may resemble rheumatoid nodules. Some patients may complain of pruritus.

Mucous membrane involvement is seen in half the cases and is most frequent on the lips and tongue; other sites are the gingiva, palate, buccal mucosa, pharynx, larynx, and sclera. One third of cases have hypercholesterolemia and xanthelasma. Rheumatoid factor is negative. In 45% of cases joint symptoms precede the appearance of the skin lesions, and in one third the skin and joint disease occurs simultaneously. The associated arthropathy is an inflammatory, symmetrical, polyarticular arthritis that can affect many joints, including the hands, knees, shoulders, wrists, hips, ankles, elbows, feet, and spine. The arthritis can be rapidly destructive and mutilating, with absorption, and telescopic shortening of the phalanges and digits—doigts en lorgnette, opera-glass fingers. In older reports at least 50% of cases develop arthritis mutilans, but this has been reduced to about 12% with aggressive early treatment. The joint

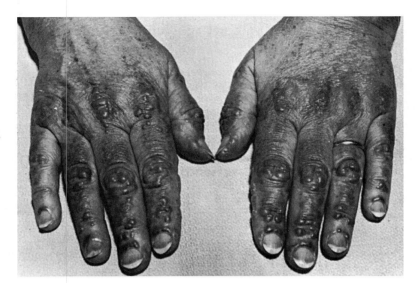

Fig. 31-23 Multicentric reticulohistiocytosis. (Courtesy Dr. T.A. Labow.)

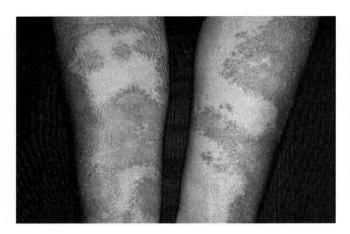

Fig. 31-24 Diffuse reticulohistiocytic granuloma.

involvement may resemble rheumatoid arthritis and psoriatic arthritis. Weight loss and fever occur in one third of patients.

Other organs and tissues may be involved, such as bone, muscle, lymph nodes, liver, myocardium, pericardium, pleura, and stomach. Myocardial involvement may be fatal. Gallium scans have been proposed as a screening method to assess the extent of disease. The clinical course varies. In many instances there is complete involution after about 8 years. The joint destruction is permanent, however, and is a cause of severe disability.

Histologically, the skin lesions are usually centered in the mid-dermis and tend to occupy much or all the dermis. The infiltrating cells are mononuclear and multinucleate monocyte-macrophages. The giant cells are most characteristic with an abundant smooth, or slightly granular,

eosinophilic or amphophilic "ground-glass" cytoplasm. Their cytoplasm is darker in the center than at the periphery. These cells stain positive for periodic-acid Schiff (PAS) after diastase digestion. The overlying epidermis may be thinned but is usually separated from the dermal process by a narrow zone of collagen (grenz zone). Characteristically, there is polymorphous infiltrate of lymphocytes, neutrophils, eosinophils, and plasma cells within the lesions.

The differential diagnosis is broad and might include rheumatoid arthritis, lepromatous leprosy, sarcoidosis, gout, xanthoma disseminatum, xanthoma tuberosum, Langerhans' cell histiocytosis, eruptive histiocytoma, lipoid proteinosis, disseminated lipogranulomatosis, and familial histiocytic dermatoarthritis. In patients with prominent myopathy and periungual lesions, the diagnosis of dermatomyositis is often initially considered.

Given the aggressive nature of the arthritis, early and adequate treatment should be considered. However, associated malignancy is frequent and can be worsened by immunosuppressive therapy. The same would be true for underlying asymptomatic tuberculosis. Initially, the patient should be screened for these two conditions and they should be adequately treated if found. In patients free of neoplasia and tuberculosis, the treatment is individualized. Spontaneous remissions are common, making efficacy of treatment hard to determine. Initially, in mild cases, low-dose prednisone with antimalarials or low-dose methotrexate could be considered. In severe cases more aggressive immunosuppressive therapy with a cytotoxic agent such as cyclophosphamide (Cytoxan), 1 to 2 mg/kg/day with or without corticosteroid treatment, could be considered. The lowest dose of cytotoxic should be used to maintain control of the arthritis and the medications discontinued as quickly as possible. For patients with skin lesions only, therapy is not required. PUVA, antimalarials, topical nitrogen mustard, and low-dose methotrexate could be considered if symptoms are severe.

Brandt F, et al: Topical nitrogen mustard in multicentric reticulohistiocytosis. *J Am Acad Dermatol* 1982, 6:260.

Campbell DA, et al: Multicentric reticulohistiocytosis. *Baillieres Clin Rheumatol* 199, 5:301.

Caputo R, et al: Solitary reticulohistiocytosis (reticulohistiocytoma) of the skin in children. *Arch Dermatol* 1992, 128:698.

Cash JM, et al: Severe multicentric reticulohistiocytosis. *J Rheumatol* 1997, 24:2250.

Chalom EC, et al: A case of multicentric reticulohistiocytosis in a 6-year-old child. *J Rheumatol* 1998, 25:794.

Conaghan P, et al: A unique presentation of multicentric reticulohistiocytosis in pregnancy. *Arthritis Rheum* 1993, 36:269.

Franck N, et al: Multicentric reticulohistiocytosis and methotrexate. *J Am Acad Dermatol* 1995, 33:524.

Gibson G, et al: Multicentric reticulohistiocytosis associated with recurrence of malignant melanoma. *J Am Acad Dermatol* 1995, 32:134.

Goette DK, et al: Diffuse cutaneous reticulohistiocytosis. *Arch Dermatol* 1982, 118:173.

Kenik JG, et al: Multicentric reticulohistiocytosis in a patient with malignant melanoma. *Arthritis Rheum* 1990, 33:1047.

Liang GC, et al: Complete remission of multicentric reticulohistiocytosis with combination therapy of steroid, cyclophosphamide and low dose pulse methotrexate. *Arthritis Rheum* 1996, 39:171.

Nakamura H, et al: A case of spontaneous femoral neck fracture associated with multicentric reticulohistiocytosis. *Arthritis Rheum* 1997, 40:2266.

Rapini R: Multicentric reticulohistiocytosis. *Clin Dermatol* 1993, 11:107.

Rentsch JL, et al: Prolonged response of multicentric reticulohistiocytosis to low dose methotrexate. *J Rheumatol* 1998, 25:1012.

Snow JL, et al: Malignancy associated multicentric reticulohistiocytosis. *Br J Dermatol* 1995, 133:71.

Tait TJ, et al: Multicentric reticulohistiocytosis. *Br J Rheumatol* 1994, 33:100.

Yee KC, et al: Cardiac and systemic complications in multicentric reticulohistiocytosis. *Clin Exp Dermatol* 1993, 18:555. _____ ▲

Generalized Eruptive Histiocytoma

The major characteristics of this rare disease are (1) widespread, essentially symmetrical papules, particularly involving the trunk and proximal extremities and rarely, the mucous membranes; (2) progressive development of new lesions over several years with eventual spontaneous involution to hyperpigmented macules; and (3) a benign histologic picture of mononuclear, histiocytic-appearing cells. Lesions appear in crops but are not grouped. They are skin colored, brown, or violaceous. Caputo reported that in affected children there was a tendency to asymmetry, sparing of mucosae, and progression to xanthomatosis. This may be difficult to distinguish from xanthoma disseminatum, if indeed it is a separate condition. Histologically, there is a dermal infiltrate of nonlipidized mononuclear histiocytes. S-100 staining is negative. It has been proposed that generalized eruptive histiocytosis is an early indeterminate stage of various non-X histiocytoses, including indeterminate cell histiocytosis, multicentric reticulohistiocytosis, xanthogranuloma, and xanthoma disseminatum.

Caputo R, et al: Generalized eruptive histiocytoma in children. *JAMA* 1987, 17:449.

Goerdt S, et al: A unique non-Langerhans cell histiocytosis with some features of generalized eruptive histiocytoma. *J Am Acad Dermatol* 1994, 31:322. _____ ▲

Necrobiotic Xanthogranuloma

Necrobiotic xanthogranuloma is a multisystem disease with prominent skin findings that affects older adults. The characteristic skin lesions are periorbital yellow (xanthomatous) plaques and nodules, which occur in 80% of cases. These lesions resemble xanthelasmas, except that they are deep, firm, and indurated and may extend into the orbit. The trunk and proximal extremities may have orange-red plaques with an active red border and an atrophic center with superficial telangiectasias. These plaques may grow to 25 cm in diameter. The skin lesions often ulcerate, leading to atrophic scarring. Acral nodules may also occur. The eyes are prominently involved with orbital masses, conjunctivitis, keratitis, scleritis, uveitis, iritis, ectropion, or proptosis. Blindness may result. Lymphadenopathy, hepatosplenomegaly, mucosal, myocardial, and pulmonary lesions may occur. There is a monoclonal IgG (usually kappa) paraproteinemia in 80% of cases, and rarely an IgA paraproteinemia. The bone marrow may show plasmacytosis, and in some cases anemia, leukopenia, myeloma, or myelodysplastic syndromes may evolve. The cause is unknown, and the course is chronic and often progressive.

Histologically, there are extensive zones of degenerated collagen surrounded by palisaded macrophages. These macrophages are of various forms—foamy, Touton cells, epithelioid, and giant cells sometimes with more than 50 nuclei. The process extends into the fat, obliterating fat lobules. Cholesterol clefts and extracelluar lipid deposits are prominent. Within this process is a perivascular and interstitial infiltrate of lymphocytes and plasma cells. Lymphoid follicles are present.

The treatment is usually directed at the paraprotein and consist of melphalan, low-dose chlorambucil, systemic corticosteroids, plasmapheresis, and local radiation therapy (for eye lesions). Alfa interferon-2b, 3 to 6 million units three times weekly in combination with systemic corticosteroids, led to dramatic improvement in one case.

Cornblath WT, et al: Varied clinical spectrum of necrobiotic xanthogranuloma. *Ophthalmology* 1992, 99:103

Johnston KA, et al: Necrobiotic xanthogranuloma with paraproteinemia. *Cutis* 1997, 59:333.

Lebey PB, et al: Periorbital papules and nodules. *Arch Dermatol* 1997, 133:97.

Mehregan DA, et al: Necrobiotic xanthogranuloma. *Arch Dermatol* 1992, 128:94.

Novak PM, et al: Necrobiotic xanthogranuloma with myocardial lesions and nodular transformation of the liver. *Hum Pathol* 1992, 23:195.

Plotnik H, et al: Periorbital necrobiotic xanthogranuloma and stage I multiple myeloma. *J Am Acad Dermatol* 1991, 25:373.

Valentine EA, et al: Necrobiotic xanthogranuloma with IgA multiple myeloma. *Am J Hematol* 1990, 35:283.

Venencie PY, et al: Recombinant interferon alfa-2b treatment of necrobiotic xanthogranuloma with parproteinemia. *J Am Acad Dermatol* 1995, 32:666. ▲

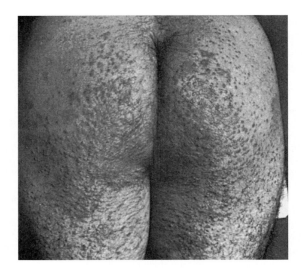

Fig. 31-25   Xanthoma disseminatum on the buttocks.

Xanthoma Disseminatum

Xanthoma disseminatum (XD), a rare normolipoproteinemic mucocutaneous xanthomatosis, is characterized by small, yellowish red to brown papules and nodules that are discrete and disseminated. They involve chiefly the axillary and inguinal folds, and the antecubital and popliteal fossae, face, neck, and flexural surfaces (Figs. 31-25 and 31-26). Diffuse xanthomatous infiltrations may involve the oral mucosa, oropharynx, larynx, and bronchi in 40% of the cases. The conjunctivae may also contain lesions. Diabetes insipidus occurs from xanthomatous involvement of the pituitary gland in 40% of cases.

The serum lipids are normal. It is hypothesized that XD is a reactive histiocytic proliferation in which lipids are secondarily deposited into the histiocytes. Histologic examination shows xanthoma cells, eosinophilic histiocytes, numerous Touton giant cells, and frequently, an inflammatory cell infiltrate.

Although its occurrence ranges between 1 and 70 years, XD appears mostly in young men. It is a chronic and benign disease, which persists indefinitely, or may involute spontaneously after some years.

Considerable speculation has been made with regard to its relationship to histiocytosis X and its variations. XD is a non-X histiocytosis and can be differentiated from Langerhans' cell histiocytosis as well as juvenile xanthogranuloma and multiple histiocytomas. A case of generalized eruptive histiocytosis has been reported to evolve into XD. Disseminated xanthosiderohistiocytosis is a variant of XD in which there is a keloidal consistency to the lesions; they have annular borders, a cephalad distribution, and extensive iron and lipid deposition in the macrophages and connective tissue. Battaglini et al reported a case in which multiple myeloma supervened.

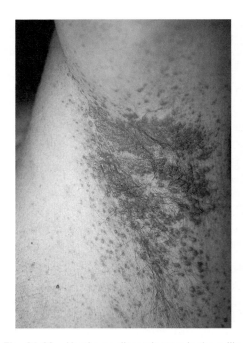

Fig. 31-26   Xanthoma disseminatum in the axilla.

Battaglini J, et al: Disseminated xanthosiderohistiocytosis, a variant of xanthoma disseminatum, in a patient with plasma cell dyscrasia. *J Am Acad Dermatol* 1984, 11:750.

Blobstein SH, et al: Bone lesions in xanthoma disseminatum. *Arch Dermatol* 1985, 121:1313.

Caputo R, et al: The various clinical patterns of xanthoma disseminatum. *Dermatology* 1995, 190:19.

Goodenberger ME, et al: Xanthoma disseminatum and Waldenstrom's macroglobulinemia. *J Am Acad Dermatol* 1990, 23:1015.

Heald P, et al: Xanthoma disseminatum. *New Engl J Med* 1998, 338:1138.

Kavalec CC, et al: Xanthoma disseminatum. *Arch Ophthalmol* 1993, 111:1428.

Repiso T, et al: Generalized eruptive histiocytoma evolving into xanthoma disseminatum in a 4-year-old boy. *Br J Dermatol* 1995, 132:978.

Soong VY, et al: Nodular lesions on the face and trunk. *Arch Dermatol* 1991, 127:1719.

Varotti C, et al: Xanthoma disseminatum. *J Am Acad Dermatol* 1991, 25:433. ▲

Papular Xanthoma

These small, usually yellowish papules, which may be localized or can occur in a generalized distribution, have no tendency to merge into plaques. There is no visceral involvement, and no abnormalities are found on lipid profile examination. Histologically, there are aggregates of foam cells in the dermis without a cellular or histiocytic phase and there is an absence of inflammatory cells.

Caputo R, et al: Papular xanthoma in children. *J Am Acad Dermatol* 1990, 22:1052.

Chen CG, et al: Primary papular xanthoma of children. *Am J Dermatopathol* 1997, 19:596.

Sanchez RL, et al: Papular xanthoma. *Arch Dermatol* 1985, 121:626. ▲

Indeterminate Cell Histiocytosis

Indeterminate cells are felt to represent dermal precursors of Langerhans' cells. They are S-100 and CD1 positive but do not contain Birbeck granules. There are rare reports of patients presenting with solitary or multiple (more than 100) papules or nodules that histologically are composed of dermal infiltrates of indeterminate cells. There is a marked clinical and histologic similarity between indeterminate cell histiocytosis and generalized eruptive histiocytoma. The course is chronic, without spontaneous remission, but systemic involvement is not found.

Levisohn D, et al: Solitary congenital indeterminate cell histiocytoma. *Arch Dermatol* 1993, 129:81.

Sidoroff A, et al: Indeterminate cell histiocytosis. *Br J Dermatol* 1996, 134:525. ▲

Progressive Nodular Histiocytoma

Progressive nodular histiocytoma is clinically characterized by eruption of two types of lesions: superficial papules and deeper nodules. The larger lesions can be up to 5 cm in diameter and be associated with pain and ulceration. The eruption is diffuse and essentially symmetrical without predilection to the flexural areas. On the face lesions may coalesce, giving the patient a leonine facies. There is no visceral, mucous membrane, or articular involvement, and the general health is good. New lesions progressively appear, and spontaneous resolution does not occur. Histologically, the lesions closely resemble dermatofibromas or fibrous histiocytomas. The smaller papules have a peripheral collarette. Touton giant cells are occasionally seen, but the typical PAS-positive giant cells of multicentric reticulohistiocytosis are not present. Local excision may be used for symptomatic lesions.

Torres L, et al: Progressive nodular histiocytosis. *J Am Acad Dermatol* 1993, 29:278. ▲

Hereditary Progressive Mucinous Histiocytosis in Women

Hereditary progressive mucinous histiocytosis is an autosomal dominant or X-linked hereditary disorder described only in women. The skin lesions consist of a few to numerous skin-colored to red-brown papules up to about 5 mm in diameter that tend to appear on the face, arms, forearms, hands, and legs. Onset is in the second decade of life, with slow progression and no tendency to spontaneous involution. Visceral and mucosal lesions have not been reported. Histologically, in the mid-dermis there is a proliferation of spindle-shaped cells with elongated nuclei and little cytoplasm. In the upper dermis the cells are more epithelioid. Superficial telangiectatic vessels and increased mast cells are found. Abundant mucin is demonstrated by alcian blue staining, indicating the presence of acid mucopolysaccharides. This condition can be distinguished from the other non-X histiocytoses by its familial pattern, the lack of lipidized and multinucleated cells, and the presence of mucin.

Schroder K, et al: Hereditary progressive mucinous histiocytosis. *J Am Acad Dermatol* 1996, 35:298. ▲

Sinus Histiocytosis with Massive Lymphadenopathy (Rosai-Dorfman Disease)

Sinus histiocytosis with massive lymphadenopathy (SHML), or Rosai-Dorfman disease, usually appears in patients in the first or second decade of life as a febrile illness accompanied by massive cervical (and commonly other) lymphadenopathy, polyclonal hyperglobulinemia, leukocytosis, anemia, and an elevated sedimentation rate. Males and blacks are especially susceptible. Extranodal involvement occurs in 43% of cases, with skin being the most common. Ten percent of patients with SHML have skin lesions, and 3% of patients have disease detectable only in the skin. The terms *cutaneous sinus histiocytosis* or *cutaneous Rosai-Dorfman disease* have been applied to these cases. Skin lesions consist of isolated or disseminated yellow-brown papules or nodules, or macular erythema. Large annular lesions, resembling granuloma annulare, may occur. Most patients with skin lesions are older (40 years) at presentation.

Histologically, there is a superficial and deep perivascular infiltrate of lymphocytes and plasma cells. Nodular and diffuse infiltration of the dermis by large, foamy histiocytes is present. A very important diagnostic feature is the finding of intact lymphocytes (and less commonly plasma cells) in the cytoplasm of the histiocytic cells. This is called *emperipolesis*. Foamy histiocytes may be seen in dermal lymphatics. The cutaneous histology in some cases may be very nonspecific (except for the finding of emperipolesis), and only on evaluation of lymph node or other organ involvement does the diagnosis become clear. Immunohistochemistry and electron microscopy may be very useful, as the infiltrating cells are CD4, Factor XIIIa, and S-100 positive but do not contain Birbeck granules.

The cause of this condition is unknown, but numerous reports have identified human herpesvirus 6 (HHV-6) in visceral and cutaneous lesions. The condition may clear spontaneously. Numerous agents have been used therapeutically with variable success. These include radiation, chemotherapy, systemic corticosteroids, and thalidomide.

Carrington PR, et al: Extranodal Rosai-Dorfman disease (RDD) of the skin. *Int J Dermatol* 1998, 37:271.

Child FJ, et al: Cutaneous Rosai-Dorfman. *Clin Exp Dermatol* 1998, 23:40.

Saenz-Santamaria MC, et al: Asymptomatic nodules on the chest. *Arch Dermatol* 1997, 133:233.

Scheel MM, et al: Sinus histiocytosis with massive lymphadenopathy. *J Am Acad Dermatol* 1997, 37:643. ⬛⬛⬛⬛⬛⬛⬛⬛ ▲

Sea-Blue Histiocytosis

Sea-blue histiocytosis may occur as a familial inherited syndrome or as an acquired secondary or systemic infiltrative process. The characteristic and diagnostic cell is a histiocytic cell containing cytoplasmic granules that stain blue-green with Giemsa stain and blue with May-Gruenwald stain. The disorder is characterized by infiltration of these cells into the marrow, spleen, liver, lymph nodes, and lungs, as well as the skin in some cases. Skin lesions include papules, eyelid swelling, and patchy gray pigmentation of the face and upper trunk. Similar histologic findings have occurred in patients with myelogenous leukemia, adult Neimann-Pick disease, and following the prolonged use of intravenous fat supplementation. The inherited form may be associated with neurologic symptoms, including ataxia, epilepsy, and dementia.

Bigorgne C, et al: Sea-blue histiocyte syndrome in the bone marrow secondary to total parenteral nutrition. *Leukemia Lymphoma* 1998, 28:523.

Zina AM, et al: Sea blue histiocyte syndrome with cutaneous involvement. *Dermatologica* 1987, 174:39. ⬛⬛⬛⬛⬛⬛⬛⬛ ▲

X-type histiocytoses

This group of disorders is caused by infiltration of the skin, and in some cases other organs, by Langerhans' cells. The spectrum of disease is similar to that seen in mastocytosis, with solitary, usually benign and autoinvoluting lesions, multicentric skin-limited disease, and visceral disease. In the Langerhans' cell histiocytoses, multicentric skin disease and systemic disease are common, and severe morbidity and mortality are unfortunately not uncommon.

CONGENITAL SELF-HEALING RETICULOHISTIOCYTOSIS (HASHIMOTO-PRITZKER)

Congenital self-healing reticulohistiocytosis is usually present at birth or appears very soon thereafter. It has been described in two forms: a solitary and a multinodular variant. Solitary or generalized lesions can affect any part of the cutaneous surface. Lesions range from 0.2 to 2.5 cm in diameter. Lesions may grow postnatally. Exceptionally large tumors up to 8 cm can occur. At presentation the lesions can be papules or nodules with or without erosion or ulceration (Fig. 31-27). Individual lesions are red, brown, pink, or dusky. Lesions greater than 1 cm characteristically ulcerate as they resolve. Lesions are asymptomatic and spontaneously involute over 8 to 24 weeks, leaving atrophic scarring from the ulcerated nodules. Internal involvement is not found.

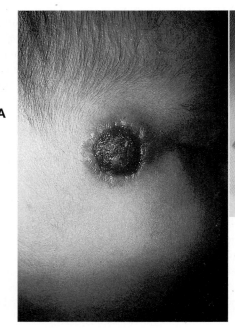
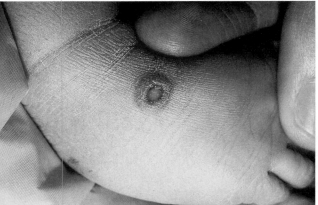

Fig. 31-27 Congenital self-healing reticulohistiocytosis **A,** on the face and **B,** on the foot.

On histologic examination large mononuclear cells and multinucleated giant cells with ground-glass or foamy cytoplasm are present in the dermis and epidermis. Immunoperoxidase staining is positive for CD1, HLA-DR, and S-100. By electron microscopy 10% to 25% of cells have Langerhans' cell granules. This histology is characteristic but cannot distinguish this entity from other forms of Langerhans' cell histiocytosis, so a definitive diagnosis cannot be made histologically.

This is a proliferation of Langerhans' cells. Because Langerhans' cell histiocytosis with systemic involvement may present in identical fashion, systemic evaluation is recommended, including a physical examination, complete blood count, liver function tests, and bone survey. Liver-spleen scan and bone marrow biopsy should be considered.

Berger TG, et al: A solitary variation of congenital self-healing reticulohistiocytosis. *Pediatr Dermatol* 1986, 3:230.

Bernstein EF, et al: Solitary congenital self-healing reticulohistiocytosis. *Br J Dermatol* 1993, 129:449.

Hashimoto K, et al: Congenital self-healing reticulohistiocytosis. *J Am Acad Dermatol* 1984, 11:447.

Herman LE, et al: Congenital self-healing reticulohistiocytosis. *Arch Dermatol* 1990, 126:210.

Schaumburg-Lever G, et al: Congenital self-healing reticulohistiocytosis. *J Cutan Pathol* 1994, 21:59.

Timpatanapong P, et al: Congenital self-healing reticulohistiocytosis. *Pediatr Dermatol* 1989, 6:28. ▲

LANGERHANS' CELL HISTIOCYTOSIS (HISTIOCYTOSIS X)

Langerhans' cell histiocytosis (LCH), or histiocytosis X, is a disease characterized by proliferation of Langerhans' cells. This group of disorders can involve many organ systems but affects primarily the bone, skin, lymph nodes, lungs, liver and spleen, endocrine glands, and nervous system. The separation of these conditions into separate entities—Letterer-Siwe disease, Hand-Schuller-Christian disease, and eosinophilic granuloma—is of historical interest. Currently, the disease is classified by the number of organ systems involved (restricted or extensive) and whether those organ systems are functionally impaired (Box 31-1). These two factors appear to be of primary importance in the eventual outcome. The disease affects primarily children from 1 to 4 years but can present from birth to the ninth decade. It is uncommon, with an incidence of 2 to 5 per million per year.

The pathogenesis of LCH is unknown. There remains debate as to whether the infiltrating cells are truly neoplastic or simply reactive. It is clear that the infiltrating Langerhans' cells are clonal. However, aneuploidy is infrequent, and histologically the cells do not appear atypical as in lymphoma. These features have led to the suggestion that the proliferation of the Langerhans' cells is cytokine related.

> **BOX 31-1**
>
> **Classification System for Langerhans' Cell Histiocytosis**
>
> **RESTRICTED LANGERHANS' CELL HISTIOCYTOSIS**
> a. Biopsy proved skin rash without any other site of involvement
> b. Monostotic lesions, with or without diabetes insipidus, adjacent lymph node enlargement, or skin rash
> c. Polyostotic lesions, consisting of lesions in several bones or more than two lesions in one bone, with or without diabetes insipidus, adjacent lymph node enlargement, or skin rash
>
> **EXTENSIVE LANGERHANS' CELL HISTIOCYTOSIS**
> a. Visceral organ involvement, with or without bone lesions, diabetes insipidus, adjacent lymph node involvement, and/or skin rash; but without signs of organ dysfunction of any of the following organ systems: lung, liver, or hematopoietic system
> b. Visceral organ involvement, with or without bone lesions, diabetes insipidus, adjacent lymph node involvement, and/or skin rash; but with signs of organ dysfunction of any of the following organ systems: lung, liver, or hematopoietic system

In addition, a viral pathogenesis has been proposed. Although HHV-6 has been found in the lesions of LCH by some investigators, this has not been reproduced by others.

Skin Lesions

Skin disease can occur as an isolated finding or can be a part of extensive multisystem disease. The pattern of skin disease does not predict the presence or extent of systemic disease. The most common form of skin disease is that described in Letterer-Siwe disease. The skin lesions are tiny red, red-brown, or yellow papules that are widespread but favor the intertriginous areas, behind the ears, and the scalp (Figs. 31-28 and 31-29). There is a superficial resemblance to seborrheic dermatitis, but on careful inspection the lesions are individual papules and there is focal hemorrhage in the lesions. Lesions may erode or weep. This pattern of disease may also rarely occur in adults, who represent about 4% of cases (Fig. 31-30). Although in children this pattern frequently is associated with multisystem disease, in adults a quarter of these patients have disease limited to the skin or skin and mucosa. A rare variant of this pattern of LCH is one in which vesicles appear. This can occur in infants or adults. The vesicles are due to large intraepidermal collections of Langerhans' cells, and a Tzanck smear may lead one to suspect the diagnosis. A less common presentation is with slightly larger papules up to 1 cm in diameter (Fig. 31-31). These lesions tend to be yellow-red and resemble xanthomas or xanthogranulomas. They can be numerous and widespread.

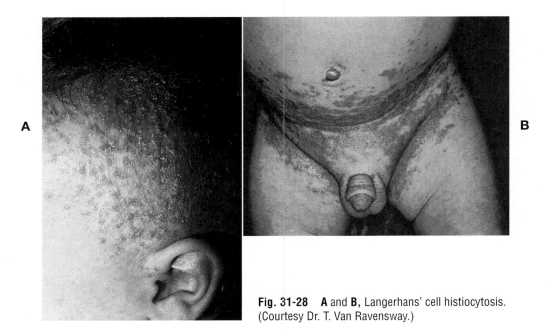

Fig. 31-28 **A** and **B**, Langerhans' cell histiocytosis. (Courtesy Dr. T. Van Ravensway.)

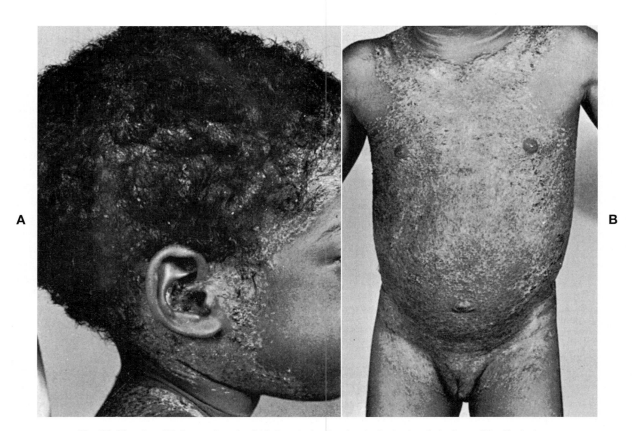

Fig. 31-29 **A** and **B**, Langerhans' cell histiocytosis showing typical seborrheic dermatitis–like lesions. (Courtesy Dr. N.B. Esterly.)

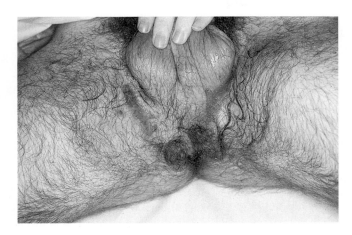

Fig. 31-30 Ulcerative lesions of Langerhans' cell histiocytosis in the inguinal folds of a young adult man.

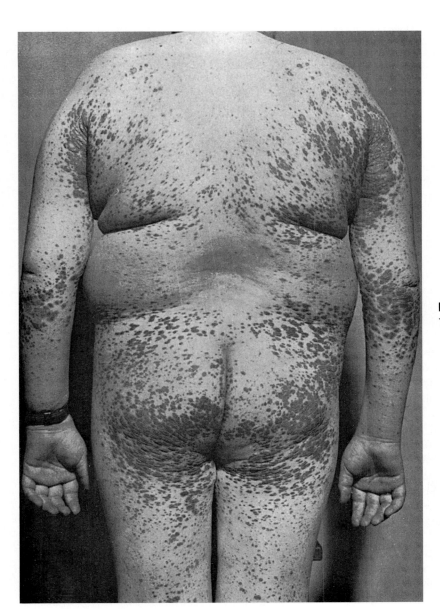

Fig. 31-31 Langerhans' cell histiocytosis in a 12-year-old boy.

Histologically, there is a dense dermal infiltrate of Langerhans' cells. This can be superficial and immediately below the epidermis (in small papular and seborrheic-like lesions) or deep and diffuse (in papular and nodular lesions). The Langerhans' cells are recognized by their abundant, amphophilic cytoplasm and round or kidney bean–shaped nucleus. There is frequently exocytosis of the abnormal cells into the overlying epidermis. If this is extensive, macroscopic vesicles can be seen, and erosion can occur secondarily. The dermal infiltrate is accompanied by many other inflammatory cells, including neutrophils, eosinophils, lymphocytes, and plasma cells. Dermal hemorrhage is characteristically present. In larger and older lesions the infiltrating histiocytic cells become foamy and fibrosis may be present.

Immunohistochemistry is useful in confirming the diagnosis. The infiltrating cells in LCH are S-100, CD1, CD4, and HLA-DR positive. Electron microscopy will detect the presence of Birbeck granules. In older lesions and in some organ systems the number of cells staining with these markers and containing Birbeck granules is much diminished.

Oral Mucosa Lesions

The oral mucosa may be involved. Nodular infiltrates, ulcerations, displaced teeth, and loss of alveolar bone are characteristic findings and represent involvement of underlying bone. Gingival lesions should be looked for, and a dental evaluation completed in all patients.

Visceral Involvement

The most commonly involved organ is the bone. In various series between one third and two thirds of patients have disease limited to one or several bones. The lesions may be asymptomatic or cause pain. The skull is most commonly involved, followed by the long bones, then the flat bones. Bony lesions tend to occur in older children and young adults. Lesions are treated with curettage, intralesional corticosteroids, or radiation. Endocrine dysfunction occurs usually in the form of diabetes insipidus, which is more common in patients with bone disease of the skull and in patients with extensive disease.

Lymph nodes are characteristically involved, especially the cervical nodes. The bone marrow may be affected, and the presence of pancytopenia is usually associated with a poor prognosis. This may present as purpura in the skin.

The liver may be involved directly by infiltration with Langerhans' cells or may be indirectly affected by enlarged nodes in the porta hepatis leading to obstructive disease. Either pattern can lead to biliary cirrhosis.

Pulmonary LCH occurs most commonly in the third decade. A diffuse micronodular pattern on chest radiograph may progress to cyst formation (honeycomb lung), large bullae, and pneumothorax. Smoking is a strong risk factor for this pattern of pulmonary LCH.

Identification of LCH in any organ is important but not as important as the function of the affected organ. Many lesions may be asymptomatic and never lead to sequelae. Simply finding involvement of an organ does not mandate treatment of that organ or lesion.

Prognosis

The outcome in any patient is determined by the extent of involvement and more importantly, the function of affected organs. Baseline and repeated evaluation are important. Lesions in one organ system may resolve while disease progresses in another organ. Skin lesions may spontaneously resolve, only for the disease to relapse, even years later, so patients must be followed regularly. In addition, if chemotherapeutic agents are used for treatment, a risk of secondary malignancies of less than 5% exists.

Differential Diagnosis

The diffuse small papular form is frequently misdiagnosed as seborrheic dermatitis. The yellow color of the lesions and the presence of hemorrhage in the small papules, if present, should suggest the diagnosis of LCH. Nodular lesions of scabies can closely simulate LCH. This includes the finding of Langerhans' cells in the dermal infiltrate by electron microscopy and S100 and CD1 staining. The larger papules resemble juvenile xanthogranulomas and xanthomas.

Treatment

Treatment of LCH is controversial. Corticosteroids, vinblastine, other chemotherapeutic agents, cyclosporine, and radiation therapy have all been helpful. In refractory cases, 2-chlorodeoxyadenosine has been successful. These treatments should be used only if required and are usually restricted to patients with extensive disease with organ dysfunction. It is unclear that aggressive treatment (beyond corticosteroids) benefits patients with extensive disease without organ dysfunction.

For disease limited to the skin, topical corticosteroids may be used. Because spontaneous remissions are frequent, palliative treatment is reasonable. Topical nitrogen mustard (as used for cutaneous T-cell lymphoma) is an effective nonsystemic approach. Some patients with superficial lesions have responded to PUVA. Interferon alfa both systemically and intralesionally has led to resolution of lesions.

Chi DH, et al: Eruptive xanthoma-like cutaneous Langerhans cell histiocytosis in an adult. *J Am Acad Dermatol* 1996, 34:688.

Dufresne RG Jr, et al: Histiocytosis X mimicking the follicular occlusion syndrome. *J Am Acad Dermatol* 1987, 16:385.

Egeler RM, et al: Langerhans cell histiocytosis. *J Pediatr* 1995, 127:1.

Esterly NB, et al: Histiocytosis X: a seven-year experience at a children's hospital. *J Am Acad Dermatol* 1985, 13:481.

Foucar E, et al: Urticating histiocytosis X. *J Am Acad Dermatol* 1986, 14:867.

Gianotti F, et al: Histiocytic syndromes. *J Am Acad Dermatol* 1985, 13:383.

Holzberg M, et al: Nail pathology in histiocytosis X. *J Am Acad Dermatol* 1985, 13:523.

Kwong YL, et al: Widespread skin-limited Langerhans cell histiocytosis. *J Am Acad Dermatol* 1997, 36:628.

Lieberman PH, et al: Langerhans cell (eosinophilic) granulomatosis. *Am J Surg Pathol* 1996, 20:519.

Longaker MA, et al: Congenital "self-healing" Langerhans cell histiocytosis. *J Am Acad Dermatol* 1994, 31:910.

McLelland J, et al: Multi-system Langerhans-cell histiocytosis in adults. *Clin Exp Dermatol* 1990, 15:79

Meja R, et al: Langerhans' cell histiocytosis in adults. *J Am Acad Dermatol* 1997, 37:314.

Nethercott JR, et al: Histiocytosis X in two adults: treatment with topical mechlorethamine. *Arch Dermatol* 1983, 119:157.

Neumann C, et al: Interferon gamma is a marker for histiocytosis X cells in the skin. *J Invest Dermatol* 1988, 91:280.

Saven A, et al: 2-chlorodeoxyadenosine-induced complete remission in Langerhans-cell histiocytosis. *Ann Intern Med* 1994, 121:430.

Stefanos CM, et al: Langerhans cell histiocytosis in the elderly. *J Am Acad Dermatol* 1998, 39:375.

Storer JS, et al: Histiocytosis X and skin scraping cytology. *J Am Acad Dermatol* 1983, 8:913.

Talanin NY, et al: Cutaneous histiocytosis with Langerhans cell features induced by scabies. *Pediatr Dermatol* 1994, 11:327.

Willman CL, et al: Langerhans'-cell histiocytosis (histiocytosis X): a clonal proliferative disease. *N Engl J Med* 1994, 331:154. ▲

CHAPTER 32

Cutaneous Lymphoid Hyperplasia, Cutaneous T-Cell Lymphoma, Other Malignant Lymphomas, and Allied Diseases

CUTANEOUS LYMPHOID HYPERPLASIA (LYMPHOCYTOMA CUTIS, LYMPHADENOSIS BENIGNA CUTIS, PSEUDOLYMPHOMA)

The term *cutaneous lymphoid hyperplasia,* originally proposed by Helwig et al, refers to an ever-expanding group of benign disorders characterized by collections of lymphocytes (and sometimes other inflammatory cells) in the skin. These processes can be considered to be caused by known stimuli (such as medications, infections, or the bites of arthropods), or they may be idiopathic. They may have a purely benign histologic appearance, or they may resemble cutaneous lymphoma. If there is a histologic resemblance to lymphoma, the term *pseudolymphoma* is sometimes used. The lesions may contain mostly T cells, mostly B cells, or may be composed of a mixed population of T and B cells. Most forms of cutaneous lymphoid hyperplasia are polyclonal in their derivation. Cases of monoclonal B- and T-cell cutaneous lymphoid hyperplasia do occur. Thus, a finding of monoclonality does not equate to the diagnosis of malignancy or lymphoma, nor does it predict biologic behavior in all cases. Some monoclonal cutaneous lymphoid hyperplasias do progress to true lymphoma.

The cutaneous lymphoid hyperplasias represent a spectrum of disease. At one end are cases that are clinically, histologically, and immunophenotypically benign. Intermediate cases are histologically atypical but with benign clinical behavior—the so-called pseudolymphomas. At the other pole are cases that are histologically or immunophenotypically ambiguous, some of which may progress to lymphoma or represent lymphoma from the onset but that we cannot reliably diagnose. This makes evaluation of some cutaneous lymphoid infiltrates very challenging histologically. The clinician must provide the dermatopathologist with accurate and complete information. Any change in clinical behavior or morphology may be an indication for repeat histologic, immunophenotypic, and immunogenetic evaluation to exclude the development of true cutaneous lymphoma. Lymphoid hyperplasias that occur in the setting of immunosuppression may behave aggressively, like lymphomas, but regress with the discontinuation of immunosuppression.

Because current classifications of lymphomas divide them into T- and B-cell types, a similar classification scheme is used here. However, in cases in which the same process may induce either a B- or T-cell phenotype, the condition is discussed under the primary pattern that it produces. Because the differential diagnosis is driven from the histologic findings primarily, the conditions are subclassified into types that are nodular and may mimic follicular lymphoma and cases that are primarily bandlike and perivascular and mimic mycosis fungoides or small cell lymphoma cutis.

Cutaneous B-Cell Lymphoid Hyperplasias (Nodular Pattern)

The nodular reaction pattern is usually idiopathic. Idiopathic B-cell lymphoid hyperplasia has been called *Speigler-Fendt sarcoid* in the past. Known causes of nodular B-cell lymphoid hyperplasias include tattoos, *Borrelia* infections, herpes zoster scars, antigen injections or acupuncture, and, in rare cases, drug reactions and persistent insect bite reactions.

Lesions that result from a known stimulus tend to be localized to the site of the original process—tattoo, injection, and so on. In idiopathic and secondary localized forms, the lesions appear as discrete firm or doughy cutaneous papules or nodules (Figs. 32-1 and 32-2). Lesions may be grouped in one area and coalesce to form a plaque. Lesions principally occur on the face, particularly on the cheek, nose, or earlobes. Less commonly, the lesions may affect the trunk (36%) or extremities (25%). The epidermis over the nodules is usually smooth and flesh colored, tan, red, or violaceous. Women are afffected three times more frequently, and two thirds of the affected patients are under age 40. Disseminated or generalized cases are unusual. They present as miliary papules.

Borrelia-induced cutaneous lymphoid hyperplasia is an uncommon manifestation of this infection, occurring in 0.6% to 1.3% of cases reported from Europe. The lack of borrelial pseudolymphoma in the United States compared with Europe may relate to the fact that there are different borrelial species in Europe, specifically *B. afzeli,* that cause

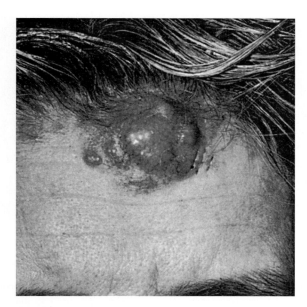

Fig. 32-1 Pseudolymphoma (lymphoid hyperplasia) of 3 years' duration in a 45-year-old woman. Complete clearing followed administration of 150 Gy (HVL 4 mm Al) at weekly intervals for four treatments.

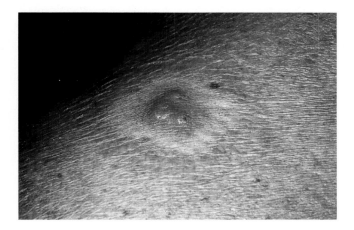

Fig. 32-2 Cutaneous B-cell lymphoid hyperplasia.

borreliosis. Lesions occur at the site of the tick bite or close to the edge of a lesion of erythema migrans. Lesions may appear up to 10 months after infection. Lesions may be multiple and favor the earlobes, nipple and areola, nose, and scrotal area and vary from 1 to 5 cm in diameter. Usually there are no symptoms, but associated regional lymphadenopathy may be present. Late manifestations of *Borrelia* infection are uncommon.

The diagnosis is suspected by a history of a tick bite or erythema migrans, the location (earlobe or nipple), and the histologic picture. The diagnosis is confirmed by an elevated anti-*Borrelia* antibody (present in 50% of cases)

and the finding of borrelial DNA in the affected tissue. The treatment is penicillin. Some cases progress to true lymphoma.

Histologic examination reveals a dense, nodular infiltrate that occupies primarily the dermis and lessens in the deeper dermis and subcutaneous fat; that is, it is "top-heavy." The process is usually separated from the epidermis by a clear grenz zone. The infiltrate is composed chiefly of mature small and large lymphocytes, histiocytes, plasma cells, and eosinophils. In the deeper portions, well-defined germinal centers are usually seen, with central large lymphoid cells with abundant cytoplasm and tingible body macrophages and a peripheral cuff of small lymphocytes.

The clinical lesions may be nondescript and the differential diagnosis quite broad, usually mandating a biopsy. Amyloidosis, sarcoidosis, and lymphoma should be considered. Histologically, the primary differential diagnosis is follicular or other cutaneous lymphoma. Histologic criteria and even immunophenotyping and immunogenetic analysis may not be sufficient to predict biologic behavior. Most cases represent B-cell or mixed B- and T-cell proliferations. Rarely, this nodular histology can occur with primarily T-cell infiltrates. This is characteristic in nodular arthropod bite reactions and nodular scabies and is rarely seen in nodular hyperplasias from anticonvulsants.

Because most lesions are asymptomatic, treatment is not required. If the process has been induced by a medication, use of the medication should be discontinued. Intralesional steroidal agents are sometimes beneficial, but lesions may recur in a few months. Potent topical steroids may also be tried for superficial lesions. Cryosurgery, interferon alfa, proquazone (an NSAID), laser ablation, or surgical excision can all be attempted. Low-dose radiation therapy is usually very effective and may be used on refractory facial lesions that cannot be satisfactorily removed surgically. If monoclonality is detected in a localized lesion, complete removal and local radiation might be recommended because of the potential risk of lymphoma. For disseminated lesions, antimalarial agents and PUVA therapy can be considered.

Cutaneous T-Cell Lymphoid Hyperplasias (Bandlike and Perivascular Patterns)

Cutaneous T-cell lymphoid hyperplasias may be idiopathic or caused by photosensitivity (formerly called *actinic reticuloid;* now called *chronic actinic dermatitis*), medications (usually anticonvulsants but also many others), contact dermatitis (so-called lymphomatoid contact dermatitis), and less commonly, by scabies or arthropod bites. Some authors consider Jessner's lymphocytic infiltrate to be in this group, whereas others consider it a condition unrelated to the cutaneous lymphoid hyperplasias.

Clinically, these patients have one of two types of lesions. The lesions in one group of patients resembles mycosis fungoides: they have widespread erythema with scaling. Thicker plaques may occur as well. These cases are frequently caused by medications. Histologically, the dermal infiltrate is bandlike, sometimes with epidermotropism. No grenz zone is present. The infiltrate may be mixed with small lymphocytes and some eosinophils. The treatment is to stop any implicated medication.

The second clinical pattern is of more papular or nodular lesions, closely resembling idiopathic B-cell lymphoid hyperplasia (Figs. 32-3 and 32-4). It is usually idiopathic (this is where we classify Jessner's lymphocytic infiltrate) but rarely may be caused by medications. The lesions are asymptomatic, smooth, and red to violaceous with no epidermal involvement or scale. Lesions resolve without scarring. Women are more commonly affected and present at a younger age.

Histologically, there is a perivascular infiltrate of small lymphocytes that is tightly cuffed around the blood vessels. There is no epidermotropism or inflammation at the dermoepidermal junction. The clinical differential diagnosis includes polymorphous light eruption, cutaneous lupus erythematosus, and cutaneous small-cell lymphoma. Histologically, the same conditions are considered, as well as a gyrate erythema. Clinicopathologic correlation will solve diagnostic difficulties in most patients. To exclude lupus erythematosus, direct immunofluorescence may be helpful, and phototesting can help to differentiate cases of polymorphous light eruption. Treatment is very difficult and not usually required except for cosmetic concerns. Topical and intralesional steroids, PUVA, and, for persistent localized lesions, radiotherapy may be considered.

The cytologic appearance of the atypical lymphocytes is usually adequate to identify the cases of small-cell lymphoma that may mimic T-cell lymphoid hyperplasia. Such lymphomas are usually of B-cell origin, so immunophenotyping is helpful. If T cells are identified, immunogenetic studies to detect T-cell receptor clonal rearrangements should be considered. If monoclonality is identified, the case must be carefully evaluated for systemic involvement (including CT scans of the chest, abdomen, and pelvis and perhaps a bone marrow biopsy). Distinguishing monoclonal T-cell lymphoid hyperplasia from small-cell lymphoma may be very difficult.

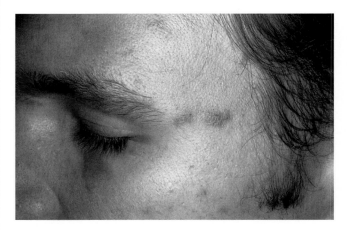

Fig. 32-3   Cutaneous T-cell lymphoid hyperplasia.

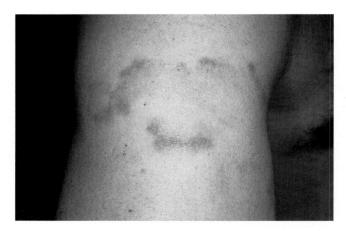

Fig. 32-4   Cutaneous T-cell lymphoid hyperplasia.

Cockerell CJ, et al: Persistent indurated plaques of the face. *Cutis* 1994, 53:49.

Goldberg NS, et al: An extensive papular eruption on the face of a 10-year-old girl. *Arch Dermatol* 1986, 122:931.

Hormark A, et al: The spirochetal etiology of lymphadenosis benigna cutis solitaria. *Acta Derm Venereol* 1986, 66:479.

Johansson EA: Proquazone. *Dermatologica* 1987, 174:117.

Landa NG, et al: Lymphoma versus pseudolymphoma of the skin. *J Am Acad Dermatol* 1993, 29:945.

Miyamoto T, et al: Lymphocytoma cutis induced by cobalt. *Br J Dermatol* 1997, 137:467.

Ploysangam T, et al: Cutaneous pseudolymphomas. *J Am Acad Dermatol* 1998, 38:877.

Rijlaarsdam U, et al: Demonstration of clonal immunoglobin gene rearrangements in cutaneous B-cell lymphomas and pseudo-B-cell lymphomas. *J Invest Dermatol* 1992, 99:749.

Spina D, et al: Distinction between diffuse cutaneous malignant follicular center cell lymphoma and lymphoid hyperplasia by computerized nuclear image analysis. *Am J Dermatopathol* 1993, 15:415.

Stoll DM: Treatment of cutaneous pseudolymphoma with hydroxychloroquine. *J Am Acad Dermatol* 1983, 8:696.

Van der Putte SCJ, et al: Immunocytoma of the skin simulating lymphadenosis benigna cutis. *Arch Dermatol Res* 1985, 26:277.

Van der Putte SCJ, et al: Solitary nonepidermotropic T cell pseudolymphomas of the skin. *J Am Acad Dermatol* 1986, 14:444.

Wantzin GL, et al: Evolution of cutaneous lymphoid hyperplasia to cutaneous T-cell lymphoma. *Clin Exp Dermatol* 1988, 13:309.

Wheeland RG, et al: Role of the argon laser in lymphocytoma cutis. *J Am Acad Dermatol* 1986, 14:267.

Willemze R, et al: Immunohistochemical studies in lymphocytic infiltration of the skin and discoid LE. *J Am Acad Dermatol* 1984, 11:832.   ▲

CUTANEOUS LYMPHOMAS

Cutaneous lymphoma can be considered to be either primary or secondary. Primary cutaneous lymphomas are those that occur in the skin and where no evidence of extracutaneous involvement is found for some period after the appearance of the cutaneous disease. Cases of simultaneous skin and lymph node involvement (except for cases of mycosis fungoides with lymph node involvement) cannot always be absolutely classified as primary, because the "origin" of the lymphoma cannot be determined. Secondary cutaneous lymphoma includes cases that have simultaneous or preceding evidence of extracutaneous involvement (especially of the lymph nodes). These cases are best classified and managed as lymph node–based lymphomas with skin involvement. This conceptual separation is not ideal, but it has been important in developing classification schemes and determining prognosis in cutaneous lymphomas.

For many years classification of lymphomas has been based on their histologic structure, and lesions from all organ systems were classified histomorphologically in an identical manner to lymphomas arising in lymph nodes. It had been recognized that these classification schemes have major shortcomings when applied to extranodal lymphomas; specifically, they did not uniformly predict clinical behavior. New classification schemes have been developed that are specific for primary cutaneous lymphomas. In the following discussion, the classification scheme of Willemze and the Dutch Cutaneous Lymphoma Working Group will be used.

Cutaneous lymphomas are classified based on their cell type of origin. There are B-cell lymphomas, T-cell lymphomas, true histiocytic lymphomas, and rarer types. Cell type is further classified by specific lymphoid markers associated with features of normal lymphocytes. Histologic features used in this classification system include cell size (large rather than small), and differentiation features (follicular center cell, immunoblast, and so on). These features are supplemented by immunophenotypic markers such as CD30. Despite these major conceptual and diagnostic advances, the diagnosis and classification of cutaneous lymphomas can still be quite difficult. Because appropriate classification may be prognostically important, experienced dermatopathology consultation should be sought in cases of cutaneous lymphoma.

Primary Cutaneous T-Cell Lymphomas

A major insight into cutaneous lymphoma was the finding that the majority of lymphomas in the skin were of T-cell origin. This is logical, since T cells normally traffic through the skin and are important in "skin-associated lymphoid tissue." Dermatologists, however, frequently use the term *cutaneous T-cell lymphoma* synonymously with mycosis fungoides (MF). Although MF represents the large majority of primary cutaneous T-cell lymphomas, it is not synonymous with cutaneous T-cell lymphoma. In fact, up to 30% of primary cutaneous T-cell lymphomas are not mycosis fungoides.

Because cutaneous Hodgkin's disease is very rare to nonexistent, the term *non-Hodgkin's lymphoma* has little meaning when speaking of a lymphoma in the skin, because virtually all cutaneous lymphomas would be "non-Hodgkin's lymphomas."

The term *non-Hodgkin's lymphoma* may sometimes also be applied in cases of secondary cutaneous lymphoma. Rather, in parallel with lymph node–based lymphoma, where the primary distinction is between Hodgkin's disease and other lymphomas, in the skin the distinction is between mycosis fungoides and other primary cutaneous T-cell lymphomas. The following discussion is divided into mycosis fungoides and related conditions, Sézary syndrome and lymphomatoid papulosis; and non-MF primary cutaneous T-cell lymphomas.

Mycosis Fungoides. Mycosis fungoides (MF) is a malignant neoplasm of T-lymphocyte origin, almost always a memory T-helper cell. The disease was once considered to be uncommon, but the incidence doubled between 1973 and 1984, and now many dermatology departments throughout the world have large clinics dedicated to managing this disorder. Mycosis fungoides affects all races. In the United States blacks are relatively more commonly affected than whites. The condition is twice as common in males as females.

NATURAL HISTORY. In general, mycosis fungoides is a chronic, slowly progressive disorder. It usually begins as flat patches (patch stage), which may or may not be histologically diagnostic of MF (hence the term *premycotic*). This inability to diagnose early cases has more to do with the limits of our diagnostic capabilities, and these cases are considered mycosis fungoides from the onset, rather than a transformation from some nonneoplastic (premycotic) condition to mycosis fungoides. Pruritus, sometimes severe, is usually present at this stage. Over time, sometimes years, the lesions become more infiltrated, and the diagnosis is usually confirmed with repeated histologic evaluation. Infiltrated plaques occur eventually; this is called the *plaque stage*. In some cases tumors may eventually appear (tumor stage). Some patients may present with or progress to erythroderma. Most rarely, patients may present with tumors de novo, the so-called *d'emblée* form. With immunophenotyping, many of these cases are now recognized as non-MF B-cell lymphomas. Eventually, in some patients, noncutaneous involvement is detected. This is most commonly first identified in lymph nodes. Peripheral blood involvement and visceral organ involvement may also occur.

In general, mycosis fungoides affects elderly patients and has a long evolution. For this reason, many patients die of other conditions rather than of MF. However, once tumors develop or lymph node involvement occurs, the prognosis is more guarded, and mycosis fungoides can be fatal. In most fatal cases the patient dies of septicemia. Early, aggressive chemotherapy in an attempt to "cure" MF is associated with excessive morbidity and mortality and is not indicated.

EVALUATION AND STAGING. The North American MF Cooperative Group has developed a staging system. Because MF is a systemic disease from the onset (as lymphocytes naturally traffic throughout the body), concepts such as used for solid tumors such as tumor burden and metastasis cannot be readily applied. The TNMB system scores involvement in the skin (T), the lymph node (N), the viscera (M), and the peripheral blood (B). Skin involvement is divided into less than 10% (T1), more than 10% (T2), tumors (T3), and erythroderma (T4). Node involvement is normal clinically and pathologically (N0), palpable but pathologically not MF (N1), not palpable but pathologically MF (N2), or clinically and pathologically involved (N3). Viscera and blood are either not involved (M0 and B0) or involved (M1 and B1). Stage IA is T1,N0,M0; stage IB is T2,N0,M0; stage IIA is T1-2,N1,M0; stage IIB is T3,N0-1,M0; stage IIIA is T4,N0,M0; stage IIIB is T4,N1,M0; stage IVA is T1-4,N2-3,M0; and stage IVB is T1-4,N0-3,M1. The "B" or blood status does not alter staging of the disease.

A staging workup would include a complete history and physical examination, with careful palpation of lymph nodes and mapping of skin lesions; a complete blood cell count with assays for circulating atypical cells (Sézary cells); serum chemistries including renal and liver function tests with lactic dehydrogenase; a chest radiograph evaluation; and a skin biopsy. If lymph nodes are palpable, they should be examined histologically. Fine-needle aspiration is not an ideal mode of evaluation, since early lymph node involvement may be localized to certain areas of the affected nodes, and architectural evaluation is often required to detect early lymph node involvement. If any abnormalities are detected through the above evaluations, they should be pursued. CT scans can be performed to assess chest, abdominal, and pelvic lymph nodes and visceral organs. These are useful in patients with stage II through IV disease but are not indicated in patients with stage IA disease. Whether patients with stage Ib disease should undergo these tests is unknown.

The value of this staging system is confirmed in large series. Stage IA patients have a life expectancy identical to a control population; only 8% to 9% progress to have more advanced disease; and only 2% die of their disease. By contrast, patients with T2 disease have a shorter survival time than control subjects (median survival, 11.7 to 15.6 years). Twenty-four percent of T2 patients progress to more advanced disease. T3 patients have a median survival of 3.2 to 8.4 years, and T4 patients have a median survival of 1.8 to 3.7 years. Palpable adenopathy is associated with a median survival of only 7.7 years, whereas patients without adenopathy had a survival of 21.8 years. The study of 144 patients at the National Institutes of Health by Epstein et al showed that lymphadenopathy, tumors, or cutaneous ulceration are cardinal prognostic factors: no patient died without having developed one of them, and patients with all three (in any order) survived a median of 1 year.

CLINICAL FEATURES. In the early patch/plaque stage, the lesions are macular or slightly infiltrated patches or plaques varying in size from a centimeter to 5 cm or more (Figs. 32-5 and 32-6). The eruption may be generalized, or begin

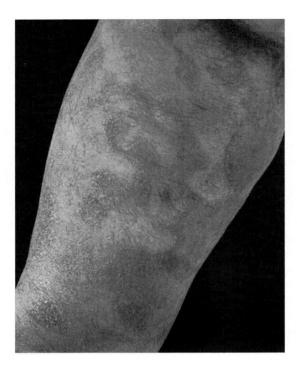

Fig. 32-5 Mycosis fungoides in patch stage, showing erythematous branny scaling patches with only slight infiltration. (Courtesy Dr. H. Shatin.)

localized to one area, then spread. The lower abdomen, buttocks, and upper thighs and the breasts of women are preferentially affected. The lesions may have an atrophic surface, or present as true poikiloderma with atrophy, mottled dyspigmentation, and telangiectasia (Fig. 32-7). Poikiloderma vasculare atrophicans is now recognized as a clinical form of patch-stage mycosis fungoides. Likewise, large-plaque parapsoriasis, and perhaps some cases of small-plaque parapsoriais represent early/patch-stage lesions of mycosis fungoides. With current diagnostic methods this can usually be confirmed. In general, the patch-stage lesions resemble an eczema, being round or ovoid, but annular, polycyclic, or arciform configurations can occur. Less common forms are the verrucous or hyperkeratotic form, the hypopigmented form, lesions resembling a pigmented purpura, and the vesicular, bullous, or pustular form. The hypopigmented form seems to be more common in persons of color and is a common presentation for adolescents and children with mycosis fungoides.

In the plaque stage, lesions are more infiltrated and may resemble psoriasis, a subacute dermatitis, or a granulomatous dermal processes such as granuloma annulare. The palms and soles may be involved with hyperkeratotic, psoriasiform, and fissuring plaques. The infiltration of the plaques, at first recognized by light palpation, may be present in only a few of the lesions. It is a manifestation of diagnostic importance. Different degrees of infiltration may exist even in the same patch, and sometimes it is more pronounced

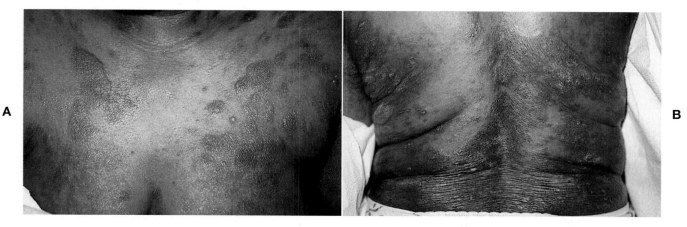

Fig. 32-6 Mycosis fungoides. **A** and **B,** Psoriasiform plaques.

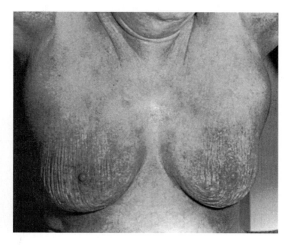

Fig. 32-7 Mycosis fungoides with generalized poikiloderma.

peripherally, the central part of the plaque being depressed to the level of the surrounding skin. The infiltration becomes more marked and leads to discoid patches or extensive plaques, which may be as much as 30 cm in width.

Eventually, through coalescence of the various plaques, the involvement becomes widespread, but there are usually patches of apparently normal skin interspersed. When the involvement is advanced, painful superficial ulcerations may occur. During this phase enlarged lymph nodes usually develop. They are nontender, firm, and freely movable.

The tumor stage is characterized by large, various sized and shaped nodules on infiltrated plaques and on apparently healthy skin (Figs. 32-8 to 32-11). These nodules have a tendency to break down early and to form deep oval ulcers, with bases covered with a necrotic grayish substance and with rolled edges (Figs. 32-12 and 32-13). The lesions generally have a predilection for the trunk, although they may be seen anywhere on the skin or may involve the mouth and upper respiratory tract. Uncommonly, tumors may be the first sign of mycosis fungoides.

The erythrodermic variety of mycosis fungoides is a generalized exfoliative process, with universal redness. The hair is scanty, nails dystrophic, palms and soles hyperkeratotic, and at times there may be generalized hyperpigmentation. Erythroderma may be the presenting feature.

Alopecia mucinosa and mycosis fungoides. The infiltrating cells of mycosis fungoides can demonstrate a predilection to involve the hair follicle. This may be observed simply by folliculotropism of the cells (pilotropic or follicular mycosis fungoides) or by the appearance of follicular mucinosis (Fig. 32-14). In all cases of follicular mucinosis, the histologic specimen should be carefully examined and the diagnosis of mycosis fungoides considered. Among patients older than 40 years of age who have follicular mucinosis, a large percentage will have mycosis fungoides or go on to develop it.

SYSTEMIC MANIFESTATIONS. Mycosis fungoides as a form of malignant lymphoma may progress to have visceral involvement. Lymph node involvement is most common; it predicts progression of the disease in at least a quarter of patients and reduces survival to about 7 years. Any other evidence of visceral involvement is a grave prognostic sign. An abnormal result on liver-spleen scan, chest radiograph or CT evaluation, abdominal or pelvic CT scans, or bone marrow biopsy is associated with a survival of about 1 year.

PATHOGENESIS. Mycosis fungoides is a neoplasm of memory helper T cells in most cases. Rare cases of suppressor cell (CD8+) mycosis fungoides have been reported. The events leading to the development of the malignant T cells are unknown. It has been speculated that it is caused by chronic exposure to an antigen, but this has yet to be confirmed. Patients with atopic dermatitis appear to be at increased risk for the development of MF, suggesting that persistent stimulation of T cells may lead to development of a malignant clone. Retroviruses have been proposed as the cause, and this theory was bolstered by the finding of a mycosis fungoides–like illness in persons infected with HTLV-1. However, the presence of retroviral infection in

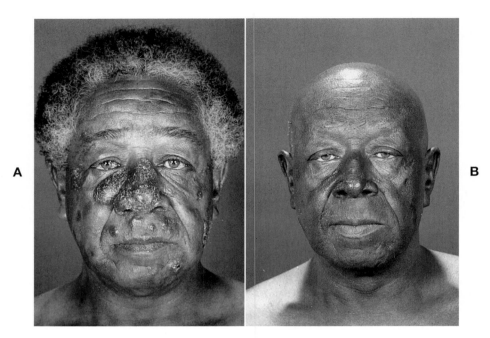

Fig. 32-8 Mycosis fungoides. **A,** Before therapy. **B,** After electron beam therapy.

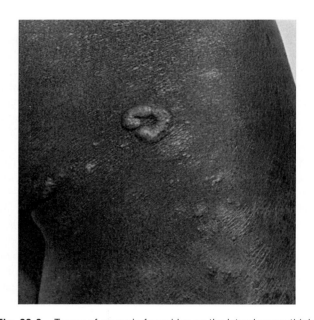

Fig. 32-9 Tumor of mycosis fungoides on the lateral upper thigh.

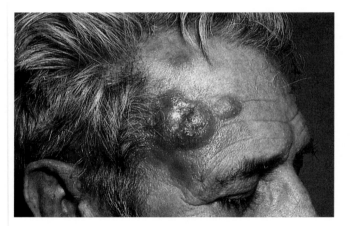

Fig. 32-10 Mycosis fungoides, tumor stages. (Courtesy Dr. Axel W. Hoke.)

MF patients has not been reproducibly confirmed and is still unproved.

The inflammatory nature of the skin lesions has led to investigation of the interactions of the malignant T cells and both keratinocytes and antigen-presenting cells (including Langerhans' cells) in MF. MF skin lesions have many features of skin that are immunologically "activated." MF cells express cutaneous lymphocyte antigen (CLA), the

ligand for E selectin, which is expressed on the endothelial cells of inflamed skin. This allows the malignant cells to traffic into the skin from the peripheral blood. Antigen-presenting cells are increased in MF lesions and have increased functional capacity to activate T cells. There is increased expression of MHC class II antigens on the surface of the antigen presenting cells. Through cytokines, infiltration of neoplastic and reactive T cells is increased. The pattern in early MF is more Th1-like, and the nonneoplastic infiltrating cells (tumor infiltrating lympho-cytes or TILs) may play a role in downregulating and controlling the neoplastic cells. There are more CD8+ cells in these early lesions, and these TILs may control the

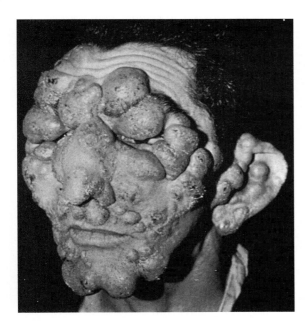

Fig. 32-11   Extensive tumors of mycosis fungoides of the face and ears.

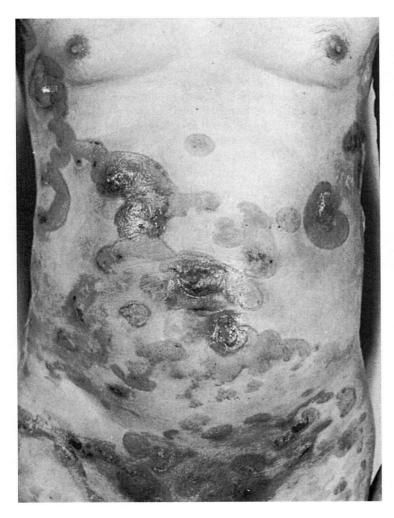

Fig. 32-12   Mycosis fungoides showing fungating tumors and plaques. Note the kidney-shaped lesions on the lateral chest.

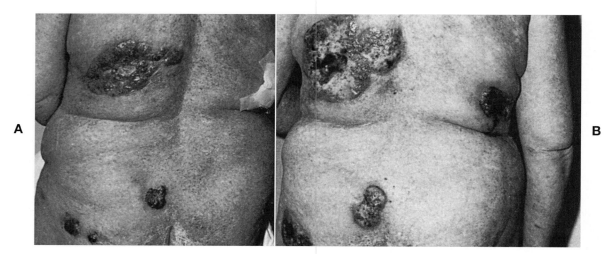

Fig. 32-13 Mycosis fungoides. **A,** Tumor stage. **B,** Three months later.

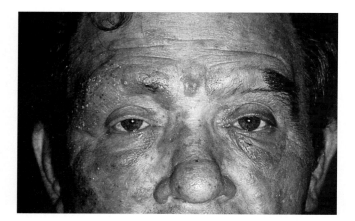

Fig. 32-14 Alopecia mucinosa and mycosis fungoides. Note loss of eyebrows.

malignant clone. In fact, MF patients with more than 20% CD8+ cells in their skin survive longer than those with less than 15%. In more advanced MF and in Sézary syndrome, perhaps through IL-4 and IL-10, a Th2 environment exists. This downregulates suppressor cell function, and the malignant clone can proliferate. Although this hypothesis has yet to be fully applied therapeutically, the response of some Sézary patients to gamma interferon treatment, which preferentially produces a Th1 environment and downregulates Th2 reactions, supports this theory.

As MF advances, the number of malignant circulating cells increases. Standard cytologic evaluation (the Sézary preparation), even when enhanced by specific labeling techniques, is expensive and not very accurate. Use of standard laboratory tests, such as the CD4/CD8 ratio test, which increases as MF progresses, and assessment of the number of CD4+CD7– circulating cells, which relatively specifically marks MF cells, yield indicators of tumor burden with advanced disease. As the number of normal helper T cells in the circulation diminishes, the patient is at

risk for complications of immunosuppression (opportunistic infections). This loss of normal T-cell function may predispose to a Th2 state.

HISTOPATHOLOGY. Perhaps more than in any other situation in dermatopathology, the ability to diagnose mycosis fungoides histologically is closely correlated to the skill, training, and experience of the reviewing pathologist. When the clinician is considering a diagnosis of MF, if original histologic reports are nonconfirmatory or nonspecific, consultation with a skilled dermatopathologist should be strongly considered.

In patch-stage lesions there is a superficial perivascular and variably interstitial infiltrate of lymphocytes. There may be a lichenoid distribution of these cells, and a few may enter into the epidermis, residing in the basal cell layer or stratum spinosum. The lymphocytes in the epidermis may be larger than those in the dermis.

Plaques of mycosis fungoides show a more prominent lichenoid pattern and a deeper perivascular dermal component than patch-stage lesions. Upper dermal collagen is altered, with horizontal fibrosis in bundles. Epidermotropism is much more marked and is typically is associated with much less spongiosis than would be expected for the amount of infiltrating cells. Vesicular variants are an exception to this rule; spongiosis is prominent and results in intraepidermal and subcorneal vesiculation. In thick plaques and tumors, epidermotropism may be substantially diminished. The diagnosis is confirmed by the presence of dense sheets of infiltrating lymphocytes in the dermis and subcutaneous fat. These cells may have cerebriform nuclei.

Cardinal features that should suggest a diagnosis of mycosis fungoides include the following:

- Solitary or small groups of lymphocytes in the basal cell layer
- Epidermotropism of lymphocytes with disproportionately scant spongiosis
- More lymphocytes within the epidermis than would normally be seen in an inflammatory dermatosis

- Lymphocytes in the epidermis larger than those in the dermis
- Lymphocytes in the stratum corneum and stratum granulosum
- Papillary dermal fibrosis with bundles of collagen arranged haphazardly
- Prominent folliculotropism of the lymphocytes, especially with intrafollicular mucin deposition (follicular mucinosis)

Features that should suggest a diagnosis of inflammatory dermatosis over mycosis fungoides include the following:

- Prominent upper dermal and papillary edema
- Marked epidermal spongiosis
- The accumulation of the intraepidermal inflammatory cells in flask-shaped collections with the top open to the stratum corneum

Immunohistochemistry is of limited value in assessing mycosis fungoides. MF cells characteristically are CD4+ but lose the CD7 antigen; that is, they are CD4+CD7–. This phenotype is very unusual for nonmalignant T cells and thus is useful in evaluating peripheral blood lymphocytes. It is more difficult to apply to early skin lesions with fewer neoplastic cells. Because most inflammatory infiltrates in benign conditions are also composed of helper T cells, and in early MF there is a component of normal helper T cells in the infiltrate, there is little distinction between MF and inflammatory disorders when using immunohistochemistry. Rather, DNA hybridization or a Southern blot test is frequently performed in equivocal cases to detect clonal rearrangement of the T-cell receptor (TCR). However, these data must be interpreted with caution; clonality does not confirm a diagnosis of malignancy. Benign processes may contain clonal TCR rearrangements. In early lesions of MF, the number of infiltrating cells may be insufficient for a clone to be detected, so a negative test does not exclude the diagnosis of MF. Similar techniques can be used to evaluate lymph nodes in MF patients. Lymph node involvement can be detected by these molecular methods, while the routine histologic evaluation yields normal results. Patients with more advanced disease are more likely to have clones in their lymph nodes, and the presence of clonality is predictive of shorter survival.

DIFFERENTIAL DIAGNOSIS. In the early patch stage, mycosis fungoides may be difficult to diagnose. The skin lesions usually resemble a nondescript form of eczema with some scale. Interestingly, despite the itching, scratch marks and lichenification are usually absent. MF presenting as papuloerythroderma of Ofuji is an obvious exception. The multiple morphologies of MF make the differential diagnosis vast. Plaquelike lesions may resemble subacute dermatitis or psoriasis. Tumors must be differentiated from other forms of lymphoreticular malignancy and metastases.

TREATMENT. Effective therapy that reliably prolongs survival has not yet been documented. Many forms of therapy induce remissions of variable length. The choice among them depends on extent of disease, the patient's overall health and physical status, the physician's experience and preference, and the availability of various options. Topical steroids, topical nitrogen mustard or 1,3-bis(2-chloroethyl)-1-nitrosourea (carmustine) (BCNU), and PUVA are generally good choices for stage IA, IB, and IIA disease. Total skin electron beam (TSEB) therapy can be used for refractory stage IIA and stage IIB cases. Single-agent chemotherapy or photophoresis can be used as initial management for stage III patients. Systemic chemotherapy, retinoids, photophoresis, and interferon alfa may be effective in stage IV disease. In general, therapies that enhance the patient's immune system are favored.

Topical corticosteroids. The availability of superpotent class I topical corticosteroids has led to a reassessment of their possible role in the management of early (patch stage, T1 and T2) mycosis fungoides. Zackheim reported a 63% complete remission for patients with T1 disease and total response rate of 94% in T1 patients. In T2 patients complete responses were only 25%, but total responses were 82%. The predominant side effect was a temporary and reversible suppression of hypothalamic-pituitary axis in about 13% of patients. The responses were short lived if therapy was stopped, but given the limited toxicity, this is not necessary in many patients. The adjunctive value of topical corticosteroids in T1 MF requires reappraisal, because the response rates are similar to other modalities used for early MF, and the toxicity is very low.

Topical nitrogen mustard (NH2). The contents of a 10-mg vial of mechlorethamine hydrochloride (Mustargen-MSD) are dissolved in 60 ml of tap water and applied to the entire skin surface except the genitalia with a 2-inch paint brush. Daily applications are made until complete clearing occurs, which usually takes several months or longer. Such treatment leads to complete responses in 80% of patients with IA disease, 68% in patients with IB, 61% in IIA, 49% in IIB, and 60% in stage III patients. About 10% of patients obtain a durable and long-lasting remission of over 8 years. The major side effect of NH2 therapy is cutaneous sensitization; this can be reduced by the use of an ointment formulation, but response rates have been reported to be inferior with the ointment form. At least half of patients will relapse when therapy is stopped, but they frequently will again respond to NH2.

The duration of maintenance therapy after achieving remission is different in different centers. Some treat for an additional 6 months, and others taper treatment over a year or more. In many centers, topical nitrogen mustard is a proven mainstay of therapy for patch or plaque stage mycosis fungoides without lymphadenopathy.

Topical BCNU (carmustine). BCNU, 2 mg/ml in 150 ml aliquots, dissolved in ethanol, is dispensed to the patient. From this stock solution, the patient takes 5 ml and adds it to 60 ml of water at room temperature. Once daily, this is applied to the whole body, sparing the folds, genitals, hands, and feet (if they do not have lesions). If the extent of disease is limited, only the affected areas are treated. The average treatment course is 8 to 12 weeks. If after 3 to 6 months the patient's condition is not responding, the concentration may be doubled and the treatment repeated for 12 weeks. For small or persistent lesions, the straight stock solution may be applied daily. Patients tolerate BCNU better than nitrogen mustard, contact sensitization is uncommon, and responses are more rapid. CBCs should be monitored monthly during treatment, but marrow suppression occurs in less than 10% of patients treated with the low concentrations. Telangiectasia, which may be persistent and severe, can occur after prolonged BCNU therapy or following an adverse cutaneous reaction to the medication.

Ultraviolet therapy. Both UVB and PUVA have been effective in the management of MF. About 75% of patients with patch-stage disease will have a complete clinical remission with UVB therapy. Home therapy is successful. PUVA has been used more extensively, and because of its deeper penetration, it is perhaps better suited to the treatment of a disorder with a dermal component. Complete clearing is seen in 88% of patients with limited patch/plaque disease and in 52% of patients with extensive disease. Tumor-stage patients do not clear. Erythrodermic patients have poor tolerance for PUVA. Remissions are short with PUVA, averaging about 1 year, so maintenance therapy is usually given. Retinoids and interferon alfa may be added to PUVA. Retinoids may reduce the total number of PUVA treatments required. Interferon plus PUVA may be used in patch-stage patients in whom topical therapy and PUVA alone are ineffective, but toxicity may be significant.

Extracorporeal photochemotherapy (photophoresis) is a therapeutic modality in which the circulating cells are extracted and treated with UVA outside the body; the patient ingests psoralen before the treatment. Complete responses are seen in a small percentage of MF patients, about 20%, and a partial response occurs in a similar percentage of patients. In the reports of Heald et al and Edelson et al, the overall improvement rate for erythrodermic patients was 80%, but many of these patients failed to have at least the 50% clearing required to be considered a partial response. In addition, survival is not prolonged by this modality. Photophoresis is very expensive, so other more economical modalities should be considered initially.

Radiation treatment. Total skin electron beam (TSEB) therapy in doses in excess of 3000 Gy is very effective in the management of MF. Stage T1 patients have a 98% complete response; stage T2, 71%; T3, 36%; and T4, 64%. Long-term remissions occur in about 50% of T1 patients and 20% of T2 patients. Erythrodermic patients tolerate TSEB poorly; other modalities should be attempted initially. Because relapses are frequent, adjuvant therapy with a topical agent or PUVA can be considered if the patient relapses. The most common side effects of TSEB are erythema, edema, worsening of lesions, alopecia, and nail loss. Persistent hyperpigmenta-

tion and chronically dry skin are problems after TSEB. Orthovoltage radiation may be used to control tumors or resistant thick plaques in patients whose condition has been otherwise controlled with another modality.

Biologic response modifiers. Interferon alfa has been shown to have efficacy against MF. It is associated with a positive response in about 60% of patients, and a complete response in 19%. Toxicity is high and includes fever, chills, myalgias, neutropenia, and depression. The dosage must be frequently adjusted. Interferon treatment may be combined with retinoid therapy.

Retinoids. Both isotretinoin and etretinate have efficacy in the treatment of MF. A clinical response is noted in about 44% of patients. Dosage is about 1 mg/kg/day to start and may be increased up to 3 mg/kg/day as tolerated. Retinoids may be effective in stage IB (T2) patients, stage III patients, and as a palliative treatment in patients with stage IVA disease. Targretin, a synthetic retinoid that is bound preferentially by the RXR receptor, induces apoptosis in a number of tumor cell lines. It may show efficacy in MF.

Systemic chemotherapy. For most forms of cancer, combinations of chemotherapeutic agents are given. These standard approaches have been used to manage MF, but the toxicity outweighs the benefit. Systemic therapy in MF is limited to patients with advanced disease, and often single agents are used. Methotrexate in doses from 5 to 125 mg weekly is effective for the management of T3 patients. In these patients, Zackheim et al demonstrated that 41% had a complete response, and an additional 17% a partial response, for a total response of 58%. The median overall survival was 8.4 years, and 69% of patients were alive at 5 years. For advanced MF, higher doses of methotrexate with citrovorum-factor rescue have been successful in obtaining a response, which was then maintained with lower doses of methotrexate, not requiring rescue. Similarly, pentostatin, etoposide, fludarabine, and 2-chlorodexoyadenosine have been used. Systemic chemotherapy beyond methotrexate, especially multiagent chemotherapy, is best managed by an oncologist. Systemic chemotherapy is indicated in stage IVA patients and can be used in stage III patients who fail more conservative approaches.

Fusion toxin. DAB389IL-2 is the fusion of a portion of the diphtheria toxin to recombinant IL-2. This selectively binds to cells expressing the IL-2 receptor and leads to their death. Saleh et al, in a series of MF cases that expressed the IL-2 receptor, demonstrated a response rate of 37%, including a complete response in 14% of cases. These patients had failed conventional therapies. Patients in stage I to III achieved response, but no patient with stage IV disease achieved a response. Fever, chills, hypotension, and nausea and vomiting were common, and at high doses a vascular-leak syndrome was produced.

Abel EA: Clinical features of cutaneous T-cell lymphoma. *Dermatol Clin* 1985, 3:647.

Abel EA, et al: Cutaneous malignancies and metastatic squamous cell carcinoma following topical therapies for mycosis fungoides. *J Am Acad Dermatol* 1986, 14:1029.

Abel EA, et al: PUVA treatment of erythrodermic and plaque-type mycosis fungoides. *Arch Dermatol* 1987, 123:897.

Bakels V, et al: Frequency and prognostic significance of clonal T-cell receptor beta-gene rearrangements in the peripheral blood of patients with mycosis fungoides. *Arch Dermatol* 1992, 128:1602.

Bergman R, et al: Immunophenotyping and T-cell receptor gamma gene rearrangement analysis as an adjunct to the histopathologic diagnosis of mycosis fungoides. *J Am Acad Dermatol* 1998, 39:554.

Braverman IM, et al: Combined total body electron beam irradiation and chemotherapy for mycosis fungoides. *J Am Acad Dermatol* 1987, 16:45.

Cather JC, et al: Unusual presentation of mycosis fungoides and pigmented purpura with malignant thymoma. *J Am Acad Dermatol* 1998, 39:858.

Costlier J, et al: Isotretinoin and cutaneous helper T-cell lymphoma (mycosis fungoides). *Arch Dermatol* 1987, 123:201.

Crowley JJ, et al: Mycosis fungoides in young patients. *J Am Acad Dermatol* 1998, 38:696.

Edelson R, et al: Treatment of cutaneous T-cell lymphoma by extracorporeal photochemotherapy. *N Engl J Med* 1987, 316:297.

Epstein EH Jr, et al: Mycosis fungoides: survival, prognostic features, response to therapy, and autopsy findings. *Medicine* 1972, 15:61.

Fitzpatrick JE, et al: Treatment of mycosis fungoides with isotretinoin. *J Dermatol Surg Oncol* 1986, 12:626.

Gibson LE, et al: Follicular mucinosis. *J Am Acad Dermatol* 1989, 20:441.

Haeffner AC, et al: Differentiation and clonality of lesional lymphocytes in small plaque parapsoriasis. *Arch Dermatol* 1995, 131:321.

Hamminga B, et al: Treatment of mycosis fungoides: total skin electron beam vs topical mechlorethamine. *Arch Dermatol* 1982, 118:150.

Hansen ER: Immunoregulatory events in the skin of patients with cutaneous T-cell lymphoma. *Arch Dermatol* 1996, 132:554.

Heald P, et al: Treatment of erythrodermic cutaneous T-cell lymphoma with extracorporeal photochemotherapy. *J Am Acad Dermatol* 1992, 27:427.

Holloway KB, et al: Therapeutic alternatives in cutaneous T-cell lymphoma. *J Am Acad Dermatol* 1992, 27:367.

Kern DE, et al: Analysis of T-cell receptor gene rearrangement in lymph nodes of patients with mycosis fungoides. *Arch Dermatol* 1998, 134:158.

Kim YH, et al: Clinical characteristics and long-term outcome of patients with generalized patch and/or plaque (T2) mycosis fungoides. *Arch Dermatol* 1999, 135:26.

Kim YH, et al: Clinical stage IA (limited patch and plaque mycosis fungoides). *Arch Dermatol* 1996, 132:1309.

Lee LA, et al: Second cutaneous malignancies in patients with mycosis fungoides treated with topical nitrogen mustard. *J Am Acad Dermatol* 1982, 7:590.

McBride SR, et al: Vesicular mycosis fungoides. *Br J Dermatol* 1998, 138:141.

Milstein HJ, et al: Home ultraviolet phototherapy of early mycosis fungoides: preliminary observations. *J Am Acad Dermatol* 1982, 6:355.

Molin L, et al: Oral retinoids in mycosis fungoides and Sézary syndrome. *Acta Derm Venereol* 1987, 67:232.

Olsen EA, et al: Interferon alfa-2a in the treatment of cutaneous T-cell lymphoma. *J Am Acad Dermatol* 1989, 20:395.

Pereyo NG, et al: Follicular mycosis fungoides. *J Am Acad Dermatol* 1997, 36:563.

Price NM, et al: Ointment-based mechlorethamine treatment for mycosis fungoides. *Cancer* 1983, 52:2214.

Ramsay DL, et al: Topical mechlorethamine therapy for early stage mycosis fungoides. *J Am Acad Dermatol* 1988, 19:684.

Rosenbaum MM, et al: Photochemotherapy in cutaneous lymphoma and parapsoriasis en plaques. *J Am Acad Dermatol* 1985, 13:613.

Saleh MN, et al: Antitumor activity of DAB389IL-2 fusion toxin in mycosis fungoides. *J Am Acad Dermatol* 1998, 39:63.

Sinha AA, et al: Advances in the management of cutaneous T-cell lymphoma. *Dermatol Clin* 1998, 16:301.

Straten PT, et al: T-cell receptor variable gene in cutaneous T-cell lymphomas. *Br J Dermatol* 1998, 138:3.

Taylor JR, et al: Mechlorethamine hydrochloride solutions and ointment: prolonged stability and biological activity. *Arch Dermatol* 1980, 116:783.

Thomsen K, et al: 13-cis-retinoic acid effective in mycosis fungoides. *Acta Derm Venereol* 1984, 64:563.

Toro JR, et al: Prognostic factors and evaluation of mycosis fungoides and Sézary syndrome. *J Am Acad Dermatol* 1997, 37:58.

Vonderheid EC: Long-term efficacy, curative potential, and carcinogenicity of topical mechlorethamine chemotherapy in cutaneous T-cell lymphoma. *J Am Acad Dermatol* 1989, 20:416.

Vonderheid EC: Recombinant interferon alfa-2b in plaque-phase mycosis fungoides. *Arch Dermatol* 1987, 123:757.

Wood GS: Using molecular biologic analysis of T-cell receptor gene rearrangements to stage cutaneous T-cell lymphoma. *Arch Dermatol* 1998, 134:221.

Zackheim HS: Treatment of cutaneous T-cell lymphoma. *Semin Dermatol* 1994, 13:207.

Zackheim HS, et al: Low-dose methotrexate to treat erythrodermic cutaneous T-cell lymphoma. *J Am Acad Dermatol* 1996, 34:626.

Zackheim HS, et al: Topical carmustine (BCNU) for cutaneous T-cell lymphoma. *J Am Acad Dermatol* 1990, 22:802.

Zackheim HS, et al: Topical corticosteroids for mycosis fungoides. *Arch Dermatol* 1998, 134:949.

Zakem MH, et al: Treatment of advanced stage mycosis fungoides with bleomycin, doxorubicin and methotrexate with topical nitrogen mustard. *Cancer* 1986, 58:2611. _____ ▲

Pagetoid Reticulosis. Localized epidermotropic reticulosis, Pagetoid reticulosis, or Woringer-Kolopp disease, is an uncommon lymphoproliferative disorder considered by some to be a form of mycosis fungoides and by others to be a separate condition. Other terms suggested for these cases have been *acral mycoses fungoides* or *mycosis fungoides palmaris et plantaris*. In large MF clinics, such cases represent about 0.6% of all MF cases. Pagetoid reticulosis is divided into classic Woringer-Kolopp, which usually describes solitary lesions, and cases with multiple lesions (Ketron-Goodman variant). The unique features of Woringer-Kolopp are clinical. The disease presents as a solitary lesion that is often located on an extremity (Fig. 32-15). If there is more than a single lesion, often there is a propensity for lesions to involve both the palms and soles. Frequently, over months to years, the lesion gradually enlarges, reaching a size of greater than 10 cm. In some cases, the lesions spontaneously come and go over many years. Twenty percent of cases occur in patients who are less than 15 years of age. The long duration without progression to frank lymphoma has been a clinical hallmark of Woringer-Kolopp, although cases may progress to more classic mycosis fungoides, so the outlook must always be guarded. Histologically, there is prominent epidermotropism of lymphocytes, with many lining up in the basal cell layer. This histologic pattern correlates with strong alphaE–beta7 and alpha 4–beta7 integrin expression by the infiltrating cells. This integrin expression is also seen in the epidermotropic cells of classic MF and contact dermatitis.

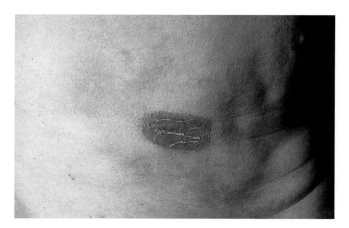

Fig. 32-15 Pagetoid reticulosis (Woringer-Kolopp).

In MF, most cases are CD4+, but in the acral MF cases, they may be CD4+, CD8+, or negative for both. T-cell receptor gene rearrangements can be detected in many cases of Woringer-Kolopp. In many ways, then, this condition is identical to mycosis fungoides, and these cases are best considered as variants of MF or true MF. Therapeutically local excision and radiation therapy have been "curative" in many cases. Topical and systemic PUVA have also proved effective. Local recurrence is possible.

Behrens S, et al: Disseminated pagetoid reticulosis. *Br J Dermatol* 1998, 139:343.

Burns MK, et al: Woringer-Kolopp disease (localized pagetoid reticulosis) or unilesional mycosis fungoides. *Arch Dermatol* 1995, 131:325.

McNiff JM, et al: Mycosis fungoides palmaris et plantaris or acral pagetoid reticulosis. *Am J Dermatopathol* 1998, 20:271.

Oliver GF, et al: Unilesional mycosis fungoides. *J Am Acad Dermatol* 1989, 20:63.

Resnik KS, et al: Mycosis fungoides palmaris et plantaris. *Arch Dermatol* 1995, 131:1052.

Zackheim HS: Is localized epidermotropic reticulosis (Woringer-Kolopp disease) benign? *J Am Acad Dermatol* 1984, 11:276. _____ ▲

Sézary Syndrome. Sézary syndrome is the leukemic phase of mycosis fungoides. The characteristic features are generalized erythroderma, superficial lymphadenopathy, and atypical cells in the circulating blood. Although patients with classic mycosis fungoides may progress to Sézary syndrome, usually patients with Sézary syndrome are erythrodermic from the onset. The skin shows a generalized erythroderma of a typical fiery red color, with leonine facies, eyelid edema, ectropion, diffuse alopecia, hyperkeratosis of the palms and soles, and dystrophic nails (Figs. 32-16 and 32-17). The symptoms are those of severe pruritus and burning, with episodes of chills and profuse perspiration.

Superficial lymphadenopathy is usually found in the cervical, axillary, and inguinal areas. Leukocytosis up to 30,000/mm^3 is usually present. In the peripheral blood, in the skin infiltrate, and in the lymph nodes, helper T cells

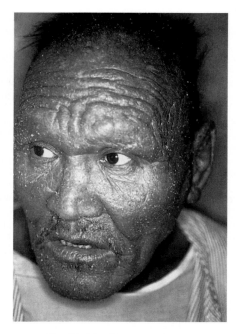

Fig. 32-16 Sézary syndrome.

with deeply convoluted nuclei are found: the so-called Sézary cells. An absolute number of greater than 1000 atypical cells, or greater than 10% of the circulating cells, is the criterion for a diagnosis of Sézary syndrome.

Histologically and by immunohistochemistry, there are no reproducible differences between cases of mycosis fungoides and Sézary syndrome. In some cases of Sézary syndrome, the cutaneous histology may be nonspecific, and additional histologic or hematologic evaluation may be necessary to confirm the diagnosis in the erythrodermic patient. T-cell gene rearrangement studies are frequently used to confirm the diagnosis of Sézary syndrome. In addition, an increased CD4/CD8 ratio in the blood with an increase in the number of CD3+/CD4+/CD7− circulating cells is suggestive of leukemic mycosis fungoides.

The erythroderma of Sézary syndrome must be distinguished from chronic lymphocytic leukemia, psoriasis, atopic dermatitis, photodermatitis, seborrheic dermatitis, contact dermatitis, drug reaction, and pityriasis rubra pilaris. This is done primarily by histopathologic and immunopathologic examination. In Sézary syndrome, the infiltrating T cells in the skin have a Th2 phenotype, and Th2 cytokines are produced by these cells. This explains the reduced delayed type hypersensitivity, elevated IgE, and eosinophilia seen in these patients.

Sézary syndrome is difficult to treat, and the median survival is approximately 3 years. Low-dose methotrexate has a reasonable response rate of about 50% and overall survival of 101 months, suggesting a survival benefit to its use. Photophoresis is effective in some patients, but the median survival time is only between 39 and 60 months. In a trial by Heald et al and Fraser-Andrews et al, no survival

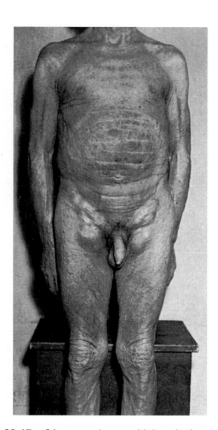

Fig. 32-17　Sézary syndrome with lymphadenopathy.

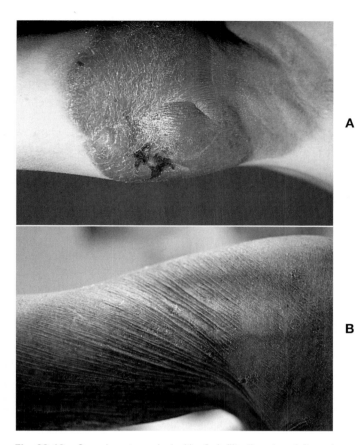

Fig. 32-18　Granulomatous slack skin. **A,** Infiltrative stage followed by **B,** atrophic stage.

benefit could be demonstrated for photophoresis therapy in Sézary syndrome. Alternative therapies include interferon alfa, retinoids, low-dose chlorambucil and prednisone, fludarabine, and systemic chemotherapy.

Bakels V, et al: Diagnostic value of the T-cell receptor beta gene rearrangement analysis on peripheral blood lymphocytes of patients with erythroderma. *J Invest Dermatol* 1991, 97:782.

Dummer R, et al: Sézary syndrome, T-helper 2 cytokines, and accessory factor-1 (AF-1). *Leuk Lymphoma* 1998, 28:515.

Fraser-Andrews E, et al: Extracorporeal photophoresis in Sézary syndrome. *Arch Dermatol* 1998, 134:1001.

Heald P, et al: Treatment of erythrodermic cutaneous T-cell lymphoma with extracorporeal photochemotherapy. *J Am Acad Dermatol* 1992, 27:427.

Kamarashev J, et al: Comparative analysis of histological and immunohistological features in mycosis fungoides and Sézary syndrome. *J Cutan Pathol* 1998, 25:407.

Winkelmann RK, et al: The treatment of Sézary syndrome. *J Am Acad Dermatol* 1984, 10:1000.

Zackheim HS, et al: Low dose methotrexate to treat erythrodermic cutaneous T-cell lymphoma. *J Am Acad Dermatol* 1996, 34:626.

▲

Granulomatous Slack Skin.

Granulomatous slack skin is a rare variant of cutaneous T-cell lymphoma that typically presents in middle-aged adults and gradually progresses over years. It occurs more often in men. Lesions are erythematous, atrophic, pendulous, and redundant plaques in the axillae and groin (Fig. 32-18). Histologically, there is a lymphohistiocytic infiltrate extending though the dermis, into the subcutaneous fat. Focal collections of large, multinucleated cells form granulomas and may completely replace fat lobules. Elastophagocytosis is prominent, and elastic tissue is absent in areas of inflammation. Lymphocytes are also found within the multinucleate giant cells and arranged around them in a wreathlike configuration. Epidermotropic lymphocytes are also seen. Immunohistologically, the cells are CD4+. T-cell gene rearrangements can be detected. About one third of patients with granulomatous slack skin develop Hodgkin's disease after years to decades.

DeGregorio R, et al: Granulomatous slack skin. *J Am Acad Dermatol* 1995, 33:1044.

Helm KF, et al: Granulomatous slack skin. *Br J Dermatol* 1992, 126:142.

Noto G, et al: Granulomatous slack skin. *Br J Dermatol* 1994, 131:275.

▲

Lymphomatoid Papulosis.

Lymphomatoid papulosis (LyP) is an uncommon but not rare disorder. It occurs at any age but is most common in adults from 20 to 40 years of age. In most typical cases, the lesions and course are very similar to that of Mucha-Haberman disease (pityriasis lichenoides et varioliformis acuta), except the lesions tend to be slightly larger, fewer in number, and have a greater propensity to necrosis. Symptoms are usually minimal. The primary lesion is a red papule up to about 1 cm in diameter (Fig. 32-19). The lesions evolve to papulovesicular, papulopustular, or hemorrhagic, then necrotic papules over days to weeks. Lesions typically heal spontaneously within 8 weeks, somewhat longer in larger lesions.

There may be crops of lesions, or a constant appearance of a few lesions. In most patients, however, the condition tends to be chronic, and lesions are present most of the time if no treatment is given. The average number of lesions present at any one time is usually 10 to 20, but cases with more than 100 lesions occur. Lesions heal with varioliform, hyperpigmented, or hypopigmented scars. Cases previously reported as solitary, large nodules of lymphomatoid papulosis would now be classified as CD30-positive large-cell lymphomas or as overlaps between LyP and lymphoma, termed *borderline cases.*

The diagnosis of LyP is confirmed histologically. There is a dermal infiltrate that is wedge-shaped, patchy, and perivascular. In larger lesions the infiltrate may occupy the whole dermis. The infiltrate may involve the epidermis, with epidermotropism of inflammatory cells. As lesions evolve, epidermal necrosis and ulceration may occur. The dermal vessels may demonstrate fibrin deposition and more rarely, a lymphocytic "vasculitis." The dermal infiltrate is composed of lymphoid cells, eosinophils, neutrophils, and larger mononuclear cells. Atypical large or small lymphoid cells are present and may represent up to 50% of the infiltrate. Histologically, lesions have been classified into type A and type B lesions.

Type A lesions contain atypical large cells with abundant cytoplasm and prominent nuclei, with prominent eosinophilic nucleoli. If these cells contain two nuclei, they closely resemble Reed-Sternberg cells. In type B lesions, the atypical cells are smaller, with a smaller cerebriform, hyperchromatic nucleus. These resemble the atypical cells of mycosis fungoides. In both types of lesions atypical mitotic figures may be observed. Immunophenotypically, the large atypical cells mark as T cells, usually of the helper type. The atypical cells, especially those of the type A lesions, stain for the activation marker Ki-1 or CD30. When clonal rearrangement studies are performed, clonal rearrangements may be found in up to 40% of LyP lesions, but this finding is not predictive of the behavior of that lesion or the case in general.

Lymphomatoid papulosis is associated with lymphoma in a substantial proportion of cases. In the general literature this number is about 5% to 10%, but some reports have documented rates as high as 20%, and at UCSF up to 40% of cases of LyP have an associated lymphoma. The lymphoma may occur before, concurrently, or after the appearance of the LyP. In most cases, the LyP precedes the development of lymphoma, sometimes by a long period—

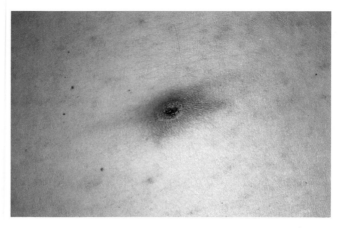

Fig. 32-19 Lymphomatoid papulosis.

up to 20 years. The associated lymphoma is most commonly mycosis fungoides (40%), a CD30-positive T-cell lymphoma (30%), or Hodgkin's disease (25%). The lymphoma and lymphomatoid papulosis may behave quite independently. If the lymphoma is successfully treated and cleared, the LyP typically continues. Despite this independent behavior, the lymphoma and the LyP may contain the same clonal T-cell receptor gene rearrangement. Patients with pure type B lesions are much less likely to develop lymphoma than patients with type A lesions.

Therapy may not be necessary; there is no evidence that treatment of LyP prevents the development of secondary lymphoma. Therefore, patients only need to be treated if they are moderately symptomatic, and the treatment has fewer potential complications than the benefits gained. Superpotent topical corticosteroids have been beneficial in some childhood cases. PUVA systemically or topically may be effective, although maintenance treatment is usually required. Topically applied carmustine (BCNU), 10 mg daily for 4 to 17 weeks, will suppress lesions without bone marrow depression. Of all the systemic oncologic agents, methotrexate gives the most dependable response, with up to 90% of LyP patients improving significantly. It is given in weekly doses similar to those used for psoriasis—usually 15 mg to 20 mg weekly. Higher doses may be required in some patients. Response is rapid. Some patients treated with oral methotrexate may have long duration remissions of the LyP. In others, maintenance therapy is required.

Basarab T, et al: Lymphomatoid papulosis in association with mycosis fungoides. *Br J Dermatol* 1998, 139:630.

Beljaards RC, et al: The prognosis of patients with lymphomatoid papulosis associated with malignant lymphoma. *Br J Dermatol* 1992, 126:596.

Karp DL, et al: Lymphomatoid papulosis. *J Am Acad Dermatol* 1994, 30:379.

Paul MA, et al: Lymphomatoid papulosis. *Pediatr Dermatol* 1996, 13:501.

Volkenandt M, et al: PUVA-bath photochemotherapy resulting in rapid clearance of lymphomatoid papulosis in a child. *Arch Dermatol* 1995, 131:1094.

Vonderheid EC, et al: Methotrexate is effective therapy for lymphomatoid papulosis and other primary cutaneous CD-30 positive lymphoproliferative disorders. *J Am Acad Dermatol* 1996, 34:470.

Wolf P, et al: Ambivalent response of lymphomatoid papulosis treated with 8-methoxypsoralen and PUVA. *J Am Acad Dermatol* 1994, 30:1018.

Zirbel GM, et al: Lymphomatoid papulosis is children. *J Am Acad Dermatol* 1995, 33:741. _____ ▲

PRIMARY CUTANEOUS T-CELL LYMPHOMAS OTHER THAN MYCOSIS FUNGOIDES

Once a cutaneous lymphoma has been identified to be of T-cell origin, and the diagnosis of mycosis fungoides and its variants has been excluded, the most important evaluation is to determine the CD30 staining pattern. CD30 is a marker found on some activated, but not resting, T and B cells. It also marks the Reed-Sternberg cells of Hodgkin's disease. Monoclonal antibodies Ki-1 and Ber H2 are used to identify CD30 positivity. A cutaneous lymphoma is considered CD30 positive if there are large clusters of CD30-positive cells or more than 75% of the anaplastic T cells are CD30 positive. Primary cutaneous T-cell lymphomas that are CD30 positive are more common and have a better prognosis than lymphomas that are CD30 negative.

CD30-Positive Cutaneous T-Cell Lymphoma

Clinically, these lymphomas present as solitary or localized skin lesions that have a tendency to ulceration (50%) and spontaneous regression (25%). These lymphomas are rare in children and occur with slightly greater frequency in males. Lesions are usually firm red to violaceous tumors, up to 10 cm in diameter. Tumors may grow in a matter of weeks. There is no favored anatomic site.

Relapses in the skin are common, but the development of extracutaneous or lymph node involvement is uncommon, and regional lymph node involvement does not impart a poor prognosis. One variant of CD30-positive cutaneous T-cell lymphoma presents with recurring and regressing cutaneous nodules that ulcerate, resembling pyoderma gangrenosum or fungating tumors. This was previously called *regressing atypical histiocytosis* but is now recognized to be a cutaneous T-cell lymphoma. A spectrum of overlap cases exists with features of both lymphomatoid papulosis and CD30-positive anaplastic T-cell lymphoma. The term *borderline cases* has been used in this setting.

Histologically, there is a dense dermal nonepidermotropic infiltrate with atypical tumor cells with large nuclei with one or several prominent nucleoli and abundant cytoplasm. The malignant cells can be further characterized as anaplastic, pleomorphic, and immunoblastic, but this distinction may be difficult and has yet to be determined to be of prognostic and therapeutic value. This form of primary cutaneous T-cell lymphoma has an excellent prognosis with a 5-year survival of 90%. Lesions are highly responsive to radiotherapy. Early individual lesions can even be surgically excised. Chemotherapy causes regression of lesions, but a rapid relapse usually occurs. The prognosis is favorable,

with about 30% of cases developing extracutaneous disease. This is in marked contrast to CD30-positive lymphoma of lymph node origin, which has a poor prognosis.

Secondary Cutaneous CD30-Positive Large-Cell Lymphoma

CD30-positive large-cell lymphomas may arise in cases of mycosis fungoides, in patients with lymphomatoid papulosis, and in patients who have documented extracutaneous disease. The prognosis is poor in patients who have extracutaneous disease preceding or near the time of cutaneous involvement. Patients with lymphomatoid papulosis who develop cutaneous CD30-positive lymphoma, and who do not have another type of lymphoma also, have a good prognosis. The prognosis for MF patients who develop CD30-positive lymphoma is poor.

Non-MF CD30-Negative Cutaneous Large T-Cell Lymphoma

Non-MF CD30-negative cutaneous large T-cell lymphomas usually present as solitary or generalized plaques, nodules, or tumors of short duration. There is no preceding patch stage that distinguishes it from MF. The prognosis is poor, with a 5-year survival rate of 15%. The malignant cells are pleomorphic large or medium cell types or are immunoblastic. The cells may be cerebriform, and epidermotropism may be present. Some cases previously called *d'emblée mycosis fungoides* are better classified in this group. Multiagent chemotherapy is recommended.

Non-MF CD30-Negative Cutaneous Pleomorphic Small or Medium-Sized Cell Lymphoma

Small or medium-sized pleomorphic cutaneous T-cell lymphoma is distinguished from the large-cell type by having less than 30% large pleomorphic cells. It is distinguished from MF by clinical features (lack of patch or plaque lesions). These primary cutaneous lymphomas usually present with one or several red-purple nodules or tumors. Immunophenotypically, they are usually of helper T-cell origin and clonal rearrangements of the T-cell receptor gene are usually present. The presence of a mixed population of suppressor cells, B cells and histiocytes, usually favors the diagnosis of reactive lymphoid hyperplasia. This form of lymphoma may demonstrate angiocentric features (Angiocentric T-cell lymphoma). The overall prognosis is good, with a 5-year survival rate exceeding 50%. Therapeutically, local radiation therapy, interferon alfa, and single agent cyclophosphamide have been reported as effective.

Subcutaneous (Panniculitis-Like) T-Cell Lymphoma

Clinically, patients present with subcutaneous nodules, usually on the lower extremities, and are frequently diagnosed as having erythema nodosum or some other form of panniculitis. Weight loss, fever, and fatigue are common.

A hemophagocytic syndrome is frequently present and is often the cause of death. Extracutaneous involvement is rare, even in fatal cases.

Histologically, there is a lacelike infiltration of the lobules of adipocytes, mimicking panniculitis. The infiltrate contains a mixture of small and large lymphoid cells. The cells are atypical, karyorrhexis is prominent, and mitotic figures are frequent. Benign histiocytes are present in large or small numbers and demonstrate erythrophagocytosis. Immunophenotypically, the neoplastic cells mark as T cells (CD2+, CD3+), usually CD4+, and are CD30 negative. This form of lymphoma must be distinguished from the benign variant of cytophagic histiocytic panniculitis, which may also have a hemophagocytic syndrome. The prognosis for a patient with subcutaneous T-cell lymphoma is poor. Multi-agent chemotherapy is recommended.

Nasal/Nasal Type T/NK Cell Lymphoma

Nasal/nasal type T/NK cell lymphoma most frequently presents in extranodal tissue and is characterized by a high incidence of nasal involvement. In some cases skin lesions precede the extracutaneous findings, suggesting this form of lymphoma may rarely be a primary cutaneous lymphoma. It occurs more frequently among Asian patients, especially women, with a mean age of about 40.

Skin lesions are generalized erythematous plaques or less commonly, localized tumors. Histologically, the dermis is infiltrated diffusely with intermediate sized, atypical lymphocytes. Epidermotropism may be present. An angiocentric pattern is common. Immunophenotypically, the lymphoma cells variably express CD2 and CD3 and the natural killer (NK) cell marker CD56. Epstein-Barr virus is often present in these lymphomas. Clonal arrangement of the T-cell receptor gene and clonal integration of the EBV genome may be present. The prognosis is poor.

Beljaards RC, et al: Primary cutaneous CD30-positive large cell lymphoma. *Cancer* 1993, 71:2097.

Camisa C, et al: Ki-1-positive anaplastic large-cell lymphoma can mimic benign dermatoses. *J Am Acad Dermatol* 1993, 29:696.

Gonzalez CL, et al: T cell lymphoma involving subcutaneous tissue. *Am J Surg Pathol* 1991, 15:17.

Miyamoto T, et al: Cutaneous presentation of nasal/nasal type T/NK cell lymphoma. *Br J Dermatol* 1998, 139:481.

Monterroso V, et al: Subcutaneous tissue involvement by T-cell lymphoma. *Arch Dermatol* 1996, 132:1345.

Motley RJ, et al: Regressing atypical histiocytosis, a regressing cutaneous phase of Ki-1-positive anaplastic large cell lymphoma. *Cancer* 1992, 70:476.

Romero LS, et al: Subcutaneous T-cell lymphoma with associated hemophagocytic syndrome and terminal leukemic transformation. *J Am Acad Dermatol* 1996, 34:904.

Willemze R, et al: EORTC classification for primary cutaneous lymphomas. *Blood* 1997, 90:354.

Willemze R, et al: Spectrum of primary cutaneous CD30 (Ki-1)-positive lymphoproliferative disorders. *J Am Acad Dermatol* 1993, 28:973. ▲

CUTANEOUS B-CELL LYMPHOMA

Primary cutaneous B-cell lymphomas occur less commonly than cutaneous T-cell lymphomas—but more frequently than generally believed. Many of the lymphoid proliferations previously classified as B-cell "pseudolymphomas" are actually low-grade B-cell lymphomas. Although the morphologic appearance of the malignant lymphocytes composing these primary cutaneous lymphomas is identical to lymphomas based in lymph nodes, they have a distinctly different clinical behavior and immunophenotypic profile. This renders the classification systems based on lymph node histology of limited benefit clinically in the diagnosis of primary cutaneous B-cell lymphomas. More simplified schemes have thus been proposed that apply to primary cutaneous lymphomas only.

The great majority of primary cutaneous B-cell lymphomas are composed of cells with the morphologic characteristics of the B cells normally found in the germinal centers of lymph nodes. Classification schemes used primarily for lymph node–based lymphomas divide these lymphomas into multiple types based on histomorphology. Fewer distinctions are made for primary cutaneous B-cell lymphomas, since the behaviors of most of the lymphomas of follicular center cell origin are similar.

Secondary cutaneous involvement can occur with all forms of B-cell lymphoma based primarily in lymph node or other sites. The clinical features are similar to those of primary cutaneous lymphoma, with violaceous papules or nodules. Typically, the histologic structure of secondary lesions in the skin is similar to that of the lymphoma at the site of origin, usually lymph nodes. The pattern in the skin may not, however, be sufficient to accurately classify the lymphoma, making lymph node biopsy necessary in most cases. The skin lesions of secondary lymphomas may be clinically and histologically identical to primary cutaneous lymphomas. In secondary cutaneous B-cell lymphomas the prognosis is, in general, poor. It is therefore critical to completely evaluate and stage any patient suspected of having primary cutaneous B-cell lymphoma to exclude involvement at another site.

Primary Cutaneous Follicular Center Cell Lymphoma (B-Cell Lymphoma of Follicular Center Cell Origin, Reticulohistiocytoma of the Dorsum)

Clinically, most patients present with a single or multiple papules or nodules in one anatomic region. About two thirds of cases present on the trunk, about one fifth on the head and neck (the vast majority of these on the scalp), and about 15% on the leg (Figs. 32-20 to 32-22). These lymphomas are twice as common in men as women. Males outnumber females four to one in trunk lesions, whereas women disproportionately have head lesions and leg lesions. Untreated the lesions gradually increase in size and number, but extracutaneous involvement is uncommon. The prognosis for trunk and head lesions is excellent, with 5-year

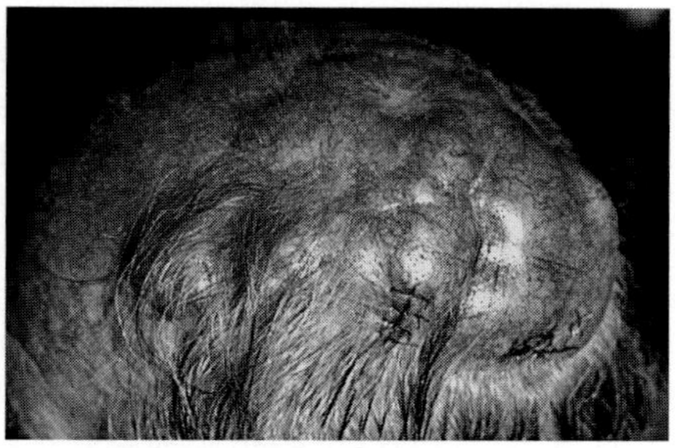

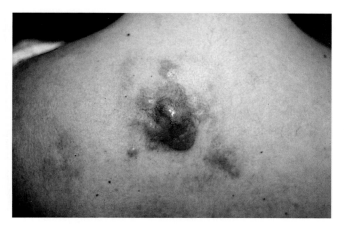

Fig. 32-22 Cutaneous B-cell lymphoma.

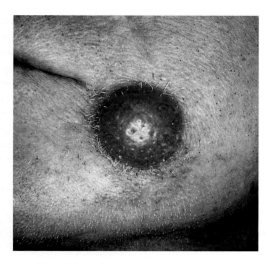

Fig. 32-20 Cutaneous B-cell lymphoma of scalp.

Fig. 32-21 Cutaneous B-cell lymphoma.

survival with treatment approaching 100%. Leg lesions occur mostly in persons over age 70, and the 5-year survival is nearly 50%. In some classifications, the primary cutaneous B-cell lymphomas of the leg are considered a separate entity because of this worse prognosis and different immunophenotypic properties.

Histologically, the infiltrate is nodular or diffuse within the dermis, and spares the epidermis. In early lesions, the neoplastic cells are of smaller size and there is a substantial portion of normal T cells surrounding and mixed with the neoplastic B cells. Over time the neoplastic B cells become a more predominant portion of the infiltrate, the neoplastic cells are larger in size, and tumor-infiltrating T cells diminish. Immunophenotypically, the neoplastic cells stain with B-cell markers (CD20 and others) and are monotypic for immunoglobulin production; that is, they stain for either kappa or lambda light chains, but not both. Immunoglobulin staining may be negative in tumorous lesions. Lymphomas of the leg, but not those of the head or trunk, express bcl-2.

Clonal rearrangement of the immunoglobulin gene can be demonstrated.

Radiation therapy totaling 30 to 40 Gy and including all erythematous skin and a 2 cm margin of normal skin is very effective for lesions of the head and trunk. For more widespread lesions, polychemotherapy with a CHOP regimen is recommended. As noted earlier, lesions on the leg have a worse prognosis, but similar treatment is recommended. In Europe some cases of primary cutaneous follicular center cell lymphoma are associated with *Borrelia* infection and may arise in lesions of acrodermatitis chronica atrophicans.

Primary Cutaneous Immunocytoma (Marginal Zone B-Cell Lymphoma, MALT Type Lymphoma)

These lymphomas present as solitary or multiple dermal or subcutaneous nodules or tumors primarily of the extremities or trunk. Histologically, the infiltrate is nodular or diffuse and composed of small lymphocytes and cells showing plasma cell differentiation. The atypical cells are often located at the periphery of aggregates of reactive T and B cells. Initially, the malignant cells may represent a very small proportion of the infiltrate and the diagnosis of pseudolymphoma is made. Over time the "marginal zone" cells predominate and the germinal centers are diminished. Immunophenotypically, the cells are monotypic for immunoglobulin, and are CD79, CD20, and bcl-2 positive. Clonal immunoglobulin gene rearrangements can be demonstrated. The prognosis is excellent, with 5-year survival near 100%. Local radiation therapy or excision if lesions are few is recommended. Some lymphomas of this type have been associated with *Borrelia* infection in Europe.

Intravascular Large B-Cell Lymphoma (Neoplastic Angioendotheliomatosis)

Clinically, these cases present with variable cutaneous morphologies. Some cases resemble classic lymphoma with violaceous papules or nodules. Other cases more closely resemble intravascular thrombotic disorders with livedo reticularis–like lesions. Sclerotic plaques may also occur. Central nervous system symptoms are prominent with progressive dementia or multiple cerebrovascular ischemic events which may precede the findings of lymphoma by many months. Histologically, the features are characteristic and diagnostic. Dermal and subcutaneous vessels are dilated and filled with large neoplastic cells. Focal extravascular accumulations may be seen. The neoplastic cells are CD20 and CD79a positive and monotypic for immunoglobulin. Clonal immunoglobulin gene rearrangements may be detected. Despite the large number of intravascular cells in the skin and other affected organs, the peripheral blood smears and bone marrow may be normal histologically. The prognosis is very poor. Multiagent chemotherapy is recommended. Rare cases of intravascular lymphoma may be of T-cell origin.

Bertero M, et al: Mantle zone lymphoma. *J Am Acad Dermatol* 1994, 30:23.

Berti E, et al: Reticulohistiocytoma of the dorsum (Crosti's disease) and other B-cell lymphomas. *Semin Diagn Pathol* 1991, 8:82.

Kerl H, et al: The morphologic spectrum of cutaneous B-cell lymphoma. *Arch Dermatol* 1996, 132:1376.

Garbe C, et al: Borrelia burgdorferi associated cutaneous B cell lymphoma. *J Am Acad Dermatol* 1991, 24:584.

Rijlaarsdam JU, et al: Treatment of primary cutaneous B-cell lymphomas of follicle center origin. *J Clin Oncol* 1996, 14:549.

Russel-Jones R: Primary cutaneous B-cell lymphoma. *Br J Dermatol* 1998, 139:945.

Vermeer MH, et al: Primary cutaneous large B-cell lymphomas of the legs. *Arch Dermatol* 1996, 132:1304.

Willemze R, et al: EORTC classification for primary cutaneous lymphomas. *Blood* 1997, 90:354.

Willemze R, et al: Primary cutaneous large-cell lymphomas of follicular center cell origin. *J Am Acad Dermatol* 1987, 16:518. _____ ▲

Plasmacytoma (Multiple Myeloma)

Plasma cells, or mature secretory B lymphocytes, when they produce neoplasms, form a spectrum from solitary plasmacytomas, to multiple plasmacytomas, to multiple myeloma, and to the rare plasma cell leukemia. Multiple myeloma is the most common of these neoplasms. Multiple myeloma is characterized by lytic bone lesions and infiltration of the bone marrow by plasma cells. In addition, it is frequently associated with anemia, hyperglobulinemia, hypercalcemia, impaired renal function, and increased susceptibility to infections.

Cutaneous plasmacytomas, or localized neoplasms of plasma cells in the skin, are seen most commonly in the setting of myeloma or as a metastasis from a primary plasmacytoma of other tissues. These cases are called *secondary cutaneous plasmacytoma.* They may also occur by direct extension from an underlying bone lesion. Most commonly, secondary cutaneous plasmacytomas occur in the setting of advanced myeloma, and the prognosis is poor. Less commonly, the skin lesions may be the initial clinical finding, leading to the diagnosis of myeloma.

More rarely, solitary or multiple skin lesions may be seen with no evidence of involvement in any other tissue. Bone films and bone marrow biopsy are normal, but the cutaneous lesions may produce a monoclonal protein. Such skin lesions are termed *primary cutaneous plasmacytomas.* The prognosis in such lesions is unpredictable. In some patients the skin lesions resolve with treatment, never to recur; these patients have an excellent prognosis. In others, the patient progresses to myeloma. Neither the clinical nor the histologic appearance of the cutaneous lesions predicts the course. In both primary and secondary cutaneous plasmacytoma, the skin lesions are relatively nonspecific in appearance, presenting as skin-colored, red, or violaceous dermal or subcutaneous nodules (Fig. 32-23). Rarely, soft-tissue extramedullary plasmacytomas may be associated with posttransplantation plasma cell dyscrasia.

Histologically, plasmacytomas are composed of diffuse infiltrates of plasma cells in the dermis and/or subcutaneous tissue. The infiltrating plasma cell may be mature and lack atypia, or may be immature and atypical with mitoses. Plasmacytomas are distinguished from other plasma cell proliferations in the skin by their monoclonality. Gene rearrangement studies are usually not required, since immunohistochemistry can often define the infiltrate as monoclonal by demonstrating the presence of only kappa or lambda chains (monotypic). Benign proliferations have a mixed population. The immunoglobulin produced may be of any type, but IgA is frequently found.

The appropriate treatment of plasmacytomas is determined by the presence or absence of associated systemic disease. Solitary or paucilesional primary cutaneous plasmacytomas have been treated successfully with local surgery and radiation therapy. Systemic chemotherapy may be required if these modalities fail. The treatment for secondary plasmacytomas and for patients with numerous primary cutaneous plasmacytomas is chemotherapy.

Numerous nonspecific skin lesions occur in patients with

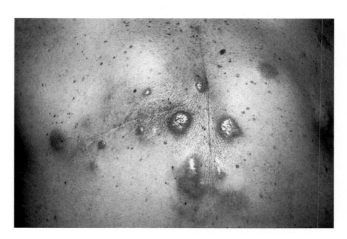

Fig. 32-23 Plasmacytomas.

multiple myeloma. These include amyloidosis, cutaneous vasculitis, thrombocytopenic purpura, alopecia, Raynaud's phenomenon, cold urticaria, pyoderma gangrenosum, planar xanthomas, and generalized anhidrosis. Anetoderma may be associated with myeloma, or may histologically show monoclonal or polyclonal plasmacytoma. Marked follicular hyperkeratosis, most prominent on the nose, is a characteristic paraneoplastic sign for myeloma, since its appearance with other malignancies is rare.

Burke WA, et al: Disseminated extramedullary plasmacytomas. *J Am Acad Dermatol* 1986, 14:335.

Green T, et al: Multiple primary cutaneous plasmacytomas. *Arch Dermatol* 1992, 128:962.

Hauschild A, et al: Multiple myeloma first presenting as cutaneous plasmacytoma. *J Am Acad Dermatol* 1996, 34:146.

James WD: Plasmacytoma. *Arch Dermatol* 1982, 118:62.

Joseph G, et al: Posttransplantation plasma cell dyscrasias. *Cancer* 1994, 74:1959.

Jubert C, et al: Anetoderma may reveal cutaneous plasmacytoma and benign cutaneous lymphoid hyperplasia. *Arch Dermatol* 1995, 131:365.

Mayr NA, et al: The role of radiation therapy in the treatment of solitary plasmacytomas. *Radiother Oncol* 1990, 17:293.

Patterson JW, et al: Cutaneous involvement of multiple myeloma and extramedullary plasmacytoma. *J Am Acad Dermatol* 1988, 18:879.

Paul C, et al: Hyperkeratotic spicules and monoclonal gammopathy. *J Am Acad Dermatol* 1995, 33:346.

Requena L, et al: Follicular spicules of the nose. *J Am Acad Dermatol* 1995, 32:834.

Shah A, et al: Multiple myeloma first observed as multiple cutaneous plasmacytomas. *Arch Dermatol* 1982, 118:922.

Shpilberg O, et al: Huge cutaneous plasmacytomas complicating multiple myeloma. *Clin Exp Dermatol* 1994, 19:324.

Torne R, et al: Clinicopathologic study of cutaneous plasmacytoma. *Int J Dermatol* 1990, 29:562.

Tuting T, et al: Primary plasmacytoma of the skin. *J Am Acad Dermatol* 1996, 34:386. —————————————————— ▲

HODGKIN'S DISEASE

The vast majority of reports of cutaneous Hodgkin's disease actually represent type A lymphomatoid papulosis. These two diseases have a considerable number of overlapping features. The type A cells of LyP have similar morphology and share immunophenotypic markers with Reed-Sternberg cells. Lymphomatoid papulosis can be seen in patients with Hodgkin's disease. Primary cutaneous Hodgkin's disease without nodal involvement is thus difficult to prove and is very, very rare.

Most cases of Hodgkin's disease of the skin usually originate in the lymph nodes, from which extension to the skin is either retrograde through the lymphatics or by direct extension. Lesions present as papules or nodules with or without ulceration. Miliary dissemination to the skin can occur in advanced disease.

Nonspecific cutaneous findings are common in patients with Hodgkin's disease. Generalized, severe pruritus may precede by many months other findings of Hodgkin's disease or may occur in patients with a known diagnosis.

Secondary prurigo nodules and pigmentation may occur as a result of scratching. An evaluation for underlying lymphoma should be considered in any patient with severe itching, no primary skin lesions, and no other cause identified for the pruritus. Acquired ichthyosis, exfoliative dermatitis, and generalized and severe herpes zoster are other cutaneous findings in patients with Hodgkin's disease.

Feiner AS, et al: Prognostic importance of pruritus in Hodgkin's disease. *JAMA* 1978, 240:2738.

Kumar S, et al: Primary cutaneous Hodgkin's disease with evolution to systemic disease. *Am J Surg Pathol* 1996, 20:754.

Moretti S, et al: In situ immunologic characterization of cutaneous involvement in Hodgkin's disease. *Cancer* 1989, 63:661.

White RM, et al: Cutaneous involvement in Hodgkin's disease. *Cancer* 1985, 55:1136. —————————————————— ▲

MALIGNANT HISTIOCYTOSIS (HISTIOCYTIC MEDULLARY RETICULOSIS)

Histiocytic medullary reticulosis is a rare, often fatal, malignant condition that occurs more commonly in men and typically presents in the second to fourth decades of life. It is characterized by the acute onset of fever, hepatosplenomegaly, and painful lymphadenopathy. Solitary or widespread papular and nodular skin lesions occur in about 10% of cases. Extensive erythrophagocytosis by histiocytes in marrow, liver, spleen, and lymph nodes is classically seen, although it is not often seen in the skin. Subcutaneous T-cell lymphoma with proliferation of histiocytes must be distinguished from malignant histiocytosis.

Morgan NE, et al: Clinical and pathological cutaneous manifestations of malignant histiocytosis. *Arch Dermatol* 1983, 119:367.

Nezelof C, et al: Malignant histiocytosis in childhood. *Semin Diagn Pathol* 1992, 9:75. —————————————————— ▲

LEUKEMIA CUTIS

CLINICAL FEATURES. Cutaneous eruptions seen in patients with leukemia may be divided into specific (leukemia cutis) and nonspecific lesions (reactive and infectious processes). Overall, about 30% of biopsies from patients with leukemia will show leukemia cutis. All forms of leukemia can be associated with cutaneous findings, but skin disease is more common in certain forms of leukemia. The vast majority of dermatologic manifestations are seen in patients with acute myelogenous leukemia (AML) or myelodysplastic syndrome (MDS). (AML includes types M1 through M5.) In AML and MDS patients, only about 25% of skin biopsies will show leukemia cutis, the remainder showing complications of the leukemia. These include infections, graft-versus-host disease, drug reactions, or the reactive conditions associated with leukemia that were formerly called *leukemids*. By contrast, in patients with acute lymphocytic leukemia, chronic myelogenous leukemia, and chronic lymphocytic leukemia about 50% of biopsies will show leukemia cutis.

Specific eruptions. The most common morphology of leukemic infiltrations of the skin in all forms of leukemia is multiple papules or nodules (60% of cases) or infiltrated plaques (26% of cases) (Figs. 32-24 and 32-25). These lesions are usually flesh colored, erythematous, or violaceous (plum colored). They are rubbery on palpation, and ulceration is uncommon. Extensive involvement of the face may lead to a leonine facies.

Less common manifestations of leukemia cutis are subcutaneous nodules resembling erythema nodosum, arciform lesions (in juvenile chronic myelogenous leukemia), ecchymoses, palpable purpura, erythroderma, ulcerations (which may resemble pyoderma gangrenosum or venous stasis ulceration), urticaria-like, urticaria pigmentosa–like (in acute lymphocytic leukemia [ALL]), and guttate psoriasis–like. Gingival infiltration causing hypertrophy is common in and relatively unique to patients with AML.

Leukemia cutis most commonly occurs concomitant with the diagnosis of leukemia or following the diagnosis of leukemia. The skin may also be a site of relapse of leukemia after chemotherapy, especially in patients who presented with leukemia cutis. Uncommonly, leukemia cutis may be identified while the bone marrow and peripheral blood are normal. Systemic involvement occurs within 3 weeks to 20 months (average, 6 months). Leukemia cutis is a poor prognostic finding in patients with leukemia, with 90% of such patients having extramedullary involvement and 40% having meningeal infiltration.

Congenital leukemia applies to cases appearing within the first 4 to 6 weeks of life. Leukemia cutis occurs in 25% to 30% of such cases, the vast majority congenital myelogenous leukemia. The typical morphology is multiple, red or plum-colored nodules. In about 10% of cases of congenital leukemia cutis (or 3% of all cases of congenital leukemia) the skin involvement occurs while the bone marrow and peripheral blood are normal. Systemic involvement is virtually always identified in 5 to 16 weeks. Unlike

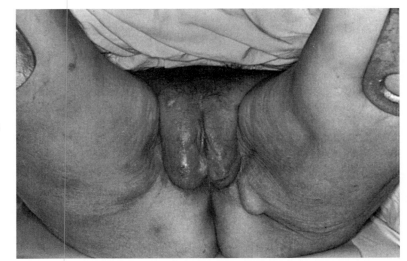

Fig. 32-24 Vulvar infiltrates of chronic lymphocytic leukemia.

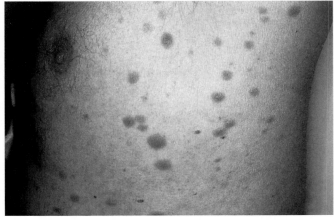

Fig. 32-25 Skin infiltrates of acute myelogenous leukemia.

other forms of leukemia, in congenital leukemia, cutaneous infiltration does not worsen prognosis.

Granulocytic Sarcoma (Chloroma)

Granulocytic sarcomas are rare tumors of immature granulocytes. They occur in about 3% of patients with myelogenous leukemia. Granulocytic sarcoma is seen in four settings: in a patient with known AML, in a patient with CGL or MDS as a sign of an impending blast crisis, in an undiagnosed patient as the first sign of AML, or after bone marrow transplantation as the initial sign of relapse. Most lesions occur in the soft tissues, periosteum, or bone. Skin lesions represent 20% to 50% of reported cases. They may be solitary or multiple. They appear as red, mahogany, or violaceous firm nodules with a predilection for the face, scalp, or trunk.

The name *chloroma* comes from the green color of fresh lesions, which can be enhanced by rubbing with alcohol; this is caused by the presence of myeloperoxidase. This appearance is variable, so the preferred term is now *granulocytic sarcoma.*

The diagnosis is not difficult if the diagnosis of leukemia has been established. Such patients are treated with appropriate chemotherapy. However, if the skin lesion is the initial manifestation of leukemia, and the blood and bone marrow are normal, the lesion may be misdiagnosed as a large-cell lymphoma. The presence of eosinophilic precursors, seen in 50% of cases of granulocytic sarcoma, suggests the correct diagnosis. Immunoperoxidase staining for lysozyme, myeloperoxidase, CD43 and CD45 characterize granulocytic sarcoma and help distinguish it from peripheral T-cell lymphoma. The treatment of such patients is controversial, but most go on to develop AML within months, so chemotherapy is often given.

Hairy-Cell Leukemia

Skin involvement is rare in hairy-cell leukemia, and violaceous papules and nodules, which are the characteristic morphology of other forms of leukemia cutis, are extremely rare in hairy-cell leukemia. Rather, often in the setting of a systemic mycobacterial infection or a drug reaction, a diffuse erythematous, nonpruritic eruption occurs. This may progress to erythroderma. Treating the underlying condition leads to resolution of the eruption. Histologically, large mononuclear cells are seen in a mixed infiltrate in the dermis. The majority of the infiltrating leukemic cells stain with tartrate-resistant acid phosphatase. In most cases the mononuclear cells also stain with B-cell markers, but a rare T-cell variant of hairy-cell leukemia occurs in HTLV-II associated leukemia.

Nonspecific Conditions Associated with Leukemia (Leukemids)

Leukemia and its treatment is associated with a series of conditions which may also be seen in patients without leukemia, but which are seen frequently enough in leukemic patients to be recognized as a complication of that condition or its treatment.

When a dermatologist or dermatopathologist is consulted to evaluate a patient with leukemia and skin lesions, the differential diagnosis usually includes four groups of conditions: drug reactions, leukemia cutis, an infectious complication, and a reactive condition. Drug reactions include all forms of reactions but are most commonly erythema multiforme, morbilliform reactions, or acral erythema. Infections may present in many ways but are usually purpuric papules, pustules, or plaques if they are caused by bacteria or fungi. Ulceration is typical. Herpes simplex and herpes zoster should be considered in all erosive, ulcerative, or vesicular lesions. The reactive conditions include a group of neutrophilic dermatoses with considerable clinical overlap. These include Sweet's syndrome, pyoderma gangrenosum, neutrophilic hidradenitis, and leukocytoclastic vasculitis.

Evaluation of these patients must be complete, and often extensive diagnostic tests and empiric treatment are pursued until the diagnosis is established. In the acute setting, a clinical diagnosis is made based on morphology. Possible infectious complications are covered by appropriate antibiotics, especially if the patient is febrile, or the diagnosis of a herpes virus infection is made. Diagnostic tests are submitted, often including a skin biopsy. For herpes infections, a direct fluorescent antibody should be done, as the results are virus specific and rapid, so appropriate treatment can be given quickly. Once the diagnostic tests return, the therapy is tailored to the appropriate condition. Except for herpes infections, a skin biopsy is often required. If infection is considered, a portion of that biopsy should be sent for culture.

In chronic lymphocytic leukemia (CLL), two unusual cutaneous manifestations occur. Vesiculobullous eruptions, some acantholytic, are rarely seen. In addition, pruritic and unremitting exfoliative erythroderma is a feature unique to CLL.

Anzai H, et al: Recurrent annular erythema in juvenile chronic myelogenous leukemia. *Br J Dermatol* 1998, 138:1058.

Bilsland D, et al: Transient leukemia cutis in hairy-cell leukemia. *Clin Exp Dermatol* 1991, 16:207.

Bourantas K, et al: Cutaneous vasculitis as the initial manifestation in acute myelomonocytic leukemia. *Ann Intern Med* 1994, 121:942.

Chan HL, et al: Cutaneous manifestations of adult T-cell leukemia/lymphoma. *J Am Acad Dermatol* 1985, 13:213.

Connelly TJ, et al: Leukemic macrocheilitis associated with hairy-cell leukemia and the Melkersson/Rosenthal syndrome. *J Am Acad Dermatol* 1986, 14:353.

Daoud MS, et al: Aleukemic monocytic leukemia cutis. *Mayo Clin Proc* 1996, 71:166.

Desch JK, et al: The spectrum of cutaneous disease in leukemias. *J Cutan Pathol* 1993, 20:407.

Flynn TC, et al: Neutrophilic eccrine hidradenitis. *J Am Acad Dermatol* 1984, 111:584.

Forjaz de Lacerda J, et al: Leukemia cutis in acute lymphoblastic leukemia. *J Am Acad Dermatol* 1994, 30:1041.

Frankel DH, et al: Acral livedosis: a sign of myeloproliferative diseases. *Arch Dermatol* 1987, 123:921.

Frix CD III, et al: Pemphigus foliaceus-like, immunologically negative dermatitis in a patient with T-cell chronic lymphocytic leukemia. *J Am Acad Dermatol* 1988, 18:1197.

Giralt S, et al: Leukemia cutis in acute promyelocytic leukemia. *Leuk Lymphoma* 1994, 14:453.

Hansen RM, et al: Aleukemic leukemia cutis. *Arch Dermatol* 1986, 122:812.

Harris DWS, et al: Cutaneous granulocytic sarcoma (chloroma) presenting as the first sign of relapse following autologous bone marrow transplantation for acute myeloid leukemia. *Br J Dermatol* 1992, 127:182.

Horan DB: Granulocytic sarcoma preceding granulocytic leukemia. *Cutis* 1984, 33:285.

Lawrence DM, et al: Cutaneous lesions in hairy-cell leukemia. *Arch Dermatol* 1983, 119:32.

Levine LL, et al: Distinctive acral erythema occurring during therapy for severe myelogenous leukemia. *Arch Dermatol* 1985, 121:102.

Longacre TA, et al: Leukemia cutis. *Am Clin Pathol* 1993, 100:276.

Margolis RJ, et al: Erythema multiforme in a patient with T-cell chronic lymphocytic leukemia. *J Am Acad Dermatol* 1986, 14:618.

O'Donnell JR, et al: Acute myelomonocytic leukemia presenting a xanthomatous skin eruption. *J Clin Pathol* 1982, 35:1200.

Ohno S, et al: Aleukemic leukemia cutis. *J Am Acad Dermatol* 1990, 22:374.

Passarini B, et al: *Cutis* verticis gyrata secondary to acute monoblastic leukemia. *Acta Derm Venereol* 1993 73:148.

Prystowsky JH, et al: Treatment of cutaneous granulocytic sarcoma in a patient with myelodysplasia. *Am J Med* 1989, 86:477.

Raj S, et al: Urticaria-pigmentosa-like lesions in acute lymphoblastic leukemia. *Dermatology* 1993, 186:226.

Ratnam KV, et al: Leukemia cutis. *Dermatol Clin* 1994, 12:419.

Resnik K, et al: Leukemia cutis in congenital leukemia. *Arch Dermatol* 1993, 129:1301.

Ritter JH, et al: Granulocytic sarcoma. *J Cutan Pathol* 1994, 21:207.

Rosen LB, et al: A characteristic vesiculobullous eruption in patients with chronic lymphocytic leukemia. *J Am Acad Dermatol* 1986, 15:943.

Schadendorf D, et al: Acute monoblastic leukemia with skin nodules in an adult. *J Am Acad Dermatol* 1993, 28:884.

Sepp N, et al: Specific skin manifestation in acute leukemia with monocytic differentiation. *Cancer* 1993, 71:124.

Spann CR, et al: Cutaneous leukocytoclastic vasculitis complicating hairy-cell leukemia. *Arch Dermatol* 1986, 122:1057.

Su WPD: Clinical, histologic, and immunohistochemical correlations in leukemia cutis. *Semin Dermatol* 1994, 13:223.

Vail JT, et al: Cutaneous xanthomas associated with chronic myelomonocytic leukemia. *Arch Dermatol* 1985, 121:1318. _____ ▲

CUTANEOUS MYELOFIBROSIS

Myelofibrosis is a chronic myeloproliferative disorder characterized by a clonal proliferation of defective multipotential stem cells in the bone marrow. Overproduction and premature death of atypical megakaryocytes in the bone marrow produce excess amounts of platelet-derived growth factor, a potent stimulus for fibroblast proliferation and collagen production. Extramedullary hematopoiesis (EMH) is a hallmark of myelofibrosis. Blast cells and committed stem cells escape the marrow in large numbers, enter the circulation, and form tumors of the same atypical clone in other organs, especially the spleen, liver, and lymph node. EMH in the skin of neonates is usually caused by intrauterine viral infections. In adults a total of 20 cases of cutaneous EMH have been reported, all associated with myelofibrosis. Skin lesions are dermal and subcutaneous nodules. Histologically, the cutaneous lesions are composed of dermal and subcutaneous infiltrates of mature and immature myeloid cells, erythroid precursors (in only half of cases), and megakaryocytic cells (which may predominate). There is marked production of reticulum fibers in the cutaneous lesions by the mechanism described above. Myelofibrosis must be distinguished from CML, since both have elevated white blood cell counts with immature myeloid forms, defective platelet production and marrow fibrosis. Both may terminate in blast crisis, and myelofibrosis may rarely convert to CML. CML is associated with the Philadelphia chromosome, whereas chromosomal abnormalities occur in 40% of myelofibrosis cases, on various chromosomes.

Hoss DM, et al: Cutaneous myelofibrosis. *J Cutan Pathol* 1992, 19:221. ▲

HYPEREOSINOPHILIC SYNDROME

Idiopathic hypereosinophilic syndrome (HES) is defined as eosinophilia with more than 1500 eosinophils per cubic millimeter for more than 6 months, with some evidence of parenchymal organ involvement; there must also be no apparent underlying disease to explain the hypereosinophilia. Ninety percent of patients reported have been men, mostly between ages 20 and 50. Childhood cases are rare. Presenting symptoms include fever (12%), cough (24%), fatigue, malaise, muscle pains and skin eruptions. Skin manifestations occur in 50% of patients and include angioedema and urticarial lesions most commonly (which are associated with a benign course), and papules and nodules. Some patients previously described as having hypereosinophilia and angioedema are now correctly diagnosed as having episodic angioedema and eosinophilia, a distinct syndrome from HES. Other cutaneous manifestations include blistering skin lesions, ulcerations, generalized erythroderma and erythema annulare centrifugum. Mucosal ulcerations can occur throughout the gastrointestinal tract and on the penis, are incapacitating, and can be seen early or late in the course of HES. Cardiac disease is the most frequent complication of HES. It occurs in three stages: necrosis of the myocardium, thrombosis overlying the necrotic areas, and eventual fibrosis of the myocardium. Cardiac disease presents as failure or arrhythmias. Neurologic abnormalities (54%), pulmonary disease (49%), splenic infarction or enlargement (43%), and hepatic involvement (30%) are other common manifestations. Cardiac disease is the most common cause of morbidity and mortality.

HES is associated with the overproduction of IL-5, a cytokine known to produce eosinophilia. In some cases it has been determined that the IL-5 is produced by a clonal proliferation of type 2 helper T cells.

No treatment is required, if there is no evidence of organ involvement. For skin-only involvement, PUVA and dapsone may be tried. Systemic steroidal agents are the first-line medications for patients with organ involvement, usually beginning at about 1 mg/kg/day or about 60 mg/day, with tapering and switching to alternate day treatment if there is a positive response. Hydroxyurea at 1 to 2 g/day is used in cases that fail to respond to treatment with prednisone. Vincristine is used to control acute flares when eosinophil counts exceed 50,000 or refractory thrombocytopenia occurs. Chemotherapy with etoposide or pulse chlorambucil may be used in refractory cases. Interferon alfa, at doses of 15 to 20 million units weekly, has controlled cases in which other treatments have failed. Cardiac surgery may be required to replace damaged cardiac valves.

Bockenstedt PL, et al: Alpha interferon treatment for idiopathic hypereosinophilic syndrome. *Am J Hematol* 1994, 45:248.

Cogan E, et al: Clonal proliferation of type 2 helper T cells in a man with the hypereosinophilic syndrome. *N Engl J Med* 1994, 330:535.

Fruehauf S, et al: Sustained remission of idiopathic hypereosinophilic syndrome following alpha interferon therapy. *Acta Haematol* 1993, 89:91.

Kazmierowski JA, et al: Dermatologic manifestations of the hypereosinophilic syndrome. *Arch Dermatol* 1978, 114:531.

Weller PF, et al: The idiopathic hypereosinophilic syndrome. *Blood* 1994, 83:2759. _____ ▲

ANGIOIMMUNOBLASTIC LYMPHADENOPATHY WITH DYSPROTEINEMIA (ANGIOIMMUNOBLASTIC T-CELL LYMPHOMA)

Angioimmunoblastic lymphadenopathy with dysproteinemia (AILD) is an uncommon lymphoproliferative disorder. Patients are middle-aged or elderly and present with fever (72%), weight loss (58%), hepatomegaly (60%), polyclonal hyperglobulinemia (65%), and generalized adenopathy (87%). Pruritus occurs in 44% and a skin rash in 46%. The skin eruption usually is morbilliform in character, resembling an exanthem or a drug reaction. Petechial, purpuric, nodular, ulcerative and erythrodermic eruptions have also been reported. In about 30% of cases the eruption is associated with the ingestion of a medication.

Histopathologically, there is a patchy and perivascular dermal infiltrate of various types of lymphoid cells, plasma cells, histiocytes, and eosinophils. Blood vessels are increased and the endothelial cells are prominent, often cuboidal. Unfortunately, these changes are non-specific, and may not be adequate to confirm the diagnosis. Lymph node biopsy is usually required.

AILD appears to develop in a stepwise fashion. Initially there is an immune response to an unknown antigen. This immune reaction persists, leading to oligoclonal T-cell proliferation. Monoclonal evolution may occur, eventuating in lymphoma in about 20% of cases over 5 years (angioimmunoblastic lymphoma or AILD-L). These are usually T-cell lymphomas, but B-cell lymphomas can also occur. In up to 50% of cases multiple unrelated neoplastic cell clones have been identified. Clones identified in the skin may be different from clones found in lymph node. Trisomy 3 or 5 or an extra X chromosome may be found. AILD is an aggressive disease, with mortality ranging from 48% to 72% in various series (average survival time, 11 to 60 months). The cause of death is usually infection. Epstein-Barr virus and human herpesviruses 6 and 8 have been implicated in AILD.

Treatment of AILD has included systemic steroids, combination chemotherapy, fludarabine, 2-chlorodeoxyadenosine, interferon alfa, and cyclosporine. Early treatment with systemic steroids during an oligoclonal or prelymphomatous stage may induce a long-lasting remission. Asymptomatic patients may not be treated initially but must be watched very closely. More aggressive chemotherapy achieves better remission. Nonetheless, recurrence rates are high.

Bernstein JE, et al: Cutaneous manifestations of angioimmunoblastic lymphadenopathy. *J Am Acad Dermatol* 1979, 1:227.

Freter CE, et al: Angioimmunoblastic lymphadenopathy with dysproteinemia. *Semin Oncol* 1993, 20:627.

Goldberg NC, et al: Cutaneous manifestations of angioimmunoblastic lymphadenopathy. *Arch Dermatol* 1980, 116:41.

Sallah S, et al: Angioimmunoblastic lymphadenopathy with dysproteinemia. *Acta Haematol* 1998, 99:57.

Schmuth M, et al: Cutaneous involvement in prelymphomatous angioimmunoblastic lymphadenopathy. *J Am Acad Dermatol* 1997, 36:290.

Seehafer JR, et al: Cutaneous manifestations of angioimmunoblastic lymphadenopathy. *Arch Dermatol* 1980, 116:41. _____ ▲

POLYCYTHEMIA VERA (ERYTHREMIA)

Polycythemia vera (PCV) is characterized by an absolute increase of circulating red blood cells, with a hematocrit level of 55% to 80%. Leukocyte and platelet counts are also increased. The skin changes are characteristic. There is a tendency for the skin to be red, especially on the face, neck, and acral areas. The mucous membranes are engorged and bluish. The phrase "red as a rose in summer and indigo blue in winter" has been ascribed to Osler in describing polycythemia. Telangiectases, bleeding gums, and epistaxis are frequently encountered. Cyanosis, purpura, petechiae, hemosiderosis, rosacea, and koilonychia may also be present.

In 50% of patients with PCV, a very distressing aquagenic pruritus occurs. This is typically triggered on emerging from a bath or shower and the feeling induced may be itching, burning, or stinging. It usually lasts 30 to 60 minutes and is independent of the water temperature. Pruritus unassociated with water exposure may also occur. There is a concurrent elevation of blood and skin histamine. Although thrombocythemia is associated with pruritus in PCV, patients with essential thrombocythemia (a disorder distinct from PCV) do not have pruritus.

The treatment of pruritus associated with PCV may be difficult. Antihistamines, such as cyproheptadine hydrochloride, alone or in combination with cimetidine, has been recommended. Other treatment measures that may help the pruritus are aspirin and PUVA.

Easton P: Cimetidine treatment of pruritus in polycythemia vera. *N Engl J Med* 1978, 299:1134.

Fjellner B, et al: Pruritus in polycythemia vera: treatment with aspirin and the possibility of platelet involvement. *Acta Dermatol* 1979, 59:505.

Kligman AM, et al: Water-induced itching without cutaneous signs. *Arch Dermatol* 1986, 122:183.

Swerlick RA: Photochemotherapy treatment of pruritus associated with polycythemia vera. *J Am Acad Dermatol* 1985, 13:675. ▲

CHAPTER 33

Diseases of the Skin Appendages

DISEASES OF THE HAIR

Normal human hairs can be classified according to cyclical phases of growth. Anagen hairs are growing hairs, catagen hairs are those undergoing transition from the growing to the resting stage, and telogen hairs are resting hairs, which remain in the follicles for variable lengths of time before they fall out.

Anagen hairs grow for about 3 years (1000 days), with the limits generally set between 2 and 6 years. The follicular cells grow, divide, and become keratinized to form growing hairs. The base of the hair shaft is soft and moist. A darkly pigmented portion is evident just above the hair bulb. Catagen hairs are in a transitional phase, lasting 1 or 2 weeks, in which all growth activity ceases, with the formation of the "club" hair. Telogen hairs, also known as *club hairs,* are resting hairs, which continue in this state some 3 to 4 months (about 100 days) before they are pushed out of the hair follicle by the hairs growing underneath them, or pulled out by a hair brush or other mechanical means.

Among human hairs plucked from a normal scalp, 85% to 90% are anagen hairs and 10% to 15% catagen or telogen hairs. It has been estimated that the scalp normally contains 100,000 hairs; therefore, the average number of hairs shed daily is 100 to 150. The hair growth rate of terminal hairs is about 0.37 mm daily. Contrary to popular belief, neither shaving nor menstruation has any effect on hair growth rate. The average uncut scalp hair length is estimated to be 25 to 100 cm, although exceptional hairs may be as long as 170 cm (70 inches).

Human hair is also designated as lanugo, vellus, or terminal hair. Lanugo hair is the fine hair present on the body of the fetus. This is replaced by the vellus and terminal hairs. Vellus hairs are fine, usually light-colored, and characteristically seen on children's faces and arms. Terminal hairs are coarse, thick, and dark, except in blondes. Hair occurs on all skin surfaces except the palms, soles, glans, and prepuce. Terminal hairs are always present on men's face, chest, and abdomen, but vellus hairs usually predominate on these sites in women.

Caserio RJ: Disorders of hair. *J Am Acad Dermatol* 1989, 19:895.
Dawber RP: An update of hair shaft disorders. *Dermatol Clin* 1996, 14:753.
Ebling FJG: The biology of hair. *Dermatol Clin* 1987, 5:467.
Headington JT: Cicatricial alopecia. *Dermatol Clin* 1996, 14:773.
Hordinsky MK: General evaluation of the patient with alopecia. *Dermatol Clin* 1987, 5:483.
Jones LN, et al: Hair keratinization in health and disease. *Dermatol Clin* 1996, 14:633.
Paus R, et al: The biology of the hair follicle. *N Engl J Med* 1999, 341:491.
Sawaya ME: Clinical updates in hair. *Dermatol Clin* 1997, 15:37.
Skelsey MA, et al: Noninfectious hair disorders in children. *Curr Opin Pediatr* 1996, 8:378.
Sperling LC: Hair density in African Americans. *Arch Dermatol* 1999, 135:656.
Stenn KS, et al: Hair follicle biology, the sebaceous gland, and scarring alopecias. *Arch Dermatol* 1999, 135:973.
Van Neste DJ: Hair problems in women. *Clin Dermatol* 1997, 15:113. ▲

Alopecia

Alopecia Areata

CLINICAL FEATURES. Alopecia areata (in French, *pelade*) is characterized by rapid and complete loss of hair in one (Fig. 33-1), or more often, several (Fig. 33-2) round or oval patches, usually on the scalp, bearded area, eyebrows, eyelashes, and less commonly, on other hairy areas of the body. Often the patches are from 1 to 5 cm in diameter. A few resting hairs may be found within the patches. Early in the course there may be sparing of gray hair. Nearly always the hair loss is patchy in distribution; however, cases may present in a diffuse pattern. At the periphery of the bald patch are loose hairs that may be broken off near the scalp, leaving short stumps. When they are pulled out a tapered, attenuated bulb is seen as a result of atrophy of that portion, hence, the term *exclamation point* hair.

In some patients there is progression of the disease, with the development of new bald patches, until there is a total loss of scalp hair (alopecia totalis). When hair has been lost over the entire body, including the scalp, the designation is alopecia universalis (Fig. 33-3). Loss may occur confluent along the temporal and occipital scalp (ophiasis) or on the entire scalp except for this area (sisaipho).

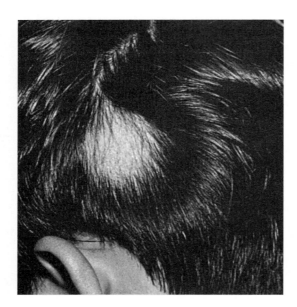

Fig. 33-1 Alopecia areata.

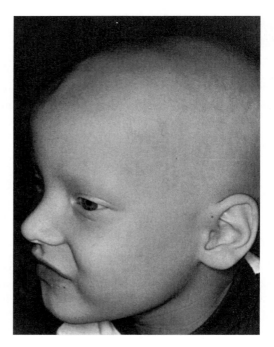

Fig. 33-3 Alopecia universalis.

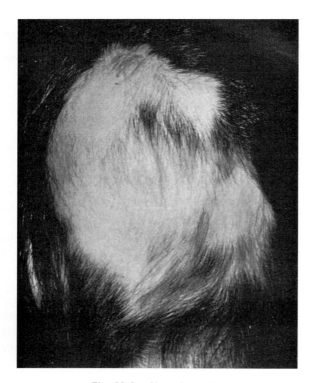

Fig. 33-2 Alopecia areata.

Alopecia areata usually occurs without associated disease. However, there is a higher incidence than usual in patients with atopic dermatitis, Down syndrome (Fig. 33-4), lichen planus, and such autoimmune diseases as systemic lupus erythematosus, thyroiditis, myasthenia gravis, and vitiligo.

In about 10% of cases of alopecia areata, especially in long-standing cases with extensive involvement, the nails develop uniform pits that may form transverse or longitudinal lines. Trachyonychia, onychomadesis, and red or spotted lunulae occur but less commonly.

ETIOLOGIC FACTORS. Although Celsus described and named alopecia areata some 20 centuries ago, its cause is still unknown. Most evidence points toward its being an autoimmune disease mediated by the cellular arm and modified by genetic factors. Many studies have documented abnormal cell-mediated immune factors in alopecia areata. In the inflammatory peribulbar infiltrate seen in active cases, helper cells predominate. There is an increased suppressor T-cell function in patients experiencing regrowth. Genetic susceptibility appears to be a factor, as suggested by a possible human leukocyte antigen (HLA) class II association. Overall, nearly 25% of patients have a positive family history; there are reports of twins with alopecia areata; and certain populations may be at higher risk. Patients with early onset, severe, familial clustering alopecia areata have a unique and highly significant association with HLA antigens DR4, DR11, and DQ7. The later onset, milder severity, better prognostic subsets of patients have a lower frequency of familial disease and do not share these HLA antigens.

HISTOLOGY. In early disease there is a helper T-cell–dominant lymphocytic infiltrate in the peribulbar area of anagen or early catagen follicles. The hair structures enter an abnormal catagen phase, followed by persistent telogen structures. The follicles miniaturize, move up into the dermis, and remain there, usually with a persistent lymphocytic peribulbar infiltrate present. Elston et al emphasized that eosinophils are common in all stages of alopecia areata,

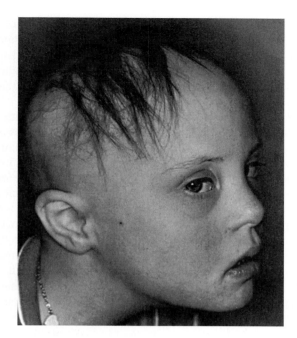

Fig. 33-4 Alopecia areata in a child with Down syndrome.

both within the peribulbar infiltrate and within fibrous tracts.

DIFFERENTIAL DIAGNOSIS. The sharply circumscribed patch of alopecia with exclamation point hairs at the periphery and the absence of scarring are indicative of alopecia areata. Tinea capitis, early lupus erythematosus, syphilis, congenital triangular alopecia, alopecia neoplastica, and trichotillomania should be kept in mind when alopecia areata is considered.

TREATMENT. It is not known why some patches will regrow in a few weeks without any treatment, whereas others will completely resist all forms of therapy. Intralesional injections of corticosteroid suspensions are the treatment of choice for localized cosmetically conspicuous patches such as those occuring in an eyebrow. Hair will usually regrow; however, pain, the need for injections to be repeated every 6 weeks, and its impracticality for more diffuse disease may limit use. High-strength topical steroid creams may also be used as first-line therapy. If there is a lack of response after several months topical anthralin 1% cream may be applied for 15 to 20 minutes and then shampooed off the treated site. Topical minoxidil may be combined with the above treatment trials or utilized as a single agent.

For extensive disease the above therapies, with the exception of intralesional steroidal therapy, are still available for trials, but treatment of the entire scalp is suggested to prevent the development of new patches while clinically evident disease is under treatment. Induction of contact sensitivity to squaric acid dibutyl ester, dinitrochlorobenzene, and diphencyprone and topical or oral methoxsalen

and ultraviolet A (PUVA) therapy are other options in this often treatment-resistant situation. However, their efficacy is not high, and there are attendant risks that will many times outweigh the use of these modalities. Several investigators have reported the use of early oral prednisone, pulse steroidal agents, or monthly high oral doses of corticosteroids in rapidly progressing widespread disease. However, long-term treatment is frequently needed to maintain growth, and the attendant risks far outweigh the benefits.

Arnold found, in his series of 63 consecutive responders to a follow-up questionnaire, that after reassurance only, hair had regrown in all but four patients after 1 year and in all but one after 2 years. The great majority had recovered in 3 months after their only office visit. So, any treatment may seem to be effective. Spontaneous recovery is extremely common. That is presumably why all treatments in uncontrolled trials yield high response rates. It is only when patients in a poor prognostic category, such as those with prepubertal onset or patients with total or universal involvement or those who have concomitant atopic disease, are considered that the real lack of efficacy surfaces.

In the widespread cases in which the remaining hair cannot cover the alopecic sites, there can be tremendous psychologic stress. Education about the disease process, cosmetically acceptable alternatives (especially information about wigs), and research into innovative therapies should all be made available to the patient. In addition to the information conveyed by the dermatologist, an excellent resource for such education, as well as a forum to allow for the sharing of feelings, is shown below:

National Alopecia Areata Foundation (NAAF)
P.O. Box 150760
San Rafael, CA 94915-0760
Phone: 415-456-4644
E-mail: NAAF@compuserve.com
Website: http://www.alopeciaareata.com

PROGNOSIS. The tendency is for spontaneous recovery in patients who are postpubertal at onset. At first, the regrowing hairs are downy and light in color; later, they are replaced by stronger and darker hair with full growth. Predictors of a poor prognosis are the presence of atopic dermatitis, childhood onset, widespread involvement, ophiasis, duration of longer than 5 years, and onychodystrophy.

Arnold HL Jr: Alopecia areata. *Arch Dermatol Syph* 1952, 66:191.

Beard HO: Social and psychological implication of alopecia areata. *J Am Acad Dermatol* 1986, 14:697.

Brown AC, et al: Ocular and testicular abnormalities in alopecia areata. *Arch Dermatol* 1982, 118:546.

Colombe BW, et al: HLA class II antigen associations help to define two types of alopecia areata. *J Am Acad Dermatol* 1995, 33:757.

Elston DM, et al: Eosinophils in fibrous tracts and near hair bulbs. *J Am Acad Dermatol* 1997, 37:101.

Fiedler VC: Alopecia areata. *Arch Dermatol* 1992, 128:1519.

Fiedler VC, et al: Treatment of alopecia areata. *Dermatol Clin* 1996, 14:733.

Hoffmann R, et al: Topical immunotherapy in alopecia areata. *Dermatol Clin* 1996, 14:739.

Kubota A, et al: Myasthenia gravis and alopecia areata. *Neurology* 1997, 48:774.

McDonagh AJ, et al: The pathogenesis of alopecia areata. *Dermatol Clin* 1996, 14:661.

Milgraum SS, et al: Alopecia areata, endocrine function, and autoantibodies in patients 16 years of age or younger. *J Am Acad Dermatol* 1987, 17:57.

Mitchell AJ: Alopecia areata. *Dermatol Clin* 1987, 5:553.

Munoz MA, et al: Sisaipho. *Arch Dermatol* 1996, 132:1255.

Nelson DA, et al: Anthralin therapy for alopecia areata. *Int J Dermatol* 1985, 24:606.

Olsen EA, et al: Systemic steroids with or without 2% topical minoxidil in the treatment of alopecia areata. *Arch Dermatol* 1992, 128:1467.

Price VH, et al: Heritable factors distinguish two types of alopecia areata. *Dermatol Clin* 1996, 14:679.

Sahn EE: Alopecia areata in childhood. *Semin Dermatol* 1995, 14:9.

Scerri L, et al: Identical twins with identical alopecia areata. *J Am Acad Dermatol* 1992, 27:766.

Schuttelaar ML, et al: Alopecia areata in children. *Br J Dermatol* 1996, 135:581.

Taylor CR, et al: PUVA treatment of alopecia areata partialis, totalis and universalis. *Br J Dermatol* 1995, 133:914.

Tosti A, et al: Long-term results of topical immunotherapy in children with alopecia totalis or alopecia universalis. *J Am Acad Dermatol* 1996, 35:199.

Tosti A, et al: Prevalence of nail abnormalities in children with alopecia areata. *Pediatr Dermatol* 1994, 11:112.

Yuen YF, et al: Scalp metastases mimicking alopecia areata. *Dermatol Surg* 1998, 24:587. ▲

Telogen Effluvium

Kligman has defined telogen effluvium as the early and excessive loss of normal club hairs from normal resting follicles in the scalp. This excessive hair loss results from traumatization of the normal hair by some stimulus, such as surgery, parturition, fever, drugs, or traction, which in short order precipitates the anagen phase into catagen and telogen phases. Kligman points out that during this process the follicle itself is not diseased, and inflammation is absent.

Headington has proposed five functional types of telogen effluvium, three of them related to events in anagen and two in telogen. In the first type, follicles that would normally complete a longer cycle by remaining in anagen prematurely enter telogen. Thus, within 3 to 5 weeks of the signal, usually a drug-related event or a period of severe physiologic stress such as a high fever, immediate anagen release is effected. Alternatively, follicles may remain in prolonged anagen rather than normally cycling into telogen. This occurs during pregnancy. On delivery, these follicles are then released into telogen, and shedding occurs some months later. The usual time interval for this delayed telogen release is 2 to 3 months but at times may take closer to 6 months.

Administration of topical minoxidil may effect telogen effluvium by initiating anagen in many telogen follicles. This causes immediate telogen release and a brief short-onset telogen effluvium. Although these three mechanisms have clinical counterparts, the other two types Headington proposes, short anagen and delayed telogen release, do not have known clinical correlates.

Whatever the cause, the hair loss is noted by the patient as "lots of hairs coming out by the roots." Loss is diffuse and only infrequently causes clinically perceptible thinning of the hair, since only rarely does it involve more than 50% of the hairs. The patient notes increased hair loss before signs of alopecia are evident. The normal telogen count is usually below 10%. It is usually estimated by the pull test: grasping 40 hairs firmly between thumb and forefinger, followed by a slow pull that causes mild discomfort to the patient. A count of greater than 4 to 6 club hairs is abnormal, but results to this test may be negative, because it is influenced by shampooing (a count of two or three hairs being abnormal in freshly shampooed scalp), combing, and the phase of telogen effluvium (whether it is resolving or entering a chronic phase). The clip test may also be useful: 25 to 30 hairs are cut just above the scalp surface and mounted. Telogen hairs are short and of small diameter, so that many hairs of this type may be present in telogen effluvium. Of course, androgenic alopecia results in miniaturization of hairs, and coexistent androgenetic change may influence the count.

Age, sex, race, and probably other genetic factors influence the normal average daily hair loss in an individual. The total number of hairs on the scalp is estimated to be about 100,000; of these, approximately 100 to 150 hairs are lost daily. In telogen effluvium, estimates of loss vary from 150 to more than 400. Patients may be instructed to collect and count the hair daily; however, they should make sure to collect all small hairs and those that come out in washing and in the bed as well as those present on the comb or brush. When the pull test is positive, daily hair shed counts are not needed.

Histologic changes are seen on horizontal sectioning. If a 4-mm punch biopsy is performed, 25 to 50 hairs are normally present for inspection. If more than 12% to 15% of terminal follicles are in telogen, this probably indicates a significant shift from anagen to telogen in most individuals. The change is noninflammatory, and no dystrophic changes in the inner sheath or signs of traction should be present. Thus traction, alopecia areata, and androgenetic alopecia all may be distinguished by histologic examination.

Postpartum telogen effluvium has been found to begin between 2 and 6 months postpartum. Often the hair loss is first noted over the anterior third of the scalp, although loss is in a diffuse pattern. The hair loss may continue for some 2 to 6 months or longer. Postnatal telogen effluvium of infants may occur between birth and the first 4 months of age. Usually, regrowth occurs by 6 months of age. Telogen counts by Kligman in six infants varied from 64% to 87%. He also found a tendency for the alopecia to occur in the male-pattern distribution.

Drug-induced telogen effluvium has been noted with the use of amphetamines, aminosalicyclic acid, bromocriptine, captopril, coumarin, carbamazepine, cimetidine, danazol, enalapril, etretinate, lithium carbonate, levodopa, metyrapone, metoprolol, propranolol, pyridostigmine, and trimethadione.

Other causes of telogen effluvium have been noted; the most dramatic has been kwashiorkor or a starvation diet. Goette and Odom have reported telogen effluvium in people on weight reduction programs and crash diets, secondary to protein deprivation. Hypothyroidism and renal dialysis with secondary hypervitaminosis A are other possible causes.

There is no specific therapy for telogen effluvium; in the majority of cases it will stop spontaneously within a few months and the hair will regrow. The prognosis is good if a specific event can be pinpointed as a probable cause. Complete reassurance is not possible, however; both Headington and Whiting warn that a chronic form of telogen effluvium may occur. Whiting reported on a group of 355 patients (346 women and 9 men) with diffuse generalized thinning of scalp hair. Most were 30 to 60 years old, and their hair loss started abruptly, with increased shedding and thinning. There was a fluctuating course and diffuse thinning of the hair all over the scalp accompanied by bitemporal recession. He found high telogen counts on horizontal sections of scalp biopsies and considers these patients to have a chronic form of telogen effluvium. In this chronic form Garcia-Hernandez et al report a 70% success rate treating men with 5% minoxidil solution; premenopausal women with 5% minoxidil solution plus cyproterone acetate, 50 mg (this drug is not available in the United States) from day 5 to 15 of their menstrual cycle taken together with ethinyl estradiol, 0.035 mg/day, and for postmenopausal women (the majority of their patients) 50 mg/day of cyproterone acetate. They recommend spironolactone, 50 to 100 mg/day, or flutamide, 125 to 250 mg/day, as alteratives to cyproterone acetate.

Although such a chronic course may occur, the vast majority of patients with telogen effluvium will recover completely and this information along with education about the basics of the hair cycle will aid in management of this anxiety-producing condition.

Garcia-Hernandez MJ, et al: Chronic telogen effluvium. *Arch Dermatol* 1999, 135:1123.

Goette DK, Odom RB: Alopecia in crash dieters. *JAMA* 1976, 235:262.

Headington JT: Telogen effluvium. *Arch Dermatol* 1993, 129:356.

Kligman AM: Pathologic dynamics of human hair loss. *Arch Dermatol* 1961, 83:175.

Rebora A: Telogen effluvium. *Dermatology* 1997, 195:209.

Sadick NS: Clinical and laboratory evaluation of AIDS trichopathy. *Int J Dermatol* 1993, 32:33.

Smith KJ, et al: Clinical and histopathologic features of hair loss in patients with HIV-1 infection. *J Am Acad Dermatol* 1996, 34:63.

Whiting DA: Chronic telogen effluvium. *Dermatol Clin* 1996, 14:723.

Whiting DA: Chronic telogen effluvium. *J Am Acad Dermatol* 1996, 35:899. ──────── ▲

Anagen Effluvium

Anagen effluvium is seen frequently following the administration of cancer chemotherapeutic agents, such as the antimetabolites, alkylating agents, and mitotic inhibitors. Severe loss is frequently seen with doxorubicin, the nitrosureas, and cyclophosphamide. When high doses are given, loss of anagen hairs becomes most apparent clinically in 1 to 2 months. The hair shafts are abruptly thinned at the time of maximum drug effect (Pohl-Pinkus constrictions), and when the very thin portion reaches the surface, the hair shafts all break at about the same time. If the bulb itself is damaged, many hairs may separate at the bulb and come out. It is to be noted that only growing (anagen) hairs are subject to this type of change. With cessation of drug therapy, the follicle resumes its normal activity within a few weeks; the process is entirely reversible. It is apparent that mitotic inhibition merely stops the reproduction of matrix cells but does not permanently destroy the hair. A pressure cuff applied around the scalp during chemotherapy and scalp hypothermia has been reported to prevent such anagen arrest. Topical minoxidil has been shown to shorten the period of baldness by an average of 50 days. In addition to the cytotoxic agents, various chemicals such as thallium and boron may induce anagen effluvium.

Bonner AK, et al: Cutaneous complications of chemotherapeutic agents. *J Am Acad Dermatol* 1983, 9:648.

Duvic M, et al: A randomized trial of minoxidil in chemotherapy-induced alopecia. *J Am Acad Dermatol* 1996, 35:74.

Johansen LV: Scalp hypothermia in the prevention of chemotherapy-induced alopecia. *Acta Radiol Oncol* 1985, 24:113. ──────── ▲

Androgenetic Alopecia

Male-Pattern Baldness. Male-pattern alopecia or male-pattern baldness (common baldness) shows itself during the twenties or early thirties by gradual loss of hair, chiefly from the vertex and frontotemporal regions. At any time after puberty the process may begin subtly, and the presence of "whisker" hair at the temples may be the first sign of impending male-pattern alopecia. The anterior hairline recedes on each side, in the Geheimratswinkeln ("professor angles"), so that the forehead becomes high. Eventually the entire top of the scalp may become devoid of hair. Several patterns of this type of hair loss occur, but the most frequent is the biparietal recession with loss of hair on the vertex. The rate of hair loss varies among individuals. Sudden hair loss may occur in the twenties and then proceed relentlessly, though very slowly, for a number of years. The follicles produce finer and lighter terminal hairs until a complete cessation of terminal hair growth results. Vellus hairs on the scalp, however, continue to grow and become more prominent because of the absence of terminal hairs. The parietal and occipital areas are usually spared permanently.

The exact mechanisms responsible for androgenetic alopecia are still unknown; however, there is no doubt that inherited factors and the effect of androgens on the hair follicle are most responsible. Arguments for regarding the inheritance as polygenic include the high prevalence, gaussian curve of distribution in the population, increased risk with number of affected relatives, increased risk in relatives of severely affected women compared with mildly affected, and greater import of an affected mother than of an affected father. The possibility that the early onset (before age 30) and later onset (after age 50) forms may be inherited separately by single genes is also hypothesized.

In addition to heredity, male-pattern alopecia is dependent on adequate androgen stimulation at a particular age of the individual. Eunuchs do not develop baldness if they are castrated before or during adolescence; if they are given androgen therapy, baldness may develop. The 5-alpha-reduction of testosterone is increased in the scalp of balding individuals, yielding increased dihydrotestosterone. Additionally, it is known that in congenital 5-alpha-reductase deficiency, in which baldness does not occur, the type 2 isoenzyme is lacking.

The pathogenesis is centered around the lengthening of the telogen phase and the shortening of the anagen phase of hair growth. The shorter the anagen phase, the shorter the hair growth. Eventually, the follicles become short and small with sclerosis of the dermis and miniaturization or a reduction in the diameter of the hairs present.

Minoxidil, an oral hypotensive drug that causes hypertrichosis when given systemically, is available in 2% and 5% topical solutions (Rogaine). Success in early cases (less than 10 years) of limited extent (less than 10 cm diameter bald area) in whom pretreatment hair density is above 20 hairs per centimeter occur; however, at best only about one third of cases grow cosmetically useful hair, and they must continue to use minoxidil indefinitely to maintain a response.

Finasteride, a type 2 5-alpha-reductase inhibitor, given as a 1-mg tablet daily, is effective in preventing further hair loss and in increasing the hair counts to the point of cosmetically appreciable results in men ages 18 to 41 with mild to moderate hair loss at the vertex, in the anterior midscalp, and the frontal region. Hair patterning on the temples is not improved. It has been shown to lower the dihydrotestosterone in the scalp and the serum of treated patients. Hair growth will begin only after 6 months or more on the drug and after 12 months, if no effect is seen, further treatment is unlikely to be of benefit. Side effects are infrequent; however, the need to take this medication indefinitely or lose the benefit completely leaves open to study long-term side effect profiles.

Hair transplantation of small plugs of scalp hair follicles from the occipital area to the anterior scalp line has been successfully developed and continually refined such that hundreds of minigrafts, even in some cases including only a single hair, may satisfactorily recreate hairlines and give excellent cosmetic results.

Androgenetic Alopecia in Women.
The pattern of hair loss is quite different in women. Women generally have diffuse hair loss throughout the midscalp (Fig. 33-5), sparing the frontal hairline except for slight recession. Although maintenance of the frontal hairline is the rule, a progressive decrease in hair density from the vertex to the front of the scalp does occur. The midline part is an important clinical clue to the diagnosis of androgenetic alopecia in women, revealing this central thinning by the appearance of the "Christmas tree pattern" of hair loss. The same basic changes—reduced hair density and diameter, and diminished anagen and increased telogen hair—occur in women as in men.

The cause is now believed to be a genetic predisposition in combination with an excessive androgen response, even though levels of circulating testosterone are as a rule not elevated. If other evidence of androgen excess is present, such as hirsutism, menstrual irregularities, or acne, or the onset is sudden, evaluation as outlined for hirsutism (see below) should be performed.

Treatment is not as satisfactory as with men as finasteride is contraindicated in women of childbearing potential and it was shown to lack efficacy in a 1-year placebo-controlled trial of postmenopausal women with androgenetic alopecia. Topical minoxidil in the lower of the two strengths may limit hair loss.

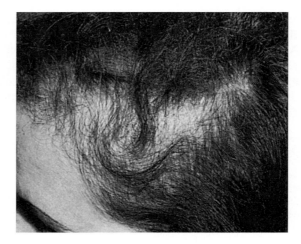

Fig. 33-5 Female diffuse alopecia in a 37-year-old woman.

Wigs or interwoven hair may give quite satisfactory cosmetic results.

Adson MH, et al: Scalp expansion in the treatment of male-pattern baldness. *Plast Reconst Surg* 1987, 79:906.

Bergfeld WF: Androgenic alopecia. *Dermatol Clin* 1987, 5:491.

Bergfeld WF: Androgenetic alopecia: an autosomal dominant disorder. *Am J Med* 1995, 98:95S.

Bergfeld WF: Etiology and diagnosis of androgenetic alopecia. *Clin Dermatol* 1988, 6:102.

Cash TF, et al: Psychological effects of androgenetic alopecia on women: comparisons with balding men and with female control subjects. *J Am Acad Dermatol* 1993, 29:568.

DeVillez RL, et al: Androgenetic alopecia in the female. *Arch Dermatol* 1994, 130:303.

Drake LA, et al: Guidelines of care for androgenetic alopecia. *J Am Acad Dermatol* 1996, 35:465.

Drake LA, et al: The effects of finasteride on scalp skin and serum androgen levels in men with androgenetic alopecia. *J Am Acad Dermatol* 1999, 41:550.

Jerums G, et al: Androgens in women: source, nature, and investigation. *Australas J Dermatol* 1985, 26:14.

Kassimir JJ: Use of topical minoxidil as a possible adjunct to hair transplant surgery. *J Am Acad Dermatol* 1987, 16:685.

Kaufman KD: Androgen metabolism as it affects hair growth in androgenetic alopecia. *Dermatol Clin* 1996, 14:697.

Kaufman KD, et al: Finasteride in the treatment of men with androgenetic alopecia. *J Am Acad Dermatol* 1998, 39:578.

Knowles WR: Hair transplantation. *Dermatol Clin* 1987, 5:515.

Leyden JJ, et al: Finasteride in the treatment of men with male pattern hair loss. *J Am Acad Dermatol* 1999, 40:930.

Norwood OT: Micrografts and minigrafts for refining grafted hairlines. *Dermatol Clin* 1987, 5:545.

Olsen EA: The midline part. *J Am Acad Dermatol* 1999, 40:106.

Olsen EA, et al: Five-year follow-up of men with androgenetic alopecia treated with topical minoxidil. *J Am Acad Dermatol* 1990, 22:643.

Olsen EA, et al: Natural history of androgenetic alopecia. *Clin Exp Dermatol* 1990, 15:34.

Pitts RL: Serum elevation of dehydroepiandrosterone sulfate associated with male-pattern baldness in young men. *J Am Acad Dermatol* 1987, 16:571.

Price VH, et al: Quantitative estimation of hair growth. *J Invest Dermatol* 1990, 95:683.

Prize VH, et al: Changes in hair weight and hair count in men with androgenetic alopecia after application of 5% and 2% topical minoxidil, placebo or no treatment. *J Am Acad Dermatol* 1999, 41:717.

Roberts JL: Androgenetic alopecia. *J Am Acad Dermatol* 1987, 16:705.

Roberts JL, et al: Clinical dose ranging studies with finasteride, a type 2 5-α reductase inhibitor, in men with male patterned hair loss. *J Am Acad Dermatol* 1999, 41:555.

Savin RC: Use of topical minoxidil in treatment of male-pattern baldness. *J Am Acad Dermatol* 1987, 16:696.

Sawaya ME: Clinical updates in hair. *Dermatol Clin* 1997, 15:37.

Sawaya ME, et al: Different levels of 5-alpha-reductase type I and II, aromatase, and androgen receptor in hair follicles of women and men with androgenetic alopecia. *J Invest Dermatol* 1997, 109:296.

Sperling LC, et al: The transverse anatomy of androgenic alopecia. *J Dermatol Surg Oncol* 1990, 16:1127.

Unger WP: What's new in hair replacement surgery. *Dermatol Clin* 1996, 14:783.

Walsh DS, et al: Improvement in androgenetic alopecia (stage V) using topical minoxidil in a retinoid vehicle and oral finasteride. *Arch Dermatol* 1995, 131:1373. ▲

Other Forms of Alopecia

Complete or partial loss of scalp hair is found in various forms and is caused by many factors. Some forms of alopecia will be described briefly.

Trichotillomania is a neurotic practice of plucking or breaking hair from the scalp or eyelashes. Usually localized, but at times widespread, areas of alopecia are seen that characteristically contain hairs of varying length. The scalp has a rough texture, resulting from the short remnants of broken-off hairs. Trichotillomania is seen mostly in girls under age 10, but boys, or adults of either sex, may engage in the practice also. It has been suggested that one ask the child not if but rather how removal of the hair is done. If this fails, shave a 3- by 3-cm area in the involved part of the scalp, and watch the hair regrow normally as the hair in this "skin window" will be too short for plucking. Finally, a biopsy, especially if cut horizontally, will confirm the diagnosis because of the high number of catagen hairs, pigmentary defects and casts, trichomalacia, and hemorrhage. Treatment of this disorder, which is usually a manifestation of an obsessive-compulsive disorder but may also be associated with depression or anxiety, is with psychotherapy, behavioral therapy, or an appropriate psychopharmacologic medication. The serotonin reuptake inhibitors are best studied with fluoxetine in doses of 20 to 60 mg being reported effective.

Hot comb alopecia was reported in the late 1960s as a scarring alopecia seen in black women who straightened their hair with hot combs for cosmetic purposes. It develops characteristically on the crown and spreads peripherally to form a large oval area of partial hair loss. The hot petrolatum used with the iron causes thermal damage to the hair follicle, leading ultimately to destruction of the entire follicle and a follicular scar. In time, significant hair loss occurs if this type of hair-straightening is continued. Sperling et al reported a similar-appearing scarring alopecia in both men and women who did not report the use of hot combs. They found that there was premature thinning of the inner root sheath, which leads to exposure of the hair shaft to the dermis and induces inflammation and scarring. Still others regard Sperling's disease (follicular degeneration syndrome or now, central centrifugal scarring alopecia), hot comb alopecia, and pseudopelade of Brocq to be all one entity.

Pseudopelade (French for pseudoalopecia areata) of Brocq, also known as *alopecia cicatrisata,* is a rare form of scarring alopecia in which destruction of the hair follicles produces multiple round, oval, or irregularly shaped, hairless, cicatricial patches of varying sizes. They are usually coin-sized and are white or slightly pink in color, with a smooth, shiny, marblelike or ivory, atrophic, "onion skin" surface. Interspersed in the patches may be a few dilated follicles with hairs growing from them. Inflammation is completely absent. No pustules, crusts, or broken-off hairs are present.

The onset is, as a rule, insidious, with one or two lesions appearing on the vertex. It affects females three times more commonly than males, and has a prolonged course. In advanced cases large patches may be formed by coalescence of some of the many small macules. The alopecia is permanent and the disease is slowly progressive. Histologically, there is no inflammation; sebaceous glands are decreased or absent; the epidermis is normal or atrophic; and fibrotic tracts are seen in the subcutaneous tissue. Direct immunofluorescence is negative.

The differential diagnosis requires the ruling out of other causes of cicatricial alopecia such as chronic suppurative folliculitis, scleroderma, sarcoidosis, favus, lichen planus, and lupus erythematosus. The inactive final stage of these conditions may be clinically identical to pseudopelade. Folliculitis decalvans is frequently accompanied by inflamed marginal follicles and marginal crusting. Alopecia areata may be simulated; however, the presence of scarring rules this out. Clinically familial focal alopecia resembles pseudopelade; however, the absence of scarring on biopsy and the pattern of inheritance distinguish it.

Topical and intralesional corticosteroids and long-term tetracycline in antiinflammatory doses may be tried but are not often successful. If hot combs are in use they should be discontinued. The disease usually reaches an inactive end stage after many years (2 to 18 in Braun-Falco's report).

Traction alopecia occurs from prolonged tension on the hair either from wearing the hair tightly braided or in a ponytail, pulling the hair to straighten it, rolling curlers too tightly, or from the habit of twisting the hairs with the fingers (Fig. 33-6).

Pressure alopecia occurs frequently on the occipital areas in babies lying on their backs. In adults it is seen most often after prolonged pressure on the scalp during general anesthesia, with the head fixed in one position (Fig. 33-7). It may also occur in chronically ill persons after prolonged bed rest in one position, which causes persistent pressure on one part of the scalp. It probably arises because of pressure-induced ischemia.

Loose anagen syndrome, described by Price in 1989, is a disorder in which anagen hairs may be pulled from the scalp with little effort. It occurs mostly in blond girls and usually improves with age.

Alopecia syphilitica may have a typical moth-eaten appearance on the occipital scalp, a generalized thinning of the hair (Fig. 33-8), or a combination of the two. Other areas such as the eyebrows and eyelashes and body hair may be involved. The alopecia may be the first sign of a syphilis infection.

Follicular mucinosis (alopecia mucinosa) (Fig. 33-9) most commonly occurs on the scalp or beard area and manifests as deposition of mucin in the outer root sheath and sebaceous glands. The inflammatory reaction produces alopecia, and at times hypopigmentation. The primary cases (i.e., unassociated with underlying disease) occur either as localized lesions of the head or neck that usually resolve

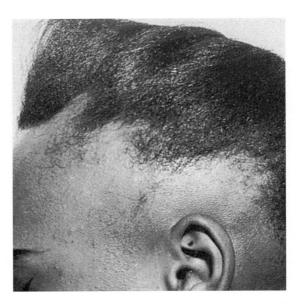

Fig. 33-6 Traction/traumatic alopecia in a 14-year-old girl.

within a year, or as more generalized lesions with a longer course. Young people are primarily affected. A secondary type exists, in which there is associated cutaneous T-cell lymphoma. Usually, in these cases, lesions are widespread and chronic, and occur in older patients.

Inflammatory alopecia may be seen in lichen simplex chronicus and various eczematous changes on the scalp, including kerion. Discoid lupus erythematosus, lichen planopilaris, sarcoidosis, and folliculitis decalvans are the commonest inflammatory causes of cicatricial alopecia. These are discussed in chapters concerning the primary disease process in other areas of this book.

Vascular or neurologic alopecia, most often of the lower extremities, may be seen in diabetes mellitus or atherosclerosis. In meralgia paresthetica there may be alopecia of the anesthetic area of the outer thigh.

Endocrinologic alopecia may occur in various endocrinologic disorders. In hypothyroidism the hair becomes coarse, dry, brittle, and sparse. Freinkel et al found in six such cases that the proportion of telogen hairs was three to seven times higher than the normal 10%. In hyperthyroidism the hair becomes extremely fine and sparse. Oral contraceptives have been implicated in some instances of androgenetic alopecia. It develops in predisposed women who are usually taking androgenic progestogens. It is advisable to discontinue the androgen-dominant pill and substitute an estrogen-dominant oral contraceptive. Some women develop telogen effluvium 2 to 4 months after discontinuing anovulatory agents, which is analogous to postpartum alopecia.

Tumor alopecia refers to hair loss in the immediate vicinity of either benign or malignant tumors of the scalp. Syringomas, nerve sheath myxomas, and steatocystoma multiplex are benign tumors that may be limited to the scalp

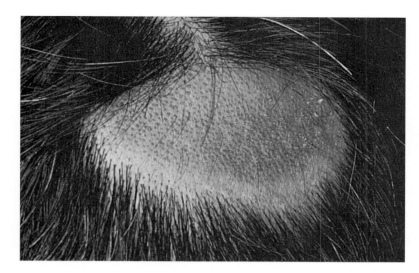

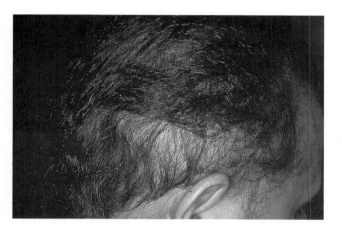

Fig. 33-7 Pressure alopecia developing after a prolonged surgical procedure.

Fig. 33-8 Alopecia syphilitica.

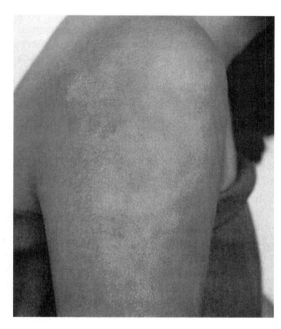

and cause alopecia. Alopecia neoplastica is the designation given to hair loss from metastatic tumors, most often from breast carcinoma.

Congenital alopecia occurs either as total or partial loss of hair or a lack of initial growth, accompanied usually by other ectodermal defects of the nails, teeth, and bone. The hair is light and sparse, and grows slowly. Congenital triangular alopecia and aplasia cutis congenita are examples of congenital localized absence of hair, while hidrotic ectodermal dysplasia is an example of a diffuse abnormality of hair associated with dental and nail changes. Further discussion of these anomalies may be found in other areas of this text.

Fig. 33-9 Follicular mucinosis (alopecia mucinosa) of arm. Note abundance of vellus hairs outside the clusters of discrete hypopigmented follicular macules.

Braun-Falco O, et al: Pseudopelade of Brocq. *Dermatologica* 1986, 172:18.

Clark J Jr, et al: Chronic alopecia: trichotillomania. *Arch Dermatol* 1995, 131:720.

Cuozzo DW, et al: Essential syphilitic alopecia revisited. *J Am Acad Dermatol* 1995, 32:840.

Freinkel RK, et al: Hair growth and alopecia in hypothyroidism. *Arch Dermatol* 1972, 106:349.

Frieden IH: Aplasia cutis congenita. *J Am Acad Dermatol* 1986, 14:646.

Headington JT, et al: Familial focal alopecia. *Arch Dermatol* 1987, 123:234.

Gibson LE, et al: Follicular mucinosis. *J Am Acad Dermatol* 1989, 20:441.

Guilln PS, et al: Aplasia cutis congenita. *J Am Acad Dermatol* 1985, 13:429.

Hamm H, et al: Loose anagen hair of childhood. *J Am Acad Dermatol* 1989, 20:242.

Headington JT: Cicatricial alopecia. *Dermatol Clin* 1996, 14:773.

Jordaan HF, et al: The moth-eaten alopecia of secondary syphilis. *Am J Dermatopathol* 1995, 17:158.

Lancer HA, et al: Follicular mucinosis. *J Am Acad Dermatol* 1984, 10:760.

Laude TA: Approach to dermatologic disorders in black children. *Semin Dermatol* 1995, 14:15.

LoPresti P: Hot comb alopecia. *Arch Dermatol* 1968, 98:234.

Muller SA: Trichotillomania. *Dermatol Clin* 1987, 5:595.

Muller SA: Trichotillomania: a histopathologic study in sixty-six patients. *J Am Acad Dermatol* 1990, 23:56.

Neuman KM, et al: Alopecia associated with syringomas. *J Am Acad Dermatol* 1985, 13:528.

O'Donnell BP, et al: Loose anagen hair syndrome. *Int J Dermatol* 1992, 31:107.

Oranje AP, et al: Trichotillomania in childhood. *J Am Acad Dermatol* 1986, 15:614.

Price VH, et al: Loose anagen syndrome. *J Am Acad Dermatol* 1989, 20:249.

Snyder RA, et al: Alopecia mucinosa. *Arch Dermatol* 1984, 120:496.

Spencer LV, et al: Hair loss in systemic disease. *Dermatol Clin* 1987, 5:565.

Sperling LC, et al: Follicular degeneration syndrome in men. *Arch Dermatol* 1994, 130:763.

Sperling LC, et al: Hair diseases. *Med Clin North Am* 1998, 82:1155.

Sperling LC, et al: The follicular degeneration syndrome in black patients: 'hot comb alopecia' revisited and revised. *Arch Dermatol* 1992, 128:68.

Tosti A: Congenital triangular alopecia. *J Am Acad Dermatol* 1987, 16:991.

Trakimas C, et al: Clinical and histologic findings in temporal triangular alopecia. *J Am Acad Dermatol* 1994, 31:205.

Trakimas C, et al: Temporal triangular alopecia acquired in an adult. *J Am Acad Dermatol* 1999, 40:842.

Wiles JC, et al: Postoperative (pressure) alopecia. *J Am Acad Dermatol* 1985, 12:195.

Wittenberg GP, et al: Follicular mucinosis presenting as an acneiform eruption: report of four cases. *J Am Acad Dermatol* 1998, 38:849. ▲

Syndromes That Include Abnormalities of the Hair

Polyostotic fibrous dysplasia (Albright's disease) may present as slowly progressive lifelong unilateral hair loss: scalp, pubic, axillary, and palpebral. Sickle cell disease is often characterized by scantiness of body and facial hair. The Cronkhite-Canada syndrome is characterized by alopecia, skin pigmentation, onychodystrophy, malabsorption, and generalized gastrointestinal polyposis.

Marinesco-Sjögren syndrome consists of cerebellar ataxia, mental retardation, congenital cataracts, inability to chew food, thin brittle fingernails, and sparse hair. The dystrophic hairs do not have the normal layers (cortex, cuticle, and medulla), and 30% of the hair shafts show narrow bands of abnormal incomplete keratinization. There is an autosomal recessive type of inheritance in this syndrome.

Trichothiodystrophy features brittle hair (Fig. 33-10) with a markedly reduced sulfur content. The hair, with sulfur reduced to 50% of the normal value, has distinctive features under polarizing, light, and scanning electron microscopy. With polarizing microscopy, the hair shows alternating bright and dark regions that give a striking striped, or tiger tail, appearance. With light microscopy, trichoschisis (clean fractures), and trichorrhexis nodosa–like fractures may be seen; in addition, the hair is markedly flattened and folds over itself like a thick ribbon, the hair

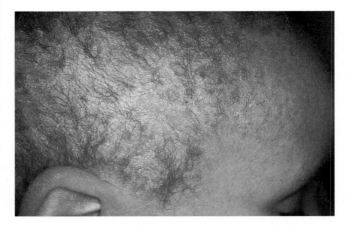

Fig. 33-10 Brittle hair in a patient with trichothiodystrophy.

shaft outline is irregular and slightly undulating, and the melanin granules are distributed in a wavy pattern. With scanning electron microscopy, the surface shows marked ridging and fluting, and the cuticle scales may be absent or greatly reduced.

In addition to the hair findings, which are present in all cases, other variable features of the syndrome include short stature, mental deficiency, ichthyosis (Fig. 33-11), nail dystrophy, ocular dysplasia, photosensitivity, and infertility. Additionally, some cases have had seizures, immune defects with recurrent infections, failure to thrive, and early death, or urologic malformations and primary hypercalcuria. Various names have been associated with differing combinations of these findings such as Brown's syndrome, brittle hair/impaired intelligence/decreased fertility/short stature (BIDS) syndrome, IBIDS (adding *I* for *ichthyosis*) syndrome, PIBIDS (adding *P* for *photosensitivity*) syndrome, and Tay's syndrome. Although the disease manifestations range from an isolated hair defect to severe life-threatening complications, Dawber proposed a classification based on the number and kind of associated disorders. To see if this grouping fits with mutational events will await further genetic analysis, but one type has now been classified. The clue was that patients were seen that had trichothiodystrophy and xeroderma pigmentosa group D overlap. The basis for those patients with trichothiodystrophy and photosensitivity is now known to be a mutation in the basal transcription factor TFIIH. This factor also plays a role in the nucleotide excision repair process and thus the link to XP. Different mutations in the ERCC2 DNA-repair gene may lead to different phenotypic expressions of disease.

Patients with trichothiodystrophy without XP do not have an increase in skin cancer formation. An autosomal recessive inheritance has been suggested in all reports involving more than one family member. The presence of brittle hair with a markedly reduced sulfur content is common to all cases and is an important clinical marker.

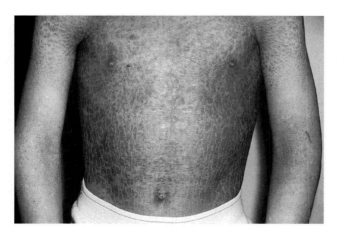

Fig. 33-11 The ichthyosis present in this patient with IBIDS syndrome.

Thus, Price and Odom proposed the term *trichothiodystrophy* (from Greek *tricho*, hair + *thio*, sulfur + *dys*, faulty + *trophe*, nourishment) as a useful designation.

Generalized trichoepitheliomas, alopecia, and myasthenia gravis was reported by Starink et al; it may be a variant of the generalized hair follicle hamartoma syndrome. There is a report of a localized variant of the hair follicle hamartoma syndrome. Histologically, there is replacement of the hair follicles by trichoepithelioma-like epithelial proliferations associated with hyperplastic sebaceous glands.

Crow-Fukase (POEMS) syndrome is characterized by *p*olyneuropathy, *o*rganomegaly, *e*ndocrinopathy, *M*-protein, and *s*kin changes such as diffuse hyperpigmentation, dependent edema, skin thickening, hyperhidrosis, and hypertrichosis.

Cartilage-hair hypoplasia encompasses short-limbed dwarfism and abnormally fine and sparse hair in children. These children are especially susceptible to viral infections and recurrent respiratory infections. A functional defect of small lymphocytes, with impaired cell-mediated immunity, may occur. Most patients are anergic to skin-test panels and have increased numbers of natural killer (NK) cells.

Many black patients with AIDS have experienced softening, straightening, lightening, and thinning of their hair. Patients with HIV-1 infection may also experience elongated eyelashes and telogen effluvium.

Tricho-rhino-phalangeal syndrome is a genetic disorder consisting of fine and sparse scalp hair, thin nails, pear-shaped broad nose, and cone-shaped epiphyses of the middle phalanges of some fingers and toes. There is an autosomal dominant and also a recessive inheritance type.

Lipedematous alopecia consists of shortened hairs, with thickening of the scalp associated with an increase in subcutaneous fat, so that the scalp may be as much as 15 mm thick. This disease appears to affect persons of color primarily.

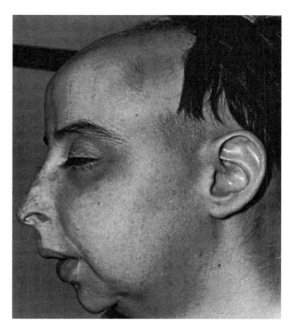

Fig. 33-12 Hallermann-Streiff syndrome.

Hallermann-Streiff syndrome (Fig. 33-12) is a rare condition characterized by birdlike facies with a pronounced beaklike nose, microphthalmia, micrognathia, congenital cataracts, and hypotrichosis. The hair is diffusely sparse and brittle. Baldness may occur frontally or at the scalp margins, but sutural alopecia—hair loss following the lines of the cranial sutures—is characteristic of this syndrome. The small face is in sharp contrast with a disproportionately large-appearing head. The lips are thin; some of the teeth may be absent while others are dystrophic, resulting in malocclusion. Nystagmus, strabismus, and other ocular abnormalities are present.

Progeria, also known as Hutchinson-Gilford syndrome, is characterized by an appearance of premature aging. It is marked by failure to develop normally in growth after the first year of life. The large bald head and lack of eyebrows and eyelashes are distinctive. The skin is wrinkled, pigmented, and atrophic. The nails are thin and atrophic. Most patients lack subcutaneous fat, which produces the appearance of premature senility. The intelligence remains intact. Arteriosclerosis, anginal attacks, and hemiplegia may occur, followed by death from coronary heart disease at an early age.

Papillon-Lefèvre syndrome is characterized by hyperkeratosis palmaris et plantaris, periodontosis, and sparsity of the hair. Hyperhidrosis and the other signs and symptoms begin early in life. Inheritance of this disease is of an autosomal recessive type.

Klippel-Feil syndrome consists of a low posterior scalp hairline extending onto the shoulders, with a short neck, limiting movement of the neck and suggestive of webbing. The cervical vertebrae are fused. This syndrome is caused by faulty segmentation of the mesodermal somites between the third and seventh weeks in utero. Strabismus, nystagmus, cleft palate, bifid uvula, and high palate are other features. This syndrome occurs mostly in girls.

McCusick's syndrome includes short-limbed dwarfism and fine, sparse, hypoplastic and dysmorphic hair.

Turner's syndrome is a distinctive clinical picture comprising short stature, webbing of the neck, low posterior hairline margin, increased carrying angle at the elbow (cubitus valgus), and infantile development of the breasts, vagina, and uterus. Coarctation of the aorta is frequently found. A triangular-shaped mouth, alopecia of the frontal area of the scalp, and cutis laxa are also seen. Turner's syndrome is caused by ovarian dysgenesis. Only 45 chromosomes are present; the sex chromosomes have an XO pattern.

Noonan's syndrome consists of short stature with typical webbing of the neck, low hairline in the back, prominent and low-set ears, and cubitus valgus. The syndrome is similar to Turner's syndrome and has been frequently termed male Turner's syndrome, in which a normal chromosome pattern is assumed. In addition to its occurrence in the male rather than the female, it is differentiated from Turner's syndrome by the absence of coarctation of the aorta; the typical heart lesion is a valvular pulmonary stenosis.

Werner's syndrome has the essential features of shortness of stature, cataracts, skin changes, premature graying and alopecia, atrophy of muscles and subcutaneous tissues, and bone atrophy of the extremities to produce spindly extremities. Osteoporosis and aseptic necrosis are frequent in the small bones of the hands. The skin changes include poikiloderma, scleroderma, atrophy, hyperkeratoses, and leg ulcers. The skin has a dark gray or blackish diffuse pigmentation. A high-pitched voice and hypogonadism in both sexes are distinctive in this syndrome. Diabetes mellitus is frequently present. Because most of these signs are not fully manifested before the age of 30, the diagnosis is usually made in middle age. These patients show marked senescence. It has an autosomal recessive mode of inheritance and is caused by a DNA helicase mutation. These patients usually die before they are 50 years of age from malignant disease or vascular accidents.

Rothmund-Thomson syndrome (Fig. 33-13) is characterized by early-onset poikiloderma, short stature, sun sensitivity, bone defects, and hypogonadism. Cataracts are seen in some families (Rothmund type), and sparseness of eyelashes, eyebrows, or scalp hair has been reported in 60% of cases. This syndrome, like Werner's syndrome and Bloom syndrome, is caused by a mutation in a DNA helicase gene.

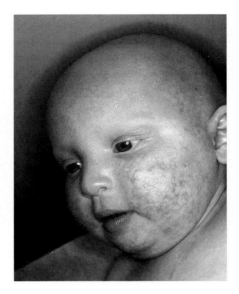

Fig. 33-13 Rothmund-Thomson syndrome.

Brusasco A, et al: The typical 'tiger tail' pattern of the hair shaft in trichothiodystrophy may not be evident at birth. *Arch Dermatol* 1997, 133:249.

Buhler EM, et al: A final word on the tricho-rhino-phalangeal syndromes. *Clin Genet* 1987, 31:273.

Chattopadhyay AK, et al: The association of hereditary neuropathies and heritable skeletal disorders. *Postgrad Med J* 1995, 71:245.

Dacou-Voutetakis C, et al: Psoriasis and blue sclerae in girls with Turner syndrome. *J Am Acad Dermatol* 1996, 35:1002.

Dawber RP: An update of hair shaft disorders. *Dermatol Clin* 1996, 14:753.

Duvic M, et al: Werner's syndrome. *Dermatol Clin* 1995, 13:163.

Ellis NA: Human genetics: mutation causing mutations. *Nature* 1996, 381:110.

Kitao S, et al: Mutations in RECQL4 cause a subset of cases of Rothmund-Thomson syndrome. *Nat Genet* 1999, 22:82.

Lee JH, et al: Lipedematous scalp. *Arch Dermatol* 1994, 130:802.

Makitie O, et al: Cartilage-hair hypoplasia. *J Med Genet* 1995, 32:39.

Malvehy J, et al: Trichothiodystrophy associated with urologic malformation and primary hypercalciuria. *Pediatr Dermatol* 1997, 14:441.

Mayou SC, et al: Generalized hair follicle hamartoma with a positive anti-acetylcholine receptor antibody. *Br J Dermatol* 1991, 125:496.

Micali G, et al: Papillon-Lefèvre syndrome. *Pediatr Dermatol* 1994, 11:354.

Ostergaard JR, et al: The central nervous system in Tay syndrome. *Neuropediatrics* 1996, 27:326.

Perniciaro C: POEMS syndrome. *Semin Dermatol* 1995, 14:162.

Pesce K, et al: The premature aging syndromes. *Clin Dermatol* 1996, 14:161.

Petrin JH, et al: A new variant of trichothiodystrophy with recurrent infections, failure to thrive, and death. *Pediatr Dermatol* 1998, 15:31.

Phillips WG, et al: Orbital oedema: an unusual presentation of Noonan's syndrome. *Br J Dermatol* 1993, 129:190.

Price VH, et al: Trichothiodystrophy: sulfur-deficient brittle hair. *Arch Dermatol* 1980, 116:1375.

Sewry CA, et al: Myopathy with unique ultrastructural feature in Marinesco-Sjögren syndrome. *Ann Neurol* 1988, 24:576.

Shelley WB, et al: Alopecia with fibrous dysplasia and osteomas of skin: sign of polyostotic fibrous dysplasia. *Arch Dermatol* 1976;112:715.

Shelley WB, et al: The skin changes in the Crow-Fukase syndrome. *Arch Dermatol* 1987, 123:85.

Smith KJ, et al: Clinical and histopathologic features of hair loss in patients with HIV-1 infection. *J Am Acad Dermatol* 1996, 34:63.

Alessi E, et al: Localized hair follicle hamartoma. *J Cutan Pathol* 1993, 20:364.

Amichai B, et al: Hallermann-Streiff syndrome. *Pediatr Dermatol* 1996, 13:255.

Brennan TE, et al: Abnormal elastic tissue in cartilage-hair hypoplasia. *Arch Dermatol* 1988, 124:1411.

Starink TM, et al: Generalized trichoepitheliomas and alopecia and myasthenia gravis. *J Am Acad Dermatol* 1986, 15:1104.

Taylor EM, et al: Xeroderma pigmentosum and trichothiodystrophy are associated with different mutations in the XPD (ERCC2) repair/transcription gene. *Proc Natl Acad Sci U S A* 1997, 94:8658.

Vennos EM. et al: Rothmund-Thomson syndrome. *J Am Acad Dermatol* 1992, 27:750.

Weeda G, et al: A mutation in the XPB/ERCC3 DNA repair transcription gene, associated with trichothiodystrophy. *Am J Hum Genet* 1997, 60:320.

Yu C-E, et al: Positional cloning of the Werner's syndrome gene. *Science* 1996, 272:258. _____ ▲

HAIR COLOR

Melanin in the hair follicles is produced in the cytoplasm of the melanocytes, in which are involved the endoplasmic reticulum, ribosomes, and the Golgi apparatus. Melanin synthesis begins on the matrix fibers of the premelanosomes, forming in the cytoplasm of the melanocytes. Hair color will depend on the degree of melanin synthesis, on matrix fibers, and on the intervening spaces between the fibers. When all tyrosinase activity halts, the premelanosome becomes a melanosome.

The pigment in black and dark brown hair is composed of eumelanin, whereas in blond and red hair it is pheomelanin. In black hair the melanocytes contain the densest melanosomes, with lightened areas that show a moth-eaten appearance. Brown hair differs only by its smaller melanosomes; light brown hair consists of a mixture of the melanosomes of dark hair and the incomplete melanosomes of blond hair. Many of the melanosomes in blond hair develop only on the matrix fibers and not in the spaces between the fibers.

Red hair shows incomplete melanin deposits on the matrix fibers to produce a splotchy-appearing melanosome. Pheomelanin is distinguished by its relatively high content of sulfur, which results from the addition of cysteine to dopaquinone along the biosynthetic pathway of melanin synthesis.

Changes in hair color occur in various metabolic disorders. The hair becomes blond in phenylketonuria because of inadequate amounts of tyrosine; in homocystinuria a bleaching effect on the hair is noted; light hair is also seen in oasthouse disease; albinism is associated with white or yellowish hair; triparanol is associated with hypopigmented hair; minoxidil (by changing vellus to terminal hairs) causes darkening of hair; another hypotensive agent, diazoxide, gives the hair a reddish tint; in Menkes' kinky hair syndrome the hair is light; in Griscelli and Chédiak-Higashi syndrome the hair has a silvery sheen; in kwashiorkor the hair assumes a red-blond color in infants; with chloroquine therapy whitening may occur, usually in redheads and blondes, not in brunettes. In vitamin B_{12} deficiency and with interferon therapy, whitening may occur. Segmental heterochromia, with alternating light and dark bands, may occur in iron-deficiency anemia. The disorder has been called *canities segmentata sideropenica*. It responds completely to iron supplementation.

In gray hair (canities), melanogenic activity is decreased as a result of fewer melanocytes and melanosomes as well as a gradual loss of tyrosinase activity. Graying of the scalp hair is genetically determined and may start at any age. Usually it begins at the temples and progresses with time. The beard usually follows, with the body hair graying last.

Early graying (before age 20 in whites or before age 30 in blacks) is usually familial; however, it may occur in progeria, in the syndrome of Rothmund-Thomson, in Böök's syndrome, and in Werner's syndrome.

In poliosis, gray hair occurs in circumscribed patches. This may occur in Waardenburg's syndrome and piebaldism and is frequent in tuberous sclerosis. Poliosis is also found in association with vitiligo and Vogt-Koyanagi syndrome and may be seen in alopecia areata when the new hairs grow. Other syndromes that include poliosis are Tietze's syndrome, Alezzandrini's syndrome, and neurofibromatosis. It may signal a regressing area of a scalp melanoma.

Green hair has been traced to copper in the water of a swimming pool. This occurs only in blond or light hair. Melnick et al recommend the following treatments: EDTA topically; penicillamine-containing shampoos; or 1.5% aqueous 1-hydroxyethyl diphosphonic acid. Tars and chrysarobin stain light-colored hair brown.

Premature whitening of scalp hair is usually caused by vitiligo, sometimes without recognized, or actually without, lesions of glabrous skin.

Cline DJ: Changes in hair color. *Dermatol Clin* 1988, 6:295.

Dunn CL, et al: Melanoma of the scalp presenting as poliosis circumscripta. *Arch Dermatol* 1995, 131:618.

Dupre A, et al: Chloroquin-induced hypopigmentation of hair and freckles. *Arch Dermatol* 1985, 121:1164.

Hann SK, et al: Segmental vitiligo. *J Am Acad Dermatol* 1996, 35:671.

Juhlin L, et al: Red scalp hair turning dark brown at 50 years of age. *Acta Dermatol Venereol* 1986, 66:71.

Lee WS, et al: Diffuse heterochromia of scalp hair. *J Am Acad Dermatol* 1996, 35:823.

Mancini AJ, et al: Partial albinism with immunodeficiency. *J Am Acad Dermatol* 1998, 38:295.

Mascaro JM Jr, et al: Green hair. *Cutis* 1995, 56:37.

Melnick BC, et al: Green hair. *J Am Acad Dermatol* 1986, 15:1065.

Mendez B, et al: Poliosis in a scalp nodule. *Arch Dermatol* 1993, 129:1333.

Ortonne JP, et al: Hair melanins and hair color. *J Invest Dermatol* 1993, 101:82S.

Rogers MJ, et al: Yellow hair discoloration due to anthralin. *J Am Acad Dermatol* 1988, 19:320.

Sato S, et al: Segmented heterochromia in black scalp hair associated with iron-deficiency anemia. *Arch Dermatol* 1989, 125:531.

Taylor JS, et al: Contact leukoderma associated with the use of hair colors. *Cutis* 1993, 52:273.

Vesper JL, et al: Hair darkening and new growth associated with etretinate therapy. *J Am Acad Dermatol* 1996, 34:860 _____ ▲

HAIR STRUCTURE DEFECTS

The examination of hairs for structural defects is greatly facilitated by a method devised by Shelley: putting a piece of double-stick tape on a microscope slide and aligning 5-cm segments of hair in parallel on it. Potassium hydroxide (KOH) examination and even gold-coating and scanning electron microscopy can be done on hairs so mounted.

Birnbaum PS, et al: Heritable disorders of the hair. *Dermatol Clin* 1987, 5:137.

Camacho-Martinez F, et al: Hair shaft dysplasias. *Int J Dermatol* 1988, 27:71.

Caserio RJ, et al: Diagnostic techniques for hair disorders. Part I. *Cutis* 1987, 40:265.

Caserio RJ, et al: Diagnostic techniques for hair disorders. Part II. *Cutis* 1987, 40:321.

Dawber RP: An update of hair shaft disorders. *Dermatol Clin* 1996, 14:753.

Rogers M: Hair shaft abnormalities. Part I. *Australas J Dermatol* 1995, 36:179.

Rogers M: Hair shaft abnormalities. Part II. *Australas J Dermatol* 1996, 37:1.

Shelley WB: Hair examination using double-stick tape. *J Am Acad Dermatol* 1983, 8:430.

Stroud JD: Hair-shaft anomalies. *Dermatol Clin* 1987, 5:581.

Whiting DA: Structural abnormalities of the hair shaft. *J Am Acad Dermatol* 1987, 16:1. _____ ▲

Hair Casts

This disorder, first described by Kligman, mimics nits so closely that it is important to be aware of it. It affects women chiefly and results from long term and frequent traction. Many scalp hairs bear a white keratinous sleeve about 3 to 5 mm long, which lies within 1 to 3 cm of the scalp surface and can, unlike a nit, be slid along the hair shaft. Their bluish yellow fluorescence under Wood's light may cause them to be confused with tinea capitis.

They are formed by retention and desquamation of segments of the root sheaths. Taeb et al reviewed 36 published cases and distinguished two groups: girls between 2 and 8 years of age with diffuse involvement and no scalp disease, and children and adults with psoriasis, lichen planus, seborrheic dermatitis, or trichotillomania. Keipert made a similar distinction, separating a large group of cases with some keratinizing disorder of the scalp and dark, oddly shaped masses of keratin adherent to or surrounding the hairs (often three or four together), which he would call parakeratotic hair casts; and lighter colored tubular casts, 2 to 4 mm long, which he would call peripilar hair casts.

Taeb et al found 0.025% tretinoin lotion effective.

Keipert JA: Hair casts. *Arch Dermatol* 1986, 122:927.

Shieh X, et al: Hair casts. *Arch Dermatol* 1992, 128:1553.

Taeb A, et al: Hair casts: a clinical and morphologic study. *Arch Dermatol* 1985, 121:1009.

Zhang W: Epidemiological and aetiological studies on hair casts. *Clin Exp Dermatol* 1995, 20:202. _____ ▲

Pili Torti

Also known as *twisted hairs,* pili torti is a malformation of hair characterized by twisting of the hair shaft on its own axis (Fig. 33-14). The hair shaft is segmentally thickened, and light and dark segments are seen. Scalp hair, eyebrows, and eyelashes may be affected. The hairs are brittle and easily broken.

In the classic type, unassociated with other disorders, onset is usually in early childhood; by puberty, it has usually improved. Clinically, it may be associated with patchy alopecia and short, broken hairs. It usually follows a dominant inheritance pattern, though recessive and sporadic cases have been reported. Acquired cases have been described in young women with anorexia nervosa.

Pili torti may be seen with associated abnormalities. The Björnstad's syndrome consists of congenital deafness of the cochlear type, with pili torti. Pili torti also may occur in citrullinemia (argininosuccinate synthetase deficiency), Menkes' kinky hair syndrome, Bazex's follicular atrophoderma syndrome, with many ectodermal defects, Crandall's syndrome (pili torti, nerve deafness, hypogonadism), with isotretinoin and etretinate therapy, and in trichothiodystrophy.

Hays SB, et al: Acquired pili torti in two patients treated with synthetic retinoids. *Cutis* 1985, 33:466.

Laub D, et al: A child with hair loss. *Arch Dermatol* 1987, 123:1071.

Lurie R, et al: Acquired pili torti: a structural hair shaft defect in anorexia nervosa. *Cutis* 1996, 57:151.

Maruyama T, et al: Pathogenesis in pili torti. *J Dermatol Sci* 1994, 7(Suppl):5.

Patel HP, et al: Pili torti in association with citrullinemia. *J Am Acad Dermatol* 1985, 12:203. _____ ▲

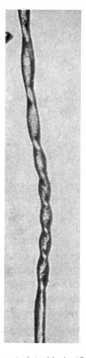

Fig. 33-14 Pilus tortus, or twisted hair. (Courtesy Dr. F. Ronchese.)

Menkes' Kinky Hair Syndrome

Pili torti, and often monilethrix and trichorrhexis nodosa, are all common in the hairs in this sex-linked recessively inherited hair disorder, seen only in boys. It has also been called *steely hair disease,* because the hair resembles steel wool. The characteristic ivory color of the hair appears between 1 and 5 months of age. Drowsiness, lethargy, convulsive seizures, and severe neurologic deterioration, with periodic hypothermia, ensue. Hairs become wiry, sparse, fragile, and twisted about their long axes. The skin is pale and the face pudgy, and the upper lip has an exaggerated "Cupid's bow" configuration. The occipital horn syndrome, primarily a connective tissue disorder, is milder variant of Menkes' syndrome.

Patients have a deficiency of serum copper and copper-dependent enzymes. A gene encoding a copper-transporting ATPase has been designated *MNK.* The Menkes protein exports intracellular copper. Loss of this protein activity, caused by mutations in the MNK gene, blocks the export of dietary copper from the gastrointestinal tract and causes the copper deficiency. There is a distinctive neurochemical pattern in the plasma that allows for early diagnosis. This allows for genetic counseling and the institution of copper histidine treatment, which is being studied and has shown promising results in some infants.

Hart DB: Menkes' syndrome. *J Am Acad Dermatol* 1983, 9:145.

Kaler SG: Diagnosis and therapy of Menkes' syndrome, a genetic form of copper deficiency. *Am J Clin Nutr* 1998, 67:1029S.

Mercer JF: Menkes' syndrome and animal models. *Am J Clin Nutr* 1998, 67:1022S.

Peterson J, et al: Menkes' kinky hair syndrome. *Pediatr Dermatol* 1998, 15:137.

Tumer Z, et al: Mutation spectrum of ATP7A, the defective gene in Menkes' disease. *Adv Exp Med Biol* 1999, 448:83. _____ ▲

Uncombable Hair Syndrome

First reported in 1973 by Dupre et al as *cheveux incoiffable* (undressable hairs) and Stroud and Mehergan as *spun-glass hair,* the microscopic abnormality of a triangular cross-sectional appearance with a longitudinal groove gives the disease its other name, *pili triangulati et canaliculi.*

Clinically, the defect is noted in the first few years of life as dry, blond, shiny hair that stands straight out from the scalp and cannot be combed (Fig. 33-15). On light microscopy it may appear quite normal when viewed lengthwise; but on horizontal sectioning and on scanning electron microscopy it shows the longitudinal grooves that make it abnormally rigid. These depressions are sometimes seen in unaffected persons so that 50% of hairs need to be affected to be clinically detectable.

An autosomal dominant inheritance has been postulated; however, most cases observed by the authors have been sporadic in nature. Kuhn et al reported a patient who acquired the abnormality at age 39 after an episode of diffuse alopecia treated with spironolactone. Although there are usually no associated ectodermal defects, isolated cases have been reported in which uncombable hair is one component of several clustered findings. Until more experience is available in the literature grouping of these cases into new syndromes is premature.

One of the Shelleys' cases responded symptomatically (although without apparent change in the hair structure) to biotin 0.3 mg orally three times daily. Some cases improve spontaneously in late childhood, however.

Kuhn CA, et al: Acquired uncombable hair. *Arch Dermatol* 1993, 129:1061.

Matis WL, et al: Uncombable-hair syndrome. *Pediatr Dermatol* 1987, 4:215.

McCullum N, et al: The uncombable hair syndrome. *Cutis* 1990, 46:479.

Ravella A, et al: Localized pili canaliculi and trianguli. *J Am Acad Dermatol* 1987, 17:377.

Rest EB, et al: Quantitative assessment of scanning electron microscope defects in uncombable-hair syndrome. *Pediatr Dermatol* 1990, 7:93.

Shelley WB, et al: Uncombable hair syndrome: observations on response to biotin and occurrence in siblings with ectodermal dysplasia. *J Am Acad Dermatol* 1985, 13:97. _____ ▲

Monilethrix

Monilethrix is a rare hereditary disease is also known as *beaded hairs.* Monilethrix is characterized by dryness, fragility, and sparseness of the scalp hair, with fusiform or spindle-shaped swellings of the hair shaft separated by narrow atrophic segments (Fig. 33-16). The hair tends to break at the delicate internodes. There is an occasional rupture at the node and longitudinal fissuring of the shaft, which also involves the nodes. Improvement of the hair may occur during pregnancy, but after delivery the hair returns to its original state. Improvement may also occur with age and there may be seasonal improvement during the summer.

The disease is often associated with keratosis pilaris of the extensor surfaces, temples, and back of the neck. Hair on regions other than the scalp may be affected. Leukonychia

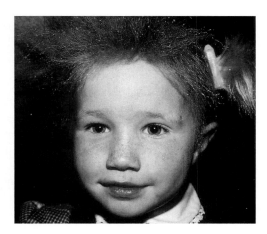

Fig. 33-15 Young girl with uncombable hair.

Fig. 33-16 **A,** Monilethrix. Sparse, short, dry hair and follicular keratosis. **B,** Monilethrix. Hair showing alternating constrictions and fusiform enlargements.

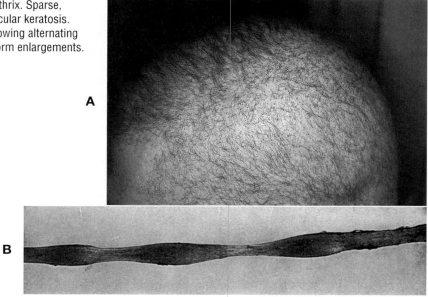

may occur. Inheritance of monilethrix is an autosomal dominant trait. It has been described in association with Menkes' syndrome. Several cases of monilethrix have been linked to the type II keratin gene cluster on chromosome 12q13. Causative heterozygous mutations of a highly conserved glutamic acid residue of the type II hair keratins hHb6 and hHb1 occur. Both hHb1 and hHb6 are largely coexpressed in cortical trichocytes of the hair shaft confirming monilethrix is a disease of the hair cortex. There is no effective treatment.

Amichai-B, et al: Hair loss in a 6-month-old child: monilethrix. *Arch Dermatol* 1996, 132:574.

Finley EM, et al: Alopecia in a 19-month-old boy. *Arch Dermatol* 1994, 130:1055.

Winter H, et al: A new mutation in the type II hair cortex keratin hHb1 involved in the inherited hair disorder monilethrix. *Hum Genet* 1997, 101:165.

Winter H, et al: Mutations in the hair cortex keratin hHb6 cause the inherited hair disease monilethrix. *Nat Genet* 1997, 16:372.

Zlotogorski A, et al: Monilethrix. *Exp Dermatol* 1998, 7:268.

▲

Trichorrhexis Nodosa

The affected hair shafts may have small white nodes arranged at irregular intervals. These nodes are the sites of fracture of the hair cortex. The splitting into strands produces a microscopic appearance suggestive of a pair of brooms stuck together end to end by their bristles (Fig. 33-17). The hairs soon break at these nodes. The number of these nodes along one hair shaft varies from one to several, depending on its length. These fractured hairs are found mostly on the scalp, often in just a small area or areas, but

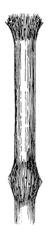

Fig. 33-17 Trichorrhexis nodosa.

other sites such as the pubic area, axillae, and chest may be involved.

Several categories or types of trichorrhexis nodosa have been described. Proximal trichorrhexis nodosa involves the proximal shafts of the hairs of blacks who traumatize their hair with styling or chemicals; involved hairs break a few centimeters from the skin surface (Fig. 33-18). It appears to occur in genetically predisposed patients. Distal trichorrhexis nodosa occurs primarily in Asians or white patients, several inches from the scalp, and is associated with trichoptilosis, or longitudinal splitting, known as *split ends*. Acquired localized trichorrhexis nodosa is a common type in which the defect occurs in a localized area, a few centimeters across. A number of diseases accompany this type of trichorrhexis nodosa in which pruritus is a prominent symptom; scratching and rubbing may be the cause. Among such diseases are circumscribed neurodermatitis, contact dermatitis, and atopic dermatitis.

The occurrence of trichorrhexis nodosa in some patients with argininosuccinicaciduria has suggested an etiologic connection. Trichorrhexis nodosa has been described in Menkes' kinky hair syndrome, Netherton's syndrome, hypothyroidism, and trichorrhexis nodosa–like fractures may be seen in trichothiodystrophy. Trichoschisis, a clean transverse fracture across the hair shaft, is more commonly present in trichothiodystrophy. The curly hair that may result from isotretinoin therapy has been attributed to extensive trichorrhexis nodosa. Because trauma may induce this hair shaft abnormality the specificity of this finding in the above conditions may simply be fortuitous.

Treatment is directed toward the avoidance of traumatization of the hair.

Camacho-Martinez F: Localized trichorrhexis nodosa. *J Am Acad Dermatol* 1989, 20:696.
Lurie R, et al: Trichorrhexis nodosa. *Cutis* 1996, 57:358.
Scott DA: Disorders of the hair and scalp in blacks. *Dermatol Clin* 1988, 6:387.
Smith RA, et al: Localized trichorrhexis nodosa. *Clin Exp Dermatol* 1994, 19:441. ▲

Trichorrhexis Invaginata

Also known as *bamboo hair,* trichorrhexis invaginata is caused by intussusception of the hair shaft at the zone where keratinization begins. The invagination is caused by softness of the cortex in the keratogenous zone. The softness may be caused by inadequate conversion of -SH to S-S proteins in the cortex. The patient with bamboo hair will have nodosa ball-and-socket deformities (Fig. 33-19), with the socket forming the proximal and the ball part forming the distal portion of the node along the hair shaft. This type of hair is associated with Netherton's syndrome. Occasionally, only the proximal half of the abnormality is seen; this has been called *golf tee hairs.*

Trichorrhexis invaginata associated with congenital ichthyosiform erythroderma or ichthyosis linearis circumflexa constitutes Netherton's syndrome (Fig. 33-20). Atopic manifestations are commonly present. The bamboo hairs may be present not only on the scalp but also on the eyebrows, eyelashes, and rarely in other hairy areas. Hair sparsity is noted all over the body. The bamboo hairs may become normal within a few years. Other reported findings include pili torti, trichorrhexis nodosa, moniliform hairs, urticaria, angioedema, growth retardation, recurrent infections, and mental retardation. An autosomal recessive mode of inheritance has been suggested although reported cases involving women far outnumber men. PUVA has been reported to help the circumflex linear ichthyosis while

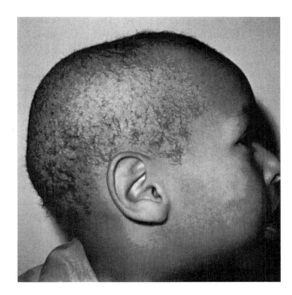

Fig. 33-18   Trichorrhexis nodosa.

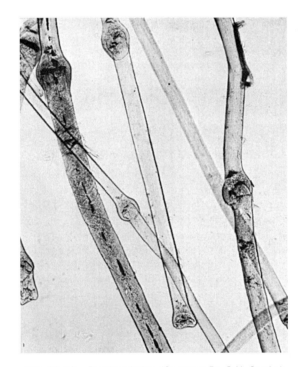

Fig. 33-19   Bamboo hairs. (Courtesy Dr. G.H. Curtis.)

etretinate has been reported to both exacerbate and improve skin findings.

Menne et al reported the bamboo hair defect in very thin, probably vellus, hairs in a 7-year-old boy with short, thin, brittle scalp hairs and no eyebrows. They termed this a *canestick* deformity.

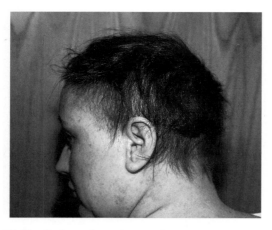

Fig. 33-20 Netherton's syndrome. (Courtesy Dr. Axel W. Hoke.)

Caputo R, et al: Netherton's syndrome in two adult patients. *Arch Dermatol* 1984, 120:220.

de Berker DA, et al: Golf tee hairs in Netherton disease. *Pediatr Dermatol* 1995, 12:7.

Greene SL, et al: Netherton's syndrome. *J Am Acad Dermatol* 1985, 13:329.

Gupta AK, et al: Hair abnormalities and a rash with a double-edged scale. *Arch Dermatol* 1986, 122:1199.

Hausser I, et al: Severe congenital generalized exfoliative erythroderma in newborns and infants. *Pediatr Dermatol* 1996, 13:183.

Menne T, et al: Canestick lesions of vellus hair in Netherton's syndrome. *Arch Dermatol* 1985, 121:451.

Smith DL, et al: Netherton's syndrome. *J Allergy Clin Immunol* 1995, 95:116. ▲

Pili Annulati (Ringed Hair)

Pili annulati is a peculiar disease in which the hair seems banded by alternating segments of light and dark color when seen in reflected light. The light bands are caused by clusters of abnormal air-filled cavities, which scatter light, as shown by the electron microscope.

Hair growth is normal in patients with pili annulati, and there are no other associated abnormalities of skin or other organ systems. It is inherited by autosomal dominant mode, begins in infancy, and requires no treatment, since the spangled appearance of the hair is not unattractive.

Amichai B, et al: Hair abnormality present since childhood. *Arch Dermatol* 1996, 132:575. ▲

Pili Pseudoannulati

This anomaly of human hair mimics pili annulati. The two differ in that the light bands in pili annulati are caused by internal effects, whereas the bright segments in pili pseudoannulati are caused by reflection and refraction of light by flattened, twisted surfaces of hair. This latter type is a variant of normal hair.

Price VH, et al: Pseudo pili annulati. *Arch Dermatol* 1970, 102:54. ▲

Kinking Hair

Acquired progressive kinking of the hair, first described and named by Wise and Sulzberger in 1932, has a structural abnormality of kinking and twisting of the hair shaft at irregular intervals. The main recognized variant of this disorder begins in men in their late teens or early twenties on the frontotemporal or vertex regions and then progresses to both the parietal and frontal areas. Usually straight, light brown hair becomes curly, frizzy, and lusterless.

When this occurs in the androgen-dependent areas of young men it is a precursor of male-pattern hair loss; usually these men have a strong family history of androgenetic alopecia. "Whisker" hairs, the short dark hairs that grow anterior to the ears in young people who eventually develop androgenic alopecia, is felt to be a variant of acquired kinking of the hair.

Acquired hair kinking has been described in other clinical situations. Some reports detail prepubertal patients or women, as well as men, in whom kinking develops in non–androgen-dependent areas. In these reports alopecia has not developed, and the curly, frizzy hair may remain present or reverse to its previous condition.

Widespread kinking of the hair may be induced by drugs, notably retinoids, and it may also occur in patients with AIDS.

Balsa RE, et al: Acquired kinking of the hair. *J Am Acad Dermatol* 1986, 15:1133.

Boudou P, et al: Increased scalp skin and serum 5-alpha-reductase reduced androgens in a man relevant to the acquired progressive kinky hair disorder and developing androgenetic alopecia. *Arch Dermatol* 1997, 133:1129.

Cullen SI, et al: Acquired progressive kinking of hair. *Arch Dermatol* 1989, 125:252.

Mortimaer PS, et al: Acquired progressive kinking of hair: report of six cases and review of the literature. *Arch Dermatol* 1985, 121:1031.

Rebora A, et al: Acquired progressive kinking of the hair. *J Am Acad Dermatol* 1985, 12:933.

Tosti a, et al: Acquired progressive kinking of the hair. *Arch Dermatol* 1999, 135:1223. ▲

Woolly Hair

Woolly hair is present at birth and is usually most severe during childhood, when it is often impossible to brush the hair. In adult life there is a variable amelioration in the condition. There is a clear distinction between the appearance of the affected and nonaffected members of a family. Four subgroups have been identified: hereditary woolly hair has evidence of autosomal dominant inheritance; familial woolly hair has a distinctive bleached appearance with a reduced diameter and a suspected autosomal recessive mode of inheritance; woolly hair nevus has partial scalp involvement by woolly hair (Fig. 33-21), which has a markedly reduced diameter; and Naxos disease, originally described in 1986 and named after a city in Greece. This autosomal recessive disease constitutes the triad of arrhythmogenic right ventricular cardiomyopathy, a heart muscle disease of unknown etiologic factors that causes arrhythmias, heart failure, and sudden death; diffuse nonepidermolytic palmoplantar keratoderma; and woolly hair. Hair abnormalities are a reliable marker for subsequent heart disease. The disease locus has been mapped to 17q21 and it appears to be caused by a mutation in keratin 9.

Woolly hairs tend to unite into locks, whereas the hairs of blacks remain individual. The hair may not grow beyond a length of 12 cm, but may attain a normal appearance in adult life. In the familial group the eyebrows and the hairs on the arms, legs, pubic and axillary regions may be short and pale. There are no associated cutaneous or systemic diseases.

The microscopic findings of the hair include an ovoid shape on cross section, a pili torti–like twisting about a longitudinal axis, trichorrhexis nodosa, and pili annulati.

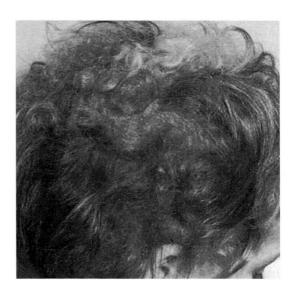

Fig. 33-21 Woolly hair nevus, with affected hairs lighter and finer than the normal hair.

al Harmozi SA, et al: Woolly hair nevus syndrome. *J Am Acad Dermatol* 1992, 27:259.

Amichai B, et al: A child with a localized hair abnormality. *Arch Dermatol* 1996, 132:573.

Coonar AS, et al: Gene for arrhythmogenic right ventricular cardiomyopathy with diffuse nonepidermolytic palmoplantar keratoderma and woolly hair (Naxos disease) maps to 17q21. *Circulation* 1998, 97:2049.

Reda AM, et al: Woolly hair nevus. *J Am Acad Dermatol* 1990, 22:377.

Tosti A, et al: Woolly hair, palmoplantar keratoderma, and cardiac abnormalities. *Arch Dermatol* 1994, 130:522. _____ ▲

Plica Neuropathica

This is a curling, looping, intertwisting, and felting or matting of the hair in localized areas of the scalp. Simpson et al reported a case occurring in a black woman who had tangled and matted hair. Predisposing factors figuring in this condition were kinky hairs and a neurotic mental state. Plica polonica is an older name of this condition.

Marshall J, et al: Felted hair untangled. *J Am Acad Dermatol* 1989, 20:688.

Ramanan C, et al: Plica neuropathica after using herbal soap. *Int J Dermatol* 1993, 32:200.

Simpson MH, et al: Plica neuropathica. *Arch Dermatol* 1969, 100:457. ▲

Pseudofolliculitis Barbae

Pseudofolliculitis barbae are hairs that, after appearing at the surface, curve back and pierce the skin as ingrowing hairs. This results in inflammatory papules and pustules, which may scar (Fig. 33-22). The chief cause is close shaving of curly hair, and the cure is to stop this. Solitary hairs may be epilated; however, many hairs are usually involved.

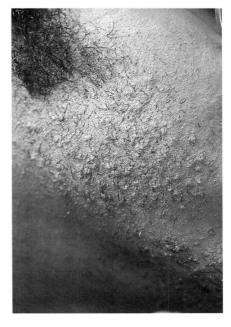

Fig. 33-22 Pseudofolliculitis barbae. (Courtesy Dr. Axel W. Hoke.)

The commonest clinical syndrome resulting is pseudofolliculitis of the beard, a serious problem seen in more than 50% of black men, who must sometimes give up shaving to alleviate the disorder. Whites are uncommonly affected; however, shaving of the pubic hair will often result in pseudofolliculitis. The use of clippers or chemical depilatories, and adjunctive antibiotic therapy are helpful. Laser hair removal holds promise for treatment in the future.

Hydrocortisone for the irritation that frequently accompanies the use of chemicals, not allowing them to be in contact with the skin longer than tolerated, and shaving only every second or third day will increase compliance with the depilatory agents. Moore has invented a tiny plastic hook for removing ingrown hairs before shaving, which is very helpful. Glycolic acid lotion has been reported to assist the affected patient to shave normally. In severe cases large deforming keloids may result in the beard area.

Brown LA Jr: Pathogenesis and treatment of pseudofolliculitis barbae. *Cutis* 1983, 32:373.

Coquilla BH, et al: Management of pseudofolliculitis barbae. *Mil Med* 1995, 160:263.

Halder RM: Pseudofolliculitis barbae and related disorders. *Dermatol Clin* 1988, 6:407.

Hall JC, et al: Pseudofolliculitis. *Cutis* 1979, 23:798.

Perricone NV: Treatment of pseudofolliculitis barbae with topical glycolic acid. *Cutis* 1993, 52:232. ▲

Pili Multigemini

This rare malformation of the pilary apparatus is characterized by the presence of bifurcated or multiple divided hair matrices and papillae, giving rise to the formation of multiple hair shafts within the individual follicles. Mehregan et al reported a patient with cleidocranial dysostosis and extensive pili multigemini over the heavily bearded chin and cheek areas. There is no treatment.

Cambiaghi S, et al: Scanning electron microscopy in the diagnosis of pili multigemini. *Acta Derm Venereol* 1995, 75:170.

Mehregan AH, et al: Pili multigemini. *Br J Dermatol* 1999, 100:315. ▲

Pili Bifurcati

Weary et al described this strange disorder in a 3-year-old child seen because of hair loss. Bifurcation was found in short segments along the shafts of several hairs. The anomaly was transient.

Breslau-Siderius LJ, et al: Pili bifurcati. *Clin Dysmorphol* 1996, 5:275.

Weary PE, et al: Pili bifurcati. *Arch Dermatol* 1973;108:403. ▲

Trichostasis Spinulosa

Trichostasis spinulosa is a common disorder of the hair follicles that clinically gives the impression of follicular keratosis, but the follicles are filled with funnel-shaped, horny plugs within which are bundles of vellus hairs. The hairs are round at their proximal ends and shredded distally (Fig. 33-23). The disease occurs on the nose and forehead of elderly persons and on the shoulders and back and manifests itself by the appearance of little black dots that look like comedones but that on closer examination are seen to be bundles of soft hairs that project 2 to 3 mm above the skin.

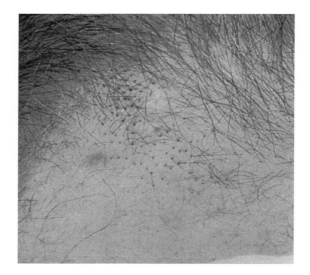

Fig. 33-23   Trichostasis spinulosa.

Microscopically, these tufts are made up of several dozen fine, stubby hairs (Fig. 33-24). Even without a magnifying glass the small tufts of vellus hair emerging from the black-dot follicle are apparent.

Trichostasis spinulosa results from retention of telogen hairs, which are derived from a single hair matrix. It is primarily caused by a hyperkeratosis of the follicular infundibulum, which leads to a partial obstruction of the follicular orifice and thus does not permit shedding of small telogen hairs.

Keratolytics are effective after using a wax depilatory. The application of 0.05% tretinoin solution, applied daily for 2 or 3 months, may also produce satisfactory results.

Harford RR, et al: Trichostasis spinulosa. *Pediatr Dermatol* 1996, 13:490.

Noel N, et al: Trichostasis spinulosa. *Arch Dermatol* 1997, 133:1579. ▲

Intermittent Hair-Follicle Dystrophy

Birnbaum et al reported in 1986 a new disorder of the hair follicle leading to increased fragility of the shaft, with no identifiable biochemical disturbance.

Birnbaum PS, et al: Heritable diseases of the hair. *Dermatol Clin* 1987, 5:137. ▲

Bubble Hair Deformity

Brown et al reported a 16-year-old girl who developed brittle, fragile hairs in localized areas of the scalp. The hairs additionally became straight and stiff. Small, bubblelike defects were found within the hair shafts on light and electron microscopy. Detwiler et al's studies proved this to be caused by heating of the hair. All hair will develop bubbles of gas when exposed to high heat. In Detwiler's

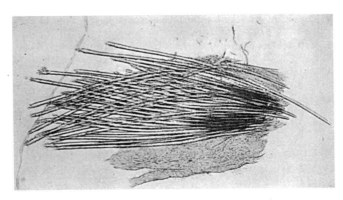

Fig. 33-24 Trichostasis spinulosa—the removed plug, full of fine hairs.

patient an old, malfunctioning, overheating hairdryer was the culprit.

Brown VM, et al: An unusual new hair shaft abnormality. *J Am Acad Dermatol* 1986, 15:1113.

Detwiler SP, et al: Bubble hair. *J Am Acad Dermatol* 1994, 30:54.

Gummer CL: Bubble hair. *Br J Dermatol* 1994, 131:901. ▲

HYPERTRICHOSIS

Hypertrichosis is an overgrowth of hair not localized to the androgen-dependent areas of the skin. Several forms exist.

Localized Acquired Hypertrichosis

Dermal tumors, such as melanocytic nevi, smooth muscle hamartoma, meningioma, or Becker's nevi, may have excessive terminal hair growth. Repeated irritation, trauma, occlusion under a cast, eczematous states, topical steroid use, linear melorheostotic scleroderma, lymphedema associated with filariasis, the Crow-Fukase (POEMS) syndrome, and pretibial myxedema may be other situations in which there is a localized increase in hair growth. Porphyrias generally show a localized hypertrichosis over the malar area such as in porphyria cutanea tarda or variegate porphyria; however, in the Gunther variety of erythropoietic porphyria it may be generalized or more diffuse in nature.

Localized Congenital Hypertrichosis

Beighton first reported a curious and rare anomaly, hairy elbows, in 1970. It is a progressive, excessive growth of lanugo hairs that often begins in infancy; the hairs may reach a length of 10 cm. Later they become coarser, but regression has been observed during adolescence. There appears to be familial cases and a sporadic form. Short stature and some developmental abnormalities are present in

some cases; however, there is no need for endocrine studies or other evaluation. The condition appears to be of only cosmetic significance.

Other causes of localized congenital hypertrichosis include congenital nevocytic nevi, anterior cervical hypertrichosis, simple nevoid hypertrichosis, or as a sign of underlying spinal dysraphism (when occurring over the sacral midline).

Generalized Congenital Hypertrichosis (Congenital Hypertrichosis Lanuginosa)

This rare type of excessive and generalized hairiness is a fully penetrant X-linked dominant trait. The entire body is covered with fine vellus hairs 2 to 10 cm long. The scalp hair appears to be normal; otherwise, except for the palms and soles, all areas were covered. Congenital hypertrichosis lanuginosa may be associated with dental anomalies and gingival fibromatosis. This type of hairiness has attracted considerable attention over the centuries. These individuals have been billed as "dog-faced boy," "human werewolf," and "human Skye terrier." In all hypertrichotic conditions, but especially this one, hair removal by laser may be quite useful because large areas may be treated, although at present repeat treatments will be necessary to maintain the results.

Other cases of congenital generalized hypertrichosis may be secondary to drug ingestion by the mother. The fetal hydantoin syndrome is characterized by hypertrichosis, depressed nasal bridge, large lips, a wide mouth, and a short, webbed neck. The fetal alcohol syndrome includes hypertrichosis, a small face, capillary hemangiomas, and physical and mental retardation. A case of generalized hypertrichosis and multiple congenital defects was reported by Kaler et al in a baby born to a mother who used minoxidil throughout pregnancy.

Generalized or Patterned Acquired Hypertrichosis

These cases include those caused by acquired hypertrichosis lanuginosa, those associated with various syndromes, and those secondary to drug intake. Acquired hypertrichosis lanuginosa has been covered earlier in this book as an ominous sign of internal malignancy. Syndromes associated with increased hair growth include lipoatrophic diabetes, stiff skin syndrome, Rubenstein-Taybi syndrome, Laband syndrome, Cornelia de Lange's syndrome, Hurler's syndrome, Morogu's syndrome, leprechaunism, Winchester's syndrome, the Schynzel-Giedier syndrome, and a newly described syndrome that includes hypertrichosis, osteochondrodysplasia, and cardiomegaly. Drugs associated with hypertrichosis include minoxidil (Fig. 33-25), cyclosporine, diphenylhydantoin, diazoxide, streptomycin, penicillamine, corticosteroids, danazol, psoralens, hexachlorobenzene, PUVA, and topical steroids or topical androgens.

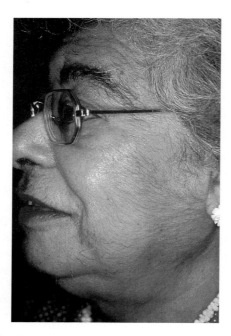

Fig. 33-25 Hypertrichosis associated with oral minoxidil.

Boffa MJ, et al: Hypertrichosis as the presenting feature of porphyria cutanea tarda. *Clin Exp Dermatol* 1995, 20:62.

Bondeson J, et al: The hairy family of Burma. *J R Soc Med* 1996, 89:403.

Braddock SR, et al: Anterior cervical hypertrichosis. *Am J Med Genet* 1995, 55:498.

Camacho F: Acquired circumscribed hypertrichosis in the "costaleros" who bear the "pasos" during Holy Week in Seville, Spain. *Arch Dermatol* 1995, 131:361.

Chang SN, et al: A case of multiple nevoid hypertrichosis. *J Dermatol* 1997, 24:337.

Escalonilla P, et al: A new case of hairy elbows syndrome (hypertrichosis cubiti). *Pediatr Dermatol* 1996, 13:303.

Garcia-Cruz D, et al: Congenital hypertrichosis, osteochondrodysplasia, and cardiomegaly. *Am J Med Genet* 1997, 69:138.

Jemec GBE: Hypertrichosis lanuginosa acquisita: report of a case and review of the literature. *Arch Dermatol* 1986, 122:805.

Kaler SG, et al: Hypertrichosis and congenital anomalies associated with maternal use of minoxidil. *Pediatrics* 1987, 79:434.

Kurzrock R, et al: Cutaneous paraneoplastic syndromes in solid tumors. *Am J Med* 1995, 99:662.

Lacombe D, et al: Congenital marked hypertrichosis and Laband syndrome in a child: overlap between the gingival fibromatosis-hypertrichosis and Laband syndromes. *Genet Couns* 1994, 5:251.

Littler CM: Laser hair removal in a patient with hypertrichosis lanuginosa congenita. *Dermatol Surg* 1997, 23:705.

McAtee-Smith J, et al: Skin lesions of the spinal axis and spinal dysraphism. *Arch Pediatr Adolesc Med* 1994, 148:740.

Miller ML, et al: Hairy elbows. *Arch Dermatol* 1995, 131:858.

Miyachi Y, et al: Linear melorheostotic scleroderma with hypertrichosis. *Arch Dermatol* 1979, 115:1233.

Nanni CA, et al: Laser hair removal. *J Am Acad Dermatol* 1999, 41:165.

Olsen EA: Methods of hair removal. *J Am Acad Dermatol* 1999, 40:143.

Penas PF, et al: Cutaneous meningioma underlying congenital localized hypertrichosis. *J Am Acad Dermatol* 1994, 30:363.

Rampen FHJ: Hypertrichosis in PUVA-treated patients. *Br J Dermatol* 1983, 109:657.

Roth SI, et al: Cutaneous manifestations of leprechaunism. *Arch Dermatol* 1981, 117:531.

Rupert LS, et al: Nevoid hypertrichosis. *Pediatr Dermatol* 1994, 11:49.

Shelley WB, et al: The skin changes in the Crow-Fukase (POEMS) syndrome. *Arch Dermatol* 1987, 123:85.

Wheeland RG: Laser-assisted hair removal. *Dermatol Clin* 1997, 15:469.

Wysocki GP, et al: Hypertrichosis in patients receiving cyclosporin therapy. *Clin Exp Dermatol* 1987, 12:191. _____ ▲

HIRSUTISM

CLINICAL FEATURES. Hirsutism is an excess of terminal hair growth in women in a pattern more typical of men (Fig. 33-26). Androgen-dependent growth areas affected include the upper lip, cheeks, chin, central chest, breasts, lower abdomen, and groin. This altered growth pattern of the hair may or may not be associated with other signs of virilization, which include temporal balding, masculine habitus, deepening of the voice, clitoral hypertrophy, and amenorrhea. Acne is an additional associated phenomenon in some cases of hirsutism. When virilization accompanies hirsutism, especially when progression is rapid, a neoplastic cause is likely. Neoplastic causes account for only a small minority of hirsute women.

PATHOGENESIS. Racial variation should be considered when evaluating hirsutism. Women of Middle Eastern, Russian, and Southern European countries commonly have facial, abdominal, and thigh hair, whereas Asian and Indian women generally have little terminal hair growth in these areas.

In women, androgen biosynthesis occurs only in the adrenal and the ovary. The potent androgen testosterone and the androgen precursor androstenedione are secreted by the ovary. The adrenal contributions are preandrogens; dehydroepiandrosterone (DHEA), DHEA sulfate, and androstenedione. They require peripheral conversion in the skin and liver to testosterone.

Testosterone is converted to dihydrotestosterone, the androgen that promotes androgen-dependent hair growth, in the hair follicle by 5-alpha-reductase. Receptor molecules in the end organ are necessary for binding and hormone action at that level. Because testosterone is normally bound to carrier molecules in the plasma at a 99% level, and it is the unbound testosterone that is active, the levels of free testosterone reflect clinical evidence of androgen excess, rather than total testosterone.

Hirsutism, then, may result either from excessive secretion of androgens from either the ovary or the adrenal gland, or from excessive stimulation by pituitary tumors. The excessive secretion may be from functional excesses or from neoplastic processes. All cases of severe or progressive hirsutism should be investigated for an endocrinopathy.

Ovarian causes include polycystic ovary disease (Stein-Leventhal syndrome), and a variety of ovarian tumors, both benign and malignant. The Stein-Leventhal syndrome is characterized by hirsutism (50%), acne (20%), and signs such as amenorrhea, uterine bleeding, anovulation, obesity,

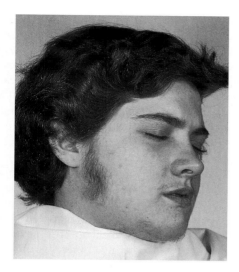

Fig. 33-26 Hirsutism.

and small breasts. The ovaries are frequently palpable on physical examination, as they are polycystic. Pelvic ultrasonography is useful; however, culdoscopy and colpotomy may be necessary for diagnosis. Serum free testosterone is generally elevated. Luteinizing hormone is also elevated, but follicle-stimulating hormone levels remain normal or may be decreased. Insulin resistance with resultant elevated insulin levels will lead to ovarian overproduction of androgens. This may be present in polycystic ovary syndrome, but also the HAIR-AN syndrome, obesity, and other states. Ovarian tumors include unilateral benign microadenomas, arrhenoblastomas, Leydig cell tumors, hilar cell tumors, granular—thecal cell tumors, and luteomas. Here the onset is usually rapid, occurs with associated virilization, and begins between the ages of 20 and 40. Again free testosterone is high (generally greater than 2 ng/ml).

Adrenal causes include congenital adrenal hyperplasia and adrenal tumors such as adrenal adenomas and carcinomas. The adrenogenital syndrome or congenital adrenal hyperplasia is an autosomal dominant disorder that may result from deficiencies of the following enzymes: 21-hydroxylase (most common form), 11β-hydroxylase, or 3β-hydroxy steroid dehydrogenase. Onset is generally in childhood, with ambiguous genitalia, precocious growth, and virilism; however, adult-onset types with partial enzyme deficiencies present generally with hirsutism as a familial trait.

Pituitary causes include Cushing's disease, acromegaly, and prolactin-secreting adenomas. Prolactin-secreting microadenomas have a 20% incidence of hirsutism and acne. Other conditions in which prolactin levels may be elevated and that may lead to hirsutism include hypothyroidism, phenothiazine intake, and hepatorenal failure.

Other causes of hirsutism include the exogenous intake of androgens and certain high-progesterone birth control pills (uncommonly). End-organ hypersensitivity may be a mechanism in patients with a normal evaluation. Drugs such as minoxidil, diazoxide, corticosteroids, and phenytoin, which have been reported to cause hirsutism, generally cause hypertrichosis—a generalized increase in hair that is not limited to the androgen-sensitive areas.

EVALUATION. A careful history and physical examination are essential. The history should focus on onset and progression, virilization, menstrual history, and family/racial background. Physical examination may reveal signs of Cushing's disease or acromegaly. Other signs to be evaluated are the distribution of muscle mass and body fat, clitoral dimensions, voice depth, and galactorrhea.

Laboratory evaluation should include a total testosterone level and a dehydroepiandrosterone sulfate level for relatively stable and mild hirsutism in patients who have no signs of virilism and infertility and menstrual disturbances are absent. If, however, severe clinical manifestations are present or the clinical findings are recent or rapid in onset or are progressively worsening an overnight dexamethasone suppression test may be utilized to screen for Cushing's disease and abnormal androgen levels should be evaluated with a 5- to 7-day dexamethasone suppression test to determine the source of the androgens. In patients with menstrual dysfunction the above tests should be considered as well as a prolactin level, which will screen for prolactin secreting tumors (this level should be obtained in any patient with galactorrhea) and an LH/FSH ratio to evaluate suspected polycystic ovarian disease. If frank virilization is present as revealed by the presence of hirsutism of the shoulders or back, clitoromegaly, a deepening of the voice, and the onset of a muscular body habitus an androgen secreting tumor is suggested. Finally a 17-hydroxyprogesterone and ACTH stimulation test will screen for late onset congenital adrenal hyperplasia. Many of these patients may have normal screening tests so that it is prudent to consider doing this test; however, it is expensive and the incidence of the disease being screened for is rare.

DIAGNOSIS. If acromegaly, Cushing's disease, or frank virilization is present clinically, referral to an internist or endocrinologist is recommended. The presence of major menstrual irregularities is also an indication for referral to a gynecologist. Although 90% of women with hirsutism have an elevated testosterone level, elevations above 2 ng/ml and rapid onset or progressive virilization suggest serious underlying disease, generally an ovarian neoplasm. Pelvic ultrasonography and referral are indicated. A major elevation in the DHEA sulfate level (above 7000 ng/ml) suggests an adrenal neoplasm, and computed tomography of the adrenal gland and referral are recommended. If the DHEA-S level is greater than 4300 ng/ml an ACTH stimulation test to exclude late onset congenital adrenal hyperplasia should be considered. Elevations of the 17-hydroxyprogesterone level (when taken between 0700 and 0900) should suggest congenital adrenal hyperplasia, and ACTH stimulation tests (for levels of 300 to 1000 ng/ml) and referral are recommended. Prolactin levels above 20 ng/ml should be likewise referred for further evaluation with and MRI or CT scan. An LH/FSH ratio of more than 3 is suspect for polycystic ovarian syndrome and an ultrasound of the ovaries and gynecologic consultation are recommended.

In other cases the cause is likely a functional disorder and treatment may be instituted. A reevaluation within 6 to 12 months should be planned.

TREATMENT. Once appropriate testing has led to diagnosis and referral of patients requiring special methods of specific treatment, such as surgical intervention, therapeutic alternatives include cosmetic (mechanical) treatments, nonspecific suppressive therapy, and specific antiandrogens. Cosmetic or mechanical methods of treatment are the cheapest and easiest methods, and expose the patient to the fewest potential side effects. Shaving, wax depilatories, chemical depilatories, bleaching of the hair, laser hair removal, and electrolysis are alternatives.

Epilating waxes, usually made of beeswax and rosin, are satisfactory for temporary removal of moderate amounts of cosmetically objectionable hair. It has been proved beyond a doubt that the temporary removal of hairs by waxes, shaving, or plucking does not stimulate their growth or coarsen subsequent growth. Depilatories containing barium sulfide corrode the projecting hair shaft but have no destructive action on the intrafollicular growing portion. The barium sulfide may irritate the skin excessively, making this procedure undesirable. Bleaching with hydrogen peroxide with or without equal parts of strong ammonia makes dark hairs less noticeable and corrodes the finer hairs. Before it is applied, the skin is cleansed with ether to remove any oiliness. It is advisable to begin with one tenth of the usual strength.

Laser hair removal is an active area of investigation. It is an effective way to remove hair from large areas quickly. Many types of lasers are available and are continuing to be studied. Epilation with the use of a high frequency or galvanic current is a safe method for the permanent removal of superfluous hair. A certain number of recurrences (20% to 35%) is inevitable even when it is done by experts. Such hairs must be removed a second time. Referral to an electrologist is suggested. These mechanical modalities should be used at least initially, even when medical treatment is planned, to achieve some early response, since medical intervention takes many months to give a noticeable response.

Attempts to cure hypertrichosis by x-rays have been proposed for almost as long as there have been x-ray devices. Permanent epilation can be effected via x-ray therapy only when sufficient exposure is given to cause subsequent permanent damage to the skin. Numerous sad cases of radiodermatitis, skin keratoses, and cancers have been produced by x-ray methods used for epilation. It should never be done.

Nonspecific suppressive therapies include oral contraceptives and glucocorticoids. Practically, these therapies suppress hirsutism resulting from adrenal or ovarian causes equally, and hence are utilized based on the individual patient's wants and needs, with particular attention to the specific side effects of each medication. In the case of a young woman who desires contraception and has no contraindications, an oral preparation with low androgenic progestins should be selected. Birth control pills are helpful in 75% of hirsute women. Glucocorticoids are indicated in the treatment of congenital adrenal hyperplasia.

Antiandrogens include cimetidine, cyproterone acetate, spironolactone, flutamide, and ketoconazole. Although generally effective, cessation of treatment is followed by recurrence. Cimetidine is a weak antiandrogen and has not been used widely. Ketoconazole improves hirsutism, but concern about hepatic toxicity and other side effects make its use impractical. The efficacy and safety of a combination of the antiandrogen cyproterone acetate combined with ethinyl estradiol has been amply proved in trials in England, Australia, France, and Holland. Cyproterone is usually given in a dose of 100 mg a day from days 5 to 14, and ethinyl estradiol 30 μg a day from day 5 through day 25. Acne and hirsutism respond best (80% to 95%) and alopecia least (50%). Strict contraception is essential. Cyproterone is not approved for use in the United States.

Spironolactone is a stronger antiandrogen than either cimetidine or cyproterone acetate. It is used in doses of 75 mg to 200 mg/day. Side effects such as metrorrhagia are commonly encountered at the higher dose levels. Used alone, it is effective in approximately half of patients, while a combination of spironolactone and oral contraceptives is effective in about three of four patients. This latter combination also limits menstrual irregularities and prevents conception. Flutamide at a dose of 250 mg/day is well tolerated and has efficacy similar to that observed with spironolactone 100 mg/day. All of the systemic treatments for hirsutism that are commonly given to women of childbearing age require strict contraception.

Finasteride, a 5-alpha-reductase inhibitor, is a useful medical therapy of hirsutism. Studies evaluating finasteride given at 5 mg per day showed it to have an effect similar to that observed with spironolactone 100 mg/day. Again this drug may cause feminization of the male fetus if exposed to the drug in utero.

Gonadotropin-releasing hormone agonists such as leuprolide and nafarelin suppress ovarian steroid production but these drugs are probably best reserved for use by gynecologists and endocrinologists.

Blankstein J, et al: Adult onset familial adrenal 21-hydroxylase deficiency. *Am J Med* 1980, 68:441.

Board JA, et al: Spironolactone and estrogen-progestin therapy for hirsutism. *South Med J* 1987, 80:483.

Braithwaite SS, et al: Hirsutism (editorial). *Arch Dermatol* 1983, 119:279.

Carpenter PC, et al: Hirsutism. *Curr Ther Endocrinol Metab* 1994, 5:237.

Chang RJ, et al: Steroid secretion in polycystic ovarian disease after ovarian suppression by long acting gonadotropin-releasing hormone agonist. *J Clin Endocrinol Metab* 1983, 56:897.

Ciotta L, et al: Treatment of hirsutism with flutamide and a low-dosage oral contraceptive in polycystic ovarian disease patients. *Fertil Steril* 1994, 62:1129.

Cusan L, et al: Comparison of flutamide and spironolactone in the treatment of hirsutism. *Fertil Steril* 1994, 61:281.

Dierickx CC, et al: Permanent hair removal by normal-mode ruby laser. *Arch Dermatol* 1998, 134:837.

Erenus M, et al: Comparison of finasteride versus spironolactone in the treatment of idiopathic hirsutism. *Fertil Steril* 1997, 68:1000.

Falsetti L, et al: Treatment of hirsutism by finasteride and flutamide in women with polycystic ovary syndrome. *Gynecol Endocrinol* 1997, 11:251.

Fine RM: Spironolactone therapy in hirsute women. *Int J Dermatol* 1989, 28:23.

Futterweit W, et al: The prevalence of hyperandrogenism in 109 consecutive female patients with diffuse alopecia. *J Am Acad Dermatol* 1988, 19:831.

Gokmen O, et al: Comparison of four different treatment regimes in hirsutism related to polycystic ovary syndrome. *Gynecol Endocrinol* 1996, 10:249.

Knochenhauer ES, et al: Advances in the diagnosis and treatment of the hirsute patient. *Curr Opin Obstet Gynecol* 1995, 7:344.

Kuttenn F, et al: Late-onset adrenal hyperplasia in hirsutism. *N Engl J Med* 1985, 313:224.

Kvedar JC, et al: Hirsutism. *J Am Acad Dermatol* 1985, 12:215.

Lucky AW: Topical antiandrogens. *Arch Dermatol* 1985, 121:55.

Lucky AW, et al: Adrenal androgen hyperresponsiveness to adrenocorticotropin in women with acne and/or hirsutism. *J Clin Endocrinol Metab* 1986, 62:840.

McKenna TJ: Pathogenesis and treatment of polycystic ovary syndrome. *N Engl J Med* 1988, 318:558.

Muderris II, et al: A comparison between two doses of flutamide (250 Mg/D and 500 Mg/D) in the treatment of hirsutism. *Fertil Steril* 1997, 68:644.

Nanni CA, et al: Laser hair removal. *J Am Acad Dermatol* 1999, 41:165.

Olsen EA: Methods of hair removal. *J Am Acad Dermatol* 1999, 40:143.

Pang S, et al: Hirsutism, polycystic ovarian disease, and ovarian 17-ketosteroid reductase deficiency. *N Engl J Med* 1987, 316:1295.

Reingold SB, et al: The relationship of mild hirsutism or acne in women to androgens. *Arch Dermatol* 1987, 123:209.

Richards RN, et al: Electroepilation (electrolysis) in hirsutism. *J Am Acad Dermatol* 1986, 15:693.

Richards RN, et al: Electrolysis. *J Am Acad Dermatol* 1995, 33:662.

Rittmaster RS: Hirsutism. *Lancet* 1997, 349:191.

Rittmaster RS, et al: Hirsutism. *Ann Intern Med* 1987, 106:95.

Schmidt JB, et al: Medroxyprogesterone acetate therapy in hirsutism. *Br J Dermatol* 1985, 113:161.

Sonino N: The use of ketoconazole as an inhibitor of steroid production. *N Engl J Med* 1987, 317:812.

Sperling LC, et al: Androgen biology as a basis for the diagnosis and treatment of androgenic disorders in women. I. *J Am Acad Dermatol* 1993, 28:669.

Sperling LC, et al: Androgen biology as a basis for the diagnosis and treatment of androgenic disorders in women. II. *J Am Acad Dermatol* 1993, 28:901.

Thomas AK, et al: The treatment of hirsutism: experience with cyproterone acetate and spironolactone. *Australas J Dermatol* 1985, 26:19.

Tope WD, et al: A hair's breath closer. *Arch Dermatol* 1998, 134:867.

Wagner RF, et al: Electrolysis and thermolysis for permanent hair removal. *J Am Acad Dermatol* 1985, 12:441.

Wheeland RG: Laser-assisted hair removal. *Dermatol Clin* 1997, 15:469.

Yucelten D, et al: Recurrence rate of hirsutism after 3 different antiandrogen therapies. *J Am Acad Dermatol* 1999, 41:64.

Zemtsov A, et al: Successful treatment of hirsutism in HAIR-AN syndrome using flutamide, spironolactone, and birth control therapy. *Arch Dermatol* 1997, 133:431. ▲

TRICHOMYCOSIS AXILLARIS

Trichomycosis axillaris is characterized by 1- to 2-mm nodules of different colors occurring on the affected hair shafts in the axillary or pubic areas (Fig. 33-27). The color of these discrete nodules attached firmly to the hair shaft may be yellow, red, or black (Fig. 33-28). Hyperhidrosis of the affected regions is usually present. A yellowish discoloration of the axillae is sometimes noted. Large numbers of corynebacterium are present in the concretions.

Treatment with topical antibiotic preparations such as topical clindamycin or erythromycin and with any modality that will decrease the hyperhidrosis is effective, but shaving is faster.

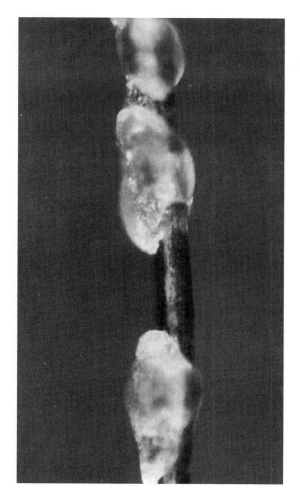

Fig. 33-27 Trichomycosis axillaris. Discrete and firmly attached nodules encircle the hair shaft. (From Freeman RG, McBride ME: *Arch Dermatol* 1969, 100:90.)

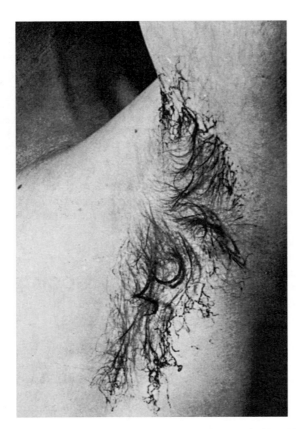

Fig. 33-28   Trichomycosis axillaris nigra of the armpit. Note black beaded hairs. (Courtesy Dr. E. Florian, Budapest.)

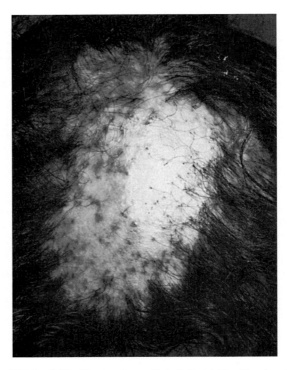

Fig. 33-29   Folliculitis decalvans. Note tufted folliculitis at periphery. (Courtesy Dr. C.P. DeFeo, Jr.)

Shelley WB, et al: Coexistent erythrasma, trichomycosis axillaris, and pitted keratolysis. *J Am Acad Dermatol* 1982, 7:752.

Shelley WB, et al: Electronmicroscopy, histochemistry, and microbiology of bacterial adhesion in trichomycosis axillaris. *J Am Acad Dermatol* 1984, 10:1005. ──────────────────────   ▲

SOME ASSOCIATED HAIR FOLLICLE DISEASES
Folliculitis Decalvans

Folliculitis decalvans is an inflammatory reaction of the hair follicles that leads to alopecia of the involved area. It is a cicatricial type of alopecia in which small pustules about the follicles, erythema, scaling, and smooth shiny depressed scars are apparent (Fig. 33-29). When the pustules have healed and scarring remains, the condition appears as pseudopelade (Fig. 33-30). This may occur not only on the scalp but on any other part of the body, such as the axillae and groin.

Tufted-hair folliculitis is a localized, inflammatory, and exudative disease of the scalp characterized by multiple hairs emerging from single follicular openings, that may result in permanent and irreversible scarring alopecia. Patients with both folliculitis decalvans and tufted hair have been reported. This latter distinctive condition is probably the end result of various inflammatory scarring processes of the scalp.

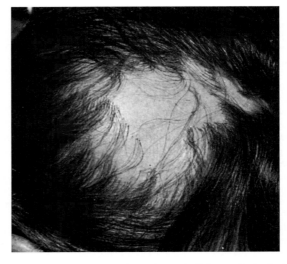

Fig. 33-30   Pseudopelade. Note intact follicles and single hairs growing.

The cause of folliculitis decalvans is unknown. Histologic findings are intrafollicular abscesses and a perifollicular infiltrate that may contain numerous plasma cells.

If a Gram stain and bacterial culture of the exudate reveals coagulase-positive staphylococci, this should be eliminated, although this may not be the primary problem; in many cases no pathogenic organism is cultured. In addition to cephalosporins, dicloxacillin, and azithromycin, rifampin may be added to the therapy to attempt to obtain better long-term control. Some feel oral zinc or vitamin C supplementation may enhance the response. Chronic inflammatory reactions may be helped by topical steroids and by the intralesional injection of triamcinolone.

Brozena SJ, et al: Folliculitis decalvans: response to rifampin. *Cutis* 1988, 42:512.
Petronic-Rosic V, et al: Tufted hair folliculitis. *J Am Acad Dermatol* 1999, 41:112.
Pujol RM, et al: Tufted-hair folliculitis. *Clin Exp Dermatol* 1991, 16:199.
Tong AK, et al: Tufted hair folliculitis. *J Am Acad Dermatol* 1989, 21:1096.

Tinea Amiantacea (Pityriasis Amiantacea)

Tinea amiantacea is an inaptly named disease manifested by thick, asbestos-like (amiantaceous), shiny scales on the scalp. The crusting may be localized or, less often, generalized over the entire scalp, and resembles psoriasis and seborrheic dermatitis. The crusts are silvery white or dull gray. The proximal parts of the hairs are matted together by the laminated crusts. There are no structural changes in the hair, but in some patches where the crusting is thick, there may be some purulent exudate under the crust and temporary alopecia such as occurs after some cases of furunculosis of the scalp.

The cause is probably a secondary infection occurring in seborrheic dermatitis or inverse psoriasis. The patient should shampoo daily or every other day with selenium sulfide suspension, or a tar shampoo, for a couple of weeks. Prior application of Baker's P & S liquid a few hours before shampooing facilitates removal of the scales and crusts. Derma-Smoothe and FS shampoo are also effective.

Ring DS, et al: Pityriasis amiantacea. *Arch Dermatol* 1993, 129:913.

Keratosis Follicularis Contagiosa

Keratosis follicularis contagiosa, also known as *epidemic acne, epidemic follicular eruption, epidemic follicular keratosis,* and *Brooke's disease,* is a disease of unknown etiologic factors that resembles keratosis follicularis and occurs in children.

The eruption is widespread and symmetrical, affecting chiefly the back of the neck, the shoulders, and the extensor surfaces of the extremities. The onset is acute, may affect large numbers of patients in a localized geographic area, and spontaneously involutes over a 3- to 6-week period. There is a horny thickening of these areas, especially pronounced about the follicles, where small black corneous plugs may be discerned. The cause has been hypothesized to be infectious but remains unproved.

Bowers RE: Epidemic follicular eruption. *Proc R Soc Med* 1952, 45:459.

Folliculitis Nares Perforans

Perforating folliculitis of the nose is characterized by small pustules near the tip of the inside of the nose. The lesion becomes crusted, and when the crust is removed it is found that the bulbous end of the affected vibrissa is embedded in the inspissated material. The affected hairs are typical of those occurring inside the nostril. *Staphylococcus aureus* may at times be cultured from the pustules. The hair should be removed, and antibiotic ointment such as mupirocin applied.

Perforating Folliculitis

Perforating folliculitis is characterized by an asymptomatic eruption of erythematous follicular papules 2 to 8 mm in diameter involving the extensor surfaces of the upper arms, the buttocks, or the upper thighs. When the small, whitish keratotic plug is removed from the follicular papule, a small bleeding crater remains behind.

The histologic examination shows a widely dilated hair follicle in which keratinous debris is encrusted. The follicular epithelium is perforated through with eosinophilic elastic fibers. Degenerated nuclei of inflammatory cells and necrotic connective tissue enter into the hair follicle just above the level of the sebaceous gland. A mild pseudoepitheliomatous hyperplasia surrounds the area of perforation.

Perforating folliculitis is resistant to treatment. Topical tretinoin (Retin-A) is reported to be effective. Rubio et al reported an HIV-infected man who responded well to thalidomide.

Patterson JW: The perforating disorders. *J Am Acad Dermatol* 1984, 10:561.
Rubio FA, et al: Perforating folliculitis. *J Am Acad Dermatol* 1999, 40:300.

Kyrle's Disease

This eponymic designation has handily supplanted the original title, hyperkeratosis follicularis et parafollicularis in cutem penetrans. Kyrle's disease is a rare disorder characterized by hyperkeratosis, which forms a horny cone that projects into the dermis, so that when it is removed a pitlike depression remains. Usually the papules are discrete, but they may coalesce to form circinate plaques. There is a predilection for the lower extremities (Figs. 33-31 and 33-32), but the upper extremities, head, and neck may also be involved. Coalescing verrucous plaques are frequently seen, especially on the lower extremities. Koebner's phenomenon may also be observed, in which case plaques or elevated verrucous streaks are formed. The latter are seen only in the antecubital and popliteal spaces. Atrophic scars are seen on involution of these lesions. The disease occurs almost exclusively in adults ages 20 to 63, with no sex or racial differences noted. Kyrle's disease has been noted to be associated especially with diabetes mellitus.

Histologically, Kyrle's disease shows large keratotic and parakeratotic plugs penetrating through the epidermis into the dermis. These plugs cause an inflammatory and foreign-body giant cell reaction about the lower end of the plug in the dermis. Mild degenerative changes in the connective tissue with no increase in the elastic tissue also occur.

Kyrle's disease remains stationary for years, with possible clearing of lesions when the associated illness has been controlled. Ultraviolet treatment, methotrexate, topical corticosteroids, 5-fluorouracil, and keratolytics are usually ineffective. Methotrexate is also ineffective. Topical retinoic acid (0.1% cream), isotretinoin, and etretinate have been effective in flattening lesions.

Cunningham SR, et al: Kyrle's disease. *J Am Acad Dermatol* 1987, 16:117.
Salomon RJ, et al: Kyrle's disease and hepatic insufficiency. *Arch Dermatol* 1986, 122:18. ————————————————— ▲

Reactive Perforating Collagenosis

Reactive perforating collagenosis is presented here because of its great similarity to perforating folliculitis and Kyrle's disease. It was described by Mehregan et al as pinhead-sized, skin-colored papules that grow to a diameter of 4 to 6 mm and develop a central area of umbilication in which keratinous material is lodged. The discrete papules may be numerous and involve sites of frequent trauma such as the backs of the hands, forearms, elbows, and knees. The lesion reaches a maximum size of about 6 mm in 4 weeks and then regresses spontaneously in 6 to 8 weeks.

It is believed that this is caused by a peculiar reaction of the skin to superficial trauma. Koebnerization is often observed. Young children are most frequently affected. Most reports support an autosomal recessive mode of inheritance; however, a family in which it appeared to be inherited by autosomal dominance has been reported.

Histologically, the epidermis becomes edematous, the granular layer disappears, and parakeratosis develops. Eventually the epidermis becomes atrophic, with disruption of the sites over the papillae. Through these sites necrobiotic connective tissue, degenerating inflammatory cells, and collagen bundles are extruded into a cup-shaped epidermal depression.

No specific treatment is indicated, since the lesions involute spontaneously. Tretinoin 0.1% cream may be effective.

Bang SW, et al: Acquired reactive perforating collagenosis. *J Am Acad Dermatol* 1997, 36:778.

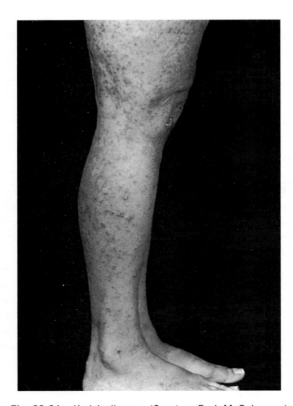

Fig. 33-31 Kyrle's disease. (Courtesy Dr. L.M. Solomon.)

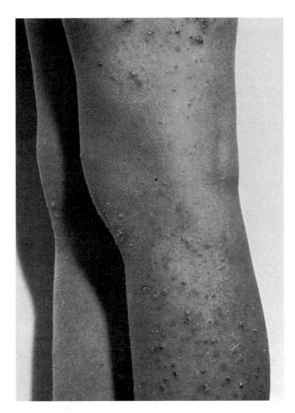

Fig. 33-32 Kyrle's disease.

Briggs PL, et al: Reactive perforating collagenosis of diabetes mellitus. *J Am Acad Dermatol* 1995, 32:521.

Faver IR, et al: Acquired reactive perforating collagenosis. *J Am Acad Dermatol* 1994, 30:575.

Kumar V, et al: Familial reactive perforating collagenosis. *J Dermatol* 1998, 25:54.

Tay YK, et al: Reactive perforating collagenosis in Treacher Collins syndrome. *J Am Acad Dermatol* 1996, 35:982. ▲

Perforating Disease of Hemodialysis

The relationship of Kyrle's disease, perforating folliculitis, and perforating collagenosis to chronic renal failure, especially of the type secondary to diabetic vasculopathy, is uncertain. Many cases of perforating lesions in patients with this condition have been reported variably as perforating folliculitis, Kyrle's disease, or reactive perforating collagenosis. Some patients may exhibit overlap of histopathologic features both between lesion and within individual lesions. Patterson, after reviewing the reports of perforating disease in chronic renal failure, proposed that they not be subclassified further, but simply placed into a category of acquired perforating disease, which would include perforating folliculitis, Kyrle's disease, and most cases of adult acquired reactive perforating collagenosis, with or without renal failure, diabetes mellitus, or both.

The reports of perforating disorders associated with chronic renal failure indicate that between 4% and 10% of dialysis patients develop them. Such lesions are characterized by dome-shaped papules on the legs, or less often on the trunk, neck, arms, or scalp, with variable itchiness (Fig. 33-33). Early lesions may be pustular; late lesions resemble prurigo nodularis both clinically and histologically. The disease may remit promptly after a renal transplant and stopping dialysis. Otherwise topical tretinoin may be tried.

Hood AF, et al: Kyrle's disease in patients with chronic renal failure. *Arch Dermatol* 1982, 118:85.

Patterson JW: The perforating disorders. *J Am Acad Dermatol* 1984, 10:561.

Rapini RP, et al: Acquired perforating dermatosis. *Arch Dermatol* 1989, 125:1074.

Sehgal VN, et al: Perforating dermatoses. *J Dermatol* 1993, 20:329. ▲

Traumatic Anserine Folliculosis

Traumatic anserine folliculosis is a curious gooseflesh-like follicular hyperkeratosis that may result from persistent pressure and lateral friction of one skin surface on another. Such friction is often caused by habitual pressure of elbows, chin or jaw, or neck, often while watching television. Two thirds of patients who develop this are atopic.

Padilha-Gonalves A: Traumatic anserine folliculosis. *J Dermatol* 1979, 6:365. ▲

Erythromelanosis Follicularis Faciei et Colli

Erythromelanosis follicularis faciei et colli is a unique erythematous pigmentary disease involving the follicles. A reddish brown, sharply demarcated, symmetrical discoloration involves the preauricular and maxillary regions. At times the pigmentation may be blotchy. In addition, follicular papules and erythema are present. Under diascopic pressure the reddish brown area, containing telangiectases, becomes pale and the light brown pigmentation becomes more apparent. Pityriasiform scaling and slight

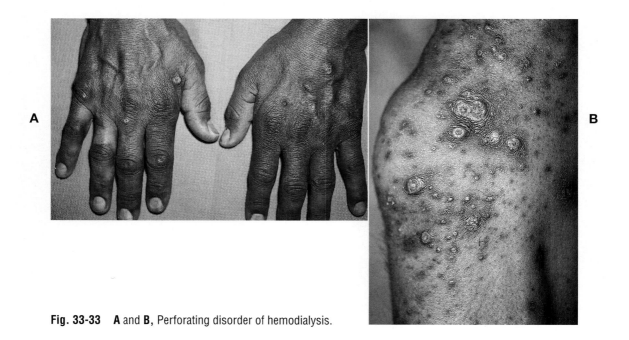

Fig. 33-33 **A** and **B**, Perforating disorder of hemodialysis.

itching may occur. Keratosis pilaris on the arms and shoulders is frequently found. It preferentially affects Asian patients.

Histologically, a slight hyperkeratosis occurs, with epidermal hyperpigmentation. The hair follicles are enlarged, especially in the infundibular areas. The sebaceous glands are also hypertrophic. A lymphocytic infiltration surrounds the adnexa.

McGillis ST, et al: Unilateral erythromelanosis follicularis faciei et colli in a young girl. *J Am Acad Dermatol* 1991, 25:430.

Sodaify M, et al: Erythromelanosis follicularis faciei et colli. *Int J Dermatol* 1994, 33:643.

Watt TL, et al: Erythromelanosis follicularis faciei et colli. *J Am Acad Dermatol* 1981, 5:533. _____ ▲

Disseminate and Recurrent Infundibulofolliculitis

Hitch and Lund described a disseminate follicular eruption on the torso of a black man that seemed to involve all the pilosebaceous structures. The lesions were irregularly shaped papules pierced by a hair. They likened the eruption to cutis anserina viewed through a magnifying glass. The eruption is mildly pruritic at times, and is chronic, with recurrent exacerbations. The papules are uniform, 1 or 2 mm in diameter, and involve all the follicles in the affected areas, which are usually the upper trunk and neck (Fig. 33-34), though the entire trunk and proximal extremities may be involved. Rarely, pustules may occur.

Histologically, the infundibular portion of the follicles was chiefly affected, and the lesions were inflammatory rather than hyperkeratotic. Edema, lymphocytic and neutrophilic infiltration, and slight fibroblastic infiltration surround the affected follicles.

Treatment with vitamin A has been reported to be effective; isotretinoin or etretinate may also be useful.

Hitch JM, et al: Disseminate and recurrent infundibulofolliculitis. *Arch Dermatol* 1968, 97:432.

Owen WR, et al: Disseminate and recurrent infundibulofolliculitis. *Arch Dermatol* 1979, 115:174. _____ ▲

Lichen Spinulosus

Lichen spinulosus (keratosis spinulosa, lichen pilaris seu spinulosus) is a disease chiefly of children and is characterized by minute filiform horny spines, which protrude from follicular openings independent of any papules (Fig. 33-35). The spines are discrete and grouped. The lesions appear in crops and are symmetrically distributed over the trunk, limbs, and buttocks (acne corne). There is a predilection for the neck, buttocks, abdominal wall, popliteal spaces, and the extensor surfaces of the arms. A generalized distribution has been reported to be a clue to underlying HIV infection. Little or no itching is present.

Histologic evaluation shows simple inflammatory changes and follicular hyperkeratosis. The lesions respond to mild keratolytics, such as 3% resorcin or salicylic acid ointment. Keralyt gel, Lac-Hydrin lotion, and tretinoin are other alternatives.

Cohen SJ, et al: Generalized lichen spinulosus in an HIV-positive man. *J Am Acad Dermatol* 1991, 25:116.

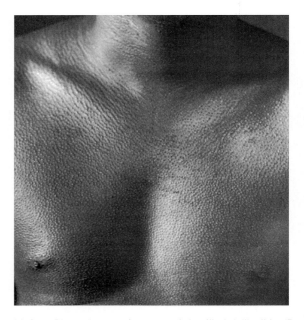

Fig. 33-34 Disseminate and recurrent infundibulofolliculitis. (From Hitch JM, Lund HZ: *Arch Dermatol* 1968, 97:432.)

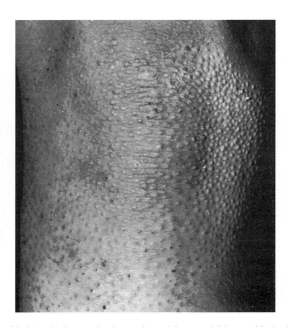

Fig. 33-35 Lichen spinulosus in a 14-year-old boy with lesions predominantly on the elbows and knees.

Friedman SJ: Lichen spinulosus. *J Am Acad Dermatol* 1990, 22:261.

Resnick SD, et al: Acne conglobata and a generalized lichen spinulosus-like eruption in a man seropositive for human immunodeficiency virus. *J Am Acad Dermatol* 1992, 26:1013. _____ ▲

DISORDERS OF THE SWEAT GLANDS
Hyperhidrosis

Hyperhidrosis, or excessive sweating, may be localized to one or several areas or it may be more generalized. True generalized hyperhidrosis is rare, and even hyperhidrosis caused by systemic diseases is usually accentuated in certain regions.

Palmoplantar Hyperhidrosis (Emotional Hyperhidrosis).
This type of hyperhidrosis is usually localized to the palms (Fig. 33-36) and soles or axillae, and may be worse during warm temperatures. Patients with palm and sole hyperhidrosis may also have axillary hyperhidrosis, but only 25% of patients with axillary hyperhidrosis have palmoplantar hyperhidrosis. The hands may be cold and show a dusky hue. The soggy keratin of the hyperhidrotic soles is frequently affected by pitted keratolysis and has a foul odor. Sweating may be constant or intermittent. If constant, usually emotion is not as important. If intermittent it may be triggered by anxiety, stress, or fear. This type of sweating can be autosomal dominantly inherited in some cases.

Gustatory Hyperhidrosis. Certain individuals regularly experience excessive sweating of the forehead, upper lip, perioral region, or sternum a few moments after eating spicy foods, tomato sauce, chocolate, coffee, tea, or hot soups. Gustatory sweating may also be caused by hyperactivity of the sympathetic nerves (Pancoast's tumor or postoperatively), sensory neuropathy (diabetes mellitus or subsequent

to zoster), parotitis or parotid abscess, and surgery or injury of the parotid gland (auriculotemporal syndrome of von Frey). Frey's syndrome occurs in one third or more of patients following parotid surgery. Fortunately, only 10% of affected patients require treatment.

Other Localized Forms of Hyperhidrosis. Localized sweating can occur over lesions of blue rubber bleb nevus, glomus tumors, hemangiomas (sudoriferous hemangioma), and in POEMS syndrome, Gopalan's syndrome, complex regional pain syndrome, as a result of spinal cord tumors (especially when unilateral palmar hyperhidrosis is the complaint), and pachydermoperiostosis.

Generalized Hyperhidrosis. Generalized hyperhidrosis may be induced by a hot, humid environment such as a tropical milieu, or by febrile diseases, or vigorous exercise. Hormonal disturbances such as hyperthyroidism, acromegaly, diabetes mellitus, pregnancy, and menopause may also produce generalized hyperhidrosis. Additional causes of hyperhidrosis include concussion, Parkinson's disease, other disturbances of the sympathetic nervous system, and metastatic tumors producing a complete transection of the spinal cord. Pheochromocytoma, hypoglycemia, salicylism, and lymphoma are other causes.

TREATMENT. The therapy of generalized hyperhidrosis is aimed at treating the underlying systemic disease. Virtually all cases of hyperhidrosis seen by dermatologists are of the palmoplantar or axillary types, and the treatments discussed below relate primarily to these conditions.

Topical medication. Topical aluminum chloride or aluminum chlorhydroxide are the most commonly used agents for hyperhidrosis. For the axillae, application of a 20% to 25% solution nightly to a very dry axilla (blown dry with a

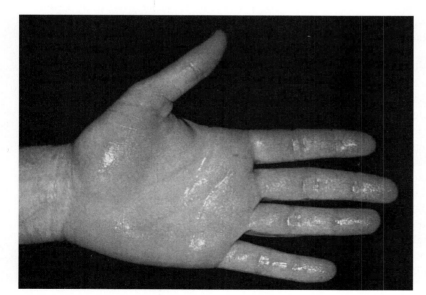

Fig. 33-36 Hyperhidrosis.

hair dryer) is usually very effective. Occlusion is usually not required. Some experts say that routine deodorant use should be avoided; baking soda should be used instead. In palmar hyperhidrosis the application of 20% aluminum chloride tincture nightly, occluded with plastic gloves, has produced good results for some patients but is less effective than the same technique in the axilla. If topical treatment is effective when performed nightly, the frequency may be reduced to as little as once or twice weekly with continued benefit. Topical formaldehyde and glutaraldehyde, which can sensitize and tan the skin respectively, are not routinely recommended.

Iontophoresis. Iontophoresis with plain tap water is an alternative for patients for whom topical treatments fail. It is frequently effective, using either a Drionic device or a Fischer unit. Treatments generally require 20- to 30-minute sessions daily or twice daily, with current flowing through water-soaked pads. Once response has occurred, treatments may be used intermittently (as little as once every 2 weeks) for maintenance. Use of glycopyrrolate 0.01% and aluminum chloride 2% in the iontophoresis medium may hasten the response.

Botulinum A toxin. Injection of Botox into 4 cm^2 areas into the palms, soles, or axillae dramatically reduces sweating at the treated areas to at least 25% and often to less than 10% of baseline rates. Complications are rare but include some grip weakness when higher doses are used. This problem, expense, and the painful injections limit its use. The hypohidrosis continues for up to 5 months. Axillary hyperhidrosis is reduced, but patients do not report reduction in axillary malodor. This form of treatment may be offered to all patients who fail topical treatments before surgical modalities are considered. This form of treatment may also be considered for other rare forms of localized hyperhidrosis.

Internal medication. The use of anticholinergic agents such as Pro-Banthine or glycopyrrolate may be helpful. The dosage of each is regulated by the patient's tolerance and response. Often, sweating is suppressed somewhat just as anticholinergic side effects reach intolerable levels, and this approach has to be abandoned. Side effects of acetylcholine-blocking agents may also cause or aggravate such conditions as glaucoma and convulsions. The effects on sweating generally last 4 to 6 hours, and many patients prefer to use the medication to ensure dryness for special occasions only rather than as continuous treatment. Other agents reported to reduce localized hyperhidrosis are diltiazem and clonidine.

Surgical treatment. Upper thoracic sympathectomy has been found to be effective in excessive palmar sweating when all other measures have failed. Sympathetic denervation of the upper extremities is performed via endoscopy by resection of the second thoracic sympathetic ganglion (for the hands). Sweating of the hands is stopped completely. Only two of three patients are satisfied, however, since

compensatory and gustatory hyperhidrosis occurs in more than two thirds of patients.

Axillary hyperhidrosis has been effectively controlled by the excision of the most actively sweating portion of the axillary skin, followed by undercutting and subcutaneous resection of the sweat glands for 1 to 2 cm on each side of the elliptical excision. This procedure is virtually always effective. The most important preoperative consideration is the accurate mapping of the most active sweating areas of the axillae. The responsible eccrine glands are not necessarily located in the same areas as the axillary hair and may be in a reasonably limited area, making the surgery less difficult.

Anhidrosis (Hypohidrosis)

Anhidrosis is the absence of sweating. Hypohidrosis, or reduced sweating, is part of the spectrum of these disorders. Dysfunction in any step in the normal physiologic process of sweating can lead to decreased or absent sweating. It may be localized or generalized. Generalized anhidrosis occurs in anhidrotic ectodermal dysplasia, quinacrine anhidrosis, miliaria profunda (tropic asthenia), Sjögren's syndrome, hereditary sensory neuropathy (type IV) with anhidrosis, and in some patients with diabetic neuropathy, and multiple myeloma. Atopic dermatitis is frequently associated with reduced sweating and pruritus when sweating is triggered. Patients with psoriasis may have similar symptoms, but less frequently.

Anhidrosis with pruritus is a rare syndrome of young adults. Patients present with severe itching whenever they attempt to sweat. No sweat is delivered to the skin surface, but when the body temperature is raised about 0.5° C, fine papules appear at each eccrine orifice. The associated pruritus is so severe that the patients feel completely incapacitated and distracted. Cooling immediately resolves the symptoms. This may represent one form of tropical asthenia. The natural history is unknown, but spontaneous resolution may occur after several years. These patients are frequently misdiagnosed as having cholinergic urticaria.

Segmental anhidrosis may be associated with tonic pupils (Holmes-Adie syndrome); this is called *Ross syndrome.* Patients have heat intolerance and segmental areas of anhidrosis on the trunk arms, or legs. Loss of deep tendon reflexes in the arms, trunk, and legs is consistently seen. Compensatory segmental hyperhidrosis of functionally intact areas may occur.

Anhidrosis localized to skin lesions occurs regularly over plaques of tuberculoid leprosy. This is also true of segmental vitiligo (but not generalized type), in the hypopigmented streaks of incontinentia pigmenti, and on the face and neck of patients with the rare syndrome of follicular atrophoderma, basal cell carcinomas, and hypotrichosis, a rare X-linked dominant disorder.

Bromidrosis

Also known as *fetid sweat* and *malodorous sweating,* bromidrosis is chiefly encountered in the axillae. It is considered to be caused by bacterial decomposition of apocrine sweat, producing fatty acids with distinctive offensive odors. Often, patients who complain of offensive axillary sweat actually have no offensive odor; the complaint represents a delusion, paranoia, phobia, or a lesion of the central nervous system. Intranasal foreign body and chronic mycotic infection in the sinuses are additional causes. True bromidrosis is usually not recognized by the patient.

Fish odor syndrome should be considered in patients presenting with complaints of offensive odor. It is caused by excretion of trimethylamine (which smells like rotten fish) in the eccrine sweat, urine, saliva, and other secretions. This chemical is produced from carnitine and choline in the diet and is normally metabolized in the liver. An autosomal dominant defect in the ability to metabolize trimethylamine is the cause of this syndrome. Dietary reduction of foods high in carnitine and choline is beneficial.

Antibacterial soaps and many commercial deodorants are quite effective in controlling axillary malodor. Frequent bathing, changing of underclothes, shaving of the axillae, and topical application of aluminum chloride (Drysol) are all helpful measures. Surgical removal of the glands is possible, as in axillary hyperhidrosis, but this is very rarely indicated.

Plantar bromidrosis is produced by bacterial action on eccrine sweat-macerated stratum corneum. Hyperhidrosis is the chief associated factor, and pitted keratolysis is often present. Careful washing with an antibacterial soap and the use of dusting powders on the feet are helpful in eliminating bromidrosis. Use of topical antibiotics, such as clindamycin, may be beneficial. Previously described measures to control plantar hyperhidrosis should be instituted.

Chromhidrosis

Chromhidrosis, or colored sweat, is an exceedingly rare functional disorder of the apocrine sweat glands, frequently localized to the face or axilla. It has been less frequently noted on the abdomen, chest, thighs, groin, genitalia, and lower eyelids. The colored sweat may be yellow (most common), blue, green, or black. The colored secretion appears in response to adrenergic stimuli, which cause myoepithelial contractions. Colored apocrine sweat fluoresces and is caused by lipofuscin.

Eccrine chromhidrosis is caused by the coloring of the clear eccrine sweat by dyes, pigments, or metals on the skin surface. Examples are the blue-green sweat seen in copper workers and the "red sweat" seen in flight attendants from the red dye in the labels in life-vests. Brownish staining of the axillae and undershirt may occur in ochronosis. Bile secretion in eccrine sweat occurs in patients with liver failure and marked hyperbilirubinemia. Small, round, brown or deep-green macules occur on the palms and soles.

Fox-Fordyce Disease

Fox-Fordyce disease is rare, occurring mostly in women during adolescence or soon afterward. It is characterized by conical, flesh-colored or grayish, intensely pruritic, discrete follicular papules in areas where apocrine glands occur. The axillae (Fig. 33-37) and areolae (Fig. 33-38) are the primary sites of involvement, but the umbilicus, pubes, labia majora, and perineum may be affected. Apocrine sweating does not occur in affected areas, and hair density may be decreased. In some cases there is no itching. Ninety percent of cases occur in women between ages 13 and 35, but cases can occur postmenopausally or in males. Pregnancy invariably leads to improvement.

Histologically, Fox-Fordyce disease is characterized by obstruction of the follicular ostia by orthokeratotic cells. An inflammatory infiltrate of lymphocytes surrounds the upper third of the hair follicles and upper dermal vessels. There is an associated spongiosis of the infundibulum at the site of entrance of the apocrine duct into the hair follicle.

Treatment of Fox-Fordyce disease is difficult, and no form of therapy is universally effective. Estrogen therapy, usually in the form of oral contraceptive pills, is most

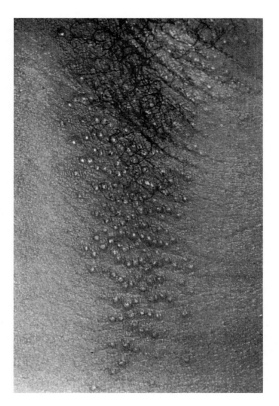

Fig. 33-37 Fox-Fordyce disease in the axilla.

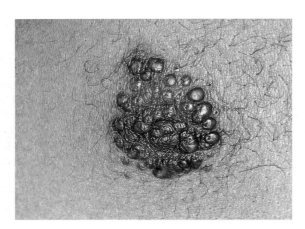

Fig. 33-38 Fox-Fordyce disease of the nipple.

uniformly effective. Topical tretinoin, topical and intralesional steroids, topical antibiotics (neomycin and clindamycin solution), oral retinoids (isotretinoin), and UV phototherapy (quartz light) have all been effective in small numbers of patients.

Granulosis Rubra Nasi

Granulosis rubra nasi is a rare familial disease of children, occurring on the nose, cheeks, and chin. It is characterized by diffuse redness, persistent hyperhidrosis, and small dark red papules that disappear on diascopic pressure. The tip of the nose is red or violet. There may be a few small pustules. The hyperhidrosis precedes the erythema. The tip of the nose is cold and is not infiltrated. The disease disappears spontaneously at puberty without leaving any traces. The cause is unknown. Histologically, blood vessels are dilated and there is an inflammatory infiltrate about the sweat ducts.

Treatment is with local preparations for relief of the inflammation, and reassurance that with puberty there is usually involution of the process.

Hidradenitis

Hidradenitis is a term used to describe diseases in which the histologic abnormality is primarily an inflammatory infiltrate around the eccrine glands. This group includes neutrophilic eccrine hidradenitis and idiopathic plantar hidradenitis (recurrent palmoplantar hidradenitis).

Neutrophilic Eccrine Hidradenitis. Neutrophilic eccrine hidradenitis (NEH) has been described primarily in patients with acute myelogenous leukemia, usually beginning about 10 days after chemotherapy begins. It has not been uniformly linked to a single chemotherapeutic agent. The lesions are typically erythematous and edematous papules and plaques of the extremities, trunk, face (periorbital), and palms (in decreasing frequency). Fever and neutropenia are often present. Lesions resolve over 1 to 4 weeks (average, 10 days). Dapsone may be therapeutic. Histologically, there

is a dense neutrophilic infiltrate around and infiltrating eccrine glands. Necrosis of sweat glands may be present, with or without the inflammatory infiltrate. Syringosquamous metaplasia may occur. This finding can also occur in fibrosing alopecia, in burn scars, adjacent to various nonmelanoma skin cancers and ischemic and surgical ulcers, in alopecia mucinosa, and in ports of radiation therapy.

Infectious neutrophilic hidradenitis may present as a recurrent, pruritic, papular eruption. *Serratia, Enterobacter cloacae,* and *Staphylococcus aureus* have been implicated, and appropriate antibiotics are curative. The diagnosis is confirmed by histologic evaluation and culture of affected tissue (surface cultures may not be adequate).

Recurrent Palmoplantar Hidradenitis. Recurrent palmoplantar hidradenitis is primarily a disorder of healthy children and young adults. Lesions are primarily painful, subcutaneous nodules on the plantar surface, resembling erythema nodosum (Fig. 33-39). Rarely, palmar lesions also occur. Children may present refusing to walk because of plantar pain. The condition is typically recurrent, and may be triggered by ambulation.

The use of oral and topical steroidal preparations may be beneficial.

Dann EJ, et al: Familial generalized anhidrosis. *Isr J Med Sci* 1990, 26:451.

Domingues JC, et al: Congenital sensory neuropathy with anhidrosis. *Pediatr Dermatol* 1994, 11:231.

Freeman R, et al: Autonomic neurodermatology. *Semin Neurol* 1992, 12:394.

Goh, CL: Aluminum chloride hexahydrate versus palmar hyperhidrosis. *Cutis* 1990, 29:368.

Heckmann M, et al: Optimizing botulinum toxin therapy for hyperhidrosis. *Br J Dermatol* 1998, 138:544.

Herbst F, et al: Endoscopic thoracic sympathectomy for primary hyperhidrosis of the upper limbs. *Ann Surg* 1994, 220:86.

Huang CL, et al: Acquired generalized hypohidrosis/anhidrosis with subclinical Sjögren's syndrome. *J Am Acad Dermatol* 1996, 35:350.

Hurt MA, et al: Eccrine squamous syringometaplasia. *Arch Dermatol* 1990, 126:73.

James WD, et al: Emotional eccrine sweating. *Arch Dermatol* 1987, 123:925.

Kanzaki T, et al: Bile pigment deposition at sweat pores of patients with liver disease. *J Am Acad Dermatol* 1992, 26:655.

Kay DM, et al: Pruritus and acquired anhidrosis. *Arch Dermatol* 1969, 100:291.

Lillis PJ, et al: Liposuction for treatment of axillary hyperhidrosis. *Dermatol Clin* 1990, 8:479.

Miller ML, et al: Fox-Fordyce disease treated with topical clindamycin solution. *Arch Dermatol* 1995, 131:1112.

Naumann M, et al: Focal hyperhidrosis. *Arch Dermatol* 1998, 134:301.

Reinauer S, et al: Ross syndrome. *J Am Acad Dermatol* 1993, 28:308.

Rufli T, et al: Localized unilateral hyperhidrosis. *Dermatology* 1992, 184:298.

Ruocco V, et al: Fish-odor syndrome. *Int J Dermatol* 1995, 34:92.

Sato K, et al: Biology of sweat glands and their disorders. I and II. *J Am Acad Dermatol* 1989, 20:537, 713.

Schnider P: Double-blind trial of botulinum A toxin for the treatment of focal hyperhidrosis of the palms. *Br J Dermatol* 1997, 136:548.

Scully RE, et al: Case records of the MGH: small unmyelinated fiber with chronic anhidrosis. *N Engl J Med* 1994, 331:259.

Seline PC, et al: Cutaneous metastases from a chondroblastoma initially presenting as unilateral palmar hyperhidrosis. *J Am Acad Dermatol* 1999, 40:325.

Shear NH, et al: Dapsone in prevention of recurrent neutrophilic hidradenitis. *J Am Acad Dermatol* 1996, 35:819.

Shen JL, et al: A new strategy of iontophoresis for hyperhidrosis. *J Am Acad Dermatol* 1990, 22:239.

Wenzel FG, et al: Nonneoplastic disorder of the eccrine glands. *J Am Acad Dermatol* 1998, 38:1. _____ ▲

DISEASES OF THE NAILS

Several general references are available that review a wide spectrum of nail changes discussed below.

Barnett JM, et al: Nail cosmetics. *Dermatol Clin* 1991, 9:9.

Bodman MA: Miscellaneous nail presentations. *Clin Podiatr Med Surg* 1995, 12:327.

Cohen PR, et al: Geriatric nail disorders: diagnosis and treatment. *J Am Acad Dermatol* 1992, 26:521.

Cohen PR, et al: Nail disease and dermatology. *J Am Acad Dermatol* 1989, 21:1020.

Cohen PR, et al: The lunula. *J Am Acad Dermatol* 1996, 34:943.

Jemec GB, et al: Nail abnormalities in nondermatologic patients: prevalence and possible role as diagnostic aids. *J Am Acad Dermatol* 1995, 32:977.

Telfer NR: Congenital and hereditary nail disorders. *Semin Dermatol* 1991, 10:2. _____ ▲

Nail-Associated Dermatoses

Numerous dermatoses are associated with characteristic, sometimes specific, nail changes. Many are considered elsewhere.

Lichen Planus of Nails. The reported incidence of nail involvement in lichen planus varies from less than 1% to 10%. Lichen planus of the nails may occur without skin changes, but 25% with nail disease will have lichen planus at other locations. Although it may occur at any age, most commonly it begins during the fifth or sixth decade of life. The various nail changes are irregular longitudinal grooving and ridging of the nail plate, thinning of the nail plate, pterygium formation, shedding of the nail plate with atrophy of the nail bed, subungual keratosis, and subungual hyperpigmentation (Figs. 33-40 and 33-41). The plate may be markedly thinned, and at times distinct papules of lichen planus may involve the nail bed. Twenty-nail dystrophy may be the sole manifestation of lichen planus.

The histologic changes of lichen planus may be evident in any individual nail constituent or a combination of them. The one most frequently involved is the matrix.

Treatment is mostly unsatisfactory. Intralesional injection of corticosteroids has been of little help in our patients. Polyethylene occlusive dressings are also inadequate in our experience. Oral prednisone (0.5 mg/kg for

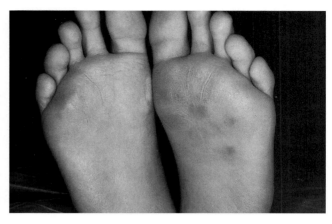

Fig. 33-39 Recurrent palmoplantar hidradenitis.

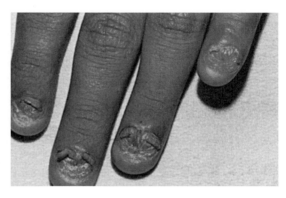

Fig. 33-40 Lichen planus of the nails in a 9-year-old boy with an atrophic patch on his scalp consistent with lichen planus. (Courtesy Dr. H. Bogaert Diaz, Dominican Republic.)

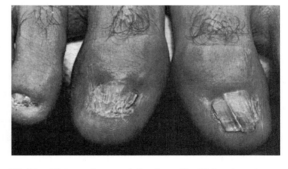

Fig. 33-41 Lichen planus of the toenails. Note almost complete absence of right great toenail, conspicuous longitudinal ridging of left great toenail. (From Ronchese F: *Arch Dermatol* 1965, 91:347.)

3 weeks) has been successful in some cases. Oral retinoids in combination with topical steroids applied to the involved sites have been successful in some. Early treatment is mandatory. (See Chapter 12 for additional therapeutic considerations.)

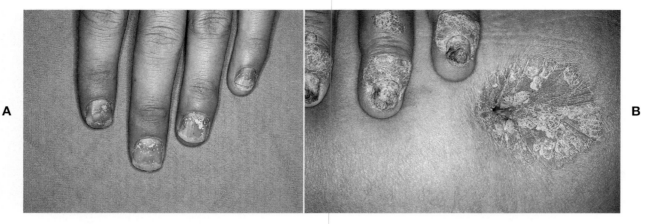

Fig. 33-42 Psoriasis of the nails. **A,** Note pitting, onycholysis, and subungual keratosis. **B,** Severe nail psoriasis and umbilical involvement.

Joshi RK, et al: Lichen planus of the nails presenting as trachyonychia. *Int J Dermatol* 1993, 32:54.

Kato N, et al: Isolated lichen planus of the nails treated with etretinate. *J Dermatol* 1993, 20:577.

Peluso AM, et al: Lichen planus limited to the nails in childhood: case report and literature review. *Pediatr Dermatol* 1993, 10:36.

Perez Oliva N, et al: Lichen planus of the nails. *Cutis* 1993, 52:171.

Taniguchi S, et al: Twenty-nail dystrophy (trachyonychia) caused by lichen planus in a patient with alopecia universalis and ichthyosis vulgaris. *J Am Acad Dermatol* 1995, 33:903.

Tosti A, et al: Nail lichen planus: clinical and pathologic study of twenty-four patients. *J Am Acad Dermatol* 1993, 28:724. ▲

Psoriatic Nails. Nail involvement in psoriasis is common, with reported incidences varying from 10% to 50%. In the nail plate there may be pits, or much less often, furrows or transverse depressions (Beau's lines), crumbling nail plate, or leukonychia, with a rough or smooth surface (Fig. 33-42). In the nail bed splinter hemorrhages are found, reddish discoloration of a part or all of the nail bed, and horny masses. In the hyponychium yellowish green discoloration may occur in the area of onycholysis. Up to 86.5% of patients with psoriatic arthritis will have psoriatic nail changes. Pustular psoriasis may produce onycholysis, with lakes of pus in the nail bed or in the perionychial areas. Rarely, anonychia may result. Other papulosquamous diseases may affect the nails like psoriasis. Reiter's disease, pityriasis rubra pilaris, Sézary syndrome, and acrokeratosis paraneoplastica produce as a rule hypertrophic nails with subungual hyperkeratosis.

Treatment of psoriatic nails is difficult; all therapies have limitations, and the condition is frequently mistaken for onychomycosis. Intralesional injection of triamcinolone acetonide suspension, 3 to 5 mg/ml, with a 30-gauge needle is frequently helpful; however, it is quite painful, and the condition soon recurs. Topical 1% 5-fluorouracil solution under the nails has been reported to be helpful. Methotrexate, PUVA, cyclosporine, or acitretin may be effective. Psoriatic nail disease may be only one area involved; the eventual treatment options selected depend on the degree of cutaneous and nail involvement. (See Chapter 10 for additional information and therapeutic options.)

de Jong EM, et al: Psoriasis of the nails associated with disability in a large number of patients: results of a recent interview with 1,728 patients. *Dermatology* 1996, 193:300.

Larko O: Problem sites: scalp, palm, and sole, and nail. *Dermatol Clin* 1995, 13:771.

Lavaroni G, et al: The nails in psoriatic arthritis. *Acta Derm Venereol Suppl* 1994, 186:113. ▲

Darier's Disease. Longitudinal, subungual, red or white streaks, associated with distal wedge-shaped subungual keratoses, are the nail signs diagnostic for Darier-White disease. Keratotic papules on the dorsal portion of the nail fold clinically may resemble acrokeratosis verruciformis but histologically have features of Darier's disease. Other nail findings include splinter hemorrhages and leukonychia. All of these findings are less pronounced on the toenails.

Clubbing

Clubbing is divided into two types: idiopathic and acquired, or secondary. The changes occur not only in the nails but also in the terminal phalanges. The nails bulge and are curved in a convex arc in both transverse and longitudinal directions, like a watch crystal. The eponychium is thickened. The angle formed by the dorsal surface of the distal phalanx and the nail plate (Lovibond's angle) is approximately 160 degrees; however, with clubbing this angle is obliterated and becomes 180 degrees or greater. The soft tissues of the terminal phalanx are bulbous, resembling drumsticks. These tissues are mobile when pressure is applied over the matrix.

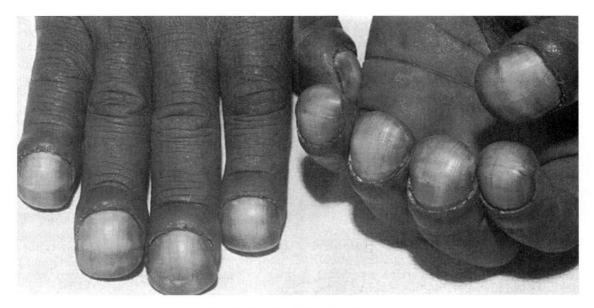

Fig. 33-43   Familial clubbed fingers.

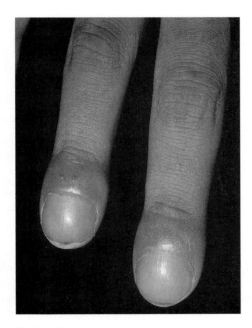

Fig. 33-44   Clubbing caused by ventricular septal defect.

Idiopathic clubbing is either of the isolated dominantly inherited type (Fig. 33-43) or of the pachydermoperiostosis type with its associated findings. Secondary (acquired) clubbing is usually a consequence of pulmonary, cardiac (Fig. 33-44), hepatic, or gastrointestinal disease. Typically, there is periostitis, with periosteal new bone formation in the phalanges, metacarpals, and distal ulna and radius. This is called *hypertrophic osteoarthropathy* and is responsible for the painful clubbing. It typically occurs in men with bronchogenic carcinoma. Unilateral or asymmetrical club-

bing may also occur, reported in cases of Takayasu's arteritis and sarcoidosis. Solitary clubbing may be associated with a digital mucous cyst.

Hashmi S, et al: Asymmetric clubbing as a manifestation of sarcoid bone disease. *Am J Med* 1992, 93:471.
Kaditis AG, et al: Takayasu's arteritis presenting with unilateral digital clubbing. *J Rheumatol* 1995, 22:2346.
Karte K, et al: Acquired clubbing of the great toenail. *Arch Dermatol* 1996, 132:225.
Richter T, et al: Idiopathic clubbing of the fingers. pathogenetic mechanisms and differential etiologic diagnosis. *Hautarzt* 1994, 45:866. ▲

Shell Nail Syndrome

Cornelius et al described a shell nail in association with bronchiectasis. The nail resembles a clubbed nail, but the nail bed is atrophic instead of being a bulbous proliferation of the soft tissue.

Cornelius CE: Shell nail syndrome. *Arch Dermatol* 1969, 100:118.
Cornelius CE, et al: Shell nail syndrome associated with bronchiectasis. *Arch Dermatol* 1967, 96:694. ▲

Koilonychia (Spoon Nails)

Spoon nails are thin and concave, with the edges everted so that if a drop of water were placed on the nail, it would not run off. Koilonychia may result from faulty iron metabolism (Fig. 33-45) and is one of the signs of Plummer-Vinson syndrome, as well as of hemochromatosis. Spoon nails have been observed in coronary disease, syphilis, polycythemia, and acanthosis nigricans. Familial forms are also known to occur.

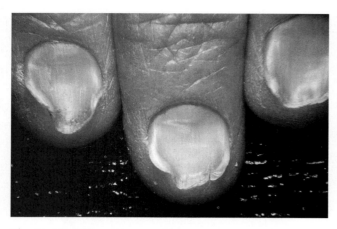

Fig. 33-45 Koilonychia associated with iron deficiency anemia. (Courtesy Dr. Axel W. Hoke.)

Other associations include psoriasis, lichen planus, Raynaud's disease, scleroderma, acromegaly, hypothyroidism and hyperthyroidism, monilethrix, palmar hyperkeratoses, and steatocystoma multiplex. A significant number of cases are idiopathic. Manual trauma in combination with cold exposure may result in seasonal disease. Sherpas are Tibetan people living in the Nepalese Himalayas who often serve as porters on mountain-climbing expeditions. Chronic cold exposure, in combination with hypoxemia, may contribute to the frequency with which koilonychia is observed among them.

Crosby DL, et al: Familial koilonychia. *Cutis* 1989, 44:209.

Dolma T, et al: Seasonal koilonychia in Ladakh. *Contact Dermatitis* 1990, 22:78.

Murdoch D: Koilonychia in Sherpas. *Br J Dermatol* 1993, 128:592. ▲

Congenital Onychodysplasia of the Index Fingers

Congenital onychodysplasia of the index fingers, a syndrome named COIF by Baran in 1980, was first observed by Iso and categorized and named by Kikuchi in 1974. Criteria for diagnosis include presence of the condition at birth, index finger involvement (unilateral or bilateral), variable distortion of the nail or lunula, and polyonychia, micronychia, anonychia, hemionychogryphosis, or malalignment. It may also involve adjacent fingers, such as the middle fingers and thumbs. A single case of second toenail dysplasia in combination with bilateral index finger disease was reported by Youn et al. Others have suggested that there are three forms—the common type, the secondary type, and the hereditary type. An abnormal hand grip and thumb sucking have been suggested as a cause of nonhereditary forms.

Kikuchi I: Congenital onychodysplasia of the index fingers: a case involving the thumbnails. *Semin Dermatol* 1991, 10:7.

Youn SH, et al: Congenital onychodysplasia of the index fingers—Iso-Kikuchi syndrome: a case involving the second toenail. *Clin Exp Dermatol* 1996, 21:457. ▲

Twenty-Nail Dystrophy (Trachyonychia)

All 20 nails may become opalescent, thin, dull, fragile, and finely longitudinally ridged (and as a result, distally notched) at any age from 1½ years to adulthood, although it is most commonly diagnosed in children. It can be idiopathic or caused by alopecia areata (Fig. 33-46), psoriasis, lichen planus, atopy, ichthyosis vulgaris, or other inflammatory dermatoses. Lichen planus is a rare cause. In a series of 23 patients reported by Tosti et al, only one case was caused by lichen planus. Familial forms exist. In some cases spongiosis may be found on nail biopsy. Psoriasis was the most frequent cause in this series. Trachyonychia has also been reported associated with autoimmune processes such as selective IgA deficiency, vitiligo, and graft-versus-host disease. Thus, twenty-nail dystrophy is caused by a heterogenous group of inflammatory conditions. Childhood cases may resolve spontaneously by the time the patient is 20 to 25 years of age.

Jerasutus S, et al: Twenty-nail dystrophy: a clinical manifestation of spongiotic inflammation of the nail matrix. *Arch Dermatol* 1990, 126:1068.

Ohta Y, et al: A case report of twenty-nail dystrophy. *J Dermatol* 1997, 24:60.

Peloro TM, et al: Twenty-nail dystrophy and vitiligo. *J Am Acad Dermatol* 1999, 40:488.

Taniguchi S, et al: Twenty-nail dystrophy (trachyonychia) caused by lichen planus in a patient with alopecia universalis and ichthyosis vulgaris. *J Am Acad Dermatol* 1995, 33:903.

Tosti A, et al: Idiopathic trachyonychia (twenty-nail dystrophy): a pathological study of 23 patients. *Br J Dermatol* 1994, 131:866.

Tosti A, et al: Prevalence of nail abnormalities in children with alopecia areata. *Pediatr Dermatol* 1994, 11:112. ▲

Onychauxis

In onychauxis the nails are thickened but without deformity (simple hypertrophy). Simple thickening of the nails may be the result of trauma, acromegaly, Darier's disease, psoriasis, or pityriasis rubra pilaris. Some cases are hereditary.

Treatment involves periodic partial or total debridement of the thickened nail plate by mechanical or chemical (40% urea paste) means.

Bartolomei FJ: Onychauxis. *Clin Podiatr Med Surg* 1995, 12:215. ▲

Onychogryphosis

Hypertrophy may produce nails resembling claws or a ram's horn (Fig. 33-47). Onychogryphosis may be caused by trauma or peripheral vascular disorders but is most often caused by neglect (failure to cut the nails for very long periods). It is most commonly seen in the elderly.

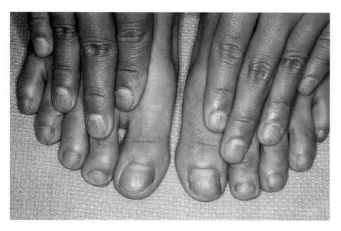

Fig. 33-46 Twenty-nail dystrophy associated with alopecia areata.

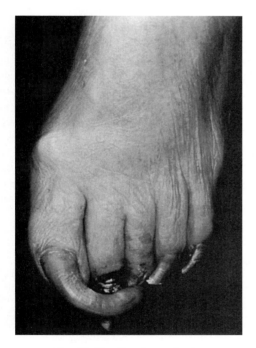

Fig. 33-47 Onychogryphosis.

Some recommend avulsion of the nail plate with surgical destruction of the matrix with phenol or the carbon dioxide laser, if the blood supply is good.

Kouskoukis CE, et al: Onychogryphosis. *J Dermatol Surg Oncol* 1982, 8:138.
Stone OJ: Resolution of onychogryphosis. *Cutis* 1984, 34:480. _____ ▲

Onychophosis

A common finding in the elderly, onychophosis is a localized or diffuse hyperkeratotic tissue that develops on the lateral or proximal nailfolds, within the space between the nailfolds and the nail plate. It may involve the subungual area, as a direct result of repeated minor trauma, and most frequently affects the first and fifth toes.

The use of comfortable shoes should be encouraged. The areas involved should be debrided and treated with keratolytics. Emollients are also helpful.

Anonychia

Absence of nails, a rare anomaly, may be the result of a congenital ectodermal defect, ichthyosis, severe infection, severe allergic contact dermatitis, self-inflicted trauma, Raynaud's phenomenon, lichen planus, or severe exfoliative diseases. Permanent anonychia has been reported as a sequel of Stevens-Johnson syndrome (Fig. 33-48). It may also be found in association with congenital developmental abnormalities such as microcephaly, and wide-spaced teeth (autosomal recessive inheritance) or Cooks syndrome (bilateral nail hypoplasia of digits 1 through 3, the absence of nails of digits 4 and 5 of the hands, total absence of all toenails, and absence or hypoplasia of the distal phalanges of the hands and feet), which is inherited in an autosomal dominant fashion.

Akoz T, et al: Congenital anonychia. *Plast Reconstr Surg* 1998, 101:551.
Hatzis J, et al: Anonychia of all toes with absence of phalangeal bones. *Australas J Dermatol* 1994, 35:83.
Hurley PT, et al: Self-inflicted anonychia. *Arch Dermatol* 1982, 118:956.
Nevin NC, et al: Anonychia and absence/hypoplasia of distal phalanges (Cooks syndrome): report of a second family. *J Med Genet* 1995, 32:638.
Teebi AS, et al: Total anonychia congenita and microcephaly with normal intelligence: a new autosomal-recessive syndrome? *Am J Med Genet* 1996, 66:257. _____ ▲

Onychoatrophy

Faulty underdevelopment of the nail may be congenital or acquired. The nail is thinned and smaller. Vascular disturbances, epidermolysis bullosa, lichen planus, Darier's disease, multicentric reticulohistiocytosis, and leprosy may cause onychatrophy. It is also seen in the nail-patella syndrome and as a side effect of etretinate therapy.

Onychomadesis

Onychomadesis is a periodic idiopathic shedding of the nail beginning at its proximal end, resulting from many systemic disorders. The temporary arrest of the function of the nail matrix may also cause onychomadesis, as may penicillin allergy. Neurologic disorders, peritoneal dialysis, and mycosis fungoides have also been reported causes. Keratosis punctata palmaris et plantaris may be associated with this type of nail loss.

Baran R, et al: Nail bleeding associated with neurological diseases: all that uncommon? *Dermatology* 1993, 187:197.

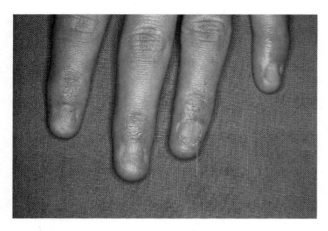

Fig. 33-48 Anonychia resulting from Stevens-Johnson syndrome.

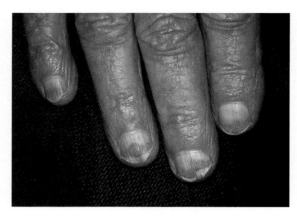

Fig. 33-49 Half and half nails associated with renal disease.

Caputo R, et al: Severe self-healing nail dystrophy in a patient on peritoneal dialysis. *Dermatology* 1997, 195:274.

Fleming CJ, et al: Mycosis fungoides with onychomadesis. *Br J Dermatol* 1996, 135:1012. _____ ▲

Beau's Lines

Beau's lines are transverse furrows that begin in the matrix and progress distally as the nail grows. They are ascribed to the temporary arrest of function of the nail matrix. Although usually found to be bilateral, unilateral Beau's lines may occur. Various systemic and local traumatic factors may cause this. Some are childbirth, measles, paronychia, acute febrile illnesses, and drug reaction. When the process is intermittent the nail plate may resemble corduroy. They may result from almost any systemic illness or major injury, such as a broken hip. Shelley's "shoreline" nails appear to be a very severe expression of essentially the same transient growth arrest. They have been reported in all 20 nails of a newborn.

Colvett KL, et al: Multiple Beau's lines in a patient with fever of unknown origin. *South Med J* 1993, 86:1424.

Harford RR, et al: Unilateral Beau's lines associated with a fractured and immobilized wrist. *Cutis* 1995, 56:263.

O'Toole EA, et al: Unilateral Beau's lines in childhood reflex sympathetic dystrophy. *Pediatr Dermatol* 1995, 12:245.

Price MA, et al: Beau's lines and pyogenic granulomas following hand trauma. *Cutis* 1994, 54:246. _____ ▲

Half and Half Nails

Half and half nails show the proximal portion of the nail white and the distal half red, pink, or brown, with a sharp line of demarcation between the two halves (Fig. 33-49). Lindsay found this condition in patients with renal disease associated with azotemia.

Lindsay PG: The half and half nail. *Arch Intern Med* 1967, 119:583. _____ ▲

Muehrcke's Lines

Narrow white transverse bands occurring in pairs were described by Muehrcke in 1956 as a sign of chronic hypoalbuminemia. In Muehrcke's experience, four patients lost the lines when serum albumin was raised to or near normal. Unlike Mees' lines, the disturbance appears to be in the nail bed, not in the nail plate. Similar lines have been reported in patients with normal albumin levels who are receiving chemotherapy. Feldman et al reported a case of unilateral Muehrcke's lines associated with trauma. The authors believe that edema effects this change by inducing microscopic separation of the normally tightly adherent nail from its bed.

Bianchi L, et al: Coexistence of apparent transverse leukonychia (Muehrcke's lines type) and longitudinal melanonychia after 5-fluorouracil/adriamycin/cyclophosphamide chemotherapy. *Dermatology* 1992, 185:216.

Feldman SR, et al: Unilateral Muehrcke's lines following trauma. *Arch Dermatol* 1989, 125:133. _____ ▲

Mees' Lines

Single or multiple white transverse bands were described by Mees in 1919 as a sign of inorganic arsenic poisoning. They have also been reported in thallium poisoning, septicemia, dissecting aortic aneurysm, parasitic infections, chemotherapy, and both acute and chronic renal failure.

Hepburn MJ, et al: Mees' lines in a patient with multiple parasitic infections. *Cutis* 1997, 59:321.

Marino MT: Mees' lines. *Arch Dermatol* 1990, 126:827.

Quecedo E, et al: Mees' lines: a clue for the diagnosis of arsenic poisoning. *Arch Dermatol* 1996, 132:349.

Shelley WB, et al: Transverse leukonychia (Mees' lines) due to daunorubicin chemotherapy. *Pediatr Dermatol* 1997, 14:144. ▲

Terry's Nails

In Terry's nails the distal 1 to 2 mm of the nail shows a normal pink color; the entire nail plate or proximal end has a white appearance as a result of changes in the nail bed (Fig. 33-50). These changes have been noted in patients with cirrhosis, chronic congestive heart failure, and adult-onset diabetes and in very elderly patients.

Onychorrhexis (Brittle Nails)

Brittleness with breakage of the nails may result from excessive strong soap and water exposure, from nail polish remover, from hypothyroidism, or after oral retinoid therapy. It affects up to 20% of the population. Fragilitas unguium (nail fragility) is part of this process. In a series by Hochman et al of 35 patients treated with B-complex vitamin biotin, 63% showed clinical improvement. The nail plate thickness in patients treated with biotin increases in thickness by 25%.

Colombo VE, et al: Treatment of brittle fingernails and onychoschizia with biotin: scanning electron microscopy. *J Am Acad Dermatol* 1990, 23:1127.

Hochman LG, et al: Brittle nails: response to daily biotin supplementation. *Cutis* 1993, 51:303.

Scher RK, et al: Brittle nails. *Semin Dermatol* 1991, 10:21. ▲

Onychoschizia

Splitting of the distal nail plate into layers at the free edge (Fig. 33-51) is a very common problem among women and represents a dyshesion of the layers of keratin, possibly as a result of dehydration. Longitudinal splits may also occur.

Nail polish should be discontinued; nail buffing can be substituted. Frequent application of emollients may be helpful. Biotin has also been shown effective in daily doses up to 2.5 mg.

Wallis MS, et al: Pathogenesis of onychoschizia (lamellar dystrophy). *J Am Acad Dermatol* 1991, 24:44. ▲

Pitted Nails (Stippled Nails)

Small, pinpoint depressions in an otherwise normal nail characterizes this type of nail change. This may be an early change seen in psoriasis. Pitted nails are also seen with some cases of alopecia areata, in early lichen planus, psoriatic or rheumatoid arthritis, chronic eczematous dermatitis, perforating granuloma annulare, and in some individuals with no apparent disease. The deeper, broader pits are more specific for psoriasis or Reiter's syndrome. The pitting in alopecia areata tends to be shallower and more regular, suggesting a "Scotch plaid" (tartan) pattern.

Racquet Nails (Nail en Raquette)

In racquet nails, the end of the thumb is widened and flattened, the nail plate is flattened as well, and the distal

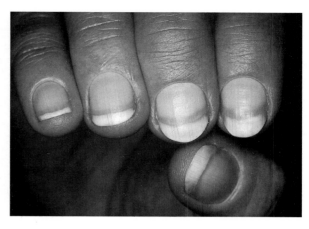

Fig. 33-50 Terry's nails associated with hepatic disease.

phalanx is abnormally short. Racquet nails occur on one or both thumbs and are apparently inherited as an autosomal dominant trait.

Chevron Nail (Herringbone Nail)

This entity appears to be a rare fingernail ridging pattern of children. The ridges arise from the proximal nail fold and converge in a V-shaped pattern toward a midpoint distally.

Parry EJ: Chevron nail/herringbone nail. *J Am Acad Dermatol* 1999, 40:497.

Zaiac MN, et al: Chevron nail. *J Am Acad Dermatol* 1998, 38:773. ▲

Hapalonychia

Softened nails result from a defect in the matrix that makes the nails thin and soft so that they can be easily bent. This type of nail change is attributed to malnutrition and debility. It may be associated with myxedema, leprosy, Raynaud's phenomenon, oral retinoid therapy, or radiodermatitis.

Platonychia

The nail is abnormally flat and broad.

Nail-Patella Syndrome (Hereditary Osteoonychodysplasia, Fong's Syndrome)

Nail-patella syndrome comprises numerous anomalies and is characterized by the absence or hypoplasia of the patella and congenital nail dystrophy. Triangular lunulae are characteristic (Fig. 33-52). Other bone features are thickened scapulae, hyperextensible joints, radial head abnormalities, and posterior iliac horns. The skin changes may also include webbing of the elbows. Eye changes such as cataracts and heterochromia of the iris may also be present. Hyperpigmentation of the pupillary margin of the iris ("Lester iris") is a characteristic finding that occurs in about

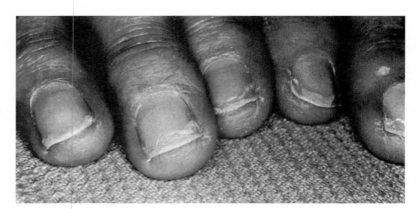

Fig. 33-51 Onychoschizia.

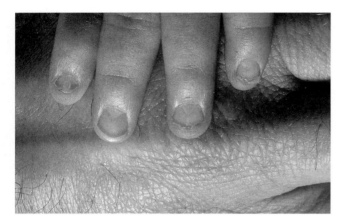

Fig. 33-52 Nail-patella syndrome. Note characteristic triangular lunulae.

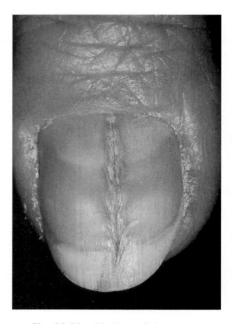

Fig. 33-53 Median nail dystrophy.

half the cases. These patients may exhibit glomerulonephritis with urinary findings of albuminuria, hematuria, and casts of all kinds, especially hyaline casts. They may be predisposed to developing hemolytic-uremic syndrome. Forty percent of patients have renal dysplasia, and 25% suffer from renal failure. It is an autosomal dominant trait localized to chromosome 9q34.1. Limb and kidney defects seen in L1M-homeodomain protein Lmx1b mutant mice are similar to those present in patients with nail-patella syndrome. Mutations of the human LMX1B gene result in this syndrome.

Chen H, et al: Limb and kidney defects in Lmx1b mutant mice suggest an involvement of LMX1B in human nail patella syndrome. *Nat Genet* 1998 19:51.

Dreyer SD, et al: Mutations in LMX1B cause abnormal skeletal patterning and renal dysplasia in nail patella syndrome. *Nat Genet* 1998 19:47.

Hussain SS, et al: Sensorineural hearing loss and nail patella syndrome. *Arch Otolaryngol Head Neck Surg* 1994, 120:674.

Robson WL, et al: Diarrhea-associated hemolytic-uremic syndrome in a child with nail-patella syndrome. *South Med J* 1995, 88:780.

Silverman RA: Diseases of the nails in infants and children. *Adv Dermatol* 1990, 5:153.

Wildfeuer T, et al: Nail-patella syndrome. *Hautarzt* 1996, 47:860.

▲

Median Nail Dystrophy (Dystrophia Unguis Mediana Canaliformis, Solenonychia)

Median nail dystrophy consists of longitudinal splitting or canal formation in the midline of the nail (Fig. 33-53). The split, which often resembles a fir tree, occurs at the cuticle and proceeds outward as the nail grows. Trauma has been suspected of being the chief cause; however, many of these cases will persist for years even with scrupulous avoidance of trauma, and this seems to be a specious explanation. The deformity may result from a papilloma in the nail matrix, forcing the production of a structure like a tube (solenos) distal to it. It does not account, however, for cases with remissions and recurrences.

Bottomley WW, et al: Median nail dystrophy associated with isotretinoin therapy. *Br J Dermatol* 1992, 127:447.

Griego RD, et al: Median nail dystrophy and habit tic deformity: are they different forms of the same disorder? *Int J Dermatol* 1995, 34:799. ▲

Pterygium Unguis

Pterygium unguis is an abnormal extension of the cuticle over the proximal nail plate. The classic example is lichen planus. It has been reported to occur as a result of sarcoidosis and Hansen's disease. Peripheral circulatory disturbances may also be causative.

Kalb RE, et al: Pterygium formation due to sarcoidosis. *Arch Dermatol* 1985, 121:276.
Lembo G, et al: Complete pterygium unguis. *Cutis* 1985, 36:427.
Patki AH, et al: Pterygium unguis in a patient with recurrent type 2 lepra reaction. *Cutis* 1989, 44:311. ▲

Pterygium Inversum Unguis

Pterygium inversum unguis is characterized by adherence of the distal portion of the nail bed to the ventral surface of the nail plate. The condition may be present at birth or acquired and may cause pain with manipulation of small objects, typing, and close manicuring of the nail. It is a condition resulting from the extension of the zone of the nail bed that normally contributes to the formation of the nail plate. This eventually leads to a more ventral and distal extension of the hyponychium, mimicking the clawnail. The most common forms of pterygium inversum unguis are the acquired secondary forms caused by systemic connective tissue diseases, particularly progressive systemic sclerosis and systemic lupus erythematosus. If a curved nail is present on the fourth toe only as a congenital lesion, this is an entity unto itself and occurs as an autosomal recessive trait.

Caputo R, et al: Pterygium inversum unguis: report of 19 cases and review of the literature. *Arch Dermatol* 1993, 129:1307.
Morimoto SS, et al: Unilateral pterygium inversum unguis. *Int J Dermatol* 1988, 27:491.
Yotsumoto S, et al: Curved nail of the fourth toe. *J Am Acad Dermatol* 1999, 40:123. ▲

Hangnail

Hangnail is an overextension of the eponychium (cuticle), which becomes split and peels away from the proximal or lateral nail fold. These lesions are painful and annoying, so that persistent cuticle biting frequently develops. Trimming these away with scissors is the best solution. The use of emollient creams to keep the cuticle soft is also recommended.

Pincer Nails

Pincer nails, trumpet nails, or omega (from the shape of the Greek letter) nails are alternative terms for a common toenail disorder in which the lateral edges of the nail slowly approach one another, compressing the nail bed and underlying dermis (Fig. 33-54). It may occur (although less

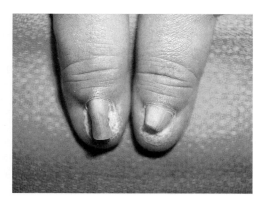

Fig. 33-54 Pincer nails.

often) in the fingernails and is (surprisingly) usually asymptomatic.

Some treatment success has been obtained with the use of commercial plastic braces after flattening of the nail. Urea ointment under occlusion has also been purported to be effective.

Effendy I, et al: Pincer nail: conservative correction by attachment of a plastic brace. *Hautarzt* 1993, 44:800.
el Bammal S, et al: Successful conservative therapy of pincer nail syndrome. *Hautarzt* 1993, 44:535.
Vanderhooft SL, et al: Pincer nail deformity after Kawasaki's disease. *J Am Acad Dermatol* 1999, 41:341. ▲

Onychophagia

Nail biting is a common compulsive behavior that may markedly shorten the nail bed, sometimes damages the matrix and leads to pterygium formation. It is a difficult habit to cure.

If there is strong motivation, application of dimethyl sulfoxide (DMSO) every day or two will provide a reminder and a mild deterrent. Psychopharmacologic intervention may be required.

Stein DJ, et al: Dermatology and conditions related to obsessive-compulsive disorder. *J Am Acad Dermatol* 1992, 26:237. ▲

Onychotillomania

Onychotillomania is a compulsive neurosis in which the patient picks constantly at the nails or tries to tear them off.

Onycholysis

Onycholysis is a spontaneous separation of the nail plate, usually beginning at the free margin and progressing proximally. Rarely the lateral borders may be involved, with spread confined to these. Less often separation may begin proximal to the free edge, in an oval area 2 to 6 mm broad, with a yellowish brown hue ("oil spot"); this is a lesion of psoriasis, as is often the case with ordinary onycholysis. The nail itself is smooth and firm with no inflammatory reaction. Underneath the nail a discoloration may occur from the accumulation of bacteria, most commonly *Pseudomonas,* or yeast, most commonly *Candida.* As a result of pyocyanin from *Pseudomonas,* color changes such as green, black, or blue may be seen. One or more nails may be affected.

Onycholysis is noted most commonly in women, probably secondary to traumatically induced separation, with rapid secondary infection with the most commonly isolated pathogen, *Candida albicans,* probably being the main reason for lack of the nail to reattach itself.

Systemic causes are many: hyperthyroidism and hypothyroidism, pregnancy, porphyria, pellagra, and syphilis. Onycholysis has been associated with psoriasis, atopic dermatitis, eczema, lichen planus, and congenital abnormalities of the nails. Other causes may be trauma induced by clawing, pinching, stabbing (manicuring), and foreign-body implantation. It may be caused by mycotic, pyogenic, or viral (herpes) infections. Women should be checked for vaginal candidiasis, because that anatomic location may be the source of the infection causing (or opportunistically invading and aggravating) onycholysis. Chemical causes may include the use of solvents, nail polish base coat, nail hardeners containing formalin derivatives, artificial fingernails, and allergic or irritant contact dermatitis from their use. Rarely, photoonycholysis may occur during or soon after therapy with tetracycline derivatives, psoralens, fluoroquinolones, or chloramphenicol, with subsequent exposure to sunlight. Chemotherapeutic agents, such as mitoxantrone, may also precipitate onycholysis. On rare occasions it may be a sign of distal metastasis. Hereditary forms are also known, inherited in an autosomal dominant fashion.

Trauma should be completely avoided and the nail bed should be kept completely dry. The affected portion of the nail should be kept clipped away. Drying by exposing the nail bed in this way will rid the area of *Pseudomonas* and assist greatly in eliminating *Candida.* For additional treatment options, refer to the text on the specific cause (see Chapter 15 for *Candida* and Chapter 10 for psoriasis).

Bazex J, et al: Hereditary distal onycholysis: a case report. *Clin Exp Dermatol* 1990, 15:146.

Creamer JD, et al: Mitoxantrone-induced onycholysis: a series of five cases. *Clin Exp Dermatol* 1995, 20:459.

Daniel CR III: Onycholysis: an overview. *Semin Dermatol* 1991, 10:34.

Daniel CR III, et al: Chronic paronychia and onycholysis: a thirteen-year experience. *Cutis* 1996, 58:397.

Lambert D, et al: Distal phalangeal metastasis of a chondrosarcoma presenting initially as bilateral onycholysis. *Clin Exp Dermatol* 1992, 17:463. ▲

Onychocryptosis (Unguis Incarnatus; Ingrown Nail)

Ingrown toenail is one of the most frequent nail complaints. It occurs chiefly on the great toes, where there is an excessive lateral nail growth into the nail fold, leading to this painful, inflammatory condition. The lateral margin of the nail acts as a foreign body and may cause exuberant granulation tissue.

Unguis incarnatus may be caused by wearing improperly fitting shoes and by improper trimming of the nail at the lateral edges so that the anterior portion cuts into the flesh as it grows distally (Fig. 33-55).

Rather than removing the nail to relieve the pressure, a simple operation in which the overhanging lateral nail fold is removed so that the nail does not cut into it is frequently successful (Fig. 33-56). When healed, the nail edge resembles that of the thumb, and an excellent functional result occurs. The nail is not altered, since it is not touched.

With the patient under local anesthesia and with use of a rubber band tourniquet at the base of the toe, a linear incision is made at the edge of the lateral nail fold perpendicular to the nail plate. A convex incision is made in a curvilinear plane parallel to the nail bed to meet the initial incision. The involved wedge of tissue is removed. The lateral flap is then approximated by one or two sutures and a petrolatum gauze dressing is applied. Healing is complete in 10 to 14 days. Another procedure is to apply saturated solution of phenol to the nail matrix after a portion of the ingrown nail has been removed surgically (phenolization). The objective is to permanently ablate the part of the nail matrix producing the nail plate that was ingrowing. Between 60% and 80% of patients treated with partial or complete nail plate avulsion have recurrence of the ingrown toenails. For such patients, partial or complete nail ablation should be considered.

In mild cases, insertion of a cotton pad beneath the distal corner of the offending nail may make surgery unnecessary. In more severe cases, use of a flexible plastic tube to splint the nail is useful. The nail may be flattened through the use of a stainless steel wire nail brace. The brace fits the over-curved nail exactly and maintains constant tension over the nail plate. Adjustments are made over a period of

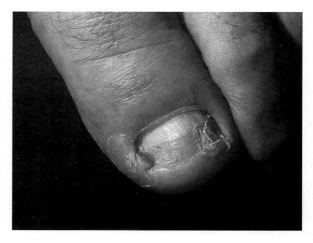

Fig. 33-55 Unguis incarnatus (ingrown nail). (Courtesy Dr. Axel W. Hoke.)

6 months. Liquid nitrogen spray to the area of tissue and nail involved for a freeze time of 20 to 30 seconds has been successful in some patients.

Schulte KW, et al: Surgical pearl: nail splinting by flexible tube. *J Am Acad Dermatol* 1998, 39:629. _____ ▲

NAIL DISCOLORATIONS

The literature on dyschromia of the nails was extensively reviewed by Jeanmougin et al. Involvement of the lunula was reviewed by Cohen.

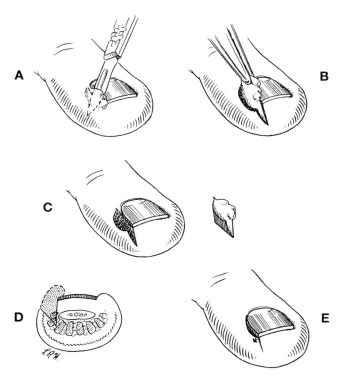

Fig. 33-56 Jansey operation. **A,** Initial linear incision parallel to nail margin. **B,** Convex portion of incision. **C,** Involved segment removed. **D,** Cross section. **E,** End result approximated with suture or adhesive, encircling the toe. (From Jansey F: *Q Bull Northwestern U Med Sch* 1955, 29:358.)

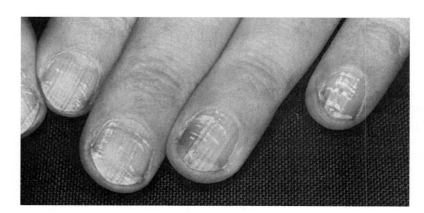

Jeanmougin M, et al: Nail dyschromia. *Int J Dermatol* 1983, 22:279.
Cohen PR: The lunula. *J Am Acad Dermatol* 1996, 34:943. _____ ▲

Leukonychia or White Nails

Four forms of white nails are recognized: leukonychia punctata, leukonychia striata, leukonychia partialis, and leukonychia totalis. The punctate variety is common in completely normal persons with otherwise normal nails. Symmetrical sympathetic punctate leukonychia in contralateral or adjacent nails following a current episode of traumatic leukonychia has been described. Leukonychia striata (Fig. 33-57) may be hereditary or of traumatic or systemic origin. Partial leukonychia may occur with tuberculosis, nephritis, Hodgkin's disease, chilblains, metastatic carcinoma, or leprosy, or idiopathic.

Leukonychia totalis may be hereditary and is of a simple autosomal dominant type (Fig. 33-58). It may also be associated with typhoid fever, leprosy, cirrhosis, ulcerative colitis, nail biting, use of emetine, cytostatic agents, and trichinosis. Leukonychia may result from abnormal keratinization, with persistence of keratohyalin granules in the nail plate.

A syndrome comprising leukonychia totalis, multiple sebaceous cysts, and renal calculi in several generations has been reported. Other reports have linked total leukonychia with deafness, or with koilonychia; however, it is most often inherited or is an isolated finding.

Unamuno P, et al: Leukonychia due to cytostatic agents. *Clin Exp Dermatol* 1992, 17:273.
Zaun H: Leukonychias. *Semin Dermatol* 1991, 10:17. _____ ▲

Melanonychia

Black or brown pigmentation of the normal nail plate is termed *melanonychia*. It may be present as a normal finding on many digits in black patients, as a result of trauma, systemic disease, or medication, or as a postinflammatory event from such localized events as lichen planus or fixed-drug reaction.

Longitudinal black or brown banding of the nails (Fig. 33-59) has been reported to occur in 77% to 96% of blacks

Fig. 33-57 Leukonychia striata.

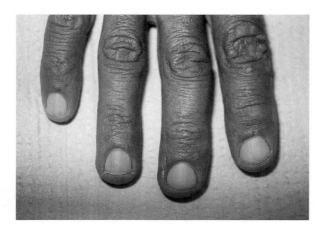

Fig. 33-58 Leukonychia totalis.

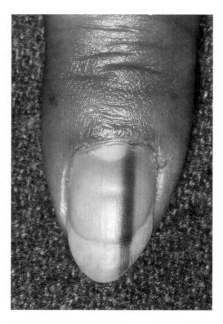

Fig. 33-59 Longitudinal melanonychia.

and 11% of Asians. It is a rare finding in white children; however, it is not uncommon in white adults. In a series by Duhard the prevalence of melanonychia in a white population was 12.6/100 in a hospitalized population and 1.4/100 in 4400 clinic-based patients. The risk increased with age, the peak occurring between ages 56 and 65.

Pigmentation of the nails may occur with acanthosis nigricans, Addison's disease, Peutz-Jeghers syndrome, vitamin B_{12} deficiency, after adrenalectomy for Cushing's syndrome, as a part of Laugier-Hunziker syndrome (pigmentation of the nails associated with buccal and lip hyperpigmentation), with PUVA or ionizing radiation treatment, and as a drug-induced melanocyte activation with such medications as chemotherapy, antimalarials, minocycline, or gold. Friction may cause longitudinal pigmented bands in the toenails, and subungual hemorrhage or black nail caused by *Proteus mirabilis* or *Trichophyton rubrum* may enter into the differential diagnosis of a dark nail.

Leaute-Labreze et al, Goettmann-Bonvallot et al, and Tosti et al found longitudinal melanonychia that appeared in children to be benign in nature, and it is recommended that since an ungual melanocytic band can appear at an age when other nevi appear, surgical excision be undertaken only in the event of a rapid change (as would be the case in acquired or small congenital nevi).

Tosti et al studied 100 white adult patients with a single band of longitudinal melanonychia of unknown cause. Biopsies revealed melanocytic activation in 65, nevi in 22, melanocytic activation in 8, and melanoma in 5. Whereas they were unable to ascertain any clear clinical criteria that would exclude melanoma, they recommended a 3-mm biopsy of any white adult with the appearance of a longitudinal band of pigment in one nail without a clear relation to a definite cause. They then excised all nevi or melanocytic hyperplasia lesions. Retracting the proximal nail fold to expose the origin of the streak at the matrix allows selection of the best biopsy site.

Baran R: Frictional longitudinal melanonychia. *Dermatologica* 1987, 174:280.

Duhard E, et al: Prevalence of longitudinal melanonychia in the white population. *Ann Dermatol Venereol* 1995, 122:586.

Goettmann-Bonvallot S, et al: Longitudinal melanonychia in children. *J Am Acad Dermatol* 1999, 41:17.

Hernandez-Martin A, et al: Longitudinal, transverse, and diffuse nail hyperpigmentation induced by hydroxy urea. *J Am Acad Dermatol* 1999, 41:333.

Leaute-Labreze C, et al: Longitudinal melanonychia in children: a study of eight cases. *Arch Dermatol* 1996, 132:167.

Perrin C, et al: Longitudinal melanonychia caused by *Trichophyton rubrum*: histochemical and ultrastructural study of two cases. *J Am Acad Dermatol* 1994, 31:311.

Tosti A, et al: Nail matrix nevi. *J Am Acad Dermatol* 1996, 34:765. ▲

Green-Striped Nails

Transverse green stripes of the fingernails are produced by a paronychial infection with *Pseudomonas aeruginosa*. The stripes are ascribed to intermittent episodes of infection.

Green Nails

When onycholysis is present, a green discoloration may occur in the onycholytic area as a result of an infection with *P. aeruginosa* (see Chapter 14).

Agger WA, et al: *Pseudomonas aeruginosa* infections of intact skin. *Clin Infect Dis* 1995, 20:302. ▲

Staining of the Nail Plate

Nail plate staining may be caused by nicotine, dyes (including hair dyes and nail polish), potassium permanganate, mercury compounds, hydroquinone, elemental iron, mepacrine, photographic developer, anthralin, chrysarobin, glutaraldehyde, or resorcin. This is only a partial list; the article by Jeanmougin et al should be consulted for a complete listing. A helpful diagnostic maneuver to distinguish nail plate staining from exogenous sources and nail plate pigmentation from melanin or endogenous chemicals is to scrape the surface of the nail plate several times firmly with a glass slide or scalpel blade. Exogenous stains frequently scrape off completely if the agent has not penetrated the entire nail plate. If the stain follows the curvature of the lunulae, it is probably endogenous; if it follows the curvature of the proximal and lateral nail folds, it is exogenous.

Coulson IH: "Fade out" photochromonychia. *Clin Exp Dermatol* 1993, 18:87.
Jeanmougin M, et al: Nail dyschromia. *Int J Dermatol* 1983, 22:279.
Olsen TG, et al: Contact exposure to elemental iron causing chromonychia. *Arch Dermatol* 1984, 120:102. _____ ▲

Red Lunulae

Dusky erythema confined to the lunulae has been reported in association with alopecia areata. It may also be seen in patients on oral prednisone for severe rheumatoid arthritis, systemic lupus, or dermatomyositis. It has also been reported in cardiac failure, cirrhosis, lymphogranuloma venereum, psoriasis, vitiligo, chronic urticaria, lichen sclerosus et atrophicus, carbon monoxide poisoning, chronic obstructive pulmonary disease, twenty-nail dystrophy, and reticulosarcoma. The cause may be vascular congestion.

Bergner T, et al: Red lunulae in severe alopecia areata. *Acta Derm Venereol* 1992, 72:203.
Cohen PR: Red lunulae: case report and literature review. *J Am Acad Dermatol* 1992, 26:292.
Garcia-Patos V, et al: Systemic lupus erythematosus presenting with red lunulae. *J Am Acad Dermatol* 1997, 36:834.
Wilkerson MG, et al: Red lunulae revisited: a clinical and histopathologic examination. *J Am Acad Dermatol* 1989, 20:453. _____ ▲

Spotted Lunulae

Shelley reported this distinctive change in a patient with alopecia areata.

Shelley WB: The spotted lunula: a neglected nail sign with alopecia areata. *J Am Acad Dermatol* 1980, 2:385. _____ ▲

Purpura of the Nail Beds

Purpura beneath the nails usually results from trauma. Causes of toe involvement include physical pressure on the toes, such as that seen in surfboarding by a windsurfer trying to maintain his balance, or exogenous pressure exerted from poorly fitting shoes. It may simulate a melanoma if the acuteness of onset is not communicated by the patient.

Gibbs RC: Toe nail disease secondary to poorly fitting shoes or abnormal biomechanics. *Cutis* 1985, 36:399.
Pierson JC, et al: Pen push purpura: iatrogenic nail bed hemorrhages in the intensive care unit. *Cutis* 1993, 51:422. _____ ▲

Blue Nails

In argyria the lunulae show a distinctive slate-blue discoloration. Lunular blue color, as well as blue discoloration of the whole nail bed, occurs with some chemotherapeutic agents, especially 5-fluorouracil and azidothymidine (Zidovudine). Blue discoloration may also result from subungual hematoma and melanotic whitlow. Mepacrine and other antimalarials may stain the nails blue. Blue nails are a normal variant finding in blacks.

A blue discoloration of the lunulae is seen in cases of hepatolenticular degeneration (Wilson's disease). The blue color is probably related to the changes in the copper metabolism of the patient. It has also been reported in hemoglobin M disease and hereditary acrolabial telangiectases.

Glaser DA, et al: Blue nails and acquired immunodeficiency syndrome: not always associated with azidothymidine use. *Cutis* 1996, 57:243.
Tanner LS, et al: Generalized argyria. *Cutis* 1990, 45:237. _____ ▲

Yellow Nail Syndrome

The yellow nail syndrome is characterized by marked thickening and yellow to yellowish green discoloration of the nails often associated with systemic disease, most commonly lymphedema and compromised respiration. The nails are typically overcurved both transversely and longitudinally, grow very slowly (less than 0.2 mm per week), are often subject to onycholysis, and lose both lunulae and cuticles. Lymphedema, pleural effusions, chronic pulmonary infections, and chronic sinusitis most commonly precede the nail changes. Clinical responses have been shown with taking 800 IU daily of D-alpha-tocopherol and topical vitamin E solution. Itraconazole (in combination with vitamin E) and oral zinc supplementation have also been used with success in individual cases.

Arroyo JF, et al: Improvement of yellow nail syndrome with oral zinc supplementation. *Clin Exp Dermatol* 1993, 18:62.
De Coste SD, et al: Yellow nail syndrome. *J Am Acad Dermatol* 1990, 22:608.
Luyten C, et al: Yellow nail syndrome and onychomycosis: experience with itraconazole pulse therapy combined with vitamin E. *Dermatology* 1996, 192:406.

Williams HC, et al: Successful use of topical vitamin E solution in the treatment of nail changes in yellow nail syndrome. *Arch Dermatol* 1991, 127:1023. _____ ▲

NEOPLASMS OF THE NAIL BED

Various benign and malignant neoplasms may occur in or overlying the nail matrix and in the nail bed. Signs heralding such neoplasms are paronychia, ingrown nail, onycholysis, pyogenic granuloma, nail plate dystrophy, bleeding, and discolorations. Symptoms of pain, itching, and throbbing may also occur with various neoplasms.

Benign tumors of the nails include verruca, pyogenic granuloma, fibromas, nevus cell nevi, myxoid cysts, angiofibromas (Koenen's tumors), and epidermoid cysts. Pyogenic granuloma–like lesions may occur during treatment with isotretinoin or indinavir. Glomangioma is readily recognized by exquisite tenderness in the nail bed. Enchondroma of the distal phalanx has been described. It often presents as a paronychia. Subungual exostoses may also present as an inflammatory process, but more commonly resemble a verruca or fibroma at the start. Most of these are on the great toe, and radiographic evaluation will aid in the diagnosis of these last two entities. Tender swelling of the distal finger with nail distortion and radiographic evidence of solitary lytic changes can be caused by intraosseous epidermoid cysts.

Squamous cell carcinoma of the nail bed is uncommon, and often mistaken for a pyogenic granuloma initially. Radiographs may reveal lytic changes in the distal phalanx. Metastases are rare. Mohs surgery is the treatment of choice. Bowen's disease may occur here, and on more than one digit. Eight such cases, seven in men, have been reported; often the condition occurred secondary to HPV-16 infection. When keratoacanthoma occurs, there is often lysis of underlying bone, which fills in after excision of the tumor.

Subungual melanoma is frequently diagnosed late in the course of growth, since it simulates onychomycosis or subungual hematoma, with which it is confused. Amelanotic melanoma may occur and may be mistaken for granuloma pyogenicum. Although melanoma is rare among Japanese, periungual and subungual melanoma is more frequently found in Japanese than in other ethnic populations. Discussion of melanoma in this location may be found in Chapter 30.

Davis DA, et al: Subungual exostosis: case report and review of the literature. *Pediatr Dermatol* 1996, 13:212.

Finley RK III, et al: Subungual melanoma: an eighteen-year review. *Surgery* 1994, 116:96.

Horton S, et al: Erythematous nodule on the nail bed. *Arch Dermatol* 1999, 135:1113.

Ishihara Y, et al: Detection of early lesions of "ungual" malignant melanoma. *Int J Dermatol* 1993, 32:44.

Kato T, et al: Epidemiology and prognosis of subungual melanoma in 34 Japanese patients. *Br J Dermatol* 1996, 134:383.

Lizuka T, et al: Subungual exostosis of the finger. *Ann Plast Surg* 1995, 35:330.

Samlaska CP, et al: Intraosseous epidermoid cysts. *J Am Acad Dermatol* 1992, 27:454.

Sau P, et al: Bowen's disease of the nail bed and periungual area. *Arch Dermatol* 1994, 130:204. _____ ▲

CHAPTER 34

Disorders of the Mucous Membranes

Lesions on the mucous membranes may be more difficult to diagnose than lesions on the skin, and not merely because they are less easily and less often seen. There is less contrast of color and greater likelihood of alterations in the original appearance because of secondary factors, such as maceration from moisture, abrasion from food and teeth, and infection. Vesicles and bullae rapidly rupture to form grayish erosions, and the epithelium covering papules becomes a soggy lactescent membrane, easily rubbed off to form an erosion. Grouping and distribution are less distinctive in the mouth than on the skin, and not infrequently it is necessary to establish the diagnosis by observing the character of associated cutaneous lesions or by noting subsequent developments.

Bouquot JE, et al: Odd lips: the prevalence of common lip lesions in 23,616 white Americans over 35 years of age. *Quintessence Int* 1987, 18:277.
Eversole LR: Clinical outline of oral pathology, Philadelphia, 1992, JB Lippincott.
Rogers RS III, et al: Diseases of the lips. *Semin Cutan Med Surg* 1997, 16:328.
Thomas JR III, et al: Factitious cheilitis. *J Am Acad Dermatol* 1983, 8:368. ▲

CHEILITIS
Cheilitis Exfoliativa

The term *cheilitis exfoliativa* has been used to designate a primarily desquamative, mildly inflammatory condition of the lips, of unknown cause, and also a clinically similar reaction secondary to other disease states. The former is a persistently recurring lesion that produces scaling and sometimes crusting; it most often affects the upper lip. The recurrent exfoliation leaves a temporarily erythematous and tender surface. In the latter form, the lips are chronically inflamed and covered with crusts that from time to time tend to desquamate, leaving a glazed surface on which new crusts form. Fissures may be present, and there may be burning, tenderness, and some pain.

The lower lip is more often involved, with the inflammation limited to the vermilion part. The cheilitis may be secondary to seborrheic dermatitis, atopic dermatitis, psoriasis, retinoid therapy, pyorrhea, habitual actinic exposure, or the habit of licking the lips. Uncommonly, the initial or only manifestation of atopic dermatitis may be a chronic cheilitis. Irritating substances in lipsticks, dentifrices, and mouthwashes may be causative factors. Dyes in lipsticks may photosensitize. Candidiasis may be present. Cheilitis may be part of the Plummer-Vinson syndrome. Allergic hypersensitivity to nail enamel, aftershave lotion, preshave lotion, lipsticks, and a wide variety of other substances may be the cause. Cheilitis is not uncommon in patients with AIDS.

The only uniformly effective treatment is the elimination of causes when they can be found. Topical corticosteroid creams are usually helpful. When there are fissures, silver nitrate or zinc oxide ointment may be useful.

Daley TD, et al: Exfoliative cheilitis. *J Oral Pathol Med* 1995, 24:177.
Freeman S, et al: Cheilitis. *Am J Contact Dermat* 1999, 10:198.
Reichert PA, et al: Exfoliative cheilitis (EC) in AIDS: association with *Candida* infection. *J Oral Pathol Med* 1997, 26:290. ▲

Allergic Contact Cheilitis

The vermilion border of the lips is much more likely to develop allergic contact sensitivity reactions than is the oral mucosa. Allergic cheilitis is characterized by dryness, fissuring, edema, crusting, and angular cheilitis (Fig. 34-1).

It may result from use of topical medications, dentifrices and other dental preparations, antichap agents, lipsticks, and sunscreening lip balms; from contact with cosmetics, nail polish, cigarette holders, rubber, and metals; or from eating such foods as oranges, lemons, artichokes, and mangoes. Exotic or occupational causes may occur, such as an allergic response to cane reed among saxophonists or clarinetists.

Treatment includes discontinuation of exposure to the offending agent and administration of topical corticosteroid preparations.

Aguirre A, et al: Allergic contact cheilitis from a lipstick containing oxybenzone. *Contact Dermatitis* 1992, 27:267.
Bruze M: Allergic contact cheilitis related to university studies. *Contact Dermatitis* 1994, 30:313.

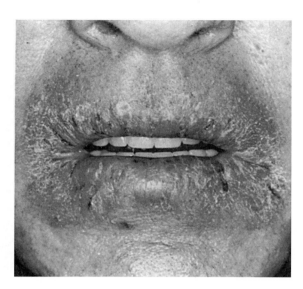

Fig. 34-1   Contact cheilitis caused by toothpaste.

Chan EF, et al: Contact dermatitis to foods and spices. *Am J Cont Dermatitis* 1998, 9:71.

Chang YC, et al: Pseudo flautist's lip: allergic contact cheilitis from geraniol. *Contact Dermatitis* 1997, 37:39.

Fisher AA: Allergic cheilitis due to castor oil in lipsticks. *Cutis* 1991, 47:389.

Freeman S, et al: Cheilitis. *Am J Contact Dermat* 1999, 10:198.

Kobayashi T, et al: Contact dermatitis due to an acrylic dental prosthesis. *Contact Dermatitis* 1996, 35:370.

Lucente P, et al: Contact cheilitis due to beeswax. *Contact Dermatitis* 1996, 35:258.

McFadden JP, et al: Contact allergy to cane reed in a clarinetist. *Contact Dermatitis* 1992, 27:117.

Ophaswongse S, et al: Allergic contact cheilitis. *Contact Dermatitis* 1995, 33:365.

Sainia EL, et al: Contact allergens in toothpaste and a review of their hypersensitivity. *Contact Dermatitis* 1995, 33:100.

Torres V, et al: Allergic contact cheilitis and stomatitis from hydroquinone in an acrylic dental prosthesis. *Contact Dermatitis* 1993, 29:102.   ▲

Actinic Cheilitis

Actinic cheilitis is an inflammatory reaction of the lips to excessive sunlight exposure over the years. The lower lip, which is usually the only one involved, becomes scaly (Fig. 34-2, *A*), fissured, and swollen; leukoplakia and even squamous cell carcinoma may develop.

Painful erosions may occur; actual ulceration is very rare unless carcinoma has developed. This type of cheilitis is caused by chronic solar radiation exposure and occurs primarily in outdoor workers and athletes. Hereditary polymorphous light eruption can resemble chronic actinic cheilitis, but it has no malignant potential.

Simply avoiding sun exposure suffices to minimize further damage in most cases; application of any of the many solar-protective lip pomades is also useful. A biopsy

should be performed on any suspicious, thickened areas that persist; preferably, a shave excision technique should be used to avoid scarring, followed by restoration of hemostasis with aluminum chloride or electrocautery.

Cryosurgical treatment may be effective, particularly for localized lesions. In severe cases with continued development of leukoplakia, application of topical 5-fluorouracil may be curative (Fig. 34-2, *B*). Treatment with a CO_2 laser may be required for severe disease and provides excellent results. Should this treatment fail, vermilionectomy of the lower lip may be necessary. Excision of the exposed vermilion mucous membrane with advancement of the labial mucosa to the skin edge of the outer lip is also effective, but this is performed less frequently since the advent of laser therapy. Photodynamic therapy using 5-aminolevulinic acid has also shown promise.

Refer to Chapter 29 for more information on actinic cheilitis.

Dufresne RG Jr, et al: Actinic cheilitis: a treatment review. *Dermatol Surg* 1997, 23:15.

Johnson TM, et al: Carbon dioxide laser treatment of actinic cheilitis: clinicohistopathologic correlation to determine the optimal depth of destruction. *J Am Acad Dermatol* 1992, 27:737.

Lustig J, et al: Bipedicled myomucosal flap for reconstruction of the lip after vermilionectomy. *Oral Surg Oral Med Oral Pathol* 1994, 77:594.

Ries WR, et al: Cutaneous applications of lasers. *Otolaryngol Clin North Am* 1996, 29:915.

Stender IM, et al: Photodynamic therapy with 5-aminolevulinic acid in the treatment of actinic cheilitis. *Br J Dermatol* 1996, 135:454.   ▲

Cheilitis Glandularis

Cheilitis glandularis is characterized by swelling and eversion of the lower lip, patulous openings of the ducts of the mucous glands, cysts, and general enlargement of the lips (Fig. 34-3).

Mucus exudes freely to form a gluey film that dries over the lips and causes them to stick together during the night. When the lip is palpated between the thumb and index finger, the enlarged mucous glands feel like pebbles beneath the surface. The lower lip is the site of predilection.

In general, two types are recognized, namely, cheilitis glandularis simplex as described by Puente and Acevedo, and cheilitis glandularis apostematosa as described by Volkman. (*Apostematosa* means "with abscess formation.") The latter type probably stems from the simplex form by the development of infection. Cheilitis glandularis is a chronic inflammatory reaction that is due to an exuberant response to chronic irritation, atopic, factitious, or actinic damage.

On biopsy, there is a moderate histiocytic, lymphocytic, and plasmocytic infiltration in and around the glands. Some believe it to be a disorder of ductal ectasia. Cheilitis glandularis has been reported to eventuate in squamous cell

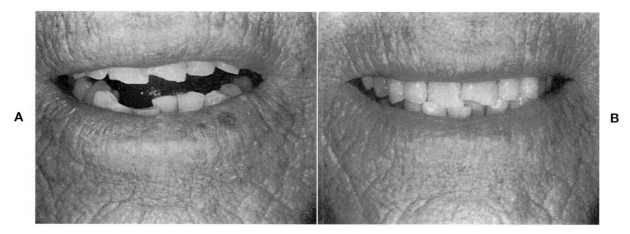

Fig. 34-2 Actinic cheilitis. **A,** Before treatment with topical 5-fluorouracil. **B,** After treatment.

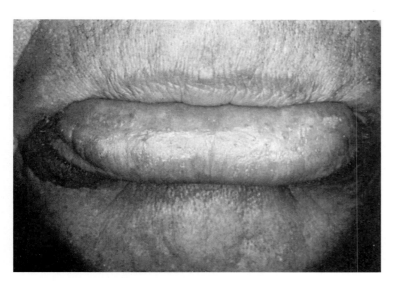

Fig. 34-3 Cheilitis glandularis.

carcinoma, but these cases may be attributed to chronic sun exposure, which frequently precedes cheilitis glandularis.

Treatment depends on the nature of the antecedent irritation; in most cases, treatment as described for actinic cheilitis is appropriate. Surgical debulking may be necessary. Intralesional triamcinolone may be beneficial in some cases.

Cohen DM, et al: Concurrent anomalies: cheilitis glandularis and double lip. Report of a case. *Oral Surg Oral Med Oral Pathol* 1988, 66:397.

Rada DC, et al: Cheilitis glandularis: a disorder of ductal ectasia. *J Dermatol Surg Oncol* 1985, 11:372.

Swerlick RA, et al: Cheilitis glandularis: a re-evaluation. *J Am Acad Dermatol* 1984, 10:466.

Winchester L, et al: Cheilitis glandularis: a case affecting the upper lip. *Oral Surg Oral Med Oral Pathol* 1986, 62:654. _____ ▲

Angular Cheilitis

Angular cheilitis is synonymous with *perlèche*, which is often complicated by infection by *Candida albicans*. Moist fissures may radiate downward and outward from the labial commissures.

The disease usually occurs in elderly people who wear dentures, but it may develop simply from an overhanging of the upper lip and cheek and recession and atrophy of the alveolar ridges in old age. Measuring the facial dimensions with a ruler and tongue blade will help one to objectively assess the importance of decreased vertical facial dimension in the development of perlèche. If the distance from the base of the nose to the lower edge of the mandible is 6 mm or more less than the distance from the center of the pupil to the parting line of the lips, the vertical dimension is decreased.

In these circumstances, drooling is usually a factor. In children, angular cheilitis occurs commonly in thumbsuckers and lollipop eaters. Other inciting factors include riboflavin deficiency, or intraoral candidiasis, especially in patients with diabetes; patients with AIDS; or patients with chronic mucocutaneous candidiasis. It may be seen in patients with tumoral calcinosis. Depletion of micronutrients (serum iron, zinc, copper, selenium, transferrin, albumin, vitamin A, vitamin E, and so on) does not appear to cause any difficulty in oral health in the elderly.

Opening the "bite" by improving denture fit, capping teeth, replacing lost teeth, or increasing denture height, combined with topical use of nystatin and iodochlorhydroxyquin (Vioform) in hydrocortisone ointment, is usually effective. Injection of collagen or insertion of Softform implants to obliterate the angular creases may be beneficial. Excision of the region, followed by a rotating flap graft, is another therapeutic option, but surgery should not be the first treatment tried.

Chernosky ME: Collagen implant in the management of perlèche. *J Am Acad Dermatol* 1985, 12:493.

Gal G, et al: Head and neck manifestations of tumoral calcinosis. *Oral Surg Oral Med Oral Pathol* 1994, 77:158.

Greenspan D: Treatment of oropharyngeal candidiasis in HIV-positive patients. *J Am Acad Dermatol* 1994, 31(Suppl):51.

Sweeney MP, et al: The relationship between micronutrient depletion and oral health in geriatrics. *J Oral Pathol Med* 1994, 23:168.

Zegarelli DJ: Fungal infections of the oral cavity. *Otolaryngol Clin North Am* 1993, 26:1069. ▲

Plasma Cell Cheilitis

Also referred to as *plasma cell orificial mucositis,* plasma cell cheilitis is characterized by a sharply outlined, infiltrated, dark red plaque with a lacquerlike glazing of the surface of the lower lip.

Luger described this lesion on the lip and believed that, histologically, it is the same lesion as Zoon's balanitis plasmacellularis. Histologic alterations include considerable plasma cell infiltration in a bandlike pattern. It has been postulated that plasma cell cheilitis is not a response that is specific for any stimulus but rather represents a reaction pattern to any one of a variety of stimuli. Successful therapies include application of clobetasol propionate ointment twice daily and administration of griseofulvin (500 mg/day).

Plasmoacanthoma. Plasma cell cheilitis and plasmoacanthoma have been reported within the same patient and are believed to represent a spectrum of the same disease. Plasmoacanthoma is a verrucous tumor with a plasma cell infiltrate involving the oral mucosa, particularly along the angles. *Candida albicans* has been found within the tissue, suggesting that it may be implicated as a cause of this disease.

Goring HD, et al: Plasmoacanthoma: a contribution to the diagnosis, etiopathogenesis and nosology. *Z Hautkr* 1985, 60:884.

Tamaki K, et al: Treatment of plasma cell cheilitis with griseofulvin. *J Am Acad Dermatol* 1994, 30:789.

van de Kerkhof PC, et al: Co-occurrence of plasma cell orificial mucositis and plasmoacanthoma. Report of a case and review of the literature. *Dermatology* 1995, 191:53. ▲

Drug-Induced Ulcer of the Lip

Mackie reported seven patients with well-defined ulcerations on the lower lip for which no cause could be found; these healed with the withdrawal of oral medications. The ulceration was tender or painful, without induration, and had been present for several weeks. The ulcers resembled those of discoid lupus erythematosus or squamous cell carcinoma. The causative drugs were phenylbutazone, chlorpromazine, phenobarbital, and methyldopa. Odom has seen several similar cases resulting from the use of thiazide diuretics (Fig. 34-4).

Solar exposure appears to be a predisposing causative influence; this reaction may represent a fixed drug photoeruption. On rare occasions, fixed drug eruptions may also involve the lip.

Mackie BS: Drug-induced ulcer of the lip. *Br J Dermatol* 1967, 79:106. ▲

Other Forms of Cheilitis

Several diseases discussed elsewhere may affect the lips, including lichen planus, lupus erythematosus, and psoriasis. A high percentage of patients with Down syndrome have cheilitis of one or both lips. Lip biting may be a factor.

ORAL AND CUTANEOUS CROHN'S DISEASE

Crohn's disease is a chronic granulomatous disease of any part or parts of the bowel, to which the names *terminal ileitis,* regional enteritis, ileocolitis, segmental colitis, and

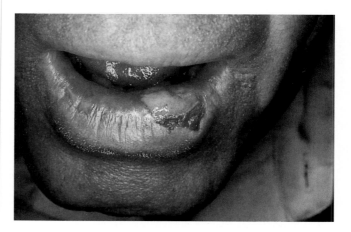

Fig. 34-4 Drug-induced ulcer of the lip.

granulomatous colitis have also been given. Patients with Crohn's disease may develop inflammatory hyperplasia of the oral mucosa, with metallic dysgeusia and gingival bleeding.

Reported typical changes include diffuse oral swelling, focal mucosal hypertrophy and fissuring (cobblestoning), persistent ulceration, polypoid lesions, indurated fissuring of the lower lip, angular cheilitis, granulomatous cheilitis, or pyostomatitis vegetans. Oral involvement occurs in 10% to 20% of cases of Crohn's disease, and 90% have granulomas on biopsy. Dupuy et al found males with early-onset disease are most often affected. Concommitant involvement of the anal and esophageal mucosa was common.

Many cases of Crohn's disease with other cutaneous manifestations have been reported, notably pyoderma gangrenosum (more closely associated with ulcerative colitis) and erythema nodosum, polyarteritis nodosa, pellagra, pernicious anemia, an acrodermatitis-like eruption, urticaria, and necrotizing vasculitis. Direct extension to perianal skin has also been reported.

Metastatic Crohn's disease denotes noncaseating granulomatous skin lesions in patients with Crohn's disease. In the absence of bowel involvement, the diagnosis cannot be made; but noncaseating granulomatous inflammatory lesions of the skin in patients with Crohn's disease are called metastatic Crohn's disease. Genital swelling, leg ulceration, pyogenic granuloma–like lesions of the retroauricular skin, or erythematous nodules, plaques, or ulcers in other locations are the morphologic appearances seen.

Treatment of the gastrointestinal manifestations with sulfasalazine, systemic corticosteroids, or immunosuppressive medications can improve the cutaneous findings. Several delivery systems use only the active ingredient of sulfasalazine, mesalamine. These include Asacol, Pentasa, Rowasa, and olsalazine, and they may be useful in treating the skin involvement of Crohn's disease. A mouthwash containing triamcinolone acetonide, tetracycline, and lidocaine may provide symptomatic and objective improvement. Budesonide, a well-absorbed oral corticosteroid that has a high rate of first-pass metabolism in the liver, has been shown to be effective in treating Crohn's disease while causing fewer long-term side effects. Cyclosporine, azathioprine, and oral metronidazole have also been shown to be effective as first-line agents. Mycophenolate mofetil may also be considered. Cutaneous ulcerated granulomas and erythematous plaques caused by Crohn's disease may respond to high-potency topical corticosteroids. Curettage and zinc by mouth have resulted in healing in several reported patients. Dietary manipulation is another measure that can be helpful in select individuals. The course is often prolonged over several years.

Dupuy A, et al: Oral Crohn disease. *Arch Dermatol* 1999, 135:439.

Gilson RT, et al: Metastatic Crohn's disese. *J Am Acad Dermatol* 1999, 41:476.

Goh M, et al: Metastatic Crohn's disease involving penile skin. *J Urol* 1998, 159:506.

Greenberg GR, et al: Oral budesonide for active Crohn's disease. *N Engl J Med* 1994, 331:873.

Halme L, et al: Oral findings in patients with active or inactive Crohn's disease. *Oral Surg Oral Med Oral Pathol* 1993, 76:175.

Nicholls S, et al: Cyclosporin as initial treatment for Crohn's disease. *Arch Dis Child* 1994, 71:243.

Nousari HC, et al: Mycophenolate mofetil in autoimmune and inflammatory skin disorders. *J Am Acad Dermatol* 1999, 40:265.

Riordan AM, et al: Treatment of active Crohn's disease by exclusion diet: East Anglian multicentre controlled trial. *Lancet* 1993, 342:1131.

Rutgeerts P, et al: A comparison of budesonide with prednisolone for active Crohn's disease. *N Engl J Med* 1994, 29:331.

Schwab RA, et al: Multiple cutaneous ulcerations. *Arch Dermatol* 1993, 129:1607.

Stark ME, et al: Maintenance of symptomatic remission in patients with Crohn's disease. *Mayo Clin Proc* 1993, 68:1183. ▲

PYOSTOMATITIS VEGETANS

Pyostomatitis vegetans, an inflammatory stomatitis, is most often seen in association with ulcerative colitis but may also occur in other inflammatory bowel diseases, such as Crohn's disease. Edema and erythema with deep folding of the buccal mucosa characterize it, together with pustules, small vegetating projections, erosions, ulcers, and fibrinopurulent exudate. Eruded pustules fuse into shallow ulcers, resulting in characteristic "snail-track" ulcers. It has also been associated with sclerosing cholangitis. Several cases have been reported without any underlying systemic disorder. Histologically, there are dense aggregates of neutrophils and eosinophils. At times, crusted erythematous papulopustules that coalesce into asymmetrical annular plaques may occur with or after the oral lesions. The associated skin lesions favor the axilla, groin, and scalp. The treatment of choice is systemic corticosteroids.

Chan SW, et al: Pyostomatitis vegetans: oral manifestation of ulcerative colitis. *Oral Surg Oral Med Oral Pathol* 1991, 72:689.

Ficarra G, et al: Oral Crohn's disease and pyostomatitis vegetans: an unusual association. *Oral Surg Oral Med Oral Pathol* 1993, 75:220.

Lewis JE, et al: Pseudo-pyostomatitis vegetans. *Int J Dermatol* 1995, 34:656.

Mehravaran M, et al: Pyodermatitis-pyostomatitis vegetans. *Br J Dermatol* 1997, 137:266.

Storwick GS, et al: Pyodermatitis-pyostomatitis vegetans: a specific marker for inflammatory bowel disease. *J Am Acad Dermatol* 1994, 31:336.

Thornhill MH, et al: Pyostomatitis vegetans: report of three cases and review of the literature. *J Oral Pathol Med* 1992, 21:128. ▲

CHEILITIS GRANULOMATOSA

Miescher in 1945 reported six cases of swelling of the lips with progressive changes resulting in permanent macrocheilia. Cheilitis granulomatosa is characterized by a sudden onset and progressive course terminating in chronic enlargement of the lips. Usually the upper lip becomes swollen first (Fig. 34-5); several months may elapse before the lower becomes swollen.

Usually, enlargement only is present, without ulceration, fissuring, or scaling. The swelling remains permanently. It may be a part of the Melkersson-Rosenthal syndrome when associated with facial paralysis and plicated tongue.

The cause is unknown. Laymon in 1961 showed that it is not sarcoidosis, nor is it a reaction to a foreign body or infectious agent. Histologically, it is characterized by an inflammatory reaction and tuberculoid granulomas. The noteworthy finding is the presence of tuberculoid granulomas consisting of epithelioid and Langerhans' giant cells. The infiltrate consists of lymphocytes, histiocytes, and plasma cells.

In the differential diagnosis solid edema, angioedema, cheilitis glandularis, sarcoidosis, oral Crohn's disease, infectious granulomas, and Ascher syndrome must be considered. This may be the presenting sign in a patient who will develop Crohn's disease or sarcoidosis at a later time.

Treatment with intralesional injections of corticosteroids is sometimes successful. In the firmly established case, plastic repair of the involved lip through a mucosal approach should be considered. In some cases, concomitant intralesional steroid treatment and surgical repair give best results.

Hines H: Facial swelling in a female adult. *Arch Dermatol* 1985, 121:127.
Krutchkoff D, et al: Cheilitis granulomatosa: successful treatment with combined local triamcinolone injections and surgery. *Arch Dermatol* 1978, 114:1203.
Venable CE, et al: Persistent swelling of the lower lip. *Arch Dermatol* 1988, 129:1705. ▲

MELKERSSON-ROSENTHAL SYNDROME

Melkersson in 1928 and Rosenthal in 1930 described a triad consisting of recurring facial paralysis or paresis, soft nonpitting edema of the lips (Fig. 34-6), and scrotal tongue.

There may be recurring edema of the upper face, buccal cavity, tongue, and other parts of the body. The facial paralysis, usually unilateral, is a peripheral seventh-nerve palsy that may be transitory or permanent. The macrocheilia may also be transitory. The syndrome may be familial.

Attacks usually start during adolescence, with paralysis of one or the other or even both facial nerves, with repeated migraine attacks and edema of the upper lip, cheeks, and occasionally the lower lip and circumoral tissues. The first symptoms are the swelling of the skin and mucous membranes of the face and mouth. In order of frequency, the swelling occurs first on the upper lip, then the lower lip, and then other regions.

Extrafacial swellings appear on the dorsal aspect of the hands and the feet and in the lumbar region. The pharynx and the respiratory tract may be involved, with thickening of the mucous membrane. The relapsing condition produces an

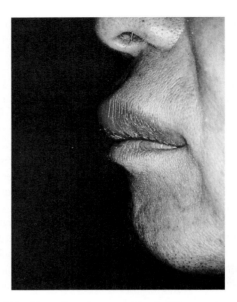

Fig. 34-5 Upper lip enlargement in cheilitis granulomatosa.

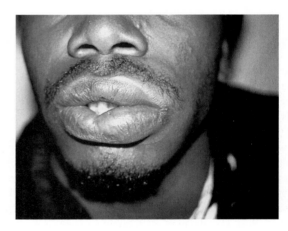

Fig. 34-6 Lip enlargement in Melkersson-Rosenthal syndrome.

overgrowth of connective tissue, edema, atrophy of the muscle fibers, and inflammatory infiltrates, with permanent deformities of the lips, cheeks, and tongue.

The cause is unknown. The association at times with megacolon, otosclerosis, and craniopharyngioma supports the theory of neurotrophic origin.

Histopathologic evaluation shows a tuberculoid type of granuloma with lymphedema and a banal perivascular infiltrate.

In the differential diagnosis, a number of diseases characterized by edema of the lips must be considered. Ascher syndrome consists of swelling of the lips with edema of the eyelids (blepharochalasis) and is inherited. Melkersson-Rosenthal syndrome must also be differentiated from the acute swellings produced by angioedema, trauma, and infections of all sorts. Lymphangioma, hemangioma, neurofibroma, and sarcoidosis are some of the diseases to be considered on a clinical basis.

Melkersson-Rosenthal syndrome is frequently seen in an incomplete form, and other granulomatous diseases may present as swellings of the lips or oral-facial tissues. It is worthwhile to consider these as a group called *orofacial granulomatosis* so that various underlying disease states or etiologic factors will not be missed when evaluating such patients. Oral Crohn's disease, patients who will develop typical Crohn's or sarcoidosis in the future, cheilitis granulomatosa, sarcoidosis, granulomatous infiltrates associated with tooth infections, and patients with food or contact allergic reactions should all be considered.

There is no satisfactory treatment, although intralesional injections of corticosteroids may be beneficial. Decompression of the facial nerve may be indicated in those patients with recurrent attacks of facial palsy. In the case of Yuzuk et al, the swollen upper lip was made much more presentable by plastic surgery. Combining surgery with intralesional steroid injections may be more successful than either alone. Worsaae et al reported that 11 of 16 patients improved on treatment of coexistent odontogenic infection. Both clofazimine and thalidomide have been reported to improve individual patients. Two children treated by Stein et al responded to a combination of prednisone and minocycline.

Daoud MS, et al: Melkersson-Rosenthal syndrome. *Semin Dermatol* 1995, 14:135.

Greene RM, et al: Melkersson-Rosenthal syndrome: a review of 36 patients. *J Am Acad Dermatol* 1989, 21:1263.

Hornstein OP: Melkersson-Rosenthal syndrome: a challenge for dermatologists to participate in the field of oral medicine. *J Dermatol* 1997, 24:281.

Minor MW, et al: Melkersson-Rosenthal syndrome. *J Allergy Clin Immunol* 1987, 80:64.

Rogers RS III: Melkersson-Rosenthal syndrome and orofacial granulomatosis. *Dermatol Clin* 1996, 14:371.

Stein SL, et al: Melkersson-Rosenthal syndrome in children. *J Am Acad Dermatol* 1999, 41:746.

Worsaae N, et al: Melkersson-Rosenthal syndrome and cheilitis granulomatosa. *Oral Surg* 1982, 54:404.

Yuzuk S, et al: Melkersson-Rosenthal syndrome. *Int J Dermatol* 1985, 24:456. ▲

FORDYCE'S DISEASE (FORDYCE'S SPOTS)

Fordyce's spots are ectopically located sebaceous glands, clinically characterized by minute orange or yellowish pinhead-sized macules or papules in the mucosa of the lips, cheeks, and, less often, the gums. Similar lesions may occur on the areola, glans penis, and labia minora. Involvement of the labial mucosa with pseudoxanthoma elasticum may simulate Fordyce's spots.

Because the anomaly is asymptomatic and inconsequential, treatment should be undertaken only if there is a significant cosmetic problem. Monk noted some success with isotretinoin therapy.

Massmanian A, et al: Fordyce spots on the glans penis. *Br J Dermatol* 1995, 133:498.

Monk BE: Fordyce spots responding to isotretinoin therapy. *Br J Dermatol* 1993, 129:355.

Tsuji T, et al: Areolar sebaceous hyperplasia with a Fordyce's spot like lesion. *J Dermatol* 1994, 21:524. ▲

STOMATITIS NICOTINA

Also known as *smoker's keratosis* and *smoker's patches*, stomatitis nicotina is characterized by distinct umbilicated papules on the palate. The ostia of the mucous ducts appear as red pinpoints surrounded by milky white, slightly umbilicated asymptomatic papules. The intervening mucosa becomes white and thick and has a tendency to desquamate in places, leaving raw, beefy red areas. Ulceration and the formation of aphthous ulcers may occur.

This condition is attributed to heavy smoking, especially pipe and cigar smoking, in middle-aged men, although it has also been reported in nonsmokers who habitually drink hot beverages. It is of interest that nicotine in some studies actually prevented recurrent aphthous stomatitis, suggesting that the heat of smoking tobacco may be the causative event. Indeed, most severe cases are associated with tobacco use, which produces intense heat, such as pipe and reverse smoking.

Treatment consists of abstaining from the use of tobacco or ingestion of hot liquids.

Bittoun R: Recurrent aphthous ulcers and nicotine. *Med J Aust* 1991, 154:471.

Grady D, et al: Smokeless tobacco use prevents apthous stomatitis. *Oral Surg Oral Med Oral Pathol* 1992, 74:463.

Rossie KM, et al: Thermally induced nicotine stomatitis: a case report. *Oral Surg Oral Med Oral Pathol* 1990, 70:597. ▲

TORUS PALATINUS

Torus palatinus is a bony protuberance in the midline of the hard palate, marking the point of junction of the two halves of the palate. It is asymptomatic.

King DR, et al: An analysis of torus palatinus in a transatlantic study. *J Oral Med* 1976, 31:44. ▲

SCROTAL TONGUE

Also known as *furrowed tongue* or *lingua plicata* (Fig. 34-7), scrotal tongue is a congenital and sometimes familial condition in which the tongue is generally larger than normal and there are plicate superficial or deep grooves (Fig, 34-8, *A*), usually arranged so that there is a longitudinal furrow along the median raphe, reminiscent of scrotal ruggae.

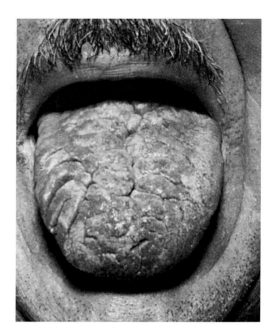

Fig. 34-7 Scrotal tongue with candidiasis.

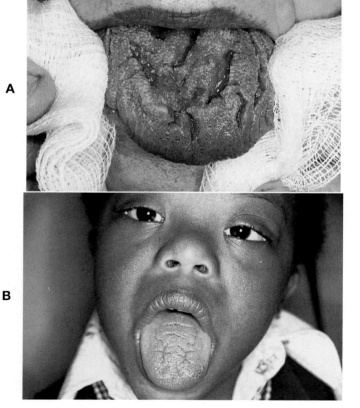

Fig. 34-8 **A,** Scrotal tongue with deep grooves. **B,** Scrotal tongue in a patient with Down syndrome.

Scrotal tongue is seen in Melkersson-Rosenthal syndrome and in most patients with Down syndrome (Fig. 34-8, *B*). Individual case reports of scrotal tongue have been seen in association with pachyonychia congenita, pemphigus vegetans, and Cowden's syndrome.

The condition gives rise to no difficulty, and treatment is not necessary, except that the deep furrows should be kept clean by use of mouthwashes. Furrowed tongue must be differentiated from the "cobblestone" tongue that develops in syphilis.

Dhar S, et al: Melkersson-Rosenthal syndrome in India: experience with six cases. *J Dermatol* 1995, 22:129.

Iraci S, et al: Pachyonychia congenita with late onset of nail dystrophy: a new clinical entity? *Clin Exp Dermatol* 1993, 18:478.

Iwata M, et al: Pemphigus vegetans presenting as scrotal tongue. *J Dermatol* 1989, 16:159.

Krasovec M, et al: Cowden's syndrome. *Hautarzt* 1995, 46:472.

GEOGRAPHIC TONGUE

Geographic tongue is also known as *lingua geographica, transitory benign plaques of the tongue, glossitis areata exfoliativa,* and *benign migratory glossitis.* In some patients it is a manifestation of atopy, and in others, of psoriasis. However, in most it is an isolated finding.

The dorsal surface of the tongue is the site usually affected. Geographic tongue begins with a small depression on the lateral border or the tip of the tongue, smoother and redder than the rest of the surface. This spreads peripherally, with the formation of sharply circumscribed ringed or gyrate red patches, each with a narrow yellowish white border, making the tongue resemble a map (Fig. 34-9). The appearance changes from day to day; patches may disappear in one place and manifest themselves in others. The disease is characterized by periods of exacerbation and quiescence. The lesion may remain unchanged in the same site for long periods. The condition is frequently unrecognized because it produces no symptoms except for the occasional complaint of glossodynia.

O'Keefe et al described two clinical variants of geographic tongue. In one type, discrete, annular "bald" patches of glistening, erythematous mucosa with absent or atrophic filiform papillae are noted. Another type shows prominent circinate or annular white raised lines that vary in width up to 2 mm. The clinical appearance and histopathologic findings of the tongue lesions in pustular psoriasis, Reiter's syndrome, and geographic tongue are identical; they suggest the name *annulus migrans* for this entity. It has been reported to be acquired in patients with AIDS or as a result of lithium therapy.

Histologically, the main features are marked transepidermal neutrophil migration with the formation of spongiform pustules in the epidermis and an upper dermal mononuclear infiltrate.

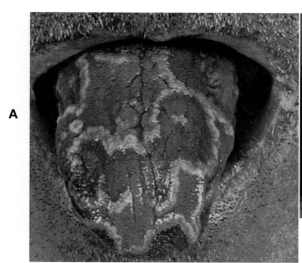

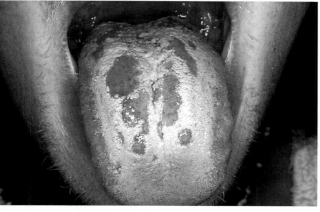

Fig. 34-9 A, Geographic tongue. **B**, Reiter's disease with annulus migrans. (**A**, Courtesy Dr. H. Shatin.)

Although treatment is not usually indicated, a 0.1% solution of tretinoin solution (Retin-A) applied topically has produced clearing within 4 to 6 days.

Fenerli A, et al: Histocompatibility antigens and geographic tongue. *Oral Surg Oral Med Oral Pathol* 1993, 76:476.

Grinspan D, et al: Ectopic geographic tongue and AIDS. *Int J Dermatol* 1990, 29:113.

O'Keefe E, et al: Annulus migrans. *Arch Dermatol* 1973, 107:240.

Patki AH: Geographic tongue developing in a patient on lithium therapy. *Int J Dermatol* 1992, 31:368. ▲

BLACK HAIRY TONGUE

Black or brown hairy tongue occurs on the dorsum of the tongue anterior to the circumvallate papillae, where black, yellowish, or brown patches form, consisting of hairlike intertwining filaments several millimeters long (Fig. 34-10).

It represents a benign hyperplasia of the filiform papillae of the anterior two thirds of the tongue, resulting in retention of long conical filaments of orthokeratotic and parakeratotic cells. It occurs far more frequently in men than in women.

Black hairy tongue may be associated with several conditions that may be predisposing factors in its causation: excessive smoking, the use of oral antibiotics, and the presence of *Candida* on the surface of the tongue.

This lesion is to be differentiated both clinically and histologically from oral hairy leukoplakia, which is seen in HIV-infected patients (see Chapter 19).

Histologically, there are elongated and stratified filaments originating from abnormal papillae within the epithelial covering of the mucous membrane. Orthokeratotic and parakeratotic cells make up the hairlike processes.

A toothbrush may be used to scrub off the projections, either alone or after application of Retin-A gel or 40%

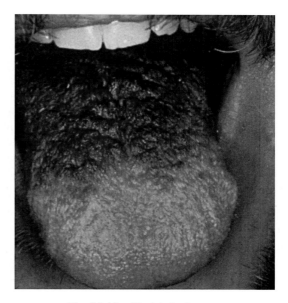

Fig. 34-10 Black hairy tongue.

aqueous solution of urea. Such predisposing local factors as smoking, antibiotics, and oxidizing agents should be eliminated, if possible, and scrupulous oral hygiene should be maintained.

Bouquot JE, et al: Odd tongues: the prevalence of common tongue lesions in 23,616 white Americans over 35 years of age. *Quintessence Int* 1986, 17:719.

Langtry JA, et al: Topical tretinoin: a new treatment for black hairy tongue. *Clin Exp Dermatol* 1992, 17:163.

McGregor JM, et al: Oral retinoids to treat black hairy tongue. *Clin Exp Dermatol* 1993, 18:291.

Newman CC, et al: Images in clinical medicine: black hairy tongue. *N Engl J Med* 1997, 337:897. ▲

GLOSSITIS
Moeller's Glossitis

Moeller's glossitis (Hunter's glossitis) occurs chiefly on the tip and lateral surfaces of the tongue as intensely red, well-defined irregular patches in which the filiform papillae are absent or thinned and the fungiform papillae are swollen. In these patches the superficial layer of the epidermis exfoliates. The disease is chronic and the patches are painful and sensitive so that eating may be difficult. With time leukoplakia results. Moeller's glossitis, painful tongue, and macrocytic anemia are signs of pernicious anemia. The histopathologic changes are those of a nonspecific inflammation.

Treatment is directed against pernicious anemia. With specific therapy, there will be improvements in the appearance and sensitivity of the tongue.

Glossitis of Pellagra

Glossitis is a distinctive sign of pellagra; it results from a deficiency of niacin or its precursor, tryptophan. The sides and tip of the tongue are erythematous and edematous, with imprints of the teeth. Eventually, the entire tongue assumes a beefy-red appearance. Small ulcers appear, and all the mucous membranes of the mouth may be involved. Later the papillae become atrophied to produce a smooth, glazed tongue, as seen in pernicious anemia. Burning or pain in the ulcers may be present. Increase salivary flow early in the disease may lead to drooling and angular cheilitis.

In malabsorption syndrome, riboflavin deficiency, anorexia nervosa, alcoholism, and sprue similar changes may be noted. Vitamin B complex is curative.

Median Rhomboid Glossitis (Glossitis Rhomboidea Mediana)

Median rhomboid glossitis is characterized by a shiny oval or diamond-shaped elevation, invariably situated on the dorsum in the midline immediately in front of the circumvallate papillae (Fig. 34-11).

The surface is abnormally red and smooth. In some instances a few pale yellow papules surmount the elevation. On palpation the lesion feels slightly firm, but it causes no symptoms. It persists indefinitely with little or no increase in size. There is no relationship to cancer.

As a result of a literature review and histologic study of 28 cases of median rhomboid glossitis, Wright suggested that this entity is the clinical expression of a localized fungal infection with *Candida* species.

Histologically, the changes are those of a simple, chronic inflammation with fibrosis, and usually with fungal hyphae in the parakeratin layer. Treatment with oral antifungals, such as itraconazole, may lead to improvement.

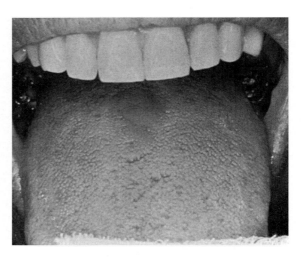

Fig. 34-11 Glossitis rhomboidea mediana.

Huber MA, et al: Glossodynia in patents with nutritional deficiencies. *Ear Nose Throat J* 1989, 68:771.

Miller SJ: Nutritional deficiency and the skin. *J Am Acad Dermatol* 1989, 21:1.

Moreno RG, et al: A painless mass on the tongue of a young man. *Arch Dermatol* 1999, 135:593.

Theaker JM, et al: Oral epithelial dysplasia in vitamin B_{12} deficiency. *Oral Surg Oral Med Oral Pathol* 1989, 67:81.

Ullmann W, et al: Glossitis rhombica mediana. *Hautarzt* 1981, 32:571.

Wright BA: Median rhomboid glossitis: not a misnomer. *Oral Surg* 1978, 46:806. ——————————————————— ▲

EOSINOPHILIC ULCER OF THE TONGUE

Eosinophilic ulcer of the tongue may occur anywhere on the tongue, including the ventral surface. It is characterized by an ulcer with indurated and elevated borders that is usually covered by a pseudomembrane. It develops rapidly, most commonly on the posterior aspect of the tongue, and spontaneously resolves in a few weeks. A traumatic cause has been postulated for this benign, self-limited disorder.

The histopathologic findings show a predominantly eosinophilic infiltrate in company with some histiocytes and neutrophils. In some multifocal, recurrent cases, CD30-positive cells have been reported. These patients may have the oral counterpart of primary cutaneous CD30-positive lymphoproliferative disease.

Liang et al reported that HIV-infected patients may develop ulcerations of the oral mucosa resulting from a variety of infectious agents, such as herpes simplex, candidiasis, and histoplasmosis. However, 5 of the 16 patients they reported had no evidence of infection and simply showed eosinophilic infiltrates below the ulcer.

Liang GS, et al: An evaluation of oral ulcers in patients with AIDS and AIDS-related complex. *J Am Acad Dermatol* 1993, 29:563.

Mezei MM, et al: Eosinophilic ulcer of the oral mucosa. *J Am Acad Dermatol* 1995;33:734.

Greenberg MS: Clinical and histological changes of the oral mucosa in pernicious anemia. *Oral Surg Oral Med Oral Pathol* 1981, 52:38.

Rosenberg A, et al: Primary extranodal CD3O-positive T-cell non-Hodgkin's lymphoma of the oral mucosa. *Int J Oral Maxillofac Surg* 1996, 25:57.

Velez A, et al: Eosinophilic ulcer of the oral mucosa. *Clin Exp Dermatol* 1997, 22:154. _____ ▲

CAVIAR TONGUE

William Bean gave the picturesque name *caviar tongue* to the small, round, purplish capillary telangiectases so commonly found on the undersurface of the tongue after age 50. They are attributed to elastic tissue deterioration incident to aging.

Kocsard E, et al: The histopathology of caviar tongue. *Dermatologica* 1970, 140:318. _____ ▲

DENTAL SINUS

In dental (or odontogenous) sinus, chronic periapical infection about a tooth produces a burrowing, practically asymptomatic sinus tract that eventually appears beneath the surface of the gum, palate, or periorificial skin and forms a fistulous opening with an inflamed red nodule at the orifice. It may appear anywhere from the inner ocular canthus to the neck but is most often seen on the chin (Fig. 34-12) or along the jawline. Bilateral involvement has been reported. The differential diagnosis from granuloma pyogenicum is accomplished by dental radiography and often by palpation of a cordlike sinus tract. Actinomycosis, squamous cell carcinoma, osteomyelitis of the mandible, congenital fistulas, the deep mycoses, and foreign-body reactions must be considered in the differential diagnosis.

Treatment requires the removal of the offending tooth or root canal therapy of the periapical abscess.

Cioffi GA, et al: Cutaneous draining sinus tract. *J Am Acad Dermatol* 1986, 14:94.

Johnson BR, et al: Diagnosis and treatment of cutaneous facial sinus tracts of dental origin. *J Am Dent Assoc* 1999, 130:832.

Palacio JE, et al: Unusual recurrent facial lesion. *Arch Dermatol* 1999, 135:593.

Spear KL, et al: Sinus tracts to the chin and jaw of dental origin. *J Am Acad Dermatol* 1983, 8:486. _____ ▲

NEOPLASMS

Many tumors may involve the oral cavity. Most are discussed elsewhere in this book, and several are uncommon entities that affect specialized oral structures, such as the many subtypes of benign and malignant proliferations that occur in the major and minor salivary glands. These will not be covered further here, and only a few selected neoplasms will be presented.

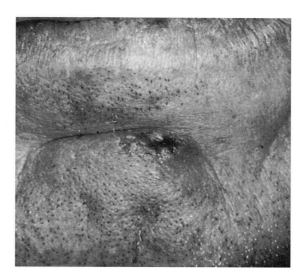

Fig. 34-12   Cutaneous sinus tract of dental origin.

Leukoplakia

Once regarded as precancerous, the term *leukoplakia* now refers only to whitish plaques or patches in mucous membranes, which may or may not show cellular atypia. See Chapter 29 for a discussion of leukoplakia.

Erythroplakia

The term *erythroplakia* is applied to leukoplakia that has lost (or has not developed) the thick keratin layer that makes leukoplakia white; it is the usual pattern in mucocutaneous junctions. A focal red patch with no apparent cause should be suspected of being precancerous when found on the floor of the mouth, soft palate, or buccal mucosa, or under the tongue. Histologically, there is cellular atypia, pleomorphism, hyperchromatism, and increased mitotic figures. Carcinoma in situ or invasive carcinoma is found in 90% of lesions.

Proliferative Verrucous Leukoplakia

Proliferative verrucous leukoplakia is a slowly progressive condition that begins as multifocal sites of hyperplasia of the oral mucous membranes and proceeds to thicken and enlarge until squamous cell carcinoma results. Women outnumber men by 4 to 1. Initially flat, usually white, patches are present, but the lesions relentlessly become warty exophytic masses. The patches may involve the lips and chin. In a series of 54 cases Silverman et al reported that 70% developed squamous cell carcinoma (most frequently of the tongue and gingiva). Twenty-one died of proliferative verrucous leukoplakia-associated carcinoma. It has been associated with human papillomavirus (HPV) 16 infection, but it remains to be proven whether this is the primary cause. Treatment is difficult because of the multifocal nature of the lesions. Most patients develop recurrence after only a short interval. Aggressive early therapy is best. Laser treatment or photodynamic therapy should be considered primary options.

Squamous Cell Carcinoma

Squamous cell carcinoma is the most common oral malignancy. It occurs primarily in older men. The most frequent sites are the lower lip, tongue, soft palate, and the floor of the mouth. Squamous cell carcinoma of the lip develops from actinic damage. Intraoral lesions frequently develop from leukoplakia or at sites of frequent irritation. Verrucous carcinomas occur in the oral mucosa as they do on the skin. Tobacco smoking, the use of smokeless tobacco, betel nut chewing, reverse smoking, and the use of alcohol are risk factors for the development of intraoral squamous cell carcinoma. They may also complicate xeroderma pigmentosa, dyskeratosis congenita, dystrophic epidermolysis bullosa, erosive lichen planus, and oral submucous fibrosis. Unfortunately, the survival rate is only 30%, because squamous cell carcinoma is often discovered late, after it has metastasized to the cervical lymph nodes.

Acquired Dyskeratotic Leukoplakia

James and Lupton reported a patient with acquired dyskeratotic leukoplakia, which manifested as distinctive white plaques on the palate, gingivae, and lips. There were similar lesions of the genitalia of the patient. Histologically, there was a unique finding of clusters of dyskeratotic cells in the prickle-cell layer in all sites.

Aggressive laser treatment was followed by recurrence. Use of etretinate afforded some improvement.

Melanocytic Oral Lesions

A wide variety of melanocytic lesions appear on the mucous membranes. Among the melanocytic nevi of the cellular type, the intramucosal type is the most frequent, with the compound nevus next and the junction nevus occurring only rarely. Nevi of the oral mucosa in general are very uncommon. Ephelis, lentigo, blue nevus, and labial melanotic macules are other types of focal hyperpigmentation. Ephelides darken on sun exposure and are usually limited to the lower lip. The blue nevus has dendritic cells in the submucosa. Lentigines show acanthosis of rete ridges on biopsy. Labial melanotic macules are solitary, sharply demarcated, flat, pigmented lesions that occur chiefly in young women (Fig. 34-13), do not change on sun exposure, and show only acanthosis and basal-layer melanin on biopsy.

Oral melanoacanthoma is a simultaneous proliferation of keratinocytes and melanocytes. They are most commonly observed in young black patients (average age, 23) on the buccal mucosa. It seems to be a reactive process, usually following trauma and resolving spontaneously in 40% of patients. Melanoma also occurs, rarely, mostly in older patients. It is recognized by being larger than the usual benign, pigmented lesion. It is more irregular in shape, with a tendency to ulcerate and bleed. A peripheral areola of erythema and satellite pigmented spots may be present.

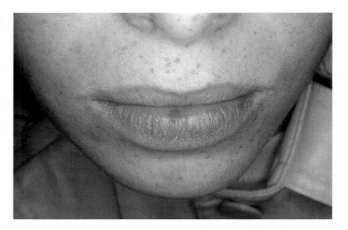

Fig. 34-13   Labial melanotic macule.

There is a striking predilection for palatal (or, less often, gingival) involvement. The overall prognosis is poor (less than 5% survival at 5 years), because the lesions are usually deeply invasive by the time they are discovered. Whereas oral nevi are uncommon, biopsy of solitary pigmented oral lesions is indicated when the clinical diagnosis is uncertain.

Oral Melanosis

Pigmentation of the oral cavity tends to occur most frequently in blacks. In other races, the darker the skin, the more mucosal pigmentation may be expected. Oral melanosis may occur with Albright's syndrome, Peutz-Jeghers syndrome, Addison's disease, or rarely, as an idiopathic process with no associated disease (Fig. 34-14).

James et al reported a patient with inflammatory acquired oral hyperpigmentation that first occurred at age 30 with numerous distinct pigmented macules, similar to those seen in Peutz-Jeghers syndrome. However, the condition progressed rapidly to a diffuse oral hyperpigmentation. This appeared to be caused by some undefined inflammation, and slow partial resolution occurred after several years of observation.

In the differential diagnosis of oral hyperpigmentation, these other entities should be included. Focal, brownish blue macules occur as amalgam tattoo incurred from fragments of dental silver or amalgam being implanted into the gums. Tar and heavy-metal poisoning may also induce such lesions. Bismuth (injected) and lead (ingested or inhaled) may produce a pigmented line along the gums near their margin. A gingival platinum line has been reported in a patient being treated for osteogenic sarcoma with *cis*-platinum.

Osseous Choristoma of the Tongue

Osseous choristoma of the tongue presents as a nodule on the dorsum of the tongue containing mature lamellar bone without osteoblastic or osteoclastic activity. This does not recur after simple excision.

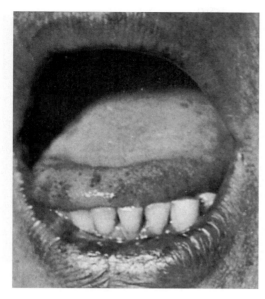

Fig. 34-14 Melanosis oris with pigmented macules on the lips and tongue but without intestinal polyposis.

Peripheral Ameloblastoma

Urmacher et al reported a case of this rare invasive neoplasm of the gingivae, which appears most often on the lower jaw. Gardner studied 21 cases, including 5 reported as basal cell carcinoma.

Bork K, et al: Diseases of the oral mucosa and the lips, Philadelphia, 1993, WB Saunders.

Buchner A, et al: Pigmented nevi of the oral mucosa. *Oral Surg* 1987, 63:676.

Buchner A, et al: Amalgam pigmentation of the oral mucosa. *Oral Surg* 1980, 49:139.

Cutright DE: The histopathologic findings in 583 cases of epulis fissuratum. *Oral Surg* 1974, 37:401.

Duffey DC, et al: Oral lichen planus and its association with squamous cell carcinoma. *Laryngoscope* 1996, 106:357.

Eisen D, et al: Oral melanoma and other pigmented lesions of the oral cavity. *J Am Acad Dermatol* 1991, 24:527.

Ettinger LJ, et al: The gingival platinum line. *Cancer* 1979, 44:1882.

Gardner DG: Peripheral ameloblastoma: a study of 21 cases, including 5 reported as basal cell carcinoma of the gingiva. *Cancer* 1977, 39:1625.

Goode RK, et al: Oral melanoacanthoma. *Oral Surg* 1983, 56:622.

Haley JC, et al: Proliferative verrucous leukoplakia with cutaneous involvement. *J Am Acad Dermatol* 1999, 41:481.

Hall JM, et al: Multiple and confluent lesions of oral leukoplakia. *Arch Dermatol* 1991, 127:887.

Horlick HP, et al: Mucosal melanotic macule, reactive type. *J Am Acad Dermatol* 1988, 19:786.

James WD, et al: Acquired dyskeratotic leukoplakia. *Arch Dermatol* 1988, 124:117.

James WD, et al: Inflammatory acquired oral hyperpigmentation. *J Am Acad Dermatol* 1987, 16:220.

Kato T, et al: Malignant melanoma of mucous membranes. *Arch Dermatol* 1987, 123:216.

Maize JC: Mucosal melanosis. *Derm Clin* 1988, 6:283.

Norton SA: Betel. *J Am Acad Dermatol* 1998, 38:81.

Palefsky JM, et al: Association between proliferative verrucous leukoplakia and infection with human papillomavirus type 16. *J Oral Pathol Med* (Denmark) 1995, 24:193.

Rapini RP, et al: Primary malignant melanoma of the oral cavity. *Cancer* 1985, 55:1543.

Schwartz RA: Verrucous carcinoma of the skin and mucosa. *J Am Acad Dermatol* 1995, 32:1.

Sexton FM, et al: Melanotic macules and melanoacanthomas of the lip. *Am J Dermatopathol* 1987, 9:438.

Silverman S Jr: Prevention, early detection and diagnosis of oral cancer. *Dermatol Clin* 1987, 5:675.

Silverman S Jr, et al: Proliferative verrucous leukoplakia. *Oral Surg Oral Med Oral Pathol Oral Radiol Endod* 1997, 84:154.

Smith JB, et al: Cutaneous manifestations and consequences of smoking. *J Am Acad Dermatol* 1996, 34:717.

Sparm CR, et al: The labial melanotic macule. *Arch Dermatol* 1987, 123:1029.

Urmacher C, et al: An uncommon neoplasm (ameloblastoma) of the oral mucosa. *Am J Dermatopathol* 1983, 5:601.

Witkop CJ, et al: Four hereditary mucosal syndromes. *Arch Dermatol* 1961, 84:762. ▲

TRUMPETER'S WART

Trumpeter's wart is a firm, fibrous, hyperkeratotic, pseudoepitheliomatous nodule on the upper lip of a trumpet player. A similar callus may grow on the lower lip of trombone players.

Fisher AA: Dermatitis in a musician. *Cutis* 1998, 62:214, 261. ▲

EPULIS

The term *epulis* means any benign lesion situated on the gingiva. The majority of these are reactive processes that display varying degrees of fibrosis, inflammation, and vascular proliferation on biopsy.

Giant cell epulis (peripheral giant cell granuloma) is a solitary, bluish red, 10- to 20-mm tumor occurring on the gingiva between or about deciduous bicuspids and incisors.

Giansanti JS, et al: Peripheral giant cell granuloma. *J Oral Surg* 1969, 27:787. ▲

Pyogenic Granuloma

Pyogenic granuloma is an exuberant overgrowth of granulation tissue, frequently occurring in the oral cavity, most often involving the gingiva. It may also involve the buccal mucosa, lips, tongue, or palate. It is a red to reddish purple, soft, nodular mass that bleeds easily and grows rapidly, but is usually not painful. When it develops during pregnancy it is called *pregnancy tumor* or *granuloma gravidarum*.

Krolls SO, et al: Denture-induced fibrous hyperplasia. *Miss Dent Assoc J* 1993, 49:18. ▲

GRANULOMA FISSURATUM

Granuloma fissuratum is a circumscribed, firm, whitish, fissured, fibrous granuloma occurring in the labioalveolar fold. The lesion is discoid, smooth, and slightly raised, about 1 cm in diameter. The growth is folded like a bent coin so that the fissure in the bend is continuous at both sides with the labioalveolar sulcus. Symptoms are slight. It is an inflammatory fibrous hyperplasia that usually results from chronic irritation from poorly fitting dentures. In the dental literature it is called *epulis fissuratum,* particularly when there is a deep cleft traversing the lesion. Treatment is by surgical extirpation or electrodesiccation, with biopsy.

ANGINA BULLOSA HAEMORRHAGICA

The sudden appearance of one or more blood blisters of the oral mucosa characterizes this entity. There is no associated skin or systemic disease. The blisters may be recurrent, occur most often in the soft palate, and usually present in middle-aged or elderly patients. No treatment is necessary.

Dominguez JD, et al: Recurrent oral blood blisters. *Arch Dermatol* 1999, 135:593. _____ ▲

MUCOCELE

The term *mucocele* refers to a lesion that occurs as a result of trauma or obstruction of the minor salivary ducts. The most common type is the mucous extravasation phenomenon, which is usually seen inside the lower lip (Fig. 34-15), but it may occur on the upper lip or in the buccal mucosa (Fig. 34-16) because it is caused by trauma from biting. It presents as a soft, rounded, translucent projection; it commonly has a bluish tint. The lesion varies from 2 to 10 mm in diameter. It is painless, fluctuant, and tense. Incision of it, or sometimes merely compression, releases sticky, straw-colored fluid (or bluish fluid if hemorrhage has occurred into it).

The cause is rupture of the mucous duct, with extravasation of sialomucin into the submucosa to produce cystic spaces with inflammation. Granulation tissue formation is followed by fibrosis. Excisional biopsy will document the diagnosis and eliminate the problem. Cryotherapy and argon laser ablation have also been reported to be successful.

There are true mucous retention cysts where there is true obstruction of the duct leading to an epithelial lined cavity. They are seen more in the posterior portions of the oral mucosa. A ranula (from *Rana,* the frog genus) is a mucocele of the floor of the mouth.

Two other cysts that may be present in the mouth are (1) the parotid duct cyst, which occurs in musicians who use wind instruments (the cyst develops opposite the upper second molar on the buccal mucosa), and (2) the dermoid cyst, which may occur on the floor of the mouth, especially in the sublingual area.

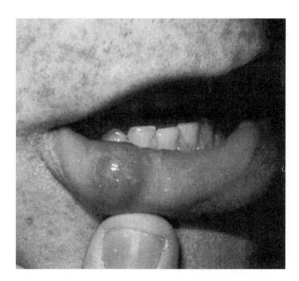

Fig. 34-15 Mucous cyst (mucocele) of the lip.

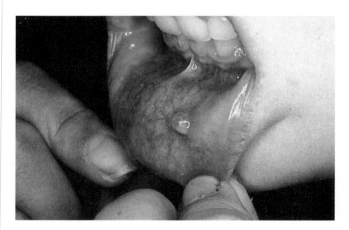

Fig. 34-16 Mucocele.

Gill D: Two simple treatments for lower lip mucocoeles. *Australas J Dermatol* 1996, 37:220.

Jensen JL: Superficial mucoceles of the oral mucosa. *Am J Dermatopathol* 1990, 12:88.

McClatchey KD, et al: Plunging ranula. *Oral Surg Oral Med Oral Pathol* 1984, 57:408.

Neumann RA, et al: Treatment of oral mucous cysts with an argon laser. *Arch Dermatol* 1990, 126:829.

Tran TA, et al: Removal of a large labial mucocele. *J Am Acad Dermatol* 1999, 40:760. _____ ▲

ACUTE NECROTIZING ULCERATIVE GINGIVOSTOMATITIS (TRENCH MOUTH, VINCENT'S DISEASE)

Acute necrotizing ulcerative gingivitis (ANUG) is characterized by a rapid onset of characteristic punched-out ulcerations appearing on the interdental papillae and marginal gingivae. A dirty white pseudomembrane may

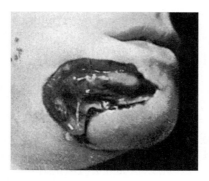

Fig. 34-17 Noma of the chin. (Courtesy Dr. L. Goldman.)

cover the ulcerations. The lesions may spread rapidly and involve the buccal mucosa, lips, and tongue as well as the tonsils, the pharynx, and the entire respiratory tract. The slightest pressure causes pain and bleeding. The outstanding finding is the characteristic foul, fetid odor that is always present.

The cause of trench mouth is thought to be necrotic tissue, which provides an anaerobic environment for the infection by fusospirochetal organisms *(Bacteroides fusiformis)* in association with *Borrelia vincentii* and other organisms. Poor dental hygiene, smoking, poor nutrition, and immunosuppression are predisposing factors. It may be seen as a component of the oral infections and inflammatory lesions that complicate the cases of HIV-infected patients.

Acute herpetic gingivostomatitis, occurring as a primary herpes simplex infection, may be confused with ANUG. Young children are susceptible to this severe febrile stomatitis with lymphadenitis. It is not primarily gingival in location and does not cause necrosis of the interdental papillae.

Noma is a form of fusospirillary gangrenous stomatitis occurring in children with low resistance and poor nutrition. At the onset there is ulceration of the buccal mucosa; this rapidly assumes a gangrenous character and extends to involve the skin and bones, with resultant necrosis (Fig. 34-17). It may end in the patient's death.

Treatment consists of thorough dental hygienic measures under the supervision of a dentist. Penicillin and debridement is the treatment of choice. Use of a 3% hydrogen peroxide mouthwash is also helpful.

Johnson BD, et al: Acute necrotizing ulcerative gingivitis: a review of diagnosis, etiology and treatment. *J Periodontol* 1986, 57:141.
Lieberman J, et al: Noma. *Cutis* 1987, 39:501.
Smith JB, et al: Cutaneous manifestations and consequences of smoking. *J Am Acad Dermatol* 1996, 34:717. _____ ▲

ACATALASEMIA

Acatalasemia (Takahara's disease) is a rare disease in which the enzyme catalase is deficient in the liver, muscles, bone marrow, erythrocytes, and skin. There are several forms. The absence of catalase leads to progressive gangrene of the mouth, with recurrent ulcerations resulting from increased susceptibility to infection by anaerobic organisms.

Nearly 60% of affected individuals develop alveolar ulcerations, beginning in childhood. The mild type of the disease is characterized by rapidly recurring ulcers. In the moderate type, alveolar gangrene develops, with atrophy and recession of the alveolar bone, so that the teeth fall out spontaneously. In the severe type, widespread destruction of the jaw occurs. After puberty all lesions heal, even in individuals who had the severe type.

There is no gross difference in appearance between the blood of an acatalasic patient and that of a normal individual, but when hydrogen peroxide is added to a sample of blood, acatalasic blood immediately turns blackish brown and the peroxide does not foam. Normal blood remains bright and causes the peroxide to foam exuberantly because of the presence of erythrocyte catalase.

Acatalasia is rare and is inherited as an autosomal recessive trait. Approximately 2 of every 100,000 Japanese have this disease.

Treatment consists of extraction of the diseased teeth and the use of antibiotics to control the harmful effects of the offending bacteria.

Ogata M: Acatalasemia. *Hum Genet* 1991, 86:331. _____ ▲

CYCLIC NEUTROPENIA

Cyclic, or periodic, neutropenia is characterized by a decrease of circulating neutrophils from the blood and dermatologic manifestations. At fairly regular intervals (21 days), neutropenia and mouth ulcerations develop, usually accompanied by fever, malaise, and arthralgia. Ulcerations of the lips, tongue, palate, gums, and buccal mucosa may be extensive. The ulcers are irregularly outlined and are covered by a grayish white necrotic slough. The anterior teeth may show a grayish brown discoloration. Premature alveolar bone loss and periodontitis occur. In addition, cutaneous infections, such as abscesses, furuncles, and cellulitis, may rarely develop. Urticaria and erythema multiforme have been reported.

There is a cyclic depression of neutrophils occurring at intervals of 12 to 30 days (average, 21 days) and lasting 5 to 8 days. The neutrophils in the peripheral blood regularly fall to low levels or disappear at this time. Some cases have been associated with agammaglobulinemia, but in other cases the globulin levels are normal. The cause of cyclic neutropenia is unknown.

Use of recombinant human granulocyte colony–stimulating factor has been successful in the treatment of some patients. If the potential side effects limit use of this therapy, cyclosporine has been reported to be effective also. Administering antibiotics during infections seems to expedite recovery. Careful attention to oral hygiene, including plaque control, helps improve mouth lesions and reduces the risk of infections. Death may occur from pneumonia, sepsis, gangrenous pyoderma, or granulocytopenia.

Fink Puches R, et al: Granulocyte colony–stimulating factor treatment of cyclic neutropenia with recurrent oral aphthae. *Arch Dermatol* 1996, 132:1399.

Rogers RS III: Recurrent aphthous stomatitis. *Semin Cutan Med Surg* 1997, 16:278.

Storek J, et al: Adult-onset cyclic neutropenia responsive to cyclosporine therapy in a patient with ankylosing spondylitis. *Am J Hematol* 1993, 43:139. _____ ▲

RECURRENT INTRAORAL HERPES SIMPLEX INFECTION

Recurrent intraoral infection with herpes simplex is characterized by numerous small vesicles occurring in one or a few clusters, almost exclusively on the palate, or, infrequently, on the gingiva. The grouped vesicles rupture rapidly to form punctate erosions with a red base. Smears from the base prepared with Wright's stain will show giant multinucleated epithelial cells. Immunofluorescent tests and viral cultures are also confirmatory.

The differential diagnosis of this uncommon manifestation of herpes simplex includes oral herpes zoster, herpangina, and oral aphthosis. The latter two involve nonattached mucosa, whereas recurrent herpes simplex involves mucosa fixed to bone. Differentiation from zoster is made on clinical grounds or by culture and immunofluorescent testing.

Chronic progressive ulcerative and nodular intraoral herpes are seen occasionally in HIV-infected patients, or those with leukemia or neutropenia.

Cohen SG, et al: Chronic oral herpes simplex virus infection in immunocompromised patients. *Oral Surg Oral Med Oral Pathol* 1985, 59:465.

Greenberg MS, et al: Oral herpes simplex infections in patients with leukemia. *J Am Dent Assoc* 1987, 114:483.

Weathers DR, et al: Intraoral ulcerations of recurrent herpes simplex and recurrent aphthae. *J Am Dent Assoc* 1970, 81:81. _____ ▲

RECURRENT APHTHOUS STOMATITIS (CANKER SORES, APHTHOSIS)

CLINICAL FEATURES. Aphthous stomatitis is a painful, recurrent disease of the oral mucous membrane. It begins as small, red, discrete or grouped papules, which in a few hours become necrotizing ulcerations. They are small, round, shallow, white ulcers (aphthae) (Fig. 34-18) generally surrounded by a ring of hyperemia. As a rule, they are tender; they may become so painful that they interfere with speech and mastication. They are mostly about 5 mm in diameter but may vary in size from 3 to 10 mm. When larger, they are called *major aphthae* (see p. 1008). Usually, one to five lesions occur per attack; however, they may occur in any number. They are located in decreasing frequency on the buccal and labial mucosa, edges of the tongue, buccal and lingual sulci, and soft palate. There is a marked predilection for the nonkeratinized mucosa (any not bound to underlying periosteum). This and the fact that they are rarely confluent, even when they occur as small crops of 1- or 2-mm lesions (herpetiform aphthae), help to distinguish them from the uncommon recurrent intraoral herpes simplex infection (see this page). Aphthae may also occur on the vagina, vulva, penis, anus, and even the conjunctiva (see the discussion of Behçet's syndrome on p. 1008).

The lesions tend to involve in 1 to 2 weeks, but recurrences are common. These recurrences may be induced by trauma, certain spicy or citrus foods, allergy, emotional

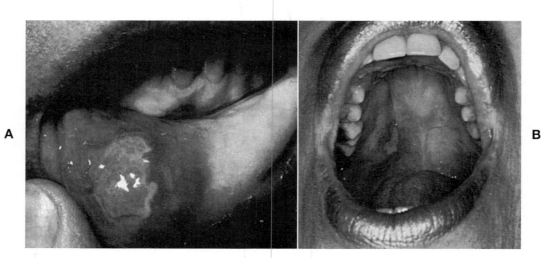

Fig. 34-18 **A** and **B**, Aphthous stomatitis.

stress, or hormonal changes in women, such as in menstruation, pregnancy, menarche, and menopause. Lesions may be induced by trauma, such as self-biting, toothbrush injury, and dental procedures. A familial predisposition has also been noted and described as familial epidemic aphthosis.

Recurrent aphthous stomatitis is the most common lesion of the oral mucosa. It affects from 10% to 20% of the population. It starts commonly in the second or third decade and patients may experience recurrent bouts of lesions several times yearly for many decades. A not uncommon presentation in children is a syndrome characterized by periodic fever, aphthous stomatitis, pharyngitis, and adenitis (PFAPA). The high fevers and associated findings occur with striking periodicity every 4 weeks, last 4 to 6 days, and resolve only to recur the following month. The children are otherwise well. A single dose of prednisone (2mg/kg) aborts the attack.

Ulcerations such as these may also be the presenting sign in Beçhet's syndrome, HIV infection. malabsorption syndromes, gluten-sensitive enteropathy, pernicious anemia, cyclic neutropenia, neutropenia, ulcerative colitis, and Crohn's disease. History, physical examination, complete blood count, and long-term follow-up documenting the recurrent course in the absence of other symptoms will secure the diagnosis. Some patients have aphthosis associated with low folate or iron levels, so testing should include evaluation of these.

ETIOLOGIC FACTORS. Although individual patients often suspect one of the factors mentioned previously was responsible for precipitating their recurrence, only infectious or immunologic mechanisms are suspected to be causative by investigators. The true cause is unknown.

Histologically, the lesion consists of a lymphocytic inflammatory infiltration with occasional plasma cells and eosinophils, which suggests delayed hypersensitivity.

DIAGNOSIS. Aphthous stomatitis must be differentiated from mucous patches of early syphilis, candidiasis, Vincent's angina, the avitaminoses (particularly pellagra and scurvy), erythema multiforme, pemphigus, cicatricial pemphigoid, lichen planus, primary herpes simplex virus infection of the mouth, recurrent labial herpes, and recurrent intraoral herpes simplex virus infection (see facing page).

TREATMENT. At present there is no permanent cure available. Several topical agents will lessen the pain. A mixture of equal parts of elixir of Benadryl and Maalox held in the mouth for 5 minutes before meals is soothing. Lidocaine (Xylocaine Viscous) 2% solution, keeping 1 teaspoonful in the mouth for several minutes, is helpful in allaying pain. Another useful topical anesthetic is dyclonine hydrochloride (Dyclone) 0.5% applied to the lesions. A large number of reasonably effective over-the-counter remedies are also available. Of course, spicy or citrus foods and other irritating substances should be avoided.

One may use other measures to shorten the course and induce healing of lesions. A mixture of equal parts of fluocinonide ointment and Orabase applied to the ulcers three or four times a day is effective in aiding the healing of existing ulcers, as shown by Pimlott et al; however, it did not prevent new ulcers. Temovate ointment may be even more effective. Intralesional steroids and short 3- or 4-day courses of oral steroids may help particularly indolent or large lesions (see the discussion of major aphthae on p. 1008). Nonsteroidal alternatives include an oral suspension of 5 ml containing 250 mg tetracycline is held in the mouth for 2 minutes and then swallowed. This is done four times daily for 1 week. 5% Amlexanox oral paste (Aphthasol) is a newly investigated, potentially useful topical therapy to both induce healing and relieve pain. Sucralfate suspension may be useful as has been described in peptic ulcer disease and the ulcerations of Behçet's disease.

To try to prevent new lesions known triggers for the individual patient should be avoided as much as possible. Dapsone in doses of 25 to 50 mg/day or colchicine, 0.6 mg two or three times daily, may be tried. Thalidomide is now available but caution regarding teratogenicity and neurotoxicity is necessary if this is to be considered. Grinspan reported 15 remissions or marked improvement in 21 severe cases and 19 mild cases—and no failures—using thalidomide, 300 mg daily to start, 200 mg/day after 10 days, and 100 mg/day after 2 months. Relapses were treated with 100 mg/day for 12 days.

Several investigators have reported finding low folate, iron, or B_{12} levels in about 20% of aphthosis patients investigated, but others do not see this with such high frequency. Still, it is worth investigating as correction of the abnormality clears or improves the condition in most cases where an abnormality exists.

Bonnetblanc JM, et al: Thalidomide and recurrent aphthous stomatitis. *Dermatology* 1996, 193:321.

Gatot A, et al: Colchicine therapy in recurrent oral ulcers. *Arch Dermatol* 1984, 120:994.

Graykowski EA, et al: Double-blind trial of tetracycline in recurrent aphthous stomatitis. *J Oral Pathol* 1978, 7:376.

Grinspan D: Significant response of oral aphthosis to thalidomide treatment. *J Am Acad Dermatol* 1985, 12:85.

Grinspan D, et al: Treatment of aphthae with thalidomide. *J Am Acad Dermatol* 1989, 20:1060.

Jacobson JM, et al: Thalidomide for the treatment of oral aphthous ulcers in patients with human immunodeficiency virus infection. *N Engl J Med* 1997, 336:1487.

Katz J, et al: Prevention of recurrent aphthous stomatitis with colchicine. *J Am Acad Dermatol* 1994, 31:459.

Khandwala A, et al: 5% Amlexanox oral paste, a new treatment for recurrent minor aphthous ulcers: I. Clinical demonstration of acceleration of healing and resolution of pain. *Oral Surg Oral Med Oral Pathol Oral Radiol Endod* 1997, 83:222.

Leiferman KM, et al: Recurrent incapacitating mucosal ulcerations: a prodrome of hypereosinophilic syndrome. *JAMA* 1982, 247:1018.

Long SS, et al: Syndrome of periodic fever, aphthous stomatitis, pharyngitis, and adenitis (PFAPA). *J Pediatr* 1999, 135:1.

MacPhail L: Topical and systemic therapy for recurrent aphthous stomatitis. *Semin Cutan Med Surg* 1997, 16:301.

Manders SM, et al: Thalidomide-resistant HIV-associated aphthae successfully treated with granulocyte colony-stimulating factor. *J Am Acad Dermatol* 1995, 33:380.

Padeh S, et al: Periodic fever, aphthous stomatitis, pharyngitis, and adenopathy syndrome. *J Pediatr* 1999, 135:98.

Piantanida EW, et al: Recurrent aphthous stomatitis. *Oral Surg Oral Med Oral Pathol Oral Radiol Endod* 1996, 82:472.

Pimlott SJ, et al: A controlled clinical trial of the efficacy of topically applied fluocinonide in the treatment of recurrent aphthous stomatitis. *Br Dent J* 1983, 154:174.

Rees TD, et al: Recurrent aphthous stomatitis. *Dermatol Clin* 1996, 14:243.

Rogers RS III: Recurrent aphthous stomatitis. *Semin Cutan Med Surg* 1997, 16:278.

Thomas KT, et al: Periodic fever in children. *J Pediatr* 1999, 135:15.

Tseng S, et al: Rediscovering thalidomide. *J Am Acad Dermatol* 1996, 35:969. _____ ▲

MAJOR APHTHOUS ULCER (PERIADENITIS MUCOSA NECROTICA RECURRENS)

In Sutton's disease, a major aphthous ulcer begins as a small shotlike nodule on the inner lip, buccal mucosa, or tongue, which breaks down into a sharply circumscribed ulcer with a deeply punched out and depressed crater (Fig. 34-19).

It is painful. It may at times begin in the faucial pillars or oropharynx. It may persist 2 to 12 weeks before healing with a soft, pliable scar. There are seldom more than one to three lesions present at one time. However, remissions tend to be short, and new lesions may appear before old ones have quite healed. The term *major aphthous ulcers* has supplanted the unwieldy Latin name of this disease.

The cause is unknown, but evidence favors an immunologic or infectious etiology, as discussed under aphthosis. These painful lesions are frequently present in HIV-infected patients.

Treatment is difficult, and the general measures discussed under recurrent aphthae should be employed. Intralesional or systemic steroids in short courses, which may be effective, are often given. If recurrences are such that systemic steroids are prescribed for more than two or three short courses per year, alternative oral medications such as colchicine or dapsone may be tried.

Chung JY, et al: Recurrent scarring ulcers of the oral mucosa. Sutton disease (periadenitis mucosa necrotica recurrens). *Arch Dermatol* 1997, 133:1162.

Grinspan D: Significant response of oral aphthosis to thalidomide treatment. *J Am Acad Dermatol* 1985, 12:85. _____ ▲

BEHÇET'S SYNDROME (OCULO-ORAL-GENITAL SYNDROME)

CLINICAL FEATURES. Behçet's syndrome consists of recurrent oral aphthous ulcerations that recur at least three times in one 12-month period in the presence of any two of the following: recurrent genital ulceration, retinal vasculitis or anterior or posterior uveitis, cutaneous lesions (erythema nodosum; pseudofolliculitis or papulopustular lesions; or acneiform nodules in postadolescent patients who are not receiving corticosteroid treatment), or a positive result to a pathergy test. In addition to these international study group criteria, O'Duffy's criteria also included synovitis or meningoencephalitis and only the more specific skin finding of vasculitis. He excluded patients with inflammatory bowel disease, collagen-vascular disease, and herpetic infection.

Oral lesions occur on the lips, tongue, buccal mucosa, soft and hard palate (Fig. 34-20), tonsils, and even in the pharynx and nasal cavity. The lesions are single or multiple, 2 to 10 mm or larger in diameter, and sharply circumscribed, with a dirty grayish base and a surrounding bright red halo. Other patients show deep ulcerations that leave scars resembling those caused by Sutton's major aphthous ulcers.

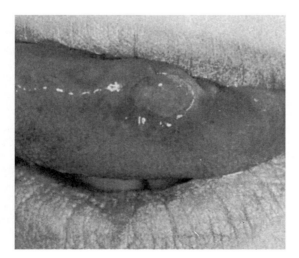

Fig. 34-19 Periadenitis mucosa necrotica recurrens on the side of the tongue. (Courtesy Dr. L. Cohen.)

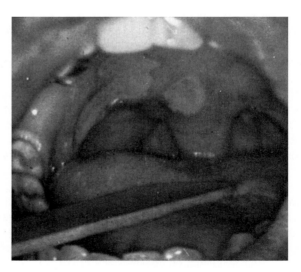

Fig. 34-20 Aphthosis in Behçet's syndrome. (Courtesy Dr. H.O. Curth.)

The lesions are so painful that eating may be difficult. A foul mouth odor is in most instances markedly noticeable.

Genital lesions occur in men on the scrotum and penis or in the urethra; in women, on the vulva (Fig. 34-21), cervix, or vagina; they may be found in both sexes on the genitocrural fold, anus, perineum, or in the rectum. These ulcerations are similar to those seen in the mouth. In addition, macules, papules, and folliculitis may develop on the scrotum. Lesions in women may lead to deep destruction of the vulva. Swellings of the regional nodes and fever may accompany oral and genital attacks.

The ocular lesions start with intense periorbital pain and photophobia. Retinal vasculitis is the most classic eye sign and the chief cause of blindness. Conjunctivitis may be an early, and hypopyon a late, accompaniment of uveitis. Iridocyclitis is frequently seen. Both eyes are eventually involved. The disease untreated leads to blindness from optic atrophy or glaucoma or cataracts.

Neurologic manifestations are mostly in the central nervous system and resemble most closely those of multiple sclerosis. Remissions and exacerbations are the rule.

Thrombophlebitis occurs with some frequency. Thrombosis of the superior vena cava may also occur. Arthralgia is present in most cases in the form of polyarthritis.

Unfortunately, the international criteria include nonspecific common cutaneous lesions (pseudofolliculitis, papulopustular or acneiform lesions). The demonstration of either leukocytoclastic vasculitis or a neutrophilic vascular reaction on histologic examination of a lesion should make the cutaneous criteria more specific.

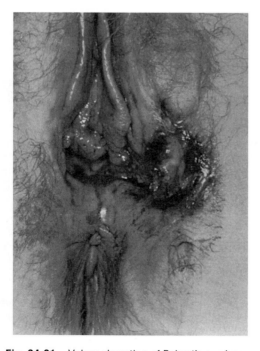

Fig. 34-21 Vulvar ulceration of Behçet's syndrome.

COURSE. Usually the disease starts with one oral ulceration, followed by others. It may take years before additional lesions develop. Therefore, the diagnosis is acceptable in patients with only two classic signs in addition to oral ulcerations. In women anal and genital lesions predominate, often with subsequent involvement of the eyes.

ETIOLOGIC FACTORS. Infectious, immunologic, and genetic causes have been postulated, but the evidence is still inconclusive for any of these. Jorizzo et al advanced a theory to explain the cutaneous pustular vasculitis (pathergy). They found five patients who developed this as a reaction to injected histamine, and also found increased neutrophil chemotaxis to Zymosan-activated serum. They postulated that this enhanced chemotaxis would bring numerous neutrophils to the site of any cutaneous or synovial trauma, in response to the release of histamine and other mediators.

INCIDENCE. There is a relatively high prevalence of Behçet's disease in the Far East and the Mediterranean countries, whereas in the United States and Western Europe it is much less common. In the large series of patients from areas of higher prevalence, men with age of onset in their thirties predominate. Mangelsdorf et al reported on 25 patients seen in a university dermatology referral practice in the United States. Twenty-two of their patients were young women who manifested by a high frequency of mucocutaneous lesions and a low prevalence of ocular involvement. This may reflect referral bias or could indicate the disease is less severe in the United States.

HISTOLOGY. The early lesions show a leukocytoclastic vasculitis. There is perivascular infiltration, which is chiefly lymphocytic in older lesions, with endothelial proliferation that obliterates the lumen.

DIFFERENTIAL DIAGNOSIS. Behçet's disease must be differentiated from herpetic or aphthous stomatitis, pemphigus, oral cancer, and Stevens-Johnson syndrome (erythema multiforme). A skin puncture or pathergy test may be used to investigate patients further; however, it is not reliable in that it may be negative in otherwise well-documented cases. It is done by injecting 0.1 ml of normal saline solution into the skin or by simply pricking the skin with a sterile needle. A pustule appears at the site within 24 hours. If results are negative, the test should be repeated at two to five points before results are accepted. Pathergy has been observed in patients with Behçet's disease, pyoderma gangrenosum, Sweet's syndrome, and bowel-associated dermatosis-arthritis syndrome.

TREATMENT. Usually the ulcerations heal spontaneously. Mild mouthwashes and toothpastes and restricted use of the toothbrush should be prescribed when there are oral lesions. With regard to treating the symptoms and healing of the aphthae, local treatments as described above may be used. Sucralfate suspension has been studied in Behçet's oral and genital ulcers and was found to decrease pain and healing time. On the whole, the therapeutic problem of aphthosis is not the healing of the individual lesions but the prevention of new attacks. For that purpose several options exist, none of which is optimal. Colchicine, 0.6 mg twice daily, may be started for 2 weeks. In the absence of response and gastrointestinal side effects, the dose may be increased to three times daily. Although this may not totally alleviate the mucocutaneous lesions, it may decrease their recurrence rate by 50% or more. Dapsone may be substituted or added to this for improvement of response. The usual therapeutic final dose is 100 mg daily. Thalidomide is now available and has been found to be effective in many patients. Saylan et al, using thalidomide 200 mg twice a day for 5 days and 100 mg twice a day for 15 to 60 days, found that it caused rapid healing of aphthae and reduced recurrences. It had no effect on iridocyclitis. Of course, long-term treatment will commonly be complicated by neurotoxicity and the teratogenicity of this medication is well known.

Methotrexate in a weekly oral dose of 7.5 to 20 mg should be reserved for severe refractory cases, as should more aggressive systemic treatments such as systemic corticosteroids, azathioprine, chlorambucil, cyclosporine, and cyclophosphamide.

Alpsoy E, et al: The use of busucralfate suspension in the treatment of oral and genital ulceration of Behçet disease: a randomized, placebo-controlled, double-blind study. *Arch Dermatol* 1999, 135:529.

Arbesfeld SJ, et al: Behçet's disease. *J Am Acad Dermatol* 1988, 19:767.

Avci O, et al: Efficacy of cyclosporine on mucocutaneous manifestations of Behçet's disease. *J Am Acad Dermatol* 1997, 36:796.

Balabanova M, et al: A study of the cutaneous manifestations of Behçet's disease in patients from the United States. *J Am Acad Dermatol* 1999, 41:540.

Chen KR, et al: Cutaneous vasculitis in Behçet's disease. *J Am Acad Dermatol* 1997, 36:689.

Dega H, et al: Mucocutaneous criteria for the diagnosis of Behçet's disease. *J Am Acad Dermatol* 1996, 35:789.

Ehrlich GE: Vasculitis in Behçet's disease. *Int Rev Immunol* 1997, 14:81.

Ghate JV, et al: Behçet's disease and complex aphthosis. *J Am Acad Dermatol* 1999, 40:1.

Jorizzo JL: Neutrophilic vascular reactions. *J Am Acad Dermatol* 1988, 19:983.

Jorizzo JL, et al: Behçet's syndrome: immune regulation, circulating immune complexes, neutrophil migration, and colchicine therapy. *J Am Acad Dermatol* 1984, 10:205.

Jorizzo JL, et al: Behçet's disease. *Arch Dermatol* 1986, 122:556.

Jorizzo JL, et al: Complex aphthosis. *J Am Acad Dermatol* 1985, 13:80.

Jorizzo JL, et al: Pustular vasculitis. *J Am Acad Dermatol* 1983, 9:160.

Kaklamani VG, et al: Behçet's disease. *Semin Arthritis Rheum* 1998, 27:197.

Kone Paut I, et al: Clinical features of Behçet's disease in children. *J Pediatr* 1998, 132:721.

Mangelsdorf HC, et al: Behçet's disease. *J Am Acad Dermatol* 1996, 34:745.

O'Duffy JD, et al: Chlorambucil in the treatment of uveitis and meningoencephalitis of Behçet's disease. *Am J Med* 1984, 76:75.

Pezzi PP, et al: Prognosis in Behçet's disease. *Ann Ophthalmol* 1985, 17:20.

Sakane T: New perspective on Behçet's disease. *Int Rev Immunol* 1997, 14:89.

Samlaska CP, et al: Superficial thrombophlebitis. II. Secondary hypercoagulable states. *J Am Acad Dermatol* 1990, 23:1.

Saylan T, et al: Thalidomide in the treatment of Behçet's syndrome. *Arch Dermatol* 1982, 118:536.

Sharquie KE: Suppression of Behçet's disease with dapsone. *Br J Dermatol* 1984, 110:493.

Tabbara KF: Chlorambucil in Behçet's disease. *Ophthalmology* 1983, 90:906. ▲

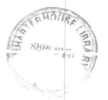

CHAPTER 35

Cutaneous Vascular Diseases

Vasomotor disorders

RAYNAUD'S PHENOMENON AND RAYNAUD'S DISEASE

Raynaud's means either Raynaud's phenomenon (in the presence of associated collagen vascular disease) or Raynaud's disease (in the absence of such disease).

Raynaud's Phenomenon

Raynaud's phenomenon is produced by an intermittent constriction of the small digital arteries and arterioles. The digits have varying but symmetrical pallor, cyanosis, and rubor. The involved parts are affected in paroxysms by the attacks of ischemia, which cause them to become pale, cold to the touch, and numb. In time the parts may fail to regain their normal circulation between attacks and become persistently cyanotic and painful. If this phenomenon persists over a long period, punctate superficial necrosis of the fingertips develops; later, even gangrene may occur.

The phenomenon is more frequently observed in cold weather. When exposed to cold the digits become white (ischemic), then blue (cyanotic), and finally red (hyperemic).

Raynaud's phenomenon occurs most frequently in young to middle-aged women. It occurs with scleroderma, dermatomyositis, lupus erythematosus, mixed connective tissue disease (MCTD), Sjögren's syndrome, rheumatoid arthritis, and paroxysmal hemoglobinuria. Occlusive arterial diseases such as embolism, thromboangiitis obliterans, and arteriosclerosis obliterans may be present. In addition, various diseases of the nervous system, or cervical rib and scalenus anticus syndrome, may produce the disorder. Physical trauma such as pneumatic hammer operation and that incurred by pianists and typists may also induce this phenomenon. Medications such as bleomycin or ergot may also be the cause. The clumping of red blood cells is believed to be responsible for the induction of Raynaud's phenomenon in cryoglobulinemia, polycythemia vera, and other disorders with high titers of circulating cold agglutinins. Scleroderma was the underlying diagnosis in more than half of patients in one series. In a series of 165 patients with Raynaud's phenomenon reported by Vayssairat et al, 51 had primary disease (Raynaud's disease) and 54 patients had incomplete connective tissue disease (35 with positive antinuclear antibody [ANA] titer). Only 2.5% of incomplete connective tissue disease will progress to fulfill the criteria for a specific rheumatologic disorder.

Simple noninvasive tests along with other clinical findings are used to distinguish between Raynaud's disease and Raynaud's phenomenon. Sclerodactyly, digital pitted scars, puffy fingers with telangiectases, positive ANA test, acrosteolysis or subcutaneous calcifications by radiograph of the hands, basilar lung fibrosis on chest radiograph, and changes on nailfold capillary microscopy ("avascular skip" areas with irregularly dilated capillary loops) are signs of connective tissue disease. Nailfold capillary changes are helpful prognostic indicators and periodic acid-Schiff (PAS)-positive globules in the proximal nailfold are frequently detected on biopsy. Anti-centromere antibody testing is part of the workup to exclude CREST syndrome.

Raynaud's Disease

Raynaud's disease is a primary disorder of cold sensitivity primarily seen in young women. It is characterized by intermittent attacks of pallor, cyanosis, hyperemia, and numbness of the fingers, precipitated by cold. The disease is bilateral, and gangrene occurs in less than 1% of cases.

Diagnosis is made by the absence of any other disease such as those enumerated under Raynaud's phenomenon. The tests outlined above are recommended. Although the current dictum is that Raynaud's disease should be present for 2 years before being classified as a primary process, it may take as long as 11 years for some systemic disorders to manifest. The prognosis is good for Raynaud's disease.

Etiology

The cause of Raynaud's phenomenon/disease is believed to be multifactorial. Increased alpha-2 sympathetic receptor activity on vessels, endothelial dysfunction, deficiency of calcitonin gene-related peptide protein–containing nerves or some central thermoregulatory defect have been implicated. Vasoconstricting and profibrotic cytokine endothelin-1 has been found elevated in patients with scleroderma, causing significant tissue damage and provoking fibrosis. Endothelin-1, -2, and -3 are a family of 21 amino acid peptides that are potent, long-acting vasoconstrictors of mammalian blood vessels. Elevated endothelin-1 has been found in many collagen vascular diseases, particularly in patients with Raynaud's phenomenon/disease and systemic sclerosis. Calcitonin gene-related peptide is a powerful vasodilator present in digital cutaneous perivascular nerves. Infusion of calcitonin gene-related peptide in patients with Raynaud's phenomenon demonstrates increased hand temperatures compared with saline controls. In addition, patients with ulcers healed with infusions compared with none of the patients with ulcerations treated with saline controls. Women receiving unopposed estrogen replacement are twice as likely to experience Raynaud's phenomenon as women not receiving estrogen replacement or women receiving estrogen and progesterone.

Treatment

The following discussion applies to both Raynaud's phenomenon and Raynaud's disease. Exposure to cold should be avoided as much as possible. This includes avoidance of exposure to cold not only of the extremities but also of other parts of the body, since vasospasm may be induced by cooling of the body alone. Warm gloves should be worn whenever possible. Residence in a warm climate is helpful. Trauma to the fingertips should be avoided. Smoking is forbidden.

Vasodilating drugs such as nifedipine, 10 to 20 mg three times a day; prazosin, 1 mg three times a day increased to 3 mg three times a day; or reserpine have been helpful in many. Nifedipine is considered to be the gold standard, and two thirds of treated patients will respond favorably. The newer second-generation dihydropyridines, such as amlodipine, isradipine, nicardipine, and felodipine, have also been shown effective and are associated with fewer side effects. Pentoxifylline and stanozolol have shown variable success. Calcitonin gene-related peptide infusions at doses of 0.6 μg/min for 3 hours per day for 5-day intervals have been shown effective. Tolazoline hydrochloride (Priscoline), 50 mg three times daily, is frequently helpful in mild cases.

The local application of 2% nitroglycerin in an ointment base (Nitro-Bid, Nitrostat) rubbed in well several times will give relief to some patients within 2 hours. Topical vasodilators may shift the blood supply to more vascularized areas and should be used cautiously. Sublingual administration of nitroglycerin was effective in only 2 of 10 patients treated by Peterson et al, while 8 of 10 were improved by biofeedback training, even 8 weeks after the

sessions were over. Sublingual nitroglycerin may be more effective if combined with oral sympatholytic agents. Additionally, sublingual nitroglycerin might be useful in patients with infrequent attacks, since it is convenient and easily administered.

In severe, disabling cases of Raynaud's with trophic changes, sympathectomy has been recommended. Sympathetic ganglionectomy with resection of the sympathetic trunk for both the upper and lower extremities has produced good or excellent results in some series. These effects are often only temporary, lasting for some 6 months to 2 years.

Bunker CB, et al: Calcitonin gene-related peptide, endothelin-1, the cutaneous microvasculature and Raynaud's phenomenon. *Br J Dermatol* 1996, 134:399.

Bunker CB, et al: Calcitonin gene-related peptide in treatment of severe peripheral vascular insufficiency in Raynaud's phenomenon. *Lancet* 1993, 342:80.

Ho M, et al: Raynaud's phenomenon: state of the art 1998. *Scand J Rheumatol* 1998, 27:319.

Isenberg DA, et al: ABC of rheumatology: Raynaud's phenomenon, scleroderma, and overlap syndromes. *BMJ* 1995, 310:795.

Kahaleh MB: Raynaud's phenomenon and the vascular disease in scleroderma. *Curr Opin Rheumatol* 1995, 7:529.

Likakis J, et al: Effect of long-term estrogen therapy on brachial arterial endothelium-dependent vasodilation in women with Raynaud's phenomenon secondary to systemic sclerosis. *Am J Cardiol* 1998, 82:1555.

Noel B, et al: Hand-arm vibration syndrome with proximal ulnar artery occlusion. *Vasa* 1998, 27:176.

Peterson LL, et al: Raynaud's syndrome: treatment with sublingual nitroglycerine, swinging arm maneuver, and biofeedback training. *Arch Dermatol* 1983, 119:396.

Sturgill MG, et al: Rational use of calcium-channel antagonists in Raynaud's phenomenon. *Curr Opin Rheumatol* 1998, 10:584.

Turton EP, et al: The aetiology of Raynaud's phenomenon. *Cardiovasc Surg* 1998, 6:431.

Vayssairat M, et al: Raynaud's phenomenon together with antinuclear antibodies: a common subset of incomplete connective tissue disease. *J Am Acad Dermatol* 1995, 32:747.

Wigley FM: Raynaud's phenomenon and other features of scleroderma, including pulmonary hypertension. *Curr Opin Rheumatol* 1996, 8:561.

Wigley FM, et al: Raynaud's phenomenon. *Rheum Dis Clin North Am* 1996, 22:765.

Yamane K: Endothelin and collagen vascular disease: a review with special reference to Raynaud's phenomenon and systemic sclerosis. *Intern Med* (Japan) 1994, 33:579.

ERYTHROMELALGIA

Also called *erythermalgia* and *acromelalgia*, this rare form of paroxysmal vasodilation affects the feet with burning, localized pain, redness, and heat, with high skin temperature (Fig. 35-1). Infrequently, the upper extremities may be involved. The burning paroxysms may last from a few minutes to several days; they are usually triggered by an increase in environmental temperature.

The disease may be primary or secondary to a myelo-

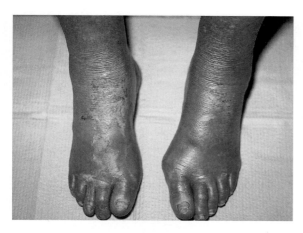

Fig. 35-1 Erythromelalgia.

proliferative disease such as polycythemia vera, thrombotic thrombocytopenic purpura, or thrombocythemia. Peripheral neuritis, myelitis, or multiple sclerosis may be present. Secondary erythromelalgia has also been associated with systemic lupus erythematosus, hypertension, and diabetes mellitus. Calcium channel blockers may exacerbate or even induce it. Childhood erythromelalgia often appears without an underlying disorder, may be familial, and tends to be resistant to aspirin.

The pathophysiology is poorly understood. Many believe the disorder is related to peripheral neurotransmission and disturbed platelet function. There has been no effective treatment for adult-onset idiopathic erythromelalgia. Erythromelalgia caused by thrombocytosis responds to aspirin. Erythromelalgia caused by underlying disease processes tend to respond to treatment of the primary disorder. The severe symptoms are relieved by measures, such as immersion in cold water, that cool the skin. Good results in difficult cases have been obtained with serotonin antagonists (methysergide, pizotifen, and sertraline), which suggests that this may be a disease of peripheral serotonin activity. Other treatment suggestions have been epinephrine, ephedrine, sublingual isoproterenol hydrochloride, nitroglycerin ointment, prednisone, phlebotomy, sodium nitroprusside, lumbar ganglionectomy, and peripheral nerve block or section.

Drenth JPH, et al: Erythromelalgia and erythermalgia. *Int J Dermatol* 1994, 13:85.

Kurzrock, et al: Paraneoplastic erythromelalgia. *Clin Dermatol* 1993, 11:73.

Nalke L, et al: Painful distal erythema and thrombocytosis: erythromelalgia secondary to thrombocytosis. *Arch Dermatol* 1993, 129:105.

Rudikoff D, et al: Erythromelalgia. *J Am Acad Dermatol* 1997, 37:281.

Yosipovitch G, et al: Erythromelalgia in a patient with thrombotic thrombocytopenic purpura. *J Am Acad Dermatol* 1992, 26:825. ▲

LIVEDO RETICULARIS

Livedo reticularis is a mottled or reticulated pink or reddish blue discoloration of the skin, mostly on the extremities (Fig. 35-2), especially the lower legs around the ankles. It also affects the feet, thighs, trunk, and forearms. Exposure to cold usually accentuates the intensity of discoloration, although the lesions may be fixed and remain present on warming (sometimes referred to as *livedo racemosa*). The lesions are often asymptomatic; in other instances, coldness, numbness, paresthesia, or a dull ache may be present.

Livedo reticularis may be a manifestation of lupus erythematosus, dermatomyositis, scleroderma, rheumatic fever, or rheumatoid arthritis. It may be seen with hepatitis C, parvovirus B19, syphilis, meningococcemia, pneumococcal sepsis, tuberculosis, pancreatitis, decompression sickness, various forms of arteritis (Wegener's granulomatosis), polycythemia vera, hypercalcemia, pheochromocytoma, mycosis fungoides, breast cancer, and thrombocytopenic purpura. It has been reported as a photosensitivity phenomenon in patients taking quinidine. It is a side effect of amantadine (Symmetrel). Some patients on long-term minocycline therapy have been shown to develop drug-induced arthritis, fever, livedo reticularis, and positive peripheral antineutrophil cytoplasmic autoantibodies (P-ANCA) titers. Livedo reticularis may be a complication of carbon dioxide arteriography. Most cases, however, are unassociated with any disease.

Necrotizing livedo reticularis may be associated with cutaneous nodules and ulcerations (Fig. 35-3). Cholesterol emboli resulting from severe atherosclerotic disease may cause unilateral or bilateral livedo reticularis. Patients frequently have concomitant cyanosis, purpura, nodules, ulceration, or gangrene. Older men with severe atherosclerotic disease are most affected. They are often on anticoagulant therapy, and many have recently undergone vascular surgery or instrumentation. The differential diagnosis includes vasculitis, septic staphylococcal emboli resulting from an infected aneurysm (usually secondary to instrumentation such as cardiac catheterization), and periarteritis nodosa. Mortality is 72%. Deep biopsy with serial sections may demonstrate the characteristic cholesterol clefts within thrombi. Livedo reticularis of recent onset in an elderly person warrants consideration of this diagnosis.

Necrotizing livedo reticularis has also been reported with leukocytoclastic vasculitis, heparin-associated thrombosis, cryoglobulinemia, calciphylaxis, calcifying panniculitis, oxalosis, compressed air injury, bismuth or pentazocine injections, atrial myxomas, Wegener's granulomatosis, systemic lupus erythematosus (SLE), and other connective tissue diseases. Although livedo reticularis with ulcerations can occur in periarteritis nodosa, most of these cases are secondary to leukocytoclastic vasculitis. Hepatitis C needs to be excluded in those patients with cryoglobulinemia.

Sneddon's syndrome is the association of livedo reticularis, usually in young to middle-aged patients who then

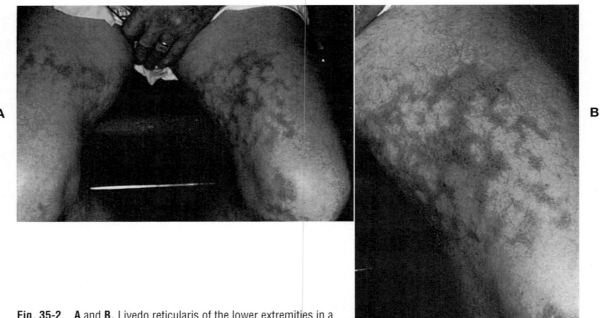

Fig. 35-2 **A** and **B,** Livedo reticularis of the lower extremities in a man with advanced arteriosclerosis of the femoral vessels.

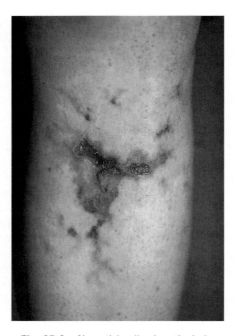

Fig. 35-3 Necrotizing livedo reticularis.

develop a cerebrovascular lesion. It may have a genetic component and is likely to be severe and progressive. Some patients have antiphospholipid antibodies and may have incipient SLE. Up to 35% will be positive for anti-endothelial cell antibodies (AECA).

Oxalosis may lead to livedo reticularis from deposition of oxalate crystals in and around blood vessel walls. The primary type comprises two rare autosomal recessive disorders, each lacking one specific enzyme. Secondary forms also occur. The characteristic crystals are seen on biopsy.

Patients with SLE may have livedo reticularis, which, when moderately severe, is apt to be associated with more severe disease manifestations such as central nervous system (CNS) disease, renal disease, vasculitis, and cardiolipin antibodies. The full spectrum of cutaneous changes are discussed under lupus erythematosus in Chapter 8.

Cutis marmorata is a term applied to skin resembling marble because of its mottled bluish discoloration. It is commonly seen on the lower extremities in young children and women exposed to cold. The mottling usually disappears when the extremities are warmed. It is a physiologic mottling of the skin.

Arnoff DM, et al: Necrosing livedo reticularis in a patient with recurrent pulmonary hemorrhage. *J Am Acad Dermatol* 1997, 37:300.

Dean SM, et al: Calciphylaxis. *Vasc Med* 1998, 3:115.

Dereure O, et al: Acute generalized livedo reticularis with myasthenialike syndrome revealing parvovirus B19 primary infection. *Arch Dermatol* 1995, 131:744.

Elkayam O, et al: Minocycline induced arthritis associated with fever, livedo reticularis, and pANCA. *Ann Rheum Dis* (England) 1996, 55:769.

Faclieru D, et al: A study of coagulation and anti-endothelial antibodies in idiopathic livedo reticularis. *Acta Derm Venereol* (Norway) 1997, 77:181.

Frances C, et al: Prevalence of anti-endothelial cell antibodies in patients with Sneddon's syndrome. *J Am Acad Dermatol* 1995, 33:64.

Gibson GE, et al: Antiphospholipid syndrome and the skin. *J Am Acad Dermatol* 1997, 36:970.

Gross AS, et al: Heparin-associated thrombocytopenia and thrombosis (HAAT) presenting with livedo reticularis. *Int J Dermatol* 1993, 32:276.

Karlsberg PL, et al: Cutaneous vasculitis and rheumatoid factor positivity as presenting signs of hepatitis C virus-induced mixed cryoglobulinemia. *Arch Dermatol* 1995, 131:1119.

Maroon M: Polycythemia rubra vera presenting as livedo reticularis. *J Am Acad Dermatol* 1992, 26:264.

McAllister SM, et al: Painful acral purpura. *Arch Dermatol* 1998, 134:789.

Rundback JH, et al: Livedo reticularis, rhabdomyolysis, massive intestinal infarction, and death after carbon dioxide arteriography. *J Vasc Surg* 1997, 26:337.

Sheehan MG, et al: Position dependent livedo reticularis in cholesterol emboli syndrome. *J Rheumatol* 1993, 20:1973.

Spiers EM, et al: Livedo reticularis and inflammatory carcinoma of the breast. *J Am Acad Dermatol* 1994, 31:689.

Triplett DA: Many faces of lupus anticoagulants. *Lupus* 1998, 7:S18.

Winship IM, et al: Primary oxalosis: an unusual cause of livedo reticularis. *Clin Exp Dermatol* 1991, 16:367.

Young PC, et al: Widespread livedo reticularis with painful ulcerations. *Arch Dermatol* 1995, 131:786. ▲

LIVEDOID VASCULITIS

Synonyms for livedoid vasculitis include *livedoid vasculopathy, atrophie blanche,* and *PURPLE (painful purpuric ulcers with reticular pattern of the lower extremities)* in which the histologic features of leukocytoclastic vasculitis are absent. The vasculopathy is characterized clinically by early, focal, painful purpuric lesions of the lower extremities that frequently ulcerate and slowly heal (Fig. 35-4). The ulcers heal with small, stellate, white scars called *atrophie blanche* but may also show telangiectasis, hemosiderin-induced hyperpigmentation, and livedo racemosa (Fig. 35-5). Patients with livedo reticularis may progress to develop livedoid vasculitis; however, not all patients with livedoid vasculitis will manifest with livedoid reticularis. *Atrophie blanche* is a nonspecific term that is best reserved to describe morphologic appearance and not as a diagnosis (venous stasis disease is the primary cause of atrophie blanche).

Livedoid vasculitis mostly represents an idiopathic disorder but may be associated with systemic diseases. Primary or secondary hypercoagulable states, particularly those associated with anticardiolipin antibody syndrome, protein C deficiency, hepatitis C, and fibrinolytic anomalies, may be the cause. Clinical evaluations should exclude these disorders, as well as venous and arterial peripheral vascular diseases.

Livedo vasculitis is a chronic, recurrent, segmental hyalinizing vasculopathy of the small blood vessels. Fibrin, C3, and IgM are often found in vessel walls. Histologically, the small vessels of the mid and lower levels of the dermis show endothelial proliferations, hyaline degeneration, fibrin plugs, and thrombosis. A perivascular hemorrhage may be present. Because of the absence of polymorphonuclear neutrophils, this is not a vasculitis but a vasculopathy. Endothelial thrombomodulin expression is elevated in patients with livedo vasculitis, while blood tests of co-

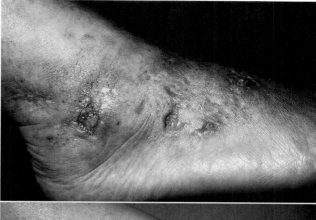
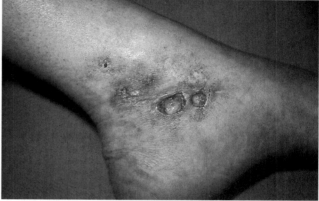

Fig. 35-4 A and B, Ulcerations in livedoid vasculitis.

agulation and fibrinolytic activity are often normal. Papi et al have demonstrated platelet (P-selectin) and lymphocyte activation, while the levels of inflammatory mediators remain normal.

Low dosage of aspirin (325 or even 162 mg once or twice daily) and dipyridamole have been effective. Addition of a third antiplatelet drug may provide additional benefit. Beraprost sodium (120 μg daily) or minidose heparin, as little as 5000 units every 3 days, has been reported to be effective. Nifedipine, 10 mg three times a day, produced healing in a patient in whom dipyridamole and aspirin had failed. Pentoxifylline, 400 mg two or three times a day, with 400 mg a day for maintenance, is another treatment option. The condition has been successfully treated with a combination of phenformin and ethylestrenol. Low–molecular-weight dextran is indicated for treating hypofibrinolytic disease, and has been shown effective in treating both livedo reticularis and livedo vasculitis. Superinfection of ulcers should be treated with systemic antibiotics, and skin grafts to large ulcers, in patients whose disease appears to be responding to therapy. PUVA has been reported useful in two patients treated by Choi et al.

Livedoid Dermatitis. Livedoid dermatitis is an embolic phenomenon (infarction) leading to temporary or prolonged

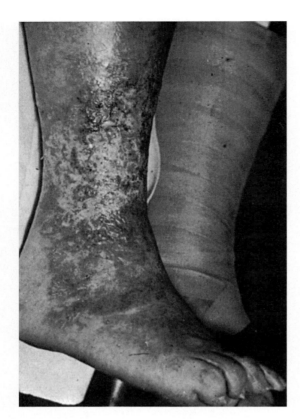

Fig. 35-5 Stellate scars and hyperpigmentation of livedoid vasculitis.

local ischemia as a result of accidental arterial obliteration from the intragluteal injections of various drugs. Refer to the discussion of injection site reactions in Chapter 6.

Perinatal Gangrene of the Buttock. Perinatal gangrene of the buttock is similar to livedoid dermatitis. It usually is a complication of umbilical artery catheterization, exchange transfusion, or cord injections by means of a syringe. It may also be a spontaneous event.

Choi H-J, et al: Livedo reticularis and livedoid vasculitis responding to PUVA therapy. *J Am Acad Dermatol* 1999, 40:204.

Fritsch P, et al: Livedo vasculitis. *Hautarzt* (Germany) 1995, 215:222.

Grattan CE, et al: Sneddon's syndrome with livedo vasculitis and anticardiolipin antibodies. *Br J Dermatol* 1989, 120:441.

Grob JJ, et al: Thrombotic skin disease as a marker of the anticardiolipin syndrome: livedo vasculitis and distal gangrene associated with abnormal serum antiphospholipid activity. *J Am Acad Dermatol* 1989, 20:1063.

Jorizzo JL: Livedoid vasculopathy: what is it (editorial)? *Arch Dermatol* 1998, 134:491.

Karlsberg PL, et al: Cutaneous vasculitis and rheumatoid factor positivity as presenting signs of hepatitis C virus-induced mixed cryoglobulinemia. *Arch Dermatol* 1995, 131:1119.

McCalmont CS, et al: Livedo vasculitis. *Clin Exp Dermatol* 1992, 17:4.

Mocan H, et al: Cutaneous polyarteritis nodosa in a child and a review of the literature. *Acta Paediatr* 1998, 87:351.

Papi M, et al: Livedo vasculopathy vs small vessel cutaneous vasculitis: cytokine and platelet P-selectin studies. *Arch Dermatol* 1998, 134:447.

Purcell SM, et al: Nifedipine treatment of idiopathic atrophie blanche (letter). *J Am Acad Dermatol* 1986, 14:851.

Serrano G, et al: Perinatal gangrene of the buttock. *Arch Dermatol* 1985, 121:23.

Tsutsui K, et al: Successful treatment of livedo vasculitis with beraprost sodium. *Dermatology* (Switzerland) 1996, 192:120.

Yamamoto M, et al: Antithrombotic treatment in livedo vasculitis. *J Am Acad Dermatol* 1988, 18:57. _____ ▲

MARSHALL-WHITE SYNDROME ("BIER'S SPOTS")

The marbled mottling produced in the forearm and hand by occluding the brachial artery with a tight sphygmomanometer cuff is characterized initially, and chiefly, by pale macules 1 or 2 cm in diameter. These were described by Bier in 1898 and are known as *Bier's spots*. Wilkin reexamined this phenomenon with laser Doppler velocimetry and concluded that the red spots that also appear (chiefly on the hand) are caused by relative vasodilatation, with vasoconstriction in the pale areas.

Marshall-White syndrome consists of Bier's spots and is associated with insomnia and tachycardia. These pale macules are cooler than the surrounding pink skin and become more apparent when the hands are lowered for some time. This syndrome has been noted in white middle-aged men.

Marshall W, et al: Dermatologic and psychosomatic aspects of Marshall-White syndrome. *Cutis* 1965, 1:184.

Wilkin JK, et al: Bier's spots reconsidered: a tale of two spots, with speculation in a humerous vein. *J Am Acad Dermatol* 1986, 14:411. ▲

Purpura

Purpura is multifocal extravasation of blood into the skin or mucous membrane. It is manifested by distinctive brownish red or purplish macules a few millimeters in diameter resulting from the rupture of the capillary walls at the arteriolar-capillary junction. Several types of purpura are recognized.

Petechiae are superficial, pinhead-sized (less than 3 mm), round, hemorrhagic macules, bright red at first, then brownish or rust colored. They are most commonly seen in the dependent areas, are evanescent, occur in crops, regress over a period of days, and most often imply a disorder of platelets, usually thrombocytopenia. They may also be a sign of a blood vessel disease such as scurvy or amyloidosis; however, they are not usually indicative of a coagulation factor disorder. These disorders typically give rise to ecchymoses or hematomas.

Ecchymoses are better known as bruises or "black and blue marks." These extravasations signify a deeper and more extensive interstitial hemorrhage, which forms a flat, irregularly shaped, bluish-purplish patch. Such patches gradually turn yellowish and finally fade away.

Vibices (singular, *vibex*) are linear purpuric lesions.

Hematoma designates a pool-like collection of extravasated blood in a dead space in tissue that, if of sufficient size, produces a swelling that fluctuates on palpation. Hematomas are usually walled off by tissue planes.

Pathogenesis

Hemorrhage may result from hyper- and hypocoagulable states, vascular dysfunction, and extravascular causes. Altered coagulation affecting platelet number or function include disorders such as idiopathic thrombocytopenic purpura, thrombotic thrombocytopenic purpura, disseminated intravascular coagulation, drug-induced thrombocytopenia, bone marrow failure, congenital or inherited platelet function defects, acquired platelet function defects (aspirin, renal or hepatic disease, or gammopathy), and thrombocytosis secondary to myeloproliferable diseases. Most of these disorders produce findings of nonpalpable purpura. Ecchymosis predominates in procoagulant defects, such as hemophilia, anticoagulants, disseminated intravascular coagulation, vitamin K deficiency, and hepatic disease resulting in poor procoagulant synthesis.

Vascular causes include both inflammatory and noninflammatory disorders. Inflammatory disorders result in inflammation within the vessel wall. Perivascular inflammation is not considered evidence of a vasculitis and does not cause palpable purpura, which is the hallmark of inflammatory hemorrhage.

Noninflammatory causes are also referred to as *bland occlusive disorders* in which fibrin, cryoglobulin, or other material occludes vessels, activating the clotting cascade and producing thrombus within the retiform (livedoid) network of the superficial dermal venules. Palpable purpura is often found. Representative causes include ecthyma gangrenosum, monoclonal cryoglobulinemia, cryofibrinogenemia, disseminated intravascular coagulation, purpura fulminans, protein C deficiency, warfarin-induced necrosis (Fig. 35-6), heparin necrosis, cholesterol emboli, oxalate crystal occlusion, antiphospholipid syndrome, and some forms of livedoid vasculitis (see necrotizing livedo vasculitis on p. 1015).

Extravascular causes often include a component of trauma. Increased frequency of ecchymotic skin can be the result of poor dermal support of blood vessels, most often localized to the area of trauma, and may result from actinic (senile) purpura, topical or systemic corticosteroid therapy (Fig. 35-7), scurvy, systemic amyloidosis, Ehlers-Danlos syndrome, or pseudoxanthoma elasticum.

Evaluation

A history and physical examination is often all that is necessary. A family history of bleeding or thrombotic disorders, duration of symptoms, use of drugs and medica-

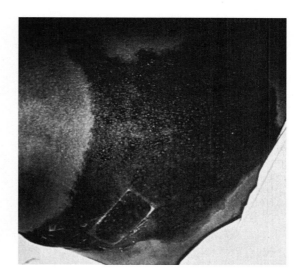

Fig. 35-6 Warfarin necrosis.

tions that might affect platelet function and coagulation, as well as a review of medical conditions that may result in altered coagulation, should be documented. Physical examination should stress the size, type, and distribution of purpura; a search for telangiectases; a joint examination; and an evaluation of skin elasticity, unusual scars, and unusual body habitus. Correlation of purpura morphology with pathogenesis allows for a more focused approach.

A complete blood cell count and differential can be used to assess for microangiopathic anemia, screen for myeloproliferative disorders, and assess the number and morphology of platelets. A bleeding time is the preferred method of assessing platelet function. Prolongations in the partial thromboplastin time (PTT) or the prothrombin time (PT) are not always indicative of abnormal coagulation states and should be correlated with the clinical findings. More detailed laboratory evaluations should be performed to investigate specific hypo- or hypercoagulable states.

Lotti T: The purpura. *Int J Dermatol* 1994, 33:1.

Piette WW: The differential diagnosis of purpura from a morphologic perspective. *Adv Dermatol* 1994, 9:3. _____ ▲

THROMBOCYTOPENIC PURPURA

Thrombocytopenic purpura may be classified into three large categories: states resulting from accelerated platelet destruction, states resulting from deficient platelet production, and states resulting from complex, often unknown pathogenesis. The latter two categories will not be discussed here because they are generally in the province of hematologists, being the result of diseases such as aplastic anemia and leukemia. Accelerated platelet destruction may be immunologic or nonimmunologic. The former may be

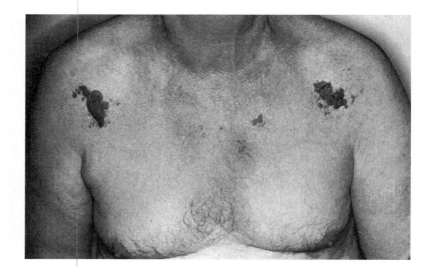

Fig. 35-7 Purpura resulting from chronic topical application of potent corticosteroids.

due to antibodies (idiopathic or drug-induced thrombocytopenia), isoantibodies (congenital, or posttransfusion), immune complex disease, or other immunologic processes such as erythroblastosis fetalis, neonatal lupus, scleroderma, other connective tissue diseases, or acquired immunodeficiency syndrome (AIDS). The group of thrombocytopenias with accelerated platelet destruction caused by nonimmunologic processes includes thrombotic thrombocytopenic purpura and disseminated intravascular coagulation.

Idiopathic Thrombocytopenic Purpura

Idiopathic thrombocytopenic purpura (ITP) is also known as *autoimmune thrombocytopenic purpura,* or *Werlhof's disease.* It is characterized by either an acute or gradual onset of petechiae or ecchymoses in the skin (Fig. 35-8) and mucous membranes, especially in the mouth. Epistaxis, conjunctival hemorrhages, hemorrhagic bullae in the mouth, and gingival bleeding may occur. Melena, hematemesis, and menorrhagia also occur, and the latter may be the first sign of this disease in young women. Chronic leg ulcers occasionally develop. The presence of splenomegaly usually, but not always, excludes the diagnosis of immune thrombocytopenic purpura.

Bleeding occurs when the platelet count drops below 50,000/mm^3. Clear-cut posttraumatic hemorrhage (Fig. 35-9), some spontaneous hemorrhage, and petechiae may appear. The risk of serious hemorrhage is greatly increased at levels below 10,000/mm^3, and the gravest complication, intracranial hemorrhage, most often occurs with counts below 2000/mm^3. Bleeding time is usually prolonged and coagulation time is normal, whereas the clot retraction is abnormal and capillary fragility is increased. Increased numbers of megakaryocytes are found in the bone marrow.

The acute variety most often occurs in children, following a seasonal viral illness in 50% of patients. The average lag between purpura and preceding infection is 2 weeks. Most of these cases resolve spontaneously or with

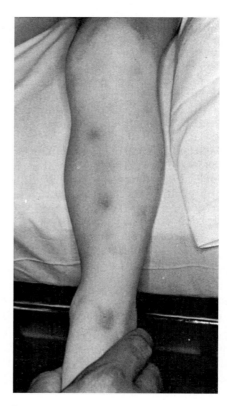

Fig. 35-8 Bruises of autoimmune thrombocytopenic purpura in a young child following a viral infection.

minimal therapy. A few patients will develop the chronic variety and a few deaths, usually from cerebral hemorrhage, have been reported in patients not treated. In the series by Medeiros et al of 332 children with ITP, 58 (17%) had episodes of major hemorrhage in which 56 were treated with corticosteroids, intravenous immunoglobulin, or both. One death resulted from sepsis. In the 427 cases reported by Bolton-Maggs et al, 323 (72%) had mild to benign disease.

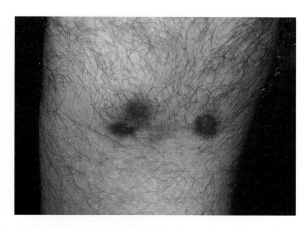

Fig. 35-9 Patient with idiopathic thrombocytopenia purpura with large ecchymotic areas after blood drawing.

There were no deaths as a result of intracranial hemorrhage. In another series analyzing chronic ITP in childhood, of 92 cases 29 of 34 (85%) patients who underwent splenectomy experienced remission. Sixty-one percent of the remaining patients developed spontaneous remission within 15 years. These results confirm the relatively benign nature of childhood ITP.

The chronic form occurs most often in adults; is persistent, lasting years to indefinitely; and has a female-male ratio of between 2:1 and 4:1. In refractory cases an evaluation for an accessory spleen should be performed using Tc99M radionuclide scan. The intermittent variety may occur in childhood or adulthood and is interrupted by intervals free from disease.

Idiopathic thrombocytopenic purpura is the result of platelet injury by antibodies of the IgG class. Antiplatelet antibodies coat the platelets, triggering their removal by the spleen after a greatly reduced survival time, which may last from minutes to a few hours.

Splenectomy and systemic corticosteroids have been the historical means of management. Platelet transfusions may be lifesaving in acutely ill patients who are actively bleeding; however, they do not increase the platelet counts and thus are not useful except in emergencies. Intravenous immunoglobulin (IVIg) is used frequently in both pediatric and adult cases in an attempt to treat and possibly postpone or eliminate the need for splenectomy. Law et al have shown that patients responsive to IVIg are more likely to respond to splenectomy. In chronic and intermittent ITP laparoscopic splenectomy has been shown as safe and effective as open splenectomy for removing spleens and accessory spleens. Additional therapeutic options include intravenous anti-D (anti-Rh$_o$), danazol, vinca alkaloids, and other immunosuppressive agents such as azathioprine and cyclophosphamide. Several therapies, such as cyclosporine, interferon-alfa, plasma exchange, staphylococcal protein A immunoadsorption, combination chemotherapy, dapsone, ascorbic acid, and colchicine have been recommended but rarely used.

Drug-Induced Thrombocytopenia

Thrombocytopenic purpura resulting from drug-induced antiplatelet antibodies may be caused by drugs such as sulfonamides, digoxin, quinine, quinidine, chlorothiazides, penicillin, phenylbutazone, acetaminophen, allopurinol, methyldopa, furosemide, gold salts, rifampin, and lidocaine. Ticlopidine, an antiplatelet agent used to reduce the occurrence of atherothrombotic arterial events, has been associated with neutropenia, aplastic anemia, thrombocytopenia, and thrombotic thrombocytopenic purpura.

Treatment consists of removal of the offending agent. Recovery usually occurs shortly thereafter. Corticosteroids are helpful in moderately high dosage (60 mg prednisone daily) and are usually only necessary as a brief course.

Thrombotic Thrombocytopenic Purpura

Also known as *Moschcowitz's syndrome,* thrombotic thrombocytopenic purpura (TTP) is a pentad of thrombocytopenia, hemolytic anemia, renal abnormalities, fever, and disturbance of the CNS. Central nervous system complaints (focal neurologic symptoms) may be the presenting feature. Multiple ecchymoses, jaundice, pallid mucous membranes, and an enlarged spleen may be found. Other associated findings include arthritis, pleuritis, Raynaud's phenomenon, abdominal pain, and hepatomegaly. Tests may show a decreased hematocrit and decreased platelets. A delay in diagnosis may lead to a mortality rate as high as 90%. Fraser et al reported a case of TTP in a young woman with a Norplant contraceptive system. Two other cases have been reported.

A positive histologic diagnosis of TTP can frequently be obtained on gingival biopsies. Diagnostic features are subendothelial hyaline deposits in capillaries and small arterioles, intraluminal deposits, and absence of inflammation in vessels or stroma. Bone marrow biopsies yield a similar percentage of diagnostic findings. Studies of plasma samples from patients with active TTP have often shown the presence of unusually large (UL) von Willebrand factor multimers, or alternatively, an absence of the largest forms during acute disease believed to be secondary to binding of UL von Willebrand to platelets with subsequent aggregation.

Until exchange plasmapheresis was instituted as the treatment of choice, 80% of these patients died; now, 80% survive. Plasma exchange of 3 to 5 liters of plasma for 4 to 10 days is required. In patients with recurrent or refractory disease, extracorporal immunoadsorption or splenectomy may be required.

Blanchette V, et al: Management of chronic immune thrombocytopenic purpura in children and adults. *Semin Hematol* 1998, 35:36.

Bolton-Maggs PH, et al: Assessment of UK practice for management of acute childhood idiopathic thrombocytopenic purpura against published guidelines. *Lancet* 1997, 350:620.

Crowther MA, et al: Splenectomy done during hematologic remission to prevent relapse in patients with thrombotic thrombocytopenic purpura. *Ann Intern Med* 1996, 125:294.

Diagnosis and treatment of idiopathic thrombocytopenic purpura: recommendations of the American Society of Hematology. *Ann Intern Med* 1997, 126:319.

Druschky A, et al: Central nervous system involvement in thrombotic thrombocytopenic purpura. *Eur Neurol* 1998, 40:220.

Fahal IH, et al: Thrombotic thrombocytopenic purpura due to rifampicin. *BMJ* 1992, 304:882.

Fraser JL, et al: Possible association between the Norplant contraceptive system and thrombotic thrombocytopenic purpura. *Obstet Gynecol* 1996, 87:860.

Katkhouda N, et al: Laparoscopic splenectomy. *Ann Surg* 1998, 228:568.

Law C, et al: High-dose intravenous immune globulin and the response to splenectomy in patients with idiopathic thrombocytopenic purpura. *N Engl J Med* 1997, 336:1494.

Love BB, et al: Adverse haematological effects of ticlopidine. *Drug Saf* 1998, 19:89.

Lozano-Salazar RR, et al: Laparoscopic versus open splenectomy for immune thrombocytopenic purpura. *Am J Surg* 1998, 176:366.

Medeiros D, et al: Major hemorrhage in children with idiopathic thrombocytopenic purpura. *J Pediatr* 1998, 133:334.

Mittelman A, et al: Response of refractory thrombotic thrombocytopenic purpura to extracorporeal immunoadsorption (letter). *N Engl J Med* 1992, 326:711.

Moake JL, et al: Thrombotic thrombocytopenic purpura. *Am J Med Sci* 1998, 316:105.

Reid MM: Chronic idiopathic thrombocytopenic purpura: incidence, treatment, and outcome. *Arch Dis Child* (England) 1995, 72:125.

Scaradavou A, et al: Clinical experience with anti-D in the treatment of idiopathic thrombocytopenic purpura. *Semin Hematol* 1998, 35:52. ▲

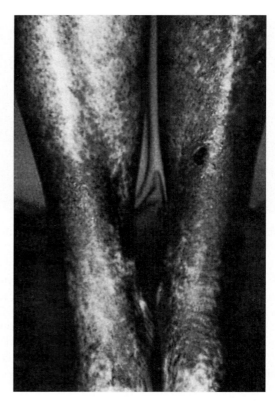

Fig. 35-10 Purpura cryoglobulinemica.

NONTHROMBOCYTOPENIC PURPURA (DYSPROTEINEMIC PURPURA)
Purpura Cryoglobulinemica and Cryofibrinogenemia

Abnormal serum proteins behaving as cryoglobulins and cryofibrinogens may be IgG, IgM, or both. Cryoglobulinemic purpura occurs most frequently in multiple myeloma and macroglobulinemia and is of a monoclonal IgM, IgG, or Bence Jones cryoglobulin form. Mixed cryoglobulinemia, in which the cryoglobulins are of various classes, may be seen in SLE, rheumatoid arthritis, Sjögren's syndrome, hepatitis B infection, and hepatitis C infection, the latter being the most common cause of mixed cryoglobulinemia.

Purpura is most apt to occur on exposed surfaces after cold exposure in monoclonal disease, and biopsy reveals amorphous eosinophilic material in the vessel lumina. In the mixed type, dependent palpable purpura is present (Fig. 35-10), which on biopsy reveals classic leukocytoclastic vasculitis. In cryocrystalglobulin syndrome, crystalline deposits are seen in the corneas and joint spaces. Vasculitic skin lesions occur. Follicular hyperkeratosis, purpura, acral blisters, and ulceration have also been reported.

Purpura secondary to these abnormal serum proteins tends to be chronic. Plasmapheresis, systemic steroids, immunosuppressors, and colchicine are some options. Prolonged remissions after treatment with high-dose gamma globulin infusion have been reported.

Abe Y, et al: Leucocytoclastic vasculitis associated with mixed cryoglobulinaemia and hepatitis C virus infection. *Br J Dermatol* 1997, 136:272.

Buezo GF, et al: Cryoglobulinemia and cutaneous leukocytoclastic vasculitis with hepatitis C virus infection. *Int J Dermatol* 1996, 35:112.

Caoud MS, et al: Chronic hepatitis C, cryoglobulinemia, and cutaneous necrotizing vasculitis. *J Am Acad Dermatol* 1996, 34:219.

Cohen SJ, et al: Cutaneous manifestations of cryoglobulinemia. *J Am Acad Dermatol* 1991, 25:21.

Gungor E, et al: Prevalence of hepatitis C virus antibodies and cryoglobulinemia in patients with leukocytoclastic vasculitis. *Dermatology* 1999, 198:26.

Klein AD, et al: Purpura and recurrent ulcers on the lower extremities: essential cryofibrinogenemia. *Arch Dermatol* 1991, 127:115. ▲

Purpura Hyperglobulinemica

Waldenström's hyperglobulinemic purpura consists of episodic showers of petechiae occurring on all parts of the body, most profusely on the lower extremities (Fig. 35-11). The dorsum of the feet are intensely involved, and the petechiae diminishes on the ascending parts of the feet. A diffuse "peppery" distribution is noted, resembling Schamberg's disease (Fig. 35-12). The petechiae may be induced or aggravated by prolonged standing or walking, or by wearing constrictive garters or stockings.

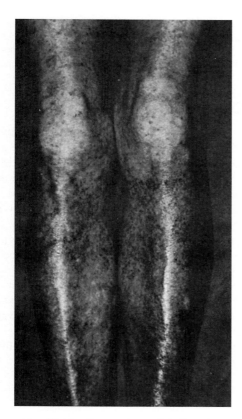

Fig. 35-11 Purpura hyperglobulinemica.

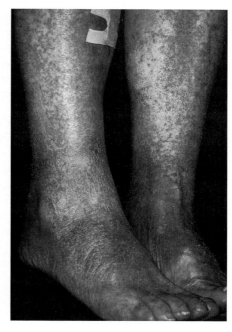

Fig. 35-12 Purpura hyperglobulinemica.

The most useful laboratory test is protein electrophoresis of the serum. The hypergammaglobulinemia is heterogeneous or polyclonal and is demonstrated as a broad-based peak. The bulk of the protein increase is IgG though occasionally, increased amounts of IgA are also found. IgM is usually normal or decreased. Rheumatoid factor in varying amounts is present in almost all patients. Antithyroglobulins, increased rate of erythrocyte sedimentation, leukopenia, antinuclear factors, and proteinuria may be found. In the series by Miyagawa et al, 7 of 9 (78%) of patients with hypergammaglobulinemic purpura of Waldenström had antibodies to Ro/SSA.

Hyperglobulinemic purpura occurs most commonly in women and is frequently seen with Sjögren's syndrome, hepatitis C, keratoconjunctivitis sicca, rheumatoid arthritis, and multiple myeloma; or it may be a primary phenomenon when it occurs as a chronic benign illness. An extensive list of associated diseases may be found in the reference by Finder et al.

Histologically, the dermal vessels have a perivascular infiltrate of mononuclear cells. In some cases a necrotizing vasculitis is present. Hypergammaglobulinemic purpura associated with hepatitis C may occur unilaterally, has a sex predilection for men, and has manifestations that usually last longer than those associated with Sjögren's syndrome. Leukocytoclastic vasculitis has correlated with high titers of Ro and La antibodies and general serohyperreactivity.

The course of the disease is essentially benign, but chronic. Hyperglobulinemic purpura may be a facet or harbinger of connective tissue diseases, and rarely, progression to myeloma has been reported. Steroids are usually not of benefit and should be reserved for severe disease. Indomethacin and hydroxychloroquine may be of value in the treatment of milder disease. Chlorambucil reduces the purpura but does not effect gross changes in the protein abnormality; therefore, response rates in combination with toxicity do not justify its use. Thioguanine, dipyridamole (Persantine) and aspirin, and colchicine have also been used with some success. Measures to obviate stasis are recommended.

Finder KA, et al: Hypergammaglobulinemic purpura of Waldenström. *J Am Acad Dermatol* 1990, 23:669.

Miyagawa S, et al: Hypergammaglobulinaemic purpura of Waldenström and Ro/SSA autoantibodies. *Br J Dermatol* 1996, 134:919.

Senecal JL, et al: Hypergammaglobulinemic purpura in systemic autoimmune rheumatic disease. *J Rheumatol* (Canada) 1995, 22:868.

Yamamoto T, et al: Hypergammaglobulinemic purpura associated with Sjögren's syndrome and chronic C type hepatitis. *J Dermatol* 1997, 24:7. ▲

Waldenström's Macroglobulinemia

In 1944, Waldenström described an entity characterized by bleeding from the mucous membranes of the mouth and nose, lymphadenopathy, hepatosplenomegaly, hemorrhage of the retina, and rarely, purpura. Gastrointestinal bleeding and anemia may occur. This disease occurs mostly in elderly white men who have oronasal bleeding and represents a plasma cell dyscrasia with lymphocytic infiltration of marrow and lymphoid organs that may be frank malignant lymphoma. Hepatitis G, a new member of the *Flaviviridae* family, and hepatitis C infection have been implicated in causing Waldenström's macroglobulinemia and B-cell lymphoma. Waldenström's macroglobulinemia has also been associated with chronic liver disease and hepatocellular carcinoma.

Two types of skin lesions may occur: violaceous to red indurated plaques, infiltrated with atypical lymphoid cells; or alternatively, translucent papules full of amorphous eosinophilic material that has proved on direct immunofluorescence to be IgM. Basement membrane deposits of IgM have also been detected. Nonspecific cutaneous findings include Raynaud's, amyloidosis, pruritus, xanthomatosis, and urticaria. Some patients with urticaria and macroglobulinemia (Schnitzler's syndrome) satisfy the criteria for Waldenström's macroglobulinemia.

The histopathologic feature in most cases is a perivascular infiltrate containing lymphocytes and in some cases neutrophils and eosinophils. Leukocytoclastic vasculitis has been rarely reported associated with Waldenström's macroglobulinemia. Large amounts of monoclonal IgM are responsible for the variable clinical pattern. Fibrinogenopenia, fibrinolysis, circulating anticoagulants, coagulation factor deficiencies, intravascular or perivascular deposition of paraprotein, or associated cryoglobulinemia or cryofibrinogenemia may result in the bleeding tendencies.

Plasmapheresis until adequate doses of chlorambucil have been administered is the recommended treatment. Cyclophosphamide and corticosteroids or 2-chlorodeoxyadenosine (cladribine) have also been shown to be effective. PUVA was used to alleviate symptoms of pruritus in the patient reported by Cobb et al.

Appenzeller P, et al: Cutaneous Waldenström macroglobulinemia in transformation. *Am J Dermatopathol* 1999, 21:151.

Cobb MW, et al: Waldenström macroglobulinemia with an IgM-kappa antiepidermal basement membrane zone antibody. *Arch Dermatol* 1992, 128:372.

Dimopoulos MA, et al: Treatment of Waldenström macroglobulinemia with 2-chlorodeoxyadenosine. *Ann Intern Med* 1993, 118:195.

Facon T, et al: Prognostic factors in Waldenström's macroglobulinemia. *J Clin Oncol* 1993, 11:1553.

Groves FD, et al: Waldenström's macroglobulinemia. *Cancer* 1998, 82:1078.

Izumi T, et al: Sequential occurrence of hepatocellular carcinoma following Waldenström's macroglobulinemia. *Intern Med* (Japan) 1996, 35:416.

Niesvizky R, et al: Epstein-Barr virus-associated lymphoma after treatment of macroglobulinemia with cladribine. *N Engl J Med* 1999, 341:55.

Tepper JL, et al: Hepatitis G and hepatitis C RNA viruses coexisting in cryoglobulinemia. *J Rheumatol* 1998, 25:925. _____ ▲

PURPURA SECONDARY TO CLOTTING DISORDERS

Hereditary disorders of blood coagulation usually result from a deficiency or qualitative abnormality of a single coagulation factor, as in hemophilia or von Willebrand's disease. Acquired disorders commonly result from multiple coagulation factor deficiencies, as in liver disease, biliary tract obstruction, malabsorption, or drug ingestion, or may also involve platelet and vascular abnormalities such as disseminated intravascular coagulation. Hemorrhagic manifestations are common and may be severe, especially in hereditary forms. Ecchymoses and subcutaneous hematomas are common, especially on the legs. Severe hemorrhage may follow trauma, and hemarthrosis is frequent. Other hemorrhagic manifestations include respiratory obstruction resulting from hemorrhage into the tongue, throat, or neck; epistaxis; gastrointestinal and genitourinary tract bleeding; and, rarely, CNS hemorrhage.

Harley JR: Disorders of coagulation misdiagnosed as nonaccidental bruising. *Pediatr Emerg Care* 1997, 13:347.

Sham RL, et al: Evaluation of mild bleeding disorders and easy bruising. *Blood Rev* 1994, 8:98. _____ ▲

DRUG- AND FOOD-INDUCED PURPURA

A list of drugs that induce antiplatelet antibodies is given on p. 1019; however, drug-induced purpura may occur without platelet destruction, as a manifestation of small-vessel vasculitis. Some purpurogenic drugs are the following: aspirin and other nonsteroidal antiinflammatory agents, allopurinol, thiazides, gold, sulfonamides, cephalosporins, hydralazine, phenytoin, quinidine, ticlopidine, and penicillin. Combinations of diphenhydramine and pyrithyldione can induce purpuric mottling and areas of necrosis. Cocaine-induced thrombosis with infarctive skin lesions is associated with skin popping. The Rumpel-Leede sign is defined as a distal shower of petechiae that occurs immediately after the release of pressure from a tourniquet or sphygmomanometer applied to an arm or leg. It is a sign of disorders that are associated with capillary fragility and has also been reported in association with drug-induced erythema multiforme.

Topical EMLA cream can induce purpura within 30 minutes of application, a result of an allergic reaction (toxic effect on capillary endothelium). Purpura has been associated with the use of acetaminophen in patients afflicted with infectious mononucleosis. Small-vessel vasculitis and urticaria-vasculitis have been caused by the ingestion of the food additives tartrazine and benzoates.

De Waard-van der Spek FB, et al: Purpura caused by EMLA is of toxic origin. *Contact Dermatitis* 1997, 36:11.

Filipe PL, et al: Drug eruption induced by acetaminophen in infectious mononucleosis (letter). *Int J Dermatol* 1995, 34:220.

Gross AS, et al: The Rumpel-Leede sign associated with drug-induced erythema multiforme. *J Am Acad Dermatol* 1992, 27:781.

Morell A, et al: Livedo reticularis and thrombotic purpura related to the use of diphenhydramine associated with pyrithyldione. *Dermatology* (Switzerland) 1996, 193:50.

Wuthrich B: Adverse reactions to food additives. *Ann Allergy* 1993, 71:379. ▲

SOLAR PURPURA (SENILE PURPURA, ACTINIC PURPURA)

Solar purpura is characterized by large, sharply outlined, 1- to 5-cm, dark purplish red ecchymoses appearing on the dorsa of the forearms and less often the hands (Fig. 35-13). Usually the skin over the forearms is thin and inelastic. Refer to Chapter 7.

PURPURA FULMINANS

Also known as *purpura gangrenosa,* this is a severe, rapidly fatal reaction occurring most commonly in children after some infectious illness. The sudden appearance of large ecchymotic areas, especially prominent over the extremities, progressing to acral hemorrhagic skin necrosis is characteristic (Fig. 35-14). Fever, shock, and disseminated intravascular coagulation usually accompany the skin lesions, which on biopsy show noninflammatory necrosis, with platelet-fibrin thrombi occluding the blood vessels.

Purpura fulminans usually follows some acute infectious disease such as scarlet fever and, rarely, streptococcal pharyngitis, meningococcal meningitis (Fig. 35-15), pneumococcal sepsis, *Capnocytophaga canimorsus* (DF-2), *Xanthomonas maltophilia* sepsis, or varicella infection. However, it may occur without any preceding illness, and adults may be affected. Asplenic patients, who are at risk for pneumococcal or meningococcal sepsis, are also predisposed to purpura fulminans. Neonates with homozygous protein C or protein S deficiencies may suffer purpura fulminans as a result of the lack of this natural anticoagulant. Some infectious or postinfectious patients develop

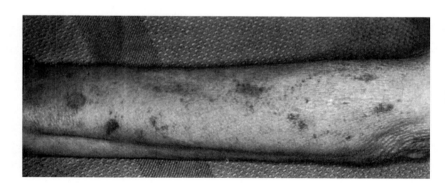

Fig. 35-13 Solar purpura.

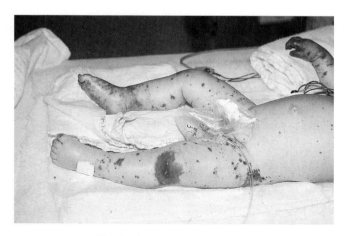

Fig. 35-14 Purpura fulminans.

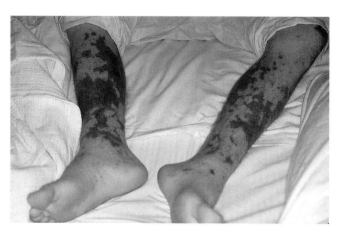

Fig. 35-15 Purpura secondary to meningococcal infection.

transient deficiencies of proteins C and S, which may be directly related to the pathogenesis of this syndrome. For example, IgG paraproteins may inhibit the functional anticoagulant activity of activated protein C. Autoimmune protein S deficiency has also been shown to be a mechanism in causing postinfectious idiopathic purpura fulminans. Other diseases, such as the fibrinolysis syndrome, may have purpura fulminans as part of the symptom complex. An acquired form has been reported secondary to alcohol and acetaminophen ingestion.

Approximately 5% of whites of European origin have a mutation in coagulation Factor V. A number of cases of purpura fulminans associated with infections and this Factor V Leiden mutation, with normal protein C and protein S levels, have been reported in children and adults. Factor V Leiden deficiency may be a more frequent cause of purpura fulminans than previously appreciated.

Management is usually supportive initially, with treatment of the underlying disease process, such as antibiotics, and replacement therapy using fresh frozen plasma. Protein C replacement is useful in treating patients shown to have protein C deficiencies. Despite these measures, however, amputations and deaths continue to occur in the severest forms of this disease.

Bick RL, et al: Syndromes of thrombosis and hypercoagulability. *Med Clin North Am* 1998, 82:409.

Darmstadt GL: Acute infectious purpura fulminans: pathogenesis and medical management. *Pediatr Dermatol* 1998, 15:169.

Guccione JL, et al: Acquired purpura fulminans induced by alcohol and acetaminophen: successful treatment with heparin and vitamin K. *Arch Dermatol* 1993, 129:1267.

Jackson RT, et al: Adult purpura fulminans and digital necrosis associated with sepsis and the Factor V mutation. *JAMA* 1998, 280:1829.

Johansen K, et al: Symmetrical peripheral gangrene (purpura fulminans) complicating pneumococcal sepsis. *Am J Surg* 1993, 165:642.

Kato N, et al: Purpura fulminans secondary to *Xanthomonas maltophilia* sepsis in an adult aplastic anemia. *J Dermatol* (Japan) 1991, 18:225.

Kullberg BJ, et al: Purpura fulminans and symmetrical peripheral gangrene caused by *Capnocytophaga canimorsus* (DF-2) septicemia complication of dog bite. *Medicine* 1991, 70:287.

Levin M, et al: Postinfectious purpura fulminans caused by an autoantibody directed against protein S. *J Pediatr* 1995, 127:355.

Manco-Johnson MJ, et al: Lupus anticoagulant and protein S deficiency in children with postvaricella purpura fulminans or thrombosis. *J Pediatr* 1996, 128:319.

Phillips WG, et al: Purpura fulminans due to protein S deficiency following chickenpox. *Br J Dermatol* 1992, 127:30.

Rivard GE, et al: Treatment of purpura fulminans in meningococcemia with protein C concentrate. *J Pediatr* 1995, 126:646.

Suss R, et al: Purpura fulminans with extensive skin necrosis. *Hautarzt* (Germany) 1996, 47:541.

Tambyah PA, et al: Streptococcus suis infection complicated by purpura fulminans and rhabdomyolysis. *Clin Infect Dis* 1997, 24:710. ▲

DISSEMINATED INTRAVASCULAR COAGULATION

Up to two thirds of patients with disseminated intravascular coagulation (DIC) have skin lesions, which may be the initial manifestation of the syndrome. Minute, widespread petechiae, ecchymoses, ischemic necrosis of the skin, and hemorrhagic bullae are the usual findings. Purpura fulminans may supervene and progress to symmetrical peripheral gangrene. DIC may be initiated by a variety of disorders, including septicemic hypotension, hypoxemia, acidosis, malignancies, chemotherapy, obstetric crises, antiphospholipid antibody syndrome, SLE, allergic reactions (Proporis), or leukemia. Children with kaposiform hemangioendotheliomas are at risk for this consumptive coagulopathy (Kasabach-Merritt syndrome). Long-term treatment with granulocyte colony–stimulating factor (G-CSF) has also been reported to precipitate DIC.

DIC is the result of widespread intravascular coagulation in which certain coagulation factors are consumed faster than they can be replaced. Laboratory findings show decreased platelets, decreased fibrinogen, elevated PT and PTT, and fibrin degradation products. Control of the underlying disease is the paramount consideration, together with correction of hemostatic abnormalities, usually through the use of intravenous heparin. However, the indications for treatment with heparin are not established, and the morbidity or mortality in treating patients with heparin remains to be proved. Some patients seem to benefit, and if initiated should be used with extreme caution and at low doses. All patients should receive vitamin K replacement, which will exclude vitamin K deficiency as a cause, and replace vitamin K stores, which are rapidly depleted in patients with DIC. Fresh frozen plasma, platelet transfusions, and, at times, select replacement of specific coagulant factors may be beneficial.

Baglin T: Disseminated intravascular coagulation: diagnosis and treatment. *BMJ* 1996, 312:683.

Bick RL: Disseminated intravascular coagulation: objective criteria for diagnosis and management. *Med Clin North Am* 1994, 78:511.

Falcini F, et al Catastrophic antiphospholipid antibody syndrome in pediatric systemic lupus erythematosus. *J Rheumatol* (Canada) 1997, 24:389.

Hadley T, et al: Disseminated intravascular coagulation after factor IX complex resolved using purified factor IX concentrate. *Ann Intern Med* 1991, 115:621.

Mueller BU, et al: Disseminated intravascular coagulation associated with granulocyte colony-stimulating factor therapy in a child with human immunodeficiency virus infection. *J Pediatr* 1995, 126:749.

Pasquini E, et al: Acute disseminated intravascular coagulation syndrome in cancer patients. *Oncology* (Switzerland) 1995, 52:505.

Takeshita A, et al: Allergic reaction involving liver dysfunction and disseminated intravascular coagulation caused by a health food, Proporis. *Intern Med* (Japan) 1995, 34:1207. _____ ▲

FIBRINOLYSIS SYNDROME (HYPOFIBRINOGENEMIA, DEFIBRINATING SYNDROME)

The fibrinolysis syndrome is characterized by an acute hemorrhagic state brought about by inability of the blood to clot. Massive hemorrhages into the skin produce blackish, purplish swellings and sloughing. There is an increased tendency to thrombosis and hemorrhage. It occurs as a complication of pregnancy in cases of placenta previa, eclampsia, and fetal death. It may be a complication in certain surgical operations, particularly in lobectomy and during extracorporeal circulation of blood. The syndrome has been repeatedly reported in amyloidosis, thrombotic thrombocytopenic purpura, liver disease, Waterhouse-Friderichsen syndrome, carcinoma of the prostate with metastases to bone marrow, and in other types of malignant disease. It may also follow snake bite. Treatment is by transfusions of fibrinogen concentrates. This disease is produced by excessive or inappropriate fibrinolysis.

Bick RL, et al: Syndromes of hypercoagulability and thrombosis: a review. *Semin Thromb Hemost* 1994, 20:109.

Funai EF, et al: Successful pregnancy outcome in a patient with both congenital hypofibrinogenemia and protein S deficiency. *Obstet Gynecol* 1997, 89:858.

Ness PM, et al: Congenital hypofibrinogenemia and recurrent placental abruption. *Obstet Gynecol* 1983, 61:519. _____ ▲

BLUEBERRY MUFFIN BABY

Originally coined to describe the characteristic appearance of the purpuric lesions observed in newborns with congenital rubella, *blueberry muffin baby* is associated with many disorders that produce extramedullary erythropoiesis. The eruption consists of generalized dark blue to magenta, nonblanchable, indurated, round to oval, hemispheric papules ranging from 1 to 7 mm. Lesions favor the head, neck, and trunk.

The differential diagnosis includes congenital infections (rubella, cytomegalovirus, and parvovirus B19), hemolytic disease of the newborn (Rh incompatibility, blood group incompatibility), hereditary spherocytosis, twin transfusion syndrome, neuroblastoma, rhabdomyosarcoma, Langerhans' cell histiocytosis, and congenital leukemia. Evaluation should include a peripheral blood cell count, hemoglobin level, TORCH serologies, viral cultures, and a Coomb's test. A skin biopsy may also be helpful in determining the cause.

Baselga E, et al: Purpura in infants and children. *J Am Acad Dermatol* 1997, 37:673.

Silver MM, et al: Anemia, blueberry-muffin rash, and hepatomegaly in a newborn infant. *J Pediatr* 1996, 128:579.

Smets K, et al: Fetomaternal haemorrhage and prenatal intracranial bleeding: two more causes of blueberry muffin baby. *Eur J Pediatr* 1998, 157:932. _____ ▲

ITCHING PURPURA

Also known as *disseminated pruriginous angiodermatitis,* punctate purpuric macules (petechiae) first appear around the ankles and then ascend to involve the entire body except the palms and face. These orange-purplish-red petechiae evolve completely and may become confluent in 2 weeks. Edema of the ankles is present, and severe pruritus is a dominant feature, producing lichenification. It is seen predominantly in men and has a seasonal predilection for spring and summer. The pruritus may be unremitting and lead to depression and sleep disturbance. The etiology is unknown. The disease usually runs its course in 3 to 6 months but may be chronic, with exacerbations over a period of months to years.

Del Pozo J, et al: Flexural purpura and Epstein-Barr virus infection. *Int J Dermatol* 1998, 37:130.

Mosto SJ, et al: Disseminated pruriginous angiodermatitis (itching purpura). *Arch Dermatol* 1965, 91:351.

Pravada DJ, et al: Itching purpura. *Cutis* 1980, 25:147. ▲

MISCELLANEOUS PURPURIC MANIFESTATIONS
Deep Venous Thrombosis

Extensive venous thrombosis, almost always affecting at least the femoral vein, can cause reversible ischemia, or frank gangrene. Patients may develop, either abruptly or gradually, severe pain, extensive edema, and cyanosis of an extremity (usually the leg). The left leg is more often affected than the right. Female patients slightly outnumber male, and the mean age is 52 years. Significant superficial vein thrombosis is considered a risk factor for deep vein thrombosis. The risk of pulmonary embolism from deep vein thrombosis is the major concern.

Malignant neoplasms are the commonest underlying condition, with bronchogenic carcinoma by far the most frequent. In 35% of cancer-associated cases, the thrombosis is the first sign of the cancer. Immobilization from surgery or travel, extensive trauma, childbirth, or congestive heart failure are other predisposing factors. In addition to the clinical signs, plethysmography, Doppler studies, or radionuclide or contrast phlebography may be required to define the extent of thrombosis. In at least 50% of patients with suspected deep vein thrombosis, the diagnosis is not confirmed by objective testing. Impedance plethysmography and real-time B-mode ultrasound with color-enhanced Doppler imaging are the preferred methods of evaluation. Treatment involves elevation of the limb, intravenous fluids, and systemic anticoagulation for deep disease.

There is a 40% mortality, often from pulmonary emboli or underlying disease. Chronic complications include venous incompetence, with stasis dermatitis or ulcers, and postphlebitic syndrome, as well as venous claudication with leg pain on exercising.

Baker WF Jr, et al: Deep vein thrombosis. *Med Clin North Am* 1994, 78:685.

Guex JJ: Thrombotic complications of varicose veins. *Dermatol Surg* 1996, 22:378. _____ ▲

Superficial Thrombophlebitis

Samlaska and James have reviewed the vast number of primary and secondary hypercoagulable states that can present with superficial vein thrombosis. Painful induration with erythema, often in a linear or branching configuration forming cords, is the classic presentation. Patients may also exhibit indurated subcutaneous nodules and overlying purpura or brown discoloration indicative of postinflammatory hyperpigmentation.

Primary hypercoagulable states that may be associated with superficial thrombophlebitis include antithrombin III, heparin cofactor II, protein C and protein S, and factor XII deficiencies; disorders of tissue plasminogen activator; abnormal plasminogen/plasminogenemia; dysfibrinogenemia; and lupus anticoagulant. Secondary hypercoagulable states include varicosities, malignancy (Trousseau's syndrome), pregnancy, oral contraceptive use, infusion of prothrombin complex concentrates, Behçet's disease, thromboangiitis obliterans, Mondor's disease, septic thrombophlebitis (aerobic and anaerobic cultures required), psittacosis, secondary syphilis, intravenous catheters, intravenous drugs (sugar solutions, protein hydrolysates, calcium, potassium, hypertonic concentrates, diazepam, nitrogen mustard, acridinylaniside, dacarbazine, and carmustine), and street drugs (cocaine, and bulking agents such as paregoric, quinine, dextrose, sucrose, and lactose).

The evaluation of superficial thrombophlebitis should consider the possibility of deep venous disease (see p. 1025). Venous duplex reports documenting "superficial femoral vein" involvement should alert the physician to deep venous disease requiring anticoagulation and treatment for deep vein thrombosis. Elliptic biopsies across the palpable cord may be required to exclude other considerations such as sarcoidal granulomas, cutaneous polyarteritis nodosa, and Kaposi's sarcoma, as well as forms of panniculitis.

Treatment is directed at the underlying cause. Leg elevation and local heat will help to promote the dissolution of clots, which may take up to 8 to 12 weeks to resolve.

Belcaro G, et al: Superficial thrombophlebitis of the legs: a randomized, controlled follow-up study. *Angiology* 1999, 50:523.

Bundens WP, et al: The superficial femoral vein: a potentially lethal misnomer. *JAMA* 1995, 274:1296.

Kohler M: Thrombogenicity of prothrombin complex concentrates. *Thromb Res* 1999, 95:S13.

Samlaska CS, James WD: Superficial thrombophlebitis. I. Primary hypercoagulable states. *J Am Acad Dermatol* 1990, 22:975.

Samlaska CS, James WD: Superficial thrombophlebitis. II. Secondary hypercoagulable states. *J Am Acad Dermatol* 1990, 23:1.

Somjen GM, et al: Duplex ultrasound examination of the acutely painful and swollen leg. *Dermatol Surg* 1996, 22:383. _____ ▲

Mondor's Disease

Mondor's disease occurs three times as frequently in women as in men, and most patients have ranged in age from 30 to 60 years. The sudden appearance of a cordlike thrombosed vein along the anterior-lateral chest wall is characteristic. It is at first red and tender and subsequently changes into a painless, tough, fibrous band. There are no systemic symptoms. Both sides of the chest have the same incidence of involvement. The cause is multifactorial and has been reported to be the result of strenuous exercise, pregnancy, intravenous drug abuse, jellyfish stings, breast cancer, and breast surgery. The condition represents a localized thrombophlebitis of the veins of the thoracoepigastric area. The veins involved are the lateral thoracic, thoracoepigastric, and superior epigastric. In the end stage a thick-walled vein remains that has a hard, ropelike appearance and on occasion may result in a furrowing of the breast. Exceptionally, a vein coursing up the inside of the upper arm may be involved. Similar string phlebitis findings have been described for the penis, antecubital fossa, groin, abdomen, and axilla.

Treatment is symptomatic, with hot, moist dressings and analgesics or nonsteroidal anti-inflammatory agents. The disease process runs its course in from 3 weeks to 6 months.

Catania S, et al: Mondor's disease and breast cancer. *Cancer* 1992, 69:2267.

Cooper RA: Mondor's disease secondary to intravenous drug abuse. *Arch Surg* 1990, 125:807.

Ganem JP, et al: Ruptured Mondor's disease of the penis mimicking penile fracture. *J Urol* 1998, 159:1302.

Hacker SM: Axillary string phlebitis in pregnancy: a variant of Mondor's disease. *J Am Acad Dermatol* 1994, 30:636.

Ingram DM, et al: Mondor's disease of the breast resulting from jellyfish sting. *Med J Aust* 1992, 157:836.

Marin-Bertolin S, et al: Mondor's disease and aesthetic breast surgery. *Aesthetic Plast Surg* 1995, 19:251.

Rubegni P, et al: Recurrent Mondor's disease after exeresis of abdominal lipoma. *Dermatol Surg* 1999, 25:563.

Samlaska CP, James WD: Superficial thrombophlebitis. II. Secondary hypercoagulable states. *J Am Acad Dermatol* 1990, 23:1. _____ ▲

Postcardiotomy Syndrome

Two to 3 weeks after pericardiotomy, fever, pleuritis, pericarditis, or arthritis may appear together with petechiae on the skin and palate. This syndrome may be confused with infectious mononucleosis and bacterial endocarditis.

Orthostatic Purpura (Stasis Purpura)

Prolonged standing or even sitting with the legs lowered (as in a bus, airplane, or train) may produce edema and a purpuric eruption on the lower extremities. Elevation of the legs and the use of elastic stockings are helpful if prevention is necessary.

Obstructive or Traumatic Purpura

Purpura may also be evoked by mechanical obstruction to the circulation, with resulting stress on the small vessels. This may be encountered in cardiac decompensation, or after convulsions, vomiting episodes, the Valsalva maneuver, pertussis, or sexual climax. Nonpalpable purpura has been reported associated with the use of a mucus-clearing device, which requires the patient to exhale forcefully through a flutter valve (flutter valve purpura). Local obstruction of the blood flow may result from compression of the veins by tumors and the gravid uterus, by occlusions from thrombosis, or by a weakening of the elastic coat as in varicose veins; in all these conditions purpura may be observed.

Purpuric lesions in children brings into question the possibility of the battered child. Bruises and ecchymoses on the genital area, buttocks, or hands are suggestive of an abused child. Linear lesions on accessible areas raises the question of factitial disease. Ecchymoses of bizarre shapes may also correspond to trauma inflicted during religious rituals or cultural practices. Coin-rubbing and cupping performed as remedies for common diseases are examples. "Passion purpura" on the palate may result from fellatio, or on the neck or upper arms (a "hickey") from biting and sucking. Facial, cheek, and periorbital purpura can occur postictal and may be mistaken as spousal abuse.

Baselga E, et al: Purpura in infants and children. *J Am Acad Dermatol* 1997, 37:673.

Knoell KA, et al: Flutter valve purpura. *J Am Acad Dermatol* 1998, 39:292.

Reis JJ, et al: Postictal hemifacial purpura. *Seizure* 1998, 7:337. ▲

Calciphylaxis

End-stage renal disease patients with metastatic calcification are almost exclusively affected by this disease. Calciphylaxis appears as reticulated, violaceous, mottled patches, later progressing to ecchymosis, cordlike nodules (usually located on the extremities), livedo reticularis, or necrosis. Progression to ecchymosis, central necrosis, and boring ulcerations frequently occur. Gangrene and self-amputation of digits or extremities has been reported. Necrosis may involve other sites, such as the penis, tongue, or breast. Ischemic myopathy may produce symptoms suggestive of dermatomyositis. Patients with diabetes and chronic renal failure have a much higher chance of developing acral gangrene.

The pathogenic mechanism is related to predisposing sensitizing conditions that create a conducive environment for calcium precipitation. Calcification occurs when an appropriate challenging factor is then introduced. Identified sensitizers include vitamin D compounds, parathyroid hormone, phosphates, and calcium salts, as well as infections, particularly granulomatous disorders, and cryofibrinogenemia. It has been reported in patients with AIDS. Challenging agents include metallic salts, local trauma, certain organic compounds (albumin and egg yolk), corticosteroids, intramuscular iron dextran complex, calcium heparinate, and intramuscular tobramycin. The sensitizing event and the challenging insult do not have to occur at the same time to cause disease. At times it may be difficult to identify the sensitizing condition and/or the precipitating

event. Crohn's disease in combination with short-bowel syndrome has been reported to cause calciphylaxis.

The prognosis is guarded, and most patients experience significant morbidity and mortality. Death is usually caused by staphylococcal sepsis after infection of the chronic ulcerations. Patients with parathyroid disease have the best prognosis after parathyroidectomy with autotransplantation of parathyroid tissue. Hyperbaric oxygen has been used with some success. Surgical intervention in patients with documented calciphylaxis is associated with an increased rate of complications such as breast necrosis after harvesting of the internal mammary artery.

Barri YM, et al: Calciphylaxis in a patient with Crohn's disease in the absence of end-stage renal disease. *Am J Kidney Dis* 1997, 29:773.

Dean SM, et al: Calciphylaxis: a favorable outcome with hyperbaric oxygen. *Vasc Med* 1998, 3:115.

Flanigan KM, et al: Calciphylaxis mimicking dermatomyositis: ischemic myopathy complicating renal failure. *Neurology* 1998, 51:1634.

Gilson RT, et al: Calciphylaxis: case report and treatment review. *Cutis* 1999, 63:149.

Hafner J, et al: Calciphylaxis: a syndrome of skin necrosis and acral gangrene in chronic renal failure. *Vasa* 1998, 27:137.

Mastruserio N, et al: Calciphylaxis associated with metastatic breast carcinoma. *J Am Acad Dermatol* 1999, 41:292.

Morris DJ, et al: Breast infarction after internal mammary artery harvest in a patient with calciphylaxis. *Ann Thorac Surg* 1997, 64:1469.

Oh DH, et al: Five cases of calciphylaxis and a review of the literature. *J Am Acad Dermatol* 1999, 40:979.

Robinson KJ, et al: The presentation and differential diagnosis of cutaneous vascular occlusion syndromes. *Adv Dermatol* 2000, 15:153.

Sankarasubbaiyan S, et al: Cryofibrinogenemia: an addition to the differential diagnosis of calciphylaxis in end-stage renal disease. *Am J Kidney Dis* 1998, 32:494.

Worth RL: Calciphylaxis. *J Cutan Med Surg* 1998, 2:245.

Young PC, et al: Widespread livedo reticularis with painful ulcerations. *Arch Dermatol* 1995, 131:786.

Zacharias JM, et al: Calcium use increases risk of calciphylaxis: a case-control study. *Perit Dial Int* 1999, 19:248. ▲

Scorbutic Purpura

In addition to the typical bleeding gums, the perifollicular purpura, and corkscrew hairs, cutaneous purpura may be extensive in scurvy. Severe dissecting subcutaneous hematomas may occur on the legs or abdomen. Deficiency of vitamin C, like solar elastosis, increases the fragility and permeability of the capillaries and accounts for the tendency to purpura and hemorrhage. This is reviewed in greater detail in Chapter 22.

Epidemic Dropsy

Epidemic dropsy manifests with eruptive angiomas, purpura, dyspnea, tachycardia, diarrhea, and fever. It occurs most frequently in parts of India, Africa, and the Fiji Islands and is the result of ingested mustard oil adulterated with oil of argemone.

Dogra J, et al: Epidemic dropsy. *Am J Med* 1986, 81:1115.

Gomber S, et al: Resurgence of epidemic dropsy (letter). *Indian J Pediatr* 1997, 34:953.

Hirschmann JV, et al: Adult scurvy. *J Am Acad Dermatol* 1999, 41:895.

Sachdev HP, et al: Electrophysiological studies of the eye, peripheral nerves and muscles in epidemic dropsy. *J Trop Med Hyg* 1989, 92:412.

Singh R, et al: Epidemic dropsy in the eastern region of Nepal. *J Trop Pediatr* 1999, 45:8. ▲

Paroxysmal Nocturnal Hemoglobinuria

This acquired intravascular hemolytic anemia usually occurs in young adults. Initial erythematous plaques progress to hemorrhagic bullae. Vascular thrombi are found on biopsy. The physiologic drop in pH that occurs with sleep appears to be responsible for the hemolysis and is the basis for the specific Ham (acid hemolysis) test.

Draelos ZK, et al: Hemorrhagic bullae in an anemic woman. *Arch Dermatol* 1986, 122:1327.

Rosse WF: Paroxysmal nocturnal hemoglobinuria as a molecular disease. *Medicine* 1997, 76:63. ▲

Purpura-Associated Diseases

Purpura may be noted at times in erythema multiforme, dermatitis medicamentosa, serum sickness, pityriasis rosea, and herpes zoster. Petechiae or ecchymoses may be associated with measles, scarlet fever, and smallpox and may appear extensively in cerebrospinal meningitis, typhus, parvovirus B19, and Rocky Mountain spotted fever. Disseminated strongyloidiasis can cause widespread purpura by the passage of the larvae through vessel walls. Purpura may occur also in septicemia, Waterhouse-Friderichsen syndrome, bacterial endocarditis, malaria, miliary tuberculosis, and anthrax.

Drolet BA, et al: Painful, purpuric plaques in a child with fever. *Arch Dermatol* 1997, 133:1500.

Pierson JC, et al: Purpuric pityriasis rosea. *J Am Acad Dermatol* 1993, 28:1021. ▲

Paroxysmal Hand Hematoma (Achenbach's Syndrome)

Spontaneous focal hemorrhage into the palm or the volar surface of a finger may result in transitory localized pain, followed by rapid swelling and localized bluish discoloration. The lesion resolves spontaneously within a few days. Spontaneous hemorrhage from an arteriole appears to be responsible. Occupational trauma may result in persistent edema of the hands, which is considered a variant of Secretan's syndrome (see p. 1056) by some. The acute nature, purpuric findings, and rapid resolution are distinguishing features of Achenbach's syndrome.

Eikenboom JC, et al: Paroxysmal finger haematoma. *Thromb Haemost* 1991, 66:266. ▲

Easy Bruising Syndrome

Young women who bruise easily despite normal coagulation profiles and normal platelet counts may have antiplatelet antibodies or increased megakaryocytes. Lackner et al have divided them into groups I (vasculitis) and II (qualitative platelet function abnormalities). A screen for bleeding time and blood eosinophilia should be performed on white children who develop easy bruising, particularly in Southeast Asia and East India. This includes white children new to these areas who develop easy bruising. They should be screened periodically for as long as 12 months after arrival. Reports have documented an acquired platelet dysfunction associated with eosinophilia of undetermined cause.

Lackner H, et al: On the "easy bruising" syndrome with normal platelet count: a study of 75 patients. *Ann Intern Med* 1975, 83:190.

Poon MC, et al: Acquired platelet dysfunction with eosinophilia in white children. *J Pediatr* 1995, 126:959. ▲

Painful Bruising Syndrome (Autoerythrocyte Sensitization, Gardner-Diamond Syndrome)

Painful bruising syndrome is a distinctive localized purpuric reaction occurring primarily in young to middle-aged women who usually manifest some emotional or personality disturbance. There may be depression, anxiety, hysterical, or masochistic character traits, or inability to deal with hostile feelings. A recurrent type of eruption, it is characterized by extremely painful and tender, ill-defined ecchymoses about the extremities (Fig. 35-16) and sometimes on the face or trunk. The lesions evolve in a few hours and resolve within 5 to 8 days. New lesions may appear in crops. Emotional upsets are generally believed to be precipitating factors in the appearance of these painful sheets of purpura. It has been noted that some patients have a premonition as to when they will develop new lesions a few hours ahead of time by the tingling and burning sensation at the site of a future lesion. Extracutaneous somatic symptoms are common, such as headache, paresthesias, transient paresis, syncope, diplopia, abdominal distress, diarrhea, nausea and vomiting, and arthralgia.

Gardner and Diamond reported that intracutaneous injections of erythrocyte stroma evoked typical lesions. Since then many have reported similar reactions to autologous whole blood, packed or washed red cells, or fractions of erythrocyte stroma. These are hard to assess, because similar reactions have been reported to substances as diverse as hemoglobin, phosphatidyl serine, histamine, histidine, trypsin, PPD, autologous serum, and platelets. Blinded, controlled testing, trying to avoid factitial trauma, has given mixed responses. Abnormalities in tissue-plasminogen activator-dependent fibrinolysis, thrombocytosis, and anticardiolipin antibodies have also been implicated. Many believe this syndrome to be artifactual, whereas other believe the lesions are spontaneous.

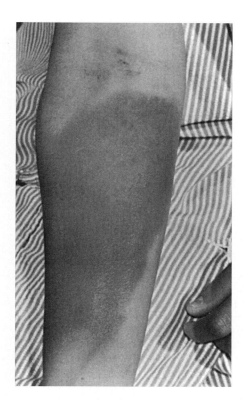

Fig. 35-16 Autoerythrocyte sensitization.

Treatment has been mostly unavailing, though psychotherapy directed at emotional problems has helped in some cases. The disease follows an irregularly intermittent course, possibly exacerbated by emotional stress or physical injury.

A similar syndrome, reported as DNA autosensitivity, has been described in eight patients who were reactive to intracutaneous injections of purified calf thymus DNA or frozen and thawed buffy coat. Further case studies are needed to fully assess this syndrome. Documentation to date suffers from the same inconsistencies and lack of controlled, blinded studies as does the Gardner-Diamond syndrome.

Archer-Dubon C, et al: Two cases of psychogenic purpura. *Rev Invest Clin* 1998, 50:145.

Berman DA, et al: Autoerythrocyte sensitization syndrome (psychogenic purpura). *J Am Acad Dermatol* 1992, 27:829.

Gomi H, et al: Autoerythrocyte sensitization syndrome with thrombocytosis. *Dermatology* 1994, 188:160.

Koblenzer PJ, et al: Psychogenic purpura. *Cutis* 1990, 45:60.

Kossard S, et al: Localised recurrent painful bruises. *Australas J Dermatol* 1993, 34:37.

Lotti T, et al: Psychogenic purpura with abnormally increased tPA dependent cutaneous fibrinolytic activity. *Int J Dermatol* 1993, 32:521.

Sudy E, et al: Autoerythrocyte sensitization syndrome with positive anticardiolipin antibodies. *Br J Dermatol* 1998, 138:367. ⎯⎯⎯⎯ ▲

Psychogenic Purpura

Psychogenic, or factitious, purpura presents a similar picture as autoerythrocyte sensitization; however, sensitivity to the erythrocytes is absent. Psychogenic purpura may be found in conversion reactions and purpura resulting from self-inflicted injury. Patients with Secretan's syndrome (factitial lymphedema of the hand) or l'oedeme bleu (factitial lymphedema of the arm) may have a purpuric component related to repetitive trauma. It is important not to confuse postictal purpura with psychogenic causes.

Moll S: Psychogenic purpura. *Am J Hematol* 1997, 55:146.

Panconesi E, et al: Stress, stigmatization and psychosomatic purpuras. *Int Angiol* 1995, 14:130. ⎯⎯⎯⎯⎯⎯⎯⎯ ▲

PIGMENTARY PURPURIC ERUPTIONS

The pigmented purpuric eruptions of the lower extremities are similar but may present in any of several clinical patterns. Clinical overlap between the various disorders may occur, and the histologies differ only by minor features that correlate with these clinical variations.

Progressive pigmentary dermatosis is better known as *Schamberg's disease*. The typical lesions are pinhead-sized, reddish puncta resembling grains of cayenne pepper, occurring in irregularly shaped patches on the lower legs (purpura and petechiae with prominent pigmentation) (Figs. 35-17 and 35-18). There is a slow proximal extension. After a few months the pinhead puncta begin to fade into the surrounding pigmented patches. These lesions seldom itch. The favored sites are around the lower shins and ankles.

Majocchi's disease is also known as *purpura annularis telangiectodes*. The early lesions are bluish-red annular macules 1 to 3 cm in diameter in which dark red telangiectatic puncta appear (Fig. 35-19). The central part of these lesions gradually fades so that the central involution and the peripheral extension form ringed or semicircular, or targetlike, concentric rings such as are seen on the cross-cut section of a tree trunk (annular pattern). The eruption begins symmetrically on the lower extremities and then spreads up the legs and may extend onto the trunk and arms. Involution usually requires as much as a year, but because of relapses the disease may be prolonged indefinitely. The lesions are asymptomatic.

Gougerot-Blum syndrome (pigmented purpuric lichenoid dermatitis) is characterized by minute, rust-colored, lichenoid papules that tend to fuse into plaques of various hues (purpura with lichenoid dermatitis) (Fig. 35-20). The plaques may contain papules of various hues. Favorite locations are on the legs, thighs, and lower trunk. The chief difference between this and Schamberg's disease is in the distribution of the lesions and the presence of lichenoid papular elevations, which in this disease are often grouped into plaques.

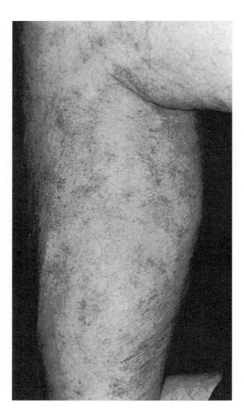

Fig. 35-17 Schamberg's disease.

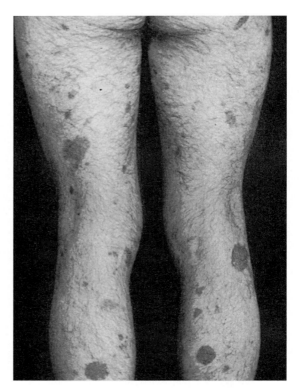

Fig. 35-19 Majocchi's disease. (Courtesy Dr. F. Daniels, Jr.)

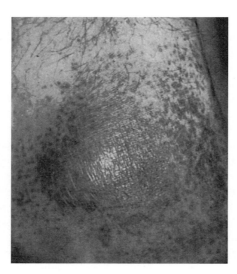

Fig. 35-18 Schamberg's progressive pigmentary dermatosis on ankle.

Lichen aureus of the skin is characterized by the sudden appearance of one or several patches of golden-hue or rusty-colored, closely packed lichenoid papules (purpura with golden patches) (Fig. 35-21). The patches vary from 2 to 30 cm in width and may occur on any part of the body.

They may be solitary or numerous. Linear segmental lesions may occasionally occur. They do not itch but may be associated with severe pain. Adults predominate among the reported cases, but children may also be affected.

Ducas and Kapetanakis' pigmented purpura is scaly and papular. It is distinguished histologically by the presence of spongiosis.

Histologically, early there is a superficial perivascular lymphocytic infiltrate with extravasation of erythrocytes. The extravasation of erythrocytes produces the purpuric aspect of the clinical lesions and should virtually always be found if such a lesion from a pigmented purpura has been biopsied. As lesions evolve the infiltrate may be more intense and become lichenoid (Gougerot-Blum type) or involve the epidermis with mild spongiosis (Ducas and Kapetanakis type). Extravasated erythrocytes are still present, but in addition hemosiderin is readily found in the upper dermis. Mild upper dermal fibrosis may eventually occur. An iron stain is sometimes used if the clinical diagnosis is a pigmented purpura, but siderophages are not readily visualized on routine sections. Lichenoid purpura must be distinguished from mycosis fungoides, which it can resemble both clinically and histologically. The absence of epidermotropism or the presence of only a few lymphocytes with spongiosis favors the diagnosis of pigmented purpura.

Anecdotal reports of benefit from topical steroids make a

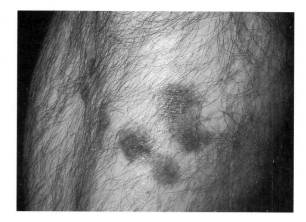

Fig. 35-21 Lichen aureus.

Ratnam KV, et al: Purpura simplex (inflammatory purpura without vasculitis): a clinicopathologic study of 174 cases. *J Am Acad Dermatol* 1991, 25:642.

Rheinhold U, et al: Treatment of progressive pigmented purpura with oral bioflavinoids and ascorbic acid: an open pilot study in 3 patients. *J Am Acad Dermatol* 1999, 41:207.

Thaipisutikul Y: Pruritic skin diseases in the elderly. *J Dermatol* 1998, 25:153.

Wahba-Yahav AV: Schamberg's purpura: association with persistent hepatitis B surface antigenemia and treatment with pentoxifylline. *Cutis* 1994, 54:205. _____ ▲

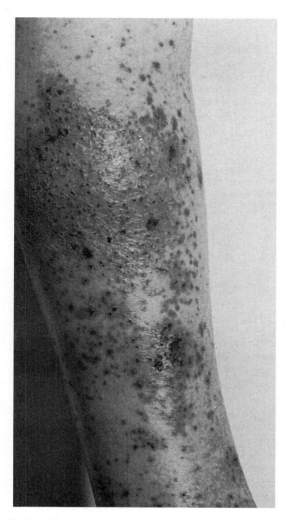

Fig. 35-20 Pigmented purpuric lichenoid dermatitis (Gougerot-Blum syndrome).

therapeutic trial for 4 to 6 weeks reasonable. Pentoxifylline, 400 mg three times daily, has also been reported to provide significant improvement within 2 to 3 weeks. Oral rutoside, 50 mg twice daily, and ascorbic acid, 500 mg twice daily, cleared 3 patients treated by Reinhold et al in 4 weeks.

Abeck D, et al: Acetaminophen-induced progressive pigmentary purpura (Schamberg's disease). *J Am Acad Dermatol* 1992, 27:123.

Gelmetti C, et al: Lichen aureus in childhood. *Pediatr Dermatol* 1996, 13:173.

Ghersetich I, et al: Cell infiltrate in progressive pigmented purpura (Schamberg's disease): immunophenotype, adhesion receptors, and intercellular relationships. *Int J Dermatol* 1995, 34:846.

Hersh CS, et al: Unilateral progressive pigmentary purpura (Schamberg's disease) in a 15-year-old boy. *J Am Acad Dermatol* 1991, 25:1098.

Kano Y, et al: Successful treatment of Schamberg's disease with pentoxifylline. *J Am Acad Dermatol* 1997, 36:827.

Vasculitis

Vasculitis is a clinicopathologic process characterized by inflammation and necrosis of blood vessels. Blood vessel size (capillaries; small, medium, and large vessels) is useful in classifying these disorders; however, some diseases may involve vessels of overlapping size. In general, small-vessel disease (venules) causes urticarial lesions and palpable purpura; small-artery disease manifests as nodules; medium-sized arteries with necrosis of major organs, livedo reticularis, purpura, and mononeuritis multiplex; and large-vessel disease with symptoms of claudication and necrosis.

Classification

Numerous classification schemes have been proposed, all of which have limitations. The 1990 American College of Rheumatology classification criteria for vasculitis have been shown to be effective in the diagnosis of 75% of the patients found to have vasculitic disorders; however, 21% of all patients sent to a university center for the consideration of vascular disease were also found to fulfill criteria for one or more entities, but not have any form of vasculitis. The following is a modified working classification proposed by Ghersetich et al:

    I. Cutaneous small-vessel disease
        A. Idiopathic cutaneous small-vessel vasculitis
        B. Henoch-Schönlein purpura
        C. Acute hemorrhagic edema of infancy

D. Urticarial vasculitis
E. Essential mixed cryoglobulinemia
F. Waldenström's hypergammaglobulinemic purpura
G. Collagen vascular associated
H. Rheumatoid nodules with vasculitis
I. Hyperimmunoglobulinemia D syndrome
J. Familial Mediterranean fever
K. Erythema elevatum diutinum
L. Granuloma faciale
M. Reactive Hansen's disease
N. Septic vasculitis
II. Medium-vessel necrotizing vasculitis
A. Polyarteritis nodosa
1. Benign cutaneous forms
2. Systemic form (including microscopic variant)
B. Granulomatous vasculitis
1. Limited Wegener's granulomatosis
2. Wegener's granulomatosis
3. Allergic granulomatosis (Churg-Strauss)
III. Large-vessel vasculitis
A. Giant-cell arteritis
B. Takayasu's arteritis

Essential mixed cryoglobulinemia, Waldenström's macroglobulinemia, collagen vascular diseases, rheumatoid nodules, and reactive Hansen's disease reactions are reviewed elsewhere.

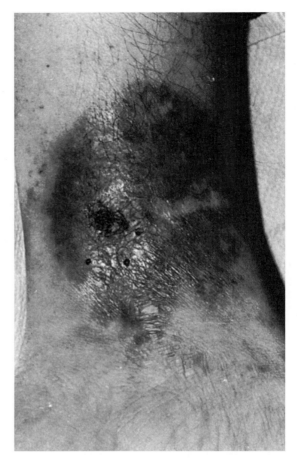

Fig. 35-22   Leukocytoclastic vasculitis.

Ghersetich I, et al: Working classification of vasculitis. *Int Angiol* 1995, 14:101.

Jennette JC, et al: Nomenclature of systemic vasculitides: proposal of an international consensus conference. *Arthitis Rheum* 1994, 37:187.

Jennette JC, et al: Small-vessel vasculitis. *N Engl J Med* 1997, 20:1512.

Jennette JC, et al: Vasculitis affecting the skin (editorial). *Arch Dermatol* 1994, 130:899.

Lotti T, et al: Cutaneous small-vessel vasculitis. *J Am Acad Dermatol* 1998, 39:667.

Rao JK, et al: Limitations of the 1990 American College of Rheumatology classification criteria in the diagnosis of vasculitis. *Ann Intern Med* 1998, 129:345. ▲

CUTANEOUS SMALL-VESSEL VASCULITIS (LEUKOCYTOCLASTIC VASCULITIS)

Palpable purpura is the hallmark of these disease processes, with lesions ranging from pinpoint to several centimeters in diameter. Early on the lesions may not be palpable. Papulonodular, vesicular, bullous, pustular, or ulcerated forms may develop. They predominate on the ankles and lower legs (Figs. 35-22 and 35-23), affecting mainly dependent areas or areas under local pressure (Fig. 35-24). Mild pruritus, fever, malaise, arthralgia, and/or myalgia may occur. The lesions usually resolve within 3 to 4 weeks with residual postinflammatory hyperpigmentation. The disease is self-limited but may recur or become chronic. Hemorrhagic vesicles or bullae may develop. Nodules with ulceration may occur and persist for months. Rarely, the face, buccal mucosae, and anogenital areas develop petechiae.

Urticaria-like lesions are next most common, having less evanescence than ordinary hives. The lesions usually resolve after a few days, leaving a residual brown discoloration. Other lesions may be pustules on a purpuric base; nodules with purpura, vesicles or bullae; erythematous plaques; and, uncommonly, livedo reticularis or necrosis.

Edema, especially of the ankles, is usually noted. Arthralgias or, less commonly, frank arthritis may be seen. The major renal manifestation is glomerulonephritis. Gastrointestinal involvement may result in hematemesis, bloody stools, ulcerations in the esophagus and stomach, anorexia, vomiting, nausea, and diarrhea. At times a pneumonitis may develop. Congestive heart failure and ocular involvement with retinal hemorrhage has been reported. Neural involvement may also be present, manifesting as peripheral neuritis, diplopia, dysphagia, hoarseness, polyneuritis, and peripheral neuritis. These findings

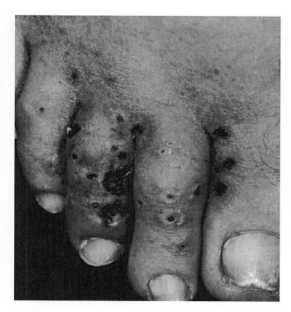

Fig. 35-23 Leukocytoclastic vasculitis. (Courtesy Dr. H. Shatin.)

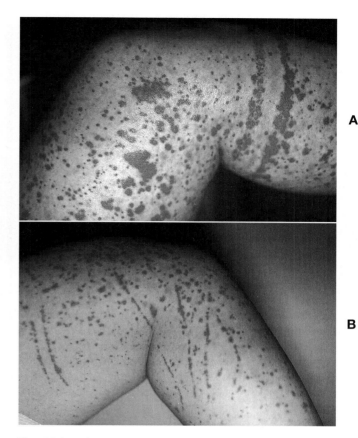

Fig. 35-24 A, Palpable purpura in leukocytoclastic vasculitis. **B,** Leukocytoclastic vasculitis with Koebner's phenomenon secondary to scratching.

and symptoms vary with the particular subset of presentation of cutaneous small-vessel vasculitis.

Histology

The histologic hallmark of patients with cutaneous small-vessel vasculitis is the presence of leukocytoclastic vasculitis. There is angiocentric segmental inflammation, endothelial cell swelling, fibrinoid necrosis of blood vessel walls, and a cellular infiltrate composed of neutrophils showing fragmentation of nuclei (karyorrhexis or leukocytoclasia). Immunofluorescence and ultrastructural studies have shown the presence of immunoglobulins, complement components, and fibrin deposits within postcapillary venule walls.

Pathogenesis

Many forms of small-vessel vasculitis are felt to be caused by circulating immune complexes. These complexes lodge in vessel walls and activate complement. Various inflammatory mediators (leukotriene B4, histamine, thrombin, IL-1, IL-6, TNF-alpha, and interferons) are produced, further contributing to endothelial injury. Abnormal fibrinolysis has also been demonstrated.

Etiology

The types of antigens inducing immune complexes vary. Some, such as infectious agents or drugs, are well defined. A host of infectious agents, such as beta-hemolytic *Streptococcus* group A, *Staphylococcus aureus*, *Mycobacterium leprae,* and *Mycobacterium tuberculosis* may cause palpable purpura. Viral infections (hepatitis A, B, C virus; herpes simplex, and influenza), fungi (*Candida albicans*),

protozoan infections *(Plasmodium malariae)* and helminthic infections *(Schistosoma haematobium, S. mansoni,* and *Onchocerca volvulus)* may also cause this form of vasculitis. Drugs (insulin, penicillin, hydantoin, streptomycin, aminosalicylic acid, sulfonamides, thiazides, phenothiazines, vitamins, phenylbutazone [Fig. 35-25], quinine, streptokinase, tamoxifen, antiinfluenza vaccines, oral contraceptives, and serum) have been reported causes. Coexisting disease, such as SLE, Sjögren's syndrome, rheumatoid arthritis, Behçet's disease, hyperglobulinemia, cryoglobulinemia, bowel bypass syndrome, ulcerative colitis, cystic fibrosis, primary biliary cirrhosis, and HIV disease, are not uncommon. Patients with lymphoproliferative neoplasms (Hodgkin's disease, mycosis fungoides, adult T-cell leukemia, and multiple myeloma) as well as solid tumors (lung, colon, ovarian, renal, prostate, head and neck, and breast cancer) may experience cutaneous small-vessel vasculitis at some time during the course of their disease.

Clinical Evaluation

Given the vast number of conditions that may result in small-vessel vasculitis a detailed history and physical exam-

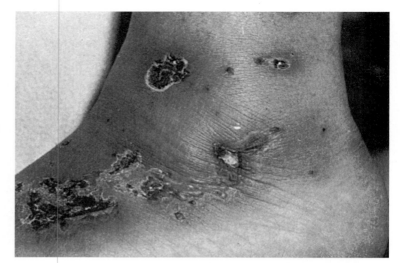

Fig. 35-25 Leukocytoclastic vasculitis from phenylbutazone.

ination is essential. The history should focus on possible infectious disorders, prior associated diseases, drugs ingested, and a thorough review of systems. Screening laboratory tests may help to elucidate the underlying cause or extent of organ involvement. A complete blood count, urinalysis, strep throat culture or ASO titer, hepatitis B and C serologies, and antinuclear antibodies are a reasonable initial screen. Serum protein electrophoresis, serum complements, and cryoglobulins may be required in some cases. A skin biopsy will confirm the diagnosis of leukocytoclastic vasculitis.

Treatment

The initial treatment of leukocytoclastic vasculitis should be nonaggressive, since the majority of cases are acute and self-limited, affect only the skin, and do not threaten progressive deterioration of internal organs. Rest and elevation of the legs is likely to be helpful. Analgesics, a good diet, and avoidance of trauma and cold are prudent general measures. An identified antigen or drug should, of course, be eliminated and any identified infectious, connective tissue or neoplastic disease treated.

A variety of systemic treatments may be required for severe, intractable, or recurrent disease. For disease limited to the skin, trials of nonsteroidal antiinflammatory agents; antihistamines; colchicine, 0.6 mg two to three times daily; or dapsone, 50 to 200 mg/day as trials of 2 to 3 weeks each, may be given. Although colchicine was ineffective in a prospective, randomized control trial, it was noted that in some patients it was clearly effective. Because of its relative safety it is worthy of a therapeutic trial. Systemic corticosteroids in doses ranging from 60 to 80 mg/day are recommended for those patients with systemic manifestations or necrotic lesions. In patients with a rapidly progressive course and severe systemic involvement, immunosuppressive agents such as cyclophosphamide, 2 mg/kg/day or as a monthly intravenous pulse; methotrexate,

5 to 25 mg/week; azathioprine, 50 to 200 mg/day; and cyclosporine, 3 to 5 mg/kg/day; have been shown effective. Pilot studies have shown promising results in treating intractable systemic vasculitis with monoclonal antibodies (Campath-1H and rat CD4 228), antiidiotypic antibodies, cytokine inhibitors or antagonists, and endothelial cell adhesion molecules (ICAM-1 or VCAM-1).

Callen JP: Cutaneous vasculitis. *Arch Dermatol* 1998, 134:355.

Dillon MJ, et al: Childhood vasculitis. *Lupus* 1998, 7:259.

Lotti T, et al: Cutaneous small-vessel vasculitis. *J Am Acad Dermatol* 1998, 39:667.

Lowry MD, et al: Leukocytoclastic vasculitis caused by drug additives. *J Am Acad Dermatol* 1994, 30:854.

Sais G, et al: Colchicine in the treatment of cutaneous leukocytoclastic vasculitis. *Arch Dermatol* 1995, 131:1399.

Sais G, et al: Prognostic factors in leukocytoclastic vasculitis. *Arch Dermatol* 1998, 134:309.

Sais G, et al: Tuberculous lymphadenitis presenting with cutaneous leukocytoclastic vasculitis. *Clin Exp Dermatol* 1996, 21:65.

Stashower ME, et al: Ovarian cancer presenting as leukocytoclastic vasculitis. *J Am Acad Dermatol* 1999, 40:287. _____ ▲

Subtypes of Small-Vessel Vasculitis

Henoch-Schönlein Purpura. Henoch-Schönlein purpura (HSP [anaphylactoid purpura]) is characterized by intermittent purpura (Fig. 35-26), arthralgia (74% to 84%), abdominal pain (61% to 76%), and renal disease (44% to 47%). Typically, palpable purpura appears on the extensor aspects of the extremities (Figs. 35-27 and 35-28), which become hemorrhagic within a day and start to fade in about 5 days. New crops may appear over a period of a few weeks. Urticarial lesions, vesicles, necrotic purpura, and hemangioma-like lesions may also be present at some stages. It occurs primarily in male children, with a peak age between 4 and 8 years; however, adults may also be affected. A viral infection or streptococcal pharyngitis are the usual triggering event. Other possibilities include other

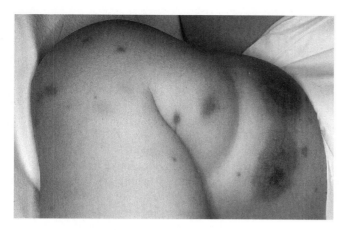

Fig. 35-26 Henoch-Schöenlein purpura.

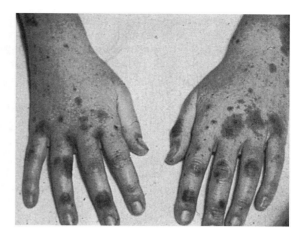

Fig. 35-28 Henoch-Schöenlein syndrome.

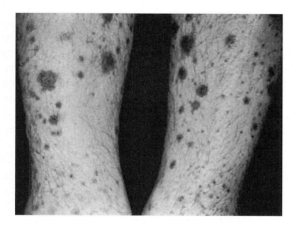

Fig. 35-27 Palpable purpuric lesions of the lower extremities of an adolescent male with Henoch-Schönlein syndrome.

bacterial infections, foods, drugs, chemical toxins, and lymphoma. Phenacetin, penicillin, phenothiazines, sulfonamides, griseofulvin, tetracycline, erythromycin, quinidine, and insect bites have all been incriminated.

In about 40% of cases the cutaneous manifestations are preceded by mild fever, headache, joint symptoms, and abdominal pain for up to 2 weeks. Arthralgia progressing to arthritis produces periarticular swelling around the knees and ankles. There may be pulmonary hemorrhage. Abdominal pain and gastrointestinal bleeding may occur at any time during the disease; severe abdominal pain may even suggest—or portend—an acute surgical abdomen. Paralytic ileus may occur. Vomiting, rebound tenderness, and distension are other manifestations. Gastrointestinal radiographs may show "spiking" or a marbled "cobblestone" appearance. Renal involvement manifests as microscopic or even gross hematuria and may occur in 25% or more of patients. The long-term prognosis in children with gross hematuria is very good; however, progressive glomerular disease and

renal failure may develop in a small percentage, so that careful follow-up supervision is necessary for those with hematuria. Guillain-Barré syndrome and mononeuropathies are uncommon but serious associated findings in a few cases of HSP.

IgA, C3, and fibrin depositions have been demonstrated in biopsies of both involved and uninvolved skin by immunofluorescence techniques. Uninvolved skin is a preferable site for biopsy because tissue morphology is better. There may be raised levels of IgA immune complexes regardless whether nephritis or purpura develops.

Treatment is supportive. The usual duration of illness is 6 to 16 weeks. Between 5% and 10% of patients will have persistent or recurrent disease. Antispasmodics, antibiotics, and antiinflammatory drugs, including systemic corticosteroids, may be helpful during the course of the disease, which will eventually clear without residua in most cases. Plasmapheresis may be used in severe, progressive cases. Other therapeutic options include dapsone. Corticosteroids or ephedrine may relieve abdominal pain more effectively than narcotic analgesia.

Andreoli SP: Renal manifestations of systemic diseases. *Semin Nephrol* 1998, 18:270.

Piette WW: What is Schönlein-Henoch purpura, and why should we care (editorial)? *Arch Dermatol* 1997, 133:438.

Tancrede-Bohin E, et al: Schönlein-Henoch purpura in adult patients. *Arch Dermatol* 1997, 133:438.

Vats KR, et al: Henoch-Schönlein purpura and pulmonary hemorrhage: a report and literature review. *Pediatr Nephrol* 1999, 13:530.

Wananukul S, et al: Henoch-Schönlein purpura presenting as hemorrhagic vesicles and bullae. *Pediatr Dermatol* 1995, 12:314.

Young PC, et al: Purpuric eruption with bloody diarrhea in an adult: Henoch-Schönlein purpura. *Arch Dermatol* 1996, 132:1241. ▲

Acute Hemorrhagic Edema of Infancy. Also known as *Finkelstein's disease, Seidlmayer syndrome,* and *purpura en* *cocarde avec oedema*, acute hemorrhagic edema of infancy affects children under age 2 with a recent history of an upper respiratory illness (75%), a course of antibiotics, or both. The children are often nontoxic in appearance. There is abrupt onset of large cockade, annular, or targetoid purpuric lesions involving the face, ears, and extremities. Scrotal purpura may also occur. Early in the course there may first be acral edema, with subsequent proximal spread. The edema is nontender and may be asymmetrical. A low-grade fever is common, and involvement of internal organ systems (joint pains, gastrointestinal symptoms, and renal involvement) is rare. Routine laboratory tests are nondiagnostic. It is considered a variant of leukocytoclastic vasculitis with many similarities to HSP. Spontaneous recovery without sequelae occurs within a few weeks. The differential diagnosis includes meningococcemia, HSP, erythema multiforme, urticaria, and Kawasaki's disease. From a clinical point of view the most urgent need is to exclude the possibility of meningococcemia.

Crowe MA, et al: Acute hemorrhagic edema of infancy. *Cutis* 1998, 62:65.

Ince E, et al: Infantile acute hemorrhagic edema: a variant of leukocytoclastic vasculitis. *Pediatr Dermatol* 1995, 12:224.

Legrain V, et al: Infantile acute hemorrhagic edema of the skin. *J Am Acad Dermatol* 1991, 24:17.

Morrison RR, et al: Acute hemorrhagic edema of infancy associated with pneumococcal bacteremia. *Pediatr Infect Dis J* 1999, 18:832. ▲

Urticarial Vasculitis. Urticarial vasculitis is a distinctive syndrome involving hypocomplementemia, arthritis, arthralgia, angioedema, abdominal or chest pain (or both), and in some cases pulmonary and renal involvement. Three clinical features distinguish the skin lesions of urticarial vasculitis from urticaria: (1) the lesions are usually painful, rather than pruritic; (2) the lesions last longer than 24 hours; and (3) on healing there is postinflammatory hyperpigmentation. Subcutaneous hemorrhage into the urticarial plaques may occur.

Underlying diseases associated with urticarial vasculitis include gammopathies (IgA multiple myeloma and IgM gammopathy), SLE, Sjögren's syndrome, serum sickness, and viral infections, such as hepatitis B, hepatitis C, and Epstein-Barr virus. Treatment options used to treat leukocytoclastic vasculitis may be helpful (see p. 1034). Additionally, plaquenil, 200 mg twice daily, may be effective in this subset of patients.

Eads TJ, et al: Pruritic, painful eruption: urticarial vasculitis. *Arch Dermatol* 1998, 134:231.

Grunwald MH, et al: Purpuric edematous lesions. *Arch Dermatol* 1999, 135:1409.

Hamid S, et al: Urticarial vasculitis caused by hepatitis C virus infection. *J Am Acad Dermatol* 1998, 39:278.

Knowles SR, et al: Serious adverse reactions induced by minocycline. *Arch Dermatol* 1996, 132:934.

Lowery N, et al: Serum sickness-like reactions associated with cefprozil therapy. *J Pediatr* 1994, 125:325.

Mehregan DR, et al: Urticarial vasculitis. *J Am Acad Dermatol* 1992, 26:441.

Nurnberg W, et al: Urticarial vasculitis syndrome effectively treated with dapsone and pentoxifylline. *Acta Derm Venereol* 1995, 75:54.

Wollenberg A, et al: Urticaria haemorrhagica profunda. *Br J Dermatol* 1997, 136:108. ▲

Hyperimmunoglobulinemia D Syndrome. Characterized by recurrent high-spiking fevers with abdominal distress, diarrhea, vomiting, headache, and arthralgias, up to 79% of patients with hyperimmunoglobulinemia D (HID) syndrome will have cutaneous findings. The most common skin eruptions include erythematous macules, erythematous papules, urticarial lesions, and erythematous nodules. Lymphadenopathy and splenomegaly are common. The age of onset is usually under 10 years, with familial clustering in individuals of European descent. Marked elevations in serum IgD are characteristic. The disorder has been found associated with erythema elevatum diutinum, and biopsies frequently demonstrate a leukocytoclastic vasculitis or features suggestive of Sweet's syndrome. Although often compared to other periodic fever syndromes, such as adult-onset Still's and familial Mediterranean fever, it has distinct clinical, serologic, and genetic features.

There is no preferred treatment although some authors believe that colchicine can prevent and ameliorate the attacks. Dapsone therapy was effective in treating the patient with associated erythema elevatum diutinum and may be therapeutic in treating HID syndrome alone.

Familial Mediterranean Fever. Familial Mediterranean fever is a periodic fever syndrome that may be confused with HID syndrome. It has been reported to affect Sephardic Jews, Armenians, and individuals of Arabian descent. Like HID syndrome its onset is usually under the age of 10 years. The cutaneous findings consist of erysipelas-like erythema showing sharp bordered, red patches with a diameter of 10 to 15 cm, affecting the lower extremities on the dorsa of the feet, over the ankles, and sometimes over the knees. Erysipelas-like erythema is considered characteristic; however, it occurs in only 3% to 46% of patients. Other associated cutaneous eruptions include purpura, angioneurotic edema, subcutaneous nodules, and bullous lesions. Arthralgias, peritonitis, and constipation may occur. There may be associated amyloidosis, eventually resulting in renal failure. Unlike HID syndrome, there is no lymphadenopathy and no elevation in serum IgD.

On skin biopsy there is most frequently a leukocytoclastic vasculitis. Genetic linkage studies have identified the defect at chromosome 16 polymorphic locus RT70, the familial Mediterranean fever susceptibility gene, which is not found in patients with HID syndrome. Treatment with colchicine significantly reduces the frequency of all cutaneous manifestations.

Boom BW, et al: IgD immune complex vasculitis in a patient with hyperimmunoglobulinemia D and periodic fever. *Arch Dermatol* 1990, 126:1621.

Cartier H, et al: Hyperimmunoglobulinemia D or periodic fever syndrome. *Ann Dermatol Venereol* 1996, 123:314.

Centola M, et al: The hereditary periodic fever syndromes: molecular analysis of a new family of inflammatory diseases. *Hum Mol Genet* 1998, 7:1581.

Drenth JP, et al: Cutaneous manifestations and histologic findings in the hyperimmunoglobulinemia D syndrome. *Arch Dermatol* 1994, 130:59.

Grateau G, et al: Hereditary fevers. *Curr Opin Rheumatol* 1999, 11:75.

Livneh A, et al: Familial Mediterranean fever and hyperimmunoglobulinemia D syndrome: two diseases with distinct clinical, serologic, and genetic features. *J Rheumatol* 1997, 24:1558.

Majaed HA, et al: The cutaneous manifestations in children with familial Mediterranean fever (recurrent hereditary polyserositis): a six-year study. *Q J Med* 1990, 37:607.

Miyagawa S, et al: Association of hyperimmunoglobulinaemia D syndrome with erythema elevatum diutinum. *Br J Dermatol* 1993, 128:572.

Ozdogan H, et al: Vasculitis in familial Mediterranean fever. *J Rheumatol* 1997, 24:323.

Pras E, et al: Mapping of a gene causing familial Mediterranean fever to the short arm of chromosome 16. *N Engl J Med* 1992, 326:1509.

▲

Erythema Elevatum Diutinum.

A rare condition, erythema elevatum diutinum (EED) is considered to be a chronic fibrosing leukocytoclastic vasculitis. Classically, multiple yellow papules develop over the joints, particularly the elbows, knees, hands, and feet (Figs. 35-29 and 35-30). Lesions may also involve the buttocks and areas over the Achilles tendon. Petechiae and purpura can be associated with early lesions. With time the papules take on a doughy to firm consistency and develop a red or purple color. Bulla formation and pyoderma gangrenosum may rarely occur. Pruritus, arthralgias, and pain have been reported; however, most patients are asymptomatic. EED has been associated with AIDS, hematologic disease (IgA monoclonal gammopathy), celiac disease, hyperimmunoglobulinemia D syndrome, Wegener's granulomatosis, and chronic and recurrent streptococcal infections.

Histologically, early lesions are a leukocytoclastic vasculitis, but with prominent interstitial neutrophils. Well-formed lesions are composed of nodular and diffuse mixed infiltrates of neutrophils and nuclear dust, eosinophils, histiocytes, and plasma cells that often extend into the subcutaneous fat. The prominence of eosinophils; the chronicity of the process, which results in perivascular dermal fibrosis; and the admixture of plasma cells and many lymphocytes are the hallmarks of EED.

Dapsone is the treatment of choice. Patients with celiac disease may respond to a gluten-free diet. Intermittent plasma exchange has been used successfully in patients with IgA paraproteinemia.

Chow RK, et al: Erythema elevatum diutinum associated with IgA paraproteinemia successfully controlled with intermittent plasma exchange. *Arch Dermatol* 1996, 132:1360.

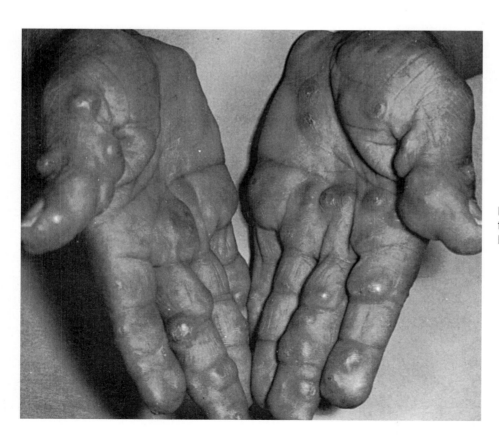

Fig. 35-29 Nodules of erythema elevatum diutinum on the palms. (Courtesy Dr. H. L. Hines.)

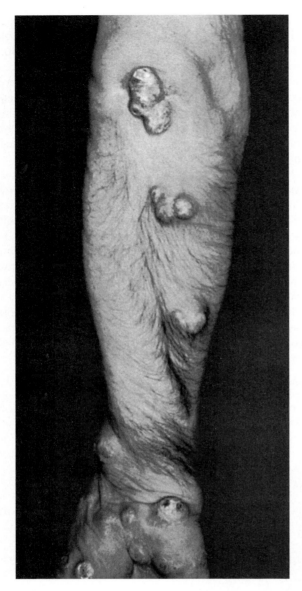

Fig. 35-30 Erythema elevatum diutinum on the hand and arm. (Courtesy Drs. J.P. Mraz and V.D. Newcomer.)

Kavanagh GM, et al: Erythema elevatum diutinum associated with Wegener's granulomatosis and IgA paraproteinemia. *J Am Acad Dermatol* 1993, 28:846.

Muratori S, et al: Erythema elevatum diutinum and HIV infection: a report of five cases. *Br J Dermatol* 1999, 141:335.

Planaguma M, et al: Pyoderma gangrenosum in association with erythema elevatum diutinum. *Cutis* 1992, 49:261.

Rodriguez-Serna M, et al: Erythema elevatum diutinum associated with celiac disease: response to a gluten-free diet. *Pediatr Dermatol* 1993, 10:125.

Shanks JH, et al: Nodular erythema elevatum diutinum mimicking cutaneous neoplasms. *Histopathology* 1997, 31:91.

Soni BP, et al: Erythematous nodules in a patient infected with the human immunodeficiency virus: erythema elevatum diutinum (EED). *Arch Dermatol* 1998, 134:232.

Tasanen K, et al: Erythema elevatum diutinum in association with coeliac disease. *Br J Dermatol* 1997, 136:624.

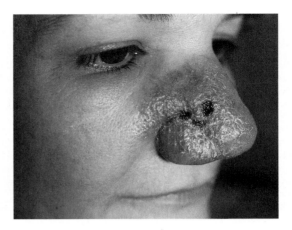

Fig. 35-31 Granuloma faciale.

Wayte JA, et al: Pyoderma gangrenosum, erythema elevatum diutinum and IgA monoclonal gammopathy. *Australas J Dermatol* 1995, 36:21. ▲

Granuloma Faciale. Characterized by brownish-red, infiltrated papules, plaques, and nodules, granuloma faciale (GF) involves the facial areas, particularly the nose (Fig. 35-31). Healthy, middle-aged white men are most typically affected; however, the lesions may also affect women and children. Extrafacial disease may occur but is rare.

The pathology of GF is identical to that of EED. Perivascular deposition of immunoglobulins (IgG) and complement are frequently found on direct immunofluorescence. The clinical differential diagnosis includes sarcoidosis, chronic cutaneous lupus erythematosus, pseudolymphoma, leukemia or lymphoma cutis, angiolymphoid hyperplasia with eosinophilia, histiocytosis X, erythema elevatum diutinum, infectious granulomas, and cutaneous T-cell lymphoma.

A variety of treatment options are available. Intralesional corticosteroids is the recommended first approach. Cryotherapy in combination with intralesional corticosteroids has been shown very effective. Topical corticosteroids may also be useful. Although controlled clinical trials are lacking, if the patient remains unresponsive, dapsone, colchicine, or antimalarials should be considered next in combination with topical and/or intralesional therapy. Topical PUVA and gold injections have also been reported effective. Surgical treatment is reserved for medical treatment failures and include dermabrasion, pulsed dye laser, electrosurgery, and cryosurgery.

Ammirati CT, et al: Treatment of granuloma faciale with the 585-nm pulsed dye laser. *Arch Dermatol* 1999, 135:903.

Dinehart SM, et al: Granuloma faciale: comparison of different treatment modalities. *Arch Otolaryngol Head Neck Surg* 1990, 116:849.

Dowlati B, et al: Granuloma faciale: successful treatment of nine cases with a combination of cryotherapy and intralesional corticosteroid injection. *Int J Dermatol* 1997, 36:548.

Konohana A: Extrafacial granuloma faciale. *J Dermatol* 1994, 21:680.

Phillips DK, et al: Recurrent facial plaques following full-thickness grafting: granuloma faciale. *Arch Dermatol* 1994, 130:1433.

Roustan G, et al: Granuloma faciale with extrafacial lesions (review). *Dermatology* 1999, 198:79.

van de Kerkhof PC: On the efficacy of dapsone in granuloma faciale. *Acta Derm Venereol* 1994, 74:61.

Welsh JH, et al: Granuloma faciale in a child successfully treated with the pulsed dye laser. *J Am Acad Dermatol* 1999, 41:351. _____ ▲

Serum Sickness. Serum sickness is a clinical syndrome resulting from circulating immune complexes that may occur after primary exposure to heterologous antisera or drugs. If the exposure is secondary, an accelerated reaction may occur in 2 to 4 days. The patients develop fever, lymphadenopathy, arthralgia, proteinuria, and skin lesions. The latter may be urticarial or morbilliform, and tend to marginate along the demarcation of the palms and soles from the dorsa of the extremities (Wallace's line). Serum sickness has been a complication of wasp venom immunotherapy, streptokinase therapy, and intravenous immune globulin, and with the use of antibiotics such as penicillin, minocycline, rifampicin, cefprozil, and cefaclor.

Comenzo RL, et al: Immune hemolysis, disseminated intravascular coagulation, and serum sickness after large doses of immune globulin given intravenously for Kawasaki disease. *J Pediatr* 1992, 120:926.

Creamer JD, et al: Serum sickness-like illness following streptokinase therapy. *Clin Exp Dermatol* 1995, 20:468.

De Bandt M, et al: Serum sickness after wasp venom immunotherapy. *J Rheumatol* 1997, 24:1195. _____ ▲

POLYARTERITIS NODOSA

Polyarteritis nodosa (PAN) is characterized by necrotizing vasculitis affecting the small and medium-sized muscular arteries of such caliber as the hepatic and coronary vessels and the arteries in the subcutaneous tissue, and sometimes adjacent veins. There are two major forms: the benign cutaneous and the systemic.

Microscopic polyangiitis is considered to be a subset of systemic PAN that may have therapeutic and prognostic implications. Patients with microscopic polyangiitis fulfill the following criteria: segmental necrotizing and crescentic glomerulonephritis associated with extrarenal vasculitis involving small-sized vessels, without granulomas or asthma. Some authors classify microscopic polyangiitis with Wegener's granulomatosis and Churg-Strauss syndrome because of similar cutaneous and histologic findings as well as the association with antineutrophil cytoplasmic autoantibodies in all three disorders.

Cutaneous Manifestations

The skin is involved in up to 40% of patients with the systemic form of PAN, with wide-ranging findings. The most striking and diagnostic lesions (15% of patients) are 5- to 10-mm subcutaneous nodules occurring singly or in groups distributed along the course of the blood vessels, above which the skin is normal or slightly erythematous. These nodules are often painful and may pulsate and, in time, ulcerate. Common sites are the lower extremities, especially below the knee. Ecchymoses and peripheral gangrene of the fingers and toes may also be present (Fig. 35-32). Livedo reticularis, bullae, papules, scarlatiniform lesions, and urticaria may also occur.

Internal Manifestations

Classic systemic periarteritis may involve the vessels throughout the entire body. Hypertension, tachycardia, fever, edema, and weight loss are cardinal signs of the disease. Hepatomegaly, icterus, lymphadenopathy, hematuria, and leukocytosis are also frequently found. Arthralgia, myocardial and intestinal infarctions, glomerulosclerosis, and peripheral neuritis are also seen. Mononeuritis multiplex, most often manifested as foot drop, is a hallmark of PAN. Involvement of the meningeal, vertebral, and carotid arteries may lead to hemiplegia and convulsions. The lungs and spleen are rarely involved. Aneurysms develop, which may result in multiorgan infarcts.

Laboratory Findings

A leukocytosis of as high as 40,000/mm^3 may occur, with neutrophilia to 80%; thrombocytosis and progressive normocytic anemia and an elevated sedimentation rate may also be found. Hypergammaglobulinemia with macroglobulins and cryoglobulins may be present. Hepatitis C studies should be performed. Urinary abnormalities such as proteinuria, hematuria, and casts are present in 70% of patients. Patients with microscopic polyangiitis have positive titers for peripheral antimyeloperoxidase (P-ANCA) as opposed to the cytoplasmic (C-ANCA) form found in systemic PAN.

Epidemiology

PAN is four times more common in men than in women, and the mean age of presentation is 45 years. It has been seen in intravenous drug abusers and in association with systemic lupus erythematosus, inflammatory bowel disease, hairy cell leukemia, and familial Mediterranean fever. Cogan's syndrome (nonsyphilitic interstitial keratitis and vestibulo-auditory symptoms) has also been reported. Infectious associations include hepatitis B, hepatitis C, and antecedent streptococcal infections.

Pathology

The histology is that of an inflammatory necrotizing and obliterative panarteritis that attacks the small and medium-sized arteries. Focal vasculitis forms nodose swellings that become necrotic, producing aneurysms and rupture of the vessels. Hemorrhage, hematoma, and ecchymosis may result. Obliteration of the lumen may occur, with ischemic

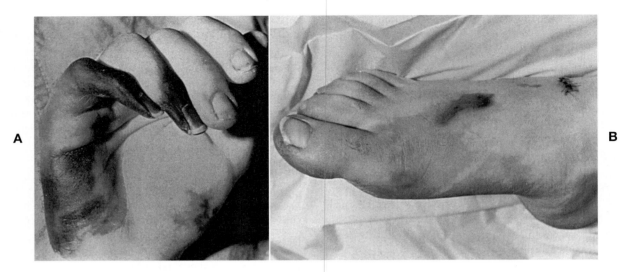

Fig. 35-32   Polyarteritis nodosa. **A,** Gangrene of fingers. **B,** Involvement of foot.

necrosis of surrounding tissue. Characteristically, the arteries are affected at their branching points.

The mainstay of diagnosis is the presence of these histologic features. The preferable site for biopsy is an accessible site such as skin, muscle, or testis. If these are not involved, angiography may detect aneurysmal dilations as small as 1 cm wide in the renal, hepatic, or other visceral vessels.

Treatment

Untreated classic PAN has a 5-year survival rate of 13%; death usually occurs from renal failure or cardiovascular or gastrointestinal complications. Treatment with corticosteroids and cytotoxic agents has increased the survival rate to more than 90%. Corticosteroids in the range of 1 mg/kg/day are given initially. Once the disease remits the dose should be reduced. After an average of 3 to 6 months, with the patient in remission, the steroids are slowly tapered to discontinuation.

Cyclophosphamide is given with steroids, or sometimes as a single agent. An initial dose of 2 mg/kg/day as a single dose is recommended. Twice this dosing may be required for severely ill patients. The oral dose is then adjusted to maintain the white blood cell count between 3000 and 3500/mm^3 and the neutrophil count above 1500 cells/mm^3. When the disease has been quiescent for at least a year, the cyclophosphamide may be tapered and stopped. On the average, 18 to 24 months of therapy is required.

Cutaneous Polyarteritis Nodosa. The cutaneous form of PAN is remarkable for an absence of visceral involvement. Patients usually have recurrent skin, joint, and muscle involvement without involvement of vital organs. The cutaneous findings are similar to those described for the systemic form. It has been associated with hepatitis B surface antigenemia, hepatitis C virus infection, Crohn's

disease, Takayasu arteritis, relapsing polychondritis, post-streptococcal infections, and tuberculosis. Most patients respond well to aspirin, prednisone, and methotrexate, alone or in combination, usually resulting in clinical responses within a few days.

Fortin PR, et al: Prognostic factors in systemic necrotizing vasculitis of the polyarteritis nodosa group: a review of 45 cases. *J Rheumatol* 1995, 22:78.

Guillevin L, et al: Distinguishing polyarteritis nodosa from microscopic polyangiitis and implications for treatment. *Curr Opin Rheumatol* 1995, 7:20.

Homas PB, et al: Microscopic polyarteritis. *Arch Dermatol* 1992, 128:1223.

Irvine AD, et al: Microscopic polyangiitis. *Arch Dermatol* 1997, 133:474.

Kumar L, et al: Benign cutaneous polyarteritis nodosa in children below 10 years of age: a clinical experience. *Ann Rheum Dis* 1995, 54:134.

Langford CA, et al: New developments in the treatment of Wegener's granulomatosis, polyarteritis nodosa, microscopic polyangiitis, and Churg-Strauss syndrome. *Curr Opin Rheumatol* 1997, 9:26.

Pak H, et al: Purpuric nodules and macules on the extremities of a young woman: cutaneous polyarteritis nodosa. *Arch Dermatol* 1998, 134:232.

Penas PF, et al: Microscopic polyangiitis: a systemic vasculitis with a positive P-ANCA. *Br J Dermatol* 1996, 134:542.

Sheth AP, et al: Cutaneous polyarteritis nodosa of childhood. *J Am Acad Dermatol* 1994, 31:561.

Siberry GK, et al: Cutaneous polyarteritis nodosa. *Arch Dermatol* 1994, 130:884.

Soufir N, et al: Hepatitis C virus infection in cutaneous polyarteritis nodosa. *Arch Dermatol* 1999, 135:1001. _____ ▲

WEGENER'S GRANULOMATOSIS

Wegener's granulomatosis is a syndrome consisting of necrotizing granulomas of the upper and lower respiratory tract, generalized necrotizing angiitis affecting the medium-sized blood vessels, and focal necrotizing glomerulitis. By far the commonest initial manifestation is the occurrence of rhinorrhea, severe sinusitis, and nasal mucosal ulcerations, with one or several nodules in the nose, larynx, trachea, or bronchi. Fever, weight loss, and malaise occur in these patients, who are usually 40 to 50 years of age and more often male than female (1.3:1). Obstruction in the nose may also block the sinuses. The nodules in the nose frequently ulcerate and bleed. The parenchymal involvement of the lungs produces cough, dyspnea, and chest pain. Granulomas may occur in the ear and mouth, where the alveolar ridge becomes necrotic and ulceration of the tongue and perforated ulcers of the palate develop. The "strawberry gums" appearance of hypertrophic gingivitis is characteristic.

Cutaneous findings occur in 45% of patients. Nodules may appear in crops, especially along the extensor surfaces of the extremities. The firm, slightly tender, flesh-colored or violaceous nodules may later ulcerate. The necrotizing angiitis of the skin may become evident as purpura in the form of a petechial or hemorrhagic pustular eruption. Livedo reticularis is rare in Wegener's granulomatosis. Patients may present with pyoderma-like lesions involving the head and neck regions, and several patients have been reported presenting with features of temporal arteritis. Limited forms involving the upper respiratory tract without renal involvement may also occur and have a better prognosis. Cutaneous findings can be associated with limited disease. The early detection of Wegener's granulomatosis has improved since the discovery of the association with cytoplasmic antineutrophil cytoplasmic autoantibodies (C-ANCA), providing a useful test. In one series of 106 patients, 88% with active disease and 43% in remission were positive for C-ANCA.

Focal necrotizing glomerulitis occurs in 85% of patients. It may be fulminant from the outset or may become more severe as the disease progresses. Renal failure was the most frequent cause of death before cyclophosphamide treatment.

Other organs frequently involved include the joints (arthralgia in two thirds); eyes (conjunctivitis, episcleritis, and proptosis) in 58%; and CNS and cardiac involvement in 22% and 12% of patients, respectively.

Histologically, the cutaneous lesions may demonstrate a leukocytoclastic vasculitis with or without granulomatous inflammation. Often, if the lesions are ulcerated, they are nonspecific histologically. Biopsy of another affected organ may be required to confirm the diagnosis.

Untreated Wegener's granulomatosis has a mean survival time of 5 months and a 90% mortality over 2 years. Cyclophosphamide therapy has dramatically changed the prognosis. Treatment recommendations are cyclophosphamide, 2 mg/kg, and prednisone, 1 mg/kg/day, followed by tapering of the prednisone to an alternate-day regimen. Complete remission is achieved in up to 93% and lasts an average of 4 years for still living patients. Pulse dose cyclophosphamide, 15 mg/kg initially every second week, gradually increasing the pulse interval, has produced remission rates of 91% after 3 months of therapy. In more limited disease some treatment success has been reported using trimethoprim-sulfamethoxazole. Trimethoprim-sulfamethoxazole may decrease the relapse rate and should be considered for long-term treatment of patients in remission. Alternative therapy includes low-dose methotrexate plus glucocorticoids, azathioprine, and cyclosporine.

De Groot K, et al: Wegener's granulomatosis: disease course, assessment of activity and extent and treatment. *Lupus* 1998, 7:285.

Frances C, et al: Wegener's granulomatosis. *Arch Dermatol* 1994, 130:861.

Harman LE, et al: Wegener's granulomatosis. *Surv Ophthalmol* 1998, 42:458.

Koldingsnes W, et al: Wegener's granulomatosis: long-term follow-up of patients treated with pulse cyclophosphamide. *Br J Rheumatol* 1998, 37:659.

Micali G, et al: Cephalic pyoderma gangrenosum (PG)-like lesions as a presenting sign of Wegener's granulomatosis. *Int J Dermatol* 1994, 33:477.

Nishino H, et al: Wegener's granulomatosis associated with vasculitis of the temporal artery. *Mayo Clin Proced* 1993, 68:194.

Sais G, et al: Antineutrophil cytoplasmic antibodies in leukocytoclastic vasculitis (letter). *Arch Dermatol* 1998, 134:239.

Stein SL, et al: Wegener's granulomatosis. *Pediatr Dermatol* 1998, 15:352.

ALLERGIC GRANULOMATOSIS (CHURG-STRAUSS SYNDROME)

Allergic granulomatosis is also known as *necrotizing angiitis with granulomata*. It is characterized by the distinctive initial manifestation of asthma. A debilitated asthmatic begins after 2 to 12 years to experience attacks of fever and eosinophilia (20% to 90%) and after a few more months or years, diffuse angiitis involves the lungs, heart, liver, spleen, kidneys, intestines, and pancreas. A fatal outcome is likely in most untreated patients, with congestive heart failure resulting from myocarditis the most frequent cause of death.

Cutaneous lesions are present in two thirds of patients. Nodules may appear on the extensor surfaces of the extremities and on the scalp. Firm, nontender papules may be present on the fingertips. Purpura or hemorrhagic bullae are present.

Laboratory studies are significant for a peripheral eosinophilia, which correlates with disease severity. Tests for ANCA are frequently positive for P-ANCA, or, less frequently, C-ANCA and tend to correlate with disease severity.

The cause is unknown; however, several drugs have been implicated in precipitating it. Zafirlukast (Accolate), a drug approved for the treatment of asthma, has been associated with acute Churg-Strauss syndrome. Azithromycin and freebase cocaine use have also been implicated. It has been reported after vaccination for hepatitis B.

Histologically, a small-vessel vasculitis is present that involves not only superficial venules but also larger and deeper vessels. The tissue is often diffusely infiltrated with eosinophils, and granulomas may be present.

Cyclophosphamide alone or in combination with corticosteroids have been the treatments of choice. Interferon-alfa has also been used successfully.

Abe-Matsuura Y, et al: Allergic granulomatosis (Churg-Strauss) associated with cutaneous manifestations. *J Dermatol* 1995, 22:46.

Cottin V, et al: Churg-Strauss syndrome. *Allergy* 1999, 54:535.

Davis MDP, et al: Cutaneous manifestations of Churg-Strauss syndrome. *J Am Acad Dermatol* 1997, 37:199.

Knoell DL, et al: Churg-Strauss syndrome with zafirlukast. *Chest* 1998, 114:332.

Kranke B, et al: Macrolide-induced Churg-Strauss syndrome in patient with atopy. *Lancet* 1997, 350:1551.

Louthrenoo W, et al: Childhood Churg-Strauss syndrome. *J Rheumatol* 1999, 26:1387.

Orriols R, et al: Cocaine-induced Churg-Strauss vasculitis. *Eur Respir J* 1996, 9:175.

Tatsis E, et al: Interferon-alpha treatment of four patients with the Churg-Strauss syndrome. *Ann Intern Med* 1998, 129:370.

Vanoli M, et al: A case of Churg-Strauss vasculitis after hepatitis B vaccination. *Ann Rheum Dis* 1998, 57:256. _____ ▲

LETHAL MIDLINE GRANULOMA

Lethal midline granuloma is a clinical term describing those entities that produce progressive destructive ulcerations of the nose, sinuses, palate, or pharynx—the central part of the face. The first sign may be a chronic mucoid nasal discharge that later becomes purulent. The necrotic ulceration usually appears first on the nasal septum. Eventually, there is necrosis of the facial bones and base of the skull. Mutilating destruction of the central face may occur. Patients are most often men between ages 20 and 50.

There are three main histologic and clinical divisions of lethal midline granuloma: (1) lymphoma, (2) nonneoplastic granulomatous tissue reaction, and (3) Wegener's granulomatosis. There are numerous reports of angiocentric T-cell lymphomas located in the midline; however, the lungs and kidneys are spared, and disseminated vasculitis rarely occurs. Epstein-Barr virus (EBV) and human T-cell leukemia/lymphoma virus-T (HTLV-I) have been implicated as a cause of these forms of T-cell lymphoma. EBV DNA was detected in 16 of 21 reported cases of lethal midline granuloma caused by angiocentric T-cell lymphoma in the series by Lee et al. A case of lethal midline granuloma developed in one patient who had lymphomatoid papulosis for more than 8 years.

Nonneoplastic granulomatous tissue reaction without evidence of arteritis is the second category, which responds to radiation therapy, as do most cases of lethal midline granuloma caused by lymphoma. Repeat biopsies of the granulomatous variety are required to exclude lymphoma.

Some authors have classified this disorder as a form of lymphomatoid granulomatosis or a variant of Wegener's granulomatosis. It is a practical classification, since lymphomatoid granulomatosis (a lymphoma) responds to radi-

ation therapy, whereas Wegener's granulomatosis responds best to chemotherapy. One-year and 5-year survival rates are 45% and 22%, respectively.

Harabuchi Y, et al: Epstein-Barr virus in nasal T-cell lymphomas in patients with lethal midline granuloma. *Lancet* 1990, 335:128.

Harabuchi Y, et al: Lethal midline granuloma (peripheral T-cell lymphoma) after lymphomatoid papulosis. *Cancer* 1992, 70:835.

Hirakawa S, et al: Nasal and nasal-type natural killer/T-cell lymphoma. *J Am Acad Dermatol* 1999, 40:268.

Lee PY, et al: Angiocentric T-cell lymphoma presenting as lethal midline granuloma. *Int J Dermatol* 1997, 36:419.

Sakata K, et al: Treatment of lethal midline granuloma type nasal T-cell lymphoma. *Acta Oncol* 1997, 36:307.

Vidal RW, et al: Sinonasal malignant lymphomas: a distinct clinicopathological category. *Ann Otol Rhinol Laryngol* 1999, 108:411.

Yamazaki M, et al: A case of angiocentric T-cell lymphoma presenting as lethal midline granuloma. *Dermatology* 1995, 191:336. _____ ▲

GIANT-CELL ARTERITIS

Giant-cell arteritis is a systemic disease of people over age 50. Its best known location is in the temporal artery, where it is known as *temporal arteritis, cranial arteritis,* and *Horton's disease*. It is characterized by a necrotizing panarteritis with granulomas and giant cells, which produce unilateral headache and exquisite tenderness in the scalp over the temporal or occipital arteries. Fever, anemia, and a high sedimentation rate are usually present. It is rarely fatal. The disease has also been shown to involve the vessels of the coronary arteries, breast, uterus, legs, abdomen, and hand. Aortic aneurysms resulting in aortic rupture have been reported.

The cutaneous manifestations may be only inflammatory. The affected artery becomes evident as a hard, pulsating, tender, tortuous bulge under red or cyanotic skin. Another manifestation is gangrene of the scalp. The lesions may first appear as ecchymoses with a zonal distribution over the affected area. Later they may become vesicular or bullous and are followed by gangrene. Urticaria, purpura, alopecia, tender nodules, and livedoid reticularis may be seen. Blindness may also develop and is the most feared complication of the disease. Lingual artery involvement may cause an accompanying red, sore tongue. The mouth may show temporomandibular pain and gangrene of the tongue.

Polymyalgia rheumatica has a significant clinical association with giant-cell arteritis. Prompt treatment may forestall serious disease. About 10% of central retinal artery occlusions are due to giant-cell arteritis. Erythrocyte sedimentation rates are elevated in more than 90% of patients with giant-cell arteritis. Temporal artery biopsy is diagnostic. Magnetic resonance angiography is a noninvasive diagnostic method that may aid in confirming the clinical suspicion and identify the best site to biopsy.

Treatment is usually begun with prednisone, 60 mg daily, continued for 1 month or until all reversible clinical and laboratory parameters (such as the sedimentation rate) have become normal. The disease is quite steroid responsive, and tapering to a dose of 7.5 to 10 mg a day is usually possible. Daily therapy seems important and is usually necessary for a minimum of 1 to 2 years. Most patients achieve complete remission that is often maintained after therapy is withdrawn.

Botella-Estrada R, et al: Magnetic resonance angiography in the diagnosis of a case of giant cell arteritis manifesting as scalp necrosis. *Arch Dermatol* 1999, 135:769.

Dudenhoefer EJ, et al: Scalp necrosis with giant cell arteritis. *Ophthalmology* 1998, 105:1875.

Evans J, et al: The implications of recognizing large-vessel involvement in elderly patients with giant cell arteritis. *Curr Opin Rheumatol* 1997, 9:37.

Hunder GG: Giant cell arteritis and polymyalgia rheumatica. *Med Clin North Am* 1997, 81:195.

Marcos O, et al: Tongue necrosis in a patient with temporal arteritis. *J Oral Maxillofac Surg* 1998, 56:1203.

Reich KA, et al: Neurologic manifestations of giant cell arteritis. *Am J Med* 1990, 89:67.

McKendry RJ, et al: Giant cell arteritis (temporal arteritis) affecting the breast. *Ann Rheum Dis* 1990, 49:1001.

Wilke WS, et al: Treatment of corticosteroid-resistant giant cell arteritis. *Rheum Dis Clin North Am* 1995, 21:59. ▲

Takayasu's Arteritis

Known also as *aortic arch syndrome* and *pulseless disease,* Takayasu's arteritis is a thromboobliterative process of the great vessels stemming from the aortic arch, occurring generally in young women. Radial and carotid pulses are typically obliterated. Skin changes are due to the disturbed circulation. There may be loss of hair and atrophy of the skin and its appendages, with underlying muscle atrophy. Occasional patients with cutaneous necrotizing or granulomatous vasculitis have been reported, and erythema nodosum may rarely occur. Like PAN, it has been reported associated with Cogan's syndrome. Treatment with corticosteroids as in temporal arteritis should be given and followed in the same way. Methotrexate may be used for its steroid-sparing effects. With active medical and surgical intervention the aggressive course of this disease can be modified.

Dillon MJ: Childhood vasculitis. *Lupus* 1998, 7:259.

Han D, et al: A review of Takayasu's arteritis in children in Gauteng, South Africa. *Pediatr Nephrol* 1998, 12:668.

Numano F, et al: Takayasu arteritis: beyond pulselessness. *Intern Med* 1999, 38:226.

Perniciaro CV, et al: Cutaneous manifestations of Takayasu's arteritis. *J Am Acad Dermatol* 1987, 17:998.

Raza K, et al: Cogan's syndrome with Takayasu's arteritis. *Br J Rheumatol* 1998, 37:369.

Shetty AK, et al: Low-dose methotrexate as a steroid-sparing agent in a child with Takayasu's arteritis. *Clin Exp Rheumatol* 1998, 16:335. ▲

MALIGNANT ATROPHIC PAPULOSIS

Papulosis atrophicans maligna, also known as *Degos' disease,* is a potentially fatal obliterative arteritis syndrome. Degos' disease occurs most frequently in men between ages 20 and 40. Patients survive untreated an average of 2 years after the disease has developed. Clinically, it is characterized by the presence of pale rose, rounded, edematous papules occurring mostly on the trunk. Similar lesions may occur on the bulbar conjunctiva and oral mucosa. Later the lesions become umbilicated, with a central depression, which enlarges. The center becomes distinctively porcelain-white, while the periphery becomes livid red and telangiectatic (Fig. 35-33). Atrophy occurs eventually. The eruption proceeds by crops in which only a few new lesions appear at any one time. One patient was reported to develop panniculitis mimicking lupus profundus.

Later, anemic infarcts involve the intestines to produce acute abdominal symptoms of epigastric pain, fever, and hematemesis. Death is usually due to fulminating peritonitis caused by multiple perforations of the intestine. Less commonly, death occurs from cerebral infarctions. Eye lesions such as episcleritis may also be present.

Wedge-shaped necroses brought on by the occlusion of arterioles and small arteries account for the clinical lesions. Proliferation of the intima with subsequent thrombosis is the typical histologic picture. On light microscopy there is extensive lymphocytic infiltration and necrotizing vasculitis of the microvasculature, with damage to cutaneous nerves by demyelination. The etiology of this disease is unknown, but viral, autoimmune, and abnormal coagulation have been suggested. Inherited forms have also been reported.

Administration of corticosteroids has not been beneficial. Ingestion of 0.5 g acetylsalicylic acid twice a day and 50 mg dipyridamole (Persantine) three times a day, for 20 months, has been shown effective in some series; however, others have found it ineffective. Anticoagulant therapy has helped on occasion, and heparin, as described by Degos, has been helpful for some patients.

Grilli R, et al: Panniculitis mimicking lupus erythematosus profundus: a new histopathologic finding in malignant atrophic papulosis (Degos' disease). *Am J Dermatopathol* 1999, 21:365.

Katz SK, et al: Malignant atrophic papulosis (Degos' disease) involving three generations of family. *J Am Acad Dermatol* 1997, 37:480.

Requena L, et al: Degos' disease in a patient with acquired immunodeficiency syndrome. *J Am Acad Dermatol* 1998, 38:852.

Yag-Howard C, et al: Multiple pink papules with white, depressed centers: malignant atrophic papulosis (Degos' disease). *Arch Dermatol* 1998, 134:233. ▲

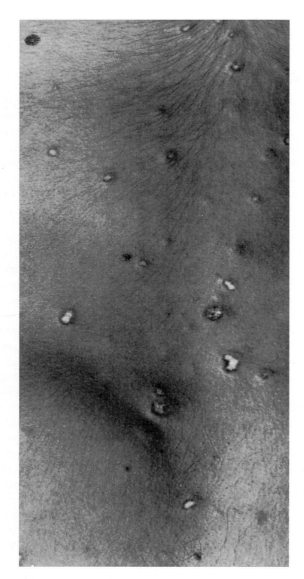

Fig. 35-33 Papulosis atrophicans maligna on mid-back. Red papules, some showing umbilication; other papules umbilicated with typical porcelaneous white centers. (From Winkelmann RK, et al: *Arch Dermatol* 1963, 87:54.)

THROMBOANGIITIS OBLITERANS (BUERGER'S DISEASE)

Thromboangiitis obliterans is an obliterative vascular disease affecting the medium- and small-sized arteries, especially those of the feet and hands. It is most often seen in men between ages 20 and 40 who smoke heavily. The vasomotor changes in early cases may be transitory or persistent; they produce blanching, cyanosis, burning, and tingling. Superficial thrombophlebitis commonly develops in the leg and foot, and attacks tend to come and go every few weeks. The color of the part may change when it is elevated or lowered below heart level, being red when dependent and white when elevated.

Pain is a constant symptom, coming only at first after exercise and subsiding on resting. Instep claudication is the classic complaint. Ultimately, pulsation in the dorsalis pedis and posterior tibial arteries, or even others, may cease. In thromboangiitis obliterans, skin supplied by affected arterioles tends to break down, with central necrosis and ulceration and eventual gangrene (Fig. 35-34). Oral lesions have also been reported. There is a strong association with cigarette smoking. Exposure to cold and dampness may have etiologic importance. Arteriography should be done to investigate for central atherosclerotic disease, which may be operable, rather than the inoperable distal damage of Buerger's disease. A characteristic tapering of the arteries with "corkscrew" collateral circulation is found in Buerger's disease on angiography.

The most important therapeutic aspect is the cessation of smoking. In a series of 69 patients in 71% the disease progressed to termination of the working life, and 83% persisted with their smoking habits. Other forms of therapy are only palliative, such as local wound care, calcium channel blockers and/or pentoxifylline, iloprost, antibiotics, and nonsteroidal antiinflammatory agents. Sympathectomy may be tried if vasodilators fail. Ultimately, serial amputations are often necessary.

Ambrosi CN, et al: A case of Buerger's disease. *Cutis* 1993, 51:180.

Borner C, et al: Long-term follow-up of thromboangiitis obliterans. *Vasa* 1998, 27:80.

Farish SE, et al: Intraoral manifestation of thromboangiitis obliterans (Buerger's disease). *Oral Surg Oral Med Oral Pathol* 1990, 69:223.

Olin JW: Thromboangiitis obliterans. *Curr Opin Rheumatol* 1994, 6:44.

Samlaska CP, et al: Superficial thrombophlebitis. II. Secondary hypercoagulable states. *J Am Acad Dermatol* 1990, 23:1.

Stvrtinova V, et al: 90 years of Buerger's disease: what has changed? *Bratisl Lek Listy* 1999, 100:123.

Zellerman GL, et al: Chronic ulcerations in the upper and lower extremities: thromboangiitis obliterans. *Arch Dermatol* 1998, 134:1020.

ARTERIOSCLEROSIS OBLITERANS

Arteriosclerosis obliterans is an occlusive arterial disease most prominently affecting the abdominal aorta and the small and medium-sized arteries of the lower extremities. The symptoms are due to ischemia of the tissues. There is intermittent claudication manifested by pain, cramping, numbness, and fatigue in the muscles on exercise; these are relieved by rest. There may be "rest pain" at nighttime when in bed. Also, sensitivity to cold, muscular weakness, stiffness of the joints, and paresthesia may be present. Sexual impotence is common, and there is an increased frequency of coronary artery disease.

Impaired to absent pulses (dorsalis pedis, posterior tibial or popliteal arteries) may be found on physical examination, confirming the diagnosis. The feet, especially the toes, may be red and cold. Striking pallor of the feet on elevation, and redness when dependent, are compatible findings. De-

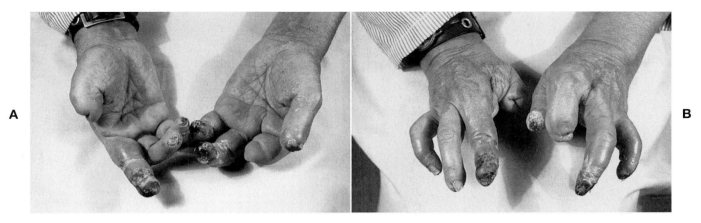

Fig. 35-34 **A** and **B**, Thromboangiitis obliterans (Buerger's disease).

creased to absent hair growth may be observed on the legs. Ulceration and gangrene may supervene. If present, they usually begin in the toes. Arteriography may be indicated as a preliminary to corrective surgery (arterial grafts). Occasionally, subclavian atherosclerosis may give rise to these signs in the distal upper extremity, producing painful nails and loss of digital skin. Diabetes and smoking appear to play a more significant role in progression of disease than hyperlipidemia.

Claudication and diminished blood pressure in the affected extremity are findings that may lead to earlier diagnosis and thus to curative surgical intervention. Usually, bypass of the affected artery, or sympathectomy, or both, are the preferred treatment. Balloon angioplasty or stint placement may also be effective.

Kerdel FA, et al: Subclavian occlusive disease presenting as a painful nail. *J Am Acad Dermatol* 1984, 10:523.

Matsumoto K, et al: Insulin resistance and arteriosclerosis obliterans in patients with NIDDM. *Diabetes Care* 1997, 20:1738. _____ ▲

MUCOCUTANEOUS LYMPH NODE SYNDROME (KAWASAKI'S DISEASE)

Irritable, febrile infants or children (or rarely, adults) with erythema multiforme–like, scarlatiniform, or morbilliform skin lesions accompanied by stomatitis, cheilitis (Fig. 35-35, *A*), edema of the hands and feet, conjunctival congestion, and cervical lymphadenitis probably have mucocutaneous lymph node syndrome (MLNS). After a week or two the fingers and toes desquamate, starting around the nails (Fig. 35-35, *B*).

Kawasaki first reported this acute febrile illness in children in 1967, in Japan. Since then it has been diagnosed in increasing numbers worldwide. More than 12,531 cases were reported in Japan in 1995-1996 (incidence of 105/10,000) with a male to female ratio of 1.37 and a peak age distribution at 6 months. A standardized mortality ratio

was 1.45, with most of the deaths occurring during the acute phase.

Diagnosis

Six criteria have been defined: fever, conjunctival congestion, oropharyngeal lesions, hand and foot lesions, an exanthem, and lymphadenopathy. To make the diagnosis the patient should have fever (above 38.3° C) of 5 days' duration plus at least four of the five following criteria: (1) peripheral extremity changes (edema, erythema, desquamation), (2) polymorphous exanthem, (3) nonpurulent bilateral conjunctival injection, (4) changes of lips and oral cavity (erythema, strawberry tongue), and (5) acute, nonpurulent cervical adenopathy. The cutaneous eruption is polymorphous and may be macular, morbilliform, urticarial, scarlatiniform, erythema multiforme–like, pustular, and resembling erythema marginatum. An early finding is the appearance of an erythematous, desquamating perianal eruption, usually within the first week of symptoms. About two thirds will manifest as perineal erythema. Periorbital and intraorbital involvement manifesting with edema and swelling has also been reported. Pincer nail deformities may resolve spontaneously. The disease lasts 10 to 20 days and then subsides. One to 2% of patients may die of myocardial infarction (MI) soon after their apparent recovery.

Pathology

The problems with MLNS are twofold. Coronary arterial disease occurs, and thrombocythemia may be present (up to 1 million). This combination of an altered endovascular surface and too many platelets leads to occlusion of the vessels and the subsequent MIs, which occur as the child is recovering from the acute illness. Although the pathogenesis of the arterial disease is not understood, this second component (thrombocythemia) is important.

Treatment

Intravenous gamma globulin (IVGG) is the cornerstone of therapy, given in doses of 400 mg/kg/day for 4 successive

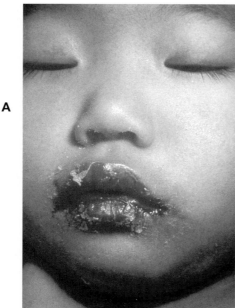

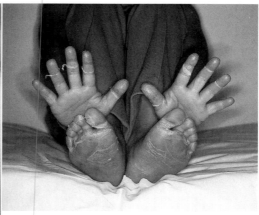

Fig. 35-35 **A,** Cheilitis of Kawasaki's disease. **B,** Late desquamation in Kawasaki's disease.

days, or as a single dose (2 g/kg). Antiplatelet therapy with aspirin is recommended, with dipyridamole used as an alternative agent for patients unable to take aspirin. Treatment with IVGG and aspirin reduces the prevalence of coronary artery abnormalities from 20% for those treated with aspirin alone, to 4%. Angioplasty, thrombolytic therapy, or coronary artery bypass surgery may be required for patients with severe disease.

Felz MW, et al: Periorbital vasculitis complicating Kawasaki syndrome in an infant. *Pediatrics* 1998, 101:E9.

Manders ST: Toxin-mediated streptococcal and staphylococcal disease. *J Am Acad Dermatol* 1998, 39:383.

Nakamura Y, et al: Mortality among patients with a history of Kawasaki disease. *Acta Paediatr* (Jpn) 1998, 40:419.

Rowley AH, et al: Kawasaki syndrome. *Clin Microbiol Rev* 1998, 11:405.

Vanderhooft SL, et al: Pincer nail deformity after Kawasaki's disease. *J Am Acad Dermatol* 1999, 41:341.

Yanagawa H, et al: Results of the nationwide Epidemiologic Survey of Kawasaki disease in 1995 and 1996 in Japan. *Pediatrics* 1998, 102:E65. ▲

TELANGIECTASIA

Telangiectases are fine linear vessels coursing on the surface of the skin; the name given to them collectively is *telangiectasia*. Telangiectasia may occur in normal skin at any age, in both sexes, and anywhere on the skin and mucous membranes. Fine telangiectases may be seen on the alae nasi of most adults. They are prominent in areas of chronic actinic damage. In addition, persons long exposed to wind, cold, or heat are subject to telangiectasia. Medications, such as nifedipine and felodipine, may lead to telangiectatic lesions in a photodistribution. Telangiectasias may also be found on the legs as a result of heredity, varicosities, pregnancy, and birth control pill use.

Telangiectases can be found in conditions such as radiodermatitis, xeroderma pigmentosum, lupus erythematosus, scleroderma and the CREST syndrome, rosacea, pregnancy, cirrhosis of the liver, AIDS, poikiloderma, basal cell carcinoma, necrobiosis lipoidica diabeticorum, lichen sclerosus et atrophicus, sarcoid, lupus vulgaris, keloid, adenoma sebaceum, Kaposiform hemangioendothelioma, angioma serpiginosum, angiokeratoma corporis diffusum, hereditary benign telangiectasia, Cockayne's syndrome, ataxia-telangiectasia, and Bloom syndrome.

Altered capillary patterns on the finger nail folds (cuticular telangiectases) are indicative of collagen vascular disease such as lupus erythematosus, scleroderma, or dermatomyositis. They may infrequently be present in rheumatoid arthritis. These disorders are reviewed in Chapter 8.

Telangiectases about the nose and cheeks from rosacea or actinic damage are best treated by touching the overlying skin at several points with the tip of the epilating needle, using either monopolar or bipolar current, or with a fine-pointed galvanocautery tip. The current should be minimal to avoid scarring. Annual touch-up treatment of old or newly developing lesions may be necessary. Sclerosing solutions are also effective in the hands of those skilled in their use, and are particularly useful in treating the legs. A variety of lasers, pulsed dye and copper vapor, for example, have shown good cosmetic results.

Beaubien ER, et al: Kaposiform hemangioendothelioma. *J Am Acad Dermatol* 1998, 38:799.

Collins P, et al: Photodistributed nifedipine-induced facial telangiectasia. *Br J Dermatol* 1993, 129:630.

Goldman MP: Sclerosing agents in the treatment of telangiectasia. *Arch Dermatol* 1987, 123:1196.

Goldman MP, et al: Treatment of facial telangiectasia with sclerotherapy, laser surgery, and/or electrodesiccation. *J Dermatol Surg Oncol* 1993, 19:899.

Goldman MP, et al: Treatment of telangiectasia: a review. *J Am Acad Dermatol* 1987, 17:167.

Green D: Photothermal removal of telangiectases of the lower extremities with Photoderm VL. *J Am Acad Dermatol* 1998, 38:61.

Huh J, et al: Localized facial telangiectasias following frostbite injury. *Cutis* 1996, 57:97.

Kanekura T, et al: Lichen sclerosus et atrophicus with prominent telangiectasia. *J Dermatol* 1994, 21:447.

Karonen T, et al: Truncal telangiectases coinciding with felodipine. *Dermatology* 1998, 196:272.

Kienle A, et al: Optimal parameters for laser treatment of leg telangiectasia. *Lasers Surg Med* 1997, 20:346.

Tan E, et al: Pulsed dye laser treatment of spider telangiectasia. *Australas J Dermatol* 1997, 38:22.

Zahorcsek Z, et al: Hereditary benign telangiectasia. *Dermatology* 1994, 189:286. ▲

Generalized Essential Telangiectasia

Generalized essential telangiectasia is characterized by the dilation of veins and capillaries over a large segment of the body without preceding or coexisting skin lesions. Characteristic features include (1) widespread cutaneous distribution, (2) progression or permanence of the lesions, (3) accentuation by dependent positioning, and (4) absence of coexisting epidermal or dermal changes such as atrophy, purpura, depigmentation, or follicular involvement. The telangiectases may be distributed over the entire body or localized to some large area such as the legs, arms, and trunk. They may be discrete or confluent. Distribution along the course of the cutaneous nerves may occur. Although Checketts et al reported a case associated with a gastrointestinal bleed from severe gastric antral vascular ectasia, generalized essential telangiectasia is usually not believed to be associated with systemic disease or a risk of bleeding.

Generalized telangiectasia develops most frequently in women in their forties and fifties. The initial onset is on the lower legs and then spreads to the upper legs, abdomen, and arms. The dilations persist indefinitely. Families with this disorder have been reported, inherited as an autosomal dominant trait.

The cause of essential telangiectasia is unknown. It is believed that estrogens, serotonin, and adrenocorticosteroids are not causative, such as would be seen in telangiectases of pregnancy, hepatic disease, metastatic carcinoid syndrome, and Cushing's syndrome. A questionable relationship with infections, particularly sinus infections, has been suggested by reported clinical responses to oral antibiotics, such as tetracycline.

Checketts SR, et al: Generalized essential telangiectasia in the presence of gastrointestinal bleeding. *J Am Acad Dermatol* 1997, 37:321.

Ossenkoppele PM, et al: Generalized essential telangiectasia. *Br J Dermatol* 1991, 125:283.

Person JR, et al: Estrogen and progesterone receptors are not increased in generalized essential telangiectasia. *Arch Dermatol* 1985, 121:836. ▲

Unilateral Nevoid Telangiectasia

In this disorder fine, threadlike telangiectases develop in a unilateral, sometimes dermatomal (or following the lines of Blaschko), distribution. The condition is rare in men and tends to correlate with increased levels of estrogen experienced during puberty or pregnancy or with cirrhosis. More recently, hepatitis C–associated unilateral nevoid telangiectasia has been documented in young men without any other known cause. The most commonly accepted theory is an increased level of estrogen receptors in involved skin. It has also been suggested that it may be the result of a localized increase in estrogen levels caused by a chromosomal mosaicism that is unmasked at times of relative estrogen excess. The latter mechanism accounts for those cases shown to follow the lines of Blaschko. Others have questioned the role of estrogen at all, since it has also been reported in young men with normal or low estrogens and normal estrogen receptors.

Hynes LR, et al: Unilateral nevoid telangiectasia: occurrence in two patients with hepatitis C. *J Am Acad Dermatol* 1997, 36:819.

Taskapan O: Acquired unilateral nevoid telangiectasia syndrome (letter). *J Am Acad Dermatol* 1998, 39:138.

Taskapan O, et al: Acquired unilateral nevoid telangiectasia syndrome. *Acta Derm Venereol* (Norway) 1997, 77:62.

Tok J, et al: Unilateral nevoid telangiectasia syndrome. *Cutis* 1994, 53:53.

Woollons A, et al: Unilateral naevoid telangiectasia syndrome in pregnancy. *Clin Exp Dermatol* 1996, 21:459. ▲

HEREDITARY HEMORRHAGIC TELANGIECTASIA (OSLER'S DISEASE)

Also known as *Osler-Weber-Rendu disease,* hereditary hemorrhagic telangiectasia (HHT) is characterized by small tufts of dilated capillaries scattered over the mucous membranes and the skin. These slightly elevated lesions develop mostly on the lips, tongue (Fig. 35-36), palate, nasal mucosa, ears, palms, fingertips, nail beds, and soles. They may closely simulate the telangiectases of the CREST variant of scleroderma, which may be distinguished by the lack of other features of CREST syndrome and by anticentromere antibodies, which are not found in HHT.

Frequent nosebleeds and melena are experienced because of the telangiectasia in the nose and gastrointestinal tract. Epistaxis is the most frequent and persistent sign. Gastrointestinal bleeding is the presenting sign in up to 25% of cases; however, 40% to 50% develop gastrointestinal bleeding sometime during the course of their disease. The spleen may be enlarged. Pulmonary and central nervous system arteriovenous fistulas may appear later in life. Retinal arteriovenous aneurysms occur only rarely. Other sites of bleeding may be the kidney, spleen, bladder, liver, meninges, and brain.

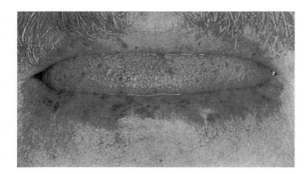

Fig. 35-36   Hereditary hemorrhagic telangiectasia.

The telangiectases tend to increase in number in middle age; however, the first appearance on the undersurface of the tongue and floor of the mouth is at puberty. Pulmonary or intracranial arteriovenous fistulas and bleeding in these areas may be a cause of death. HHT has been reported associated with von Willebrand's disease, further promoting a risk of bleeding. It may also be associated with polycystic kidney disease and fibropolycystic liver disease.

Osler's disease is inherited as an autosomal dominant trait. The vascular abnormalities found in HHT consist of direct arteriovenous connections without an intervening capillary bed. Germline mutations in one of two different genes, endoglin or ALK-1, can cause HHT. Endoglin encodes a 95-kDa membrane-bound proteoglycan that binds TGF beta 1 and regulates signaling via the type I and II TGF beta receptors on the surface of vascular endothelial cells.

Several treatment methods have been recommended. The tendency to epistaxis has been reduced by estrogen therapy. Dermoplasty of the bleeding nasal septum may be performed by replacing the mucous membrane with skin from the thigh or buttock. Aminocaproic acid has been used to treat acute bleeding episodes; however, most bleeding episodes are treated supportively.

Adam PJ, et al: Expression of endoglin mRNA and protein in human vascular smooth muscle cells. *Biochem Biophys Res Commun* 1998, 247:33.

Kjeldsen AD, et al: Hereditary hemorrhagic telangiectasia. *N Engl J Med* 1995, 333:918.

Marchiuk DA: Genetic abnormalities in hereditary hemorrhagic telangiectasia. *Curr Opin Hematol* 1998, 5:332.

Rebeiz EE, et al: Surgical management of life-threatening epistaxis in Osler-Weber-Rendu disease. *Ann Plast Surg* 1995, 35:208.

Saxena R, et al: Coexistence of hereditary hemorrhagic telangiectasia and fibropolycystic liver disease. *Am J Surg Pathol* 1998, 22:368.

Sharma VK, et al: Gastrointestinal and hepatic manifestations of hereditary hemorrhagic telangiectasia. *Dig Dis* 1998, 16:169.

Swanson DL, et al: Embolic abscesses in hereditary hemorrhagic telangiectasia. *J Am Acad Dermatol* 1991, 24:580. _____ ▲

Bloom Syndrome (Bloom-Torre-Machacek Syndrome)

Bloom syndrome is transmitted as an autosomal recessive trait, chiefly among Jews of eastern European origin. It is characterized by telangiectatic erythema in the butterfly area of the face, photosensitivity, and dwarfism.

Telangiectatic erythematous patches resembling lupus erythematosus (Fig. 35-37) develop in the first two years of life. Bullous, crusted lesions may be present on the lips. Exacerbation of skin lesions occurs during the summer. Other changes that may be noted are café au lait spots, ichthyosis, acanthosis nigricans, syndactyly, irregular dentition, prominent ears, hypospadias, and cryptorchidism.

The stunted growth is characterized by normal body proportions, no endocrine abnormalities, and low birth weight at full term. Dolichocephaly and narrow, delicate facies are present. Immune functions are abnormal, and gastrointestinal and respiratory infections occur frequently. The gene (BML) defect has been localized to 15q26.1, resulting in a deficient ATP-dependent DNA-helicase activity. Leukemia, lymphoma, adenocarcinoma of the sigmoid colon, and oral and esophageal squamous cell carcinoma, as well as other malignancies, have been associated with Bloom syndrome. About one fourth of patients under age 20 develop a neoplasm. Regular use of a sunscreen is recommended.

Bahr A, et al: Point mutations causing Bloom's syndrome abolish ATPase and DNA helicase activities of the BLM protein. *Oncogene* 1998, 19:2565.

Ellis NA, et al: Molecular genetics of Bloom's syndrome. *Hum Mol Genet* 1996, 5:1457.

Gretzula JC, et al: Bloom's syndrome. *J Am Acad Dermatol* 1987, 17:479.

Straughen JE, et al: A rapid method for detecting the predominant Ashkenazi Jewish mutation in the Bloom's syndrome. *Hum Mutat* 1998, 11:175. _____ ▲

Hereditary Sclerosing Poikiloderma and Mandibuloacral Dysplasia

Weary et al have described a heritable, widespread poikilodermatous and sclerotic disorder called hereditary sclerosing poikiloderma (HSP). It was found in seven members of two unrelated black families. The skin changes consist of generalized poikiloderma with hyperkeratotic and sclerotic cutaneous bands extending across the antecubital spaces, axillary vaults, and popliteal fossae. In addition, the palms and soles may show sclerosis resembling shiny scotch-grain leather. Clubbing of the fingers and localized calcinosis of the skin have also been noted. There is no treatment.

The same cases reported by Weary et al have subsequently been reported later in life as mandibuloacral dysplasia (MAD), a rare autosomal recessive syndrome characterized by mandibular hypoplasia; delayed cranial

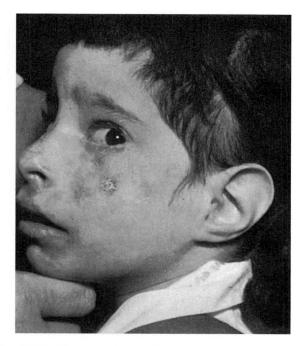

Fig. 35-37 Bloom syndrome with telangiectatic patches resembling discoid lupus erythematosus in a female dwarf. (Courtesy Dr. D. Bloom.)

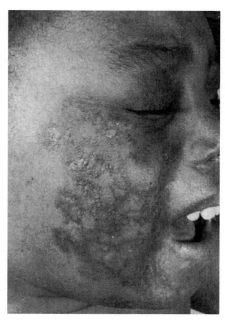

Fig. 35-38 Poikiloderma congenitale. (Courtesy Dr. J.L. Burton, Bristol, England.)

suture closure; dysplastic clavicles; abbreviated, club-shaped terminal phalanges; acroosteolysis; atrophy of the skin of the hands and feet; and typical facial changes. MAD must be distinguished from progeria and Werner's syndrome.

Fazio M, et al: Weary hereditary sclerosing poikiloderma. *Ann Dermatol Venereol* 1995, 122:618.

Fryburg JS, et al: Long-term follow-up of cutaneous changes in siblings with mandibuloacral dysplasia who were originally considered to have hereditary sclerosing poikiloderma. *J Am Acad Dermatol* 1995, 33:900.

Weary PE, et al: Hereditary sclerosing poikiloderma. *Arch Dermatol* 1969, 100:413. ▲

SCLEROATROPHIC SYNDROME OF HURIEZ

Characterized by (1) scleroatrophy, (2) ridging or hypoplasia of the nails, and (3) lamellar keratoderma of the hands and, to a lesser extent, the soles, patients with Huriez syndrome may also have poikiloderma-like changes of the nose, telangiectasias of the lips, flexion contractures of the little finger, and a distinctive little finger nodule. There is a risk of the development of aggressive cutaneous squamous cell carcinoma.

Hamm H, et al: The scleroatrophic syndrome of Huriez: a cancer prone genodermatosis. *Br J Dermatol* 1996, 134:512.

Kavanagh GM, et al: The scleroatrophic syndrome of Huriez. *Br J Dermatol* 1997, 137:114. ▲

POIKILODERMA CONGENITALE

Poikiloderma congenitale is also known as *Thomson's disease* and *Rothmund-Thomson syndrome*. It is a rare familial syndrome transmitted as an autosomal recessive trait. It occurs predominantly in girls. Poikiloderma begins at 3 to 6 months of age, with tense, pink, edematous patches on the cheeks (Fig. 35-38), hands, feet, and buttocks; there follows fine reticulated or punctate atrophy associated with telangiectasia and reticulated pigmentation.

Short stature, small hands, absence or sparseness of eyebrows and eyelashes, alopecia of the scalp, and congenital bone defects are frequently observed. Hypogonadism, dystrophic nails, and defective dentition are seen in less than 30% of cases. Juvenile cataracts occur between ages 3 and 6 in 50% of patients. Sensitivity to sunlight may be manifested by the development of bullae or intense erythema after brief sun exposure.

Squamous and basal cell carcinoma of the skin occasionally occur, and osteosarcoma of bone has been reported. Pronounced chromosomal instability in fibroblasts is believed to be the cause of increased risk of mesenchymal tumors. Several patients with compound heterozygous mutations in RECQL4, a human helicase gene, have been reported. Thus at least a subset of patients with Rothmund-Thomson syndrome have abnormal DNA helicase activity, as do patients with Werner and Bloom syndromes. DNA helicase unwinds double-stranded DNA into single-stranded DNA.

Drouin CA, et al: Rothmund-Thomson syndrome with osteosarcoma. *J Am Acad Dermatol* 1993, 28:301.

Judge MR, et al: Rothmund-Thomson syndrome and osteosarcoma. *Br J Dermatol* 1993, 129:723.

Kerr B, et al: Rothmund-Thomson syndrome. *J Med Genet* 1996, 33:928.

Kitao S, et al: Mutations in RECQL4 cause a subset of cases of Rothmund-Thomson syndrome. *Nat Genet* 1999, 22:82.

Miozzo M, et al: Chromosomal instability in fibroblasts and mesenchymal tumors from 2 sibs with Rothmund-Thomson syndrome. *Int J Cancer* 1998, 77:504.

Spurney C, et al: Multicentric osteosarcoma, Rothmund-Thomson syndrome, and secondary nasopharyngeal non-Hodgkin's lymphoma. *J Pediatr Hematol Oncol* 1998, 20:494.

Tong M: Rothmund-Thomson syndrome in fraternal twins. *Pediatr Dermatol* 1995, 12:134.

Vennos EM, et al: Rothmund-Thomson syndrome: review of the world literature. *J Am Acad Dermatol* 1992, 27:750. _____ ▲

LEG ULCERS

Much progress has been made in understanding the cellular and biochemical constituents that are required for normal wound healing. This complex response involves intricate interactions between different cell types, structural proteins, growth factors, and proteinases. Normal wound repair consists of three phases—inflammation, proliferation, and remodeling—that occur in a predictable sequence and comprise a series of cellular and biochemical events. Abnormalities in any one of these components can produce delayed or ineffectual wound healing.

VENOUS DISEASES OF THE EXTREMITIES

Stasis Dermatitis. Stasis dermatitis, also known as *dermatitis hemostatica* and *erythromelia,* is a blotchy red mottling and a yellowish or light brown pigmentation of the lower third of the lower legs due to venous insufficiency (Fig. 35-39). An associated eczematous dermatitis may occur and is a frequent finding in the elderly (Fig. 35-40). Stasis dermatitis is often associated with obesity and other disease states, such as congestive heart failure, that promote lower extremity edema, and may be a presenting manifestation of Budd-Chiari syndrome (hepatic vein thrombosis).

The approach to management should be twofold: relief of symptoms and treatment of the underlying cause. Patients with pruritus and an eczematous component should be treated with emollients and class IV or V topical corticosteroids. Pretibial edema requires leg elevation and support stockings. Underlying conditions, such as congestive heart failure, obesity, or Budd-Chiari syndrome, should be effectively managed. Vascular surgical intervention to promote venous outflow and decrease pooling may be helpful in some instances.

Venous Ulcer ("Varicose" Ulcer, "Stasis" Ulcer). Chronic venous insufficiency in the deep veins of the legs leads to shunting the venous return into the superficial veins,

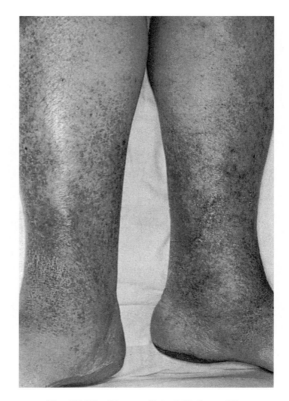

Fig. 35-39   Venous ("stasis") dermatitis.

in which pressure, oxygen content, and flow rate are increased. The dermatitis that results is called *stasis dermatitis.*

Edema and fibrosis develop in the skin over the medial aspect of the ankle and lower third of the shin, and eventually, often as a result of minor trauma, an ulcer (Figs. 35-41 and 35-42). The dermatitis may be weepy or dry, scaling or lichenified; it is almost invariably hyperpigmented by melanin and hemosiderin. Varicose veins are usually present, though they need not be numerous or conspicuous.

The cause of varicose veins is multifactorial and there is no doubt about an inherited tendency. Standing in one position for long periods promotes the development of varicosities. Any condition causing prolonged intraabdominal pressure against the iliac veins may also cause them; the commonest cause of this is pregnancy. Thrombophlebitis may also cause incompetence of the veins.

Venous ulcers usually occur on the lower medial aspect of the leg. Usually there is preceding venous ("stasis") dermatitis with lipodermatosclerosis. Ninety percent of all leg ulcers result from chronic venous insufficiency, and perhaps 5% from arteriosclerosis obliterans, with the majority of remaining cases occurring as a complication of diabetes. Patients with venous leg ulceration have a higher prevalence of Factor V Leiden mutation compared with controls and the general population.

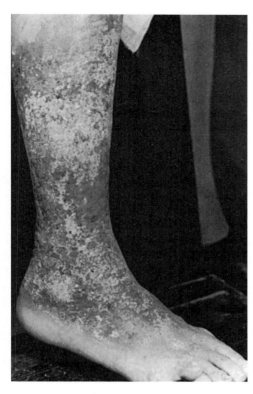

Fig. 35-40   Venous eczema. (Courtesy Dr. F. Daniels, Jr.)

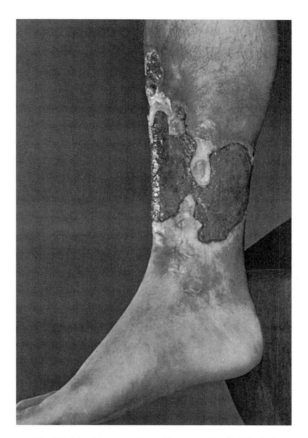

Fig. 35-41   Venous ulcer. (Courtesy Dr. H. Shatin.)

In most cases the diagnosis of a venous ulceration can be made on clinical grounds. If there is no clear history or physical findings of venous insufficiency, venous rheography can be performed. Lesions in atypical locations or those that do not respond appropriately to therapy, but that have normal venous rheography, may require a biopsy to exclude neoplasm. Additional workup may also be required to identify other, less common causes of leg ulcers, such as cryoglobulins, sickle cell disease, vasculitis, and myeloma. Diabetes should always be considered in any nonhealing leg ulceration.

Treatment is primarily to improve venous return. This involves elevation of the leg above the heart as much of the time as possible. Elastic support to the legs and exercise to improve calf muscle strength are recommended. The avoidance of long, cramped sitting (in airplanes or vehicles) or prolonged standing is advisable. Avoidance of trauma is important. Compression therapy is the mainstay of treatment. In some cases venous reconstruction is helpful. A cooperative patient and a patient physician are necessary in the long-term management of venous disease.

Many treatment options have been developed for chronic ulcers; unfortunately, conclusive comparative studies between the various treatment alternatives are lacking. Occlusive permeable biosynthetic wound dressings have been shown very effective. They speed healing, reduce pain, make dressing changes infrequent, help debridement, exclude microorganisms, and improve cosmetic results. Advance preparation consists of reduction of edema by leg elevation and use of dextranomer, to reduce the rate of exudation. If a hard eschar is present over the ulcer when first seen, a dressing will assist in its removal. Cultured epidermal allografts have been shown to produce a more rapid healing and greater reduction in ulcer size than hydrocolloid dressings. Various skin substitutes are becoming available for the treatment of chronic wounds, including leg ulcers. The human skin equivalent (Apligraf) is a bilayer constituent of type I bovine collagen, live allogeneic human skin fibroblasts, and keratinocytes. The place of this product and other newly developed skin substitutes in the treatment of leg ulcers is under investigation.

In the acute setting, graded compression with Unna boots and graded elastic bandages are extremely helpful. Support hose is inappropriate because of the leg edema that is usually present, since the size of the extremity will change. Leg ulcers are frequently contaminated with microorganisms. Metronidazole gel applied in the ulcer bed before dressing may be useful in reducing the foul odor in leg ulcers. If healing is slow or there is substantial peripheral erythema or tenderness suggesting a cellulitis, a

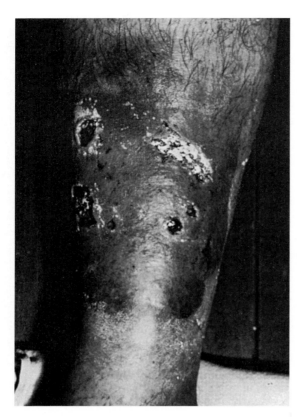

Fig. 35-42 Venous ulcers.

culture should be performed. The topical antibiotic applied may then be modified. Chronic oral antibiotics may be required.

Risk factors that predict failure to heal within 24 weeks of limb-compression therapy include a large wound area, history of venous ligation or stripping, history of hip or knee replacement, ankle brachial index of less that 0.80, fibrin on 50% or more of the wound surface, and the presence of the ulcer for an extended time. Patients who present with many such risk factors may be best considered for other or adjunctive therapies. Randomized trials of 300 mg of oral aspirin versus placebo showed significantly improved wound healing at 2 and 4 months. Oral zinc sulfate, 220 mg three times a day, has been shown to be useful adjunctive therapy. A trial of stanazol, 2 to 4 mg a day for 6 to 9 months, in patients with recurrent ulcerations is effective, but its use is limited by several contraindications. Grafting may ultimately be necessary in some cases. Pinch grafts or use of a meshed graft are good choices as are cultured autologous epidermal cells.

ISCHEMIC ULCER

Ischemic ulcers are mostly located on the lateral surface of the ankle or digits. The initial red, painful plaque breaks down into a painful superficial ulcer with a surrounding zone of purpuric erythema. Granulation tissue is minimal, little or no infection is present, and a membranous inactive eschar forms over the ulcer. Patients at risk are those with long-standing hypertension or other signs and risk factors of arteriosclerotic disease.

Signs and symptoms indicative that arterial disease is the cause of the ulceration include thinning of the skin, absence of hair, decreased or absent pulses, pallor on elevation, coolness of the extremity, dependent rubor, claudication on exercise, and pain on elevation (especially at night) relieved on dependency. In progressive disease the diagnosis of thromboangiitis obliterans, or Buerger's disease, should be considered.

The diagnosis of arterial insufficiency can usually be confirmed by physical examination and careful palpation of the pulses in the legs. For more accurate evaluation, take the blood pressure in the arm and leg. They should be nearly identical. The ratio of the popliteal to brachial pressure is called the ABI. If it is less than 0.75 arterial insufficiency exists, and if less than 0.5, the insufficiency is substantial.

Treatment with topical antibiotic ointments and protection of the affected area from injury, plus avoidance of cold, smoking, and tight socks, are important. Enhancement of the blood supply by raising the head of the bed on 6-inch blocks is advisable.

A vascular surgeon should be asked to consult and advise with regard to arteriography, Doppler arterial flow studies, and ankle and arm blood pressure evaluation. Lumbar sympathectomy may be considered.

If the blood supply can be improved, local wound care (perhaps with a DuoDERM dressing) will heal the ulcer. If the blood supply cannot be improved, little can be done except to prevent infection by the measures described under venous ulcers. Hyperbaric oxygen is another useful therapeutic option but is limited by availability and cost.

LEG ULCERS OF OTHER CAUSES

One of the commonest causes of leg ulcers is diabetic microangiopathy. Hematopoietic ulcers are those occurring with sickle cell anemia (Fig. 35-43), Cooley's anemia (thalassemia), congenital hemolytic anemia, polycythemia vera, thrombocytopenic purpura, macroglobulinemia, and cryoglobulinemia. In addition, cryofibrinogenemia may also be manifested by ulcerations on the lower extremities.

The diagnosis is usually established by the accompanying signs and symptoms of the original disease. Treatment of the underlying disease should be maximal, and then general measures used for leg ulcers should be followed—avoidance of trauma and dressings to provide a moist, infection-free local environment, or use of compression dressings or consideration of cultured epidermal allografts.

Leg ulcers resulting from collagen vascular disease may be seen with systemic lupus erythematosus, Felty's syndrome, rheumatoid arthritis, scleroderma, and dermatomy-

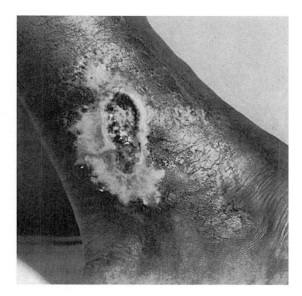

Fig. 35-43 Ulcer on ankle in sickle cell anemia.

ositis. The ulcers are deep, indolent, and dry. Basal cell and squamous cell carcinoma, malignant melanoma, Kaposi's sarcoma, and malignant lymphomas may be the cause of leg ulcers. Diagnosis of neoplastic causes of leg ulcers requires biopsy of the ulcer margin. Burns, radiodermatitis, decubitus ulcers, neurotic excoriations, factitial ulcers, and chrome ulcers are in this category.

Necrobiosis lipoidica, gout, diabetes, pellagra, prolidase deficiency, Gaucher's disease, Klinefelter's syndrome, ulcerative colitis, and primary amyloidosis form another group in which leg ulcers also may be found. The ulcers of lupus vulgaris, mycobacterial ulcers (Buruli ulcers), sporotrichosis, blastomycosis, coccidioidomycosis, cryptococcosis, histoplasmosis, and schistosomiasis are some of the more important infectious leg ulcers. The gummatous ulcers of late syphilis should not be forgotten.

Baldursson B, et al: Venous leg ulcers and squamous cell carcinoma. *Br J Dermatol* 1995, 133:571.

Choucair M, et al: Compression therapy. *Dermatol Surg* 1998, 24:141.

Falanga V, et al: Rapid healing of venous ulcers and lack of clinical rejection with an allogeneic cultured human skin equivalent. *Arch Dermatol* 1998, 134:293.

Fletcher A, et al: A systematic review of compression treatment for venous leg ulcers. *BMJ* 1997, 315:576.

Grey JE, et al: The chronic non-healing wound: how to make it better. *Hosp Med* 1998, 59:557.

Grossman D, et al: Activated protein C resistance and anticardiolipin antibodies in patients with venous leg ulcers. *J Am Acad Dermatol* 1997, 37:409.

Hafner J, et al: Management of venous leg ulcers. *Vasa* 1996, 25:161.

Herrick SE, et al: Venous ulcer fibroblasts compared with normal fibroblasts show differences in collagen but not fibronectin production under both normal and hypoxic conditions. *J Invest Dermatol* 1996, 106:187.

Korstanje MJ: Venous stasis ulcers: diagnostic and surgical considerations. *Dermatol Surg* 1995, 21:635.

Maessen-Visch MB, et al: The prevalence of Factor V Leiden mutation in patients with leg ulcers and venous insufficiency. *Arch Dermatol* 1999, 135:41.

Margolis DJ, et al: Risk factors associated with failure of a venous leg ulcer to heal. *Arch Dermatol* 1999, 135:920.

Miller OF III: Essentials of pressure ulcer treatment: the diabetic experience. *J Dermatol Surg Oncol* 1993, 19:759.

Munkvad S, et al: Resistance to activated protein C: a common anticoagulant deficiency in patients with venous leg ulceration. *Br J Dermatol* 1996, 134:296.

Peus D, et al: Activated protein C resistance caused by factor V gene mutation. *J Am Acad Dermatol* 1997, 36:616.

Phillips TJ: New skin for old. *Arch Dermatol* 1998, 134:344.

Phillips TJ: Tissue-engineerred skin. *Arch Dermatol* 1999, 135:977.

Pryce DW, et al: Hemodynamics of leg ulceration assessed by laser Doppler flowmetry. *J Am Acad Dermatol* 1993, 29:708.

Samson RH, et al: Stockings and the prevention of recurrent venous ulcers. *Dermatol Surg* 1996, 22:373.

Sivaram M, et al: Stasis dermatitis: a new cutaneous manifestation of Budd-Chiari syndrome. *Int J Dermatol* 1998, 37:397.

Stadelmann WK, et al: Physiology and healing dynamics of chronic cutaneous wounds. *Am J Surg* 1998, 176:26S.

Taylor LM Jr, et al: Limb salvage vs amputation for critical ischemia: the role of vascular surgery. *Arch Surg* 1991, 126:1251.

Teepe RG, et al: Randomized trial comparing cryopreserved cultured epidermal allografts with hydrocolloid dressings in healing chronic venous ulcers. *J Am Acad Dermatol* 1993, 29:982.

Torrence BP, et al: Stasis dermatitis: practical pearls for the dermatologic nurse. *Dermatol Nurs* 1993, 5:186.

Zeegelaar JE, et al: Local treatment of venous ulcers with tissue type plasminogen activator containing ointment. *Vasa* 1997, 26:81. ▲

Lymphedema

Lymphedema is the swelling of soft tissues in which an excess amount of lymph has accumulated. Chronic lymphedema is characterized by long-standing nonpitting edema. The following is a working classification of lymphedema:

Primary lymphedema
Congenital lymphedema (Milroy's disease)
Lymphedema praecox
Lymphedema tarda
Syndromes associated with primary lymphedema
    Yellow nail syndrome
    Turner's syndrome
    Noonan's syndrome
    Pes cavus
    Phakomatosis pigmentovascularis
Cutaneous disorders sometimes associated with primary lymphedema
    Yellow nails
    Capillary hemangiomas
    Xanthomatosis and chylous lymphedema
    Congenital absence of nails
Secondary lymphedema
    Postmastectomy lymphedema
    Melphalan isolated limb perfusion

Malignant occlusion with obstruction
Extrinsic pressure
Factitial lymphedema
Postradiation therapy
Following recurrent lymphangitis/cellulitis
Lymphedema of upper limb in recurrent eczema
Granulomatous disease
Rosaceous lymphedema
Primary amyloidosis
Complications of lymphedema
Cellulitis of lymphedema
Elephantiasis nostras verrucosa
Ulceration
Lymphangiosarcoma

To these complications lymphangioma circumscriptum, localized neurodermatitis, and pseudoacanthosis nigricans may also occur. The most prevalent worldwide cause of lymphedema is filariasis. In the United States the most common cause is postsurgical.

Types

The primary noninflammatory types include lymphedema praecox and congenital lymphedema (Milroy's disease and "simple" type). The secondary noninflammatory type consists of lymphedema caused by malignant occlusion, surgical removal of lymph nodes, pressure, or ionizing radiation therapy.

The inflammatory types may be caused by recurrent lymphangitis or cellulitis, systemic granulomatous disease, or filariasis.

Lymphedema Praecox. Lymphedema praecox develops in females between ages 9 and 25. A puffiness appears around the ankle and then extends upward to involve the entire leg (Fig. 35-44). With the passage of time the leg becomes painful, with a dull, heavy sensation. Once this has evolved the swollen limb remains swollen. Primary lymphedema is caused by a defect in the lymphatic system. Lymphangiography demonstrates hypoplastic lymphatics in 87%, aplasia in approximately 5%, and hyperplasia with varicose dilation of the lymphatic vessels in 8%. Distichiasis is defined as a double row of eyelashes. Association of distichiasis and late-onset lymphedema is believed by some authors to be a form of hereditary lymphedema called *lymphedema-distichiasis syndrome.*

Nonne-Milroy-Meige Syndrome (Hereditary Lymphedema). Milroy's hereditary edema of the lower legs is characterized by a unilateral or bilateral lymphedema present at birth and inherited as an autosomal dominant trait. The edema is painless, pits on pressure, is not associated with any other disorder, and persists throughout life. It may involve the genitalia and produce lymphangiectasias superficially (Fig. 35-45). Chylous discharge can occur. Most

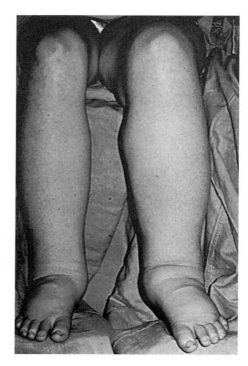

Fig. 35-44   Lymphedema.

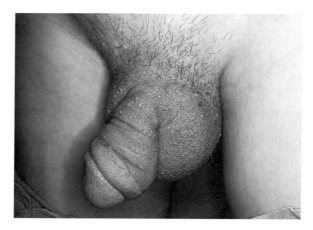

Fig. 35-45   Penile and scrotal lymphedema with lymphangiectases in a patient with Milroy's disease.

frequently the affection is unilateral, and females are predominantly affected.

This type of lymphedema is differentiated from the acquired type, which occurs not only on the lower extremities but also on the lips, lower eyelids (Fig. 35-46), or other areas where lymph stasis has been produced secondary to other areas of involvement. If lymphedema is long-standing a verrucous appearance to the affected extremity develops (Fig. 35-47).

Treatment of this particular type of edema is extremely difficult since the disease is an anomaly of the lymph-

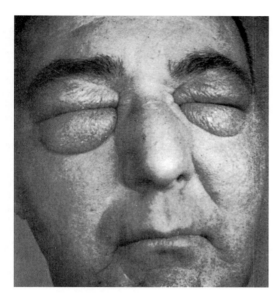

Fig. 35-46 Chronic lymphedema, solid.

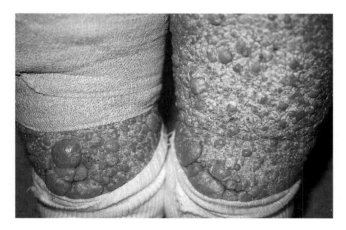

Fig. 35-47 Chronic lymphedema with verrucous surface of the legs.

draining vessels. The Pratt procedure, consisting of the excision of edematous, fibrotic, cutaneous and subcutaneous tissue and fascia, has had varying degrees of success. The Kondoleon operation is similar to the Pratt procedure. Other forms of treatment of lymphedema, such as decongestive physiotherapy, should be considered.

Primary Lymphedema Associated with Yellow Nails and Pleural Effusion (Yellow Nail Syndrome).
Primary lymphedema is confined mostly to the ankles, although other areas may be involved. The nails show a distinct yellowish discoloration and thickening. Recurrent pleural effusion requiring thoracocentesis may be a feature.

Phakomatosis Pigmentovascularis.
Bielsa et al reported a patient with generalized nevus spilus associated with a nevus anemicus and primary lymphedema. The authors believe the three findings are not coincidental and that the disorder represents a new type of phakomatosis pigmentovascularis.

Secondary Lymphedema.
In some malignant diseases involvement of the lymph nodes will produce blockage and lymphedema. Malignant disease of the breast, uterus, prostate, skin, bones, or other tissues may cause such changes. Hodgkin's disease and, especially, Kaposi's sarcoma may be accompanied by chronic lymphedema. Chronic lymphedema is frequently seen after mastectomy and the removal of the axillary nodes; it may occur after varying lengths of time. Occasionally, it is a result of metastatic basal cell carcinoma or infiltrating primary amyloidosis. A rare form of rosaceous lymphedema produces disfiguring facial edema.

Postmastectomy Lymphangiosarcoma (Stewart-Treves Syndrome).
This type may arise in chronic postmastectomy lymphedema. Stewart and Treves were the first to describe this complication of simple or radical mastectomy. The lesions are bluish or reddish nodules arising on the arms. Numerous localized lesions of lymphangiosarcoma may occur, and pulmonary metastasis is frequent. The prognosis is extremely poor.

Isolated Limb Perfusion.
Advanced chemotherapeutic options for patients with organ-limited cancer is the use of organ or limb perfusion. Melphalan when used for treatment of malignancies with isolated limb perfusion has been reported to result in an increased chance of developing regional toxicity and lymphedema. The risk of developing lymphedema has been strongly linked to regional lymph node dissections, and if this therapeutic option is being considered, lymph node dissection should be performed after the infusions have occurred.

Inflammatory Lymphedema.
The inflammatory reaction is caused by recurrent bouts of acute cellulitis and lymphangitis. Chills, high fever, and swelling and redness of the involved extremity are severe and may last for as long as 3 or 4 days. Recurrent attacks of streptococcal infections increases the likelihood of lymphedema. It is these recurrent attacks, when they complicate filariasis, that eventuate in elephantiasis. Non-group A beta-hemolytic streptococcal cellulitis following venectomy in patients who had undergone coronary bypass surgery is a well-documented cause. However, almost any chronic or recurrent cellulitis can cause this.

Factitial Lymphedema.
Also known as *hysterical edema*, lymphedema can be produced by wrapping an elastic bandage, cord, or shirt around an extremity and/or holding the extremity in a dependent and immobile state.

Self-inflicted causes of lymphedema are usually difficult to prove and may occur in settings of known causes of lymphedema, such as postphlebitic syndrome or surgical injury to the brachial plexus.

Factitial lymphedema caused by blunt trauma localized to the dorsum of the hand or forearm is referred to as *Secretan's syndrome* and *l'oedeme bleu*, respectively. It often is unilateral, and there may be significant purpura. Occupational causes must be excluded. Angelini et al reported four cases of occupational persistent hand edema in fishing divers related to the constrictive action of the divers' suits and pricks from sea urchin spines. Biopsy of Secretan's syndrome often shows organizing hematoma and amorphous polysaccharide masses commingled with iron pigment within the dermis.

Effective care of such patients requires psychiatric intervention.

Evaluation

The diagnosis is usually based on a classic presentation; however, in the early stages the disease may require further investigation. Considerations include isotopic lymphoscintigraphy, indirect and direct lymphography, magnetic resonance imaging, computed tomography, and ultrasonography.

Treatment

Most cases are treated conservatively, by means of various forms of compression therapy, complex physical therapy, pneumatic pumps, and compressive garments. Volume-reducing surgery and lymphatic microsurgery are rarely performed, although a few centers consistently report favorable results. It is best to refer these patients to a center versed in the treatment of these complicated conditions, to optimize patient compliance, and customize therapy to the patient's lifestyle.

Allen PJ, et al: Lower extremity lymphedema caused by acquired immune deficient syndrome-related Kaposi's sarcoma. *J Vasc Surg* 1995, 22:178.

Angelini G, et al: Occupational traumatic lymphedema of the hands. *Dermatol Clin* 1990, 8:205.

Bastien MR, et al: Treatment of lymphedema with a multicompartmental pneumatic compression device. *J Am Acad Dermatol* 1989, 20:853.

Bielsa I, et al: Generalized nevus spilus and nevus anemicus in a patient with a primary lymphedema: a new type of phakomatosis pigmentovascularis? *Pediatr Dermatol* 1998, 15:293.

Christian MM, et al: Metastatic basal cell carcinoma presenting as unilateral lymphedema. *Dermatol Surg* 1998, 24:1151.

Cook W, et al: Milroy's disease. *JAMA* 1951, 147:650.

Halm U, et al: Primary amyloidosis of the mesentery and the retroperitoneum presenting with lymphedema. *Am J Gastroenterol* 1998, 93:2299.

Harel L, et al: Lymphedema praecox seen as isolated unilateral arm involvement. *J Pediatr* 1997, 130:492.

Harvey DT, et al: Rosaceous lymphedema. *Cutis* 1998, 61:321.

Johnson SM, et al: Lymphedema-distichiasis syndrome: report of a case and review. *Arch Dermatol* 1999, 135:347.

Ko DS, et al: Effective treatment of lymphedema of the extremities. *Arch Surg* 1998, 133:452.

Lee MW, et al: Mycobacterium marinum: chronic and extensive infections of the lower limbs in south Pacific islanders. *Australas J Dermatol* 1998, 39:173.

Miller TA, et al: Staged skin and subcutaneous excision for lymphedema: a favorable report of long-term results. *Plast Reconstr Surg* 1998, 102:1486.

Mortimer PS: Managing lymphedema. *Clin Dermatol* 1995, 13:499.

Schissel DJ, et al: Elephantiasis nostras verrucosa. *Cutis* 1998, 62:77.

Sinclair SA, et al: Angiosarcoma arising in a chronically lymphoedematous leg. *Br J Dermatol* 1998, 138:692.

Stoberl C, et al: Artifical edema of the extremity. *Hautarzt* 1994, 45:149.

Szuba A: Lymphedema: anatomy, physiology and pathogenesis. *Vasc Med* 1997, 2:321.

Szuba A, et al: Lymphedema: classification, diagnosis and therapy. *Vasc Med* 1998, 3:145.

Tunkel RS, et al: Lymphedema of the limb. *Postgrad Med* 1998, 104:131.

Vrouenraets BC, et al: Toxicity and morbidity of isolated limb perfusion. *Semin Surg Oncol* 1998, 14:224.

Winkelmann RK, et al: Factitial traumatic panniculitis. *J Am Acad Dermatol* 1985, 13:988. ▲

CHAPTER 36

Disturbances of Pigmentation

Melanin is the primary pigment producing brown coloration of the skin. Melanin is formed from tyrosine, via the action of tyrosinase, in the melanosomes of melanocytes. The melanosomes are transferred from a melanocyte to a group of keratinocytes called the epidermal melanin unit.

The variations in skin color between persons and between races are related to the degree of melanization of melanosomes, their number, and their distribution in the epidermal melanin unit.

Abdel-Malek ZA, et al: The nature and biological effects of factors responsible for proliferation and differentiation of melanocytes. *Pigment Cell Res* 1992, 2(Suppl):43.

Barrett AW, et al: Human oral melanocytes. *J Oral Pathol Med* 1994, 23:97.

Jimbow K, et al: Melanin pigments and melanosomal proteins as differentiation markers unique to normal and neoplastic melanocytes. *J Invest Dermatol* 1993, 100(Suppl):259.

Pavel S: Dynamics of melanogenesis intermediates. *J Invest Dermatol* 1993, 100(Suppl):162. ⎯⎯⎯⎯⎯⎯⎯⎯⎯⎯ ▲

PIGMENTARY DEMARCATION LINES

Pigmentary demarcation boundaries of the skin can be classified in five groups, as follows:

1. Group A: Lines along the outer upper arms with variable extension across the chest
2. Group B: Lines along the posteromedial aspect of the lower limb
3. Group C: Paired median or paramedian lines on the chest, with midline abdominal extension
4. Group D: Medial, over the spine
5. Group E: Bilaterally symmetrical, obliquely oriented, hypopigmented macules on the chest

More than 70% of black patients have one or more lines; they are much less common in whites. Type B lines often appear for the first time during pregnancy.

James WD, et al: Pigmentary demarcation lines. *J Am Acad Dermatol* 1987, 16:584.

Ozawa H, et al: Pigmentary demarcation lines of pregnancy with erythema. *Dermatology* 1993, 187:134. ⎯⎯⎯⎯⎯⎯⎯⎯⎯⎯ ▲

ABNORMAL PIGMENTATION

Normal pigmentation of the skin is influenced by the amount and location of melanin, by the degree of vascularity, by the presence of carotene, and by the thickness of the horny layer. The amount of melanin produced is influenced by genetic factors, the amount and wavelengths of ultraviolet light received, the amount of melanocyte-stimulating hormone (MSH) secreted, and the effect of melanocyte-stimulating chemicals such as furocoumarins (psoralens).

Hemosiderin Hyperpigmentation

Pigmentation due to deposits of hemosiderin occurs in purpura, hemochromatosis, hemorrhagic diseases, and stasis ulcers. Clinically, hemosiderin hyperpigmentation is difficult to distinguish from postinflammatory dermal melanosis.

Postinflammatory Hyperpigmentation

Any inflammatory condition can result in hyperpigmentation or hypopigmentation. This is also a complication of medical intervention, such as chemical peels, dermabrasions, laser therapy, or liposuction. Histologically, there is melanin in the upper dermis and around upper dermal vessels, located primarily in macrophages (melanophages).

Industrial Hyperpigmentation

In industrial dermatoses, melanosis is an important feature. It occurs in coal miners, anthracene workers, pitch workers, and those in similar occupations. Pigmentation of the face may occur from the incorporation in cosmetics of derivatives of coal tar, petroleum, or picric acid, as well as mercury, lead, bismuth, or furocoumarins (psoralens).

Systemic Diseases

Among the causes may be mentioned syphilis, malaria, pellagra, and diabetes, in which there may be a diffuse bronzing of the skin, as well as Addison's disease, in which there is a diffuse melanosis that is pronounced in the axillae and in the palmar creases, about the nipples and the genitals, and on the buccal mucosa. In cases of virilizing adrenal tumors, hyperpigmentation and hypertrichosis usually develop. In Cushing's syndrome treated by bilateral adrenalectomy, some patients, after a good initial response, later develop extreme hyperpigmentation despite corticosteroid therapy. A pituitary MSH-producing tumor should be suspected. This condition is called *Nelson's syndrome*. Pheochromocytoma, hemochromatosis, amyloidosis, scurvy, pregnancy, menopause, porphyria cutanea tarda, vitamin B_{12} deficiency, kwashiorkor, and vitamin A deficiency are some other conditions in which hyperpigmentation is seen.

Primary biliary cirrhosis produces a diffuse hyperpigmentation. The triad of diffuse hyperpigmentation, pruritus, and xanthomas is quite specific for this disease. The pigmentation is similar to that seen in Whipple's. In abdominal carcinoma, tuberculosis, severe anemias, hepatic and pancreatic disease, hyperthyroidism, chronic encephalitis, and Gaucher's disease various degrees of melanoderma may be present.

Betts CM, et al: Progressive hyperpigmentation. *Dermatology* 1994, 189:384.

Bohler-Sommeregger K, et al: Reactive lentiginous hyperpigmentation after cryosurgery for lentigo maligna. *J Am Acad Dermatol* 1992, 27:523.

Bottomley WW, et al: A case of dermatomyositis presenting as localized hyperpigmentation of the hands and face (letter). *Br J Dermatol* 1995, 132:670.

Bu TS, et al: A case of dermatopathia pigmentosa reticularis. *J Dermatol* 1997, 24:266.

Burns RL, et al: Glycolic acid peels for postinflammatory hyperpigmentation in black patients. *Dermatol Surg* 1997, 23:171.

Chung AD, et al: Cutaneous hyperpigmentation and polyglandular autoimmune syndrome type II. *Cutis* 1997, 59:77.

Jones D, et al: Coal-black hyperpigmentation at birth in a child with congenital adrenal hypoplasia. *J Am Acad Dermatol* 1995, 33:323.

Kikuchi A, et al: Mycosis fungoides with marked hyperpigmentation. *Dermatology* 1996, 192:360.

Mateu LP, et al: Cutaneous hyperpigmentation caused by liposuction. *Aesthetic Plast Surg* 1997, 21:230. _____ ▲

HEMOCHROMATOSIS (BRONZE DIABETES)

Hemochromatosis is characterized by gray to brown mucocutaneous hyperpigmentation, diabetes mellitus, and hepatomegaly. In addition, heart disease, cirrhosis of the liver, and hypogonadism are usually present. The skin pigmentation is usually generalized, although more pronounced on the face, the extensor surfaces of the forearms, the backs of the hands, and the genitocrural area. Iron is deposited in the skin, being present as granules around blood vessels and sweat glands and within macrophages. The pigmentation, however, is caused by increased basal-layer melanin. The mucous membranes are pigmented in up to 20% of patients.

Koilonychia occurs in 50%, and localized ichthyosis in 40%. Alopecia is common.

Hemochromatosis occurs mostly in men in their sixties. Women with genetic hemochromatosis can have full phenotypic expression of the disease, and the belief that it is less severe in women due to iron loss associated with menses and pregnancy is unfounded. It is extremely rare in the young. Neonatal hemochromatosis has been shown to be associated with intrauterine infections, such as cytomegalovirus. Adults with hemochromatosis are susceptible to *Yersinia enterocolitica* infection, producing multiple liver abscesses. *Y. enterocolitica* is an iron-dependent bacterium that relies entirely on exogenous iron for growth.

Levels of plasma iron and the serum iron-binding protein are elevated. High serum ferritin levels in the absence of an obvious cause should prompt investigation for both hemochromatosis and porphyria cutanea tarda. The cause is either an inborn error of metabolism of iron, or an excessive number of blood transfusions. The autosomal recessive gene for hereditary hemochromatosis is linked to the HLA-A locus on chromosome 6p. Mutations in C282Y have been associated with hemochromatosis and porphyria cutanea tarda. A second less prevalent mutation is called H63D.

Treatment is by phlebotomy until satisfactory iron levels are attained. Extracorporeal chelation has also been used successfully. Associated diabetes may require additional medical management. Hepatomas occur not infrequently as a long-term complication of cirrhosis.

Andrews NC: Disorders of iron metabolism. *N Engl J Med* 1999, 341:1986.

Burke W, et al: Hemochromatosis: genetics helps to define a multifactorial disease. *Clin Genet* 1998, 54:1.

Held JL, et al: Hyperpigmentation and secondary hemochromatosis: a novel treatment with extracorporeal chelation. *J Am Acad Dermatol* 1993, 28:253.

Kershisnik MM, et al: Cytomegalovirus infection, fetal liver disease, and neonatal hemochromatosis. *Hum Pathol* 1992, 23:1075.

Leal-Khouri S, et al: Jaundice and bleeding from peripheral intravenous sites in a neonate. *Arch Dermatol* 1996, 132:1507.

Moirand R, et al: Clinical features of genetic hemochromatosis in women compared with men. *Ann Intern Med* 1997, 127:105.

O'Reilly FM, et al: Screening of patients with iron overload to identify hemochromatosis and porphyria cutanea tarda. *Arch Dermatol* 1997, 133:1098.

Rouault TA: Hereditary hemochromatosis. *JAMA* 1993, 269:3152.

Vadillo M, et al: Multiple liver abscesses due to *Yersinia enterocolitica* discloses primary hemochromatosis. *Clin Infect Dis* 1994, 18:938. ▲

MELASMA (CHLOASMA FACIEI)

Melasma is characterized by brown patches, typically on the malar prominences and forehead (Figs. 36-1 and 36-2). There are three clinical patterns: (1) centrofacial, (2) malar, and (3) mandibular. The pigmented patches are usually quite sharply demarcated. Increased pigmentation may also occur at the same time on the nipples and about the external

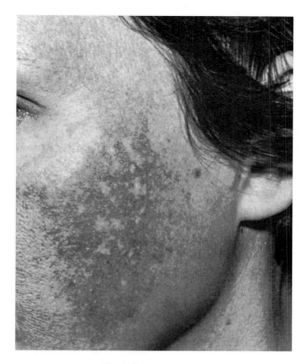

Fig. 36-1 Melasma.

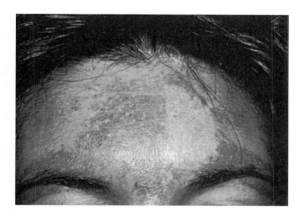

Fig. 36-2 Melasma.

Bleaching creams with hydroquinone are the standard treatment and are moderately efficacious; they contain from 2% (available over the counter) to 4% hydroquinone. Tretinoin cream may be added to increase efficacy. This combination, administered in conjunction with a mild topical steroid, has been called "Kligman's formula" and is excellent. At times 4% is insufficient, and higher doses of hydroquinone must be compounded. Satellite pigmentation and local ochronosis are potential complications from use of these higher-concentration preparations. Glycolic acid may be added to tretinoin/hydroquinone therapy to further enhance efficacy. Jessner's solution, glycolic acid peels, azelaic acid, kojic acid, and cystamine and buthionine sulfoximine are additional considerations. Laser treatment has a limited role because of the risk of postinflammatory hyperpigmentation.

Bolognia JL, et al: Enhancement of the depigmenting effect of hydroquinone by cystamine and bythionine sulfoximine. *Br J Dermatol* 1995, 133:349.

Breathnach AS: Melanin hyperpigmentation of skin: melasma, topical treatment with azelaic acid, and other therapies. *Cutis* 1996, 57:36.

Garcia A, et al: The combination of glycolic acid and hydroquinone or kojic acid for the treatment of melasma and related conditions. *Dermatol Surg* 1996, 22:443.

Goldberg DJ: Laser treatment of pigmented lesions. *Dermatol Clin* 1997, 15:397.

Grimes PE: Melasma. Etiologic and therapeutic considerations. *Arch Dermatol* 1995, 131:1453.

Hassan I, et al: Hormonal milieu in the maintenance of melasma in fertile women. *J Dermatol* 1998, 25:510.

Kang WH, et al: Intermittent therapy for melasma in Asian patients with combined topical agents (retinoic acid, hydroquinone and hydrocortisone). *J Dermatol* 1998, 25:587.

Kim NY, et al: Pigmentary diseases. *Med Clin North Am* 1998, 82:1185.

Lawrence N, et al: Treatment of melasma with Jessner's solution versus glycolic acid. *J Am Acad Dermatol* 1997, 36:589.

Lim JT, et al: Glycolic acid peels in the treatment of melasma among Asian women. *Dermatol Surg* 1997, 23:177.

O'Brien TJ, et al: Melasma of the forearms. *Australas J Dermatol* 1997, 38:35. _____ ▲

ACROMELANOSIS PROGRESSIVA

Acromelanosis progressiva, also known as *acropigmentation,* is a progressive pigmentary disorder that was first described by Furuya and Mishima in a Japanese infant. A diffuse black pigmentation on the dorsum of all the fingers and toes became progressively more widespread and more intensely pigmented. By the time the child was age 4 to 5, the perineum, extremities, and areas of the head and neck were involved. Epileptiform seizures also occurred. The history revealed consanguinity.

Gonzalez JR, et al: Acromelanosis. *J Am Acad Dermatol* 1980, 2:128. ▲

genitals. It tends to affect darker-complexioned individuals. It may at times be found on the forearms.

Melasma occurs frequently during pregnancy and at menopause. It may also be seen in ovarian disorders and other endocrinologic disorders. It is seen most frequently in young women, men making up 10% of reported cases. There is a strong association with birth control pill use. Use of dilantin may induce melasma. Discontinuing the use of contraceptives rarely clears the pigmentation, and it may last for many years after discontinuing them. Melasma of pregnancy usually clears within a few months of delivery.

A number of topical therapies are available. Exposure to sunlight should be avoided, and a complete sun block with broad-spectrum UVA coverage should be used daily.

PIGMENTED ANOMALIES OF THE EXTREMITIES
Acropigmentation of Dohi

Originally described in 12 patients from Japan, acropigmentation of Dohi has been found to affect individuals from Europe, India, and the Caribbean. It is also referred to as *dyschromatosis symmetrica hereditaria* or *symmetrical dyschromatosis of the extremities*. Patients develop progressive pigmented and depigmented macules, often mixed in a reticulate pattern. Many investigators believe this disorder to be a variation of acropigmentation of Kitamura.

Dhar S, et al: Spectrum of reticulate flexural and acral pigmentary disorders in northern India. *J Dermatol* 1994, 21:598.

Ostlere LS, et al: Reticulate acropigmentation of Dohi. *Clin Exp Dermatol* 1995, 20:477.

Tan HH, et al: Neurofibromatosis and reticulate acropigmentation of Dohi. *Pediatr Dermatol* 1997, 14:296. ▲

Reticular Pigmented Anomaly of the Flexures

Reticular pigmented anomaly of the flexures is a rare pigmentary adult-onset disorder; it is sometimes called *Dowling-Degos disease* or *dark dot disease*. The disorder should be part of the differential diagnosis whenever acanthosis nigricans is considered in a patient who is not obese and is not known to have internal cancer. Clinically, it does not look velvety: it looks smooth. The pigmentation is reticular; at the periphery, discrete, brownish black macules surround the partly confluent central pigmented area (Fig. 36-3). Typically, axillae, inframammary folds, and intercrural folds are involved. It begins when an individual is 20 to 30 years of age and progresses very gradually. There are frequently pits, sometimes pigmented, about the mouth. Rarely, comedonal and cystic lesions have been described.

Although the cause is unknown, it is an autosomal dominant genodermatosis with variable penetrance and expressivity, and delayed onset. Many authors believe Kitamura's reticulate acropigmentation is a spectrum of the same disease. Familial rosacea-like dermatitis with warty keratotic plaques on the trunk and limbs is believed to be another manifestation of this disorder.

Histologically, the appearance is distinctive—elongation, tufting, and deep hyperpigmentation of the rete ridges, with protrusion of similar tufts even from the sides of the follicles. In Dowling's original case (which was initially thought to be atypical acanthosis nigricans), there was even a trichoepithelioma in one of the areas subjected to biopsy. There is no treatment.

Bedlow AJ, et al: Dowling-Degos disease associated with hidradenitis suppurativa. *Clin Exp Dermatol* 1996, 21:305.

Kershenovich J, et al: Dowling-Degos' disease mimicking chloracne. *J Am Acad Dermatol* 1992, 27:345.

Thami GP, et al: Overlap of reticulate acropigmentation of Kitamura, acropigmentation of Dohi and Dowling-Degos disease in four generations. *Dermatology* 1998, 196:350.

Weber LA, et al: Reticulate pigmented anomaly of the flexures (Dowling-Degos disease): a case report associated with hidradenitis suppurativa and squamous cell carcinoma. *Cutis* 1990, 45:446. ▲

Reticulate Acropigmentation of Kitamura

Reticulate acropigmentation of Kitamura consists of linear palmar pits and pigmented macules 1 to 4 mm in diameter on the volar and dorsal aspects of the hands and feet. It is usually an autosomal dominantly inherited disorder. It has been argued that the pitting and the absence of hypopigmented lesions distinguishes it from acropigmentation of Dohi; however, this argument has been challenged, and families with features of both disease have been reported. It is likely that acropigmentation of Dohi, Dowling-Degos disease, and reticulate acropigmentation of Kitamura are

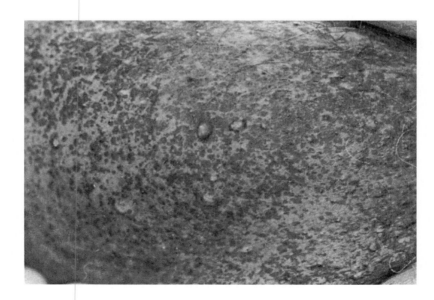

Fig. 36-3 Reticulated pigmented anomaly of the flexures. (Courtesy Dr. James B. Howell, Dallas.)

various expressions of the same disease. A patient with bony abnormalities consisting of absence of terminal phalanges of the second, third, and fourth toes was reported by el-Hoshy et al. Some treatment success for the cutaneous lesions has been reported using azelaic acid ointment.

Cox NH, et al: Dowling-Degos disease and Kitamura's reticulate acropigmentation: support for the concept of a single disease. *Br J Dermatol* 1991, 125:169.

el-Hoshy K, et al: Bony anomalies in a patient with reticulate acropigmentation of Kitamura. *J Dermatol* 1996, 23:713.

Erel A, et al: Reticulate acropigmentation of Kitamura. *Int J Dermatol* 1993, 32:726.

Kameyama K, et al: Treatment of reticulate acropigmentation of Kitamura with azelaic acid. *J Am Acad Dermatol* 1992, 26:817.

Ostlere L, et al: Dowling-Degos disease associated with Kitamura's reticulate acropigmentation. *Clin Exp Dermatol* 1994, 19:492.

Singal A, et al: Is the heredity of reticulate acropigmentation of Kitamura always autosomal dominant? *J Dermatol* 1998, 25:57. _____ ▲

DERMATOPATHIA PIGMENTOSA RETICULARIS

Dermatopathia pigmentosa reticularis is composed of the triad of generalized reticulate hyperpigmentation, noncicatricial alopecia, and onychodystrophy. Additional associations include adermatoglyphia, hypohidrosis or hyperhidrosis, palmoplantar hyperkeratosis, and nonscarring blisters on the dorsa of the hands and feet. An autosomal dominant inheritance pattern has been reported.

Bu TS, et al: A case of dermatopathia pigmentosa reticularis. *J Dermatol* 1997, 24:266.

Heimer WL II, et al: Dermatopathia pigmentosa reticularis. *J Am Acad Dermatol* 1992, 26:298.

Maso MJ, et al: Dermatopathis pigmentosa reticularis. *Arch Dermatol* 1990, 126:935. _____ ▲

TRANSIENT NEONATAL PUSTULAR MELANOSIS

Infants develop 2- to 3-mm macules, pustules, and ruptured pustules at birth, predominantly involving the face. Pigmentation may persist for weeks or months after the pustules have healed. The condition is observed in 4.4% of black and 0.6% of white newborns.

Histologically, there are intracorneal or subcorneal aggregates of predominantly neutrophils, but eosinophils may also be found. Dermal inflammation is composed of an admixture of neutrophils and eosinophils. The differential diagnosis includes erythema toxicum neonatorum, neonatal acne, and acropustulosis of infancy.

Laude TA: Approach to dermatologic disorders in black children. *Semin Dermatol* 1995, 14:15.

Treadwell PA: Dermatoses in newborns. *Am Fam Physician* 1997, 56:443.

Van Praag MC, et al: Diagnosis and treatment of pustular disorders in the neonate. *Pediatr Dermatol* 1997, 14:131.

Wagner A: Distinguishing vesicular and pustular disorders in the neonate. *Curr Opin Pediatr* 1997, 9:396. _____ ▲

PEUTZ-JEGHERS SYNDROME

Peutz-Jeghers syndrome is characterized by hyperpigmented macules on the lips and oral mucosa and polyposis of the small intestine. The dark brown or black macules appear typically on the lips, especially the lower lip, in infancy or early childhood (Fig. 36-4). Similar lesions may appear on the buccal mucosa, tongue, gingiva, and genital mucosa; macules may also occur around the mouth, on the central face, and on the backs of the hands, especially the fingers, and on the toes and tops of the feet.

The associated polyposis involves the small intestine by preference, but hamartomatous polyps may also occur in the stomach and colon. The polyposis of the small intestine may cause repeated bouts of abdominal pain and vomiting. Bleeding is common. Intussusception is frequent. Cosmetic treatment of labial macules in Peutz-Jeghers syndrome has been accomplished with the use of a 694-nm ruby laser.

The incidence of malignancy within the polyps is about 2% to 3%. Although the incidence of gastrointestinal malignancy is low, patients with Peutz-Jeghers syndrome have an increased risk of developing other kinds of cancer, particularly breast cancer and gynecologic malignancies in women.

The syndrome is inherited and is transmitted as a simple mendelian dominant trait. However, sporadic noninherited cases may also occur. The gene (STK11) has been localized to 19p13.3, which is believed to be a tumor suppressor gene. Although Carney complex (2p16), Cowden disease (10q23), and Bannayan-Zonana syndrome (10q23) share similar cutaneous and endocrine manifestations, their gene loci differ from Peutz-Jeghers syndrome.

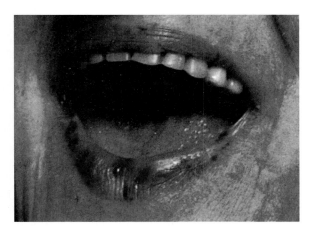

Fig. 36-4 Peutz-Jeghers syndrome. Note melanin-pigmented macules on lips. (Courtesy Dr. A. Kaminsky.)

Cronkhite-Canada syndrome should be considered in the differential diagnosis. It consists of melanotic macules on the fingers and gastrointestinal polyposis. Also there is generalized, uniform darkening of the skin, extensive alopecia, and onychodystrophy. The polyps that occur are usually benign adenomas and may involve the entire gastrointestinal tract. A protein-losing enteropathy may develop and is associated with the degree of intestinal polyposis. Onset is typically after age 30 in this sporadically occurring, generally benign condition. Hypogeusia is the dominant initial symptom, followed by diarrhea and ectodermal changes. Seventy-five percent of all cases have been reported from Japan (see Chapter 33).

Allbritton J, et al: Cronkhite-Canada syndrome. *Cutis* 1998, 61:229.
Boardman LA, et al: Increased risk for cancer in patients with the Peutz-Jeghers syndrome. *Ann Intern Med* 1998, 128:896.
Goto A: Cronkhite-Canada syndrome. *Nippon Geka Hokan* 1995, 64:3.
Gruber SB, et al: Pathogenesis of adenocarcinoma in Peutz-Jeghers syndrome. *Cancer Res* 1998, 58:5267.
Hanada K, et al: Successful treatment of mucosal melanosis of the lip with normal pulsed ruby laser. *J Dermatol* 1996, 23:263.
Hanzawa M, et al: Surgical treatment of Cronkhite-Canada syndrome associated with protein-losing enteropathy. *Dis Colon Rectum* 1998, 41:932.
Herzberg AJ, et al: Cronkhite-Canada syndrome. *Int J Dermatol* 1990, 29:121.
Katz SK, et al: The cutaneous manifestations of gastrointestinal disease. *Prim Care* 1996, 23:455.
Resta N, et al: STK11 mutations in Peutz-Jeghers syndrome and sporadic colon cancer. *Cancer Res* 1998, 58:4799.
Stratakis CA, et al: Carney complex, Peutz-Jeghers syndrome, Cowden disease, and Bannayan-Zonana syndrome share cutaneous and endocrine manifestations, but not genetic loci. *J Clin Endocrinol Metab* 1998, 83:2972.
Wong SS, et al: Peutz-Jeghers syndrome associated with primary malignant melanoma of the rectum. *Br J Dermatol* 1996, 135:439. ▲

RIEHL'S MELANOSIS

This pigmentary disease, first described by Riehl, is a photosensitivity, probably a phototoxic dermatitis. It begins with pruritus, erythema, and pigmentation, gradually spreads and, after reaching a certain extent, becomes stationary. The melanosis occurs mostly in women and develops slowly over the course of several months. Most reported cases occur in Japan.

The characteristic feature is spotty light to dark brown pigmentation. This is most intense on the forehead, on the malar regions, behind the ears, on the sides of the neck, and on other sun-exposed areas. Pigmentation on covered parts of the body is only on areas exposed to friction, such as the anterior axillary folds and the umbilicus. In addition to the melanosis, there may be circumscribed telangiectasia and temporary hyperemia. Diffuse hyperkeratosis occurs, making the skin appear as if dusted with flour.

The pathogenesis of Riehl's melanosis is believed to be sun exposure following the use of some perfume or cream (a photocontact dermatitis). Serrano et al reported positive patch test results to lemon oil, geraniol, and hydroxy-citronellal. In other reported patients patch test and photopatch test results have been negative. Riehl's melanosis has been reported in patients with AIDS and Sjögren's syndrome. All treatment methods are of no avail unless the cause of photosensitivity is determined. Eventually the hyperkeratosis and pigmentation disappear spontaneously.

Hanada K, et al: Melanosis Riehl-like facial pigmentation in a Japanese case of AIDS. *J Dermatol* 1994, 21:363.
Miyoshi K, et al: Riehl's melanosis-like eruption associated with Sjögren's syndrome. *J Dermatol* 1997, 24:784.
Serrano G, et al: Riehl's melanosis. *J Am Acad Dermatol* 1989, 21:1057. ▲

TAR MELANOSIS (MELANODERMATITIS TOXICA LICHENOIDES)

Tar melanosis is an occupational dermatosis that occurs among tar handlers after several years' exposure. Severe widespread itching develops and is soon followed by the appearance of reticular pigmentation, telangiectases, and a shiny appearance of the skin. In addition, there is a hyperhidrotic tendency. Small, dark, lichenoid, follicular papules become profuse on the extremities, particularly the forearms. Bullae are sometimes observed. This represents a photosensitivity or phototoxicity induced by tar.

Lehowhl M, et al: Tar melanosis. *Mt Sinai J Med* 1995, 62:412. ▲

FAMILIAL PROGRESSIVE HYPERPIGMENTATION

Familial progressive hyperpigmentation (FPH) is characterized by patches of hyperpigmentation, present at birth, which increase in size and number with age. Later, hyperpigmentation appears in the conjunctivae and the buccal mucosa. Eventually a large portion of the skin and mucous membranes becomes involved. Inheritance is believed to be of a dominant mode.

Histologically, the most distinctive finding is the increase of melanin in the basal cell layer, especially at the tips of the rete ridges. In addition, pigmented granules were scattered diffusely throughout the epidermal layers, including the stratum corneum. FPH is differentiated from other hyperpigmentations mainly by the presence of bizarre, sharply marginated patterns of hyperpigmented skin.

Chernosky ME, et al: Familial progressive hyperpigmentation. *Arch Dermatol* 1971, 103:581.
Ling DB, et al: Familial progressive hyperpigmentation. *Br J Dermatol* 1991, 125:607. ▲

UNIVERSAL ACQUIRED MELANOSIS (CARBON BABY)

Ruiz-Maldonado et al reported the case of a Mexican child, born white, who progressively became black, with pigmentation of palms, soles, and the mucous membranes. Electron microscopy showed a negroid pattern in the melanosomes of the epidermal melanocytes and keratinocytes. Melanocytes were not increased in number.

Ruiz-Maldonado R, et al: Universal acquired melanosis: a carbon baby. *Arch Dermatol* 1978, 114:775. _____ ▲

ZEBRALIKE HYPERPIGMENTATION

Alimurung et al reported an unusual pattern of hyperpigmentation in a black male infant with congenital defects that included an atrial septal defect, dextrocardia, auricular atresia, deafness, and growth retardation. The hyperpigmentation was strikingly linear and symmetrical, with involvement of the trunk and extremities. An increased number of melanocytes in the bands of hyperpigmentation has been demonstrated. The pigmentary anomaly fades spontaneously. It may be a variant of incontinentia pigmenti. The differential diagnosis includes incontinentia pigmenti, Franceschetti-Jadassohn syndrome and Naegeli's reticular pigmented dermatosis.

Alimurung FM, et al: Zebra-like hyperpigmentation in an infant with multiple congenital defects. *Arch Dermatol* 1979, 115:878. _____ ▲

PERIORBITAL HYPERPIGMENTATION

Many disorders and conditions can produce discoloration around the eyes. The hyperpigmentation of familial periorbital melanosis, an autosomal dominant disorder, usually involves all four eyelids and may extend to involve the eyebrows and the cheekbones. Erythema dyschromicum perstans is a rare cause. Dark circles around the eyes are not uncommon, often familial, and are frequently found in individuals with dark pigmentation or Mediterranean ancestry.

Hacker SM: Common disorders of pigmentation: when are more than cosmetic cover-ups required? *Postgrad Med* 1996, 99:177.

Ing EB, et al: Periorbital hyperpigmentation and erythema dyschromicum perstans. *Can J Ophthalmol* 1992, 27:353. _____ ▲

METALLIC DISCOLORATIONS

Pigmentation may develop from the deposit of fine metallic particles in the skin. The metal may be carried to the skin by the blood stream or may permeate into it from surface applications.

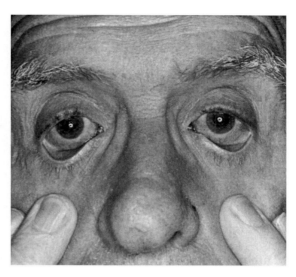

Fig. 36-5 Diffuse pigmentation of the sclerae in a man with argyria.

Argyria

Argyria is a localized or widespread slate-colored pigmentation resulting from the presence of silver in the skin. The pigmentation is most noticeable in parts exposed to sunlight (the face and hands) and spares the skin folds; however, it also occurs in the conjunctivae, sclerae, mucous membranes, and nails (Fig. 36-5). Tissue silver is felt to stimulate melanocytes, explaining the photoaccentuation. At first the discoloration is hardly perceptible: it has a faint bluish gray tone, but as it becomes more pronounced, a slate-gray color develops. The oral mucous membranes and the sclerae are usually pigmented in a distinctive diffuse manner. Local treatment with a silver-containing product may produce argyria localized to the region of use; for example, the conjunctivae, from eye drops; a wound, from silver sulfadiazine cream; the earlobes, from silver earrings; and from silver acupuncture needles. It can also occur from occupational exposure, usually in silversmiths. In these localized exposures, the appearance may be separated by many years from the exposure.

Histologically, systemic argyria and localized argyria have the same features. The skin appears relatively normal at lower magnifications. Fine black granules are found in the basement membrane zone of the sweat glands, as well as blood vessel walls, the dermoepidermal junction, and along the arrector pili muscles. Examination of an unstained biopsy section by darkfield illumination demonstrates silver granules outlining the basement membrane of the epidermis and the eccrine sweat glands. Electron probe microanalysis can be used to confirm the diagnosis.

Bismuth

When bismuth compounds were used intramuscularly or orally for a long time, it rarely was associated with the deposition of metallic particles in the gums. This was

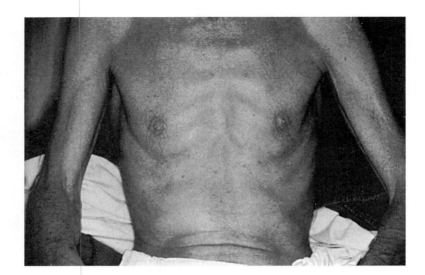

Fig. 36-6 Generalized hyperpigmentation caused by chronic arsenic ingestion.

known as the *bismuth line*. The presence of stomatitis or periodontitis increased the risk of this complication. Generalized cutaneous discoloration, as well as oral mucous membrane and conjunctival pigmentation resembling argyria, has rarely occurred but has not been reported in the past 50 years.

Arsenic

Chronic exposure to inorganic arsenic may lead to cutaneous hyperpigmentation. It is often accentuated in the inguinal folds and the areolae. Areas of hypopigmentation may be scattered in the hyperpigmented areas, giving a "raindrop" appearance (Fig. 36-6). The pigmentation may resolve or persist indefinitely. Punctate keratoses on the palms and soles are characteristic. Diffuse palmoplantar keratoderma may rarely occur. The most common source of current exposure is from drinking water contaminated with arsenic (hydroarsenicism). Histologically, the arsenical keratosis on the palms and soles show hyperkeratosis, acanthosis, and minimal to moderate basilar atypia. Arsenic exposure leads to the development of nonmelanoma skin cancers 2 to 20 years after exposure. Bowen's disease represents 54% of arsenic-induced skin cancers and may appear on sun-exposed or sun-protected skin. Basal cell carcinomas are frequent, usually multiple, most common on the trunk, and can be in sun-protected sites. Squamous cell carcinoma may also occur.

Lead

Chronic lead poisoning can produce a "lead hue," with lividity and pallor, and a deposit of lead in the gums may occur: the "lead line."

Iron

In the past, soluble iron compounds were used in the treatment of allergic contact and other dermatitides. In eroded areas iron was sometimes deposited in the skin, like a tattoo. The use of Monsel's solution can produce similar tattooing, so aluminum chloride is now preferred.

Titanium

A titanium-containing ointment caused yellowish papules on the penis in a patient.

Gold

Chrysiasis may be induced by the parenteral administration of gold salts, usually for the treatment of rheumatoid arthritis. It appears to be more commonly recognized in white patients. A mauve, blue, or slate/gray pigmentation develops initially on the eyelids, spreading to the face, dorsal hands, and other areas. The severity of chrysiasis is related to the total dose received, and it is rare below a total dose of 20 mg/kg of elemental gold. The pigmentation is accentuated in light-exposed areas, and sun-protected areas do not histologically demonstrate gold, even when the patient has documented chrysiasis at other sites. Localized chrysiasis has been induced by Q-switched ruby laser treatment in a patient on parenteral gold therapy. Melanin is not increased in the areas of hyperpigmentation. Therefore, it appears, the gold itself contributes to the visible hyperpigmentation. Mucous membrane and scleral pigmentation is very uncommon.

Histologically, there is no inflammation in the skin, and gold is deposited in the dermis predominantly in a perivascular pattern. The epidermis and dermoepidermal junction are spared, but the granules are accentuated in the basement membrane zone of sweat glands. Darkfield examination will demonstrate the granules and electron probe microanalysis can be used to confirm the presence of gold. Patients with chrysiasis are not at increased risk of developing other gold-related cutaneous complications, namely lichenoid and psoriasiform drug eruptions.

Mercury

Mercurial pigmentation in the skin is rare, especially since the use of mercurials in cosmetics has been strictly controlled. The most common presentation is subcutaneous nodules that result from accidental implantation of elemental mercury from a thermometer into the skin.

Burge JM, et al: Mercury pigmentation. *Arch Dermatol* 1979, 102:51.

Dupre A, et al: Titanium pigmentation. *Arch Dermatol* 1985, 121:656.

Dupuis LL, et al: Hyperpigmentation due to topical application of silver sulfadiazine cream. *J Am Acad Dermatol* 1985, 12:1112.

Fleming CJ, et al: Chrysiasis after low-dose gold and UV exposure. *J Am Acad Dermatol* 1996, 34:349.

Granstein RD, et al: Drug- and heavy-metal induced hyperpigmentation. *J Am Acad Dermatol* 1981, 5:1.

Legat FJ, et al: Argyria after short-contact acupuncture. *Lancet* 1998, 352:241.

Morton CA, et al: Localized argyria caused by silver earrings. *Br J Dermatol* 1996, 135:484.

Prescott, RJ, et al: Systemic argyria. *J Clin Pathol* 1994, 47:556.

Smith RW, et al: Chrysiasis revisited. *Br J Dermatol* 1995, 133:671.

Suchard J, et al: Cutaneous nodular reaction to oral mercury. *J Am Acad Dermatol* 1998, 784.

Tanita Y, et al: Blue macules of localized argyria caused by implanted acupuncture needles. *Arch Dermatol* 1985, 121:1550.

Trotter MJ, et al: Localized chrysiasis induced by laser therapy. *Arch Dermatol* 1995, 131:1411.

Woollons A, et al: Chronic endemic hydroarsenicism. *Br J Dermatol* 1998, 139:1092 ▲

CANTHAXANTHIN

The orange-red pigment canthaxanthin is present in many plants (notably algae and mushrooms) and in bacteria, crustaceans, sea trout, and feathers. When ingested for the purpose of simulating a tan, its deposition in the panniculus imparts a golden orange hue to the skin. Stools become brick red and the plasma orange, and golden deposits appear in the retina.

Lober CW: Canthaxanthin: the "tanning" pill. *J Am Acad Dermatol* 1985, 13:660. ▲

DYE DISCOLORATION

Blue hands from accidental dyeing were reported by Albert in 1976. A man's hands were dyed as a result of warming them in his armpits while wearing a new blue flannel shirt. The dye, which was insoluble in water, was soluble in sweat.

Albert BL: Blue dye, blue hands, and sweat. *Ann Intern Med* 1976, 85:541. ▲

RUBEOSIS

Rubeosis is a rosy coloration of the face occurring in young people with uncontrolled diabetes mellitus. It may be associated with xanthochromia to produce a "peaches and cream" complexion.

VITILIGO

Vitiligo usually begins in childhood or young adulthood, with about half of cases beginning before age 20. The prevalence ranges from 0.5% to 1%. Although females are disproportionately represented among patients seeking care, it is not known whether they are actually more commonly affected or simply are more likely to seek medical care.

CLINICAL FEATURES. Vitiligo is an acquired pigmentary anomaly of the skin manifested by depigmented white patches surrounded by a normal or a hyperpigmented border (Figs. 36-7 and 36-8). There may be intermediate tan zones or lesions, halfway between the normal skin color and depigmentation—so-called trichrome vitiligo. The hairs in the vitiliginous areas usually become white also. Very rarely, the patches may have a red, inflammatory border. The patches are of various sizes and configurations.

Four types have been described according to the extent and distribution of the involved areas: localized or focal (including segmental), generalized, universal, and acrofacial. The generalized pattern is most common. Involvement is symmetrical. The most commonly affected sites are the face, upper part of the chest, dorsal aspects of the hands, axillae, and groin. There is a tendency for the skin around orifices to be affected, namely the eyes, nose, mouth, ears, nipples, umbilicus, penis, vulva, and anus. Lesions appear at areas of trauma, so vitiligo favors the elbows and knees. Universal vitiligo applies to cases where the entire body surface is depigmented. The acrofacial type affects the distal fingers and the facial orifices. Focal vitiligo may affect one nondermatomal site (such as the glans penis) or asymmetrically affect a single dermatome. This form of vitiligo is treatment resistant, has an earlier onset, and is less frequently associated with other autoimmune phenomena. It represents 5% of adult vitiligo and 20% of childhood vitiligo. The trigeminal area is most commonly affected.

Local loss of pigment may occur around nevi and melanomas, the so-called halo phenomenon. Vitiligo-like leukoderma occurs in about 1% of melanoma patients. In those with previously diagnosed melanoma, it suggests metastatic disease. Paradoxically, however, as the reaction indicates an autoimmune response against melanocytes, patients who develop it have a better prognosis than patients without leukoderma. Halo nevi are also common in patients with vitiligo. Lesions of vitiligo are hypersensitive to ultraviolet light and burn readily when exposed to the sun. It is not unusual to note the onset of vitiligo after a severe sunburn.

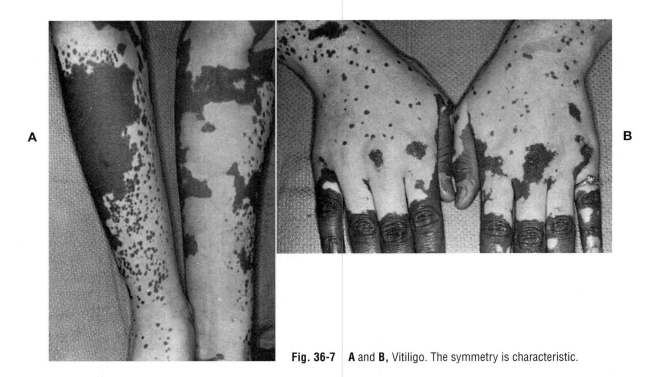

Fig. 36-7   **A** and **B**, Vitiligo. The symmetry is characteristic.

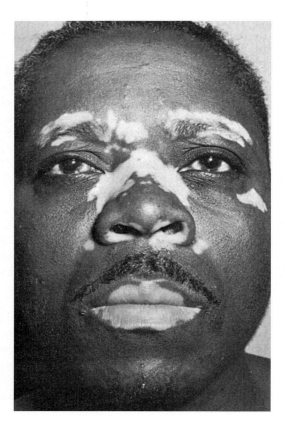

Fig. 36-8   Vitiligo.

Ocular abnormalities are increased in patients with vitiligo, including iritis and retinal pigmentary abnormalities. Patients have no visual complaints. Eight percent of patients with idiopathic uveitis have vitiligo or poliosis. The most frequent associations, however, are with other "autoimmune" diseases. These include insulin-dependent diabetes mellitus, pernicious anemia, Hashimoto's thyroiditis, Graves' disease, Addison's disease, and alopecia areata. Vitiligo occurs in 13% of patients with the autoimmune polyendocrinopathy-candidiasis-ectodermal dystrophy (APECED) syndrome.

Although familial aggregation of vitiligo is seen—up to 30% of vitiligo patients have an affected relative—it is not inherited as an autosomal dominant or recessive trait, but rather seems to have a multifactorial genetic basis. Vitiligo in childhood shows an increased segmental presentation, more frequent autoimmune or endocrine anomalies, high incidence of premature graying in the families, and a poor response to PUVA therapy.

The psychologic effect of vitiligo should not be underestimated. Patients are frequently anxious or depressed because of the appearance of their skin and the way it affects their social interactions. Referring the patient to a mental health professional or the Vitiligo Foundation may be helpful in this situation.

Occupational Vitiligo

Thiols, phenolic compounds, catechol, derivatives of catechol, mercaptoamines, and several quinones produce depigmentation. All of the intermediates in the biosynthesis of melanin are phenolic compounds, and it has been suggested that accumulation of these within the melanocyte may damage or kill the cell. The clinical pattern may be very similar to idiopathic vitiligo, but lesions tend to be concentrated in areas of contact with the incriminated substance. Occupational vitiligo may occur in individuals who work in rubber garments or wear gloves that contain an antioxidant, monobenzyl ether of hydroquinone. Many phenolic compounds can produce leukoderma, with or without antecedent dermatitis. Examples are paratertiary butylphenol, amylphenol, and butylcatechol; alkyl phenols; sulfhydryls; and monobenzyl ether of hydroquinone. One source of these is phenolic antiseptic detergents used in hospitals. Adhesives and glues containing them may be found in shoes, wristbands, and adhesive tape, and rubber products used in brassieres, girdles, panties, or condoms may also be at fault. Self-sticking bindis (the cosmetic used by many Indian women on the forehead) has been reported to induce leukoderma from the adhesive material. Also, electrocardiograph electrodes may cause similar round hypopigmented spots at the site of contact. A similar pattern of postinflammatory hypopigmentation simulating vitiligo is observed around the mouth, in persons with no prior history of allergic dermatitis but with a positive patch test to cinnamates.

PATHOGENESIS. Three possible mechanisms that have been proposed as inducing vitiligo are autoimmunity, neurohumoral factors, and autocytotoxicity. None of these mechanisms has been conclusively proven.

HISTOPATHOLOGY. There is a complete absence of melanocytes. Usually there is no inflammatory component.

DIFFERENTIAL DIAGNOSIS. Vitiligo must be differentiated from morphea and lichen sclerosis, both of which are hypopigmented but associated with a change in the skin texture. Pityriasis alba has a fine scale, is slightly papular, and is poorly defined. Tinea versicolor favors the center back and chest, has a fine scale, and yeast and hyphal forms are demonstrable with potassium hydroxide (KOH) examination. The tertiary stage of pinta might easily lead to diagnostic confusion, but a travel history and serologic testing will help elucidate the diagnosis.

TREATMENT. Vitiligo is a frustrating condition to treat. Spontaneous repigmentation occurs in no more than 15% to 25% of cases. Response is slow, and response rates are low. In addition, some forms of treatment, such as PUVA, actually worsen the appearance of the vitiligo initially by pigmenting surrounding skin, accentuating the depigmented areas.

Because the major concern is cosmetic, various cover-up strategies have been developed. There are various brands of make-up available to temporarily conceal the lesions. Topical dyes are more resistant to washing off and are very acceptable to some patients. The newer self-tanning creams are useful for light-skinned patients with acral lesions.

Fair-skinned patients with vitiligo may sometimes effec-

tively manage their disease with sunblock. If the patient can prevent tanning of the skin around the vitiligo lesions, the lesions will appear similar to the untanned skin and require no additional treatment. Sun protection is mandatory in all patients with vitiligo because of the loss of protection from UV radiation in the depigmented skin.

Topical steroids may be useful on focal or limited lesions. The thinner skinned areas of the face seem to respond best. Trunk and acral lesions are often resistant to this treatment. Mid to super high–potency steroids are often required, with the strength tapered as the lesions respond. A 2-month trial should be attempted. Although systemic steroids lead to temporary repigmentation, this is usually lost as the steroidal agents are tapered, so this is usually not a viable long-term strategy.

PUVA therapy has been used topically and systemically to treat vitiligo for centuries and is the most commonly used treatment for generalized vitiligo. Topical application of 8-methoxypsoralen at a concentration of 0.05% to 0.1%, followed by UVA exposure, may lead to repigmentation. Topical PUVA is used for focal or limited lesions. Inadvertent burns with blistering are frequent during treatment, even when the patient is treated by professionals. For this reason, topical PUVA is very difficult for the patient to do at home.

Trioxsalen, at a dose of up to 20 to 40 mg (not the 10 mg recommended in the PDR and package insert), is taken a few hours before natural sun exposure. The risk of phototoxicity is low, so the patient can do this form of treatment at home. Ocular protection must be worn from the ingestion of the drug through the whole treatment day.

Most commonly, 8-methoxypsoralen is used. Initially, treatment is every other day (because of the delayed erythema of PUVA) but may be increased to daily once the dose is defined. An hour to an hour and a half before UVA exposure, 8-methoxypsoralen 0.5 mg/kg is ingested. The initial UVA dose is 1 or 2 J/cm^2, which is gradually increased; 5-MOP has an efficacy equal to that of 8-MOP and has less risk of phototoxicity. Two or three treatments are done per week. In 20% of patients, total repigmentation occurs; another 30% to 40% have a partial response. Acral, periorificial, and segmental lesions respond less well. Darker-skinned patients have a better result, since they tolerate higher UV doses. Repigmentation may begin after 15 to 25 treatments; however, significant improvement may take as many as 100 to 300 treatments. If follicular repigmentation has not appeared after 3 to 6 months or approximately 50 treatments, PUVA treatments should be discontinued. Known photosensitivity, porphyria, liver disease, and systemic lupus erythematosus are contraindications to psoralen therapy.

Phenylalanine/UVA (PAUVA) is substantially less effective than PUVA. UVB therapy alone with 311-nm irradiation is associated with a higher rate of acute phototoxic events but may also be successful. UVA plus topical steroids is superior to either agent alone, but only 24% to 36% repigmentation can be achieved after 9 months of therapy.

Surgical treatments can be applied to limited lesions if the above methods have not proved beneficial, but these are time consuming. Epidermal grafting, autologous minigrafts, and transplantation of cultured and noncultured melanocytes have all been reported to be effective. The vitiligo should be stable if surgical approaches are to be undertaken.

Total depigmentation. If more than 50% of the body surface area is affected by vitiligo, the patient can consider depigmentation. This form of treatment should be considered permanent, and the goal of treatment is total depigmentation. Limited areas (such as those exposed daily) may be treated, but satellite and distant depigmentation may occur, so the action of the medication cannot be limited to the applied area. Monobenzone (monobenzyl ether of hydroquinone) 20% is applied twice daily for 3 to 6 months to residual pigmented areas. Up to 10 months may be required to complete the treatment. About one in six patients so treated experiences acute dermatitis, usually confined to the still-pigmented areas, but this rarely limits treatment.

Bajaj AK, et al: Bindi depigmentation. *Arch Dermatol* 1983, 119:629.

Behl PN: Repigmentation of segmental vitiligo by autologous minigrafting. *J Am Acad Dermatol* 1985, 12:19.

Berterle C, et al: Incidence and significance of organ-specific autoimmune disorders (clinical, latent or only autoantibodies) in patients with vitiligo. *Dermatologica* 1985, 171:419.

Doersma BR: Repigmentation in vitiligo vulgaris by autologous minigrafting. *J Am Acad Dermatol* 1995, 33:990.

Cormane RH, et al: Phenylalanine and UV light in vitiligo. *Arch Dermatol Res* 1985, 277:176.

Cowan CI, et al: Ocular disturbances in vitiligo. *J Am Acad Dermatol* 1986, 15:17.

el-Mofty AM, et al: Clinical study of a new preparation of 8-methoxypsoralen in photochemotherapy. *Int J Dermatol* 1994, 33:588.

Falabella R, et al: The minigrafting test for vitiligo. *J Am Acad Dermatol* 1995, 32:228.

Gould IM: Vitiligo in diabetes mellitus. *Br J Dermatol* 1985, 113:153.

Grimes PE, et al: Determination of optimal topical photochemotherapy for vitiligo. *J Am Acad Dermatol* 1982, 7:771.

Halder RM, et al: Childhood vitiligo. *J Am Acad Dermatol* 1987, 16:948.

Hann SK, et al: Treatment of vitiligo with oral 5-methyoxypsoralen. *J Dermatol* 1991, 18:324.

Koga M: Epidermal grafting using the tops of suction blisters in the treatment of vitiligo. *Arch Dermatol* 1988, 124:1656.

Koh HK, et al: Malignant melanoma and vitiligo-like leukoderma. *J Am Acad Dermatol* 1983, 9:696.

Kovacs SO: Vitiligo. *J Am Acad Dermatol* 1998, 38:647.

Kumari J: Vitiligo treated with topical clobetasol propionate. *Arch Dermatol* 1984, 120:6.

Lerner AB, et al: Repopulation of pigment cells in patients with vitiligo. *Arch Dermatol* 1988, 124:1701.

Mathias CGT, et al: Perioral leukoderma simulating vitiligo from use of a toothpaste containing cinnamic aldehyde. *Arch Dermatol* 1980, 116:1172.

Monk B: Topical fluorouracil in vitiligo. *Arch Dermatol* 1985, 121:25.

Mosher DB, et al: Monobenzyl ether of hydroquinone: a retrospective study of treatment of 18 vitiligo patients and a review of literature. *Br J Dermatol* 1977, 97:669.

Naughton GK, et al: Correlation between vitiligo autoantibodies and extent of depigmentation in vitiligo. *J Am Acad Dermatol* 1986, 15:978.

Naughton GK, et al: Detection of autoantibodies to melanocytes in vitiligo by specific immunoprecipitation. *J Invest Dermatol* 1983, 81:540.

Nordlund JJ, et al: Dermatitis produced by applications of monobenzone in patients with active vitiligo. *Arch Dermatol* 1985, 121:1141.

Olsson MJ, et al: Transplantation of melanocytes in vitiligo. *Br J Dermatol* 1995, 132:587.

Ortel B, et al: Treatment of vitiligo with khellin and ultraviolet A. *J Am Acad Dermatol* 1988, 18:693.

Suvanprakorn P, et al: Melanocyte autologous grafting for treatment of leukoderma. *J Am Acad Dermatol* 1985, 13:968.

Urbauck RW: Tar vitiligo therapy. *J Am Acad Dermatol* 1983, 8:755.

Weigand DA: Contact hypopigmentation from electrocardiograph electrodes. *J Am Acad Dermatol* 1986, 15:1048.

Westerhof W, et al: Left-Right comparison study of the combination of fluticasone propionate and UVA vs either fluticasone propionate or UVA alone for the long-term treatment of vitiligo. *Arch Dermatol* 1999, 135:1061.

Westerhof W, et al: Treatment of vitiligo with UV-B radiation vs. topical psoralen plus UV-A. *Arch Dermatol* 1997, 133:1525. _____ ▲

VOGT-KOYANAGI-HARADA SYNDROME

Vogt-Koyanagi-Harada (VKHS) syndrome is a disease complex characterized by marked bilateral uveitis, symmetrical vitiligo, alopecia, white scalp hair, eyelashes and brows (poliosis), and dysacousia (diminished hearing). The disease usually occurs in adults in their third decade of life. The initial or meningoencephalitic phase occurs with prodromata of fever, malaise, headache, nausea, and vomiting. Variable involvement including psychosis, paraplegia, hemiparesis, aphasia, and nuchal rigidity occur. Recovery is usually complete. The second phase, the ophthalmic-auditory stage, is characterized by uveitis, which may appear rapidly and last for up to 10 years. Decreased visual acuity, photophobia (worse with anterior than posterior uveitis), and decreased hearing (in 50% of cases) may also occur. The convalescent phase begins 3 weeks to 3 months after the uveitis appears or after it begins to improve.

The condition is characterized by vitiligo, plus alopecia and poliosis of the scalp, eyebrows, eyelashes, and hairs of the axillae. Alopecia invariably occurs; poliosis occurs in about 90% of patients; vitiligo and temporary deafness occur in about half. Treatment of the ocular inflammatory disease with systemic steroidal agents may prevent blindness.

Heier JS, et al: Vision loss in a woman of American Indian heritage: Vogt-Koyanagi-Harada (VKH) syndrome (uveoencephalitis). *Arch Dermatol* 1995, 131:83.

Ikeda K, et al: How high is high in steroid treatment of Vogt-Koyanagi-Harada syndrome? *Neurology* 1997, 48:537.

Rathinam SR, et al: Vogt-Koyanagi-Harada syndrome after cutaneous injury. *Ophthalmology* 1999, 106:635.

Wong SS, Ng SK, Lee HM: Vogt-Koyanagi-Harada disease: extensive vitiligo with prodromal generalized erythroderma. *Dermatology* 1999, 198:65. _____ ▲

ALEZZANDRINI'S SYNDROME

Alezzandrini's syndrome is a very rare syndrome characterized by a unilateral degenerative retinitis, followed after several months by ipsilateral vitiligo on the face and ipsilateral poliosis. Deafness may also be present.

Hoffman MD, Dudley C: Suspected Alezzandrini's syndrome in a diabetic patient with unilateral retinal detachment and ipsilateral vitiligo and poliosis. *J Am Acad Dermatol* 1992, 26:496. _____ ▲

LEUKODERMA

Postinflammatory leukoderma may result from many inflammatory dermatoses, such as pityriasis rosea, psoriasis, herpes zoster, secondary syphilis, and morphea. Sarcoidosis, tinea versicolor, mycosis fungoides, scleroderma, and pityriasis lichenoides chronica may all present with hypopigmented (only rarely, actually depigmented) lesions, as may leprosy. Burns, scars, postdermabrasion, and intralesional steroid injections with depigmentation are other examples of leukoderma.

Friedman SJ, et al: Perilesional linear atrophy and hypopigmentation after intralesional corticosteroid therapy. *J Am Acad Dermatol* 1988, 19:537. _____ ▲

ALBINISM

Albinism is a partial or complete congenital absence of pigment in the skin, hair, and eyes (oculocutaneous albinism), or the eyes alone (ocular albinism) (Fig. 36-9). The cutaneous phenotype of the various forms of albinism is broad, but the ocular phenotype is reasonably constant in most forms. This includes decreased visual acuity, nystagmus, pale irides that transilluminate, hypopigmented fundi, hypoplastic foveae, and lack of stereopsis. The recent discovery of the genetic basis of many of the forms of albinism has dramatically changed the classification scheme.

Oculocutaneous Albinism 1

Oculocutaneous albinism 1 (OCA 1) results from mutations in the tyrosinase gene. Affected patients are homozygous for the mutant gene or are compound heterozygotes for different mutations in the tyrosinase gene. It is therefore an autosomal recessive disorder. OCA 1 is divided into two forms: OCA 1A and OCA 1B. At birth they are indistinguishable. OCA 1A is the most severe form, with complete absence of tyrosinase activity and complete absence of melanin in the skin and eyes. Visual acuity is decreased to 20/400. With OCA 1B, tyrosinase activity is greatly reduced but not absent. Affected patients may show increase in skin, hair, and eye color with age, and can tan. OCA 1B was

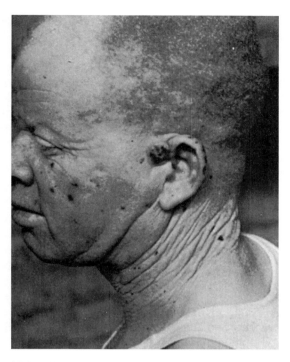

Fig. 36-9 Albinism with numerous basal cell carcinomas and squamous cell carcinoma on the ear. (Courtesy Dr. S.F. Rosen.)

originally called "yellow mutant" albinism. Temperature-sensitive OCA (OCA 1-TS) results from mutations in the tyrosinase gene that produce an enzyme with limited activity below 35° C (95° F) and no activity above this temperature. Affected patients have white hair, skin, and eyes at birth. At puberty, dark hair develops in cooler acral areas.

Oculocutaneous Albinism 2

Oculocutaneous albinism 2 (OCA 2) has a prevalence of 1:15,000. Patients were formerly called "tyrosinase-positive" albinos. Inheritance is autosomal recessive and results from mutations in the P gene. The P gene codes a membrane transport protein that is present in the melanosome membrane. The cutaneous phenotype of OCA 2 patients is broad, from nearly normal pigmentation to virtually no pigment. Pigmentation increases with age, and visual acuity improves from infancy to adolescence. Prader-Willi and Angleman syndromes are caused by deletions in the same chromosomal region as the P gene. One percent of patients with these syndromes also have OCA 2.

Oculocutaneous Albinism 3

Oculocutaneous albinism 3 (OCA 3) is an autosomal recessive disorder caused by mutations in the tyrosine-related protein 1 (TRP-1), located on chromosome 9. OCA 3 has been described only in black patients and is characterized by light brown hair, light brown skin, blue/brown irides, nystagmus, and decreased visual activity. Brown rather than black melanin is formed.

Ocular Albinism

There are multiple forms of ocular albinism. OA 1 may present with lighter skin than expected. It is X linked. Female carriers have "mud-splattered" fundi. Macromelanosomes are found in the skin, so skin biopsy may be used to help establish this diagnosis. Many cases of autosomal recessive ocular albinism have been reclassified as OCA 1 or OCA 2.

Syndromes Associated with Albinism

Chédiak-Higashi Syndrome. Chédiak-Higashi syndrome is an autosomal recessive disorder characterized by oculocutaneous albinism and immunologic deficiency, including defective phagocyte, lymphocyte, and natural killer (NK) cell function. Antibody-dependent cellular cytotoxicity is also defective. Eighty-five percent of CHS patients develop an accelerated phase characterized by a lymphocyte and macrophage activation syndrome. The results of liver function tests will be abnormal, and fever, hepatosplenomegaly, lymphadenopathy, pancytopenia, and infiltration of the central nervous system occur.

Although the accelerated phase may respond to etoposide plus systemic steroid and intrathecal methotrexate, relapses invariably occur. These relapses are less responsive to treatment and are eventually fatal.

Giant intracytoplasmic inclusion bodies are seen in most granulated cells. The gene is located on chromosome 1. Lysosomal transport is defective. Giant melanosomes cause pigment dilution, with hypopigmentation of skin, hair, and fundi. The hair is a frosted, metallic gray color. Unless they undergo bone marrow transplantation, most patients die in childhood.

Hermansky-Pudlak Syndrome

Hermansky-Pudlak syndrome is a rare autosomal recessive disorder consisting of oculocutaneous albinism, a hemorrhagic diathesis secondary to the absence of dense bodies in platelets, and accumulation of a ceroidlike material in the reticuloendothelial system, visceral organs, oral mucosa, and urine. Patients with this disorder have a history of easy bruisability, epistaxis, gingival bleeding, hemoptysis, and bleeding after various surgical procedures and childbirth. Interstitial pulmonary fibrosis, inflammatory bowel disease, renal failure, and cardiomyopathy are late complications. One in 21 Puerto Ricans has a mutation (usually a 16-bp duplication) in the HPS gene (HPS1), which is located at 10q23. HPS accounts for 80% of albinos in Puerto Rico, and 1 in 1800 Puerto Ricans has HPS. Patients may have completely absent to normal pigmentation, and the majority have the ocular findings typical of albinism. Atypical nevi, acanthosis nigricans–like lesions in the axillae and neck and

trichomegaly also occur. Solar damage as evidenced by solar lentigines, actinic keratoses, and nonmelanoma skin cancers occurs in 80% of patients with the 16-bp duplication in HPS1.

Griscelli Syndrome (Partial Albinism with Immunodeficiency)

Griscelli syndrome is a rare autosomal recessive syndrome characterized by variable pigmentary dilution, silvery metallic hair, frequent pyogenic infections, neutropenia, and thrombocytopenia. Defective NK cell function, impaired delayed type hypersensitivity, and hypogammaglobulinemia are present. The giant cytoplasmic granules seen in Chédiak-Higashi syndrome are absent. Neurologic features are prominent. Patients develop an accelerated phase similar to patients with Chédiak-Higashi disease.

Histologically, melanocytes are hyperpigmented and filled with stage IV melanosomes, whereas adjacent keratinocytes contain only sparse melanosomes. Giant melanosomes are not seen. Hair bulbs reveal uneven clusters of aggregated melanin pigment in the medulla of the shaft.

Elejalde Syndrome

Elejalde syndrome is a rare autosomal recessive syndrome consisting of moderate pigment dilution with silvery, metallic hair, prominent neurologic defects, but no immune defects. Hair findings are similar to those of Griscelli syndrome, but a skin biopsy reveals a normal histologic picture. Incomplete melanization of melanosomes in melanocytes is present.

Cross-McKusick-Breen Syndrome

Also known as *Cross syndrome, oculocerebral-hypopigmentation syndrome,* or *hypopigmentation and microphthalmia,* this extremely rare disorder is characterized by white skin, blond hair with a yellow-gray metallic sheen, small eyes with cloudy corneas, jerky nystagmus, gingival fibromatosis, and severe mental and physical retardation.

Cuna Moon Children

The Cuna Indians live on the San Blas islands and on the nearby Atlantic coast in Colombia. The Cuna are a pure race among whom there is frequent inbreeding. The frequency of albinism among these Indians is about 1 in 100. Cuna Indian albinos are called "moon children" because they have photophobia and prefer to go outdoors only at night. About the age of 10, the skin of the moon children becomes wrinkled, freckled, and easily blistered by sunshine. The scalp hair is silky and white to straw-colored, sometimes with a reddish tinge. The irides are yellow, gray, or light blue. Nystagmus and other visual anomalies are common. Benign and malignant tumors are common; consequently, their life expectancy is shorter than that of other Cuna Indians.

Selenium Deficiency

Selenium deficiency in the setting of total parenteral nutrition can lead to pseudoalbinism. Skin and hair pigmentation return to normal with supplementation.

Waardenburg's Syndrome

Four genotypic variants of Waardenburg's syndrome exist, with overlapping phenotypic features. Types 1 and 3 are caused by mutations in the PAX gene on chromosome 2. Type 2 is caused by mutations in the MITF gene on chromosome 3, and type 4 is due to mutations in the ENDRB gene on chromosome 13. Patients with this syndrome have some features of piebaldism, with a white forelock, hypopigmentation, premature graying, and other characteristic findings including synophrys, congenital deafness, a broad nasal root, and ocular changes including heterochromia irides. Apparently, melanoblasts fail to reach the target sites during embryogenesis (see Chapter 27).

PIEBALDISM

Piebaldism is a rare, autosomal dominant syndrome with variable phenotype, presenting at birth. The characteristic clinical features are a white forelock, and patchy absence of skin pigment (Fig. 36-10). The depigmented lesions are static and characteristically occur on the anterior and posterior trunk, mid upper arm to wrist, mid-thigh to mid-calf, and shins. A characteristic feature of piebaldism is the presence of hyperpigmented macules within the areas of lack of pigmentation and also on normally pigmented skin. The white forelock arises from a triangular or diamond-shaped midline white macule on the frontal scalp or forehead. The medial portions of the eyebrows, and eyelashes, may be white. Histologically, melanocytes are completely absent in the white macules.

Piebaldism is caused by mutations in the c-kit proto-oncogene. The phenotypic differences between families is caused by different locations of mutations in the gene. A mild phenotype occurs in cases associated with mutations in the ligand binding region, whereas more severe phenotypes occur from mutations in the tyrosine-kinase end of the genome. The white lesions may respond to surgical corrections (see discussion under vitiligo).

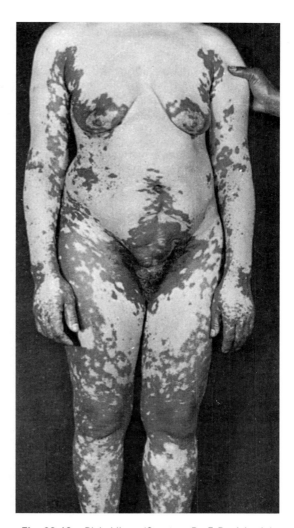

Fig. 36-10   Piebaldism. (Courtesy Dr. F. Daniels, Jr.)

Spritz RA: Molecular basis of human piebaldism. *J Invest Dermatol* 1994 103(Suppl):137.

Spritz RA, Oh J: HPS gene mutations in Hermansky-Pudlak syndrome (letter). *Am J Hum Genet* 1999, 64:658.

Tomita Y: The molecular genetics of albinism and piebaldism. *Arch Dermatol* 1994, 130:355.

Toro J, Turner M, Gahl WA: Dermatologic manifestations of Hermansky-Pudlak syndrome in patients with and without a 16-base pair duplication in the HPS1 gene. *Arch Dermatol* 1999, 135:774.

Vinton NE, et al: Macrocytosis and pseudoalbinism. *J Pediatr* 1987, 111:711.

Yoshiike T, et al: Macromelanosomes in x-linked ocular albinism. *Acta Derm Venereol* 1985, 65:66. _____ ▲

Bolognia JL, et al: Biology of hypopigmentation. *J Am Acad Dermatol* 1988, 19:217.

Carden SM, et al: Albinism. *Br J Ophthal* 1998, 82:189.

Haddad E, et al: Treatment of Chédiak-Higashi syndrome by allogenic bone marrow transplantation. *Blood* 1995, 85:3328.

Leal I, et al: Chédiak-Higashi syndrome in a Venezuelan black child. *J Am Acad Dermatol* 1985, 13:337.

Mancini AJ, et al: Partial albinism with immunodeficiency: Griscelli syndrome. *J Am Acad Dermatol* 1998, 38:295.

IDIOPATHIC GUTTATE HYPOMELANOSIS (LEUKOPATHIA SYMMETRICA PROGRESSIVA)

Idiopathic guttate hypomelanosis is a very common acquired disorder that affects women more frequently than men; it usually occurs after age 40. In a study that examined 400 patients, prevalence was 46%. The lesions occur chiefly on the shins and forearms; they are small (6 or 8 mm), rarely become very numerous (a dozen or two at most), and never occur on the trunk or face. The lesions are irregularly shaped and very sharply defined, like depigmented ephelides, and are of only minor cosmetic significance.

Falabella R, et al: On the pathogenesis of idiopathic guttate hypomelanosis. *J Am Acad Dermatol* 1987, 16:35. _____ ▲

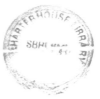

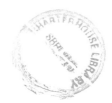

CHAPTER 37

Dermatologic Surgery

The practice of dermatology has always included surgical procedures, but with the advent of the twenty-first century the surgical side of dermatology is growing. The basic foundation of correct biopsy, including simple destructive and excisional technique, has not changed since this text's last edition. In contrast, the more specialized fields of cutaneous laser and aesthetic surgery continue to change rapidly. Nonetheless, as the trend within the specialty of dermatology toward increasingly complex surgical and cosmetic procedures grows, the diagnosis and treatment of skin cancer continues to be the cornerstone of dermatologic surgery. In this chapter we will discuss the simpler procedures that all dermatologists should be competent to perform, as well as the basics of more complex surgical procedures with which dermatologists may wish to be familiar.

PREPARATION FOR SURGERY

Before any surgical procedure, preoperative evaluation should include questions about drug allergies (especially to local anesthetics), medications (including aspirin and warfarin [Coumadin]), the presence of pacemakers, and any prior wound infections or medical history of recently implanted prosthetics, or endocarditis. True allergy to local anesthetics is extremely rare, but vasovagal reactions are relatively common. If extensive surgery is planned, aspirin should be discontinued 2 weeks before the procedure when possible. If a procedure is performed within a few centimeters of a pacemaker, electrosurgery should be executed with extreme care or possibly replaced by true cautery (heat only, no electric transmission). Although modern devices are better shielded and less likely to respond to external electrical interference, it is always prudent to consult with the patient's cardiologist and deliver current in short bursts of less than 5 seconds. If possible, one should consider postponing surgery on a recently infected wound, or prescribe antibiotics to decrease the risk of wound infection (Box 37-1).

The workhorse anesthetic of dermatologic surgery is lidocaine (Xylocaine). Longer-acting anesthetics, such as bupivacaine (Marcaine/Sensorcaine), are also employed for special procedures such as nerve and digital blocks. Epinephrine is often added to decrease bleeding and increase duration of anesthetic if appropriate for the procedure planned. Effective topical anesthetics, including EMLA cream and ELA-Max cream, are now available to make the pinprick from local anesthetic more bearable, and can be especially helpful in children.

The thoughtful choice of instruments and suture depends on the procedure being performed. Most simple, in-office biopsies are performed in a "clean" rather than sterile manner, and require minimal instruments. More complex excisional and reconstructive surgery is generally performed with sterile technique and employs a "standard" surgical tray with a wider range of instruments (Box 37-2). For procedures requiring sutures, absorbable material is used for deeper, layered closures, whereas surface sutures are generally nonabsorbable or fast-absorbing (Box 37-3). Facial sutures are often taken out in 4 to 7 days to decrease the chance of forming track marks from epithelialization of the suture puncture site, whereas sutures on the scalp, neck, and body are often left in for 2 weeks. Running subcuticular sutures can be left in for 3 weeks to add tensile strength to wounds without the risk of track marks.

Many surgical preparations are available, including isopropyl alcohol, hexachlorophene (pHisoHex), Phisoderm, chlorhexidine (Hibiclens), Techni-Care, and Betadine. Alcohol is the most common skin antiseptic agent for clean, but not sterile procedures since it has only weak antimicrobial activity. Hexachlorophene should not be used on children or pregnant women, because of potential neurotoxicity and teratogenicity, respectively. Chlorhexidine can cause keratitis if direct ocular contact occurs, and should therefore be avoided around the eyes. Hydrogen peroxide has no significant antiseptic properties, and thus it is not suitable for sterile skin preparation. Betadine and all iodine-containing preparations are often irritating to the skin, leave a residual

---

BOX 37-1

Preparations Checklist for Cutaneous Surgery

PATIENT HISTORY
Medications
Pacemakers
Need for antibiotic prophylaxis
Allergies

PREOPERATIVE DISCUSSION
Explain techniques, benefits, alternative, and risks of procedure
Obtain written informed consent for procedure

SUPPLIES
Surgical scrub
Anesthetic
Appropriate instruments
Sutures, if needed
Dressing material

BOX 37-2

Basic Cutaneous Surgical Tray

Scalpel handle (flat No. 3)
Blade (No. 15)
Curettes (3 and 5 mm)
Needle holder (appropriate for suture material)
Iris scissors, curved and straight
Undermining scissors
Skin hook (double prong)
Hemostats (curved and straight)
Forceps (toothed)
Skin preparatory scrub in sterile basin
Sterile towels and cotton-tipped swabs
Sterile gauze (4 × 4 and 2 × 2 cm)
Hyfrecator cover (penrose or sanisleeve)
Appropriate suture material
Suture scissors
Towel clamps

BOX 37-3

Common Skin Suture Material

ABSORBABLE
Gut (chromic, fast absorbing,* plain)
Polyglycolic acid (Dexon)
Polyglactin 910 (Vicryl)
Polydioxanone (PDS)
Polytrimethylylene carbonate (Maxon)
Poliglecaprone 25 (Monocryl)

NONABSORBABLE
Silk
Nylon (Dermalon, Ethilon, Surgilon)
Polypropylene (Prolene, Surgilene)
Polyester (Dacron, Ethibond, Mersilene)
Polybutester (Novafil)

*Fast-absorbing gut is used as a surface suture since it loses tensile strength within days.

BOX 37-4

Indications for Antibiotic Prophylaxis in Patients Undergoing Cutaneous Surgery

ABSOLUTE
Artificial heart valve
Recent artificial joint placement (within 6 months)
Past history of endocarditis or rheumatic fever
Mitral valve prolapse with a holosystolic murmur

DISCRETIONARY
Surgery involving mucous membranes
Wounds open longer than 24 hours during prolonged surgery
Immunosuppressed patients

---

color, can be absorbed in very premature infants, and must dry before the procedure to act as an effective antimicrobial agent.

Antibiotic prophylaxis is not generally given for small punch-and-shave biopsies but is considered for larger excisions and any procedure on mucous membranes in appropriate patients (Box 37-4). Although prophylactic antibiotics are warranted when operating in certain high-risk anatomic sites, in patients at risk for endocarditis or with recently implanted prosthetics, the literature does not support routine perioperative antibiotics without specific indications. Cephalexin (Keflex) is the preferred antibiotic. The dose is 1 g orally 1 hour before the procedure or intramuscularly a few minutes before the procedure, with a second dose of 500 mg taken orally 6 hours after the procedure. For penicillin-allergic patients, erythromycin at the same dose is adequate.

BIOPSIES

When performing a skin biopsy, the clinician should consider the lesion, reason for biopsy (e.g., diagnostic versus cosmetic), and site. Shave biopsies can range from a superficial snip of an epidermal growth to deep shave excisions of papillary dermal processes. Punch biopsies are most often used for dermal lesions, sampling deeper than shave biopsies, but requiring sutures. Excisional biopsies remove an entire clinical lesion and are the biopsy of choice for pigmented lesions suspicious for melanoma. Incisional biopsies remove a portion of a clinical lesion and are often performed on larger plaques or patches when an excisional biopsy is not cosmetically acceptable or feasible. A wedge biopsy is a deep incisional biopsy that can sample pathologic tissue and adjacent normal tissue, and is especially useful for pathologic diagnosis of certain inflammatory conditions (e.g., panniculitis, fasciitis).

Shave biopsy or shave excision is a simple and quick technique with high applicability to dermatology. With proper selection of lesion and location, cosmetically acceptable cure or the rapid procurement of adequate biopsy material can be achieved. The lack of sutures and the speed of the procedure may be of great importance in children or anxious adults.

This technique is best suited to pedunculated, papular, or otherwise exophytic lesions. However, using a deep or rolled shave, one can also use this procedure to obtain samples of macular or indurated lesions for biopsy, provided the necessary histologic changes reside in the epidermis or papillary dermis. Examples of lesions that are amenable to shave excision include seborrheic and actinic keratoses, intradermal nevi, pyogenic granulomas, warts, and superficial basal and squamous cell carcinomas.

Local anesthesia is required before a shave excision, for pain control and to facilitate the procedure. The intradermal instillation of anesthetic distends and elevates the lesion, increases skin turgor, and affords greater resistance to the blade, giving better control to the operator. It also facilitates undercutting the lesion.

The shave excision is generally performed with a No. 15 blade on a handle. Bigger lesions may require a No. 10 blade. After injection of the anesthetic, the skin surrounding the lesion is pinched up with the thumb and third finger. This stabilizes the lesion and aids hemostasis. With the blade edge parallel to the skin surface, the excision is then performed with one or more sweeping strokes. A rapid sawing motion may damage the specimen and impair the cosmetic result. Just before the blade exits the skin, the lesion should be stabilized with the index finger to avoid tearing the last bit of tissue. Hemostasis is easily attained with 35% aluminum chloride solution. Monsel's solution may stain the skin with iron deposition, and electrofulguration may make the scar less cosmetically acceptable and prolong healing.

A variation of this procedure may be performed with a Gillette Blue Blade razor. Cut in half longitudinally by twisting between two hemostats or with a heavy scissors, this tool is extremely sharp and also bends enough to follow the skin's or the lesion's contour. It is particularly useful for shave removal of lesions on convex surfaces such as the nasal tip or alae, jaw line, or helix of the ear (Fig. 37-1).

Sharp scissors excisions are a variant of shave excisions. In this procedure, two scissors blades are used simultaneously in opposing directions to remove a lesion parallel to

the skin surface. As with the scalpel, an open wound is left that, depending on its depth, may have an excellent cosmetic outcome. The scissors excision is very quickly performed. It is best suited for pedunculated lesions such as skin tags, filiform warts, and baggy (Unna's) nevi. However, it is also an excellent technique for debulking lesions of softer consistency, such as basal cell carcinomas and large warts, providing good-quality biopsy specimens before performing curettage and electrodesiccation. It has its greatest value in very flaccid, elastotic skin.

For smaller or pedunculated lesions, sharp scissors excision may not require anesthesia, since the sting of the scissors is fleeting and less painful than the injection. The distal lesion is grasped with a fine-toothed forceps (e.g., Adson's toothed forceps) and gently elevated. Using the tips of a sharp, curved iris scissors or small tenotomy scissors, the base is quickly cut flush with the skin surface. Hemostasis may not be necessary, but can easily be obtained with pressure or aluminum chloride.

The dermatologic punch is a round knife with great versatility. In the experienced hand it can perform many different tasks with speed and cosmetic acceptability. Punches are available in sizes ranging from 2 to 10 mm. Most punches now used are disposable.

The most common use of punches is for skin biopsy. These tools generally provide adequate epidermal and dermal specimens when 3- or 4-mm punches are employed. To diagnose scalp alopecia, a 6-mm punch is preferred to ensure that an appropriate number of follicles can be examined. Punches are generally not suitable for biopsy of conditions involving the subcutaneous tissue, since they do not go deep enough to adequately sample the subcutis. A superior cosmetic result can be obtained compared with all but the most superficial shave biopsies, and a far better histologic specimen is the rule. The procedure is more quickly performed than fusiform excision and requires less expertise.

Punches may also be used to completely excise lesions, to treat acne scars, and for hair transplantation. The dermatologic punch is an easy tool to use, but some finesse is necessary to obtain optimal specimens and cosmetic results. It is important to choose the right size punch depending on the lesion's size, type, and location. After properly cleansing the skin, an intradermal wheal is raised by injection of local anesthetic. Anesthesia will be achieved immediately, and the quality of the biopsy specimen is improved by firming up the skin. Care must be taken when using the punch not to apply too much downward pressure. Too much pressure may result in a tapering or conical shape of the specimen removed. This will limit the tissue for histologic examination and may cause artifact.

Before performing a punch excision or biopsy the normal skin tension lines should be determined. Using the thumb and forefinger, stretch the skin perpendicular to these lines. After the punch incision is performed, release of the stretch will result in the formation of an elliptical wound, which

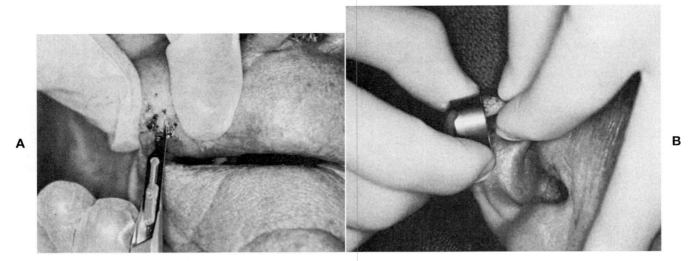

Fig. 37-1   Shave biopsy techniques. **A**, Technique for shave excision, using smooth, sweeping strokes. **B**, Shave excision using a blue blade razor.

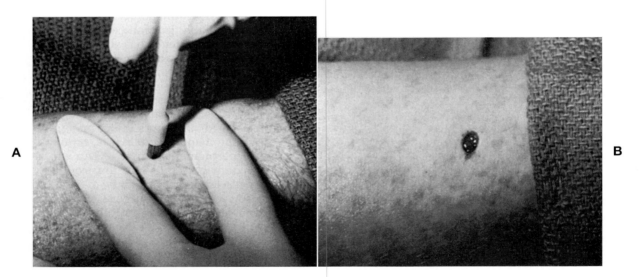

Fig. 37-2   **A** and **B**, Technique for performing a punch.

can be closed within normal skin tension lines without "dog ears."

Grasped between the thumb and first two fingers, the punch is placed on the skin perpendicular to the surface. While applying gentle pressure, it is rotated back and forth and advanced to the hub. The edge of the specimen is then gently grasped with a toothed forceps or "scooped" out with the punch so as not to crush the skin. If the base of the specimen is tethered to the underlying fatty tissue, an iris scissors is used to snip the tissue free. Hemostasis can be obtained by a styptic solution, light electrofulguration, or pressure. Closure should be performed with one or two sutures to avoid a depressed scar (Fig. 37-2).

Narrow hole extrusion is a surgical technique that uses a punch biopsy to make a small cutaneous portal through which larger benign growths (e.g., lipoma, cyst) can be extruded. This technique allows the evacuation of large subcutaneous growths with a relatively small surface incision, leading to improved final cosmetic outcome (Fig. 37-3).

DESTRUCTIVE TECHNIQUES

Curettage, cryosurgery, and electrosurgery are the mainstays of dermatologic techniques for destruction of both benign and malignant lesions. If pathologic examination of tissue

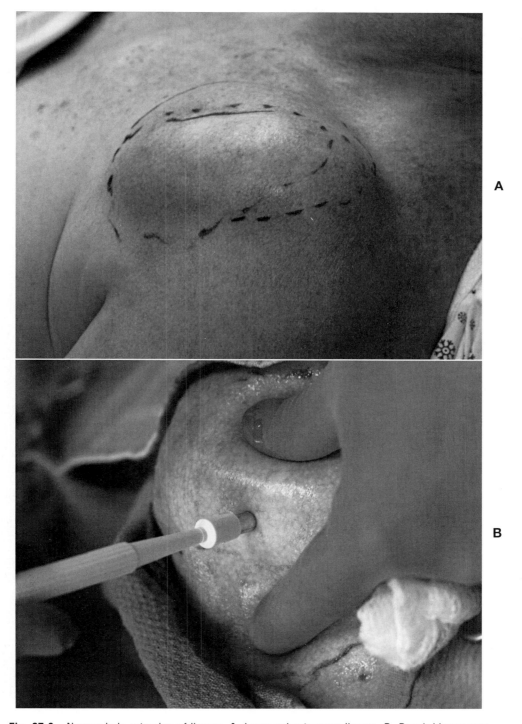

Fig. 37-3   Narrow hole extrusion of lipoma. **A,** Large subcutaneous lipoma. **B,** Punch biopsy over center of subcutaneous mass.   *Continued*

is required, an excisional rather than destructive technique should be employed. With the increasing diversity and availability of lasers, many benign and malignant lesions can be destroyed with equal or superior cosmesis to these basic destructive techniques (see following discussion).

Curettage

The curette has long been a standard tool in the dermatologist's surgical armamentarium. This round, semisharp knife is available in sizes from 0.5 to 10 mm, allowing for the removal of a variety of lesions. The proper selection of

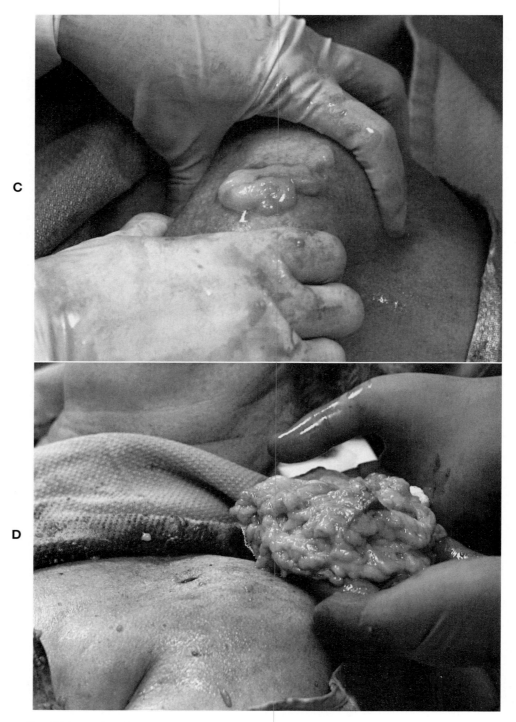

Fig. 37-3, cont'd C, Extrusion of lipoma through narrow hole of punch biopsy. **D,** Entire lipoma extruded through small cutaneous incision.

lesion, its location, and the size of the curette, combined with the surgeon's technique, all play a role in both the therapeutic and cosmetic outcome.

Because it is not as sharp as a scalpel, the curette does not easily cut through normal epidermis and will not enter the dermis. Therefore, it is best suited for use on soft or friable lesions such as warts, seborrheic and actinic keratoses, the papules of molluscum contagiosum, or selected basal and squamous cell carcinomas.

Appropriate choice of curette size is important. Too

small a diameter may cause severe fragmentation of a biopsy specimen and is inefficient. A curette that is too large may cause unnecessary damage to normal tissue, as well as miss small extensions of tumor growth into the deeper dermis.

Use of the curette is simple, and the technique is quickly learned by first-year residents. Nonetheless, a necessary degree of expertise must be achieved. In 1977, Kopf et al showed that recurrence rates of basal cell carcinomas were far higher when residents rather than attending physicians performed curettage and electrodesiccation.

Except for treatment of extremely small or superficial lesions, anesthesia must be used to ensure patient comfort when using the curette. The skin should be stabilized with the nondominant hand while the curette is held like a pencil or a potato-peeler in the dominant hand (Fig. 37-4). Because the most power is delivered toward the surgeon, initial debulking is done in this direction. However, for completeness of excision, the area should be repeatedly curetted in all directions. This also aids in producing symmetrical wound margins. Particularly with malignant lesions, initial debulking should be followed by curettage with a smaller curette, 1 to 3 mm, to eradicate any fine, fingerlike tumor extensions.

The consistency of the normal dermis has a "gritty," firm sensation when curetted, thereby indicating the necessary depth of curettage. A slight amount of punctate dermal bleeding is easily controlled by 35% aluminum chloride or electrodesiccation, if needed.

When treating appropriately selected basal and squamous cell carcinomas (see the section on skin cancer management), curettage must be followed by electrodesiccation. The bulk of the tumor should be removed by vigorous curettage followed by light electrodesiccation of the entire base of the lesion with a 2- to 3-mm margin of surrounding skin. There is little agreement regarding the requisite number of cycles of curettage and electrodesiccation. Indeed, treating all lesions identically with a particular number of cycles may lead to overtreatment of some lesions and undertreatment of others. In general, we employ three cycles to treat selected malignant lesions. Nonetheless, the success of curettage and electrodesiccation (C&D) relies on the operator's ability to identify by feel and appearance the tissue to be ablated. Finally, C&D should be replaced by excision if curettage extends into subcutaneous tissue.

Cryosurgery

Over the past 60 years, especially since the ready availability of liquid nitrogen, cryosurgery has become deeply ingrained in the practice of dermatology. This technique offers several advantages to both physician and patient. It is technically easy to perform, and the reactions heal relatively quickly. Postoperative wound care is simple, and complications are infrequent. Cryosurgery is useful in patients afraid of more directly invasive surgery and electrosurgery.

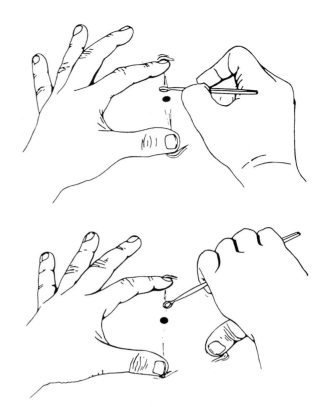

Fig. 37-4 Two techniques for holding the curette: the "pencil" method and the "potato-peeler" method.

The first true cryosurgery was performed in the late nineteenth century by dermatologist A. Campbell White, using solid carbon dioxide. Its use did not become widespread within dermatology, however, until modern apparatus was developed by a neurosurgeon, Irving Cooper, in 1962. Although a number of cryogens are available (including ethyl chloride, Freon, carbon dioxide, and nitrous oxide), liquid nitrogen, with a boiling point of −195.6° C, is most widely used.

The mechanism of cell death following cryosurgery is not completely understood. Several factors are thought to be important, including mechanical damage to cells resulting from rapid crystal formation, exposure to high electrolyte concentrations in surrounding nonfrozen or thawing fluids, recrystallization patterns during thaw, and ischemia caused by vascular stasis and damage. Experience has shown that rapid freezing, followed by a slow thaw, results in increased damage, as do repeated freeze-thaw cycles.

It is known that different cells and tissues demonstrate a range of sensitivities to freezing. Melanocytes are more sensitive than keratinocytes, which is advantageous in treating lentigos, but may produce permanent hypopigmentation in darkly complected patients, or long-lasting reactive hyperpigmentation in Asian patients. Nerves can be damaged, and care must be taken to avoid sensory or functional defects, especially in areas where nerves are relatively superficial (e.g., lateral aspects of the fingers, ulnar groove of the elbow). Hair follicles are also sensitive as demonstrated by the excellent response of trichiasis to cryosurgery. Vascular endothelial cells are also sensitive to freezing. Fibroblasts and stromal structures are less sensitive to the effects of cryosurgery, and this may be an important factor in the lack of scarring seen following superficial procedures.

It is important to grasp the concept of the expanding "ice ball" forming in the tissue during cryosurgery. This must reach an appropriate size in both horizontal and vertical dimensions to effect adequate treatment. A reasonable estimate of depth of freeze can be made by an experienced operator, based on the surface area of ice formation. However, when treating malignant lesions such as basal and squamous cell carcinomas, it is advisable to employ thermocouples to directly measure the depth and duration of the desired isotherm (temperature level) and ensure adequate treatment. In treating benign superficial lesions, some authors believe it is better to undertreat initially. It is better to have to retreat a lesion than to overfreeze the first time and increase the risk of scarring and hypopigmentation.

Liquid nitrogen may be delivered to the skin in numerous ways. The simplest is to use a cotton-tipped applicator. The size may be altered to fit the lesion by removing or adding cotton. The depth of freeze may also be controlled by varying the amount of pressure applied by applicator to the skin; depth of the ice ball increases with increasing pressure. Longer contact will also increase the depth of freeze. Several models of handheld liquid nitrogen spray units are made. These come with a changeable nozzle to vary the size of the stream so that very fine control can be achieved.

Cryoprobes are sophisticated instruments that allow for a very precise delivery of liquid nitrogen to the lesion and fine control of tissue temperature over a wide range. The equipment one selects should reflect the experience and training of the cryosurgeon and the complexity of the cryosurgical procedure.

Numerous lesions, benign or malignant, can be effectively treated by cryosurgery (Box 37-5), either alone or in combination therapy. The bias toward selecting cryosurgery for a particular lesion will certainly be influenced by a physician's training and past experience. It is important to reiterate that cryosurgical treatment of malignant lesions should be carefully monitored with thermocouples and the patient closely followed postoperatively to ensure complete tumor extirpation, since no specimen is created to examine for clear margins.

Side effects of cryosurgery are generally not severe but cause some patient discomfort. Pain is associated with the application of liquid nitrogen. Occasionally, patients will suffer a vasovagal response, so it is advisable to have them lie down, even for small procedures. Postoperatively, there will be a throbbing or burning sensation, the duration and intensity of which will depend on the depth of freeze. Postoperative inflammation and edema are a function of the intensity of the freeze and the location. Areas with

---

BOX 37-5

Lesions Responding to Cryosurgery

Acne (pustules, small cysts)
Actinic cheilitis
Actinic keratosis
Adenoma sebaceum
Angiomas
Basal cell carcinoma (especially superficial)
Bowen's disease
Chondrodermatitis nodularis helicis
Condyloma acuminatum
Dermatofibroma
Elastosis perforans serpiginosa
Epidermal nevi
Granuloma annulare
Keloid (also acne keloidalis)
Keratoacanthoma
Leiomyoma
Leishmaniasis
Lentigo
Molluscum contagiosum
Mucocele
Myxoid cyst
Porokeratosis (including DSAP)
Prurigo nodularis
Sebaceous hyperplasia
Seborrheic keratosis
Skin tags
Steatocystoma
Syringoma
Trichoepithelioma
Venous lakes
Warts
Xanthelasma

---

low-tissue turgor, such as the eyelids and genitalia, will swell more. Bulla formation is common, and the fluid may be quite bloody. If the patient is warned, it should pose no problems. If it is painful, evacuation may help. Infection is uncommon, especially with good wound care.

From 2 to 4 weeks after freezing, a hyperplastic or pseudoepitheliomatous healing response may occur. This is self-limited. Hypertrophic scarring can occur, particularly with very deep freezes. However, mildly atrophic scarring is more common. As melanocytes are quite sensitive to freezing, temporary or permanent hypopigmentation or depigmentation can occur. Patients must be warned about the risk of postcryosurgical pigmentary changes, emphasizing the increasing risk for darker skin tones.

Nerve damage is probably the most worrisome adverse reaction. In areas at risk (e.g., fingers), care should be taken to avoid this reaction. Tenting the skin up and away from the nerve, ballooning the skin with lidocaine, or sliding the skin back and forth over the underlying fascia during treatment can help prevent nerve damage, which may rarely be permanent.

Electrosurgery

Electrosurgery comprises a variety of surgical techniques, applications, and apparatus. In general, the tissue effect is created by heat delivered to or generated in the tissue as a result of an electrical current. Because of this heat, local anesthesia is required for all but the simplest procedures. Some type of electrosurgery is routinely used by dermatologists for destruction, hemostasis, or simple or complex excisions. An understanding of the different modalities and their applications can improve the surgical outcome.

Electrocautery. With electrocautery a step-down transformer is used to pass current through thin platinum tips of various configurations. Resistance to the flow of current through the tip causes heat to be generated. The amount of heat can be controlled by the intensity of the current. No electrical current passes through the patient. The heated electrode can be used to destroy lesions such as verrucae by carbonization, to coagulate small vascular lesions, or to shave-excise small papular or pedunculated lesions such as nevi, seborrheic keratoses, and skin tags. Hemostasis is generally excellent. The current should be controlled to produce a heated surgical tip that cuts easily without accumulating charred tissue while limiting destruction of surrounding tissue. Anesthesia is required only if the lesions are large. Today, this is most often performed with battery-powered, handheld, disposable units.

Electro-epilation. One of the first applications of electrical current in surgery was the use of direct (galvanic) current to destroy hair follicles (electrolysis). In this technique heat is actually not a factor. A chemical reaction at the electrode tip, as a result of direct current passing through, causes the production of sodium hydroxide (lye) at the hair root. The lye is responsible for follicular destruction. Although this is a safe technique, with minimal pain or risk of scarring, it is very slow, requiring 1 minute or more for hair root destruction.

Thermolysis is a form of diathermy in which resistance to a high-frequency current causes heat in the follicle, resulting in tissue destruction. Thermolysis is more painful, may have a higher regrowth rate, and is more likely to cause scarring if not properly used. However, it is very fast in its effect and 100 to 200 hairs may be treated in a half-hour session. For this reason it has generally replaced electrolysis.

Electrodesiccation, Electrofulguration. Electrodesiccation and electrofulguration represent the most commonly employed uses of electrosurgery in dermatology. Although often used to denote the same procedure, there is a subtle technical difference between the two. With electrodesicca-

tion the electrode tip is in contact with the tissue; with electrofulguration there is a 1- to 2-mm separation.

The current is produced by a spark-gap generator. With this device, current is supplied to a capacitor, which builds sufficient charge to overcome air resistance, allowing current to cross the spark gap and flow to the patient. A highly damped (decreasing amplitude) waveform is produced, of high voltage and low amperage. This limits the depth of tissue destruction. As this is a monoterminal current, a grounding electrode on the patient is not required. This type of electrosurgery has numerous applications in the daily practice of dermatology.

Using a low-power setting and a fine needle, electroepilation may be performed. Although slightly painful, it can also be used to treat a small number of coarse dark hairs that may trouble the patient, particularly in nevi. Fine telangiectases may also be blanched with this technique. It is important not to overtreat telangiectases, to avoid creating pitted scars. Superficial, small dermal tumors, such as syringomas, may be treated with electrodesiccation. Insertion of the fine epilating needle into the tumor is followed by the application of low current until a surface bubbling occurs. The small amount of char is then removed with a curette, resulting in a smooth surface appearance.

Higher power electrofulguration may be used to destroy seborrheic keratoses, skin tags, or warts. These lesions are then curetted to appropriate depths to ensure their removal.

Electrodesiccation or fulguration is commonly employed in treatment of many basal cell and squamous cell carcinomas under 2 cm in diameter. Following thorough, vigorous curettage of the lesion, the base and margins of the defect created should be electrodesiccated for both hemostasis and extension of treatment margins. It is these authors' bias that the cycle be carried out three times, but electrodesiccation of the final cycle should be for hemostasis only.

Electrodesiccation/fulguration is very useful in excisional surgery to provide hemostasis. It is important that the field be dry for this to be effective, since the destruction by this current is rather superficial and will not be transmitted through blood.

Electrosection (Cutting Current). The biterminal current used for electrosection is produced by a vacuum tube, resulting in waves with a frequency similar to that of radiowaves. For cutting purposes a sinusoidal, undamped (equal amplitude) waveform is generated. The active electrode is cool. Cellular disruption (cutting) occurs as a result of heat produced in response to the wave at the point of contact with the electrode.

When properly used, fine surgical excisions can be produced with minimal trauma to surrounding tissue and excellent hemostasis. Various attachments to the handpiece, including scalpels, needles, wire loops, and balls, can further adapt the instrument to the specific procedure. Most of these devices are able to have their waveform altered to produce a current that also electrocoagulates and electrofulgurates like spark-gap machines. This makes these instruments quite versatile. It is important to note that because the treatment tips used in electrofulguration, electrodesiccation, electrocoagulation, and electrosection are cool, they are not self-sterilizing.

EXCISIONAL TECHNIQUE

The fusiform or elliptical excision is the workhorse procedure used to treat invasive skin cancers as well as benign skin lesions needing extirpation. This technique is indicated for all low-risk squamous cell carcinoma and basal cell carcinomas (see skin cancer management section on p. 1086 for discussion of low- versus high-risk tumors). The basic principle of the fusiform ellipse is excision of a specimen oriented with its longest axis along skin tension lines and its width not exceeding one third of its length. The ellipse can be curved in a crescentic or "lazy-S" pattern to better align the final scar with skin tension lines. If performed with the correct dimensions (usually length:width ratio of 3:1) and a 30-degree angle at each pole, redundant tissue (dog ears, standing cones) at the two extremes of the excision is generally avoided. Dog ears represent excess tissue bunching at the poles of a skin closure and should be excised or "sewn out," if needed. *Undermining* refers to the practice of sharp or blunt dissection of the skin from underlying subcutaneous tissue to reduce wound tension and create wound edge eversion. Most excisional surgery involves some degree of undermining. An in-depth discussion of excisional technique can be found elsewhere (see Wheeland or Zachary references) (Fig. 37-5).

MOHS' MICROSURGERY

Mohs' microsurgery was initially developed by Dr. Frederick Mohs in the 1930s as a fixed-tissue technique for treating various tumors. Drs. Tromovitch and Stegman in the 1970s modified the technique to a fresh-frozen tissue variant offering the relatively rapid treatment of high-risk skin cancers with excellent cure rates. Mohs' microsurgery is a tissue-sparing technique that entails frozen-section control of 100% of surgical margins. Because all margins are examined microscopically, smaller margins can be taken. This is especially important in cosmetically sensitive areas where sparing of normal adjacent tissue can improve final cosmesis and decrease the risk of functional defects. In addition, microscopic control of all margins results in higher cure rates than for simple excision or destructive techniques, especially in tumors that may grow asymmetrically.

ACUTE SURGICAL COMPLICATIONS

The major acute surgical complications are often described as the "terrible tetrad" of hematoma, infection, dehiscence, and necrosis. The most common causes for these complications are persistent bleeding and excessive wound edge tension. Unfortunately, these complications are often interrelated, such that one triggers a cascade leading to several. The most important factor in preventing persistent bleeding is meticulous intraoperative hemostasis. Dermatologic surgeons often discontinue aspirin (2 weeks), warfarin (2 days), and nonsteroidal antiinflammatory drugs (1 week) before surgery to decrease intraoperative bleeding. Nonetheless, controlled studies have failed to show a significant increase in postoperative hematoma in patients taking these medications. Excessive wound edge tension is a function of surgical planning (e.g., incorrect assessment of skin tension and extensibility, poorly designed flap, or inadequate undermining) and can lead to ischemia and necrosis. In addition, postoperative edema can significantly increase wound edge tension, and should be considered when placing surface sutures to avoid wound edge ischemia. The predicted infection rate for "clean" surgical procedures is 1% to 3%, but it increases dramatically once hematoma and/or necrosis are present. Finally, the infection rate for Mohs' microsurgery performed on the ear may be significantly increased, especially when cartilage is involved.

RADIATION THERAPY OF SKIN CANCER

Radiation therapy in dermatology has a long history of being used to treat both benign and malignant conditions of the skin. Nonetheless, the use of ionizing radiation in dermatologic therapy of benign conditions has decreased markedly owing to highly effective medical therapies balanced against the potential genetic and somatic hazards of radiation. Radiation therapy for malignant skin conditions, however, continues to play an important primary and adjunctive role in cutaneous oncology despite the development of highly effective ablative and surgical treatments for skin cancer. A discussion of the physics and techniques of administering radiation therapy is beyond the scope of this text, but modern indications, as well as disadvantages, of radiation therapy will be examined.

Radiation therapy (XRT) can be used as primary treatment for skin cancers, especially in patients who are excessively fearful of surgery or too frail to undergo extensive surgery. Nonetheless, if the patient is relatively young, other primary treatments should be considered because of the increased risk of developing new primary tumors within the radiation port in 15 to 20 years. A prospective, randomized trial by Avril et al found that 4-year recurrence rates of 347 primary facial basal cell carcinomas (BCCs) less than 4 cm in diameter were 0.7% in those tumors treated surgically, whereas 7.5% of the radiation-treated tumors recurred. In addition, cosmesis was judged to be "good" or better in 87% of surgically treated tumors versus only 69% of XRT-treated patients. Differences in both recurrence rates and cosmesis were statistically significant. Meta-analyses by Rowe et al examining literature

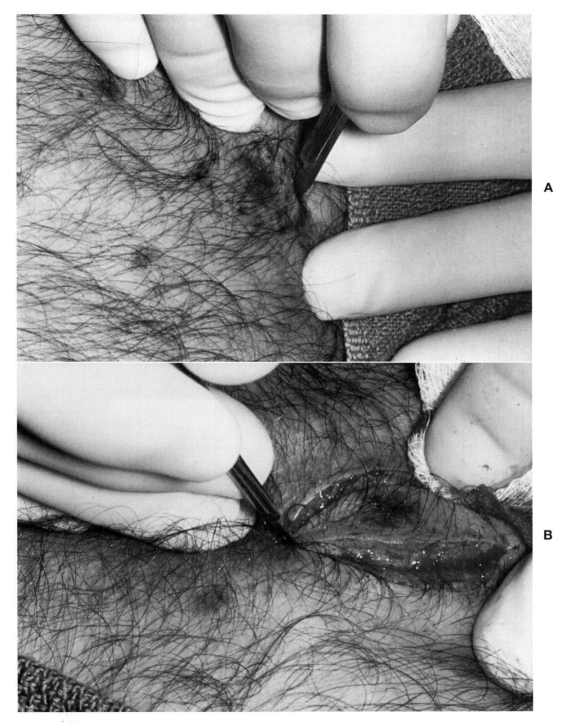

Fig. 37-5 Fusiform elliptical excision. **A,** Fusiform ellipse delineated along normal skin tension lines with a 3:1 length-to-width ratio. **B,** Incision to fat of fusiform ellipse. *Continued*

since 1947 show 5-year recurrence rates of primary BCCs as follows: Mohs' microsurgery 1.0%, surgical excision 10.1%, C&D 7.7%, and XRT 8.7%. Recurrent BCCs showed higher recurrence rates in all treatment categories. Primary squamous cell carcinoma (SCC) showed 5-year

recurrence rates as follows: Mohs' microsurgery 3.1%, surgical excision 8.1%, C&D 3.7%, and XRT 10%. The literature in general supports the conclusions that XRT has lower cure rates than Mohs' microsurgery (but not necessarily surgical excision), and cosmesis of XRT-treated areas

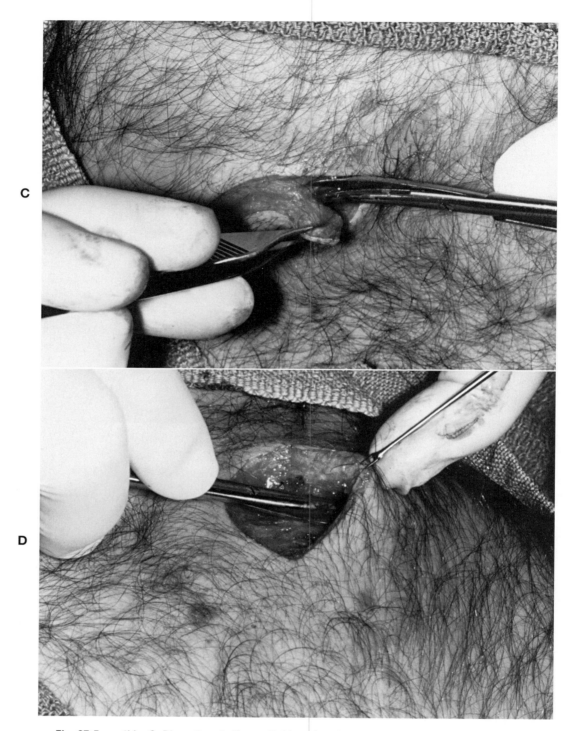

Fig. 37-5, cont'd   C, Dissection of ellipse with blunt-tipped scissors along even subcutaneous plane.
D, Undermining skin edge margins in subcutaneous plane, gently cradling skin edges with skin hooks.

tends to be slightly inferior to surgically treated sites, which often improve over time.

Several studies indicate that recurrence of nonmelanoma skin cancer (NMSC) after primary XRT may be more aggressive and invasive than recurrence after primary surgical treatment. Smith et al demonstrated a statistically significant percentage area increase and extension of tumor beyond subcutaneous fat in tumors treated with XRT compared with tumors treated with surgery. Robins et al have suggested that XRT-treated recurrent periocular BCCs

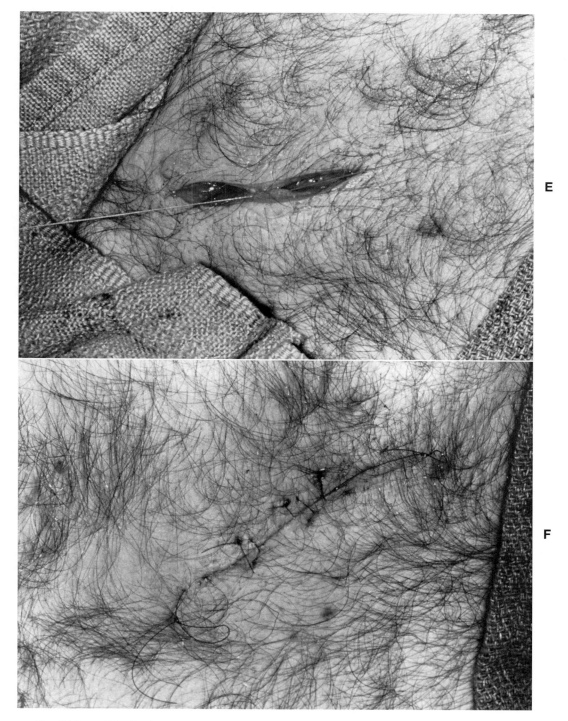

Fig. 37-5, cont'd   **E,** Placement of subcutaneous tension-bearing sutures. **F,** Surface placement of nonabsorbable sutures for wound edge alignment.

demonstrate wider subclinical tumor extension as illustrated by more Mohs stages to clearance compared with tumors recurring after primary surgical therapy. The mechanism behind increased tumor aggressiveness following XRT is unclear, but Boothman et al have hypothesized that radi-

ation may induce genes (such as that for tissue plasminogen activator expression) leading to neoplastic progression, changes in tissue remodeling, or increased metastatic ability.

Radiation therapy offers a valuable adjunctive treatment option for particularly aggressive perineural SCC and BCC.

Because of the increased risk of this subset of NMSC to metastasize and recur, adjuvant XRT should be considered after surgical excision. It is particularly difficult to detect single-cell spread of tumor during excisional surgery, including Mohs' microsurgery, and perineural NMSC may spread more rapidly along nerve sheaths than by contiguous growth. Thus, perineural involvement of large nerves by NMSC warrants consideration of adjuvant XRT. Finally, XRT may also be considered after surgical excision if margins show microscopic evidence of tumor residual. This is especially valuable in patients who do not wish to undergo surgical reexcision.

PHOTODYNAMIC THERAPY

Photodynamic therapy (PDT) involves the uptake of photo-sensitizer by diseased cells that are preferentially destroyed through the interaction of light and photosensitizer forming highly reactive oxygen intermediates. These free oxygen radicals damage cell membranes and vascular endothelium. Several photosensitizers have been used in dermatology, including hematoporphyrin derivative, porfimer sodium (Photofrin), 5-aminolevulinic acid, benzoporphyrin derivative, tin ethyl etiopurpurin (SnET2), and mono-L-aspartyl chlorin e6. Current systemic photosensitizers have prolonged photosensitivity, limiting their use. PDT has been used to treat a wide gamut of neoplastic and inflammatory conditions of the skin, including NMSC, actinic keratoses, and mycosis fungoides. Clinical trials using PDT for NMSC vary from 50% to 100% cure rates, but definitive large, controlled studies are needed to establish the efficacy of PDT compared with other treatment modalities. The technique may best be suited to conditions such as Gorlin's disease (nevoid BCC syndrome), where multiple, relatively superficial lesions can be treated more quickly and less painfully than with conventional surgical therapy. Unfortunately, until better photosensitizers and light sources become easily accessible, PDT will remain a somewhat obscure secondary treatment for NMSC in North America.

SKIN FLAPS AND GRAFTS

Local skin flaps are geometric segments of tissue contiguous with a skin defect that are rotated, advanced, or transposed over tissue to close a wound. Skin grafts are full or partial dermal thickness skin harvested from a site distant and without vascular connection to the skin defect to be closed. Choosing whether to close a wound by second intention, linear closure, skin flap, or skin graft is complex. Important considerations include local tissue movement, adjacent anatomic structural preservation, cosmesis, and risk of recurrence of the extirpated tumor. A full discussion of skin flap and graft repair is beyond the scope of this text and can be found in the cutaneous surgical texts referenced at the end of this chapter.

SKIN CANCER MANAGEMENT

The dermatologist is uniquely trained to diagnose and treat skin cancer. Early diagnosis of skin cancer can affect prognosis dramatically. Once diagnosed, the subsequent treatment of skin cancer is a function of tumor biology and patient characteristics, but treatment most often involves some form of surgery. Because of the unique biology of melanoma, skin cancer is often divided into two groups: melanoma and nonmelanoma skin cancer (NMSC). Although the list of nonmelanoma malignant cutaneous tumors is extensive, the overwhelming majority of these tumors are basal and squamous cell carcinoma. In an attempt to standardize treatment of NMSC, the National Comprehensive Cancer Network has developed guidelines for treatment of these tumors (Fig. 37-6). This algorithm is based on classification of tumors as either low or high risk for recurrence (Table 37-1). Once the clinician has determined whether a tumor is of low or high risk, the therapy best indicated for a particular tumor and patient can be selected (Box 37-6).

CUTANEOUS LASER SURGERY

Almost no area of dermatology is changing as rapidly as that of cutaneous laser surgery. Development of new lasers, as well as improvements in existing lasers, have advanced the field to the point that laser therapy is by far the best treatment for many dermatologic conditions.

The first laser (light amplification by stimulated emission of radiation) was operated in 1960 by Maiman. Medical applications were quickly recognized, and Leon Goldman pioneered their dermatologic use. Lasers produce a light beam that is described as "coherent." This means a beam of one or a very few wavelengths (temporal coherence), travels in a highly collimated fashion (spatial coherence). The beam produces its effect as a result of heat generated following the beam's absorption by specific tissue elements or chromophores. A chromophore is a component of tissue that preferentially absorbs specific wavelengths of light. Oxyhemoglobin, hemoglobin, and melanin are the main chromophores exploited by dermatologic lasers. Cutaneous laser surgery is largely based on the theory of selective photothermolysis, which was introduced by Anderson and Parrish in 1983. This theory states that destruction of tissue by laser energy absorption leads to selective damage of the chromophore while relatively sparing adjacent tissue. The depth to which light penetrates into the skin increases with wavelength, beam diameter, and energy delivered. The wavelength produced by a laser depends on its active medium (Table 37-2).

The laser is a technologically advanced instrument. However, as with any surgery, side effects can occur. Hypertrophic scarring and pigmentary changes are the most common, but infection, pain, and lack of efficacy are possible. It is essential that appropriate instruction and

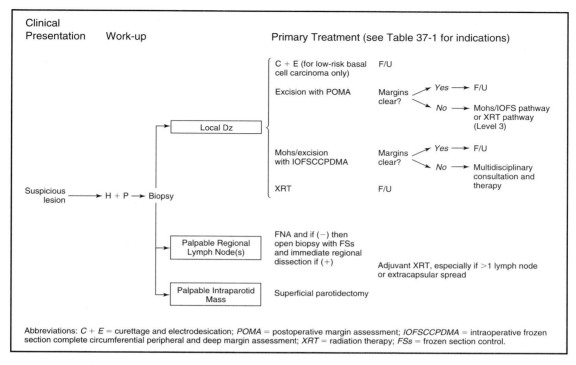

Fig. 37-6 Treatment algorithm for tumors. (Modified with permission from the National Comprehensive Cancer Network.)

TABLE 37-1

Risk Factors for Recurrence of Nonmelanoma Skin Cancer

History and Physical	Low	High
Location/size	Area L <20 mm	Area L >20 mm
	Area M <10 mm	Aream M >10 mm
	Area H <6 mm	Area H >6 mm
Borders	Well-defined	Ill-defined
Primary versus recurrent	Primary	Recurrent
Age	>40	<40
Immunosuppression	−	+
Site of prior XRT or chronic inflammatory process	−	+
Rapidly growing tumor	−	+
Palpable regional lymphadenopathy	−	+
Neurologic symptoms: pain, paresthesia, paralysis	−	+
PATHOLOGY (SCC)		
Poorly differentiated	−	+
Adenoid or desmoplastic subtype	−	+
Clark's level	I, II, III	IV, V
Perineural involvement	−	+
PATHOLOGY (BCC)		
Nodular, superficial	+	−
Morpheic, infiltrative, micronodular	−	+

Area H = "Mask areas" of face, genitalia, hands, feet.
Area M = Cheeks, forehead, scalp.
Area L = Trunk, neck, extremities.

Indications for Therapy

C + E
Low-risk* tumors in non–hair-bearing sites

EXCISION WITH POMA
Low-risk tumors excised with 6-mm margins and primary repair
High-risk primary tumors in area L excised with 10-mm margins and primary repair

MOHS/EXCISION WITH IOFSCCPDMA
High-risk tumors

XRT
Low risk-tumors in areas M and H in patients older than 55
(1.0 to 1.5 cm margins = 4000 to 6000 cGy in 10 to 30 fractions or 3000 to 4000 cGy in 5 to 10 fractions)
High-risk tumors in which surgery is contraindicated or not desired
(>2-cm margins = 700 cGy in 35 fractions)
Adjunctive therapy for high-risk tumors with perineural invasion after excision
Maximize fractions to maximize cosmesis

POMA = Postoperative margin assessment; IOFSCCPDMA = Intraoperative frozen section complete circumferential peripheral and deep margin assessment.
*See Table 37-1 to determine low- versus high-risk tumors.
Area H = "Mask areas" of face, genitalia, hands, feet.
Area M = Cheeks, forehead, scalp.
Area L = Trunk, neck, extremities.
Modified with permission from the National Comprehensive Cancer Network.

supervision in the use of lasers be obtained by prospective surgeons to ensure that optimum safety is provided and the best surgical results are achieved.

Argon Laser

The argon laser is best suited to treatment of vascular and pigmented lesions. Because its wavelengths (488 to 514 nm) do not correspond to absorption peaks of either hemoglobin or melanin, and also because of its continuous-wave nature, thermal damage to surrounding tissue may be significant. By carefully tracing (under magnification) the individual vessels in a port-wine stain with a 0.1-mm beam diameter, the risk of scarring can be minimized. However, hypopigmentation may still occur. The argon laser is not advised for use before puberty, since the risk of scarring is greater in children. Indeed, this laser is rapidly being replaced by more effective lasers with less risk of scarring and hypopigmentation.

Flashlamp Pumped Pulsed Dye Laser

The pulsed dye laser is an extremely useful instrument for treating port-wine stains, telangiectases, and other small,

flat, or minimally elevated vascular lesions. Older flashlamp pumped rhodamine dye lasers emit a beam of yellow light at a wavelength of 585 nm with a 450- to 500-ms pulse duration. More recently, lasers emitting wavelengths of 590, 595, and 600 nm with pulse durations that can be increased up to1500 μsec have increased the depth and diameter of vessel that can be treated with these lasers while decreasing the concomitant absorption by melanin. The risk of scarring and pigment change is very slight, and infants as young as a few weeks old can be treated. Disadvantages include the black/gray discoloration caused by intravascular coagulation associated with therapy with the pulsed dye laser.

Q-Switched Ruby Laser

The Q-switched ruby laser emits a red 694-nm beam with melanin and darkly pigmented (black, blue, green) tattoo pigments as its main chromophore. Q-switching allows for production of extremely high energies and short nanosecond pulses. This laser successfully treats benign pigmented lesions as well as tattoos with minimal side effects other than transient hypopigmentation. The treatment of melanoma-in-situ is controversial, but early clinical trials indicate some success in treating frail elderly patients who could not tolerate large surgical excisions. The longer wavelength of this laser permits greater depth of penetration, making it an excellent option for deep, dermal pigmented lesions such as nevus of Ota.

Neodymium:Yttrium-Aluminum-Garnet Lasers

The neodymium:yttrium-aluminum-garnet (Nd:YAG) lasers can be used in three modes: continuous wave, Q-switched, and frequency doubled. Both continuous and Q-switched modes emit an invisible near-infrared beam (1064 nm) for which there is no specific chromophore. In the continuous mode, nonspecific thermal damage can penetrate to 8 mm and has been used to treat exophytic port-wine stains or venous malformations. In the Q-switched mode, it is highly effective for black and blue tattoos. The Q-switched Nd:YAG laser beam is modified by passage through either a potassium diphosphate or potassium titanyl phosphate (KTP) crystal, doubling the frequency and halving the wavelength. In a quasi-continuous mode, the green 532-nm beam can be used to treat vascular and superficial pigmented lesions as well as red tattoo.

Potassium Titanyl Phosphate Laser

The potassium titanyl phosphate (KTP) laser produces a visible green beam of 532 nm, which is useful for treating both vascular and superficial pigmented lesions because of significant hemoglobin and melanin absorption at this wavelength. The KTP laser is equivalent to the copper vapor laser (578 nm quasi-continuous wave) for superficial vascular lesions, and some KTP lasers can be adjusted to pulse durations as high as 50 ms to better treat larger vessels. KTP lasers can be quite compact. With few moving parts they

TABLE 37-2

Dermatologic Lasers

Laser	Wavelength (nm)	Color	Applications
Argon	488-514	Blue-green	Vascular lesions
PhotoDerm	515-1000	Green-red and infrared	Vascular lesions, pigmented lesions, epilation
Potassium titanyl phosphate (KTP)	532	Green	Vascular lesions, pigmented lesions
Q-switched Nd:YAG (frequency doubled)	532	Green	Vascular lesions, pigmented lesions; tattoo—red
Copper vapor	578/511	Yellow/green	Vascular lesions, pigmented lesions
Flashlamp pumped pulsed dye (PDL)	585-600	Yellow	Vascular lesions
Q-switched ruby	694	Red	Deep and superficial pigmented lesions; tattoo—black, blue, green
Long-pulse ruby	694	Red	Epilation
Q-switched alexandrite	755	Infrared	Tattoo—black, blue, green
Long-pulse alexandrite	755	Infrared	Epilation
Diode	810	Infrared	Epilation
Q-switched Nd:YAG	1064	Invisible	Deep dermal pigment; tattoo—black, blue
Er:YAG	2940	Invisible	Superficial skin resurfacing and destruction of superficial growths
Carbon dioxide	10,600	Invisible	Skin resurfacing and destruction of warts, keloids, superficial cancers, and benign growths

are relatively maintenance free. Because of their quasi-continuous mode, they must be delivered by way of a narrow beam to limit skin heat damage. Many employ a cooling tip to limit surface epidermal damage. This permits delivery of a wider beam diameter and pulse duration, allowing for deeper penetration and more rapid treatment of a larger area.

Q-Switched Alexandrite Laser

In addition to the Q-switched ruby and Q-switched Nd:YAG lasers, the Q-switched alexandrite laser effectively treats tattoos. The long wavelength (755 nm) penetrates deeply into the dermis with absorption by blue, black, and green tattoo pigment. These lasers show a similar therapeutic profile to the Q-switched ruby laser. One advantage, however, is the ability to deliver the alexandrite laser at 10 pulses/second, allowing for more rapid therapy compared with the single pulse/second delivery with the ruby laser.

Intense Pulsed Noncoherent Light (PhotoDerm)

PhotoDerm is an intense pulsed light source that emits a continuous spectrum of light between 515 and 1200 nm. Filters can be used to more specifically tailor the wavelength of emitted light to the chromophore being treated (e.g., vascular versus pigment versus pigment of hair follicles). With computer-controlled adjustments to pulse duration, fluence, and spot size, the PhotoDerm is extremely versatile but may also be more difficult to learn to use effectively.

Epilating Lasers

Market demand for safe, long-term hair removal has led to the development of several effective epilating lasers. Most epilating lasers use melanin of the hair follicle as a chromophore, such that light or gray hair responds poorly. In addition, more superficial melanin can be affected leading to hypopigmentation, especially in more darkly pigmented patients. Currently available are normal-mode ruby lasers, an alexandrite laser, filtered flashlamp pulsed light sources, high-powered diode arrays, and a Q-switched Nd:YAG laser. Although all of these systems show efficacy, the field is too new to claim fully reliable and predictable permanent hair removal.

Carbon Dioxide Lasers

The carbon dioxide (CO_2) laser emits an invisible infrared beam of 10,600 nm and can be used in continuous-wave mode, super-pulsed mode, and scanning mode. Water nonselectively absorbs laser energy, producing ablative and thermal damage. Used in the continuous-wave mode, it is an excellent therapeutic choice for very large plantar and periungual warts, which have failed to respond to routine office modalities. However, the presence of human papillomaviral DNA in the smoke plume is well documented, necessitating proper safety precautions to limit exposure to the laser operator and assistants. The CO_2 laser is also an excellent treatment option for ear lobe keloids but may not be as successful for keloids elsewhere. Other lesions amenable to CO_2 laser ablation include actinic cheilitis, xanthelasma, rhinophyma, syringomas, and superficial basal and squamous cell carcinomas.

Used in the super-pulsed mode the laser beam can be delivered in short bursts, allowing thermal destruction of the epidermis and papillary dermis while limiting deeper thermal damage. Delivery in this mode is more uniform and markedly faster when the optomechanical scanner is employed. Super-pulsed CO_2 lasers are extremely useful in the treatment of actinic damage and photoaging. Side effects include postinflammatory pigmentary changes, scarring and textural changes, and prolonged erythema.

Erbium:Yttrium-Aluminum-Garnet Laser

The erbium:yttrium-aluminum-garnet (Er:YAG) laser emits an invisible near-infrared beam of 2940 nm, which allows for tissue ablation with less thermal injury than seen with CO_2 laser because of more efficient absorption by water of the 2940-nm beam. This decreased thermal injury is an advantage for treatment of superficial facial photoaging, scars, and treatment of photodamaged skin below the jawline. Healing may be faster, with less risk of prolonged erythema and scarring (especially below the jawline). Nonetheless, depth of injury is the primary determinant for prolonged erythema and scarring. The lack of thermal damage can also be a disadvantage, resulting in poor hemostasis with the Er:YAG laser. In addition, the collagen-tightening effect may not be as pronounced as with the CO_2 laser. Thus, the Er:YAG laser may be the ideal resurfacing laser for very early photodamage, but the CO_2 laser remains the premier treatment for more severe photodamage needing new collagen formation and collagen remodeling.

Adams JE: The technique of curettage surgery. *J Am Acad Dermatol* 1986, 15:697.

Anderson RR, Parrish JA: Selective photothermolysis: precise microsurgery by selective absorption of pulsed radiation. *Science* 1983, 220:524.

Avril MF, et al: Basal cell carcinoma of the face: surgery or radiotherapy? Results of a randomized study. *Br J Cancer* 1997, 76:100.

Barrett TL, et al: Treatment of basal cell carcinoma and squamous cell carcinoma with perineural invasion. *Adv Dermatol* 1993, 8:277.

Billingsley EM, Maloney ME: Intraoperative and postoperative bleeding problems in patients taking warfarin, aspirin, and nonsteroidal antiinflammatory agents. *Dermatol Surg* 1997, 23:381.

Bissonnette R, Liu H: Current status of photodynamic therapy in dermatology. *Dermatol Clin* 1997, 15:507.

Boothman DA, et al: Immediate x-ray-inducible responses from mammalian cells. *Radiat Res* 1994, 138:S44.

Chao CKS, et al: Reirradiation of recurrent skin cancer of the face: a successful salvage modality. *Cancer* 1995, 75:2351.

Childers J, et al: Long-term results of irradiation for basal cell carcinoma of the skin of the nose. *Plast Reconst Surg* 1994, 93:1169.

Futoryan T, Grande D: Postoperative wound infection rates in dermatologic surgery. *Dermatol Surg* 1995, 21:509.

Goldman MP, Fitzpatrick RE: Cutaneous laser surgery: the art and science of selective photothermolysis, ed 2, St Louis, 1999, Mosby.

Haas AF, Grekin RC: Antibiotic prophylaxis in dermatologic surgery. *J Am Acad Dermatol* 1995, 32:155.

Haas AF, Grekin RC: Practical thoughts on antibiotic prophylaxis. *Arch Dermatol* 1998, 134:872.

Johnson TM, et al: Squamous cell carcinoma of the skin (excluding lip and oral mucosa). *J Am Acad Dermatol* 1992, 26: 467.

Kopf AW, et al: Curettage-electrodesiccation treatment of basal cell carcinomas. *Arch Dermatol* 1977, 113:439.

Kuflik EG: Cryosurgery updated. *J Am Acad Dermatol* 1994, 31(6):925.

Leffell DJ, Brown MD: Manual of skin surgery: a practical guide to dermatologic procedures, New York, 1997, Wiley-Liss.

LeVasseur JG, et al: Dermatologic electrosurgery in patients with implantable cardioverter-defibrillators and pacemakers. *Dermatol Surg* 1998, 24:233.

Lovett RD, et al: External irradiation of epithelial skin cancer. *Int J Radiat Oncol Biol Phys* 1990, 19:235.

Maiman T: Stimulated optical radiation in ruby. *Nature* 1960, 187:493.

Mazeron JJ, et al: Radiation therapy of carcinomas of the skin of the nose and nasal vestibule: a report of 1676 cases by the Groupe Europeen de Curietherapie. *Radiother Oncol* 1989, 13:165.

Otley CC, et al: Complications of cutaneous surgery in patients who are taking warfarin, aspirin, or nonsteroidal anti-inflammatory drugs. *Arch Dermatol* 1996, 132:161.

Petrovich Z, et al: Carcinoma of the lip and selected sites of head and neck skin: a clinical study of 896 patients. *Radiother Oncol* 1987, 8:11.

Petrovich Z, et al: Treatment results and patterns of failure in 646 patients with carcinoma of the eyelids, pinna, and nose. *Am J Surg* 1987, 154:447.

Pollack SV: Electrosurgery of the skin, New York, 1991, Churchill Livingstone.

Robins P, et al: Mohs surgery for periocular basal cell carcinomas. *J Dermatol Surg Oncol* 1985, 11:1203.

Robinson JK: Fundamentals of skin biopsy, Chicago, 1986, Year Book Medical Publishers.

Rowe DE, et al: Long-term recurrence rates in previously untreated (primary) basal cell carcinoma: implications for patient follow-up. *J Dermatol Surg Oncol* 1989, 15:315.

Rowe DE, et al: Mohs surgery is the treatment of choice for recurrent (previously treated) basal cell carcinoma. *J Dermatol Surg Oncol* 1989, 15:424.

Rowe DE, et al: Prognostic factors for local recurrence, metastasis, and survival rates in squamous cell carcinoma of the skin, ear, and lip. *J Am Acad Dermatol* 1992, 26:976.

Salasche SJ: Acute surgical complications: cause, prevention, and treatment. *J Am Acad Dermatol* 1986, 15:1163.

Salasche SJ: Status of curettage and desiccation in the treatment of primary basal cell carcinoma. *J Am Acad Dermatol* 1984, 10:285.

Silverman MK, et al: Recurrence rates of treated basal cell carcinomas. Part I: Overview. *J Dermatol Surg Oncol* 1991, 17:713.

Silverman MK, et al: Recurrence rates of treated basal cell carcinomas. Part II: Curettage-electrodesiccation. *J Dermatol Surg Oncol* 1991, 17:720.

Silverman MK, et al: Recurrence rates of treated basal cell carcinomas. Part III: Surgical excision. *J Dermatol Surg Oncol* 1992, 18:471.

Silverman MK, et al: Recurrence rates of treated basal cell carcinomas. Part IV: X-ray therapy. *J Dermatol Surg Oncol* 1992, 18:549.

Smith SP, et al: Use of Mohs micrographic surgery to establish quantitative proof of heightened tumor spread in basal cell carcinoma recurrent following radiotherapy. *J Dermatol Surg Oncol* 1990, 16:1012.

Smith SP, Grande DJ: Basal cell carcinoma recurring after radiotherapy: a unique, difficult treatment subclass of recurrent basal cell carcinoma. *J Dermatol Surg Oncol* 1991, 17:26.

Spicer MS, Goldberg DJ: Lasers in dermatology. *J Am Acad Dermatol* 1996, 34:1.

Wheeland RG: Cutaneous surgery, Philadelphia, 1994, WB Saunders.

Wilder RB, et al: Basal cell carcinoma treated with radiation therapy. *Cancer* 1991, 68:2134.

Wilder RB, et al: Recurrent basal cell carcinoma treated with radiation therapy. *Arch Dermatol* 1991, 127:1668.

Zachary CB: Basic cutaneous surgery: a primer in technique, New York, 1991, Churchill Livingstone. ▲

Index

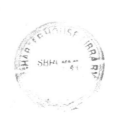

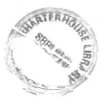

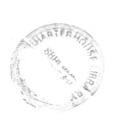

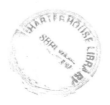